MEDICAL PHYSIOLOGY

MEDICAL PHYSIOLOGY

A Cellular and Molecular Approach

UPDATED-EDITION

Walter F. Boron, MD, PhD
Professor
Department of Cellular and Molecular Physiology
Yale University School of Medicine
New Haven, Connecticut

■

Emile L. Boulpaep, MD
Professor
Department of Cellular and Molecular Physiology
Yale University School of Medicine
New Haven, Connecticut

ELSEVIER
SAUNDERS

ELSEVIER
SAUNDERS

The Curtis Center
170 S Independence Mall W 300E
Philadelphia, Pennsylvania 19106

MEDICAL PHYSIOLOGY

Permissions may be sought directly from Elsevier's Health Sciences Rights
Department in Philadelphia, PA, USA: phone: (+1) 215 239 3804, fax: (+1) 215 239 3805,
e-mail: healthpermissions@elsevier.com. You may also complete your request on-line
via the Elsevier homepage (http://www.elsevier.com), by selecting 'Customer Support'
and then 'Obtaining Permissions'.

NOTICE

Medicine is an ever-changing field. Standard safety precautions must be followed, but as new research and clinical experience broaden our knowledge, changes in treatment and drug therapy may become necessary or appropriate. Readers are advised to check the most current product information provided by the manufacturer of each drug to be administered to verify the recommended dose, the method and duration of administration, and contraindications. It is the responsibility of the licensed prescriber, relying on experience and knowledge of the patient, to determine dosages and the best treatment for each individual patient. Neither the publisher nor the author assumes any liability for any injury and/or damage to persons or property arising from this publication.

Library of Congress Cataloging-in-Publication Data

Boron, Walter F.
  Medical physiology: a cellular and molecular approach / Walter F. Boron, Emile L.
Boulpaep—Updated ed.
    p. ;   cm.
  Includes bibliographical references and index.
    ISBN -13: 978-1-4160-2328-9   ISBN -10: 1-4160-2328-3
  1. Human physiology.   I. Boulpaep, Emile L.   II. Title.
  [DNLM: 1. Physiology.   QT 104 B7356M 2005]
  QP34.5.B65 2005
  612—dc22   2004051158

ISBN -13: 978-1-4160-2328-9

ISBN -10: 1-4160-2328-3

Acquisitions Editor: William R. Schmitt
Developmental Editor: Melissa Dudlick
Publishing Services Manager: Frank Polizzano
Design Manager: Ellen Zanolle

Printed in the United States of America

Last digit is the print number: 9 8 7 6 5 4 3

Contributors

Michael Apkon, MD, PhD
Associate Professor and Vice Chairman, Department of
  Pediatrics, Yale University School of Medicine, New
  Haven, Connecticut
  *Cellular Physiology of Skeletal, Cardiac, and Smooth
  Muscle*

Peter S. Aronson, MD
C.N.H. Long Professor of Internal Medicine, Chief,
  Section of Nephrology, and Professor Department of
  Cellular and Molecular Physiology, Yale University
  School of Medicine, New Haven, Connecticut
  Physiology of Membranes

Eugene J. Barrett, MD, PhD
Professor of Medicine and Pediatrics and Vice Chairman,
  Department of Internal Medicine, University of Virginia
  School of Medicine, Charlottesville, Virginia
  *Organization of Endocrine Control; The Endocrine
  Regulation of Growth; The Thyroid Gland; The Adrenal
  Gland; The Endocrine Pancreas; The Parathyroid Glands
  and Vitamin D*

Paula Barrett, PhD
Professor of Pharmacology, Department of Pharmacology,
  University of Virginia School of Medicine,
  Charlottesville, Virginia
  The Parathyroid Glands and Vitamin D

Henry J. Binder, MD
Professor of Medicine and Professor Department of
  Cellular and Molecular Physiology, Yale University
  School of Medicine, New Haven, Connecticut
  *Organization of the Gastrointestinal System; Gastric
  Function; Intestinal Fluid and Electrolyte Movement;
  Nutrient Digestion and Absorption*

Walter F. Boron, MD, PhD
Professor, Department of Cellular and Molecular
  Physiology, Yale University School of Medicine, New
  Haven, Connecticut
  *Foundations of Physiology; Physiology of Membranes;
  Organization of the Respiratory System; Mechanics of
  Respiration; Acid-Base Physiology; Transport of Oxygen
  and Carbon Dioxide in the Blood; Gas Exchange in the
  Lungs; Ventilation and Perfusion of the Lungs; Control of
  Ventilation*

Emile L. Boulpaep, MD
Professor, Department of Cellular and Molecular
  Physiology, Yale University School of Medicine, New
  Haven, Connecticut
  *Foundations of Physiology; Physiology of Membranes;
  Organization of the Cardiovascular System; Arteries and
  Veins; The Microcirculation; The Heart As a Pump;
  Regulation of Arterial Pressure and Cardiac Output;
  Integrated Control of the Cardiovascular System*

Michael J. Caplan, MD, PhD
Professor Department of Cellular and Molecular
  Physiology, Yale University School of Medicine, New
  Haven, Connecticut
  Functional Organization of the Cell

Barry W. Connors, PhD
Professor of Neuroscience, Division of Biology and
  Medicine, Brown University, Providence, Rhode Island
  *Physiology of Neurons; Synaptic Transmission in the
  Nervous System; Sensory Transduction; Circuits of the
  Central Nervous System*

Alan H. DeCherney, MD
Department of Obstetrics and Gynecology, Professor,
  University of California–Los Angeles School of
  Medicine, Los Angeles, California
  *Sexual Differentiation; The Male Reproductive System; The
  Female Reproductive System; Fertilization, Pregnancy, and
  Lactation; Fetal and Neonatal Physiology*

Gerhard Giebisch, MD
Sterling Professor Emeritus, Department of Cellular and
  Molecular Physiology, Yale University School of
  Medicine, New Haven, Connecticut
  *Organization of the Urinary System; Glomerular Filtration
  and Renal Blood Flow; Transport of Sodium and Chloride;
  Transport of Urea, Glucose, Phosphate, Calcium,
  Magnesium, and Organic Solutes; Transport of Potassium
  by the Tubules; Urine Concentration and Dilution;
  Transport of Acids and Bases; Integration of Salt and
  Water Balance*

Fred S. Gorelick, MD
Professor of Medicine and Cell Biology, Yale University
    School of Medicine, New Haven; Staff Physician,
    Veterans Administration Medical Center, West Haven,
    Connecticut
Pancreatic and Salivary Glands

Winita Hardikar, MBBS, PhD
Paediatric Hepatologist and Senior Research Officer,
    Department of Gastroenterology, Royal Children's
    Hospital, Melbourne, Victoria, Australia
Hepatobiliary Function

Peter Igarashi, MD
Professor of Internal Medicine, Chief of Division of
    Nephrology, and Robert Tucker Hayes Distinguished
    Chair in Nephrology in Honor of Dr. Floyd C. Rector,
    Jr., University of Texas Southwestern Medical Center at
    Dallas; Chief of Nephrology, Parkland Memorial
    Hospital and Zale Lipshy University Hospital, Dallas,
    Texas
Regulation of Gene Expression

Ervin E. Jones, MD, PhD
Professor, Department of Obstetrics and Gynecology,
    Division of Reproductive Endocrinology and Infertility,
    Yale University School of Medicine, New Haven,
    Connecticut
*Sexual Differentiation; The Male Reproductive System; The
    Female Reproductive System; Fertilization, Pregnancy, and
    Lactation; Fetal and Neonatal Physiology*

W. Jonathan Lederer, MD, PhD
Professor and Director, Medical Biotechnology Center,
    University of Maryland Biotechnology Center; Professor
    of Physiology, University of Maryland Medical School,
    Baltimore, Maryland
Cardiac Electrophysiology and the Electrocardiogram

Christopher R. Marino, MD
Professor of Medicine and Associate Professor of
    Physiology and Biophysics, University of Tennessee
    Health Science Center; Chief, Gastroenterology Section,
    Veterans Administration Medical Center, Memphis,
    Tennessee
Pancreatic and Salivary Glands

Edward G. Moczydlowski, PhD
Baynard & Virginia Clarkson Chair and Department
    Chair, Department of Biology, Clarkson University,
    Potsdam, New York
*Electrophysiology of the Cell Membrane; Electrical
    Excitability and Action Potentials; Synaptic Transmission
    and the Neuromuscular Junction*

Ethan Nadel, PhD†
Director, John B. Pierce Laboratories, and Professor,
    Department of Cellular and Molecular Physiology, Yale
    University School of Medicine, New Haven,
    Connecticut
*Metabolism and Nutrition; Regulation of Body
    Temperature; Exercise Physiology and Sports Science;
    Environmental Physiology: Diving, Altitude, and Space*

Bruce R. Ransom, MD, PhD
Professor and Chairman, Department of Neurology,
    University of Washington School of Medicine, Seattle,
    Washington
*Organization of the Nervous System; The Neuronal
    Microenvironment*

Adrian Reuben, MBBS
Professor of Medicine and Director of Liver Studies,
    Medical University of South Carolina, Charleston,
    South Carolina
Nutrient Digestion and Absorption

George B. Richerson, MD, PhD
Associate Professor, Departments of Neurology and
    Cellular and Molecular Physiology, Yale University
    School of Medicine, New Haven, Connecticut
The Autonomic Nervous System; Control of Ventilation

Laura M. Roman, PhD
Assistant Professor, Department of Physiology, Johns
    Hopkins University School of Medicine, Baltimore,
    Maryland
Signal Transduction

Steven S. Segal, PhD
Professor of Cellular and Molecular Physiology, Yale
    University School of Medicine; Fellow, John B. Pierce
    Laboratories, New Haven, Connecticut
Special Circulations

Frederick J. Suchy, MD
Herbert H. Lehman Professor of Pediatrics and Chairman,
    Jack and Lucy Clark Department of Pediatrics, Mount
    Sinai School of Medicine, Pediatrician-in-Chief, Mount
    Sinai Medical Center, New York, New York
Hepatobiliary Function

Erich Windhager, MD
Upson Professor, Department of Physiology, Weill
    Medical College of Cornell University, New York, New
    York
*Organization of the Urinary System; Glomerular Filtration
    and Renal Blood Flow; Transport of Sodium and Chloride;
    Transport of Urea, Glucose, Phosphate, Calcium,
    Magnesium, and Organic Solutes; Transport of Potassium
    by the Tubules; Urine Concentration and Dilution;
    Transport of Acids and Bases; Integration of Salt and
    Water Balance*

---

†Deceased

Preface

We were intrigued by an idea suggested to us by W.B. Saunders: write a modern textbook of physiology that combines the expertise of a multi-author book with the consistency of a single pen. Our approach has been, first, to recruit as writers mainly professors who teach medical physiology at the Yale University School of Medicine, and then to recast the professors' manuscripts in a uniform style. After much effort, we now present our book, which we hope will bring physiology to life and at the same time be a reliable resource for students.

Target Audience. We wrote *Medical Physiology* primarily as an introductory text for medical students, although it should also be valuable for students in the allied health professions and for graduate students in the physiological sciences. The book should continue to be useful for the advanced medical student who is learning pathophysiology and clinical medicine. Finally, we hope that physicians in training, clinical fellows, and clinical faculty will find the book worthwhile for reviewing principles and becoming updated on new information pertinent for understanding the physiological basis of human disease.

Content of the Textbook. Aside from Part I, which is a brief introduction to the discipline of physiology, the book consists of nine major Parts. Part II (Physiology of Cells and Molecules) reflects that, increasingly, the underpinnings of modern physiology have become cellular and molecular. Chapters 2, 4, and 5 would not be present in a traditional physiology text. Chapter 2 (Functional Organization of the Cell), Chapter 4 (Signal Transduction), and Chapter 5 (Regulation of Gene Expression) provide the essentials of cell biology and molecular biology necessary for understanding cell and organ function. The other chapters in Part II cover the *cellular* physiology of transport, excitability, and muscle—all of which are classic topics for traditional physiology texts. In this book we have extended each of these subjects to the *molecular* level. The remainder of the book will frequently send the reader back to the principles introduced in Part II.

Parts III to IX address individual organ systems. In each case, the first chapter provides a general introduction to the system. Part III (Cellular Physiology of the Nervous System) is untraditional in that it deliberately omits those aspects of the physiology of the central nervous system that neuroscience courses generally treat and that require extensive knowledge of neuroanatomical pathways. Rather, Part III focuses on cellular neurophysiology, including synaptic transmission in the nervous system, sensory transduction, and neural circuits. In addition, Part III also treats two subjects—the autonomic nervous system and the neuronal microenvironment—that are important for understanding other physiological systems. Finally, Part X (The Physiology of Everyday Life) is an integrated, multisystem approach to metabolism, temperature regulation, exercise, and adaptations to special environments.

Emphasis of the textbook. Some important aspects of physiology remain as fundamentally important today as when the pioneers of physiology discovered them a century or more ago. These early observations were generally phenomenological descriptions that physiologists have since been trying to understand at a mechanistic level. Where possible, a goal of this textbook is to extend this understanding all the way to the cell and molecule. Moreover, although some areas are evolving rapidly, we have tried to be as up to date as practical. To make room for the cellular and molecular bricks, we have omitted some classic experimental observations, especially when they were of a "black-box" nature.

Just as each major Part of the textbook begins with an introductory chapter, each chapter generally first describes—at the level of the whole body or organ system (e.g., the kidney)—how the body performs a certain task and/or controls a certain parameter (e.g., plasma K^+ concentration). As appropriate, our discussion then progresses in a reductionistic fashion from organ to tissue to cell and organelles, and ultimately to the molecules that underlie the physiology. Finally, most chapters include a discussion of how the body regulates the parameter of interest at all levels of integration, from molecules to the whole body.

Creating the Textbook. The first draft of each chapter was written by authors with extensive research and/or teaching experience in that field. The editors, sitting shoulder to shoulder at a computer, then largely rewrote all chapters line by line. The goal of this exercise was for the reader to recognize, throughout the entire book, a single voice—a unity provided by consistency in style, in organization, in the sequence for presenting concepts, and in terminology and notation, as well as in consistency in the expression of standard values (e.g., a cardiac output of 5 liters/min). The editors also attempted to minimize overlap among chapters by making extensive use of cross references (by page, figure, or table number) to principles introduced elsewhere in the book.

After the first round of editing, Dr. Malcolm Thaler—a practicing physician and accomplished author in his own right—improved the readability of the text and sometimes added clinical examples. Afterwards, the editors again went through the entire text line by line to decide on the material to be included in specific illustrations, and to match the main text of the book with the content of each figure. The editors then traveled to Philadelphia to visit the art studio of JB Woolsey and Associates. Over many visits, John Woolsey and the editors together developed the content and format for each of the approximately 760 full-color illustrations used in the textbook. These meetings were unique intellectual and pedagogical dialogues concerning the design of the figures. To a large extent, the figures owe their pedagogical style to the creativity of John Woolsey.

The illustrations evolved through several iterations of figure editing, based on suggestions from both the editors and authors. This evolution, as well as text changes requested by authors, led to yet a third round of editing of the entire book, often line by line. Throughout this seemingly endless process, our goal has been to achieve the proper balance among reader friendliness, depth, and accuracy.

Special features. Compared with other major textbooks of physiology, a much larger fraction of the space in this book is devoted to illustrations. Thus, although our textbook may appear thick, it actually has fewer text words than most other leading medical physiology books. Virtually all illustrations in our book are in full color, conceived de novo, with consistent style and pedagogy. Many of the figures feature "dialogue balloons" that tell a story. The illustrations are also available in digital format on an Electronic Image Collection CD-ROM for use in the classroom.

The textbook makes considerable use of clinical boxes—highlighted on a color background—that present examples of diseases illustrating important physiological principles. The text includes over 2000 cross references that send the reader from the current page to specific pages, figures, or tables elsewhere in the book for relevant concepts or data.

The website **www.StudentConsult.com** offers the reader access to the online edition of the textbook, with the ability to search, bookmark, post notes, download highlighted text to a handheld device, access all of the images in the book, and more. The hundreds of "spider-web" icons 🕸 in the text direct the reader to "webnotes" that are also available on **Student Consult**. These webnotes provide derivations of mathematical equations, amplification of concepts, material that was deleted for the sake of brevity from earlier drafts of the textbook, and illustrations not included in the clinical boxes.

The **Student Consult** website also contains several other features not included in the printed text, including summaries for each subchapter, an expanded list of references with direct links to the primary literature (as available), other links that may be of interest to the physiol-ogy student (e.g., biographies of famous physiologists), late-breaking scientific developments that occur after publication of the book, and—alas—the correction of errors.

Acknowledgements. A textbook is the culmination of successful collaborations among many individuals. First, we would like to thank our authors. Second, we acknowledge the expert input of Dr. Malcolm Thaler, both in terms of style and clinical insight. We also thank Dr. Thaler for emphasizing the importance of telling a "good story." The textbook's aesthetic appeal is largely attributable to JB Woolsey and Associates, particularly John Woolsey and Joel Dubin.

At W.B. Saunders, we are especially thankful to William R. Schmitt—Acquisitions Editor—for his trust and patience over the years that this book has been in gestation. At the times when the seas were rough, he steered a safe course. Melissa Dudlick—Developmental Editor at W.B. Saunders—was the project's nerve center, responsible for day-to-day communication among all parties working on the textbook, and for assembling all of the many components that went into making the final product. Her good humor and careful attention to detail greatly facilitated the creation of the textbook. We thank Frank Polizzano—Publishing Services Manager at W.B. Saunders—for overseeing production of the textbook.

Before this textbook was completed, the author of Part X (The Physiology of Everyday Life), Ethan Nadel, passed away. We are indebted to those who generously stepped up to carefully check the nearly finished manuscripts for the final four chapters: Dr. Gerald Shulman for Chapter 57, Dr. John Stitt for Chapter 58, the late Dr. Carl Gisolfi for Chapter 59, and Dr. Arthur DuBois for Chapter 60. In addition, Dr. George Lister provided expert advice for Chapter 56. We are also grateful to Dr. Bruce Davis for researching the sequences of the polypeptide hormones, to Mr. Duncan Wong for expert information-technology services, and to Mrs. Leisa Strohmaier for administrative assistance.

Preface to the 2005 Updated Edition. We are very grateful for the enthusiastic reception with which the academic community has received our book. Inevitably, errors creep into a textbook as part of both the preproduction and production processes. We thank our readers for pointing out many of these errors. In this Updated Edition, we have corrected all errors (of which we are aware) in both the text and the figures. In addition, we have updated information and also improved the text and several figures. Finally, we have added new text on Hemostasis and Fibrinolysis, which appears at the end of Chapter 17. In all, we have made text changes to a total of 302 pages (nearly a quarter of the book), made changes to 63 figures (approximately 8% of the figures), and for the new Hemostasis subchapter, we have added 7 pages and three new figures.

We now invite the reader to enjoy the experience of learning physiology. If you are pleased with our effort, tell others. If not, tell us.

Contents

I

Introduction

CHAPTER 1

Foundations of Physiology

Emile L. Boulpaep and Walter F. Boron

What Is Physiology?

Physiology is the dynamic study of life. Physiology describes the "vital" functions of living organisms and their organs, cells, and molecules. For centuries, the discipline of physiology has been closely intertwined with medicine. Although physiology is not primarily concerned with structure—as is the case of anatomy, histology, and structural biology—structure and function are inextricably linked because the living structures perform the functions.

For some, physiology is the function of the whole person (e.g., exercise physiology). For many practicing clinicians, physiology may be the function of an individual organ system, such as the cardiovascular, respiratory, or gastrointestinal system. For still others, physiology may focus on the cellular principles that are common to the function of all organs and tissues. This last field has traditionally been called "general physiology," a term that is now supplanted by "cellular and molecular physiology." Although one can divide up physiology according to varying degrees of reductionism, it is also possible to define a branch of physiology—for example, comparative physiology—that focuses on differences and similarities among different species. Indeed, comparative physiology may deal with all degrees of reductionism, from molecule to whole organism. In a similar way, medical physiology deals with how the human body functions, which depends on how the individual organ systems function, which depends on how the component cells function, which in turn depends on the interactions among subcellular organelles and countless molecules. Thus, medical physiology takes a global view of the human body, but in doing so requires an integrated understanding of events at the level of molecules, cells, and organs.

Physiology is the mother of several biological sciences, having given birth to the disciplines of biochemistry, biophysics, and neuroscience, as well as their corresponding scientific societies and journals. Thus, it should come as no surprise that the boundaries of physiology are not sharply delineated. Conversely, physiology has its own unique attributes. For example, physiology has evolved over the centuries from a more qualitative to a more quantitative science. Indeed, many of the leading physiologists were—and still are—trained as chemists, physicists, mathematicians, or engineers.

3

Physiological Genomics Is the Link Between the Organ and the Gene

The life of the human body requires not only that individual organ systems do their jobs but also that these organ systems work "hand-in-hand" with each other. They must share information. Their actions must be interdependent. The cells within an organ or a tissue often share information, and certainly the individual cells must act in concert to perform the proper function of the organ or tissue. In fact, cells in one organ must often share information with cells in another organ and make decisions that are appropriate for the health of the individual cell as well as for the health of the whole person.

In the vast majority of cases, the sharing of information between organs and between cells takes place at the level of atoms or molecules. Cell-to-cell messengers or intracellular messengers may be atoms such as H^+ or K^+ or Ca^{2+}. The messengers may also be more complex chemicals. A cell may release a molecule that acts on a neighboring cell or that enters the bloodstream and acts on other cells a great distance away. In other cases, a neuron may send an axon a centimeter or even a meter away and rapidly modulate, via a neurotransmitter molecule, the activity of another cell or another organ. Cells and organs must interact with one another, and the method of communication is almost always molecular.

The grand organizer—that master that controls the molecules, the cells, and the organs and the way they interact—is the genome. Traditionally, the discipline of physiology has, in its reductionistic journey, always stopped at about the level of cells and certain subcellular organelles, as well as their component and controlling molecules. The discipline of physiology left to molecular biology and molecular genetics the business of how the cell controls itself through its DNA. The modern discipline of physiology, however, has become closely intertwined with molecular biology because the proteins encoded by DNA are often the proteins in which physiologists are most interested. Very often, physiologists painstakingly develop elegant strategies for cloning the genes relevant to physiology. But sometimes brute-force approaches, such as the Human Genome Project in the United States, hand the physiologist a candidate gene, homologous to one of known function, on a silver platter. In still other cases, molecular biologists may clone a gene with no known function. In this case it may be up to the physiologist to determine the *function* of the gene product, that is, to determine its *physiology*.

Physiological genomics (or functional genomics) is a new branch of physiology devoted to understanding the roles genes play in physiology. Traditionally, physiologists have moved in a reductionistic direction from organ to cell to molecule to gene. One of the most fascinating aspects of physiological genomics is that it has closed the circle and linked organ physiology directly with molecular biology. Perhaps one of the most striking examples is the knockout mouse. Knocking out the gene encoding a protein that, according to conventional wisdom, is very important will sometimes have no obvious effect or sometimes very unexpected effects. It is up to the physiologist, at least in part, to figure out why. It is perhaps rather sobering to consider that to truly understand the impact of a trans-gene or a knockout on the physiology of a mouse, one would have to carefully re-evaluate the totality of mouse physiology. In order to grasp the function of a gene product, the physiologist must retrace his steps back up the reductionistic road and achieve an integrated understanding of that gene's function at the level of the cells, organs, and whole body. Physiology is unique among the basic medical sciences in that it is both broad in its scope (i.e., it deals with multiple systems) and integrative in its outlook.

Cells Live in a Highly Protected "Milieu Intérieur"

In his lectures on the phenomena of life, Claude Bernard wrote in 1878 on the conditions of the constancy of life, which he considered a property of higher forms of life. According to Bernard, animals have two environments: the "milieu extérieur" that physically surrounds the whole organism and the "milieu intérieur," in which the tissues and cells of the organism live. This internal environment is neither the air nor the fresh or salt water of less developed organisms. Instead, the internal environment of the human body is a well-controlled liquid environment that Bernard called "the organic liquid that circulates and bathes all the anatomic elements of the tissues, the lymph or the plasma"; in short, what we call today the extracellular fluid. He argued that physiological functions continue in a manner indifferent to the changing environment because the milieu intérieur isolates the organs and tissues of the body from the vagaries of the physical conditions of the environment. Indeed, Bernard described the milieu intérieur as if an organism had placed itself in a greenhouse.

According to Bernard's concept of "milieu intérieur," some fluids contained within the body are not really inside the body at all. For example, the *contents* of the gastrointestinal tract, sweat ducts, and renal tubules are all outside the body. They are all continuous with the "milieu extérieur."

Bernard compares a complex organism to an ensemble of anatomic elements that live together inside the "milieu interieur." Therefore, in Part II of this textbook, we examine the physiology of these cells and molecules. In Chapter 2 ("Functional Organization of the Cell"), we begin our journey through physiology with a discussion of the biology of the cells that are the individual elements of the body. Chapter 3 ("Physiology of Membranes") discusses how the plasma membrane determines the composition of the cell interior and separates the cell interior from Bernard's milieu intérieur. In Chapter 4 ("Signal Transduction"), we address how cells can communicate *directly* via gap junctions or *indirectly* via molecules released into the extracellular fluid. These released molecules can bind to receptors on the cell membrane and initiate signal-transduction cascades that can modify gene transcription (a genomic response) and a wide range of other cell functions (nongenomic responses). Alternatively, these released molecules can bind to receptors in the cytoplasm or nucleus and alter the transcription of genes. Chapter 5

("Regulation of Gene Expression") examines the response of the nucleus. In addition to the "chemical" transmission of information via the extracellular fluid, and indeed among cells, the body relies on "electrical" transmission of information through electrical signals in excitable tissues such as nerve and muscle. The property of "excitability," which requires both the perception of a change (a signal) as well as the reaction to it, is the topic of Chapters 6 to 9. The elements of the function of the nervous system are further developed in Part III.

Another theme developed by Bernard was that the "fixité du milieu intérieur" (the constancy of the extracellular fluid) is the condition of "free, independent life." He explains that organ differentiation is the exclusive property of higher organisms and that each organ contributes to "compensate and equilibrate" against changes in the external environment. In that sense each of the systems discussed in Parts IV to VIII permit the body to live within an adverse external environment because the cardiovascular system, the respiratory system, the urinary system, the gastrointestinal system, and the endocrine system create and maintain a constant internal environment. Individual cell types in various organ systems act in concert to support the constancy of the internal milieu, and in turn the internal milieu provides these cells with a culture medium in which they can thrive.

The discipline of physiology also deals with those characteristics that are the property of a living organism as opposed to a nonliving organism. Four fundamental properties distinguish the living body. First, only living organisms exchange matter and energy with the environment in order to continue their existence. Several organ systems of the body participate in these exchanges. Second, only living organisms can receive signals from their environment and react accordingly. The principles of sensory perception, processing by the nervous system, and reaction are discussed in the chapters on excitability and the nervous system. Third, what distinguishes a living organism is the life cycle of growth and reproduction, as discussed in the chapters on reproduction (Part IX). Finally, the living organism is able to adapt to changing circumstances. This is a theme that is developed throughout this textbook, but especially in the chapters on everyday life (Part X).

Homeostatic Mechanisms—Operating Through Sophisticated Feedback Control Mechanisms—Are Responsible for Maintaining the Constancy of the "Milieu Intérieur"

Homeostasis is the control of a vital parameter. The body carefully controls a seemingly endless list of vital parameters. Examples of tightly controlled parameters that affect nearly the whole body are arterial pressure and blood volume. At the level of the "milieu intérieur," tightly regulated parameters include body core temperature and plasma levels of oxygen, glucose, potassium ions (K^+), calcium ions (Ca^{2+}), and hydrogen ions (H^+). Homeostasis also occurs at the level of the single cell. Thus, cells regulate many of the same parameters that the body as a whole regulates: volume, the concentrations of many small inorganic ions (e.g., Na^+, Ca^{2+}), and energy levels (e.g., ATP).

One of the most common themes in physiology is the **negative-feedback mechanism** responsible for homeostasis. Negative feedback requires at least three elements. First, the system must be able to sense the vital parameter (e.g., glucose) or something related to it. Second, the system must be able to respond to changes in that vital parameter by producing some sort of signal (e.g., releasing insulin). Third, the signal must be able to act in such a way as to produce an effect that controls the parameter (e.g., a decrease in blood glucose levels). Sometimes the body controls a parameter, in part, by cleverly employing positive feedback loops.

A single feedback loop often does not operate in isolation, but rather as part of a larger network of controls. Thus, a complex interplay may exist among feedback loops within single cells, within a tissue, within an organ or organ system, or at the level of the whole body. After studying these individual feedback loops in isolation, the physiologist may find that two feedback loops act either synergistically or antagonistically. For example, insulin lowers blood glucose levels, whereas epinephrine and cortisol have the opposite effect. Thus, the physiologist must determine the relative weights of feedback loops in **competition** with one another. Finally, the physiologist must also establish **hierarchy** among various feedback loops. For example, the hypothalamus controls the anterior pituitary, which controls the adrenal cortex, which releases cortisol, which helps control blood glucose levels.

Another theme of homeostasis is **redundancy.** The more vital a parameter is, the more systems that the body mobilizes to regulate it. If one system should fail, others are there to help maintain homeostasis. It is probably for this reason that genetic knockouts sometimes fail to have their expected deleterious effects. The result of many homeostatic systems controlling many vital parameters is a "milieu intérieur" with a stable composition.

It is important to recognize that, whether at the level of the "milieu intérieur" or the cytoplasm of a single cell, homeostasis occurs at a price: energy. When a vital parameter (e.g., the blood glucose level) is well regulated, that parameter is not in equilibrium. Equilibrium is a state that does not involve energy consumption. Instead, a well-regulated parameter is generally in a **steady state.** That is, its value is constant because the body or the cell carefully matches actions that lower the parameter value with other actions that raise it. The net effect is that the vital parameter is held at a constant value.

An important principle in physiology, to which we have already alluded, is that each cell plays a specialized role in the overall function of the body. In return, the body—which is the sum of all these cells—provides the "milieu intérieur" appropriate for the life of each cell. As part of the bargain, each cell or organ must respect the needs of the body as a whole and not run amok for its own greedy interests. For example, during exercise, the system that controls body core temperature sheds heat by elaborating sweat for evaporation. However, the production of sweat ultimately reduces blood volume. Because the body as a whole places a higher **priority** on the control of blood volume than on the control of body core temperature, at some point the system that controls blood volume will instruct the system that controls body core temperature to reduce the production of sweat. Unfortunately, this juggling of priorities only works if the individual stops exercising; if not, the result may be heat stroke.

The **adaptability** of an organism depends on its ability to alter its response. Indeed, flexible feedback loops are at the root of many forms of physiological adaptation. For instance, at sea level, experimentally lowering the level of oxygen (the sensory stimulus) in the inspired air causes an increase in breathing (the response). However, after adapting to low oxygen levels at high altitude, the same low level of oxygen (the same sensory stimulus) causes one to breathe much faster (a greater response). Thus, the response may depend on the previous history and therefore the "state" of the system.

Medicine Is the Study of "Physiology Gone Awry"

Medicine borrows its physicochemical principles from physiology. Medicine also uses physiology as a reference state: it is essential to know how organs and systems function in the healthy person in order to grasp which components may be malfunctioning in a patient. A large part of clinical medicine is simply dealing with the abnormal physiology brought about by a disease process. One malfunction (e.g., heart failure) can lead to a *primary* pathologic effect (e.g., a decrease in cardiac output) that—in chain-reaction style—leads to a series of *secondary* effects (e.g., fluid overload) that are the appropriate responses of physiological feedback loops. Indeed, as clinician/physiologists have explored the basis of disease, they have discovered a great deal about physiology. For this reason, we have tried to illustrate physiological principles with clinical examples, some of which are displayed in clinical boxes in this text.

Physiologists have developed many tools and tests to examine normal function. A large number of functional tests—used in diagnosing a disease, monitoring the evolution of an illness, and evaluating the progress of therapy—are direct transfers of technology developed in the physiology laboratory. Typical examples are cardiac monitoring, pulmonary function tests, and renal clearance tests, as well as the assays used to measure plasma levels of various ions, gases, and hormones. Refinements of such technology in the hospital environment, in turn, benefit the study of physiology. Thus, the exchange of information between medicine and physiology is a two-way street. The understanding of physiology summarized in this book comes from some experiments on humans, but mostly from research on other mammals and even on squids and slime molds. However, our ultimate focus is on the human body.

REFERENCES

Bernard C: Leçons sur les phénomènes de la vie communs aux animaux et aux végétaux. Cours de Physiologie générale du Museum d'Histoire Naturelle. Paris, Baillière et fils, 1878.
Cannon WB: The Wisdom of the Body. New York, Norton, 1932.
Smith HW: From Fish to Philosopher. New York, Doubleday, 1961.

II

Physiology of Cells and Molecules

CHAPTER 2

Functional Organization of the Cell

Michael J. Caplan

In the minds of many students, the discipline of physiology is linked inextricably to images from its past. This prejudice is not surprising, because many experiments from physiology's proud history, such as those of Pavlov and his dogs, have transcended mere scientific renown and entered the realm of popular culture. Some might believe that the science of physiology devotes itself exclusively to the study of whole animals and is, therefore, an antique relic in this era of molecular reductionism. Nothing could be further from the truth. Physiology is and always has been the study of the homeostatic mechanisms that allow an organism to persist despite the ever-changing pressures imposed by a hostile environment. These mechanisms can be appreciated at many different levels of resolution.

Certainly it would be difficult to understand how the body operates unless one appreciates the functions of its organs and the communication between these organs that allows them to influence one another's behaviors. It would also be difficult to understand how an organ performs its particular tasks unless one is familiar with the properties of its constituent cells and molecules.

The modern treatment of physiology that is presented in this textbook is as much about the interactions of molecules in cells as it is about the interactions of organs in organisms. It is necessary, therefore, at the outset to discuss the structure and characteristics of the cell. Our discussion focuses first on the architectural and dynamic features of a generic cell. We will then examine how this generic cell can be adapted to serve in diverse physiological capacities. Through adaptations at the cellular level, organs acquire the machinery necessary to perform their individual metabolic tasks.

STRUCTURE OF BIOLOGIC MEMBRANES

The Surface of the Cell Is Defined by a Membrane

The chemical composition of the cell interior is very different from that of its surroundings. This observation applies equally to unicellular paramecia that swim freely in a freshwater pond and to neurons that are densely packed in the cerebral cortex of the human brain. The biochemical processes involved in cell function require the maintenance of a precisely regulated intracellular environment. The cytoplasm is an extraordinarily complex solution, the constituents of which include myriad proteins, nu-

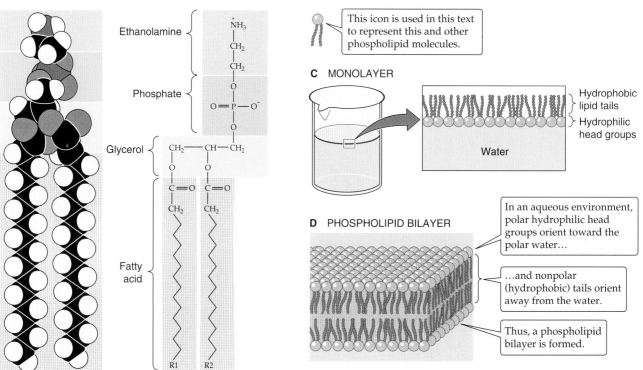

FIGURE 2–1. Phospholipids.

cleic acids, nucleotides, and sugars that the cell synthesizes or accumulates at great metabolic cost. The cell also expends tremendous energy to regulate the intracellular concentrations of numerous ions. If there were no barrier surrounding the cell to prevent exchange between the intracellular and extracellular spaces, all of the cytoplasm's hard-won compositional uniqueness would be lost by diffusion in a few seconds.

The requisite barrier is provided by the **plasma membrane**, which forms the cell's outer skin. The plasma membrane is *impermeable* to large molecules such as proteins and nucleic acids, thus ensuring their retention within the cytosol. It is *selectively permeable* to small molecules such as ions and metabolites. However, the metabolic requirements of the cell demand a plasma membrane that is much more sophisticated than a simple passive barrier that allows various substances to leak through at different rates. Frequently, the concentration of a nutrient in the extracellular fluid is several orders of magnitude lower than required inside the cell. If the cell wishes to use such a substance, therefore, it must be able to *accumulate* it against a concentration gradient. A simple pore in the membrane cannot concentrate anything; it can only modulate the rate at which a gradient dissipates. To accomplish the more sophisticated feat of creating a concentration gradient, the membrane must be endowed with special machinery that uses metabolic energy to drive the *uphill* movements of substances—**active transport**—into or out of the cell. In addition, it would be useful to rapidly modulate the permeability properties of the plasma membrane in response to various metabolic stimuli. Active transport and the ability to control passive

permeabilities underlie a wide range of physiological processes, from the electric excitability of neurons to the resorptive and secretory functions of the kidney. In Chapter 3, we will explore how cells actively transport solutes across the plasma membrane. The mechanisms through which the plasma membrane's dynamic selectivity is achieved, modified, and regulated are discussed briefly later in this chapter and in greater detail in Chapter 6.

The Cell Membrane Is Composed Primarily of Phospholipids

Our understanding of biologic membrane structure is based on studies of red blood cells, or erythrocytes, that were conducted in the early part of the 20th century. The erythrocyte lacks the nucleus and other complicated intracellular structures that are characteristic of most animal cells. It consists of a plasma membrane surrounding a cytoplasm that is rich in hemoglobin. It is possible to break open erythrocytes and release their cytoplasmic contents. The plasma membranes can then be recovered by centrifugation, providing a remarkably pure preparation of cell-surface membrane. Biochemical analysis reveals that this membrane is composed of two principal constituents: lipid and protein.

Most of the lipid associated with erythrocyte plasma membranes belongs to the molecular family of **phospholipids**. Generally, phospholipids share a **glycerol** backbone, two hydroxyl groups of which are esterified to molecules of **fatty acid** (Fig. 2–1A). However, in the case of another phospholipid—sphingomyelin—the backbone is *serine* rather than glycerol. For glycerol-based phospholipids, the third glycerolic hydroxyl group is esterified to a **phosphate** group, which is in turn esterified to a small molecule that is referred to as a **head group**. The identity of the head group determines the name as well as many of the properties of the individual phospholipids. A glycerol-based phospholipid that bears an ethanolamine molecule in the head group position is categorized as a **phosphatidylethanolamine** (see Fig. 2–1*A*), and one with a choline head group is known as a **phosphatidylcholine**.

Phospholipids Form Complex Structures in Aqueous Solution

The unique structure and physical chemistry of each phospholipid (see Fig. 2–1*B*) underlies the formation of biologic membranes and explains many of their most important properties. Fatty acids are nonpolar molecules. Their long carbon chains lack the charged groups that would facilitate interactions with water, which is polar. Consequently, fatty acids dissolve poorly in water but readily in organic solvents; thus, fatty acids are **hydrophobic**. On the other hand, the head groups of most phospholipids are charged or polar. These head groups interact well with water and, consequently, are very water soluble. Thus, the head groups are **hydrophilic**. Because phospholipids combine hydrophilic heads with hydrophobic tails, their interaction with water is referred to as **amphipathic**.

When mixed with water, phospholipids organize themselves into structures that prevent their hydrophobic tails from making contact with water while simultaneously permitting their hydrophilic head groups to be fully dissolved. When added to water at fairly low concentrations, phospholipids form a **monolayer** (see Fig. 2–1*C*) on the water's surface at the air-water interface. It is energetically less costly to the system for the hydrophobic tails to stick up in the air than to interact with the solvent.

At higher concentrations, phospholipids assemble into **micelles**. The hydrophilic head groups form the surfaces of these small spheres, whereas the hydrophobic tails point toward their centers. In this geometry, the tails are protected from any contact with water and instead are able to participate in energetically favorable interactions among themselves. At still higher concentrations, phospholipids spontaneously form **bilayers** (see Fig. 2–1*D*). In these structures, the phospholipid molecules arrange themselves into two parallel sheets or **leaflets** that face each other tail to tail. The surfaces of the bilayer are composed of hydrophilic head groups, whereas the hydrophobic tails form the center of the sandwich. The hydrophilic surfaces insulate the hydrophobic tails from contact with the solvent, leaving the tails free to associate exclusively with one another.

The physical characteristics of a lipid bilayer largely depend on the chemical composition of its constituent phospholipid molecules. For example, the width of the bilayer is determined by the length of the fatty-acid side chains. Dihexadecanoic phospholipids (whose two fatty-acid chains are each 16 carbons long) produce bilayers that are 2.47 nm wide, whereas ditetradecanoic phospholipids (bearing 14-carbon fatty acids) generate 2.3-nm bilayers. Similarly, the nature of the head groups determines how densely packed adjacent phospholipid molecules are in each leaflet of the membrane.

Detergents can dissolve phospholipid membranes because, like the phospholipids themselves, they are amphipathic. They possess very hydrophilic head groups and hydrophobic tails and are water soluble at much higher concentrations than are the phospholipids. When mixed together in aqueous solutions, detergent and phospholipid molecules interact through their hydrophobic tails, and the resulting complexes are water soluble, either as individual dimers or in mixed micelles. Therefore, adding sufficient concentrations of detergent to phospholipid bilayer membranes disrupts the membranes and dissolves the lipids. Detergents are extremely useful tools in research into the structure and composition of lipid membranes.

The Diffusion of Individual Lipids Within a Leaflet of a Bilayer Is Determined by the Chemical Make-Up of Its Constituents

Despite its highly organized appearance, a phospholipid bilayer is a fluid structure. An individual phospholipid molecule is free to diffuse within the entire leaflet in which it resides. The rate at which this two-dimensional diffusion occurs is extremely temperature dependent. At high temperatures, the thermal energy of any given lipid molecule is greater than the interaction energy that would tend to hold adjacent lipid molecules together. Under these conditions, lateral diffusion can proceed rapidly, and the lipid is said to be in the **sol state**. At lower temperatures, interaction energies exceed the thermal energies of most individual molecules. Thus, phospholipids diffuse slowly because they lack the energy to free themselves from the embraces of their neighbors. This behavior is characteristic of the **gel state**.

The temperature at which the bilayer membrane converts from the gel to sol phases (and vice versa) is referred to as the **transition temperature**. The transition temperature is another characteristic that depends on the chemical make-up of the phospholipids in the bilayer. Phospholipids with long, saturated fatty-acid chains can extensively interact with one another. Consequently, a fair amount of thermal energy is required to overcome these interactions and permit diffusion. Not surprisingly, such bilayers have relatively high transition temperatures. For example, the transition temperature for dioctadecanoic phosphatidylcholine (which has two 18-carbon fatty-acid chains, fully saturated) is 55.5°C. In contrast, phospholipids that have shorter fatty-acid chains or double bonds (which introduce kinks) cannot line up next to each other as well and, hence, do not interact as well. Considerably less energy is required to induce them to participate in diffusion. For example, if we reduce the length of the carbon chain from 18 to 14, the transition temperature falls to 23°C. If we retain 18 carbons, but introduce a single, double bond (making the fatty-acid chains

FIGURE 2–2. Structures of some common membrane lipids.

monounsaturated), the transition temperature also falls dramatically.

By mixing other types of lipid molecules into phospholipid bilayers, we can markedly alter the membrane's fluidity properties. In addition to the glycerol-based phospholipids that were described earlier—such as phosphatidylethanolamine (see Fig. 2–1A), phosphatidylinositol (Fig. 2–2A), phosphatidylserine (see Fig. 2–2B) and phosphatidylcholine (see Fig. 2–2C)—the plasma membranes of animal cells can contain other structurally distinct classes of lipids, including sphingomyelin (see Fig. 2–2D), glycosphingolipids such as galactocerebroside (see

Fig. 2–2E), and cholesterol (see Fig. 2–2F). Because these latter three classes of molecules are not shaped exactly like the glycerol-based phospholipids, they participate to different degrees in intermolecular interactions with phospholipid side chains. The presence of these alternative lipids (Fig. 2–3A) changes the strength of the interactions that prevents lipid molecules from diffusing. Consequently, the membrane has a different fluidity and a different transition temperature. This behavior is especially characteristic of the cholesterol molecule, whose rigid steroid ring binds to and partially immobilizes fatty-acid side chains. Therefore, at modest concentrations,

A DIVERSITY OF LIPIDS IN A BILAYER

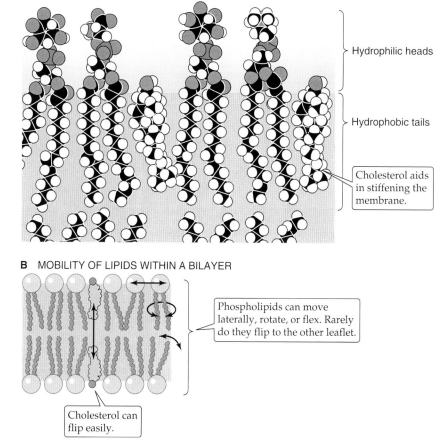

Hydrophilic heads

Hydrophobic tails

Cholesterol aids
in stiffening the
membrane.

FIGURE 2–3. Interaction among lipids in a bilayer. In *A*, the upper leaflet of this lipid bilayer contains, from left to right, phosphatidylinositol, phosphatidylserine, cholesterol, phosphatidylinositol, phosphatidylcholine, and cholesterol.

B MOBILITY OF LIPIDS WITHIN A BILAYER

Phospholipids can move
laterally, rotate, or flex. Rarely
do they flip to the other leaflet.

Cholesterol can
flip easily.

cholesterol decreases fluidity. However, when present in high concentrations, cholesterol can substantially disrupt the phospholipids' ability to interact among themselves, which increases fluidity and lowers the gel-sol transition temperature. This issue is significant because animal cell plasma membranes can contain substantial quantities of cholesterol.

Bilayers composed of several different lipids do not undergo the transition from gel to sol at a single, well-defined temperature. Instead, they interconvert more gradually over a temperature range that is defined by the composition of the mixture. Within this transition range in such multicomponent bilayers, the membrane can become divided into compositionally distinct zones. The phospholipids with long-chain, saturated fatty acids will adhere to one another relatively tightly, which results in the formation of regions with "gel-like" properties. Phospholipids bearing short-chain, unsaturated fatty acids will be excluded from these regions and migrate to sol-like regions. Hence, "lakes" of lipids with markedly different physical properties can exist side-by-side in the plane of a phospholipid membrane. Thus, the same thermodynamic forces that form the elegant bilayer structure can partition distinct lipid domains within the bilayer. As discussed later, the segregation of lipid lakes in the plane of the membrane may be important for sorting membrane proteins to different parts of the cell.

Although phospholipids can diffuse in the plane of a lipid bilayer membrane, they do not diffuse between adjacent leaflets (see Fig. 2–3*B*). The rate at which phospholipids spontaneously "flip-flop" from one leaflet of a bilayer to the other is extremely low. As mentioned earlier, the center of a bilayer membrane consists of the fatty-acid tails of the phospholipid molecules and is an extremely hydrophobic environment. For a phospholipid molecule to jump from one leaflet to the other, its highly hydrophilic head group would have to transit this central hydrophobic core, which would have an extremely high energy cost. This caveat does not apply to cholesterol (see Fig. 2–3*B*), whose polar head is a single hydroxyl group. The energy cost of dragging this small polar hydroxyl group through the bilayer is relatively low, thus permitting relatively rapid cholesterol flip-flop.

Phospholipid-Bilayer Membranes Are Impermeable to Charged Molecules

The lipid bilayer is ideally suited to separate two aqueous compartments. Its hydrophilic head groups interact well with water at both membrane surfaces, whereas the hydrophobic center ensures that the energetic cost of crossing the membrane is prohibitive for charged atoms or molecules. Pure phospholipid-bilayer membranes are extremely impermeable to almost any charged, water-soluble substance. Ions, such as Na^+, K^+, Cl^-, and Ca^{2+}, are

FIGURE 2–4. Transmission electron micrograph of a cell membrane. The photograph shows two adjacent cells of the pancreas of a frog at a magnification of ×43,000. The inset is a high-magnification view (×216,000) of the plasma membranes of the cells. Note that each membrane includes two dense layers with an intermediate layer of lower density. The dense layers represent the interaction of the polar head groups of the phospholipids with the OsO_4 used to stain the preparation. (From Porter KR, Bonneville MR: Fine Structure of Cells and Tissues, 4th ed., Philadelphia, Lea & Febiger, 1973.)

insoluble in the hydrophobic membrane core and, consequently, cannot travel from the aqueous environment on one side of the membrane to the aqueous environment on the opposite side. The same is true of large water-soluble molecules, such as proteins, nucleic acids, sugars, and nucleotides.

Whereas phospholipid membranes are impermeable to water-soluble molecules, small *uncharged* polar molecules can cross fairly freely. This is often true for O_2, CO_2, NH_3, and, remarkably, for water itself. Water molecules may, at least in part, traverse the membrane through transient cracks between the hydrophobic tails of the phospholipids, without having to surmount an enormous energetic barrier. The degree of water permeability (and perhaps that of CO_2 and NH_3 as well) varies extensively with lipid composition; some phospholipids (especially those with short or kinked fatty-acid chains) permit a much greater rate of transbilayer water diffusion than others.

The Plasma Membrane Is a Bilayer

As may be inferred from the preceding discussion, the membrane at the cell surface is, in fact, a phospholipid bilayer. The truth of this statement was established by a remarkably straightforward experiment. In 1925, Gorter and Grendel measured the surface area of the lipids they extracted from erythrocyte plasma membranes. They used a device called a Langmuir trough in which the lipids are allowed to line up at an air-water interface (see Fig. 2–1C) and are then packed together into a continuous monolayer by a sliding bar that decreases the surface that is available to them. The area of the monolayer that was created by the erythrocyte lipids was exactly twice the surface area of the erythrocytes from which they were derived. Therefore, the plasma membrane must be a bilayer.

Confirmation of the bilayer structure of biologic membranes has come from x-ray diffraction studies that were performed on the repetitive whorls of membrane that form the myelin sheaths that surround neuronal axons (p. 417). The membrane's bilayer structure can be visualized directly in the high-magnification electron micrograph that is depicted in Figure 2–4. The osmium tetraoxide molecule (OsO_4), with which the membrane is stained, binds to the head groups of phospholipids. Thus, both surfaces of a phospholipid bilayer appear black in electron micrographs, whereas the membrane's unstained central core appears white.

The phospholipid compositions of the two leaflets of the plasma membrane are not identical. Labeling studies performed on erythrocyte plasma membranes reveal that the surface that faces the cytoplasm contains phosphatidylethanolamine and phosphatidylserine, whereas the outward-facing leaflet is composed almost exclusively of phosphatidylcholine. As is discussed later in this chapter, this asymmetry is created during the biosynthesis of the phospholipid molecules. It is not entirely clear what advantage this distribution provides to the cell. It appears likely that the interactions between certain proteins and the plasma membrane may require this segregation. The lipid asymmetry may be especially important for those phospholipids that are involved in second-messenger cascades (p. 100 & 103). Finally, it should be noted that the phospholipids that are characteristic of animal-cell plasma membranes generally have one saturated and one unsaturated fatty-acid residue. Consequently, they are less likely

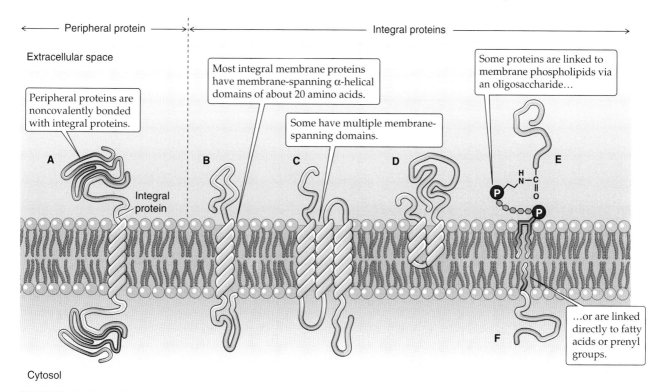

FIGURE 2–5. Classes of membrane proteins. In *E*, protein is coupled via a glycosylphosphatidylinositol (GPI) linkage.

to partition into sol-like or gel-like lipid domains than are phospholipids that bear identical fatty-acid chains.

Membrane Proteins Can Be Integrally or Peripherally Associated with the Plasma Membrane

The demonstration that the plasma membrane's lipid components form a bilayer leaves open the question of how the membrane's protein constituents are organized. Membrane proteins can belong to either of two broad classes: peripheral or integral. **Peripherally associated membrane proteins** are neither embedded within the membrane nor attached to it by covalent bonds; instead, they adhere tightly to the cytoplasmic or extracellular surfaces of the plasma membrane (Fig. 2–5A). They can be removed from the membrane, however, by mild treatments that disrupt ionic bonds (very high salt concentrations) or hydrogen bonds (very low salt concentrations).

In contrast, **integral membrane proteins** are very intimately associated with the lipid bilayer. They cannot be eluted from the membrane by these high- or low-salt washes. To dislodge integral membrane proteins, the membrane itself must be dissolved by adding detergents. Integral membrane proteins can be associated with the lipid bilayer in any of three ways. First, some proteins actually span the lipid bilayer once or several times (see Fig. 2–5B and C) and, hence, are referred to as **transmembrane proteins**. Experiments performed on erythrocyte membranes reveal that these proteins can be labeled with protein-tagging reagents that are applied to either side of the bilayer.

The second group of integral membrane proteins is embedded in the bilayer without actually crossing it (see Fig. 2–5D). A third group of membrane-associated proteins is not actually embedded in the bilayer at all. Instead, these lipid-anchored proteins are attached to the membrane by a covalent bond that links them either to a lipid component of the membrane or to a fatty-acid derivative that intercalates into the membrane. For example, proteins can be linked to a special type of glycosylated phospholipid molecule (see Fig. 2–5E), which is most often glycosylphosphatidylinositol (**GPI**), on the outer leaflet of the membrane. This family is referred to collectively as the **glycophospholipid-linked proteins**. Another example is a direct linkage to a fatty acid (e.g., a myristyl group) or a prenyl (e.g., farnesyl) group that intercalates into the inner leaflet of the membrane (see Fig. 2–5F).

The Membrane-Spanning Portions of Transmembrane Proteins Are Usually Hydrophobic α Helices

How can membrane-spanning proteins remain stably associated with the bilayer in a conformation that requires that at least some portion of their amino acid sequence be in continuous contact with the membrane's hydrophobic central core? The answer to this question can be found in the special structures of those protein domains that actually span the membrane.

Table 2–1

CLASSIFICATION OF THE AMINO ACIDS BASED ON THE CHEMISTRY OF THEIR SIDE CHAINS

	NAME	3-LETTER CODE	SINGLE-LETTER CODE	STRUCTURE OF SIDE CHAIN	HYDROPATHY INDEX*
Nonpolar	Alanine	Ala	A	—CH₃	+1.8
	Valine	Val	V	—CH(CH₃)₂	+4.2
	Leucine	Leu	L	—CH₂CH(CH₃)₂	+3.8
	Isoleucine	Ile	I	—CH—CH₂—CH₃ / CH₃	+4.5
	Proline	Pro	P		−1.6
	Phenylalanine	Phe	F	—CH₂—	+2.8
	Tryptophan	Trp	W	—CH₂—	−0.9
	Methionine	Met	M	—CH₂—CH₂—S—CH₃	+1.9
Polar uncharged	Glycine	Gly	G	—H	−0.4
	Serine	Ser	S	—CH₂—OH	−0.8
	Threonine	Thr	T	—CH—CH₃ / OH	−0.7
	Cysteine	Cys	C	—CH₂—SH	+2.5
	Tyrosine	Tyr	Y	—CH₂— —OH	−1.3
	Asparagine	Asn	N	—CH₂—C=O / NH₂	−3.5
	Glutamine	Gln	Q	—CH₂—CH₂—C=O / NH₂	−3.5
Polar, charged, acidic	Aspartate	Asp	D	—CH₂—C=O / O⁻	−3.5
	Glutamate	Glu	E	—CH₂—CH₂—C=O / O⁻	−3.5
Polar, charged, basic	Lysine	Lys	K	—CH₂—CH₂—CH₂—CH₂—NH₃⁺	−3.9
	Arginine	Arg	R	—CH₂—CH₂—CH₂—NH—C—NH₂ / NH₂⁺	−4.5
	Histidine	His	H	—CH₂—	−3.2

* Kyte and Doolittle generated these values (arbitrary scale from −4.5 to +4.5) by averaging two kinds of data. The first is an index of the energy that is required to transfer the side chain from the vapor phase into water. The second indicates how likely it is to find the side chain buried in (as opposed to being on the surface of) 12 globular proteins, whose structures were solved by X-ray crystallography. A positive value indicates that the side chain is hydrophobic. (From Kyte J, Doolittle RF: A simple method for displaying the hydropathic character of a protein. J Mol Biol 157:105–132, 1982.)

Note: The portion shown in red is part of the peptide backbone.

The side chains of the eight amino acids listed in the upper portion of Table 2–1 are hydrophobic. These aromatic or uncharged aliphatic groups are almost as difficult to solvate in water as are the fatty-acid side chains of the membrane phospholipids themselves. Not surprisingly, therefore, these hydrophobic side chains are quite comfortable in the hydrophobic environment of the bilayer core. Most **membrane-spanning segments**—that is, the short stretch of amino acids that passes through the membrane once—are composed mainly of these nonpolar amino acids, in concert with polar, uncharged amino acids.

The hydrophobic, membrane-spanning segments of transmembrane proteins are specially adapted to the hydrophobic milieu in which they reside. The phospholipid molecules of the membrane bilayer actually protect these portions of transmembrane proteins from energetically unfavorable interactions with the aqueous environment. Transmembrane proteins tend to be extremely insoluble in water. If we separate the membrane-spanning segments of these proteins from the amphipathic phospholipids that surround them, these hydrophobic sequences tend to interact tightly with one another rather than with water. The resulting large protein aggregates are generally insoluble, and precipitate out of solution. If, however, we disrupt the phospholipid membrane by adding detergent, the amphipathic detergent molecules can substitute for the phospholipids. The hydrophobic membrane-spanning sequences remain insulated from interactions with the aqueous solvent, and the proteins remain soluble as components of **detergent micelles**. This ability of detergents to remove transmembrane proteins from the lipid bilayer—while maintaining the solubility and native architectures of these proteins—has proved important for purifying individual membrane proteins.

Transmembrane proteins can have a single membrane-spanning segment (see Fig. 2–5B) or several (see Fig. 2–5C). Those with a single transmembrane segment can be oriented with either their amino (N) or their carboxy (C) termini facing the extracellular space. Multispanning membrane proteins weave through the membrane like a thread through cloth. Again, the N or C termini can be exposed to either the cytoplasmic or extracellular compartments. The pattern with which the transmembrane protein weaves across the lipid bilayer defines its membrane **topology**.

The amino-acid sequences of membrane-spanning segments tend to form α-helices, with approximately 3.6 amino acids per turn of the helix (see Fig. 2–5B). In this conformation, the polar atoms of the peptide backbone are maximally hydrogen bonded to one another—from one turn of the helix to the next—so they do not require the solvent to contribute hydrogen-bond partners. Hence, this structure ensures the solubility of the membrane-spanning sequence in the hydrophobic environment of the membrane. Whereas the vast majority of transmembrane proteins appears to traverse the membrane with α-helical spans, it is clear that an intriguing subset of membrane polypeptides makes use of a very different structure. The best-studied member of this class is the porin protein, which serves as a channel in bacterial membranes (p. 58). As discussed in Chapter 3, the membrane-spanning portions of porin are arranged as a β-barrel.

In the case of multispanning membrane proteins, their transmembrane helices probably pack together tightly (Fig. 2–5C). Molecular analysis of a number of known membrane-spanning sequences has helped in developing algorithms that predict the likelihood that a given amino-acid sequence can span the membrane. These algorithms are widely used to assess the likelihood that newly identified genes encode transmembrane proteins, and to predict the number and location of membrane-spanning segments.

Many membrane proteins form tight, noncovalent associations with other membrane proteins in the plane of the bilayer. These **multimeric proteins** can be composed of a single type of polypeptide or of mixtures of two or more different proteins. The side-to-side interactions that hold these complexes together can involve the membrane-spanning segments or regions of the proteins that protrude at either surface of the bilayer. By assembling into multimeric complexes, membrane proteins can increase their stability. They can also increase the variety and complexity of the functions that they are capable of performing (Fig. 2–6).

Some Membrane Proteins Are Mobile in the Plane of the Bilayer

As is true for phospholipid molecules (see Fig. 2–3B), some transmembrane proteins can also diffuse within the surface of the membrane. In the absence of any protein-protein attachments, transmembrane proteins are free to diffuse over the entire surface of a membrane. This fact was demonstrated by Frye and Edidin in 1970 (Fig. 2–7). They labeled the surface proteins of a population of *mouse* lymphocytes with a lectin (a plant sugar that binds strongly to certain proteins) that was linked to the fluorescent dye fluorescein. They also tagged the surface proteins of a second population of *human* lymphocytes with a lectin that was conjugated to a different fluorescent dye, rhodamine. Because fluorescein glows green and rhodamine glows red when excited by the light of the appropriate wavelengths, these labeling molecules can be easily distinguished from one another in a fluorescence microscope. Frye and Edidin mixed the two lymphocyte populations and treated them with a reagent that caused the cells to fuse to each other. Immediately following fusion, the labeled surface proteins of the newly joined cells remained separate: half of the fused cell surface appeared red, whereas the other half appeared green. Over a period of approximately 30 minutes, however, the green and red protein labels intermixed until the entire surface of the fused cell was covered with both labeling molecules. The rate at which this intermingling occurred increased with temperature, which is not surprising, given the temperature dependence of membrane fluidity.

Because transmembrane proteins are large molecules, their diffusion in the plane of the membrane is much slower than that of lipids. Even the fastest proteins diffuse approximately 1000 times more slowly than the average phospholipid. The diffusion of many transmembrane proteins appears to be further impeded by their attachments

Rhodamine-tagged
membrane proteins

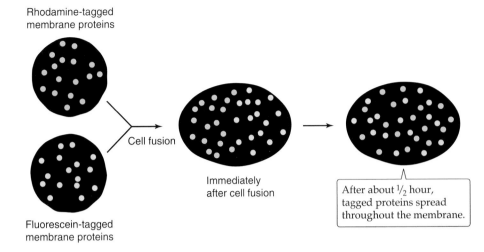

Fluorescein-tagged
membrane proteins

Cell fusion

Immediately
after cell fusion

After about ½ hour,
tagged proteins spread
throughout the membrane.

FIGURE 2–6. Diffusion of membrane proteins within the plane of the cell membrane. The surface proteins of a *human* lymphocyte are tagged with a lectin conjugated to rhodamine, a fluorescent dye, whereas the surface proteins of a *mouse* lymphocyte are tagged with a lectin linked to fluorescein, another fluorescent dye. Immediately after fusion of the two cells, the labeled surface proteins remained segregated. However, the membrane proteins intermingle over a period of approximately 30 minutes.

to the cytoskeleton, just below the surface of the membrane. Tight binding to this meshwork can render proteins essentially immobile. Other transmembrane proteins appear to travel in the plane of the membrane via directed processes that are much faster and less directionally random than diffusion is. Motor proteins that are associated with the cytoplasmic cytoskeleton (discussed later) appear to grab on to certain transmembrane proteins, dragging them in the plane of the membrane like toy boats on strings. Finally, it should be noted that, like phospholipids, proteins can only diffuse in the plane of the bilayer. They cannot flip-flop across it. The energetic barrier to dragging a transmembrane protein's hydrophilic cytoplasmic and extracellular domains across the bilayer's

hydrophobic core is very difficult to surmount. Thus, a membrane protein's topology does not change over its life span.

FUNCTION OF MEMBRANE PROTEINS

Integral-Membrane Proteins Can Serve as Receptors

All communication between a cell and its environment must involve or at least pass through the plasma membrane. For the purposes of this discussion, we define communication rather broadly as the exchange of any

A   LIGAND-BINDING RECEPTOR

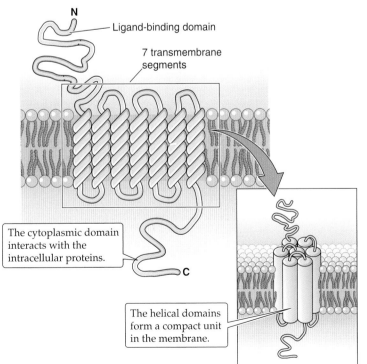

N

Ligand-binding domain

7 transmembrane
segments

The cytoplasmic domain
interacts with the
intracellular proteins.

C

The helical domains
form a compact unit
in the membrane.

B   CELL-MATRIX ADHESION MOLECULE (INTEGRIN)

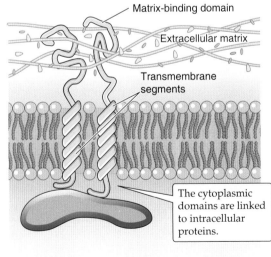

Matrix-binding domain

Extracellular matrix

Transmembrane
segments

The cytoplasmic
domains are linked
to intracellular
proteins.

FIGURE 2–7. Integral membrane proteins that transmit signals from the outside to the inside of a cell. *A,* The ligand may be a hormone, a growth factor, a neurotransmitter, an odorant, or another local mediator. *B,* An integrin is an adhesion molecule that attaches the cell to the extracellular matrix.

signal between the cell and its surroundings. Except for lipid-soluble signaling molecules such as steroid hormones, essentially all communication functions served by the plasma membrane occur via membrane proteins. From an engineering perspective, membrane proteins are perfectly situated to transmit signals because they form a single, continuous link between the two compartments that are separated by the membrane.

Ligand-binding receptors comprise the group of transmembrane proteins that perhaps most clearly illustrate the concept of transmembrane signaling (see Fig. 2–7A). For water-soluble hormones such as epinephrine to influence cellular behavior, their presence in the extracellular fluid compartment must be made known to the various intracellular mechanisms whose behaviors they modulate. The interaction of a hormone with the extracellular portion of the hormone receptor, which forms a high-affinity binding site, produces conformational changes within the receptor protein that extend through the membrane-spanning domain to the intracellular domain of the receptor. As a consequence, the intracellular domain either becomes enzymatically active or can interact with cytoplasmic proteins that are involved in the generation of so-called second messengers. Either mechanism completes the transmission of the hormone signal across the membrane. The transmembrane disposition of a hormone receptor thus creates a single, continuous communication medium that is capable of conveying, through its own structural modifications, information from the environment to the cellular interior. The process of transmembrane signal transduction is discussed in Chapter 4.

Integral-Membrane Proteins Can Serve as Adhesion Molecules

Cells can also exploit integral membrane proteins as **adhesion molecules** that form physical contacts with the surrounding extracellular matrix (i.e., cell-matrix adhesion molecules) or with their cellular neighbors (i.e., cell-cell adhesion molecules). These attachments can be extremely important in regulating the shape, growth, and differentiation of cells. The nature and extent of these attachments must be communicated to the cell interior so that the cell can adapt appropriately to the physical constraints and cues that are provided by its immediate surroundings. Numerous classes of transmembrane proteins are involved in these communication processes. The **integrins** are examples of matrix receptors or **cell-matrix adhesion molecules**. They comprise a large family of transmembrane proteins that link cells to components of the extracellular matrix (e.g., fibronectin, laminin) at adhesion plaques (see Fig. 2–7B). These linkages produce conformational changes in the integrin molecules that are transmitted to their cytoplasmic tails. These tails, in turn, communicate the linkage events to various structural and signaling molecules that participate in formulating a cell's response to its physical environment.

In contrast to matrix receptors, which attach cells to the extracellular matrix, several enormous superfamilies of **cell-cell adhesion molecules** attach cells to each other. These cell-cell adhesion molecules include the Ca^{2+}-dependent cell-adhesion molecules (cadherins) and Ca^{2+}-independent neuronal cell-adhesion molecules (N-CAMs). The **cadherins** are glycoproteins (i.e., proteins with sugars attached) with one membrane-spanning segment and a large extracellular domain that binds Ca^{2+}. The **N-CAMs**, on the other hand, generally are members of the immunoglobulin superfamily. The two classes of cell-cell adhesion molecules mediate similar sorts of transmembrane signals that help to organize the cytoplasm and control gene expression in response to intercellular contacts. Some cell-cell adhesion molecules belong to the **GPI-linked class** of membrane proteins (p. 15). These polypeptides lack a transmembrane and cytoplasmic tail. It is not clear, therefore, how (or if) interactions mediated by this unique class of adhesion molecules are communicated to the cell interior.

Adhesion molecules orchestrate processes that are as diverse as the directed migration of immune cells and the guidance of axons in the developing nervous system. Loss of cell-cell and cell-matrix adhesion is a hallmark of metastatic tumor cells.

Integral-Membrane Proteins Can Carry Out the Transmembrane Movement of Water-Soluble Substances

Earlier in this discussion, we noted that a pure phospholipid bilayer does not have the permeability properties that are normally associated with animal-cell plasma membranes. Pure phospholipid bilayers also lack the ability to transport substances uphill. Transmembrane proteins endow biologic membranes with these capabilities. Ions and other membrane-impermeable substances can cross the bilayer with the assistance of transmembrane proteins that serve as pores, channels, carriers, and pumps. **Pores** and **channels** serve as conduits that allow water, specific ions, or even very large proteins to flow passively through the bilayer. **Carriers** can either facilitate the transport of a specific molecule across the membrane or couple the transport of a molecule to that of other solutes. **Pumps** use the energy that is released through the hydrolysis of adenosine triphosphate (ATP) to drive the transport of substances into or out of cells against energy gradients. Each of these important classes of proteins is discussed in Chapter 3.

Channels, carriers, and pumps succeed in allowing hydrophilic substances to cross the membrane by creating a hydrophilic pathway in the bilayer. Previously, we asserted that membrane-spanning segments are as hydrophobic as the fatty acids that surround them. How is it possible for these *hydrophobic* membrane-spanning domains to produce the *hydrophilic* pathways that permit the passage of ions through the membrane? The solution to this puzzle appears to be that the α helices that make up these membrane-spanning segments are amphipathic. That is, they possesses both hydrophobic and hydrophilic domains.

For each α helix, the helical turns produce alignments of amino acids that are spaced at regular intervals in the sequence. Thus, it is possible to align all the hydrophilic or hydrophobic amino acids along a single edge of the helix. In **amphipathic helices**, hydrophobic amino acids alternate with hydrophilic residues at regular intervals of approximately 3 or 4 amino acids (recall that there are ~3.6 amino acids per turn of the helix). Thus, as the helices pack together—side-by-side—the resultant membrane protein has distinct hydrophilic and hydrophobic surfaces. The hydrophobic surfaces of each helix will face either the membrane lipid or the hydrophobic surfaces of neighboring helices. Similarly, the hydrophilic surfaces of each helix will face a common central pore through which water-soluble particles can move. Depending on how the protein regulates access to this pore, the protein could be a channel, a carrier, or a pump. The mix of hydrophilic amino acids that line the pore presumably determines, at least in part, the nature of the substances that the pore can accommodate. In some instances, the amphipathic helices that line the pore are contributed by several distinct proteins—or subunits—that assemble into a single multimeric complex. Figure 2–8 shows an example of a type of K$^+$ channel that is discussed in Chapter 7. This channel is formed by the apposition of four identical subunits, each of which has six membrane-spanning segments. The pore of this channel is created by the amphipathic helices as well as by short, hydrophilic loops ("P loops") contributed by each of the four subunits.

Integral Membrane Proteins Can Also Be Enzymes

Ion pumps are actually enzymes. They catalyze the hydrolysis of ATP and use the energy released by that reaction to drive ion transport. Many other classes of proteins that are embedded in cell membranes function as enzymes as well. Membrane-bound enzymes are especially prevalent in the cells of the intestine, which participate in the final stages of nutrient digestion and absorption (p. 951 & 955). These enzymes—located on the side of the intestinal cells that faces the lumen of the intestine—break down small polysaccharides into single sugars, or break down polypeptides into shorter polypeptides or amino acids, so that they can be imported into the cells. By embedding these enzymes in the plasma membrane, the cell can generate the final products of digestion close to the transport proteins that mediate the uptake of these nutrient molecules. This theme is repeated in numerous other cell types. Thus, the membrane can serve as an extremely efficient two-dimensional reaction center for multistep processes that involve enzymatic reactions or transport.

Many of the GPI-linked proteins are enzymes. Several of the enzymatic activities that are classically thought of as extracellular markers of the plasma membrane, such as **alkaline phosphatase** and **5′-nucleotidase**, are anchored to the external leaflet of the bilayer by covalent attachment to a GPI. The biologic utility of this arrangement has yet to be determined. However, the GPI linkage is itself a substrate for enzymatic cleavage. Phospholipase C, which is present at appreciable levels in the serum, can cleave the covalent bond between the protein and its lipid anchor, thereby releasing the protein from the membrane.

The released protein subsequently behaves like a soluble polypeptide.

Integral Membrane Proteins Can Participate in Intracellular Signaling

Some integral proteins associate with the cytoplasmic surface of the plasma membrane by covalently attaching to fatty acids or prenyl groups that in turn intercalate into the lipid bilayer (see Fig. 2–5F). The fatty acids or prenyl groups act as hydrophobic tails that anchor an otherwise soluble protein to the bilayer. These proteins are all located at the *intra*cellular leaflet of the membrane bilayer, and often participate in intracellular-signaling and growth-regulation pathways. The family of lipid-linked proteins includes the small and heterotrimeric guanosine triphosphate–binding (GTP–binding) proteins, kinases, and oncogene products (Chapter 4). Many of these proteins are involved in relaying the signals that are received at the cell surface to the effector machinery within the cell interior. Their association with the membrane, therefore, brings these proteins close to the cytoplasmic sides of receptors that transmit signals from the cell exterior across the bilayer. The medical relevance of this type of membrane association is beginning to be appreciated. For example, denying certain oncogene products their lipid modifications—and hence their membrane attachment—eliminates their ability to induce tumorigenic transformation.

Peripheral Membrane Proteins Participate in Intracellular Signaling and Can Form a Submembranous Cytoskeleton

Peripheral membrane proteins attach loosely to the lipid bilayer but are not embedded within it (p. 15). Their association with the membrane can take one of two forms. First, some proteins interact via **ionic interactions** with phospholipid head groups. Many of these head groups are positively or negatively charged and thus can participate in salt bridges with adherent proteins.

For a second group of peripheral membrane proteins, attachment is based on the direct binding of peripheral membrane proteins to the extracellular or cytoplasmic surfaces of integral membrane proteins (see Fig. 2–5A). This form of attachment is epitomized by the cytoskeleton. For instance, the cytoplasmic surface of the erythrocyte plasma membrane is in close apposition to a dense meshwork of interlocking protein strands known as the **subcortical cytoskeleton**. It consists of a long, fibrillar molecule called spectrin, short polymers of the cytoskeletal protein actin, and other proteins, including ankyrin and band 4.1 (Fig. 2–9).

Two closely related isoforms of **spectrin** (α and β) form dimers, and two of these dimers assemble head-to-head with one another to form spectrin heterotetramers. The tail regions of spectrin bind the globular protein **band 4.1**, which in turn can bind to actin fibrils. Each **actin** fibril can associate with more than one molecule of band 4.1 so that, together, spectrin, actin, and band 4.1 assemble into an extensive interlocking matrix. The pro-

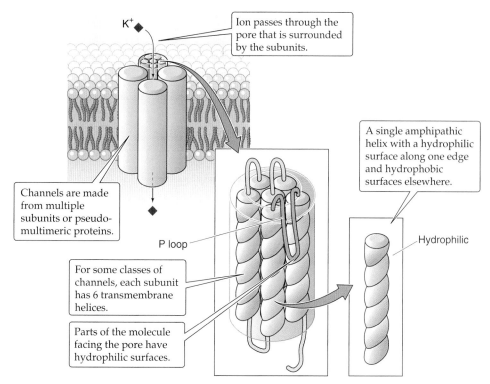

FIGURE 2–8. Amphipathic α helices interacting to form a channel through the cell membrane. This is an example of a potassium channel.

tein known as **ankyrin** binds to spectrin as well as to the cytoplasmic domain of **band 3**, the integral-membrane protein responsible for transporting Cl^- and HCO_3^- ions across the erythrocyte membrane. Thus, ankyrin is a *peripheral* membrane protein that anchors the spectrin-actin meshwork directly to an *integral* membrane protein of the erythrocyte.

The subcortical cytoskeleton provides the erythrocyte plasma membrane with strength and resilience. People who carry mutations in genes that encode their components have erythrocytes that do not have the characteristic biconcave disc morphology. These erythrocytes are ex-

tremely fragile and are easily torn apart by the shear stresses (p. 429) associated with circulation through capillaries. It would appear, therefore, that the subcortical cytoskeleton forms a scaffolding of peripheral membrane proteins whose direct attachment to transmembrane proteins enhances the bilayer's structural integrity.

The subcortical cytoskeleton is not unique to erythrocytes. Numerous cell types, including neurons and epithelia cells, have submembranous meshworks that consist of proteins that are very similar to those first described in the erythrocyte. In addition to band 3, transmembrane proteins found in a wide variety of cells (including ion

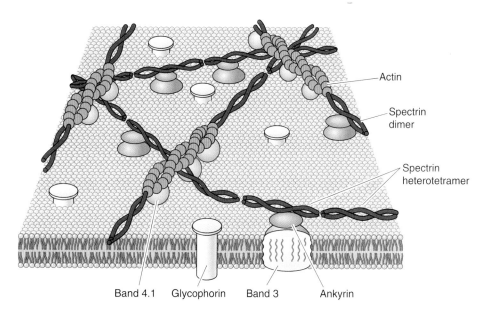

FIGURE 2–9. Attachments of the cell membrane to the submembranous cytoskeleton in red blood cells. Integral membrane proteins form the bridges that link the cell membrane to the interlocking system of proteins that form the subcortical cytoskeleton.

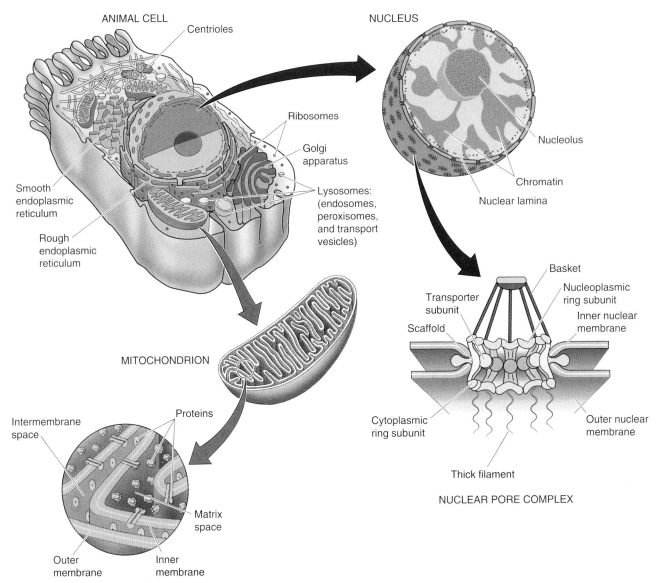

FIGURE 2–10. Ultrastructure of a typical animal cell.

pumps, ion channels, and cell-adhesion molecules) bind ankyrin and can thus serve as focal points of cytoskeletal attachment. In polarized cells (e.g., neurons and epithelial cells), the subcortical cytoskeleton appears to play a critically important role in organizing the plasma membrane into morphologically and functionally distinct domains.

CELLULAR ORGANELLES AND THE CYTOSKELETON

The Cell Is Composed of Discrete Organelles That Subserve Distinct Functions

When a eukaryotic cell is viewed through a light microscope, a handful of recognizable intracellular structures can be discerned. The intracellular matrix, or cytoplasm, appears grainy, suggesting the presence of components that are too small to be discriminated by this technique. With the much higher magnifications available with an electron microscope, the graininess gives way to clarity that reveals the cell interior to be remarkably complex. Even the simplest nucleated animal cell possesses a wide variety of intricate structures with specific shapes and sizes. These structures are the **membrane-enclosed organelles,** the functional building blocks of cells.

Figure 2–10 illustrates the interior of a typical cell. The largest organelle in this picture is the **nucleus,** which houses the cell's complement of genetic information. This structure, which is visible in the light microscope, is usually round or oblong, although in some cells it displays a complex, lobulated morphology. Depending on the cell type, the nucleus can range in diameter from 2 to 20 μm. With some exceptions, including skeletal muscle and certain specialized cells of the immune system, each animal cell has a single nucleus.

Surrounding the nucleus is a web of tubules or saccules known as the **endoplasmic reticulum** (ER). This organelle can exist in either of two forms: "rough" or "smooth." The surfaces of the rough ER tubules are studded with **ribosomes**, the major sites of protein synthesis. Ribosomes can also exist free in the cytosol. The surfaces of the smooth ER, which participates in lipid synthesis, are not similarly endowed. The ER also serves as a major reservoir for calcium ions. The ER membrane is endowed with a Ca^{2+} pump that uses the energy released through ATP hydrolysis to drive the transport of Ca^{2+} from the cytoplasm into the ER lumen (p. 64). This Ca^{2+} can be rapidly released in response to messenger molecules and plays a major role in intracellular signaling (p. 100).

The **Golgi complex** resembles a stack of pancakes. Each pancake in the stack represents a discrete, flat saccule. The number and size of the saccules in the Golgi stack varies among cell types. The Golgi complex is a processing station that participates in protein maturation and targets newly synthesized proteins to their appropriate subcellular destinations.

Perhaps the most intriguing morphology belongs to the **mitochondrion**, which is essentially a balloon within a balloon. The outer membrane and inner membrane define two distinct internal compartments: the intermembrane space and the matrix space. The surface of the inner membrane is thrown into dramatic folds called *cristae*. This organelle is approximately 0.2 μm in diameter, placing it at the limit of resolution of the light microscope. The mitochondrion is the power plant of the cell, a critical manufacturer of ATP. Many cellular reactions are also catalyzed within the mitochondrion.

The cell's digestive organelle is the **lysosome**, which is also referred to as a multivesicular body, because this large structure frequently contains several smaller round vesicles within its internal space.

The cytoplasm contains numerous other organelles whose shapes are not quite as distinguishing, including **endosomes**, **peroxisomes**, and **transport vesicles**.

Despite their diversity, all cellular organelles are constructed from the same building blocks. Each is composed of a membrane that forms the entire extent of its surface. The membranes of the subcellular organelles are what can be visualized in electron micrographs. The biochemical and physical properties of an organelle's limiting membrane dictate many of its functional properties.

The Nucleus Stores, Replicates, and Reads the Cell's Genetic Information

The nucleus serves as a cell's repository for its complement of chromosomal DNA. To conceive of the nucleus as simply a hermetically sealed vault for genetic information, however, is a gross oversimplification. All of the machinery necessary to maintain, copy, and transcribe DNA is in the nucleus, which is the focus of all of the cellular pathways that regulate gene expression and cell division. Transcriptional control is discussed in Chapter 5. The focus of this section is nuclear structure.

The nucleus is surrounded by a double membrane (see Fig. 2–10). The **outer membrane** is studded with ribosomes and is continuous with the membranes of the rough ER. The **inner membrane** is smooth and faces the intranuclear space, or nucleoplasm. The space between these concentric membranes is continuous with the lumen

of the rough ER. The inner and outer nuclear membranes meet at specialized structures known as **nuclear pores**, which penetrate the nuclear envelope and provide a transport pathway between the cytoplasm to the nuclear interior (p. 58). All RNA transcripts that are produced in the nucleus must pass through nuclear pores to be translated in the cytoplasm. Similarly, all the signaling molecules that influence nuclear function, as well as all proteins of the nuclear interior (which are synthesized in the cytoplasm), enter the nucleus through nuclear pores.

Nuclear pores are selective in choosing the molecules that they allow to pass. Cytoplasmic proteins destined for the nuclear interior must be endowed with a **nuclear-localization sequence** to gain entry. Several nuclear localization sequences have been characterized, and all seem to share common structural elements. For example, they all have short stretches of four to eight basic amino acids that can be located anywhere in the protein's sequence. Evidence implies that the ability of these signals to mediate nuclear localization can be modulated by phosphorylation, which suggests that the entry of proteins into the nucleus may be under the control of the cell's second-messenger systems.

The selectivity of the nuclear pore is surprising, considering its size. The outer diameter of the entire nuclear pore is approximately 100 nm, considerably larger than the proteins whose passage it controls. The nuclear pore's specificity is provided by the **nuclear-pore complex** (NPC), an intricate matrix of protein that is distributed in a highly organized octagonal array. In its resting state, the NPC forms an aqueous channel that is approximately 9 nm in diameter, restricting the movement of any protein larger than 60 kDa. However, when confronted with a protein bearing a nuclear-localization signal or a messenger RNA (mRNA) transcript, the pore complex can dilate to many times this size. The mechanisms by which the pore's permeability is regulated remain unknown. The NPC has a barrier that prevents the diffusion of intrinsic-membrane proteins between the outer and inner membranes of the nuclear envelope. Thus, although the inner and outer nuclear membranes are continuous with one another at nuclear pores, their protein contents remain distinct.

Between mitoses, the chromosomal DNA is present in the nucleus as densely packed heterochromatin and more loosely arrayed euchromatin. **Chromatin** is a complex between DNA and numerous DNA-binding proteins, which organize the chromosome into a chain of tightly folded DNA-protein assemblies called **nucleosomes** (p. 136). Interspersed within the nucleoplasm are round, dense **nucleoli**, where the transcription of ribosomal RNA and the assembly of ribosomal subunits appear to occur.

The interior surface of the inner nuclear membrane is apposed to a fibrillar protein skeleton that is referred to as the **nuclear lamina**. Presumably this meshwork, composed of proteins known as *lamins*, is involved in providing structural support to the nuclear envelope. The nuclear lamina may also play a role in orchestrating **nuclear re-assembly**. During mitosis, the nuclear envelope breaks down into small vesicles, and the contents of the nucleoplasm mix with the cytoplasm. Following mitosis, these vesicles fuse with one another to regenerate the double-walled nuclear membrane. The means by which these vesicles find one another and assemble correctly is the subject of intense study. Similarly, the mechanisms involved in maintaining the compositional discreteness of the inner and outer membranes during vesiculation and re-assembly have yet to be determined. Following reconstitution of the nuclear envelope, the proteins of the nucleoplasm are re-imported from the cytoplasm through the nuclear pores by virtue of their nuclear-localization sequences.

Lysosomes Digest Material That Is Derived from the Interior and Exterior of the Cell

In the course of normal daily living, cells accumulate waste. Organelles become damaged and dysfunctional. Proteins denature and aggregate. New materials are constantly being brought into the cells from the extracellular environment through the process of endocytosis (discussed later). In specialized cells of the immune system, such as macrophages, the collection of foreign materials (in the form of pathogens) from the extracellular milieu is the cellular raison d'être. If this material were allowed to accumulate indefinitely, it would ultimately fill the cell and essentially choke it to death. Clearly, cells must have mechanisms for disposing of this waste material.

The lysosome is the cell's trash incinerator. It is filled with a broad assortment of degradative enzymes that can break down most forms of cellular debris. **Proton pumps** embedded within the lysosome's limiting membrane ensure that this space is an extremely acidic environment, which aids in protein hydrolysis. A rare group of inherited disorders, called lysosomal storage diseases (see box on p. 43), result from the deficiency of lysosomal enzymes that are involved in the degradation of a variety of substances.

The lysosomal membrane is specially adapted to resist digestion by the enzymes and the acid that it encapsulates, thus ensuring that the harsh conditions that are necessary for efficient degradation are effectively contained. Loss of lysosomal-membrane integrity may underlie some clinically important inflammatory conditions, such as gout.

Material that has been internalized from the cell exterior by endocytosis is surrounded by the membrane of an **endocytic vesicle**. To deliver this material to the lysosome, the membranes of the endocytic vesicles fuse with the lysosomal membrane and discharge their cargo into the lysosomal milieu.

Intracellular structures that are destined for degradation, such as fragments of organelles, are engulfed by the lysosome in a process called **autophagy**. Autophagy results in the formation of membrane-enclosed structures within the lysosomal lumen; hence, the lysosome is often referred to as a "multivesicular body."

The Mitochondrion Is the Site of Oxidative Energy Production

Oxygen-dependent ATP production—or oxidative phosphorylation—occurs in the mitochondrion. Like the nucleus, the mitochondrion (see Fig. 2–10) is a double-membrane structure. The inner mitochondrial membrane contains the proteins that constitute the electron-transport chain, which generates pH and voltage gradients across this membrane. According to the "chemiosmotic" model (p. 64), the inner membrane uses the energy in these gradients to generate ATP from adenosine diphosphate (ADP) and inorganic phosphate.

The mitochondrion maintains and replicates its own genome. This circular DNA strand encodes **mitochondrial transfer RNAs** (tRNAs) and (in humans) 13 **mitochondrial proteins**. Several copies of the mitochondrial genome are located in the inner mitochondrial matrix, which also has all of the machinery necessary to transcribe and translate this DNA, including ribosomes. Whereas the proteins encoded in mitochondrial DNA contribute to the structure and function of the mitochondrion, they account for a relatively small fraction of total mitochondrial protein. Most *mitochondrial* proteins are specified by nuclear DNA and are synthesized on *cytoplasmic* ribosomes.

The two mitochondrial membranes enclose two distinct compartments: the intermembrane space and the inner mitochondrial matrix space. The **intermembrane space** lies between the two membranes, whereas the **inner mitochondrial matrix space** is completely enclosed by the inner mitochondrial membrane. These compartments have completely different complements of soluble proteins, and the two membranes themselves have extremely different proteins.

In addition to its role in energy metabolism, the mitochondrion also serves as a reservoir for intracellular Ca^{2+}. It is not clear whether—under physiological conditions—the mitochondrion releases Ca^{2+} from this reservoir. The mitochondrial Ca^{2+} stores are released as a consequence of energy starvation, which leads to cell injury and death.

The Cytoplasm Is Not Amorphous But Is Organized by the Cytoskeleton

Our discussion thus far has focused almost exclusively on the cell's membranous elements. We have treated the cytoplasm as if it were a homogeneous solution in which the organelles and vesicles carry out their functions while floating about unimpeded and at random. Rather, the cytoplasm is enormously complex with an intricate local structure and the capacity for locomotion.

The cytoplasmic **cytoskeleton** is composed of protein filaments that radiate throughout the cell, serving as the beams, struts, and stays that determine cell shape and resilience. On the basis of their appearances in the electron microscope, these filaments were initially divided into several classes (Table 2–2): thick, thin, and intermediate filaments as well as microtubules. Subsequent biochemical analysis has revealed that each of these varieties is composed of distinct polypeptides and differs with respect to its formation, stability, and biologic function.

Intermediate Filaments Provide Cells with Structural Support

Intermediate filaments are so named because their 8- to 10-nm diameters, as measured in the electron micro-

Table 2–2

COMPONENTS OF THE CYTOSKELETON

	SUBUNITS	DIAMETER (nm)
Intermediate filaments	Tetramer of two coiled dimers	8–10
Microtubules	Heterodimers of α and β tubulin form long protofilaments, 5 nm in diameter	25
Thin filaments	Globular or G-actin, 5 nm in diameter, arranged in a double helix to form fibrous or F-actin	5–8
Thick filaments	Assembly of myosin molecules	10

scope, are intermediate between those of the actin *thin* filaments and the myosin *thick* filaments. As with all of the cytoskeletal filaments that we will discuss, intermediate filaments are polymers that are assembled from individual protein subunits. There is a very large variety of biochemically distinct subunit proteins that are all structurally related to one another and that derive from a single gene family. The expression of these subunit polypeptides can be cell-type specific, or can be restricted to specific regions within a cell. Thus, **vimentin** is found in cells that are derived from mesenchyme, and the closely related **glial fibrillary acidic protein** is expressed exclusively in glial cells (p. 413). **Neurofilament proteins** are present in neuronal processes. The **keratins** are present in epithelial cells as well as in certain epithelially derived structures. The **nuclear lamins** (p. 23) that form the structural scaffolding of the nuclear envelope are also members of the intermediate-filament family.

Intermediate-filament monomers are themselves fibrillar in structure. They assemble to form long, intercoiled dimers that in turn assemble side-to-side to form the tetrameric subunits. Finally, these tetrameric subunits pack together, end-to-end and side-to-side, to form intermediate filaments. Filament assembly can be regulated by the cell and in some cases appears to be governed by phosphorylation of the subunit polypeptides. Intermediate filaments appear to radiate from and reinforce areas of a cell that are subject to tensile stress. They emanate from the **adhesion plaques** that attach cells to their substrata. In epithelial cells, they insert at the **desmosomal junctions** that attach neighboring cells to one another. The toughness and resilience of the meshworks formed by these filaments is perhaps best illustrated by the **keratins**, the primary constituents of nails, hair, and the outer layers of skin.

Microtubules Provide Structural Support and Provide the Basis for Several Types of Subcellular Motility

Microtubules are polymers that are formed from heterodimers of the proteins α and β **tubulin** (Fig. 2–11A).

These heterodimers assemble head to tail, creating a circumferential wall of a microtubule, which surrounds an empty lumen. Because the tubulin heterodimers assemble with a specific orientation, microtubules are polar structures, and their ends manifest distinct biochemical properties. At one tip of the tubule, designated the "**plus end**," tubulin heterodimers can be added to the growing polymer at three times the rate that this process occurs at the opposite "**minus end**." The relative rates of microtubule growth and depolymerization are controlled in part by an enzymatic activity that is inherent in the tubulin dimer. Tubulin dimers bind to **GTP**, and in this GTP-bound state they associate more tightly with the growing ends of microtubules. Once a tubulin dimer becomes part of the microtubule, it hydrolyzes the GTP to GDP, which lowers the binding affinity of the dimer for the tubule and helps to hasten disassembly. Consequently, the microtubules can undergo rapid rounds of growth and shrinkage, a behavior termed *dynamic instability*. Various cytosolic proteins can bind to the ends of microtubules and serve as caps that prevent assembly and disassembly and thus stabilize the structures of the microtubules. A large and diverse family of **microtubule-associated proteins** appears to modulate not only the stability of the tubules but also their capacity to interact with other intracellular components.

In most cells, all of the microtubules originate from the microtubule-organizing center or **centrosome**. This structure generally consists of two **centrioles**, each of which is a small ($\sim$0.5 μm) assembly of nine triplet microtubules that are arranged obliquely along the wall of a cylinder (see Fig. 2–11B). The two centrioles in a centrosome are oriented at right angles to one another. The minus ends of all of a cell's microtubules are associated with proteins that surround the centrosome, whereas the rapidly growing "plus ends" radiate throughout the cytoplasm in a star-like arrangement ("astral" microtubules).

Microtubules participate in a multitude of cellular functions and structures. For example, microtubules project down the axon of neurons. Microtubules also provide the framework for the lacy membranes of the ER and Golgi complex. Disruption of microtubules causes these organelles to undergo dramatic morphologic rearrangements and vesicularization. During cell division, the microtubules form the **spindle fibers** that align the chromosomes (see Fig. 2–11C). Their coordinated growth and dissolution at either side of the chromosomes may provide the force for separating the genetic material during the anaphase of mitosis. During mitosis, these centrioles are replicated, and a pair remains with each daughter cell.

The architectural and mechanical capacities of microtubules are perhaps best illustrated by their role in motility. An electron microscopic cross section of a cilium demonstrates the elegance, symmetry, and intricacy of this structure (Fig. 2–12A). Every cilium arises out of its own **basal body**, which is essentially a centriole that is situated at the ciliary root. **Cilia** are found on the surfaces of many types of epithelial cells, including those that line the larger pulmonary airways (p. 601). Their oar-like beating motions help to propel foreign bodies and pathogens toward their ultimate expulsion at the pharynx. At the center of a cilium is a structure called the **axoneme**,

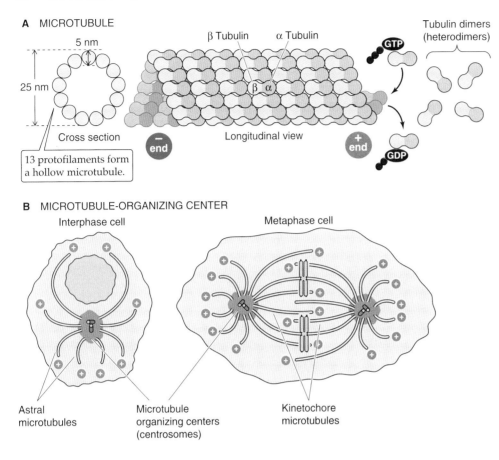

A MICROTUBULE

β Tubulin   α Tubulin

Tubulin dimers (heterodimers)

5 nm

25 nm

Cross section

13 protofilaments form a hollow microtubule.

– end

Longitudinal view

+ end

GTP

GDP

B MICROTUBULE-ORGANIZING CENTER

Interphase cell

Metaphase cell

Astral microtubules

Microtubule organizing centers (centrosomes)

Kinetochore microtubules

FIGURE 2–11. Microtubule structure. *A,* Heterodimers of *α-* and *β-*tubulin form long protofilaments, 13 of which surround the hollow core of a microtubule. The microtubule grows more rapidly at its "plus" end. *B,* The microtubules originate from a microtubule-organizing center or centrosome, which generally consists of two centrioles (*green cylinders*).

which is composed of a precisely defined "9 + 2" array of microtubules. Each of the "9" (which are also called "outer tubules") consists of a complete microtubule with 13 tubulin monomers in cross section (the "A" tubule) to which is fused an incomplete microtubule with 11 tubulin monomers in cross section (the "B" tubule). Each of the "2," which lie at the core of the cilium, is a complete microtubule. This entire "9 + 2" structure runs the entire length of the cilium. The same array forms the core of a flagellum, the serpentine motions of which propel sperm cells (p. 1169).

Radial spokes connect the outer tubules to the central pair, and outer tubules attach to their neighbors by two types of linkages. One is composed of the protein dynein, which acts as a **molecular motor** to power ciliary and flagellar motions. **Dynein** is an ATPase that converts the energy released through ATP hydrolysis into a conformational change that produces a bending motion. Because dynein attached to one outer tubule interacts with a neighboring outer tubule, this bending of the dynein molecule causes the adjacent outer tubules to slide past one another. It is this sliding-filament motion that gives rise to the coordinated movements of the entire structure. To some extent, this coordination is accomplished through the action of the second linkage protein, called nexin. The **nexin** arms restrict the extent to which neighboring outer tubules can move with respect to each other and thus prevent the dynein motor from driving the dissolution of the entire complex.

The utility of the dynein motor protein is not restricted to its function in cilia and flagella. Cytoplasmic dynein, which is a close relative of the motor molecule found in cilia, and a second motor protein called kinesin provide the force necessary to move membrane-bound organelles through the cytoplasm along microtubular tracks (see Fig. 2–12*B*). The ability of vesicular organelles to move rapidly along microtubules was first noted in neurons, where vesicles carrying newly synthesized proteins must be transported over extremely long distances from the cell body to the axon tip. Rather than trust this critical process to the vagaries of slow, non-directed diffusion, the neuron makes use of the kinesin motor, which links a vesicle to a microtubule. **Kinesin** hydrolyzes ATP and, like dynein, converts this energy into mechanical transitions that cause it to "walk" along the microtubule. Kinesin will only move along microtubules and thereby transport vesicles in the **minus-to-plus direction**. Thus, in neurons, kinesin-bound vesicles move from the microtubular minus ends, originating at the centrosome in the cell body, toward the plus ends in the axons. This direction of motion is referred to as "anterograde fast axonal transport." **Cytoplasmic dynein** moves in the opposite **plus-to-minus** (or retrograde) direction.

The motor-driven movement of cellular organelles along microtubular tracks is not unique to neurons. This process, involving both kinesin and cytoplasmic dynein, appears to occur in almost every cell and may control the vast majority of subcellular vesicular traffic.

A CILIUM

Nine outer microtubule doublets

Two central microtubules

Dynein arms

Cell membrane

Radial spokes

Tubulin dimers

A   B

13   11

Microtubule

Dynein arms

ATP

Axoneme

Cilium

FIGURE 2–12. The role of microtubules and molecular motors in motility. *A,* A cilium can bend as its microtubules slide past each other. The molecular motor dynein produces this motion, fueled by adenosine triphosphate (ATP). *B,* The molecular motor dynein moves along the microtubule in the plus-to-minus direction, whereas the molecular motor kinesin moves in the opposite direction. ATP is the fuel for each of these motors. ADP, adenosine diphosphate.

B MOLECULAR MOTORS MOVING ALONG A MICROTUBULE

Dynein

Light and intermediate chains

Base

Head domain

Kinesin

Tail

Light chain

Coiled-coil

Head domain

– end

+ end

Thin Filaments (Actin) and Thick Filaments (Myosin) Are Present in Almost Every Cell Type

Thin filaments, also called microfilaments, are 5 to 8 nm in diameter. They are helical polymers composed of a single polypeptide called globular actin or **G-actin**. Thin filaments are functionally similar to microtubules in two respects: (1) the actin polymers are polar and grow at different rates at their two ends, and (2) actin binds and then hydrolyzes a nucleotide. However, whereas tubulin binds GTP and then hydrolyzes it to GDP, actin binds ATP and then hydrolyzes it to ADP. After G-actin binds ATP, it may interact with another ATP-bound monomer

to form an unstable dimer (see Fig. 2–13*A*). Adding a third ATP-bound monomer, however, yields a stable trimer that serves as a nucleus for assembly of the polymer of fibrous actin or **F-actin**. Once it is part of F-actin, the actin monomer hydrolyzes its bound ATP, retaining the ADP and releasing the inorganic phosphate. The ADP-bound actin monomer is more likely to disengage itself from its neighbors, just as GDP-bound tubulin dimers are more likely to disassemble from tubulin (p. 25). Even though the length of the F-actin filament may remain more or less constant, the polymer may continually grow at its "plus end" but disassemble at its "minus end" (Fig. 2–13*B*). This "treadmilling" requires the continuous input of energy (i.e., hydrolysis of ATP) and illustrates the

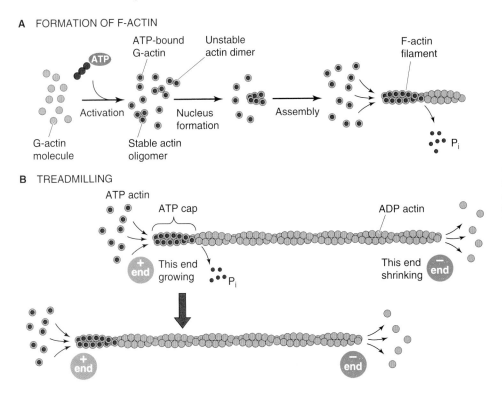

A FORMATION OF F-ACTIN

B TREADMILLING

FIGURE 2–13. Thin filaments. *A,* Single molecules of G-actin form F-actin filaments. *B,* F-actin can grow at the "plus" end while shrinking at the "minus" end, with no change in length.

unique dynamic properties of actin filament elongation and disassembly.

Thick filaments are composed of dimers of a remarkable force-generating protein called myosin. All **myosin** molecules have helical tails and globular head groups that hydrolyze ATP and act as motors to move along an actin filament. The energy liberated by ATP hydrolysis is invested in bending the myosin molecule around a pivot point called the "hinge region," which marks the junction between the globular and tail regions. By means of this bending, myosin, like the dynein and kinesin that interact with microtubules, acts as a molecular motor that converts chemical into mechanical energy.

In muscle, the myosin molecules are in the **myosin-II** subfamily and exist as dimers with their long tails intertwined (Fig. 2–14*A*). In muscle, each of the two myosin-II heads binds two additional protein subunits that are referred to as myosin **light chains**. Non-muscle cells, in addition to myosin-II, may have a variety of other, smaller myosin molecules. These other myosins, the most widely studied of which is **myosin-I**, have shorter tails and, at least in some cases, act as molecular motors that move vesicles along actin filaments.

In muscle, the myosin-II dimers stack as antiparallel arrays to form a bipolar structure with a bare central region that contains only tails (see Fig. 2–14*A*). The ends of the thick filament contain the heads that bend toward the filament's central region. The pivoting action of the myosin head groups drags the neighboring thin filament (see Fig. 2–14*B*), which includes other molecules besides actin. This sliding-filament phenomenon underlies muscle contraction and force generation (see Fig. 2–14*C*).

Actin, as well as an ever-growing list of myosin iso-forms is present in essentially every cell type. The functions of these proteins are easy to imagine in some cases and are less obvious in many others. Many cells, including all of the fibroblast-like cells, possess actin filaments that are arranged in **stress fibers**. These linear arrays of fibers interconnect adhesion plaques to one another and to interior structures in the cell. They orient themselves along lines of tension and can, in turn, exert contractile force on the substratum that underlies the cell. Stress-fiber contractions may be involved in the macroscopic contractions that are associated with wound healing. Frequently, actin filaments in non-muscle cells are held together in bundles by cross-linking proteins. Numerous classes of cross-linking proteins have been identified, several of which can respond to physiological changes by either stabilizing or severing filaments and filament bundles.

In motile cells, such as fibroblasts and macrophages, arrays of actin-myosin filaments are responsible for **cell locomotion**. A Ca^{2+}-stimulated, myosin light chain kinase regulates the assembly of myosin and actin filaments and thus governs the generation of contractile force. The precise mechanism by which these fibers cooperate in causing the cell to crawl along a substrate remains poorly understood.

In contrast to fibroblasts and circulating cells of the immune system, cells such as neurons and epithelial cells generally do not move much after their differentiation is complete. Despite this lack of movement, however, these cells are equipped with remarkably intricate actin- and myosin-filament networks. In some cases, these cytoskeletal elements permit the cell to extend processes to distant locations. This is the case in neurons, in which the growth and migration of axons during development or

A MYOSIN

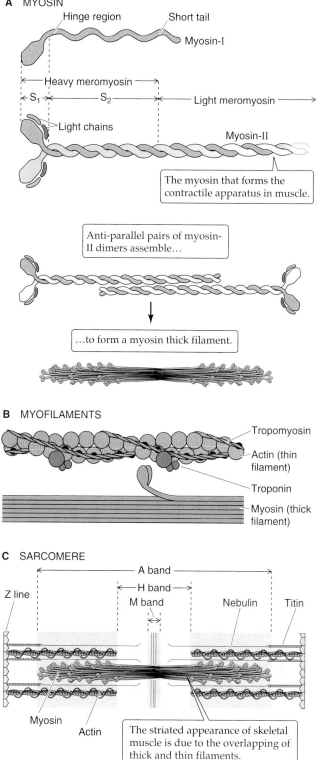

Hinge region   Short tail
                                    Myosin-I

Heavy meromyosin
←S₁→←   S₂   →   Light meromyosin →

Light chains
                          Myosin-II

The myosin that forms the contractile apparatus in muscle.

Anti-parallel pairs of myosin-II dimers assemble...

...to form a myosin thick filament.

B MYOFILAMENTS

Tropomyosin
Actin (thin filament)
Troponin
Myosin (thick filament)

C SARCOMERE

A band
H band
M band
Z line   Nebulin   Titin

Myosin
Actin

The striated appearance of skeletal muscle is due to the overlapping of thick and thin filaments.

FIGURE 2–14. Thick filaments. *A,* Myosin-I is one of a large number of widely distributed myosins that have short tails. Myosin-II is the myosin that participates in muscle contraction. *B,* The pivoting action of the myosin head, fueled by adenosine triphosphate, moves the thick filament past the thin filament. *C,* In skeletal and cardiac muscle, the sarcomere is the fundamental contractile unit.

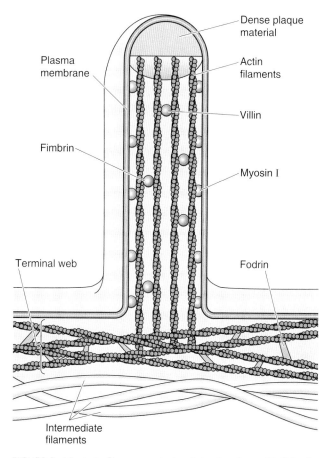

Dense plaque material
Plasma membrane   Actin filaments
                          Villin
Fimbrin   Myosin I
Terminal web   Fodrin
Intermediate filaments

FIGURE 2–15. Actin filaments at the brush border of an epithelial cell.

regeneration of the nervous system bears a striking morphologic resemblance to the crawling of free-living amebae. The tip of a growing axon, known as a **growth cone,** is richly endowed with contractile fibers and is capable of the same types of crawling motions that characterize motile cells.

In **epithelial cells,** the role of the actin-myosin cytoskeleton is somewhat less obvious but still important to normal physiologic function. The **microvilli** at the apical surfaces of many epithelial cell types (e.g., those that line the renal proximal tubule and the small intestine) are supported by an intricate scaffolding of actin filaments that form their cores (Fig. 2–15). This bundle of actin fibers is held together and anchored to the overlying plasma membrane by a variety of cross-linking proteins, including various myosin isoforms. The roots of the microvillar actin filament bundles emerge from the bases of the microvilli into a dense meshwork of cytoskeletal filaments known as the **terminal web.** Included among the components of the terminal-web network are **fodrin** (the nonerythroid homologue of spectrin) and myosin. It remains unclear whether the myosin in the terminal web is present simply to interconnect the actin filaments of neighboring microvilli or if this actin-myosin complex is capable of generating contractile movements.

Actin and myosin filaments also form an **adhesion belt** that encircles the cytoplasmic surface of the epithelial plasma membrane at the level of the **tight junctions** that interconnect neighboring cells. These adhesion belts are apparently capable of contraction and thus cause epithelial cells that normally form a continuous sheet to pull away from one another, temporarily loosening tight junctions and creating direct passages that connect the luminal space to the extracellular fluid compartment.

Actin and myosin also participate in processes common to most, if not all, cell types. The process of cytokinesis, in which the cytoplasm of a dividing cell physically separates into two daughter cells, is driven by actin and myosin filaments. Beneath the cleavage furrow that forms in the membrane of the dividing cell is a contractile ring of actin and myosin filaments. Contraction of this ring deepens the cleavage furrow; this invagination ultimately severs the cell and produces the two progeny.

SYNTHESIS AND RECYCLING OF MEMBRANE PROTEINS

Secretory and Membrane Proteins Are Synthesized in Association with the Rough Endoplasmic Reticulum

As noted, transmembrane proteins are composed of hydrophobic domains that are embedded within the phospholipid bilayer and hydrophilic domains that are exposed at the intra- and extracellular surfaces (p. 15). We also pointed out that these proteins do not "flip" through the membrane. How, then, do intrinsic membrane proteins overcome the enormous energetic barriers that should logically prevent them from getting inserted into the membrane in the first place?

The cell has developed several schemes to address this problem. Mammalian cells have at least three different membrane-insertion pathways, each associated with specific organelles. The first two are mechanisms for inserting membrane proteins into peroxisomes and mitochondria (p. 33). The third mechanism inserts membrane proteins destined for delivery to the plasma membrane and to the membranes of organelles (the "endomembranous system") other than the peroxisome and mitochondrion. This same mechanism is involved in the biogenesis of essentially all proteins that mammalian cells secrete, and is the focus of the following discussion.

The critical work in this field centered on studies of the rough ER. The membrane of the **rough ER** (p. 22) is notable for the presence of numerous ribosomes that are bound to its cytosol-facing surface. Whereas all nucleated mammalian cells have at least some rough ER, cells that produce large quantities of secretory proteins—such as the exocrine cells of the pancreas, which function as factories for digestive enzymes (p. 909)—are endowed with an abundance of rough ER. Roughly half of the cytoplasmic space in an exocrine pancreatic-acinar cell is occupied by rough ER.

In early experiments exploring cell-fractionation techniques, membranes that were derived from the rough ER were separated from the other membranous and cytoplasmic components of pancreatic-acinar cells. The mRNAs associated with rough-ER membranes were isolated and the proteins they encoded were synthesized by in vitro

translation. Analysis of the resultant polypeptides revealed that they included the cell's entire repertoire of *secretory* proteins. It is now appreciated that the mRNA that is associated with the ER also encodes the cell's entire repertoire of *membrane* proteins, with the exception of those destined for either the peroxisome or mitochondrion. When the same experiment was performed with mRNAs isolated from ribosomes that are freely distributed throughout the cytoplasm, the products were not *secretory* proteins, but rather the soluble *cytosolic* proteins. Later work showed that the ribosomes bound to the ER are biochemically identical to, and in equilibrium with, those that are free in the cytosol. Therefore, a ribosome's subcellular localization—that is, whether it is free in the cytosol or bound to the rough ER—is somehow dictated by the mRNA that the ribosome is currently translating. A ribosome that is involved in assembling a secretory or membrane protein will associate with the membrane of the rough ER, whereas the same ribosome will be free in the cytosol when it is producing cytosolic proteins. Clearly, some **localization signal** that resides in the mRNA or in the protein that is being synthesized must tell the ribosome what kind of protein is being produced and where in the cell that production should occur.

The nature of this signal was discovered in 1972 during studies on the biosynthesis of immunoglobulin light chains. Light chains synthesized in vitro—in the absence of rough-ER membranes—have a 15–amino acid extension at their amino terminus that is absent from the same light chains synthesized and secreted in vivo by B lymphocytes. Similar **amino-terminal extensions** are present on most secretory or membrane proteins, but never with the soluble proteins of the cytosol. Although they vary in length and composition, these extensions are present on most acids that are interspersed with occasional basic residues. These "**signal sequences**," as they have come to be known, serve as the localization devices discussed earlier. As it emerges from a ribosome and is freely floating in the cytosol, the signal sequence of a nascent protein (Fig. 2–16, *stage 1*) targets the ribosome-mRNA complex to the surface of the rough ER where the protein's biogenesis will be completed. Ribosome-mRNA complexes that lack a signal sequence complete the translation of the mRNA—which encodes neither secretory nor membrane proteins—without attaching to the rough ER. For his work on signal sequences, Günter Blobel received the 1999 Nobel Prize for Physiology or Medicine.

Why does the cell bother to segregate the synthesis of different protein populations to different cellular locales? Proteins that are destined either to reside in a membrane, or to be secreted, are inserted into or across the membrane of the rough ER at the same time that they are translated; this is called **cotranslational translocation**. As the nascent polypeptide chain emerges from the ribosome, it traverses the rough-ER membrane and ultimately appears at the ER's luminal face. There, an enzyme cleaves the amino-terminal signal sequence while the protein is still being translocated. This is why proteins that are synthesized in vitro in the absence of membranes are longer than the same proteins that are produced by intact cells.

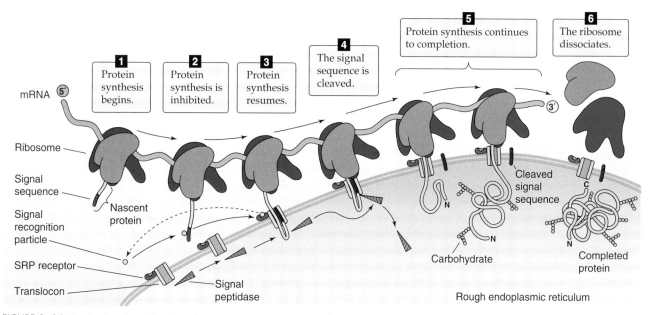

FIGURE 2–16. Synthesis and translocation of a secretory protein. SRP, signal recognition particle.

Simultaneous Protein Synthesis and Translocation Through the Rough Endoplasmic Reticulum Membrane Requires Signal-Recognition and Protein-Translocation Machinery

The information embodied within a signal sequence explains how a nascent protein can direct a cell to complete that protein's translation at the time of translocation in the rough ER. However, the signal sequence by itself is not sufficient. Two critical pieces of targeting machinery are also necessary to direct the ribosome and its attached nascent peptide to the ER. The first is a ribonucleoprotein complex called the **signal-recognition particle** (SRP), which binds to the signal sequence on the nascent peptide (see Fig. 2–16, *stage* 2). The SRP is composed of seven distinct polypeptides and a short strand of RNA. When the SRP binds to a nascent chain, it also binds a GTP molecule. The second vital piece of targeting machinery is a transmembrane component of the rough ER, the **SRP receptor**, also called the **docking protein**. Interaction between a signal sequence and the SRP, and subsequently between the SRP–nascent peptide–ribosome complex and the docking protein, directs the nascent chain to the rough ER's translocation apparatus.

Because the membrane of the rough ER has a finite number of docking sites, the cell must coordinate the synthesis of secretory and membrane proteins with the availability of docking sites. If all docking sites were occupied, and if the synthesis of nascent secretory and membrane proteins were allowed to continue unabated, these nascent peptides would be synthesized entirely in the cytoplasm on free ribosomes. As a consequence, these newly synthesized proteins would never arrive at their proper destination. The SRP serves as a regulatory system that matches the rate of secretory- and membrane-protein syntheses to the number of unoccupied translocation sites. By associating with a nascent signal sequence, the

SRP causes the ribosome to halt further protein synthesis (Fig. 2–16, *stage* 2). This state of **translation arrest** persists until the SRP–nascent peptide–ribosome complex finds an unoccupied docking protein with which to interact. Thus, SRP prevents secretory and membrane proteins from being translated until their cotranslational translocation can be ensured. Because SRP only interacts with nascent chains that bear signal sequences, ribosomes that synthesize proteins that are destined for release into the cytosol never associate with SRP, and their translation is never arrested. Thus, SRP serves as a highly specific spatial and temporal sorting machine, guaranteeing the accurate and efficient targeting of secretory and membrane proteins.

How does the cell terminate the translation arrest of the SRP–nascent peptide–ribosome complex? When this complex interacts with a docking protein (see Fig. 2–16, *stage* 3), one of the SRP's subunits hydrolyzes the previously bound GTP, thereby releasing the SRP from a successfully targeted nascent peptide–ribosome complex. In this way, the docking protein informs the SRP that its mission has been accomplished and it can return to the cytosol to find another ribosome with a signal peptide. A second GTP-hydrolysis step transfers the nascent peptide from the docking protein to the actual translocation-tunnel complex. GTP hydrolysis is a common event and is involved in the transmission of numerous cellular messages (Chapter 4). In this case, the two separate instances of GTP hydrolysis serve a quality-control function, because the activation of the GTPase activity depends on the delivery of the nascent peptide to the appropriate component in the translocation apparatus.

Adjacent to the docking protein in the membrane of the rough ER is a protein translocator termed a **translocon** (see Fig. 2–16, *stage* 3), which contains a tunnel through which the nascent protein will pass across the rough-ER membrane. It appears that delivery of a nascent chain to the translocon causes the entrance of the translocator's tunnel, which is normally closed, to open. This

A SINGLE MEMBRANE-SPANNING SEGMENT, CYTOPLASMIC C TERMINUS

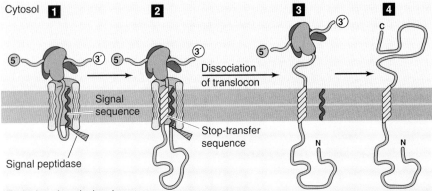

Cytosol

Signal sequence

Dissociation of translocon

Stop-transfer sequence

Signal peptidase

Endoplasmic reticulum lumen

B SINGLE MEMBRANE-SPANNING SEGMENT, CYTOPLASMIC C TERMINUS (ALTERNATE MECHANISM)

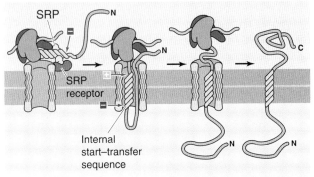

SRP

SRP receptor

Internal start–transfer sequence

C SINGLE MEMBRANE-SPANNING SEGMENT, CYTOPLASMIC N TERMINUS

Internal start–transfer sequence

D MULTIPLE MEMBRANE-SPANNING SEGMENTS

Internal start–transfer sequence

Stop-transfer sequence

SRP

Reinsertion into membrane

Second signal sequence

FIGURE 2–17. Synthesis of integral membrane proteins. *A,* Like a secreted protein, the membrane protein can have a cleavable signal sequence. In addition, it has a stop-transfer sequence that remains in the membrane as a membrane-spanning segment. *B,* The emerging protein lacks a signal sequence but instead has an *internal start–transfer sequence,* which is a bifunctional sequence that serves both as a signal sequence that binds signal recognition particles (SRP) and as a hydrophobic membrane-spanning segment. In this example, the positively charged region flanking the internal start–transfer sequence is on the *carboxy* terminal end of the internal start–transfer sequence. Therefore, the C-terminal end is in the cytoplasm. *C,* The example is similar to that in *B* except that the positively charged region flanking the internal start–transfer sequence is on the *amino* terminal end of the internal start–transfer sequence. *D,* The emerging peptide has alternating internal start–transfer and stop–transfer sequences.

opening of the translocon also allows the flow of small ions. The electrical current carried by these ions can be measured using the "patch-clamp" technique (p. 159). By "gating" the translocon so that it opens only when it is occupied by a nascent protein, the cell keeps the tunnel's entrance closed when it is not in use. This gating prevents the Ca^{2+} stored in the ER from leaking into the cytoplasm.

Because the tunnel of the translocon is an aqueous pore, the nascent secretory or membrane protein does not come into contact with the hydrophobic core of the ER membrane's lipid bilayer during cotranslational translocation. Thus, this tunnel allows hydrophilic proteins to cross the membrane. As translation and translocation continue and the nascent protein enters the lumen of the rough ER, an enzyme called **signal peptidase** cleaves the signal peptide, which remains in the membrane of the rough ER (see Fig. 2–16, *stage 4*). Meanwhile, translation and translocation of the protein continue (see Fig. 2–16, *stage 5*). In the case of **secretory proteins** (i.e., *not* membrane proteins), the peptide translocates completely through the membrane. The ribosome releases the complete protein into the lumen of the rough ER, and then dissociates from the rough ER (see Fig. 2–16, *stage 6*).

Proper Insertion of Membrane Proteins Requires Start- and Stop-Transfer Sequences

Unlike soluble proteins, nascent *membrane proteins* do not translocate completely through the membrane of the rough ER (Fig. 2–17A, *stage 1*). The current concept is that the hydrophobic amino-acid residues that will ultimately become the transmembrane segment of a membrane protein also function as a "**stop-transfer sequence**" (see Fig. 2–17A, *stage 2*). When a stop-transfer sequence emerges from a ribosome, it causes the translocon to disassemble, releasing the hydrophobic membrane-spanning segment into the hospitable environment of the rough-ER membrane's hydrophobic core (see Fig. 2–17A, *stage 3*). In the meantime, the ribosomal machinery continues to translate the rest of the nascent protein. If the signal peptidase cleaves the amino terminus at this time, the end result is a protein with a *single transmembrane segment*, with the amino terminus in the lumen of the rough-ER and the carboxy terminus in the cytoplasm (see Fig. 2–17A, *stage 4*).

There is another way of generating a protein with a single transmembrane segment. In this case, the protein lacks a signal sequence at the N terminus, but instead has—somewhere in the middle of the nascent peptide— a bifunctional sequence that serves both as a signal sequence that binds SRP and as a hydrophobic membrane-spanning segment. This special sequence is called an **internal start-transfer sequence**. The SRP binds to the internal start-transfer sequence and brings the nascent protein to the rough ER where the internal start-transfer sequence binds to the translocon in such a way that the more positively charged residues that flank the start-transfer sequence face the cytosol. Because these positively charged flanking residues can either precede or follow the hydrophobic residues of the internal start-transfer se-

quence, either the C terminus or the N terminus can end up in the cytosol. If the more positively charged flanking residues are at the *carboxy*-terminal end of the internal start-transfer sequence (see Fig. 2–17B), the protein will be oriented with its *carboxy* terminus in the cytosol. If the more positively charged flanking residues are at the *amino*-terminal end of the internal start-transfer sequence (see Fig. 2–17C), the protein will be oriented with its *amino* terminus in the cytosol.

By alternating both *stop-transfer* sequences (see Fig. 2–17A) and *internal start-transfer* sequences (see Fig. 2–17B, C), the cell can fabricate membrane proteins that span the membrane more than once. Figure 2–17D shows how the cell could synthesize a multispanning protein with its N terminus in the cytosol. The process starts just as in Figure 2–17C, as the translation machinery binds to the rough ER (see Fig. 2–17D, *stage 1*) and the protein's first internal start-transfer sequence inserts into the translocon (see Fig. 2–17D, *stage 2*). However, when the first stop-transfer sequence reaches the translocon (see Fig. 2–17D, *stage 3*), the translocon disassembles, releasing the protein's first two membrane-spanning segments into the membrane of the rough ER. Note that the first membrane-spanning segment is the internal start-transfer sequence, and the second is the stop-transfer sequence. In the meantime, an SRP binds to the second internal start-transfer sequence (see Fig. 2–17D, *stage 4*), and directs it to the rough ER (see Fig. 2–17D, *stage 5*) so that cotranslational translocation can once again continue (see Fig. 2–17D, *stage 6*). If there are no further stop-transfer sequences, we will end up with a protein with three membrane-spanning segments.

Several points from the preceding discussion deserve special emphasis. First, translocation through the ER membrane can only occur cotranslationally. If a secretory or membrane protein were synthesized completely on a cytoplasmic ribosome, it would be unable to interact with the translocation machinery and, consequently, would not be inserted across or into the bilayer. As discussed later, this is not true for the insertion of either peroxisomal or mitochondrial proteins. Second, once a signal sequence emerges from a ribosome, there is only a brief time period during which it is competent to mediate the ribosome's association with the ER and to initiate translocation. This time constraint is presumably due to the tendency of nascent polypeptide chains to begin to fold and acquire tertiary structure very soon after exiting the ribosome. This folding quickly buries hydrophobic residues of a signal sequence so that they cannot be recognized by the translocation machinery. Third, because the translocation channel appears to be fairly narrow, the nascent protein cannot begin to acquire tertiary structure until after it has exited at the ER's luminal face. Thus, the peptide must enter the translocation tunnel as a thin thread immediately after emerging from the ribosome. These facts explain why translocation is cotranslational. In systems in which post-translational translocation occurs (e.g., peroxisomes and mitochondria), special adaptations keep the newly synthesized protein in an unfolded state until its translocation can be consummated.

Finally, because the protein cannot flip once it is in the membrane, the scheme just outlined results in proteins

A N-LINKED GLYCOSYLATION

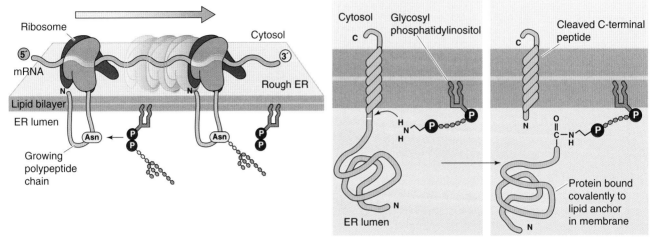

B FORMATION OF A GPI LINKAGE

FIGURE 2–18. Post-translational modifications of integral membrane proteins. *A,* An enzyme in the endoplasmic reticulum (ER) lumen attaches a preassembled, branched, oligosaccharide chain to an asparagine (Asn or N) residue on the nascent protein. *B,* An enzyme in the ER lumen cleaves the protein and couples the protein's new terminal carboxy group to the terminal amino group on the glycosyl phosphatidylinositol (GPI) molecule.

that are inserted into the rough-ER membrane in their final or "mature" topology. The number and location of a membrane protein's transmembrane segments, as well as its cytoplasmic and extracytoplasmic loops, are entirely determined during the course of its cotranslational insertion into the ER membrane. The order in which signal, internal start-transfer, and stop-transfer sequences appear in a membrane protein's primary structure completely determine how that protein will be arrayed across whatever membrane it ultimately comes to occupy.

Newly Synthesized Secretory and Membrane Proteins Undergo Post-Translational Modification and Folding in the Lumen of the Rough Endoplasmic Reticulum

As a newly synthesized secretory or membrane protein exits the tunnel of the translocon and enters the lumen of the rough ER, it may undergo a series of **post-translational modifications** that will help it to acquire its mature conformation. The first alteration, as discussed earlier, is cleavage of the signal sequence (if present), and is accomplished very soon after the signal sequence has completed its translocation. Other covalent modifications that occur as translocation continues include glycosylation and formation of intramolecular disulfide bonds. **Glycosylation** refers here to the enzymatic, en-bloc coupling of preassembled, branched oligosaccharide chains that contain 14 sugar molecules (Fig. 2–18*A*) to asparagine (Asn) residues that appear in the sequence Asn-X-Ser or Asn-X-Thr (X can be any amino acid except proline). These **N-linked sugars** (*N* is the single-letter amino-acid code for asparagine) will go on to be extensively modified as the protein passes through other organellar compartments. The addition of sugar groups to proteins can serve numerous functions, which include increasing the protein's stability and endowing it with specific antigenic, adhesive, or receptor properties.

Disulfide bond formation is catalyzed by **protein disul-**fide isomerase, an enzyme that is retained in the ER lumen through noncovalent interactions with ER membrane proteins. Because the cytoplasm is a reducing environment, disulfide bonds can only form between proteins or protein domains that have been removed from the cytosolic compartment through translocation to the ER's interior. Other, more specialized, modifications also take place in the lumen of the rough ER. For example, the ER contains the enzymes responsible for the **hydroxylation** of the proline residues that are present in newly synthesized collagen chains.

The ER also catalyzes the formation of **GPI linkages** to membrane proteins (see Fig. 2–18*B*). GPI-linked proteins are synthesized as transmembrane polypeptides, with a typical membrane-spanning region. Shortly after their translation, however, their lumen-facing domains are cleaved from the membrane-spanning segments and covalently transferred to the GPI phospholipid. They retain this structure and orientation throughout the remainder of their journey to the cell surface. A defect in the synthesis of GPI-linked proteins underlies the human disease paroxysmal nocturnal hematuria (see box titled Paraoxysmal Nocturnal Hematuria).

Perhaps the most important maturational process for a nascent chain emerging into the ER lumen is the acquisition of **tertiary structure**. The folding of a secretory or membrane protein is determined during and immediately following its cotranslational translocation. The progress of protein folding influences—and is influenced by—the addition of sugar residues and the formation of disulfide bridges. Proteins fold into conformations that minimize their overall free energies. Their extramembranous surfaces are composed of hydrophilic residues that interact easily with the aqueous solvent. Hydrophobic residues are hidden in internal globular domains where they can be effectively isolated from contact with water or charged molecules. Left to its own devices, a linear strand of denatured protein will spontaneously fold to form a structure that reflects these thermodynamic considerations.

PAROXYSMAL NOCTURNAL HEMATURIA

The list of proteins embedded in the plasma membrane via a GPI linkage is remarkably long and ever-growing. In red blood cells, the inventory of GPI-linked proteins includes a pair of polypeptides, decay-accelerating factor (DAF), and CD59, which help to protect the erythrocytes from being accidentally injured by constituents of the immune system. One of the mechanisms that the immune system uses to rid the body of invading bacteria involves the activation of the **complement cascade**. Complement is a complex collection of proteins that circulate in the blood plasma. The complement system recognizes antibodies that are bound to the surface of a bacterium or polysaccharides in the bacterial membrane. This recognition initiates a cascade of enzymatic cleavages that results in the assembly of a subset of complement proteins to form the membrane attack complex, which inserts itself into the membrane of the target organism and forms a large pore that allows water to rush in (p. 58). The target bacterium swells and undergoes osmotic lysis. Unfortunately, the complement system's lethal efficiency is not matched by its capacity to discriminate between genuine targets and normal host cells. Consequently, almost every cell type in the body is equipped with surface proteins that guard against a misdirected complement attack.

DAF and CD59 are two such proteins that interfere with distinct steps in the complement-activation pathway. Because GPI linkages couple both proteins to the membrane, any dysfunction of the enzymes that participate in the transfer of GPI-linked proteins from their transmembrane precursors to their GPI tails in the endoplasmic reticulum would interfere with the delivery of DAF and CD59 to their sites of functional residence at the cell surface. One of the proteins that participates in the synthesis of the GPI anchor is a sugar transferase that is encoded by the phosphatidylinositol glycan-class *A* (PIG-A) gene. This gene is located on the X chromosome.

Because every cell has only one working copy of the X chromosome (although female cells are genetically XX, one of the two X chromosomes is inactivated in every cell), if a spontaneous mutation occurs in the PIG-A gene in a particular cell, that cell and all of its progeny will lose the ability to synthesize GPI-linked proteins.

In **paroxysmal nocturnal hemoglobinuria** (i.e., hemoglobin appearing in the urine at night, with a sharp onset), a spontaneous mutation occurs in the PIG-A gene in just one of the many precursor cells that give rise to erythrocytes. All of the erythrocytes that arise from this particular precursor, therefore, are deficient in GPI-linked protein synthesis. Consequently, these cells lack DAF and CD59 expression and are susceptible to complement attack and lysis. For reasons that are largely unknown, the complement system is somewhat more active during sleep, so the hemolysis (lysis of erythrocytes) occurs more frequently at night in these patients. Some of the hemoglobin released by this lysis is excreted in the urine.

Because the PIG-A gene product is required for the synthesis of *all* GPI-linked proteins, the plasma membranes of affected red blood cells in paroxysmal nocturnal hemoglobinuria patients are missing a number of different proteins that are found in the surface membranes of their normal counterparts. It is the lack of DAF and CD59, however, that renders the cells vulnerable to complement-mediated killing and that creates the symptoms of the disease. Paroxysmal nocturnal hemoglobinuria is an uncommon disease. Because it is the result of an acquired mutation, it is much more likely to occur in people of middle age rather than in children. Patients with paroxysmal nocturnal hemoglobinuria are likely to become anemic and can suffer life-threatening disorders of clotting and bone marrow function. It is, however, a chronic condition, and more than half of patients survive at least 15 years after diagnosis.

Thus, protein folding requires no catalysis and can occur without help from any cellular machinery. However, the cell is not content to allow protein folding to follow a random course and instead orchestrates the process through the actions of molecular chaperones.

The **chaperones** constitute a large class of ATP-hydrolyzing proteins that appear to participate in a wide variety of polypeptide-folding phenomena, including the initial folding of newly synthesized proteins, as well as the refolding of proteins whose tertiary structures have been damaged by exposure to high temperature (i.e., "heat shock") or other denaturing conditions. Chaperones bind to unfolded protein chains and stabilize them in an unfolded conformation, thus preventing them from spontaneously folding into what might be an energetically favorable but biologically useless arrangement. Using energy that is provided through ATP hydrolysis, the chaperones sequentially release domains of unfolded proteins, and thus allow them to fold in an ordered fashion. Distinct subclasses of chaperones are present in several cell compartments, including the cytoplasm, the mitochondrion,

and the lumen of the rough ER. Newly synthesized secretory and membrane proteins appear to interact with ER chaperones as they exit from the tunnel of the translocon and subsequently disengage from the chaperones to assume their mature tertiary structure.

The acquisition of tertiary structure is followed quickly by the acquisition of **quaternary structure**. As noted earlier in this chapter, many membrane proteins assemble into oligomeric complexes in which several identical or distinct polypeptides interact with one another to form a macromolecular structure. Assembly of these multimers occurs in the ER. It is unknown whether the oligomeric assembly process occurs entirely spontaneously or if, like folding, it is orchestrated by specialized cellular mechanisms. Cells clearly go to great trouble to ensure that proteins inserted into or across their ER membranes are appropriately folded and oligomerized before allowing them to continue with their postsynthetic processing. As discussed later, proteins destined for secretion from the cell, or for residence in the cell membrane or other organellar membranes, depart the ER for further processing in

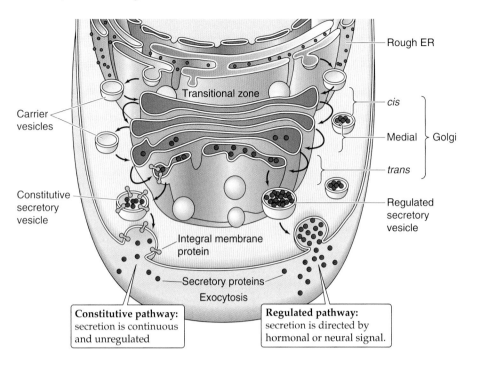

FIGURE 2–19. The secretory pathway. After their synthesis in the rough endoplasmic reticulum (ER), secretory and membrane proteins destined for the plasma membrane move through the Golgi stacks and secretory vesicles. In the constitutive pathway, vesicles fuse spontaneously with the plasma membrane. In the regulated pathway, the vesicles fuse only when triggered by a signal such as a hormone.

the membranous stacks of the **Golgi complex**. This departure is entirely contingent upon successful completion of the protein folding and assembly operations. Misfolded or unassembled proteins are retained in the ER and ultimately degraded. The ER chaperone proteins appear to play a role both in identifying proteins with incorrect tertiary or quaternary structures and in actively preventing their egress to the Golgi complex.

Secretory and Membrane Proteins Follow the Secretory Pathway Through the Cell

The rough ER is the common point of origin for the cell's secretory and membrane proteins. Most of these proteins are not retained in the rough ER, but depart for distribution to their sites of ultimate functional residence throughout the cell. As is true for their arrival in the rough ER, the departure of these proteins is a highly organized and regimented affair. In fact, the rough ER is the first station along the **secretory pathway**, which is the route followed (at least in part) by all secretory and membrane proteins as they undergo their post-translational modifications (Fig. 2–19).

The elucidation of the secretory pathway occurred in the 1960s, mainly in the laboratory of George Palade. For his contribution, Palade was awarded the 1975 Nobel Prize in Physiology or Medicine. This work also exploited the unique properties of pancreatic acinar cells to illuminate the central themes of secretory-protein biogenesis. Because approximately 95% of the protein that is synthesized by pancreatic acinar cells are digestive enzymes destined for secretion (p. 909), when these cells are fed radioactively labeled amino acids, the vast majority of these tracer molecules are incorporated into secretory polypeptides. Within a few minutes after the tracer is added, most of the label is associated with a specialized

subregion of the rough ER. Known as **transitional zones**, these membranous saccules are ribosome-studded on one surface and smooth at the opposite face (see Fig. 2–19). The smooth side is directly apposed to one pole of the pancake-like membrane stacks (or cisternae) of the **Golgi complex**. Smooth-surfaced carrier vesicles crowd the narrow moat of cytoplasm that separates the transitional zone from the Golgi. These vesicles "pinch off" from the transitional zone and fuse with a Golgi stack. From this first, or *cis*-Golgi stack, **carrier vesicles** ferry the newly synthesized proteins sequentially and vectorially through each Golgi stack, ultimately delivering them to the *trans*-most saccule of the Golgi. Finally, the newly synthesized secretory proteins appear in **secretory vesicles** (also called secretory granules in many tissues).

The journey from the rough ER to the secretory vesicle takes about 45 minutes in pancreatic acinar cells and requires the expenditure of metabolic energy. Each nucleated eukaryotic cell possesses a secretory pathway that shares this same general outline, although the specific features reflect the cell's particular function. The secretory pathway of the pancreatic acinar cell, for example, is specially adapted to accommodate the controlled secretion of protein via the so-called **regulated pathway**. Instead of being released from the cell continuously as they are produced, newly synthesized secretory proteins are held in *specialized secretory vesicles* that serve as an intracellular storage depot. This type of storage occurs in several cells, including those of endocrine and exocrine secretory tissues, and neurons. When the cells receive the requisite message, the storage vesicles fuse with the plasma membrane in a process known as **exocytosis**. The vesicles then dump their contents into the extracellular space. In the case of the pancreatic acinar cells, the enzymes are secreted into the pancreatic ductules and then make their way to the site of digestion in the duodenum (p. 911).

Most cell types, however, deliver newly synthesized secretory and membrane proteins to the cell surface in a *continuous* and *unregulated* fashion, which is referred to as the **constitutive pathway**. Specialized cells that have the capacity for regulated delivery also send an important subset of their secretory and membrane protein synthetic products to the cell surface constitutively. The regulated and constitutive secretory pathways are identical except for the final station of the Golgi complex. At this point, the "regulated" proteins divert to the specialized secretory vesicles described in the previous paragraph. The "constitutive" proteins, at the *trans*-most cisterna of the Golgi complex, sort into other secretory vesicles, which move directly to the cell surface. There, the constitutive *membrane proteins* are delivered to the plasma membrane, and the constitutive *secretory proteins* are immediately exocytosed.

This section has provided a broad overview of the secretory pathway. In the following sections, we examine the details of how newly synthesized proteins move between organellar compartments of the secretory pathway, how the proteins are processed during this transit, and how they are sorted to their final destination.

Carrier Vesicles Control the Traffic Between the Organelles of the Secretory Pathway

As the preceding discussion suggests, the secretory pathway is not a single, smooth, continuous highway but rather a series of saltatory translocations from one discrete organellar compartment to the next. Each of these steps requires some orchestration to ensure that the newly synthesized proteins arrive at their next terminus.

The cell solves the problem of moving newly synthesized proteins between membranous organelles by using membrane-enclosed carrier vesicles (or vesicular carriers). Each time proteins are to be moved from one compartment to the next, they are gathered together within or beneath specialized regions of membrane that subsequently evaginate, or "pinch off," to produce a carrier vesicle (see Fig. 2–19). Secretory proteins reside within the lumen of the carrier vesicle, whereas membrane proteins span the vesicle's own encapsulating bilayer. Upon arrival at the appropriate destination, the carrier vesicle fuses with the membrane of the acceptor organelle, thus delivering its contents of *soluble* proteins to the organelle's lumen and its cargo of *membrane* proteins to the organelle's own membrane. Carrier vesicles mediate the transport of secretory and membrane proteins across the space between the ER's transition zone and the *cis*-Golgi stack and also between the rims of the Golgi stacks themselves. The movement between one vesicular compartment and the next is mediated by the cytoskeleton and molecular motors that were discussed earlier.

A few critical facts deserve emphasis. First, throughout the formation, transit, and fusion of a carrier vesicle, no mixing occurs between the vesicle lumen and cytosol. The same principle applies to the carrier vesicle's membrane-protein passengers, which were inserted into the membrane of the rough ER with a particular topology. Those domains of a membrane protein that are exposed to the cytosol in the rough ER remain exposed to the cytosol as the protein completes its journey through the secretory pathway.

Second, the flow of vesicular membranes is not unidirectional. The rate of synthesis of new membrane lipid and protein in the ER is less than the rate at which carrier vesicles bud off of the ER that is bound for the Golgi. Because the sizes of the ER and Golgi are relatively constant, the membrane that moves to the Golgi via carrier vesicles must return to the ER. This return is again accomplished by vesicular carriers. Each discrete step of the secretory pathway must maintain vesicle-mediated back flow of membrane from the acceptor to the donor compartment so that each compartment can retain a constant size.

Finally, we have already noted that each organelle along the secretory pathway is endowed with a specific set of "resident" membrane proteins that determines the properties of the organelle. Despite the rapid forward and backward flow of carrier vesicles between successive stations of the secretory pathway, the resident membrane proteins do not get swept along in the flow. They are either actively retained in their home organelles' membranes or actively retrieved by the returning "retrograde" carrier vesicles. Thus, not only the size but also the composition of each organelle of the secretory pathway remains essentially constant despite the rapid flux of newly synthesized proteins that it constantly handles.

Specialized Protein Complexes, Such as Clathrin and Coatamers, Mediate the Formation and Fusion of Vesicles in the Secretory Pathway

The formation of a vesicle through evagination appears to be geometrically indistinguishable from its fusion with a target membrane. In both cases, a cross-sectional view in the electron microscope reveals an "omega" profile, which is so-named because the vesicle maintains a narrow opening to the organellar lumen that resembles the shape of the Greek letter omega (Ω). However, different problems are confronted during the formation and fusion of membrane vesicles.

VESICLE FORMATION IN THE SECRETORY PATHWAY. To form a spherical vesicle from a planar membrane, the mechanism that pulls the vesicle off from the larger membrane must grab on to the membrane over the entire surface of the nascent vesicle. The mechanism that achieves this makes use of a scaffolding that is composed of coat proteins. The cell has at least two and probably more varieties of coat proteins. The best characterized of these is clathrin, which mediates the formation of secretory vesicles from the *trans* Golgi. Clathrin also mediates the internalization of membrane from the cell surface during the process of endocytosis, which is the reverse of exocytosis. Another major protein coat, which is involved in nonselective trafficking of vesicles between the ER and Golgi, and between the stacks of the Golgi, is a protein complex known as *coatamer*. Both clathrin and coatamer proteins form the borders of a cage-like lattice.

In the case of **clathrin**, the coat proteins preassemble

A   FORMATION OF CLATHRIN-COATED VESICLES

FIGURE 2–20. Vesicle formation and fusion. *A,* Clathrin mediates the formation of secretory vesicles that bud off from the *trans* Golgi, as well as the internalization of membrane from the cell surface during the process of endocytosis. *B,* A complex of proteins forms a bridge between the vesicle and the target membranes. Adenosine triphosphate provides the fuel for fusion. The Rab appears to be a molecular switch. GTP, guanosine triphosphate; NSF, *N*-ethyl maleimide–sensitive factor; SNAP, soluble NSF-attachment protein; SNARE, SNAP receptor.

in the cytoplasm to form three-armed "triskelions" (Fig. 2–20A). A triskelion is not planar but resembles the three adjoining edges of a tetrahedron. As triskelions attach to one another, they produce a three-dimensional structure resembling a geodesic dome with a roughly spherical shape. A triskelion constitutes each vertex in the lattice of hexagons and pentagons that form the cage.

The triskelions of clathrin attach indirectly to the surface of the membrane that is to be excised by binding to the cytosolic tails of membrane proteins. Mediating this binding are adapter proteins, called adaptins, that link the membrane protein tails to the triskelion scaffold. The specificity for particular membrane proteins is apparently conferred by specialized adaptins. Triskelions assemble spontaneously to form a complete cage that attaches to the underlying membrane and pulls it up into a spherical configuration. Completion of the cage occurs simultaneously with the pinching off of the evaginated membrane from the planar surface, forming a closed sphere.

The pinching-off, or fission, process appears to involve the action of a GTP-binding protein called dynamin, which forms a collar around the neck of the forming vesicle, and may sever it. The fission process must include an intermediate that resembles the structure depicted in Figure 2–20A. According to the prevalent view, each of the lumen-facing leaflets of membrane lipids fuse, leaving only the cytoplasmic leaflets to form a continuous bridge from the vesicle to the donor membrane. This bridge then breaks and fission is complete.

Once formed, the clathrin-coated vesicle cannot fuse with its target membrane until it loses its cage, which prevents the two membranes from achieving the close contact required to permit fusion. Because formation of the clathrin cage is spontaneous and energetically favorable, dissolution of the cage requires energy. Uncoating is accomplished by a special class of cytoplasmic enzymes that hydrolyze ATP and use the energy thus liberated to disassemble the scaffold (see Fig. 2–20A).

The function of **coatamers** is similar to that of clathrin in that coatamer forms a cage around the budding membrane. However, coatamer coats differ from clathrin in several respects. First, coatamer coats are composed of several coatamer proteins or COPs, one of which is related to the adaptins. Second, unlike the spontaneous assembly of the clathrin triskelions, assembly of the coatamer coat around the budding vesicle requires ATP. Third, a coatamer-coated vesicle retains its coat until it docks with its target membrane.

VESICLE FUSION IN THE SECRETORY PATHWAY. Membrane fusion occurs when the hydrophobic cores of two bilayers come into contact with one another, a process that requires that the two membranes be very closely apposed. Because the cytoplasmic leaflets of most cellular membranes are predominantly composed of negatively charged phospholipids, electrostatic repulsion prevents this close apposition from occurring spontaneously. To overcome this charge barrier, and perhaps to assist in targeting as well, a multicomponent protein complex forms and acts as a bridge, linking vesicular membrane proteins to membrane proteins in the target bilayer (see Fig. 2–20B). Investigators have established the components of this complex using three approaches: studies of the membrane-fusion steps involved in vesicular transport between successive Golgi stacks, genetic analysis of protein secretion in yeast, and molecular dissection of the protein constituents of the synaptic vesicles of nerve terminals. In each case, the same proteins are instrumental in attaching the donor and target membranes to one another.

The central components of the bridge are proteins known as **SNAREs** (so named because they act as receptors for the SNAPs discussed in the next paragraph). There are SNAREs in both the vesicular membrane (v-SNAREs) and in the membrane of the target organelle (t-SNAREs). The best studied SNARE family members are those that participate in the fusion of neurotransmitter-containing synaptic vesicles with the plasma membrane of the axons in neurons (p. 222). In that setting, the v-SNARE is known as synaptobrevin, and proteins known as syntaxin and SNAP-25 together act as t-SNAREs. The t-SNAREs and v-SNAREs bind to each other extremely tightly, pulling the vesicular and target membranes very close together. This proximity alone may be sufficient to initiate fusion, although this point remains controversial. Although the nature of the fusion event itself remains unclear, clues have emerged regarding its regulation. Fusion requires the participation of a class of small GTP-binding proteins called **Rabs** that are important for signaling. Rabs appear to act as molecular switches that assemble with the SNARE fusion complex when they are binding GTP, but dissociate from the complex after they hydrolyze the GTP to GDP. Rab-GTP must associate with the fusion complex for fusion to occur. Numerous Rab isoforms exist, each isoform associated with a different vesicular compartment and a distinct membrane-transport step.

Once fusion occurs, the former vesicle generally loses its spherical shape rapidly as it becomes incorporated into the target membrane. This "flattening out" is the result of surface tension, inasmuch as the narrow radius of curvature demanded by a small spherical vesicle is energetically unfavorable. Following fusion, it is also necessary to disassemble the v-SNARE/t-SNARE complex so that its components can be reused in subsequent fusion events. The dissociation step involves the activity of two additional components that participate in the SNARE complex. The first is an ATP-hydrolyzing enzyme; because it is inhibited by the alkylating agent N-ethyl maleimide (NEM), it was named NEM-Sensitive Factor (NSF). The second are soluble NSF-attachment proteins (the SNAPs mentioned above), which target NSF to the SNARE complex. Hydrolysis of ATP by NSF causes dissociation of the SNARE complex, thus regenerating the fusion machinery. Homologues of the neuronal t-SNARE and v-SNARE proteins are found in almost every cell type in the body and are thought to participate in most, if not all, membrane fusion events.

Newly Synthesized Secretory and Membrane Proteins Are Processed During Their Passage Through the Secretory Pathway

While in the rough ER, newly synthesized secretory and membrane proteins undergo the first in a series of post-translational modifications. As discussed earlier, this first group includes glycosylation, disulfide-bond formation, and the acquisition of tertiary structure. Upon delivery to the *cis* stack of the Golgi complex, these proteins begin a new phase in their post-synthetic maturation. For many proteins, the most visible byproduct of this second phase is the complete remodeling of their N-linked sugar chains, originally attached in the rough ER.

Of the 14 sugar residues transferred en bloc to newly synthesized proteins during N-linked glycosylation (p. 34), nine are mannose and three are glucose (see Fig. 2–21A). Enzymes called glucosidases and one called a mannosidase are associated with the luminal face of the ER; these enzymes remove the three glucose residues and one mannose. As proteins arrive from the ER, mannosidases in the *cis* Golgi attack the N-linked sugar trees, thereby shearing off all except two N-acetylglucosamine and five mannose residues. As the proteins pass from the *cis* to the medial and ultimately to the *trans*-Golgi cisterna, another mannosidase removes two additional mannose residues, and other enzymes add sugars to the stump of the original sugar tree in a process referred to as **complex glycosylation**.

The addition of new sugars occurs one residue at a time and is accomplished by enzymes called **sugar transferases** that face the lumens of the Golgi stacks. Each sugar is transported from the cytoplasm to the Golgi lumen by a carrier protein that spans the Golgi membrane. Throughout the maturation process, the N-linked sugar chains are always exposed only to the luminal face of the Golgi.

Each cisterna of the Golgi is characterized by a different set of sugar transferases and sugar transporters. Thus, each Golgi compartment catalyzes a distinct step in the maturation of the N-linked chains. Complex glycosylation, therefore, proceeds like an assembly line from one modification station to the next. Because proteins have different shapes and sizes, however, the degree to which a sugar chain of any given polypeptide has access to each transferase can vary quite extensively. Thus, each protein emerges from the assembly line with its own particular pattern of complex glycosylation. The Golgi's *trans*-most cisterna houses the enzymes responsible for adding the terminal sugars, which cap the N-linked chain. The final residue of these terminal sugars is frequently N-acetyl neuraminic acid, also known as sialic acid. At neutral pH, sialic acid is negatively charged. This acidic sugar residue, therefore, is responsible for the net negative electrostatic charge that is frequently carried by **glycoproteins**.

The Golgi's function is not limited to creating N-linked sugar-tree topiaries. It oversees a number of other post-

FIGURE 2–21. Modification and assembly of the sugar chains on proteins in the Golgi. *A*, Remodeling of N-linked sugars. *B*, Proteoglycans. A trisaccharide links glycosaminoglycan chains to the protein via the −OH group of a serine residue. The glycosaminoglycan (or "GAG") is made up of "n" repeating disaccharide units, one of which is always an *amino* sugar. Asn, asparagine; ER, endoplasmic reticulum.

translational modifications, including the assembly of O-linked sugars. Many proteins possess **O-linked sugar chains**, which attach not to asparagine residues but to the hydroxyl groups (hence the "O") of serine and threonine residues. The O-linked sugars are not preassembled for en bloc transfer the way that the original 14-sugar tree is added in the rough ER in the case of their N-linked counterparts. Instead, the O-linked sugars are added one residue at a time by sugar transferases such as those that participate in the remodeling of complex N-linked glycosylation. O-linked chains frequently carry a great deal of negatively charged sialic acid.

Proteoglycans contain a very large number of a special class of O-linked sugar chains that are extremely long (see Fig. 2–21B). Unlike other O-linked sugars that attach to the protein core via an N-acetylglucosamine, the sugar chain in a proteoglycan attaches via a xylose-containing three-sugar "linker" to a serine residue on the protein backbone. One or more glycosaminoglycan side chains are added to this linker, one sugar at a time, to form the mature proteoglycan.

As the sugar chains grow, enzymes can add sulfate groups and greatly increase the quantity of negative charge that they carry. **Sulfated proteoglycans** that are secreted proteins become important components of the extracellular matrix and are also constituents of mucus. Proteoglycan chains can also be attached to membrane proteins that eventually reach the plasma membrane. The negatively charged sugars that are associated with the glycosaminoglycan groups, which are present both in mucus and on cell-surface glycoproteins, can help to form a barrier that protects cells from harsh environmental conditions such as those inside the stomach (p. 903). In the upper portion of the respiratory tract, the mucus assists in the removal of foreign bodies (p. 601).

Newly Synthesized Proteins Are Sorted in the *Trans*-Golgi Network

From their common point of origin at the rough ER, newly synthesized secretory and membrane proteins must

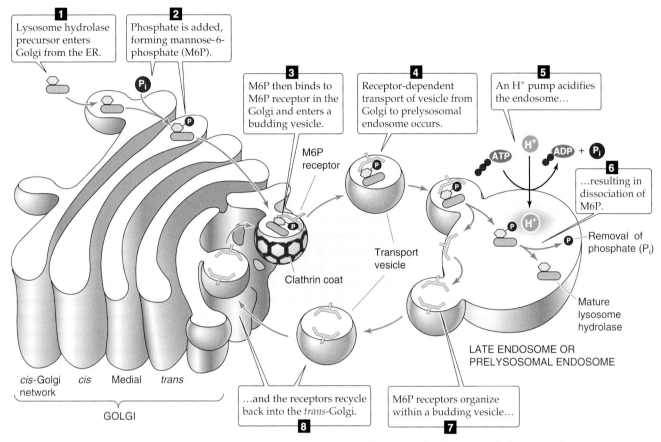

1 Lysosome hydrolase precursor enters Golgi from the ER.

2 Phosphate is added, forming mannose-6-phosphate (M6P).

3 M6P then binds to M6P receptor in the Golgi and enters a budding vesicle.

4 Receptor-dependent transport of vesicle from Golgi to prelysosomal endosome occurs.

5 An H⁺ pump acidifies the endosome...

6 ...resulting in dissociation of M6P.

M6P receptor

Clathrin coat

Transport vesicle

Removal of phosphate (Pᵢ)

Mature lysosome hydrolase

LATE ENDOSOME OR PRELYSOSOMAL ENDOSOME

cis-Golgi network   *cis*   Medial   *trans*

GOLGI

8 ...and the receptors recycle back into the *trans*-Golgi.

7 M6P receptors organize within a budding vesicle...

FIGURE 2–22. Sorting of lysosomal enzymes. ADP, adenosine diphosphate; ATP, adenosine triphosphate; ER, endoplasmic reticulum.

be distributed to a wide variety of different subcellular destinations. How can a cell recognize an individual protein from among the multitudes that are inserted into or across the membranes of the rough ER, and ensure its delivery to the site of its ultimate functional residence? Such a sorting operation has two prerequisites: (1) each protein to be sorted must carry some manner of address or "sorting signal" that communicates its destination, and (2) the cell must possess machinery capable of reading this sorting signal and acting on the information it embodies.

Little is known about the molecular correlates of sorting signals, and even less is established regarding the sorting machinery. However, for many proteins it is clear that sorting occurs in the *trans*-Golgi network (TGN). The *trans*-most cisterna of the Golgi complex is morphologically and biochemically distinct from the other Golgi stacks. Viewed in cross section, it appears as a complex web of membranous tubules and vesicles (Fig. 2–22). This structure befits the TGN's apparent function as a staging area from which carrier vesicles depart to transport their specific protein cargoes to one of many distinct subcellular locales.

Sorting machinery within or at the TGN appears to segregate classes of proteins—each bound for a common destination—into small discrete clusters. Each cluster is subsequently incorporated into a separate carrier vesicle, which evaginates from the TGN membrane and mediates the final stage of delivery. In the case of *secretory proteins*, this clustering happens within the lumen of the TGN. In

fact, such clusters of secretory proteins can be directly visualized in the electron microscope. *Membrane proteins* gather into two-dimensional clusters in the plane of the TGN membrane. Carrier vesicles incorporate these clusters into their own bilayers. Proteins bound for different destinations co-cluster in different subdomains of the TGN. Secretory and membrane proteins that are earmarked for the same destination can cluster in the same subdomain of the TGN and can be incorporated into the same carrier vesicle. Therefore, the TGN appears to function as a cellular transportation terminal that is able to direct groups of passengers who are carrying the same tickets to a common waiting area and ultimately to load them onto a common shuttle. Ticket agents herd passengers bearing different tickets into different waiting lounges.

A Mannose-6-Phosphate Recognition Marker Is Required to Target Newly Synthesized Hydrolytic Enzymes to Lysosomes

The most thoroughly established sorting paradigm is the pathway for newly synthesized lysosomal enzymes. Like secretory proteins, lysosomal enzymes carry amino-terminal signal sequences that direct their cotranslational translocation across the membrane of the rough ER. Their N-linked glycosylation and folding proceeds in the usual fashion, after which they join all of the other simultaneously synthesized proteins in the Golgi complex (see Fig. 2–22, *stage 1*).

A special sugar transferase in the *cis*-Golgi cisterna recognizes newly synthesized lysosomal enzymes, and adds a unique sugar. This enzyme adds N-acetylglucosamine phosphate to the mannose residues at the termini of the lysosomal enzymes' N-linked sugar trees. This enzyme differs from the usual sugar transferases (p. 39) in that it adds a *phospho*sugar group to the mannose residue, rather than just a sugar. This enzyme is also unique in recognizing specific amino-acid sequences that are exclusively in these lysosomal enzymes. A second *cis*-Golgi enzyme removes the additional N-acetylglucosamine sugar, leaving its phosphate group behind. As a result, the sugar trees of the lysosomal enzymes terminate in mannose-6-phosphate residues (see Fig. 2-22, *stage 2*).

A special class of mannose-6-phosphate receptors, localized predominantly in the elements of the *trans* Golgi, recognize proteins that carry mannose-6-phosphate groups (see Fig. 2–22, *stage 3*). This recognition step constitutes the first stage of the co-segregation and clustering process that was discussed earlier. The mannose-6-phosphate receptors are transmembrane proteins. Their luminal portions bind to the newly synthesized lysosomal enzymes, whereas their cytoplasmically facing tails possess a particular signal that allows them to interact with adaptins and hence to be incorporated into clathrin-coated vesicles. The assembly of the clathrin lattice causes the mannose-6-phosphate receptors to cluster, along with their associated lysosomal enzymes, in the plane of the TGN membrane. Completion of the clathrin cage results in the formation of a vesicle, whose membrane contains the mannose-6-phosphate receptors that bind their cargo of lysosomal enzymes.

After departing the TGN, these transport vesicles lose their clathrin coats (see Fig. 2–22, *stage 4*) and fuse with structures that are referred to as late endosomes or **prelysosomal endosomes**. Proton pumps in the membranes of these organelles ensure that their luminal pH is acidic (see Fig. 2–22, *stage 5*). When exposed to this acidic environment, the mannose-6-phosphate receptors undergo a conformational change that releases the mannose-6-phosphate-bearing lysosomal enzymes (see Fig. 2–22, *stage 6*). Consequently, the newly synthesized enzymes are dumped into the lumen of the prelysosomal endosome, which will go on to fuse with or mature into a lysosome. The empty mannose-6-phosphate receptors join vesicles that bud off from the lysosome (see Fig. 2–22, *stage 7*) and return to the TGN (see Fig. 2–22, *stage 8*). The luminal environment of the TGN allows the receptors to recover their affinity for mannose-6-phosphate, thus allowing them to participate in subsequent rounds of sorting.

Disruption of lysosomal sorting can be produced in several ways. For example, a drug called **tunicamycin** blocks the addition of N-linked sugars to newly synthesized proteins and thereby prevents attachment of the mannose-6-phosphate recognition marker. Compounds that elevate the luminal pH of the prelysosomal endosomes prevent newly synthesized enzymes from dissociating from the mannose-6-phosphate receptors and consequently block recycling of the receptor pool back to the TGN. The resulting shortage of unoccupied receptors allows mannose-6-phosphate–bearing proteins to pass through the

TGN unrecognized (see box titled Lysosomal Storage Diseases). Thus, instead of diverting to the lysosomes, these lysosomal enzymes continue along the secretory pathway and are ultimately released from the cell by constitutive secretion.

Cells Internalize Extracellular Material Through the Process of Endocytosis

The same fundamental mechanisms in the secretory pathway that produce vesicles by evaginating regions of Golgi membrane can also move material in the opposite direction by inducing vesicle formation through the invagination of regions of the plasma membrane. Vesicles created in this fashion are delimited by membrane that had formerly been part of the cell surface, and their luminal contents derive from the extracellular compartment.

This internalization process, referred to as **endocytosis**, serves the cell in at least four ways. First, certain nutrients are too large to be imported from the extracellular fluid into the cytoplasm via transmembrane carrier proteins; they are instead carried into the cell by endocytosis. Second, endocytosis of hormone-receptor complexes can terminate the signaling processes that are initiated by numerous hormones. Third, endocytosis is the first step in remodeling or degrading portions of the plasma membrane. Membrane that is delivered to the surface during exocytosis must be retrieved and ultimately returned to the TGN. Fourth, proteins or pathogens that need to be cleared from the extracellular compartment are brought into the cell by endocytosis and subsequently condemned to degradation in the lysosomes. Because endocytosed material can pursue a number of very different destinies, there must be sorting mechanisms in the endocytic pathway, just as in the secretory pathway, that allow the cell to direct the endocytosed material to its appropriate destination.

Fluid-phase endocytosis is the uptake of the materials that are dissolved in the extracellular fluid (Fig. 2–23, *stage 1*) and not specifically bound to receptors on the cell surface. This process begins when a clathrin cage starts to assemble on the cytoplasmic surface of the plasma membrane. Earlier we discussed the physiology of clathrin-coated vesicles in the *secretory* pathway (see Fig. 2–20). The clathrin attaches to the membrane through interactions with adaptin proteins, which in turn adhere to the cytoplasmic tail domains of certain transmembrane polypeptides. Construction of the cage causes its adherent underlying membrane to invaginate and form a coated pit (see Fig. 2–23, *stage 2A*). Completion of the cage creates a closed vesicle, which detaches from the cell surface through the process of membrane fission (see Fig. 2–23, *stage 3*). The resultant vesicle quickly loses its clathrin coat through the action of the uncoating ATPase and fuses with an organelle called an **endosome**.

Receptor-Mediated Endocytosis Is Responsible for Internalizing Specific Proteins

Most of the proteins that a cell seeks to import via endocytosis are present in the extracellular fluid in extremely centrating specific proteins at the site of endocytosis prior to initiating their uptake.

This concentration is achieved in a process known as **receptor-mediated endocytosis**, in which molecules to be internalized (see Fig. 2–23, *stage 1*) bind to cell-surface receptors with high affinity (see Fig. 2–23, *stage 2B*). Through this interaction, the substrates for endocytosis become physically associated with the plasma membrane, thus greatly enhancing the probability that they will be successfully internalized. Cells increase this probability even further by ensuring that the receptors themselves cluster in regions of the membrane destined to be endocytosed. The cytoplasmic tails of these receptors are endowed with recognition sequences that allow them to serve as binding sites for adaptins. Consequently, these receptors congregate in regions of the cell membrane where clathrin cages are assembling, and are incorporated into coated pits as they are forming. The affinity of these receptors for the endocytic machinery ensures that their ligands are internalized with maximum efficiency.

Most endocytic receptors are constitutively associated with coated pits and are endocytosed whether or not they have bound their specific ligands. The cytoplasmic tails of certain receptors, however, interact with adaptins only when the receptor is in the bound state. For example, in the absence of epidermal growth factor (EGF), the EGF receptor is excluded from regions of the membrane in which coated pits are assembling. Modifications induced by ligand binding alter these receptors' tails, which allows them to participate in coated vesicle formation and hence in endocytosis.

After the clathrin-coated vesicle forms (see Fig. 2-23, *stage 3*), it quickly loses its clathrin coat, as described earlier for fluid-phase endocytosis, and fuses with an endosome. Although endosomes can be wildly pleiomorphic, they frequently manifest a frying-pan–like appearance in which a round vesicular body is attached to a long tubular "handle" (see Fig. 2–23, *stage 4*). Often the cytoplasmic surfaces of the handles are decorated with forming clathrin lattices and are the sites of vesicular budding.

Endocytosed Proteins Can Be Targeted to Lysosomes or Recycled to the Cell Surface

In many cell types, endocytosis is so rapid that, each hour, the cell internalizes a quantity of membrane that is equivalent in area to the entire cell surface. To persist in the face of this tremendous flux of membrane, the cell must retrieve most of the endocytosed membrane components and return them to the plasmalemma. However, substances that a cell wishes to degrade must be routed to lysosomes and prevented from escaping back to the surface. The sophisticated sorting operation required to satisfy both of these conditions takes place in the endosome.

Proton pumps embedded in its membrane ensure that, like the lysosome, the endosome maintains an acidic luminal pH (see Fig. 2–23, *stage 4*). This acidic environment initiates the separation of material that is destined for lysosomal destruction from those proteins that are to

---

LYSOSOMAL STORAGE DISEASES

The experimental elucidation of lysosomal-enzyme sorting was achieved only because of the existence of a remarkable, naturally occurring human disease that was traced to a genetic defect in the sorting machinery. In lysosomal storage diseases, the absence of a particular hydrolase—or group of hydrolases—from the lysosome prevents the lysosomes from degrading certain substances, resulting in the formation of overstuffed lysosomes that crowd the cytoplasm and impede cell function.

In **I-cell disease,** most hydrolases are missing from the lysosomes of many cell types. As a result, lysosomes become engorged with massive quantities of undigested substrates. The enormously swollen lysosomes that characterize this disease were named "inclusion bodies," and the cells that possess them were designated "inclusion cells," or "I-cells," for short. Whereas I-cells lack most lysosomal enzymes, the genes that encode all of the hydrolases are completely normal. The mutation responsible for I-cell disease resides in the gene for the **phosphosugar transferase** that creates the mannose-6-phosphate recognition marker (Fig. 2–22). Without this enzyme, the cell cannot sort any of the hydrolases to the lysosomes. Instead, the hydrolases pass through the *trans*-Galgi network unnoticed by the mannose-6-phosphate receptors and are secreted constitutively from the affected cells. It is interesting to note that certain cell types from I-cell individuals can sort newly synthesized hydrolases normally, suggesting that alternative, as yet unelucidated pathways for the targeting of lysosomal enzymes must also exist.

In some other lysosomal storage diseases, *specific* hydrolases are not missorted, but rather are genetically defective. For example, children who suffer from **Tay-Sachs disease** carry a homozygous mutation in the gene that encodes the lysosomal enzyme **hexosaminidase A** (HEX A). Consequently, their lysosomes are unable to degrade substances that contain certain specific sugar linkages. Because they cannot be broken down, these substances accumulate in lysosomes. Over time, these substances fill the lysosomes, which swell and crowd the cytoplasm. The resulting derangements of cellular function are toxic to a number of cell types and ultimately underlie this disease's uniform fatality within the first few years of life. Carriers of the Tay-Sachs trait can be detected either by HEX A enzyme testing, or by DNA analysis of the HEX A gene. Among the Ashkenazi Jewish population, in which 1 in 27 individuals is a carrier, three distinct HEX A mutations account for 98% of all carrier mutations.

---

low concentrations. Furthermore, the volume of extracellular fluid that is internalized by an individual coated vesicle is very small. Consequently, the probability that any particular target molecule will enter the cell during a given round of fluid-phase endocytosis is low. To improve the efficiency of endocytosis and ensure that the desired extracellular components are gathered in every endocytic cycle, the cell has devised a method for con-

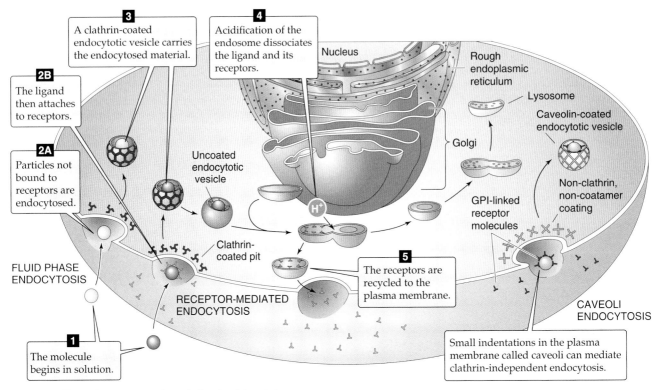

3 A clathrin-coated endocytotic vesicle carries the endocytosed material.

4 Acidification of the endosome dissociates the ligand and its receptors.

2B The ligand then attaches to receptors.

2A Particles not bound to receptors are endocytosed.

Nucleus

Rough endoplasmic reticulum

Lysosome

Caveolin-coated endocytotic vesicle

Uncoated endocytotic vesicle

Golgi

Non-clathrin, non-coatamer coating

GPI-linked receptor molecules

Clathrin-coated pit

FLUID PHASE ENDOCYTOSIS

H⁺

5 The receptors are recycled to the plasma membrane.

RECEPTOR-MEDIATED ENDOCYTOSIS

CAVEOLI ENDOCYTOSIS

1 The molecule begins in solution.

Small indentations in the plasma membrane called caveoli can mediate clathrin-independent endocytosis.

FIGURE 2–23. Endocytosis. GPI, glycosyl phosphatidylinositol.

be recycled. Most endocytic receptors bind their ligands tightly at neutral pH but release them rapidly at pH values below 6.0. Therefore, as soon as a surface-derived vesicle fuses with an endosome, proteins that are bound to receptors fall off and enter the endosomal lumen. The receptor proteins segregate in the membranes of the "handles" of the frying-pan–shaped endosomes and are ultimately removed from the endosome in vesicles that shuttle them back to the cell surface (see Fig. 2–23, stage 5). The soluble proteins of the endosome lumen, which include the receptors' former ligands, are ultimately delivered to the lysosome. This sorting scheme allows the receptors to avoid the fate of their cargo and ensures that the receptors are used in many rounds of endocytosis.

The low-density lipoprotein (LDL) receptor follows this regimen precisely. Upon arrival of the LDL-laden receptor at the endosome, the acidic environment of the endosome induces the LDL to dissociate from its receptor, which then promptly recycles to the cell surface. The LDL travels on to the lysosome, where enzymes destroy the LDL and liberate its bound cholesterol.

A variation on this paradigm is responsible for the cellular uptake of iron. Iron circulates in the plasma bound to a protein called **transferrin**. At the mildly alkaline pH of extracellular fluid, the iron-transferrin complex binds with high affinity to a transferrin receptor in the plasma membranes of almost every cell type. Bound transferrin is internalized by endocytosis and delivered to endosomes. Instead of inducing *transferrin* to fall off its receptor, the acid environment of the endosome lumen causes *iron* to fall off transferrin. **Apotransferrin** (i.e., transferrin without bound iron) remains tightly bound to

the transferrin receptor at an acidic pH. The released iron is transported across the endosomal membrane for use in the cytosol. The complex of apotransferrin and the transferrin receptor recycles to the cell surface where it is again exposed to the extracellular fluid. The mildly alkaline extracellular pH causes the transferrin receptor to lose its affinity for apotransferrin and promptly releases it. Thus, the cell uses the pH-dependent sorting trick twice to ensure that both the transferrin receptor and apotransferrin recycle for subsequent rounds of iron uptake.

Certain Molecules Are Internalized Through an Alternative Process That Involves Caveoli

Clathrin-coated pits are not the only cellular structures involved in receptor-mediated internalization. Electron microscopic examination of vascular endothelial cells that line blood vessels long ago revealed the presence of clusters of small vesicles that display a characteristic appearance, in close association with the plasma membrane. These **caveoli** were thought to be involved in the transfer of large molecules across the endothelial cells, from the blood space to the tissue compartment. Actually, caveoli are present in most cell types. The caveoli carry a coat that is morphologically distinct from the clathrin lattice (see Fig. 2–23). Caveoli appear to be rich in membrane-associated polypeptides that participate in intracellular signaling, such as the Ras-like proteins (p. 97) as well as heterotrimeric GTP-binding proteins (p. 92). They are also enriched in the receptor for folate, a vitamin required by several metabolic pathways (p. 967). Unlike the receptors in the plasma membrane discussed earlier, the **folate receptor** has no cytoplasmic tail that might allow it to associate with coated pits. Instead, it belongs to the GPI-linked class of proteins (p. 15) that are anchored to the membrane through covalent attachment to phospholipid molecules. It appears that caveoli mediate the internalization of folate. In fact, a large number and variety of GPI-linked proteins are embedded in the leaflet of the caveolar membrane that faces its lumen.

The role of caveoli in the uptake of other substances, the significance of the large inventory of GPI-linked proteins in caveoli, and the functions served by their cache of signaling molecules all remain to be determined. It is clear, however, that the caveoli comprise a novel endocytic structure that participates in pathways that are distinct from those involving coated vesicles and endosomes.

SPECIALIZED CELL TYPES

All cells are constructed of the same basic elements and share the same basic metabolic and biosynthesic machinery. What distinguishes one cell type from another? Certainly, cells have different shapes and molecular structures. In addition, out of an extensive repertory of molecules that cells are capable of making, each cell type chooses which molecules to express, how to organize these molecules, and how to regulate them. It is this combination of choices that endows them with specific physiological functions. These specializations are the product of cell differentiation. Each of these cell types arises from a **stem cell**. Stem cells are mitotically active and can give rise to multiple, distinct cellular lineages; thus, they are referred to as *pluri*potent. Clearly the zygote is the ultimate stem cell, because through its divisions it gives rise to every cell lineage present in the complete organism. Specific cell types arise from stem cells by activating a differentiation-specific program of gene expression. The interplay of environmental signals, temporal cues, and transcription factors that control the processes of cellular differentiation constitutes one of the great unravelling mysteries of modern biologic science.

The Actin-Myosin Based Cytoskeleton Is Responsible for Contractility in Cardiac and Skeletal Muscle Cells

The physiology of muscle contraction is the topic of Chapter 9. Two common cytoskeletal elements, actin and myosin, are structurally organized in **striated muscle**. In skeletal- and cardiac-muscle cells, the thin filaments, which are composed primarily of actin, are aligned in parallel arrays that interdigitate with arrays of thick filaments, which are composed primarily of myosin. Actin filaments serve as the structural scaffolding against which myosin can exert its tensile force. The array of actin filaments, which runs parallel to the long axis of the cell, inserts into a filamentous meshwork referred to as the **Z line** or **Z disk** (Fig. 2–24), which lies perpendicular to the long axis of the cell and is composed of the actin-

binding protein α **actinin**. The structural unit of *skeletal* and *cardiac* muscle is the **sarcomere**, which consists of the actin and myosin filaments between two consecutive Z lines. A single **myofibril** may be composed of hundreds or thousands of sarcomeres that are joined end-to-end. The cytoplasm of each muscle cell is filled with parallel arrays of myofibrils, the Z lines of which are more or less aligned in register. Consequently, when a myocyte is viewed in the light microscope, its cytoplasm is characterized by a repetitive pattern of stripes that are arranged perpendicular to the cell's long axis. These successive dark and light regions correspond to the distributions and overlaps of the filaments that comprise the sarcomeres. In *cardiac* myocytes, the "registration" of sarcomeres is not as pronounced.

Myosin is a molecular motor that can "walk" along actin filaments in non-muscle cells. What is unique about muscle cells is that the actin and myosin are in parallel arrays, so that the myosin literally pulls the actin—and therefore two neighboring Z lines—toward each other. For this mechanism to work productively, the "head" of the myosin molecule must sequentially relax and flex at its "hinge" in a cycle that requires ATP hydrolysis (Fig. 9–7).

If ATP were the only factor that regulates the actin-myosin interaction, then muscle contraction would occur continuously and would not subside until ATP supplies had been exhausted. In Chapter 9, we discuss a more elegant and responsive control system that modulates contractility and makes it responsive to neuronal cues. However, it is worth noting here that the striated-muscle cell achieves this control through the intercession of actin-binding proteins. Under resting conditions, a long fibrillar protein called **tropomyosin** overlies the actin filaments and obscures the myosin-binding sites. Tropomyosin is held in place by a small, globular, calcium-binding protein called **troponin**, which attaches simultaneously to both actin and tropomyosin. When the cytosolic Ca^{2+} concentration ($[Ca^{2+}]_i$) increases, troponin alters its conformation, displaces the tropomyosin, and thereby exposes the myosin-binding sites on the actin strands. Thus, the addition of regulatory proteins to the cytoskeletal framework allows intracellular second messengers to regulate contraction in striated muscle.

Less Ordered Arrays of Actin and Myosin Filaments Participate in Smooth Muscle Contraction

Smooth muscle cells are responsible for the contractile capabilities of blood vessels, airways, the gastrointestinal tract, and the uterus. These cells generate slow but sustained contractions that persist for many minutes or hours. Chapter 9 includes an overview of the physiology of smooth muscle. Here we will discuss the specialized adaptations of smooth-muscle cells in terms of both architecture and physiological regulation.

There are no sarcomeres in smooth muscle cells. Instead, actin and myosin filaments are arrayed in a roughly parallel meshwork that is oriented at an angle to the long

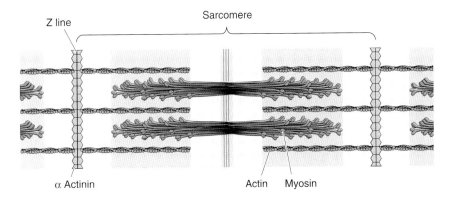

FIGURE 2–24. A sarcomere in striated muscle. In skeletal and cardiac muscle, the actin and myosin filaments are highly ordered. The fundamental unit is the sarcomere, the structures between two adjacent Z lines.

axis of the cell. These filaments insert onto the plasma membrane, and when they shorten, the cell contracts.

As in skeletal and cardiac muscle, the trigger for contraction is an elevation in $[Ca^{2+}]_i$. However, the whole chain of events that leads to the increase in $[Ca^{2+}]_i$, as well as the mechanism by which Ca^{2+} triggers contraction, is different from that in striated muscle. Rather than interacting with troponin, the Ca^{2+} in smooth muscle binds to regulatory proteins that activate **myosin light chain kinase**, an enzyme that phosphorylates the light chains of smooth-muscle myosin. With its light chains phosphorylated, myosin is able to bind to actin and produce contraction. The myosin ATPase in smooth muscle hydrolyzes ATP much more slowly than its striated muscle counterpart, and thus smooth muscle can maintain tension over time at considerably less energy expense than would be required in skeletal or cardiac muscle. Dephosphorylation, which is catalyzed by a family of tightly regulated enzymes called **phosphatases**, causes the actin-myosin complex to disassemble and contraction to cease. Thus, skeletal muscle and smooth muscle represent two very different means by which the structural and biochemical features of the actin-myosin cytoskeleton have been adapted to produce distinct types of force generation.

Epithelial Cells Form a Barrier Between the Internal and External Milieu

How can an organism tightly regulate its internal fluid environment (i.e., internal milieu) without allowing this environment to come into direct and disastrous contact with the external world (i.e., external milieu)? The body has solved these problems by arranging a sheet of cells— an **epithelium**—between two disparate solutions. Because of their unique subcellular designs and intercellular relationships, epithelial cells form a dynamic barrier that can import or expel substances, sometimes against steep concentration gradients.

Two structural features of epithelia permit them to function as useful barriers between two very different solutions (Fig. 2–25). First, epithelial cells connect to one another via tight junctions, which constrain the free diffusion of solutes and fluids around the epithelial cells, between the internal and external compartments. Second, the tight junctions define a boundary between an apical

and a basolateral domain of the plasma membrane. Each of these two domains is endowed with distinct protein and lipid components, and each subserves a distinct function. Thus, the surface membranes of epithelial cells are polarized. In Chapter 3, we discuss the mechanisms by which polarized epithelial cells exploit their unique geometry to transport salts and water from one solution to the other. However, it is worth touching on a few of the cellular specializations that characterize polarized epithelia and permit them to perform their critical roles.

The **apical membranes** of the epithelial cells (see Fig. 2–25) face the lumen of a compartment that is often topologically continuous with the outside world. For example, in the stomach and intestine, apical membranes form the inner surface of the organs that come into contact with ingested matter. The **basolateral membranes** of epithelial cells face the extracellular fluid compartment— which indirectly makes contact with the blood—and rest on a basement membrane. The **basement membrane** is composed of extracellular-matrix proteins that the epithelial cells themselves secrete, and include collagens, laminin, and proteoglycans. The basement membrane provides the epithelium with structural support and, most importantly, serves as an organizing foundation that helps the epithelial cells to establish their remarkable architecture.

Each epithelial cell is interconnected to its neighbors by a variety of **junctional complexes** (see Fig. 2–25). The lateral surfaces of epithelial cells participate in numerous types of cell-cell contacts, including tight junctions, adhering junctions, gap junctions, and desmosomes.

TIGHT JUNCTIONS. A **tight junction** (or *zonula occludens*) is a complex structure that impedes the passage of molecules and ions *between* the cells of the epithelial monolayer. This pathway between the cells is termed the **paracellular pathway**. Although the complete molecular structure of the tight junction has yet to be elucidated, it is clear that its functional properties are related to its intriguing architecture (see Fig. 2–25). When viewed by transmission electron microscopy, tight junctions include regions of apparent fusion between the outer leaflets of the lipid bilayer membranes of neighboring epithelial cells. Freeze-fracture electron microscopy reveals that the tight junction is composed of parallel strands of closely packed particles that presumably represent the transmembrane proteins that participate in the junction's formation.

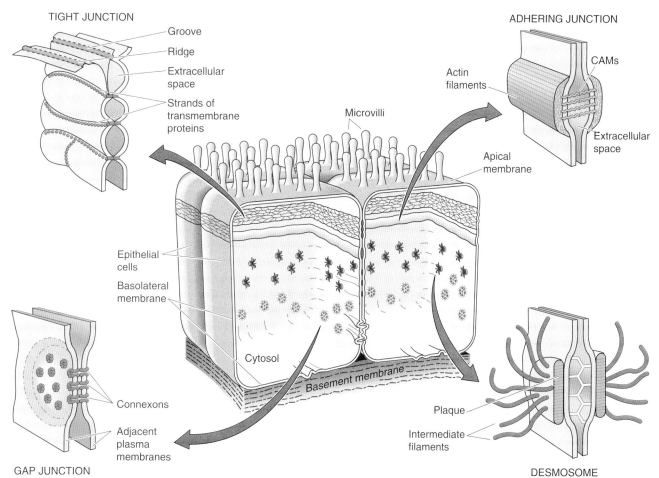

FIGURE 2–25. Epithelial cells. In an epithelial cell, the tight junction separates the cell membrane into apical and basolateral domains that have very different functional properties. CAM, cell adhesion molecule.

The degree of an epithelium's impermeability—or "tightness"—is roughly proportional to the number of these parallel strands.

Tight junctions play several roles. First, they are **barriers** in that they separate one compartment from another. In some epithelial cells, such as those of the renal thick ascending limb, the tight junctions form an essentially impenetrable boundary that completely blocks the flow of ions and water between cells. In contrast, the tight junctions of the renal proximal tubule are leaky, permitting significant transepithelial movement of fluid and solutes.

Second, tight junctions can act as selective **gates** in that they permit certain solutes to flow more easily than others. Examples are the leaky tight junctions of tissues such as the proximal tubule. As discussed in Chapter 3, the permeability and selectivity of an epithelium's tight junctions are critical variables for determining that epithelium's transport characteristics. Moreover, the permeability properties of the gate function of tight junctions can be modulated in response to various physiological stimuli.

Third, tight junctions act as **fences** that separate the polarized surfaces of the epithelial plasma membrane into apical and basolateral domains. The presence of distinct populations of proteins and lipids in each plasma membrane domain is absolutely essential for an epithelium to mediate transepithelial fluid and solute transport (p. 84).

ADHERING JUNCTION. An **adhering junction** (or *zonula adherens*) is a belt that encircles an entire epithelial cell just below the level of the tight junction. Epithelial cells need two pieces of information to build themselves into a coherent epithelium. First, the cells must know which end is up. The extracellular matrix (see earlier) provides this information by defining which side will be basolateral. Second, the cells must know that there are like neighbors with which to establish cell-to-cell contacts. Adhering junctions provide epithelial cells with clues regarding the nature and proximity of their neighbors. These cell-cell contacts are mediated by cell-cell adhesion molecules (CAMs), which are members of a large class of membrane proteins that participate in intercellular interactions (p. 19). Epithelial cells will only organize themselves into a properly polarized epithelium—with differentiated apical and basolateral plasma membranes—if the CAMs of neighboring cells have come into close enough apposition to form an adhering junction. Formation of these junctions initiates the assembly of a subcortical cytoskeleton (particularly actin) that is associated with the cytosolic surfaces of the lateral membranes. Conversely, the disruption of adhering junctions can lead to a loss of epithelial organization. In epithelial tumors, for example, loss of expression of the adhering-junction CAMs tends to correlate with the tumor cell's loss of controlled growth and its ability to **metastasize**—that is, to leave the epithelial monolayer and form a new tumor at a distant site in the body.

GAP JUNCTIONS. Gap junctions, which are discussed in Chapter 6, are channels that interconnect the cytosols of neighboring cells. They allow small molecules (less than ~1000 in molecular weight) to diffuse freely between cells. In some organs, epithelial cells are interconnected by an enormous number of gap junctions, which organize into paracrystalline hexagonal arrays. Because ions can flow through gap junctions, cells that communicate through gap junctions are electrically coupled. The permeability of gap junctions, and hence, the extent to which the cytoplasmic compartments of neighboring cells are coupled, can be regulated in response to a variety of physiological stimuli.

DESMOSOME. A **desmosome** (or *macula adherens*) holds adjacent cells together tightly at a single, round spot where the plasma membranes of the two cells are in close apposition. Desmosomes are easily recognized in thin-section electron micrographs by the characteristic dense plaques of intermediate filaments (p. 24) that radiate into the cytoplasm from the point of intercellular contact (see Fig. 2–25). These filaments interact with and organize the cytoplasmic intermediate filaments, thus coupling the structurally stabilizing elements of neighboring cells to one another. Epithelial cells are often coupled to adjacent cells by numerous desmosomes, especially in regions where the epithelium is subject to physical stress.

Epithelial Cells Are Polarized

In many epithelia, the apical surface area is amplified by the presence of a **brush border** that is composed of hundreds of finger-like, microvillar projections (see Fig. 2–25). In the case of the small intestine and the renal proximal tubule, the membrane covering each microvillus is richly endowed with enzymes that digest sugars and proteins, as well as with transporters that carry the products of these digestions into the cells. The presence of a microvillar brush border can amplify the apical surface area of a polarized epithelial cell by as much as 20-fold, thus greatly enhancing its capacity to interact with, modify, and transport substances present in the luminal fluid.

The basolateral surface area of certain epithelial cells is amplified by the presence of **lateral interdigitations** and **basal infoldings** (see Fig. 2–25). Although they are not as elegantly constructed as microvilli, these structures can greatly increase the basolateral surface area. In epithelial cells that are involved in large volumes of transport—or in transport against steep gradients—amplifying the basolateral membrane can greatly increase the number of basolateral Na-K pumps that a single cell can place at its basolateral membrane.

Although the morphologic differences between apical and basolateral membranes can be dramatic, the most important distinction between these surfaces is their protein composition. As noted earlier, the "fence" function of the tight junction separates completely different rosters of membrane proteins between the apical and basolateral membranes. For example, the Na-K pump is restricted to the basolateral membrane in almost all epithelial cells, and the membrane-bound enzymes that hydrolyze complex sugars and peptides are restricted to apical membranes in intestinal epithelial cells. The polarized distribution of transport proteins is absolutely necessary for the directed movement of solutes and water across epithelia. Furthermore, the restriction of certain enzymes to the apical domain limits their actions to the lumen of the epithelium and, therefore, offers the advantage of not wasting energy putting enzymes where they are not needed. The polarity of epithelial membrane proteins also plays a critical role in detecting antigens present in the external milieu and in transmitting signals between the external and internal compartments.

Maintaining epithelial polarity involves complex intermolecular interactions that are only beginning to be understood. When tight junctions are disrupted, diffusion in the plane of the membrane leads to intermingling of apical- and basolateral-membrane components, and thus a loss of polarity. The subcortical cytoskeleton beneath the basolateral surface may play a similar role by physically restraining a subset of membrane proteins at the basolateral surface.

However, such mechanisms for stabilizing the polarized distributions of membrane proteins do not explain how newly synthesized proteins come to be distributed at the appropriate plasma-membrane domain. We will give two examples of mechanisms that cells can use to direct membrane proteins to either the basolateral or apical membrane. The first example focuses on protein-protein interactions. As noted during our discussion of the secretory-protein pathway, the sorting operation that separates apically from basolaterally directed proteins apparently occurs in the TGN (p. 41). Some proteins destined for the basolateral membrane have special amino acid motifs that act as sorting signals. Some of these motifs are similar to those that allow membrane proteins to participate in endocytosis. Members of the adaptin family may recognize these motifs during the formation of clathrin-coated vesicles at the TGN, and segregate the basolateral proteins into a vesicle destined for the basolateral membrane.

Another example of mechanisms that cells use to generate a polarized distribution of membrane proteins focuses on lipid-lipid interactions. In many epithelia, GPI-linked proteins are concentrated exclusively at the apical surface. It appears that the phospholipid components of GPI-linked proteins are unusual in that they cluster into complexes of fairly immobile gel-phase lipids during their passage through the Golgi apparatus. We saw earlier how "lakes" of phospholipids with different physical properties may segregate within a membrane (p. 13). The "glycolipid rafts" of GPI-linked proteins incorporate into apically directed vesicles so that sorting can occur through lipid-lipid interactions in the plane of the membrane rather than through protein-protein interactions occurring at the cytoplasmic surface of the Golgi membrane. From these two examples, it should be clear that a number of different mechanisms may contribute to protein sorting and the maintenance of epithelial polarity.

REFERENCES

Books and Reviews

Goldstein JL, Brown MS, Anderson RGW, et al: Receptor-mediated endocytosis: Concepts emerging from the LDL receptor system. Annu Rev Cell Dev Biol 1:1–39, 1985.

Mellman I: Endocytosis and molecular sorting. Annu Rev Cell Dev Biol 12:575–625, 1996.

Palade GE: Intracellular aspects of the process of protein synthesis. Science 189:347–358, 1985.

Rodriguez-Boulan E, Powell SK: Polarity of epithelial and neuronal cells. Annu Rev Cell Dev Biol 8:395–427, 1992.

Rothman JE: The protein machinery of vesicle budding and fusion. Protein Sci 5:185–194, 1995.

Sheetz MP: Microtubule motor complexes moving membranous organelles. Cell Struct Funct 21:369–373, 1996.

Journal Articles

Frye LD, Edidin M: The rapid intermixing of cell surface antigens after formation of mouse-human heterokaryons. J Cell Sci 7:319–335, 1970.

Griffiths G, Hoflack B, Simons K, et al: The mannose-6-phosphate receptor and the biogenesis of lysosomes. Cell 52:329–341, 1988.

Kyte J, Doolittle RF: A simple method for displaying the hydropathic character of a protein. J Mol Biol 157:105–132, 1982.

Walter P, Ibrahimi I, Blobel G: Translocation of proteins across the endoplasmic reticulum. I. Signal recognition protein (SRP) binds to in vitro assembled polysomes synthesizing secretory protein. J Cell Biol 91:545–550, 1981.

CHAPTER 3

Physiology of Membranes

Peter S. Aronson, Walter F. Boron, and
Emile L. Boulpaep

The cells of the human body live in a carefully regulated fluid environment. The fluid inside the cells, the **intracellular fluid** (ICF), occupies what is called the intracellular compartment, and the fluid outside the cells, the **extracellular fluid** (ECF), occupies the extracellular compartment. The barriers that separate these two compartments are the **cell membranes**. For life to be sustained, the body must rigorously maintain the volume and composition of the intracellular and extracellular compartments. To a large extent, such regulation is the result of transport across the cell membrane. In this chapter we discuss how cell membranes regulate the distribution of ions and water in the intracellular and extracellular compartments.

THE INTRACELLULAR AND EXTRACELLULAR FLUIDS

Total Body Water Is the Sum of the Intracellular and Extracellular Fluid Volumes

Total body water (TBW) is approximately 60% of total body weight in a young adult human male, approximately 50% of total body weight in a young adult human female (Table 3–1), and 65% to 75% of total body weight in an infant. TBW accounts for a lower percentage of weight in females because they typically have more adipose tissue, and fat cells have a lower water content than muscle. Even if gender and age are taken into consideration, the fraction of total body weight contributed by water is not constant for all individuals under all conditions. For example, variability in the amount of adipose tissue can influence the fraction. Because water represents such a large fraction of body weight, acute changes in TBW can be detected simply by monitoring body weight.

The anatomy of the body fluid compartments is illustrated in Figure 3–1. The prototypic 70-kg male has approximately 42 liters of TBW (60% of 70 kg). Of these 42 liters, approximately 60% (~25 liters) is intracellular and 40% (~17 liters) is extracellular. *Extracellular fluid* is composed of blood plasma, interstitial fluid, and transcellular fluid.

PLASMA VOLUME. Of the approximately 17 liters of ECF, only approximately 20% (~3 liters) is contained within the cardiac chambers and blood vessels, that is, within the intravascular compartment. The *total* volume of this intravascular compartment is the **blood volume**, approximately 5.5 liters. The extracellular 3 liters of the blood volume is the plasma volume.

TABLE 3–1

APPROXIMATE WATER DISTRIBUTION IN ADULT HUMANS*

	MEN	TYPICAL VOLUME (liters)	WOMEN	TYPICAL VOLUME (liters)
Total-body water (TBW)	60% of BW	42	50% of BW	35
Intracellular fluid (ICF)	60% of TBW	25	60% of TBW	21
Extracellular fluid (ECF)	40% of TBW	17	40% of TBW	14
Interstitial fluid	75% of ECF	13	75% of ECF	10
Plasma (PV)	20% of ECF	3	20% of ECF	3
Blood (BV)	PV/(1 − Hct)	5.5	PV/(1 − Hct)	5
Transcellular fluid	5% of ECF	1	5% of ECF	1

*Assuming a body weight (BW) of 70 kg for both sexes, a hematocrit (Hct) for men of 45%, and an Hct for women of 40%.

The balance, approximately 2.5 liters, consists of the cellular elements of blood: erythrocytes, leukocytes, and platelets. The fraction of blood volume that is occupied by these cells is called the **hematocrit**. The hematocrit is determined by centrifuging blood that is treated with an anticoagulant and measuring the fraction of the total volume that is occupied by the packed cells.

INTERSTITIAL FLUID. About 75% (~13 liters) of the ECF is located outside the intravascular compartment, where it bathes the nonblood cells of the body. Within this interstitial fluid are two smaller compartments that communicate only slowly with the bulk of the interstitial fluid: dense connective tissue, such as cartilage and tendons, and bone matrix.

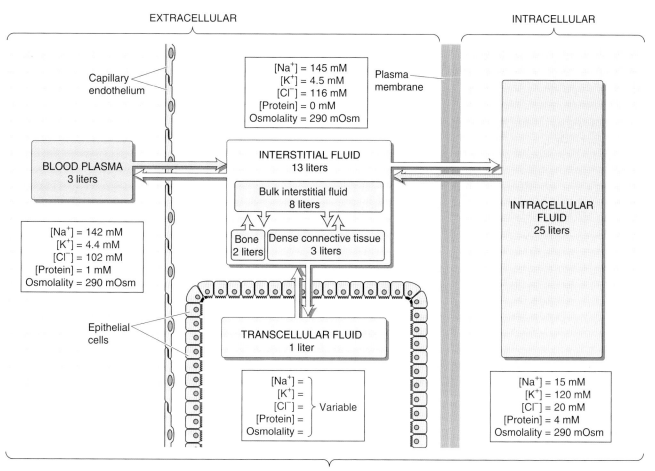

FIGURE 3–1. The fluid compartments of a prototypical adult human weighing 70 kg. Total body water is divided into four major compartments: intracellular fluid (*green*), interstitial fluid (*blue*), blood plasma (*red*), and transcellular water such as synovial fluid (*"sand" color*). Color codes for each of these compartments are maintained throughout this book.

TABLE 3-2

APPROXIMATE SOLUTE COMPOSITION OF KEY FLUID COMPARTMENTS

SOLUTE	PLASMA	PROTEIN-FREE PLASMA	INTERSTITIUM	CELL
Na^+ (mM)	142	153	145	15
K^+ (mM)	4.4	4.7	4.5	120
Ca^{2+} (mM)	1.2 (ionized)	1.3 (ionized)	1.2 (ionized)	0.0001 (ionized)
	2.5 (total)*			
Mg^{2+} (mM)	0.6 (ionized)	0.6 (ionized)	0.55 (ionized)	1 (ionized)
	0.9 (total)*			18 (total)
Cl^- (mM)	102	110	116	20
HCO_3^- (mM)	22†	24	25	15
$H_2PO_4^-$ and HPO_4^{2-} (mM)	0.7 (ionized)	0.75 (ionized)	0.8 (ionized)	0.7 (free)
	1.4 (total)‡			
Proteins	7 g/dl	—	1 g/dl	30 g/dl
	1 mmole/liter			
	14 meq/liter			
Glucose (mM)	5.5	5.9	5.9	Very low
pH	7.4	7.4	7.4	~7.2
Osmolality (mosmole/kg H_2O)	291	290	290	290

* Total includes amounts ionized, complexed to small solutes, and protein-bound.
† Arterial value. The value in mixed-venous blood would be approximately 24 mM.
‡ As discussed in Chapter 51, levels of total plasma inorganic phosphate are not tightly regulated and vary between 0.8 and 1.5 mM.

The barriers that separate the intravascular and interstitial compartments are the walls of **capillaries.** Water and solutes can move between the interstitium and blood plasma by crossing capillary walls, and between the interstitium and cytoplasm by crossing cell membranes.

TRANSCELLULAR FLUID. Finally, approximately 5% (~1 liter) of ECF is trapped within spaces that are completely surrounded by epithelial cells. This transcellular fluid includes the synovial fluid within joints and the cerebrospinal fluid surrounding the brain and spinal cord. Transcellular fluid does *not* include fluids that are, strictly speaking, outside the body, such as the contents of the gastrointestinal (GI) tract or urinary bladder.

The Intracellular Fluid Is Rich in K^+, Whereas the Extracellular Fluid Is Rich in Na^+ and Cl^-

Not only do the various body fluid compartments have very different volumes, they also have radically different compositions, as summarized in Figure 3–1. Table 3–2 is a more exhaustive listing of these values. *Intracellular fluid* is high in K^+ and low in Na^+ and Cl^-; *extracellular fluids* (interstitial and plasma) are high in Na^+ and Cl^- and low in K^+. The cell maintains a relatively high K^+ concentration ($[K^+]_i$) and low Na^+ concentration ($[Na^+]_i$), not by making its membrane totally impermeable to these ions, but by using an Na-K pump to actively extrude Na^+ from the cell and actively transport K^+ into the cell.

The composition of transcellular fluids differs greatly both from each other and from plasma because they are secreted by different epithelia. The two major constituents of ECF, the plasma and interstitial fluid, have very similar composition as far as small solutes are concerned. For most cells, it is the composition of the interstitial fluid enveloping the cells that is the relevant parameter. The major difference between plasma and interstitial fluid is the absence of plasma proteins from the interstitium. These plasma proteins, which cannot equilibrate across the walls of most capillaries, are responsible for the usually slight difference in small-solute concentrations between plasma and interstitial fluid. Plasma proteins affect solute distribution because of the volume they occupy and the electrical charge they carry.

VOLUME OCCUPIED BY PLASMA PROTEINS. The proteins and, to a much lesser extent, the lipids in plasma ordinarily occupy approximately 7% of the total plasma volume. Clinical laboratories report the plasma composition of ions (e.g., Na^+, K^+) in units of milliequivalents (meq) per liter of plasma solution. However, for cells bathed by interstitial fluid, more meaningful units would be **milliequivalents per liter of protein-free plasma solution** because it is only the protein-free portion of plasma—and not the proteins dissolved in this water—that can equilibrate across the capillary wall. For example, we can obtain $[Na^+]$ in protein-free plasma (which clinicians call "plasma water") by dividing the laboratory value for plasma $[Na^+]$ by the plasma water content (usually 93%):

Equation 3–1

$$[Na^+]_{plasma\ water} = \frac{142\ meq/liter\ plasma}{0.93}$$

$$= 153\ meq/liter\ plasma\ water$$

Similarly, for Cl^-,

$$\text{Equation 3-2}$$

$$[Cl^-]_{\text{plasma water}} = \frac{102 \text{ meq/liter plasma}}{0.93}$$

$$= 110 \text{ meq/liter plasma water}$$

Table 3–2 lists solute concentrations in terms of both liters of *plasma* and liters of *plasma water*. If the plasma water fraction is less than 93% because of hyperproteinemia (high levels of protein in blood) or hyperlipemia (high levels of lipid in blood), the values that the clinical laboratory reports for electrolytes may appear abnormal even though the physiologically important concentration (solute concentration per liter of plasma water) is normal. For example, if a patient's plasma proteins and lipids occupy 20% of plasma volume and, consequently, plasma water is only 80% of plasma, a correction factor of 0.80 (rather than 0.93) should be used in Equation 3–1. If the clinical laboratory were to report a very low plasma $[Na^+]$ of 122 meq/liter plasma, the patient's $[Na^+]$ relevant to interstitial fluid would be 122/0.80 = 153 meq/liter plasma water, which is quite normal.

EFFECT OF PROTEIN CHARGE. For noncharged solutes such as glucose, the correction for protein and lipid volume is the only correction needed to predict interstitial concentrations from plasma concentrations. Because plasma proteins carry a net negative charge and because the capillary wall confines them to the plasma, they tend to retain cations in plasma. Thus, the **cation** concentration of the protein-free solution of the interstitium is lower by approximately 5%. Conversely, because these negatively charged plasma proteins repel anions, the **anion** concentration of the protein-free solution of the interstitium is higher by approximately 5%. We consider the basis for these 5% corrections in the discussion of the Gibbs-Donnan equilibrium (p. 73).

Thus, for a monovalent cation such as Na^+, the interstitial concentration is 95% of the $[Na^+]$ of the protein-free plasma water, the value from Equation 3–1:

$$\text{Equation 3-3}$$

$$[Na^+]_{\text{interstitium}} = 153 \text{ meq/liter plasma water} \times 0.95$$

$$= 145 \text{ meq/liter interstitial fluid}$$

For a monovalent anion such as Cl^-, the interstitial concentration is 105% of the $[Cl^-]$ of the protein-free water of plasma, a value already obtained in Equation 3–2:

$$\text{Equation 3-4}$$

$$[Cl^-]_{\text{interstitium}} = 110 \text{ meq/liter plasma water} \times 1.05$$

$$= 116 \text{ meq/liter interstitial fluid}$$

Thus, for cations (e.g., Na^+), the two corrections (0.95/0.93) nearly cancel each other. On the other hand, for anions (e.g., Cl^-), the two corrections (1.05/0.93) are cumulative and yield a total correction of approximately 13%.

All Body Fluids Have Approximately the Same Osmolality, and Each Fluid Has Equal Numbers of Positive and Negative Charges

OSMOLALITY. Despite the differences in solute composition among the intracellular, interstitial, and plasma compartments, they all have approximately the same osmolality. Osmolality describes the total concentration of all particles that are free in a solution. Thus, glucose contributes one particle, whereas fully dissociated NaCl contributes two. Particles bound to macromolecules do not contribute at all to osmolality. In all body fluid compartments, humans have an osmolality—expressed as the number of osmotically active particles per kilogram of water—of approximately 290 mosmoles/kg water (290 mOsm).

Plasma proteins contribute approximately 14 meq/liter (Table 3–2). However, because these proteins usually have many negative charges per molecule, not many particles (~1 mM) are necessary to account for these milliequivalents. Moreover, even though the protein concentration—measured in terms of grams per liter—may be high, the high molecular weight of the average protein means that the protein concentration—measured in terms of moles per liter—is very low. Thus, proteins actually contribute only slightly to the total number of osmotically active particles (~1 mOsm).

Summing the *total* concentrations of all the solutes in the cells and interstitial fluid (including metabolites not listed in Table 3–2), we would see that the *total* solute concentration of the intracellular compartment is higher than that of the interstitium. Because the flow of water across cell membranes is governed by differences in osmolality across the membrane, and because the net flow is normally zero, intracellular and extracellular osmolality must be the same. How, then, do we make sense of this discrepancy? For some ions, a considerable fraction of their total intracellular store is bound to cellular proteins or complexed to other small solutes. In addition, some of the proteins are themselves attached to other materials that are out of solution. In computing osmolality, we count each particle once, whether it is a free ion, a complex of two ions, or several ions bound to a protein. For example, most of the intracellular Mg^{2+} and phosphate and virtually all the Ca^{2+} are either complexed or bound. Some of the electrolytes in blood plasma are also bound to plasma proteins; however, the bound fraction is generally much lower than the fraction in the cytosol.

ELECTRONEUTRALITY. All solutions must respect the principle of bulk electroneutrality: the number of positive charges in the overall solution must be the same as the number of negative charges. If we add up the major cations and anions in the cytosol (Table 3–2), we see that the sum of $[Na^+]_i$ and $[K^+]_i$ greatly exceeds the sum of $[Cl^-]_i$ and $[HCO_3^-]_i$. The excess positive charge reflected by this difference is balanced by the negative charge on intracellular macromolecules (e.g., proteins), as well as smaller anions such as organic phosphates.

There is a similar difference between major cations and anions in blood plasma, where it is often referred to as the **anion gap**. The clinical definition of anion gap is:

Equation 3–5

$$\text{Anion gap}_{plasma} = [Na^+]_{plasma}$$
$$- ([Cl^-]_{plasma} + [HCO_3^-]_{plasma})$$

Note that plasma $[K^+]$ is ignored. The anion gap, usually 9–14 meq/liters, is the difference between ignored anions and ignored cations. Among the ignored anions are anionic proteins, as well as small anionic metabolites. Levels of anionic metabolites, such as acetoacetate and β-hydroxybutyrate, can become extremely high, for example, in type 1 diabetic patients with very low levels of insulin. Thus, the anion gap increases under these conditions.

The differences in ionic composition between the ICF and ECF compartments are extremely important for normal functioning of the body. For example, because the K^+ gradient across cell membranes is a major determinant of electrical excitability, clinical disorders of extracellular $[K^+]$ can cause life-threatening disturbances in the heart rhythm. Disorders of extracellular $[Na^+]$ cause abnormal extracellular osmolality, with water being shifted into or out of brain cells; if uncorrected, such disorders lead to seizures, coma, or death.

These examples of clinical disorders emphasize the absolute necessity of understanding the processes that control the volume and composition of the body fluid compartments. These processes are the ones that move water and solutes between the compartments and between the body and the outside world.

TRANSPORT OF SOLUTES AND WATER ACROSS CELL MEMBRANES

In Passive, Noncoupled Transport Across a Permeable Membrane, a Solute Moves Down Its Electrochemical Gradient

We are all familiar with the way that water can flow from one side of a dike to another, provided that the water levels between the two sides of the dike are different and the water has an open pathway (a breach in the dike) to move from one side to the other. In much the same way, a substance can passively move across a membrane that separates two compartments when there is both a favorable driving force and an open pathway through which the driving force can exert its effect.

When a pathway exists for transfer of a substance across a membrane, the membrane is said to be **permeable** to that substance. The **driving force** that determines the passive transport of solutes across a membrane is the **electrochemical gradient** or electrochemical potential difference acting on the solute between the two compartments. This **electrochemical potential difference** includes a contribution from the concentration gradient for the solute (the chemical potential difference) and, for charged solutes (e.g., Na^+, Cl^-), a contribution from any difference in electrical potential that exists between the two compartments (the electrical potential difference).

This concept of how force and pathway determine passive movement of solutes is most easily illustrated by the example of passive, noncoupled transport. **Noncoupled**

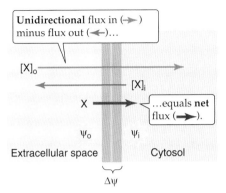

FIGURE 3–2. Uncoupled transport of a solute across a cell membrane. The net passive movement of a solute (X) depends on both the difference in concentrations between the inside of the cell ($[X]_i$) and the outside of the cell ($[X]_o$) and the difference in electrical potential between the inside of the cell (Ψ_i) and the outside of the cell (Ψ_o).

transport of a substance X means that movement of X across the membrane is not directly coupled to the movement of any other solute or to any chemical reaction (e.g., the hydrolysis of adenosine triphosphate [ATP]). What, then, are the driving forces for the net movement of X? Clearly, if the concentration of X is higher in the outside compartment ($[X]_o$) than the inside compartment ($[X]_i$), and assuming no voltage difference, the concentration gradient will act as the driving force to bring about the net movement of X across the membrane from outside to inside (Fig. 3–2). If $[X]$ is the same on both sides but there is an electrical potential difference across the membrane—that is, the electrical potential on the outside (Ψ_o) is not the same as on the inside (Ψ_i)—this electrical potential difference will also drive the net movement of X, provided that X is charged. The concentration gradient for X and the electrical potential difference across the membrane are the two determinants of the electrochemical potential difference for X between the two compartments. Because the movement of X by such a noncoupled mechanism is not directly coupled to the movement of other solutes or to any chemical reactions, the electrochemical gradient for X is the only driving force that contributes to the transport of X. Thus, the transport of X by a noncoupled, passive mechanism must always proceed "downhill"—in the direction down the electrochemical potential difference for X.

Regardless of *how* X moves passively through the membrane—whether X moves through lipid or through a membrane protein—the direction of the overall driving force acting on X determines the direction of net transport. In the example in Figure 3–2, the overall driving force favors net transport from outside to inside (influx). However, X may still move from inside to outside (efflux). Movement of X across the membrane in one direction or the other is known as **unidirectional flux**. The algebraic sum of the two unidirectional fluxes is the **net flux**, or the net transport rate. Net transport occurs only when the unidirectional fluxes are unequal. In Figure 3–2, the overall driving force makes unidirectional influx greater than unidirectional efflux, resulting in net influx.

When no net driving force is acting on X, we say that X is at **equilibrium** across the membrane and there is no net transport of X across the membrane. However, even when X is in equilibrium, there may be and usually are equal and opposite movements of X across the membrane. Net transport takes place only when the net driving force acting on X is displaced from the equilibrium point, and transport proceeds in the direction that would bring X back to equilibrium.

Equilibrium is actually a special case of a **steady state**. In a steady state, by definition, the conditions related to X do not change with time. Thus, a transport system is in a steady state when both the driving forces acting on it and the rate of transport are constant with time. Equilibrium is the particular steady state in which there is no net driving force and thus no net transport.

How can a steady state persist when X is not in equilibrium? Returning to the dike analogy, the downhill flow of water can be constant only if some device, such as a pump, keeps the water levels constant on both sides of the dike. A cell can maintain a nonequilibrium steady state for X only when some device, such as a mechanism for actively transporting X, can compensate for the passive movement of X and prevent the intracellular and extracellular concentrations of X from changing with time. This combination of a pump and a leak maintains both the concentrations of X and the passive flux of X.

At Equilibrium, the Chemical and Electrical Potential Differences Across the Membrane Are Equal, but Opposite

As noted in the previous section, the driving force for the passive, uncoupled transport of a solute is the electrochemical potential (i.e., energy) difference for that solute across the membrane that separates the inside (i) from the outside (o). We define the electrochemical potential difference as

Equation 3–6

$$\Delta \bar{\mu}_X \quad = \quad RT\,ln\,\frac{[X]_i}{[X]_o} \quad + \quad z_X\,F(\Psi_i - \Psi_o)$$

Electrochemical energy difference = Chemical energy difference + Electrical energy difference

where z_X is the valence of X, T is absolute temperature, R is the gas constant, and F is Faraday's constant. The first term on the right-hand side of Equation 3–6, the difference in chemical energy, describes the energy (joules/mole) change as X moves across the membrane if we disregard the charge—if any—on X. The second term, the difference in electrical energy, describes the energy change as a mole of charged particles (each with a valence of z_X) moves across the membrane. The difference $(\Psi_i - \Psi_o)$ is the voltage difference across the membrane, also known as the **membrane potential difference** (V_m).

By definition, X is at equilibrium when the electrochemical potential difference for X across the membrane is zero:

Equation 3–7

$$\Delta \bar{\mu}_X = 0$$

Thus, $\Delta \bar{\mu}_X$ is the *net driving force*. When $\Delta \bar{\mu}_X$ is *not* zero, X is *not* in equilibrium and will obviously tend to either enter the cell or leave the cell, provided that a pathway exists for X to cross the membrane.

It is worthwhile to consider two special cases of the equilibrium state (Equation 3–7). First, when either the chemical or the electrical term in Equation 3–6 is zero, the other must also be zero. For example, when X is uncharged ($z_X = 0$), as in the case of glucose, equilibrium can occur only when [X] is equal on the two sides of the membrane. Alternatively, when X is charged, as in the case of Na^+, but the electrical potential difference and thus V_m is zero, equilibrium likewise can occur only when [X] is equal on the two sides of the membrane. Second, when neither the chemical nor the electrical term in Equation 3–6 is zero, equilibrium can occur only when the two terms are equal, but of opposite sign. Thus, if we set $\Delta \bar{\mu}_X$ in Equation 3–6 to zero, as necessary for a state of equilibrium,

Equation 3–8

$$0 = RT\,ln\,\frac{[X]_i}{[X]_o} + z_X F V_m$$

$$-\frac{RT}{z_X F}\,ln\,\frac{[X]_i}{[X]_o} = V_m$$

$$V_m = E_X = -\frac{RT}{z_X F}\,ln\,\frac{[X]_i}{[X]_o}$$

This relationship is the **Nernst equation**, which describes the conditions when an ion is in equilibrium across a membrane. Given values for $[X]_i$ and $[X]_o$, X can be in equilibrium only when the voltage difference across the membrane equals the **equilibrium potential** (E_X), also known as the Nernst potential. Stated somewhat differently, E_X is the value that the membrane potential *would have to have* for X to be in equilibrium. If we express the logarithm to the base 10, then for the special case in which the temperature is 29.5°C:

Equation 3–9

$$V_m = E_X = -\frac{60\ mV}{z_X}\,log_{10}\,\frac{[X]_i}{[X]_o}$$

At normal body temperature (37°C), the coefficient is approximately 61.5 mV instead of 60 mV. At 20°C, it is approximately 58.1 mV.

To illustrate the use of Equation 3–9 we will compute E_X for a monovalent cation, such as K^+. If $[K^+]_i$ were 100 mM and $[K^+]_o$ were 10 mM, a 10-fold concentration gradient, then

Equation 3–10

$$E_K = -\frac{60\ mV}{1}\,log_{10}\,\frac{100}{10} = -60\ mV$$

Thus, a 10-fold gradient of a monovalent ion such as K^+ is equivalent, as a driving force, to an electrical potential difference of 60 mV. For a divalent ion such as Ca^{2+}, a 10-fold concentration gradient can be balanced as a driving force by an electrical potential difference of 60 mV/2, or only 30 mV.

In Simple Diffusion, the Flux of an Uncharged Substance Through Membrane Lipid Is Directly Proportional to its Concentration Difference

The difference in electrochemical potential of a solute X across the membrane is a useful parameter because it allows us to predict whether X is in equilibrium across the cell membrane (i.e., Is $\Delta\bar{\mu}_X = 0$?) or, if not, whether X would tend to passively move into the cell or out of the cell. As long as the movement of X is not coupled to the movement of another substance or to some biochemical reaction, the only factor that determines the direction of net transport is the driving force $\Delta\bar{\mu}_X$. The ability to predict the movement of X is independent of any detailed knowledge of the actual transport pathway mediating its passive transport. In other words, we can understand the overall *energetics* of X transport without knowing anything about the transport mechanism itself, other than knowing that it is passive.

So far, we have discussed only the *direction* of net transport, not the *rate*. How will the rate of X transport vary if we vary the driving force $\Delta\bar{\mu}_X$? Unlike the issue of direction, determining the rate—that is, the **kinetics**—of transport requires knowing the peculiarities of the actual mechanism that mediates passive X transport.

Most transport systems are so complicated that a straightforward relationship between transport rate and $\Delta\bar{\mu}_X$ may not exist. Here we will examine the simplest case, which is **simple diffusion.** How fast does an uncharged, hydrophobic solute move through a lipid bilayer? Gases (e.g., CO_2), a few endogenous compounds (e.g., steroid hormones), and many drugs (e.g., anesthetics) are both uncharged and hydrophobic. Imagine that such a solute is present on both sides of the membrane, but at a higher concentration on the outside (Fig. 3–2). Because X has no electrical charge and because $[X]_o$ is greater than $[X]_i$, the net movement of X will be *into* the cell. How *fast* X moves is described by its **flux** (J_X), namely, the number of moles of X crossing a unit area of membrane (typically 1 cm^2) per unit time (typically 1 second). Thus J_X has the units moles/($cm^2 \cdot s$). The better that X can dissolve in the membrane lipid (i.e., the higher the lipid water **partition coefficient** of X), the more easily X will be able to traverse the membrane-lipid barrier. The flux of X will also be greater if X moves more readily once it is in the membrane (i.e., a higher **diffusion coefficient**) and if the distance that it must traverse is short (i.e., a smaller **membrane thickness**). We can combine these three factors into a single parameter called the **permeability coefficient** of X (P_X). Finally, the flux of X will be greater as the difference in [X] between the two sides of the membrane increases (a large **gradient**).

These concepts governing the simple diffusion of an electrically neutral substance were quantified by Adolf Fick in the 1800s and applied by others to the special case of a cell membrane. They are embodied in the fol-

lowing equation, which is a simplified version of **Fick's Law:**

Equation 3–11

$$J_X = P_X([X]_o - [X]_i)$$

As already illustrated in Figure 3–2, we can separate the *net* flux of X into a *unidirectional influx* ($J_X^{o \rightarrow i}$) and a *unidirectional efflux* ($J_X^{i \rightarrow o}$). The net flux of X into the cell is simply the difference between the unidirectional fluxes:

Equation 3–12

Unidirectional influx:	$J_X^{o \rightarrow i} = P_X[X]_o$
Unidirectional efflux:	$J_X^{i \rightarrow o} = P_X[X]_i$
Net flux:	$J_X = P_X([X]_o - [X]_i)$

Thus, unidirectional influx is proportional to the outside concentration, unidirectional efflux is proportional to the inside concentration, and net flux is proportional to the concentration *difference* (not the *ratio* $[X]_o/[X]_i$, but the *difference* $[X]_o - [X]_i$). In all cases, the proportionality constant is P_X.

A description of the *kinetic* behavior of a transport system (Equation 3–12)—that is, how fast things move—cannot violate the laws of *energetics*, or thermodynamics (Equation 3–6)—that is, the direction in which things move to restore equilibrium. For example, the laws of thermodynamics (Equation 3–6) predict that when the concentration gradient for a neutral substance is zero (i.e., when $[X]_o/[X]_i = 1$), the system is in equilibrium and therefore the net flux must be zero. The law of simple diffusion (Equation 3–12), which is a kinetic description, also predicts that when the concentration gradient for a neutral substance is zero (i.e., $[X]_o - [X]_i = 0$), the flux is zero.

Some Substances Cross the Membrane Passively Through Intrinsic-Membrane Proteins That Can Form Either Pores, Channels, or Carriers

Because most ions and hydrophilic solutes of biologic interest partition poorly into the lipid bilayer, simple passive diffusion of these solutes through the lipid portion of the membrane is negligible. Noncoupled transport across the plasma membrane generally requires specialized pathways that allow particular substances to cross the lipid bilayer. In all known cases, such pathways are formed from **integral membrane proteins**. Three types of protein pathways through the membrane are recognized:

1. The membrane protein forms a **pore** that is always open (Fig. 3–3A). Physiological examples are the porins in the outer membranes of mitochondria, cytotoxic pore-forming proteins such as the perforin released by lymphocytes, and perhaps the aquaporin water channels. A physical equivalent would be a straight, open tube. If you look though this tube, you always see light coming through from the opposite side.

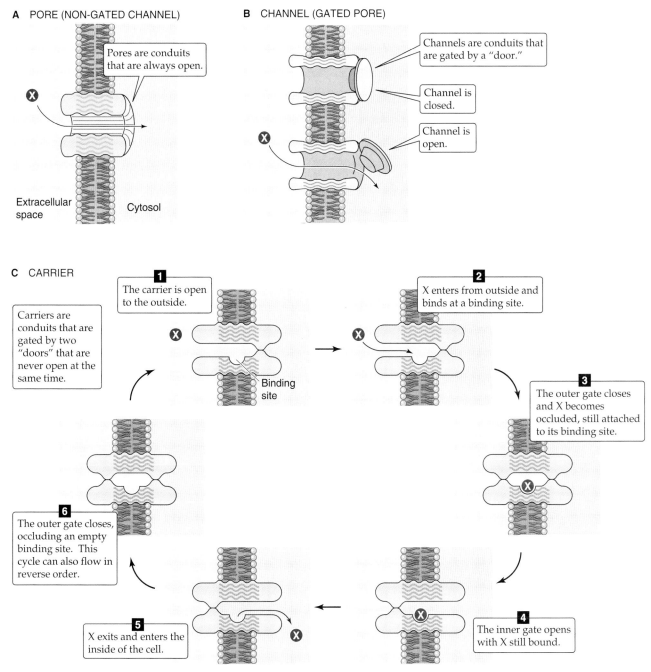

A PORE (NON-GATED CHANNEL)

Pores are conduits that are always open.

Extracellular space

Cytosol

B CHANNEL (GATED PORE)

Channels are conduits that are gated by a "door."

Channel is closed.

Channel is open.

C CARRIER

Carriers are conduits that are gated by two "doors" that are never open at the same time.

1 The carrier is open to the outside.

Binding site

2 X enters from outside and binds at a binding site.

3 The outer gate closes and X becomes occluded, still attached to its binding site.

4 The inner gate opens with X still bound.

5 X exits and enters the inside of the cell.

6 The outer gate closes, occluding an empty binding site. This cycle can also flow in reverse order.

FIGURE 3–3. Three types of passive, non-coupled transport through integral membrane proteins.

2. The membrane protein forms a **channel** that is alternately open and closed because it is equipped with a movable barrier or gate (Fig. 3–3B). Physiological examples include virtually all ion channels, such as the ones that allow Na^+, Cl^-, K^+, and Ca^{2+} to cross the membrane. The process of opening and closing of the barrier is referred to as **gating**. Thus, a channel is a gated pore, and a pore is a nongated channel. A physical equivalent would be a tube with a shutter near one end. As you look through this tube, you see the light flickering as the shutter opens and closes.

3. The membrane protein forms a **carrier** surrounding a conduit that never offers a continuous transmembrane path because it is equipped with at least two gates that are never open at the same time (Fig. 3–3C). Between the two gates is a compartment that can contain one or more binding sites for the solute. If the two gates are both closed, one (or more) of the transiting particles is trapped, or **occluded**, in that compartment. Physiological examples include carriers that move single solutes through the membrane by a process known as facilitated diffusion, which is discussed in the next section. A physical equivalent would be a tube with shutters at both ends. As you look through this tube,

FIGURE 3–4. Structure of the PhoE porin of *Escherichia coli*. *A,* Top view of a porin trimer that shows the backbones of the polypeptide chains. Each of the three identical monomers, which are shown in different colors, contains 330 amino acids. The center of each monomer is a pore. *B,* Side view of a porin trimer. The extracellular surface is shown at the top. Each monomer consists of a "β barrel" with 16 antiparallel β sheets (i.e., adjacent polypeptide strands are oriented in opposite directions) surrounding a large cavity that, at its narrowest point, has an oval cross sectin (internal diameter, 0.7 × 1.1 nm). The images are based on high-resolution electron microscopy, at a resolution of 3.5 Å (0.35 nm). (Reproduced from Jap BK, Walian PJ: Structure and functional mechanisms of porins. Physiol Rev 76:1073–1088, 1996.)

you never see any light passing through because both shutters are never open simultaneously.

Water-Filled Pores Can Allow Molecules, Some as Large as 45 kDa, to Cross Membranes Passively

As discussed, some membrane proteins form **pores** that provide an aqueous transmembrane conduit that is always open (Fig. 3–3A). Among the large-size pores are the

porins (Fig. 3–4) found in the outer membranes of gram-negative bacteria and mitochondria. Mitochondrial porin allows solutes as large as 5 kDa to diffuse passively from the cytosol into the mitochondria's intermembrane space.

One mechanism by which cytotoxic T lymphocytes kill their target cells is by releasing monomers of a pore-forming protein known as **perforin**. Perforin monomers polymerize within the target cell membrane and assemble like staves of a barrel to form large, doughnut-like channels with an internal diameter of 16 nm. The passive flow of ions, water, and other small molecules through these pores kills the target cell. A similar pore plays a crucial role in the defense against bacterial infections. The binding of antibodies to an invading bacterium ("classic" pathway), or simply the presence of native polysaccharides on bacteria ("alternative" pathway), triggers a cascade of reactions known as the **complement cascade**. This cascade culminates in the formation of a doughnut-like structure with an internal diameter of 10 nm. This pore is made up of monomers of C9, the final component of the complement cascade.

The **nuclear-pore complex** (NPC), which regulates traffic into and out of the nucleus (p. 22), is remarkably large. The NPC is made up of at least 30 different proteins and has a molecular mass of 10^8 Da and an outer diameter of approximately 100 nm. It can transport huge molecules (approaching 10^6 Da) in a complicated process that involves ATP hydrolysis. In addition to this active component of transport, the NPC also has a passive component. Contained within the massive NPC is a simple aqueous pore with an internal diameter of approximately 9 nm that allows molecules smaller than 45 kDa to move between the cytoplasm and nucleus, but almost completely restricts the movement of globular proteins that are larger than approximately 60 kDa.

The plasma membranes of many types of cells have proteins that form channels that are just large enough to allow water molecules to pass through. The first water channel to be studied was **aquaporin** 1 (AQP1), 28-kDa protein. AQP1 belongs to a larger family of aquaporins that has representatives in organisms as diverse as bacteria, plants, and animals. In mammals, the various aquaporin isoforms have different tissue distributions, different mechanisms of regulation, and varying abilities to transport small neutral molecules other than water. In the lipid bilayer, AQP1 (Fig. 3–5) exists as tetramers. Each monomer consists of six membrane-spanning helices as well as two shorter helices that dip into the plane of the membrane. These structures form a permeation pathway for the single-file diffusion of water. Peter Agre shared the 2003 Nobel Prize in Chemistry for his discovery of the aquaporins.

Gated Channels, Which Alternately Open and Close, Allow Ions to Cross the Membrane Passively

Gated **ion channels**, like the aquaporins just discussed, consist of one or more polypeptide subunits with α helical membrane-spanning segments. These channels have several functional components (see Fig. 3–3B). The first

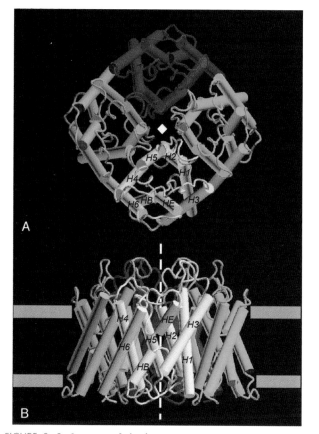

FIGURE 3–5. Structure of the human AQP1 water channel. *A,* Top view of an aquaporin tetramer. Each of the four identical monomers is made up of 269 amino acids and has a pore at its center. *B,* Side view of aquaporin. The extracellular surface is shown at the top. The images are based on high-resolution electron microscopy at a resolution of 3.8 Å (0.38 nm). (Reproduced from Murata K, Mitsuoka K, Hirai T, et al: Structural determinants of water permeation through aquaporin-1. Nature 407:599–605, 2000. Copyright 2000 Macmillan Magazines Limited.)

is a **gate** that determines whether the channel is open or closed, each state reflecting a different conformation of the membrane protein. Second, the channel generally has one or more **sensors** that can respond to one of several different types of signals: (1) changes in membrane potential, (2) second messenger systems that act at the cytoplasmic face of the membrane protein, or (3) ligands, such as neurohumoral agonists, that bind to the extracellular face of the membrane protein. These signals regulate transitions between the open and closed states. A third functional component is a **selectivity filter**, which determines the *classes* of ions (e.g., anions or cations) or the *particular* ions (e.g., Na^+, K^+, Ca^{2+}) that have access to the channel pore. The fourth component is the actual **open-channel pore** (see Fig. 3–3*B*). Each time that a channel assumes the open conformation, it provides a continuous pathway between the two sides of the membrane so that ions can flow through it passively by diffusion until the channel closes again. During each channel opening, many ions flow through the channel pore, usually a sufficient number to be detected as a small current by sensitive "patch-clamping" techniques (p. 159).

Na⁺ CHANNELS. Because the electrochemical potential difference for Na^+ ($\Delta\bar{\mu}_{Na}$) is always strongly *negative*, a large, inwardly directed net driving force or gradient favors the passive movement of Na^+ into virtually every cell of the body. Therefore, an open Na^+ channel will act as a conduit for the passive entry of Na^+. One physiological use for channel-mediated Na^+ entry is the transmission of information. Thus, voltage-gated Na^+ channels are responsible for generating the action potential (e.g., "nerve impulse") in many excitable cells. Another physiological use of Na^+ channels can be found in epithelial cells such as those in certain segments of the renal tubule and intestine. In this case, ENaC Na^+ channels are largely restricted to the apical surface of the cell, where they allow Na^+ to enter the epithelial cell from the renal tubule lumen or intestinal lumen. This passive influx is a key step in the movement of Na^+ across the entire epithelium, from lumen to blood.

K⁺ CHANNELS. The electrochemical potential difference for K^+ ($\Delta\bar{\mu}_{K}$) is usually fairly close to zero or somewhat *positive*, so K^+ is either at equilibrium or tends to move *out* of the cell. In virtually all cells, K^+ channels play a major role in generating a resting membrane potential that is inside-negative. Other kinds of K^+ channels play a key role in excitable cells, where these channels help terminate action potentials.

Ca²⁺ CHANNELS. The electrochemical potential difference for Ca^{2+} ($\Delta\bar{\mu}_{Ca}$) is always strongly *negative*, so Ca^{2+} tends to move *into* the cell. When Ca^{2+} channels are open, Ca^{2+} rapidly enters the cell down a steep electrochemical gradient. This inward movement of Ca^{2+} plays a vital role in transmembrane signalling for both excitable and nonexcitable cells, as well as in generating action potentials in some excitable cells.

ANION CHANNELS. Most cells contain one or more types of anion-selective channels through which the passive, noncoupled transport of Cl^-—and, to a lesser extent, HCO_3^-—can take place. The electrochemical potential difference for Cl^- ($\Delta\bar{\mu}_{Cl}$) in most cells is modestly *positive*, so Cl^- tends to move *out of* these cells. In certain epithelial cells with Cl^- channels on their basolateral membranes, the passive movement of Cl^- through these channels plays a role in the transepithelial movement of Cl^- from lumen to blood.

Some Carriers Facilitate the Passive Diffusion of Small Solutes Such as Glucose

Carrier-mediated transport systems transfer a broad range of ions and organic solutes across the plasma membrane. Each carrier protein has a specific affinity for binding one or a small number of solutes, and transporting them across the bilayer. Later, we will introduce *cotransporters* (which carry two or more solutes in the same direction) and *exchangers* (which move them in opposite directions). The simplest carrier-mediated transporter is one that mediates *facilitated diffusion.*

Carrier-mediated transport systems behave according to a general kinetic scheme for facilitated diffusion that is outlined in Figure 3–3*C*. This model illustrates how, in a cycle of six steps, a carrier could passively move a solute X into the cell.

A SIMPLE DIFFUSION   **B** CARRIER-MEDIATED OR
                              FACILITATED DIFFUSION

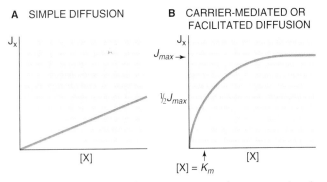

FIGURE 3–6. Dependence of transport rates on solute concentration. *A*, The net flux of the solute X through the cell menbrane is J_X. *B*, The maximal flux of X (J_{max}) occurs when the carriers are saturated. The flux is half of its maximal value ($\frac{1}{2}J_{max}$) when the concentration of X is equal to the K_m.

This mechanism can mediate only the downhill, or passive, transport of X. Therefore, it mediates a type of diffusion called **facilitated diffusion**. When [X] is equal on the two sides of the membrane, no *net* transport will take place, although equal and opposite *unidirectional* fluxes of X may still occur.

In a cell membrane, a fixed number of carriers is available to transport X. Furthermore, each carrier has a limited speed with which it can cycle through the steps illustrated in Figure 3–3C. Thus, if the extracellular X concentration is gradually increased, for example, the influx of X will eventually reach a maximal value once all the carriers have become loaded with X. This situation is very different from the one that exists with simple diffusion, that is, the movement of a solute through the lipid phase of the membrane. Influx by simple diffusion increases linearly with increases in $[X]_o$, with no maximal rate of transport. As an example, if X is initially absent on *both* sides of the membrane and we gradually increase [X] on *one* side, the net flux of X (J_X) is described by a straight line that passes through the origin (Fig. 3–6A). However, with carrier-mediated transport, J_X reaches a maximum (J_{max}) when [X] is high enough to occupy all the carriers in the membrane (Fig. 3–6B). Thus the relationship describing carrier-mediated transport follows the same Michaelis-Menten kinetics as enzymes:

Equation 3–13

$$V = \frac{[S]\,V_{max}}{K_m + [S]}$$

This equation describes how the velocity of an enzymatic reaction (V) depends on the substrate concentration ([S]), the Michaelis constant (K_m), and the maximal velocity (V_{max}). The comparable equation for carrier-mediated transport is identical, except that fluxes replace reaction velocities:

Equation 3–14

$$J_X = \frac{[X]\,J_{max}}{K_m + [X]}$$

Thus, K_m is the solute concentration at which J_X is half

of the maximal flux (J_{max}). The lower the K_m, the higher the apparent **affinity** of the transporter for the solute.

Historically, the name "carrier" suggested that carrier-mediated transport occurs as the solute binds to a miniature ferryboat that shuttles back and forth across the membrane. Small polypeptides that act as shuttling carriers exist in nature, as exemplified by the antibiotic valinomycin. Such "ion carriers," or **ionophores**, bind to an ion on one side of the membrane, diffuse across the lipid phase of the membrane, and release the ion on the opposite side of the membrane. Valinomycin is a K^+ ionophore that certain bacteria produce to achieve a selective advantage over their neighbors. However, none of the known carrier-mediated transport pathways in animal cell membranes are ferries.

An example of a membrane protein that mediates facilitated diffusion is the glucose transporter **GLUT1** (Fig. 3–7). This membrane protein has 12 membrane-spanning segments, as well as multiple hydrophilic polypeptide loops facing either the ECF or ICF. It could not possibly act as a ferryboat shuttling back and forth across the membrane. Instead, some of the membrane-spanning segments of carrier-mediated transport proteins most likely form a permeation pathway through the lipid bilayer, as illustrated by the amphipathic membrane-spanning segments 7, 8, and 11 in Figure 3–7. These membrane-spanning segments, as well as other portions of the protein, probably also act as the gates and solute-binding sites that allow transport to proceed in the manner outlined in Figure 3–3C.

Molecular cloning studies have revealed that a given carrier-mediated transporter often has several variants or isoforms with a relatively high amino acid sequence similarity among the isoforms. Variants of a transporter may differ in kinetic properties (e.g., affinity for solute), regulation (e.g., phosphorylation), sites of membrane targeting (e.g., plasma membrane versus intracellular organelles), or tissues in which they are expressed (e.g., kidney versus

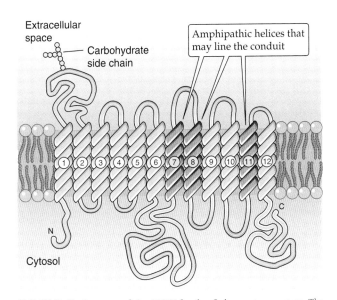

FIGURE 3–7. Structure of the GLUT family of glucose transporters. The 12 membrane-spanning segments are connected to each other by intracellular and extracellular loops.

TABLE 3–3

COMPARISON OF PROPERTIES OF PORES, CHANNELS, AND CARRIERS			
	PORES	**CHANNELS**	**CARRIERS**
Example	Water channel (AQP1)	Shaker K^+ channel	Glucose transporter (GLUT1)
Conduit through membrane	Always open	Intermittently open	Never open
Unitary event	None (continuously open)	Opening	Cycle of conformational changes
Particles translocated per "event"	—	6×10^4 *	1–5
Particles translocated per second	up to 2×10^9	10^6–10^8 when open	200–50,000

* Assuming a 100-pS channel, a driving force of 100 mV, and an opening time of 1 ms.

brain). For example, there are multiple structurally related isoforms of the GLUT family. Whereas GLUT1 is constitutively expressed on the cell surface, GLUT4 in the basal state is predominantly present in the membranes of intracellular vesicles, which represent a storage pool for the transporters. Because a solute such as glucose permeates the lipid bilayer so poorly, its uptake by the cell depends strictly on the activity of a carrier-mediated transport system for glucose. Insulin increases the rate of carrier-mediated glucose transport into certain cells by recruiting the GLUT4 isoform to the plasma membrane from the storage pool (p. 1078).

Two other examples of transporters that mediate facilitated diffusion are the UT (<u>u</u>rea <u>t</u>ransporter) family and the OCT (<u>o</u>rganic <u>c</u>ation <u>t</u>ransporter) family. Because OCT moves an electrical charge (i.e., carries current), it is said to be **electrogenic**.

The Physical Structure of Pores, Channels, and Carriers Is Quite Similar

Pores, ion channels, and carriers all have multiple transmembrane segments surrounding a solute-permeation pathway. Moreover, some channels also contain binding sites within their permeation pathways, so transport is saturable with respect to ion concentration. However, pores, channels, and carriers are fundamentally distinct kinetically (Table 3–3). *Pores*, such as the porins, are thought to be continuously open and allow vast numbers of particles to cross the membrane. No evidence suggests that pores have conformational states. *Channels* undergo conformational transitions between closed and open states. When they are open, they are open to both intracellular and extracellular solutions simultaneously. Thus, while the channel is open, it allows multiple ions, perhaps millions, to cross the membrane per "open" event. Because the length of time that a particular channel remains open varies from one "open" event to the next, the number of ions flowing through that channel per "open" event is not fixed. *Carriers* have a permeation pathway that is virtually never open simultaneously to both intracellular and extracellular solutions. Whereas the fundamental event for a channel is "opening," the fundamental event for a carrier is a complete cycle of conformational changes. Because the binding sites in a carrier are limited, each cycle of a carrier can transport only one or a *small, fixed* number of solute particles. Thus the number of particles per second that can move across the membrane

is generally several orders of magnitude lower for a single carrier than for a single channel.

We have seen how carriers can mediate facilitated diffusion of glucose, which is a passive or downhill process. However, carriers can also mediate **coupled** modes of transport. The remainder of this subchapter is devoted to these carriers, which act as pumps, cotransporters, and exchangers.

The Na-K Pump, the Most Important Primary Active Transporter in Animal Cells, Uses the Energy of ATP to Extrude Na^+ and Take Up K^+

Active transport is a process that can transfer a solute uphill across a membrane—that is, against its electrochemical potential difference. In **primary active transport**, the driving force needed to cause net transfer of a solute against its electrochemical gradient comes from the favorable energy change that is associated with an exergonic chemical reaction, such as ATP hydrolysis. In **secondary active transport**, the driving force is provided by coupling the *uphill* movement of that solute to the *downhill* movement of one or more other solutes for which a favorable electrochemical potential difference exists. A physical example would be to use a motor-driven winch to lift a large weight into the air (primary active transport) and then to transfer this large weight to a seesaw, on the other end of which is a lighter child. The potential energy stored in the elevated weight will then lift the child (secondary active transport). For transporters, it is commonly the favorable inwardly directed Na^+ electrochemical gradient, which itself is set up by a *primary* active transporter, that drives the *secondary* active transport of another solute. In this and the next section, we discuss primary active transporters, which are also referred to as **pumps**. The pumps discussed here are all energized by ATP hydrolysis and hence are **ATPases**.

As a prototypical example of a primary active transporter, consider the nearly ubiquitous **Na-K pump** (or Na,K-ATPase). This substance was the first enzyme recognized to be an ion pump, a discovery for which Jens Skou shared the 1997 Nobel Prize in Chemistry. The Na-K pump is located in the plasma membrane and has both α and β subunits (Fig. 3–8A). The α subunit, which has 10 transmembrane segments, is the catalytic subunit that mediates active transport. The β subunit, which has one transmembrane segment, is essential for proper assembly and membrane targeting of the Na-K

A   Na–K PUMP

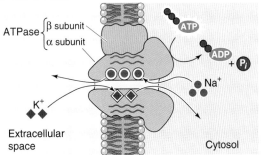

FIGURE 3–8. Model of the sodium pump. *A*, Schematic representation of the α and β subunits of the pump. *B*, The protein cycles through at least 8 identifiable stages as it moves 3 Na$^+$ out of the cell, and 2 K$^+$ into the cell. ADP, adenosine diphosphate. ATP, adenosine triphosphate; P$_i$, inorganic phosphate.

B   ENZYMATIC CYCLE OF THE Na–K PUMP

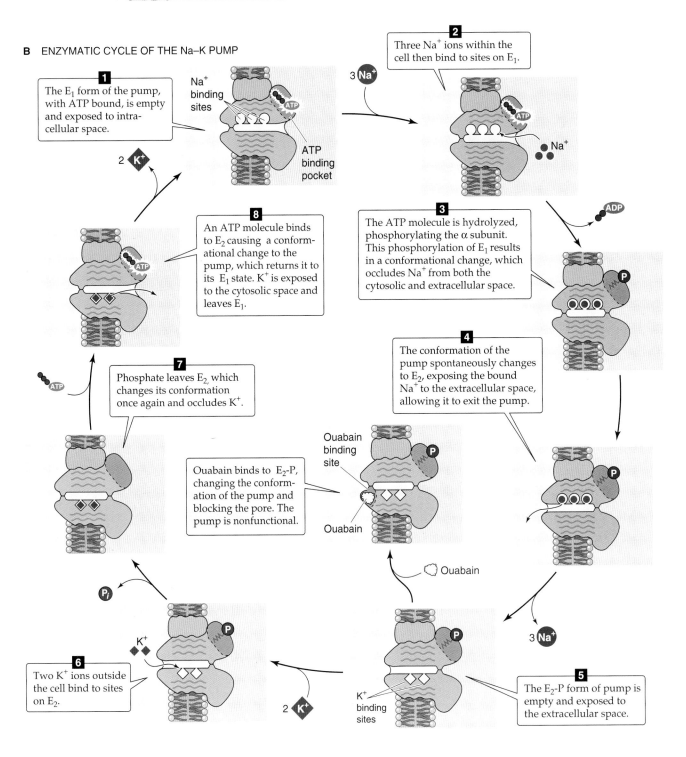

1 The E$_1$ form of the pump, with ATP bound, is empty and exposed to intracellular space.

2 Three Na$^+$ ions within the cell then bind to sites on E$_1$.

3 The ATP molecule is hydrolyzed, phosphorylating the α subunit. This phosphorylation of E$_1$ results in a conformational change, which occludes Na$^+$ from both the cytosolic and extracellular space.

4 The conformation of the pump spontaneously changes to E$_2$, exposing the bound Na$^+$ to the extracellular space, allowing it to exit the pump.

5 The E$_2$-P form of pump is empty and exposed to the extracellular space.

6 Two K$^+$ ions outside the cell bind to sites on E$_2$.

7 Phosphate leaves E$_2$, which changes its conformation once again and occludes K$^+$.

8 An ATP molecule binds to E$_2$ causing a conformational change to the pump, which returns it to its E$_1$ state. K$^+$ is exposed to the cytosolic space and leaves E$_1$.

Ouabain binds to E$_2$-P, changing the conformation of the pump and blocking the pore. The pump is nonfunctional.

pump. Four α isoforms and two β isoforms have been described. These isoforms have different tissue and developmental patterns of expression, as well as different kinetic properties.

With each forward cycle, the pump couples the extrusion of three Na^+ and the uptake of two K^+ to the intracellular hydrolysis of one ATP. By themselves, the transport steps of the Na-K pump are energetically uphill; that is, if the pump were not an ATPase, the transporter would run in reverse, with Na^+ leaking into the cell and K^+ leaking out. Indeed, under extreme experimental conditions, the Na-K pump can be reversed and forced to synthesize ATP! However, under physiological conditions, hydrolyzing one ATP molecule releases so much free energy—relative to the aggregate free energy needed to fuel the uphill movement of three Na^+ and two K^+—that the pump is poised far from its equilibrium and brings about the net active exchange of Na^+ for K^+ in the desired directions.

Although animal cells may have other pumps in their plasma membranes, the Na-K pump is the only primary active transport process for Na^+. The Na-K pump is also the most important primary active transport mechanism for K^+. In cells throughout the body, the Na-K pump is responsible for maintaining a low $[Na^+]_i$ and a high $[K^+]_i$ relative to ECF. In most epithelial cells, the Na-K pump is restricted to the basolateral side of the cell.

The Na-K pump exists in two major conformational states: E_1, in which the binding sites for the ions face the inside of the cell, and E_2, in which the binding sites face the outside. The Na-K pump is a member of a larger superfamily of pumps known as **E_1-E_2 ATPases** or **P-type ATPases**. It is the ordered cycling between these two states that underlies the action of the pump. Figure 3–8*B* is a simplified model showing the eight stages of this catalytic cycle of the α subunit:

Stage 1: **ATP-bound "$E_1 \cdot ATP$" state.** The cycle starts with the ATP-bound E_1 conformation, just after the pump has released its bound K^+ to the ICF. The Na^+-binding sites face the ICF and have high affinities for Na^+.

Stage 2: **Na^+-bound "$E_1 \cdot ATP \cdot 3Na^+$" state.** Three intracellular Na^+ ions bind.

Stage 3: **Occluded "E_1-P·($3Na^+$)" state.** The ATP previously bound to the pump phosphorylates the pump at an aspartate residue. Simultaneously, adenosine diphosphate (ADP) leaves. This phosphorylation triggers a minor conformational change in which the E_1 form of the pump now occludes the three bound Na^+ ions within the permeation pathway. In this state the Na^+ binding sites are inaccessible to both the ICF and ECF.

Stage 4: **Deoccluded "E_2-P · $3Na^+$" state.** A major conformational change shifts the pump from the E_1 to the E_2 conformation and has two effects. First, the pump becomes **deoccluded**, so that the Na^+-binding sites now communicate with the *extracellular* solution. Second, the Na^+ affinities of these binding sites decrease.

Stage 5: **Empty "E_2-P" state.** The three bound Na^+ ions dissociate into the external solution, and the protein undergoes a minor conformational change to the empty E_2-P form, which has high affinity for binding of extra-

cellular K^+. However, the pore still communicates with the extracellular solution.

Stage 6: **K^+-bound "E_2-P·$2K^+$" state.** Two K^+ ions bind to the pump.

Stage 7: **Occluded "$E_2 \cdot (2K^+)$" state.** Hydrolysis of the acylphosphate bond, which links the phosphate group to the aspartate residue, releases the inorganic phosphate into the intracellular solution and causes a minor conformational change. In this $E_2 \cdot (2K^+)$ state, the pump occludes the two bound K^+ ions within the permeation pathway so that the K^+-binding sites are inaccessible to both the ECF and ICF.

Stage 8: **Deoccluded "$E_1 \cdot ATP \cdot 2K^+$" state.** Binding of intracellular ATP causes a major conformational change that shifts the pump from the E_2 back to the E_1 state. This conformational change has two effects. First, the pump becomes **deoccluded**, so that the K^+-binding sites now communicate with the *intracellular* solution. Second, the K^+ affinities of these binding sites decrease.

Stage 1: **ATP-bound "$E_1 \cdot ATP$" state.** Dissociation of the two bound K^+ ion into the intracellular solution returns the pump to its original $E_1 \cdot ATP$ state, ready to begin another cycle.

Because each cycle of hydrolysis of one ATP is coupled to the extrusion of three Na^+ from the cell and the uptake of two K^+, the *stoichiometry* of the pump is three Na^+ to two K^+, and each cycle of the pump is associated with the net extrusion of one positive charge from the cell. Thus, the Na-K pump is *electrogenic*.

Just as glucose flux through the GLUT1 transporter is a saturable function of [glucose], the rate of active transport by the Na-K pump is a saturable function of $[Na^+]_i$ and $[K^+]_o$. The reason is that the number of pumps is finite and each must bind three Na^+ and two K^+. The transport rate is also a saturable function of $[ATP]_i$ and, therefore, depends on the metabolic state of the cell. In cells with high Na-K pump rates, such as renal proximal tubules, a third or more of cellular energy metabolism is devoted to supplying ATP to the Na-K pump.

A hallmark of the Na-K pump is that it is blocked by a class of compounds known as **cardiac glycosides**, examples of which are ouabain and digoxin, the latter widely used for a variety of cardiac conditions. These compounds have a high affinity for the extracellular side of the E_2-P state of the pump, which also has a high affinity for extracellular K^+. Thus, the binding of extracellular K^+ competitively antagonizes the binding of cardiac glycosides. An important clinical correlate is that hypokalemia (a low $[K^+]$ in blood plasma) potentiates digitalis toxicity in patients.

Other Primary Active Transporters on the Plasma Membranes Are Also ATPases

THE H-K PUMP. Other than the Na-K pump, relatively few primary active transporters are located on the plasma membranes of animal cells. In the parietal cells of the gastric gland, an H-K pump extrudes H^+ across the apical membrane into the gland lumen. Similar pumps are present in the kidney and intestines. The H-K pump mediates the active extrusion of H^+ and the uptake of K^+, all fueled by ATP hydrolysis, probably in the ratio of two

H^+, two K^+, and one ATP. Like the Na-K pump, the H-K pump is composed of α and β subunits with multiple isoforms. The α subunit of the H-K pump also undergoes phosphorylation through E_1 and E_2 intermediates during its catalytic cycle (Fig. 3–8B). Moreover, the α and β subunits of the Na-K pump and the H-K pump share significant sequence similarity. Thus the H-K pump is also a member of the superfamily of E_1-E_2 or P-type ATPases.

Ca²⁺ PUMPS. Most, if not all cells have a primary active transporter at the plasma membrane that extrudes Ca^{2+} from the cell. These pumps are abbreviated PMCA (for **plasma-membrane Ca²⁺-ATPase**), and there are at least four PMCA isoforms. These pumps exchange one H^+ for one Ca^{2+} for each molecule of ATP that is hydrolyzed. Ca^{2+} pumps (or Ca^{2+}-ATPases) also exist on the membrane surrounding such intracellular organelles as the sarcoplasmic reticulum (SR) in muscle cells and the endoplasmic reticulum (ER) in other cells, where they play a role in the active sequestration of Ca^{2+} into intracellular stores. The three known ER/SR Ca^{2+} pumps are expressed in different muscle types. The SERCAs (for **sarcoplasmic and endoplasmic reticulum calcium ATPase**) appear to transport two H^+ and two Ca^{2+} ions for each ATP hydrolyzed. The PMCA isoforms and the SERCA Ca^{2+} pumps are additional examples of E_1-E_2 or P-type ATPases. They share significant sequence similarity with the α subunits of the Na-K and H-K pumps. β subunits have yet to be identified for these Ca^{2+} pumps.

F-TYPE OR F₀F₁ ATPases. The ATP synthase of the inner membrane of mitochondria, also known as an F-type or F_oF_1 or F-type ATPase, catalyzes the final step in the ATP synthesis pathway.

The F_oF_1 ATPase of mitochondria (Fig. 3–9A) looks a little like a lollipop held in your hand. The "hand-like" F_o portion is embedded in the membrane and serves as the pathway for H^+ transport. The F_o portion has at least three different subunits (a, b, and c), for an overall stoichiometry of ab_2c_{10-12}. The lollipop-like F_1 portion is outside the plane of the membrane and points into the mitochondrial matrix. The "stick" consists of a γ subunit, with an attached ϵ subunit. The "candy" portion of F_1, which has the ATPase activity, consists of three alternating pairs of α and β subunits, as well as an attached δ subunit. Thus, the overall stoichiometry of F_1 is $\alpha_3\beta_3\gamma\delta\epsilon$. The entire F_oF_1 complex has a molecular weight of approximately 500 kDa.

A fascinating property of the F_oF_1 ATPase is that parts of it undergo substantial rotational movements. We can think of the "hand," "stick," and "candy" portions of the F_oF_1 ATPase as having three distinct functions: (1) The "hand" (the "c" proteins of F_o) acts as a turbine that rotates in the plane of the membrane, driven by the H^+ ions that flow through the turbine—down the H^+ electrochemical gradient—into the mitochondrion. (2) The "stick" is an axle (γ and ϵ subunits of F_1) that rotates with the turbine. And (3) the "candy" (the α and β subunits of F_1) is a chemical factory—energized by the rotating axle—that synthesizes one ATP for each 120-degree turn of the turbine/axle complex. In addition, the a and b subunits of F_o, and possibly the δ subunit of F_1, form a stator that holds the "candy" in place while the turbine/axle complex turns. Paul Boyer and John Walker shared part of the 1997 Nobel Prize in Chemistry for elucidating this "rotary catalysis" mechanism.

Under physiological conditions, the mitochondrial F_oF_1 ATPase runs as an ATP synthase (i.e., "backward" for an H^+ pump)—the final step in oxidative phosphorylation—because of a large, inwardly directed H^+ gradient across the inner mitochondrial membrane (Fig. 3–9B). The citric acid cycle captures energy as electrons and transfers these electrons to reduced nicotinamide adenine dinucleotide (NADH) and reduced flavin adenine dinucleotide (FADH$_2$). NADH and FADH$_2$ transfer their high-energy electrons to the "**respiratory chain**," which consists of four major complexes on the inner membrane of the mitochondrion (Fig. 3–9B). As this respiratory chain transfers the electrons from one electron carrier to another, the electrons gradually lose energy until they finally combine with two H^+ and $\frac{1}{2}$ O_2 to form H_2O. Along the way, three of the four major complexes of the respiratory chain (I, III, IV) pump H^+ across the inner membrane into the intermembrane space (i.e., the space between the inner and outer mitochondrial membranes). These "pumps" are *not* ATPases. The net result is that electron transport has established a large out-to-in H^+ gradient across the mitochondrial inner membrane.

The F_oF_1 ATPase—which is complex V in the respiratory chain—can now use this large electrochemical potential difference for H^+. The H^+ ions then flow "backward" (i.e., down their electrochemical gradient) into the mitochondrion through the F_oF_1 ATPase, which generates ATP in the matrix space of the mitochondrion from ADP and inorganic phosphate. The entire process by which electron transport generates an H^+ gradient and the F_oF_1 ATPase harnesses this H^+ gradient to synthesize ATP is known as the "chemiosmotic" hypothesis. Peter Mitchell, who proposed this hypothesis in 1961, received the Nobel Prize in Chemistry for his work in 1978.

The precise stoichiometry is unknown, but may be one ATP molecule synthesized for every three H^+ flowing downhill into the mitochondrion (one H^+ for each pair of $\alpha\beta$ subunits of F_1). If the H^+ gradient across the mitochondrial inner membrane reverses, the F_oF_1 ATPase will actually function as an ATPase and use the energy of ATP hydrolysis to pump H^+ out of the mitochondrion. Similar F_oF_1 ATPases are also present in bacteria and chloroplasts.

V-TYPE H⁺ PUMP. The membranes surrounding such intracellular organelles as lysosomes, endosomes, secretory vesicles, storage vesicles, and the Golgi apparatus contain a so-called vacuolar-type (or V-type) H^+-ATPase that pumps H^+ from the cytoplasm to the interior of the organelles. The low pH generated inside these organelles is important for sorting proteins, dissociating ligands from receptors, optimizing the activity of acid hydrolases, and accumulating neurotransmitters in vesicles. The apical membranes of certain renal-tubule cells, as well as the plasma membranes of certain other cells, also have V-type H^+ pumps that extrude H^+ from the cell. These V-type H^+ pumps, unlike the gastric H-K pump, are independent of K^+. Instead, the V-type H^+ pump is similar to the hand-held, lollipop-like structure of the F-type ATPase, with which it shares a significant—though low—level of amino-acid homology. For example, the "hand" of the V-

B MODEL OF THE CHEMIOSMOTIC HYPOTHESIS

FIGURE 3–9. The F_oF_1 ATPase and its role as the ATP synthase in the mitochondrial synthesis of ATP. *A*, A cartoon of the F_oF_1 ATPase. The pump has two functional units, F_o (which historically stood for oligomycin-sensitive factor) and F_1 (which historically stood for factor #1). F_o is the transmembrane portion that contains the ion channel through which the H^+ passes. The F_1 is the ATPase. In one complete cycle, the downhill movement of H^+ ions causes the c subunits of F_o and the axle formed by the $\gamma\epsilon$ subunits of F_1 to rotate 360 degrees in three 120-degree steps, causing the α and β subunits to sequentially synthesize and release 3 ATP molecules, for a synthase stoichiometry of ~3 H^+ per ATP. However, the mitochondrion uses ~1 additional H^+ to import inorganic phosphate, and to exchange cytosolic ADP for mitochondrial ATP. Thus, a total of ~4 H^+ would be needed per ATP. *B*, Complexes I, III, and IV of the respiratory chain use the energy of one NADH to pump H^+ out of the mitochondrial matrix; the consensus is 10 H^+ per NADH. The resulting H^+ gradient causes the mitochondrial F_oF_1 ATPase to run as an ATP synthase. Thus, the mitochondrion synthesizes (10 H^+/NADH) × (1 ATP/4 H^+) = 2.5 ATP/NADH. Similarly, the consensus is that complexes III and IV use the energy of one $FADH_2$ to pump six H^+ out of the mitochondrial matrix (*not shown*). Thus, the mitochondrion synthesizes (6 H^+/$FADH_2$) × (1 ATP/4 H^+) = 1.5 ATP/$FADH_2$. ADP, adenosine diphosphate; ATP, adenosine triphosphate; ATPase, adenosine triphosphatase; NAD^+, nicotinamide adenine dinucleotide; NADH, reduced NAD^+; P_i, inorganic phosphate.

type pump has only six subunits, but each is twice as large as a "c" subunit in the F-type ATPase.

ABC TRANSPORTERS. The so-called ABC proteins all have a motif in their amino acid sequence that is an ATP-binding cassette (ABC). Over 50 diverse members of this superfamily are pumps that presumably hydrolyze ATP to provide energy for solute transport. Some may hydrolyze ATP, but they do not couple the liberated energy to perform active transport. In other cases, ATP regulates ABC proteins that function as ion channels or regulators of ion channels or transporters.

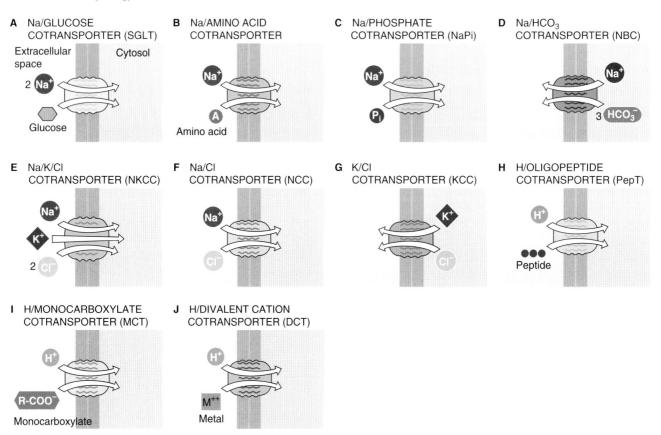

FIGURE 3–10. Representative cotransporters. In *A*, the isoform shown transports 2 Na$^+$ ions for each glucose. In *D*, the isoform shown transports 1 Na$^+$ ion and 3 HCO$_3^-$ ions.

One ABC family that functions as an ATPase is the family of **multidrug resistance transporters** (MDRs). MDR1, also called P-glycoprotein, is a primary active transporter. It extrudes cationic metabolites and drugs across the cell membrane. The substrates of MDR appear to have little in common structurally, except that they are hydrophobic. A wide variety of cells express MDRs, including those of the liver, kidney, and GI tract. MDR1 plays an important and clinically antagonistic role in cancer patients in that it pumps a wide range of anticancer drugs out of cancer cells, thereby rendering cells resistant to these drugs. The MDR protein is a tandem repeat of two structures, each of which has six membrane-spanning segments and a nucleotide-binding domain (NBD).

Another member of the ABC superfamily that is of physiologic interest is the cystic fibrosis transmembrane regulator (CFTR), which is mutated in the hereditary disease **cystic fibrosis** (p. 925). CFTR is a Cl$^-$ channel, as well as a regulator of other ion channels (p. 916).

Cotransporters, One Class of Secondary Active Transporters, Are Generally Driven by the Energy of the Inwardly Directed Na$^+$ Gradient

Like pumps or primary active transporters, secondary active transporters can move a solute uphill (against its electrochemical gradient). However, unlike the pumps, which fuel the process by hydrolyzing ATP, the secondary active transporters fuel it by coupling the uphill movement of one or more solutes to the downhill movement of other solutes. The two major classes of secondary active transporters are cotransporters (or symporters) and exchangers (or antiporters). Cotransporters are intrinsic membrane proteins that move the "driving" solute (the one whose gradient provides the energy) and the "driven" solutes (which move uphill) in the *same* direction.

Na/GLUCOSE COTRANSPORTER. The sodium/glucose cotransporter (SGLT) is located at the apical membrane of the cells that line the proximal tubule and small intestine (Fig. 3–10A). The SGLTs consist of a single subunit, probably with 14 membrane-spanning segments. The SGLT2 and SGLT3 isoforms move one Na$^+$ with each glucose (i.e., 1:1 stoichiometry of Na$^+$ to glucose), whereas the SGLT1 isoform moves two Na$^+$ ions with each glucose.

For a Na/glucose cotransporter with 1:1 stoichiometry, the overall driving force is the sum of the electrochemical potential difference for Na$^+$ and the chemical potential difference for glucose. Thus, the highly favorable, inwardly directed Na$^+$ electrochemical gradient can drive the uphill accumulation of glucose from the lumen of the kidney tubule or gut into the cell. Equilibrium is achieved when the electrochemical potential difference for Na$^+$ in one direction is balanced by the chemical potential difference for glucose in the opposite direction:

$$Equation\ 3{-}15$$
$$-\Delta\tilde{\mu}_{Na} = \Delta\mu_{glucose}$$

We can express $\Delta\tilde{\mu}_{Na}$ in terms of the Na$^+$ concentrations and membrane potential and can express $\Delta\mu_{Glucose}$

in terms of the glucose concentrations. If we substitute these expressions into Equation 3–15, we derive the following relationship for the maximal glucose concentration gradient that can be generated by a given electrochemical potential difference for Na^+:

Equation 3–16

$$\frac{[Glucose]_i}{[Glucose]_o} = \frac{[Na^+]_o}{[Na^+]_i} \times 10^{-V_m/(60\ mV)}$$

In an epithelial cell that has a 10-fold Na^+ concentration gradient and a 60-mV inside-negative voltage across the apical membrane, the Na^+ electrochemical gradient can generate a 10×10^1, or 100-fold, glucose concentration gradient across the plasma membrane. In other words, the 10:1 Na^+ concentration gradient buys a 10-fold glucose gradient, and the V_m of −60 mV buys another 10-fold. However, the leakage of glucose out of the cell by other pathways at the basolateral membrane prevents the Na^+-glucose cotransporter from coming to equilibrium.

A Na/glucose cotransporter with 2:1 stoichiometry is capable of generating an even larger concentration gradient for glucose across the plasma membrane. Such a cotransporter would be in equilibrium when

Equation 3–17

$$2\Delta\tilde{\mu}_{Na} = -\Delta\mu_{glucose}$$

The maximal glucose gradient is

Equation 3–18

$$\frac{[Glucose]_i}{[Glucose]_o} = \left(\frac{[Na^+]_o}{[Na^+]_i}\right)^2 \times 10^{-2V_m/(60\ mV)}$$

In the same epithelial cell with a 10-fold Na^+ concentration gradient and a V_m of −60 mV, the Na^+ electrochemical gradient can generate a glucose concentration gradient of $10^2 \times 10^2$, or 10,000-fold! In other words, the 10:1 Na^+ concentration gradient—when squared for two Na^+ ions—buys a 100-fold glucose gradient, and the −60 mV membrane potential—when multiplied by two for the effective charge on two Na^+ ions—buys another 100-fold.

Because the cotransporter protein has specific sites for binding Na^+ and glucose and because the number of transporters is fixed, the rate of transport by SGLT is a saturable function of the glucose and Na^+ concentrations.

Na^+-DRIVEN COTRANSPORTERS FOR ORGANIC SOLUTES. Functionally similar, but structurally distinct from one another, are a variety of Na^+ cotransporters in the proximal tubule and small intestine. These transporters mediate the absorption of amino acids (Fig. 3–10B), as well as monocarboxylates, dicarboxylates, and tricarboxylates. Na/amino acid cotransport can also take place in nonepithelial cells.

Na^+-DRIVEN COTRANSPORTERS FOR INORGANIC ANIONS. Important examples include the cotransporters for inorganic phosphate (NaPi; Fig. 3–10C) and sulfate. The **Na/HCO₃ cotransporters** (NBCs; Fig. 3–10D) are a key group of acid-base transporters. Multiple forms of Na/HCO₃ cotransporters exist with different Na^+:HCO_3^- stoichiometries. Because of the ion and voltage gradients for typical cells, the form with a 1:3 stoichiometry mediates electrogenic HCO_3^- efflux (NBCe for electrogenic). The forms with stoichiometries of 1:2 (electrogenic) and 1:1 (NBCn for electroneutral) both mediate HCO_3^- influx.

Na/K/Cl COTRANSPORTER. Two Na^+-driven cotransport systems have been identified that mediate the uptake of Cl^- across the plasma membrane by secondary active transport. The first is the Na/K/Cl cotransporter (NKCC), which harnesses the energy of the inwardly directed Na^+ electrochemical gradient to drive the accumulation of Cl^- and K^+ (Fig. 3–10E). One variant of this cotransporter, NKCC1, is present in a wide variety of nonepithelial cells (p. 76), as well as in the *basolateral* membranes of some epithelial cells. Another variant of the Na/K/Cl cotransporter, NKCC2, is present on the *apical* membrane of cells lining the thick ascending limb of the loop of Henle in the kidney (p. 778). A characteristic of the NKCCs is that they are inhibited by **furosemide** and bumetanide, which are called "loop diuretics" because they increase urine flow by inhibiting transport at the loop of Henle. Because of its sensitivity to bumetanide, NKCC is sometimes called the bumetanide-sensitive cotransporter (BSC).

Na/Cl COTRANSPORTER. The second Na^+-driven cotransport system that can move Cl^- across the membrane is found in the apical membrane of the early distal tubule of the kidney (p. 779). This K^+-*independent* Na/Cl cotransport system (NCC) is blocked by **thiazide** diuretics rather than by loop diuretics (Fig. 3–10F). For this reason, NCC has also been called the thiazide-sensitive cotransporter (TSC). NCC and the NKCCs are members of the same gene family.

K/Cl COTRANSPORTER. Another important cotransport mechanism for Cl^- transport across the plasma membrane is Na^+-*independent* K/Cl cotransport (Fig. 3–10G). Because the Na-K pump causes K^+ to accumulate inside the cell, the K^+ electrochemical gradient is outwardly directed across the plasma membrane. In addition, pathways such as the NKCC and the Cl-HCO₃ anion exchanger (see later) bring Cl^- into the cell, so that in most cells the Cl^- electrochemical gradient is also outwardly directed. Thus, the net driving force acting on the K/Cl cotransporter (KCC) favors the exit of K^+ and Cl^- from the cell (p. 77). KCC shares a high degree of amino acid homology with the NKCC and NCC transporters, and belongs to the same gene family.

H⁺-DRIVEN COTRANSPORTERS. Although the majority of known cotransporters in animal cells are driven by the inward movement of Na^+, some are instead driven by the downhill, inward movement of H^+. The **H/oligopeptide cotransporter** (PepT, Fig. 3–10H), which is electrogenic, is responsible for the uptake of small peptides from the lumen into the cells of the renal proximal tubule (p. 797) and small intestine (p. 956). The **monocarboxylate transporter** (MCT, Fig. 3–10I), which is electroneutral, mediates the H^+-coupled flux of lactate, pyruvate, or other monocarboxylates across the cell membranes of most tissues in the body. In the case of lactate, MCT can operate

FIGURE 3–11. Representative exchangers.

in either the net inward or net outward direction, depending on the lactate and H⁺ gradients across the cell membrane. MCT probably moves lactate out of cells that produce lactate by glycolysis but into cells that consume lactate. The **divalent metal cation cotransporter** (DCT, Fig. 3–10*J*) couples the influx of H⁺ to the influx of ferrous iron (Fe²⁺), as well as a variety of other divalent metals, some of which (Cd²⁺, Pb²⁺) are toxic to cells. DCT is expressed at high levels in the kidney and proximal portions of the small intestine.

Exchangers, Another Class of Secondary Active Transporters, Exchange Ions for One Another

The other major class of secondary active transporters is the exchangers, or antiporters. Exchangers are intrinsic membrane proteins that move one or more "driving" solutes in one direction and one or more "driven" solutes in the *opposite* direction. In general, these transporters exchange cations for cations or anions for anions.

Na-Ca EXCHANGER. A nearly ubiquitous cation exchanger is the Na-Ca exchanger (NCX) (Fig. 3–11*A*), which most likely mediates the exchange of three Na⁺ per Ca²⁺. NCX is electrogenic and moves net positive charge in the same direction as Na⁺. Under most circumstances, the inwardly directed Na⁺ electrochemical gradient across the plasma membrane drives the uphill extrusion of Ca²⁺ from the cell. Thus, in concert with the plasma membrane Ca²⁺ pump, this transport system helps maintain the steep, inwardly directed electrochemical potential difference for Ca²⁺ that is normally present across the plasma membrane of all cells.

NCX uses the inwardly directed Na⁺ electrochemical gradient to drive the secondary active efflux of Ca²⁺. With a presumed stoichiometry of three Na⁺ per Ca²⁺, the effectiveness of the Na⁺ electrochemical gradient as a driving force is magnified, thus NCX is at equilibrium

when the Ca²⁺ electrochemical gradient is balanced by three times the Na⁺ electrochemical gradient:

$$\Delta\bar{\mu}_{Ca} = 3\Delta\bar{\mu}_{Na}$$

Equation 3–19

Alternatively,

$$\frac{[Ca^{2+}]_o}{[Ca^{2+}]_i} = \left(\frac{[Na^+]_o}{[Na^+]_i}\right)^3 \cdot 10^{-V_m/60\ mV}$$

Equation 3–20

In a cell with a 10-fold Na⁺ concentration gradient and a V_m of −60 mV, the electrochemical potential difference for Na⁺ can buy a Ca²⁺ concentration gradient of $10^3 \times 10^1$, or 10,000-fold, which is the Ca²⁺ gradient across most cell membranes. Thus the effect of the 10-fold inward Na⁺ concentration gradient is cubed and can account for a 10^3-fold Ca²⁺ concentration gradient across the plasma membrane. In addition, the stoichiometry of three Na⁺ per Ca²⁺ produces a net inflow of one positive charge per transport cycle. Thus the 60-mV inside-negative V_m acts as the equivalent driving force to another 10-fold concentration gradient.

Na-H EXCHANGER. The Na-H exchanger (NHE) mediates the 1:1 exchange of extracellular Na⁺ for intracellular H⁺ across the plasma membrane (Fig. 3–11*B*). One or more of the nine known NHE isoforms are present on the plasma membrane of almost every cell in the body. Through operation of the NHE, the inwardly directed Na⁺ electrochemical gradient can drive the uphill extrusion of H⁺ from the cell and raise intracellular pH (pH$_i$). The ubiquitous NHE1 isoform, which is present in non-epithelial cells, as well as on the basolateral membranes of epithelia, plays a major role in the regulation of pH$_i$ (p. 72) and cell volume (p. 76). The NHE3 isoform is present at the apical membranes of several epithelia, where it plays a major role in acid secretion (p. 852) or Na$^+$ absorption.

Additional cation exchange processes that involve H$^+$ include the organic cation–H$^+$ exchanger that secretes cationic metabolites and drugs across the apical membrane of renal proximal tubule cells and hepatocytes.

Na$^+$-DRIVEN CI-HCO$_3$ EXCHANGER. A second Na$^+$-coupled exchanger that is involved in intracellular pH regulation is the Na$^+$-driven Cl-HCO$_3$ exchanger (NDCBE). This electroneutral transporter couples the movement of one Na$^+$ and the equivalent of two HCO$_3^-$ ions in one direction to the movement of one Cl$^-$ in the opposite direction (Fig. 3–11C). This exchanger uses the inwardly directed Na$^+$ electrochemical gradient to drive the uphill entry of HCO$_3^-$ into the cell. Thus, like NHE, NDCBE helps keep pH$_i$ more alkaline than would be the case if H$^+$ were passively distributed across the plasma membrane. NDCBE is in the same gene superfamily as the NBCs.

CI-HCO$_3$ EXCHANGER. A third exchanger that is involved in the transport of acid-base equivalents is a Cl-HCO$_3$ exchanger (Fig. 3–11D) that functions independently of Na$^+$. Virtually all cells in the body express one or more of the three known isoforms of the Cl-HCO$_3$ exchanger, also known as the anion exchanger (AE). Cl-HCO$_3$ exchangers are physiologically important for transporting HCO$_3^-$ out of the red blood cell in the peripheral tissues, and into the red blood cell within the lungs (p. 664). In other cells, the inwardly directed Cl$^-$ gradient almost always drives HCO$_3^-$ out of the cell. The efflux of HCO$_3^-$ plays an important role in pH$_i$ regulation (p. 72), whereas the uptake of Cl$^-$ often plays a role in cell-volume regulation (p. 76). The AEs share a high degree of amino-acid homology with the NBCs and NDCBE, and belong to the same gene superfamily.

OTHER ANION EXCHANGERS. In addition to the Cl-HCO$_3$ exchangers, several other anion exchangers are known. A **sulfate exchanger** (sulfate-anion transporter [SAT]) exchanges one divalent anion (e.g., sulfate, oxalate) for another of the same group (Fig. 3–11E). In the small intestine and proximal tubule, SAT moves sulfate across the basolateral membrane from the cell to the blood. One member of the SAT family is the "downregulated in adenoma" (DRA) protein, which is in fact a Cl-HCO$_3$ exchanger that is structurally quite different from the Cl-HCO$_3$ exchangers of the AE family.

Distinct anion exchangers with affinities for specific organic anions mediate the secretion of organic anions in various tissues. For example, in the liver, **organic anion transport protein** (OATP) mediates the uptake of bile acids, bilirubin, and the test substrate bromosulphthalein. Another member of the OATP family is the **prostaglandin transporter** (PGT), which mediates the uptake of prostanoids (e.g., prostaglandins E$_2$ and F$_{2\alpha}$ and thromboxane B$_2$). In the kidney, **renal organic anion transporter** (ROAT) mediates the active uptake of endogenous organic anions (Fig. 3–11F), as well as drugs, including penicillin and the test substrate para-aminohippurate. Surprisingly, ROAT is a member of the same superfamily as

OCT, an organic *cation* transporter. In addition to the aforementioned transporters, which have all been cloned, other anion exchangers have been detected from physiological studies on various tissues. For example, the **Cl-formate exchanger** (Fig. 3–11G) and the **Cl-oxalate exchanger** (Fig. 3–11H), which are present in the apical membranes of renal proximal tubule cells, play a role in the secondary active uptake of Cl$^-$. These exchange processes are both likely to be mediated by members of the SAT family. Other anion exchangers are involved in the reabsorption of urate in the kidney.

REGULATION OF INTRACELLULAR ION CONCENTRATIONS

Figure 3–12 illustrates the tools at the disposal of a prototypic cell for managing its intracellular composition. Cells in different tissues—and even different cell types within the same tissue—have different complements of channels and transporters. Epithelial cells and neurons may segregate specific channels and transporters to different parts of the cell (e.g., apical versus basolateral membrane or axon versus soma/dendrite). Thus, different cells may have somewhat different intracellular ionic compositions.

The Na-K Pump Keeps [Na$^+$] Inside the Cell Low and [K$^+$] High

The most striking and important gradients across the cell membrane are those for Na$^+$ and K$^+$. **Sodium** is the predominant cation in ECF, where it is present at a concentration of approximately 145 mM (Fig. 3–12). Na$^+$ is relatively excluded from the intracellular space, where it is present at only a fraction of the extracellular concentration. This Na$^+$ gradient is maintained primarily by active extrusion of Na$^+$ from the cell by the Na-K pump (Fig. 3–12, *no. 1*). In contrast, **potassium** is present at a concentration of only approximately 4.5 mM in ECF, but it is the predominant cation in the intracellular space, where it is accumulated approximately 25- to 30-fold above the outside concentration. Again, this gradient is the direct result of primary active uptake of K$^+$ into the cell by the Na-K pump. When the Na-K pump is inhibited with ouabain, [Na$^+$]$_i$ rises and [K$^+$]$_i$ falls.

In addition to generating concentration gradients for Na$^+$ and K$^+$, the Na-K pump plays an important role in generating the inside-negative membrane potential, which is approximately 60 mV in a typical cell. The Na-K pump accomplishes this task in two ways. First, because the Na-K pump transports three Na$^+$ out of the cell for every two K$^+$, the pump itself is **electrogenic**. This electrogenicity causes a net outward current of positive charge across the plasma membrane and tends to generate an inside-negative V$_m$. However, the pump current itself usually makes only a small contribution to the negative V$_m$. Second, and quantitatively much more important, the active K$^+$ accumulation by the Na-K pump creates a concentration gradient that favors the exit of K$^+$ from the cell through K$^+$ channels (Figure 3–12, *no. 2*). The tendency

FIGURE 3–12. Ion gradients, channels, and transporters in a typical cell.

of K^+ to *exit* through these channels, with unmatched negative charges left behind, is the main cause of the inside-negative membrane potential. When K^+ channels are blocked with an inhibitor such as Ba^{2+}, V_m becomes considerably less negative (i.e., the cell depolarizes). In most cells, the principal pathway for current flow across the plasma membrane (i.e., the principal ionic conductance) is via K^+ channels. We discuss the generation of membrane potentials in Chapter 6.

The inside-negative V_m, together with the large concentration gradient for Na^+, summates to create a large, inwardly directed Na^+ electrochemical gradient, which strongly favors passive Na^+ entry. Given the large amount of energy that is devoted to generating this favorable driving force for Na^+ entry, one might expect that the cell would permit Na^+ to move into the cell only through pathways serving important physiological purposes. The simple passive entry of Na^+ via channels—without harnessing this Na^+ entry for some physiological purpose—would complete a futile cycle that culminates in active Na^+ extrusion. It would make little teleologic sense for the cell to use up considerable energy stores to extrude Na^+ only to let it passively diffuse back in with no effect. Rather, cells harness the energy of Na^+ entry for three major purposes:

1. In certain **epithelial cells**, amiloride-sensitive Na^+ channels (ENaC) are largely restricted to the *apical* or *luminal* surface of the cell (Fig. 3–12, *no. 3*), and the Na-K pumps are restricted to the *basolateral* surface of the cell. In this way, *transepithelial* Na^+ transport takes place rather than a futile cycling of Na^+ back and forth across a single plasma membrane.

2. In **excitable cells**, passive Na^+ entry occurs through voltage-dependent Na^+ channels (Fig. 3–12, *no. 4*) and plays a critical role in generation of the action potential. In such cells, Na^+ is cycled at high energy cost across the plasma membrane for the important physiological purpose of information transfer.

3. Virtually **every cell** in the body uses the electrochemical Na^+ gradient across the plasma membrane to drive the secondary active transport of nutrients and ions (Fig. 3–12, *no. 5*).

The Ca²⁺ Pump and the Na-Ca Exchanger Keep Intracellular [Ca²⁺] Four Orders of Magnitude Lower Than Extracellular [Ca²⁺]

Whereas the concentration of Ca^{2+} in the extracellular space is about 1 mM (10^{-3} M), that in the ICF is only approximately 100 nM (10^{-7} M), a concentration gradient of 10^4-fold. Because of the inside-negative membrane potential of a typical cell and the large chemical gradient for Ca^{2+}, the inwardly directed electrochemical gradient for Ca^{2+} across the plasma membrane is enormous, far larger than that for any other ion. Many cells have a variety of Ca^{2+} channels through which Ca^{2+} can enter the cell (Fig. 3–12, *no. 6*). In general, Ca^{2+} channels are gated by voltage (p. 189) or by humoral agents (p. 313) so that rapid Ca^{2+} entry into the cell occurs only in short bursts. However, given the existence of pathways for passive Ca^{2+} transport *into* cells, we may ask what transport mechanisms keep $[Ca^{2+}]_i$ low and thus maintain the enormous Ca^{2+} electrochemical gradient across the plasma membrane.

Ca²⁺ PUMPS (SERCA) IN ORGANELLE MEMBRANES. Ca^{2+} pumps (ATPases) are present on the membranes that sur-

In most cells, [Cl⁻] is modestly above equilibrium because Cl⁻ uptake via the Cl–HCO₃ exchanger and Na/K/Cl cotransporter balances passive Cl⁻ efflux through channels of magnitude lower than extracellular [Ca²⁺].

The Na⁺–H⁺ exchanger and Na⁺-driven Cl–HCO₃ keep intracellular pH and [HCO₃⁻] above their equilibrium values.

10 Cl⁻ channel

11 Cl–HCO₃ exchanger

12 Na/K/2Cl cotransporter

13 K–Cl cotransporter

14 Cation channel for H⁺ entry

15 Cl⁻ channel for HCO₃⁻ exit

16 Na–H exchanger

17 Na-driven Cl–HCO₃ exchanger

19 Na/HCO₃ cotransporter

18 V–type H⁺ pump

round various intracellular organelles, such as the SR and ER (Fig. 3–12, *no. 7*). These pumps actively sequester cytosolic Ca^{2+} in intracellular stores. These stores of Ca^{2+} can later be released into the cytoplasm in bursts as part of a signal-transduction process in response to membrane depolarization or humoral agents. Even though Ca^{2+} sequestration in intracellular stores is an important mechanism for regulating $[Ca^{2+}]_i$ in the short term, there is a limit to how much Ca^{2+} a cell can store. Therefore, in the steady state, Ca^{2+} extrusion across the cell membrane must balance the passive influx of Ca^{2+}.

Ca²⁺ PUMP (PMCA) ON THE PLASMA MEMBRANE. The plasma membranes of most cells contain a Ca^{2+} pump that plays a major role in extruding Ca^{2+} from the cell (Fig. 3–12, *no. 8*). It would seem that rising levels of intracellular Ca^{2+} would stimulate the Ca^{2+} pump to extrude Ca^{2+} and thereby return $[Ca^{2+}]_i$ toward normal. Actually, the pump *itself* is incapable of this type of feedback control because it has such a high K_m for $[Ca^{2+}]_i$ that the pump is virtually inactive at physiological $[Ca^{2+}]_i$. However, as $[Ca^{2+}]_i$ rises, the Ca^{2+} binds to a protein known as **calmodulin** (CaM, p. 102), which has a high affinity for Ca^{2+}. The newly formed Ca^{2+}-CaM binds to the Ca^{2+} pump, lowers the pump's K_m for $[Ca^{2+}]_i$ into the physiological range, and thus stimulates Ca^{2+} extrusion. As $[Ca^{2+}]_i$ falls, Ca^{2+}-CaM levels inside the cell also fall so that Ca^{2+}-CaM dissociates from the Ca^{2+} pump, thereby returning the pump to its inactive state. At resting $[Ca^{2+}]_i$ levels of approximately 100 nM, the Ca^{2+} pump is the major route of Ca^{2+} extrusion.

Na-Ca EXCHANGER (NCX) ON THE PLASMA MEMBRANE. NCX (Fig. 3–12, *no. 9*) plays a key role in extruding Ca^{2+} only when $[Ca^{2+}]_i$ rises substantially above

normal levels. Thus, NCX is especially important in restoring low $[Ca^{2+}]_i$ when large influxes of Ca^{2+} occur. This property is most notable in excitable cells such as neurons and cardiac muscle, which may be challenged with vast Ca^{2+} influxes through voltage-gated Ca^{2+} channels during action potentials.

In Most Cells, [Cl⁻] Is Modestly Above Equilibrium Because Cl⁻ Uptake via the Cl-HCO₃ Exchanger and Na/K/Cl Cotransporter Balances Passive Cl⁻ Efflux Through Channels

The $[Cl^-]$ in all cells is below the $[Cl^-]$ in the extracellular space. Virtually all cells have **anion-selective channels** (Fig. 3–12, *no. 10*) through which Cl^- can permeate passively. In a typical cell with a 60-mV inside-negative membrane potential, $[Cl^-]_i$ would be a tenth that of $[Cl^-]_o$ if Cl^- were passively distributed across the plasma membrane. Such is the case for skeletal muscle. However, for most cell types, $[Cl^-]_i$ is approximately twice as high as that predicted for passive distribution alone, which indicates the presence of transport pathways that mediate the active uptake of Cl^- into the cell. Probably the most common pathway for Cl^- uptake is the **Cl-HCO₃ exchanger** (Fig. 3–12, *no. 11*). Because $[HCO_3^-]_i$ is several-fold higher than if it were passively distributed across the cell membrane, the outwardly directed electrochemical potential difference for HCO_3^- can act as a driving force for the uphill entry of Cl^- via Cl-HCO₃ exchange. Another pathway that can mediate uphill Cl^- transport into the cell is the **Na/K/Cl cotransporter** (Fig. 3–12, *no. 12*), which is stimulated by low $[Cl^-]_i$.

Given the presence of these transport pathways mediating Cl^- uptake, why is $[Cl^-]_i$ only about 2-fold above that predicted for passive distribution? The answer is that the passive Cl⁻ efflux through anion-selective channels in the plasma membrane opposes Cl⁻-uptake mechanisms. Another factor that tends to keep Cl⁻ low in some cells is the **K/Cl cotransporter**. KCC (Fig. 3–12, *no. 13*), driven by the outward K⁺ gradient, tends to move K⁺ and Cl⁻ out of cells. Thus, the K⁺ gradient promotes Cl⁻ efflux both by generating the inside-negative V_m that drives Cl⁻ out of the cell via channels, and by driving K/Cl cotransport.

The Na-H Exchanger and Na-Driven HCO_3^- Transporters Keep the Intracellular pH and $[HCO_3^-]$ Above Their Equilibrium Values

H⁺, HCO_3^-, and CO_2 within a particular compartment are generally in equilibrium with one another. Extracellular pH is normally approximately 7.4, $[HCO_3^-]_o$ is 24 mM, and P_{CO_2} is approximately 40 mm Hg. In a typical cell, intracellular pH is approximately 7.2. Because $[CO_2]$ is usually the same on both sides of the cell membrane, $[HCO_3^-]_i$ can be calculated to be approximately 15 mM. Even though the ICF is slightly more acidic than the ECF, pH_i is actually much more alkaline than it would be if H⁺ and HCO_3^- were passively distributed across the cell membrane. H⁺ can enter the cell passively and HCO_3^- can exit the cell passively, although both processes occur at a rather low rate. H⁺ can permeate certain **cation channels** (Fig. 3–12, *no. 14*), and HCO_3^- moves fairly easily through most **Cl⁻ channels** (Fig. 3–12, *no. 15*). Because a membrane potential of −60 mV is equivalent as a driving force to a 10-fold concentration gradient of a monovalent ion, one would expect [H⁺] to be 10-fold higher within the cell than in the ECF, which corresponds to a pH_i that is 1 pH unit more acidic than pH_o. Similarly, one would expect $[HCO_3^-]_i$ to be only one tenth of $[HCO_3^-]_o$. The observation that pH_i and $[HCO_3^-]_i$ are maintained higher than predicted for passive distribution across the plasma membrane indicates that cells must actively extrude H⁺ or take up HCO_3^-.

The transport of acid out of the cell or base into the cell is collectively termed "acid extrusion." In most cells, the **acid extruders** are secondary active transporters that are energized by the electrochemical Na⁺ gradient across the cell membrane. The most important acid extruders are the **Na-H** (Fig. 3–12, *no. 16*) and the **Na-driven Cl-HCO3 exchangers** (Fig. 3–12, *no. 17*) as well as the **Na/HCO3 cotransporters** with Na⁺:HCO_3^- stoichiometries of 1:2 and 1:1 (p. 67). These transport systems are generally sensitive to changes in pH_i; they are stimulated when the cell is acidified and inhibited when the cell is alkalinized. Thus, these transporters maintain pH_i in a range that is optimal for cell functioning. Less commonly, certain epithelial cells that are specialized for acid secretion use **V-type H⁺ pumps** (Fig. 3–12, *no. 18*) or **H-K pumps** on their apical membranes to extrude acid. These epithelia include the renal collecting duct and the stomach. As noted earlier, virtually all cells have V-type H⁺ pumps on the membranes surrounding such intracellular organelles as lysosomes, endosomes, and Golgi.

Because most cells have powerful acid-extrusion systems, one might ask why the pH_i is not far more alkaline than approximately 7.2. Part of the answer is that trans-

port processes that act as **acid loaders** balance acid extrusion. Passive leakage of H⁺ and HCO_3^- through *channels*, as noted earlier, tends to acidify the cell. Cells also have *transporters* that generally move HCO_3^- out of cells. The most common is the Cl-HCO3 exchanger (Fig. 3–12, *no. 11*). Another is the electrogenic NBC with an Na⁺:HCO_3^- stoichiometry of 1:3 (Fig. 3–12, *no. 19*), which moves HCO_3^- out of the cell across the basolateral membrane of renal proximal tubules.

WATER TRANSPORT AND THE REGULATION OF CELL VOLUME

Water Transport Is Driven by Osmotic and Hydrostatic Pressure Differences Across Membranes

Transport of water across biologic membranes is always passive. No water pumps have ever been described. To a certain extent, single water molecules can dissolve in lipid bilayers and thus move across cell membranes at a low, but finite rate by simple diffusion. The ease with which H_2O diffuses through the lipid bilayer depends on the lipid composition of the bilayer. Membranes with low fluidity (p. 12), that is, those whose phospholipids have long saturated fatty acid chains with few double bonds (i.e., few kinks), exhibit lower H_2O permeability. The addition of other lipids that decrease fluidity (e.g., cholesterol) may further reduce H_2O permeability. Therefore, it is not surprising that the plasma membranes of many types of cells have specialized water channels—the aquaporins—that serve as passive conduits for water transport. The presence of aquaporins greatly increases membrane water permeability. In some cells, such as erythrocytes or the renal proximal tubule, AQP1 is always present in the membrane. The collecting-duct cells of the kidney regulate the H_2O permeability of their apical membranes by inserting AQP2 water channels into their apical membranes under the control of arginine vasopressin.

Water transport across a membrane is always a linear, nonsaturable function of its net driving force. The direction of net passive transport of an uncharged solute is always down its chemical potential difference. For water, we must consider two passive driving forces. The first is the familiar chemical potential difference ($\Delta\mu_{H_2O}$), which depends on the difference in **water concentration** on the two sides of the membrane. The second is the energy difference, per mole of water, that results from the difference in **hydrostatic pressure** ($\Delta\mu_{H_2O,Pressure}$) across the membrane. Thus, the relevant energy difference across the membrane is the sum of the chemical and pressure potential differences:

Equation 3–21

$$\Delta\mu_{H_2O,Total} = \Delta\mu_{H_2O} + \Delta\mu_{H_2O,Pressure}$$

$$\Delta\mu_{H_2O,Total} = RT\, ln\, \frac{[H_2O]_i}{[H_2O]_o} + \overline{V}_W(P_i - P_o)$$

$$\underbrace{\text{Total energy difference}} = \underbrace{\text{Chemical part}} + \underbrace{\text{Pressure part}}$$

P is the hydrostatic pressure and $\overline{V}_w$ is the partial molar volume of water (i.e., volume occupied by 1 mole of water). Because the product of pressure and volume is work, the second term in Equation 3–21 is work per mole. Dealing with water concentrations is cumbersome and imprecise because [H_2O] is very high (i.e., ~ 56 M) and does not change substantially in the dilute solutions that physiologists are interested in. Therefore, it is more practical to work with the inverse of [H_2O], namely, the concentration of osmotically active solutes, or **osmolality.** The units of osmolality are osmoles per kilogram H_2O, or Osm. In dilute solutions, the H_2O gradient across the cell membrane is roughly proportional to the difference in osmolalities across the membrane:

Equation 3–22

$$ln \frac{[H_2O]_i}{[H_2O]_o} \cong \overline{V}_W(Osm_o - Osm_i)$$

Osm is the total concentration of all osmotically active solutes in the indicated compartment (e.g., Na^+ + Cl^- + K^+ + ...). Substituting Equation 3–22 into Equation 3–21 yields a more useful expression for the total energy difference across the membrane:

Equation 3–23

$$\underbrace{\Delta\mu_{H_2O,Total}}_{\dfrac{Energy}{mole}} \cong \underbrace{\overline{V}_W}_{\dfrac{Volume}{mole}} \underbrace{[RT(Osm_o - Osm_i) + (P_i - P_o)]}_{Pressure}$$

In this equation, the terms inside the brackets have the units of pressure (force/area) and thus describe the *driving force* for water movement from the inside to the outside of the cell. This driving force determines the flux of water across the membrane:

Equation 3–24

$$J_V = L_p[RT(Osm_o - Osm_i) + (P_i - P_o)]$$

J_V is positive when water flows out of the cell and has the units liters/($cm^2 \cdot s$). The proportionality constant L_p is the **hydraulic conductivity.**

Water is in equilibrium across the membrane when the net driving force for water transport is nil. If we set $\Delta\mu_{H_2O, Total}$ to zero in Equation 3–23:

Equation 3–25

$$\underbrace{RT(Osm_i - Osm_o)}_{\substack{\text{Osmotic pressure} \\ \text{difference} \\ \Delta\pi}} = \underbrace{(P_i - P_o)}_{\substack{\text{Hydrostatic pressure} \\ \text{difference} \\ \Delta P}}$$

The term on the left is referred to as the **osmotic pressure difference** ($\Delta\pi$). Thus, at equilibrium the osmotic pressure difference is equal to the hydrostatic pressure difference (ΔP). An osmotic pressure difference of 1 mosmole/kg H_2O (or 1 mOsm) is equivalent to a hy-

drostatic pressure difference of 19.3 mm Hg at normal body temperature.

The plasma membranes of animal cells are not very rigid (unlike the walls of plant cells) and cannot tolerate any significant hydrostatic pressure difference without deforming. Therefore, the hydrostatic pressure difference *across a cell membrane* is virtually always near zero and is therefore not a significant driving force for water transport.

Movement of water in and out of cells is driven by osmotic gradients only, that is, by differences in osmolality across the membrane. For example, if the osmolality is greater outside the cell than inside, water will flow out of the cell and the cell will shrink. Such a movement of water driven by osmotic gradients is called **osmosis.** Water is at equilibrium across *cell membranes* only when the osmolality inside and outside the cell is the same.

Hydrostatic pressure differences are an important driving force for driving fluid out across the *walls of capillaries* (p. 469). Small solutes permeate freely across most capillaries. Thus, any difference in *osmotic* pressure as a result of these small solutes does not exert a driving force for water flow across that capillary. The situation is quite different for plasma proteins, which are too large to penetrate the capillary wall freely. As a result, the presence of a greater concentration of plasma proteins in the intravascular compartment than in interstitial fluid sets up a difference in osmotic pressure that tends to pull fluid back into the capillary. This difference is called the **colloid osmotic pressure** or **oncotic pressure.** Water is at equilibrium across the wall of a *capillary* when the colloid osmotic and hydrostatic pressure differences are equal. When the hydrostatic pressure difference exceeds the colloid osmotic pressure difference, the resulting movement of water out of the capillary is called **ultrafiltration.**

Because of the Presence of Impermeant, Negatively Charged Proteins Within the Cell, Donnan Forces Will Lead to Cell Swelling

NaCl, the most abundant salt in ECF, is largely excluded from the intracellular compartment by the direct and indirect actions of the Na-K pump. This relative exclusion of NaCl from the intracellular space is vital for maintaining normal cell water content (i.e., cell volume). In the absence of Na-K pumps, cells tend to swell even when both the intracellular and extracellular osmolalities are normal and identical. This statement may appear to contradict the principle that there can be no water flux without a difference in osmolality across the cell membrane (Equation 3–24). To understand this apparent paradox, consider a simplified model that illustrates the key role played by **negatively charged, impermeant macromolecules** (i.e., proteins) inside the cell (Fig. 3–13).

Imagine that a semipermeable membrane separates a left compartment (analogous to the *extra*cellular space) and a right compartment (analogous to the *intra*cellular space). The two compartments are rigid and have equal volumes throughout the experiment. The right compartment is fitted with a pressure gauge. The membrane is nondeformable and permeable to Na^+, Cl^-, and water, but is not permeable to a negatively charged macromole-

A   INITIAL CONDITION

B   INTERMEDIATE STATE
(after 10 mM NaCl has moved to cytosol)

C   FINAL EQUILIBRIUM

FIGURE 3–13. Gibbs-Donnan equilibrium. A semipermeable membrane separates two compartments that have rigid walls and equal volumes. The membrane is permeable to Na^+, Cl^-, and water, but not to the macromolecule Y, which carries 150 negative charges.

cule (Y). For the sake of simplicity, assume that each Y carries 150 negative charges and is restricted to the intracellular solution. Figure 3–13A illustrates the ionic conditions at the beginning of the experiment. At this initial condition, the system is far out of equilibrium: although $[Na^+]$ is the same on both sides of the membrane, $[Cl^-]$ and $[Y^{-150}]$ have opposing concentration gradients of 150 mM.

What will happen now? The system will tend toward equilibrium. Cl^- will move down its concentration gradient into the cell. This entry of negatively charged particles will generate an inside-negative membrane potential, which in turn will attract Na^+ and cause Na^+ to move into the cell. In the final equilibrium condition, both Na^+ and Cl^- will be distributed so that the concentration of each is balanced against the same V_m, which is given by the Nernst equation (Equation 3–8):

Equation 3–26

$$V_m = -\frac{RT}{F} \ln \frac{[Na^+]_i}{[Na^+]_o}$$

Equation 3–27

$$V_m = -\frac{RT}{(-1) F} \ln \frac{[Cl^-]_i}{[Cl^-]_o}$$

Because V_m must be the same in the two cases, we combine the two equations, obtaining

Equation 3–28

$$-\ln \frac{[Na^+]_i}{[Na^+]_o} = \ln \frac{[Cl^-]_i}{[Cl^-]_o}$$

$$\frac{[Na^+]_o}{[Na^+]_i} = \frac{[Cl^-]_i}{[Cl^-]_o} = r$$

where r is the Donnan ratio because this equilibrium state is a **Gibbs-Donnan equilibrium** (often shortened to Donnan equilibrium). All the values for ionic concentrations in Equation 3–28 are *new* values. As Na^+ entered the cell, not only did $[Na^+]_i$ rise, but $[Na^+]_o$ also fell, by identical amounts. The same is true for Cl^-. How much did the Na^+ and Cl^- concentrations have to change before the system achieved equilibrium? An important constraint on the system as it approaches equilibrium is that in each compartment, the total number of positive charges must balance the total number of negative charges (bulk electroneutrality) at all times. Imagine an *intermediate* state, between the initial condition and the final equilibrium state, in which 10 mM of Na^+ and 10 mM of Cl^- have moved into the cell (Fig. 3–13B). This condition is still far from equilibrium because the Na^+ ratio in Equation 3–28 is 0.875, whereas the Cl^- ratio is only 0.071; thus, these ratios are not equal. Therefore, Na^+ and Cl^- continue to move into the cell until the Na^+ ratio and the Cl^- ratio are both 0.5, the Donnan r ratio (Fig. 3–13C). This ratio corresponds to Nernst potentials of -18.4 mV for both Na^+ and Cl^-.

However, although the ions are in equilibrium, far more osmotically active particles are now on the inside than on the outside. Ignoring the osmotic effect of Y^{-150}, the sum of $[Na^+]$ and $[Cl^-]$ on the inside is 250 mM, whereas on the outside it is only 200 mM. Because of this 50-mOsm gradient (ΔOsm) across the membrane, water cannot be at equilibrium and will therefore move into the cell. In our example, the right (inside) compartment is surrounded by a rigid wall so that only a minuscule amount of water needs to enter the cell to generate a hydrostatic pressure of 967 mm Hg to oppose the additional net entry of water. This equilibrium hydrostatic pressure difference (ΔP) opposes the osmotic pressure difference ($\Delta\pi$):

Equation 3–29

$$\begin{aligned}
\Delta P &= \Delta\pi \\
&= RT\Delta Osm \\
&= RT[([Na^+]_i + [Cl^-]_i) - ([Na^+]_o + [Cl^-]_o)] \\
&= RT(50 \text{ mM}) \\
&= 967 \text{ mm Hg} \\
&= 1.3 \text{ atm}
\end{aligned}$$

Thus, in the rigid "cell" of our example, achieving Gibbs-Donnan equilibrium would require developing

Osmotic equilibrium is maintained by an equal number of positive and negative ions moving in and out of the cell.

After inhibition of the Na–K pump with ouabain, continued passive leakage disrupts the osmotic equilibrium. As a result, water flows into the cell causing it to swell.

FIGURE 3–14. Role of the Na-K pump in maintaining cell volume.

within the model cell a hydrostatic pressure that is 1.3 atm greater than the pressure in the left compartment (outside).

The Na-K Pump Maintains Cell Volume by Doing Osmotic Work That Counteracts the Passive Donnan Forces

Unlike the preceding example, the plasma membranes of animal cells are not rigid, but deformable, so that transmembrane hydrostatic pressure gradients cannot exist. Thus, in animal cells the distribution of ions toward the Donnan-equilibrium condition would, it appears, inevitably lead to progressive water entry, cell swelling, and ultimately, bursting. Although the Donnan-equilibrium model is very artificial (for example, ignoring all ions other than Na^+, Cl^-, and Y^{-150}), it nevertheless illustrates a point that is important for real cells: the negative charge on impermeant intracellular solutes (e.g., proteins and organic phosphates) will lead to bursting unless the cell does "osmotic work" to counteract the passive Donnan-like swelling. The net effect of this osmotic work is to largely exclude NaCl from the cell and thereby make the cell functionally impermeable to NaCl. In a sense, NaCl acts as a functionally impermeant solute in the extracellular space that offsets the osmotic effects of intracellular negative charges. This state of affairs is not an equilibrium, but a *steady state* maintained by active transport.

To illustrate the role of active transport, consider a somewhat more realistic model of a cell (Fig. 3–14). Under "normal" conditions, $[Na^+]_i$, $[K^+]_i$, and $[Cl^-]_i$ are constant because (1) the active extrusion of three Na^+ in exchange for two K^+ is balanced by the passive influx of three Na^+ and the passive efflux of two K^+, and (2) the net flux of Cl^- is zero (i.e., we assume that Cl^- is in equilibrium). When the Na-K pump is inhibited, the passive entry of three Na^+ exceeds the net passive efflux of two K^+ and thereby results in a gain of one intracellular cation and an immediate, small depolarization (i.e., cell becomes less negative inside). In addition, as intracellular $[K^+]$ slowly declines after inhibition of the Na-K pump, the cell depolarizes even further because the outward K^+ gradient is the predominant determinant of the membrane potential. The inside-negative V_m is the driving force that is largely responsible for excluding Cl^- from the cell, and depolarization of the cell causes Cl^- to enter through anion channels. Cl^- influx results in the gain of one intracellular anion. The net gain of one intracellular cation and one anion increases the number of osmotically active particles and in so doing creates the inward osmotic gradient that leads to cell swelling. Thus, in the normal environment in which cells are bathed, the action of the Na-K pump is required to prevent the cell swelling that would otherwise occur.

A real cell, of course, is far more complex than the idealized cell in Figure 3–14, having a myriad of interrelated channels and transporters (Fig. 3–12). These other pathways, together with the Na-K pump, have the net effect of excluding NaCl and other solutes from the cell. Because the solute gradients that drive transport through these other pathways ultimately depend on the Na-K pump, inhibiting the Na-K pump will de-energize these other pathways and lead to cell swelling.

Cells Respond to Short-Term Volume Changes by Activating Ion Channels or Transporters and Thereby Returning Volume Toward Normal

The joint efforts of the Na-K pump and other transport pathways are necessary for maintaining normal cell volume. What happens if cell volume is acutely challenged? A subset of "other pathways" respond to the cell-volume

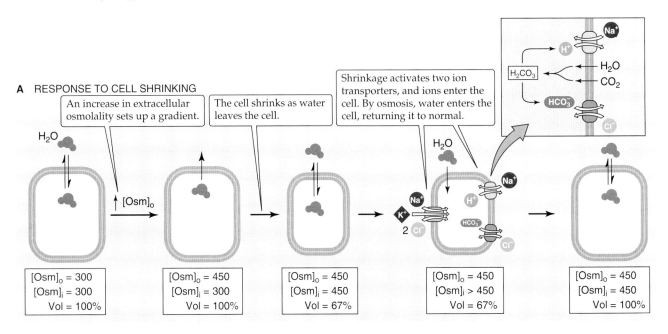

A   RESPONSE TO CELL SHRINKING

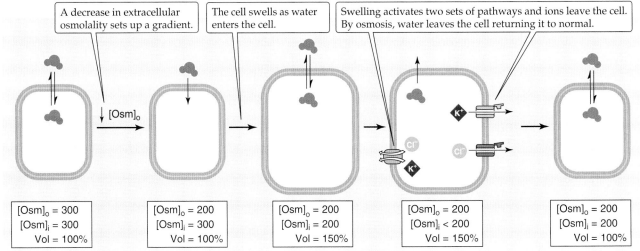

B   RESPONSE TO CELL SWELLING

FIGURE 3–15. Short-term regulation of cell volume.

change by transferring solutes across the membrane, thereby returning the volume toward normal.

RESPONSE TO CELL SHRINKAGE. If we increase extracellular osmolality by adding an impermeant solute such as mannitol (Fig. 3–15A), the extracellular solution becomes **hyperosmolal** and exerts an osmotic force that draws water out of the cell. The cell continues to shrink until the osmolality inside and out become the same. Many types of cells respond to this shrinkage by activating solute-uptake processes to increase cell solute and water content. This response is known as a **regulatory volume increase (RVI)**. Depending on the cell type, cell shrinkage activates different types of solute-uptake mechanisms. In many types of cells, shrinkage activates the ubiquitous NHE1 isoform of the *Na-H exchanger*. In addition to me-

diating increased uptake of Na^+, extrusion of H^+ alkalinizes the cell and consequently activates *Cl-HCO_3 exchange*. The net effect is thus the entry of Na^+ and Cl^-. The resulting increase in intracellular osmoles then draws water into the cell to restore cell volume toward normal. Alternatively, the RVI response may be mediated by activation of the NKCC1 isoform of the *Na/K/Cl cotransporter*.

RESPONSE TO CELL SWELLING. If extracellular osmolality is decreased by the addition of water (Fig. 3–15B), the extracellular solution becomes **hypo-osmolal** and exerts a lesser osmotic force so that water moves into the cell. The cell continues to swell until the osmolality inside and out becomes the same. Many cell types respond to this swelling by activating solute-efflux pathways to decrease cell solute and water content and thereby return cell volume

DISORDERS OF EXTRACELLULAR OSMOLALITY

Regulatory adjustments in cell volume can be extremely important clinically. In major disorders of extracellular osmolality, the principal signs and symptoms arise from abnormal brain function, which can be fatal. For example, it is all too common for the elderly or infirm, unable to maintain proper fluid intake because of excessive heat or disability, to be brought to the emergency room in a state of severe dehydration. The hyperosmolality that results from dehydration can lead to brain shrinkage, which in extreme cases can cause intracerebral hemorrhage from tearing of blood vessels. However, if the brain cells compensate for this hyperosmolality by the long-term mechanisms discussed before (e.g., manufacturing idiogenic osmoles), cell shrinkage may be minimized. However, consider the consequence if an unsuspecting physician, unaware of the nuances of cell volume regulation, rapidly corrects the elevated extracellular hyperosmolality back down to normal. Rapid water entry into the brain cells will cause cerebral edema (i.e., brain swelling) and may cause death from herniation of the brain stem through the tentorium. For this reason, severe disturbances in extracellular-fluid osmolality must usually be corrected slowly.

toward normal. This response is known as a **regulatory volume decrease (RVD)**. Depending on the cell type, swelling activates different types of solute-efflux mechanisms. In many types of cells, swelling activates *Cl⁻ or K⁺ channels* (or both). Because the electrochemical gradients for these two ions are generally directed outward across the plasma membrane, activating these channels causes a net efflux of K⁺ and Cl⁻, which lowers the intracellular solute content and causes water to flow out of the cell. The result is restoration of cell volume toward normal. Alternatively, the RVD response may be initiated by activating the *K/Cl cotransporter*.

In the normal steady state, the transport mechanisms that are responsible for RVI and RVD are usually not fully quiescent. Not only does cell shrinkage activate the transport pathways involved in RVI (i.e., solute loaders), it also appears to inhibit at least some of the transport pathways involved in RVD (i.e., solute extruders). The opposite is true of cell swelling. In all cases, it is the Na-K pump that ultimately generates the ion gradients that drive the movements of NaCl and KCl that regulate cell volume when extracellular osmolality is altered.

Cells Respond to Long-Term Hyperosmolality by Accumulating New Intracellular Organic Solutes

Whereas the acute response (seconds to minutes) to hyperosmolality (i.e., RVI) involves the uptake of salts, chronic adaptation (hours to days) to hyperosmolality involves accumulating organic solutes (*osmolytes*) within the

cell. Examples of such intracellularly accumulated osmolytes include two relatively impermeant alcohol derivatives of common sugars (i.e., sorbitol and inositol), as well as two amines (betaine and taurine). Generation of organic solutes (*idiogenic osmoles*) within the cell plays a major role in raising intracellular osmolality and restoring cell volume during chronic adaptation to hyperosmolality—a response that is particularly true in brain cells. Sorbitol is produced from glucose by a reaction that is catalyzed by the enzyme **aldose reductase**. Cell shrinkage is a powerful stimulus for the synthesis of aldose reductase.

In addition to synthesizing organic solutes, cells can also transport them into the cytosol from the outside. For example, cells use distinct Na⁺-coupled cotransport systems to accumulate inositol, betaine, and taurine. In some types of cells, shrinkage induces greatly enhanced expression of these transporters, thereby leading to the accumulation of these intracellular solutes.

The Gradient in Tonicity—or *Effective Osmolality*—Determines the Osmotic Flow of Water Across a Cell Membrane

Total body water is distributed among blood plasma, the interstitial, intracellular, and transcellular fluids. The mechanisms by which water exchanges between interstitial fluid and ICF, and between interstitial fluid and plasma, rely on the principles that we have just discussed.

WATER EXCHANGE ACROSS CELL MEMBRANES. Because cell membranes are not rigid, hydrostatic pressure differences never arise between cell water and interstitial fluid. Increasing the *hydrostatic* pressure in the interstitial space will cause the cell to compress so that the intracellular hydrostatic pressure increases to a similar extent. Thus, water does not enter the cell under these conditions. However, increasing the interstitial *osmotic* pressure, thus generating a $\Delta\pi$, is quite a different matter. If we suddenly increase ECF osmolality by adding an *impermeant* solute such as mannitol, the resulting osmotic gradient across the cell membrane causes water to move out of the cell. If the cell does not have an RVI mechanism or if the RVI mechanism is blocked, cell volume will remain reduced indefinitely.

On the other hand, consider what would happen if we suddenly increase ECF osmolality by adding a *permeant* solute such as urea. Urea can rapidly penetrate cell membranes by facilitated diffusion via members of the UT family of transporters; however, cells have no mechanism for extruding urea. Because urea penetrates the membrane more slowly than water does, the initial effect of applying urea is to shrink the cell (Fig. 3–16). However, as urea gradually equilibrates across the cell membrane and abolishes the initially imposed osmotic gradient, the cell reswells to its initial volume. Thus, sustained changes in cell volume do not occur with a change in the extracellular concentration of a permeant solute.

The difference between the effects of mannitol and urea on the final cell volume illustrates the need to distinguish between total osmolality and **effective osmolality** (also known as **tonicity**). In terms of clinically measured sol-

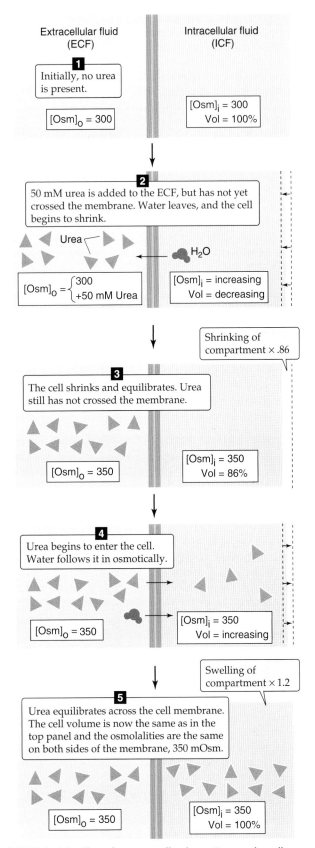

Extracellular fluid (ECF) | **Intracellular fluid (ICF)**

1 Initially, no urea is present.

[Osm]$_o$ = 300

[Osm]$_i$ = 300
Vol = 100%

2 50 mM urea is added to the ECF, but has not yet crossed the membrane. Water leaves, and the cell begins to shrink.

Urea   H$_2$O

[Osm]$_o$ = { 300, +50 mM Urea }

[Osm]$_i$ = increasing
Vol = decreasing

Shrinking of compartment × .86

3 The cell shrinks and equilibrates. Urea still has not crossed the membrane.

[Osm]$_o$ = 350

[Osm]$_i$ = 350
Vol = 86%

4 Urea begins to enter the cell. Water follows it in osmotically.

[Osm]$_o$ = 350

[Osm]$_i$ = 350
Vol = increasing

Swelling of compartment × 1.2

5 Urea equilibrates across the cell membrane. The cell volume is now the same as in the top panel and the osmolalities are the same on both sides of the membrane, 350 mOsm.

[Osm]$_o$ = 350

[Osm]$_i$ = 350
Vol = 100%

FIGURE 3–16. Effect of urea on cell volume. Because the cell membrane is far more permeable to water than to urea, we will assume that, during the initial moments in *steps 2* and *3*, the cell membrane is permeable only to water. Later, during *steps 4* and *5*, we assume that the membrane is permeable to both water and urea.

utes, total and effective osmolality of the ECF can be approximated as

Equation 3–30

$$\text{Total osmolality (mOsm)} = 2 \cdot [\text{Na}^+] + \frac{\text{Glucose (mg/dl)}}{18} + \frac{\text{BUN (mg/dl)}}{2.8}$$

$$\text{Tonicity or Effective osmolality (mOsm)} = 2 \cdot [\text{Na}^+] + \frac{\text{Glucose (mg/dl)}}{18}$$

BUN stands for blood urea nitrogen, that is, the concentration of the nitrogen that is contained in the plasma as urea. In Equation 3–30, the clinical laboratory reports [Na$^+$] in milliequivalents per liter. Because the laboratory reports the glucose and BUN concentrations in terms of milligrams per deciliter, we divide "glucose" by one tenth of the molecular weight of glucose and "BUN" by one tenth of the summed atomic weights of the two nitrogen atoms in urea. The computed "tonicity" does not include BUN because—as we saw earlier—urea easily equilibrates across most cell membranes. On the other hand, the computed tonicity includes both Na$^+$ and glucose. It includes Na$^+$ because Na$^+$ is *functionally* impermeant owing to its extrusion by the Na-K pump. Tonicity includes glucose because this solute does not appreciably accumulate in most cells as a result of metabolism. In some clinical situations, the infusion of impermeant solutes, such as radiographic contrast agents or mannitol, can also contribute to tonicity of the ECF.

Osmolality describes the number of osmotically active solutes in a single solution. If we regard a plasma osmolality of 290 mOsm as being normal, solutions having an osmolality of 290 mOsm are **isosmolal**, solutions with osmolalities above 290 mOsm are hyperosmolal, and those with osmolalities below 290 mOsm are hypo-osmolal. On the other hand, when we use the terms *isotonic*, *hypertonic*, and *hypotonic*, we are comparing one solution with another solution (e.g., ICF) across a well-defined membrane (e.g., a cell membrane). A solution is **isotonic** when its *effective* osmolality is the same as that of the reference solution, which for our purposes is the ICF. A **hypertonic** solution is one that has a higher effective osmolality than the reference solution, and a **hypotonic** solution has a lower effective osmolality.

Shifts of water between the intracellular and interstitial compartments result from alterations in *effective* ECF osmolality, or *tonicity*. Clinically, such changes in tonicity are usually caused by decreases in [Na$^+$] in the plasma and ECF (hyponatremia); increases in [Na$^+$] (hypernatremia); or increases in glucose concentration (hyperglycemia). Changes in the concentration of a highly permeant solute such as urea, which accumulates in patients with kidney failure, have no effect on tonicity.

WATER EXCHANGE ACROSS THE CAPILLARY WALL. The barrier separating the blood plasma and interstitial compartments, the capillary wall, is—to a first approximation—freely permeable to solutes that are smaller than plasma proteins. Thus, the only *net* osmotic force that acts across the capillary wall is that caused by the asymmetric distribution of proteins in plasma versus interstitial fluid. Several terms may be used for the osmotic force that is generated by these impermeant plasma proteins, such as protein osmotic pressure, colloid osmotic pressure, and oncotic pressure. These terms are synonymous and can be represented by the symbol $\pi_{oncotic}$. The **oncotic pressure difference** ($\Delta\pi_{oncotic}$), which tends to pull water from the interstitium to the plasma, is opposed by the hydrostatic pressure difference across the capillary wall (ΔP), which drives fluid from plasma into the interstitium. All net movements of water across the capillary wall are accompanied by the small solutes dissolved in this water, at their ECF concentrations; that is, the pathways taken by the water across the capillary wall are so large that small solutes are not *sieved* out.

To summarize, fluid shifts between plasma and the interstitium respond only to changes in the balance between ΔP and $\Delta\pi_{oncotic}$. Small solutes such as Na^+, which freely cross the capillary wall, do not contribute significantly to osmotic driving forces across this barrier and move along with the water in which they are dissolved. We will return to this subject when we discuss the physiology of capillaries in Chapter 19.

Adding Isotonic Saline, Pure Water, or Pure NaCl to the ECF Will All Increase ECF Volume but Will Have Divergent Effects on ICF Volume and ECF Osmolality

Adding various combinations of NaCl and solute-free water to the ECF will alter the volume and composition of the body-fluid compartments. Three examples illustrate the effects seen with intravenous therapy. In Figure 3–17A, we start with a TBW of 42 liters (60% of a 70-kg person), subdivided into an ICF volume of 25 liters (60% of TBW) and an ECF volume of 17 liters (40% of TBW). These numerical values are the same as those in Figure 3–1 and Table 3–1.

INFUSION OF ISOTONIC SALINE. Consider the case in which we infuse or ingest 1.5 liters of "isotonic saline," which is a 0.9% solution of NaCl in water (Fig. 3–17B). This solution has an effective osmolality of 290 mOsm in the ECF. This 1.5 liters is initially distributed throughout the ECF and raises ECF volume by 1.5 liters. Because the effective osmolality of the ECF is unaltered, no change occurs in the effective osmotic gradient across the cell membranes, and the added water neither moves into nor out of the ICF. This outcome is, of course, in accord with the definition of an *isotonic* solution. Thus, we see that adding isotonic saline to the body is a very efficient way to expand the ECF without affecting the ICF. Similarly, if it were possible to remove isotonic saline from the body, we would see that this measure would efficiently contract the ECF and again have no effect on the ICF.

INFUSION OF "SOLUTE-FREE" WATER. Now consider a case in which we either ingest 1.5 liters of pure water or infuse 1.5 liters of an isotonic ("5%") glucose solution (Fig. 3–17C). Infusing the glucose solution intravenously is equivalent, in the long run, to infusing pure water because the glucose is metabolized to CO_2 and water,

with no solutes left behind in the ECF. Infusing pure water would be unwise inasmuch as it would cause the cells near the point of infusion to burst.

How do the effects of adding 1.5 liters of pure water compare with those of the previous example? At first, the 1.5 liters of pure water will be rapidly distributed throughout the ECF and increase its volume from 17 to 18.5 liters (see Fig. 3–17C, *Early*). This added water will also dilute the pre-existing solutes in the ECF, thereby lowering ECF osmolality to 290 mOsm × 17/18.5 = 266 mOsm. Because intracellular osmolality remains at 290 mOsm at this imaginary, intermediate stage, a large osmotic gradient is created that favors the entry of water from the ECF into the ICF. Water will move into the ICF and consequently lower the osmolality of the ICF and simultaneously raise the osmolality of the ECF until osmotic equilibrium is restored (see Fig. 3–17C, *Final*). Because the added water is distributed between the ICF and ECF according to the initial ICF/ECF ratio of 60%/40%, the final ECF volume is 17.6 liters (i.e., 17 liters expanded by 40% of 1.5 liters). Thus infusion of solute-free water is a relatively *ineffective* means of expanding the ECF. More of the added water has ended up intracellularly (60% of 1.5 liters = 0.9 liter of expansion). The major effect of the water has been to dilute the osmolality of body fluids. The initial total body solute content was 290 mOsm × 42 liters = 12,180 milliosmoles. This same solute has now been diluted in 42 + 1.5 or 43.5 liters, so the final osmolality is 12,180/43.5 = 280 mOsm.

INGESTION OF PURE NaCl SALT. The above two "experiments" illustrate two extremely important principles that govern fluid and electrolyte homeostasis, namely, that adding or removing Na^+ will mainly affect ECF volume (see Fig. 3–17B), whereas adding or removing solute-free water will mainly affect the *osmolality* of body fluids (see Fig. 3–17C). The first point can be further appreciated by considering a third case, one in which we add the same amount of NaCl that is contained in 1.5 liters of isotonic (i.e., 0.9%) saline: 1.5 liters × 290 mOsm = 435 milliosmoles. However, we will not add any water. At first, this 435 milliosmoles of NaCl will rapidly distribute throughout the 17 liters of ECF and increase the osmolality of the ECF (Fig. 3–17D, *Early*). The initial, total osmolal content of the ECF was 290 mOsm × 17 liters = 4930 milliosmoles. Because we added 435 milliosmoles, we now have 5365 milliosmoles in the ECF. Thus, the ECF osmolality is 5365/17 = 316 mOsm. The resulting hyperosmolality draws water out of the ICF into the ECF until osmotic equilibrium is re-established. What is the final osmolality? The total number of milliosmoles dissolved in TBW is the original 12,180 milliosmoles plus the added 435 milliosmoles, for a total of 12,615 milliosmoles. Because these milliosmoles are dissolved in 42 liters of TBW, the final osmolality of the ICF and ECF is 12,615/42 = 300 mOsm. In the new equilibrium state, the ECF volume has increased by 0.9 liter even though no water at all was added to the body. Because the added ECF volume has come from the ICF, the ICF shrinks by 0.9 liter. This example further illustrates the principle that the total body content of Na^+ is the major determinant of ECF volume.

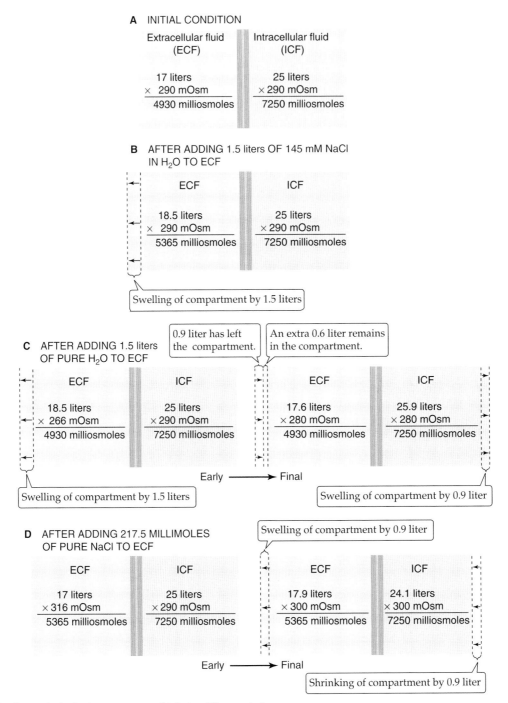

FIGURE 3–17. Effect on body fluid compartments of infusing different solutions.

Whole-Body Na+ Content Determines ECF Volume, Whereas Whole-Body Water Content Determines Osmolality

Changes in ECF volume are important because they are accompanied by proportional changes in the volume of blood plasma, which in turn affects the adequacy with which the circulatory system can perfuse vital organs with blood. The blood volume that is necessary to achieve adequate perfusion of key organs is sometimes referred to as the **effective circulating volume**. Because the body

generally stabilizes osmolality, an increase in extracellular Na+ content will increase ECF volume:

Equation 3–31

$$\underbrace{\text{Extracellular Na}^+ \text{ content}}_{\text{millimoles}} = \underbrace{[\text{Na}^+]_o}_{\text{millimoles/liter}} \times \underbrace{\text{ECF volume}}_{\text{liters}}$$

$$\cong \left(\frac{\text{Osmolality}}{2}\right) \times \underbrace{\text{ECF volume}}_{\text{liters}}$$

Because cells contain very little Na^+, extracellular Na^+ content is nearly the same as **total-body Na^+ content.**

We will see in Chapter 39 how the body regulates effective circulating volume—increases in effective circulating volume, which reflect increases in ECF volume or total-body Na^+ *content*, stimulate the renal excretion of Na^+. In contrast, the plasma Na^+ *concentration* does *not* regulate renal excretion of Na^+. It makes sense that regulation of Na^+ excretion is not sensitive to the plasma Na^+ concentration because the concentration is not an indicator of ECF volume.

As discussed, when we hold osmolality constant, Na^+ content determines ECF volume. What would happen if we held constant the Na^+ content, which is a major part of total-body osmoles? An increase in **total-body water** would decrease **osmolality**.

$$\underbrace{\text{Total-body osmoles}}_{\text{milliosmoles}} = \underbrace{[\text{Osmolality}]}_{\text{milliosmoles/liter}} \times \underbrace{\text{Total-body water}}_{\text{liters}}$$

Equation 3–32

Thus, a net gain or loss of solute-free water has a major impact on the *osmolality* and [Na^+] of the ECF. Moreover, because a large part (~60%) of the added solute-free water distributes into the ICF, a gain or loss of solute-free water affects ICF more than ECF. We will see in Chapter 39 how the body regulates osmolality: a small decrease in osmolality triggers osmoreceptors to diminish thirst (resulting in diminished intake of solute-free water) and increase renal water excretion. In emergency states of very low ECF and effective circulating volume, some crosstalk occurs between the volume- and osmolality-control systems. As a result, the body will not only try to conserve Na^+ but will also seek water (by triggering thirst) and conserve water (by concentrating the urine). Although water (in comparison to saline) is not a very good expander of plasma and ECF volume, it is better than nothing.

EPITHELIAL TRANSPORT

Thus far we have examined how cells transport solutes and water across their membranes and thereby control their intracellular composition. We now turn our attention to how the body controls the "milieu interieur," namely, the ECF that bathes the cells. Just as the cell membrane is the barrier between the ICF and ECF, epithelia are the barriers that separate the ECF from the outside world. In this subchapter we will examine the fundamental principles of how epithelial cells transport solutes and water across epithelial barriers.

An epithelium is an uninterrupted sheet of cells that are joined together by junctional complexes (p. 46). These junctions serve as a selectively permeable barrier between the solutions on either side of the epithelium and demarcate the boundary between the apical and basolateral regions of the cell membrane. The apical and basolateral membranes are remarkably different in their transport function. This polarization allows the epithelial cell to transport water and selected solutes from one compartment to another. In other words, the epithelium is capable of vectorial transport. In many cases, transport of solutes across an epithelium is an active process.

Membranes may be called by different names in different epithelia: the **apical membrane** can be known as the brush border, the mucosal membrane, or the luminal membrane; the **basolateral membrane** is also known as the serosal or peritubular membrane.

The Epithelial Cell Generally Has Different Electrochemical Gradients Across Its Apical and Basolateral Membranes

Imagine an artificial situation in which an epithelium separates two identical solutions. Furthermore, imagine that there is no difference in voltage across the epithelium, and no difference in hydrostatic pressure. Under these circumstances, the driving forces for the *passive movement* of solutes or water across the epithelium would be nil. Because the apical and basolateral membranes of the cell share the same cytosol, the electrochemical gradients across the apical and basolateral membranes would be identical.

However, this example is virtually never realistic for two reasons. First, because the composition of the "outside world" is not the same as that of ECF, transepithelial concentration differences occur. Second, transepithelial voltage is not zero. Thus, the electrochemical gradients across the apical and basolateral membranes of an epithelial cell are generally very different.

Electrophysiologic methods provide two major types of information about ion transport by epithelial cells. First, electrophysiologic techniques can define the electrical driving forces that act on ions either across the entire epithelium or across the individual apical and basolateral cell membranes. Second, these electrical measurements can define the overall electrical resistance of the epithelium or the electrical resistance of the individual apical and basolateral cell membranes.

The voltage difference between the solutions on either side of the epithelium is the **transepithelial voltage** (V_{te}). We can measure V_{te} by placing one microelectrode in the lumen of the organ or duct of which the epithelium is the wall and a second "reference" electrode in the blood or interstitial space (Fig. 3–18A). If we instead insert the first microelectrode directly into an epithelial cell (Fig. 3–18B), the voltage difference between this cell and the "reference" electrode in blood or the interstitial space measures the **basolateral cell membrane potential** (V_{bl}). Finally, if we compare the intracellular electrode with a reference electrode in the lumen (Fig. 3–18C), the voltage difference is the **apical cell membrane potential** (V_a). Obviously, the sum of V_a and V_{bl} is equal to the transepithelial voltage. It is also possible to insert ion-sensitive microelectrodes into the lumen or the epithelial cells and thereby determine the local activity of ions such as Na^+, K^+, H^+, Ca^{2+}, and Cl^-.

By using the same voltage electrodes that we introduced in the previous paragraph, we can pass electrical

A TRANSEPITHELIAL VOLTAGE

V_{te}

Lumen

Interstitial space

Cell

B BASOLATERAL MEMBRANE POTENTIAL

V_{bl}

Lumen

Interstitial space

Cell

C APICAL MEMBRANE POTENTIAL

V_a

Lumen

Interstitial space

Cell

D ELECTRICAL PROFILE ACROSS AN EPITHELIAL CELL

Lumen   Cell   Interstitial space

0 mV

V_{te}

−3 mV

V_a V_{bl}

−70 mV

FIGURE 3–18. Measurement of voltage in an epithelium. *A,* The voltage difference between electrodes placed in the lumen and interstitial space (or blood) is V_{te}. *B,* The voltage difference between electrodes placed in the cell and interstitial space is V_{bl}. *C,* The voltage difference between electrodes placed in the lumen and cell is V_a. *D,* Relative to the reference voltage of zero in the interstitial space, the voltage inside the cell in this example is −70 millivolts (mV), and the voltage in the lumen is −3 mV. These values are typical of a cell in the renal proximal tubule or a small intestine.

current across either the whole epithelium or the individual apical and basolateral membranes. From Ohm's law it is thus possible to calculate the **electrical resistance** of the entire wall of the epithelium, or transepithelial resistance (R_{te}); that of the apical membrane, or apical resistance (R_a); or that of the basolateral membrane, or basolateral resistance (R_{bl}).

Tight and Leaky Epithelia Differ in the Permeabilities of Their Tight Junctions

One measure of how tightly an epithelium separates one compartment from another is its resistance to the flow of electrical current. The range of transepithelial electrical resistance is quite large. For example, 1 cm^2 of a rat

proximal tubule has a resistance of only 6 Ω, whereas 1 cm^2 of a rabbit urinary bladder has a resistance of 70,000 Ω. Why is the range of R_{te} values so great? The cells of these epithelia do not differ greatly in either their apical- or basolateral-membrane resistances. Instead, the epithelia with low electrical resistances have a low-resistance pathway located in their tight junctions. Epithelia are thus classified as either "tight" (high electrical resistance) or "leaky," depending on the relative resistance of their tight junctions. In other words, the tight junctions of leaky epithelia are relatively more permeant to the diffusion of ions than the tight junctions of tight epithelia.

Now that we have introduced the concept that solutes and water can move between epithelial cells via tight junctions, we can define two distinct pathways by which

A Na⁺ ABSORPTION ("USSING MODEL")

Na⁺ enters across apical membrane via channels, but is pumped out across basolateral membrane.

The K⁺ pumped into cell recycles back out.

3 Na⁺

3 Na⁺

2 K⁺

Epithelial cell

ATP

Apical membrane

Basolateral membrane

Tight junction

2 K⁺

Exterior milieu (lumen)

3 Cl⁻

Interstitial space

The lumen is negative compared with interstitium.

B K⁺ SECRETION

3 Na⁺

3 Na⁺

2 K⁺

ATP

K⁺

K⁺

2 Cl⁻

C GLUCOSE ABSORPTION

This cotransporter cycles three times.

3 Na⁺

2 K⁺

ATP

3 Na⁺

3 Glucose

2 K⁺

3 Glucose

3 Cl⁻

D Cl⁻ SECRETION

3 Na⁺

2 K⁺

6 Cl⁻

ATP

5 K⁺

3 K⁺

3 Na⁺

6 Na⁺

6 Cl⁻

This cotransporter cycles three times.

FIGURE 3–19. Models of epithelial solute transport.

substances can cross epithelia. First, a substance can cross through the cell by sequentially passing across the apical and then the basolateral membranes, or vice versa. This route is called the **transcellular pathway**. Second, a substance can bypass the cell entirely and cross the epithelium via the tight junctions and lateral intercellular spaces. This route is called the **paracellular pathway**.

As might be expected, leaky epithelia are not very good at maintaining large transepithelial ion or osmotic gradients. Generally, **leaky epithelia** perform bulk transepithelial transport of solutes and water in a nearly isosmotic fashion (i.e., the transported fluid has about the same osmolality as the fluid from which it came). Examples include the small intestine and the proximal tubule of the kidney. As a general rule, **tight epithelia** generate or maintain large transepithelial ion-concentration or osmotic gradients. Examples include the distal nephron of the

kidney, the large intestine, and the tightest of all epithelia, the urinary bladder (whose function is to be an absolutely impermeable storage vessel).

In addition to tight junctions, epithelia share a number of basic properties First, the Na-K pump is located exclusively on the basolateral membrane (Fig. 3–19). The only known exception is the choroid plexus, where the Na-K pump is located on the apical membrane.

Second, most of the K⁺ that is taken up by the Na⁺ pump generally recycles back out across the basolateral membrane through K⁺ channels (see Fig. 3–19). A consequence of the abundance of these K⁺ channels is that the K⁺ gradient predominantly determines V_{bl}, which is usually 50 to 60 mV, inside negative.

Third, as in other cells, $[Na^+]_i$, typically 10 to 30 mM, is much lower in an epithelial cell than the ECF. This low $[Na^+]_i$ is a consequence of the active extrusion of Na⁺ by the Na-K pump. The large, inwardly directed Na^+ electrochemical gradient serves as a driving force for Na^+ entry through apical Na^+ channels and for the secondary active transport of other solutes across the apical membrane (e.g., via Na/glucose cotransport, Na-H exchange, Na/K/Cl cotransport) or basolateral membrane (e.g., via Na-Ca exchange).

Epithelial Cells Can Absorb or Secrete Different Solutes by Inserting Specific Channels or Transporters at Either the Apical or Basolateral Membrane

By placing different transporters at the apical and basolateral membranes, epithelia can accomplish net transepithelial transport of different solutes in either the absorptive or secretory direction. For example, the renal proximal tubule moves glucose from the tubule lumen to the blood by using an Na/glucose cotransporter (SGLT) to move glucose into the cell across the apical membrane, but it uses facilitated diffusion of glucose (GLUT) to move glucose out of the cell across the basolateral membrane. Clearly, the proximal tubule cell could not use the same Na/glucose cotransporter at both the apical and basolateral membranes because the electrochemical Na^+ gradient is very similar across both membranes.

We will now look at four examples to illustrate how epithelia can absorb or secrete various solutes by using the transporters discussed earlier in this chapter.

Na^+ **ABSORPTION.** Consider the model in Figure 3–19A, which is similar to that first proposed by Hans Ussing and coworkers to explain NaCl absorption across the frog skin. The basolateral Na-K pump pumps Na^+ out of the cell, thereby lowering $[Na^+]_i$ and generating an inward Na^+ electrochemical gradient across the apical membrane. This apical Na^+ gradient in turn provides the driving force for Na^+ to enter the cell passively across the apical membrane through ENaC Na^+ channels. The Na^+ that enters the cell in this way is pumped out across the basolateral membrane in exchange for K^+, which recycles back out across the basolateral membrane. Note that the Na-K pump generates a current of positive charge across the cell from lumen to interstitium. This current, in turn, creates a lumen-negative transepithelial voltage that can then provide a driving force for passive Cl^- absorption across the tight junctions—via the so-called paracellular pathway. The net result is NaCl absorption. This process is the mechanism for NaCl reabsorption in the collecting tubule of the kidney.

K^+ **SECRETION.** With slight alterations, the same basic cell model can perform K^+ secretion as well as Na^+ absorption (Fig. 3–19B). Adding K^+ channels to the apical membrane allows some of the K^+ that is taken up by the Na-K pump across the basolateral membrane to be secreted across the apical membrane. This mechanism is the basis of K^+ secretion in the collecting tubule of the kidney. Such a model accurately predicts that drugs such as amiloride, which blocks apical ENaC Na^+ channels in these cells, will inhibit K^+ secretion as well as Na^+ reabsorption.

GLUCOSE ABSORPTION. The small intestine and proximal tubule absorb nutrients that are present in the luminal compartment by secondary active cotransport of Na^+ with organic solutes. An example is Na^+ cotransport with glucose via SGLT (Fig. 3–19C). The inwardly directed electrochemical Na^+ gradient across the apical membrane, generated by the Na-K pump, now drives the entry of both Na^+ and glucose. Glucose, which has accumulated in the cell against its concentration gradient, exits passively across the basolateral membrane by a carrier-mediated transporter (GLUT) that is not coupled to Na^+. Again, the flow of positive current across the cell generates a lumen-negative transepithelial voltage that can drive passive Cl^- absorption across the tight junctions. The net effect is to absorb both NaCl and glucose.

Cl^- **SECRETION.** If the cell places an Na^+-coupled Cl^--entry mechanism on the basolateral membrane, the same basic cell model can mediate NaCl *secretion* into the lumen (Fig. 3–19D). The inwardly directed Na^+ electrochemical gradient now drives secondary active Cl^- uptake across the basolateral membrane via the Na/K/Cl cotransporter NKCC1. Cl^- accumulated in the cell in this way can then exit across the apical membrane passively through Cl^- channels such as CFTR. Notice that negative charges now move across the cell from interstitium to lumen and generate a lumen-negative voltage that can drive passive Na^+ secretion across the tight junctions (paracellular pathway). The net process is NaCl secretion, even though the primary active transporter, the Na-K pump, is pumping Na^+ from the cell to the interstitium. Secretory cells in the intestine and pulmonary-airway epithelium use this mechanism for secreting NaCl.

Water Transport Across Epithelia Passively Follows Solute Transport

In general, water moves passively across an epithelium in response to osmotic gradients. An epithelium that secretes salt will secrete fluid, and one that absorbs salt will absorb fluid.

The finite permeability of the bare lipid bilayer to water, and the presence of water channels in most cells, ensure that osmotic equilibration for most cells is rapid. Additionally, particularly in "leaky epithelia," tight junctions provide a pathway for water movement between the epithelial cells. However, epithelial water permeability ("hydraulic conductivity") varies widely because of differences in membrane-lipid composition and in abundance of water channels. The presence of water channels in the plasma membrane may be either constitutive or highly regulated. Some epithelia have a high salt-transport rate and low water permeability (approximately equal to that of the bare lipid bilayer), and thus can generate a large transepithelial osmotic gradient. An example is the thick ascending limb of the loop of Henle in the kidney, which reabsorbs a large amount of salt but relatively little water. As a result, dilute fluid is left behind in the lumen. In contrast, the water permeability of the renal collecting duct is variable and under hormonal control via arginine vasopressin, which regulates insertion of AQP2 water channels into the apical membrane.

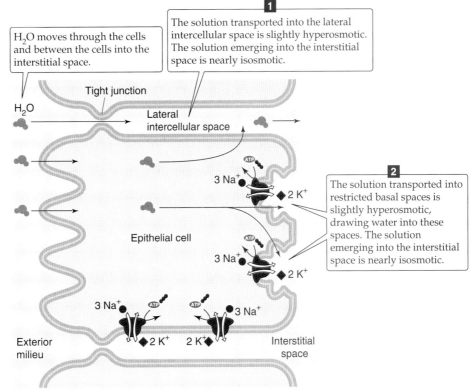

> **1**
> The solution transported into the lateral intercellular space is slightly hyperosmotic. The solution emerging into the interstitial space is nearly isosmotic.

> H₂O moves through the cells and between the cells into the interstitial space.

> **2**
> The solution transported into restricted basal spaces is slightly hyperosmotic, drawing water into these spaces. The solution emerging into the interstitial space is nearly isosmotic.

FIGURE 3–20. Model of "isotonic" water transport in a leaky epithelium. Na-K pumps present on the lateral and basal membrane pump Na⁺ into two restricted spaces: the lateral intercellular space and restricted spaces formed by infoldings of the basal membrane. The locally high osmolality in the lateral intercellular space pulls water from the lumen and the cell. Similarly, the locally high osmolality in the restricted basal spaces pulls water from the cell. The solution that emerges from these two restricted spaces—and enters the interstitial space—is only slightly hypertonic (virtually "isotonic") compared with the luminal solution. ATP, Adenosine triphosphate.

In certain epithelia, such as the renal proximal tubule and small intestine, net water movement occurs with no detectable osmotic gradients across the epithelium (Fig. 3–20). Moreover, the reabsorbed fluid appears to be isosmotic with respect to luminal fluid. Of course, fluid absorption could not really occur without the requisite solute driving force across the epithelium. Two explanations, which are not exclusive, have been offered.

First, the water permeability of epithelia performing "isosmotic" water reabsorption might be extremely high because of the high constitutive expression of aquaporin water channels in the apical and basolateral membranes. Thus, very modest trans-epithelial osmotic gradients (perhaps only 1 to 2 mOsm), which are the product of solute absorption, are sufficient to drive water transport at the rates observed. Measurements cannot distinguish such small osmotic gradients from no gradient at all.

Second, the lateral intercellular spaces between the epithelial cells ("lateral interspaces"—Fig. 3–20, *option 1*), as well as the spaces between the infoldings of the basal membrane ("basal labyrinth"—Fig. 3–20, *option 2*), might be modestly hyperosmotic as a consequence of the accumulation of absorbed solutes in a localized region. The resulting localized osmotic gradient would pull water into the lateral interspaces from the cell (across the lateral portion of the basolateral membrane) or from the lumen (across the tight junction). Similarly, a localized osmotic gradient would pull water into the basal labyrinth from the cell (across the basal portion of the basolateral membrane). By the time that the fluid emerges from these spaces and reaches the interstitium, it would have become nearly isosmotic.

Epithelia Can Regulate Transport by Controlling Transport Proteins, Tight Junctions, and the Supply of the Transported Substances

A large range of physiological stimuli regulate the rates at which specific epithelia transport specific solutes. Virtually all known intracellular signalling cascades (see Chapter 4) have been implicated in mediating these regulatory effects. Ultimately, these cascades must affect the rates at which specific solutes move through transporters and/or channels.

INCREASED SYNTHESIS (OR DEGRADATION) OF TRANSPORT PROTEINS. One approach for modifying transport activity is to change the number of transport molecules in the cell. For example, the hormone aldosterone directly or indirectly increases the transcription rate of genes that encode Na-K pump subunits, thereby increasing Na-K pump synthesis in the distal nephron of the kidney.

RECRUITMENT OF TRANSPORT PROTEINS TO THE CELL MEMBRANE. Cells can also change the functional activity of transporters by storing some of them in an intracellular organelle "pool" and then inserting them into the cell membrane. For example, histamine causes cytoplasmic "tubulovesicles" containing H-K pumps (the "pool") to fuse with the apical membrane of gastric parietal cells, thereby initiating gastric-acid secretion.

POST-TRANSLATIONAL MODIFICATION OF PRE-EXISTING TRANSPORT PROTEINS. Another approach for modulating the transporter rate is to change the activity of pre-existing transport proteins. For example, increases in the level of intracellular cyclic adenosine monophosphate (cAMP) enhance the phosphorylation of apical-membrane Cl^- channels that are involved in NaCl secretion by intestinal and airway epithelia. The cystic fibrosis gene product (CFTR) is a Cl^- channel whose function is regulated by phosphorylation. A defect in the regulation of apical-membrane Cl^- channels is the primary physiologic abnormality in cystic fibrosis.

CHANGES IN THE PARACELLULAR PATHWAY. The passive movement of solutes across the tight junction can contribute to either "forward" transepithelial movement of the solute or backleak of the solute, depending on the solute gradients. Thus, the epithelium can modulate net transport by changing the permeability of the paracellular pathway. For example, the Na^+ permeability of the tight junctions of the proximal tubule increases when ECF volume increases. This increase in the permeability of the paracellular pathway may lower net Na^+ reabsorption because of increased backleak of absorbed Na^+ from the lateral interspace, across the tight junction, and into the lumen.

LUMINAL SUPPLY OF TRANSPORTED SPECIES. Changes in the concentration of transported solutes can have profound effects on rates of net solute transport. As fluid moves along the renal proximal tubule, for example, the very process of glucose absorption depletes glucose from the lumen, thereby slowing further glucose absorption. Increasing the rate at which fresh, high-glucose fluid enters the proximal-tubule lumen raises the glucose concentration at the site of glucose uptake, and thus increases the rate of glucose absorption.

REFERENCES

Books and Reviews

Alper SL: The band 3–related anion exchanger (AE) gene family. Annu Rev Physiol 53:549–564, 1991.

Boyer PD: The ATP synthase—a splendid molecular machine. Annu Rev Biochem 66:717–749, 1997.

Kaplan MR, Mount DB, Delpire E, et al: Molecular mechanisms of NaCl cotransport. Annu Rev Physiol 58:649–668, 1996.

Lang F, Busch GL, Ritter M, et al: Functional significance of cell volume regulatory mechanisms. Physiol Rev 78:247–306, 1998.

Palacin M, Estevez R, Bertran J, Zorzano A: Molecular biology of mammalian plasma membrane amino acid transporters. Physiol Rev 78:969–1054, 1998.

Steel A, Hediger MA: The molecular physiology of sodium- and proton-coupled solute transporters. News Physiol Sci 13:123–131, 1998.

Journal Articles

Canessa CM, Schild L, Buell G, et al: Amiloride-sensitive epithelial Na^+ channel is made of three homologous subunits. Nature 367:463–467, 1994.

Hediger MA, Coady MJ, Ikeda IS, Wright EM: Expression cloning and cDNA sequencing of the Na^+/glucose transporter. Nature 330:379–381, 1987.

Preston GM, Agre P: Isolation of the cDNA for erythrocyte integral membrane protein of 28 kilodaltons: Member of an ancient channel family. Proc Natl Acad Sci U S A 88:1110–1114, 1991.

Skou JC: The influence of some cations on an adenosine triphosphatase from peripheral nerves. Biochim Biophys Acta 23:394–401, 1957.

CHAPTER 4

Signal Transduction

Laura M. Roman

The evolution of multicellular organisms necessitated the development of mechanisms to tightly coordinate the activities among cells. Such **communication** is fundamental to all biological processes, ranging from the induction of embryonic development to the integration of physiological responses in the face of environmental challenges.

Classically, neural and endocrine tissues have been considered the major signalling systems. However, as our understanding of cellular and molecular physiology has increased, it has become evident that all cells can receive and process information. External **signals** such as odorants, chemicals that reflect metabolic status, ions, hormones, growth factors, and neurotransmitters can all serve as **chemical messengers** linking neighboring or distant cells. Even external signals that are not considered chemical in nature (e.g., light and mechanical or thermal stimuli) may ultimately be transduced into a chemical messenger. Most chemical messengers interact with specific **cell-surface receptors** and trigger a cascade of secondary events, including the mobilization of diffusible intracellular **second-messenger systems** that mediate the cell's response to that stimulus. However, hydrophobic messengers, such as steroid hormones and some vitamins, can diffuse across the plasma membrane and interact with **cytosolic or nuclear receptors**. It is now clear that cells use a number of different, often intersecting, intracellular signalling pathways to ensure that the cell's response to a stimulus is tightly controlled.

MECHANISMS OF CELLULAR COMMUNICATION

Some Cells Communicate with Each Other by Direct Contact Through Gap Junctions

Neighboring cells can be electrically and metabolically coupled by means of **gap junctions** formed between apposing cell membranes (p. 164). These water-filled channels facilitate the passage of inorganic ions and small molecules, such as Ca^{2+} and $3',5'$-cyclic adenosine monophosphate (cAMP), from the cytoplasm of one cell into the cytoplasm of an adjacent cell. Mammalian gap junctions permit the passage of molecules that are less than approximately 1200 Da but restrict the movement of molecules that are greater than approximately 2000 Da. Gap junctions are also excellent pathways for the flow of electrical current, which plays a critical role in coordinating the electrical activity in cardiac and smooth muscle.

FIGURE 4–1. Modes of cell communication.

A gap junction consists of two "half" channels that are arranged end to end in the membranes of adjacent cells (see Fig. 6–18). Each half channel has six **connexin** molecules surrounding a hollow core. Gap junctions alternate between an open and closed state. The permeability of gap junctions can be rapidly regulated by changes in cytosolic concentrations of Ca^{2+}, cAMP, and H^+, as well as the voltage across the cell membrane or membrane potential (V_m) (p. 55). This type of modulation is physiologically important for cell-to-cell communication. For example, the extracellular Ca^{2+} concentration ($[Ca^{2+}]_o$) is approximately 10^{-3} M, whereas the intracellular concentration ($[Ca^{2+}]_i$) is approximately 10^{-7} M. If a cell's plasma membrane is damaged, Ca^{2+} will passively move into the cell and raise $[Ca^{2+}]_i$ to toxic levels. Elevated *intra*cellular $[Ca^{2+}]$ in the damaged cell triggers closure of the gap junctions, thus preventing the flow of excessive amounts of Ca^{2+} into the adjacent cell.

Cells Can Communicate with One Another via Chemical Signals

Early insight into signal-transduction pathways was obtained from studies of the endocrine system. The classic definition of a **hormone** is *a substance that is produced in one tissue or organ and released into the blood and carried to other organs (targets), where it acts to produce a specific response.* The idea of endocrine or ductless glands developed from the recognition that certain organs—such as the pituitary, adrenal, and thyroid gland—can synthesize and release specific chemical messengers in response to particular physiological states. However, many other cells and tissues—not classically thought of as endocrine in nature—also produce hormones. For example, the kidney produces 1,25-dihydroxyvitamin D_3, and the salivary gland synthesizes nerve growth factor (NGF).

It is now recognized that intercellular communication can involve the production of a "hormone" or chemical signal by one cell type that acts in any (or all) of three ways, as illustrated in Figure 4–1: on distant tissues (**en-docrine**), on a neighboring cell in the same tissue (**para-crine**), or on the same cell that released the signalling molecule (**autocrine**). For paracrine and autocrine signals to be delivered to their proper targets, their diffusion must be limited. This restriction can be accomplished by rapid endocytosis of the chemical signal by neighboring cells, its destruction by extracellular enzymes, or its immobilization by the extracellular matrix. The events that take place at the neuromuscular junction are excellent examples of paracrine signalling. When an electrical impulse travels down an axon and reaches the nerve terminal (Fig. 4–2), it stimulates release of the neurotransmitter acetylcholine (ACh). In turn, ACh transiently activates a ligand-gated cation channel on the muscle cell membrane. The resultant transient influx of Na^+ causes a localized positive shift of V_m (i.e., depolarization), initiating events that result in propagation of an action potential along the muscle cell. The ACh signal is rapidly terminated by the action of acetylcholinesterase, which is present in the synaptic cleft. This enzyme degrades the ACh that is released by the neuron.

Chemical Signals Interact with Target Cells by Binding to Surface or Intracellular Receptors

Four types of chemicals can serve as extracellular signalling molecules: **amines**, such as epinephrine; **peptides and proteins**, such as angiotensin II and insulin; **steroids**, including aldosterone, estrogens, and retinoic acid; and other **small molecules**, such as amino acids, nucleotides, ions (e.g., Ca^{2+}), and gases (e.g., nitric oxide).

For a molecule to act as a signal, it must bind to a **receptor**. A receptor is a protein (or in some cases a lipoprotein) on the cell surface or within the cell that specifically binds a signalling molecule (the ligand). In some cases, the receptor is itself an ion channel, and ligand binding produces a change in V_m. Thus, the cell can transduce a signal with no machinery other than the receptor. In most cases, however, interaction of the ligand with one or more specific receptors results in an associa-

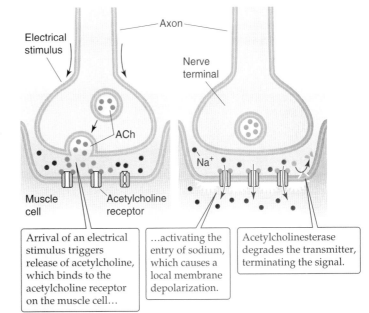

FIGURE 4–2. Example of paracrine signalling. The release of acetylcholine at the neuromuscular junction is a form of paracrine signalling because the nerve terminal releases a chemical (i.e., acetylcholine) that acts on a neighboring cell (i.e., the muscle). ACh, acetylcholine.

tion of the receptor with an effector molecule that initiates a cellular response. Effectors include enzymes, channels, transport proteins, contractile elements, and transcription factors. The ability of a cell or tissue to respond to a specific signal is dictated by the complement of receptors it possesses and by the chain of intracellular reactions that are initiated by the binding of any one ligand to its receptor. Receptors can be divided into four categories based on their associated mechanisms of signal transduction (Table 4–1), in addition to a fifth class of membrane-signalling molecules that do not fit the classic definition of a receptor.

1. **Ligand-gated ion channels**. Integral membrane proteins, these hybrid receptor/channels are involved in signalling between electrically excitable cells. The binding of a neurotransmitter such as ACh to its receptor—which in fact is merely part of the channel—results in transient opening of the channel, thus altering the ion permeability of the cell.
2. **G-protein–coupled receptors**. These integral plasma membrane proteins work indirectly—through an intermediary—to activate or inactivate a separate membrane-associated enzyme or channel. The intermediary is a heterotrimeric guanosine triphosphate (GTP)-binding complex called a G protein.
3. **Catalytic receptors**. When activated by a ligand, these integral plasma membrane proteins are either enzymes themselves or part of an enzymatic complex.
4. **Intracellular (or steroid-type) receptors**. These proteins, located in the cytosol or nucleus, are ligand-activated transcription factors (see p. 116). These receptors link extracellular signals to gene transcription.
5. **Transmembrane proteins that release transcription factors**. These signalling molecules are all transmembrane proteins that undergo proteolytic cleavage within the plane of the membrane, liberating cytosolic fragments that enter the nucleus to modulate gene expression.

Sometimes, the same signalling molecule can bind to more than one kind of receptor and thus trigger parallel signal-transduction pathways. For example, ACh can bind to both ligand-gated channels and G-protein–coupled receptors. Signalling events initiated by plasma membrane receptors can generally be divided into six steps:

Step 1: **Recognition** of the signal by its receptor. Binding of a ligand to its receptor involves the same three types of weak, noncovalent interactions that characterize substrate-enzyme interactions. *Ionic bonds* are formed between groups of opposite charge. In *van der Waals* interactions, a transient dipole in one atom generates the opposite dipole in an adjacent atom, thereby creating an electrostatic interaction. *Hydrophobic interactions* occur between nonpolar groups.

Step 2: **Transduction** of the extracellular message into an intracellular signal or second messenger. Ligand binding causes a conformational change in the receptor that triggers the catalytic activities intrinsic to the receptor or causes the receptor to interact with membrane or cytoplasmic enzymes. The final consequence is the generation of a **second messenger** or the activation of a catalytic cascade.

Step 3: **Transmission** of the second messenger's signal to the appropriate effector. These effectors represent a diverse array of molecules, such as enzymes, ion channels, and transcription factors.

Step 4: **Modulation of the effector**. These events often result in the activation of protein **kinases** (which put phosphate groups on proteins) and **phosphatases** (which take them off), thereby altering the activity of other enzymes and proteins.

Step 5: **Response** of the cell to the initial stimulus. This

TABLE 4–1

CLASSIFICATION OF RECEPTORS AND ASSOCIATED SIGNAL TRANSDUCTION PATHWAYS

CLASS OF RECEPTOR	SUBUNIT COMPOSITION OF RECEPTOR	LIGAND	SIGNAL TRANSDUCTION PATHWAY DOWNSTREAM FROM RECEPTOR
Ligand-gated ion channels (ionotropic receptors)	Heteromeric or homomeric oligomers	*Extracellular*	*Ion Current*
		GABA	$Cl^- > HCO_3^-$
		Glycine	$Cl^- > HCO_3^-$
		ACh: muscle	Na^+, K^+, Ca^{2+}
		ACh: nerve	Na^+, K^+, Ca^{2+}
		5-HT	Na^+, K^+
		Glutamate: non-NMDA	Na^+, K^+, Ca^{2+}
		Glutamate: NMDA	Na^+, K^+, Ca^{2+}
		ATP (opening)	Ca^{2+}, Na^+, Mg^{2+}
		Intracellular	
		cGMP (vision)	Na^+, K^+
		cAMP, cGTP (olf)	Na^+, K^+
		ATP (closes channel)	K^+
		IP_3	Ca^{2+}
		Ca^{2+} or ryanodine	Ca^{2+}
Receptors coupled to heterotrimeric ($\alpha\beta\gamma$) G proteins	Single polypeptide that crosses the membrane seven times	*Small transmitter molecules*	$\beta\gamma$ Directly activates downstream effector:
		ACh	Muscarinic ACh receptor activates atrial K^+ channel
		Norepinephrine	
		Peptides	α Activates an enzyme:
		Oxytocin	Cyclases that make cyclic nucleotides (cAMP, cGMP)
		PTH	
		NPY	Phospholipases that generate IP_3 and diacylglycerols
		Gastrin	
		CCK	Phospholipases that generate arachidonic acid and its metabolites
		Odorants	
		Certain cytokines, lipids, and related molecules	
Catalytic receptors	Single polypeptide that crosses the membrane once. May be dimeric or may dimerize after activation	ANP	Receptor guanylyl cyclase
		NGF, EGF, PDGF, FGF, insulin, IGF-I	Receptor tyrosine kinase
		IL-3, -5, -6, EPO, LIF, CNTF, GH, interferon-α, -β, and -γ, GM-CSF	Tyrosine kinase–associated receptor
		CD-45	Receptor tyrosine phosphatase
		TGF-β	Receptor serine/threonine kinases
Intracellular (or nuclear) receptors	Homodimers of polypeptides, each with multiple functional domains	*Steroid hormones*	Bind to regulatory DNA sequences and directly or indirectly increase or decrease the transcription of specific genes
		Mineralocorticoids	
		Glucocorticoids	
		Androgens	
		Estrogens	
		Progestins	
	Heterodimers of polypeptides, each with multiple functional domains	*Others*	
		Thyroid hormones	
		Retinoic acid	
		Vitamin D	
		Prostaglandins	

ACh, acetylcholine; ANP, atrial natriuretic peptide; ATP, adenosine triphosphate; cAMP, cyclic adenosine monophosphate; CCK, cholecystokinin; cGMP, cyclic guanosine monophosphate; GTP, guanosine triphosphate; CNTF, ciliary neurotrophin factor; EGF, epidermal growth factor; EPO, erythropoietin; FGF, fibroblast growth factor; GABA, γ-aminobutyric acid; GH, growth hormone; GM-CSF, granulocyte-macrophage colony-stimulating factor; 5-HT, 5-hydroxytryptamine or serotonin; IGF-I, insulin-like growth factor type I; IL-3, interleukin-3; IP_3, inositol 1,4,5-triphosphate; LIF, leukocyte inhibitory factor; NGF, nerve growth factor; NPY, neuropeptide Y; PDGF, platelet-derived growth factor; PTH, parathyroid hormone; TGF, transforming growth factor.

collection of actions represents the summation and integration of input from multiple signalling pathways.

Step 6: **Termination** of the response by feedback mechanisms at any or all levels of the signalling pathway.

Second-Messenger Systems Amplify Signals and Integrate Responses Among Cell Types

For a molecule to function as a second messenger, its concentration, or window of activity, must be finely regulated. The cell achieves this control by rapidly producing or activating the second messenger and then inactivating or degrading it. To ensure that the system returns to a resting state when the stimulus is removed, counterbalancing activities function at each step of the cascade.

The involvement of second messengers in catalytic cascades provides numerous opportunities to **amplify** a signal. For example, the binding of a ligand to its receptor can generate hundreds of second-messenger molecules, which can in turn alter the activity of thousands of downstream effectors. Usually, this modulation involves the conversion of an inactive species into an active molecule or vice versa. An example of such a cascade is the increased intracellular concentration of the second messenger **cyclic AMP**. Receptor occupancy activates a G protein, which in turn stimulates a membrane-bound enzyme, **adenylyl cyclase**. This enzyme catalyzes the synthesis of cAMP from adenosine triphosphate (ATP), and a 5-fold increase in the intracellular concentration of cAMP is achieved in approximately 5 seconds. This sudden rise in cAMP levels is rapidly counteracted by its breakdown to adenosine 5′-monophosphate by **cAMP phosphodiesterase**.

Second-messenger systems also allow for **specificity** and **diversity**. Ligands that activate the same signalling pathways in cells usually produce the same effect. For example, epinephrine, adrenocorticotropic hormone (ACTH), glucagon, and thyroid-stimulating hormone (TSH) induce triglyceride breakdown via the cAMP messenger system. However, the same signalling molecule can produce distinct responses in different cells, depending on the complement of receptors and signal-transduction pathways that are available in the cell, as well as the specialized function that the cell carries out in the organism. For example, ACh induces contraction of skeletal muscle cells but inhibits contraction of heart muscle. It also facilitates the exocytosis of secretory granules in pancreatic acinar cells. This signalling molecule achieves these different end points by interacting with distinct receptors.

The diversity and specialization of second-messenger systems are important to a multicellular organism, as can be seen in the coordinated response of an organism to a stressful situation. Under these conditions, the adrenal gland releases epinephrine. Different organ systems respond to epinephrine in a distinct manner, such as activation of glycogen breakdown in the liver, constriction of the blood vessels of the skin, dilation of the blood vessels in skeletal muscle, and increased rate and force of heart contraction. The overall effect is an **integrated response** that readies the organism for attack, defense, or escape. In contrast, complex cell behaviors, such as proliferation and differentiation, are generally stimulated by combinations of signals rather than a single signal. Integration of these stimuli requires **crosstalk** among the various signalling cascades.

As discussed later, most signal-transduction pathways use elaborate cascades of signalling proteins to relay information from the cell surface to effectors in the cell membrane, the cytoplasm, or even the nucleus. In Chapter 5, we discuss how signal-transduction pathways that lead to the nucleus can affect the cell by modulating gene transcription. These are **genomic** effects. Signal-transduction systems that project to the cell membrane or to the cytoplasm produce **nongenomic** effects, the focus of this chapter.

Regulated Intramembrane Proteolysis of Certain Transmembrane Proteins Releases Transcription Factors

Several intrinsic membrane proteins do not fit the classic definition of a receptor but do appear to serve as critical sentinels for a diverse array of biologic processes, including cellular differentiation, lipid metabolism, and the response of the cell to unfolded proteins. By a process called **regulated intramembrane proteolysis** (RIP), these membrane proteins undergo proteolytic cleavage within the plane of the membrane to liberate cytosolic fragments that enter the nucleus to affect gene expression. This group of membrane proteins includes SREBP, Notch, Irel, ATF6, and APP. These proteins share several features. They all span the membrane bilayer at least once. For SREBP, Notch, and APP, the intramembrane cleavage does not take place until a primary cleavage event removes the bulk of the protein on the extracytoplasmic face. Although the cleaved bonds differ in the three cases, the net effect of the first step is to shorten the extracytoplasmic domain to less than 30 amino acids. The second cleavage releases a portion of the cytoplasmic domain. It remains to be determined how enzymes recognize and cleave their specific substrates within the bilayer.

The best characterized is SREBP (sterol regulatory element–binding proteins), which serves an essential role in the control of cholesterol homeostasis. SREBP is a resident protein of the ER membrane, whose cytoplasmic transcription factor domain is liberated when cells are depleted of sterols. The translocation of this peptide to the nucleus results in the transcriptional activation of the genes needed for cholesterol biosynthesis as well as the plasma membrane receptor for low-density lipoproteins.

Notch is a plasma membrane receptor whose cytoplasmic domain is released in response to Delta, a membrane-bound ligand that dictates cell fate throughout development. The most recently recognized examples of RIP are Ire1 and ATF6, transmembrane ER proteins that release their cytoplasmic domains in response to the presence of unfolded secretory proteins in the ER. A final example is APP (amyloid precursor protein), a protein of unknown function that is cleaved in the membrane to produce the extracellular amyloid β peptide implicated in Alzheimer's disease.

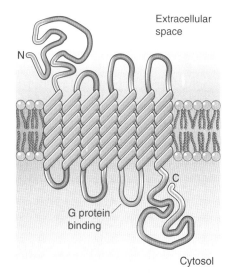

FIGURE 4–3. Receptor coupled to a G protein.

RECEPTORS THAT ARE ION CHANNELS

Ligand-Gated Ion Channels Transduce a Chemical Signal into an Electrical Signal

The property that defines this class of multisubunit membrane-spanning receptors is that the signalling molecule itself controls the opening and closing of an ion channel by binding to a site on the receptor. Thus, these receptors are also called **ionotropic receptors** to distinguish them from the metabotropic receptors, which act via "metabolic" pathways. One superfamily of ligand-gated channels includes the ionotropic receptors for ACh, serotonin, γ-aminobutyric acid (GABA), and glycine. Most structural and functional information for ionotropic receptors comes from the *nicotinic* ACh receptor (AChR) present in skeletal muscle (see Fig. 4–2). The *nicotinic* AChR is a cation channel that consists of four membrane-spanning subunits, α, β, γ, and δ, in a stoichiometry of 2:1:1:1. This receptor is called "nicotinic" because the nicotine contained in tobacco can activate or open the channel and thereby alter V_m. Note that the nicotinic AChR is very different from the *muscarinic* AChR discussed later, which is not a ligand-gated channel. Additional examples of ligand-gated channels are the IP_3 receptor and the Ca^{2+}-release channel (also known as the ryanodine receptor). Both receptors are located in the membranes of intracellular organelles. They are tetramers that function as Ca^{2+} channels.

RECEPTORS LINKED TO G PROTEINS

G-protein–linked receptors constitute the largest family of receptors on the cell surface, with more than 1000 members. These receptors mediate cellular responses to a diverse array of signalling molecules, such as hormones, neurotransmitters, vasoactive peptides, odorants, tastants,

and other local mediators. Despite the chemical diversity of their ligands, most receptors of this class have a similar structure (Fig. 4–3). They consist of a single polypeptide chain with seven membrane-spanning α helical segments, an extracellular N terminus that is glycosylated, a large cytoplasmic loop that is composed mainly of hydrophilic amino acids between helices 5 and 6, and a hydrophilic domain at the cytoplasmic C terminus. Most small ligands (e.g., epinephrine) bind in the plane of the membrane at a site that involves several membrane-spanning segments. In the case of larger protein ligands, a portion of the extracellular N terminus also participates in ligand binding. The 5,6-cytoplasmic loop appears to be the major site of interaction with the G protein, although the 3,4-cytoplasmic loop and the cytoplasmic C terminus also contribute to binding in some cases. G proteins couple cell-surface receptors to downstream effectors. In the next four sections of this subchapter, we discuss the general principles of how G proteins function and then consider three major second-messenger systems that are triggered by G proteins.

GENERAL PROPERTIES OF G PROTEINS

G Proteins Are Heterotrimers That Exist in Many Combinations of Different α, β, and γ Subunits

G proteins are members of a superfamily of **GTP-binding proteins**. This superfamily includes the classic heterotrimeric proteins, as well as the so-called small GTP-binding proteins, such as Ras. Both the heterotrimeric and small G proteins can hydrolyze GTP and switch between an active GTP-bound state and an inactive guanosine diphosphate (GDP)-bound state.

Heterotrimeric G proteins are composed of three subunits, α, β, and γ. At least 16 different α subunits (~42 to 50 kDa), 5 β subunits (~33 to 35 kDa), and 11 γ subunits (~8 to 10 kDa) are present in mammalian tissue. The α subunit binds and hydrolyzes GTP, and also interacts with "downstream" effector proteins such as adenylyl cyclase. Historically, the α subunits were thought to provide the principal specificity to each type of G protein, with the βγ complex functioning to anchor the trimeric complex to the membrane. However, it is now clear that the βγ complex also functions in signal transduction by interacting with certain effector molecules. Moreover, both the α and γ subunits are involved in anchoring the complex to the membrane. The α subunit is held to the membrane by either a myristyl or a palmitoyl group, whereas the γ subunit is held via a prenyl group.

The multiple α, β, and γ subunits demonstrate distinct tissue distributions and interact with different receptors and effectors (Table 4–2). Because of the potential for several hundred combinations of the known α, β, and γ subunits, G proteins are ideally suited to link a diversity of receptors to a diversity of effectors. The many classes of G proteins, in conjunction with the presence of several receptor types for a single ligand, provide a mechanism whereby a common signal can elicit the appropriate physiological changes in different tissues. For example, when epinephrine binds $β_1$-adrenergic receptors in the heart, it

TABLE 4–2

FAMILIES OF G PROTEINS

FAMILY/SUBUNIT	% IDENTITY	TOXIN	DISTRIBUTION	RECEPTOR	EFFECTOR/ROLE
G_s					
$\alpha_{s(s)}$	100	CTX	Ubiquitous	βAR, TSH, glucagon, etc.	↑ AC
$\alpha_{s(l)}$					↑ Ca^{2+} channel
					↓ Na^+ channel
α_{olf}	88	CTX	Olfactory epithe-lium	Odorant	↑ AC
					Open K^+ channel
G_i					
α_{i1}	100	PTX	~Ubiquitous	M_2, α_2AR, others	↑ IP_3, DAG, Ca^{2+}
α_{i2}	88	PTX	Ubiquitous		and AA release,
α_{i3}		PTX	~Ubiquitous		↓ AC
α_{O1A}	73	PTX	Brain, others	Met-Enk, α_2AR, others	
α_{O1B}	73	PTX	Brain, others		
α_{t1}	68	PTX, CTX	Retinal rods	Rhodopsin	↑ cGMP-phos-phodiesterase
α_{t2}	68	PTX, CTX	Retinal cones	Cone opsin	
α_g	67	PTX, CTX (?)	Taste buds	Taste (?)	?
α_z	60		Brain, adrenal, platelet	M_2 (?), others (?)	↓ AC
G_q					
α_q	100		~Ubiquitous	M_1, α_1AR, others	↑ PLCβ1, β2, β3
α_{11}	88		~Ubiquitous		
α_{14}	79		Lung, kidney, liver		
α_{15}	57		B cell, myeloid		
α_{16}	58		T cell, myeloid	Several receptors	↑ PLCβ1, β2, β3
G_{12}					
α_{12}	100		Ubiquitous		
α_{13}	67		Ubiquitous		

AA, arachidonic acid; AC, adenylyl cylase; α_2AR, α_2-adrenergic receptor; βAR, β-adrenergic receptor; CTX, cholera toxin; DAG, diacylglycerol; GMP, guanosine monophosphate, IP_3, inositol 1,4,5-triphosphate; M_1 or M_2, muscarinic cholinergic receptors; Met-Enk, metenkephalin; PTX, pertussis toxin; TSH, thyrotropin (thyroid-stimulating hormone).

stimulates adenylyl cyclase, which increases heart rate and the force of contraction. However, in the periphery, epinephrine acts on α_2-adrenergic receptors that are coupled to a G protein that *inhibits* adenylyl cyclase, thereby increasing peripheral vascular resistance and consequently increasing venous return and blood pressure.

Among the first effectors found to be sensitive to G proteins was the enzyme adenylyl cyclase. The heterotrimeric G protein known as **G**$_s$ was so named because it stimulates adenylyl cyclase. A separate class of G proteins was given the name **G**$_i$ because it is responsible for the hormone-dependent inhibition of adenylyl cyclase. Identification of these classes of G proteins was greatly facilitated by the observation that the α subunits of individual G proteins are substrates for adenosine diphosphate (ADP) ribosylation catalyzed by bacterial toxins. The toxin from *Vibrio cholerae* activates G_s, whereas the toxin from *Bordetella pertussis* inactivates the cyclase-inhibiting G_i (see the box titled Action of Toxins on Heterotrimeric G Proteins).

For their work in identifying G proteins and elucidating the physiologic role of these proteins, Alfred Gilman and Martin Rodbell received the 1994 Nobel Prize in Physiology or Medicine.

G-Protein Activation Follows a Cycle

In their inactive state, heterotrimeric G proteins are a complex of α, β, and γ subunits in which GDP occupies the guanine nucleotide binding site of the α subunit. On ligand binding (Fig. 4–4, *step 1*), the activated receptor interacts with the $\alpha\beta\gamma$ heterotrimer to promote a conformational change that facilitates the release of bound GDP and simultaneous binding of GTP (*step 2*). This GDP-GTP exchange stimulates dissociation of the complex from the receptor (*step 3*) and causes disassembly of the trimer into a free α subunit and $\beta\gamma$ complex (*step 4*). The free, active GTP-bound α subunit can now interact in the plane of the membrane with downstream effectors such as adenylyl cyclase and phospholipases (*step 5*). Similarly, the $\beta\gamma$ subunit can now activate ion channels or other effectors.

The α subunit terminates the signalling events that are mediated by the α and $\beta\gamma$ subunits by hydrolyzing GTP to GDP and inorganic phosphate (P_i). The result is an

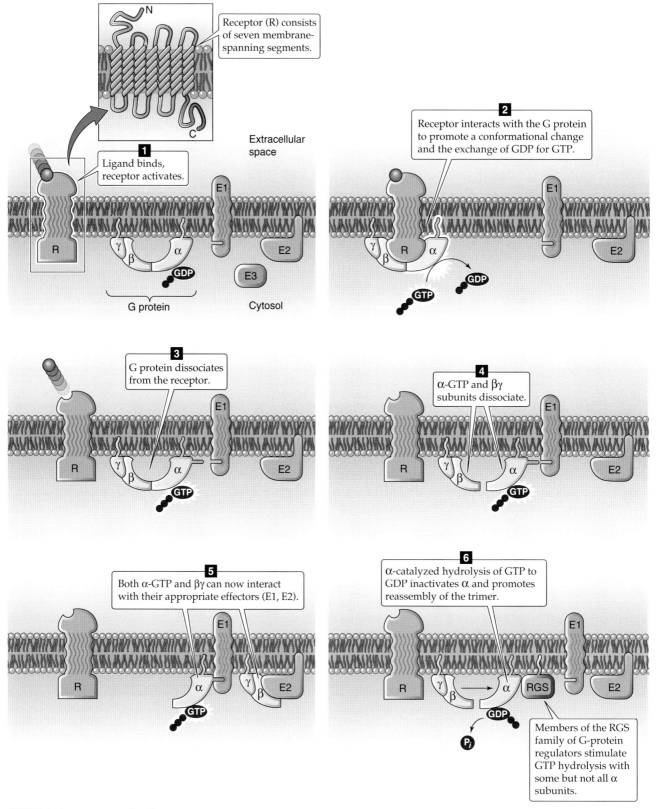

Receptor (R) consists of seven membrane-spanning segments.

1 Ligand binds, receptor activates.

Extracellular space

G protein

Cytosol

2 Receptor interacts with the G protein to promote a conformational change and the exchange of GDP for GTP.

3 G protein dissociates from the receptor.

4 α-GTP and βγ subunits dissociate.

5 Both α-GTP and βγ can now interact with their appropriate effectors (E1, E2).

6 α-catalyzed hydrolysis of GTP to GDP inactivates α and promotes reassembly of the trimer.

Members of the RGS family of G-protein regulators stimulate GTP hydrolysis with some but not all α subunits.

FIGURE 4–4. Enzymatic cycle of heterotrimeric G proteins. GDP, guanosine diphosphate; GTP, guanosine triphosphate; P_i, inorganic phosphate.

inactive α-GDP complex that dissociates from its downstream effector and reassociates with a $\beta\gamma$ subunit (Fig. 4–4, *step* 6), thus completing the cycle (*step* 1). The $\beta\gamma$ subunit stabilizes α-GDP and thereby substantially slows the rate of GDP-GTP exchange (*step* 2) and dampens signal transmission in the resting state.

The RGS (for "regulation of G-protein signalling") family of proteins appears to enhance the intrinsic GTPase activity of some, but not all, α subunits. Investigators have identified at least 15 mammalian RGS proteins and shown that they interact with specific α subunits. RGS proteins bind the complex $G\alpha$/GDP/AlF$_4^-$, which is the structural analog of the GTPase transition state. By stabilizing the transition state, RGS proteins may promote GTP hydrolysis and thus the termination of signalling.

As noted earlier, α subunits can be anchored to the cell membrane via myristyl or palmitoyl groups. Activation can result in the removal of these groups, and the release of the α subunit into the cytosol. Loss of the α subunit from the membrane may decrease the interaction of G proteins with receptors and downstream effectors (e.g., adenylyl cyclase).

Activated α Subunits Couple to a Variety of Downstream Effectors, Including Enzymes, Ion Channels, and Membrane-Trafficking Machinery

Activated α subunits can be coupled to a variety of enzymes. On one hand, **adenylyl cyclase**, which is activated by $G\alpha_s$, catalyzes the production of cAMP from ATP (Fig. 4–5A). On the other hand, $G\alpha_i$ inhibits adenylyl cyclase and thus decreases [cAMP]$_i$. Thus, different hormones—acting through different G-protein complexes—can have opposing effects on the same intracellular messenger.

G proteins can also activate enzymes that break down cyclic nucleotides. For example, the G protein called **transducin**, which plays a key role in phototransduction (p. 339), activates the cyclic guanosine monophosphate (cGMP) **phosphodiesterase**, which catalyzes the breakdown of cGMP to GMP (Fig. 4–5B). Thus, light leads to a decrease in [cGMP]$_i$.

G proteins can also be coupled to **phospholipases**. These enzymes catabolize phospholipids, as discussed in detail later in the section on G-protein second messengers. This superfamily of phospholipases can be grouped into phospholipases A$_2$, C, or D, based on the site at which the enzyme cleaves the phospholipid. The G-protein α_q subunit activates phospholipase C (PLC), which breaks phosphoinositol bisphosphate (PIP$_2$) into two intracellular messengers, membrane-associated DAG and cytosolic IP$_3$ (Fig. 4–5C). DAG stimulates protein kinase C (PKC), whereas IP$_3$ binds to a receptor on the endoplasmic reticulum (ER) membrane and triggers the release of Ca^{2+} from intracellular stores.

Some G proteins interact with **ion channels**. Agonists that bind to the β-adrenergic receptor activate the L-type Ca^{2+} channel in the heart and skeletal muscle (p. 190). The G protein G$_s$ directly stimulates this channel as the α subunit of G$_s$ binds to the channel, and G$_s$ also indirectly stimulates this channel via a signal-transduction cascade that involves cAMP-dependent protein kinase.

ACTION OF TOXINS ON HETEROTRIMERIC G PROTEINS

Infectious diarrheal disease has a multitude of causes. **Cholera toxin**, a secretory product of the bacterium *Vibrio cholerae,* is responsible in part for the devastating characteristics of cholera. The toxin is an oligomeric protein composed of one A subunit and five B subunits (AB$_5$). After cholera toxin enters intestinal epithelial cells, the A subunit separates from the B subunits and becomes activated by proteolytic cleavage. The resulting active A1 fragment catalyzes the adenosine diphosphate (ADP) ribosylation of Gα_s. This ribosylation, which involves transfer of the ADP-ribose moiety from the oxidized form of nicotinamide adenine dinucleotide (NAD$^+$) to the α subunit, inhibits the guanosine triphosphatase (GTPase) activity of Gα_s. As a result of this modification, Gα_s remains in its activated, GTP-bound form and can activate adenylyl cyclase. In intestinal epithelial cells, the constitutively activated Gα_s elevates levels of cyclic adenosine monophosphate (cAMP), which causes an increase in Cl$^-$ conductance and water flow and thereby contributes to the large fluid loss characteristic of this disease.

A related bacterial product is **pertussis toxin,** which is also an AB$_5$ protein. It is produced by *Bordetella pertussis,* the causative agent of whooping cough. Pertussis toxin ADP-ribosylates Gα_i. This ADP-ribosylated Gα_i cannot exchange its bound guanosine diphosphate (GDP) (inactive state) for GTP. Thus, α_i remains in its GDP-bound inactive state. As a result, receptor occupancy can no longer release the active α_i-GTP, so adenylyl cyclase cannot be inhibited. Thus, both cholera toxin and pertussis toxin increase the generation of cAMP.

A clue that G proteins serve additional functions in **membrane trafficking** (p. 37) in the cell comes from the observation that many cells contain intracellular pools of heterotrimeric G proteins, some bound to internal membranes and some free in the cytosol. Experiments involving toxins, inhibitors, and cell lines harboring mutations in G-protein subunits have demonstrated that these intracellular G proteins are involved in vesicular transport. G proteins have been implicated in the budding of secretory vesicles from the *trans*-Golgi network, fusion of endosomes, recruitment of nonclathrin coat proteins, and transcytosis and apical secretion in polarized epithelial cells. The receptors and effectors that interact with these intracellular G proteins have not been determined.

The $\beta\gamma$ Subunits of G Proteins Can Also Activate Downstream Effectors

Considerable evidence now indicates that the $\beta\gamma$ subunits can also interact with downstream effectors. The neurotransmitter ACh released from the vagus nerve reduces the rate and strength of heart contraction. This action in the atria of the heart is mediated by *muscarinic* M$_2$ AChRs (p. 387). These receptors can be activated by muscarine, an alkaloid found in certain poisonous mushrooms. *Mus-*

A G PROTEINS ACTING VIA ADENYLYL CYCLASE

B G PROTEIN ACTING VIA A PHOSPHODIESTERASE

C G PROTEIN ACTING VIA A PHOSPHOLIPASE

FIGURE 4–5. Downstream effects of activated G-protein α subunits. *A,* When a ligand binds to a receptor coupled to α_s, adenylyl cyclase is activated, whereas when a ligand binds to a receptor coupled to α_i, the enzyme is inhibited. The activated enzyme converts ATP to cAMP, which then can activate protein kinase A. *B,* In phototransduction, a photon interacts with the receptor and activates the G protein transducin. The α_t activates phosphodiesterase, which in turn hydrolyzes cGMP and lowers the intracellular concentrations of cGMP and, therefore, closes the cGMP-activated channels. *C,* In this example, the ligand binds to a receptor that is coupled to α_q, which activates phospholipase C. This enzyme converts PIP$_2$ to IP$_3$ and DAG. The IP$_3$ leads to the release of Ca^{2+} from intracellular stores, whereas the DAG activates protein kinase C. AMP, adenosine monophosphate; ATP, adenosine triphosphate; cGMP, cyclic guanosine monophosphate; DAG, diacylglycerol; ER, endoplasmic reticulum; GMP, guanosine monophosphate; IP$_3$, 1,4,5-inositol triphosphate; PIP$_2$, phosphatidyl inositol 4,5-biphosphate.

carinic AChRs are very different from the *nicotinic* AChRs discussed earlier, which are ligand-gated channels. Binding of ACh to the muscarinic M$_2$ receptor in the atria activates a heterotrimeric G protein and liberates the $\beta\gamma$ subunit complex. The $\beta\gamma$ complex then interacts with a particular class of K$^+$ channels, increasing their permeability. This increase in K$^+$ permeability keeps the V_m relatively negative, and thus renders the cell more resistant to excitation. The $\beta\gamma$ subunit complex also modulates the activity of adenylyl cyclase and PLC and stimulates PLA$_2$. Such effects of $\beta\gamma$ can be independent of, synergize with, or antagonize the action of the α subunit.

For example, studies using various isoforms of adenylyl cyclase have demonstrated that purified $\beta\gamma$ stimulates some isoforms, inhibits others, and has no effect on still others. Different combinations of $\beta\gamma$ isoforms may have different activities. For example, $\beta_1\gamma_1$ is one tenth as efficient at stimulating type II adenylyl cyclase as is $\beta_1\gamma_2$.

An interesting action of some $\beta\gamma$ complexes is that they bind to a special protein kinase called the β-adrenergic receptor kinase (βARK). As a result of this interaction, βARK translocates to the plasma membrane, where it phosphorylates the ligand-receptor complex (but not the unbound receptor). This phosphorylation attenuates the activity of the same β-adrenergic receptors that gave rise to the $\beta\gamma$ complex in the first place. This action is an example of **receptor desensitization**. These phosphorylated receptors eventually undergo endocytosis, which transiently reduces the number of receptors that are available on the cell surface. This endocytosis is an important step in **resensitization** of the receptor system.

Small GTP-Binding Proteins Are Involved in a Vast Number of Cellular Processes

Small GTP-binding proteins, such as the Ras proteins, are 21-kDa membrane-associated proteins that bind guanine nucleotides. The three isoforms of Ras (N, Ha, and Ki) relay signals from the plasma membrane to the nucleus via an elaborate kinase cascade (p. 133). Like the structurally related α subunit of heterotrimeric G proteins, members of the Ras family are GTPases that switch between an inactive GDP-bound form and an active GTP-bound form. Two classes of regulatory proteins modulate Ras activity. The first of these includes the **GTPase-activating proteins** GAP and neurofibromin (a product of the neurofibromatosis type 1 gene). These proteins increase the rate at which Ras hydrolyzes bound GTP and thus becomes inactive. Counteracting the activity of GAP are **guanine nucleotide exchange proteins** such as "son of sevenless" or SOS (p. 134), which promote the conversion of inactive Ras-GDP to active Ras-GTP. In some tumors, mutation of the genes encoding Ras proteins results in constitutively active Ras. These mutated genes are called **oncogenes** because the altered Ras gene product promotes the malignant transformation of a cell and can contribute to the development of cancer (oncogenesis).

G-PROTEIN SECOND MESSENGERS: CYCLIC NUCLEOTIDES

cAMP Usually Exerts Its Effect by Increasing the Activity of Protein Kinase A

Activation of G_s-coupled receptors results in the stimulation of adenylyl cyclase and a rise in intracellular concentrations of cAMP (see Fig. 4–5A). The downstream effects of this increase in $[cAMP]_i$ depend on the specialized functions that the responding cell carries out in the organism. For example, in the adrenal cortex, ACTH stimulation of cAMP production results in the secretion of aldosterone and cortisol (p. 1056), whereas in the kidney, vasopressin-induced changes in cAMP levels facilitate water reabsorption (p. 842). Excess cAMP is also responsible

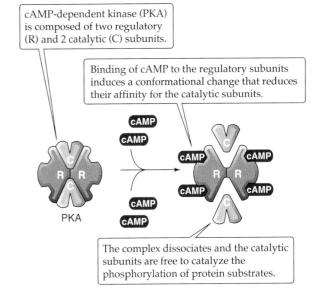

FIGURE 4–6. Activation of protein kinase A by cyclic adenosine monophosphate (cAMP).

for certain pathologic conditions. One is **cholera** (see box titled Action of Toxins on Heterotrimeric G Proteins). Another is **McCune-Albright syndrome**, which is characterized by a triad of (1) variable hyperfunction of multiple endocrine glands, including precocious puberty in girls; (2) bone lesions; and (3) pigmented skin lesions (café au lait spots). This disorder is caused by a somatic mutation that constitutively activates the G protein α_s subunit in a mosaic pattern.

cAMP exerts many of its effects through **cAMP-dependent protein kinase A (PKA)**. This enzyme catalyzes transfer of the terminal phosphate of ATP to certain **serine or threonine residues** within selected proteins. PKA is involved in many cell-signalling pathways. To ensure firm regulation of phosphorylation events, the cell tightly controls the activity of PKA so that the enzyme can respond to subtle variations in cAMP levels. One important control mechanism is the use of **regulatory subunits** that constitutively inhibit PKA. In the absence of cAMP, PKA is composed of four subunits—two regulatory and two catalytic subunits (Fig. 4–6)—so the complex has a low level of catalytic activity. Although most cells use the same catalytic subunit, different regulatory subunits are found in different cell types. Binding of cAMP to the regulatory subunits induces a conformational change in these proteins that diminishes their affinity for the catalytic subunits. Dissociation of the complex results in activation of the enzyme.

Another mechanism that contributes to regulation of PKA is the targeting of the enzyme to specific subcellular locations. Such targeting promotes the preferential phosphorylation of substrates that are confined to precise locations within the cell. PKA targeting is achieved by the association of a PKA regulatory subunit with an **A kinase anchoring protein** (AKAP), which in turn binds to cytoskeletal elements or to components of cellular subcompartments. Over 35 AKAPs are known. The specificity of PKA targeting is highlighted by the observation that, in neurons, PKA is localized to postsynaptic densities through its association with AKAP79. This anchoring protein also targets calcineurin—a protein phosphatase—to the same site. This targeting of both PKA and calcineurin to the same postsynaptic site makes it possible for the cell to tightly regulate the phosphorylation state of important neuronal substrates.

In addition to the short-term effects just discussed, elevation of cAMP levels can activate the transcription of specific genes via PKA (p. 133).

The cAMP generated by adenylyl cyclase does not necessarily interact only with PKA. For example, olfactory receptors (p. 330) interact with a member of the G_s family called G_{olf}. The rise in $[cAMP]_i$ that results from activation of the olfactory receptor activates a cation channel. Na^+ influx through this channel leads to membrane depolarization and the initiation of a nerve impulse.

For his work in elucidating the role played by cAMP as a second messenger in signal transduction, Earl Sutherland received the 1971 Nobel Prize in Physiology or Medicine. In 1992, Edmond Fischer and Edwin Krebs shared the prize for their part in demonstrating the role of protein phosphorylation in the signal-transduction process.

Epinephrine Stimulates Glycogen Breakdown and Inhibits Glycogen Synthesis via cAMP

The importance of cAMP-dependent protein phosphorylation was first demonstrated for glycogen catabolism in skeletal muscle. **Glycogen**, a glucose polymer stored primarily in liver and muscle cells, is the major storage form of carbohydrate in the body (p. 1214). Epinephrine plays a major role in regulating both the synthesis and degradation of glycogen. In muscle cells, for example, epinephrine induces glycogen breakdown and inhibits glycogen synthesis (Fig. 4–7) by controlling a series of phosphorylation and dephosphorylation events. The ultimate effect is release of glucose for use by the muscle cell.

Binding of epinephrine to its "adrenergic" receptor results in activation of PKA, which phosphorylates three enzymes (see Fig. 4–7). First, PKA phosphorylates the regulatory α and β subunits of inactive **glycogen phosphorylase kinase (PK)**, a massive enzyme that has the subunit structure $(\alpha\beta\gamma\delta)_4$. The δ subunit is also "regulatory," as discussed later. Thus, only the γ subunits are involved in catalysis. The net effect of this phosphorylation by PKA is to activate the enzyme, which allows PK to phosphorylate a second inactive enzyme, glycogen phosphorylase *b* (GPb). The now-active glycogen phosphorylase *a* (GPa) then catalyzes the stepwise removal of glucose 1-phosphate residues from glycogen. This intermediate is converted to glucose 6-phosphate, which in turn can enter the glycolytic pathway.

Second, PKA phosphorylates the active form of **glycogen synthase (GS)** and renders it inactive. Normally, the active GS transfers the glucose residue from uridine diphosphate (UDP)-glucose to a free 4-OH group of a glucose residue at the end of the growing glycogen chain. Thus, phosphorylation of GS inhibits glycogen synthesis.

Third, PKA also inactivates **phosphoprotein phosphatase-1 (PP1)**, the enzyme that is responsible for removing the phosphates added in the PKA reactions just discussed. The mechanism of this inactivation is indirect: PKA phosphorylates and thus activates an inhibitor of PP1, thus

ensuring that the phosphate groups added to the other enzymes are not removed. The entire process is reversed when epinephrine is removed and the levels of cAMP fall.

This coordinated set of phosphorylation and dephosphorylation reactions has several physiological advantages. First, it allows a single molecule (e.g., cAMP) to regulate a range of enzymatic reactions. Second, it affords a large amplification to a small signal. The concentration of epinephrine needed to stimulate glycogenolysis in muscle is approximately 10^{-10} M. This subnanomolar level of hormone can raise $[cAMP]_i$ to approximately 10^{-6} M. As a consequence of the catalytic cascades, a further 10,000-fold amplification occurs, and enough glucose is liberated to raise blood glucose levels from approximately 5 to 8 mM. Although the effects of cAMP on the synthesis and degradation of glycogen are confined to muscle and liver, cAMP-mediated activation cascades are used in the response of cells to a wide variety of hormones.

Protein Phosphatases Reverse the Action of Kinases

As discussed, one way that the cell can terminate a cAMP signal is to use a phosphodiesterase to degrade cAMP. In this way, the subsequent steps along the signalling pathway can also be terminated. However, because the downstream effects of cAMP usually involve phosphorylation at serine and threonine residues of effector proteins, another powerful way to terminate the action of cAMP is to dephosphorylate these effector proteins. Such dephosphorylation events are mediated by enzymes called serine/threonine phosphoprotein phosphatases.

Four groups of **serine/threonine phosphoprotein phosphatases** (PP) are known. 1, 2a, 2b, and 2c. These enzymes themselves are regulated by phosphorylation at their serine, threonine, and tyrosine residues. The balance between kinase and phosphatase activity plays a major role in the control of signalling events. PP1 dephosphorylates many proteins phosphorylated by PKA, including those phosphorylated in response to epinephrine (above). PP2a, which is less specific than PP1, appears to be the main phosphatase responsible for reversing the action of other protein kinases. The Ca^{2+}-dependent PP2b—also known as **calcineurin**—is most prevalent in the brain. Calcineurin is also the target of the immunosuppressive reagents FK-506 and cyclosporine. PP2c appears to be of relatively minor importance.

As discussed later in this chapter, growth factors often act via receptors that themselves are tyrosine kinases. That is, the receptor phosphorylates target proteins or themselves at *tyrosine* residues rather than at serine or threonine residues. The enzymes that remove phosphates from these tyrosine residues are much more variable than the serine and threonine phosphatases. The first **phosphotyrosine phosphatase** (PTP) to be characterized was the cytosolic enzyme PTP1B from human placenta. PTP1B has a high degree of homology with **CD45**, a membrane protein that is both a receptor and a phosphatase. cDNA sequence analysis has identified a large number of PTPs that can be divided into two classes: membrane-spanning receptor-like proteins such as CD45 and cytosolic forms such as PTP1B. A number of intracellular PTPs contain so-called Src homology-2 (SH2) domains, a peptide se-

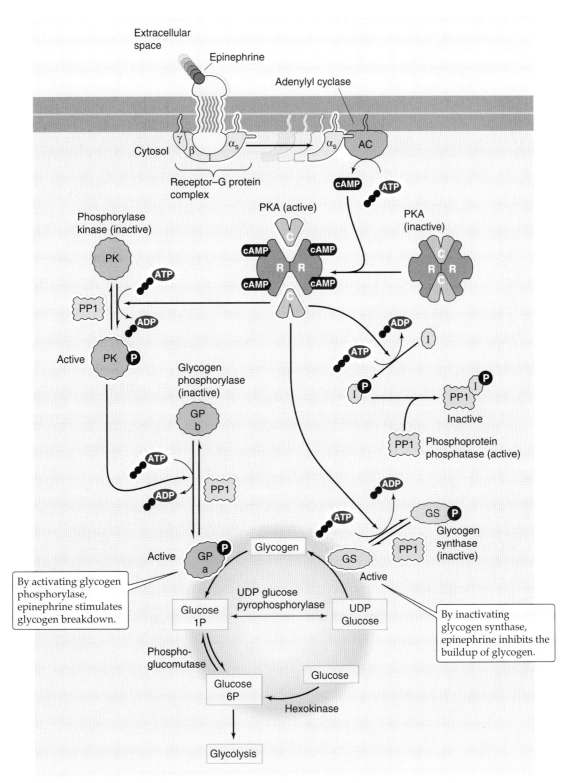

FIGURE 4–7. Regulation of glycogen breakdown and synthesis in muscle by cAMP. When epinephrine binds to the appropriate receptor, the activation of α_s stimulates adenylyl cyclase (AC), which in turn increases $[cAMP]_i$. This cAMP activates protein kinase A (PKA), which—via phosphorylation—has three major downstream effects: (1) PKA *activates* glycogen phosphorylase kinase (PK), which phosphorylates and activates glycogen phosphorylase (GP), which in turn breaks down glycogen. (2) PKA *inactivates* glycogen synthase (GS) and thus diminishes the formation of glycogen. (3) PKA activates an inhibitor of phosphoprotein phosphatase-1 (PP1) and thus inhibits the phosphatase that would otherwise reverse the phosphorylations in (1) and (2). The net effect is a coordinated series of changes that increase the availability of glucose. ADP, adenosine diphosphate; ATP, adenosine triphosphate; cAMP, cyclic adenosine monophosphate; Glucose 1P, glucose-1-phosphate; Glucose 6P, glucose-6-phosphate; PKA, protein kinase A; UDP glucose, uridine diphosphate glucose.

quence or motif that interacts with phosphorylated tyrosine groups. Several of the PTPs are themselves regulated by phosphorylation.

During Phototransduction, a Decrease in [cGMP]$_i$ Inhibits a Nonselective Cation Channel

cGMP is another cyclic nucleotide that is involved in G-protein signalling events. A classic example is phototransduction in the outer segments of rods and cones in the visual system (p. 339). The light sensor is **rhodopsin**, a member of the family of G-protein–coupled receptors that pass through the membrane seven times. A key difference between the adrenergic receptor that binds epinephrine and rhodopsin is that the rhodopsin molecule consists of two parts: a receptor—the **opsin**—and a covalently attached ligand, the chromophore 11-*cis* retinal. When it absorbs a photon of light, this chromophore isomerizes to all-*trans* retinal. This isomerization alters the conformation of the protein (opsin) in a way that is analogous to the conformational change that a ligand such as epinephrine produces when it binds to its G-protein–coupled receptor. The conformational change of the opsin acts through a special G protein (**transducin**) to activate **cGMP phosphodiesterase**. This enzyme in turn decreases [cGMP]$_i$. The plasma membrane surrounding the outer segment contains nonselective cation channels that are kept open, in the dark, by a bound cGMP. The major effect of keeping these channels open in the dark is an inwardly directed Na$^+$ current that tends to make V_m more positive. As a consequence of the light-induced decrease in [cGMP]$_i$, cGMP dissociates from the channels, which allows them to close. This channel closure results in a more negative V_m.

G-PROTEIN SECOND MESSENGERS: PRODUCTS OF PHOSPHOINOSITIDE BREAKDOWN

Many Messengers Bind to Receptors That Activate Phosphoinositide Breakdown

Although the phosphatidylinositols (PIs) are minor constituents of cell membranes, they play an important role in signal transduction. PI phospholipids contain the sugar inositol (see Fig. 2–2A). The inositol moiety of PI molecules, which are largely distributed in the internal leaflet of the membrane, can be phosphorylated to yield the two major phosphoinositides that are involved in signal transduction, phosphatidylinositol bisphosphate (PI$_{4,5}$P$_2$) and PI$_{3,4,5}$P$_3$.

Extracellular signals that activate receptors linked to certain G proteins (e.g., G$_q$) stimulate phospholipase Cβ (PLCβ), which breaks down PIP$_2$ into IP$_3$ and DAG (Fig. 4–8A). PLCs are classified into three families (β, γ, δ) that differ in their catalytic properties, cell-type–specific expression, and modes of activation. Stimulation of PLCβ by G proteins causes the hydrolysis of PIP$_2$. The result is a rapid increase in cytosolic IP$_3$ levels as well as an *early* peak in DAG levels (see Fig. 4–8B). Both products are second messengers. DAG remains in the plane of the membrane to activate PKC, which migrates from the cytosol and binds to DAG in the membrane. The water-soluble IP$_3$ travels through the cytosol to stimulate Ca^{2+} release from intracellular stores. It is within this system that Ca^{2+} was first identified as a messenger that mediates the stimulus-response coupling of endocrine cells.

Phosphatidylcholine (PC), which—unlike PI—is an abundant phospholipid in the cell membrane, is also a source of DAG. The cell can produce DAG from PC by either of two mechanisms (Fig. 4–8C). First, PLC can directly convert PC to phosphocholine and DAG. Second, **phospholipase D**, by cleaving the phosphoester bond on the other side of the phosphate, converts PC to choline and phosphatidic acid (PA; also phospho-DAG). This PA can then be converted to DAG via PA-phosphohydrolase. Production of DAG from PC, either directly (via PLC) or indirectly (via PLD), produces the *slow* wave of increasing cytosolic DAG shown in Figure 4–8B. Thus, in some systems the formation of DAG is biphasic and consists of an early peak that is transient and rapid and parallels the formation of IP$_3$, followed by a late phase that is slow in onset but sustained over several minutes.

Factors such as **tumor necrosis factor–α** (TNF-α), **interleukin-1** (IL-1), **interleukin-3** (IL-3), **interferon-α** (IFN-α), and **colony-stimulating factor** stimulate the production of DAG from PC. Once generated, DAG can be further cleaved by DAG lipase to **arachidonic acid** (AA), which can have signalling activity itself or can be metabolized to other signalling molecules, the **eicosanoids**. We will cover AA metabolism later in this chapter.

Inositol Triphosphate Liberates Ca^{2+} from Intracellular Stores

As discussed earlier, IP$_3$ is generated by the metabolism of membrane phospholipids and then travels through the cytosol to release Ca^{2+} from intracellular stores. The receptor for IP$_3$ is a ligand-gated Ca^{2+} channel located in the membrane of the *endoplasmic* reticulum (see Fig. 4–8A). This Ca^{2+} channel is structurally related to the Ca^{2+} release channel (or ryanodine receptor), which is responsible for releasing Ca^{2+} from the *sarcoplasmic* reticulum (SR) of muscle and thereby switching on muscle contraction (p. 241). The IP$_3$ receptor is a tetramer that is composed of subunits of approximately 260 kDa. At least three genes encode the subunits of the receptor. These genes are subject to alternative splicing, which further increases the potential for receptor diversity. The receptor is a substrate for phosphorylation by PKA, PKC, and Ca^{2+}/calmodulin (CaM)-dependent protein kinases.

Interaction of IP$_3$ with its receptor results in passive efflux of Ca^{2+} from the ER and thus a rapid rise in the free cytosolic Ca^{2+} concentration. The IP$_3$-induced changes in [Ca^{2+}]$_i$ exhibit complex temporal and spatial patterns. The rise in [Ca^{2+}]$_i$ can be brief or persistent and can oscillate repetitively, spread in spirals or waves within a cell, or spread across groups of cells that are coupled by gap junctions. In at least some systems, the frequency of [Ca^{2+}]$_i$ oscillations seems to be physiologically important. For example, in isolated pancreatic acinar cells, graded increases in the concentration of ACh produce graded increases in the *frequency*—but not the *magnitude*—of repetitive [Ca^{2+}]$_i$ spikes. The mechanisms responsible for [Ca^{2+}]$_i$ oscillations and waves are complex.

FIGURE 4–8. Second messengers in the DAG/IP$_3$ pathway. ATP, adenosine triphosphate; DAG, diacylglycerol; ER, endoplasmic reticulum; PIP$_2$, phosphatidylinositol 4,5-biphosphate; PKC, protein kinase C; PLC, phospholipase C; PLD, phospholipase D; SERCA, sarcoplasmic and endoplasmic reticulum Ca^{2+} ATPase.

It appears that both propagation and oscillation depend on positive feedback mechanisms in which low $[Ca^{2+}]_i$ facilitates Ca^{2+} release, as well as negative feedback mechanisms in which high $[Ca^{2+}]_i$ inhibits further Ca^{2+} release.

Release of Ca^{2+} from intracellular stores is terminated by dephosphorylation of IP_3. An ATP-fueled Ca^{2+} pump (SERCA; p. 64) then moves the Ca^{2+} back into the ER. Some of the IP_3 is further phosphorylated to IP_4, which may mediate a slower and more prolonged response of the cell or may promote the refilling of intracellular stores. In addition to IP_3, **cyclic ADP ribose** (cADPR) can mobilize Ca^{2+} from intracellular stores. Although the details of these interactions have not been fully elucidated, cADPR appears to bind to the Ca^{2+} release channel (ryanodine receptor) in a CaM-dependent manner.

In addition to the increase in $[Ca^{2+}]_i$ produced by the release of Ca^{2+} from intracellular stores, $[Ca^{2+}]_i$ can also rise as a result of enhanced influx of this ion through Ca^{2+} channels in the plasma membrane. For Ca^{2+} to function as a second messenger, it is critical that $[Ca^{2+}]_i$ be normally maintained at relatively low levels (at or below ~100 nM). Leakage of Ca^{2+} into the cell via Ca^{2+} channels is opposed by the extrusion of Ca^{2+} across the plasma membrane by both an ATP-dependent Ca^{2+} pump and the Na-Ca exchanger (p. 70).

As discussed later, increased $[Ca^{2+}]_i$ exerts its effect by binding to cellular proteins and changing their activity. Some Ca^{2+}-dependent signalling events are so sensitive to Ca^{2+} that a $[Ca^{2+}]_i$ increase of as little as 100 nM can trigger a vast array of cellular responses. These responses include secretion of digestive enzymes by pancreatic acinar cells, release of insulin by β cells, contraction of vascular smooth muscle, conversion of glycogen to glucose in the liver, release of histamine by mast cells, aggregation of platelets, and DNA synthesis and cell division in fibroblasts.

Calcium Activates Calmodulin-Dependent Protein Kinases

How does an increase in $[Ca^{2+}]_i$ lead to downstream responses in the signal-transduction cascade? The effects of changes in $[Ca^{2+}]_i$ are mediated by Ca^{2+}-binding proteins, the most important of which is **calmodulin (CaM)**. CaM is a high-affinity cytoplasmic Ca^{2+}-binding protein of 148 amino acids. Each molecule of CaM cooperatively binds four calcium ions. Ca^{2+} binding induces a major conformational change in CaM that allows it to bind to other proteins (Fig. 4–9). Although CaM does not have intrinsic enzymatic activity, it forms a complex with a number of enzymes and thereby confers a Ca^{2+} dependence on their activity. For example, binding of the Ca^{2+}-CaM complex activates the enzyme that degrades cAMP, cAMP phosphodiesterase.

Many of the effects of CaM are mediated by protein phosphorylation that is catalyzed by a family of Ca^{2+}-CaM–dependent kinases (**CaM kinases**). These kinases phosphorylate certain serine and threonine residues of a variety of proteins. An important CaM kinase in smooth muscle cells is myosin light chain kinase (MLCK) (p. 238). Earlier in this chapter we introduced glycogen PK, which

has the subunit structure $(\alpha\beta\gamma\delta)_4$. Whereas the α and β subunits are substrates for PKA, the δ subunits are in fact CaM (i.e., PK is also a CaM kinase). Thus, an increase in $[Ca^{2+}]_i$ can also activate PK.

MLCK, PK, and some other CaM kinases have a rather narrow substrate specificity. The ubiquitous CaM kinase II, on the other hand, has a broad substrate specificity. Especially high levels of this multifunctional enzyme are present at the synaptic terminals of neurons. One of the actions of CaM kinase II is to phosphorylate and thereby activate the rate-limiting enzyme (tyrosine hydroxylase; see Fig. 12–9C) in the synthesis of catecholamine neurotransmitters. CaM kinase can also phosphorylate itself, which allows it to remain active in the absence of Ca^{2+}.

Diacylglycerols and Ca^{2+} Activate Protein Kinase C

As noted earlier, hydrolysis of PIP_2 by PLC yields two products, the IP_3 that leads to Ca^{2+} release from internal stores and DAG (Fig. 4–8A). The most important function of DAG is to activate **protein kinase C (PKC)**, a Ca^{2+}-dependent serine/threonine kinase. In mammals, the PKC family comprises at least 10 members that differ in their tissue and cellular localization. This family is further subdivided into three groups that are all dependent on membrane-associated phosphatidylserine but have different requirements for Ca^{2+} and DAG. As a consequence, the signals generated by the PKC pathway depend on the isoforms of the enzyme that a cell expresses, as well as the levels of Ca^{2+} and DAG within the cell.

In its basal state, PKC is an inactive, soluble cytosolic protein. When Ca^{2+} binds to cytosolic PKC, PKC can interact with DAG, which is located in the inner leaflet of the plasma membrane. This interaction with DAG activates PKC by raising its affinity for Ca^{2+}. This process is often referred to as "translocation" of PKC from the cytoplasm to the membrane. In most cells, the Ca^{2+} signal is transient, whereas the resulting physiologic responses, such as proliferation or differentiation, often persist substantially longer. Sustained activation of PKC may be essential for maintaining these responses. Elevated levels of active PKC are maintained by a slow wave of elevated DAG (see Fig. 4–8B), which is due to the hydrolysis of PC by PLC and PLD.

Physiological stimulation of PKC by DAG can be mimicked by the exogenous application of a class of tumor promoters called **phorbol esters**. These plant products bind to PKC, cause it to translocate to the plasma membrane, and thus specifically activate this enzyme even in the absence of DAG.

Among the major substrates of PKC are the myristoylated, alanine-rich C kinase substrate (**MARCKS**) proteins. These acidic proteins contain consensus sites for PKC phosphorylation as well as CaM- and actin-binding sites. MARCKS proteins cross-link actin filaments and thus appear to play a role in translating extracellular signals into actin plasticity and changes in cell shape. Unphosphorylated MARCKS proteins are associated with the plasma membrane, and they cross-link actin. Phosphorylation of the MARCKS proteins causes them to translocate

FIGURE 4–9. Calmodulin. After four intracellular Ca^{2+} ions bind to calmodulin (CaM), the Ca^{2+}-CaM complex can bind to and activate another protein. In this example, the activated protein is a Ca^{2+}-CaM–dependent kinase.

Calmodulin

Ca^{2+}/Calmodulin

Ca^{2+}/Calmodulin-dependent protein kinase

Inactive protein

Active protein

Ca^{2+}

into the cytosol, where they are no longer able to cross-link actin. Thus, mitogenic growth factors that activate PKC may produce morphologic changes and anchorage-independent cell proliferation, in part by modifying the activity of MARCKS proteins.

PKC can also directly or indirectly modulate transcription factors and thereby enhance the transcription of specific genes (p. 116). Such genomic actions of PKC explain why phorbol esters are tumor promoters.

cAMP and Ca^{2+} Pathways Intersect at the Level of Second Messengers, Downstream Enzymes, and Target Molecules

A cell's response to an environmental change often involves two or more signalling pathways that interact with one another. Such interactions can occur at three levels. First, second messengers themselves can modulate each other's levels. For example, cAMP activates PKA, which in turn can phosphorylate IP_3 receptors, Ca^{2+} channels, and Ca^{2+} pumps, thereby affecting $[Ca^{2+}]_i$. On the other hand, Ca^{2+}-CaM can modulate some forms of adenylyl cyclase and phosphodiesterase and thereby affect $[cAMP]_i$.

At a second level of interaction, signalling pathways can modulate each other's downstream enzymes. For example, PKA (cAMP cascade) can phosphorylate CaM kinases (Ca^{2+} cascade).

At a third level of interaction, multiple signal transduction pathways may modify the same target molecules. For example, PKA, PKC, and CaM kinases often phosphorylate sites on the same proteins. We have already noted that glycogen PK is the target of both PKA (cAMP pathway), which phosphorylates the α and β subunits, and Ca^{2+}, which activates the δ subunit (i.e., CaM).

G-PROTEIN SECOND MESSENGERS: ARACHIDONIC ACID METABOLITES

As previously discussed, PLC can hydrolyze PIP_2 and thereby release two important signalling molecules, IP_3 and DAG. In addition, both PLC and PLD can release

DAG from PC. However, other hydrolysis products of membrane phospholipids can also act as signalling molecules. The best characterized of these hydrolysis products is **arachidonic acid,** which is found esterified at the second carbon of the glycerol backbone of membrane phospholipids (Fig. 4–10). PLA_2 initiates the cellular actions of AA by releasing this fatty acid from glycerol-based phospholipids. A series of enzymes subsequently convert AA into a family of biologically active metabolites that are collectively called **eicosanoids** (from the Greek eikosi for 20) because, like AA, they all have 20 carbon atoms. Three major pathways can convert AA into these eicosanoids (Fig. 4–11). In the first pathway, cyclooxygenase (COX) enzymes produce *thromboxanes*, *prostaglandins*, and *prostacyclins*. In the second pathway, 5-lipoxygenase enzymes produce *leukotrienes* and some hydroxyeicosatetraenoic acid (*HETE*) compounds. In the third pathway, the epoxygenase enzymes, which are members of the cytochrome P-450 class, produce other *HETE* compounds, as well as *cis*-epoxy-eicosatrienoic acid (*EET*) compounds. These three enzymes catalyze the stereospecific insertion of molecular oxygen into various positions in AA. The COXs, lipoxygenases, and epoxygenases are selectively distributed in different cell types, further increasing the complexity of eicosanoid biology. Eicosanoids have powerful biologic activities, including effects on allergic and inflammatory processes, platelet aggregation, vascular smooth muscle, and gastric acid secretion.

Phospholipase A_2 Is the Primary Enzyme Responsible for Releasing Arachidonic Acid

The first step in the PLA_2 signal-transduction cascade is binding of an extracellular agonist to a membrane receptor (see Fig. 4–11). These receptors include those for serotonin (5-HT_2 receptors), glutamate (mGLUR1 receptors), fibroblast growth factor–β (FGF-β), INF-α, and INF-γ. Once the receptor is occupied by its agonist, it can activate a G protein that belongs to the G_i/G_o family. The mechanism by which this activated G protein stimulates PLA_2 is not well understood. It does not appear that

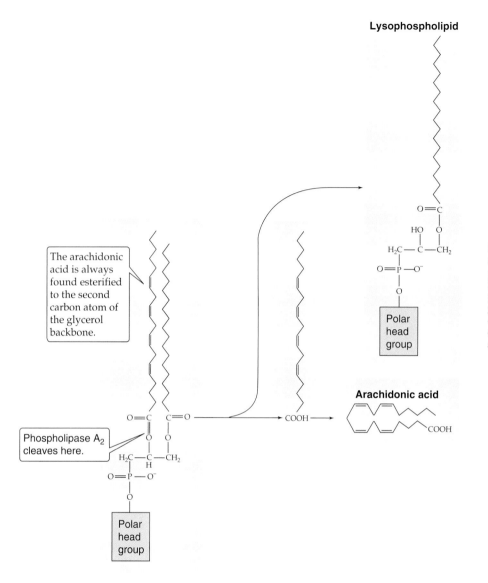

FIGURE 4–10. Release of arachidonic acid from membrane phospholipids by phospholipase A_2. Arachidonic acid (AA) is esterified to membrane phospholipids at the second carbon of the glycerol backbone. Phospholipase A_2 cleaves the phospholipid at the indicated position and releases AA as well as a lysophospholipid.

a G-protein α subunit is involved. The G-protein $\beta\gamma$ dimer may stimulate PLA_2 either directly or via mitogen-activated protein **(MAP) kinase** (p. 134), which phosphorylates PLA_2 at a serine residue. The result is rapid hydrolysis of phospholipids that contain AA.

In contrast to the *direct* pathway just mentioned, agonists acting on other receptors may promote AA release indirectly. First, a ligand may bind to a receptor coupled to PLC, which would lead to the release of DAG (see Fig. 4–11). As noted earlier, DAG lipase can cleave DAG to yield AA and a monoacylglycerol (MAG). Agonists that act via this pathway include dopamine (D_2 receptors), adenosine (A1 receptors), norepinephrine (α_2-adrenergic receptors), and serotonin ($5-HT_1$ receptors). Second, any agonist that raises $[Ca^{2+}]_i$ can promote AA formation because Ca^{2+} can stimulate some cytosolic forms of PLA_2. Third, any signal-transduction pathway that activates MAP kinase can also enhance AA release because, as discussed, MAP kinase phosphorylates PLA_2 on a serine residue. For example, two growth factors that we discuss later—plate-let-derived growth factor (PDGF) and epidermal growth factor (EGF)—also activate MAP kinase.

Cyclooxygenases, Lipoxygenases, and Epoxygenases Mediate the Formation of Biologically Active Eicosanoids

Once released from the membrane, AA can diffuse out of the cell, be reincorporated into membrane phospholipids, or be metabolized (see Fig. 4–11). The eicosanoids formed from AA can act as second messengers and affect the activity of other intracellular enzymes and ion channels in the same cell as well as act as local mediators and have profound paracrine effects on neighboring cells, as seen in the inflammatory response.

In the first pathway of AA metabolism (see Fig. 4–11), **cyclooxygenases** catalyze the stepwise conversion of AA into the intermediates prostaglandin G_2 (PGG_2) and prostaglandin H_2 (PGH_2). As noted in the box titled Inhibition of Cyclooxygenase Isoforms by Aspirin, COX exists in

FIGURE 4–11. Arachidonic acid: signalling pathways. In the direct pathway, an agonist binds to a receptor that activates phospholipase A_2 (PLA_2), which releases arachidonic acid (AA) from a membrane phospholipid (see Fig. 4–10). In one of three indirect pathways, an agonist binds to a different receptor that activates PLC and thereby leads to the formation of diacylglycerol (DAG) and IP_3, as in Fig. 4–8; DAG lipase then releases the AA from DAG. In a second indirect pathway, the IP_3 releases Ca^{2+} from internal stores, which leads to the activation of PLA_2 (see "direct pathway"). In a third indirect pathway (*not shown*), mitogen-activated protein (MAP) kinase stimulates PLA_2. Regardless of its source, the AA may follow any of three pathways to form a wide array of eicosanoids. The cyclooxygenase (COX) pathway produces thromboxanes, prostacyclins, and prostaglandins. The 5-lipoxygenase pathway produces 5-HETE and the leukotrienes. The epoxygenase pathway leads to the production of other HETEs and EETs. ASA, acetylsalicylic acid; EET, *cis*-epoxyeicosatrienoic acid; ER, endoplasmic reticulum; HETE, hydroxyeicosatetraenoic acid; MAG, monoacylglycerol.

INHIBITION OF CYCLOOXYGENASE ISOFORMS BY ASPIRIN

Cyclooxygenase (COX) is a bifunctional enzyme that first oxidizes arachidonic acid to prostaglandin G_2 (PGG_2) through its *cyclooxygenase* activity and then *peroxidizes* this compound to PGH_2. COX exists in two forms, COX-1 and COX-2. X-ray crystallographic studies of **COX-1** reveal that the sites for the two enzymatic activities (i.e., COX and peroxidase) are adjacent but spatially distinct. The COX site is a long hydrophobic channel. **Aspirin** (acetylsalicylic acid) irreversibly inhibits COX-1 by acetylating a serine residue at the top of this channel. Several of the other nonsteroidal anti-inflammatory drugs interact, via their carboxyl groups, with other amino acids in the same region. COX-1 is constitutively expressed. When activated, COX-1 produces **prostacyclins.** In the case of endothelial cells, prostacyclins inhibit the formation of blood clots ("thrombi"). In the case of gastric mucosa, prostacyclins are cytoprotective.

COX-2 is induced in a number of cell types by inflammatory stimuli. Thus, the anti-inflammatory actions of aspirin are probably due to inhibition of COX-2, whereas the unwanted side effects (e.g., irritation of the stomach lining and toxic effects on the kidney) are due to inhibition of COX-1. Fortunately, the two enzymes are only 60% homologous, and pharmaceutical companies have generated compounds that specifically inhibit COX-2. In addition, because low doses of aspirin are very efficient at inhibiting thromboxane A_2 production by platelets, use of this compound in the prevention of heart attack and stroke is likely to increase.

two isoforms, COX-1 and COX-2. In monocytes stimulated by inflammatory agents such as IL-1β, only levels of COX-2 increase. Thus, the induction of COX-2 may participate in the inflammatory response. PGH_2 is the precursor of the other **prostaglandins**, the **prostacyclins** and the **thromboxanes**. The nomenclature of the eicosanoids is not as arcane as it might first appear. The numerical subscript "2" (as in PGH_2) or "4" (as in leukotriene A_4 [LTA_4]) refers to the number of double bonds in the eicosanoid backbone. For example, AA has four double bonds, as do the leukotrienes. For the COX metabolites, the letter (A to I) immediately preceding the "2" refers to the structure of the 5-carbon ring that is formed about halfway along the 20-carbon chain of the eicosanoid.

In the second pathway of AA metabolism, **5-lipoxygenase** initiates the conversion of AA into biologically active **leukotrienes**. For example, in myeloid cells, 5-lipoxygenase converts AA to 5-HPETE, which is short lived and rapidly degraded by a peroxidase to the corresponding alcohol 5-HETE. Alternatively, a dehydrase can convert 5-HPETE to an unstable epoxide, LTA_4, which can either be further metabolized by LTA_4 hydrolase to LTB_4 or coupled ("conjugated") to the tripeptide glutathione (p. 987). This conjugation—via the cysteine residue of glutathione—yields LTC_4. This product is the substrate for several proteases, which generate LTD_4 and LTE_4. LTC_4, D_4,

and E_4 are the "cysteinyl" leukotrienes; they participate in allergic and inflammatory responses and make up the mixture previously described as the "**slow-reacting substance of anaphylaxis**." As far as nomenclature of the leukotrienes is concerned, the letters A, B, or C through F, which immediately precede the "4," refer to differences in the backbone of the eicosanoid. For the cysteinyl leukotrienes, the letters C through F refer to different derivatives of the conjugated cysteine.

The third pathway of AA metabolism begins with the transformation of AA by **epoxygenase** (a cytochrome P-450 oxidase). Molecular oxygen is a substrate in this reaction. The epoxygenase pathway converts AA into two major products, **HETEs** and **EETs**. Members of both groups display a diverse array of biologic activities. Moreover, the cells of different tissues (e.g., liver, kidney, eye, and pituitary) use different biosynthetic pathways to generate different epoxygenase products.

Prostaglandins, Prostacyclins, and Thromboxanes (COX Products) Are Vasoactive, Regulate Platelet Action, and Modulate Ion Transport

The metabolism of PGH_2 is cell-specific. Many cells produce prostaglandins. Acting locally in a paracrine or autocrine fashion, **prostaglandins** are involved in such processes as platelet aggregation, constriction of the airways, renin release, and inflammation. Prostaglandins also are vasoactive and are important in the regulation of renal blood flow. Platelets convert PGH_2 to **thromboxane A_2**, a short-lived compound that can aggregate platelets, bring about the platelet release reaction, and constrict small blood vessels. On the other hand, endothelial cells convert PGH_2 to **prostacyclin I_2** (also known as PGI_2), which inhibits platelet aggregation and dilates blood vessels.

The eicosanoids may participate in regulation of the Na-K pump, which plays a central role in salt and water transport in the kidney and the maintenance of ion gradients in all cell types. For example, the inhibition of the Na-K pump produced by IL-1 appears to be mediated by the formation of PGE_2. Indeed, IL-1 stimulates the formation of PGE_2, and application of exogenous PGE_2 inhibits Na-K pump activity directly. Moreover, COX blockers prevent the Na-K pump inhibition induced by IL-1. This action on the Na-K pump is not limited to the kidney; AA metabolites also inhibit the pump in the brain.

Prostaglandin synthesis has also been implicated in the pathophysiology of cardiovascular disease, cancer, and inflammatory diseases. Nonsteroidal anti-inflammatory drugs (NSAIDs) such as aspirin, acetaminophen, ibuprofen, indomethacin, and naproxen directly target COX. NSAID inhibition of COX is a useful tool in the treatment of inflammation and fever and, more recently, in the prevention of heart disease.

The Leukotrienes (5-Lipoxygenase Products) Play a Major Role in Inflammatory Responses

Both free AA and its metabolites can influence the activity of many ion channels, either directly or by regulating

TABLE 4–3

INVOLVEMENT OF LEUKOTRIENES IN HUMAN DISEASE

DISEASE	EVIDENCE
Asthma	Bronchoconstriction from inhaled LTE$_4$; identification of LTC$_4$, LTD$_4$, and LTE$_4$ in the serum or urine or both of patients with asthma
Psoriasis	LTB$_4$ and LTE$_2$ found in fluids from psoriatic lesions
Adult respiratory distress syndrome	Elevated levels of LTB$_4$ detected in the plasma of patients with ARDS
Allergic rhinitis	Elevated levels of LTB$_4$ found in nasal fluids
Gout	LTB$_4$ detected in joint fluid
Rheumatoid arthritis	Elevated LTB$_4$ found in joint fluids and serum
Inflammatory bowel disease (ulcerative colitis and Crohn's disease)	Identification of LTB$_4$ in GI fluids and LTE$_4$ in urine

LT, leukotriene.

intracellular protein kinases. For example, in synaptic nerve endings, lipoxygenase metabolites of AA decrease the excitability of cells by activating K$^+$ channels. In addition to their effects on channels, lipoxygenase products may also regulate secretion. In pancreatic islet cells, free AA generated in response to glucose appears to be part of a negative feedback loop that prevents excess insulin secretion by inhibiting CaM kinase II.

The biologic effects of many AA metabolites have led to the suggestion that they have a role in allergic and inflammatory diseases (Table 4–3).

The HETEs and EETs (Epoxygenase Products) Tend to Enhance Ca^{2+} Release from Intracellular Stores and to Enhance Cell Proliferation

The epoxygenase pathway leads to the production of HETEs other than 5-HETE as well as EETs. HETEs and EETs have been implicated in a wide variety of processes, some of which are summarized in Table 4–4. For example, in stimulated mononuclear leukocytes, HETEs enhance Ca^{2+} release from intracellular stores and promote cell proliferation. In smooth muscle cells, HETEs increase proliferation and migration; these AA metabolites may be one of the primary factors involved in the formation of atherosclerotic plaque. In blood vessels, HETEs can be potent vasoconstrictors.

EETs generally tend to enhance the release of Ca^{2+} from intracellular stores, Na-H exchange, and cell proliferation. In blood vessels, EETs cause vasodilation and angiogenesis.

Degradation of the Eicosanoids Terminates Their Activity

Inactivation of the products of eicosanoids is an important mechanism for terminating their biologic action. In the case of COX products, the enzyme 15-hydroxyprostaglandin dehydrogenase catalyzes the initial reactions that convert biologically active prostaglandins into their inactive 15-keto metabolites. This enzyme also appears to be active in the catabolism of thromboxanes.

As far as the 5-lipoxygenase products are concerned, the specificity and cellular distribution of the enzymes that metabolize leukotrienes parallel the diversity of the enzymes involved in their synthesis. For example, 20-hydrolase-LTB$_4$, a member of the P-450 family, catalyzes the ω oxidation of LTB$_4$, thereby terminating its biologic activity. LTC$_4$ is metabolized through two pathways. One oxidizes the LTC$_4$. The other pathway first removes the glutamic acid residue of the conjugated glutathione, which yields LTD$_4$, and then removes the glycine residue, which yields LTE$_4$, which is readily excreted into the urine.

In the case of epoxygenase (cytochrome P-450) products, it has been difficult to characterize their metabolic

ROLE OF LEUKOTRIENES IN DISEASE

Since the original description of the "slow-reacting substance of anaphylaxis," which is generated during antigenic challenge of a sensitized lung, leukotrienes have been presumed to play a part in allergic disease of the airways (Table 4–3). The involvement of cells (mast cells, basophils, and eosinophils) that produce cysteinyl leukotrienes (LTC$_4$ through LTF$_4$) in these pathobiologic processes supports this concept. In addition, LTC$_4$, LTD$_4$, and LTE$_4$ are found in lavage fluid from the nares of patients with allergic rhinitis after the application of specific antigens to the nasal airways. The pharmacologic effects of the leukotrienes on human airways give further credence to the idea that these compounds are important mediators of **allergic asthma.** In normal subjects, introducing LTC$_4$ or LTD$_4$ into the airways as an aerosol (nebulizer concentration of only 10 μM) causes maximal expiratory airflow (a rough measure of airway resistance; see p. 621) to decline by 30%. This bronchoconstrictor effect is 1000-fold more potent than that of histamine, the "reference" agonist. Leukotrienes affect both large and small airways, whereas histamine affects relatively smaller airways.

In addition to their involvement in allergic disease, several of the leukotrienes are associated with other inflammatory disorders. Synovial fluid from patients with **rheumatoid arthritis** contains 5-lipoxygenase products. Another example is the skin disease **psoriasis.** In patients with active psoriasis, LTB$_4$, LTC$_4$, and LTD$_4$ have been recovered from skin chambers overlying abraded lesions. Leukotrienes also appear to be involved in inflammatory bowel disease. LTB$_4$ and other leukotrienes are generated and released *in vitro* from intestinal mucosa obtained from patients with **ulcerative colitis** or **Crohn disease.**

TABLE 4–4

ACTIONS OF EPOXYGENASE PRODUCTS

	CELL/TISSUE	ACTION
HETEs	Stimulated mono-nuclear leukocytes	↑ Cell proliferation ↑ Ca²⁺ release from intracellular stores ↓ TNF production
	β Cells of pancreatic islets	Implicated in the destruction of these cells in type 1 (juvenile-onset) diabetes mellitus
	Endothelial cells	↓ Release of fibrinolytic factors ↓ Binding of anti-thrombin
	Vascular smooth muscle cells	↑ Cell proliferation ↑ Migration Formation of athero-sclerotic plaque?
	Blood vessels	Potent vasoconstrictors "Myogenic" vasoconstrictive response of renal and cerebral arteries
EETs	Cells, general	↑ Ca²⁺ release from intracellular stores ↑ Na-H exchange ↑ Cell proliferation ↓ COX activity
	Endocrine cells	↓ Release of somatostatin, insulin, glucagon
	Toad bladder	↓ Vasopressin-stimulated H₂O permeability ↓ Renin release
	Blood vessels	Vasodilation Angiogenesis
	Endothelium Platelets	↑ Tumor cell adhesion ↓ Aggregation

COX, cyclooxygenase; EETs, cis-epoxyeicosatrienoic acids; HETEs, hydroxyeicosatetraenoic acids; TNF, tumor necrosis factor.

breakdown because the reactions are so rapid and complex. Both enzymatic and nonenzymatic hydration reactions convert these molecules to the corresponding vicinyl diols. Some members of this group can form conjugates with reduced glutathione (GSH).

Platelet-Activating Factor Is a Lipid Mediator Unrelated to Arachidonic Acid

Although it is not a member of the AA family, platelet-activating factor (PAF) is an important lipid signalling molecule. PAF is an *ether* lipid that the cell synthesizes either de novo or by remodeling a membrane-bound precursor. PAF occurs in a wide variety of organisms and mediates many biologic activities. In mammals, PAF is a

potent inducer of platelet aggregation and stimulates the chemotaxis and degranulation of neutrophils, thereby facilitating the release of LTB₄ and 5-HETE. PAF is involved in several aspects of allergic reactions; for example, it stimulates histamine release and enhances the secretion of IgE, IgA, and TNF. Endothelial cells are also an important target of PAF; PAF causes a negative shift of V_m in these cells by activating Ca²⁺-dependent K⁺ channels. PAF also enhances vascular permeability and the adhesion of neutrophils and platelets to endothelial cells.

PAF exerts its effects by binding to a specific receptor on the plasma membrane. A major consequence of PAF binding to its G-protein–coupled receptor is formation of IP₃ and stimulation of a group of MAP kinases. PAF acetylhydrolase terminates the action of this signalling lipid.

RECEPTORS THAT ARE CATALYTIC

A number of hormones and growth factors bind to cell-surface proteins that have—or are associated with—enzymatic activity on the cytoplasmic side of the membrane. Five classes of such catalytic receptors are discussed here (Fig. 4–12):

Receptor guanylyl cyclases catalyze the generation of cGMP from GTP.

Receptor serine/threonine kinases phosphorylate serine and/or threonine residues on cellular proteins

Receptor tyrosine kinases (RTKs) phosphorylate tyrosine residues on themselves and other proteins.

Tyrosine kinase–associated receptors interact with cytosolic (i.e., non–membrane-bound) tyrosine kinases.

Receptor tyrosine phosphatases cleave phosphate groups from tyrosine groups of cellular proteins.

The Receptor Guanylyl Cyclase Transduces the Activity of Atrial Natriuretic Peptide, Whereas a Soluble Guanylyl Cyclase Transduces the Activity of Nitric Oxide

RECEPTOR (i.e., MEMBRANE-BOUND) GUANYLYL CYCLASE. Some of the best characterized examples of a transmembrane protein with guanylyl cyclase activity (Fig. 4–12A) are the receptors for **atrial natriuretic peptide (ANP)**. The ANP hormones are a family of related peptides of approximately 28 amino acids that myocytes of the cardiac atria release in response to stretch. ANP has two major effects. First, it acts on vascular smooth muscle to dilate blood vessels (p. 555). Second, it enhances Na⁺ excretion into urine, which is termed "natriuresis" (p. 867). Both activities contribute to lowering blood pressure and effective circulating blood volume (p. 80).

The receptor for ANP is a membrane protein with a single membrane-spanning segment. The extracellular domain binds the ligand. The intracellular domain has two consensus catalytic domains for guanylyl cyclase activity. Binding of ANP induces a conformational change in the receptor that causes receptor dimerization and activation. Thus, binding of ANP to its receptor causes the conversion of GTP to cGMP and raises intracellular levels of

A RECEPTOR GUANYLYL CYCLASES

Extracellular space

N   N

Guanylyl cyclase domains

Cytosol   **ANP RECEPTOR**

B RECEPTOR SERINE/THREONINE KINASES

Ligand

N   N

Serine-threonine kinase domain

Type I

Type II

This is the kinase that phosphorylates downstream effectors.

TGF-β RECEPTOR

C RECEPTOR TYROSINE KINASES (RTKs)

Ligand

N   N

N   N   α

S S   S ─ S   S S
S   S

β

Tyrosine kinase domains

NGF RECEPTOR   **INSULIN RECEPTOR**

D TYROSINE-KINASE–ASSOCIATED RECEPTORS

N   N

JAK   JAK

Tyrosine kinase domains

LIF RECEPTOR

E RECEPTOR TYROSINE PHOSPHATASES

Carbohydrate groups

Tyrosine phosphatase domain

CD45

FIGURE 4–12. Catalytic receptors. *A,* Receptor of guanylyl cyclases has an extracellular ligand-binding domain. Ligand binding leads to receptor dimerization and activation of guanylyl cyclase activity, which converts GTP to cGMP. *B,* Receptor serine/threonine kinases have two subunits, each of which has intrinsic serine/threonine kinase activity. The ligand (e.g., TGFβ) binds to the type II subunit, causing it to transphosphorylate the type I subunit at serine and threonine residues. This phosphorylation, in turn, activates the type I subunit, which phosphorylates intracellular proteins at serine and/or threonine residues. *C,* There are two classes of receptor tyrosine kinases (RTKs). Ligand binding to two NGF receptors leads to receptor dimerization and activation of tyrosine kinase activity. The monomers in the dimer phosphorylate each other as well as downstream effectors. Ligand binding to the insulin receptor causes conformational changes in each of the two *αβ* pairs, which leads to activation of the tyrosine kinases on the *β* subunits. The activated *β* subunits then phosphorylate each other as well as downstream effectors. *D,* The tyrosine-kinase–associated receptors have *no* intrinsic enzyme activity. However, tyrosine kinases of the Src and Janus families associate noncovalently with these receptors. Ligand binding leads to the formation of receptor homodimers, heterodimers, or trimers. This aggregation stimulates the associated tyrosine kinases. An example is the receptor for LIF. *E,* Receptor tyrosine phosphatases have intrinsic tyrosine phosphatase activity. An example is the CD45 protein. Antibody binding to CD45 stimulates its phosphatase activity. ANP, atrial natriuretic peptide; cGMP, cyclic guanosine monophosphate; GTP, guanosine triphosphate; JAK, Janus kinase (originally "just another kinase"); LIF, leukemia inhibitory factor; NGF, nerve growth factor; TGF, transforming growth factor.

cGMP. In turn, cGMP activates a **cGMP-dependent kinase** ("G kinase" or PKG) that phosphorylates proteins at certain serine and threonine residues. In the renal medullary collecting duct, the cGMP generated in response to ANP may act not only via PKG but also by directly modulating ion channels (p. 788).

SOLUBLE GUANYLYL CYCLASE. In contrast to the receptor for ANP, which is an intrinsic membrane protein with guanylyl cyclase activity, the receptor for **nitric oxide** is a soluble (i.e., cytosolic) guanylyl cyclase. This soluble guanylyl cyclase (sGC) is totally unrelated to the receptor guanylyl cyclase and contains a heme moiety that binds NO.

NO plays an important role in the control of blood flow and blood pressure. Vascular endothelial cells use the enzyme **NO synthase** (NOS) to cleave arginine into citrulline plus NO in response to stimuli such as ACh, bradykinin, substance P, thrombin, adenine nucleotides, and Ca^{2+}. These agents trigger the entry of Ca^{2+}, which binds to cytosolic CaM and then stimulates NOS. Activation of NOS also requires the cofactors tetrahydrobiopterin and NADPH. The newly synthesized NO rapidly diffuses out of the endothelial cell and crosses the membrane of a neighboring smooth muscle cell. In smooth muscle, NO stimulates its "receptor," soluble guanylyl cyclase, which then converts GTP to cGMP. As a result, $[cGMP]_i$ may increase 50-fold and relax the smooth muscle.

The importance of NO in the control of blood flow had long been exploited unwittingly to treat **angina pectoris**. Angina is the classic chest pain that accompanies inadequate blood flow to the heart muscle, usually as a result of coronary artery atherosclerosis. Nitroglycerin relieves this pain by spontaneously breaking down and releasing NO. NO relaxes the smooth muscles of peripheral arterioles, thereby reducing the work of the heart and relieving the associated pain.

In addition to its role as a chemical signal in blood vessels, NO appears to play an important role in the destruction of invading organisms by macrophages and neutrophils. NO also serves as a neurotransmitter (p. 304) and may play a role in learning and memory (p. 322). Some of these actions may involve different forms of NOS.

The importance of the NO signalling pathway was recognized by the awarding of the 1998 Nobel Prize for Physiology or Medicine to Drs. R.F. Furchgott, L.J. Ignarro, and F. Murad for their discoveries concerning nitric oxide as a signalling molecule in the cardiovascular system.

Some Catalytic Receptors Are Serine/Threonine Kinases

Earlier in this chapter we discuss how activation of various G-protein–linked receptors can initiate a cascade that eventually activates kinases that phosphorylate proteins at serine and threonine residues. Examples of such serine/threonine kinases are PKA, PKC, and the CaM-dependent protein kinases. Some receptors, such as the one for transforming growth factor-β (TGF-β), are also serine/threonine kinases and are thus catalytic receptors.

The TGF-β superfamily includes a large group of cytokines, including five TGF-βs, anti-Müllerian hormone (AMH), the inhibins, the activins, bone morphogenic proteins, and other glycoproteins, all of which control cell growth and differentiation. Members of this family participate in establishing the basic body plan during embryogenesis and also play key roles in suppressing epithelial cell growth, promoting wound repair, and influencing important immune and endocrine functions. The roles of AMH, inhibins, and activins in differentiation and regulation of the male and female reproductive systems are discussed in Chapters 52 through 54.

The receptors for TGF-β and related factors are glycoproteins with a single membrane-spanning segment and intrinsic serine/threonine-kinase activity. Receptor types I and II (see Fig. 4–12B) are required for ligand binding and catalytic activity. Although the **type II receptor** binds the ligand, this receptor by itself does not transmit the signal downstream. Although the **type I receptor** cannot bind TGF-β, it recognizes that the ligand has bound to the type II receptor and forms a very stable ternary ligand/type I receptor/type II receptor complex. Recruitment of the type I receptor into the complex results in phosphorylation of the type I receptor at serine and threonine residues, which in turn activates the kinase activity of the type I receptor and propagates the signal to downstream effectors.

Substrates of activated type I kinase include the SMAD family of transcription factors. The TGF-β receptor complex specifically phosphorylates members of the SMAD family, which then translocate to the nucleus and contribute to the formation of transcriptional complexes (p. 127).

Receptor Tyrosine Kinases Produce Phosphotyrosine Motifs Recognized by SH Domains of Downstream Effectors

In addition to the class of receptors with intrinsic *serine/threonine* kinase activity, other plasma membrane receptors have intrinsic *tyrosine* kinase activity. All **receptor tyrosine kinases** discovered to date phosphorylate themselves in addition to other cellular proteins. EGF, PDGF, insulin and insulin-related growth factor type I (IGF-1), FGF, and NGF can all bind to receptors that possess intrinsic tyrosine kinase activity.

Most RTKs are single-pass transmembrane proteins that contain a single intracellular kinase domain (see Fig. 4–12C, left receptor). Binding of a ligand, such as **NGF**, induces a conformational change in the receptor that facilitates the formation of receptor dimers. Dimerization allows the two cytoplasmic catalytic domains to phosphorylate each other ("autophosphorylation") and thereby activate the receptor complex. The activated receptors also catalyze the addition of phosphate to tyrosine residues on specific cytoplasmic proteins. The resulting phosphotyrosines of the receptor and other protein substrates serve as high-affinity binding sites for a number of intracellular signalling molecules. These interactions lead to the formation of a signalling complex and the activation of downstream effectors.

Activation of **insulin** and **IGF-I** receptors (see Fig. 4–12C, right receptor) occurs by a somewhat different

TABLE 4–5

THE TYROSINE PHOSPHOPEPTIDES OF THE PDGF RECEPTOR THAT ARE RECOGNIZED BY SH2 DOMAINS ON VARIOUS PROTEINS		
TYROSINE (Y) THAT IS PHOSPHORYLATED IN THE PDGF RECEPTOR	**PHOSPHOTYROSINE (pY) MOTIF RECOGNIZED BY THE SH2-CONTAINING PROTEIN**	**SH2-CONTAINING PROTEIN**
Y579	pYIYVD	Src family kinases
Y708	pYMDMS	p85
Y719	pYVPML	p85
Y739	pYNAPY	GAP
Y1021	pYIIPY	PLCγ

GAP, guanosine triphosphatase–activating protein; PDGF, platelet-derived growth factor; PLCγ, phospholipase Cγ; SH2, *Src* homology domain 2.

mechanism. These receptors are tetrameric; they are composed of two α and two β subunits. The α subunit contains a cysteine-rich region and functions in ligand binding. The β subunit is a single-pass transmembrane protein with a cytoplasmic tyrosine kinase domain. The α and β subunits are held together by disulfide bonds (as are the two α subunits), forming a heterotetramer. Ligand binding produces conformational changes that appear to cause allosteric interactions between the two α and β pairs, as opposed to the dimerization characteristic of the first class of RTKs (see Fig. 4–12C, *left*). Thus, insulin binding results in the autophosphorylation of tyrosine residues in the catalytic domains of the β subunits. The activated insulin receptor also phosphorylates cytoplasmic substrates such as **IRS-1** (insulin-receptor substrate-1; p. 1074), which, once phosphorylated, serves as a docking site for additional signalling proteins.

We have seen that an RTK, when activated by its ligand, produces phosphotyrosines either on the RTK itself or on other proteins. How are these phosphotyrosine "signals" transmitted to the subsequent steps in the signal-transduction cascade? These phosphotyrosines bind to a large number of cytoplasmic proteins that have in common two highly conserved motifs called SH2 and SH3. These names are a shorthand for Src homology domains 2 and 3, which were first identified in the *src* oncogene. These SH2 and SH3 motifs are critical in the signalling pathways downstream of tyrosine kinase activating growth factors. **SH2** domains are approximately 100 amino acids in length. They are composed of relatively well-conserved residues that form the binding pocket for phosphotyrosine motifs, as well as more variable residues that are implicated in binding specificity. These SH2 domains recognize the three amino acids on the C-terminal side of the phosphotyrosine. For example, the activated PDGF receptor has five such phosphotyrosine regions (Table 4–5), each of which interacts with a specific SH2-containing protein. **SH3** domains are approximately 50 amino acids in length. They are also modular and appear to be responsible for targeting signalling molecules to specific subcellular locations.

SH2- or SH3-containing proteins include growth factor receptor–bound protein-2 (GRB2), PLCγ, and the receptor-associated tyrosine kinases of the Src family. **GRB2** (p. 134) is the first step in activating the Ras-dependent signalling pathway, the targets of which are transcription factors that modulate gene transcription. As we will see in the next section, members of the Src family represent some of the tyrosine kinases that are activated by tyrosine kinase–associated receptors. Thus, the phosphorylation of Src by RTKs is an example of crosstalk between RTKs and the tyrosine kinase–associated receptors.

Tyrosine Kinase–Associated Receptors Activate Loosely Associated Tyrosine Kinases Such as Src and JAK

Some of the receptors for cytokines and growth factors that regulate cell proliferation and differentiation trigger tyrosine kinase activity, even though they themselves do not have *intrinsic* tyrosine kinase activity (see Fig. 4–12D). Receptors in this class include those for several cytokines, including IL-2, IL-3, IL-4, IL-5, IL-6, leukemia inhibitory factor (LIF), granulocyte-macrophage colony-stimulating factor (GM-CSF), and erythropoietin (EPO). The family also includes receptors for growth hormone (GH), prolactin (PRL), ciliary neurotrophin factor (CNTF), oncostatin M, and INF-α, INF-β, and INF-γ. The **tyrosine kinase–associated receptors** comprise multiple subunits that form homodimers (αα), heterodimers (αβ), or heterotrimers (αβγ). For example, the IL-3 and the GM-CSF receptors are heterodimers (αβ) that share common β subunits with transducing activity. However, none of the cytoplasmic portions of the receptor subunits contains kinase domains or other sequences with recognized catalytic function. Instead, tyrosine kinases of the Src family and Janus family (JAK or Janus kinases) associate noncovalently with the cytoplasmic domains of these receptors. Thus, these are **receptor-associated tyrosine kinases**. Ligand binding to these receptors results in receptor dimerization and tyrosine kinase activity. The activated kinase then phosphorylates tyrosines on both itself and the receptor. Thus, tyrosine kinase–associated receptors, together with their tyrosine kinases, function much like the RTKs discussed in the previous section. A key difference is that for the tyrosine kinase–*associated* receptors, the receptors and kinases are encoded by separate genes and the proteins are only loosely associated with one another.

The **Src** family of receptor-associated tyrosine kinases includes at least nine members. Alternative initiation codons and tissue-specific splicing (p. 139) result in at least 14 related gene products. Many of these gene products were first identified in transformed cells or tumors. However, these Src proteins are important in normal cells. When a member of the Src family becomes mutated in such a way that it is spontaneously active, it may function as an **oncogene**. The normal, unaltered physiological counterpart of an oncogene is called a **proto-oncogene**. The conserved regions of Src-related proteins can be divided into five domains: (1) an N-terminal myristylation site, through which the kinase is tethered to the membrane; (2) an SH3 domain, which binds to proline-rich regions of cytosolic proteins; (3) an

SH2 domain, which binds phosphorylated tyrosines; (4) the catalytic domain, which has tyrosine kinase activity; and (5) a noncatalytic C terminus. Members of this family are regulated by tyrosine phosphorylation as well as by allosteric mechanisms.

The **Janus family** of receptor-associated tyrosine kinases includes **JAK1, JAK2, and Tyk2**. JAK stands for "just another kinase." One of the major downstream targets of the JAKs is one or more of the members of the so-called STAT (signal transducers and activators of transcription) family. When phosphorylated, STATs interact with other STAT family members to form a complex that translocates to the nucleus (p. 135). There, the complex facilitates the transcription of specific genes that seem to be specialized for a rapid response, such as those that are characterized by the **acute-phase response** of inflammation (p. 1240). For example, after IL-6 binds to hepatocytes, the STAT pathway is responsible for producing **acute phase proteins**. During inflammation, these acute phase proteins function to limit tissue damage by inhibiting the proteases that attack healthy cells as well as diseased ones. The *pattern* of STAT activation provides a mechanism for cytokine individuality. For example, EPO activates STAT5a and STAT5b as part of the early events in erythropoiesis, whereas IL-4 or IL-12 activates STAT4 and STAT6.

Attenuation of the cytokine JAK-STAT signalling cascade involves the production of **inhibitors** that suppress tyrosine phosphorylation and activation of the STATs. For example, IL-6 and LIF both induce expression of the inhibitor SST-1, which contains an SH2 domain and prevents JAK2 or Tyk2 from activating STAT3 in M1 myeloid leukemia cells.

Receptor Tyrosine Phosphatases Are Required for Lymphocyte Activation

Tyrosine residues that are phosphorylated by the tyrosine kinases described in the previous two sections are *dephosphorylated* by phosphotyrosine phosphatases (PTPs), which can be either cytosolic or membrane bound (i.e., the receptor tyrosine phosphatases). We discussed the cytosolic PTPs earlier. Both classes of *tyrosine* phosphatases have very different structures from the ones that dephosphorylate *serine* and *threonine* residues. Because the tyrosine phosphatases are extremely active, phosphotyrosine groups tend to have brief life spans and are relatively few in number.

The **CD45** protein, found at the cell surface of T and B lymphocytes, is an example of a receptor tyrosine phosphatase. CD45 makes a single pass through the membrane. Its glycosylated extracellular domain functions as a receptor for antibodies, whereas its cytoplasmic domain is a catalytic site with tyrosine phosphatase activity (see Fig. 4–12*E*). During their maturation, lymphocytes express several variants of CD45 characterized by different patterns of alternative splicing and glycosylation. CD45 plays a critical role in signal transduction in lymphocytes. For instance, CD45 dephosphorylates and thereby activates *lck* and *fyn* (two receptor-associated tyrosine kinases of the Src family) and triggers the phosphorylation of other proteins downstream in the signal transduction cascade. This interaction between receptor tyrosine phosphatases and

ONCOGENES

The ability of certain viral proteins (**oncogenes**) to transform a cell from a normal to a malignant phenotype was initially thought to occur because these viral proteins acted as transcriptional activators or repressors. However, over the last 20 years only a few of these viral proteins have been found to work in this manner. The majority of these oncogenes harbor mutations that transform them into constitutively active forms of normal cellular signalling proteins called **proto-oncogenes.** Most of these aberrant proteins (i.e., the oncogenes) encode proteins important in a key signal transduction pathway. For example, expression of the viral protein v-erb B is involved in fibrosarcomas, and both v-erb A and v-erb B are associated with leukemias. **v-erb B** resembles a constitutively activated receptor tyrosine kinase (epidermal growth factor receptor), and the retroviral **v-erb A** is derived from a cellular gene encoding a thyroid hormone receptor. Other receptors and signalling molecules implicated in cell transformation include Src, Ras, and platelet-derived growth factor receptor. A mutation in protein tyrosine phosphatase 1C results in abnormal hematopoiesis and an increased incidence of lymphoreticular tumors.

tyrosine kinase–associated receptors is another example of crosstalk between signalling pathways.

INTRACELLULAR (OR NUCLEAR) RECEPTORS

Steroid and Thyroid Hormones Enter the Cell and Bind to Members of the Intracellular Receptor Superfamily in the Cytoplasm or Nucleus

A number of important signalling molecules produce their effects not by binding to receptors on the cell membrane but by binding to **intracellular receptors** (also called **nuclear receptors**) that are transcription factors. This family includes receptors for steroid hormones, prostaglandins, vitamin D, thyroid hormones, and retinoic acid. In addition, this family includes related receptors—known as "orphan receptors"—whose ligands have yet to be identified. Steroid hormones, vitamin D, and retinoic acid appear to enter the cell by diffusing through the lipid phase of the cell membrane. Thyroid hormones, which are charged amino acid derivatives, may cross the cell membrane either by diffusion or by carrier-mediated transport. Once inside the cell, these substances bind to intracellular receptors. The ligand-bound receptors are activated **transcription factors** that regulate the expression of target genes by binding to specific DNA sequences.

The family of nuclear receptors contains at least 32 genes and has been classically divided into two subfamilies based on structural homology. One subfamily consists of receptors for **retinoic acid** (p. 133), **thyroid hormone** (p. 1035), and **vitamin D** (p. 1095). These receptors

FIGURE 4–13. Modular construction of intracellular (or nuclear) receptors. Members of this family exist in the cytoplasm or nucleus and include receptors for several ligands, including retinoic acid, vitamin D, thyroid hormones, and steroid hormones. These receptors have modular construction, with up to six elements. The "%" figures listed inside the A/B, C, and E domains refer to the degrees of amino acid identity, referenced to the glucocorticoid receptor. Thus, the DNA-binding or C domain of the retinoic acid receptor is 45% identical to the corresponding domain on the glucocorticoid receptor.

appear to act as *heterodimers*. The other group includes receptors for **steroid hormones**. These hormones include the glucocorticoids (p. 1049), mineralocorticoids (pp. 787 and 1057), androgens (p. 1131), estrogens (p. 1156), and progesterone (p. 1161). These receptors function primarily as *homodimers*.

The intracellular localization of the different unoccupied receptors varies. The glucocorticoid (GR) and mineralocorticoid (MR) receptors are mainly cytoplasmic, the estrogen (ER) and progesterone (PR) receptors are primarily nuclear, and the thyroid hormone (THR) and retinoic acid (RAR/RXR) receptors are bound to DNA in the nucleus. Cytoplasmic receptors are complexed to chaperone (or "heat shock") proteins. Hormone binding induces a conformational change in these receptors that causes dissociation from the cytoplasmic chaperone and unmasks a nuclear transport signal that allows the hormone-receptor complex to translocate into the nucleus.

All nuclear receptors contain six functionally distinct domains—designated A through F from the N to C terminus (Fig. 4–13)—that are differentially conserved among the various proteins. The N-terminal A/B region differs widely among receptors and contains the first of two transactivation domains. **Transactivation** is the process by which a ligand-induced conformational change of the receptor results in a change in conformation of the DNA, thus initiating transcription (p. 116). The C region, the most highly conserved among receptor types, contains the DNA-binding domain and is also involved in dimerization. It is composed of two "zinc-finger" structures (p. 126). The D, or hinge, region contains the "nuclear localization signal" and may also contain transactivation sequences. The E domain is responsible for hormone binding. Like the C region, it is involved in dimerization via its "basic zipper" region (p. 126). Finally, like the A/B region, the E region contains a transactivation domain. The small C-terminal F domain is of unknown function.

Activated Nuclear Receptors Bind to Sequence Elements in the Regulatory Region of Responsive Genes and Either Activate or Repress DNA Transcription

One of the remarkable features of nuclear receptors is that they bind to specific DNA sequences—called **hormone response elements**—in the regulatory region of responsive genes. The various nuclear receptors display specific cell and tissue distributions. Thus, the battery of genes affected by a particular ligand depends on the complement of receptors in the cell, the ability of these receptors to form homodimers or heterodimers, and the affinity of these receptor-ligand complexes for a particular response element on the DNA.

In addition to their ability to affect transcription by directly binding to specific regulatory elements, several nuclear receptors modulate gene expression by acting as transcriptional repressors (p. 129). For example, the glucocorticoids—acting via their receptor—can attenuate components of the inflammatory response by interacting with or "quenching" the transcription factor activator protein-1 (AP-1) and nuclear factor κB (NF-κB).

REFERENCES

Books and Reviews

Clapham DE, Neer EJ: New roles of G protein $\beta\gamma$ dimers in transmembrane signalling. Nature 365:403–406, 1993.

Exton JH: Phosphoinositide phospholipases and G proteins in hormone action. Annu Rev Physiol 56:349–369, 1994.

Gilman AG: G proteins: Transducers of receptor-generated signals. Annu Rev Biochem 56:615–649, 1987.

Lefkowitz RJ: G protein–coupled receptor kinases. Cell 74:409–412, 1993.

Nakamura S, Nishizuka Y: Lipid mediators and protein kinase C activation for the intracellular signaling network. J Biochem 115:1029–1034, 1994.

Vane JR, Botting RM: Mechanism of action of nonsteroidal anti-inflammatory drugs. Am J Med 104 (Suppl):S2–S8, 1998.

Journal Articles

Conklin BR, Bourne HR: Structural elements of Gα subunits that interact with $G_{\beta\gamma}$, receptors, and effectors. Cell 73:631–641, 1993.

Fraser ID, Tavalin SJ, Lester LB, et al: A novel lipid-anchored A-kinase anchoring protein facilitates cAMP-responsive membrane events. EMBO J 17:2261–2272, 1998.

Hildebrandt JD: Role of subunit diversity in signaling by heterotrimeric G proteins. Biochem Pharmacol 54:325–339, 1997.

Rodig SJ, Meraz MA, White JM, et al: Disruption of the Jak1 gene demonstrates obligatory and nonredundant roles of the Jaks in cytokine induced biological responses. Cell 93:373–383, 1998.

CHAPTER 5

Regulation of Gene Expression

Peter Igarashi

With few exceptions, all cells in the body share the same genetic information. This information is contained in the sequence of DNA, most of which is packaged into chromosomes within the nucleus of each cell (a small, but important fraction of a cell's DNA is carried in the mitochondria). DNA has two functions. The first is to serve as a self-renewing data repository that maintains a constant source of genetic information for the cell. This role is achieved by DNA replication, which ensures that when cells divide, exact copies of the DNA are transmitted to the progeny cells. The second purpose of DNA is to serve as a template so that genetic information can be translated into the functional units of the cell. These functional units are mostly proteins, but they also include structural and catalytic RNA. This second purpose, which is broadly defined as **gene expression**, is the subject of this chapter.

FROM GENES TO PROTEINS

Gene Expression Differs among Tissues and—In Any Tissue—May Vary in Response to External Stimuli

The necessity for regulation of gene expression can be appreciated if one considers a simple fact: although the haploid human genome contains 30,000 to 40,000 distinct genes, only a fraction of that number—10,000 or so—is actively translated into proteins in any individual cell. Cells from different tissues have distinct morphologies and functions and respond differently to external stimuli, even though their DNA content is identical. For example, although all cells of the body contain an albumin gene, only liver cells (hepatocyte) can synthesize and secrete albumin into the bloodstream. Conversely, hepatocytes cannot synthesize myosin and some other contractile proteins that skeletal muscle cells produce. The explanation for these observations is that expression of genes is regulated so that some genes are active in hepatocytes, whereas others are silent. In skeletal muscle cells, a different set of genes is active, whereas others—such as those expressed only in the liver—are silent. How is one cell type programmed to express liver-specific genes whereas another cell type expresses a set of genes that are appropriate for skeletal muscle? This is the phenomenon of **tissue-specific gene expression**.

A second issue is that genes in individual cells are generally not expressed at constant, unchanging levels (constitutive expression). Rather, their expression levels often vary widely in response to environmental stimuli. For example, when blood glucose levels decrease, α cells in the pancreas secrete the hormone glucagon (p. 1081). Glucagon circulates in the blood until it reaches the liver, where it causes a 15-fold increase in expression of the gene that encodes phosphoenolpyruvate carboxykinase (PEPCK), an enzyme that catalyzes the rate-limiting step in gluconeogenesis (p. 1082). Increased gluconeogenesis then contributes to restoring blood-glucose levels toward normal. This simple regulatory loop, which necessitates that the liver cells perceive the presence of glucagon and stimulate PEPCK gene expression, illustrates the phenomenon of **inducible gene expression**.

In this chapter, we discuss the mechanisms underlying the regulation of tissue-specific and inducible gene expression, some general principles of gene structure and expression, and regulatory elements in DNA that control gene expression. Also, this chapter examines the proteins (transcription factors) that regulate gene expression and their participation in signal-transduction pathways. Finally, we will describe the important roles of chromatin structure and post-transcriptional regulation of gene expression.

Because many of the proteins and DNA sequences are known by abbreviations, the Glossary at the end of the chapter identifies these entities.

Gene Expression May Be Regulated at Multiple Steps

According to James Watson, the "central dogma of molecular biology" is that genetic information flows unidirectionally from DNA to proteins. This process requires an intermediary, called messenger RNA (mRNA), that transports the genetic information from the nucleus, where DNA is stored, to the cytoplasm, where proteins are synthesized (p. 30). The synthesis of RNA from DNA is referred to as **transcription**, and the synthesis of protein from mRNA is called **translation**. The complete process, proceeding from DNA in the nucleus to protein in the cytoplasm, constitutes **gene expression**.

Gene expression involves eight steps (Fig. 5–1):

Step 1: **Alteration in chromatin structure**. As is discussed later, chromosomal DNA is packaged into a higher-order structure called chromatin, which contains DNA, histones, and other nuclear proteins. This condensed structure is required for DNA to fit into the nucleus. However, before genes can be transcribed, some local alteration in chromatin structure must occur so that the enzymes that mediate transcription can gain access to the DNA.

Step 2: **Initiation of transcription**. An enzyme called RNA polymerase II (pol II) mediates transcription. In this step, RNA polymerase binds to DNA and begins to synthesize RNA that is complementary in sequence to one of the strands of the template DNA. For most eukaryotic genes, initiation of transcription is the critical, rate-limiting step in gene expression.

Step 3: **Transcript elongation**. During transcript elongation, RNA polymerase proceeds down the DNA strand and sequentially adds ribonucleotides to the elongating strand of RNA.

Step 4: **Termination of transcription**. After producing a full-length RNA, the enzyme halts elongation.

Step 5: **RNA processing**. The RNA that is transcribed from DNA is called the primary transcript or heterogeneous nuclear RNA (hnRNA). In eukaryotes, the primary transcript must undergo processing to produce a mature mRNA that can be translated into protein. RNA processing involves the following steps, which occur while the primary transcript still resides within the nucleus: (1) the addition of a 5′ methylguanosine cap, (2) cleavage of the RNA strand, (3) polyadenylation at the cleavage site, and (4) pre-mRNA splicing.

Step 6: **Nucleocytoplasmic transport**. The next step in gene expression is the regulated export of the mature mRNA from the nucleus into the cytoplasm.

Step 7: **Translation**. The mRNA is translated into proteins on ribosomes. During translation, the genetic code on the mRNA is "read" by transfer RNA (tRNA), and then amino acids carried by the tRNA are added to the nascent polypeptide chain.

Step 8: **mRNA degradation**. Finally, the mRNA is degraded in the cytoplasm by a combination of endonucleases and exonucleases.

Each of these steps is potentially a target for regulation (see Fig. 5–1, *rightmost column*): (1) Gene expression may be regulated by global as well as local alterations in chromatin structure. (2) An important, related alteration in chromatin structure is the state of methylation of the DNA. (3) Initiation of transcription can be regulated by transcriptional activators and transcriptional repressors. (4) Transcript elongation may be regulated by premature termination in which the polymerase falls off (or is displaced from) the template DNA strand; such termination results in the synthesis of truncated transcripts. (5) Pre-mRNA splicing may be regulated by alternative splicing, which generates different mRNA species from the same primary transcript. (6) Expression of certain genes, especially those with premature stop codons, is prevented at the step of nucleocytoplasmic transport. (7) In eukaryotes, control of translation of specific mRNA is less common than in bacteria, but there are noteworthy exceptions (e.g., expression of the transferrin receptor). (8) Control of mRNA stability contributes to steady-state levels of mRNA in the cytoplasm and is important for the overall expression of many genes.

Although any of these steps may be critical for regulating a particular gene, transcription initiation is the most frequently regulated (step 2) and is the focus of this chapter. At the end of the chapter, we describe examples of control of gene expression at steps that are subsequent to the initiation of transcription—post-transcriptional regulation.

Transcription Factors Are Proteins That Regulate Gene Transcription

A general principle is that gene transcription is regulated by interactions of specific proteins with specific DNA elements. Proteins that are involved in the regulation of transcription are called **transcription factors**. These proteins are referred to as *trans-acting* factors because they

FIGURE 5–1. Steps in gene expression. Nearly all of the eight steps in gene expression are potential targets for regulation. mRNA, messenger RNA.

are encoded by genes that reside elsewhere in the genome from the genes that they regulate. Many transcription factors reside in the nucleus. These proteins recognize specific DNA sequences to which they bind, although certain transcription factors do not interact with DNA directly. Transcription factors exist in two classes: general transcription factors, which are defined as proteins that are essential for the transcription of all genes, and specific transcription factors, which are required for the transcription of only certain genes but not others. The binding sites for these transcription factors are specific DNA sequences called **regulatory elements**. Because they are located on the same piece of DNA as the genes that they

regulate, these regulatory elements are referred to as *cis-acting* factors.

Figure 5–2 illustrates the overall scheme for the regulation of gene expression. Transcription requires proteins (transcription factors) that bind to specific DNA sequences (regulatory elements) that are located near the genes that they regulate (target genes). Once the proteins bind to DNA, something happens to stimulate (or inhibit) transcription of the target gene. Regulation of gene expression can therefore occur at the level of either transcription factors or regulatory elements. Examples of regulation at the transcription-factor level include variation in the concentration of the proteins, their DNA-binding

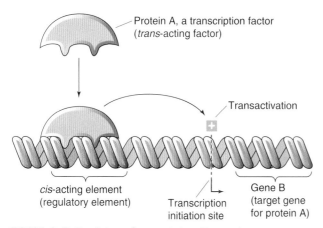

FIGURE 5–2. Regulation of transcription. Protein A, a transcription factor that is encoded by Gene A (not shown), regulates another gene, Gene B. Thus, Protein A is a *trans*-acting factor. Protein A binds to a DNA sequence that is upstream from Gene B; this DNA sequence is a *cis*-acting element because it is close to Gene B. In this example, Protein A stimulates (transactivates) the transcription of Gene B. Transcription factors also can inhibit transcription.

activities, and their ability to stimulate (or inhibit) transcription. Examples of regulation at the regulatory-element level include alterations in chromatin structure (which influences accessibility to transcription factors) and covalent modifications, especially methylation.

GENE STRUCTURE

The Gene Consists of a Transcription Unit

Defining exactly what is meant by a "gene" is not as simple as it might seem. Historically, the gene, originally called a **cistron**, was defined functionally based on its capacity to complement mutations. If crosses between animals—each homozygous for a recessive mutation—could produce progeny of normal phenotype, the two mutations were considered to affect different cistrons or genes. If the crosses could not produce a normal phenotype, the mutations affected the same gene. Later, a gene was defined as a transcription unit that gives rise to a single mRNA that is translated into a unique polypeptide. This explanation was in accordance with the "one gene–one polypeptide" rule. The situation in vivo is somewhat more complex because a gene can often produce multiple, distinct types of mRNA as a result of alternative splicing, alternative promoter selection, or alternative polyadenylation. The proteins encoded by these transcript variants may exhibit sequence differences, but they will all be structurally related. Such is not the case in bacteria, which are polycistronic; that is, bacteria can produce multiple, unrelated polypeptides from a single transcription unit that contains multiple reading frames.

We will define the **gene** as a transcription unit consisting of the *segment of DNA that extends from the site of transcription initiation to the site of transcription termination.* As it turns out, in eukaryotes this structural definition is similar, although not quite identical to the functional definition that was provided earlier. In particular, regions of

DNA that are outside the transcription unit—but contain regulatory elements that are necessary for expression of the gene—would be included in the definition of a cistron. We consider these regulatory regions to be formally outside the gene itself because they may be located at great distances from the protein-coding region, and different genes may share common regulatory elements.

Figure 5–3 depicts the structure of a typical eukaryotic gene and its products. The region of DNA that is immediately adjacent and upstream (i.e., in the 5′ direction) to the gene is called the **5′ flanking region**. The corresponding domain that is downstream (3′) to the gene is called the **3′ flanking region**. (Recall that DNA strands have directionality because of the 5′-to-3′ orientation of the phosphodiester bonds in the sugar-phosphate backbone of DNA. By convention, the DNA strand that has the same sequence as the mRNA is called the "coding" strand, and the complementary strand is called the "noncoding" strand. The 5′-to-3′ orientation refers to the coding strand.) Although the 5′ and 3′ flanking regions are not transcribed into RNA, they frequently contain regulatory elements that control gene transcription. In the 5′ flanking region, immediately upstream from the transcription initiation site, is the gene **promoter**. Frequently, other regulatory elements are located further upstream. The site where transcription of the gene begins, sometimes called the "cap site," may have a variant of the nucleotide sequence 5′-ACTT(T/C)TG-3′ (called the cap sequence), where T/C means T *or* C. The 'A' is the **transcription initiation site**. Transcription proceeds to the **transcription termination site**, which has a less defined sequence and location in eukaryotic genes. Slightly upstream from the termination site is another sequence called the **polyadenylation signal**, which often has the sequence 5′-AATAAA-3′.

The **primary transcript** that is synthesized from the gene is colinear with the coding strand of the DNA template; that is, the primary RNA transcript has exactly the same number of nucleotides as the DNA template. As previously mentioned, the sequence of the primary transcript differs from that of the mature mRNA. Mature mRNA is produced by a number of processing steps. In the first of these processing steps, an unusual guanosine base, which is methylated at the 7 position (m^7G), is added via a 5′-5′ phosphodiester bond to the 5′ end of the transcript. The result is a 5′ methyl **cap**. The presence of the 5′ methyl cap is required for export of the mRNA from the nucleus to the cytoplasm, as well as for translation of the mRNA.

A second processing step is cleavage of the RNA transcript about 20 nucleotides downstream from the polyadenylation signal, near the 3′ end of the transcript. A third step is the addition of a string of 100 to 200 adenine bases at the site of the cleavage to form a **poly(A) tail**. This tail contributes to mRNA stability.

The fourth processing step may be RNA splicing. In eukaryotic genes, the DNA sequences that are ultimately translated into proteins (i.e., the **exons**) may be interrupted by **introns**. Pre-mRNA splicing removes the introns. As a result, mature mRNA is shorter and not colinear with the coding strand of the DNA template.

The mRNA produced by RNA processing contains a

FIGURE 5–3. The structure of a eukaryotic gene and its products. The figure depicts a gene, a primary RNA transcript, the mature messenger RNA (mRNA), and the resulting protein. m⁷G, 7-methyl guanosine; ATG, AATAAA, etc., are nucleotide sequences.

coding region that is translated into protein, as well as sequences at the 5′ and 3′ ends that are not translated into protein (the 5′ and 3′ untranslated regions, respectively). Translation of the mRNA on ribosomes always begins at the codon AUG, which encodes methionine, and proceeds until one of the three stop codons (UAG, UAA, or UGA) is encountered. Thus, the 5′ end of the mRNA is the first to be translated and provides the N terminus of the protein, whereas the 3′ end is the last to be translated and contributes the C terminus.

The Promoter Determines the Initiation Site and Direction of Transcription

As will be discussed later, initiation of DNA transcription requires assembly of a complex of proteins that contains pol II and is known as the basal transcriptional ma-

chinery. Assembly of the basal transcriptional machinery does not occur at random sites on the DNA template. Rather, genes have specific boundaries that correspond to sites of initiation and termination of transcription. The basal transcription machinery assembles at a region of DNA that is immediately upstream from and includes the transcription initiation site. This region is called the **gene promoter**. The promoter is a *cis*-acting regulatory element because it is located on the same piece of DNA as the gene and is required for expression of the gene. In addition to locating the *site* for initiation of transcription, the promoter also determines the *direction* of transcription.

Perhaps somewhat surprisingly, no unique sequence defines the gene promoter. Instead, the promoter consists of modules of simple sequences (elements). Figure 5–4 depicts the structure of two typical eukaryotic gene promoters. The most important element in promoters is the

FIGURE 5–4. Typical eukaryotic gene promoters. A promoter consists of modules of simple DNA sequences or "elements."

Goldberg-Hogness **TATA box**. Examination of the sequences of a large number of genes reveals that the TATA box has the consensus sequence 5′-GNGTATA(A/T)A(A/T)-3′, where N is any nucleotide. The TATA box is analogous to the Pribnow box in bacterial genes, which is an RNA polymerase binding site located about 10 bp upstream from the transcription initiation site. In eukaryotes, the TATA box is usually located approximately 30 bp upstream (5′) to the site of transcription initiation. As discussed on p. 123, a transcription factor known as TFIID binds specifically to the TATA box and is the first component of the basal transcriptional machinery to assemble. Thus the TATA box is believed to determine the site of transcription initiation.

Many eukaryotic genes, especially the ubiquitously expressed "housekeeping" genes, do not contain a TATA box in their promoters. What determines the site of transcription initiation in TATA-less genes? At least part of the answer appears to be a series of small DNA sequence elements, collectively called the **initiator** (Inr). Inr functions analogously to the TATA box to position the basal transcriptional machinery in these genes. Interestingly, it appears that TFIID can also bind to the Inr element, so it may function to establish assembly of the basal transcriptional machinery on both TATA-containing and TATA-less genes. However, in TATA-less genes, the site of transcription initiation appears to be less precisely defined, and often several transcripts that originate at several distinct, but neighboring sites are produced.

In addition to the TATA box, gene promoters contain additional DNA elements that are necessary for initiating transcription. These elements consist of short DNA sequences and are often called **promoter-proximal sequences** because they lie approximately 100 bp upstream from the transcription initiation site. Promoter-proximal sequences are required for the transcription of specific genes. Well-characterized examples include the GC box (5′-GGGCGG-3′) and the CAAT box (5′-CCAAT-3′) shown in Figure 5–4A, as well as the CACCC box and octamer motif (5′-ATGCAAAT-3′). These DNA elements

function as binding sites for the additional proteins that are necessary for initiating transcription of particular genes. Although they are present in many cells, the proteins that bind to these sites are not necessary for the transcription of *all* genes, so they are not included in the class of general transcription factors. Each of these proteins, called a **specific transcription factor**, binds to a site on the DNA that is physically close to the site of transcription initiation. These specific transcription factors are believed to interact with the basal transcriptional machinery. Examples of specific transcription factors, as well as the DNA sequences to which they bind, are discussed later. Multiple GC boxes are frequently found in the promoters of genes that lack a TATA box. Some promoter-proximal sequences are present in genes that are only active in certain cell types. For example, the CACCC box is found in β globin, immunoglobulins, and apolipoprotein A-II gene promoters.

Positive and Negative Regulatory Elements Modulate Gene Transcription

Although the promoter is the site where pol II binds and initiates transcription, the promoter alone is not generally sufficient to initiate transcription at a physiologically significant rate. High-level gene expression generally requires activation of the basal transcriptional machinery by additional proteins—the *specific transcription factors* introduced in the previous section—which function by binding to specific sites in DNA. The DNA binding sites for transcription factors are called **regulatory elements**. They are *cis*-acting factors because they reside on the same piece of DNA as the gene that they regulate. Two general types of regulatory elements are recognized. The first type, called **positive regulatory elements** or **enhancers**, includes DNA binding sites for proteins that activate transcription; the proteins that bind to these DNA elements are called **activators**. The second type, called **negative regulatory elements** (NREs) and sometimes called **silenc-**

ers, includes DNA binding sites for proteins that inhibit transcription; the proteins that bind to these DNA elements are called **repressors**.

A general property of enhancers and NREs is that they consist of modules of relatively short sequences of DNA, generally 6 to 12 bp. Sometimes they contain distinct sequences, such as direct or inverted repeats, but often they do not. Typically, regulatory elements do not reside within the portion of the gene that encodes protein, but rather are located in noncoding regions, most frequently in the 5′ flanking region that is upstream from the promoter. However, some enhancers and NREs are located downstream from the transcription initiation site and are embedded either in introns or in the 3′ flanking region of the gene. In fact, enhancers and NREs can function at great physical distances from the gene promoter, many hundreds of base pairs away. Moreover, the distance between the enhancer or silencer and the promoter can often be varied experimentally without substantially affecting transcriptional activity. In addition, many regulatory elements work equally well if their orientation is inverted. Thus in contrast to the gene promoter, enhancers and NREs exhibit position independence and orientation independence. Another property of regulatory elements is that they are active on heterologous promoters; that is, if enhancers and NREs from one gene are placed near a promoter for a different gene, they can stimulate or inhibit transcription of the second gene.

How do transcription factors (activators or repressors), when they bind to regulatory elements (enhancers or NREs) that are physically distant from the promoter, interact with components of the basal transcriptional machinery? Regulatory elements may be located hundreds of base pairs from the promoter. This distance is much too great to permit proteins that are bound at the enhancer and promoter to come into contact along a two-dimensional linear strand of DNA. Two models have been proposed to explain the long-range effects of transcription factors. The first is the **sliding model**, in which the transcription factor first binds to the regulatory element and then translocates along the DNA toward the promoter. The second model, which is currently favored, is the **DNA looping** model. According to this model, the transcription factor attaches to the regulatory element, thereby inducing conformational changes in the DNA that allow the transcription factor and promoter-bound proteins to become juxtaposed.

Locus-Control Regions and Boundary Elements Influence Transcription within Multigene Chromosomal Domains

In addition to enhancers and NREs, which regulate the expression of *neighboring* genes, some *cis*-acting regulatory elements are involved in the regulation of chromosomal domains containing multiple genes.

The first of this type of element to be discovered was the **locus-control region (LCR)**, also called the locus-activating region or dominant control region. The LCR is a dominant, positive-acting *cis*-element that regulates the expression of several genes within a chromosomal do-

main. LCRs were first identified at the β-globin gene locus, which encodes the β-type subunits of hemoglobin. Together with α-type subunits, these β-globin–like subunits form embryonic, fetal, and adult hemoglobin (see box on p. 657). As shown in Figure 5–5, the β-globin gene locus consists of a cluster of five genes (ϵ, γ_G, γ_A, δ, β) that are distributed over 90 kb on chromosome 11 (see the box titled Abnormalities of Regulatory Elements in β Thalassemias). During ontogeny, the genes exhibit highly regulated patterns of expression in which they are transcribed only in certain tissues and only at precise developmental stages. Moreover, there is a *temporal colinearity* in the expression of these genes. In other words, the genes at the 5′ end of the cluster are transcribed early in ontogeny, whereas genes at the 3′ end are expressed later. Thus, embryonic globin (ϵ) is expressed in the yolk sac, fetal globins (γ_G, γ_A) are expressed in fetal liver, and adult globins (δ, β) are expressed in adult bone marrow. Although the mechanism by which this tightly regulated expression pattern is achieved remains uncertain, it is clear that a regulatory region that is located far from the structural genes is needed. This region, designated as the LCR, extends from 6 to 18 kb upstream from the ϵ-globin gene. The LCR is essential for high-level expression of the β-globin–like genes within red blood cell precursors because the promoters and enhancers near the individual genes permit only low-level expression. Moreover, the LCR can direct erythrocyte-specific expression of unrelated genes that are not normally expressed in this tissue.

The β-globin LCR contains five DNase-hypersensitive sites, each with an enhancer-like structure that consists of modules of simple sequence elements that are binding sites for the erythrocyte-specific transcription factors GATA-1 and NF-E2. It is believed that the LCRs perform two functions: one is to alter the chromatin structure of the β-globin gene locus so that it is more accessible to transcription factors, and the second is to serve as a powerful enhancer of transcription of the individual genes. In one model, temporal-dependent expression of β-type globin genes is achieved by sequential interactions that involve activator proteins that bind to the LCR and promoters of individual genes (see Fig. 5–5).

A potential problem that is associated with the existence of LCRs that can exert transcriptional effects over long distances is that the LCRs may interfere with the expression of nearby genes. One solution to this problem is provided by **boundary elements**, which function to insulate genes from neighboring regulatory elements. Boundary elements (or matrix-attachment regions) were first observed in *Drosophila* but have subsequently been found in many organisms, including mammals. Expression of foreign genes in transgenic mice is sometimes influenced by regulatory elements in the host genome that are adjacent to the site of integration of the foreign gene. However, when the foreign gene is flanked by boundary elements, the effects of these nearby regulatory elements are eliminated. Boundary elements are believed to represent sites of attachment of DNA to the chromosome scaffold, and loops of physically separated DNA are generated that may correspond to discrete functional domains.

A β-GLOBIN FAMILY OF GENES ON CHROMOSOME 11

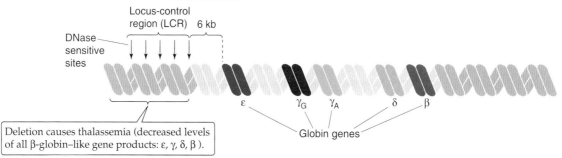

B TIME COURSE OF EXPRESSION OF β-GLOBIN–LIKE GENE PRODUCTS

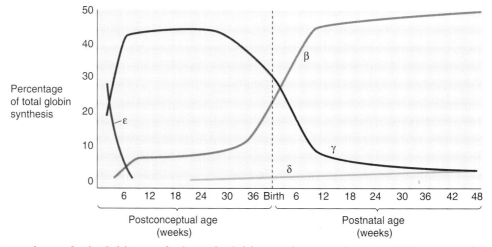

FIGURE 5–5. Locus-control region for the β-globin gene family. *A,* The β-globin gene locus control region (LCR) lies upstream from the genes that encode the ε, γ_G, γ_A, δ, and β globin subunits. The five *vertical arrows* indicate sites at which the DNA is unusually sensitive to degradation by deoxyribonuclease (DNase). *B,* The LCR ensures that the genes are expressed in a temporally colinear manner, with ε and γ expressed early during development and δ and β expressed later.

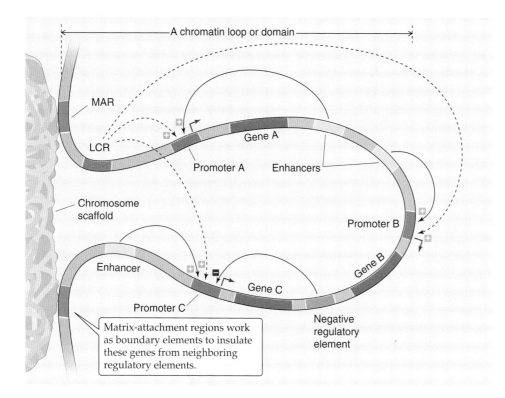

FIGURE 5–6. *cis*-acting elements that regulate gene transcription. This model shows a loop of chromatin that contains Genes A, B, and C. Matrix-attachment regions (MARs) are boundary elements on the DNA that attach to the chromosome scaffold and thus isolate this loop of chromatin from other chromosomal domains. Contained within this loop are several *cis*-acting elements (i.e., DNA sequences that regulate genes on the same piece of DNA), including promoters, enhancers, negative regulatory elements, and a locus-control region.

ABNORMALITIES OF REGULATORY ELEMENTS IN β THALASSEMIAS

The best characterized examples of mutations affecting DNA regulatory elements occur at the gene cluster encoding the β-globin–like chains of hemoglobin. Some of these mutations result in thalassemia, whereas other cause hereditary persistence of fetal hemoglobin. The β **thalassemias** are a heterogeneous group of disorders characterized by anemia caused by a deficiency in production of the β chain of hemoglobin. The anemia can be mild and inconsequential or severe and life threatening. The thalassemias were among the first diseases to be characterized at the molecular level. As described in the text and shown in Figure 5–5, the β-globin gene locus consists of five β-globin–like genes that are exclusively expressed in hematopoietic cells and exhibit temporal colinearity. As expected, many patients with β thalassemia have mutations or deletions that affect the coding region of the β-globin gene. These patients presumably have

thalassemia because the β-globin gene product is functionally abnormal or absent. In addition, some patients have a deficiency in β globin as a result of inadequate levels of expression of the gene. Of particular interest are patients with the Hispanic and Dutch forms of β thalassemia. These patients have deletions of portions of chromosome 11, as shown in Figure 5–5. However, the deletions do not extend to include the β-globin gene itself. Why, then, do these patients have β-globin deficiency? It turns out that the deletions involve the region 50 to 65 kb upstream from the β-globin gene, which contains the locus-control region (LCR). In these cases, deletion of the LCR results in failure of expression of the β-globin gene, even though the *structural gene* and its *promoter* are completely normal. These results underscore the essential role that the LCR plays in β-globin gene expression.

However, this physical separation has not yet been proved directly.

Figure 5–6 summarizes our understanding of the arrangement of *cis*-acting regulatory elements and their functions. Each gene has its own promoter where transcription is initiated. Enhancers are positive-acting regulatory elements that may be located either near or distant from the transcription initiation site, whereas NREs are regulatory elements that inhibit gene expression. A cluster of genes within a chromosomal domain may be under the control of an LCR. Finally, boundary elements (or matrix-attachment regions) functionally insulate one chromosomal domain from another. This functional arrangement corresponds to physical loops of chromatin that are anchored to the chromosome scaffolding.

TRANSCRIPTION FACTORS

The Basal Transcriptional Machinery Consists of RNA Polymerase II and General Transcription Factors

The preceding discussion has emphasized the structure of the gene and the *cis*-acting elements that regulate gene expression. We will now turn to the proteins that interact with these DNA elements and thus regulate gene transcription. Transcription is mediated by **RNA polymerase**, an enzyme that catalyzes the DNA-dependent synthesis of RNA. Eukaryotes have three distinct RNA polymerases: RNA polymerase I (pol I) transcribes genes encoding ribosomal RNA. RNA polymerase II (pol II or RNAPII) transcribes genes into mRNA, which is later translated into protein. Finally, RNA polymerase III (pol III) transcribes genes that encode tRNA and small-nuclear RNA. This discussion is confined to the protein-encoding genes transcribed by pol II (so-called class II genes).

Pol II is a large protein (molecular weight of 600 kDa) comprising 10 to 12 subunits (the largest of which is structurally related to bacterial RNA polymerase) and is

capable of transcribing RNA from synthetic DNA templates in vitro. Although pol II catalyzes mRNA synthesis, when acting alone it is incapable of initiating transcription at specific sites. Such directed initiation of transcription requires an assembly of proteins—*general transcription factors*—that enable RNA polymerase to bind to DNA and initiate transcription. Together with pol II, the general transcription factors constitute the **basal transcriptional machinery**, which is also known as the **RNA polymerase holoenzyme** or **preinitiation complex** because its assembly is required before transcription can begin. In vitro, the general transcription factors and pol II assemble in a stepwise, ordered fashion on the gene promoter (Fig. 5–7A). The first protein that binds to DNA is transcription factor IID (TFIID), followed, in order, by the other general transcription factors. Each of these proteins is essential for transcription. Once TFIID binds to the DNA, the other transcription factors assemble spontaneously by protein-protein interactions. Although this stepwise assembly of pol II and general transcription factors occurs in vitro, the situation in vivo may be different. In vivo, pol II has been observed in a multiprotein complex containing general transcription factors and other proteins. Promoters may recruit this preformed complex to initiate transcription.

TFIID is a general transcription factor that has sequence-specific DNA-binding activity. The recognition site for TFIID is usually the TATA box, although it may also recognize the Inr element (p. 120). TFIID is a multisubunit protein composed of **TATA-binding protein (TBP)** and at least 10 TBP-associated factors. The TBP subunit is a 38-kDa protein that binds to the TATA box. Reconstitution studies indicate that recombinant TBP can replace TFIID in basal transcription, but it fails to support elevated levels of transcription in the presence of transcriptional activators. Thus, **TBP-associated factors** (TAFs) are involved in transcriptional activation (see later).

The next general transcription factor that binds is **TFIIA**, which interacts with TBP and stabilizes its interaction with DNA. TFIIA is thought to compete with nega-

A GENERAL TRANSCRIPTION FACTORS

B SPECIFIC TRANSCRIPTION FACTORS

FIGURE 5–7. The action of general and specific transcription factors. *A,* The sequential assembly of general transcription factors and RNA polymerase II (pol II) results in the formation of the basal transcriptional machinery. *B,* In this example, specific transcription factors bind to enhancer elements on the DNA and interact with the basal transcriptional machinery to increase the efficiency of gene transcription.

tive cofactors that bind to TBP and block further assembly of the complex (this process has been called antirepression). Assembly of TFIIA is followed by assembly of **TFIIB**, which is important because it interacts with transcriptional activators. Moreover, TFIIB is a bridging protein that interacts with the TBP component of TFIID and recruits a preassembled complex of **pol II and TFIIF**. Entry of pol II–TFIIF into the basal transcriptional machinery is followed by binding of TFIIE, TFIIH, and TFIIJ. **TFIIE** is a protein kinase whose substrates remain unidentified. **TFIIH** is also a kinase and can phosphorylate pol II in vitro. **TFIIJ** increases the phosphorylation of pol II. TFIIE and TFIIH may assist in the transition from basal transcriptional machinery to an elongation complex, which may involve unwinding of the DNA that is mediated by the helicase activity of TFIIH.

Specific Transcription Factors Are Proteins That Regulate the Rate of Transcription

Because the basal transcriptional machinery—pol II and the general transcription factors (Fig. 5–7A)—is incapable of efficient gene transcription alone, additional proteins are required to stimulate the activity of the enzyme complex. Most of these *specific transcription factors* are located within the nucleus and bind to specific sequences of DNA (Table 5–1). The general mechanism of action of a specific transcription factor is depicted in Figure 5–7B. After the basal transcriptional machinery assembles on the gene promoter, it can interact with a transcription factor that binds to a specific DNA element, the enhancer. Looping out of the intervening DNA permits physical interaction between the transcription factor and the basal transcriptional machinery, which subsequently leads to stimulation of gene transcription.

The specificity with which transcription factors bind to DNA depends on the interactions between the amino-acid side chains of the transcription factor and the purine and pyrimidine bases in DNA. Most of these interactions consist of noncovalent hydrogen bonds between amino acids and DNA bases. A peptide capable of a specific pattern of hydrogen bonding can recognize and bind to the reciprocal pattern in the major (and to a lesser extent the minor) groove of DNA. Interaction with the DNA backbone may also occur and involves electrostatic interactions (salt-bridge formation) with anionic phosphate groups. The site that a transcription factor recognizes (see Table 5–1) is generally short, usually less than a dozen or so base pairs.

Many specific transcription factors do not recognize unique DNA sequences, but rather a *family* of closely related sequences. For example, the transcription factor AP-1 (activator protein-1) recognizes the sequences

5′-TGACTCA-3′

5′-TGAGTCA-3′

5′-TGAGTCT-3′

and so on, as well as each of the complementary sequences. That is, some *redundancy* is usually built into the

TABLE 5–1

SPECIFIC TRANSCRIPTION FACTORS AND THE DNA SEQUENCES THAT THEY RECOGNIZE*

NAME	TYPE	RECOGNITION SITE	BINDS AS
SP1	Zinc finger	5'-GGGCGG-3'	Monomer
AP-1 (c-Fos and c-Jun)	Basic zipper	5'-TGASTCA-3'	Dimer
C/EBP	Basic zipper	5'-ATTGCGCAAT-3'	Dimer
Heat shock factor	Basic zipper	5'-NGAAN-3'	Trimer
ATF/CREB	Basic zipper	5'-TGACGTCA-3'	Dimer
c-Myc	Basic-HLH	5'-CACGTG-3'	Dimer
Oct-1	HTH	5'-ATGCAAAT-3'	Monomer
NF-1	Novel	5'-TTGGCN$_5$GCCAA-3'	Dimer

*N, any nucleotide; S, G or C; W, A or T.

recognition sequence for a transcription factor. An important consequence of these properties is that the recognition site for a transcription factor may occur many times in the genome. For example, if a transcription factor recognizes a 6-bp sequence, the sequence would be expected to occur once every 4^6 (or 4096) base pairs, that is, 7×10^5 times in the human genome. If redundancy is permitted, recognition sites will occur even more frequently. Of course, most of these sites will not be relevant to gene regulation but will instead have occurred simply by chance. This high frequency of recognition sites leads to an important concept: *transcription factors act in combination*. Thus, high-level expression of a gene, requires that a combination of multiple transcription factors binds to multiple regulatory elements. Although it is complicated, this system ensures that transcription activation occurs only at appropriate locations. Moreover, this system permits greater "fine tuning" of the system, inasmuch as the activity of individual transcription factors can be altered to modulate the overall level of transcription of a gene.

An important general feature of specific transcription factors is their **modular** construction (Fig. 5–8A). Transcription factors may be divided into discrete domains that bind DNA and domains that activate transcription (i.e., "**transactivation domains**"). This property was first directly demonstrated for a yeast transcription factor known as GAL4, which activates certain genes when yeast grows in galactose-containing media. GAL4 has two domains. One is a so-called zinc-finger domain (discussed later) that mediates sequence-specific binding to DNA. The other domain is an "acidic blob" that is enriched in acidic amino acids (i.e., glutamate and aspartate) and is necessary for transcriptional activation. Two lines of evidence suggest that these two domains are physically distinct and separable.

The first line of evidence is that mutations of the acidic domain in GAL4 can abolish transcriptional activation and yet have no effect on DNA binding (see Fig. 5–8B). The transactivation domains often fall into one of several categories. In addition to the "acidic blob," these other transcriptional activation domains are proline rich, glutamine rich, or serine/threonine rich.

The second line of evidence for the modular structure of specific transcription factors comes from experiments with chimeric molecules that are composed of the DNA-binding domain of GAL4 and the **transactivation domain** of the herpesvirus transcription factor VP16 (see Fig. 5–8C). The transactivation domain of VP16 has an acidic domain similar to that of GAL4. The GAL4-VP16 chimera binds to the same DNA sequence as normal GAL4, but mediates transcriptional activation via the VP16 transactivation domain. This type of "domain-swapping" experiment has been repeated for many transcription factors and has led to the notion that transcription factors have a modular construction in which physically distinct domains mediate binding to DNA and transcriptional activation (or repression).

Some transcription factors do not recognize specific DNA sequences. These factors are collectively termed **coactivators**, **mediators**, or **adapters**. The first protein of this type found in eukaryotes was the VP16 herpesvirus protein discussed earlier. We have already seen that the transactivation domain of VP16 contains a region of acidic amino acids. The other domain of VP16 does not bind to DNA directly, but interacts with the nuclear protein Oct-1, which is a ubiquitous DNA-binding protein that recognizes a DNA sequence called the octamer motif. Thus, transcriptional activation by VP16 first involves the binding of a host protein, Oct-1, to the octamer motif (see Table 5–1). VP16 then binds to Oct-1, and the acidic domain of VP16 mediates transcriptional activation.

Specific Transcription Factors That Bind DNA Can Be Grouped into Families Based on Tertiary Structure

Based on sequence conservation, as well as structural determinations from x-ray crystallography and nuclear magnetic resonance spectroscopy, DNA-binding transcription factors have been grouped into families. Members of the same family use common structural motifs for binding DNA (see Table 5–1). These structures include the zinc finger, basic zipper (bZIP), basic helix-loop-helix (bHLH), helix-turn-helix (HTH), and β sheet. Each of these motifs

A DNA-BINDING AND TRANSACTIVATION DOMAINS

B SELECTIVE MUTATION OF TRANSACTIVATION DOMAIN

C CHIMERIC TRANSCRIPTION FACTOR

FIGURE 5–8. Modular design of specific transcription factors. *A,* Specific transcription factors have independent domains for binding to DNA regulatory sequences and for activating transcription. In this example, amino acids 1 through 147 of the GAL4 transcription factor bind to DNA, whereas amino acids 768 through 881 activate basal transcriptional machinery. *B,* Mutations in the transactivation domain can abolish the activation of transcription without altering the ability of the mutant protein to bind to the DNA. *C,* Replacing the transactivation domain of GAL4 with that of VP16 results in a chimera that is a functional transcription factor.

consists of a particular tertiary protein structure in which a component, usually an α helix, interacts with DNA, especially the major groove of the DNA.

ZINC FINGER. The term **zinc finger** describes a loop of protein that is held together at its base by a Zn^{2+} ion that tetrahedrally coordinates to either two histidine residues and two cysteine residues or to four cysteine residues. Sometimes two Zn^{2+} ions coordinate to six cysteine groups. Figure 5–9A shows a zinc finger in which the Zn^{2+} coordinates to two residues on an α helix and two residues on a β sheet of the protein. The loop (or finger) of protein can protrude into the major groove of DNA, where amino-acid side chains can interact with the base pairs and thereby confer the capacity for sequence-specific DNA binding. Zinc fingers consist of 30 amino acids with the consensus sequences $Cys-X_{2-4}-Cys-X_{12}-His-X_{3-5}-His$, where X can be any amino acid. However, not all proteins that contain this sequence bind DNA. Transcription factors of this family contain at least two zinc fingers and may contain dozens. Three amino acid residues at the tips of each zinc finger contact a DNA subsite that consists of three bases in the major groove of DNA; these residues are responsible for site recognition and binding (see Table 5–1). The zinc finger was first identified in the *Xenopus* transcription factor TFIIIA, which is necessary for transcription of the 5S RNA gene by pol III. Zinc fingers are also found in many mammalian transcription factors including several that we discuss in this chapter: Egr-1,

Wilms-tumor protein (WT-1), and stimulating protein-1 (SP1; see Table 5–1), as well as the steroid-hormone receptors (p. 131).

BASIC ZIPPER. This bZIP family (also known as the "leucine zipper" family) consists of transcription factors that bind to DNA as dimers (Fig. 5–9B). Members include C/EBP β (CCAAT/enhancer-binding protein β), c-Fos, c-Jun, and CREB (cyclic adenosine monophosphate response element–binding protein). Each monomer consist of two domains, a basic region that contacts DNA and a leucine zipper region that mediates dimerization. The "basic" region contains about 30 amino acids and is enriched in arginine and lysine residues. This region is responsible for sequence-specific binding to DNA via an α helix that inserts into the major groove of DNA. The leucine zipper consists of a region of about 30 amino acids in which every seventh residue is a leucine. Because of this spacing, the leucine residues align on a common face every second turn of an α helix. Two protein subunits that both contain leucine zippers can associate because of hydrophobic interactions between the leucine side chains; they form a tertiary structure called a *coiled coil.* Proteins of this family interact with DNA as *homo*dimers or as structurally related *hetero*dimers. Dimerization is essential for transcriptional activity because mutations of the leucine residues abolish both dimer formation and the ability to bind DNA and activate transcription. The crystal structure reveals that these transcription factors

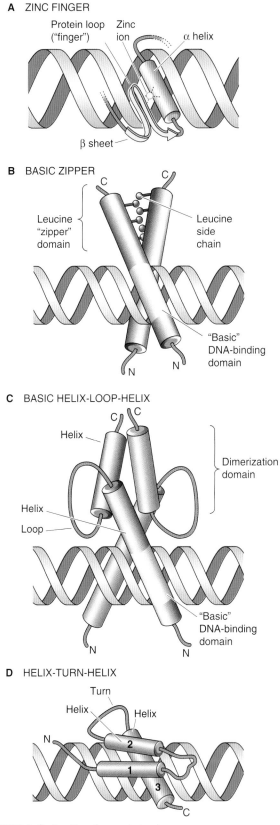

A ZINC FINGER

Protein loop ("finger") Zinc ion α helix

β sheet

B BASIC ZIPPER

C   C

Leucine "zipper" domain

Leucine side chain

"Basic" DNA-binding domain

N   N

C BASIC HELIX-LOOP-HELIX

C   C

Helix

Dimerization domain

Helix

Loop

"Basic" DNA-binding domain

N   N

D HELIX-TURN-HELIX

Turn

Helix   Helix

N

2

1

3

C

FIGURE 5–9. Families of transcription factors.

resemble scissors in which the blades represent the leucine zipper domains and the handles represent the DNA-binding domains (see Fig. 5–9*B*).

BASIC HELIX-LOOP-HELIX. Similar to the bZIP family, members of the bHLH family of transcription factors also bind to DNA as dimers. Each monomer has an extended α-helical segment containing the "basic" region that contacts DNA, linked by a loop to a second α helix that mediates dimer formation (see Fig. 5–9*C*). Thus the bHLH transcription factor forms by association of four amphipathic α helices (two from each monomer) into a bundle. The basic domains of each monomer protrude into the major grooves on opposite sides of the DNA. bHLH proteins include the MyoD family, which is involved in muscle differentiation, and E proteins (E12 and E47). MyoD and an E protein generally bind to DNA as heterodimers. In addition to mediating DNA binding, the basic region of the MyoD family contains two amino acids that are essential for muscle-specific transactivation.

HELIX-TURN-HELIX. In prokaryotes such as *Escherichia coli*, the HTH family consists of two α helices that are separated by a β turn. In eukaryotes, a modified HTH structure is represented by the so-called homeodomain (see Fig. 5–9*D*), which is present in some transcription factors that regulate development. The homeodomain consists of a 60–amino-acid sequence that forms three α helices. Helices 1 and 2 lie adjacent to one another, and helix 3 is perpendicular and forms the DNA-recognition helix. Particular amino acids protrude from the recognition helix and contact bases in the major groove of the DNA. Examples of homeodomain proteins include the Hox proteins, which are involved in mammalian pattern formation, engrailed homologs that are important in nervous system development, and the POU family members Pit-1, Oct-1, and unc-86.

Transcriptional Activators Physically Interact with the Basal Transcriptional Machinery

As we have already seen, specific transcription factors that stimulate transcription are called activators. Once transcriptional activators bind to enhancers (i.e., positive regulatory elements on the DNA), how do they stimulate gene transcription? Unfortunately, the answer to this question is not completely known, but some clues are available. We discuss three possible mechanisms by which transactivation might be achieved and the experimental evidence that supports each of these three possibilities.

First, **transcriptional activators may directly facilitate assembly of the basal transcriptional machinery**. Evidence supporting this hypothesis comes both from experiments demonstrating that transcriptional activators directly bind to components of the preinitiation complex and from experiments in which purified general transcription factors and activators are added stepwise to in vitro transcription assays. We have already introduced the concept by which looping out of DNA permits proteins that are bound to distant DNA enhancer elements to become

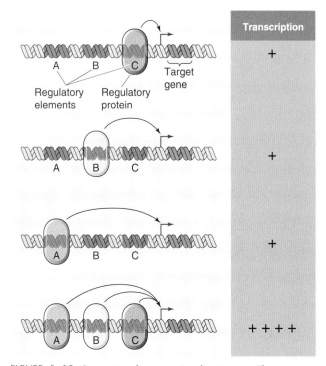

FIGURE 5–10. Synergism of transcriptional activators. The promoter contains three DNA enhancer elements—A, B, and C. Binding of a transcription factor to only one of the enhancer elements (A, B, or C) causes a modest activation of transcription. Simultaneous binding of different transcription factors to each of the three enhancer elements can produce a supra-additive increase in transcription (i.e., synergy).

physically juxtaposed to proteins that are bound to the gene promoter (see Fig. 5–7B). It is believed that this interaction occurs between the transactivation domain of the transcription factor (e.g., an "acidic blob") and components of the preinitiation complex, perhaps including pol II itself (see Fig. 5–8). Two general transcription factors, TFIID and TFIIB, are candidates for targeting by the acidic components of transcriptional activators. We have already introduced VP16, a herpesvirus transcriptional activator (p. 125). The acidic blob of VP16 binds to TFIIB. Mutations of the acidic-activation domain of VP16 that destroy the interaction between VP16 and TFIIB also abolish transcriptional activation. Conversely, mutations of TFIIB that eliminate the interaction with an acidic activator also abolish transactivation but have little effect on *basal* transcription. Because assembly of the basal transcriptional machinery may stall at TFIIB unless activating proteins are present, acidic activators may play a crucial role in the recruitment of TFIIB and thus in the assembly of the preinitiation complex.

A second mechanism by which transcriptional activators may function is to influence general transcription factors **indirectly via protein intermediaries** called **coactivators, mediators,** or **adapters.** Excellent candidates for adapters include the TBP-associated factors or TAFs (p. 123). TFIID consists of TBP and approximately 10 associated TAFs. TAFs are essential for transcriptional activation by an activator protein, although they are not required for basal transcription. Direct physical interaction between transcriptional activators and TAFs has been demon-

strated. For example, the transcriptional activator SP1 (p. 126) binds to a 250-kDa TAF called TAF_{250}. TAF_{250} binds to a smaller TAF_{110}, which in turn binds to TBP. This sequence establishes an uninterrupted linkage between SP1 and the TBP component of the TFIID that is being recruited to the transcription initiation site.

A third mechanism by which transcriptional activators may function is **by stimulating RNA polymerase II.** The C-terminal domain (CTD) of the largest subunit of pol II has a remarkable feature: it contains 52 repeats of the sequence Tyr-Ser-Pro-Thr-Ser-Pro-Ser, which can be phosphorylated at multiple Ser and Thr residues. A novel, cyclin-dependent kinase called positive transcription elongation factor b (P-TEFb) phosphorylates the CTD and thereby converts the initiation complex into an **elongation complex.** Only the dephosphorylated form of pol II can efficiently *enter* the preinitiation complex. Phosphorylation of the CTD occurs coincident with initiation of transcription and is required for chain elongation in vitro. Thus, when the CTD is dephosphorylated, elongation pauses and restarts only when the CTD is rephosphorylated.

Taken together, these three mechanisms of interaction lead to an attractive model for activation of transcription. The transcriptional activator that is bound to an enhancer presents a functional domain (e.g., an acidic blob) that either directly or via coactivators interacts with components of the basal transcriptional machinery and facilitates their assembly. Subsequent interactions—with the CTD of pol II, for example—may also contribute to transcriptional activation.

Transcriptional Activators Act in Combination

Two or more activators may increase the rate of transcription by an amount that is greater than the sum of each of the activators alone. Almost all naturally occurring promoters contain more than one site for binding transcriptional activators. A promoter region that contains only a single copy of an enhancer element shows only weak stimulation, whereas a promoter containing multiple copies of an enhancer exhibits substantial activation (Fig. 5–10). Two mechanisms for synergy have been proposed.

In the first, synergy may reflect **cooperative binding to DNA**; that is, binding of one transcription factor to its recognition site enhances binding of a second transcription factor to a different site. This phenomenon occurs with the glucocorticoid receptor (GR), which binds to a site on DNA known as the **glucocorticoid response element** (GRE). Binding of GRs to the multiple GREs is cooperative in that binding of the first receptor promotes binding of additional receptors. Thus the presence of multiple copies of the GRE greatly stimulates gene expression in comparison to a single copy of the GRE.

In the second case, synergy reflects **cooperative protein-protein interactions** between transcription factors and multiple sites on the basal transcriptional machinery. For example, a transcriptional activator that recruits TFIID could synergize with another activator that recruits TFIIB. Here, the effect on transcription depends on the

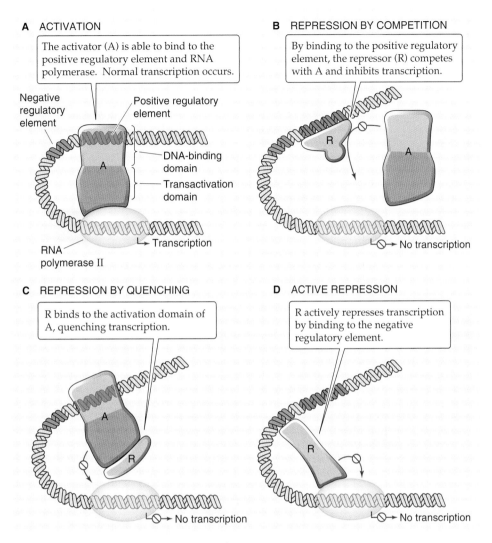

A ACTIVATION

The activator (A) is able to bind to the positive regulatory element and RNA polymerase. Normal transcription occurs.

Negative regulatory element

Positive regulatory element

DNA-binding domain

Transactivation domain

A

RNA polymerase II

⤷ Transcription

B REPRESSION BY COMPETITION

By binding to the positive regulatory element, the repressor (R) competes with A and inhibits transcription.

R

A

⤷ No transcription

C REPRESSION BY QUENCHING

R binds to the activation domain of A, quenching transcription.

A

R

⤷ No transcription

D ACTIVE REPRESSION

R actively represses transcription by binding to the negative regulatory element.

R

⤷ No transcription

FIGURE 5–11. Transcriptional repressor modes of action.

cumulative effects of multiple transcription factors, each bound to its cognate recognition site and interacting with the basal transcriptional machinery.

Transcription factors may act in combination by binding to DNA as **homodimers** or **heterodimers**. This synergism is particularly true for members of the bZIP and bHLH families, but also for steroid and thyroid hormone receptors. Often, different combinations of monomers have different DNA binding *affinities*. For example, the thyroid hormone receptor (THR) can bind to DNA as a homodimer, but the heterodimer formed from the thyroid receptor and the 9-*cis*-retinoic acid receptor has much higher binding affinity. As we saw earlier (p. 127), the transcription factor MyoD, which is involved in muscle differentiation, requires heterodimerization with the ubiquitous proteins E12 or E47 for maximal DNA binding. Different combinations of monomers may also have different DNA binding *specificities* and thus be targeted to different sites on the DNA. Finally, different combinations of monomers may have different *transactivational properties*. For example, the c-Myc protein can bind to DNA as a

homodimer or as a heterodimer with Max, but c-Myc/Max heterodimers have greater transcriptional activity.

Transcriptional Repressors Act by Competition, Quenching, or Active Repression

Not only can cells regulate transcription *positively* via transcriptional activators (Fig. 5–11A), they can also regulate transcription *negatively* via transcriptional repressors. Repression of transcription is important for tissue specificity in that it allows cells to silence certain genes where they should not be expressed. Repression is also important for regulating inducible gene expression by rapidly turning off transcription after removal of the inducing stimulus.

Transcriptional repressors may act by three mechanisms. First, some repressors inhibit the binding of transcriptional activators because they **compete** for DNA binding sites that are identical to, or overlap with, those

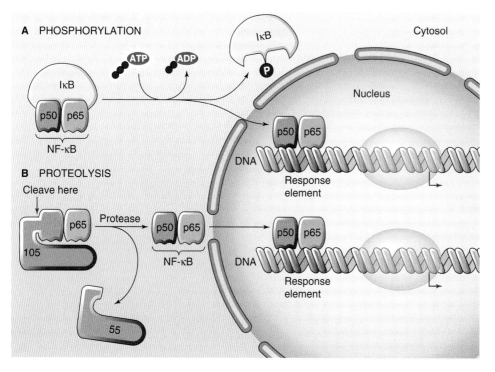

FIGURE 5–12. Regulating transcription factors by post-translational modification. *A,* The phosphorylation of the cytoplasmic anchor IκB releases the p50 and p65 subunits of NF-κB, allowing them to translocate into the nucleus. *B,* Proteolytic cleavage of a 105-kDa precursor releases the p50 subunit of NF-κB. Together with the p65 subunit, the p50 subunit can now translocate to the nucleus.

for activators (see Fig. 5–11B). An example is the CCAAT displacement protein (CDP), which binds to the CAAT box in the promoter of the γ-globin gene and thereby prevents binding of the transcriptional activator CP1. This action helps prevent inappropriate expression of the fetal globin gene in adults.

Second, some repressors inhibit the activity of transcriptional activators not by interfering with DNA binding, but by a direct protein-protein interaction with activators. This form of repression is termed **quenching** (see Fig. 5–11C). A classic example in yeast is the GAL80 repressor, which inhibits transcriptional activation by GAL4. By binding to the activation domain of GAL4, GAL80 blocks transcriptional activation. Dissociation of GAL80 (which occurs in the presence of galactose) relieves the inhibition of GAL4, which can then induce expression of galactose-metabolizing genes. Transcriptional repression can also be mediated by proteins that prevent transcriptional activators from entering the nucleus. For example, the heat shock protein hsp90 binds to GR and prevents this transcriptional activator from entering the nucleus.

A third class of repressors binds to an NRE (or silencer) and then interacts directly with the basal transcriptional machinery. This mechanism is referred to as **active repression** (see Fig. 5–11D). The opposite of transcriptional activators, these proteins contain domains that mediate repression, presumably by interacting with and inhibiting the assembly or activity of the basal transcriptional machinery. Some repressors act via multiple mechanisms. For example, the Wilms tumor protein WT-1 (p. 126) inhibits transcription by competing with the transcriptional activator Egr-1 for binding to a common sequence and also contains a domain that mediates active repression.

The nuclear milieu, particularly the presence of protein

"partners," also can influence the activity of a transcription factor. For instance, heterodimerization of the basic zipper protein CREB with the alternate partner CREM (cAMP-response element modifier) reduces transcriptional activity. We have seen that MyoD—a basic-HLH transcription factor—requires heterodimer formation with E12 or E47 for maximal activity. If MyoD dimerizes instead with Id, an HLH protein that lacks a basic region and cannot bind DNA, MyoD is inactive.

The Activity of Transcription Factors May Be Regulated by Post-Translational Modifications

Cells can regulate the activity of transcription factors by controlling the amount of transcription factor they synthesize. In addition, cells can modulate the activity of preformed transcription factors by "post-translational modification" (p. 34). Examples include phosphorylation and proteolysis.

Phosphorylation (p. 91) is the most important post-translational modification affecting transcription-factor activity, which it can affect by increasing or decreasing (1) transport of the transcription factor from the cytoplasm into the nucleus, (2) the affinity with which the transcription factor binds to DNA, and (3) transcriptional activation.

For transcription factors that reside in the cytoplasm under basal conditions, migration from the cytoplasm into the nucleus is a necessary step. Many proteins that are transported into the nucleus contain a sequence that is relatively enriched in basic amino-acid residues (i.e., arginine and lysine). This sequence, the **nuclear-localization signal,** is required for transport of the protein into the nucleus. Phosphorylation at sites within or near the nuclear localization signal can dramatically change the rate of nuclear translocation. Phosphorylation can also modulate import into the nucleus by regulating the binding of transcription factors to cytoplasmic anchors. In the case of the transcription factor NF-κB (Fig. 5–12A), binding to the cytoplasmic anchor IκB conceals the nuclear localization signal on the p50 and p65 subunits of NF-κB from the nuclear translocation machinery. Only after these two other subunits dissociate from the phosphorylated IκB is the transcription factor dimer free to enter the nucleus.

Phosphorylation can also regulate transcription-factor activity by altering the *affinity* of the transcription factor for its target-recognition sequences on DNA. As a result, phosphorylation increases or decreases DNA-binding activity. For example, casein kinase II phosphorylates SRF (serum response factor), a transcription factor that activates the *c-Fos* gene in response to growth factors, thereby enhancing DNA binding. In contrast, phosphorylation of the transcription factor c-Jun by casein kinase II inhibits binding to DNA.

Phosphorylation can greatly influence the *transactivation properties* of transcription factors. c-Jun is an example in which transcriptional activity is increased by the phosphorylation of serine residues located within the transactivation domain near the N terminus of the protein. Phosphorylation can also *inhibit* transcriptional activation by reducing transcriptional activation or stimulating active transcriptional repression.

Effects of phosphorylation on nuclear translocation, DNA binding, and transactivation are not mutually exclusive. Moreover, in addition to phosphorylation by protein kinases, dephosphorylation by protein phosphatases may also regulate transcriptional activity.

Site-specific proteolysis is the second post-translational process that is important for regulating some transcription factors. Although phosphorylation can regulate NF-κB by controlling its binding to IκB (see Fig. 5–12A), proteolysis can also regulate NF-κB (see Fig. 5–12B). A 105-kDa precursor of the 50-kDa subunit of NF-κB (p50), which we mentioned earlier, binds to and thereby retains the 65-kDa subunit of NF-κB (p65) in the cytoplasm. Proteolysis of this larger precursor yields the 50-kDa subunit that, together with the 65-kDa subunit, constitutes the active NF-κB transcription factor.

REGULATION OF INDUCIBLE GENE EXPRESSION BY SIGNAL-TRANSDUCTION PATHWAYS

How do cells activate previously quiescent genes in response to environmental cues? How are such external signals transduced to the cell nucleus to stimulate the transcription of specific genes? Transcription factors may be thought of as effector molecules in signal-transduction pathways (Chapter 4) that modulate gene expression. Several such signalling pathways have been defined. Lipid-soluble steroid and thyroid hormones can enter the cell and interact with specific receptors that are themselves transcription factors. However, most cytokines, hormones, and mitogens cannot diffuse into the cell interior and instead bind to specific receptors that are located on the cell surface. After examining the mechanisms by which

steroid or thyroid hormones act via transcription factors, we will consider three pathways for transducing signals from cell-surface receptors into the nucleus: a cAMP-dependent pathway, a Ras-dependent pathway, and the JAK (Janus kinase) pathway.

Steroid and Thyroid Hormone Receptors Are Transcription Factors

Steroid and thyroid hormones are examples of ligands that activate gene expression by binding to cellular receptors that are themselves transcription factors. Members of the steroid- and thyroid-hormone receptor superfamily, also called the intracellular or nuclear receptor superfamily, are grouped together because they are structurally similar and have similar mechanisms of action. After these hormones enter the cell, they bind to receptors in the cytoplasm or nucleus. Ligand binding converts the receptors into active transcription factors. The transcription factors bind to specific regulatory elements on the DNA called **hormone response elements** and activate the transcription of *cis*-linked genes. This family of hormone receptors includes receptors that are specific for glucocorticoids (GR), mineralocorticoids (MR), estrogens (ER), progesterone (PR), androgens (AR), thyroid hormone (THR), vitamin D (VDR), retinoic acid (RAR), and 9-*cis*-retinoic acid (retinoid X receptor, RXR).

With the exception of the thyroid hormones, the hormones that bind to these receptors are low-molecular-weight, lipophilic molecules that enter cells by diffusion and do not require interaction with cell-surface receptors. The thyroid hormones differ in that they are electrically charged and may cross the cell membrane via transporters (p. 1040). The steroid/thyroid-hormone *receptors* have a modular construction (p. 113). These receptors bind to specific DNA sequences via two *zinc fingers* (p. 126), each of which contains four cysteine residues rather than the two histidines and two cysteines that are typical of many other zinc-finger proteins (see Fig. 5–9A). Particularly important for DNA recognition is the P-box motif in the hormone receptor, a sequence of six amino acids at the C-terminal end of each finger. These P-boxes make base-pair contacts in the major groove of DNA and determine the DNA binding specificities of the zinc finger.

GR, MR, PR, ER, and AR bind to DNA as **homodimers** (Table 5–2). The recognition sites for these receptors (except for ER) consist of two 6-bp DNA sequences that are separated by three other base pairs. The 6-bp DNA sequences, commonly called **half-sites**, represent binding sites for each zinc-finger monomer.

In contrast, the other "steroid" receptors (VDR, THR, RAR) preferentially bind to DNA as **heterodimers** formed with RXR, the receptor for 9-*cis*-retinoic acid. Thus the dimers are VDR/RXR, THR/RXR, and RAR/RXR. Interestingly, these heterodimers work even in the absence of the ligand of RXR (i.e., 9-*cis*-retinoic acid). Only the VDR, THR, or RAR part of the dimer needs to be occupied by its hormone ligand. These heterodimers recognize a family of DNA sites containing a DNA sequence such as 5′-AGGTCA-3′, followed by a DNA spacer and then by a direct repeat of the previous 6-bp DNA sequence. Moreover, because each of the three heterodimers may recog-

TABLE 5–2

STEROID AND THYROID HORMONE RECEPTORS

RECEPTOR	FULL NAME	DIMERIC ARRANGEMENT
GR	Glucocorticoid receptor	GR/GR
MR	Mineralocorticoid receptor	MR/MR
PR	Progesterone receptor	PR/PR
ER	Estrogen receptor	ER/ER
AR	Androgen receptor	AR/AR
VDR	Vitamin D receptor	VDR/RXR
THR	Thyroid hormone receptor	THR/RXR
RAR	Retinoic acid receptor	RAR/RXR

nize the *same* 6-bp sequences, binding specificity also depends on the length of the spacer between the direct repeats. The VDR/RXR, THR/RXR, and RAR/RXR heterodimers preferentially recognize separations of 3 bp, 4 bp, and 5 bp, respectively, between the repeats of 5′-AGGTCA-3′. This relationship forms the basis for the so-called **3-4-5 rule.**

The mechanism by which ligand binding activates the receptors remains controversial. The receptors are located in the nucleus or cytoplasm, and the mechanism of hormone-dependent activation may differ, depending on the location of the receptor. Receptors that are normally located in the cytoplasm, such as GR, are maintained in an inactive state by association with a cytoplasmic anchoring protein (Fig. 5–13A). The protein that retains GR in the cytoplasm is a molecular chaperone, the 90-kDa heat shock protein **hsp90**. GR must bind to hsp90 to have a high affinity for a glucocorticoid hormone. When glucocorticoids bind to the GR, hsp90 dissociates from the GR and exposes a nuclear localization signal that permits the transport of GR into the nucleus. The receptor must remain hormone bound for receptor dimerization, which is a prerequisite for binding to the GRE response element on the DNA. Other receptors, such as THR, are normally already present in the nucleus before binding the hormone (see Fig. 5–13B). For these receptors, binding of hormone is evidently not essential for dimerization or binding to DNA. However, ligand binding is necessary for transactivation.

Steroid hormone receptors *stimulate gene expression* by interacting with the basal transcriptional machinery. Direct protein-protein interactions occur between the N terminus of the THR and the C terminus of TFIIB. Thus, steroid hormone receptors may function like acidic activators by recruiting TFIIB to the preinitiation complex. Receptors may also interact with other components of the basal transcriptional machinery such as TBP, and some interactions may be indirect and involve coactivators. Al-

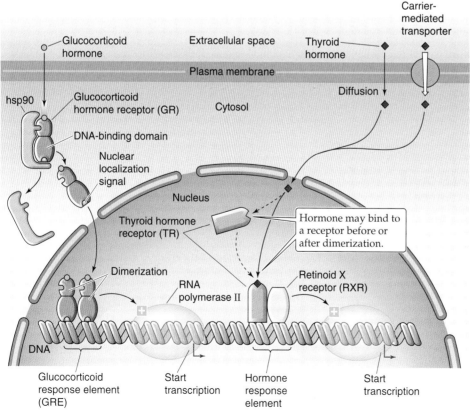

A TRANSCRIPTIONAL ACTIVATION BY GLUCOCORTICOID HORMONE

B TRANSCRIPTIONAL ACTIVATION BY THYROID HORMONE

FIGURE 5–13. Transcriptional activation by glucocorticoid and thyroid hormones. *A,* The binding of a glucocorticoid hormone to a cytoplasmic receptor causes the receptor to dissociate from the chaperone hsp90 (90-kDa heat shock protein). The free hormone-receptor complex can then translocate to the nucleus, where dimerization leads to transactivation. *B,* The binding of thyroid hormone to a receptor in the nucleus leads to transactivation. The active transcription factor is a heterodimer of the thyroid hormone receptor and the retinoid X receptor.

though steroid hormone receptors usually function as transcriptional activators, they sometimes *function as active repressors*. THRs may also act as repressors, and a number of alternative mechanisms have been proposed for this repression. First, the receptor may form inactive heterodimers with other receptors. Second, the receptor may compete with other transcription factors for DNA binding sites. For example, when the THR—without bound thyroid hormone—interacts with its own DNA response element, the THR acts as a repressor. In addition, the receptor THR_α can dimerize with one of the retinoic acid receptors (RXR_β) to interfere with binding of ER to its response element. This competition may be one of the mechanisms that retinoids use to inhibit estrogen-induced alterations in gene expression and growth in mammary tissue.

The intracellular receptor pathway can communicate with other signalling pathways that also affect transcription. The result is that cooperative interaction between unrelated transcriptional activators can produce novel patterns of gene regulation. Such interaction can occur by at least two mechanisms. First, an intracellular receptor can interact with an unrelated transcription factor, thus modulating the latter's activity. For example, RAR can interact with members of the AP-1 family and prevent AP-1 from interacting with its response element. A second mechanism by which unrelated transcription factors can interact is by jointly binding to a response element. A good example is the interaction between AP-1 and GR. In addition to binding to their individual DNA binding sites (or *simple* hormone response elements), AP-1 and GR together can bind to a 25-bp sequence of DNA known as the "composite site," which neither can recognize alone. Although the GR and MR have similar effects when bound to simple hormone-response elements, they have differential effects at the composite site. Joint binding of GR and AP-1 to the composite site inhibits transactivation, whereas the individual binding of MR or AP-1 has no effect.

cAMP Regulates Transcription via the Transcription Factors CREB and CBP

cAMP is an important second messenger (p. 97) in the response to agonists binding to specific cell-surface receptors. Increases in $[cAMP]_i$ stimulate the transcription of certain genes, including those that encode a variety of hormones, such as somatostatin (p. 1026), the enkephalins (p. 304), glucagon (p. 1081), and vasoactive intestinal polypeptide (p. 884). Many genes that are activated in response to cAMP contain within their regulatory regions a common DNA element called **CRE** (cAMP response element) that has the consensus sequence 5'-TGACGTCA-3'. Several different transcription factors bind to CRE, among them **CREB**, a 43-kDa member of the bZIP family (p. 126). As shown in Figure 5–14, increases in $[cAMP]_i$ stimulate protein kinase A (PKA) by causing dissociation of the PKA regulatory subunit. The catalytic subunit of PKA then translocates into the nucleus, where it phosphorylates CREB and other proteins. Activation of CREB is rapid (30 minutes) and declines gradually over a 24-hour period. This phosphorylation greatly increases the

ROLE OF A CHIMERIC TRANSCRIPTION FACTOR IN ACUTE PROMYELOCYTIC LEUKEMIA

Correct regulation of gene expression involves both transcription factors and the DNA regulatory elements to which they bind. Abnormalities of either could and do result in abnormal regulation of gene expression, which is often manifested as disease. An example of a transcription factor abnormality is acute promyelocytic leukemia (APL), a hematologic malignancy in which cells of the granulocyte lineage (promyelocytes) fail to differentiate. Normally, retinoic acid (RA) binds to **retinoic acid receptor** α (RAR_α), a member of the steroid-thyroid hormone receptor superfamily. RAR_α/RA then binds to retinoic-acid response elements (RAREs), thereby promoting expression of RARE-containing genes involved in cell differentiation. Ninety percent of patients with APL have a translocation affecting chromosomes 15 and 17, t(15;17), that results in a chimeric transcription factor. Such a chimera is formed by chromosomal translocations that produce a novel gene product with properties derived from both parental genes. In APL, the translocation breakpoint on chromosome 17 occurs within the first intron of the gene encoding RAR_α so the RAR_α gene is fused to a gene on chromosome 15 that encodes the **nuclear protein PML**. The protein encoded by this novel chimeric gene contains both the DNA- and hormone-binding domains of RAR_α as well as most of the PML protein. The PML/RAR_α chimeric protein interferes with function by nonchimeric RAR_α and thus interferes with promyelocytic differentiation. Because the chimeric protein also contains the hormone-binding domain of RAR_α, the chimeric protein is responsive to high concentrations of RA. Indeed, it is possible to induce clinical remissions in patients with APL by administering exogenous RA.

affinity of CREB for another nuclear protein called **CBP** (CREB-binding protein). CBP is a 245-kDa protein that contains two domains, one that binds to phosphorylated CREB and another that activates components of the basal transcriptional machinery. Thus CBP serves as a "bridge" protein that communicates the transcriptional activation signal from CREB to the basal transcriptional machinery. The result of phosphorylating CREB is a 10- to 20-fold stimulation of CREB's ability to induce the transcription of genes containing a CRE.

How is the transcriptional signal terminated? When $[cAMP]_i$ is high, PKA phosphorylates and activates phosphoprotein phosphatase 1 (p. 98) in the nucleus. When cAMP levels fall, the still-active phosphatase dephosphorylates CREB.

Receptor Tyrosine Kinases Regulate Transcription via a Ras-Dependent Cascade of Protein Kinases

Many growth factors bind to cell-surface receptors that—when activated by the ligand—have tyrosine kinase activ-

FIGURE 5–14. Regulation of gene transcription by cyclic adenosine monophosphate (cAMP). Phosphorylated CREB binds CBP, which has a transactivation domain that stimulates the basal transcriptional machinery. In parallel, phosphorylation activates PP1, which dephosphorylates CREB, terminating the activation of transcription. ADP, adenosine diphosphate; ATP, adenosine triphosphate.

Step 1: A ligand binds to the extracellular domain of a specific **RTK**, thus causing receptor dimerization.

Step 2: The now-activated RTK phosphorylates itself on tyrosine residues of the cytoplasmic domain (autophosphorylation).

Step 3: **GRB2** (growth factor receptor–bound protein-2), an SH2 (Src homology domain 2)-containing protein (p. 98), recognizes the phosphotyrosine residues on the activated receptor.

Step 4: Binding of GRB2 recruits **SOS** (son of sevenless), a guanine nucleotide exchange protein (see p. 97).

Step 5: SOS activates **Ras** by causing GTP to replace guanosine diphosphate (GDP) on Ras.

Step 6: The activated GTP-Ras complex activates other proteins by physically recruiting them to the plasma membrane. In particular, the active GTP-Ras complex interacts with the N-terminal portion of the serine-threonine kinase **Raf-1** (also known as **mitogen-activated protein [MAP] kinase kinase kinase**), which is the first in a series of sequentially activated protein kinases that ultimately transmits the activation signal to the cell nucleus.

Step 7: Raf-1 phosphorylates and activates a protein kinase called **MEK**, also known as MAP kinase kinase (MAPKK). MEK is a multifunctional protein kinase that phosphorylates substrates on both tyrosine and serine/threonine residues. MEK is also activated by the JAK system (see the next section).

Step 8: MEK phosphorylates **MAP kinase** (MAPK), which is also called extracellular signal–regulated kinase (ERK1, ERK2). Activation of MAPK requires dual phosphorylation on neighboring serine and tyrosine residues.

Step 9: MAPK is an important effector molecule in Ras-dependent signal transduction because it phosphorylates many cellular proteins after mitogenic stimulation.

Step 10: Activated MAPK also translocates to the nucleus, where it phosphorylates a number of nuclear proteins that are transcription factors. Phosphorylation of a transcription factor by MAPK can enhance or inhibit binding to DNA and can stimulate either transactivation or transrepression (Table 5–3).

Two other signal-transduction pathways (cAMP and Ca^{2+}) can also modulate the activity of some of the protein intermediates in this cascade. In addition, some of the same transcription factors activated via the Ras cascade are also affected by these other pathways, thus suggesting multiple points of integration for the various signalling systems.

Tyrosine Kinase–Associated Receptors Can Regulate Transcription via JAK-STAT, a More Direct Pathway to the Nucleus

A group of cell-surface receptors termed tyrosine kinase–associated receptors lack *intrinsic* tyrosine kinase activity (p. 111). The ligands that bind to these receptors include several cytokines, growth hormone, prolactin, and interferon-α (IFN-α), IFN-β, and IFN-γ. Although the receptors themselves lack catalytic activity, their cytoplasmic domains are associated with the Janus family of protein

ity (p. 110). Examples of growth factors that act through such receptor tyrosine kinases (RTKs) are epidermal growth factor (EGF), platelet-derived growth factor (PDGF), insulin, insulin-like growth factor type I (IGF-I), fibroblast growth factor (FGF), and nerve growth factor (NGF). The common pathway by which activation of RTKs is transduced into the nucleus is a cascade of events that increase the activity of the small guanosine triphosphate (GTP)–binding protein Ras (p. 97). This **Ras-dependent signalling pathway** involves the following steps (Fig. 5–15):

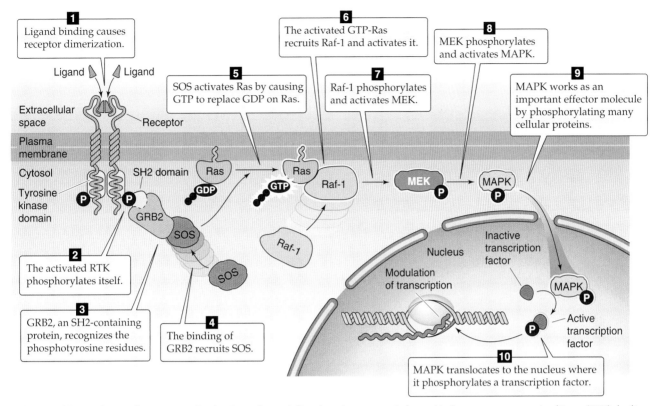

FIGURE 5–15. Regulation of transcription by the *Ras* pathway. A ligand, such as a growth factor, binds to a receptor tyrosine kinase (RTK), leading to an increase in gene transcription in a ten-step process. GDP, guanosine diphosphate; GTP, guanosine triphosphate.

tyrosine kinases. The Janus family is also called **JAK** (originally named "just another kinase").

Binding of ligand to certain tyrosine-kinase–associated receptors activates a member of the Janus family, which results in phosphorylation of cytoplasmic proteins, among which are believed to be latent cytoplasmic transcription factors called **STATs** (signal transducers and activators of transcription). When phosphorylated on tyrosine residues, the STAT proteins dimerize and thereby become competent to enter the nucleus and induce transcription.

A well-characterized example of the JAK-STAT pathway is the activation of **interferon-responsive genes** by IFN-α and IFN-γ. IFN-α activates the JAK1 and Tyk2 kinases that are associated with its receptor (Fig. 5–16A). Subsequent phosphorylation of two different STAT monomers causes the monomers to dimerize. This STAT heterodimer enters the nucleus, where it combines with a third, 48-kDa protein to form a transcription factor that binds to a DNA sequence called the IFN-α–stimulated response element (ISRE). In the case of IFN-γ (see Fig. 5–16B), the

TABLE 5–3

TRANSCRIPTION FACTORS PHOSPHORYLATED BY MITOGEN-ACTIVATED PROTEIN KINASE

TRANSCRIPTION FACTOR	SITE	EFFECT
c-Myc	Ser-62	Stabilizes protein
c-Jun	Ser-243 (Ser-63/Ser-73 in activation domain are phosphorylated by distinct Ras-dependent kinase)	Inhibits DNA binding
c-Fos	Ser-374 (direct) Ser-362 (indirect via ribosomal S6 kinase, which is activated by MAP kinase)	Stimulates transrepression
p62TCF (Elk-1)	Multiple	Stimulates transactivation and possibly also DNA binding
C/EBPβ (LAP, NF–IL-6)	Thr-235	Stimulates transactivation
ATF-2	Thr-69 & Thr-71 (via p38 & JNK MAP kinases)	Stimulates transactivation

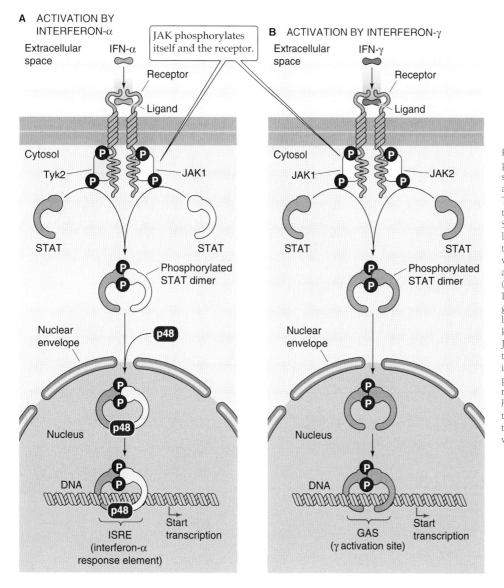

A ACTIVATION BY INTERFERON-α

JAK phosphorylates itself and the receptor.

Extracellular space   IFN-α
Receptor
Ligand
Cytosol
Tyk2   JAK1
STAT   STAT
Phosphorylated STAT dimer
Nuclear envelope
p48
Nucleus
p48
DNA
p48
ISRE (interferon-α response element)
Start transcription

B ACTIVATION BY INTERFERON-γ

Extracellular space   IFN-γ
Receptor
Ligand
Cytosol
JAK1   JAK2
STAT   STAT
Phosphorylated STAT dimer
Nuclear envelope
Nucleus
DNA
GAS (γ activation site)
Start transcription

FIGURE 5–16. The JAK-STAT pathway. *A,* Binding of a ligand such as IFN-α to a tyrosine-kinase–associated receptor causes JAK1 and Tyk2 to phosphorylate themselves, the receptor, and two different STAT monomers. The phosphorylation of the STAT monomers leads to the formation of a *hetero*dimer, which translocates to the nucleus and combines with a third protein (p48). The complex binds to the ISRE response element and activates gene transcription. *B,* Binding of a ligand such as IFN-γ to a tyrosine-kinase–associated receptor causes JAK1 and JAK2 to phosphorylate themselves, the receptor, and two identical STAT monomers. The phosphorylation of the STAT monomers leads to the formation of a *homo*dimer, which translocates to the nucleus. The complex binds to the GAS response element and activates gene transcription.

receptor associates with the JAK1 and JAK2 (rather than Tyk2) kinases, and subsequent phosphorylation of a *single* kind of STAT monomer causes these monomers to dimerize. These STAT homodimers also enter the nucleus, where they bind to the DNA at IFN-γ response elements called γ activation sites (GAS), without requiring the 48-kDa protein.

REGULATION OF GENE EXPRESSION BY CHANGES IN DNA STRUCTURE

You might recall that at the outset of this chapter we noted that gene expression entails several steps, beginning with alteration of chromatin structure (see Fig. 5–1, *step 1*). Having already discussed the control of transcription (see Fig. 5–1, *step 2*) in the previous three subchapters, in this penultimate subchapter we return to the first step and consider how changes in chromatin structure and the

methylation of DNA affect gene transcription. In the last subchapter, we will examine several of the later steps.

Chromatin Structure Influences the Initiation of Transcription

Although DNA is commonly depicted as linear, DNA in the nucleus is actually organized into a higher-order structure called chromatin. **Chromatin** consists of DNA and associated nuclear proteins, the best characterized of which are the **histones**. The basic building block of chromatin is the **nucleosome** (Fig. 5–17). Each nucleosome consists of a protein core and approximately 200 bp of associated DNA. The protein core is an octamer of the histones H2A, H2B, H3, and H4. Negatively supercoiled DNA wraps around the core histones to form a solenoid-like structure. A linker histone, H1, associates with segments of DNA between nucleosomes. Regular arrays of nucleosomes have a beads-on-a-string appearance and constitute the so-called 11-nm fiber of chromatin, which

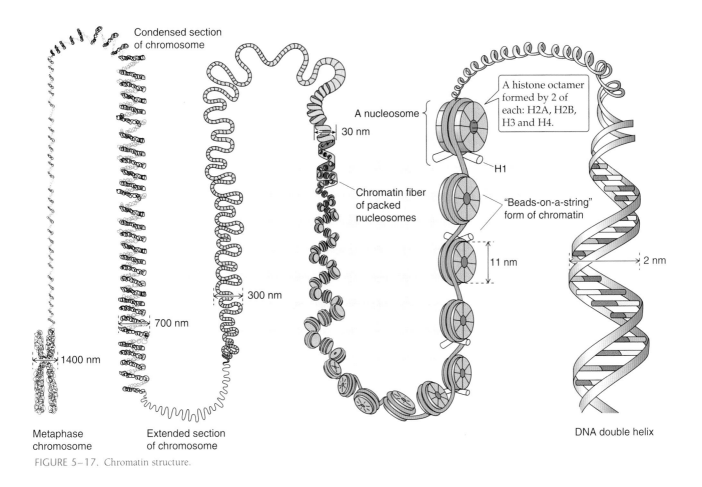

Condensed section of chromosome

A nucleosome

30 nm

A histone octamer formed by 2 of each: H2A, H2B, H3 and H4.

H1

Chromatin fiber of packed nucleosomes

"Beads-on-a-string" form of chromatin

11 nm

300 nm

700 nm

1400 nm

2 nm

Metaphase chromosome

Extended section of chromosome

DNA double helix

FIGURE 5–17. Chromatin structure.

can condense to form the 30-nm fiber. Transcription from DNA in active chromatin probably requires partial disruption of the regular nucleosome structure and some unwinding of the DNA (more on this later).

Chromatin exists in two general forms that can be distinguished cytologically by their different degrees of condensation. **Heterochromatin** is a highly condensed form of chromatin that is transcriptionally inactive, probably because its DNA is unable to bind to transcription factors. Heterochromatin contains mostly repetitive sequences and relatively few genes. Even in the transcriptionally active "open" chromatin (**euchromatin**), local chromatin structure may influence the activity of individual genes. In general, highly organized chromatin structure is associated with *repression* of gene transcription.

Activation of gene expression is accompanied by a change in chromatin structure that can be detected by using enzymes that digest the DNA of euchromatin (i.e., DNase). Genes being actively transcribed are more sensitive to digestion by exogenous DNase than genes that are transcriptionally silent. These data suggest that transcriptionally active chromatin has a less condensed structure that renders the DNA more accessible to enzymatic digestion.

In addition to a *generalized* increase in the sensitivity to DNase that accompanies transcriptional activation, there are also *specific* sites that exhibit unusually high sensitivity to exogenous DNase, so-called **DNase hypersensitive sites.** These sites are frequently located in the 5′ flanking regions of actively transcribed genes and correspond to locations of enhancers. This relationship implies that binding of transcription factors to regulatory elements is associated with almost complete local disruption of chromatin structure, which results in DNase hypersensitivity. In vitro studies have provided direct evidence that the binding of transcription factors to DNA in chromatin causes the appearance of DNase hypersensitive sites. Thus, the transcription of genes, which requires binding of proteins, leads to disruption of chromatin structure. However, it is also clear that transcription of a gene does not require complete dissolution of the chromatin structure. How the transcriptional machinery assembles and translocates down the DNA even in the presence of histones remains an unanswered question.

Histones are not mere bystanders in transcription. Rather, interactions among transcription factors and histones may be involved in regulating particular genes. The role of histone acetylation is of particular interest (Fig. 5–18). The N termini of core histone proteins contain many lysine residues that impart a highly positive charge. These positively charged domains can bind tightly to the negatively charged DNA via electrostatic interactions. Tight binding between DNA and histones is associated with gene inactivity. However, if the ϵ-amino groups of the lysine side chains are chemically modified by **acetylation,**

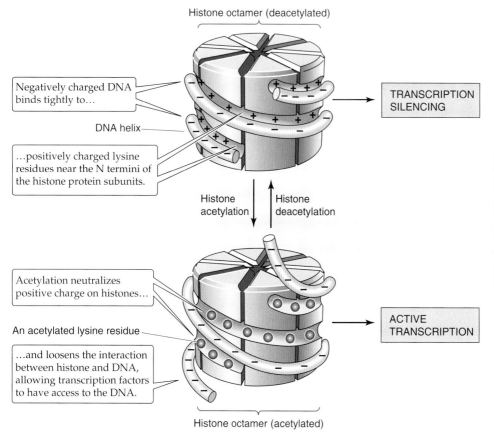

Histone octamer (deacetylated)

Negatively charged DNA binds tightly to...

DNA helix

...positively charged lysine residues near the N termini of the histone protein subunits.

TRANSCRIPTION SILENCING

Histone acetylation

Histone deacetylation

Acetylation neutralizes positive charge on histones...

An acetylated lysine residue

...and loosens the interaction between histone and DNA, allowing transcription factors to have access to the DNA.

ACTIVE TRANSCRIPTION

Histone octamer (acetylated)

FIGURE 5–18. Effect of histone acetylation on the interaction between histone proteins and DNA. When the histone octamer is deacetylated (*top*), positively charged lysine groups on the histone strongly attract a strand of DNA. When the histone octamer becomes acetylated (*bottom*), the acetyl groups neutralize the positive charge on the histone and allow the DNA strand to loosen.

the positive charge is neutralized and the interaction with DNA is weakened. This modification is believed to result in a loosening of chromatin structure that permits transcriptional regulatory proteins to gain access to the DNA. Recently, enzymes have been identified that can acetylate histones (histone acetylases) or deacetylate histones (histone deacetylases). Interestingly, several coactivator proteins that mediate transcriptional activation, such as CBP (p. 133), possess intrinsic histone acetylase activity. In addition, some transcriptional corepressors, such as the N-Cor adapter protein that mediates repression by steroid hormone receptors, can interact with histone deacetylase. These observations lead to a model in which transcriptional activation is mediated by **coactivator proteins** that not only bind to components of the basal transcriptional machinery but also acetylate histones and thus produce local alterations in chromatin structure that are more favorable for transcription. Conversely, **repressors** may function in part through proteins that remove the acetyl groups, leading to tighter binding between DNA and histones and inhibition of transcription.

Methylation of DNA Is Associated with Gene Inactivation

Methylation of cytosine residues at the N^5 position is the only well-documented postsynthetic modification of DNA in higher eukaryotes. Approximately 5% of cytosine residues are methylated in mammalian DNA. Methylation usually occurs on cytosine residues that are immediately upstream from guanosines (i.e., CpG dinucleotides).

Several lines of evidence implicate DNA methylation in the control of gene expression: (1) Although CpG dinucleotides are relatively underrepresented in mammalian genomes, they are frequently clustered near the 5' ends of genes (forming so-called **CpG islands**). Moreover, methylation of cytosines in these locations is associated with inhibition of gene expression. For example, during female development, X inactivation (lyonization) inactivates one X chromosome. Examination of the inactive X chromosome reveals that the genes are heavily methylated. (2) Methylation/demethylation may explain tissue-specific and stage-dependent gene expression. For example, globin genes are methylated in nonexpressing tissues but hypomethylated in erythroid cells. During fetal development, fetal globin genes are demethylated and then become methylated in the adult. (3) Foreign genes that are introduced into cells are transcriptionally inactive if they are methylated but active if demethylated at the 5' end. (4) Chemical demethylating agents, such as 5-azacytidine, can activate previously inactive genes.

How does DNA methylation cause gene inactivation? Cells contain a protein called MeCP2 that binds specifically to methylated CpG dinucleotides, as well as to the *histone deacetylase* discussed in the previous section. Thus, methylation may cause gene silencing by promoting histone deacetylation.

A ABSENCE OF Tat

RNA polymerase II

Bulge

"TAR"

RNA polymerase II released prematurely

Bulge

Short RNA

B PRESENCE OF Tat

RNA polymerase II

Coactivator

Tat

RNA polymerase II released normally

Long RNA

FIGURE 5–19. Role of Tat in transcript elongation. *A,* The TAR (*trans*-activation response element) of the newly transcribed RNA forms a hairpin loop with a bulge. In the absence of Tat, transcription terminates prematurely and releases a short strand of RNA. *B,* Tat binds to the bulge and recruits a coactivator that allows transcript elongation to form full-length RNAs.

POST-TRANSCRIPTIONAL REGULATION OF GENE EXPRESSION

Although initiation of transcription (Fig. 5–1, *step* 2) is the most frequently regulated step in gene expression, for certain genes subsequent steps are more important for determining the overall level of expression. These processes are generally classified as **post-transcriptional regulation**. The mechanisms for regulating these steps are less well understood than are those for regulating transcription initiation, but some information comes from the study of model genes. Post-transcriptional processes that we will review here are transcript elongation (*step* 3) and termination (*step* 4), pre-mRNA splicing (*step* 5), and transcript degradation (*step* 8). We will not discuss nucleocytoplasmic transport (*step* 6). Nor will we discuss regulation of translation (*step* 7), although regulation at this step can also be important for the expression of certain genes.

Eukaryotes Regulate Termination of Transcription

The next step after initiation of transcription is **transcript elongation**, which involves proteins known as **elongation factors** such as TFIIF. Regulation of elongation appears to be critical for the expression of certain genes, such as some genes of the human immunodeficiency virus (HIV-1), the causative agent of acquired immunodeficiency syndrome (AIDS). HIV-1 is a retrovirus (RNA virus) that preferentially infects cells of the immune system. After

infection, the RNA viral genome is "reverse" transcribed into double-stranded DNA, which integrates into the host genome. A viral promoter that is located in the long terminal repeat of the viral genome then drives expression of the viral genes. Immediately downstream from the promoter—and within the 5′ untranslated region—is a regulatory element known as the **_trans_-activation response element (TAR)**. Unlike the regulatory elements that we have discussed previously, this element is active in *transcribed RNA*. The sequence of TAR contains an inverted repeat, and a stretch of nucleotides on one part of the TAR pairs with nucleotides on the other part to create a hairpin structure in this viral transcript (Fig. 5–19). Because the inverted repeat is imperfect, the hairpin contains a "bulge." Elongation of transcription cannot occur unless a virally encoded protein called **Tat** binds to this bulge in the TAR portion of the RNA transcript. In the absence of Tat, transcription initiates but elongation does not proceed past the TAR; the resulting truncated transcripts do not encode proteins. In the presence of Tat, pol II can read through the TAR and elongation proceeds normally, producing full-length RNA. It appears that the function of TAR is to recruit Tat to the promoter. Tat, in turn, associates with P-TEFb, a kinase that phosphorylates the CTD of pol II (p. 128) and stimulates transcription elongation.

Alternative Splicing Generates Diversity from Single Genes

Eukaryotic genes contain introns (p. 118) that must be removed from the primary transcript to create mature

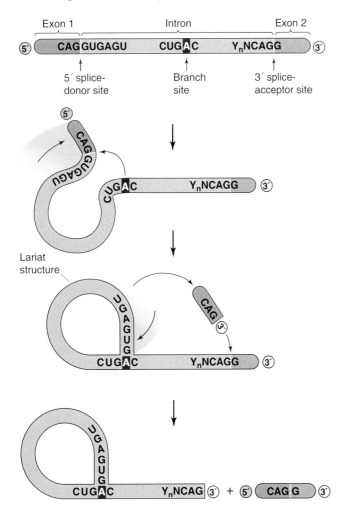

FIGURE 5–20. Mechanism of pre-mRNA splicing. This example illustrates how a 5′ splice-donor site at one end of Exon 1 can link to the 3′ splice-acceptor site at the end of Exon 2, thereby splicing out the intervening intron. The process can be divided into three steps: (1) cleavage of the pre-mRNA at the 5′ splice-donor site; (2) joining of the 5′ end of the intron to an adenosine residue that is located within the intron, forming a "lariat" structure; and (3) ligation of the 5′ and 3′ splice sites and release of the lariat intron. mRNA, messenger RNA; N, any nucleotide; Y_n, polypyrimidine tract.

mRNA; this process is called **pre-mRNA splicing**. Splicing involves the joining of two sites on the RNA transcript, the **5′ splice-donor site** and the **3′ splice-acceptor site**, and removal of the intervening intron (Fig. 5–20). The first step involves cleavage of the pre-mRNA at the 5′ splice-donor site. Second, joining of the 5′ end of the intron to an adenine residue located within the intron forms a "lariat" structure. Third, ligation of the 5′ and 3′ splice sites releases the lariat intron.

The location of the 5′ and 3′ splice sites is based, at least in part, on the sequences at the ends of the introns. The 5′ splice-donor site has the consensus sequence 5′-(C/A)AG ↓ GU(G/A)AGU-3′; the vertical arrow represents the boundary between the exon and the intron. The 3′ splice-acceptor site has the consensus sequence 5′-Y_nNCAG ↓ G-3′; Y_n represents a polypyrimidine tract (i.e., a long sequence of only C and U) and N represents any nucleotide. An intronic site located more than 17 nucleotides upstream from the 3′ acceptor site (5′-YNCUGAC-3′), called the branch point, is also present and contains the adenosine (red background in Fig. 5–20) that contributes to formation of the lariat structure. The splicing reaction is mediated by ribonucleoprotein particles (snRNPs, pronounced "snurps") that are composed of proteins and small nuclear RNA (snRNA). Together, the assembly of pre-mRNA and snRNPs forms a large complex called the **spliceosome**.

Many genes undergo **alternative splicing**, which refers to differential splicing of the same primary transcript to produce mature transcripts that contain different combinations of exons. If the coding region is affected, the resulting splicing variants will encode proteins with distinct primary structures, which may have different physiologic functions. Thus, alternative splicing is a mechanism for increasing the diversity of proteins that a single gene can produce. Figure 5–21 summarizes seven patterns of alternative splicing.

RETAINED INTRON. In some cases, the cell may choose whether to splice out a segment of RNA. For example, the γA isoform of rat γ-fibrinogen lacks the seventh intron, whereas the γB isoform retains the intron (see Fig. 5–21A). The retained intron encodes a unique 12–amino-acid C terminus in γB-fibrinogen.

ALTERNATIVE 3′ SPLICE SITES. In this case, the length of an intron is variable because the *downstream* boundary of the intron can be at either of two or more different 3′ splice acceptor sites (see Fig. 5–21B). For example, in rat fibronectin, a single donor site may be spliced to any of

TYPES OF ALTERNATIVE SPLICING	mRNA	EXAMPLES

A Retained intron — γ-Fibrinogen

B Alternative 3′ splice sites — Fibronectin

C Alternative 5′ splice sites — HMG–CoA reductase

D Cassette exons — α-Tropomyosin Troponin

E Mutually exclusive exons — Na/K/Cl cotransporter (NKCC) α-Tropomyosin

F Alternative 5′ ends — Myosin light chain α-Amylase

G Alternative 3′ ends — α-Tropomyosin Calcitonin/CGRP

FIGURE 5–21. Types of alternative splicing. CGRP, calcitonin gene-related peptide; HMG CoA, 3-hydroxy-3-methylglutaryl coenzyme A; Poly-A, polyadenylic acid.

three acceptor sites. The presence or absence of the amino acids encoded by the sequence between the different splice acceptor sites results in fibronectin isoforms with different cell adhesion properties.

ALTERNATIVE 5′ SPLICE SITES. Here also, the length of the intron is variable. However, in this case it is the *upstream* boundary of the intron that can be at either of two or more different 5′ splice-donor sites (see Fig. 5–21C). For example, cells can generate mRNA encoding 3-hydroxy-3-methylglutaryl-coenzyme A (HMG-CoA) reductase (p. 999) with different 5′ untranslated regions by splicing from multiple donor sites for the first intron to a single acceptor site.

CASSETTE EXONS. In some cases, the cell may choose either to splice in an exon or group of exons ("**cassette exons**") or to not splice them in (see Fig. 5–21D). An example is the α-tropomyosin gene, which contains 12 exons. All α-tropomyosin transcripts contain the invariant

exons 1, 4 to 6, 8, and 9. All muscle-like cells splice in exon 7, but hepatoma (i.e., liver tumor) cells do not splice in exon 7; they directly link exon 6 to exon 8.

MUTUALLY EXCLUSIVE EXONS. In yet other cases, the cell may splice in **mutually exclusive exons** (see Fig. 5–21E). One of the Na/K/Cl cotransporter genes (*NKCC2*) is an example. Isoforms containing distinct 96-bp exons are differentially expressed in the kidney cortex and medulla. Because the encoded amino-acid sequence is predicted to reside in the membrane, the isoforms may have different kinetic properties. The α-tropomyosin gene again is another example. Smooth muscle cells splice in exon 2 but not 3. Striated muscle cells and myoblasts splice in exon 3 but not 2. Fibroblasts and hepatoma cells do not splice in either of these two exons.

ALTERNATIVE 5′ ENDS. Cells may differentially splice the 5′ end of the gene (see Fig. 5–21F) and thereby select

FIGURE 5–22. The role of iron in regulating the stability of the mRNA for the transferrin receptor. The mRNA that encodes the transferrin receptor has a series of iron response elements (IREs) in its 3′ untranslated region. mRNA, messenger RNA.

different promoters. In the case of the myosin light chain (MLC) gene (p. 236), which consists of nine exons, one transcript is initiated from a promoter that is located upstream from exon 1, skips exons 2 and 3, and includes exons 4 to 9. The other transcript is initiated instead at a promoter located in the first *intron* and consists of exons 2, 3, and 5 to 9. Because the coding region is affected, the two transcripts encode proteins that differ at their N-terminal ends. These splice variants are found in different cells or different developmental stages. α-Amylase (p. 949) is another example. Transcription can begin from two different sites and produce mRNA that contains different first exons. Because the two mRNAs have different promoters, this alternative splicing permits differential regulation of gene expression in liver and salivary glands.

ALTERNATIVE 3′ ENDS. Finally, cells may differentially splice the transcript near the 3′ end of the gene (see Fig. 5–21G) and thereby alter the site of cleavage and poly-adenylation. Such splicing may also affect the coding region. Again, α-tropomyosin is an example. Striated muscle cells splice in exon 11, which contains one alternative 3′ untranslated region. Smooth muscle cells splice in exon 12 instead of 11. Another example is the calcitonin gene, which encodes both the hormone calcitonin (p. 1099) and calcitonin gene–related peptide α (CGRPα). Thyroid C cells produce one splice variant that includes exons 1 to 4 and encodes calcitonin. Sensory neurons, on the other hand, produce another splice variant that excludes exon 4 but includes exons 5 and 6. It encodes a different protein, CGRPα.

These examples illustrate that some splicing variants are expressed in only certain cell types but not in others. Clearly, control of alternative splicing must involve steps other than initiation of transcription because many splice variants have identical 5′ ends. In some genes, the control elements that are required for alternative splicing have been identified, largely on the basis of deletion mutations that result in aberrant splicing. These control elements can reside in either introns or exons and are lo-

cated within or near the splice sites. The proteins that interact with such elements remain largely unknown, although some RNA-binding proteins that may be involved in regulating splicing have been identified.

Regulatory Elements in the 3′ Untranslated Region Control RNA Stability

The stability of mRNA in cytoplasm varies widely for different transcripts. Transcripts that encode cytokines and immediate-early genes are frequently short lived, with half-lives measured in minutes. Other transcripts are much more stable, with half-lives that exceed 24 hours. Moreover, cells can modulate the stability of individual transcripts and thus use this mechanism to affect the overall level of expression of the gene.

Degradation of mRNA is mediated by enzymes called **ribonucleases**. These enzymes include 3′-5′ exonucleases, which digest RNA from the 3′ end, 5′-3′ exonucleases, which digest from the 5′ end, and endonucleases, which digest at internal sites. Structural features of typical mRNA that contribute to its stability in cytoplasm include the 5′ methyl cap, in which the presence of the 5′-5′ phosphodiester bond makes it resistant to digestion by 5′-3′ exonucleases. Similarly, the poly(A) tail at the 3′ end of the transcript often protects messages from degradation. Deadenylation (i.e., removal of the tail) is often a prerequisite for mRNA degradation. Accordingly, transcripts with long poly(A) tails may be more stable in cytoplasm than are transcripts with short poly(A) tails.

Regulatory elements that stabilize mRNA, as well as elements that accelerate its degradation, are frequently located in the 3′ untranslated region of the transcripts. A well-characterized example of a gene that is primarily regulated by transcript stability is the **transferrin receptor** (Fig. 5–22). The transferrin receptor is required for uptake of iron into most of the cells of the body (p. 44). During states of iron deprivation, transferrin receptor mRNA levels increase, whereas transcript levels decrease when iron is plentiful. Regulation of transferrin-receptor gene expression is primarily post-transcriptional; these alterations in the level of transferrin receptor mRNA are achieved through changes in the half-life of the message.

Regulation of transferrin receptor mRNA stability depends on elements that are located in the 3′ untranslated region called **iron-responsive elements (IREs)**. Similar to the TAR near the HIV promoter, an IRE is a stem-loop structure that is created by intramolecular hydrogen bond formation. The human transferrin receptor transcript contains five IREs in the 3′ untranslated region. The IRE binds a cellular protein called IRE-binding protein (IRE-BP), which stabilizes transferrin-receptor mRNA in the cytoplasm. When IRE-BP dissociates, the transcript is rapidly degraded. IRE-BP can also bind to iron, and the presence of iron decreases its affinity for the IRE. During states of iron deficiency, less iron binds to IRE-BP, and thus more IRE-BP binds to the IRE on the mRNA. The increased stability of the transcript allows the cell to produce more transferrin receptors. Conversely, when iron is plentiful and binds to IRE-BP, IRE-BP dissociates from the IRE, and the transferrin receptor transcript is rapidly degraded. This design prevents cellular iron overload.

REFERENCES

Books and Reviews

Conaway RC, Conaway JW: General initiation factors for RNA polymerase II. Annu Rev Biochem 63:161–190, 1993.
Karin M: Signal transduction from the cell surface to the nucleus through the phosphorylation of transcription factors. Curr Opin Cell Biol 6:415–424, 1994.
Maniatis T, Goodbourn S, Fischer JA: Regulation of inducible and tissue-specific gene expression. Science 236:1237–1245, 1987.
McKeown M: Alternative mRNA splicing. Annu Rev Cell Biol 8:133–155, 1992.
Pabo CO, Sauer RT: Transcription factors: Structural families and principles of DNA recognition. Annu Rev Biochem 61:1053–1095, 1992.
Ptashne M, Gann A: Transcriptional activation by recruitment. Nature 386:569–577, 1997.

Journal Articles

Casey JL, Koeller DM, Ramin VC, et al: Iron regulation of transferrin receptor mRNA levels requires iron-responsive elements and a rapid turnover determinant in the 3′ untranslated region of the mRNA. EMBO J 8:3693–3699, 1989.
Gillies SD, Morrison SL, Oi VT, Tonegawa S: A tissue-specific transcription enhancer element is located in the major intron of a rearranged immunoglobulin heavy chain gene. Cell 33:717–728, 1983.
Koleske AJ, Young RA: An RNA polymerase II holoenzyme responsive to activators. Nature 368:466–469, 1994.
Schindler C, Shuai K, Prezioso VR, Darnell JE Jr: Interferon-dependent tyrosine phosphorylation of a latent cytoplasmic transcription factor. Science 257:809–813, 1992.
van der Ploeg LHT, Flavell RA: DNA methylation in the human $\gamma\delta\beta$-globin locus in erythroid and nonerythroid tissues. Cell 19:947–958, 1980.

GLOSSARY

AP-1–activator protein-1, a Jun/Fos heterodimer that is a transcription factor
AR–androgen receptor
ATF-2–activating transcription factor-2, a transcription factor

bZIP–basic zipper family of transcription factors
C/EBPβ–CCAAT/enhancer-binding protein β, a transcription factor.
cAMP–cyclic adenosine monophosphate
CBP–CREB binding protein, 245 kDa
c-Fos–a transcription factor
c-Jun–a transcription factor
c-Myc–a transcription factor
CRE–cAMP response element, a DNA sequence
CREB–CRE-binding protein, 43 kDa
CREM–cAMP response element modifier. A transcriptional repressor
CTD–C-terminal domain of the largest subunit of pol II
DNA–deoxyribonucleic acid
EGF–epidermal growth factor
Egr-1–A transcription factor (activator) that binds via zinc fingers to the same DNA site as WT-1 (repressor)
ER–estrogen receptor
FGF–fibroblast growth factor
GAL4–A yeast transcription factor that activates certain genes when yeast grows in galactose-containing media.
GAS–interferon-γ activation site
GR–glucocorticoid receptor
GRB2–growth factor receptor–bound protein-2, a protein that contains SH2 domains that bind to phosphotyrosine residues on an activated receptor tyrosine kinase. GRB2 also contains SH3 domains that bind to proline-rich regions of SOS
GRE–glucocorticoid response element
hnRNA–heterogeneous nuclear RNA, primary transcript of DNA, unprocessed
hsp90–90-kDa heat shock protein, a molecular chaperone
IFN-α, β, γ–interferon-α, β, and γ
IGF-I–insulin-related growth factor-I
Inr–"initiator," a promoter sequence in both TATA-containing and TATA-less genes
ISRE–interferon-stimulated response element
JAK1, JAK2–Janus kinase, a protein tyrosine kinase
LCR–locus-control region, a site distant from the structural genes
MAP kinase–mitogen-activated protein kinase. Also known as ERK-1, ERK-2 for extracellular signal–regulated kinase
MEK–MAP kinase kinase (MAPKK). In the Ras cascade it is phosphorylated by Raf-1 (MAPKKK) and it phosphorylates MAP kinase (MAPK). It is also activated by JAK, part of the receptor-associated tyrosine kinase pathway
mRNA–messenger RNA
MR–mineralocorticoid receptor
N-Cor–a corepressor of transcription. Also known as SMRT
NF-1–nuclear factor-1, a transcription factor. See Table 5–1
NGF–nerve growth factor
NRE–negative regulatory element
Oct-1–ubiquitous DNA-binding protein that recognizes a DNA sequence called the octamer motif
P-box–sequence of six amino acids at the C terminus of a zinc finger
p62TCF–ternary complex factor, a transcription factor
PDGF–platelet-derived growth factor

PEPCK – phosphoenolpyruvate carboxykinase, the enzyme that catalyzes the rate-limiting step in gluconeogenesis

pol II – RNA polymerase II, the polymerase that transcribes DNA to mRNA

PR – progesterone receptor

P-TEFb – positive transcription elongation factor b. A kinase that phosphorylates the CTD of pol II

Raf-1 – a Ser/Thr kinase, also known as MAP kinase kinase kinase (MAPKKK)

RAR – retinoic acid receptor

Ras – a low-molecular-weight GTP-binding protein

RNA – ribonucleic acid

RNAPII – an alternative designation for RNA polymerase II (pol II)

RTK – receptor tyrosine kinase

RXR – retinoid X receptor

SH2 – Src homology domain 2. A domain on a protein that binds to phosphotyrosine-containing sites

SH3 – Src homology domain 3. A domain on a protein that binds to proline-rich sequences

SOS – son of "sevenless" protein. A guanine nucleotide exchange protein that is part of the Ras signalling cascade. It becomes active when it binds to GRB2. It promotes the conversion of inactive GDP-Ras to active GTP-Ras

SP1 – stimulating protein 1. A transcription factor

SRF – serum response factor, a transcription factor

STAT – signal transducer and activator of transcription

TAFs – TBP-associated factors

TAR – *trans*-activation response element, active only in the transcribed RNA.

Tat – A protein that is encoded by the HIV-1 virus and binds to TAR. Tat prevents premature termination of the RNA transcript

TATA box – common gene promoter sequence

TBP – TATA-binding protein

TFIIA – transcription factor IIA

TFIIB – transcription factor IIB

TFIID – transcription factor IID

TFIIE – transcription factor IIE

TFIIF – transcription factor IIF

TFIIH – transcription factor IIH

TFIIJ – transcription factor IIJ

THR – thyroid hormone receptor

tRNA – transfer RNA

Tyk – a protein tyrosine kinase related to JAK

UTR – untranslated region of mRNA

VDR – vitamin D receptor

WT-1 – Wilms-tumor protein. A transcriptional repressor that binds via zinc fingers to the same DNA site as Egr-1 (activator)

zinc finger – a zinc-containing protein domain that binds to DNA. Part of a transcription factor

CHAPTER 6

Electrophysiology of the Cell Membrane

Edward G. Moczydlowski

Physics is concerned with the fundamental nature of matter and energy, whereas the goal of medical physiology is to understand the function of biologic tissue. Despite their different perspectives, physics and physiology share common historical roots in the early investigations of charge and electricity. In the late 1700s, Luigi Galvani, a professor of anatomy in Bologna, Italy, used the leg muscles of a dissected frog to assay the presence of electrical charge stored in various ingenious devices that were the predecessors of modern capacitors and batteries. He observed that frog legs vigorously contracted when electrical stimulation was applied either directly to the leg muscle or to the nerves leading to the muscle (Fig. 6–1). Such early physiological experiments contributed to the development of electromagnetic theory in physics and electrophysiological theory in biology.

The phenomenon of "animal electricity" is central to the understanding of physiological processes. Throughout this book, we will describe many basic functions of tissues and organs in terms of electrical events mediated by cell membranes. Whereas electrical currents in a metallic wire are conducted by the flow of electrons, electrical currents across cell membranes are carried by the major inorganic ions of physiological fluids: Ca^{2+}, Na^+, K^+, Cl^-, and HCO_3^-. Many of the concepts and much of the terminology used in cellular electrophysiology are the same as those used with electrical circuits. At the molecular level, electrical current across cell membranes flows through three unique classes of integral membrane proteins (p. 56): ion channels, electrogenic ion transporters, and electrogenic ion pumps. The flow of ions through specific types of channels is the basis of the electrical events that determine animal behavior. The activity of such channels is the fundamental process behind electrical phenomena such as the nerve impulse, the heartbeat, and sensory perception. Channel proteins are also intimately involved in hormone secretion, ionic homeostasis, osmoregulation, and the regulation of muscle contractility.

This chapter begins with a review of the basic principles of electricity and introduces the essentials of electrophysiology. We also discuss the molecular biology of ion channels and provide an overview of channel structure and function.

A

B

IONIC BASIS OF MEMBRANE POTENTIALS

Principles of Electrostatics Explain Why Ions Such as Na⁺ Cannot Diffuse Across Phospholipid Membranes without Aqueous Pores Formed by Channel Proteins

The plasma membranes of most living cells are electrically polarized, as indicated by the presence of a transmembrane voltage—or a **membrane potential**—in the range of 0.1 V. In Chapter 3, we discussed how the energy stored in this miniature battery can drive a variety of transmembrane transport processes. Electrically excitable cells such as brain neurons and heart myocytes also use this energy for signalling purposes. The brief electrical impulses produced by such cells are called **action potentials**. To explain these electrophysiological phenomena, we begin with a basic review of electrical energy.

Atoms consist of negatively (−) and positively (+) charged elementary particles, such as electrons (e⁻) and protons (H⁺), as well as electrically neutral particles (neutrons). Charges of the same sign repel each other, and those of opposite sign attract. Charge is measured in units of **coulombs** (C). The **unitary charge** of one electron or proton is denoted by e_0 and is equal to 1.6022×10^{-19} C. Ions in solution have a charge valence (z) that is an integral number of elementary charges: for example, $z = +2$ for Ca^{2+}, $z = +1$ for K^+, and $z = -1$ for Cl^-. The charge of a single ion (q_0), measured in coulombs, is the product of its valence and the elementary charge:

Equation 6–1

$$q_0 = z\, e_0$$

In an aqueous solution or a bulk volume of matter, the number of positive and negative charges is always equal. Charge is also conserved in any chemical reaction.

The attractive electrostatic force between two ions that have valences of z_1 and z_2 can be obtained from Coulomb's law. This force (F) is proportional to the product of these valences and inversely proportional to the square of the distance (r) between the two. The force is also inversely proportional to a dimensionless term called the **dielectric constant** (ϵ):

Equation 6–2

$$F \propto \frac{z_1 \times z_2}{\epsilon\, r^2}$$

Because the dielectric constant of water is approximately 40-fold greater than that of the hydrocarbon interior of the cell membrane, the electrostatic force between ions is reduced by a factor of about 40 in water compared with membrane lipid.

If we were to move a Na⁺ ion from the extracellular to the intracellular fluid without the aid of any proteins, the Na⁺ would have to cross the membrane by "dissolving" in the lipids of the bilayer. However, the energy required to transfer an Na⁺ ion from water (high ϵ) to the interior of a phospholipid membrane (low ϵ) is approximately 36 kcal/mol. This value is 60-fold higher than molecular thermal energy at room temperature. Thus, the probability that an ion would dissolve in the bilayer (i.e., partition from an aqueous solution into the lipid interior of a cell membrane) is essentially zero. This analysis explains why inorganic ions cannot readily cross a phospholipid membrane without the aid of other molecules such as specialized transporters or channel proteins, which provide a favorable polar environment for the ion as it moves across the membrane (Fig. 6–2).

Cell Membrane Potentials Can Be Measured by Using Microelectrodes and Voltage-Sensitive Dyes

The voltage difference across the cell membrane, or the **membrane potential** (V_m), is the difference between the electrical potential in the cytoplasm (Ψ_i) and the electrical potential in the extracellular space (Ψ_o). Figure 6–3A shows how to measure V_m with an intracellular electrode. One gently inserts the sharp tip of a microelectrode into the cell and measures the transmembrane potential with respect to the electrical potential of the extracellular solution, which is defined as ground (i.e., $\Psi_o = 0$). If the cell membrane is not damaged by electrode impalement and the impaled membrane seals tightly around the glass, this technique provides an accurate measurement of V_m. Such a voltage measurement is called an **intracellular recording**.

FIGURE 6–1. Early electrophysiological experiments of Galvani. *A*, Electrical stimulation of a dissected frog with diverse sources of electricity. On the center of the table is a board with a dissected frog that has been prepared for an experiment (Fig. Ω). A hand with a charged metal rod (G) is about to touch the sacral nerves (D), contracting the limbs (C). A metal wire (F) penetrates the spinal cord; a second metal wire (K) grounds the first wire to the floor. On the left side of the table (Fig. 1) is a large "electrical machine" with a rotating disk (A), a conductor (C), and a hand holding a metal rod (B) that is about to be charged. On the extreme left of the room (Fig. 2), a dissected frog is suspended from an iron wire that penetrates the spinal cord (F); the wire is attached to the wall by a hook. A hand with a charged metal rod (G) is touching the wire, stimulating the sacral nerves (D) and causing the legs (C) to twitch. Outside the room, on the extreme right side (Fig. 3) is a frog in a glass jar (A). Emerging from the glass jar is an iron wire (B) that is attached at one end to a hook on the frog and ends in a hook (C) in the air. A silk loop (D) near this hook connects to a long conductor (F) that runs near the ceiling to a hook in the wall at the extreme left of the main room. At the far right/front of the table in the main room (Fig. 4) is a dissected frog with one conductor connected to a nerve (C) and another connected to a muscle (D). Just behind this frog (Fig. 5) is a "Leiden Jar" (A) containing small lead shot used by hunters. A hand with a charged metal rod (C) is about to touch a conductor (B) emerging from the jar. To the left of the Leiden Jar (Fig. 6) is an inverted jar (A) with lead shot (C). This jar sits on top of a similar jar (B) containing a suspended, dissected frog and is connected by a conductor to the lead shot in the upper jar. The legs of the frog are grounded to lead shot near the bottom of the jar. *B*, Electrical stimulation of the leg muscles of a dissected frog by "natural electricity" (i.e., lightning). In one experiment (Fig. 7), an iron wire (A) runs from near the roof, through several insulating glass tubes (B), to a flask (C) that contains a freshly dissected frog. A second wire (D) grounds the frog's legs to the water in the well. In a second experiment (Fig. 8), a non-insulated wire extends from an iron hook fastened to the wall and to the spinal cord of a frog (E), which is on a table coated with oil. (From Galvani L: De viribus electricitatis in motu musculari commentarius Aloysii Galvani, Bononiae. New Haven, CT, Yale University, Harvey Cushing/John Hay Whitney Medical Library, 1791.)

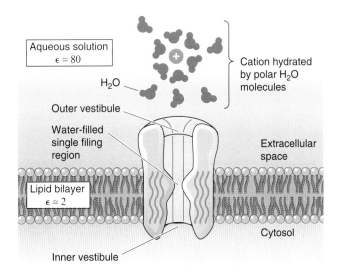

FIGURE 6–2. Formation of an aqueous pore by an ion channel. The dielectric constant of water ($\epsilon = 80$) is about 40-fold higher than the dielectric constant of the lipid bilayer ($\epsilon = 2$).

For an amphibian or mammalian skeletal muscle cell, the resting V_m is typically about -90 mV, which is an indication of separation of charge across the membrane. The interior of the resting cell is about 90 mV more negative than the exterior. There is a simple relationship between the electrical potential difference across a membrane and another parameter, namely, the **electrical field** (E) across that membrane:

Equation 6–3

$$E = \frac{V_m}{d}$$

V_m = Electrical potential difference across membrane

d = Distance across membrane

Accordingly, for a V_m of -0.1 V and a membrane thickness of $d = 4$ nm (i.e., 40×10^{-8} cm), the magnitude of the electrical field is about 250,000 V/cm. Thus, despite the small transmembrane *voltage*, cell membranes actually sustain a very large electrical *field*. Later, we discuss how this electrical field influences the activity of a particular class of membrane signalling proteins called voltage-sensitive ion channels (p. 182).

Skeletal muscle cells, cardiac cells, and neurons typically have resting membrane potentials of approximately -60 to -90 mV, smooth-muscle cells have membrane

FIGURE 6–3. Recording of membrane potential. (Panels *C* and *D*: data modified from Grinvald A: Real-time optical mapping of neuronal activity: From single growth cones to the intact mammalian brain. Annu Rev Neurosci 8:26–305, 1985. © by Annual Reviews www.annualreviews.org)

potentials in the range of -55 mV, and the V_m of the human erythrocyte is only about -9 mV; however, certain bacteria and plant cells have transmembrane voltages as large as -200 mV. For very small cells such as erythrocytes, small intracellular organelles such as mitochondria, and fine processes such as the synaptic endings of neurons, V_m cannot be directly measured with a microelectrode. Instead, spectroscopic techniques allow the membrane potentials of such inaccessible membranes to be measured indirectly (see Fig. 6–3B). This technique involves labeling the cell or membrane with an appropriate organic dye molecule and monitoring the absorption or fluorescence of the dye. The optical signal of the dye molecule can be independently calibrated as a function of V_m. Whether V_m is measured directly by a microelectrode or indirectly by a spectroscopic technique, virtually all biologic membranes have a nonzero membrane potential. This transmembrane voltage is an important determinant of physiological transport processes that involve the movement of charge.

Measurements of V_m have shown that many types of cells are electrically excitable. Examples of excitable cells are neurons, muscle fibers, heart cells, and secretory cells of the pancreas. In such cells, V_m exhibits characteristic time-dependent changes in response to electrical or chemical stimulation. When the cell body, or "soma," of a neuron is electrically stimulated, the electrical and optical methods for measuring V_m detect an almost identical response at the cell body (see Fig. 6–3C). The optical method provides the additional insight that the V_m changes are similar but delayed in the more distant neuronal processes that are inaccessible to a microelectrode (see Fig. 6–3D). When the cell is not undergoing such active responses, V_m usually remains at a steady value that is called the **resting potential**. In the next section, we discuss the origin of the membrane potential and lay the groundwork for understanding its active responses.

The Membrane Potential Is Generated By Ion Gradients, Not Directly by Ion Pumps

In Chapter 3, we introduced the concept that some integral membrane proteins are electrogenic transporters in that they generate an electrical current that sets up an electrical potential across the membrane. One class of electrogenic transporters includes the adenosine triphosphate (ATP)-dependent *ion pumps*. These proteins use the energy of ATP hydrolysis to produce and maintain concentration gradients of ions across cell membranes. In animal cells, the Na-K pump and Ca^{2+} pump are responsible for maintaining normal gradients of Na^+, K^+, and Ca^{2+}. The reactions catalyzed by these ion transport enzymes are electrogenic because they lead to separation of charge across the membrane. For example, enzymatic turnover of the Na-K pump (p. 61) results in the translocation of three Na^+ ions out of the cell and two K^+ ions into the cell, with a net movement of one positive charge out of the cell. In addition to electrogenic pumps, cells may express *secondary active transporters* that are electrogenic, such as the Na/glucose cotransporter (p. 66).

It may seem that the inside negative V_m originates from

the continuous pumping of positive charges out of the cell by the electrogenic Na-K pump. The resting potential of large cells—whose surface-to-volume ratio is so large that ion gradients run down slowly—is maintained for a long time even when metabolic poisons block ATP-dependent energy metabolism. This finding implies that an ATP-dependent pump is not the immediate energy source underlying the membrane potential. Indeed, the squid giant axon normally has a resting potential of -60 mV. When the Na-K pump in the giant axon membrane is specifically inhibited with a cardiac glycoside (p. 63), the immediate positive shift in V_m is only 1.4 mV. Thus, in most cases the direct contribution of the Na-K pump to the resting V_m is very small.

In contrast, many experiments have shown that cell membrane potentials depend on ionic **concentration gradients**. In a classic experiment, Paul Horowicz and Alan Hodgkin measured the V_m of a frog muscle fiber with an intracellular microelectrode. The muscle fiber was bathed in a modified physiologic solution in which SO_4^{2-} replaced Cl^-, a manipulation that eliminates the contribution of anions to V_m. In the presence of normal extracellular concentrations of K^+ for amphibians ($[K^+]_o = 2.5$ mM) and Na^+ ($[Na^+]_o = 120$ mM), the frog muscle fiber has a resting V_m of approximately -94 mV. As $[K^+]_o$ is increased above 2.5 mM by substituting K^+ for Na^+, V_m shifts in the positive direction. As $[K^+]_o$ is decreased below 2.5 mM, V_m becomes more negative (Fig. 6–4). For $[K^+]_o$ values greater than 10 mM, the V_m measured in Figure 6–4 is approximately a linear function of the *logarithm* of $[K^+]_o$. Numerous experiments of this kind have demonstrated that the *immediate* energy source of the membrane potential is not the active pumping of ions, but rather the potential energy stored in the ion concentration gradients themselves. Of course, it is the ion pumps—and the secondary active transporters that derive their energy from these pumps—that are responsible for generating and maintaining these ion gradients.

One way to investigate the role of ion gradients in determining V_m is to study this phenomenon in an in vitro (cell-free) system. Many investigators have used an artificial model of a cell membrane called a **planar lipid bilayer**. This system consists of a partition with a hole approximately 200 μm in diameter that separates two chambers filled with aqueous solutions (Fig. 6–5). It is possible to paint a planar lipid bilayer having a thickness of only approximately 4 nm across the hole, thereby sealing the partition. By incorporating membrane proteins and other molecules into planar bilayers, one can study the essential characteristics of their function in isolation from the complex metabolism of living cells. Transmembrane voltage can be measured across a planar bilayer with a voltmeter that is connected to a pair of Ag/AgCl electrodes that are in electrical contact with the solution on each side of the membrane via salt bridges. This experimental arrangement is much like an intracellular voltage recording, except that both sides of the membrane are completely accessible to manipulation.

The ionic composition of the two chambers on opposite sides of the bilayer can be adjusted to simulate cellular concentration gradients. Suppose that we put 4 mM KCl on the left side of the bilayer and 155 mM KCl on the right side to mimic, respectively, the external and

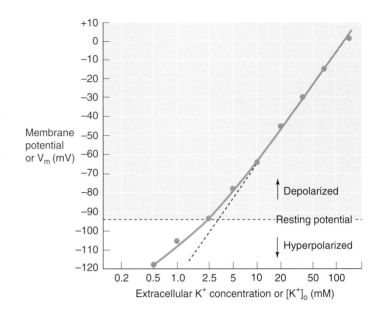

FIGURE 6–4. Dependence of resting potential on extracellular K^+ concentration. The resting V_m of a frog muscle fiber (measured with a microelectrode) depolarizes with increasing $[K^+]_o$. The slope of the linear part of the curve is 58 mV for a 10-fold increase in $[K^+]_o$. (Data from Hodgkin AL, Horowicz P: The influence of potassium and chloride ions on the membrane potential of single muscle fibers. J Physiol (Lond) 148:127–160, 1959.)

FIGURE 6–5. Diffusion potential across a planar lipid bilayer containing a K^+-selective channel.

internal concentrations of K^+ for a mammalian muscle cell. To eliminate the osmotic flow of water between the two compartments (p. 73), we add a sufficient amount of a nonelectrolyte (e.g., mannitol) to the side with 4 mM KCl. If a bilayer were *not* separating the two solutions, the unequal concentrations of KCl would lead to diffusion of the salt in the direction of high to low [KCl]. However, by sealing the hole in the partition with a pure lipid bilayer having no permeability to K^+ or Cl^-, we ensure that the system does not have any separation of charge, and therefore the measured transmembrane voltage is 0 mV.

We can make the membrane selectively permeable to K^+ by introducing purified K^+ channels or K^+ ionophores into the membrane. Assuming that the K^+ channels are in an open state and are impermeable to Cl^-, the right ("internal") compartment would become electrically negative with respect to the left ("external") compartment. The reason that the right compartment becomes negative is that K^+ is more likely to leave the right compartment (155 mM K^+) than the left compartment (4 mM K^+). However, as the right compartment becomes more and more negative, the developing negative voltage opposes further efflux of K^+ from the right compartment. Eventually, the voltage difference across the membrane becomes so negative that no further net movement of K^+ occurs. At this point, the system is in **equilibrium**, and the transmembrane voltage reaches a value of 92.4 mV, right side negative. This value is the one predicted by the Nernst equation (p. 55) for a transmembrane K^+ gradient of 4 mM versus 155 mM at 20°C. In the process of generating the transmembrane voltage, a separation of charge has occurred in such a way that the excess *positive* charge on the left side (low $[K^+]$) is balancing the same excess *negative* charge on the right side (high $[K^+]$). Thus, the voltage difference arises from the separation of K^+ ions from their counterions (in this case Cl^-) across the bilayer membrane. The final observed voltage (−92.4 mV) remains stable in this experiment, thus confirming that equilibrium has indeed been reached.

Nernst Potentials of Physiological Ions Across Cell Membranes Can Be as Negative as −100 mV in the Case of K⁺ or More Positive Than +100 mV in the Case of Ca²⁺

The model system of a planar bilayer (impermeable membrane), unequal salt solutions (ionic gradient), and an ion-selective channel (conductance pathway) contains the minimal components essential for generating a membrane potential. The hydrophobic membrane bilayer is a formidable barrier to inorganic ions and is also a poor conductor of electricity. Poor conductors are said to have a high **resistance** to electrical current, in this case, ionic current. On the other hand, ion channels act as molecular conductors of ions. They introduce a **conductance pathway** into the membrane and lower its resistance.

The membrane potential recorded in the planar bilayer experiment (see Fig. 6–5) is close to the resting V_m of a skeletal muscle cell that has a similar $[K^+]$ gradient. What determines the value of V_m? In the bilayer experiment, the V_m reflects the diffusion of K^+ down its concentration gradient. Membrane potentials that arise by this mechanism are called **diffusion potentials**. At equilibrium, the diffusion potential of an ion is the same as its equilibrium potential (E_X), as described by the **Nernst equation** already introduced as Equation 3–8.

Equation 6–4

$$E_X = -\frac{RT}{z_X F} \, ln \, \frac{[X]_i}{[X]_o}$$

The Nernst equation predicts the equilibrium membrane potential for any concentration gradient of a particular ion across a membrane. E_X is often simply referred to as the **Nernst potential**. The Nernst potentials for K^+, Na^+, Ca^{2+}, and Cl^-, respectively, are written as E_K, E_{Na}, E_{Ca}, and E_{Cl}.

The linear portion of the plot of V_m versus the logarithm of $[K^+]_o$ in Figure 6–4 has a **slope** that is approximately 58.1 mV for a 10-fold change in $[K^+]$. This figure is the same value predicted by the Nernst equation. Indeed, if we insert the appropriate values for R and F into Equation 6–4, select a temperature of 20°C, and convert the logarithm base e (ln) to the logarithm base 10 (log_{10}), we obtain a coefficient of 58.1, and the Nernst equation becomes

Equation 6–5

$$E_K = (-58.1 \text{ mV}) log_{10} \frac{[K^+]_i}{[K^+]_o}$$

For a negative ion such as Cl^-, where $z = -1$, the sign in front of the slope is positive:

Equation 6–6

$$E_{Cl} = (+58.1 \text{ mV}) log_{10} \frac{[Cl^-]_i}{[Cl^-]_o}$$

For Ca^{2+} ($z = +2$), the slope is half of −58.1 mV, or approximately −30 mV. Note that a Nernst slope of 58.1 mV is the value for a univalent ion at 20°C. For mammalian cells at 37°C, this value is 61.5 mV.

TABLE 6–1

ION CONCENTRATION GRADIENTS IN MAMMALIAN CELLS

ION	OUT (mM)	IN (mM)	OUT/IN	E_{Nernst}* (mV)
Skeletal Muscle				
Na^+	145	12	12	+67
K^+	4.5	155	0.026	−95
Ca^{2+}	1.0	10^{-4}	10,000	+123
Cl^-	116	4.2	29	−89
HCO_3^-	24	12	2	−19
Most Other Cells				
Na^+	145	15	9.67	+61
K^+	4.5	120	0.038	−88
Ca^{2+}	1.0	10^{-4}	10,000	+123
Cl^-	116	20	5.8	−47
HCO_3^-	24	15	1.6	−13

*At 37°C.

At $[K^+]_o$ values above approximately 10 mM, the magnitude of V_m and the slope of the plot in Figure 6–4 are essentially what we would predict from the Nernst equation for K^+ (Equation 6–5), which suggests that the resting V_m of the muscle cell is almost equal to the K^+ diffusion potential. When V_m follows the Nernst equation for K^+, the membrane is said to behave like a potassium electrode because ion-specific electrodes monitor ion concentrations according to the Nernst equation.

Table 6–1 lists the expected Nernst potentials for K^+, Na^+, Ca^{2+}, Cl^-, and HCO_3^- as calculated from the known concentration gradients of these physiologically important inorganic ions for mammalian skeletal muscle and a typical nonmuscle cell. For a mammalian muscle cell with a V_m of −80 mV, E_K is about 15 mV more negative than V_m. E_{Cl} is also negative, 9 mV more negative than V_m in muscle cells but slightly more positive than the V_m of −60 mV in most other cells. On the other hand, for the two positive ions with large inward gradients, the equilibrium potentials are much more positive. In muscle, E_{Na} and E_{Ca} are approximately +67 and +123 mV, respectively.

What determines whether the cell membrane potential follows the Nernst equation for K^+ or Cl^- rather than that for Na^+ or Ca^{2+}? As we shall see in the next two sections, the membrane potential is determined by the relative permeabilities of the various ions.

Currents Carried by Ions Across Membranes Depend on the Concentration of Ions on Both Sides of the Membrane, Membrane Potential, and the Permeability of the Membrane to Each Ion

Years before ion channel proteins were discovered, physiologists devised a simple but powerful way to predict the

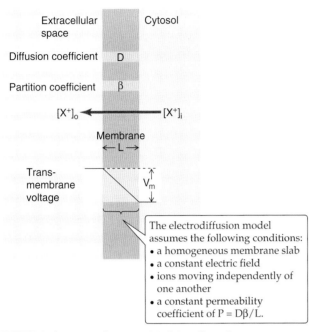

Extracellular space   Cytosol

Diffusion coefficient   D

Partition coefficient   β

$[X^+]_o \leftarrow [X^+]_i$

Membrane
$\leftarrow L \rightarrow$

Trans-membrane voltage V_m

The electrodiffusion model assumes the following conditions:
• a homogeneous membrane slab
• a constant electric field
• ions moving independently of one another
• a constant permeability coefficient of P = Dβ/L.

FIGURE 6–6. Electrodiffusion model of the cell membrane.

membrane potential, even if several different kinds of permeable ions are present at the same time. The first step, which we discuss in this section, is to compute an ionic current—that is, the movement of a single ion species through the membrane. The second step, which we describe in the following section, is to obtain V_m by summating the currents carried by each species of ion present, assuming that each species moves independently of the others.

The process of ion permeation through the membrane is called **electrodiffusion** because both electrical and concentration gradients are responsible for the ionic current. To a first approximation, the permeation of ions through most channel proteins behaves as though the flow of these ions follows a model based on the Nernst-Planck electrodiffusion theory, which was first applied to the diffusion of ions in simple solutions. This theory leads to an important equation in medical physiology called the constant-field equation, which predicts how V_m will respond to changes in ion concentration gradients or membrane permeability. Before introducing this equation, we first consider some important underlying concepts and assumptions.

Without knowing the molecular basis for ion movement through the membrane, we can treat the membrane as a "black box" characterized by a few fundamental parameters (Fig. 6–6). We must assume that the rate of ion movement through the membrane depends on (1) the external and internal concentrations of the ion X ($[X]_o$ and $[X]_i$, respectively), (2) the transmembrane voltage (V_m), and (3) a permeability coefficient for the ion X (P_X). In addition, we make four major assumptions about how the ion X behaves in the membrane:

The membrane is a homogeneous medium with a thickness L.

The voltage difference varies linearly with distance across the membrane (see Fig. 6–6). This assumption is equivalent to stating that the *electrical field*—that is, the change in voltage with distance—is constant throughout the thickness of the membrane. This requirement is therefore called the **constant-field assumption**.

The movement of an ion through the membrane is independent of the movement of any other ions. This assumption is called the **independence principle**.

The permeability coefficient P_X is a constant (i.e., it does not vary with the chemical or electrical driving forces). P_X (units: cm/s) is defined as $P_X = D_X\beta/L$. D_X is the diffusion coefficient for the ion in the membrane, β is the membrane/water partition coefficient for the ion, and L is the thickness of the membrane. Thus, P_X describes the ability of an ion to dissolve in the membrane (as described by β) and diffuse from one side to the other (as described by D_X) over the distance L.

With these assumptions, we can calculate the current carried by a single ion X (I_X) through the membrane by using the basic physical laws that govern (1) the movement of molecules in solution (Fick's law of diffusion; see Equation 3–11), (2) the movement of charged particles in an **electrical** field (electrophoresis), and (3) the direct proportionality of current to voltage (Ohm's law). The result is the **Goldman-Hodgkin-Katz (GHK)** *current* **equation**, named after the pioneering electrophysiologists who applied the constant-field assumption to Nernst-Planck electrodiffusion:

Equation 6–7

$$I_X = \frac{z^2 F^2 V_m P_X}{RT}\left(\frac{[X]_i - [X]_o e^{(-zFV_m/RT)}}{1 - e^{(-zFV_m/RT)}}\right)$$

I_X, or the rate of ions moving through the membrane, has the same units as electrical current: amperes (coulombs per second). Thus, the GHK current equation relates the current of ion X through the membrane to the internal and external concentrations of X, the transmembrane voltage, and the permeability of the membrane to X. The GHK equation thus allows us to predict how the current carried by X depends on V_m. This **current-voltage (I-V) relationship** is important for understanding how ionic currents flow into and out of cells.

Figure 6–7A shows how the K^+ current (I_K) depends on V_m, as predicted by Equation 6–7 for the normal internal (155 mM) and external (4.5 mM) concentrations of K^+. By convention, a current of ions flowing into the cell (**inward current**) is defined in electrophysiology as a negative-going current, and a current flowing out of the cell (**outward current**) is defined as a positive current. (As in physics, the direction of current is always the direction of movement of positive charge. This convention means that an inward flow of Cl^- is an outward current.) For the case of 155 mM K^+ inside the cell and 4.5 mM K^+ outside the cell, an inward current is predicted at voltages that are more negative than −95 mV and an outward current is predicted at voltages that are more positive than −95 mV (see Fig. 6–7A). The value of −95

A POTASSIUM CURRENT

B SODIUM CURRENT

FIGURE 6–7. Current–voltage relationships predicted by the GHK current equation. *A*, The *solid curve* is the K⁺ current predicted from the GHK equation (Equation 6–7)—assuming that the membrane is perfectly selective for K⁺—for a [K⁺]ᵢ of 155 mM and a [K⁺]ₒ of 4.5 mM. The *dashed line* represents the current that can be expected if both [K⁺]ᵢ and [K⁺]ₒ were 155 mM (Ohm's law). *B*, The *solid curve* is the Na⁺ current predicted from the GHK equation—assuming that the membrane is perfectly selective for Na⁺—for a [Na⁺]ᵢ of 12 mM and a [Na⁺]ₒ of 145 mM. The *dashed line* represents the current that can be expected if both [Na⁺]ᵢ and [Na⁺]ₒ were 145 mM.

mV is called the **reversal potential** (V_{rev}), because it is precisely at this voltage that the direction of current reverses (i.e., the net current equals zero). If we set I_K equal to zero in Equation 6–7 and solve for V_{rev}, we find that the GHK current equation reduces to the Nernst equation for K⁺ (see Equation 6–5). Thus, the GHK current equation for an ion X predicts a reversal potential (V_{rev}) equal to the Nernst potential (E_X) for that ion; that is, the current is zero when the ion is in electrochemical equilibrium. At V_m values more negative than V_{rev}, the net driving force on a cation is inward; at voltages that are more positive than V_{rev}, the net driving force is outward.

Figure 6–7B shows the analogous *I-V* relationship predicted by Equation 6–7 for physiological concentrations of Na⁺. In this case, the Na⁺ current (I_{Na}) is inward at V_m values more negative than V_{rev} (+67 mV) and outward at voltages that are more positive than this reversal potential. Here again, V_{rev} is the same as the Nernst potential, in this case, E_{Na}.

Membrane Potential Depends on Ionic Concentration Gradients and Permeabilities

In the previous section, we discuss how to use the GHK current equation to predict the current carried by any *single* ion, such as K⁺ or Na⁺. If the membrane is permeable to the monovalent ions K⁺, Na⁺, and Cl⁻—and only to these ions—the **total ionic current** carried by these ions across the membrane is the sum of the individual ionic currents:

Equation 6–8

$$I_{total} = I_K + I_{Na} + I_{Cl}$$

The individual ionic currents given by Equation 6–7 can be substituted into the right-hand side of Equation 6–8. Note that for the sake of simplicity, we have not considered currents carried by electrogenic pumps or other ion transporters; we could have added extra "current" terms for such electrogenic transporters. At the resting membrane potential (i.e., V_m is equal to V_{rev}), the sum of all ion currents is zero (i.e., $I_{total} = 0$). When we set I_{total} to zero in the expanded Equation 6–8 and solve for V_{rev}, we get an expression known as the **GHK *voltage* equation** or the **constant-field equation**:

Equation 6–9

$$V_{rev} = -\frac{RT}{F} \ln\left(\frac{P_K[K^+]_i + P_{Na}[Na^+]_i + P_{Cl}[Cl^-]_o}{P_K[K^+]_o + P_{Na}[Na^+]_o + P_{Cl}[Cl^-]_i}\right)$$

Because we derived Equation 6–9 for the case of $I_{total} = 0$, it is only valid when zero net current is flowing across the membrane. This zero net current flow is the steady-state condition that exists for the cellular *resting* potential, that is, when V_m equals V_{rev}. The logarithmic term of Equation 6–9 indicates that the resting V_m depends on the concentration gradients and the permeabilities of the various ions. However, the resting V_m depends mainly on the concentrations of the most permeant ion.

The principles underlying Equation 6–9 show why the plot of V_m versus [K⁺]ₒ in Figure 6–4—which summarizes data obtained from a frog muscle cell—bends away from the idealized Nernst slope at very low values of [K⁺]ₒ. Imagine that we expose a mammalian muscle cell to a range of [K⁺]ₒ values, always substituting extracellular K⁺ for Na⁺—or vice versa—so that the sum of [K⁺]ₒ

FIGURE 6–8. Dependence of the resting membrane potential on $[K^+]_o$ and on the P_{Na}/P_K ratio, α. The *blue line* describes an instance in which there is no Na^+ permeability (i.e., $P_{Na}/P_K = 0$). The three *orange curves* describe the V_m predicted by Equation 6–10 for α values greater than zero. The deviation of these orange curves from linearity is greater at low values of $[K^+]_o$, where the $[K^+]_o$ is relatively larger.

and $[Na^+]_o$ is kept fixed at its physiologic value of 4.5 + 145 = 149.5 mM. To simplify matters, we assume that the membrane permeability to Cl^- is very small (i.e., $P_{Cl} \cong 0$). We can also rearrange Equation 6–9 by dividing the numerator and denominator by P_K and representing the ratio P_{Na}/P_K as α. At 37°C, this simplified equation becomes

Equation 6–10

$$V_{rev} = (61.5 \text{ mV}) \times log_{10} \left(\frac{[K^+]_o + \alpha[Na^+]_o}{[K^+]_i + \alpha[Na^+]_i} \right)$$

Figure 6–8 shows that when α is zero—that is, when the membrane has no permeability to Na^+—Equation 6–10 reduces to the Nernst equation for K^+ (see Equation 6–4), and the plot of V_m versus the logarithm of $[K^+]_o$ is linear. If we choose an α of 0.01, however, the plot bends away from the ideal at low $[K^+]_o$ values. This bend reflects the introduction of a slight permeability to Na^+. As we increase this P_{Na} further by increasing α to 0.03 and 0.1, the curvature becomes even more pronounced. Thus, as predicted by Equation 6–10, increasing the permeability of Na^+ relative to K^+ tends to shift V_m in a positive direction, toward E_{Na}. In some skeletal muscle cells, an α of 0.01 best explains the experimental data.

The constant-field equation (see Equation 6–9), as well as simplified relationships derived from it (e.g., Equation 6–10), shows that steady-state V_m depends on the concentrations of all permeant ions, weighted according to their relative permeabilities. Another very useful application of the constant-field equation is for determining the ionic selectivity of channels. If the *I-V* relationship of a particular channel is determined in the presence of known gradients of two different ions, one can solve Equation 6–10 to obtain the permeability ratio, α, of the two ions from the measured value of the reversal potential, V_{rev}.

In general, the resting potential of most vertebrate cells is dominated by high permeability to K^+, which accounts for the observation that the resting V_m is typically close to E_K. The resting permeability to Na^+ and Ca^{2+} is normally very low. For example, the value of P_{Na}/P_K at rest is usually 0.01 to 0.1, and P_{Ca}/P_K at rest is essentially zero. Skeletal muscle cells, cardiac cells, and neurons typically have resting membrane potentials ranging from −60 to −90 mV. As discussed in Chapter 7, excitable cells generate action potentials by transiently increasing Na^+ or Ca^{2+} permeability and thus driving V_m in a positive direction toward E_{Na} or E_{Ca}. A few cells, such as vertebrate skeletal muscle fibers, have high permeability to Cl^-, which therefore contributes to the resting V_m. This high permeability also explains why the Cl^- equilibrium potential in skeletal muscle is essentially equivalent to the resting potential (see Table 6–1).

ELECTRICAL MODEL OF A CELL MEMBRANE

The Cell Membrane Model Includes Various Ionic Conductances and Electromotive Forces in Parallel with a Capacitor

The current carried by a particular ion varies with membrane voltage, as described by the *I-V* relationship for that ion (e.g., Fig. 6–7). This observation suggests that the contribution of each ion to the electrical properties of the cell membrane may be represented by elements of an electrical circuit. The various ionic gradients across the membrane provide a form of stored electrical energy, much like that of a battery. In physics, the voltage source of a battery is known as an **emf** (electromotive force). The equilibrium potential of a given ion can be considered an emf for that ion. Each of these batteries produces its own ionic **current** across the membrane, and the sum of these individual ionic currents is the total ionic current (see Equation 6–8). According to **Ohm's law**, the emf or voltage (V) and current (I) are related to each other by the **resistance** (R) or by its reciprocal, **conductance** (G):

Equation 6–11

$$\begin{aligned} V &= I\,R \quad \text{Ohm's law} \\ &= I/G \end{aligned}$$

Thus, the slopes of the broken lines in Figure 6–7 represent conductances. In a membrane, we can represent each ionic permeability pathway with an electrical conductance. Ions with high permeability or conductance move through a low-resistance pathway; ions with low permeability move through a high-resistance pathway. For cell membranes, V_m is measured in millivolts, membrane current (I_m) is given in amps per square centimeter of membrane area, and membrane resistance (R_m) has the units of ohms × square centimeter. Membrane conductance (G_m), the reciprocal of membrane resistance, is thus measured in units of ohms^{-1} per square centimeter, which is equivalent to siemens per square centimeter.

Currents of Na^+, K^+, Ca^{2+}, and Cl^- generally flow across the cell membrane through distinct pathways. At the molecular level, these pathways correspond to specific

A   MODEL OF A CELL MEMBRANE

Extracellular space

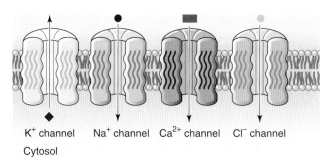

K+ channel   Na+ channel   Ca²+ channel   Cl⁻ channel

Cytosol

B   EQUIVALENT CIRCUIT MODEL

C   PARALLEL–PLATE CAPACITOR   LIPID MEMBRANE

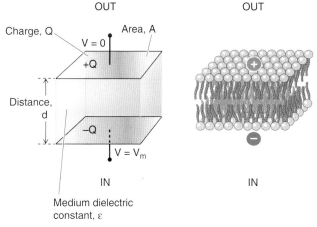

FIGURE 6–9. Electrical properties of model cell membranes. *A*, Four different ion channels are arranged in parallel in the cell membrane. *B*, The model represents each channel in *A* with a variable resistor. The model represents the Nernst potential for each ion as a battery. Notice that the four parallel current paths correspond to the four parallel channels in *A*. Also shown is the membrane capacitance, which is parallel with each of the channels. *C*, On the left is an idealized capacitor, which is formed by two parallel plates, each with an area, A, and separated by a distance, d. On the right is a capacitor that is formed by a piece of lipid membrane. The two *plates* are, in fact, the electrolyte solutions on either side of the membrane.

types of ion channel proteins (Fig. 6–9A). It is helpful to model the electrical behavior of cell membranes by a circuit diagram (Fig. 6–9B). The electrical current carried by each ion flows through a separate parallel branch of the circuit that is under the control of a **variable resistor**

and an emf. For instance, the variable resistor for K^+ represents the conductance provided by K^+ channels in the membrane (G_K). The emf for K^+ corresponds to E_K. Similar parallel branches of the circuit in Figure 6–9B represent the other physiologically important ions. Each ion provides a component of the total conductance of the membrane, so $G_K + G_{Na} + G_{Ca} + G_{Cl}$ sum to G_m.

The GHK voltage equation (see Equation 6–9) predicts steady-state V_m, provided that the underlying assumptions are valid. It turns out that a more general equation that does not depend on these assumptions also predicts V_m:

Equation 6–12

$$V_m = \frac{G_K}{G_m} E_K + \frac{G_{Na}}{G_m} E_{Na} + \frac{G_{Ca}}{G_m} E_{Ca} + \frac{G_{Cl}}{G_m} E_{Cl} \ldots$$

Thus, V_m is the sum of equilibrium potentials (E_X), each weighted by the ion's fractional conductance (e.g., G_X/G_m).

One more parallel element, a **capacitor**, is needed to complete our model of the cell membrane as an electrical circuit. A capacitor is a device that is capable of storing separated charge. Because the lipid bilayer can maintain a separation of charge (i.e., a voltage) across its approximately 4-nm width, it effectively functions as a capacitor. In physics, a capacitor that is formed by two parallel plates separated by a distance d can be represented by the diagram in Figure 6–9C. When the capacitor is charged, one of the plates bears a charge of $+Q$ and the other plate has a charge of $-Q$. Charge is measured in units of coulombs. Such a capacitor maintains a potential difference (V) between the plates. **Capacitance** (C) is the magnitude of the charge stored per unit potential difference:

Equation 6–13

$$C = \frac{Q}{V}$$

Capacitance is measured in units of farads (F). For the particular geometry of the parallel-plate capacitor in Figure 6–9C, capacitance is directly proportional to the surface area (A) of one side of a plate, to the dielectric constant of the medium between the two plates (ϵ), and to the permittivity constant (ϵ_0), and it is inversely proportional to the distance (d) separating the plates.

Equation 6–14

$$C = \frac{A\epsilon\epsilon_0}{d}$$

Because of its similar geometry, the cell membrane has a capacitance that is analogous to that of the parallel-plate capacitor. The capacitance of 1 cm² of most cell membranes is approximately 1 μF; that is, most membranes have a specific capacitance of 1 μF/cm². We can use Equation 6–14 to estimate the thickness of the membrane. If we assume that the average dielectric constant of a biological membrane is $\epsilon = 5$ (slightly greater than the value of 2 for pure hydrocarbon), Equation 6–14 gives a value of 4.4 nm for d—that is, the thickness of

FIGURE 6–10. Electrochemical driving forces acting on various ions. For each of the four ions represented in Figure 6–9, we represent both the equilibrium potential (e.g., E_{Na} = +67 mV) and the net driving force for that ion (e.g., $V_m - E_{Na}$ = −147 mV). The values for the equilibrium potentials are those for mammalian skeletal muscle in Table 6–1. We also give a typical value for E_{Cl} in a non-muscle cell, as also shown in Table 6–1. For Na$^+$ and Ca^{2+}, the arrows—which indicate the driving force—point down, indicating that the driving force favors the passive *influx* of these ions. For K$^+$, the arrow points up, indicating that the driving force favors the passive *efflux* of K$^+$. For Cl$^-$ in skeletal muscle cells, the arrow points up, indicating that the driving force favors a small passive *influx*. In other cells, the arrow for Cl$^-$ points down, indicating that the driving force favors passive efflux.

the membrane. This value is quite close to estimates of membrane thickness that have been obtained by other physical techniques.

The Separation of Relatively Few Charges Across the Bilayer Capacitance Maintains the Membrane Potential

We can also use the capacitance of the cell membrane to estimate the amount of charge that the membrane actually separates in generating a typical membrane potential. For example, consider a spherical cell with a diameter of 10 μm and a [K$^+$]$_i$ of 100 mM. This cell needs to lose only 0.004% of its K$^+$ to charge the capacitance of the membrane to a voltage of −61.5 mV. This small loss of K$^+$ is clearly insignificant in comparison with a cell's total ionic composition and does not significantly perturb concentration gradients. In general, cell membrane potentials are sustained by a very small separation of charge.

Because of the existence of membrane capacitance, total membrane current has two components (see Fig. 6–9), one carried by ions through channels and the other carried by ions as they charge the membrane capacitance.

Ionic Current, the First of Two Components of the Total Membrane Current, Is Directly Proportional to the Electrochemical Driving Force (Ohm's Law)

Figure 6–10 compares the equilibrium potentials for Na$^+$, K$^+$, Ca^{2+}, and Cl$^-$ with a membrane potential of −80 mV. In our discussion of Figure 6–7, we saw that I_K or I_{Na} becomes zero when V_m equals the V_{rev}, which is the same as the E_X or emf for that ion. When V_m is more

negative than E_X, the current is negative or inward, whereas when V_m is more positive than E_X, the current is positive or outward. Thus, the ionic current depends on the difference between the actual V_m and E_X. In fact, the ionic current through a given conductance pathway is proportional to the difference ($V_m - E_X$), and the proportionality constant is the ionic conductance (G_X):

Equation 6–15
$$I_X = G_X(V_m - E_X)$$

This equation simply restates Ohm's law (Equation 6–11). The term ($V_m - E_X$) is often referred to as the **driving force** in electrophysiology. In our electrical model of the cell membrane (see Fig. 6–9), this driving force is represented by the difference between V_m and the emf of the battery. The larger the driving force, the larger the observed current.

Returning to the *I-V* relationship for K$^+$ in Figure 6–7A, we see that I_K is zero when V_m is equal to E_K (i.e., when the driving force is zero). At V_m values more positive than E_K, the driving force is positive, producing an outward (i.e., positive) current. Conversely, at V_m values more negative than E_K, the negative driving force produces an inward current. If G_K were constant, the *I-V* relationship in Figure 6–7A would be linear, like the dashed line in that figure. The reason that the *I-V* relationship is curvilinear is that G_K is not constant but varies with the deviation of V_m from E_K, as predicted by the GHK current equation.

In Figure 6–10, the *arrows* represent the magnitudes and directions of the driving forces for the various ions. For a typical value of the resting potential (−80 mV), the driving force on Ca^{2+} is the largest of the four ions, followed by the driving force on Na$^+$. In both cases, V_m is

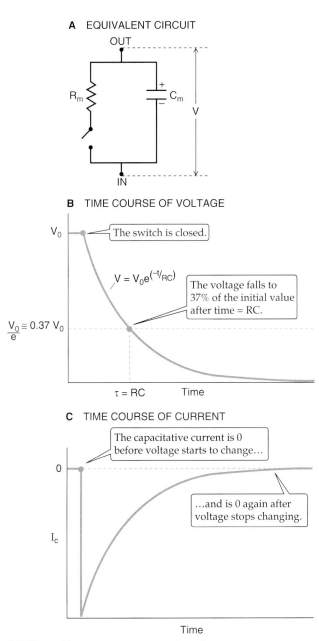

A EQUIVALENT CIRCUIT

OUT

R_m C_m

V

IN

B TIME COURSE OF VOLTAGE

V_0 The switch is closed.

$V = V_0 e^{(-t/RC)}$

The voltage falls to 37% of the initial value after time = RC.

$\frac{V_0}{e} \cong 0.37\, V_0$

$\tau = RC$ Time

C TIME COURSE OF CURRENT

The capacitative current is 0 before voltage starts to change...

0

...and is 0 again after voltage stops changing.

I_c

Time

FIGURE 6–11. Capacitative current through a resistance-capacitance (RC) circuit.

more negative than the equilibrium potential and thus draws the positive ion *into* the cell. The driving force on K^+ is small. V_m is more positive than E_K and thus pushes K^+ out of the cell. In muscle, V_m is slightly more positive than E_{Cl} and thus draws the anion inward. In most other cells, however, V_m is more negative than E_{Cl} and pushes the Cl^- out.

Capacitative Current, the Second Component of the Total Membrane Current, Is Proportional to the Rate of Voltage Change

The idea that ionic channels can be thought of as conductance elements (G_X) and that ionic current (I_X) is proportional to driving force ($V_m - E_X$) provides a frame-

work for understanding the electrical properties of cell membranes. These ionic currents are the only currents that flow across the membrane in the steady state, that is, when V_m is constant. However, if V_m changes—as it does during an action potential—current also flows across the membrane because of the presence of an additional component, membrane capacitance. This second current, which flows only while V_m is changing, is called the capacitative current. How does a capacitor produce a current? When voltage across a capacitor changes, the capacitor either gains or loses charge. This movement of charge onto or off the capacitor is an electrical (i.e., the "capacitative") current.

The simple membrane circuit of Figure 6–11A, which is composed of a capacitor (C_m) parallel with a resistor (R_m) and a switch, can help to illustrate how capacitative currents arise. Assume that the switch is open and that the capacitor is initially charged to a voltage of V_0, causing a separation of charge (Q) across the capacitor. According to the definition of capacitance (Equation 6–13), the charge stored by the capacitor is a product of capacitance and voltage.

Equation 6–16

$$Q = C_m V_0$$

As long as the switch in the circuit remains open, the capacitor maintains this charge. However, when the switch is closed, the charge on the capacitor discharges through the resistor, and the voltage difference between the circuit points labeled "In" and "Out" decays from V_0 to a final value of zero (see Fig. 6–11B). This voltage decay follows an exponential time course. The time required for the voltage to fall to 37% of its initial value is a characteristic parameter called the **time constant** (τ), which has units of time:

Equation 6–17

$$\tau = R_m \times C_m$$

Thus, the time course of the decay in voltage is

Equation 6–18

$$V = V_0 e^{-t/RC}$$

Figure 6–11C shows that the **capacitative current** (I_C) is zero before the switch is closed, when the voltage is stable at V_0. When we close the switch, charge begins to flow rapidly off the capacitor, and the magnitude of I_C is maximal. As the charge on the capacitor gradually falls, the rate at which charge flows off the capacitor gradually falls as well until I_C is zero at "infinite" time. Note, however, that V and I_C relax with the same time constant.

In Figure 6–11, current and voltage change freely. Figure 6–12 shows two simpler examples in which either current or voltage is abruptly changed to a fixed value, held constant for a certain time, and returned to the original value. This pattern is called a "square pulse." In Figure 6–12A, we control, or "clamp," the current and allow the voltage to follow. When we inject a square pulse of current across the membrane, the voltage changes to a new value with a rounded time course

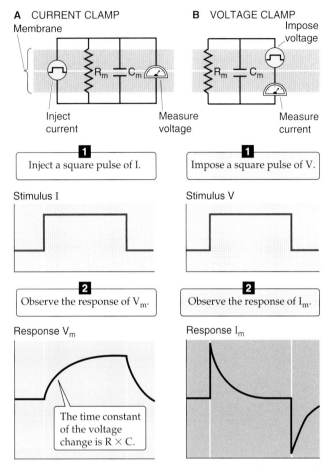

FIGURE 6–12. Voltage and current responses caused by the presence of a membrane capacitance.

determined by the *RC* value of the membrane. In Figure 6–12B, we clamp voltage and allow the current to follow. When we suddenly change voltage to a new value, a transient capacitative current flows as charge flows onto the capacitor. The capacitative current is maximal at the beginning of the square pulse, when charge flows most rapidly onto the capacitor, and then falls off exponentially with a time constant of RC. When we suddenly decrease the voltage to its original value, I_C flows in the direction opposite that observed at the beginning of the pulse. Thus, I_C appears as brief spikes at the beginning and end of the voltage pulse.

A Voltage Clamp Measures Currents Across Cell Membranes

Electrophysiologists use a technique called **voltage clamping** to deduce the properties of ion channels. In this method, specialized electronics are used to inject current into the cell to set the membrane voltage to a value that is different from the resting potential. The device then measures the total current required to clamp V_m to this value. A typical method of voltage clamping involves impaling a cell with two sharp electrodes, one for monitoring V_m and one for injecting the current. Figure 6–13A illustrates how the technique can be used with a *Xenopus*

(i.e., frog) oocyte. When the voltage-sensing electrode detects a difference from the intended voltage, called the command voltage, a feedback amplifier rapidly injects opposing current to maintain a constant V_m. The magnitude of the injected current needed to keep V_m constant is equal, but opposite in sign, to the membrane current and is thus an accurate measurement of the **total membrane current** (I_m).

I_m is the sum of the individual currents through each of the parallel branches of the circuit in Figure 6–9B. For a simple case in which only one type of ionic current (I_X) flows through the membrane, I_m is simply the sum of the capacitative current and the ionic current:

Equation 6–19

$$I_m = \underset{\substack{\text{Capacitative} \\ \text{current}}}{I_C} + \underset{\substack{\text{Ionic} \\ \text{current}}}{I_X}$$
$$= I_C + G_X(V_m - E_X)$$

Equation 6–19 suggests a powerful way to analyze how ionic conductance (G_X) changes with time. For instance, if we abruptly change V_m to another value and then hold V_m constant (i.e., we *clamp* the voltage), the capacitative current flows for only a brief time at the voltage transition and disappears by the time that V_m reaches its new steady value (see Fig. 6–12B). Therefore, after I_C has decayed to zero, any additional changes in I_m must be due to changes in I_X. Because V_m is clamped and the ion concentrations do not change (i.e., E_X is constant), only one parameter on the right side of Equation 6–19 is left free to vary, G_X. In other words, we can directly monitor changes in G_X because this conductance parameter is directly proportional to I_m when V_m is constant (i.e., clamped).

Figure 6–13B shows examples of records from a typical voltage-clamp experiment on an oocyte expressing voltage-gated Na^+ channels. In this experiment, a cell membrane is initially clamped at a resting potential of −80 mV. V_m is then stepped to −120 mV for 10 ms (a step of −40 mV) and finally returned to −80 mV. Such a negative-going V_m change is called a **hyperpolarization**. With this protocol, only brief spikes of current are observed at the beginning and end of the voltage step and are due to the charging of membrane capacitance. No current flows in between these two spikes.

What happens if we rapidly change V_m in the opposite direction by shifting the voltage from −80 to −40 mV (a step of +40 mV)? Such a positive-going change in V_m from a reference voltage is called a **depolarization**. In addition to the expected transient *capacitative* current, a large, inward, time-dependent current flows. This current is an *ionic* current and is due to the opening and closing kinetics of a particular class of channels called voltage-gated Na^+ channels, which open only when V_m is made sufficiently positive. We can remove the contribution of the capacitative current to the total current by subtracting the inverse of the rapid transient current recorded during the hyperpolarizing pulse of the same magnitude. The remaining slower current is inward (i.e., downward) and

A OOCYTE TWO-ELECTRODE VOLTAGE CLAMP

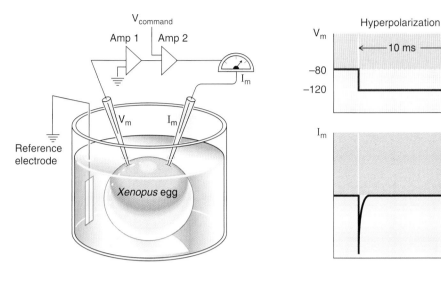

B VOLTAGE CLAMP METHOD OF MEASURING IONIC CURRENT

FIGURE 6–13. Two-electrode voltage clamp. *A,* Two microelectrodes impale a *Xenopus* oocyte. One electrode monitors membrane potential (V_m) and the other passes enough current (I_m) through the membrane to clamp V_m to a predetermined command voltage ($V_{command}$). *B,* In the left panel, the membrane is clamped for 10 ms to a hyperpolarized potential (40 mV more negative). Because a hyperpolarization does not activate channels, no ionic currents flow. Only transient capacitative currents flow after the beginning and end of the pulse. In the right panel, the membrane is clamped for 10 ms to a depolarized potential (40 mV more positive). Because the depolarization opens voltage-gated Na^+ channels, a large inward Na^+ current flows, in addition to the transient capacitative current. Adding the transient capacitative currents in the left panel to the total current in the right panel, thereby canceling the transient capacitative currents (I_c), yields the pure Na^+ current shown at the bottom in the right panel.

represents I_{Na}, which is directly proportional to G_{Na} (Equation 6–19).

The ionic current in Figure 6–13*B* (*lower right panel*) is called a **macroscopic current**, because it is due to the activity of a large population of channels sampled from a whole cell. Why did we observe an Na^+ current only when we shifted V_m in a positive direction from the resting potential? As described later, such Na^+ channels are actually members of a large family of voltage-sensitive ion channels that are activated by *depolarization*. A current activated by depolarization is commonly observed when an electrically excitable cell, such as a neuron, is voltage-clamped under conditions in which Na^+ is the sole extracellular cation.

A modern electrophysiologic method called **whole-cell voltage clamping** involves the use of a single microelectrode to both monitor V_m and pass current into the cell. In this method, a glass micropipette electrode with a smooth, fire-polished tip that is approximately 1 μm in diameter is pressed onto the surface of a cell (Fig. 6–14*A*). One then applies slight suction to the inside of the pipette, forming a high-resistance seal between the circular rim of the pipette tip and the cell membrane. The piece of sealed membrane is called a **patch**, and the pipette is called a **patch pipette**. Subsequently applying stronger suction causes the patch to rupture, creating a continuous, low-resistance pathway between the inside of the cell and the pipette. In this configuration, **whole-cell currents** can be recorded (see Fig. 6–14*B*). Because single cells can be dissociated from many different tissues and studied in culture, this method has proved very pow-

erful for analyzing the physiologic roles of various types of ion channels and their regulation at the cellular level. The approach for recording whole-cell currents with a patch pipette was introduced by Erwin Neher and Bert Sakmann, who received the Nobel Prize in Physiology or Medicine in 1991.

The Patch-Clamp Technique Resolves Unitary Currents Through Single-Channel Molecules

Voltage-clamp studies of ionic currents at the whole-cell (i.e., macroscopic) level led to the question of how many channels are involved in the production of a macroscopic current. Electrophysiologists realized that if the area of a voltage-clamped membrane was reduced to a very small fraction of the cell surface area, it might be possible to observe the activity of a single channel.

This goal was realized when Neher and Sakmann developed the **patch-clamp technique**. Applying suction to a patch pipette creates a high-resistance seal between the glass and the cell membrane, as described in the previous section for whole-cell voltage clamping. However, instead of rupturing the enclosed membrane patch as in the whole-cell approach, the tiny membrane area within the patch is kept intact so that one can record current from channels within the patch. A current recording made with the patch pipette attached to a cell is called a **cell-attached recording** (see Fig. 6–14*A*). After establishing a cell-attached patch, it is also possible to withdraw the pipette from the cell membrane to produce an **inside-out**

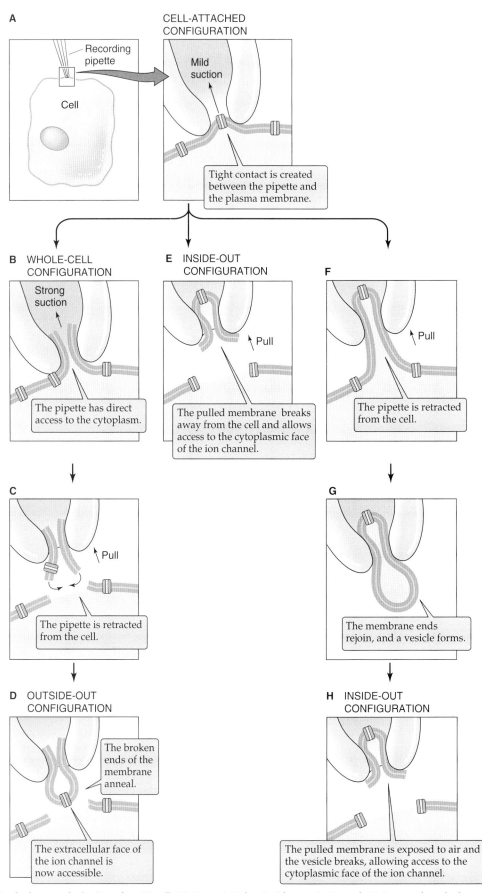

FIGURE 6–14. Patch clamp methods. (Data from Hamill OP, Marty A, Neher E, Sakmann B, Sigworth FJ: Improved patch-clamp techniques for high-resolution current recording from cells and cell-free membrane patches. Pflugers Arch 391:85–100, 1981.)

A

Single channel currents from outside-out patches (pA)

B

Average current (pA)

Tetrodotoxin, which blocks Na⁺ channels, abolishes the current.

FIGURE 6–15. Outside-out patch recordings of Na⁺ channels. *A*, Eight single-current responses—in the same patch on a myotube (a cultured skeletal muscle cell)—to a depolarizing step in voltage (cytosolic side of patch negative). *B*, Average current. The *record in black* shows the average of many single traces, such as those in *A*. The *blue record* shows the average current when tetrodotoxin blocks the Na⁺ channels. (Data from Weiss RE, Horn R: Single-channel studies of TTX-sensitive and TTX-resistant sodium channels in developing rat muscle reveal different open channel properties. Ann N Y Acad Sci 479:152–161, 1986.)

patch configuration by either of two methods (Fig. 6–14E or 6–14F to H). In this configuration, the *intracellular* surface of the patch membrane faces the bath solution. One can also arrive at the opposite orientation of the patch of membrane by starting in the cell-attached configuration (see Fig. 6–14A), rupturing the cell-attached patch to produce a whole-cell configuration (see Fig. 6–14B), and then pulling the pipette away from the cell (see Fig. 6–14C). When the membranes reseal, the result is an **outside-out patch configuration** in which the *extracellular* patch surface faces the bath solution (see Fig. 6–14D).

The different patch configurations summarized in Figure 6–14 are useful for studying drug-channel interactions, receptor-mediated processes, and biochemical regulatory mechanisms that take place at either the inner or external surface of cell membranes.

Single-Channel Currents Sum to Produce Macroscopic Membrane Currents

Figure 6–15 illustrates the results of a patch-clamp experiment that is analogous to the macroscopic experiment on the *right-hand side* of Figure 6–13B. Under the diagram of the voltage step in Figure 6–15A are eight current records, each of which is the response to an identical step of depolarization lasting 45 ms. The smallest, nearly rectangular transitions of current correspond to the opening and closing of a single Na⁺ channel. When two or three channels in the patch are open simultaneously, the measured current level is an integral multiple of the single-channel or "unitary" transition.

The opening and closing process of ion channels is called **gating**. Patch-clamp experiments have demonstrated that macroscopic ionic currents represent the gating of single channels that have discrete unitary currents. Averaging consecutive, microscopic Na⁺ current records produces a time-dependent current (see Fig. 6–15B) that has the same shape as the macroscopic I_m shown in Figure 6–13B. If one does the experiment in the same way, but blocks the Na⁺ channels with tetrodotoxin, the averaged time-dependent current is no different from "noise."

Measuring the current from a single channel in a patch at different clamp voltages reveals that the size of the discrete current steps depends on voltage (Fig. 6–16A). Plotting the **unitary current** (*i*) of single channels versus the voltage at which they were measured yields a single-channel *I-V* relationship (see Fig. 6–16B) that is similar to the one we discussed earlier for macroscopic currents (see Fig. 6–7). This single-channel *I-V* relationship reverses direction at a certain potential (V_{rev}), just like a macroscopic current does. If a channel is permeable to only one type of ion present in the solution, the V_{rev} equals the equilibrium potential for that ion (E_X). However, if the channel is permeable to more than one ion, the single-channel reversal potential depends on the relative permeabilities of the various ions, as described by the GHK voltage equation (Equation 6–9).

The slope of a single-channel *I-V* relationship is a measure of the conductance of a single channel—the *unitary*

FIGURE 6–16. Voltage dependence of currents through single Cl⁻ channels in outside-out patches. *A*, The channel is a gamma-aminobutyric acid-A (GABA_A) receptor channel, which is a Cl⁻ channel activated by GABA. Identical solutions, containing 145 mM Cl⁻, were present on both sides of the patch. *B*, The magnitudes of the single-channel current transitions (y-axis) vary linearly with voltage (x-axis). (Data from Bormann J, Hamill OP, Sakmann B: Mechanism of anion permeation through channels gated by glycine and γ-aminobutyric acid in mouse cultured spinal neurones. J Physiol (Lond) 385:243–286, 1987.)

conductance (g). Every type of ion channel has a characteristic value of g under a defined set of ionic conditions. The single-channel conductance of most known channel proteins is in the range of 1 to 500 picosiemens (pS), where 1 pS is equal to 10^{-12} ohms⁻¹.

How do we know that the unitary current in fact corresponds to just a single channel? One good indication is that such conductance measurements are close to the theoretical value expected for ion diffusion through a cylindrical, water-filled pore that is long enough to span a phospholipid membrane and that has a diameter large enough to accept an ion. The unitary conductance of typical channels corresponds to rates of ion movement in the range of 10^6 to 10^8 ions per second per channel at 100 mV of driving force. These rates of ion transport through single ion channels are many orders of magnitude greater than typical rates of ion transport by ion pumps (~500 ions per second) or by the fastest ion cotransporters and exchangers (~50,000 ions/sec). The high ionic flux through channels places them in a unique class of transport proteins whose unitary activity can be resolved by patch-clamp current recordings.

Single Ion Channels Can Exist In Open and Closed States

When a channel has opened from the **closed state** (zero current) to its full unitary conductance value, the channel is said to be in the **open state**. Channel gating thus represents the transition between closed and open states. A single-channel record is actually a record of the conformational changes of a single protein molecule as monitored by the duration of opening and closing events.

Examining the consecutive records of a patch recording, such as that in Figure 6–15A, shows that the gating of a single channel is a probabilistic process. On average, there is a certain probability that a channel will open at any given time, but such openings occur randomly. For example, the average record in Figure 6–15B indicates that the probability that the channels will open is highest approximately 4 ms after the start of the depolarization.

The process of channel gating can be represented by kinetic models that are similar to the following hypothetical two-state scheme.

Equation 6–20

$$C \underset{k_c}{\overset{k_o}{\rightleftharpoons}} O$$

This scheme indicates that a channel can reversibly change its conformation between closed (C) and open (O) states according to first-order reactions that are determined by an opening rate constant (k_o) and a closing rate constant (k_c). The **probability of channel opening** (P_o) is the fraction of total time that the channel is in the open state.

We already have seen in Figure 6–15 that the *average* of many single-channel records from a given patch produces a time course that is similar to a macroscopic current recorded from the same cell. The same is true for the *sum* of the individual single-channel current records. This conclusion leads to an important principle: macroscopic ionic current is equal to the product of the **number of channels** (N) within the membrane area, the unitary current of single channels, and the probability of channel opening:

Equation 6–21

$$I = N P_o i$$

Comparison of the magnitude of macroscopic currents recorded from large areas of voltage-clamped membrane with the magnitude of unitary current measured by patch techniques indicates that the surface density of ion channels typically falls into the range of 1 to 1000 channels per square micrometer of cell membrane, depending on the channel and cell type.

MOLECULAR PHYSIOLOGY OF ION CHANNELS

Classes of Ion Channels Can Be Distinguished on the Basis of Electrophysiology, Pharmacology, Extracellular Agonists, Intracellular Messengers, and Sequence Homology

Mammalian cells express a remarkable array of ion channels. One way of making sense of this diversity is to classify channels according to their functional characteristics. Among these characteristics are electrophysiologic behavior, inhibition or stimulation by various pharmacologic agents, activation by extracellular agonists, and modulation by intracellular regulatory molecules. In addition, we can classify channels by structural characteristics, such as amino-acid sequence homology and the kinds of subunits of which they are composed.

ELECTROPHYSIOLOGY. This approach consists of analyzing ionic currents by voltage-clamp techniques and then characterizing the channels on the basis of their ionic selectivity, dependence of gating on membrane potential, and the kinetics of their opening and closing.

One of the most striking differences among channels is their **selectivity** for various ions. Indeed, channels are generally named according to which ion they are most permeable to—for example, Na^+ channels, Ca^{2+} channels, K^+ channels, and Cl^- channels.

Another major electrophysiological characteristic of channels is their **voltage dependence**. In electrically excitable cells (e.g., nerve, skeletal muscle, heart), a major class of channels becomes activated—and often inactivated—as a steep function of V_m. For example, the Na^+ channel in nerve and muscle cells becomes increasingly more active as V_m becomes more positive (p. 186). Such voltage-gated channels are generally highly selective for Na^+, Ca^{2+}, or K^+.

A final electrophysiological characteristic of channels is the timing of their **gating** behavior. For example, imagine two channels, each with an open probability (P_o) of 0.5. One channel might exhibit openings and closures with a duration of 1 sec each on average, whereas the other could achieve the same P_o with openings and closures of 1 ms each on average. Finally, the gating pattern of some channels is characterized by bursts of activity, followed by periods of relative inactivity.

PHARMACOLOGY. Currents that are virtually indistinguishable by electrophysiological criteria can sometimes be distinguished pharmacologically. For example, subtypes of voltage-gated Na^+ channels can be distinguished by their sensitivity to the peptide toxin μ-conotoxin, which is produced by *Conus geographus*, a venomous marine mollusk. This toxin strongly inhibits the Na^+ channels of adult skeletal muscle but has little effect on the Na^+ channels of neurons and cardiac myocytes.

EXTRACELLULAR AGONISTS. Some channels are characterized by their unique ability to be activated by the binding of a particular molecule termed an **agonist**. For example, at the vertebrate neuromuscular junction, a channel called the nicotinic acetylcholine (ACh) receptor opens in response to the binding of ACh released from a presynaptic nerve terminal. Other agonist-gated channels respond to different chemical activators such as glutamate, serotonin (5-hydroxytryptamine [5-HT]), gamma-aminobutyric acid (GABA), and glycine. The types of agonist-gated channels are numerous and diverse, and they differ on the basis of electrophysiological and pharmacological criteria.

INTRACELLULAR MESSENGERS. Channels can be categorized by their physiological regulation via intracellular messengers. For example, increases in $[Ca^{2+}]_i$ stimulate some ionic currents, in particular K^+ and Cl^- currents. Channels underlying such currents are known as Ca^{2+}-gated K^+ channels and Ca^{2+}-gated Cl^- channels, respectively. Another example is seen in the plasma membrane of light-sensitive rod cells of the retina, in which a certain type of channel is directly activated by intracellular cyclic guanosine monophosphate (cGMP).

Now that we have presented four functional criteria (electrophysiology, pharmacology, extracellular agonists, and intracellular regulators) for characterizing channels, it should be kept in mind that these criteria are not mutually exclusive. For example, the Ca^{2+}-gated K^+ channel is also voltage gated. So how should we classify such channels? From an evolutionary point of view, Ca^{2+}-gated K^+ channels and cGMP-activated channels are both structurally related to the family of voltage-gated channels.

SEQUENCE HOMOLOGY. Because of the diversity of channels anticipated on the basis of functional criteria, a molecular biologic approach is ultimately required to classify ion channels. Such an approach began in the 1970s and 1980s with the biochemical purification of channel proteins. Membrane biochemists used rich, natural sources of ion channels—such as the electrical organs of the Torpedo ray and *Electrophorus* eel—to isolate channel proteins such as the nicotinic ACh receptor (p. 213) and the voltage-gated Na^+ channel, respectively. Amino acid sequencing of purified channel proteins provided the information needed to prepare oligonucleotide probes that could be used to isolate the coding sequences of channels from cDNA clones derived from mRNA. This approach has led to the cloning of many different types of ion channels and has confirmed that the diversity of channels foreshadowed by physiological assays corresponds to an enormous diversity at the molecular level.

When annotation of the human genome is completed, it will eventually be possible to provide a definitive survey

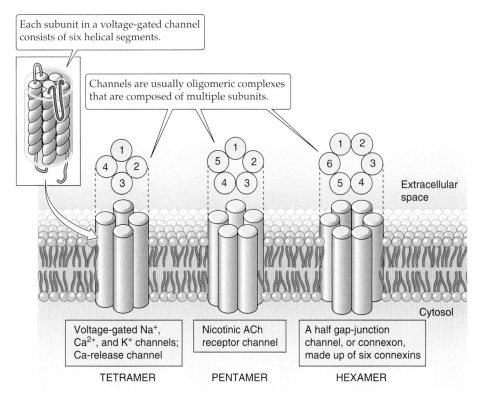

Each subunit in a voltage-gated channel consists of six helical segments.

Channels are usually oligomeric complexes that are composed of multiple subunits.

Extracellular space

Cytosol

Voltage-gated Na⁺, Ca²⁺, and K⁺ channels; Ca-release channel

TETRAMER

Nicotinic ACh receptor channel

PENTAMER

A half gap-junction channel, or connexon, made up of six connexins

HEXAMER

FIGURE 6–17. Structure of ion channels. Most ion channels consist of four to six subunits that are arranged like a rosette in the plane of the membrane. The channel can be made up of (1) identical, distinct subunits (homo-oligomer); (2) distinct subunits that are homologous but not identical (hetero-oligomer); or (3) repetitive subunit-like domains within a single polypeptide (pseudo-oligomer). In any case, these "subunits" surround the central pore of the ion channel. Note that each "subunit" is itself made up of several transmembrane segments.

of channel types and functions. On the basis of the data bank of mammalian channel-protein sequences derived from cloning methods, we recognize at least 18 distinct families of channel proteins (Table 6–2 on pp. 168–169). Despite rapid progress in the cloning of channels, detailed knowledge of the three-dimensional structures of channels is emerging more slowly because of the difficulty in crystallizing membrane proteins for x-ray crystallographic analysis. However, molecular information gleaned from sequence analysis and structural information on several channel proteins has revealed a number of important themes that we discuss in the remainder of this subchapter.

Many Channels Are Formed by a Radially Symmetric Arrangement of Subunits or Domains Around a Central Pore

The essential function of a channel is to facilitate the passive flow of ions across the hydrophobic membrane bilayer according to the electrochemical gradient. This task requires the channel protein to form an aqueous pore. The ionophore gramicidin is a small peptide that forms a unique helix dimer that spans the membrane; the hollow cylindrical region inside the helix is the channel pore. Another interesting type of channel structure is that of the **porin** channel proteins (p. 58), which are present in the outer membranes of mitochondria and gram-negative bacteria. This protein forms a large pore through the center of a barrel-like structure; the 16 staves of the barrel are formed by 16 strands of the protein, each of which are in a β-sheet conformation. However, the structural motifs of a hole through a helix (gramicidin) or a

hole through a 16-stranded β barrel (porin) appear to be exceptions rather than the rule.

For the vast majority of eukaryotic channels, the aqueous pores are located at the center of an oligomeric rosette-like arrangement of homologous subunits in the plane of the membrane (Fig. 6–17). Each of these subunits, in turn, is a polypeptide that weaves through the membrane several times. In some cases, the channel is not a true homo-oligomer or hetero-oligomer, but rather a pseudo-oligomer: the subunits are replaced by a single polypeptide composed of repetitive homologous domains. The rosette-like arrangement of these domains surrounds a central pore. In the case of gap junction channels and ACh receptor channels, which we discuss in the following two sections, it has been possible to use cryoelectron microscopy to construct images of the channel from membrane preparations in which the proteins exist in a densely packed two-dimensional crystalline array. Such analyses have provided low-resolution pictures that show how the polypeptide chains of the channel proteins weave through the membrane, although they have not yet identified individual atoms.

Gap-Junction Channels Are Made Up of Two Connexons, Each of Which Has Six Identical Subunits Called Connexins

Gap junctions are protein channels that connect two cells with a large, unselective pore (about 1.5 nm in diameter) that allows ions and small molecules as large as 1 kDa to pass between cells. These channels have been found in practically all mammalian cells with only a few exceptions, such as adult skeletal muscle and erythrocytes. For example, gap junctions interconnect hepatocytes of the liver, cardiac muscle fibers of the heart and smooth muscle of the gut, β cells of the pancreas, and epithelial cells in the cornea of the eye, to name just a few. Gap junctions provide pathways for chemical communication and electrical coupling between cells. The basic structure deduced for a gap junction from the liver is shown in Figure 6–18A. The gap junction comprises two apposed hexameric structures called **connexons**, one contributed by each cell. These connexons contact each other to bridge a gap of approximately 3 nm between the two cell membranes. Each connexon has six identical subunits surrounding a central pore, so-called radial hexameric symmetry. Each of these subunits is an integral membrane protein called **connexin** (Cx) that has a molecular mass of 26 to 46 kDa. The aqueous pore formed at the center of the six connexin subunits has a diameter that is estimated to be 1.2 to 2 nm. At the cytoplasmic end of the connexon, the pore appears to open to a wider funnel-shaped entrance.

In one mode of regulation, increases in $[Ca^{2+}]_i$ can cause gap junctions to close. For Ca^{2+}-dependent gating, it is possible to visualize a structural change in the conformation of the connexon. In the absence of Ca^{2+}, the pore is in an open configuration and the connexin subunits are tilted 7 to 8 degrees from an axis perpendicular to the plane of the membrane. After the addition of Ca^{2+}, the pore closes and the subunits move to a more parallel alignment (see Fig. 6–18B). The gating of the gap-junction channel may thus correspond to a conformational change that involves concerted tilting of the six connexin subunits to widen (open) or constrict (close) the pore.

The gating properties of gap junctions can be studied by measuring electrical currents through gap junctions, using two patch electrodes simultaneously placed in a pair of coupled cells (Fig. 6–18C). When the two cells are clamped at different values of V_m, so that current flows from one cell to the other through the gap junctions, the current measured in either cell fluctuates as a result of the opening and closing of individual gap-junction channels. Because the amount of current that enters one cell is the same as the amount of current that leaves the other cell, the current fluctuations in the two cells are mirror images of one another. Studies of this type have shown that increases in $[Ca^{2+}]_i$ or decreases in intracellular pH generally favor the closing of gap-junction channels. In addition, gating of gap-junction channels can be regulated by the voltage difference between the coupled cells, as well as by phosphorylation.

Nicotinic Acetylcholine Receptor Channels Are $\alpha_2\beta\gamma\delta$ Pentamers Made Up of Four Homologous Subunits

In contrast to the gap-junction channel, which is a hexamer made up of six identical subunits, the nicotinic ACh receptor is a channel that is a pentamer that comprises four different homologous subunits. The α subunit is represented twice; therefore, the pentamer has a subunit composition of $\alpha_2\beta\gamma\delta$. The nicotinic ACh receptor channel is located in a specialized region of the skeletal mus-

cle membrane, at the postsynaptic nerve terminal. The receptor responds to ACh released from the nerve terminals by opening and allowing cations to flow through its pore (p. 212). Images of the ACh receptor show a pentameric radial symmetry that corresponds to a rosette-like arrangement of the five subunits (Fig. 6–19). When viewed from the extracellular face of the membrane, a hole with a diameter of 2 to 2.5 nm is observed in the center of the rosette and corresponds to the extracellular entrance to the cation-selective channel. The structural changes induced by ACh binding that control opening and closing of the channel appear to occur in a central region of the protein that lies within the plane of the lipid bilayer. We discuss the structure and function of this particular class of channels, an example of **ligand-gated channels** (or agonist-gated channels), in Chapter 8.

An Evolutionary Tree Called a Dendrogram Illustrates the Relatedness of Ion Channels

It is possible to gain insight into the molecular evolution of proteins by comparing their deduced primary amino-acid sequences, as well as the nucleotide sequences of genes that encode them. Although the data bank of channel sequences is characterized by great diversity, one can discern numerous evolutionary inter-relationships.

Humans have hundreds of distinct channel genes. Like other proteins, specific isoforms of channels are differentially expressed in different parts of cells in various tissues and at certain stages of development. In particular, many different kinds of channels are expressed in the brain. In the central nervous system, the great diversity of ion channels provides a means of specifically and precisely regulating the complex electrical activity of a huge number of neurons that are connected in numerous functional pathways.

As an example of the diversity and inter-relatedness of a channel family, consider the connexins. Figure 6–20 compares 14 sequences of homologous proteins that are members of the connexin family. Like many other proteins, connexins are encoded by a family of related genes that evolved by gene duplication and divergence. In the connexin family, various subtypes are named according to their protein molecular weights. Thus, rat Cx32 refers to a rat connexin with a protein molecular weight of about 32 kDa. The various connexins differ primarily in the length of the intracellular C-terminal domain.

By aligning various connexin sequences according to identical amino acids and computing the relative similarity of each pair of connexin sequences, it is possible to reconstruct a hypothetical family tree of evolutionary relationships. Such a tree is called a **dendrogram**. The one in Figure 6–20 includes 9 rat, 2 human, 1 chicken, and 2 frog (*Xenopus*) connexins. The branch lengths of the tree correspond to relative evolutionary distances as measured by sequence similarity. Clusters of sequences in the tree represent highly related groups of proteins. The connexin tree indicates that the Cx32 from rats and humans is very closely related, only differing by 4 amino acids out of a total of 284 residues. Thus, these Cx32 proteins probably represent the same functional genes in these two species.

A GAP-JUNCTION CHANNELS IN APPOSING MEMBRANES

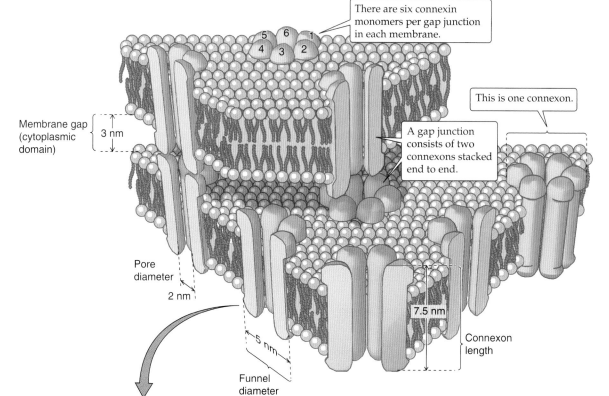

There are six connexin monomers per gap junction in each membrane.

This is one connexon.

A gap junction consists of two connexons stacked end to end.

Membrane gap (cytoplasmic domain) 3 nm

Pore diameter 2 nm

5 nm

Funnel diameter

7.5 nm

Connexon length

B OPEN AND CLOSED CONFIGURATIONS OF A CONNEXON

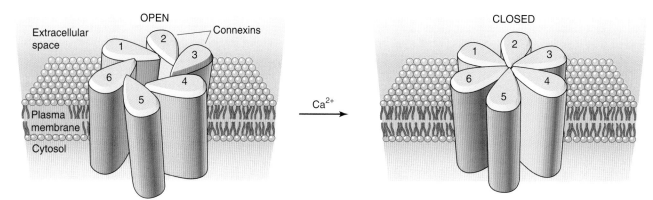

OPEN

Extracellular space

Connexins

Plasma membrane

Cytosol

Ca^{2+}

CLOSED

C ELECTRICAL COUPLING OF TWO CELLS CONNECTED BY GAP JUNCTIONS

I_1 is the sum of the fluctuating current through the gap junction (I_g) and the stable membrane current (I_m).

I_1

I_2

V_m clamped to -40 mV

V_m clamped to -80 mV

Gap junction

I_j

Cell 1

Cell 2

Patch pipette in whole-cell configuration

I_m

I_m

Current through membrane (I_m) is steady.

Current through gap junction (I_j).

5 pA

500 milliseconds

FIGURE 6–18. Gap-junction channels. In *C*, left panel shows the preparation of the two cells, each of which is voltage clamped by means of a patch pipette in the whole-cell configuration (see Fig. 6–14). Because Cell 1 is clamped to −40 mV and Cell 2 is clamped to −80 mV, current flows through the gap junctions from Cell 1 to Cell 2. The right panel shows that the current recorded by the electrode in Cell 1 is the mirror image of the current recorded in Cell 2. The fluctuating current transitions represent the openings and closings of individual gap-junction channels. (Data from Veenstra RD, DeHaan RL: Measurement of single channel currents from cardiac gap junctions. Science 233:972–974, 1986.)

The same is likely to be true of the closely related Cx43 from the rat and human. Sequence analysis of the connexin family also reveals the presence of two major subfamilies called class I (or β group) and class II (or α group). Sometimes, members of a family of channel proteins can be distinguished by patterns of tissue expression. For example, rat Cx32 (class I) is expressed in the liver and rat Cx43 (class II) is expressed in the heart. However, both these proteins are also expressed at various levels in a number of other tissues.

The connexin tree illustrates how we can systematically classify ion-channel proteins based on sequence-homology relationships. In cases where the functional properties of cloned channel genes are known from their behavior in expression systems, such as *Xenopus* oocytes, their function is consistent with the classification of channel subtypes based on molecular evolution. For example, ion channels that share the property of being voltage gated also share sequence homology of their voltage-sensing domain. We discuss the superfamily of voltage-gated channels in Chapter 7. Similarly, members of a channel family or subfamily generally have similar ion selectivity, common gating characteristics, or shared pharmacologic sensi-

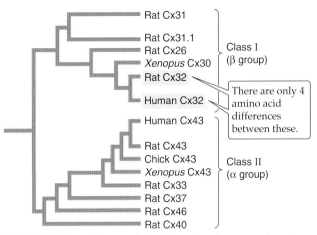

FIGURE 6–20. Family tree of hypothetical evolutionary relationships among connexin sequences of gap-junction channels. This dendrogram is based on amino-acid sequence differences among 14 connexins. The summed length of the horizontal line segments connecting two connexins is a measure of the degree of difference between the two connexins. (Data from Dermietzel R, Spray DC: Gap junctions in the brain: where, what type, how many and why? Trends Neurosci 16:186–192, 1993.)

tivity to particular drugs and toxins. Divergent members of a channel superfamily exhibit numerous differences in functional properties.

Hydrophobic Domains of Channel Proteins Can Predict How These Proteins Weave Through the Membrane

From the sequence information of many ion channels that have now been cloned, a number of common structural principles emerge. Like other integral membrane proteins (p. 15), channel proteins generally have several segments of hydrophobic amino acids, each long enough ($\sim$20 amino acids) to span the lipid bilayer as an α helix. If the channel has N membrane-spanning segments, it also has $N + 1$ hydrophilic domains of variable length that connect or terminate the membrane spans. Putative transmembrane segments are normally identified by hydropathy analysis (see Table 2–1), which identifies long segments of hydrophobic amino-acid residues. In some cases, supporting biochemical evidence indicates that such domains are actually embedded in the membrane. By analogy to a few membrane proteins of known three-dimensional structure, such as the bacterial photosynthetic reaction center, it is generally presumed that such hydrophobic transmembrane domains have an α-helical conformation. The intervening hydrophilic segments that link the transmembrane regions together are presumed to form extracellular and intracellular protein domains that contact the aqueous solution.

The primary sequences of channel proteins are often schematically represented by hypothetical folding diagrams, such as that shown in Figure 6–21 for Cx32, one of the connexins that we have already discussed. Cx32 is a polypeptide of 284 amino acids that contains four identifiable hydrophobic transmembrane segments. In connexins, these transmembrane segments are known as M1,

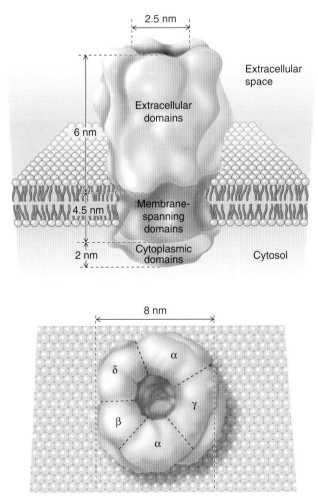

FIGURE 6–19. Three-dimensional image of the nicotinic acetylcholine receptor channel. (Data from Toyoshima C, Unwin N: Ion channel of acetylcholine receptor reconstructed from images of postsynaptic membranes. Nature 336:247–250, 1988.)

TABLE 6–2

MAJOR STRUCTURAL FEATURES OF THE KNOWN FAMILIES OF ION CHANNELS

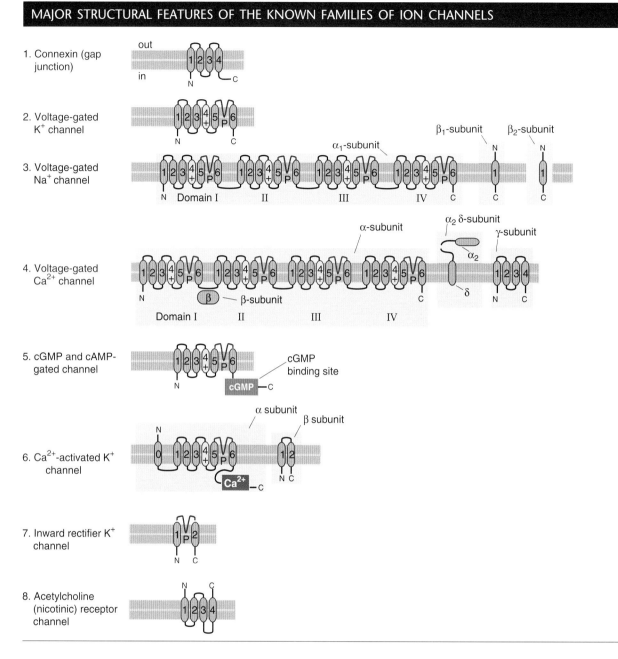

1. Connexin (gap junction)

2. Voltage-gated K⁺ channel

3. Voltage-gated Na⁺ channel

4. Voltage-gated Ca²⁺ channel

5. cGMP and cAMP-gated channel

6. Ca²⁺-activated K⁺ channel

7. Inward rectifier K⁺ channel

8. Acetylcholine (nicotinic) receptor channel

M2, M3, and M4. Biochemical evidence indicates that the N-terminal and C-terminal hydrophilic segments of connexin are located on the cytoplasmic side of the membrane and that the M3 domain is involved in forming part of the gap-junction pore. Mutations in Cx32 can lead to a rare hereditary neuropathy known as Charcot-Marie-Tooth disease (see the box on this disease).

Protein Superfamilies, Subfamilies, and Subtypes Are the Structural Bases of Channel Diversity

Table 6–2 summarizes the major structural features of the known families of ion channels that have been identified in mammals by cloning of their pore-forming sub-units. In most cases, the hypothetical membrane topologies are based primarily on hydropathy analysis. Thus, the folding diagrams should be considered a "best-guess" representation.

CONNEXINS. As we have already noted, the connexins have four transmembrane segments. Six connexins surround a central pore to form a connexon. Two connexons from neighboring cells stack end to end to form a gap-junction channel (Table 6–2, #1).

VOLTAGE-GATED CATION CHANNELS. Some families of channel proteins are so large and diverse that they are known as **superfamilies**. The superfamily of **voltage-gated channels** consists of K⁺, Na⁺, and Ca²⁺ channels that have a common structural motif (p. 182). The main

TABLE 6-2

MAJOR STRUCTURAL FEATURES OF THE KNOWN FAMILIES OF ION CHANNELS *Continued*

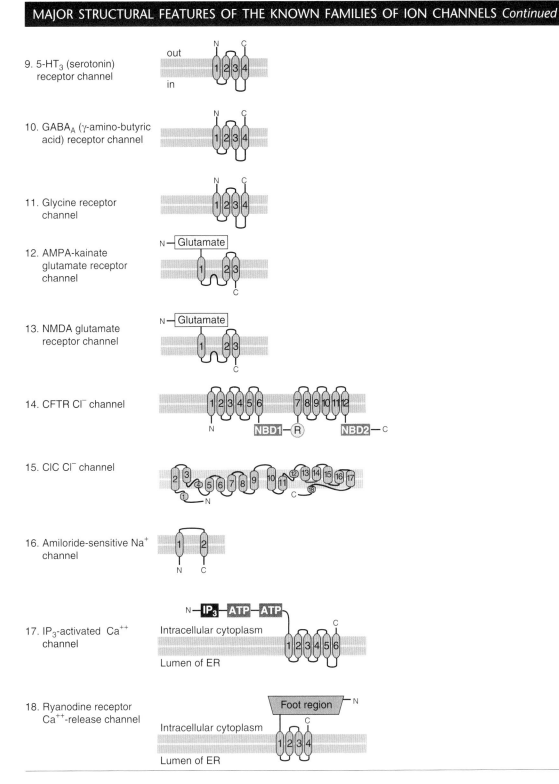

9. 5-HT$_3$ (serotonin) receptor channel

10. GABA$_A$ (γ-amino-butyric acid) receptor channel

11. Glycine receptor channel

12. AMPA-kainate glutamate receptor channel

13. NMDA glutamate receptor channel

14. CFTR Cl$^-$ channel

15. ClC Cl$^-$ channel

16. Amiloride-sensitive Na$^+$ channel

17. IP$_3$-activated Ca^{++} channel

18. Ryanodine receptor Ca^{++}-release channel

part of each of these channels consists of four subunits or domains, each of which contains six transmembrane segments denoted as S1 through S6. **K$^+$ channels** are believed to represent the evolutionary precursor form of these channels because their pore-forming subunit contains only one S1 through S6 domain (Table 6–2, #2). As mentioned earlier, several types of voltage-gated K$^+$ channels are tetramers of these simple subunits. The pore-forming subunits of **Na$^+$ and Ca^{2+} channels** (Table 6–2, #3 and #4) both comprise four domains (I, II, III, and IV), each of which contains the S1 through S6 structural motif that is homologous to the basic K$^+$ channel subunit.

Extracellular
space

Plasma
membrane

Cytosol

Mutation

N

M1   M2   M3   M4

↑ Frameshift
  mutation

C

FIGURE 6–21. Membrane folding of connexin-32, one of the gap-junction proteins. Mutations of the human Cx32 can cause Charcot-Marie-Tooth disease. The locations of six such identified, single-point mutations are indicated in *red*. (Data from Bergoffen J, Scherer SS, Wang S, et al: Connexin mutations in X-linked Charcot-Marie-Tooth disease. Science 262:2039–2042, 1993.)

Because domains I through IV are apparently organized to form four repeats within the membrane, these domains are referred to as **pseudosubunits**. The molecular evolution of the four-repeat structure of Na$^+$ and Ca^{2+} channels is believed to have occurred by a process involving consecutive gene duplication from a primordial gene containing S1 through S6. Members of the voltage-gated superfamily of channels are also recognized by a characteristic structure of the S4 domain in which four to seven positively charged residues (lysine or arginine) are located at every third position. This unique S4 domain appears to function as the protein's voltage sensor (p. 184).

Voltage-gated Ca^{2+} channels also illustrate another feature of some ion channels: they are multisubunit complexes consisting of **accessory proteins** in addition to the channel-forming subunits. For example, voltage-gated Ca^{2+} channels are composed of a large pseudotetrameric α_1 subunit with domains I through IV that form the pore, plus four additional structurally unrelated subunits known as α_2, β, γ, and δ (Table 6–2, #4). Like the homologous α subunit of Na$^+$ channels, the large α_1 subunit of Ca^{2+} channels specifies most of the basic channel functions, including ionic selectivity, voltage sensitivity, and the binding sites of various drugs. It appears that the β, γ, and δ subunits are important for modulating the activity of Ca^{2+} channels, but their exact functional role is largely unknown. It is possible that such accessory subunits of channels may help target newly synthesized channels to their proper cellular locations. In any case, the example of the Ca^{2+} channel illustrates that the identification of channel-forming subunits alone does not provide a comprehensive picture of channel physiology.

CYCLIC NUCLEOTIDE–GATED CHANNELS. Several other types of channels that are not considered to be voltage gated (i.e., they are not activated—physiologically—by a shift in V_m) are nevertheless clearly evolutionarily related to the voltage-gated superfamily. One example is a family of cation-selective channels that are directly activated by intracellular cGMP or cyclic adenosine monophosphate (cAMP). These channels play an important role in visual and olfactory sensory transduction (see Chapter 13). The cyclic nucleotide–gated channels have the same basic S1 through S6 motif as K$^+$ channels, but they contain a unique cyclic nucleotide binding domain at the C terminus (Table 6–2, #5).

Ca^{2+}-ACTIVATED K$^+$ CHANNELS. A second gene family of K$^+$ channels—large-conductance **Ca^{2+}-activated K$^+$ channels** (Table 6–2, #6)—is also structurally related to the superfamily of voltage-gated channels. The pore-forming subunit of these Ca^{2+}-activated K$^+$ channels has the basic S1 through S6 structure; however, it also has a transmembrane segment named S0 at the N terminus, plus a large C-terminal region that contains binding sites for Ca^{2+}.

INWARD RECTIFIER K$^+$ CHANNELS. A third family of K$^+$ channels consists of the **inward rectifier K$^+$ channels** (Table 6–2, #7). The basic pore-forming subunit of this family of channels contains only two membrane-spanning segments, and these are structurally related to the S5-S6 portion of the S1 through S6 domain of the voltage-gated K$^+$ channels (Table 6–2, #2). Because the linker between the S5 and S6 segments of voltage-gated channels forms the external vestibule of the channel and part of the pore region, it appears that inward rectifier K$^+$ channels contain the minimal structural unit required for forming a K$^+$-selective pore.

AGONIST-ACTIVATED CHANNELS. In addition to the voltage-gated superfamily, the agonist-activated channels—discussed earlier in regard to synaptic transmission—are also represented by two large and diverse gene superfamilies. Table 6–2 lists receptor channels that are gated by the binding of ACh (#8), serotonin (#9), GABA (#10), glycine (#11), and glutamate (#12 and #13).

OTHERS. Other important channels listed in Table 6–2 are two types of plasma membrane channels selective for Cl$^-$, the cystic fibrosis transmembrane conductance regulator (CFTR; #14) and ClC (#15). Amiloride-sensitive Na$^+$ channels (#16) are prominent in Na$^+$-transporting epithelia. Finally, Table 6–2 includes two types of Ca^{2+} release channels. One is present in the endoplasmic reticulum membrane and is gated by the intracellular messenger inositol 1,4,5-triphosphate (IP$_3$; #17). The second is located in the sarcoplasmic reticulum membrane of muscle and plays a critical role in the release of Ca^{2+} during muscle contraction (#18). It should be noted that Table 6–2 lists the major families of channel proteins that are rather well understood from a functional standpoint. Based on data from the Human Genome Project, we anticipate that several more channel families will be added to this compendium.

In conclusion, sequence information derived from the molecular biology of channel proteins complements the four categories of functional criteria that we discussed

CHARCOT-MARIE-TOOTH DISEASE

Many human genetic diseases have been identified in which the primary defect has been mapped to mutations of ion channel proteins. For example, Charcot-Marie-Tooth disease is a rare form of hereditary neuropathy that involves the progressive degeneration of peripheral nerves. Patients with this inherited disease have been found to have various mutations in the human gene for one of the gap junction proteins, connexin 32 (Cx32), which is located on the X chromosome. Cx32 appears to be involved in forming gap junctions between the folds of Schwann cell membranes. These **Schwann cells** wrap around the axons of peripheral nerves and form a layer of insulating material called **myelin,** which is critical for the conduction of nerve impulses. Apparently, mutations in Cx32 interfere with the normal function of these cells and result in the disruption of myelin and axonal degeneration. Some of these mutations have been identified at the amino acid level by gene sequencing. The protein folding diagram of Cx32 in Figure 6–21 indicates the locations of six point mutations, as well as a frameshift mutation, that have been observed in patients with this disease. Many other human diseases involve either a genetic defect of a particular channel protein or an autoimmune response directed against a channel protein.

earlier: electrophysiological characteristics, pharmacology, agonists, and intracellular messengers. This information can ultimately be used by the physician to treat human disease with pharmacologic agents designed on the basis of knowledge at the molecular level.

REFERENCES

Books and Reviews

Aidley DJ, Stanfield PR: Ion Channels: Molecules in Action. Cambridge, UK, Cambridge University Press, 1996.

Andersen OS, Koeppe RE: Molecular determinants of channel function. Physiol Rev 72 (Suppl):S89–S158, 1992.

Catterall WA: Cellular and molecular biology of voltage-gated sodium channels. Physiol Rev 72 (Suppl):S15–S48, 1992.

Hille B: Ionic Channels of Excitable Membranes, 3rd ed. Sunderland, MA, Sinauer Associates, 2001.

Neher E: Ion channels for communication between and within cells. Science 256:498–502, 1992.

Sakmann B, Neher E (eds): Single Channel Recording, 2nd ed. New York, Plenum Press, 1995.

Journal Articles

Bergoffen J, Scherer SS, Wang S, et al: Connexin mutations in X-linked Charcot-Marie-Tooth disease. Science 262:2039–2042, 1993.

Hamill OP, Marty A, Neher E, et al: Improved patch-clamp techniques for high resolution current recording from cells and cell-free membrane patches. Pflugers Arch 391:85–100, 1981.

Ho K, Nichols CG, Lederer J, et al: Cloning and expression of an inwardly rectifying ATP-regulated potassium channel. Nature 362:31–38, 1993.

Sigworth FJ, Neher E: Single Na-channel currents observed in cultured rat muscle cells. Nature 287:447–449, 1980.

CHAPTER 7

Electrical Excitability and Action Potentials

Edward G. Moczydlowski

Cellular communication in the nervous system is based on electrical and chemical signalling events that are mediated by ion channels. Certain types of cells, including neurons and myocytes, have a remarkable property called **electrical excitability**. In cells with this property, a spontaneous action potential is generated if the membrane is depolarized above a certain **threshold** voltage. An **action potential** is a transient, regenerative electrical impulse in which the membrane potential (V_m) rapidly rises to a peak that is approximately 100 mV more positive than the normal, negative resting voltage (V_{rest}). Such signals, also called spikes, can propagate for long distances along nerve or muscle fibers. Conduction of action potentials allows information from sensory organs to be transmitted along afferent nerves leading to the brain. Conversely, the brain exerts voluntary and involuntary control of muscles and other effector organs by efferent nerves leading away from it.

In the first part of this chapter, we examine the biophysical and molecular basis of action potentials and the mechanisms that underlie their genesis and propagation. The second part deals with the structure and function of voltage-gated ion-channel proteins. Finally, we examine the conduction properties of neurons—called cable properties—and how they determine the spread of action potentials along the axon.

MECHANISMS OF NERVE AND MUSCLE ACTION POTENTIALS

An Action Potential Is an All-or-None Response That Consists of Rapid Depolarization Followed by Slow Repolarization

The change in membrane potential that occurs during an action potential can be accurately measured by recording the V_m with an intracellular microelectrode. Figure 7–1A is a diagram illustrating various features of a typical action potential recorded from an electrically stimulated nerve or muscle cell. If the depolarizing stimulus causes V_m to become more positive than a **threshold** voltage, it triggers an action potential. The initial depolarizing (positive-going) phase of an action potential consists of a rapid and smooth increase in V_m from the negative resting potential to a maximum positive value that typically lies between +10 and +40 mV. This sharp rise in V_m to the peak voltage of the action potential is then followed by a slower repolarizing (negative-going) phase. The part of the action potential

FIGURE 7–1. The action potential.

that lies above 0 mV is sometimes called the **overshoot**. As we will see, the time course and shape of the repolarization phase vary considerably among different excitable tissues and cells. The repolarization phase may lead directly back to V_{rest}, or it may undershoot and give rise to a voltage minimum that is more negative than V_{rest} before relaxing back to V_{rest}. Such an undershoot is called an **afterhyperpolarization**.

The threshold, amplitude, time course, and duration of the action potential depend on the following factors:

1. The gating (opening and closing) and permeability properties of specific types of ion channels. These properties depend on both V_m and time.
2. The intracellular and extracellular concentrations of the ions that pass through these channels, such as Na^+, K^+, Ca^{2+}, and Cl^-.
3. Membrane properties that do not depend on V_m or time, such as membrane capacitance, membrane resistance, and the geometry of the cell.

The shape of the action potential in a given cell reflects the specialized functions of that cell. For example, the brief action potentials of a nerve axon permit rapid signalling, whereas the prolonged, repetitive action potentials of cardiac and certain types of smooth muscle cells mediate the slow, rhythmic contractions of these tissues. Figure 7–1B compares action potentials recorded from an invertebrate nerve fiber (unmyelinated squid axon), a ver-

tebrate nerve fiber (myelinated rabbit axon), a skeletal muscle fiber, and a cardiac atrial myocyte. This comparison illustrates the diversity in the duration and shape of the repolarizing phase of action potentials. The shape of the action potential is subject to hormonal modulation in certain cell types. As one example, the peptide hormone endothelin, produced by vascular endothelial cells, shortens the duration of the action potential when it is applied to a guinea pig atrial myocyte. Modulation of the shape and frequency of action potentials occurs by various biochemical regulatory mechanisms that affect the function of ion channels.

A Graded Response Is Proportional to the Stimulus and Decays with Distance Along the Axon, Whereas an Action Potential Maintains a Fixed Magnitude Along the Entire Length of the Axon

Not all electrical activity in nerve or muscle cells is characterized by an all-or-none response. As shown earlier in Figure 6–12A, when we apply a small square pulse of hyperpolarizing current to a cell membrane, V_m gradually becomes more negative and then stabilizes (Fig. 7–2A). In such an experiment, the observed change in V_m follows an exponential time course, with a time constant (p. 157) that is determined by the product of membrane resistance and capacitance ($\tau = RC$). This electrical response is an

A RESPONSE TO GRADED CURRENT STIMULI

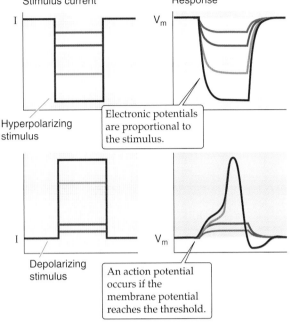

Stimulus current   Response

Electronic potentials are proportional to the stimulus.

Hyperpolarizing stimulus

Depolarizing stimulus

An action potential occurs if the membrane potential reaches the threshold.

FIGURE 7–2. Basic properties of action potentials. *A,* The *upper panels* show four graded hyperpolarizing stimuli and the V_m responses. The *lower panels* show four graded depolarizing stimuli and the V_m responses. Note that the two largest stimuli evoke identical action potentials. *B,* A stimulating electrode injects current at the *extreme left* of the cell. Four recording electrodes monitor V_m at equidistant sites to the *right.* If the stimulus is hyperpolarizing, the graded V_m responses decay with distance from the stimulus site. If the stimulus is depolarizing and large enough to evoke an action potential, a full action potential appears at each of the recording sites. However, the action potential arrives at the most distant sites with increasing delay.

B RESPONSE TO STIMULI AS A FUNCTION OF DISTANCE

Stimulating electrode

Recording electrodes

Nerve axon or muscle fiber

Stimulus current

Hyperpolarizing stimulus

The electrotonic potential decays as a function of the distance from the stimulus.

Depolarizing stimulus

The action potential remains constant in magnitude and shape...

...but the delay between stimulus and response increases with distance.

inherent property of phospholipid membranes, regardless of whether ion-channel proteins are present. Figure 7–2A also shows that progressively greater hyperpolarizing currents produce progressively larger V_m responses, but the time constant is always the same. The size of the **graded**

voltage change (i.e., the steady-state ΔV_m) is proportional to the strength of the stimulus (i.e., the current), in accord with Ohm's law.

If instead of imposing a hyperpolarizing stimulus we impose a small *depolarizing* stimulus, V_m changes to the

A STRENGTH-DURATION CURVE

If the duration of the stimulus is short, the intensity must be high...

...whereas if the duration is long, a lower-intensity stimulus can trigger an action potential.

Intensity of stimulus

0   Duration of stimulus

B REFRACTORY PERIODS

Absolute refractory period

Relative refractory period

Absolute refractory period: A second response is not possible regardless of strength or duration of the stimulus.

Relative refractory period: A second response can be elicited, but at a greater "cost" (i.e., strength and/or duration).

Voltage

Time

FIGURE 7–3. Nerve and muscle excitability. The curve in *A* represents the combination of the minimum stimulus intensity and duration that is required to reach threshold and evoke an action potential.

same extent and with the same time course as we described for the hyperpolarizing stimulus, but in the opposite direction (see Fig. 7–2A). The size of ΔV_m is also proportional to the size of the depolarizing stimulus—up to a point. If the membrane is excitable, a square-wave depolarization above the threshold triggers an action potential, or voltage spike. Smaller or **subthreshold depolarizations** will not elicit an action potential. *Hyperpolarizations* are always ineffective. Thus, both hyperpolarizations and subthreshold depolarizations behave as graded voltage changes. That is, the magnitude of a cell's voltage change increases proportionally with the size of the stimulus. Such graded responses can be seen in the response of certain cells to synaptic transmitters, to sensory stimuli (e.g., light), or in the laboratory, to the injection of current into cells through a microelectrode.

Why do excitable cells exhibit threshold behavior? As V_m becomes progressively more and more positive, the **gating** process (i.e., transitions from closed to open states) of certain types of voltage-gated ion channels becomes activated. When V_m passes the threshold, opening of these voltage-gated channels initiates the runaway depolarization that characterizes the rising phase of the action potential. Thus, the firing of an action potential is an all-or-none event; that is, the spike has a constant, nongraded voltage peak that occurs only if the depolarizing stimulus exceeds the threshold.

Thus far we have seen that graded responses and action potentials differ markedly from one another if we examine the cell at one particular site. However, graded responses and action potentials also behave very differently in the way that they spread along the membrane from the site of origin. Figure 7–2B illustrates how a graded hyperpolarizing response spreads along the axon of a neuron or along a skeletal muscle fiber. As the graded response spreads, its magnitude decays exponentially with the distance from the site of stimulation because of loss of energy to the medium. This decay is called **electrotonic conduction**. We see the same kind of

electrotonic spread for a subthreshold, depolarizing stimulus. The electrotonic spread of graded responses is governed by the same physical principles that determine the spread of electrical current in an electric cable. We briefly discuss "cable theory" at the end of this chapter.

Migration of an action potential signal is very different from the spread of a graded signal. In a healthy axon or muscle fiber, action potentials propagate at a constant velocity (up to ~130 ms), without change in amplitude or shape. The amplitude of a propagating action potential does not diminish with distance, as would a graded, subthreshold response, because excitation of voltage-gated channels in adjacent regions of the excitable membrane progressively regenerates the original response. Because the action potential in a given nerve fiber propagates at a constant velocity, the time between the stimulus and the peak of the action potential increases linearly with distance from the point of stimulus.

The Excitability of a Nerve or Muscle Cell Depends on the Product of the Strength and Duration of the Stimulus, as Well as on the Refractory Period

In the previous section, the importance of the *magnitude* (intensity) of the depolarizing stimulus emerged as a critical factor for firing an action potential. However, the *duration* of the stimulus pulse is also important. A large stimulus is effective in triggering an action potential even at short duration, and a small stimulus may be effective at long duration (Fig. 7–3A). This strength-duration relationship arises because the same minimum electric charge necessary to excite an action potential can come either from a brief, but large or from a prolonged, but small depolarizing current. It is the *product* of strength and duration that determines excitability, and thus these two parameters are inversely related in their effectiveness. However, regardless of the stimulus strength, successful

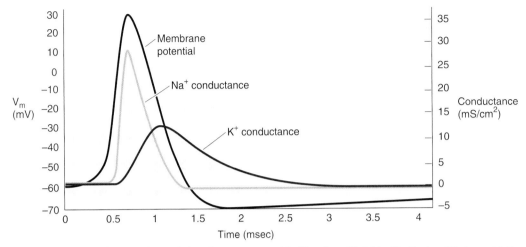

FIGURE 7–4. Changes in ionic conductance that underlies the action potential. (Data from Hodgkin AL, Huxley AF: A quantitative description of membrane current and its application to conduction and excitation in nerve. J Physiol (Lond) 117:500–544, 1952.)

stimulation requires a minimum duration (vertical asymptote in Fig. 7–3A). Conversely, regardless of the stimulus duration, successful stimulation requires a minimum strength (horizontal asymptote in Fig. 7–3A).

An important feature of excitable cells is their ability to fire repetitive action potentials. Once a cell fires an action potential, how quickly can it fire a second? If we were to impose a current step that produced a graded response, we could immediately add a second current step while the first persisted. As long as V_m did not exceed the threshold, the result would be a simple algebraic and instantaneous summation of the two graded responses. The situation for action potentials is quite different. First, action potentials never summate. Second, after one action potential fires, a finite period of time must lapse before it is possible to trigger a second. The time after initiation of an action potential when it is impossible or difficult to produce a second spike is the **refractory period** (see Fig. 7–3B). The **absolute refractory period** lasts from initiation of the spike to a time after the peak when repolarization is almost complete. During this time, a second action potential cannot be elicited, regardless of the stimulus strength or duration. After this period, a second action potential can be evoked during the **relative refractory period**, but the minimal stimulus necessary for activation is stronger or longer than predicted by the strength-duration curve for the first action potential. The two phases of the refractory period arise from the gating properties of particular Na+ and K+ channels and the overlapping time course of their currents.

Changes in Membrane Conductance to Na+ and K+ Underlie the Action Potential

Approximately 200 years after Luigi Galvani (1737–1798) discovered "animal electricity" (p. 145), the electrochemical basis of the nerve action potential was finally elucidated by the combined application of modern electrical recording techniques and the theory of electrodiffusion (p. 152). We now understand that the nerve action potential is a phenomenon that involves voltage-dependent currents of Na+ and K+ that flow through distinct molec-

ular pathways called Na+ channels and K+ channels. In 1963, the Nobel Prize in Physiology or Medicine was awarded to A.L. Hodgkin and A.F. Huxley for their quantitative description of these ionic currents in the squid giant axon in studies involving two-electrode voltage-clamp recordings. Invertebrate axons are unmyelinated, and axons in certain squid nerves have an unusually large diameter (500 to 1000 μm), which allows both external and internal ionic concentrations to be manipulated experimentally. The basic concepts underlying the Hodgkin-Huxley analysis have since been extended to a wide variety of voltage-dependent ionic currents.

The squid axon generates a very brief action potential signal without a significant plateau phase (Fig. 7–4). Ionic permeability changes underlying this impulse can be interpreted with a form of the constant-field equation (see Equation 6–9) that includes only Na+ and K+:

Equation 7–1

$$V_m = -\frac{RT}{F} \ln \left(\frac{P_K[K^+]_i + P_{Na}[Na^+]_i}{P_K[K^+]_o + P_{Na}[Na^+]_o} \right)$$

According to Equation 7–1, the negative resting potential (about −60 mV) of the axon membrane corresponds to a K+/Na+ permeability ratio (P_K/P_{Na}) of about 14:1. The change in V_m to a value near +40 mV at the peak of the action potential must involve a transient and selective increase in the permeability to either Na+ or Ca2+ because the equilibrium potential of these cations lies in the positive voltage range (see Fig. 6–10). Experimentally, if [Na+]$_o$ is reduced by replacing it with a nonelectrolyte such as sucrose, the nerve action potential decreases in amplitude. Complementary experiments measuring radioactive tracer fluxes of Na+ and K+ also demonstrate that action potentials are accompanied by a small influx of Na+ and an efflux of K+. These and related findings showed that the waveform of the squid action potential is produced by separate permeability pathways for Na+ and K+.

The time course of the action potential (see Fig. 7–4) can be dissected into an initial, transient increase in Na+ conductance (and thus permeability), followed by a similar

FIGURE 7–5. Dissection of Na$^+$ and K$^+$ currents by voltage-clamp analysis and pharmacology. *A,* In a typical voltage-clamp experiment, a sudden *hyper*polarization from −80 to −140 mV results in a transient capacitative current, but no ionic currents. *B,* In a voltage-clamp experiment, a sudden *de*polarization from −80 to −20 mV results in a transient capacitative current followed first by an inward ionic current and then by an outward ionic current. *C,* Blockade of the outward current by tetraethylammonium leaves only the inward current, which is carried by Na$^+$. Conversely, a blockade of the inward current by tetrodotoxin or saxitoxin leaves only the outward current, which is carried by K$^+$.

but delayed increase in K$^+$ conductance. As one would predict from our discussion of Equation 6–12, a transient increase in Na$^+$ conductance—relative to K$^+$—would shift V_m toward the positive Na$^+$ equilibrium potential (E_{Na}), whereas the subsequent increase in K$^+$ conductance would restore the original negative resting potential, which approaches the K$^+$ equilibrium potential (E_K). We can thus attribute the depolarizing and repolarizing phases of the action potential to a transient reversal of the large resting conductance of K$^+$ relative to Na$^+$.

The Na$^+$ and K$^+$ Currents That Flow during the Action Potential Are Time and Voltage Dependent

The assumption of independent permeability pathways—or distinct channels for Na$^+$ and K$^+$—has been verified by ionic substitution and pharmacologic experiments. Figure 7–5 illustrates the use of inhibitors to pharmacologically dissect Na$^+$ and K$^+$ currents (I_{Na} and I_K) from the total membrane current (I_m) in a typical excitable membrane preparation, such as a myelinated vertebrate nerve fiber bathed in a normal physiological solution. In a myelinated nerve, these currents flow through small segments

of the axon that are *not* covered with myelin; these segments are called nodes of Ranvier. As we shall see, pharmacologic dissection of Na$^+$ and K$^+$ currents allows us to determine how they vary with time and how they depend on V_m.

TIME DEPENDENCE OF Na$^+$ AND K$^+$ CURRENTS. Stepwise *hyperpolarization* of the nerve membrane (from a "holding potential" of −80 to −140 mV) by a voltage-clamp technique produces a transient capacitative current (p. 157), but little or no ionic current (see Fig. 7–5A). However, a step *depolarization* of equivalent magnitude produces a capacitative transient current that is followed by a large, time-dependent ionic current (Fig. 7–5B). This ionic current first flows inward, reaches a maximum in the inward direction, and then reverses to the outward direction. The initial inward current corresponds to a movement of cations into the axon. After the reversal of I_m, the outward current corresponds to an outward movement of cations. Ion substitution experiments—in which selected ions are removed from either the outside or the inside of the cell—have shown that the inward current corresponds to Na$^+$ current and the outward current corresponds to K$^+$ current. Applying a particular organic cation, tetraethylammonium (TEA), to an axon prevents the outward I_K

and reveals the isolated inward I_{Na} (see Fig. 7–5C, top I_m record). Conversely, adding either tetrodotoxin (TTX) or saxitoxin (STX)—which we will discuss later—abolishes the inward I_{Na} and reveals the isolated outward I_K (see Fig. 7–5C, bottom I_m record). TEA, TTX, and STX are cationic molecules that act as specific ion channel blockers. Millimolar concentrations of TEA block the outer entrance of certain neuronal K^+ channels, and nanomolar concentrations of TTX (or STX) block the outer entrance of neuronal Na^+ channels. Biophysical evidence suggests that these particular molecules act by binding in the outer vestibule of their respective channels, thus occluding the channel pore to permeant ions. Thus, the terms "channel block" and "blocking agent" are often used to describe their effect.

VOLTAGE DEPENDENCE OF Na⁺ AND K⁺ CURRENTS. The ability to use specific inhibitors to resolve separate pathways for Na^+ and K^+ current in excitable membranes makes it possible to characterize how these ionic currents depend on V_m. Figure 7–6A illustrates an idealized family of records of total membrane current (I_m) recorded from a myelinated nerve axon. In each case, V_m was initially clamped to −60 mV and then rapidly shifted to a more positive value. The five traces in Figure 7–6A show the current evoked by depolarizations to −45, −30, 0, +30, and +60 mV, respectively. By repeating the same experiment in the presence of TEA or TTX, one can obtain the unique time course and voltage dependence of I_{Na} and I_K.

The time course of I_{Na} obtained in the presence of TEA to block K^+ channels, is distinctly biphasic (see Fig. 7–6B). Immediately after a depolarizing voltage step to a V_m of −30 mV, for example, the inward I_{Na} (downward-going) reaches a "peak" value and then returns to zero. The initial phase of this time course (before the "peak") is called **activation**, and the later phase (after the "peak") is called **inactivation**.

In contrast to I_{Na}, a depolarizing voltage step to a V_m of +60 mV, for example, causes the outward I_K to activate with a definite lag time that gives rise to a sigmoidal time course (see Fig. 7–6C). Moreover, I_K takes longer to reach its maximal value ("peak"). Notice that the K^+ current is sustained even at the end of the depolarizing pulse. Thus, I_K does not show significant inactivation over the same rapid time scale as does I_{Na}.

If we measure the peak Na^+ and K^+ currents obtained at each of the clamped voltages in experiments such as those in Figure 7–6B and C, we can plot these peak values of I_{Na} and I_K as a function of the clamped V_m values at which they were obtained. The result is the two I-V relationships shown in Figure 7–6D. Because the currents in Figure 7–6B and C represent the activity of many individual ion channels, the plots in Figure 7–6D are **macroscopic current-voltage relationships.** The I-V relationship for K^+ is the more straightforward of the two. If we step V_m from −60 mV to increasingly more positive values, the peak I_K is outward and increases with voltage in a monotonic fashion, as expected from Ohm's law ($\Delta I = \Delta V/R$). Because such nerve K^+ channels pass current in the outward direction and activate with a time delay (see Fig. 7–6C) under physiological conditions, the term **delayed rectifier K⁺** current (or delayed, outwardly rectify-

ing K^+ channel) has been coined. We discuss this delayed outward rectifying K^+ current and the K^+ channel responsible for it in more detail later.

The voltage dependence of the peak Na^+ current is biphasic. Stepping V_m from −60 mV to more positive values at first causes I_{Na} to become increasingly negative (i.e., inward) and then reach a "peak." This portion of the Na^+ I-V relationship is sometimes referred to as the "negative resistance region" because the negative slope corresponds to an anomalous or negative resistance value according to Ohm's law ($\Delta I = \Delta V/R$). At more positive values of V_m, the peak I_{Na} reverses direction and becomes more positive, with a nearly linear or "ohmic" dependence on voltage.

The Macroscopic Na⁺ and K⁺ Currents During an Action Potential Are the Result of Opening and Closing of Single Channels

The complex macroscopic I-V relationships of the Na^+ and K^+ currents (see Fig. 7–6D) reflect the single-channel conductance and gating of Na^+ and K^+ channels. The pore of an open channel is expected to have a linear or "ohmic" I-V relationship:

Equation 7–2

$$i_X = g_X(V_m - E_X)$$

Here, i_X is the single-channel current and g_X is the single-channel conductance. We already introduced a similar relationship as Equation 6–15. Figure 7–7A illustrates the predicted linear behavior of single-channel currents as a function of V_m for hypothetical Na^+ and K^+ channels. Because we assumed a Na^+ reversal potential (E_{Na}) of +50 mV, the Na^+ current is zero at a V_m of +50 mV. Similarly, because we assumed an E_K of −80 mV, the K^+ current is zero at a V_m of −80 mV. Because we assumed a unitary conductance of 20 pS for each channel, the two I-V relationships have the same slope. Note that these idealized single-channel I-V plots for Na^+ and K^+ approximate the shape of the macroscopic peak I-V relationships of Figure 7–6D for the positive V_m range (i.e., in the right upper quadrant of Fig. 7–6D). In this V_m range, both the Na^+ and K^+ channels through which the currents flow are maximally activated at the peaks of their respective time courses. Thus the macroscopic peak I-V relationships (see Fig. 7–6D) are nearly linear in this range, just as they would be for idealized, fully open channels (see Fig. 7–7A).

However, in the *negative* voltage range, the macroscopic peak I-V relationships for Na^+ and K^+ in Figure 7–6D deviate from the linear (or ohmic) behavior in Figure 7–7A. Why, as the voltage is made more negative, does the inward Na^+ current fail to increase further, and even decrease ("negative resistance")? Similarly, why, as the voltage becomes more negative, does the outward K^+ current fall to zero long before the voltage reaches an E_K of −80 mV? The answer is that the probability that the Na^+ and K^+ channels are "open" (P_o)—and therefore able to conduct current—depends on voltage. We introduced the

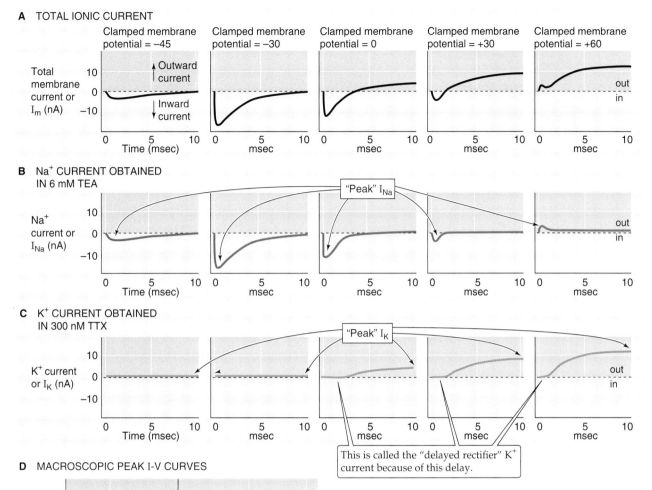

A TOTAL IONIC CURRENT

B Na$^+$ CURRENT OBTAINED IN 6 mM TEA

C K$^+$ CURRENT OBTAINED IN 300 nM TTX

This is called the "delayed rectifier" K$^+$ current because of this delay.

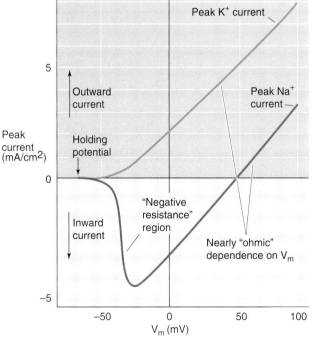

D MACROSCOPIC PEAK I-V CURVES

FIGURE 7–6. Voltage dependence of ionic currents. *A*, The *top panels* show the time course of the total ionic current. This is a voltage-clamp experiment on a frog node of Ranvier. Suddenly shifting V_m from a holding potential of −60 mV to −45, −30, 0, +30, and +60 mV elicits ionic currents that depend on V_m. *B*, These results are comparable to those in *A*, except that TEA abolished the outward K$^+$ currents, leaving the Na$^+$ current. Notice that the "peak" Na$^+$ current varies with V_m. *C*, These results are comparable to those in *A*, except that TTX abolished the inward Na$^+$ currents, leaving the K$^+$ current. Notice that the "peak" K$^+$ current varies with V_m. *D*, The *blue curve* is a plot of peak Na$^+$ currents from experiments that are similar to those in *B*. The *green curve* is a plot of peak K$^+$ currents from experiments that are similar to those in *C*. Notice that both the Na$^+$ and the K$^+$ currents are linear or "ohmic" in the positive voltage range. In a more negative V_m range, the Na$^+$ current exhibits "negative resistance"; that is, the magnitude of the current becomes more negative rather than positive as V_m increases in the positive direction. TEA, tetraethylammonium; TTX, tetrodotoxin. *A–C*, data from Hille B: Common mode of action of three agents that decrease the transient change in sodium permeability in nerves. Nature 210:1220–1222, 1966 and Hille B: The selective inhibition of delayed potassium currents in nerve by tetraethylammonium ions. J Gen Physiol 50:1287–1302, 1967. *D*, data from Cole KS, Moore JW: Ionic current measurements in the squid giant axon membrane. J Gen Physiol 44:123–167, 1960.)

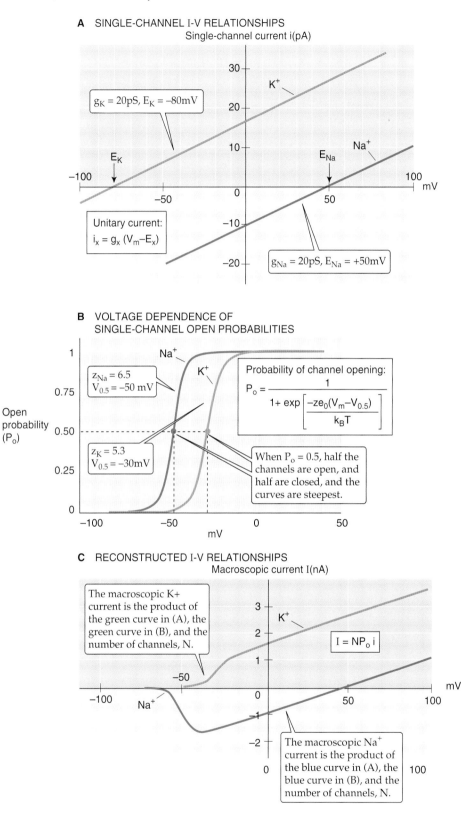

A   SINGLE-CHANNEL I-V RELATIONSHIPS

Single-channel current i(pA)

$g_K = 20pS, E_K = -80mV$

K^+

E_K

E_{Na} Na^+

Unitary current:
$i_x = g_x (V_m - E_x)$

$g_{Na} = 20pS, E_{Na} = +50mV$

**B   VOLTAGE DEPENDENCE OF
SINGLE-CHANNEL OPEN PROBABILITIES**

Open probability (P_o)

Na^+

$z_{Na} = 6.5$
$V_{0.5} = -50$ mV

K^+

Probability of channel opening:
$$P_o = \frac{1}{1 + \exp\left[\dfrac{-ze_0(V_m - V_{0.5})}{k_B T}\right]}$$

$z_K = 5.3$
$V_{0.5} = -30mV$

When $P_o = 0.5$, half the channels are open, and half are closed, and the curves are steepest.

C   RECONSTRUCTED I-V RELATIONSHIPS

Macroscopic current I(nA)

The macroscopic K+ current is the product of the green curve in (A), the green curve in (B), and the number of channels, N.

K^+

$I = NP_o i$

Na^+

The macroscopic Na^+ current is the product of the blue curve in (A), the blue curve in (B), and the number of channels, N.

FIGURE 7–7. The microscopic basis of macroscopic I-V relationships. *A,* The *blue line* represents the I-V relationship of an idealized, open Na^+ channel. The *green line* represents the I-V relationship of an idealized, open K^+ channel. Because the channels are assumed to always be fully open (i.e., the conductance does not change with voltage), the current through them is linear or "ohmic." *B,* The *blue curve* shows the open probability of Na^+ channels. The equation shown in the *inset* will generate this curve if the values $z_{Na} = 6.5$ and $V_{0.5} = -50$ mV are inserted. The *green curve* shows the open probability of K^+ channels. The equation in the *inset* will generate this curve if the values $z_K = 5.3$, and $V_{0.5} = -30$ mV are inserted. *C,* We can obtain a reasonable estimate for the macroscopic Na^+ current and the macroscopic K^+ current by multiplying the single-channel current in A, the P_O in B, and the number of channels (N). We assume that there are 100 Na^+ and 100 K^+ channels.

concept of open probability on p. 162. To see why V_m might affect P_o, we consider a simplified model.

Assume that a channel protein molecule may exist in either of two conformational states, closed (C) and open (O), and that these two conformational states are in equilibrium with one another:

$$C \rightleftharpoons O$$

The equilibrium constant K_{eq} for this reaction is the ratio of the concentrations of open to closed channels, which can also be expressed as the ratio of the probability that the channel is open (P_o) to the probability that the channel is closed (P_c):

Equation 7−3

$$K_{eq} = \frac{[Open]}{[Closed]} = \frac{P_o}{P_c}$$

In the case of voltage-gated channel proteins, V_m changes affect K_{eq} and thus the distribution of channels between the open and closed states. The probability of a channel's being open depends on V_m, according to a Boltzmann distribution (see Fig. 7−7B).

If the valence (z) of the voltage-sensing part of the channel protein (i.e., the "gating charge") is positive, the probability of channel opening should increase from 0 to 1 in a sigmoid fashion as V_m becomes more positive. Figure 7−7B shows the behavior of P_o for hypothetical Na^+ and K^+ channels that simulate Na^+ and K^+ channels in real cells.

To summarize, Figure 7−7A shows that once a single channel is open, the current flowing through the open channel is linearly related to V_m. Figure 7−7B shows that the likelihood that the channel is open depends on V_m in a sigmoid fashion. The actual macroscopic current (I_x) depends on the number of channels (N) in the area being sampled, the open probability, and the single-channel current, as we already pointed out in Equation 6−21:

Equation 7−4

$$I_X = N \, P_o \, i_X$$

Thus, we can use Equation 7−5 to compute the macroscopic currents (I) contributed by our hypothetical Na^+ and K^+ channels. We merely multiply the number of channels (which we assume to be 100 for both cations), the open probability for Na^+ and K^+ channels in Figure 7−7B, and the single-channel currents for Na^+ and K^+ in Figure 7−7A. If we compare the resulting hypothetical I_{Na} and I_K curves in Figure 7−7C, which are based on a simple theory, with actual data on macroscopic I-V relationships (see Fig. 7−6D), we see that this model provides a reasonable description of voltage-sensitive ionic currents.

Hodgkin and Huxley Used Voltage- and Time-Dependent Parameters to Accurately Predict Macroscopic Currents and the Shape of the Action Potential

Even before the concepts of single channels and channel proteins emerged, Hodgkin and Huxley in 1952 formulated voltage-dependent and time-dependent parameters to predict the ionic currents that underlie the action potential of the squid giant axon. Hodgkin and Huxley defined a series of three dimensionless parameters, n, m, and h, each of which can have a value between 0 and 1. The activation parameter n describes the probability that the K^+ channels are open (Fig. 7−8A). The activation parameter m describes the probability that the Na^+ channels are open (Fig. 7−8B, *blue curve*). Because Hodgkin and Huxley observed that the Na^+ current **inactivates**, they

introduced the inactivation parameter h to describe this process (Fig. 7−8B, *violet curve*).

Hodgkin and Huxley developed an equation for total membrane current (I_m) and used it to predict the shape of the action potential in the squid giant axon. Figure 7−8C shows their *predicted* action potential, which is triggered by a brief depolarization. Figure 7−8D shows an actual recording. The close agreement between the Hodgkin-Huxley (HH) theory and experiment indicates that this model provides a reasonable description of nerve excitation. The fundamental observation of Hodgkin and Huxley was that a rapid increase in Na^+ conductance causes the upswing or depolarizing phase of the action potential as V_m approaches E_{Na}, whereas inactivation of Na^+ conductance and delayed activation of K^+ conductance underlie the repolarization of V_m to its resting value near E_K. The importance of the HH model in electrophysiology is that it was the first analysis that accurately described the time course and voltage dependence of ionic currents that occur during an action potential.

In addition to delineating the basis of the action potential waveform, the HH model also explains threshold behavior and the refractory period. For an action potential to fire, an external stimulus must depolarize the membrane above threshold to activate a sufficient number of Na^+ channels. The external stimulus can come from an electrode, a synaptic event, or propagation of a depolarizing wave along the cell membrane. What determines whether a stimulus will be sufficient to reach the threshold V_m for firing an action potential? The number of Na^+ channels activated by the stimulus is determined by the voltage dependence of the *activation* process (i.e., m parameter). Opposing the local depolarization that is produced by the current flowing through these Na^+ channels are current losses that occur because of passive spread of the current through intracellular and extracellular fluid (see discussion of cable theory on p. 200). Also opposing depolarization is the hyperpolarizing effect of currents through any open K^+ or Cl^- channels in the membrane. Thus, the **threshold** is the level of depolarization at which the depolarizing effect of the open Na^+ channels becomes sufficiently self-reinforcing to overcome these opposing influences. Once threshold is reached, further activation of Na^+ channels rapidly drives V_m toward E_{Na}.

The basis of the **absolute refractory period**, the time during which a second action potential cannot occur under any circumstances, is *Na^+ channel inactivation*. In other words, it is impossible to recruit a sufficient number of Na^+ channels to generate a second spike unless previously activated Na^+ channels have recovered from inactivation (i.e., h parameter), a process that takes several milliseconds. The **relative refractory period**, during which a stronger-than-normal stimulus is required to elicit a second action potential, depends largely on delayed K^+ *channel opening* (i.e., n parameter). In other words, for a certain period after the peak of the action potential, the increased K^+ conductance tends to hyperpolarize the membrane, so a stronger depolarizing stimulus is required to activate the population of Na^+ channels that in the meantime have reprimed for activation.

Another key feature of the HH model is that it implies that V_m activates a channel by inducing the movement of

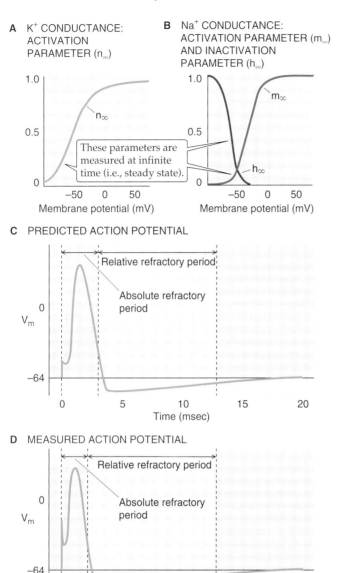

A K⁺ CONDUCTANCE: ACTIVATION PARAMETER (n_∞)

B Na⁺ CONDUCTANCE: ACTIVATION PARAMETER (m_∞) AND INACTIVATION PARAMETER (h_∞)

These parameters are measured at infinite time (i.e., steady state).

C PREDICTED ACTION POTENTIAL

D MEASURED ACTION POTENTIAL

FIGURE 7–8. Voltage-dependent parameters of the Hodgkin-Huxley model and their use in predicting the shape of the action potential. *A,* The *n* parameter describes the probability that each of four particles in the K⁺ channel are in the proper state for channel opening. It is believed that these four "particles" are the gates of the four K⁺-channel subunits. The parameter plotted here is the value of n at infinite time. *B,* The *m* parameter describes the probability that each of three particles in the Na⁺ channel are in the proper state for channel opening. The *h* parameter describes the probability that an inactivation particle is *not* in the proper state for inactivating the Na⁺ channel. Thus, a high *h* favors the open state of the channel. The parameters plotted here are the values of *m* and *h* at infinite time. *C,* Hodgkin and Huxley used data similar to those in *A* and *B,* to compute the time course of an action potential in the squid giant axon. *D,* The actual data are very similar to the computed action potential in *C.* (Data from Hodgkin AL, Huxley AF: A quantitative description of membrane current and its application to conduction and excitation in nerve. J Physiol 117:500–544, 1952.)

an electrically charged gating particle or voltage sensor across the membrane. Physically, this gating could occur by the movement of a charged portion of the channel protein through all or part of the transmembrane electric field or by the reorientation of an electric dipole (a neutral structure with positive and negative polarity) within the electrical field of the membrane. Thus the HH model correctly predicted that activation of a voltage-gated Na⁺ channel or K⁺ channel should be accompanied by a small movement of gating charge, which should produce a **gating current**. This prediction was satisfied in 1973 when Armstrong and Bezanilla recorded a very small, rapid outward current that is activated by depolarization in a voltage-clamped squid axon in which the ionic current of the Na⁺ channels was completely blocked by TTX (see Fig. 7–5C, bottom I_m record). This tiny, transient gating current is almost finished by the time that the slower K⁺ current begins to flow. The properties of such gating currents account for the voltage dependence of channel-

activation kinetics. Although the key features of the HH theory are correct, modern patch-clamp studies of single Na⁺ and K⁺ channels have revealed that the kinetics of channel gating are much more complicated than originally assumed. Such complexity is to be expected inasmuch as the conformational dynamics of large protein molecules cannot generally be adequately described by simple models that incorporate only a few discrete states.

PHYSIOLOGY OF VOLTAGE-GATED CHANNELS

Voltage-Gated Channels Belong to a Large Superfamily of Structurally Related Membrane Proteins

As outlined in Chapter 6, voltage-gated ion channels are a large and diverse family of evolutionarily related proteins

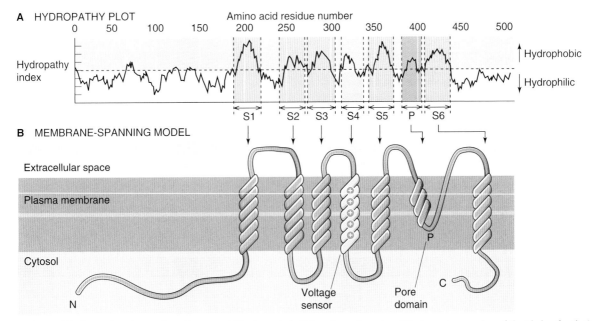

FIGURE 7–9. Model of a single subunit of a voltage-gated K⁺ channel. *A,* This voltage-dependent K⁺ channel, a member of the Shaker family (Kv1.1), has six domains (S1–S6) with a high hydropathy index. Each of these six domains (highlighted in *green* or *yellow*) is presumed to traverse the membrane completely. In addition, the channel also has a smaller region (highlighted in *red*) with a somewhat lower hydropathy index, the P domain. *B,* This model is based on the hydropathy data in A. The six membrane-spanning segments are assumed to be α helices. The S4 segment (highlighted in *yellow*) has a large number of positively charged lysine and arginine residues and appears to be the voltage sensor. The linker between the S5 and S6 segments is known as the P region, which lines the pore of the channel. (Data from Shen NV, Pfaffinger PJ: Conservation of K⁺ channel properties in gene subfamilies. In Peracchia C [ed]: Handbook of Membrane Channels: Molecular and Cellular Physiology. New York, Academic Press, 1994, pp 5–16.)

that includes Na⁺ channels, Ca²⁺ channels, K⁺ channels, and more distant relatives, such as the cyclic nucleotide–gated (CNG) channels. Initial progress toward biochemical characterization of the voltage-gated ion channels responsible for the action potential began with the discovery of naturally occurring, specific, high-affinity neurotoxins such as TTX and STX and their use as biochemical probes. Tritium-labeled derivatives of TTX and STX were prepared chemically and used in radioligand-binding assays to directly measure the number of voltage-gated Na⁺ channels in excitable tissues.

The electroplax organ of the electric eel (*Electrophorus electricus*) proved to be a convenient source of tissue for the first successful biochemical purification of the Na⁺ channel protein by Agnew and coworkers in 1978. These Na⁺ channels consist of a large glycosylated α subunit of about 200 kDa that contains the TTX binding site. Reconstitution experiments revealed that this subunit—by itself—mediates ionic selectivity for Na⁺, voltage-dependent gating, and pharmacologic sensitivity to various neurotoxins. Thus, the α subunit is the channel-forming protein.

Similar biochemical purification procedures on rat skeletal muscle and brain led to the identification of analogous mammalian Na⁺ channel α subunits. In addition to the α subunit, the rat skeletal muscle Na⁺ channel also contains a 38-kDa subunit, and the rat brain Na⁺ channel contains both a 33- and a 36-kDa subunit. These smaller subunits of mammalian Na⁺ channels are called β subunits. Although the exact function of the auxiliary β subunits is still under investigation, they appear to play a role in modulating channel gating or channel expression.

Molecular biologic studies of voltage-gated channels began in 1984 with the cloning of the *Electrophorus* **Na⁺ channel** α subunit by the laboratory of Shosaku Numa. These investigators used antibodies raised against the purified α subunit to screen a cDNA library, and they isolated the cDNA encoding the electroplax Na⁺ channel. In addition, direct sequencing of channel peptides provided partial amino-acid sequence information. Similar strategies led to the purification and cloning of voltage-gated **Ca²⁺ channel** proteins from skeletal muscle and brain tissue. The primary sequence of the α₁ subunit of the Ca²⁺ channel is structurally homologous to the α subunit of the Na⁺ channel.

In contrast to the biochemical approach used for Na⁺ and Ca²⁺ channels, the initial breakthrough in the molecular biology of **K⁺ channels** came with the study of *Shaker* mutants of the fruit fly *Drosophila*. These mutants are called "Shaker" because their bodies literally shake under the influence of ether anesthesia. This phenotype is due to defective voltage-gated K⁺ channels. The laboratory of L.Y. Jan and Y.N. Jan, and those of O. Pongs and M. Tanouye, used molecular genetic techniques to identify and clone the first K⁺ channel genes in 1987.

The hydropathy plot of the amino-acid sequence of a voltage-gated K⁺ channel (Fig. 7–9A) provides a relative scale of the hydrophobic or hydrophilic nature of domains of the channel molecule (p. 15). Such plots for voltage-gated K⁺ channels typically reveal six distinct peaks of hydrophobicity, corresponding to transmembrane segments S1 through S6—a conserved structural feature of all voltage-gated K⁺ channels. Transmembrane segments S1 through S6 are thought to have an α-helical

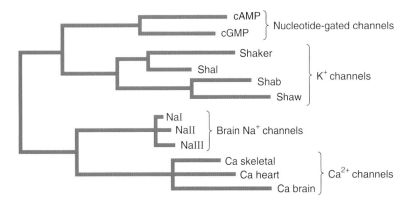

FIGURE 7–10. Family tree of hypothetical evolutionary relationships among voltage-gated cation channels based on sequences of the S4 segments. This dendrogram of the superfamily of voltage-gated channels shows four distinct branches or families. Only a few examples of each are depicted. The family of nucleotide-gated channels is represented by mammalian channels that are gated by cAMP and cGMP. The family of K⁺ channels is presented by four types of *Drosophila* channels. The family of Na⁺ channels is represented by three types of Na⁺ channels from mammalian brain. Finally, the family of Ca²⁺ channels is represented by mammalian channels from skeletal muscle, heart, and brain. (Data from Strong M, Chandy KG, Gutman GA: Molecular evolution of voltage-sensitive ion channel genes: On the origin of electrical excitability. Mol Biol Evol 10:221–242, 1993.)

secondary structure and to be connected by cytoplasmic and extracellular linker regions that are drawn as extended loops (see Fig. 7–9B).

Sequence analysis and biochemical studies can help identify sites of post-translational protein modification, such as extracellular glycosylation sites and intracellular phosphorylation sites, which provide additional topologic information. Extensive mutagenesis studies on cloned channel genes have associated various channel functions and binding sites with particular domains. The **S4 segment** is of particular interest because it has 4 to 7 lysine or arginine residues that occur at every third position. Because an α helix completes one turn every 3.6 residues, these positively charged residues may form a charged edge of the S4 segment (p. 20). Functional evidence indicates that these positively charged residues of the S4 segment play an important role in the **voltage-sensing mechanism** of channel activation.

The extracellular linker region between the S5 and S6 segments is termed the **P region** (for pore region) and is of special significance inasmuch as it contains residues that form the binding sites for toxins and external blocking molecules such as TEA. The P region also contains residues that are critical determinants of the ionic selectivity for permeant cations. Compelling evidence indicates that the S6 transmembrane segment is associated with the internal aspect of the ion conduction pathway.

The initial identification of genes encoding Na⁺, Ca²⁺, and K⁺ channels has led to the discovery of many related channel genes from numerous animal species, including humans. Sequence analysis indicates that they constitute a large protein superfamily.

Figure 7–10 shows a phylogenetic tree of related channel proteins that is based on a comparison of the nucleotide sequences of the S4 segment of the channel. This tree contains four branches corresponding to four distinct subfamilies of channels: K⁺ channels, Na⁺ channels, Ca²⁺ channels, and CNG channels.

In 1998, a major breakthrough in the structure of ion channel proteins was achieved when MacKinnon and col-

A   TOP VIEW

B   LATERAL VIEW

C   LATERAL VIEW (SPACE-FILLING)

FIGURE 7–11. Structure of the *Streptomyces* K⁺ channel (KcsA). *A,* KcsA is a homotetramer. Each monomer is represented in a different color and contains only two membrane-spanning elements, which is analogous to the S5-P-S6 portion of Shaker-type K⁺ channels. *B,* This view more clearly shows the P region, which is very similar to the P region of the Shaker K⁺ channel. The P region appears to form the selectivity filter of the channel. *C,* This is a cut-away view of the pore that shows three K⁺ ions. The top two K⁺ ions are bound in a tight cage that is formed by the peptide backbones of the P regions of each of the four channel subunits. (Data from Doyle DA, Morais Cabral J, Pfuetzner RA, et al: The structure of the potassium channel: Molecular basis of K⁺ conduction and selectivity. Science 280:69–77, 1998.)

A Na$^+$ CHANNEL

FIGURE 7–12. Subunit structure and membrane-folding models of voltage-gated channels. *A*, A voltage-gated Na$^+$ channel is made up of a pseudo-oligomeric α subunit, as well as membrane-spanning β_1 and β_2 subunits. Note that the domains I through IV of the α subunit are homologous to a single subunit of a voltage-gated K$^+$ channel (see *C*). *B*, A voltage-gated Ca^{2+} channel is made up of a pseudo-oligomeric α_1 subunit, as well as an extracellular α_2 subunit, a cytoplasmic β subunit, and membrane-spanning γ and δ subunits. Note that the domains I through IV of the α subunit are homologous to a single subunit of a voltage-gated K$^+$ channel (see *C*). *C*, A voltage-gated K$^+$ channel is made up of four α subunits, as well as a cytoplasmic β subunit. (Data from Isom LL, De Jongh KS, Catterall WA: Auxiliary subunits of voltage-gated ion channels. Neuron 12:1183–1194, 1994.)

CRYSTAL STRUCTURE OF A K⁺ CHANNEL

In 1998, the laboratory of Roderick MacKinnon at Rockefeller University solved the three-dimensional structure of a small K⁺ channel protein. To accomplish this feat they first expressed a recombinant version of a K⁺ channel protein from the actinomycete bacterium *Streptomyces lividans* in the host bacterium *Escherichia coli*. They solubilized the bacteria in detergent and purified large amounts of the expressed recombinant K⁺ channel protein KcsA. They also found conditions suitable for growing protein crystals, which they analyzed by x-ray diffraction analysis to a resolution of approximately 3.2 Å.

The KcsA channel is a prokaryotic homolog of the vertebrate inward rectifier K⁺ channel gene family, which we discuss later in this chapter. As is the case for the Shaker-type K⁺ channels, KcsA is a homotetramer. However, each monomer of KcsA contains only two membrane-spanning elements and a P region, analogous to the S5-P-S6 portion of K_V channels. The P-region sequence of KcsA is very similar to the P region of the Shaker K⁺ channel, which contains amino acid residues critical for K⁺ selectivity, as well as extracellular sensitivity to blockade by tetraethylammonium (TEA) and charybdotoxin. Figure 7–11 shows a ribbon diagram representation of the structure of KcsA, in one view looking down from the top of the membrane (Fig. 7–11A) and in a second view looking from the side (Fig. 7–11B). Each of the four subunits of the protein is shown in a different color. Starting from the intracellular N terminus, the first transmembrane span ("outer helix," corresponding to Shaker S5) forms an α helix that serves as the periphery of the channel. After crossing the membrane to the extracellular side, the peptide backbone then forms a loop that corresponds to the **P region.** The first half of this loop is a short α helix that folds back a short distance into the plane of the membrane and then immediately exits the extracellular side of the membrane. In the tetrameric complex that constitutes the channel protein, this latter portion of the P loop forms a narrow region called the **ion selectivity filter.** After exiting the extracellular face of the membrane, the peptide backbone turns again to form a third α helix ("inner helix," corresponding to Shaker S6) that crosses the membrane to the intracellular side. The four inner helices of the tetramer form the scaffold of the ion channel pore. These four inner helices are tilted in a remarkable flower-like configuration that has also been likened to four poles of an inverted teepee tent dwelling.

This structure reveals the basis for K⁺ selectivity by showing that the selectivity filter region is lined not by the side chains of amino acids, but rather by the carbonyl oxygen atoms contributed by the peptide backbone of several amino acid residues in the P region. Two K⁺ ions in the selectivity filter (near the extracellular surface of the channel) appear to be coordinated in a tight cage by oxygen atoms contributed by each of the four subunits. The size of this cage is just the right size for a K⁺ ion. A smaller Na⁺ ion would fit too loosely, so its binding in the cage would not be energetically favorable in comparison to its binding to water in its normal hydrated state.

Figure 7–11C is a cutaway surface view of the pore showing the probable location of three K⁺ ions in the crystal structure. The presence of three K⁺ ions in the pore is consistent with many electrophysiologic studies, which suggested that multiple K⁺ ions move through the channel in single file.

For his work on the structural biology of ion channels, Roderick MacKinnon shared the 2003 Nobel Prize in Chemistry.

leagues first reported the crystal structure of a K⁺ channel protein. This work revealed the three-dimensional structure of a protein that contained segments analogous to the S5–P–S6 part of voltage-gated channels (see Fig. 7–11 and the box entitled "Crystal Structure of a K⁺ Channel").

Figure 7–12 is a schematic representation of the predicted membrane-folding diagrams of the superfamily of voltage-gated ion channels. In keeping with the nomenclature that was first established for Na⁺ channels, the channel-forming subunit of each type of channel is called the α subunit for Na⁺ and K⁺ channels and the α_1 subunit in the case of Ca²⁺ channels. Other identified accessory subunits are designated as β_1 and β_2 for Na⁺ channels; α_2, β, γ, and δ for Ca²⁺ channels; and β for K⁺ channels.

The α and α_1 subunits of this protein superfamily all contain the common S1 through S6 domain that was described earlier for K⁺ channels. The α subunit of Na⁺ channels (see Fig. 7–12A) and the α_1 subunit of Ca²⁺ channels (see Fig. 7–12B) consist of four internally homologous repeats—domains I, II, III, and IV—each containing an S1 through S6 motif. K⁺ channels (see Fig. 7–12C) are believed to represent an evolutionary precursor of this voltage-gated channel superfamily inasmuch as their pore-forming α subunit is smaller in size, ranging from 60 to 100 kDa, and contains only one S1 through S6 motif. Voltage-gated K⁺ channels are formed by a rosette-like association of four α subunits. Because Na⁺ and Ca²⁺ channels are composed of four internally homologous repeats of S1 through S6, all α subunits of this channel superfamily presumably function as tetrameric (K⁺ channels) or pseudotetrameric (Na⁺ and Ca²⁺ channels) units. Molecular evolution of the pseudotetrameric structure of Na⁺ and Ca²⁺ channels is believed to have occurred by consecutive gene duplication of a primordial gene containing the basic S1 through S6 motif.

Na⁺ Channels Are Responsible for the Rapid Depolarization During the Action Potential

Because the equilibrium potential for Na⁺ and Ca²⁺ is in the positive voltage range for normal cellular ionic gradients, channels that are selectively permeable to these ions mediate electrical depolarization. However, prolonged cellular depolarization is an adverse condition inasmuch as it results in sustained contraction and rigor of muscle fibers, cardiac dysfunction, and abnormally elevated levels of intracellular Ca²⁺, which leads to cell death. Thus, Na⁺ and

FIGURE 7–13. Effect of extracellular Ca^{2+} concentration on Na^+-channel activation. High $[Ca^{2+}]_o$ shifts the P_o versus V_m to more positive voltages (i.e., less excitable). Thus, *hypo*calcemia leads to *hyper*excitability.

Ca^{2+} channels normally reside in a closed conformation at the resting membrane potential. Their opening is an intrinsically transient process that is determined by the kinetics of channel activation and inactivation.

The primary role of voltage-gated Na^+ channels is to produce the initial depolarizing phase of fast action potentials in neurons and skeletal and cardiac muscle. The selectivity of Na^+ channels to Na^+ is much higher than that for other alkali cations. The permeability ratio of Na^+ relative to K^+ (P_{Na}/P_K) lies in the range of 11 to 20 under physiological conditions. Voltage-gated Na^+ channels are virtually impermeable to Ca^{2+} and other divalent cations under normal physiological conditions.

Although Na^+ channels do not significantly conduct Ca^{2+} ions across the cell membrane, the voltage dependence of Na^+ channel gating is nevertheless dependent on the extracellular Ca^{2+} concentration ($[Ca^{2+}]_o$). If $[Ca^{2+}]_o$ is progressively increased above the normal physiological level, the voltage activation range of Na^+ channels progressively shifts to a more positive range. In Figure 7–13 this change is represented as a shift in the P_o versus V_m relationship. Similarly, if $[Ca^{2+}]_o$ is decreased, the voltage activation range is shifted to more negative voltages. This

phenomenon has important clinical implications because a negative shift corresponds to a **reduced voltage threshold** for action potential firing and results in hyperexcitability and spontaneous muscle twitching. Similarly, a positive voltage shift of Na^+ channel gating corresponds to decreased electrical excitability (i.e., the threshold is now further away from resting V_m) and muscle weakness. Thus, metabolic disorders that result in abnormal plasma $[Ca^{2+}]$, such as hypoparathyroidism (low $[Ca^{2+}]$) and hyperparathyroidism (high $[Ca^{2+}]$), can cause marked neurologic and neuromuscular symptoms. The mechanism of this voltage shift in Na^+ channel gating by extracellular divalent cations such as Ca^{2+} is thought to involve an alteration in the transmembrane electric field that is sensed by the channel protein. Presumably, this alteration is caused by Ca^{2+} binding or electrostatic screening of negative charges at the membrane surface.

Mammals have at least nine homologous genes that encode the pore-forming α subunit of Na^+ channels (Table 7–1). The isoforms encoded by these genes are expressed in different excitable tissues and can be partially discriminated on the basis of their sensitivity to TTX. Four of the isoforms (Nav 1.1, 1.2, 1.3, and 1.6) are differentially expressed in various regions of the brain. One isoform (Nav 1.4) is the major isoform in skeletal muscle. This muscle Na^+ channel is also uniquely sensitive to blockade by a peptide toxin called μ-conotoxin from a venomous marine snail. Natural mutations in the human gene for this last Na^+ channel result in a variety of human genetic diseases, such as hyperkalemic periodic paralysis, and in several types of myotonia (see box titled "Na^+ Channel Genetic Defects"). Heart ventricular muscle expresses a TTX-insensitive isoform (Nav 1.5) that also appears in skeletal muscle after denervation. Various natural mutations in the heart Na^+ channel cause irregularities in heartbeat characterized by a particular type of long QT syndrome. Neurons from the dorsal root ganglia express Nav 1.6, 1.7, 1.8, and 1.9 Na^+-channel isoforms, the latter two of which are TTX insensitive. In addition to this major family of Na^+ channels, there also appears to be another distinct subfamily that is expressed in the uterus and brain.

TABLE 7–1

Na^+ CHANNEL α-SUBUNIT ISOFORMS

ISOFORM	HUMAN GENE	TISSUE	SENSITIVITY TO TTX (MOLAR)
Nav 1.1	SCN1A	Central nervous system, heart	10^{-9}
Nav 1.2	SCN2A	Central nervous system	10^{-9}
Nav 1.3	SCN3A	Central nervous system, heart	10^{-9}
Nav 1.4	SCN4A	Skeletal muscle	10^{-9}
Nav 1.5	SCN5A	Heart, denervated skeletal muscle	Insensitive, 10^{-6}
Nav 1.6	SCN8A	Central and peripheral nervous system	10^{-9}
Nav 1.7	SCN9A	Peripheral nervous system	10^{-9}
Nav 1.8	SCN10A	Peripheral and sensory neurons	Insensitive, 10^{-6}
Nav 1.9	SCN11A	Peripheral nervous system	Insensitive, 10^{-6}

TTX, tetrodotoxin.

Na⁺ Channels Are Blocked by Neurotoxins and Local Anesthetics

Studies of the mechanism of action of neurotoxins have provided important insight into channel function and structure. The guanidinium **toxins** TTX and STX (see Fig. 7–5C) are specific blocking agents of Na⁺ channels that act on the extracellular side of the cell membrane.

TTX is produced by certain marine bacteria and is apparently accumulated in some tissues of various invertebrates, amphibians, and fish. The internal organs of certain fish, such as the puffer fish that is consumed in Japan, often contain lethal amounts of TTX. The flesh of such fish must be carefully prepared to prevent food poisoning.

STX is produced by specific species of marine dinoflagellates that are responsible for "red tide" in the ocean, as well as by freshwater cyanobacteria, which can poison ponds and rivers. It is the agent responsible for "paralytic shellfish poisoning," which is caused by human ingestion of toxic shellfish that have accumulated STX-producing plankton. Death from TTX and STX intoxication, which ultimately results from respiratory paralysis, can be pre-

vented by the timely administration of mechanical respiration.

As mentioned earlier, the snail peptide μ-conotoxin similarly blocks muscle Na⁺ channels by binding near the external binding site for TTX and STX.

TTX, STX, and μ-conotoxin are important pharmacologic probes because they can be used to functionally discriminate among several distinct isoforms of Na⁺ channels (see Table 7–1). Other important neurotoxins that act on Na⁺ channels include batrachotoxin (a steroidal alkaloid from certain tropical frogs and birds), various plant alkaloids (veratridine, grayanotoxin, aconitine), natural plant insecticides (pyrethrins), brevetoxins (cyclic polyethers from dinoflagellates), and two distinct classes (α and β) of peptide scorpion toxins. Members of this diverse group of neurotoxins act primarily by altering the gating kinetics of Na⁺ channels by promoting both a longer duration of channel opening and channel opening under voltage conditions in which Na⁺ channels are normally closed or inactivated.

Local anesthetics are a large group of synthetic drugs that are generally characterized by an aromatic moiety that is linked to a tertiary amine substituent via an ester

A   STRUCTURES OF SOME LOCAL ANESTHETICS

B   USE DEPENDENCE OF INHIBITION BY LIDOCAINE

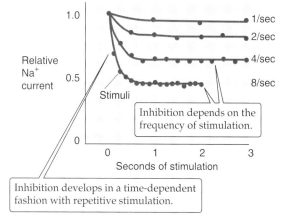

FIGURE 7–14. Effect of local anesthetics. *A,* The three clinically useful local anesthetics shown here are all synthetic analogues of the plant alkaloid cocaine. *B,* In the presence of lidocaine, the relative Na⁺ current decays with time. However, the inhibition becomes more pronounced as the rate of stimulation increases from 1/sec to 8/sec. (Data from Hille B: Local anesthetics: Hydrophilic and hydrophobic pathways for the drug-receptor reaction. J Gen Physiol 69:497–515, 1977.)

Na+ CHANNEL GENETIC DEFECTS

Several human genetic diseases have been traced to inheritable defects in the genes for skeletal and cardiac muscle Na+ channels. The skeletal muscle gene *SCN4A* is located on human chromosome 17, and the cardiac muscle gene *SCN5A* is located on chromosome 3. One of the muscle disorders is called **hyperkalemic periodic paralysis** (HYPP) because muscle weakness is triggered by an elevation in serum [K+] that may occur after vigorous exercise or ingestion of foods rich in K+. A second muscle disorder is called **paramyotonia congenita** (PC). This form of periodic paralysis may be induced in afflicted individuals by exposure to cold temperature and results in symptoms of myotonia (muscle stiffness) associated with abnormal repetitive firing of muscle action potentials. **Long QT syndrome** is an inherited defect in heart rhythm that can lead to sudden death from cardiac arrhythmia. A deletion of three amino acids, ΔKPQ, in the linker region between repetitive domains III and IV of the heart Na+ channel is the cause of this disease. We will see later in the box titled "Human Heart Defects Linked to Mutations of K+ Channels" that defects in cardiac K+ channels can also cause a long QT syndrome. As shown in Figure 7–15, a number of mutations responsible for skeletal muscle diseases have also been identified and mapped within the folding diagram of the muscle Na+ channel α subunit. These mutations generally occur in one of the putative membrane-spanning segments (S3, S4, S5, and S6). Two PC mutations have also been located in the intracellular linker segment between repeats III and IV; this linker plays an important role in Na+ channel inactivation. Electrophysiologic analysis of some of these mutations suggests that abnormal kinetics of Na+ channel gating is the underlying cause of the profound symptoms associated with these diseases. For example, the occasional failure of the mutant heart Na+ channel to inactivate results in long bursts of openings and abnormal prolongation of the action potential.

or amide linkage (Fig. 7–14A). Drug development of local anesthetics began with the recognition by Carl Koller in 1884 that the plant alkaloid **cocaine** numbs sensation in the tongue, in addition to producing psychoactive effects via its actions on the central nervous system (CNS). Attempts to synthesize safer alternatives to cocaine led to **procaine**, which mimics the local anesthetic effect of cocaine without the CNS effects.

Local anesthetics that are used clinically, such as procaine, **lidocaine**, and **tetracaine**, reversibly block nerve impulse generation and propagation by inhibiting voltage-gated Na+ channels. The action of these drugs is "use dependent," which means that inhibition of Na+ current progresses in a time-dependent manner with increasing repetitive stimulation or firing of action potentials (see Fig. 7–14B). **Use dependence** occurs because the drug binds most effectively only after the Na+ channel has already opened. This use-dependent action of the drug further enhances inhibition of nerve impulses at sites

where repetitive firing of action potentials takes place. Local anesthetics are used to control pain during dentistry, many types of minor surgery, and labor during childbirth.

Ca²⁺ Channels Contribute to Action Potentials in Some Cells and also Function in Electrical and Chemical Coupling Mechanisms

Calcium channels play important roles in the depolarization phase of certain action potentials, in coupling electrical excitation to secretion or muscle contraction, and in other signal-transduction processes. Because $[Ca^{2+}]_o$ is approximately 1.2 mM, whereas $[Ca^{2+}]_i$ is only about 10^{-7} M, a huge gradient favors the passive influx of Ca^{2+} into cells. At the relatively high $[Ca^{2+}]_o$ that prevails under physiological conditions, voltage-gated Ca^{2+} channels are highly selective for Ca^{2+}, with permeability to Ca^{2+} being about 1000-fold greater than permeability to Na+. Other alkaline earth divalent cations such as Sr^{2+} and Ba^{2+} also readily permeate through Ca^{2+} channels and are often used as substitute ions for recording the activity of Ca^{2+} channels in electrophysiologic studies. However, if $[Ca^{2+}]_o$ is reduced to a *nonphysiological* level of less than 10^{-6} M with the use of chelating agents, Ca^{2+} channels can also conduct large currents of monovalent alkali cations, such as Na+ and K+. Thus, in terms of its intrinsic ionic selectivity, the Ca^{2+} channel is functionally similar to the Na+ channel, except that high-affinity binding of Ca^{2+} in the pore effectively prevents permeation of all other physiological ions except Ca^{2+}.

The mechanism of this extraordinary selectivity behavior is based on ion-ion interactions within the pore. For the Ca^{2+} channel to conduct current, at least two Ca^{2+} ions must bind simultaneously in close proximity to sites within the channel. Interactions between individual ions within the narrow region of the channel pore appear to control ion selectivity and the ionic flux. Variations on this general mechanism, referred to as **multi-ion conduction**, have also been described for many other classes of ion channels, notably K+ channels. Multi-ion conduction generally appears to play an important role in determining the permeation properties of channels that have a very high degree of ionic selectivity, such as Ca^{2+} channels and K+ channels.

One of the major functions of voltage-gated Ca^{2+} is to contribute to the depolarizing phase of **action potentials** in certain cell types. The gating of voltage-gated Ca^{2+} channels is slower than that of Na+ channels. Whereas Na+ channels are most important in initiating action potentials and generating rapidly propagating spikes in axons, Ca^{2+} channels often give rise to a more sustained depolarizing current, which is the basis for the long-lived action potentials observed in cardiac cells, smooth muscle cells, secretory cells, and many types of neurons.

The exquisite selectivity of Ca^{2+} channels under physiological conditions endows them with special roles in **cellular regulation**. If a depolarizing electrical stimulus or a signal-transduction cascade activates these Ca^{2+} channels, the subsequent influx of Ca^{2+} raises $[Ca^{2+}]_i$, and Ca^{2+} can thereby serve as an important second messenger

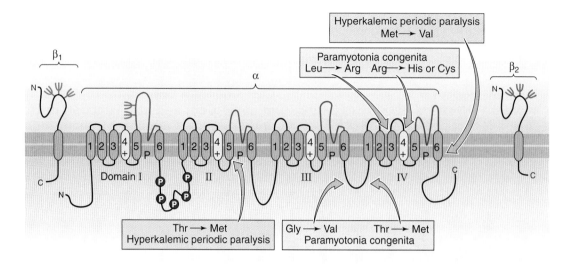

FIGURE 7–15. Some mutations of human Na$^+$ channels. At least two genetic diseases are caused by mutations in the Na$^+$ channel of human skeletal muscle. Hyperkalemic periodic paralysis can be caused by mutations in membrane-spanning segment S5 of domain II and S6 of domain IV. Paramyotonia congenita can be caused by mutations in membrane-spanning segment S3 of domain IV and S4 of domain IV. The disease can also be caused by mutations in the intracellular segment that links domains III and IV. (Data from Catterall WA: Cellular and molecular biology of voltage-gated sodium channels. Physiol Rev 72:S15–S48, 1992.)

in regulating the activity of a multitude of intracellular proteins and enzymes. Thus in serving as a major gateway for Ca^{2+} influx across the plasma membrane, Ca^{2+} channels not only have an electrical function in membrane depolarization but also have an important biochemical function in signal transduction.

Ca^{2+} channels also play a pivotal role in a special subset of signal-transduction processes known as excitation-contraction (EC) coupling and excitation-secretion (ES) coupling. **Excitation-contraction coupling** refers to the process by which an electrical depolarization at the cell membrane leads to cell contraction, such as the contraction of a skeletal muscle fiber. In EC coupling of skeletal muscle (p. 241), one class of plasma membrane Ca^{2+} channel that is located in the transverse tubule membrane of skeletal muscle serves as the voltage sensor and forms a direct structural linkage to intracellular Ca^{2+} release channels that are located in the sarcoplasmic reticulum (SR) membrane. In contrast, Ca^{2+} channels play a different role in EC coupling in cardiac muscle, where Ca^{2+} channels in the plasma membrane mediate an initial influx of Ca^{2+}. The resultant increase in [Ca^{2+}]$_i$ triggers an additional release of Ca^{2+} stored in the SR by a process known as Ca^{2+}-induced Ca^{2+} release (p. 242).

Excitation-secretion coupling is the process by which depolarization of the plasma membrane causes release of neurotransmitters in the nervous system and the secretion of hormones in the endocrine system. Such processes require an increase in [Ca^{2+}]$_i$ via the plasma membrane to trigger exocytosis of synaptic and secretory vesicles. Thus, in providing a primary signal for the initiation of cellular contraction and neurotransmitter/hormone release, Ca^{2+} channels are a fundamental locus of control.

Because Ca^{2+} channels must fulfill diverse roles, higher vertebrates use a family of genes that encode structurally homologous, but functionally diverse Ca^{2+} channels. Mammals have at least ten distinct genes for the channel-forming α_1 subunit of Ca^{2+} channels (Table 7–2). Biochemical and cloning work has also identified four accessory subunits of Ca^{2+} channels: α_2, δ, β, and γ (see Fig. 7–12B). The α_2 and δ subunits are the products of a single gene; after translation, proteolytic cleavage of the polypeptide yields α_2 and δ. Coexpression studies have shown that these latter accessory subunits can greatly influence the kinetics, voltage sensitivity, and peak currents that are exhibited by various α_1 channel subunits. This structural complexity and diversity at the genetic level are mirrored by a diversity of Ca^{2+} currents that have been differentiated in various cell types on the basis of their functional characteristics. However, complete correspondence between known structural isoforms and functional current types has not yet been achieved.

Ca^{2+} Channels Are Characterized as L-, T-, P/Q-, N-, and R-Type Channels Based on Kinetic Properties and Inhibitor Sensitivity

An example of the functional diversity of Ca^{2+} channels is illustrated in Figure 7–16, which shows two different types of voltage-gated Ca^{2+} channels that have been identified in cardiac ventricular cells by the patch-clamp technique. If the cell-attached patch, initially clamped at −50 mV, is suddenly depolarized to +10 mV, currents appear from a large-conductance (18 to 25 pS), slowly inactivating Ca^{2+} channel (see Fig. 7–16A). However, if the same patch is initially clamped at −70 mV and depolarized to only −20 mV, currents appear instead from a small-

TABLE 7–2

PROPERTIES AND CLASSIFICATION OF VOLTAGE-GATED Ca^{2+} CHANNELS

PROPERTY	CHANNEL				
	L	**T**	**N**	**P/Q**	**R**
Kinetics	Long duration	Transient	Intermediate–long duration	Intermediate–long duration	Intermediate
Voltage activation	High threshold $(> -30$ mV$)$	Low threshold $(< -30$ mV$)$	High threshold $(> -30$ mV$)$	High threshold $(> -30$ mV$)$	High threshold $(> -30$ mV$)$
Pharmacology	Blocked by DHPs	Less sensitive to DHPs	Insensitive to DHPs, blocked by ω-conotoxin GVIA	Insensitive to DHPs, blocked by ω-agatoxin IVA	Insensitive to DHPs, ω-conotoxin GVIA, and ω-agatoxin IVA
Location	Heart, skeletal muscle, neurons, vascular smooth muscle, uterus, neuroendocrine cells	SA node of heart, brain neurons	Presynaptic terminals, dendrites, and cell bodies of neurons	Cerebellar Purkinje and granule cells, cell bodies of central neurons	Cerebellar granule cells, neurons
Function	EC coupling in skeletal muscle, link membrane depolarization to intracellular Ca signalling	Repetitive firing of action potentials in heart and many neurons	Exocytotic neurotransmitter release	Exocytotic neurotransmitter release	Exocytotic neurotransmitter release
Genes	Cav 1.1 Cav 1.2 Cav 1.3 Cav 1.4	Cav 3.1 Cav 3.2 Cav 3.3	Cav 2.2	Cav 2.1	Cav 2.3

DHP, 1,4-dihydropyridine; EC, excitation-contraction; SA, sinoatrial.

conductance (8 pS), rapidly inactivating Ca^{2+} channel (see Fig. 7–16*B*). These two types of Ca^{2+} channels are respectively named **L-type** (for long lived) and **T-type** (for transient) channels. T-type channels are activated at a lower voltage threshold (more negative than -30 mV) than other types of Ca^{2+} channels are and are also inactivated over a more negative voltage range. These characteristics of T-type channels permit them to function briefly in the initiation of action potentials and to play a role in the repetitive firing of cardiac cells and neurons. Other types of Ca^{2+} channels, including L-, N-, P/Q-, and R-type channels—which are activated at a higher voltage threshold (more positive than -30 mV)—mediate the long-lived plateau phase of slow action potentials and provide a more substantial influx of Ca^{2+} for contractile and secretory responses.

In addition to discrimination on the basis of gating behavior, Ca^{2+} channel isoforms can also be distinguished by their sensitivity to different drugs and toxins (see Table 7–2). Ca^{2+} **channel blockers** are an important group of therapeutic agents. Figure 7–17 shows the structures of representatives of three different classes of Ca^{2+} channel blockers: 1,4-dihydropyridines (DHPs), phenylalkylamines, and benzothiazepines. These synthetic compounds are used in the treatment of cardiovascular disorders such as angina pectoris (p. 562) and hypertension and also are being evaluated for their potential in treating various diseases of the CNS.

DHPs such as nitrendipine selectively block L-type

Ca^{2+} channels. Phenylalkylamines (e.g., verapamil) and benzothiazepines (e.g., diltiazem) also inhibit L-type Ca^{2+} channels; however, these other two classes of drugs act at sites that are distinct from the site that binds DHPs. Particular DHP derivatives, such as Bay K8644, actually *enhance* rather than inhibit Ca^{2+} channel currents. DHPs can have the contrasting effects of either inhibitors (antagonists) or activators (agonists) because they act not by plugging the channel pore directly but by binding to a site composed of transmembrane helices S5 and S6 in domain III and S6 in domain IV. Drug binding in this region probably induces various conformational changes in channel structure and thereby perturbs Ca^{2+} permeation and gating behavior.

Other molecules that are useful in discriminating Ca^{2+} channel isoforms are present in the venom of the marine snail *Conus geographus* and the funnel web spider *Agelenopsis aperta*. The snail produces a peptide called ω-conotoxin GVIA, which selectively blocks N-type Ca^{2+} channels, whereas the spider produces the peptide ω-agatoxin IVA, which selectively blocks P/Q-type Ca^{2+} channels. N-, P/Q-, and R-type Ca^{2+} channels appear to mediate the entry of Ca^{2+} into certain types of presynaptic nerve terminals and thus play an important role in facilitating the release of neurotransmitters.

The summary of the basic properties of L-, T-, N-, P/Q-, and R-type Ca^{2+} channels contained in Table 7–2 indicates their presumed correspondence to ten known genes that encode α_1 subunits.

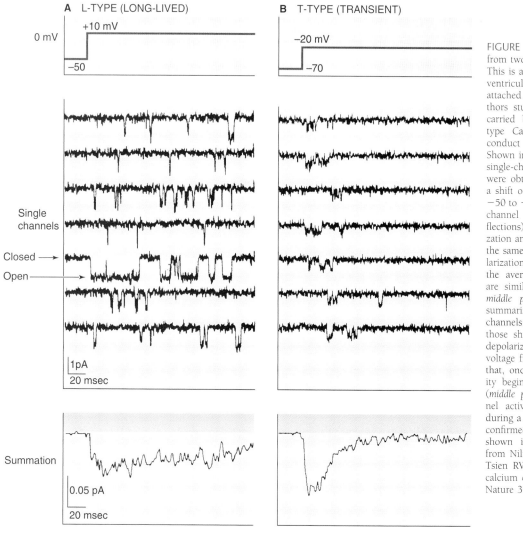

A L-TYPE (LONG-LIVED)

B T-TYPE (TRANSIENT)

FIGURE 7–16. Current records from two types of Ca²⁺ channels. *A,* This is an experiment on guinea-pig ventricular myocytes in which cell-attached patches were used. The authors studied the currents that are carried by Ba²⁺ through these L-type Ca²⁺ channels because they conduct Ba²⁺ even better than Ca²⁺. Shown in the *middle panel* are seven single-channel current records that were obtained during and following a shift of the cytosolic voltage from −50 to +10 mV. Note that the channel activity (i.e., downward deflections) only begins after depolarization and continues more or less at the same level throughout the depolarization. The *lower panel* shows the average of many records that are similar to those shown in the *middle panel. B,* The experiments summarized for these T-type Ca²⁺ channels were identical in design to those shown in *A,* except that the depolarizing step shifted cytosolic voltage from −70 to −20 mV. Note that, once again, the channel activity begins only after depolarization (*middle panel*). However, the channel activity is transient; it wanes during a sustained depolarization, as confirmed by the average current shown in the *lower panel.* (Data from Nilius B, Hess P, Lansman JB, Tsien RW: A novel type of cardiac calcium channel in ventricular cells. Nature 316:443–446, 1985.)

A 1,4-DIHYDROPYRIDINES

B PHENYLALKYLAMINES

Nitrendipene
Inhibitor
(antagonist)

Bay K 8644
Activator
(agonist)

Verapamil

C BENZOTHIAZEPINES

Diltiazem

FIGURE 7–17. Antagonists and agonists of L-type Ca²⁺-channels. *A,* 1,4-Dihydropyridines (DHPs). One DHP, nitrendipine, is an antagonist. Another DHP, Bay K8644, is an agonist. *B,* Phenylalkylamines. Verapamil is an antagonist. *C,* Benzothiazepines. Diltiazem is an antagonist.

Ca²⁺ CHANNEL GENETIC DEFECTS

Ca^{2+} channels have now yet been linked to a large variety of genetic diseases. In mice, an interesting mutation results in **muscular dysgenesis,** or failure of normal skeletal muscle to develop. These mice lack a functional Ca^{2+} channel α_1 subunit in their skeletal muscle. They die shortly after birth, but their cultured muscle cells provide an assay system to investigate the mechanism of excitation-contraction (EC) coupling. Contraction of such defective muscle cells can be rescued by expressing cloned genes for either the skeletal α_{1S} or cardiac α_{1C} isoforms of L-type Ca channels. As discussed in Chapter 9 a physiologically distinguishing feature of EC coupling in normal skeletal versus cardiac muscle is that skeletal muscle does not require extracellular Ca^{2+} whereas cardiac muscle does. Indeed, when the rescue is accomplished with skeletal α_{1S}, contraction does not require extracellular Ca^{2+}, whereas when the rescue is accomplished with cardiac α_{1C}, contraction *does* require extracellular Ca^{2+}. Such studies have provided strong support for the concept that EC coupling in skeletal muscle takes places by direct coupling of α_{1S} to the Ca^{2+} release channels of the sarcoplasmic reticulum whereas in cardiac muscle, EC coupling occurs as Ca^{2+} entering through α_{1C}-containing channels induces the release of Ca^{2+} from internal stores. Mutagenesis experiments with chimeric α_1 subunits containing artificially spliced segments of the cardiac and skeletal channel isoforms have shown that the intracellular linker region between repeats II and III is the domain of the α_1 subunit that determines the skeletal versus the cardiac type of EC coupling.

A human pathologic condition called **Lambert-Eaton syndrome** has been characterized as a impairment of presynaptic Ca^{2+} channels at motor nerve terminals. Lambert-Eaton syndrome is an autoimmune disorder that is most often seen in patients with certain types of cancer, such as small-cell lung carcinoma. Patients afflicted with this condition produce antibodies against presynaptic Ca^{2+} channels that somehow reduce the number of such channels able to function in the depolarization-induced influx of Ca^{2+} for neurotransmitter release.

Hypokalemic periodic paralysis (not to be confused with hyperkalemic periodic paralysis, discussed earlier in the box titled "Na⁺ Channel Genetic Defects") is an autosomal dominant muscle disease of humans. Affected family members have a point mutation in the α_{1S} Ca^{2+} channel gene, located in transmembrane segment S4 of domain II. This finding explains the basis for a human disorder involving defective EC coupling of skeletal muscle. Certain other rare human genetic diseases result in neurologic symptoms of migraine (severe headache) and ataxia (a movement disorder). One of these diseases, **familial hemiplegic migraine,** is caused by point mutations at various locations in the human α_{1A} Ca^{2+} channel gene. These locations include the S4 region of domain I, the P region of domain II, and the S6 helices of domains I and IV. Another such genetic disease caused by mutations in the human α_{1A} Ca^{2+} channel gene is called **episodic ataxia type 2**, a condition associated with the occurrence of ataxia originating from the cerebellum. Discovery of the genetic origin of such diseases has led to the realization that delicate perturbations of Ca^{2+} channel activity can have profound consequences on proper function of the human nervous system.

K⁺ Channels Determine Resting Potential, Modulate Electrical Excitability, and Terminate Action Potentials

K⁺ channels are the largest and most diverse family of voltage-gated ion channels. Vertebrates have at least 38 distinct genes encoding K⁺ channels with the complete S1 through S6 motif. Ion conduction through most types of K⁺ channels is very selective for K⁺ according to the permeability sequence $K^+ > Rb^+ > NH_4^+ \gg Cs^+ > Li^+$, Na^+, Ca^{2+}. Under normal physiological conditions, the permeability ratio P_K/P_{Na} is greater than 100 and Na⁺ can block some K⁺ channels. Some K⁺ channels can pass Na⁺ current in the complete absence of K⁺. This finding is analogous to the behavior of Ca²⁺ channels, which can pass Na⁺ and K⁺ currents in the absence of Ca²⁺.

Given such strong K⁺ selectivity and an equilibrium potential near -80 mV, the primary role of K⁺ channels in excitable cells is inhibitory. K⁺ channels oppose the action of excitatory Na⁺ and Ca²⁺ channels and stabilize the resting, nonexcited state. Whereas some K⁺ channels are major determinants of the resting potential, the voltage dependence and kinetics of other K⁺ channels in excitable cells have specialized functions, such as mediating the repolarization and shaping of action potentials, controlling firing frequency, and defining the bursting be-

havior of rhythmic firing. Such functions are broadly important in regulating the strength and frequency of all types of muscle contraction, in terminating transmitter release at nerve terminals, and in attenuating the strength of synaptic connections. Finally, in epithelia, K⁺ channels also function in K⁺ absorption and secretion.

Before molecular cloning revealed the structural relationships among the various kinds of K⁺ channels, electrophysiologists classified K⁺ currents according to their functional properties and gating behavior. They grouped the macroscopic K⁺ currents into four major types:

1. Delayed outward rectifiers
2. Transient outward rectifiers (A-type currents)
3. Ca²⁺-activated K⁺ currents
4. Inward rectifiers

We now know that these four fundamental K⁺ currents are the macroscopic manifestation of at least three distinct families of genes:

1. Kv channels (voltage-gated K⁺ channels related to the Shaker family)
2. K_{Ca} channels (Ca²⁺-activated K⁺ channels)
3. IR channels (inward rectifier K⁺ channels)

In the next three sections, we discuss each of these three families of K+ channels and their associated macroscopic currents.

The Kv (or Shaker-Related) Family of K+ Channels Mediates Both the Delayed Outward Rectifier Current and the Transient A-Type Current

The K+ current in the HH voltage-clamp analysis of the squid giant axon (p. 181) is an example of a **delayed outward rectifier**. Figure 7–18A shows that the current activates with a sigmoidal lag phase (i.e., it is *delayed* in time, as in Figure 7–6C). Figure 7–18B is an *I-V* plot of peak currents obtained in experiments such as that in Figure 7–18A, and shows that the outward current rises steeply at positive voltages (i.e., it is an *outward rectifier*).

A second variety of K+ current, which is also outwardly rectifying, is the **transient A-type** K+ current. This current was first characterized in mollusk neurons, but similar currents are common in the vertebrate nervous system. A-type currents are activated and inactivated over a relatively rapid time scale. Because their voltage activation range is typically more negative than that of other K+ currents, they are activated in the negative V_m range that prevails during the afterhyperpolarizing phase of action potentials. In neurons that spike repetitively, this A-type current can be very important in determining the interval between successive spikes, and thus the timing of repetitive action potentials. For example, if the A-type current is small, V_m rises relatively quickly toward the threshold, and consequently, the interspike interval is short and the firing frequency is high (see Fig. 7–18C). However, if the A-type current is large, V_m rises slowly toward the threshold and therefore the interspike interval is long and the firing frequency is low (see Fig. 7–18D). Because the nervous system often encodes information as a frequency-modulated signal, these A-type currents play a critical role.

The channels responsible for both the delayed outward rectifier and the transient A-type currents are a closely related group of voltage-gated K+ channels, which in mammals is called the **Kv-channel family** (which stands for "K+, voltage-gated"). The prototypic protein subunit of these channels is the *Shaker* channel of *Drosophila* (p. 183). All channels belonging to this family contain the conserved S1 through S6 core that is characteristic of the Shaker channel (see Fig. 7–9), but may differ extensively in the length and sequence of their intracellular N-terminal and C-terminal domains. The voltage-sensing element in the S4 segment underlies activation by depolarization; the S4 region actually moves outward across the membrane with depolarizing voltage, thus increasing the probability of the channel's being open.

The Kv channel family has four subclasses, Kv1, Kv2, Kv3, and Kv4, that correspond to the *Shaker, Shab, Shaw,* and *Shal* genes of *Drosophila*. Individual members of this Kv channel family, whether in *Drosophila* or humans, exhibit profound differences in gating kinetics that are analogous to delayed rectifier (slow activation) or A-type

(rapid inactivation) currents. For example, Figure 7–18E shows the macroscopic currents of four subtypes of rat brain Kv1 (or "Shaker") channels heterologously expressed in frog oocytes. All these Kv1 channel subtypes (Kv1.1 through Kv1.4) exhibit sigmoidal activation kinetics when examined on a brief time scale—in the millisecond range (*left side* of Fig. 7–18E). That is, these channels display some degree of "delayed" activation. Different Kv channels exhibit different rates of activation. Thus, these currents can modulate action potential duration by either keeping it *short* (e.g., in nerve and skeletal muscle) when the delayed rectifier turns on quickly or keeping it *long* (e.g., in heart) when the delayed rectifier turns on slowly.

Kv1 channels also differ markedly in their *inactivation* kinetics when observed over a long time scale—in the range of seconds (*right side* of Fig. 7–18E). Kv1.1 exhibits little time-dependent inactivation (i.e., the current is sustained throughout the stimulus). On the other hand, the Kv1.4 channel completely inactivates in less than 1 second. Kv1.2 and Kv1.3 show intermediate behavior.

How are Kv channels inactivated? The structural basis for one particular type of K+ channel inactivation, known as **N-type inactivation,** is a stretch of approximately 20 amino acid residues at the N terminus of some fast-inactivating Kv channels. This domain acts like a "ball" to block or plug the internal mouth of the channel after it opens, thereby resulting in inactivation (see Fig. 7–18F). Thus, this process is also known as the **"ball-and-chain" mechanism** of K+ channel inactivation. Particular kinds of β subunits that are physically associated with some isoforms of Kv channels have structural elements that mimic this N-terminal ball domain and rapidly inactivate K+ channel α subunits that lack their own inactivation ball domain.

Particular types of delayed rectifier K+ channels are blocked by either internal or external application of quaternary ammonium ions such as **TEA**. We already have described an example of how TEA can inhibit the outward rectifier K+ current (see Fig. 7–5C) in pharmacologic dissection of the currents underlying the action potential. Many transient A-type K+ currents are inhibited by another organic cation, **4-aminopyridine**. Two distinct families of peptide toxins—**charybdotoxins** of scorpion venom and **dendrotoxins** of mamba snake venom—can discriminate particular subtypes of Kv and K_{Ca} channels, depending on the particular amino acids present in the P region.

The K_{Ca} Family of K+ Channels Mediates Ca²⁺-Activated K+ Currents

Calcium-activated K+ channels—K_{Ca} channels—appear to be present in the plasma membrane of cells in virtually every tissue. In patch-clamp experiments, they are easily recognized because the opening probability of individual channels increases at positive values of V_m (Fig. 7–19A). P_o also increases with increasing [Ca²⁺] on the *intracellular* surface of the membrane patch (see Fig. 7–19B). Figure 7–19C shows how increasing [Ca²⁺]$_i$ causes a negative shift in the P_o versus V_m plot for these channels. A particular type of K_{Ca} channel called the maxi-K_{Ca} or BK

FIGURE 7–18. Outwardly rectifying K⁺ channels. *A,* Note that in a voltage-clamp experiment, a depolarizing step in V_m activates the current, but with a delay. *B,* The current-voltage relationship is shown for a delayed outward-rectifying K⁺ channel, as in *A. C,* This A-type K⁺ current is active at relatively negative values of V_m and tends to hyperpolarize the cell. In a spontaneously spiking neuron, a low level of the A-type current allows V_m to rise relatively quickly toward the threshold, which produces a relatively short interspike interval, and thus a high firing rate. *D,* In a spontaneously spiking neuron, a high level of the A-type current causes V_m to rise relatively slowly toward the threshold, which produces a relatively long interspike interval, and thus a low firing rate. *E,* These experiments were performed on four different types of K⁺ channels (Kv1.1, 1.2, 1.3, and 1.4) from mammalian brain and expressed in *Xenopus* oocytes. Shown are the results of voltage-clamp experiments in which V_m was stepped from −80 mV to 0 mV. The *left panel,* at high time resolution, shows that some of these channels activate more slowly than others. The *right panel,* at a longer time scale, shows that inactivation gradually speeds up from Kv1.1 to Kv1.4. *F,* The *left panel* shows "N-type" inactivation, so called because the "N" or amino terminus of the protein is essential for inactivation. Each of the four subunits is thought to have an N-terminal "ball" that is tethered by a "chain" and can swing into place and block the pore. The *right panel* shows a variant in which certain β subunits can provide the ball-and-chain for Kv-channel α subunits that themselves lack this capability at their N termini. (Data from Stühmer W, Ruppersberg JP, Schroter KH, et al: Molecular basis of functional diversity of voltage-gated potassium channels in mammalian brain. EMBO J 8:3235–3244, 1989.)

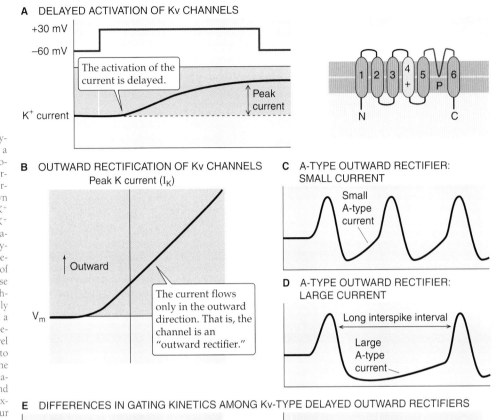

A DELAYED ACTIVATION OF Kv CHANNELS

B OUTWARD RECTIFICATION OF Kv CHANNELS
Peak K current (I_K)

C A-TYPE OUTWARD RECTIFIER: SMALL CURRENT

D A-TYPE OUTWARD RECTIFIER: LARGE CURRENT

E DIFFERENCES IN GATING KINETICS AMONG Kv-TYPE DELAYED OUTWARD RECTIFIERS

F INACTIVATION OF Kv-TYPE CHANNELS

HUMAN HEART DEFECTS LINKED TO MUTATIONS OF K⁺ CHANNELS

A congenital cardiac abnormality in some people results in lengthening of the QT interval of the electrocardiogram signal—**long QT syndrome**—which corresponds to a prolonged cardiac action potential. Affected children and young adults can exhibit an arrhythmic disturbance of the ventricular heartbeat that results in sudden death. As we have already seen in the box entitled "Na⁺ Channel Genetic Defects," one form of a long QT syndrome involves defects in cardiac Na⁺ channels. However, several forms of this syndrome are caused by mutations in cardiac K⁺ channel proteins. Some families have mutations in a gene encoding KvLQT1, a 581-residue protein belonging to the K_V family of voltage-gated K⁺ channels. Another form of this disease involves mutations in a K⁺ channel gene called *HERG,* which is a more distant relative of the Kv channel family. Both KvLQT1 and HERG K⁺ channels participate in repolarization of the cardiac action potential. Such defective repolarization can lead to premature heartbeats or asynchronous ventricular contraction, with subsequent death. The KvLQT1 K⁺ channel also physically associates with another small membrane protein called minK. Mutations in minK also cause a form of long QT syndrome. K⁺ channels are also crucial for proper function of the auditory system. Thus, congenital deafness is commonly associated with mutations in some of these K⁺ channels.

(for "Big" K⁺) channel is noted for its large unitary conductance (~300 pS) and distinctive gating activity.

In principle, K_{Ca} channels provide a stabilizing mechanism to counteract repetitive excitation and intracellular Ca^{2+} loading. K_{Ca} channels mediate the afterhyperpolarizing phase of action potentials (see Fig. 7–1A) in cell bodies of various neurons. They have also been implicated in terminating bursts of action potentials in bursting neuronal pacemaker cells. Thus, the gradual increase in $[Ca^{2+}]_i$ that occurs during repetitive firing triggers the opening of K_{Ca} channels, which results in hyperpolarization and a quiescent interburst period that lasts until intracellular Ca^{2+} accumulation is reversed by the action of Ca^{2+} pumps (p. 64). K_{Ca} channels are also present at high density in many types of smooth muscle cells, where they appear to contribute to the relaxation of tension by providing a hyperpolarizing counterbalance to Ca^{2+}-dependent contraction. In a number of nonexcitable cells, K_{Ca} channels are activated during cell swelling and contribute to regulatory volume decrease (p. 77).

Drosophila genetics also led the way to identification of the first of several genes that encode members of the **K_{Ca} channel family**. Electrophysiologic studies of the *Slowpoke* mutation in flies showed that this mutation eliminated a fast, Ca^{2+}-activated K⁺ current that is present in larval muscle and neurons. Subsequent cloning and sequencing of the *Slowpoke* gene product revealed a channel-forming subunit that has an S1 through S6 core domain that is similar to that of the Kv family, but it also contains a

unique C-terminal domain of around 850 residues (see Fig. 7–19). Because K_{Ca} channels—like Kv channels—have a voltage-sensing domain that is analogous to S4, they are also activated by positive voltage. A homologous *Slowpoke* gene in mammals encodes a BK-type K_{Ca} channel. Structure-function studies on this class of K⁺ channel indicate that the unique C-terminal domain contains the Ca^{2+}-binding sites that function in channel activation.

Besides the BK channel, recent work has identified a distinct gene family of small-conductance Ca^{2+}-activated K⁺ channels known as SK channels (for "small" K⁺). Unlike BK channels, SK channels are voltage *insensitive* and are regulated by the Ca^{2+}-binding protein calmodulin (p. 102). SK channels function in the regulation of neuronal excitation, hormone secretion, and activation of lymphocytes.

The IR Family of K⁺ Channels Mediates Inward Rectifier K⁺ Currents

In contrast to delayed rectifiers and A-type currents—which are *outwardly* rectifying K⁺ currents—the inward rectifier K⁺ current (also known as the "anomalous rectifier") actually conducts more K⁺ current in the *inward* direction than in the outward direction. Such inwardly rectifying, steady-state K⁺ currents have been recorded in many types of cells, including heart, skeletal muscle, and epithelia. Physiologically, these channels help clamp the resting membrane potential close to the K⁺ equilibrium potential and prevent excessive loss of intracellular K⁺ during repetitive activity and long-duration action potentials. In epithelial cells, these inwardly rectifying K⁺ currents are important because they stabilize V_m in the face of electrogenic ion transporters that tend to depolarize the cell (see Chapter 3).

In contrast to the Kv and K_{Ca} channel families, the channel-forming subunits of the inward rectifier (IR) K⁺ channel family are smaller proteins (~400 to 500 residues) that do not contain a complete S1 through S6 core domain. However, they do have a conserved region that is similar to the S5–P–S6 segment of Kv channels (Fig. 7–20A). It appears that the conserved P region is the most basic structural element that is common to all K⁺ channels. The lack of an S4 voltage-sensing domain in IR channels accounts for the observation that unlike Kv channels, IR K⁺ channels are not steeply activated by voltage.

Figure 7–20B shows a series of single-channel currents that were obtained from an IR K⁺ channel, with equal concentrations of K⁺ on both sides of the membrane, as well as Mg^{2+} on the cytosolic side. Under these conditions, the channel conducts K⁺ current only in the inward direction. An *I-V* plot (see Fig. 7–20C) derived from data such as these shows typical inward rectification of the unitary current. At negative values of V_m, the inward current decreases linearly as voltage becomes more positive, and no outward current is present at positive values of V_m. However, when Mg^{2+} is omitted from the cytosolic side of the membrane, the channel now exhibits a linear or **ohmic *I-V* curve** even over the positive range of V_m values. Thus, the inward rectification is due to

A VOLTAGE DEPENDENCE

$V_m = -60$ mV   ← Closed

← Open

← Two channels open

$V_m = +80$ mV   ← One channel open

← Closed

40pA

60 msec

α subunit

β subunit

N

0 1 2 3 4+ 5 P 6   1 2

N C

Ca^{2+} — C

B CALCIUM DEPENDENCE

1 μM Ca^{2+}
$V_m = +40$ mV

← Closed

10 μM Ca^{2+}
$V_m = +40$ mV

← Open

← Closed

100 μM Ca^{2+}
$V_m = +40$ mV

← Open

← Closed

20 pA

150 ms

C COMBINED EFFECTS OF CHANGING V_m AND $[Ca^{2+}]_i$

1.0

100 μM Ca^{2+}

Relative P_o

0.5

10 μM Ca^{2+}

1 μM Ca^{2+}

0

−60   −40   0   40

Membrane potential (mV)

FIGURE 7–19. Ca^{2+}-activated K^+ channels (K_{Ca}). *A,* Shown is an experiment on K_{Ca} channels that are expressed in *Xenopus* oocytes and studied using a patch pipette in an inside-out configuration (see Fig. 6–14*E* or *H*). When V_m is held at −60 mV, there is very little channel activity. On the other hand, when V_m is +80 mV, both channels in the patch are open most of the time. *B,* The experiment is the same as in *A* except that V_m is always held at +40 mV and the $[Ca^{2+}]$ on the cytosolic side of the patch varies from 1 to 10 to 100 μM. Note that channel activity increases with increasing $[Ca^{2+}]_i$. *C,* Combined effects of changing V_m and $[Ca^{2+}]_i$. Shown is a plot of relative open probability (P_o) of the K_{Ca} channels versus V_m at three different levels of Ca^{2+}. The data come from experiments such as those shown in *B*. (Data from Butler A, Tsunoda S, McCobb DP, et al: mSlo, a complex mouse gene encoding "maxi" calcium-activated potassium channels. Science 261:221–224, 1993.)

intracellular block of the channel by Mg^{2+}. Inhibition of outward K^+ current in the presence of intracellular Mg^{2+} results from voltage-dependent binding of this divalent metal ion. Positive internal voltage favors the binding of Mg^{2+} to the inner mouth of this channel (see Fig. 7–20*D*), as would be expected if the Mg^{2+}-binding site is located within the transmembrane electric field. Because Mg^{2+} is impermeant, it essentially blocks outward K^+ current. However, negative values of V_m pull the Mg^{2+} out of the channel. Moreover, incoming K^+ tends to displace any remaining Mg^{2+}. Thus, the IR channel favors K^+ influx over efflux. Intracellular polyamines such as spermine and spermidine—which, like Mg^{2+}, carry a positive charge—also produce inward rectification of IR

channels. These organic cations are important channel-modulating factors that also determine the current-voltage behavior of this particular class of ion channels.

The IR family of K^+ channels can be classified according to their mode of regulation. One subfamily of IR K^+ channels (the G-protein–activated, inwardly rectifying K^+ channels [**GIRKs**]) is regulated by the βγ subunits of heterotrimeric **G proteins** (p. 95). For example, stimulation of the vagus nerve slows the heartbeat because the vagal neurotransmitter, acetylcholine, binds to postsynaptic muscarinic receptors in the heart that are coupled to G proteins. The binding of acetylcholine to its receptor causes the release of G-protein βγ subunits, which apparently diffuse to a site on neighboring GIRK channels to

FIGURE 7–20. Inwardly rectifying K⁺ channels. *A,* This family of channels has only two membrane-spanning segments that correspond to the S5-P-S6 domain of the voltage-gated K⁺ channels. *B,* The GIRK1 channels were expressed in *Xenopus* oocytes and studied using a patch pipette in the inside-out configuration (see Fig. 6–14E or H). V_m was clamped to values between −100 mV and +60 mV, and [Mg²⁺] was 2.5 mM on the cytosolic side. Note that channel activity increases at more negative voltages, but is virtually inactive at positive voltages. *C,* The I-V plot shows that there is inward rectification only in the presence of Mg²⁺ on the cytosolic side. In the absence of Mg²⁺, the I-V relationship is nearly linear, or "ohmic." *D,* As shown in the *left panel,* cytosolic Mg²⁺ occludes the channel pore and prevents the *exit* of K⁺. However, even in the presence of Mg²⁺, K⁺ can move into the cell by displacing the Mg²⁺. (Data from Kubo Y, Reuveny E, Slesinger PA, et al: Primary structure and functional expression of a rat G-protein-coupled muscarinic potassium channel. Nature 364:802–806, 1993.)

activate their opening. The resulting increase in inward current hyperpolarizes the cardiac cell, thereby slowing the rate at which V_m approaches the threshold for firing action potentials and lowering the heart rate.

The members of another subfamily of IR K⁺ channels, the **K_{ATP} channels,** are directly regulated by adenine nucleotides. K_{ATP} channels are present in the plasma membrane of many cell types, including skeletal muscle, heart, neurons, the insulin-secreting β cell of the pancreas, and renal tubule. These channels are inhibited by intracellular adenosine triphosphate (ATP) and activated by adenosine diphosphate (ADP) in a complex fashion. They are believed to provide a direct link between cellular metabolism on the one hand and membrane excitability and K⁺ transport on the other. For example, if cellular ATP levels fall because of oxygen deprivation, such channels could theoretically open and hyperpolarize the cell to suppress firing of action potentials and further reduce energy expenditure. In the pancreatic β cell, an increase

in glucose metabolism increases the ATP/ADP ratio. This increased ratio inhibits enough K_{ATP} channels to cause a small depolarization, which in turn activates voltage-gated Ca²⁺ channels and results in insulin secretion (p. 1070).

K_{ATP} channels are the target of a group of synthetic drugs called **sulfonylureas** that include tolbutamide and glibenclamide. Sulfonylureas are used in the treatment of type 2 (or non–insulin-dependent) diabetes mellitus because they inhibit pancreatic K_{ATP} channels and stimulate insulin release. Newer and chemically diverse synthetic drugs called K⁺ channel openers (e.g., pinacidil and cromakalim) activate K_{ATP} channels. The therapeutic potential of K⁺ channel openers is being explored in light of their ability to relax various types of smooth muscle. The ability of sulfonylurea drugs to inhibit K_{ATP} channels depends on an accessory subunit called SUR (for sulfonylurea receptor). This latter protein is a member of the ATP-binding cassette family of proteins (p. 65), which includes two nucleotide-binding domains.

PROPAGATION OF ACTION POTENTIALS

The Propagation of Electrical Signals in the Nervous System Involves Local Current Loops

The extraordinary functional diversity of ion channel proteins provides a large array of mechanisms by which the membrane potential of a cell can be changed to evoke an electrical signal or biochemical response. However, channels alone do not control the spread of electrical current. Like electricity in a copper wire, the passive spread of current in biologic tissue depends on the nature of the conducting and insulating medium. Important factors include the geometry (i.e., anatomy), electrical resistance of the aqueous solutions and cell membrane, and membrane capacitance. Furthermore, the electrotonic spread of electrical signals is not limited to excitable cells.

Efficient propagation of a change in V_m is essential for the *local* integration of electrical signals at the level of a single cell and for the *global* transmission of signals across large distances in the body. As we discussed earlier in this chapter (see Fig. 7–2), *action potentials* propagate in a regenerative manner without loss of amplitude as long as the depolarization spreads to an adjacent region of excitable membrane and does so with sufficient strength to depolarize the membrane above its threshold. However, many types of *nonregenerative*, subthreshold potentials also occur and spread for short distances along cell membranes. These **graded responses**, which we also discussed earlier, contrast with the all-or-nothing nature of action potentials. Such nonregenerative signals include **receptor potentials** generated during the transduction of sensory stimuli and **synaptic potentials** generated by the opening of agonist-activated channels.

With a graded response, the greater the stimulus, the greater the voltage response. For example, the greater the intensity of light that is shined on a mammalian photoreceptor cell in the retina, the greater the hyperpolarization produced by the cell. Similarly, the greater the concentration of acetylcholine that is applied at a postsynaptic neuromuscular junction, the greater the resulting depolarization (i.e., synaptic potential). Of course, if this depolarization exceeds the threshold in an excitable cell, an all-or-nothing action potential is initiated. The generation of a physiological response from a graded potential change critically depends on its **electrotonic** spread to other regions of the cell. Like the subthreshold voltage responses produced by injecting a current into a cell through a microelectrode, the electrotonic spread of graded responses declines with distance from the site of initiation. Graded signals dissipate over distances of a few millimeters and thus have only local effects; propagated action potentials can travel long distances via nerve axons.

Electrotonic spread of voltage changes along the cell occurs by the flow of electrical current that is carried by ions in the intracellular and extracellular medium along pathways of the least electrical resistance. Both depolarizations and hyperpolarizations of a small area of membrane produce **local circuit currents**. Figure 7–21A illustrates how the transient voltage change that occurs during an action potential at a particular "active" site results in local

current flow. The cytosol of the active region, where the membrane is depolarized, has a slight excess of positive charge when compared with the adjacent "inactive" regions of the cytosol, which have a slight excess of negative charge. This charge imbalance within the cytosol causes currents of ions to flow from the electrically excited region to adjacent regions of the cytoplasm. Because current always flows in a complete circuit along pathways of least resistance, the current spreads longitudinally from positive to negative regions along the cytoplasm, moves outward across membrane conductance pathways ("leak channels"), and flows along the extracellular medium back to the site of origin, thereby closing the current loop. Because of this flow of current (i.e., positive charge), the region of membrane immediately adjacent to the "active" region becomes more depolarized, and V_m eventually reaches threshold. Thus, an action potential is generated in this adjacent region as well. Nerve and muscle fibers conduct impulses in both directions if an inactive fiber is excited at a central location, as in this example. However, if an action potential is initiated at one end of a nerve fiber, it will travel only to the opposite end and stop because the refractory period prevents backward movement of the impulse. Likewise, currents generated by subthreshold responses migrate equally in both directions.

Myelin Improves the Efficiency with Which Axons Conduct Action Potentials

The flow of electrical current along a cylindric nerve axon has often been compared to electrical flow through an undersea cable. Similar principles apply to both types of conducting fiber. An underwater cable is designed to carry an electrical current for long distances with little current loss; therefore, it is constructed of a highly conductive (low resistance) metal in its core and a thick plastic insulation wrapped around the core to prevent loss of current to the surrounding seawater. In contrast, the axoplasm of a nerve fiber has much higher resistance than a copper wire, and the nerve membrane is inherently electrically leaky because of background channel conductance. Therefore, in a biologic fiber such as a nerve or muscle cell, some current is passively lost into the surrounding medium, and the amplitude of the signal rapidly dissipates over a short distance.

Animal nervous systems use two basic strategies to improve the conduction properties of nerve fibers: (1) increasing the diameter of the axon, thus decreasing the internal resistance of the cable, and (2) myelination, which increases the electrical insulation around the cable. As **axon diameter** increases, the conduction velocity of action potentials increases because the internal resistance of the axoplasm is inversely related to the internal cross-sectional area of the axon. Unmyelinated nerve fibers of the invertebrate squid giant axon (as large as ~1000 μm in diameter) are a good example of this type of size adaptation. These nerve axons mediate the escape response of the squid from its predators and can propagate action potentials at a velocity of about 25 m/s.

In vertebrates, **myelination** of smaller-diameter (~1 to

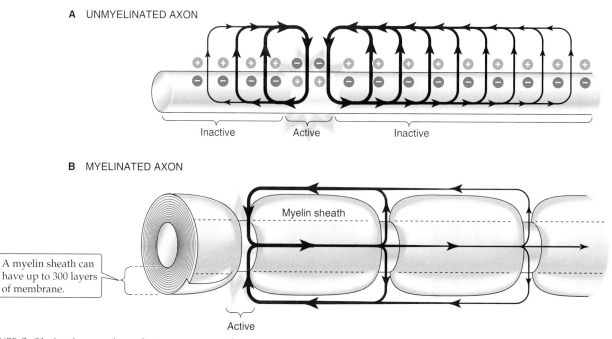

A UNMYELINATED AXON

Inactive   Active   Inactive

B MYELINATED AXON

Myelin sheath

A myelin sheath can
have up to 300 layers
of membrane.

Active

FIGURE 7–21. Local current loops during action-potential propagation. *A,* The currents flow at one instant in time as a result of the action potential ("active" zone). In the "inactive" zones that are adjacent to the active zone, the outward currents lead to a depolarization. If the membrane is not in an absolute refractory period and if the depolarization is large enough to reach threshold, the immediately adjacent inactive zones will become active and fire their own action potential. In the more distant inactive zones, the outward current is not intense enough to cause V_m to reach threshold. Thus, the magnitudes of the outward currents decrease smoothly with increasing distance from the active zone. *B,* In this example, the "active" zone consists of a single node of Ranvier. In a myelinated axon, the currents flow only through the nodes, where there is no myelin and the density of Na^+ channels is very high. Current does not flow through the internodal membrane because of the high resistance of myelin. As a result, the current flowing down the axon is conserved, and the current density at the nodes is very high. This high current density results in the generation of an action potential at the node. Thus, the active zones jump in a "saltatory" manner from one node to another. The internodal membrane (i.e., underneath the myelin) may not ever fire an action potential.

5 μm) nerve axons serves to improve the efficiency of impulse propagation, especially over the long distances that nerves traverse between the brain and the extremities. Axons are literally embedded in myelin, which consists of concentrically wound wrappings of the membranes of glial cells (p. 417). The thickness of the myelin sheath may amount to 20% to 40% of the diameter of a nerve fiber, and the sheath may consist of as many as 300 membrane layers. The glial cells that produce myelin are called Schwann cells in the periphery and oligodendrocytes in the brain. Because resistors in series add directly and capacitors in series add as the sum of the reciprocal, the insulating resistance of a myelinated fiber with 300 membrane layers is increased by a factor of 300 and the capacitance is decreased to 1/300 that of a single membrane. This large increase in membrane resistance minimizes loss of current across the leaky axonal membrane and forces the current to flow longitudinally along the inside of the fiber.

In myelinated peripheral nerves, the myelin sheath is interrupted at regular intervals, forming short ($\sim$1 μm) uncovered regions called **nodes of Ranvier**. The length of the myelinated axon segments between adjacent unmyelinated nodes ranges from 0.2 to 2 mm. In mammalian axons, the density of voltage-gated Na^+ channels is very high in the nodal membrane. The unique anatomy of myelinated axons results in a mode of impulse propagation known as **saltatory conduction**. Current flow that is initiated at an excited node flows directly to adjacent

nodes with little loss of transmembrane current through the internode region (see Fig. 7–21*B*). In other words, the high membrane resistance in the internode region effectively forces the current to travel from node to node.

The high efficiency of impulse conduction in such axons allows several adjacent nodes in the same fiber to fire an action potential virtually simultaneously as it is being propagated. Thus, saltatory conduction in a myelinated nerve can reach a very high velocity, up to 130 m/s. The action potential velocity in a myelinated nerve fiber can thus be several-fold greater than that in a giant unmyelinated axon, even though the axon diameter in the myelinated fiber may be more than two orders of magnitude smaller. During conduction of an action potential in a myelinated axon, the intracellular regions between nodes also depolarize. However, no transmembrane current flows in these internodal regions, and therefore no dissipation of ion gradients occurs. The nodal localization of Na^+ channels conserves ionic concentration gradients that must be maintained at the expense of ATP hydrolysis by the Na-K pump.

The Cable Properties of the Membrane and Cytoplasm Determine the Velocity of Signal Propagation

Following the analogy of a nerve fiber as an underwater cable, **cable theory** allows one to model the pathways of electric current flow along biomembranes. The approach

A   EQUIVALENT-CIRCUIT MODEL

Membrane

r_m c_m

Axoplasm

Extracellular fluid

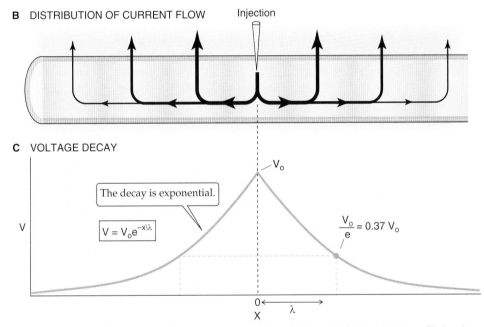

B   DISTRIBUTION OF CURRENT FLOW

Injection

C   VOLTAGE DECAY

V_o

The decay is exponential.

$V = V_o e^{-x/\lambda}$

$\dfrac{V_o}{e} = 0.37\ V_o$

V

0

X

λ

FIGURE 7–22. Passive cable properties of an axon. *A,* The axon is represented as a hollow, cylindric "cable" that is filled with an electrolyte solution. All of the electrical properties of the axon are represented by discrete elements that are expressed in terms of the length of the axon. r_i is the resistance of the internal medium. Similarly, r_o is the resistance of the external medium. r_m and c_m are the membrane resistance and capacitance per discrete element of axon length. *B,* When current is injected into the axon, the current flows away from the injection site in both directions. The current density smoothly decays with increasing distance from the site of injection. *C,* Because the current density decreases with distance from the site of current injection in *B,* the electrotonic potential (V) also decays exponentially with distance in both directions. V_o is the maximum change in V_m that is at the site of current injection.

is to use circuit diagrams that were first employed to describe the properties of electric cables. Figure 7–22A illustrates the equivalent circuit diagram of a cylindrical electric cable or membrane that is filled and bathed in a conductive electrolyte solution. The membrane itself is represented by discrete elements, each with a transverse membrane resistance (r_m) and capacitance (c_m) connected in parallel (a representation we used earlier, in Fig. 6–11A). Consecutive membrane elements are connected in series by discrete resistors, each of which represents the electrical resistance of a finite length of the external medium (r_o) or internal medium (r_i). The parameters r_m, c_m, r_o, and r_i refer to a unit length of axon (Table 7–3).

How do the various electrical components of the cable model influence the electrotonic spread of current along an axon? To answer this question, we inject a steady electric current into an axon with a microelectrode to produce a constant voltage (V_0) at a particular point (x = 0) along the length of the axon (see Fig. 7–22B). This

injection of current results in the longitudinal spread of current in both directions from point x = 0. The voltage (V) at various points along the axon decays exponentially with distance (x) from the point of current injection (Fig. 7–22C), according to the following equation:

Equation 7–5

$$V = V_0 \exp(-x/\lambda)$$

The parameter λ has units of *distance* and is referred to as the **length constant** or the **space constant**. One length constant away from the point of current injection, V is $1/e$, or about 37% of the maximum value of V_0. The decaying *currents* that spread away from the location of a current-passing electrode are called **electrotonic currents**. Similarly, the spread of subthreshold *voltage* changes away from a site of origin is referred to as electrotonic spread, unlike the regenerative propagation of action potentials.

TABLE 7–3

CABLE PARAMETERS

PARAMETER	UNITS	DEFINITION OR RELATIONSHIP
r_m	ohm × cm	Membrane resistance (per unit length of axon)
r_o	ohm/cm	Extracellular resistance (per unit length of axon)
r_i	ohm/cm	Intracellular resistance (per unit length of axon)
c_m	μF/cm	Membrane capacitance (per unit length of axon)
$R_m = r_m \times 2\pi a$	ohm × cm²	Specific membrane reistance (per unit area of membrane)
$R_i = r_i \times \pi a^2$	ohm × cm	Specific internal resistance (per unit cross-sectional area of axoplasm)
$C_m = c_m/(2\pi a)$	μF/cm²	Specific membrane capacitance (per unit area of membrane)

a, radius of the axon.

The length constant depends on the three resistance elements in Figure 7–22A:

$$\lambda = \sqrt{\frac{r_m}{r_o + r_i}}$$

Equation 7–6

We can simplify this expression by noting that internal resistance is much larger than external resistance, so the contribution of r_o to the denominator can be ignored. Thus,

$$\lambda = \sqrt{\frac{r_m}{r_i}}$$

Equation 7–7

The significance of the length constant is that it determines how far the electrotonic spread of a local change in membrane potential is able to influence neighboring regions of membrane. The longer the length constant, the further down the axon a voltage change spreads.

How does the diameter of an axon affect the length constant? To answer this question, we must replace r_m and r_i (expressed in terms of axon length) in Equation 7–7 with the **specific resistances** R_m and R_i (expressed in terms of the area of axon membrane or cross-sectional

area of axoplasm). Making the substitutions according to the definitions in Table 7–3, we have:

$$\lambda = \sqrt{\frac{aR_m}{2R_i}}$$

Equation 7–8

Thus, the length constant (λ) is directly proportional to the square root of the axon radius (a). Equation 7–8 confirms basic intuitive notions about what makes an efficiently conducting electric cable: (1) The greater the specific membrane resistance (R_m) and cable radius, the greater the length constant and the less the loss of signal. (2) The greater the resistance of the internal conductor (R_i), the smaller the length constant and the greater the loss of signal. These relationships also confirm measurements of length constants in different biologic preparations. For example, the length constant of a squid axon with a diameter of about 1 mm is approximately 13 mm, whereas that of a mammalian nerve fiber with a diameter of about 1 μm is approximately 0.2 mm.

So far, we have been discussing the *spatial* spread of voltage changes that are stable in *time*. In other words, we assumed that the amount of injected current was steady. What happens if the current is not steady? For example, what happens at the beginning of a stimulus when we (or a physiological receptor) first turn the current "on"? To answer these questions, we need to know how rapidly V_m changes in time at a particular site, which is described by a second cable parameter called the membrane **time constant** (τ_m). Rather than determining the spread of voltage changes in space, as the length constant does, the time constant influences the spread of voltage changes in *time* and thus the *velocity* of signal propagation. We previously discussed the time constant with respect to the time course of the change in V_m caused by a stepwise pulse of current (see Fig. 6–12A). Because the membrane behaves as an RC circuit, the voltage response to a square current pulse across a small piece of membrane follows an exponential time course with a time constant that is equal to the product of membrane resistance and capacitance:

$$\tau_m = R_m \times C_m$$

Equation 7–9

We introduced this expression earlier as Equation 6–17. The shorter the time constant, the more quickly a neighboring region of membrane will be brought to threshold and the sooner the region will fire an action potential. Thus, the shorter the time constant, the faster the speed of impulse propagation and vice versa. In contrast, conduction velocity is directly proportional to the length constant. The greater the length constant, the further a signal can spread before decaying below threshold and the greater the area of membrane that the stimulus can excite. These relationships explain why, in terms of relative conduction velocity, a high-resistance, low-capacitance *myelinated* axon has a distinct advantage over an *unmyelinated* axon of the same diameter for all but the smallest axons (<1 μm in diameter; p. 289).

In summary, the cable parameters of length constant and time constant determine the way in which graded potentials and action potentials propagate over space and time in biologic tissue. These parameters are in turn a function of material properties that include resistance, capacitance, and geometric considerations. The dependence of impulse conduction velocity on fiber diameter has been studied experimentally and analyzed theoretically for unmyelinated and myelinated nerve axons. For *unmyelinated* axons, conduction velocity increases roughly with the square root of the axon's diameter, just as the length constant increases with the square root of the axon's diameter or radius (see Equation 7–8). In contrast, the conduction velocity of *myelinated* fibers is a linear function of diameter and increases approximately 6 m/s per 1-μm increase in outer diameter. Thus, a mammalian myelinated axon with an outer diameter of about 4 μm has roughly the same impulse velocity as a squid giant axon with a diameter of 500 μm! However, for myelinated fibers with a very small diameter ($<$1 μm), the adverse effect of high internal resistance of the axoplasm predominates, and conduction is slower than in unmyelinated axons of the same outer diameter. For outer diameters that are greater than approximately 1 μm, the increased membrane resistance and reduced capacitance caused by myelination result in much faster conduction velocities.

The physiologic importance of myelin in action potential propagation is most dramatically illustrated in the pathology that underlies human demyelinating diseases such as **multiple sclerosis**. As discussed more fully in Chapter 11, MS is an autoimmune disorder in which the myelin sheath surrounding CNS axons is progressively lost (see box on p. 292). Gradual demyelination is responsible for an array of neurologic symptoms that involve various degrees of paralysis and altered or lost sensation. As myelin is eliminated, the loss of membrane resistance and increased capacitance mean that propagated action potentials may ultimately fail to reach the next node of Ranvier and thus result in nerve blockage.

REFERENCES

Books and Reviews

Ackerman MJ, Clapham DE: Ion channels—basic science and clinical disease. N Engl J Med 336:1575–1586, 1997.

Catterall WA: Cellular and molecular biology of voltage-gated sodium channels. Physiol Rev 72 (Suppl):S15–S48, 1992.

Chandy KG, Gutman GA: Voltage-gated K$^+$ channel genes. In North RA (ed): Handbook of Receptors and Channels: Ligand and Voltage-Gated Ion Channels. Boca Raton, FL, CRC Press, 1995, pp 1–71.

Hille B: Ionic Channels of Excitable Membranes, 3rd ed. Sunderland, MA, Sinauer Associates, 2001.

Pallotta BS, Wagoner PK: Voltage-dependent potassium channels since Hodgkin and Huxley. Physiol Rev 72 (Suppl):S49–S67, 1992.

Tsien RW, Wheeler DB: Voltage-gated calcium channels. In Carafoli E, Klee CB (eds): Calcium as a Cellular Regulator. New York, Oxford University Press, 1999, pp 171–199.

Journal Articles

Cole KS, Moore JW: Ionic current measurements in the squid giant axon membrane. J Gen Physiol 44:123–167, 1960.

Hille B: The selective inhibition of delayed potassium currents in nerve by tetraethylammonium ions. J Gen Physiol 50:1287–1302, 1967.

Ho K, Nichols CG, Lederer WJ, et al: Cloning and expression of an inwardly rectifying ATP-regulated potassium channel. Nature 362:31–38, 1993.

Hodgkin AL, Huxley AF: A quantitative description of membrane current and its application to conduction and excitation in nerve. J Physiol (Lond) 117:500–544, 1952.

Kim YI, Neher E: IgG from patients with Lambert-Eaton syndrome blocks voltage-dependent calcium channels. Science 239:405–408, 1988.

Kubo Y, Reuveny E, Slesinger PA, et al: Primary structure and functional expression of a rat G-protein coupled muscarinic potassium channel. Nature 364:802–806, 1993.

Ptacek LJ, Gouw L, Kwiecinski H, et al: Sodium channel mutations in paramyotonia congenita and hyperkalemic periodic paralysis. Ann Neurol 33:300–307, 1993.

CHAPTER 8

Synaptic Transmission and the Neuromuscular Junction

Edward G. Moczydlowski

The ionic gradients that cells maintain across their membranes provide a form of stored electrochemical energy cells can use for electrical signalling. The combination of a resting membrane potential of −60 to −90 mV and a diverse array of voltage-gated ion channels allows excitable cells to generate action potentials that propagate over long distances along the surface membrane of a *single* nerve axon or muscle fiber. However, another class of mechanisms is necessary to transmit such electrical information from cell to cell throughout the myriad of neuronal networks that link the brain with sensory and effector organs. Electrical signals must pass across the specialized gap region between two apposing cell membranes that is called a **synapse.** The process underlying this cell-to-cell transfer of electrical signals is termed **synaptic transmission.** Communication between cells at a synapse can be either electrical or chemical. Electrical synapses provide direct electrical continuity between cells by means of gap junctions, whereas chemical synapses link two cells together by a chemical **neurotransmitter** that is released from one cell and diffuses to another.

In this chapter we discuss the general properties of synaptic transmission and then focus mainly on synaptic transmission between a motor neuron and a skeletal muscle fiber. This interface between the motor neuron and the muscle cell is called the neuromuscular junction. In Chapter 12, the focus is on synaptic transmission between neurons in the central nervous system (CNS).

MECHANISMS OF SYNAPTIC TRANSMISSION

Electrical Continuity Between Cells Is Established Either by Direct Flow of Current Through Gap Junction Channels at an Electrical Synapse or by Diffusion of a Neurotransmitter across a Chemical Synapse

Once the concept of bioelectricity had taken hold among physiologists of the 19th century, it became clear that the question of how electrical signals flow between cells posed a fundamental biologic problem. Imagine that two cells lie side by side without any specialized device for communicating between them. Furthermore, imagine that a flat, 20-μm^2 membrane area of the first, or **presynaptic,** cell is separated—by 15 nm—from a similar area of the second, or **postsynaptic,** cell. In his classic book on electrophysiology, Katz calculated that a voltage signal at the presynaptic membrane would suffer 10,000-fold attenuation in the postsynaptic membrane.

204

TABLE 8–1

SUMMARY OF PROPERTIES OF ELECTRICAL AND CHEMICAL SYNAPSES

| | ELECTRICAL | CHEMICAL | |
		Ionotropic	Metabotropic
Agonist	None	e.g., ACh	e.g., ACh
Membrane protein	Connexon	Receptor/ channel	Receptor/G protein
Speed	Instantaneous	1 msec	sec to min
Effect	V_m	V_m	V_m, etc.

ACh, acetylcholine; V_m, membrane potential.

A similar calculation based on the geometry and cable properties of a typical nerve-muscle synapse suggests that an action potential arriving at a nerve terminal could depolarize the postsynaptic membrane by only 1 μV after crossing the synaptic gap—an attenuation of 10^5. Clearly, the evolution of complex multicellular organisms required the development of special synaptic mechanisms for electrical signalling to serve as a workable means of intercellular communication.

Two competing hypotheses emerged in the 19th century to explain how closely apposed cells could communicate electrically. One school of thought proposed that cells are directly linked by microscopic connecting bridges that enable electrical signals to flow directly. Other pioneering physiologists used pharmacologic observations to infer that cell-to-cell transmission was chemical in nature. Ultimate resolution of this question awaited both the development of electron microscopic techniques, which permitted visualization of the intimate contact region between cells, and further studies in neurochemistry, which identified the small, organic molecules that are responsible for neurotransmission. By 1960, accumulated evidence led to the general recognition that cells use *both* direct electrical and indirect chemical modes of transmission to communicate with one another.

The essential structural element of intercellular communication, the synapse, is a specialized point of contact between the membranes of two different, but connected, cells. Electrical and chemical synapses have unique morphologies, distinguishable by electron microscopy. One major distinction is the distance of separation between the two apposing cell membranes. At **electrical synapses**, the adjacent cell membranes are separated by about 3 nm and appear to be nearly sealed together by a plate-like structure that is a fraction of a micrometer in diameter. Freeze-fracture images of the intramembrane plane in this region reveal a cluster of closely packed intramembranous particles that represent a **gap junction**. As described in Chapter 6, a gap junction corresponds to planar arrays of connexons, each of which is made up of six connexin monomers (see Fig. 6–18). The multiple connexons from apposing cells physically connect the two cells together via multiple aqueous channels.

In contrast to the gap junction, the apposing cell membranes of the **chemical synapse** are separated by a much larger gap. Approximately 30 nm separates the two cell membranes at a neuronal chemical synapse, and the gap is as large as 50 nm at the vertebrate nerve-muscle synapse. An additional characteristic of a chemical synapse is the presence of numerous synaptic vesicles on the side of the synapse that initiates the signal transmission, termed the *pre*synaptic side. These vesicles are sealed, spherical membrane-bound structures that range in diameter from 40 to 200 nm and contain a high concentration of chemical neurotransmitter.

The contrasting morphologies of electrical and chemical synapses underline the contrasting mechanisms by which they function (Table 8–1). Electrical synapses pass voltage changes directly from one cell to another across the low-resistance continuity that is provided by the connexon channels. On the other hand, chemical synapses link two cells by the diffusion of a chemical transmitter across the large gap separating them. The neurotransmitter that is stored in the synaptic vesicles is released into the synaptic space, diffuses across the cleft of the synapse, and activates the postsynaptic cell by binding to a specific receptor protein on the postsynaptic cell membrane.

Direct evidence for the existence of chemical transmission predated the experimental confirmation of electrical synapses. The foundations of synaptic physiology can be traced back to early studies of the autonomic nervous system. Early in the 1900s, researchers noted that adrenal gland extracts, which contain epinephrine, elicited physiological effects (e.g., an increase in heart rate) that were similar to those elicited by stimulation of sympathetic nerve fibers. In 1904, Elliot proposed that sympathetic nerves might release a substance that is analogous to epinephrine that would function in chemical transmission between a nerve and its target organ. Similar studies suggested that the vagus nerve, which is parasympathetic, produces a related substance that is responsible for depression of the heartbeat.

A classic experiment performed by Loewi in 1921 is widely cited as the first definitive evidence for chemical neurotransmission. Loewi used an ingenious bioassay to test for the release of a chemical substance by the vagus nerve. He repeatedly stimulated the vagus nerve of a cannulated frog heart and observed a slowing of the heartbeat. At the same time, he collected the artificial saline that emerged from the ventricle of this overstimulated heart. When he later perfused the same heart with the fluid he had previously collected while stimulating the vagus, he observed that this perfusate itself slowed the heart rate in a manner that was identical to direct vagal stimulation. He also later identified the active compound in the perfusion fluid, originally called *Vagusstoff*, as acetylcholine (ACh).

Efforts by Dale and coworkers to understand the basis of neurotransmission between motor nerves and skeletal muscle culminated in the identification of ACh as the endogenous excitatory neurotransmitter. Thus, the inherent complexity of chemical synaptic transmission was evident from these earliest investigations, which indicated that the same neurotransmitter (ACh) could have an inhibitory action at one synapse (vagus nerve—heart) and an excitatory action at another synapse (motor nerve—skeletal muscle). For their work on nerve transmission across chemical synapses, Otto Loewi and Sir Henry Dale received the Nobel Prize in Medicine in 1936.

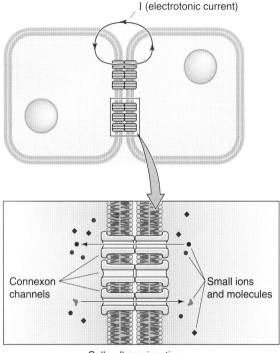

I (electrotonic current)

Connexon channels

Small ions and molecules

Cell-cell gap junction

FIGURE 8–1. An electrical synapse. An electrical synapse consists of one or more gap-junction channels permeable to small ions and molecules.

Electrical and Chemical Synapses Both Convey Signals From One Cell to Another, but Differ Greatly in the Particulars

ELECTRICAL SYNAPSES. Whereas overwhelming support for chemical synaptic transmission accumulated in the first half of the 20th century, the first direct evidence for electrical transmission came much later from electrophysiologic recordings of a crayfish nerve preparation. In 1959, Furshpan and Potter used two pairs of stimulating and recording electrodes to show that depolarization of a presynaptic nerve fiber (the crayfish abdominal nerve) resulted in excitation of a postsynaptic nerve cell (the motor nerve to the tail muscle) with virtually no time delay. In contrast, chemical synapses exhibit a characteristic delay of approximately 1 ms in the postsynaptic voltage signal after excitation of the presynaptic cell. The demonstration of an electrical synapse between two nerve membranes highlighted an important functional difference between electrical and chemical synapses—immediate signal propagation (electrical) versus briefly delayed communication (chemical) through the junction.

An electrical synapse is a true structural connection between two cells, mediated by the connexon channels of gap junctions that link the cytoplasm of the two cells (Fig. 8–1). These channels thus provide a low-resistance path for electrotonic current flow, and allow voltage signals to flow with little attenuation and no delay between two or more coupled cells. Many types of gap junctions pass electrical current with equal efficiency in both directions (**reciprocal synapses**). In other words, the current passing through the gap junction is "ohmic"; it varies

linearly with the transjunctional voltage (i.e., the V_m difference between the two cells). However, the crayfish synapse described by Furshpan and Potter allows depolarizing current to pass readily only in one direction, from the presynaptic cell to the postsynaptic cell. Such electrical synapses are called **rectifying synapses** to indicate that the underlying junctional conductance is voltage dependent. Studies of cloned and expressed connexins have shown that the voltage dependence of electrical synapses arises from unique gating properties of different connexin isoforms. Some isoforms are voltage dependent, whereas others are voltage independent. Intrinsic rectification can also be altered by the formation of a gap junction that is composed of two hemichannels, each made up of a different connexin monomer. Such hybrid connexins are called heterotypic channels.

CHEMICAL SYNAPSES. By their very nature, chemical synapses are inherently rectifying or polarized. They propagate current in one direction: from the presynaptic cell that releases the transmitter to the postsynaptic cell that contains the receptors that recognize and bind the transmitter. However, the essentially vectorial nature of chemical synaptic transmission belies the possibility that the postsynaptic cell can influence synapse formation or transmitter release by the presynaptic cell. Studies of synapse development and regulation have shown that postsynaptic cells also play an active role in synapse formation. In the CNS, postsynaptic cells may also produce retrograde signalling molecules, such as nitric oxide (NO), that diffuse back into the presynaptic terminal and modulate the strength of the synaptic connection (p. 322). Furthermore, the presynaptic membrane at some synapses contains receptors that may either inhibit or facilitate the release of transmitter by biochemical mechanisms. Thus, chemical synapses should be considered a unidirectional pathway for signal propagation that can be modulated by bidirectional chemical communication between two interacting cells.

The process of chemical transmission can be summarized by the following series of steps (Fig. 8–2):

Step 1: Neurotransmitter molecules are packaged into synaptic vesicles. Specific transport proteins in the vesicle membrane use the energy of an H^+ gradient to energize uptake of the neurotransmitter in the vesicle.

Step 2: An action potential, which involves voltage-gated Na^+ and K^+ channels (p. 182), arrives at the presynaptic nerve terminal.

Step 3: Depolarization opens voltage-gated Ca^{2+} channels, which allows Ca^{2+} to enter the presynaptic terminal.

Step 4: The increase in intracellular Ca^{2+} concentration ($[Ca^{2+}]_i$) triggers the fusion of synaptic vesicles with the presynaptic membrane. As a result, packets (quanta) of transmitter molecules are released into the synaptic cleft.

Step 5: The transmitter molecules diffuse across the synaptic cleft and bind to specific receptors on the membrane of the postsynaptic cell.

Step 6: The binding of transmitter activates the receptor, which in turn activates the postsynaptic cell.

Step 7: The process is terminated by (1) enzymatic de-

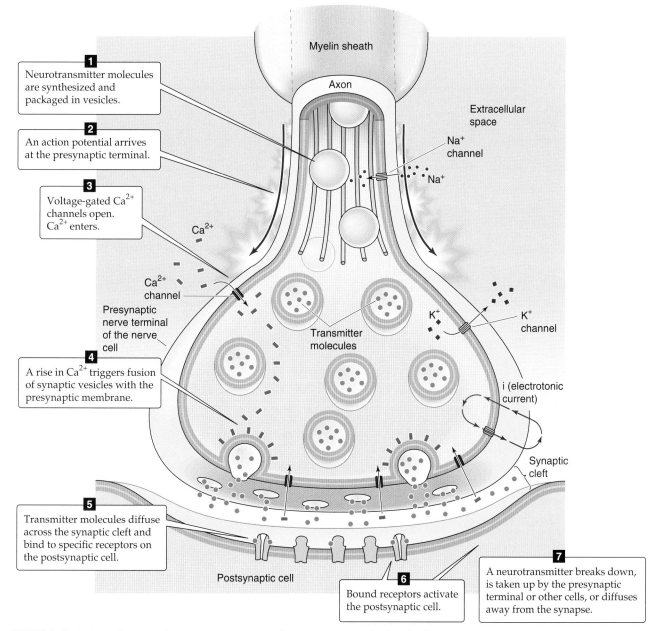

1 Neurotransmitter molecules are synthesized and packaged in vesicles.

2 An action potential arrives at the presynaptic terminal.

3 Voltage-gated Ca^{2+} channels open. Ca^{2+} enters.

4 A rise in Ca^{2+} triggers fusion of synaptic vesicles with the presynaptic membrane.

5 Transmitter molecules diffuse across the synaptic cleft and bind to specific receptors on the postsynaptic cell.

6 Bound receptors activate the postsynaptic cell.

7 A neurotransmitter breaks down, is taken up by the presynaptic terminal or other cells, or diffuses away from the synapse.

Myelin sheath

Axon

Extracellular space

Na^+ channel

Na^+

Ca^{2+}

Ca^{2+} channel

Presynaptic nerve terminal of the nerve cell

Transmitter molecules

K^+

K^+ channel

i (electrotonic current)

Synaptic cleft

Postsynaptic cell

FIGURE 8–2. A chemical synapse. Synaptic transmission at a chemical synapse can be thought of as occurring in seven steps.

struction of the transmitter (e.g., hydrolysis of ACh by acetylcholinesterase [AChE]), (2) uptake of transmitter into the presynaptic nerve terminal or into other cells by Na^+-dependent transport systems, or (3) diffusion of the transmitter molecules away from the synapse.

The molecular nature of chemical synapses permits enormous diversity in functional specialization and regulation. Functional diversity occurs at the level of the transmitter substance, receptor protein, postsynaptic response, and subsequent electrical and biochemical processes. Many different small molecules are known—or proposed—to serve as neurotransmitters (p. 304). These molecules include both small organic molecules such as norepinephrine, ACh, serotonin (5-hydroxytryptamine [5-HT]), glutamate, gamma-aminobutyric acid (GABA), glycine, and peptides such as endorphins and enkephalins.

The Transmitter at a Chemical Synapse Can Activate Either an Ionotropic Receptor that Is Itself a Channel or a Metabotropic Receptor that Is Linked to a G Protein

The two basic categories of neurotransmitter receptors are ligand-gated ion channel proteins and G protein–linked receptor proteins (also called seven–transmembrane-helix receptors; p. 92). Several neurotransmitter molecules, such as glutamate and ACh, serve as ligands (agonists) for both types of receptors. In the particular case of gluta-

A   IONOTROPIC RECEPTOR

B   METABOTROPIC RECEPTOR

Axon

Electrical stimulus

Na-driven cotransport of choline occurs.

Na⁺

Choline

Acetylcholinesterase

Axon

Electrical stimulus

Acetylcholine

Acetylcholine

Na⁺   K⁺

Acetylcholinesterase breaks down acetylcholine.

Atrial muscle cell membrane

Skeletal muscle fiber membrane

G protein complex

α

γ

β

K⁺

GTP

Nicotinic ACh receptor channel activation

Muscarinic ACh receptor activation

Membrane depolarization

Release of α-GTP + βγ from the heterotrimeric G protein

Action potential excitation

Activation of inward rectifier K⁺ channel by βγ

Muscle contraction

Membrane hyperpolarization

Decrease in heart rate

FIGURE 8–3. Ionotropic and metabotropic acetylcholine receptors. *A,* This example illustrates a "nicotinic" acetylcholine receptor, which is a ligand-gated channel on the postsynaptic membrane. In a skeletal muscle, the end result is muscle contraction. *B,* This example illustrates a "muscarinic" acetylcholine receptor, which is coupled to a heterotrimeric G protein. In a cardiac muscle, the end result is decreased heart rate. Note that the presynaptic release of ACh is very similar here and in A. ACh, acetylcholine; GTP, guanosine triphosphate.

mate, glutamate receptors that are ion channels are known as **ionotropic receptors**, and glutamate receptors coupled to G proteins are called **metabotropic receptors**. This nomenclature is being increasingly used to describe the two major types of receptors for transmitters other than glutamate.

Ionotropic and metabotropic receptors determine the ultimate functional response to transmitter release. Activation of an ionotropic receptor causes rapid opening of ion channels. This channel activation in turn results in depolarization or hyperpolarization of the postsynaptic membrane, the choice depending on the ionic selectivity of the conductance change. Activation of a metabotropic G protein–linked receptor results in the production of active α and βγ subunits, which initiate a wide variety of cellular responses by direct interaction with either ion channel proteins or other second-messenger effector proteins (p.

95). By their very nature, ionotropic receptors mediate fast ionic synaptic responses that occur on a millisecond time scale, whereas metabotropic receptors mediate slow, biochemically mediated synaptic responses in the range of seconds to minutes.

Figure 8–3 compares the basic processes mediated by two prototypic ACh receptors (AChRs): (1) the ACh-activated ion channel at the neuromuscular junction of skeletal muscle, an ionotropic receptor also known as the **nicotinic** AChR (Fig. 8–3*A*), and (2) the G protein–linked AChR at the atrial parasympathetic synapse of the heart, a metabotropic receptor also known as the **muscarinic** AChR (Fig. 8–3*B*). The nicotinic versus muscarinic distinction was a classic *pharmacologic* classification based on whether the AChR is activated by nicotine or muscarine. The molecular basis for this distinction was discovered only much later. In the case of the ionotropic (nicotinic) receptor, opening of the AChR channel results in a transient increase in permeability to Na^+ and K^+, which directly produces a brief depolarization that activates the muscle fiber. In the case of the metabotropic (muscarinic) receptor, activation of the G protein–coupled receptor opens an inward rectifier K^+ channel, or GIRK (p. 197), via $\beta\gamma$ subunits released from an activated heterotrimeric G protein. Enhanced opening of these GIRKs produces membrane hyperpolarization and leads to inhibition of cardiac excitation (p. 488). These two functionally distinct mechanisms are the molecular basis for the seemingly conflicting observations of early physiologists that ACh (*Vagusstoff*) activates skeletal muscle but inhibits heart muscle.

SYNAPTIC TRANSMISSION AT THE NEUROMUSCULAR JUNCTION

Neuromuscular Junctions are Specialized Synapses with Active Zones of Synaptic Vesicles on Presynaptic (Neuronal) Membranes and Highly Amplified Junctional Folds on Postsynaptic (Muscle) Membrane

The chemical synapse between peripheral nerve terminals and skeletal muscle fibers is the most intensely studied synaptic connection in the nervous system. Even though the detailed morphology and the specific molecular components (e.g., neurotransmitters and receptors) differ considerably among different types of synapses, the basic electrophysiologic principles of the neuromuscular junction are applicable to many other types of chemical synapses, including neuronal synaptic connections in the brain, to which we will return in Chapter 12. In this chapter, we focus on the neuromuscular junction in discussing the basic principles of synaptic transmission.

Motor neurons with cell bodies in the spinal cord have long axons that branch extensively near the point of contact with the target muscle (Fig. 8–4). These axon processes each innervate a separate fiber of skeletal muscle. The whole assembly of muscle fibers innervated by the axon from one motor neuron is called a **motor unit**.

Typically, an axon makes a single point of synaptic contact with a skeletal muscle fiber, midway along the length of the muscle fiber. This specialized synaptic region is called the **neuromuscular junction** or the **end plate** (Fig. 8–4). An individual end plate consists of a small tree-like patch of unmyelinated nerve processes that are referred to as terminal arborizations. The bulb-shaped endings that finally contact the muscle fiber are called **boutons**. Schwann cells are intimately associated with the nerve terminal and form a cap over the face of the nerve membrane that is located away from the muscle membrane. The postsynaptic membrane of the skeletal muscle fiber lying directly under the nerve terminal is characterized by extensive invaginations known as **postjunctional folds**. These membrane infoldings greatly increase the surface area of the muscle plasma membrane in the postsynaptic region. The intervening space of the **synaptic cleft**, which is approximately 50 nm wide, is filled with a meshwork of proteins and proteoglycans that are part of

the extracellular matrix. A particular region of the muscle basement membrane called the synaptic basal lamina contains various proteins (e.g., collagen, laminin, agrin) that mediate adhesion of the neuromuscular junction and play important roles in synapse development and regeneration. The synaptic basal lamina also contains a high concentration of the enzyme **acetylcholinesterase** (AChE), which ultimately terminates synaptic transmission by rapidly hydrolyzing free ACh to choline and acetate.

Electron micrographs of the bouton region demonstrate the presence of numerous spherical synaptic vesicles, each with a diameter of 50 to 60 nm. The cell bodies of motor neurons in the spinal cord produce these vesicles, and the microtubule-mediated process of fast axonal transport (p. 26) translocates them to the nerve terminal. The quantal nature of transmitter release (described later in more detail) reflects the fusion of individual synaptic vesicles with the plasma membrane of the presynaptic terminal. Each synaptic vesicle contains 6000 to 10,000 molecules of ACh. The ACh concentration in synaptic vesicles is approximately 150 mM. ACh is synthesized in the nerve terminal—outside the vesicle—from choline and acetyl-coenzyme A by the enzyme **choline acetyltransferase**. The ACh moves into the synaptic vesicle via a specific ACh-H exchanger, which couples the inward transport of ACh to the efflux of H^+. Energetically, this process is driven by the vesicular proton electrochemical gradient (positive voltage and low pH inside), which in turn is produced by a vacuolar-type H^+ pump fueled by adenosine triphosphate (ATP) (p. 64). The nerve terminal also contains numerous mitochondria that produce the ATP required to fuel energy metabolism.

The process of fusion of synaptic vesicles and release of ACh occurs at differentiated regions of the presynaptic membrane called **active zones.** In electron micrographs, active zones appear as dense spots over which synaptic vesicles are closely clustered in apposition to the membrane. High-resolution images of active zones reveal a double, linear array of synaptic vesicles and intramembranous particles. These zones are oriented directly over secondary *post*synaptic clefts that lie between adjacent postjunctional folds. Molecular localization studies have shown that the density of ionotropic (nicotinic) AChRs is very high at the crests of postjunctional folds. Examination of the detailed microarchitecture of the neuromuscular synapse thus reveals a highly specialized structure for delivering neurotransmitter molecules to a precise location on the postsynaptic membrane.

Acetylcholine Activates the Ionotropic (Nicotinic) Acetylcholine Receptor to Produce an End-Plate Current and Thus an Excitatory Postsynaptic Potential

Electrophysiological experiments on muscle fibers have characterized the electrical nature of the postsynaptic response at the muscle end plate. Figure 8–5 illustrates results obtained from a classic experiment performed by Fatt and Katz in 1951. Their work is the first description of how stimulation of the motor nerve affects the membrane potential (V_m) at the postsynaptic region (i.e., mus-

FIGURE 8–4. The vertebrate neuromuscular junction or motor end plate. A motor neuron, with its cell body in the ventral horn of the spinal cord, sends out an axon that progressively bifurcates to innervate several muscle fibers (a "motor unit"). The neuron contacts a muscle fiber at exactly one spot called a neuromuscular junction or motor end plate. The end plate consists of an arborization of the nerve into many presynaptic terminals, or boutons, as well as the specializations of the postsynaptic membrane. A high-magnification view of a bouton shows that the synaptic vesicles containing the neurotransmitter acetylcholine (ACh) cluster and line up at the active zone of the presynaptic membrane. The active zones on the presynaptic membrane are directly opposite the secondary postsynaptic clefts that are created by infoldings of the postsynaptic membrane (postjunctional folds). Depolarization of the bouton causes the vesicles to fuse with the presynaptic membrane and to release their contents into the synaptic cleft. The ACh molecules must diffuse at least 50 nm before reaching nicotinic ACh receptors. Note the high density of ACh receptors at the crests of the postjunctional folds. The activity of the released ACh is terminated mainly by an acetylcholinesterase. The bouton reloads its discharged synaptic vesicles by resynthesizing ACh and transporting this ACh into the vesicle via an ACh-H exchanger.

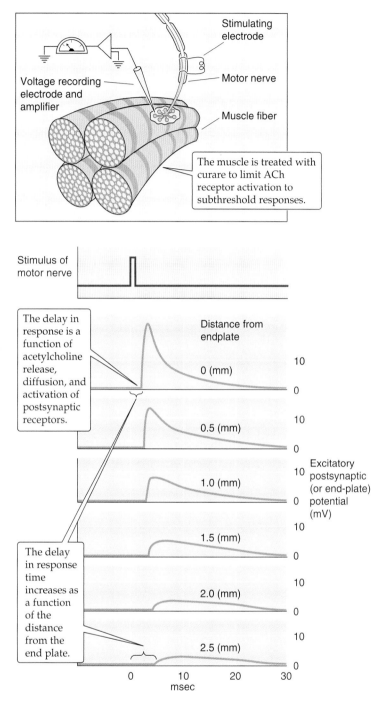

FIGURE 8-5. End-plate potentials elicited at the frog neuromuscular junction by stimulating the motor neuron. The magnitude of the excitatory postsynaptic potential (EPP) is greatest near the end plate and decays farther away. (Data from Fatt P, Katz B: An analysis of the end-plate potential recorded with an intracellular electrode. J Physiol 115:320–370, 1951.)

cle cell) of the neuromuscular junction. Normally, nerve stimulation would drive the V_m of the muscle above threshold and elicit an action potential (p. 172). However, Fatt and Katz were interested not in seeing the action potential, but in studying the small, graded electrical responses that are produced as ACh binds to receptors on the muscle cell membrane. Therefore, Fatt and Katz greatly reduced the response of the AChRs by blocking most of them with a carefully selected concentration of *d*-tubocurarine, which we discuss later. They inserted a KCl-filled microelectrode into the end-plate region of a frog sartorius muscle fiber. This arrangement allowed

them to measure tiny changes in V_m at one particular spot of the muscle cell.

When Fatt and Katz electrically excited the motor nerve axon, they observed a transient depolarization in the muscle membrane after a delay of a few milliseconds. The delay represents the time required for the release of ACh, its diffusion across the synapse, and activation of postsynaptic AChRs. The positive voltage change follows a biphasic time course: V_m rapidly rises to a peak and then more slowly relaxes back to the resting value, consistent with an exponential time course. This signal, known as the **end-plate potential** (EPP), is an example of an **excit-**

A EXPERIMENTAL PREPARATION

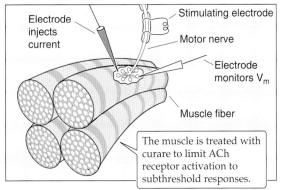

Electrode injects current

Stimulating electrode

Motor nerve

Electrode monitors V_m

Muscle fiber

The muscle is treated with curare to limit ACh receptor activation to subthreshold responses.

B END-PLATE CURRENTS OBTAINED AT VARIOUS HOLDING POTENTIALS

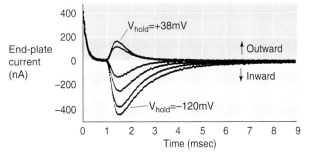

End-plate current (nA)

V_{hold}=+38mV

↑ Outward

↓ Inward

V_{hold}=−120mV

Time (msec)

C I-V RELATIONSHIP FOR PEAK END-PLATE CURRENT

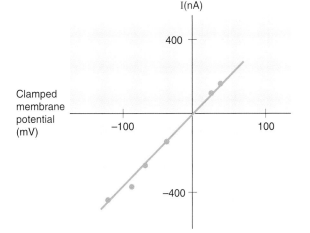

I(nA)

Clamped membrane potential (mV)

FIGURE 8–6. End-plate currents obtained at different membrane potentials in a voltage-clamp experiment. *A,* Two-electrode voltage clamp is used to measure the end-plate current in a frog muscle fiber. The tips of the two microelectrodes are in the muscle fiber. *B,* The six records represent end-plate currents that were obtained while the motor nerve was stimulated and the postsynaptic membrane was clamped to V_m values of −120, −91, −68, −37, +24, +38 mV. Notice that the peak current reverses from inward to outward as the holding potential shifts from −37 to +24 mV. *C,* The reversal potential is near 0 mV because the nicotinic ACh receptor has a poor selectivity for Na⁺ versus K⁺. (Data from Magleby KL, Stevens CF: The effect of voltage on the time course of end-plate current. J Physiol 223:151–171, 1972.)

atory postsynaptic potential. It is produced by the transient opening of AChR channels, which are selectively permeable to monovalent cations such as Na⁺ and K⁺. The increase in Na⁺ conductance drives V_m to a more positive value in the vicinity of the end-plate region. In this experiment, curare blockade allows only a small number of AChR channels to open, so that the EPP does not reach the threshold to produce an action potential. If the experiment is repeated by inserting the microelectrode at various distances from the end plate, the amplitude of the potential change is successively diminished and its peak is increasingly delayed. This decrement with distance occurs because the EPP originates at the end-plate region and spreads away from this site according to the passive cable properties (p. 200) of the muscle fiber. Thus, the EPP in Figure 8–5 is an example of a propagated, graded response. However, without the curare blockade, more AChR channels would open and a larger EPP would ensue, which would drive V_m above threshold and consequently trigger a regenerating action potential (p. 172).

What ions pass through the AChR channels during generation of the EPP? This question can be answered by using the same voltage-clamp technique that was also used to study the basis of the action potential (see Fig. 7–5B). Figure 8–6A illustrates the experimental preparation for a two-electrode voltage-clamp experiment in which the motor nerve is stimulated while the muscle fiber in the region of its end plate is voltage-clamped to a chosen V_m. The recorded current, which is proportional to the conductance change at the muscle end plate, is called the **end-plate current** (EPC). The EPC has a characteristic time course that rises to a peak within 2 ms after stimulation of the motor nerve and falls exponentially back to zero (Fig. 8–6B). The time course of the EPC corresponds to the opening and closing of a population of AChR channels, governed by the rapid binding and disappearance of ACh as it diffuses to the postsynaptic membrane and is hydrolyzed by AChE.

As shown in Figure 8–6B, when the muscle fiber is clamped to a "holding potential" of −120 mV, we observe a large inward current (i.e., the EPC). This inward current decreases in magnitude as V_m is made more positive, and the current reverses direction to become an outward current at positive values of V_m. A plot of the peak current versus the clamped V_m shows that the reversal potential for the EPC is close to 0 mV (Fig. 8–6C). Because the EPC specifically corresponds to current through AChR channels, this reversal potential reflects the ionic selectivity of these channels when extracellular Na⁺ and K⁺ concentrations ($[Na^+]_o$ and $[K^+]_o$) are normal.

By varying the concentrations of the extracellular ions while monitoring the shift in the reversal potential of the EPC, researchers found that the AChR channel is permeable to Na⁺, K⁺, and Ca²⁺, but not to anions such as Cl⁻. Because of its low extracellular concentration, the current attributable to Ca²⁺ is small under physiological conditions and its contribution can be ignored. By plugging the values for the various cations into the Goldman-Hodgkin-Katz voltage equation (Equation 6–9), one can obtain the permeability of the AChR channel to various alkali monovalent ions, relative to Na⁺ permeability. The result is the

ACh RECEPTOR VIEWED FROM ABOVE

α SUBUNIT OF ACh RECEPTOR

CROSS SECTION OF ACh RECEPTOR

The α subunit of an ACh receptor is composed of 4 transmembrane regions, M1, M2, M3, M4, with extramembrane sequences above and below.

FIGURE 8–7. Structure of the nicotinic acetylcholine (ACh) receptor. The nicotinic ACh receptor is a heteropentamer with the subunit composition of $\alpha_2\beta\gamma\delta$. These subunits are homologous to one another, and each has four membrane-spanning segments (M1–M4).

following sequence of relative permeability: 0.87 (Li$^+$), 1.00 (Na$^+$), 1.11 (K$^+$), and 1.42 (Cs$^+$). This weak ionic selectivity stands in marked contrast to typical voltage-gated Na$^+$ channels, which have P_{Na}/P_K ratios of approximately 20, and voltage-gated K$^+$ channels, which have P_K/P_{Na} ratios greater than 100. On this basis, the ionotropic (nicotinic) AChR channel at the muscle end plate is often classified as **a nonselective cation channel**. Nevertheless, the weak ionic selectivity of the AChR is well suited to its basic function of raising V_m above the threshold of about -50 mV, which is necessary for firing an action potential. When the nicotinic AChR channel at the muscle end plate opens, the normally high resting permeability of the muscle plasma membrane for K$^+$ relative to Na$^+$ falls so that Na$^+$ and K$^+$ become equally permeant and V_m shifts to a value between E_K (approximately -80 mV) and E_{Na} (approximately $+50$ mV).

As we shall see in Chapter 12, which focuses on synaptic transmission in the CNS, similar principles hold for generating postsynaptic currents by other types of agonist-gated channels. For example, the receptor-gated channels for serotonin and glutamate are cation selective and give rise to *depolarizing* **excitatory postsynaptic potentials**. In contrast, the receptor-gated channels for glycine and GABA are anion selective and drive V_m in the hyperpolarizing direction, toward the equilibrium potential for Cl$^-$. These *hyperpolarizing* postsynaptic responses are called **inhibitory postsynaptic potentials**.

The Ionotropic (Nicotinic) Acetylcholine Receptor Is a Member of a Superfamily of Pentameric Ligand-Gated Ion Channels

The molecular nature of the nicotinic AChR channel was revealed by studies that included protein purification,

amino acid sequencing of isolated subunits, and molecular cloning. Purification of the receptor was aided by the recognition that the electric organs of certain fish are a particularly rich source of the nicotinic AChR. In the electric eel and *Torpedo* ray, the electric organs are embryologically derived from skeletal muscle. The *Torpedo* ray can deliver large electrical discharges by summating the simultaneous depolarizations of a stack of many disk-like cells called electrocytes. These cells have the skeletal muscle isoform of the nicotinic AChR, which is activated by ACh released from presynaptic terminals.

The purified *Torpedo* AChR consists of four subunits (α, β, γ, and δ) in a pentameric stoichiometry of $2\alpha:1\beta:1\gamma:1\delta$ (Fig. 8–7). Each subunit has a molecular mass of approximately 50 kDa and exhibits relatively high homology to the other subunits. The primary sequences of nicotinic AChR subunits are also highly conserved in evolutionary terms: the skeletal muscle isoforms of the α subunit are approximately 90% identical among the *Torpedo* ray, frog, chicken, mouse, and human.

The α, β, γ, and δ subunits each have four distinct hydrophobic regions known as M1 through M4, which correspond to membrane-spanning segments. The agonist-binding site for ACh is in the extracellular N-terminal domain of the α subunit. For each of the subunits, the M2 transmembrane segment lines the aqueous pore of the pentameric channel protein. It is through this pore that Na$^+$ and K$^+$ cross the membrane.

AChRs of normal adult *muscle fibers* are present in high density in the junctional folds of the postsynaptic membrane. However, in developing muscle fibers of the mammalian embryo and in denervated fibers of adult skeletal muscle, AChRs are also widely distributed in the membrane outside the end-plate region. The two types of AChRs, called junctional and nonjunctional receptors,

A SINGLE-CHANNEL CURRENTS

FIGURE 8–8. Properties of embryonic and adult acetylcholine (ACh) receptors from skeletal muscle. *A,* The results of patch-clamp experiments, with the patch pipettes in the outside-out configuration and the patch exposed to 0.5 μM ACh, are summarized. In the *upper panel,* the investigators expressed the embryonic AChR, which has the subunit composition $\alpha_2\beta\gamma\delta$, in *Xenopus* oocytes. In the *lower panel,* the investigators expressed the adult AChR, which has the subunit composition $\alpha_2\beta\epsilon\delta$. Notice that the mean open times are greater for the embryonic form, whereas the unitary currents are greater for the adult form. *B,* The *two lines* summarize data that are similar to those obtained in *A.* The single-channel conductance of the adult form (59 pS) is higher than that of the embryonic form (40 pS). (Data from Mishina M, Takai T, Imoto K, et al: Molecular distinction between fetal and adult forms of muscle acetylcholine receptor. Nature 321:406–411, 1986.)

have different functional properties. The unitary conductance of junctional receptors is approximately 50% larger and the single-channel lifetime is shorter in duration than that of nonjunctional receptors. The basis for this phenomenon is a difference in subunit composition. The *nonjunctional* (or embryonic) receptors are a pentameric complex with a subunit composition of $\alpha_2\beta\gamma\delta$ in mammals, just as in the electric organ of the *Torpedo* ray. For the *junctional* AChR in adult skeletal muscle, substitution of an ϵ subunit for the fetal γ subunit results in a complex with the composition $\alpha_2\beta\epsilon\delta$.

The functional properties of the two types of receptors have been studied by coexpressing the cloned subunits in *Xenopus* oocytes. Figure 8–8A shows patch-clamp recordings of single ACh-activated channels in oocytes that had been injected with mRNA encoding either α, β, γ, δ or α, β, ϵ, δ. Measurements of currents at different voltages yielded single-channel I-V curves (Fig. 8–8B) showing that the channel formed with the ϵ subunit had a unitary conductance of 59 pS whereas that formed with the γ subunit had a conductance of 40 pS. The mean lifetime of single-channel openings at 0 mV was 1.6 msec for ϵ-type and 4.4 msec for γ-type receptors, closely corresponding to values found in native adult and fetal muscle, respectively. The different functional properties of junctional and nonjunctional nicotinic ACh receptors presum-

ably reflect their specialized roles in synaptic transmission versus development and synapse formation.

Molecular cloning of genes that encode AChR subunits of the *Torpedo* ray electric organ and mammalian skeletal muscle led to the identification of a large number of related genes for AChR channel proteins. For example, mammals have a family of at least eight genes that encode homologous α subunits of nicotinic ACh-activated receptors. The α subunit of the skeletal muscle receptor is the product of a gene called α1. Seven additional genes designated α2 through α8 encode α subunits that are expressed in neuronal tissues. Only the protein products of genes α1, α7, and α8 bind the snake venom protein called α-bungarotoxin. In addition, at least four β subunits exist. Besides the β subunit of the skeletal muscle AChR—which is called β1—there are three neuronal homologs (β2, β3, β4). Heteromeric association of different combinations of these subunits could potentially produce a large number of functional receptor isoforms. Although the exact physiological role of nicotinic AChR channels in various *neuronal* pathways remains to be established, it is likely that AChRs in the brain play a role in addiction to the nicotine contained in tobacco.

Besides nicotinic AChRs, three other related classes of agonist-activated channels are recognized, including ionotropic receptor channels that are activated by **serotonin**

FIGURE 8–9. Currents activated by glycine and γ-aminobutyric acid (GABA). *A,* These experiments were performed on cultured mouse spinal cord neurons using patch-clamp techniques. The *left panel* shows the macroscopic Cl^- current, which is measured in the whole-cell configuration and carried by glycine receptor (GlyR) channels when exposed to glycine. The *right panel* shows single-channel currents that are recorded in the outside-out patch configuration. In both scenarios, the holding potential was −70 mV. *B,* The *left panel* shows the macroscopic Cl^- current that is carried by $GABA_A$ receptor channels when exposed to GABA. The *right panel* shows single-channel currents. (Data from Bormann J, Hamill OP, Sakmann B: Mechanism of anion permeation through channels gated by glycine and γ-aminobutyric acid in mouse spinal neurones. J Physiol 385:243–286, 1987.)

(5-HT₃ receptor), glycine (GlyR), and **GABA** ($GABA_A$ receptor). As mentioned previously, AChR and 5-HT₃ receptor channels are both permeable to cations and thus produce excitatory currents, whereas glycine-activated and $GABA_A$ channels are permeable to anions such as Cl^- and produce inhibitory currents. Figure 8–9 shows examples of macroscopic and unitary Cl^- currents mediated by glycine-activated and $GABA_A$ channels. Cloned genes encoding subunits of these latter receptor channels encode proteins that are homologous to AChR subunits. Their primary amino acid sequences share a common arrangement of M1, M2, M3, and M4 transmembrane segments, as described earlier for the nicotinic AChR (see Fig. 8–7). These proteins thus all belong to a large gene family that is known as the **ligand-gated ion channel superfamily** (p. 170). Sequence analysis of these genes suggests that they evolved from a common ancestor. The basis for cation versus anion selectivity appears to reside solely within the M2 segment. Mutation of only three residues within the M2 segment of a cation-selective α subunit of a neuronal nicotinic AChR is sufficient to convert it to an anion-selective channel activated by ACh.

Acetylcholine Receptor Channels Cannot Open Until Two Acetylcholine Molecules Bind

The EPC is the sum of many single-channel currents, each representing the opening of a single AChR channel at the neuromuscular junction. Earlier we described the random opening and closing of an idealized channel in a two-state model in which the channel could be either closed or open (p. 181):

$$\text{Equation 8–1}$$

$$C \rightleftharpoons O$$

In the case of an *agonist*-activated channel, such as the AChR channel, at least one additional state must be present because the closed channel can either bind agonist or not:

$$\text{Equation 8–2}$$

C		AC		AO
Closed channel		Closed channel		Open channel
No agonist		Agonist bound		Agonist bound

In this two-step scheme, the closed state (C) of the channel must bind one molecule of the agonist ACh to form an agonist-bound channel that is closed (AC) before it can convert to an agonist-bound channel that is open (AO). However, even this scheme is overly simplistic because we know that each of the two α subunits of the AChR channel must bind ACh simultaneously for the channel to open:

$$\text{Equation 8–3}$$

$$C \rightleftharpoons A_1C \rightleftharpoons A_2C \rightleftharpoons A_2O$$

1 agonist   2 agonists   Open

Understanding the kinetics of channel opening can be very important for clarifying the mechanism by which certain channel inhibitors work. For example, a competitive inhibitor could prevent binding of the agonist ACh. However, many noncompetitive antagonists of the AChR channel, including some local anesthetics, act by entering the lumen of the channel and blocking the flow of ionic current. Figure 8–10A shows the results of a patch-clamp experiment in which a single AChR channel opened and closed in response to its agonist, ACh. After adding QX-222, an analog of the local anesthetic agent lidocaine (p. 189), to the extracellular side, the channel exhibits a rapidly flickering behavior. This flickering represents a series of brief interruptions of the open state by numerous closures (Fig. 8–10B). This type of flickering block is caused by rapid binding and unbinding of the anesthetic drug to a site in the mouth of the *open* channel. When the drug binds, it blocks the channel to the flow of ions (A_2B). Conversely, when the drug dissociates, the channel becomes unblocked (A_2O):

Equation 8–4

$$C \rightleftharpoons A_1C \rightleftharpoons A_2C \rightleftharpoons A_2O \rightleftharpoons A_2B$$

$$\text{Blocked}$$

Channel blockers have proved to be effective tools to study the mechanism of ion permeation. For example, QX-222 helped in locating amino acid residues on the M2 transmembrane segment that form part of the blocker binding site, thus identifying residues that line the aqueous pore.

Miniature End-Plate Potentials Reveal the Quantal Nature of Transmitter Release from the Presynaptic Terminals

Under physiological conditions, an action potential in a *presynaptic* motor nerve axon produces a depolarizing *postsynaptic* EPP that peaks at approximately 40 mV more positive than the resting V_m. This large signal results from the release of ACh from only about 200 synaptic vesicles, each containing 6000 to 10,000 molecules of ACh. The neuromuscular junction is clearly designed for excess capacity inasmuch as a single end plate is composed of numerous synaptic contacts (~1000 at the frog muscle end plate), each with an active zone that is lined with dozens of mature synaptic vesicles. Thus, a large inventory of ready vesicles ($>10^4$), together with the ability to synthesize ACh and package it into new vesicles, allows the neuromuscular junction to maintain a high rate of successful transmission without significant loss of function as a result of presynaptic depletion of vesicles or ACh.

The original notion of a vesicular mode of transmitter delivery is based on classic observations of EPPs under conditions of reduced ACh release. In 1950, Fatt and Katz observed an interesting kind of electrophysiologic "noise" in their continuous, high-resolution recordings of V_m with a microelectrode inserted at the end-plate region of a frog muscle fiber. Their recordings from resting muscle fibers that were not subjected to nerve stimulation revealed the occurrence of tiny depolarizations of approximately 0.4 mV that appeared at random intervals. These small depolarizations were blocked by curare, an antagonist of AChR channels, and they increased in size and duration with the application of neostigmine, an inhibitor of AChE. Because the spontaneous V_m fluctuations also exhibited a time course that is similar to that of the normal EPP, they were named **miniature end-plate potentials** (also known as "MEPPs" or "minis"). These observations suggested that even in the absence of nerve stimulation, there is a certain low probability of transmitter release at the presynaptic terminal, resulting in the opening of a small number of AChRs in the postsynaptic membrane. An examination of the size of individual MEPPs suggested that they occur in discrete multiples of a unitary amplitude. This finding led to the notion that ACh release is *quantized*, with the quantum event corresponding to ACh release from one synaptic vesicle.

Another way of studying the quantal release of ACh is to stimulate the presynaptic motor neuron and monitor V_m at the end plate under conditions when the probability of ACh release is greatly decreased. How can we decrease the probability of ACh release? The amplitude of the EPP that is evoked in response to nerve stimulation is decreased by lowering $[Ca^{2+}]_o$ and increasing $[Mg^{2+}]_o$. A low $[Ca^{2+}]_o$ decreases Ca^{2+} entry into the presynaptic terminal (Fig. 8–2, *step 3*). A high $[Mg^{2+}]_o$ partially blocks the presynaptic Ca^{2+} channels and thus also decreases Ca^{2+} entry. Therefore, the consequence of either decreased $[Ca^{2+}]_o$ or increased $[Mg^{2+}]_o$ is a fall in $[Ca^{2+}]_i$ in the presynaptic terminal, which reduces transmitter release and thus the amplitude of the EPP (Fig. 8–11). Del Castillo and Katz exploited this suppression of transmitter release under conditions of low $[Ca^{2+}]_o$ and high $[Mg^{2+}]_o$ to observe the V_m changes caused by the quantal release of transmitter. Figure 8–12A shows seven superimposed records of MEPPs that were recorded from a frog muscle fiber during seven repetitive trials of nerve stimulation under conditions of reduced $[Ca^{2+}]_o$ and elevated $[Mg^{2+}]_o$. The records are aligned at the position of the nerve stimulus artifact. The amplitudes of the peak responses occur in discrete multiples of approximately 0.4 mV. Among the seven records were one "nonresponse," two responses of approximately 0.4 mV, three responses of approximately 0.8 mV, and one response of approximately 1.2 mV. One of the recordings also revealed a spontaneous MEPP with a quantal amplitude of approximately 0.4 mV that appeared later in the trace. Del Castillo and Katz proposed that the macroscopic EPP is the sum of many unitary events, each having a magnitude of approximately 0.4 mV. Microscopic observation of numerous vesicles in the synaptic terminal naturally led to the supposition that a single vesicle releases a relatively fixed amount of ACh and thereby produces a unitary MEPP. According to this view, the quantized MEPPs thus correspond to the fusion of discrete numbers of synaptic vesicles: 0, 1, 2, 3, and so on.

For elucidating the mechanism of synaptic transmission at the neuromuscular junction, Bernard Katz shared the 1970 Nobel Prize in Physiology or Medicine.

Direct Measurements of Extracellular Transmitter Levels Also Show That Transmitter Release is Quantal

Instead of using the postsynaptic AChR as a biologic detector of quantum release, one can use a microscopic electrochemical sensor to measure neurotransmitter levels directly. Figure 8–13 shows results from an experiment in which a fine carbon-fiber electrode was placed very

FIGURE 8–10. The effect of a local anesthetic on the acetylcholine receptor channel (AChR). *A,* Single-channel recording of nicotinic ACh receptor expressed in a *Xenopus* oocyte. The patch was in the outside-out configuration, and the holding potential was −150 mV. The continuous presence of 1 μM ACh caused brief channel openings. *B,* This experiment is similar to that in *A,* except that in addition to the ACh, the lidocaine analog QX-222 (20 μM) was present at the extracellular surface of the receptor channel. Note that the channel opening is accompanied by rapid flickering caused by many brief channel closures. The time scale of the lower panel is expanded 10-fold. (Data from Leonard RJ, Labarca CG, Charnet P, et al: Evidence that the M2 membrane-spanning region lines the ion channel pore of the nicotinic receptor. Science 242:1578–1581, 1988.)

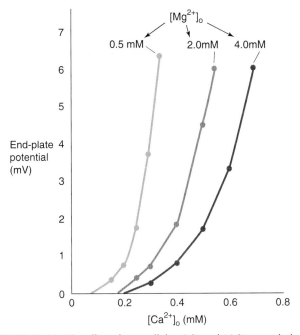

FIGURE 8–11. The effect of extracellular Ca^{2+} and Mg^{2+} on end-plate potentials. The data, obtained by stimulating the motor neuron and monitoring the evoked subthreshold EPP, show that the EPP is stimulated by increasing levels of Ca^{2+} but inhibited by increasing levels of Mg^{2+}. (Data from Dodge FA Jr, Rahaminoff R: Co-operative action of calcium ions in transmitter release at the neuromuscular junction. J Physiol 193:419–432, 1967.)

close to the presynaptic terminal membrane of a leech neuron that uses serotonin as its only neurotransmitter. The carbon fiber is an electrochemical detector of serotonin (see Fig. 8–13A); the current measured by this electrode corresponds to four electrons per serotonin molecule oxidized at the tip. Stimulating the leech neuron to produce an action potential also elicits an oxidation current, as measured by the carbon fiber, that corresponds to the release of serotonin. At a $[Ca^{2+}]_o$ of 5 mM, the current is large and composed of many small spikes (see Fig. 8–13B, *top*). On the other hand, reducing $[Ca^{2+}]_o$ to 1 mM—presumably reducing Ca^{2+} influx into the nerve terminal and thus reducing the number of quanta released—reveals individual spikes of serotonin release. The release spikes come in two sizes, small and large (see Fig. 8–13B, *bottom*), corresponding to two separate classes of synaptic vesicles that are evident on electron micrographs. Injecting the cell with tetanus toxin, which blocks the release of synaptic vesicles, abolishes the serotonin release spikes. Thus, the spikes represent genuine events of synaptic exocytosis.

The nearly immediate appearance of the small release spikes after electrical stimulation of the cell shows that this type of vesicular release is extremely rapid. From the height and duration of the small and large spikes in Figure 8–13B, one can estimate the amount of electrical charge and thus the number of serotonin molecules oxidized at the carbon fiber per spike. A unitary *small* event corresponds to the release of approximately 4700 serotonin molecules, whereas a unitary *large* event corresponds to the release of 15,000 to 300,000 serotonin

A MINIATURE END-PLATE POTENTIALS (MEPPs)

B DISTRIBUTION OF MEPP AMPLITUDES

FIGURE 8–12. Evoked and spontaneous miniature end-plate potentials (MEPPs). *A,* The investigators recorded V_m in frog skeletal muscle fibers that were exposed to extracellular solutions having a $[Ca^{2+}]$ of 0.5 mM and a $[Mg^{2+}]$ of 5 mM. These values minimize transmitter release, and therefore it was possible to resolve the smallest possible MEPP, which corresponds to the release of a single synaptic vesicle (i.e., 1 quantum). The investigators stimulated the motor neuron seven consecutive times and recorded the evoked MEPPs. In one trial, the stimulus evoked no response (0 quanta). In two trials, the peak MEPP was about 0.4 mV (1 quantum). In three others, the peak response was about 0.8 mV (2 quanta). Finally, in one, the peak was about 1.2 mV (3 quanta). In once case, a MEPP of the smallest magnitude appeared spontaneously. *B,* The histogram summarizes data from 198 trials on a cat neuromuscular junction in the presence of 12.5-mM extracellular Mg^{2+}. The data are in bins with a width of 0.1 mV. The distribution has eight peaks. The first represents stimuli that evoked no responses. The other seven represent stimuli that evoked MEPPs that were roughly integral multiples of the smallest MEPP. The curve overlying each cluster of bins is a gaussian or "normal" function and facilitates calculation of the average MEPP for each cluster of bins. The peak values of these gaussians follow a Poisson distribution. (Data from Magleby KL: Neuromuscular transmission. In Engel AG, Franzini-Armstrong C (eds): Myology, Basic and Clinical, 2nd ed. New York, McGraw-Hill, pp 442–463, 1994.)

molecules. Thus, the amount of serotonin released by the small synaptic vesicles of the leech neuron is about half the number of ACh molecules contained in a synaptic vesicle at the frog neuromuscular junction. These and other observations of the synaptic function of nerve-muscle and nerve-nerve synapses have led to the conclusion that *chemical neurotransmission operates by a fundamentally similar mechanism* at many types of synapses in different animal species (Chapter 12).

Short-term or long-term changes in the relative efficiency of neurotransmitter release can increase or decrease the *strength* of a particular synapse and thereby give rise to an alteration in behavior. Three types of synaptic modulation occur at the neuromuscular junction, and they differ in how they affect the quantal release of neurotransmitter:

Facilitation is a *short-lived* enhancement of the end-plate potential in response to a *brief* increase in the frequency of nerve stimulation. One way that facilitation may occur is by a transient increase in the mean number of quanta per nerve stimulus.

Potentiation (or post-tetanic potentiation) is a *long-*

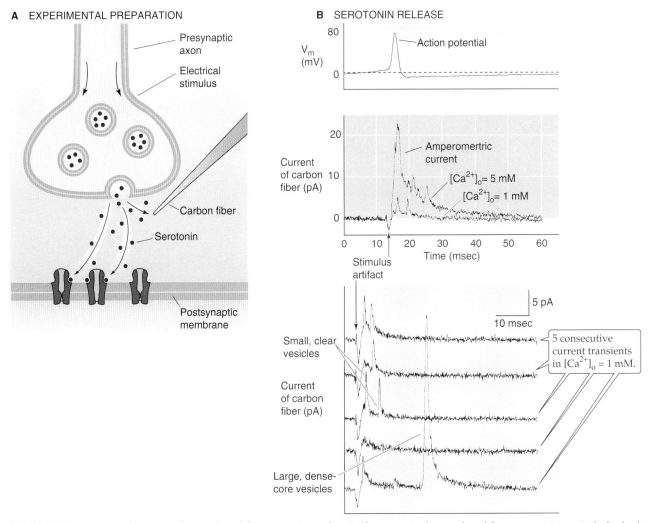

FIGURE 8–13. Detection of serotonin that is released from synaptic vesicles. *A,* The serotonin that is released from a synaptic terminal of a leech neuron can be detected electrochemically using a carbon-fiber microelectrode. The current carried by the carbon fiber increases with the amount of serotonin that is released, reflecting the oxidation of serotonin molecules on the surface of the carbon fiber. *B,* The *top panel* shows the action potential recorded from the stimulated motor neuron. The *middle panel* shows the evoked serotonin release (measured as a current) at both a $[Ca^{2+}]_o$ of 5 mM (high level of serotonin release) and a $[Ca^{2+}]_o$ of 1 mM (lower level or release). The *bottom panel* shows five consecutive trials at a $[Ca^{2+}]_o$ of 1 mM and illustrates that the release of serotonin can occur in either small quanta or very large quanta. These two sizes of quanta correspond to small clear vesicles and large dense-core vesicles, both of which can be observed by electron microscopy. (Data from Bruns D, Jahn R: Real-time measurement of transmitter release from single synaptic vesicles. Nature 377:62–65, 1995.)

lived and pronounced increase in transmitter release that occurs after a *long* period of high-frequency nerve stimulation. This effect can last for minutes after the conditioning stimulus. Potentiation may be caused by a period of intense nerve firing, which increases $[Ca^{2+}]_i$ in the presynaptic terminal and thus increases the probability of exocytosis.

Synaptic **depression** is a *transient* decrease in the efficiency of transmitter release and, consequently, a reduction in the end-plate potential in response to a period of frequent nerve stimulation. Depression may result from temporary depletion of transmitter-loaded vesicles from the presynaptic terminal, that is, a reduction in the number of available quanta. Thus, these three temporal changes in synaptic strength and efficiency appear to reflect changes at different steps of synaptic transmission. Similar modulation of synaptic strength in the CNS pro-

vides a mechanistic paradigm for understanding how individual nerve terminals may "learn" (p. 318).

Synaptic Vesicles Package, Store, and Deliver Neurotransmitters

The physiology of synaptic vesicles in the nervous system is a variation on the universal theme used by endocrine-like cells in animals from the most primitive invertebrates up to mammals (p. 88). Many of the proteins involved in synaptic vesicle movement and turnover are related to those involved in the intracellular membrane trafficking processes that take place in almost all eukaryotic cells. This trafficking involves vesicular translocation from the endoplasmic reticulum to the Golgi network and fusion with the plasma membrane. Genetic analysis of the yeast

A   BIOGENESIS

1 Vesicle and peptide neurotransmitter precursors and enzymes are synthesized in the cell and are released from Golgi.

2 Vesicles travel through the axon on microtubule tracks via fast axonal transport. Peptide neurotransmitters are already in some vesicles.

3 Nonpeptide neurotransmitters are synthesized and transported into vesicles the in nerve terminal.

Endoplasmic reticulum

Myelin sheath   Microtubules

Synaptic cleft

Nucleus

cis Golgi   *trans* Golgi

Endosomes (vesicles)

CELL BODY   AXON   Nerve Terminal

B   EXOCYTOSIS

A nonpeptide neurotransmitter is synthesized in the nerve terminal and transported into a vesicle.

Active zone

H⁺

H⁺   ATP

Transporter

FIGURE 8–14. Synthesis and recycling of synaptic vesicles and their content.

secretory pathway has identified various gene products that are homologous to those associated with synaptic vesicles of higher vertebrates. Thus, the processes underlying synaptic function are inherently quite similar to cellular exocytosis and endocytosis.

Synaptic vesicles are spherical organelles with a diameter of 40 to 200 nm. As shown in Figure 8–14A, synaptic vesicles are produced in the neuronal cell body by a process similar to the **secretory pathway** (p. 36). Thus, the membrane proteins of synaptic vesicles are synthesized in the rough endoplasmic reticulum and are then directed to the Golgi network, where processing, maturation, and sorting occur. Nascent synaptic vesicles—which are, in fact, secretory vesicles destined to become synaptic vesicles once they reach the nerve terminal—are then transported to the nerve terminal by **fast axonal trans-**port (p. 26) mediated by the microtubule system, which also carries mitochondria to the terminal.

Vesicles destined to contain *peptide* neurotransmitters travel down the axon with the presynthesized peptides or peptide precursors already inside. On arrival at the nerve terminal (Fig. 8–14B), the vesicles—now called synaptic vesicles—that carry peptide neurotransmitters become attached to the actin-based cytoskeletal network. Other vesicles are loaded with nonpeptide neurotransmitters (e.g., ACh) that are synthesized locally in the nerve terminal and likewise attach to the actin-based cytoskeletal network. At this point, the mature synaptic vesicles are functionally ready for Ca²⁺-dependent transmitter release and become docked at specific release sites in the active zones of the presynaptic membrane. After exocytotic fusion of the synaptic vesicles, endocytosis via clathrin-coated vesi-

OUTSIDE SYNAPTIC VESICLE   INSIDE SYNAPTIC VESICLE

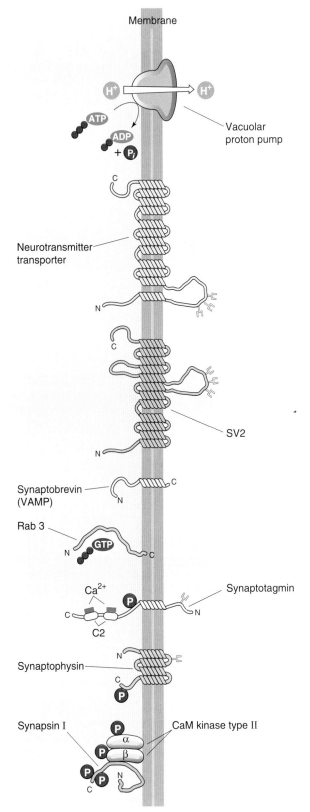

FIGURE 8–15. Membrane-associated proteins of synaptic vesicles.

cles (p. 42) recovers membrane components and recycles them to an endosome compartment in the terminal. Synaptic vesicles may then be reformed within the terminal for reuse in neurotransmission, or they may be transported back to the cell body for turnover and degradation.

Given their ubiquitous distribution in the nervous system and their relatively uniform size and molecular composition, synaptic vesicles can be obtained in large quantities from various sources such as the rat brain and the electric organ of the *Torpedo* ray. The purification of synaptic vesicles has made it possible to analyze their composition, which has facilitated gene cloning and the molecular characterization of many proteins that are intrinsic to synaptic vesicle function. Figure 8–15 summarizes a number of the major classes of synaptic vesicle proteins.

The uptake of nonpeptide neurotransmitters is accomplished by the combination of a vacuolar-type H$^+$-ATPase and a neurotransmitter transport protein. The **vacuolar-type H$^+$ pump** is a large, multisubunit complex that catalyzes the inward movement of H$^+$ into the vesicle, coupled to the hydrolysis of cytosolic ATP to adenosine diphosphate (ADP) and inorganic phosphate (p. 64). The resulting pH and voltage gradients across the vesicle membrane energize the uptake of neurotransmitters into the vesicle by a unique family of **neurotransmitter transport proteins** that exchange neurotransmitters in the cytosol for H$^+$ in the vesicle. This family of transporters includes members specific for ACh, monoamines (e.g., serotonin), catecholamines (e.g., norepinephrine), glutamate, and GABA/glycine.

Another cloned synaptic vesicle protein named **SV2** (for synaptic vesicle protein-2) structurally resembles a transport protein; however, a transport substrate for SV2 has not been identified and its function is unknown.

Synaptobrevin is an 19-kDa synaptic vesicle protein containing one transmembrane segment. Synaptobrevin, which is a v-SNARE (p. 39), is essential for transmitter release. As discussed in the next section, synaptobrevin on the *vesicle* membrane forms a complex with two proteins on the *presynaptic* membrane and helps drive vesicle fusion. *Tetanus toxin* or *botulinum toxins B, D, F,* and *G* are endoproteinases that digest synaptobrevin and are potent inhibitors of synaptic vesicle exocytosis.

Rab3 is a member of a large family of low-molecular-weight GTP-binding proteins that appears to be universally involved in cellular membrane trafficking (p. 39) via the binding and hydrolysis of GTP. **Synaptotagmin** is the synaptic vesicle Ca^{2+} receptor, a protein with two external repetitive domains that are homologous to the C2 domain of protein kinase C. The C2 domains appear to mediate binding of Ca^{2+}, a process that also depends on the presence of acidic phospholipids. Synaptotagmin senses a local rise in [Ca^{2+}]$_i$ and triggers the exocytosis of docked vesicles.

Another major constituent, **synaptophysin**, is an integral membrane protein with four transmembrane segments that exhibits channel-forming activity in planar bilayers. It may be involved in the formation of a fusion pore during exocytosis. The **synapsins** are a group of synaptic vesicle proteins that are phosphorylated by both cyclic adenosine monophosphate (cAMP)-dependent and calmodulin-dependent protein kinases. Interactions of synapsins with cytoskeletal proteins and their inhibition by phosphorylation have led to the notion that synapsins normally mediate the attachment of synaptic vesicles to the actin cytoskeleton. With an increase in $[Ca^{2+}]_i$ and subsequent phosphorylation, the synapsin detaches and permits vesicles to move to active sites at the synaptic membrane.

Neurotransmitter Release Occurs by Exocytosis of Synaptic Vesicles

Although the mechanism by which synaptic vesicles fuse with the plasma membrane and release their contents is far from fully understood, we have working models (Fig. 8–16) for the function of various key components and steps involved in synaptic vesicle release. These models are based on a variety of in vitro experiments. The use of specific toxins that act at nerve synapses and elegant functional studies of genetic mutants in *Drosphilia*, *C. elegans*, and gene knockout mice have provided important information on the role of various components.

We have already introduced the key proteins located in the synaptic vesicle. Of these, we now focus on the v-SNARE synaptobrevin and the Ca^{2+} sensor synaptotagmin. In addition, several other proteins—located in the target area of the presynaptic membrane of the nerve terminal—play an important role in the fusion process. **Syntaxin** is anchored in the presynaptic membrane by a single membrane-spanning segment. **SNAP-25** (synaptosome-associated protein −25 kDa) is tethered to the presynaptic membrane via palmitoyl side chains. Both syntaxin and SNAP-25 are t-SNARES (p. 39). *Botulinum toxins A and E*, which are endoproteinases, specifically cleave SNAP-25, whereas another endoproteinase, *botulinum toxin C1*, specifically cleaves syntaxin. These toxins block the fusion of synaptic vesicles.

According to the model shown in Figure 8–16, docking of the vesicle to the presynaptic membrane occurs as n-Sec1 dissociates from syntaxin. The free ends of synaptobrevin, syntaxin, and SNAP-25 begin to coil around each other. The result is a ternary complex, an extraordinarily stable rod-shaped structure of α helices. As the energetically favorable coiling of the three SNAREs continues, the vesicle membrane is pulled ever closer to the presynaptic membrane. Ca^{2+} enters through voltage-gated Ca^{2+} channels located in register with the active zone of the presynaptic membrane. A local increase in $[Ca^{2+}]_i$ triggers the final event, fusion and exocytosis. The synaptic vesicle protein synaptotagmin is believed to be the actual sensor of increased $[Ca^{2+}]_i$ because knockout mice and *Drosophila* mutants lacking the appropriate isoform of this protein have impaired Ca^{2+}-dependent transmitter release. The soluble α-SNAP (soluble NSF attachment protein) binds to the ternary complex formed by the intertwined SNAREs and promotes the binding of NSF (an ATPase), which uses the energy of ATP hydrolysis to disassemble the three tightly wound SNAREs. The now-free synaptobrevin presumably undergoes endocytosis,

whereas the syntaxin and SNAP-25 on the presynaptic membrane are available for the next round of vesicle fusion.

The model just presented leaves unanswered some important questions. For example, what is the structure of the fusion pore detected by electrophysiological measurements as a primary event in membrane fusion? Also, the model does not fully explain the basis for the rapid catalysis of fusion by Ca^{2+}. Neuroscientists are very interested in the details of synaptic vesicle fusion because this exocytotic process might be a target for controlling synaptic strength and may thus play a role in the synaptic plasticity that is responsible for changes in animal behavior.

Re-Uptake or Cleavage of the Neurotransmitter Terminates Its Action

Effective transmission across chemical synapses requires not only release of the neurotransmitter and activation of the receptor on the postsynaptic membrane but also rapid and efficient mechanisms for removing the transmitter. At synapses where ACh is released, this removal is accomplished by enzymatic destruction of the neurotransmitter. However, the more general mechanism in the nervous system involves re-uptake of the neurotransmitter mediated by specific, high-affinity transport systems located in the presynaptic plasma membrane and surrounding glial cells. These secondary active transport systems use the normal ionic gradients of Na^+, K^+, H^+, or Cl^- to achieve concentrative uptake of transmitter. Vertebrates have two distinct families of neurotransmitter transport proteins. The first family is characterized by a common motif of 12 membrane-spanning segments and includes transporters with specificity for catecholamines, serotonin, GABA, glycine, and choline. Energy coupling of transport in this class of systems is generally based on cotransport of the substrate with Na^+ and Cl^-. The second family is represented by transporters for the excitatory amino acids glutamate and aspartate. In these latter systems, substrate transport generally couples to cotransport of Na^+ and H^+, and to exchange of K^+.

At the neuromuscular junction and other cholinergic synapses, immediate termination of the action of ACh is accomplished enzymatically by the action of **acetylcholinesterase** (AChE). Although AChE is primarily found at the neuromuscular junction, AChE activity can be detected throughout the nervous system. The enzyme occurs in a variety of physical forms. The **globular** or **G forms** exist as monomers, dimers, or tetramers of a common, approximately 72-kDa glycoprotein catalytic subunit. These molecules can be found either in soluble form or bound to cell membranes via a GPI linkage (p. 15) in which a post-translational modification attaches the C terminus of the protein to a glycolipid moiety. The **asymmetric** or **A forms** consist of one to three tetramers of the globular enzyme coupled through disulfide bond linkage to a collagen-like structural protein. The largest asymmetric form, which has 12 catalytic subunits attached to the collagen-like tail, is the major species located at the neuromuscular junction. The triple-helical, collagen-like

1
Vesicles with synaptotagmin and synaptobrevin (a v-SNARE) move to the nerve terminal membrane, which contains syntaxin and SNAP-25 (both t-SNAREs).

2
n-sec-1 dissociates from syntaxin, allowing the syntaxin and SNAP-25 to form a complex. The distal end of synaptobrevin begins to wind around the syntaxin/SNAP-25 complex, forming a ternary complex.

3
The three SNAREs—synaptobrevin, syntaxin and SNAP-25—continue to form a tight bundle of α helices, drawing the vesicle and presynaptic membranes into close apposition.

INITIAL STATE

FORMATION OF TERNARY COMPLEX OF SNARES

TIGHTENING OF TERNARY SNARE COMPLEX

RECYCLING OF SNAREs

DISASSEMBLY OF TERNARY SNARE COMPLEX

FUSION AND EXOCYTOSIS

6
With the endocytosis of the vesicle, the synaptobrevin is effectively recycled. The syntaxin and SNAP-25 are now free for an additional cycle of vesicle fusion.

5
α-SNAP and the ATPase NSF bind to the ternary SNARE complex and use the energy of ATP hydrolysis to disassemble the SNAREs.

4
The entry of Ca^{2+} and its binding to synaptotagmin triggers fusion.

FIGURE 8–16. Model of synaptic-vesicle fusion and exocytosis. ADP, adenosine diphosphate; ATP, adenosine triphosphate; NSF, N-ethyl maleimide–sensitive factor; SNAP-25, synaptosome-associated protein–25 kDa; α-SNAP, soluble NSF-attachment protein; SNARE, SNAP receptor.

tail attaches the asymmetric AChE complex to extracellular matrix components of the synaptic basal lamina. The various physical forms of AChE are a result of the alternative splicing that occurs in the transcription of a single AChE gene.

The enzyme AChE rapidly hydrolyzes ACh to choline and acetate in a two-step process:

Equation 8–5

$$AChE + ACh \longrightarrow \underset{\text{choline}}{\text{acetyl-AChE}} \longrightarrow acetate + AChE$$

In the first step of the reaction, the enzyme cleaves choline from ACh, which results in the formation of an

DISEASES OF THE HUMAN ACETYLCHOLINE RECEPTOR: MYASTHENIA GRAVIS AND A CONGENITAL MYASTHENIC SYNDROME

The term "myasthenia" means muscle weakness (from the Greek *mys* and *asthenia*) and is used clinically to usually mean weakness in the absence of primary muscle disease, neuropathy, or central nervous system disorder. **Myasthenia gravis,** one specific type of myasthenia and the most common adult form, afflicts 25 to 125 of every 1 million people. It can occur at any age but has a bimodal distribution, with peak incidences occurring among people in their 20s and 60s. Those afflicted at an early age tend to be women with hyperplasia of the thymus, whereas those who are older are more likely to be men with coexisting cancer of the thymus gland. The cells of the thymus possess nicotinic acetylcholine receptors (AChRs), and the disease arises as a result of antibodies directed against these receptors. The antibodies then lead to skeletal muscle weakness caused in part by competitive antagonism of AChRs. Symptoms include fatigue and weakness of skeletal muscle. Two major forms of the disease are recognized: one that involves weakness of only the extraocular muscles and another that results in generalized weakness of all skeletal muscles. In either case, myasthenia gravis is typified by fluctuating symptoms, with weakness greatest toward the end of the day or after exertion. In severe cases, paralysis of the respiratory muscles can lead to death. Treatment directed at enhancing cholinergic transmission, alone or combined with thymectomy or immunosuppression, is highly effective in most patients.

Progress toward achieving an understanding of the cause of myasthenia gravis was first made when electrophysiologic analysis of involved muscle revealed that the amplitude of the miniature end-plate potential was decreased, although the frequency of quantal events was normal. This finding suggested either a defect in the postsynaptic response to ACh or a reduced concentration of ACh in the synaptic vesicles. A major breakthrough occurred in 1973, when Patrick and Lindstrom found that symptoms similar to those of humans with myasthenia developed in rabbits immunized with AChR protein purified from the electric eel. This finding was shortly followed by the demonstration of anti-AChR antibodies in human patients with myasthenia gravis and a severe reduction in the surface density of AChR in the junctional folds. These anti-AChR antibodies are directed against one or more subunits of the receptor, where they bind and activate complement and accelerate destruction of the receptors. The most common target of these antibodies is a region of the AChR α subunit called MIR (main immunogenic region).

Myasthenia gravis is now recognized to be an acquired autoimmune disorder in which the spontaneous production of anti-AChR antibodies results in progressive loss of muscle AChRs and degeneration of postjunctional folds. Treatment is aimed at either reducing the potency of the immunologic attack or enhancing cholinergic activity within the synapse. The former is achieved by the use of immunosuppressants (most commonly corticosteroids) or plasmapheresis (removal of antibodies from the patient's serum). Some patients with myasthenia gravis have a thymoma (a tumor of the thymus gland) that is often readily seen on routine chest radiographs. In these patients, removal of the thymoma leads to clinical improvement in nearly 75% of the cases. Enhancement of cholinergic activity is achieved through the use of AChE inhibitors, with pyridostigmine being the most widely used agent. The dosage of these drugs must be carefully monitored to prevent *over*exposure of the remaining AChRs to ACh. Overexposure can lead to overstimulation of the postsynaptic receptors, prolonged depolarization of the postsynaptic membrane, inactivation of neighboring Na^+ channels, and thus synaptic blockade.

Another condition characterized by progressive muscle weakness and fatigue is the **Lambert-Eaton syndrome** (see box on p. 193). Lambert-Eaton syndrome is caused by antibodies that attack the presynaptic Ca^{2+} channel and can be distinguished from myasthenia gravis in several ways. First, it primarily attacks the limb muscles, not the ocular and bulbar muscles. Second, repetitive stimulation of a particular muscle leads to enhanced amplitude of the postsynaptic action potential, whereas in patients with myasthenia, repetitive stimulation leads to progressive lessening of the action potential. Thus, repeated muscle stimulation leads to increasing contractile strength in patients with Lambert-Eaton syndrome and to decreasing strength in patients with myasthenia.

The term **congenital myasthenic syndromes** (CMS) refers to a variety of inherited disorders, present at birth, that affect neuromuscular transmission in a variety of ways. Because specific cases can involve acetylcholinesterase deficiency, abnormal presynaptic release of ACh, or defective AChR function (without the presence of antireceptor antibodies), the signs and symptoms can also vary widely. In 1995, an unusual example of a CMS disorder was traced to a mutation in the ε subunit of the human AChR. Single-channel recordings from biopsied muscle fibers of a young myasthenic patient revealed a profound alteration in AChR kinetics. The burst duration of AChR openings was greatly prolonged in comparison with that of normal human AChR channels. The molecular defect is a point mutation of Thr to Pro at position 264 in the adult ε subunit of the AChR. This amino acid residue corresponds to an evolutionarily conserved position in the M2 membrane-spanning segment, which is involved in formation of the channel pore. Thus, a human mutation in the pore region of the AChR protein results in failure of the channel to close normally, thereby causing excessive depolarization and pathologic consequences at the muscle end plate.

The aforementioned mutation is only one of at least 53 mutations in 55 different kinships that have been identified in the AChR. Some of the other mutations result in electrophysiologic changes similar to those described earlier. Thus, failure of neuromuscular transmission may be induced by multiple mechanisms, and even those related to the AChR can have many causes.

FIGURE 8–17. Pharmacology of the vertebrate neuromuscular junction. Many of the proteins that are involved in synaptic transmission at the mammalian neuromuscular junction are the targets of naturally occurring or synthetic drugs. The antagonists are shown as "−" signs highlighted in *red*. The agonists are shown as "+" signs highlighted in *green*.

intermediate in which the acetate group is covalently coupled to a serine group on the enzyme. The second step is the hydrolysis and release of this acetate, as well as the free enzyme. Via a high-affinity, Na^+-coupled uptake system, the nerve terminal recovers the choline formed in this reaction and uses it for the synthesis of ACh.

TOXINS AND DRUGS AFFECTING SYNAPTIC TRANSMISSION

Much of our knowledge of the synaptic physiology of the neuromuscular junction and the identities of its various molecular components have been derived from experiments using specific pharmacologic agents and toxins that permit functional dissection of the system. Figure 8–17 illustrates the relative synaptic location and corresponding pharmacology of AChE, as well as several ion channels and proteins involved in exocytosis.

Guanidinium Neurotoxins Such as Tetrodotoxin Prevent Depolarization of the Nerve Terminal, Whereas Dendrotoxins Inhibit Repolarization

The action potential is the first step in transmission: a nerve action potential arriving at the terminal initiates the

entire process. As discussed in Chapter 7, the depolarizing phase of the action potential is mediated by voltage-dependent Na^+ channels that are specifically blocked by nanomolar concentrations of the small guanidinium neurotoxins **tetrodotoxin** (TTX) and **saxitoxin** (STX) (see Fig. 7–5C).

The mamba snake toxin **dendrotoxin** (p. 194) has an effect that is precisely opposite that of TTX: it facilitates the release of ACh that is evoked by nerve stimulation. Dendrotoxins are a family of approximately 59-residue proteins with three disulfide bonds that block certain isoforms of voltage-gated K^+ channels by binding to an extracellular site in the P-region domain with high affinity. These toxins reveal the important role of K^+ channels in terminating the process of transmitter release. Blockade of presynaptic K^+ channels by dendrotoxin inhibits repolarization of the presynaptic membrane, thereby prolonging the duration of the action potential and facilitating the release of transmitter in response to the entry of extra Ca^{2+} into the nerve terminal.

By Inhibiting Ca²⁺ Channels in the Active Zone of the Nerve Terminal, Molluscan Toxins Such as ω-Conotoxin Prevent the Triggering of Exocytosis by Intracellular Ca²⁺

The exocytotic fusion of mature synaptic vesicles positioned at presynaptic active zones and the subsequent

TABLE 8–2

NEUROTOXINS THAT BLOCK FUSION OF SYNAPTIC VESICLES	
TOXIN	**TARGET**
Tetanus	Synaptobrevin
Botulinum B, D, F, G	Synaptobrevin
Botulinum A/E	SNAP-25
Botulinum C1	Syntaxin

SNAP-25, synaptosome-associated protein–25 kDa.

release of ACh require the entry of Ca^{2+} into the nerve terminal. Ca^{2+} enters the presynaptic terminal through voltage-gated Ca^{2+} channels that are activated by the depolarization of an incoming action potential. One type of voltage-gated Ca^{2+} channel, the N-type isoform, has been localized to the region of the active zone of the frog neuromuscular junction. Voltage-clamp experiments demonstrate that a class of molluscan peptide toxins called ω-conotoxins (p. 191) block N-type Ca^{2+} currents in a practically irreversible fashion. Exposure of a frog nerve-muscle preparation to ω-conotoxin thus inhibits the release of neurotransmitter. This effect is manifested as an abolition of muscle EPP when the preparation is stimulated via the nerve. The ω-conotoxins are 24 to 29 residues long and contain three disulfide bonds. Imaging with confocal laser scanning microscopy has shown that ω-conotoxin binds at highest density to voltage-dependent Ca^{2+} channels in the presynaptic nerve terminal, directly across the synaptic cleft from AChR channels. This observation implies that Ca^{2+} channels are located precisely at the active zones of synaptic vesicle fusion. This arrangement provides for focal entry and short-range diffusion of Ca^{2+} entering the nerve terminal to the exact sites involved in promoting Ca^{2+}-dependent transmitter release.

By Cleaving Proteins Involved in Exocytosis, Bacterial Toxins Such as Tetanus and Botulinum Toxins Prevent Fusion of the Synaptic Vesicles

Another class of neurotoxins that specifically inhibits neurotransmitter release includes the tetanus and botulinum toxins. These large protein toxins (~150 kDa) are respectively produced by the bacteria *Clostridium tetani* and *C. botulinum* (see the box titled Clostridial Catastrophes). *C. tetani* is the causative agent of tetanus ("lockjaw"), which is characterized by a general increase in muscle tension and muscle rigidity, beginning most often with the muscles of mastication. The reason for this paradoxical enhancement of muscle action is that the toxins have their greatest effect on *inhibition* of synaptic transmission by inhibitory neurons in the spinal cord, neurons that would normally *inhibit* muscle contraction. *C. botulinum* causes botulism, which is characterized by weakness and paralysis of skeletal muscle, as well as a variety of symptoms that are related to inhibition of cholinergic nerve endings in the autonomic nervous system.

In humans, infection by these bacteria can lead to death because the toxins that they synthesize are potent inhibitors of neurotransmitter release. This inhibition occurs because both tetanus and botulinum toxin proteins have zinc-dependent endoproteinase activity (Table 8–2). These toxins enter nerve terminals and specifically cleave three different proteins required for synaptic vesicle exocytosis. **Tetanus toxin** and **botulinum toxins** B, D, F, and G cleave synaptobrevin, an integral membrane protein of the synaptic vesicle membrane. Botulinum toxins C1 and A/E respectively cleave syntaxin and SNAP-25, two proteins associated with the presynaptic membrane. These neurotoxins can have useful medical applications. For example, botulinum toxin is used to treat certain disorders characterized by muscle spasms. Injection of a small amount of botulinum toxin into the eye muscles of a patient with strabismus (a condition in which both eyes cannot focus on the same object because of abnormal hyperactivity of particular eye muscles) is able to suppress aberrant muscle spasms and restore normal vision.

Both Agonists and Antagonists of the Nicotinic Acetylcholine Receptor Can Prevent Synaptic Transmission

The ionotropic (nicotinic) AChR channel located in the postsynaptic muscle membrane (see Fig. 8–17) also has a rich and diverse pharmacology that can be exploited for clinical applications, as well as for elucidating many functional aspects of the neuromuscular junction. Figure 8–18 shows the chemical structures of two classes of agents that act on the nicotinic AChR. These agents are classified as agonists or antagonists according to whether they activate opening of the channel or prevent its activation. Many **agonists** have a structure similar to that of the natural neurotransmitter ACh. In general, such agonists activate the opening of AChR channels with the same unitary conductance as those activated by ACh, but with different kinetics of channel opening and closing. The synthetic drugs **carbamylcholine** (or carbachol) and **succinylcholine** contain the choline moiety of ACh that is required for receptor activation. Carbamylcholine is a carbamyl ester of choline, whereas succinylcholine (or succinyldicholine) is dimer of ACh linked together via the acetyl methyl group. Both of these agents are resistant to hydrolysis by muscle AChE, but succinylcholine is susceptible to hydrolysis by plasma and liver esterases. This property allows for prolonged activation of AChRs.

Succinylcholine is used to produce sustained muscle relaxation or "flaccid paralysis," which is useful in certain types of surgery in which it is important to prevent excitation and contraction of skeletal muscles. This paralytic action occurs because succinylcholine prolongs the opening of AChR channels and thereby depolarizes the muscle membrane in the vicinity of the end plate. Such depolarization results in initial repetitive muscle excitation and tremors, followed by relaxation secondary to **inactivation of Na^+ channels** in the vicinity of the end plate. This latter effect prevents the spread of muscle action potentials beyond the end-plate region. On a longer time scale, such agents also lead to **desensitization of the AChR** to

CLOSTRIDIAL CATASTROPHES

Botulism, although hardly one of the most common causes of food poisoning today, is still the illness that many people think of when food-borne disorders are discussed. The neurotoxin of *Clostridium botulinum* is very potent, and only a small amount of contamination can lead to death. The most common source of botulism is homemade foods. The spores of this organism can survive boiling temperatures for a number of hours, and if the cooked food is allowed to stand at room temperature for more than 16 hours, the clostridial spores can germinate and produce toxin. Symptoms of the illness may appear from several hours to more than a week after ingestion, although most cases occur within 18 to 36 hours. Patients begin to complain of symptoms attributable to inhibition of synaptic vesicle release in the autonomic nervous system (see Chapter 15), such as dry mouth, double vision, and difficulty swallowing and speaking, and later begin to experience gastrointestinal complications, including vomiting, pain, and diarrhea. Symptoms attributable to inhibition of synaptic vesicle release at the neuromuscular junction such as weakness and paralysis of the limbs may soon follow; ultimately, paralysis of the respiratory muscles (see Chapter 26) can be fatal. Prompt intervention with mechanical ventilation has reduced the mortality from botulism dramatically, and the figure today stands at about 20%. Almost all deaths occur among the first victims of a contaminated ingestion because the disease is not quickly recognized; those who fall victim later, when the diagnosis is much easier, do much better.

Vaccination has reduced the number of cases of **tetanus** reported in the United States to only about 100 each year, almost all occurring in inadequately vaccinated individuals. The disease is caused by a neurotoxin (tetanospasmin) produced by *Clostridium tetani*. The organism gains entry to its host through a cut or puncture wound. The toxin then travels along the peripheral nerves to the spinal cord, the major site of its attack. There, the toxin inhibits synaptic-vesicle release by interneurons that normally inhibit firing of the motor neurons that, in turn, activate skeletal muscle. Thus, because the toxin suppresses inhibition of the normal reflex arc, muscular contraction leads to profound spasms, most characteristically of the jaw muscles but potentially affecting any muscle in the body. Symptoms can commence on the day of the injury or as long as 2 months later. Complications include respiratory arrest, aspiration pneumonia, rib fractures caused by the severe spasms, and a host of other pulmonary and cardiac manifestations.

agonist, which further inhibits neuromuscular transmission.

Another important agent acting on AChRs is **nicotine,** a natural constituent of tobacco that is responsible for the stimulant action and at least some of the addictive effects of smoking. The selective ability of nicotine to activate AChR channels is the basis of the classification scheme of "nicotinic" AChRs versus "muscarinic" AChRs (see Fig. 8–3). Nicotine is not an agonist of the muscarinic or G protein–linked receptors, which instead are activated by the mushroom alkaloid muscarine. Although nicotine is able to activate the AChR at the neuromuscular junction, the physiological effects of smoking are primarily manifested in the CNS and autonomic ganglia, where other neuronal isoforms of nicotinic AChRs are located.

A classic example of a nicotinic AChR **antagonist** is *d*-tubocurarine (see Fig. 8–18), the active ingredient of curare, a poison extracted from plants of the genus *Strychnos*. The indigenous tribes of the Amazon region used curare to poison arrows for hunting. *d*-Tubocurarine is a competitive inhibitor of ACh binding to two activation sites on the α subunits of the AChR. This action leads to flaccid paralysis of skeletal muscle from inhibition of the nicotinic AChR. However, curare does not cause depolarization. A hallmark of the action of *d*-tubocurarine is that it can be reversed by an increase in concentration of the natural agonist ACh by binding competition. A large increase in local ACh concentration can be produced indirectly by an inhibitor of AChE such as neostigmine (see later).

Figure 8–18 also shows the structure of **pancuronium,** which is a synthetic bis-quaternary ammonium steroid derivative. This drug is also useful for the production of neuromuscular blockade in surgery, and it is actually a more potent, selective competitive antagonist of the muscle nicotinic AChR than D-tubocurarine is.

Another class of nicotinic AChR inhibitors is a family of approximately 8-kDa proteins present in the venom of Elapidae snakes (e.g., cobras). These toxins include α-bungarotoxin (α-Bgt) and homologous α toxins, which bind very strongly to nicotinic receptors. The specific binding of α-Bgt to the nicotinic AChR of skeletal muscle is virtually irreversible. When α-Bgt binds to the nicotinic AChR, it obstructs the agonist-binding site and prevents activation of the receptor by ACh. The radioiodinated derivative ^{125}I-labeled α-Bgt has been widely used as a ligand for purifying the nicotinic AChR from various tissues. Fluorescent derivatives of α-Bgt can also be used as specific labels for localizing AChRs at the muscle end plate. The same snake venom (*Bungarus multicinctus*) that contains α-Bgt also contains a homologous protein toxin called κ-bungarotoxin (κ-Bgt). This toxin has little effect on nicotinic AChR channels at the neuromuscular junction, but it does inhibit AChR channels in neuronal tissue. The differential effect of α-Bgt and κ-Bgt on muscle and neuronal currents activated by both ACh and nicotine led to the recognition that different classes of nicotinic receptors exist in the CNS versus skeletal muscle. The basis for these isoforms is the differential expression of multiple genes for homologous nicotinic AChR subunits.

Inhibitors of Acetylcholinesterase Prolong and Magnify the End-Plate Potential

A variety of specific inhibitors of anticholinesterase have been helpful in defining the contribution of AChE to responses at the muscle end plate. Inhibition of AChE generally increases the amplitude and prolongs the duration of the postsynaptic response to ACh; thus, the en-

AGONISTS

FIGURE 8–18. Agonists and antagonists of the nicotinic acetylcholine receptor (AChR).

zyme plays an important role in limiting the excitatory action of ACh under normal physiological conditions. In the absence of ACh breakdown by AChE, the prolonged decay of the EPP reflects the underlying kinetics of activated receptors and slow depletion of the agonist in the vicinity of the junctional folds by diffusion of ACh.

The plant alkaloid **physostigmine** (also known as eserine) is the prototypic anticholinesterase (Fig. 8–19). **Neostigmine** (also called prostigmine), a synthetic anti-AChE drug that is partially analogous to physostigmine, is used to treat myasthenia gravis. As discussed in the box on p. 224, this disease is caused by the autoimmune destruction and loss of nicotinic AChRs at the muscle end plate. Because ACh is an acetyl ester, the catalytic cycle of AChE results in the formation of an intermediate in which a serine group of the AChE is acetylated. Physostigmine and neostigmine, on the other hand, have a carbamyl ester linkage that produces a carbamoylated intermediate form of AChE. However, slow hydrolysis of the carbamoylated enzyme results in an approximately 4-hour duration of esterase inhibition.

Another important class of synthetic AChE inhibitors consists of **organophosphorus compounds**, which are *irreversible* inhibitors. This group is typified by diisopropyl-

fluorophosphate (**DFP**) (see Fig. 8–19). These compounds react with the aforementioned serine residue of AChE and form an essentially irreversible covalent modification of the enzyme. Such agents rank highly among the most potent and lethal of toxic chemicals. Their devastating effect is caused by excessive enhancement of cholinergic neurotransmission, mediated by both muscarinic and nicotinic receptor pathways throughout the body. For example, exposure to toxic organophosphorus agents results in the flaccid paralysis of respiratory muscles because of initial muscle stimulation followed by depolarization blockade. The devastating action of these compounds dramatically underlines the essential role of AChE in terminating cholinergic neurotransmission. A tragic application of various volatile forms of these compounds is their use as chemical warfare agents (i.e., "nerve gas" such as sarin). Related compounds, such as malathion (see Fig. 8–19), which are selectively toxic to insects, are widely used as agricultural insecticides.

A natural organophosphorus neurotoxin is produced by *Anaebena flos-aquae*, a toxic cyanobacterium (blue-green alga). Known as **anatoxin-a(s)**, this toxin is a potent inhibitor of AChE and is responsible for the poisoning of dogs and farm animals that drink from contaminated

REVERSIBLE

Physostigmine (eserine)

Neostigmine (prostigmine)

IRREVERSIBLE

Diisopropylfluorophosphate (DFP)

O,O-dimethyl S-(1,2-dicarbethoxyethyl) phosphorodithioate (Malathion)

FIGURE 8–19. Structures of acetylcholinesterase (AChE) inhibitors.

ponds. Another interesting class of natural inhibitors includes the **fasciculins**, a family of small protein toxins present in mamba snake venom that inhibit AChE with very high affinity and specificity.

By Inhibiting Muscle Na⁺ Channels, Certain Neurotoxins Block Spread of the Postsynaptic Action Potential and Muscle Contraction

An action potential is not only the first but also the last step in transmission at the neuromuscular junction: the production of an action potential in the muscle fiber membrane signals the successful completion of synaptic transmission. As discussed earlier, action potentials, including those in muscle, can be blocked by TTX and STX. Selective blockade of the muscle action potential can be achieved with a unique toxin called **μ-conotoxin** (p. 187), which is obtained from a marine snail (*Conus geographus*). μ-Conotoxin is a 22-residue, basic peptide with a discoidal, star-like three-dimensional structure that is stabilized by three disulfide bonds. It is an especially potent blocker of the particular isoform of the voltage-dependent Na⁺ channel that is present in adult mammalian skeletal muscle, but it has little effect on the Na⁺ channel isoforms of nerve or heart. If an intact nerve-muscle preparation is exposed to μ-conotoxin, stimulation of the nerve still evokes the release of ACh, but the muscle action potential is completely eliminated.

REFERENCES

Books and Reviews

Engel AG: Acquired autoimmune myasthenia gravis. In Engel AG, Franzini-Armstrong C (eds): Myology, Basic and Clinical, 2nd ed. New York, McGraw-Hill, 1994, pp 1769–1797.

Hall ZW, Sanes JR: Synaptic structure and development: The neuromuscular junction. Cell 10 (Suppl):99–121, 1993.

Jahn R, Hanson PI: SNAREs line up in new environment. Nature 393: 14–15, 1998.

Katz B: Nerve, Muscle, and Synapse. New York, McGraw-Hill, 1966.

Nicholls JG, Martin AR, Wallace BG: From Neuron to Brain, 3rd ed. Sunderland, MA, Sinauer Associates, 1992.

Südhof T: The synaptic vesicle cycle: A cascade of protein-protein interactions. Nature 375:645–653, 1995.

Van der Kloot W, Molgó J: Quantal acetylcholine release at the vertebrate neuromuscular junction. Physiol Rev 74:899–989, 1994.

Journal Articles

Del Castillo J, Katz B: Interaction at end-plate receptors between different choline derivatives. Proc R Soc Lond B Biol Sci 146:369–381, 1957.

Fatt P, Katz B: Spontaneous subthreshold activity at motor nerve endings. J Physiol 117:109–128, 1952.

Furshpan EJ, Potter DD: Transmission at the giant motor synapse of the crayfish. J Physiol 145:289–325, 1959.

Magleby KL, Stevens CF: A quantitative description of end-plate currents. J Physiol 233:173–197, 1972.

Noda M, Takahashi H, Tanabe T, et al: Structural homology of *Torpedo californica* acetylcholine receptor subunits. Nature 302:528, 1983.

Ohno K, Hutchinson DO, Milone M, et al: Congenital myasthenic syndrome caused by prolonged acetylcholine receptor channel openings due to a mutation in the M2 domain of the epsilon subunit. Proc Natl Acad Sci U S A 92:758–762, 1995.

CHAPTER 9

Cellular Physiology of Skeletal, Cardiac, and Smooth Muscle

Michael Apkon

The primary function of each of the three fundamental types of muscle—skeletal, cardiac, and smooth muscle—is to generate force or movement in response to a physiological stimulus. All muscles transduce a chemical or electrical command into a mechanical response. However, the unique physiological role of each of the three basic muscle types dictates inherent differences in the rate and duration of contraction, metabolism, fatigability, and the ability to regulate contractile strength. For example, both skeletal and cardiac muscle must be capable of rapid force development and shortening. However, skeletal muscle must be able to maintain contractile force for relatively long periods, whereas cardiac muscle need only contract briefly with each heartbeat, although it must sustain this periodic activity for an entire lifetime. Smooth muscle, like skeletal muscle, must be able to regulate contraction over a wide range of force. However, in some tissues (e.g., sphincters), smooth muscle must be able to sustain contraction without fatigue for very long periods. In spite of these differences, the trigger for muscle contraction is the same for all three types of muscle: a rise in the free cytosolic Ca^{2+} concentration ($[Ca^{2+}]_i$).

In muscle of all types, certain components of the muscle cell are highly specialized to accomplish the muscle's unique function. Given the disparity in their physiological roles, it is not surprising that each muscle type has evolved unique anatomic structures and functional mechanisms. Thus, the various types of muscle cells have specialized plasma membranes, cytoskeletons, endoplasmic reticulum, and metabolic pathways for energy generation and utilization.

EXCITATION OF MUSCLE CELLS

The plasma membrane—or sarcolemma—of each of the types of muscle cells has regions that are specialized to facilitate communication between cells. In skeletal muscle, this specialization takes the form of the postsynaptic portion of the neuromuscular junction. Neuromuscular junctions (i.e., chemical synapses) are also present in cardiac and smooth muscle. In cardiac muscle, neuromuscular transmission does not initiate contraction; it only *modulates* it. On the other hand, neuromuscular transmission may initiate contraction in smooth muscle cells, or it may modulate contraction that has been initiated by another mechanism. In both smooth and cardiac muscle cells, gap junctions (i.e., electrical synapses) couple the sarcolemma of neighboring cells; these also play an important role in intercellular communication.

Branched structure of cardiac muscle

Intercalated disk

Myosin Actin Microfibril Intercalated disk

Z-line

Desmosome

Mitochondrion

Gap junction

Z-line

FIGURE 9–1. Electrical coupling of cardiac myocytes.

Skeletal Muscle Contracts in Response to Neuromuscular Synaptic Transmission

The mature skeletal muscle cell has a single neuromuscular junction where acetylcholine (ACh) receptors are concentrated (p. 209). A single muscle cell responds to only a single neuron. However, a single neuronal axon may bifurcate to innervate several individual muscle cells. The group of muscle cells innervated by a single neuron is referred to as a **motor unit**.

The neuromuscular junction is the focus of Chapter 8. Briefly, the ACh released by the presynaptic nerve terminal binds to inotropic (nicotinic) ACh receptors at the neuromuscular junction. These receptors are nonselective cation channels that open when ACh binds to a specific site on the channel, and a depolarization known as the **end-plate potential** is produced. If this end-plate potential exceeds the threshold for activating Na^+ channels, an action potential results. Generation of an action potential initiates the sequence of processes leading to contraction. The ACh is rapidly inactivated by acetylcholinesterase, an enzyme that is manufactured by the muscle cell, and muscle contraction stops a few milliseconds after neuronal activity ceases.

Cardiac Muscle Contracts in Response to the Propagation of Electrical Signals from One Cardiac Cell to Another Across Gap Junctions

Cardiac muscle cells also have chemical synapses, but the sympathetic and parasympathetic branches of the autonomic nervous system (see Chapter 15) use these synap-

ses to *modulate*, rather than to *initiate*, cardiac muscle function. In contrast to skeletal muscle, cardiac muscle contraction is triggered by electrical signals from neighboring cardiac muscle cells. These electrical impulses originate in the **pacemaker** region of the heart, the sinoatrial node (p. 489), which spontaneously and periodically generates action potentials. To facilitate direct electrical communication between cardiac muscle cells, the sarcolemma of cardiac muscle is specialized to contain gap junctions (p. 164), electrical synapses that couple neighboring cells (Fig. 9–1). When an action potential is initiated in one cell, current flows through the gap junctions and depolarizes neighboring cells. If depolarization causes the membrane potential (V_m) to be more positive than threshold, self-propagating action potentials occur in the neighboring cells as well. Thus, the generation of an action potential is just as critical for initiating contraction in cardiac muscle as it is in skeletal muscle.

Smooth Muscles May Contract in Response to Either Neuromuscular Synaptic Transmission or Electrical Coupling

Like skeletal muscle, smooth muscle receives synaptic input from the nervous system. However, the synaptic input to smooth muscle differs from that to skeletal muscle in two ways. First, the neurons are part of the autonomic nervous system rather than the somatic nervous system (see Chapter 15). Second, the neuron makes multiple contacts with a smooth muscle cell. At each contact point, the axon diameter expands to form a varicosity that contains the presynaptic machinery. The varicosity is in close proximity to the postsynaptic membrane of the smooth muscle cell, but there is relatively little specialization of the postsynaptic membrane. Rather than the neurotransmitter receptors being closely clustered at the neuromuscular junction, as in skeletal muscle, in smooth muscle the receptors are spread more widely across the postsynaptic membrane.

The mechanisms of intercellular communication among smooth muscle cells are more diverse than are those of skeletal or cardiac muscle. In some organs, smooth muscle is innervated in a manner similar to skeletal muscle in that each smooth muscle cell receives synaptic input. However, a difference is that a smooth muscle cell may receive input from more than one neuron. Moreover, there is little electrical coupling among these smooth muscle cells (i.e., few gap junctions). As a result, each smooth muscle cell may contract independently of its neighbor. Because this type of smooth muscle behaves as multiple, independent cells or groups of cells, it is called **multiunit smooth muscle** (Fig. 9–2A). Note that the "multi" in "multiunit" refers to the muscle fibers' acting independently of one another as multiple units. Multiunit smooth muscles are capable of finer control. Indeed, multiunit smooth muscle is found in the iris and ciliary body of the eye, the piloerector muscles of the skin, and some blood vessels.

In contrast to multiunit smooth muscle, the smooth muscle cells of most organs have extensive intercellular communication in the manner of cardiac muscle cells. In

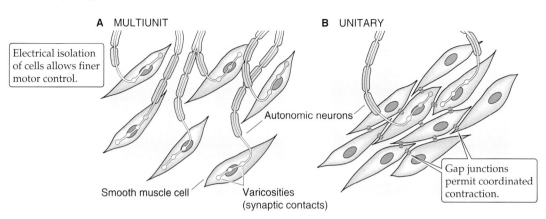

FIGURE 9–2. Smooth-muscle organization. *A,* Each smooth muscle cell receives its own synaptic input. *B,* Only a few of the smooth muscle cells receive direct synaptic input.

this type of smooth muscle, gap junctions permit electrical communication between neighboring cells. This communication allows coordinated contraction of many cells. Because these cells contract as a single unit, this type of smooth muscle is called **unitary smooth muscle** (Fig. 9–2*B*). Unitary smooth muscle is the predominant smooth muscle type within the walls of visceral organs such as the gastrointestinal tract, the uterus, and many blood vessels. For this reason, unitary smooth muscle is often referred to as **visceral smooth muscle**. Among unitary smooth muscles, variation in the strength of intercellular coupling from organ to organ leads to variation in the spatial extent of a single unit. For example, in the bladder, extensive coupling among cells defines large functional units, which allows the muscular wall of the bladder to contract in synchrony. On the other hand, the smooth muscle cells of blood vessels couple to form smaller, independently functioning units that are more akin to multiunit smooth muscle. In fact, electrical coupling of smooth muscle units exhibits a tissue-specific continuum from multiunit to unitary coupling.

Action Potentials of Smooth Muscles May Be Brief or Prolonged

Whereas both skeletal muscle and cardiac muscle produce action potentials that initiate contraction, smooth muscle cells produce a wide range of V_m variations that can either initiate or modulate contraction. Action potentials that are similar to those seen in skeletal muscle are observed in unitary smooth muscle and in some multiunit muscle. Like cardiac muscle cells, some smooth muscle cells exhibit prolonged action potentials that are characterized by a prominent plateau. Still other smooth muscle cells cannot generate action potentials at all. In these cells, V_m changes in a graded fashion (p. 173) rather than in the all-or-none manner of action potentials. The stimuli that produce a **graded response** of V_m include many circulating and local humoral factors, as well as mechanical stimuli such as stretching the cell. These graded V_m changes may be either hyperpolarizing or depolarizing; they sum temporally as well as spatially. If the summation of graded depolarizations brings V_m above threshold—in

a smooth muscle cell capable of producing an action potential—an action potential will then ensue.

Action potentials are usually seen in unitary (visceral) smooth muscle. These action potentials typically have a slower upstroke and longer duration (up to ~100 ms) than do skeletal muscle action potentials (~2 ms). The action potential in a smooth muscle cell can be a simple spike, a spike followed by a plateau, or a series of spikes on top of slow waves of V_m (Fig. 9–3*A*). In any case, the upstroke or depolarizing phase of the action potential reflects opening of voltage-gated Ca^{2+} channels. The inward Ca^{2+} current further depolarizes the cell and thereby causes still more voltage-gated Ca^{2+} channels to open. Thus, some smooth muscle cells can undergo the same type of regenerative depolarization that is seen in skeletal muscle. However, the rate of rise of the action potential in smooth muscle is lower because Ca^{2+} channels open more slowly than do Na^+ channels in skeletal and cardiac muscle (p. 189). Repolarization of the smooth muscle cell is also relatively slow. Two explanations may be offered for this slower repolarization. First, voltage-gated Ca^{2+} channels, which are responsible for the depolarization phase of the action potential, inactivate slowly. Second, the repolarization phase of the action potential reflects the delayed activation of voltage-gated K^+ channels and, in some cases, Ca^{2+}-activated K^+ channels.

Some smooth muscle cells have fast, voltage-gated Na^+ channels. However, even when these channels are present, they do not appear to be necessary for generating an action potential. Their main role may be to allow more rapid activation of voltage-gated Ca^{2+} channels and thus contribute to a faster rate of depolarization.

In some unitary smooth muscle, repolarization is so delayed that the action potential contour displays a prominent plateau. These plateau potentials may be several hundred milliseconds in duration, as in cardiac muscle. Plateau action potentials occur in smooth muscle of the genitourinary tract, including the ureters, bladder, and uterus. The long V_m plateau allows the entry of Ca^{2+} to continue for a longer period and thus allows $[Ca^{2+}]_i$ to remain high for a longer period, thereby prolonging the contraction.

A TYPES OF SMOOTH-MUSCLE ACTION POTENTIALS

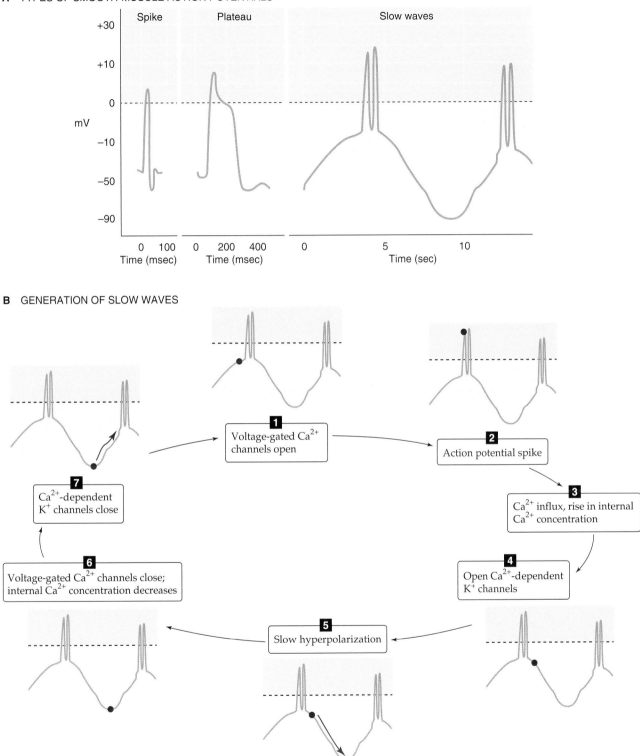

FIGURE 9–3. Action potentials and slow waves in smooth muscle.

Some Smooth Muscle Cells Can Initiate Spontaneous Electrical Activity

Although smooth muscle cells undergo changes in V_m in response to neural, hormonal, or mechanical stimulation, many smooth muscle cells are capable of initiating spontaneous electrical activity. In some cells, this spontaneous activity results from pacemaker currents. These currents result from time- and voltage-dependent properties of ion currents that produce either a spontaneous increase in inward, or depolarizing, currents (e.g., voltage-gated Ca^{2+} currents) or a spontaneous decrease in outward, or hyperpolarizing, currents (e.g., voltage-gated K^+ currents). The pacemaker currents cause the cell to depolarize until V_m reaches threshold, triggering an action potential.

In other smooth muscle cells, this spontaneous electrical activity results in regular, repetitive oscillations in V_m. These V_m oscillations occur at a frequency of several oscillations per minute and are referred to as **slow waves** (Fig. 9–3B). One hypothesis for the origin of slow-wave potentials suggests that voltage-gated Ca^{2+} channels—active at the resting V_m—depolarize the cell enough to activate more voltage-gated Ca^{2+} channels. This activation results in progressive depolarization and Ca^{2+} influx. The increase in $[Ca^{2+}]_i$ activates Ca^{2+}-dependent K^+ channels, which leads to progressive hyperpolarization and termination of the depolarization phase of the wave. These periodic depolarizations and $[Ca^{2+}]_i$ increases cause periodic, tonic contractions of the smooth muscle. When the amplitude of the slow V_m waves is sufficient to depolarize the cell to threshold, the ensuing action potentials lead to further Ca^{2+} influx and phasic contractions.

Other hypotheses to explain spontaneous electrical and mechanical activity in smooth muscle cells are based on oscillatory changes in other intracellular ions or molecules. For example, increased $[Ca^{2+}]_i$ during an action potential might stimulate Na-Ca exchange and lead to a cyclic increase in $[Na^+]_i$ and thus an increase in the rate of Na^+ extrusion by the electrogenic Na-K pump. Alternatively, the inositol 1,4,5-triphosphate (IP_3) receptor channel (p. 100) might spontaneously open and release Ca^{2+}. The effect on $[Ca^{2+}]_i$ would be self-reinforcing because of Ca^{2+}-activated Ca^{2+} release via the IP_3 receptor. At high $[Ca^{2+}]_i$, this channel is inhibited and the Ca^{2+} release event is terminated, followed by re-uptake of Ca^{2+} into the sarcoplasmic reticulum (SR). The $[Ca^{2+}]_i$ increases may themselves lead to periodic electrical activity by stimulating Ca^{2+}-activated inward and outward currents.

Some Smooth Muscles Contract Without Action Potentials

Whereas action-potential generation is essential for initiating contraction of skeletal and cardiac muscle, many smooth muscle cells contract despite being unable to generate an action potential. As discussed previously, V_m oscillations can lead to tonic contractions in the absence of action potentials. Action potentials usually do not occur in **multiunit** smooth muscle. For example, in the smooth muscle that regulates the iris, excitatory neurotransmitters such as norepinephrine or ACh cause a local depolarization, the **junctional potential**, which is similar to the

end-plate potential in skeletal muscle. Junctional potentials spread electrotonically (i.e., in a graded fashion) throughout the muscle fiber, thereby altering V_m and affecting the entry of Ca^{2+} through voltage-gated slow (L-type) Ca^{2+} channels. Changes in V_m—by an unknown mechanism—may also modulate the activity of the enzyme phospholipase C, which cleaves phosphoinositides to release the intracellular second messengers diacylglycerol (DAG) and IP_3 (p. 100). Both these second messengers are modulators of contractile force. In the absence of action potentials, some unitary smooth muscle, including some vascular smooth muscle, also contracts as a result of graded V_m changes.

Some smooth muscle cells contract without any change in V_m. For example, a neurotransmitter can bind to a receptor, activate a G protein, and lead to the generation of IP_3, which in turn leads to the release of Ca^{2+} from the SR. The eventual depletion of Ca^{2+} stores in the SR may in turn stimulate Ca^{2+} influx across the cell membrane via so-called **store-operated Ca^{2+} channels**.

MUSCLE CONTRACTION

Striated Muscle Cells Are Densely Packed with Myofibrils That Contain Ordered Arrays of Thick and Thin Filaments

As summarized in Figure 9–4A, each individual skeletal muscle cell (or *myocyte* or *fiber*) contains a dense parallel array of smaller, cylindrical elements called **myofibrils** that have the diameter of a Z disk (p. 45). Each of these myofibrils comprises repeating units, or **sarcomeres**, that consist of smaller interdigitating filaments called **myofilaments**. These myofilaments come in two types (see Fig. 9–4B), thick filaments composed primarily of myosin and thin filaments composed primarily of actin (p. 27). The sarcomere extends from one Z disk to another. Sarcomeres stacked end to end make up a myofibril. The repeating **sarcomeres** are most highly organized within skeletal and cardiac muscle and impart a striped appearance. Thus, both skeletal and cardiac muscle are referred to as **striated muscle**.

In **smooth muscle**, striations are not visible. Although actin and myosin are present in smooth muscle cells, the relationship between actin and myosin (thin and thick filaments) is less highly organized. The actin filaments are oriented mainly parallel or oblique to the long axis of the cell. Multiple actin filaments appear to join at electron-dense regions called **dense bodies**, which are found immediately beneath the cell membrane, as well as within the interior of the myocyte. The thick filaments are interspersed among the thin filaments in smooth muscle, and are far less abundant than in skeletal or cardiac muscle.

Thin filaments are 5 to 8 nm in diameter and, in striated muscle, 1 μm in length. In striated muscle, the thin filaments are tethered together at one end, where they project from a dense disk known as the **Z disk**. The Z disk is oriented perpendicular to the axis of the muscle fiber; thin filaments project from both its faces. Not only do Z disks tether the thin filaments of a single myofibril together, but connections between the Z disks also tether

A FROM MUSCLE TO MYOFILAMENTS

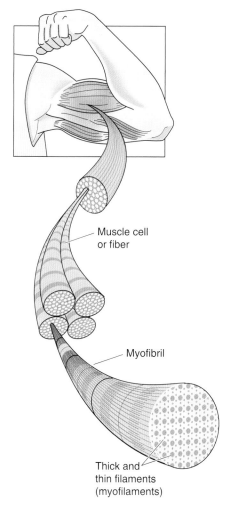

Muscle cell
or fiber

Myofibril

Thick and
thin filaments
(myofilaments)

B MODEL OF A SARCOMERE

A band

Z line

H band

I band

α-Actinin

M line

Actin

Myosin

One sarcomere

C ELECTRON MICROGRAPH OF SARCOMERE

A band

I band

H band

One sarcomere

FIGURE 9–4. Structure of the sarcomere.

each myofibril to its neighbors. These interconnections align the sarcomeres and give skeletal and, to a lesser extent, cardiac muscle its striated appearance.

The **thick filaments** are 10 nm in diameter and, in striated muscle, 1.6 μm in length. They lie between and partially interdigitate with the thin filaments. This partial interdigitation results in alternating light and dark bands along the axis of the myofibril (see Fig. 9–4C). The light bands, which represent regions of the thin filament that do not lie alongside thick filaments, are known as **I bands** because they are *isotropic* to polarized light. The Z disk is visible as a dark perpendicular line at the center of the I band. The dark bands, which represent the myosin filaments, are known as **A bands** because they are *aniso-tropic* to polarized light. During contraction, the A bands are unchanged in length whereas the I bands shorten.

Within the A bands, the pivoting heads of the thick myosin filaments, the molecular motors, establish cross-bridges to the thin actin filaments. As discussed later, the adenosine triphosphate (ATP)–dependent cycle of making and breaking cross-bridges causes the actin filament to be drawn over the myosin filament and thereby results in muscle contraction.

The Thin and Thick Filaments Are Supramolecular Assemblies of Protein Subunits

THIN FILAMENTS. Thin filaments (Fig. 9–5A) consist of actin, tropomyosin, and troponin. The backbone of the filament is a double-stranded α-helical polymer of **actin** molecules. Each helical turn of a single strand of filamentous or F-actin consists of 13 individual actin monomers and is approximately 70 nm long. F-actin is associated with two important regulatory, actin-binding proteins: tropomyosin and troponin.

Individual **tropomyosin** molecules consist of two identical α helices that coil around each other and sit near the two grooves that are formed by the two helical actin strands. Head-to-tail contact between neighboring tropo-myosin molecules results in two nearly continuous helical

A THIN FILAMENT

B MYOSIN MOLECULE

C INTERACTION OF THIN AND THICK FILAMENTS

FIGURE 9–5. Structure of thin and thick filaments.

myosin-II molecules. Each myosin-II molecule is a hexamer (actually a double trimer) composed of two intertwined *heavy chains*, two *regulatory light chains*, and two *alkali* (or *essential*) *light chains*. The two **heavy chains** have three regions: a rod, a hinge, and a head region. The *rod* portions are α helices that wrap around each other. At the *hinge* regions, the molecule flares open to form two globular *heads*, which are the cross-bridges between the thick and thin filaments of the sarcomere. The heads of the heavy chains—also called S1 fragments—each possess a site for binding actin as well as a site for binding and hydrolyzing ATP. The head portion of each myosin forms a complex with two light chains, one regulatory and one alkali. The **alkali light chain** plays an essential role in stabilizing the myosin head region. The **regulatory light chain**, as its name implies, regulates the ATPase activity of myosin. The activity of the myosin regulatory light chain is in turn regulated via phosphorylation by Ca^{2+}-dependent and Ca^{2+}-independent kinases.

Figure 9–5C summarizes the interaction between a thin filament and a single pair of head groups from the myosin of a thick filament.

In All Three Muscle Types, An Increase in $[Ca^{2+}]_i$ Triggers Contraction By Removing the Inhibition of Cross-Bridge Cycling

Underlying muscle contraction is a cycle in which myosin-II heads bind to actin, these cross-bridges become distorted, and finally the myosin heads detach from actin. Energy for this cycling comes from the hydrolysis of ATP. However, if unregulated, the cycling would continue until the myocyte was depleted of ATP. It is not surprising, then, that skeletal, cardiac, and smooth muscle each have mechanisms for regulating cross-bridge cycling. In all three cell types, an increase in $[Ca^{2+}]_i$ initiates and allows cross-bridge cycling to continue. During this excitatory increase, $[Ca^{2+}]_i$ may rise from its resting level of less than 10^{-7} M to greater than 10^{-5} M. The subsequent decrease in $[Ca^{2+}]_i$ is the signal to cease cross-bridge cycling and relax.

Regardless of the muscle type, Ca^{2+} modulates contraction through regulatory proteins rather than interacting directly with the contractile proteins. In the absence of Ca^{2+}, these regulatory proteins act in concert to inhibit actin-myosin interactions, thus inhibiting the contractile process. When Ca^{2+} binds to one or more of these proteins, a conformational change takes place in the regulatory complex that releases the inhibition of contraction.

SKELETAL MUSCLE. The heterotrimeric troponin molecule contains the key Ca^{2+}-sensitive regulator troponin C (Fig. 9–6A). Each **troponin C** molecule in skeletal muscle has two high-affinity Ca^{2+}-binding sites that participate in binding of troponin C to the thin filament. Ca^{2+} binding to these high-affinity sites does not change during muscle activation. Each troponin C molecule in skeletal muscle also has two *additional*, low-affinity Ca^{2+}-binding sites. Binding of Ca^{2+} to these low-affinity sites induces a conformational change in the troponin complex that has two effects. The first effect is that the C terminus of the

filaments that shadow the actin double helix. The length of a single tropomyosin molecule corresponds to about seven actin monomers (i.e., a half turn of the actin helix). As we shall see later, the role of tropomyosin is to interfere with the binding of myosin to actin.

Troponin is a heterotrimer consisting of troponin *T* (which binds to a single molecule of *tropomyosin*), troponin *C* (which binds *Ca^{2+}*), and troponin *I* (which binds to actin and inhibits contraction). Troponin C is closely related to another Ca^{2+}-binding protein, calmodulin (CaM; p. 102). Thus, each troponin heterotrimer interacts with a single tropomyosin molecule, which in turn interacts with seven actin monomers. The troponin complex also interacts directly with the actin filaments. The coordinated interaction among troponin, tropomyosin, and actin allows actin-myosin interactions to be regulated by changes in $[Ca^{2+}]_i$.

THICK FILAMENTS. Like thin actin filaments, thick filaments are polymers of proteins (see Fig. 9–5B). Thick filaments are bipolar assemblies composed of multiple

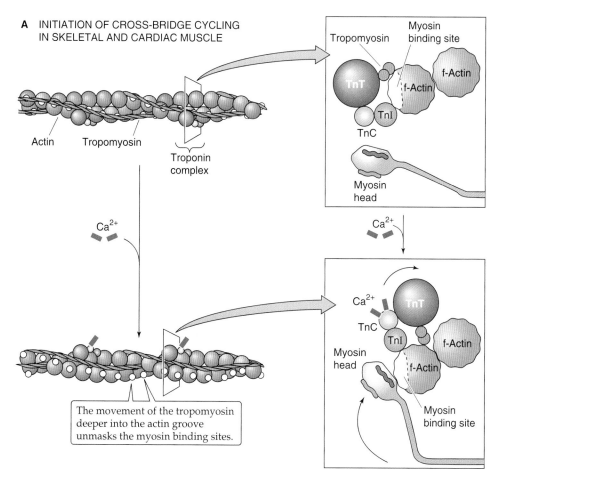

A INITIATION OF CROSS-BRIDGE CYCLING IN SKELETAL AND CARDIAC MUSCLE

The movement of the tropomyosin deeper into the actin groove unmasks the myosin binding sites.

B INITIATION OF CROSS-BRIDGE CYCLING IN SMOOTH MUSCLE

FIGURE 9–6. The role of Ca^{2+} in triggering muscle contraction. MLCK, myosin light chain kinase.

inhibitory troponin I moves away from the actin/tropomyosin filament, thereby permitting the tropomyosin molecule to move. According to one hypothesis, the other effect, transmitted through **troponin T**, is to push tropomyosin away from the myosin-binding site on the actin and into the actin groove. With the steric hindrance removed, the myosin head is able to interact with actin and engage in cross-bridge cycling.

CARDIAC MUSCLE. The regulatory mechanism within cardiac muscle is similar to that of skeletal muscle, although troponin C from cardiac muscle has just a single, active low-affinity Ca^{2+}-binding site.

SMOOTH MUSCLE. An entirely different mechanism controls cross-bridge turnover in smooth muscle. Here, an increase in $[Ca^{2+}]_i$ initiates a slow chain of events that ultimately increases the ATPase activity of the myosin (see Fig. 9–6*B*). The first step is the binding of four Ca^{2+} ions to **calmodulin**, which, as we noted earlier, is closely related to troponin C. Next, the Ca^{2+}-CaM complex activates an enzyme known as **myosin light chain kinase** (MLCK), which in turn phosphorylates the regulatory light chain that is associated with the myosin-II molecule. Phosphorylation of the light chain alters the conformation of the myosin head, which greatly increases its ATPase activity and allows it to interact with actin and act as a molecular motor. Thus, in smooth muscle, CaM rather than troponin C is the Ca^{2+}-binding protein responsible for transducing the contraction-triggering increases in $[Ca^{2+}]_i$. Note that in smooth muscle, contraction cannot begin until MLCK increases the ATPase activity of myosin, which is a time-consuming process. In skeletal and cardiac muscle, on the other hand, the ATPase activity of the myosin head is constitutively high, and cross-bridge cycling can begin as soon as the tropomyosin is moved out of the way.

The mechanism just outlined activates the *thick* filaments in smooth muscle. Other mechanisms act on the thin filaments of smooth muscle to remove the tonic inhibition to actin-myosin interactions that are caused by steric hindrance. Two proteins—caldesmon and calponin—tonically inhibit the interaction between actin and myosin. Both are Ca^{2+}-CaM–binding proteins, and both bind to actin and tropomyosin. **Calponin**, which is found in a fixed stoichiometry with tropomyosin and actin (one calponin—one tropomyosin—seven actin monomers), tonically inhibits the ATPase activity of myosin. As we saw earlier, the increase in $[Ca^{2+}]_i$ that triggers smooth muscle contraction activates Ca^{2+}-CaM. Besides activating MLCK, this Ca^{2+}-CaM complex has two effects on calponin. First, Ca^{2+}-CaM binds to calponin. Second, Ca^{2+}-CaM activates Ca^{2+}-CaM–dependent protein kinase, which phosphorylates calponin. Both effects reduce calponin's inhibition of myosin's ATPase activity. Like calponin, **caldesmon** also tonically inhibits the ATPase activity of myosin in smooth muscle.

During the Cross-Bridge Cycle, Contractile Proteins Convert the Energy of ATP Hydrolysis Into Mechanical Energy

The cross-bridge cycle that we introduced in the previous section occurs in five steps (Fig. 9–7). Initially, the myosin head is attached to an actin filament after the "power stroke" from the previous cycle and after the actomyosin complex has released adenosine diphosphate (ADP). In the absence of ATP, the system could remain in this rigid state for an indefinitely long period, as is indeed the case in rigor mortis. In this rigid state, the myosin head is at a 45-degree angle with respect to the actin and myosin filaments.

Step 1: **ATP binding**. ATP binding to the head of the myosin heavy chain (MHC) reduces the affinity of myosin for actin, causing the myosin head to release from the actin filament. If all cross-bridges in a muscle were in this state, the muscle would be fully relaxed.

Step 2: **ATP hydrolysis**. The breakdown of ATP to ADP and inorganic phosphate (P_i) occurs on the myosin head; the products of hydrolysis are retained on the myosin. As a result of hydrolysis, the myosin head pivots around the hinge into a "cocked" position (perpendicular or at a 90-degree angle to the thick and thin filaments). This rotation causes the tip of the myosin to move about 11 nm along the actin filament so that it now lines up with a new actin monomer two monomers further along the actin filament (see the box titled Measuring the Force of a Single Cross-Bridge Cycle). Once again, if all cross-bridges in a muscle were in this state, the muscle would be fully relaxed.

Step 3: **Cross-bridge formation**. The cocked myosin head now binds to its new position on the actin filament. This binding reflects the increased affinity of the myosin-ADP-P_i complex for actin.

Step 4: **Release of P_i from the myosin**. Dissociation of P_i from the myosin head triggers the power stroke, a conformational change in which the myosin head bends approximately 45 degrees about the hinge and pulls the actin filament about 11 nm toward the tail of the myosin molecule. This conformational change causes the actin filament to be drawn along the myosin filament, thereby generating force and motion.

Step 5: **ADP release**. Dissociation of ADP from myosin completes the cycle, and the actomyosin complex is left in a rigid state. The myosin head remains in the same position and at a 45-degree angle with respect to the thick and thin filaments. The ADP–free myosin complex remains bound to actin until another ATP binds and initiates another cycle.

The ADP–free myosin complex ("attached state" in Fig. 9–7) would quickly bind ATP at the concentrations of ATP normally found within cells. If unrestrained, this cross-bridge cycling would continue until depleting the cytoplasm of ATP. At that time, the muscle would remain in the stiff "attached state" because release of the cross-bridges from actin requires binding of ATP to myosin.

As discussed earlier, muscle cells do not regulate cross-bridge cycling by modifying $[ATP]_i$. Instead, skeletal muscle and cardiac muscle control this cycle at the third step by preventing cross-bridge formation until the tropomyosin moves out of the way in response to an increase in $[Ca^{2+}]_i$. Smooth muscle controls the cycle at the second step by preventing ATP hydrolysis until the ATPase activity of the myosin head increases in response to an increase in $[Ca^{2+}]_i$.

Although this general schema of cross-bridge cycling occurs in smooth muscle as well as skeletal and cardiac muscle, the frequency of cross-bridge cycling in smooth muscle is less than one tenth the frequency encountered in skeletal muscle. This variation reflects differences in the properties of the various myosin isoforms that are expressed in various cell types. Even though cross-bridge cycling occurs less frequently in smooth muscle, force generation may be as great or greater, perhaps because the cross-bridges remain intact for a longer period with each cycle. It is likely that this longer period during which the cross-bridges are intact reflects a lower rate of ADP release from the smooth muscle isoform of myosin.

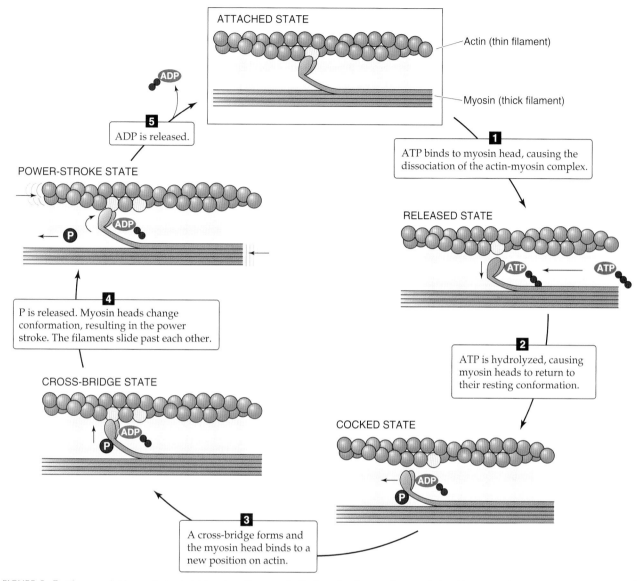

ATTACHED STATE

Actin (thin filament)

Myosin (thick filament)

5 ADP is released.

1 ATP binds to myosin head, causing the dissociation of the actin-myosin complex.

POWER-STROKE STATE

ADP

P

RELEASED STATE

ATP   ATP

4 P is released. Myosin heads change conformation, resulting in the power stroke. The filaments slide past each other.

2 ATP is hydrolyzed, causing myosin heads to return to their resting conformation.

CROSS-BRIDGE STATE

ADP

P

COCKED STATE

ADP

P

3 A cross-bridge forms and the myosin head binds to a new position on actin.

FIGURE 9–7. The cross-bridge cycle in skeletal and cardiac muscle. Each cycle advances the myosin head by two actin monomers, or approximately 11 nm.

Because ATP Stores Are Small, the Cell Must Regenerate the ATP Needed For Muscle Contraction

Each cross-bridge cycle consumes one molecule of ATP. In skeletal muscle, the entire cellular store of ATP is sufficient to allow only a few seconds of continuous maximal contraction. Therefore, the muscle cell must resynthesize ATP from ADP at a rate comparable to the rate of ATP consumption. Skeletal muscle has specialized energy stores that permit rapid regeneration of ATP. The most readily available pool of this energy is the high-energy phosphate bond of **phosphocreatine**. The enzyme *creatine phosphotransferase* transfers the high-energy phosphate of phosphocreatine to ADP, thereby rephosphorylating ADP to ATP. The phosphocreatine content of skeletal muscle is adequate to replenish the ATP pool several times, but it is still inadequate for sustaining the energy needs of contracting muscle for more than 10 seconds.

In comparison with the energy stored as phosphocreatine, glycogen is a far more abundant energy source within skeletal muscle. **Glycogen** that has been previously stored by muscle can be enzymatically degraded to pyruvic acid. Degradation of glycogen to pyruvate is rapid and liberates energy that the cell invests in phosphorylating ADP to yield ATP. Pyruvate can be further degraded along with other foodstuffs by *oxidative metabolism*, which over the long term is the primary mechanism for the regeneration of ATP (p. 1220). The rate of ATP generation by oxidative metabolism is limited by the rate of oxygen delivery to the muscle. However, glycolytic formation of pyruvate occurs independently of oxygen, as does the conversion of pyruvate to lactate. This *anaerobic metabolism* of muscle glycogen ensures that energy stores are sufficient to sustain muscle activity for nearly a minute even when oxygen is unavailable. In Chapter 59 we will discuss the aerobic and anaerobic metabolism of exercising muscle in more depth.

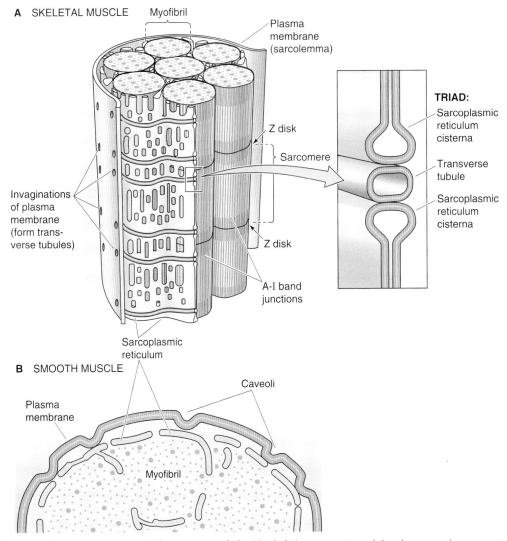

FIGURE 9–8. Plasma-membrane invaginations. *A*, The transverse tubules (T tubules) are extensions of the plasma membrane, penetrating the muscle cell at two points in each sarcomere: the junctions of the A and I bands. *B*, Smooth-muscle cells have rudimentary invaginations of the plasma membrane, called caveoli, contacting with the sarcoplasmic reticulum.

EXCITATION-CONTRACTION COUPLING

In our discussion of the mechanism of muscle contraction, we saw that regardless of whether the muscle is skeletal, cardiac, or smooth, it is an increase in $[Ca^{2+}]_i$ that triggers muscle contraction. The time during which $[Ca^{2+}]_i$ remains elevated determines the duration of muscle contraction. The process by which "excitation" triggers the increase in $[Ca^{2+}]_i$ is known as *excitation-contraction coupling*. Different kinds of myocytes have specialized mechanisms that regulate the entry of Ca^{2+} into the cytoplasm, as well as remove Ca^{2+} from the cytoplasm once the stimulus for muscle contraction subsides. Ca^{2+} can enter the cytoplasm from the extracellular space through voltage-gated or ligand-gated ion channels, or alternatively, Ca^{2+} can be released into the cytoplasm from the SR. Thus, both extracellular and intracellular sources contribute to the increase in $[Ca^{2+}]_i$. However, the relative importance of these two sources varies among the different muscle types.

Invaginations of the Sarcolemma Facilitate Communication Between the Surface of the Cell and Its Interior

The plasma membranes of muscle cells display invaginations that extend the surface membrane into the muscle cell. In skeletal and cardiac muscle, these invaginations take the form of radially projecting tubes called **transverse tubules** or T tubules (Fig. 9–8A). T tubules are highly organized and penetrate the muscle at two points in each sarcomere: at the junctions of the A and I bands. A cross section through the A-I junction would show a complex, branching array of T tubules penetrating to the center of the muscle cell and surrounding the individual myofibrils. Along its length the tubule associates with two **cisternae**, which are specialized regions of the SR. The **sarcoplasmic reticulum** is the muscle equivalent of the endoplasmic reticulum, and it serves as a storage organelle for intracellular Ca^{2+}. The combination of the T-tubule membrane and its two neighboring cisternae is called a **triad**; this structure plays a crucial role in the

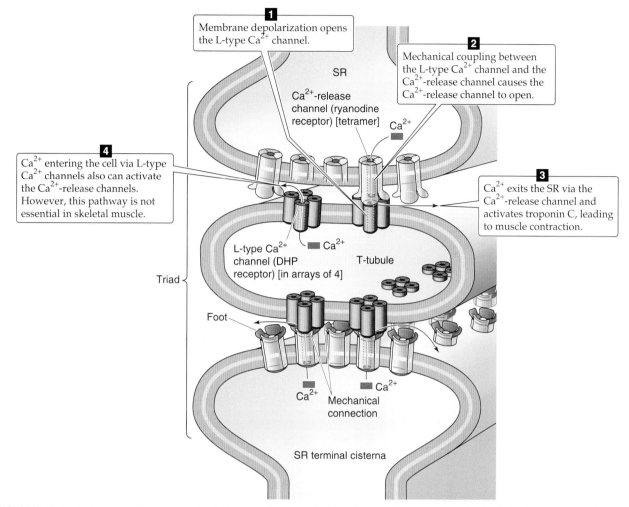

1 Membrane depolarization opens the L-type Ca^{2+} channel.

2 Mechanical coupling between the L-type Ca^{2+} channel and the Ca^{2+}-release channel causes the Ca^{2+}-release channel to open.

4 Ca^{2+} entering the cell via L-type Ca^{2+} channels also can activate the Ca^{2+}-release channels. However, this pathway is not essential in skeletal muscle.

3 Ca^{2+} exits the SR via the Ca^{2+}-release channel and activates troponin C, leading to muscle contraction.

SR

Ca^{2+}-release channel (ryanodine receptor) [tetramer] Ca^{2+}

L-type Ca^{2+} channel (DHP receptor) [in arrays of 4] Ca^{2+}

T-tubule

Triad

Foot

Ca^{2+}

Ca^{2+} Mechanical connection

SR terminal cisterna

FIGURE 9–9. Excitation-contraction coupling in skeletal muscle. A tetrad of four L-type Ca^{2+} channels on the T tubules faces a single Ca^{2+}-release channel of the SR, so that each L-type Ca^{2+} channel interacts with the foot of one of the four subunits of the Ca^{2+}-release channel. Note that half of the Ca^{2+}-release channels lack associations with L-type Ca^{2+} channels. DHP, dihydropyridine; SR, sarcoplasmic reticulum.

coupling of excitation to contraction in skeletal and cardiac muscle. *Smooth* muscle, in contrast, has more rudimentary and shallow invaginations called **caveoli** (see Fig. 9–8*B*).

In Skeletal Muscle, Depolarization of the T-Tubule Membrane Leads to Ca^{2+} Release from the Sarcoplasmic Reticulum at the Triad

Action potentials originating from depolarizations at the motor end plate propagate along the skeletal muscle membrane and down the T tubules. Depolarization of the triad region of the T tubules activates **L-type Ca^{2+} channels** (p. 190), which are clustered in groups of four called "tetrads" (Fig. 9–9). These voltage-gated channels play a pivotal role in coupling electrical excitation to contraction because they function as the **voltage sensor** in EC coupling. Electron microscopy reveals a checkerboard pattern of projections arising from the T-tubule membrane and extending toward the cisternae of the SR; these projections probably represent the cytoplasmic face of these L-type Ca^{2+} channels. Each of the four voltage-gated Ca^{2+} channels in a tetrad is in fact a heteropenta-

meric protein (see Fig. 7–12*B*). Each of the four Ca^{2+} channels is also called a **DHP receptor**, because it is inhibited by a class of antihypertensive drugs known as dihydropyridines. Depolarization of the T-tubule membrane evokes conformational changes in each of the four L-type Ca^{2+} channels and has two effects. First, the conformational changes allow Ca^{2+} to enter through the four channel pores. Second, and much more important, the conformational changes in the four L-type Ca^{2+} channels induce a conformational change in each of the four subunits of another channel—the Ca^{2+}-release channel—that is located in the SR membrane.

The **Ca^{2+}-release channel** (Table 6–2, #18) has a homotetrameric structure quite different from that of the L-type Ca^{2+} channel that constitutes the voltage sensor. The Ca^{2+}-release channel in the SR is also known as the **ryanodine receptor** because it is inhibited by a class of drugs that include the plant alkaloids *ryanodine* and *caffeine*. Ca^{2+}-release channels cluster in the portion of the SR membrane that faces the T tubules. Each of the four subunits of these channels has a large extension—also known as a "foot." These feet project as a regular array into the cytosol. The foot of each of the four Ca^{2+}-release channel subunits is complementary to the cytoplasmic projection of one of the four L-type Ca^{2+} channels in a tetrad on the T tubule (see Fig. 9–9). The close physical proximity of these two proteins, as well as the ability of both DHP and ryanodine to block muscle contraction, suggests that interaction between these two different Ca^{2+} channels underlies EC coupling. The precise mechanism of interaction between these proteins is not yet fully understood, although we know that it is not electrical inasmuch as ion conductance of the Ca^{2+}-release channel is not strongly voltage dependent. A large cytoplasmic projection on the α_1 subunit of the L-type Ca^{2+} channel appears to be necessary for interaction between the two Ca^{2+} channels on opposing T-tubule and SR membranes. Thus, it is possible that direct *mechanical* coupling exists between this projection and the Ca^{2+}-release channel.

As the L-type Ca^{2+} channel on the T-tubule membrane mechanically opens the Ca^{2+}-release channel in the SR, Ca^{2+} sequestered in the SR rapidly leaves via the Ca^{2+}-release channel. The resultant rapid increase in $[Ca^{2+}]_i$ activates troponin C, thus initiating cross-bridge cycling as described earlier. The entire process, extending from depolarization of the T-tubule membrane to the initiation of cross-bridge cycling, is termed **excitation-contraction coupling**.

Although we have stressed activation of the Ca^{2+}-release channel in the SR by *mechanical* coupling between it and the L-type Ca^{2+} channel in the T-tubule membrane, local elevations in $[Ca^{2+}]_i$ can also activate the Ca^{2+}-release channel in skeletal muscle. When the L-type Ca^{2+} channel opens during depolarization, it allows an influx of Ca^{2+} that locally increases $[Ca^{2+}]_i$. This mechanism of activating the Ca^{2+}-release channel in the SR is known as **Ca^{2+}-induced Ca^{2+} release** (CICR). Although L-type Ca^{2+} channels allow $[Ca^{2+}]_i$ to rise during action potentials in skeletal muscle, CICR is not necessary for contraction. Indeed, skeletal muscle contraction persists even when Ca^{2+} is absent from the extracellular fluid. However, as we will see later, CICR plays a critical role in EC coupling in *cardiac* muscle.

In Cardiac Muscle, Ca^{2+} Entry Through L-Type Ca^{2+} Channels Is Amplified By Ca^{2+}-Induced Ca^{2+} Release from the Sarcoplasmic Reticulum

Whereas EC coupling in skeletal muscle does not require Ca^{2+} influx through L-type Ca^{2+} channels, cardiac contraction has an *absolute requirement* for Ca^{2+} influx through these channels during the action potential. Because the T-tubule lumen is an extension of the extracellular space, it facilitates the diffusion of Ca^{2+} from bulk extracellular fluid to the site of the L-type Ca^{2+} channels on the T-tubule membrane. Thus, the Ca^{2+} can simultaneously reach superficial and deep regions of the muscle. The increase in $[Ca^{2+}]_i$ resulting from Ca^{2+} influx alone is not, however, sufficient to initiate contraction. Rather, the increase in $[Ca^{2+}]_i$ that is produced by the L-type Ca^{2+} channels is greatly amplified by CICR from the SR via the Ca^{2+}-release channels. Indeed, because the Ca^{2+}-release channels remain open for a longer period than do L-type

Ca^{2+} channels, the contribution of CICR to the rise in $[Ca^{2+}]_i$ is greater than the flux contributed by the L-type Ca^{2+} channels of the T tubules.

It appears that each L-type Ca^{2+} channel controls only one SR Ca^{2+}-release channel. The close physical proximity of L-type Ca^{2+} channels of the T-tubule membrane and the Ca^{2+}-release channel in the SR at the triad junctions allows for this tight local control. Although Ca^{2+} diffuses in the cytosol away from its SR release site, Ca^{2+} release at one site does not appear to be able to induce Ca^{2+} release from a neighboring SR Ca^{2+}-release channel. Thus, Ca^{2+} release events are not propagated along the myocyte. In fact, the SR Ca^{2+}-release channel does not appear to respond to generalized increases in cytoplasmic $[Ca^{2+}]_i$. Generalized cardiac muscle contractions occur as a result of the spatial and temporal summation of individual CICR events.

In Smooth Muscle, Both Extracellular and Intracellular Ca^{2+} Activate Contraction

In smooth muscle cells, three major pathways—which are not mutually exclusive—can lead to the increase in $[Ca^{2+}]_i$ that triggers contraction: (1) Ca^{2+} entry through voltage-gated channels in response to cell depolarization, (2) Ca^{2+} release from the SR, and (3) Ca^{2+} entry through voltage-independent channels.

Ca^{2+} ENTRY THROUGH VOLTAGE-GATED CHANNELS. As noted earlier, smooth muscle cells respond to stimulation with graded depolarizations or action potentials. In either case, depolarization may produce an influx of Ca^{2+} through voltage-gated L-type Ca^{2+} channels (Fig. 9–10).

Ca^{2+} RELEASE FROM THE SR. This Ca^{2+} release may occur by either of two mechanisms: CICR or IP_3-mediated Ca^{2+} release. As we have already seen, CICR plays a key role in EC coupling in cardiac muscle, where the L-type Ca^{2+} channels are highly ordered and in close proximity to the Ca^{2+}-release channels in the SR. Thus, Ca^{2+} influx through L-type Ca^{2+} channels can trigger CICR. In smooth muscle, the relationship between the plasma membrane and the SR is not as regularly organized as it is in striated muscle. Nevertheless, electron-dense couplings have been observed bridging the 8- to 10-nm gap between the cell membranes and elements of the SR in smooth muscle. Although CICR occurs in smooth muscle cells under some conditions, it requires $[Ca^{2+}]_i$ levels that are higher than those that typically occur under physiological conditions, and its role remains unclear.

A more important mechanism for Ca^{2+} release from the SR of smooth muscle is the IP_3 pathway. The existence of this pathway is supported by the observation that some extracellular agonists can elicit smooth muscle contraction with minimal depolarization and negligible Ca^{2+} influx. Furthermore, even for agonists such as serotonin or norepinephrine, which activate a Ca^{2+}-influx pathway, the observed increase in $[Ca^{2+}]_i$ is out of proportion to that expected from Ca^{2+} influx alone. Thus, another pathway must exist for increasing $[Ca^{2+}]_i$. Some agonists cause smooth muscle contraction by triggering the production of IP_3 (p. 100), which binds to a specific receptor on the

MALIGNANT HYPERTHERMIA

Malignant hyperthermia (MH) is a genetic disorder affecting between 1 in 10,000 and 1 in 50,000 individuals. Affected individuals are at risk for a potentially life-threatening syndrome when exposed to any of the various inhalation anesthetic agents, particularly halothane. Administration of succinylcholine can also trigger or exaggerate MH. This drug is a short-acting inotropic (nicotinic) acetylcholine-receptor antagonist that acts by first opening the acetylcholine receptor channel and then blocking it, thereby resulting in a burst of muscle activity, followed by paralysis. Onset of the syndrome in the setting of the operating room is typified by the development of tachypnea (rapid breathing), low plasma [O_2], high plasma [CO_2], tachycardia (rapid heart rate), and *hyperthermia* (rising body temperature), as well as rigidity, sweating, and dramatic swings in blood pressure. The patient's temperature may rise as rapidly as 1°C every 5 minutes. The onset of MH is usually during anesthesia, but it can occur up to several hours later. If untreated, the patient will develop respiratory and lactic acidosis, muscular rigidity, and a breakdown of muscle tissue that leads to the release of K^+ and thus profound hyperkalemia. These episodes reflect a progressively severe hypermetabolic state in the muscle tissues. Fortunately, our evolving understanding of the physiology of MH has led to the development of a therapeutic regimen that has greatly improved the once-dismal prognosis.

The major features of the syndrome—hyperthermia, muscular rigidity, and an increased metabolic rate—led early investigators to suggest that MH was a disease of abnormal regulation of muscle contraction. According to this hypothesis, uncontrolled muscle contraction—somehow triggered by the administration of halothane and succinylcholine—causes excessive adenosine triphosphate (ATP) hydrolysis to provide energy for contraction. The increased rate of ATP hydrolysis leads to an increased metabolic rate as muscle tries to replenish and sustain its ATP stores. Hyperthermia develops because of the heat liberated by the hydrolysis of ATP.

Further support for this hypothesis came from the observation that more tension developed in muscle fibers obtained by biopsy from susceptible individuals than in fibers from normal individuals when the fibers were exposed to halothane. In muscle fibers from both humans and a strain of swine susceptible to MH, Ca^{2+}-induced Ca^{2+} release from the sarcoplasmic reticulum (SR) is enhanced when compared with fibers from unaffected subjects. Furthermore, caffeine, which causes the Ca^{2+}-release channels to open, induced greater contractions in fibers from susceptible subjects. Taken together, these observations suggested the possibility that MH results from an abnormality in the Ca^{2+}-release channel in the SR membrane.

In both humans and animals, inheritance of MH follows a mendelian autosomal-dominant pattern. Cloning of the gene (*RyR1*) encoding the Ca^{2+}-release channel (ryanodine receptor) allowed genetic linkage analysis to demonstrate that human MH is closely linked in some families to the *RyR1* gene on chromosome 19. In swine, MH results from a single amino-acid substitution in *RyR1* (Cys for Arg at position 614). An analogous substitution is present in some human kindreds as well. This substitution increases the probability that the Ca^{2+}-release channel will be open. In other families, MH has been associated with other genetic abnormalities in the *RyR1* gene. In still others, MH does not appear to be genetically linked to the *RyR1* gene. It is possible that defects in other steps along the excitation-contraction cascade can result in abnormal regulation of muscle contraction and the MH phenotype. For example, when under anesthesia, patients with some forms of muscular dystrophy may have metabolic crises that resemble MH.

MH also occurs in domestic livestock. The incidence of MH is particularly high in swine, where episodes are triggered by a variety of physical and environmental stresses (porcine stress syndrome). MH in animals has significant economic importance in view of the potential loss from fatal episodes and the devaluation of meat as a result of muscle destruction during non-fatal episodes.

In humans, a condition similar to MH may occur in patients treated with neuroleptic agents such as the phenothiazines or haloperidol. It is called the *neuroleptic malignant syndrome* and appears to result from abnormally high neuronal input to the muscle cells.

Therapy for MH now involves administration of the drug dantrolene, cessation of anesthesia, and aggressive efforts aimed at cooling the body. **Dantrolene** is an effective therapeutic agent because it blocks excitation-contraction coupling between T tubules and the SR, thus interrupting the otherwise uncontrolled progression of muscular contractions. The drug can be given acutely in an effort to abort an ongoing attack or, in a person known to be at risk, it can be given before the initiation of anesthesia in order to prevent onset of the syndrome. Therapy also includes intravenous hydration and the judicious use of diuretics to keep the urine flowing. The latter lessens damage to the kidneys from the release of breakdown products, such as myoglobin from the damaged muscles. Sodium bicarbonate is given to counter the lactic acidosis, and patients may be mechanically hyperventilated to blow off the excess CO_2.

Despite the intensive protocol just outlined, MH is still associated with high mortality. The relatives of a patient with a documented history of one episode of MH should be carefully screened to see whether they, too, carry the inherited trait; many of the affected relatives may demonstrate baseline elevations in muscle enzyme levels in their blood (e.g., an increase in creatine kinase levels).

---

membrane of the smooth muscle SR (p. 100). This IP_3 receptor is itself a ligand-gated Ca^{2+} channel. Thus, a receptor in the plasma membrane can indirectly induce Ca^{2+} release from the SR and hence contraction.

Ca^{2+} ENTRY THROUGH VOLTAGE-*INDEPENDENT* CHANNELS. In smooth muscle it is possible that extracellular ligands may trigger the influx of Ca^{2+} through either ligand-gated channels (p. 170) or channels that are activated via G-protein–coupled receptors. Nevertheless, it is not clear to what extent, if any, these types of Ca^{2+} channels contribute to [Ca^{2+}]$_i$ increases in smooth muscle. However, another class of channels—**store-operated Ca^{2+} channels**—appears to play an important role. Neu-

FIGURE 9-10. Excitation-contraction (E-C) coupling in smooth muscle. DAG, diacylglycerol; IP$_3$, inositol 1,4,5-triphosphate; PIP$_2$, phosphatidyl inositol 4,5-biphosphate; SR, sarcoplasmic reticulum.

rotransmitters that lead to the discharge—and thus the depletion—of SR Ca^{2+} stores (i.e., second pathway) somehow lead to the activation of store-operated Ca^{2+} channels in the plasma membrane. The Ca^{2+} entering through these channels allows [Ca^{2+}]$_i$ to remain elevated even after SR depletion and also appears to replenish SR Ca^{2+} stores.

Together, the second pathway for increasing [Ca^{2+}]$_i$ (Ca^{2+} release from the SR) and the third pathway (Ca^{2+} influx through store-operated channels) have been called **pharmacomechanical coupling** because these excitatory neurotransmitters and hormones can induce smooth muscle contraction that is independent of action-potential generation. Regardless of the source of the Ca^{2+}, the resultant increase in [Ca^{2+}]$_i$ leads to contraction via a Ca^{2+}-CaM–dependent increase in MLCK activity and myosin phosphorylation.

Smooth Muscle Contraction May Also Occur Independently of Increases in [Ca^{2+}]$_i$

Whereas many excitatory stimuli rely on increases in [Ca^{2+}]$_i$ to evoke contraction, some stimuli appear to cause contraction without a measurable increase in [Ca^{2+}]$_i$. One mechanism by which excitatory stimuli might induce Ca^{2+}-independent contractions is by modulating the activity of contractile or regulatory proteins directly. Thus, the

amount of force developed at any given [Ca^{2+}]$_i$ may vary. This force/[Ca^{2+}]$_i$ ratio may be increased or decreased and is generally higher during pharmacomechanical activation than during depolarization-activated contractions. Because phosphorylation of the myosin light chain (MLC) is a major determinant of contractile force in smooth muscle, Ca^{2+}-independent contractions may result either from an increase in the rate of MLC phosphorylation by MLCK or from a decrease in the rate of MLC dephosphorylation by MLC phosphatase. One second-messenger system that can decrease the activity of phosphatases is protein kinase C (PKC) (p. 102). Some excitatory stimuli are therefore capable of initiating smooth muscle contraction by inducing IP$_3$-mediated release of Ca^{2+} from intracellular stores, as well as by producing PKC-mediated decreases in MLC phosphatase activity. These pathways are further examples of pharmacomechanical coupling.

TERMINATING CONTRACTION

In Skeletal, Cardiac, and Smooth Muscle, Terminating Contraction Requires Re-Uptake of Ca^{2+} Into the Sarcoplasmic Reticulum

After the contraction-activating stimulus has subsided, Ca^{2+} must be removed from the cytoplasm for contrac-

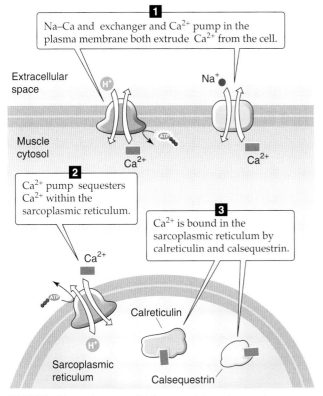

FIGURE 9–11. Mechanisms of Ca²⁺ removal from the cytoplasm.

The boxes in the figure read:

1 Na–Ca and exchanger and Ca^{2+} pump in the plasma membrane both extrude Ca^{2+} from the cell.

2 Ca^{2+} pump sequesters Ca^{2+} within the sarcoplasmic reticulum.

3 Ca^{2+} is bound in the sarcoplasmic reticulum by calreticulin and calsequestrin.

Labels: Extracellular space; Muscle cytosol; Sarcoplasmic reticulum; Calreticulin; Calsequestrin

tion to cease and for relaxation to occur. Ca^{2+} may be extruded across the cell membrane or sequestered within intracellular compartments (Fig. 9–11).

The cell may extrude Ca^{2+} using either an Na-Ca exchanger (NCX, p. 68) or a Ca^{2+} pump at the plasma membrane (PMCA, p. 64). Extrusion across the cell membrane, however, would eventually deplete the cell of Ca^{2+} and is therefore a minor mechanism for Ca^{2+} removal from the cytoplasm. Instead, Ca^{2+} re-uptake into the SR is the most important mechanism by which the cell returns $[Ca^{2+}]_i$ to resting levels. Ca^{2+} re-uptake by the SR is mediated by a SERCA-type Ca^{2+} pump (p. 64).

It is possible that the rate of Ca^{2+} re-uptake into the SR may be regulated by modulating the activity of the SR Ca^{2+} pump. For example, in cardiac muscle, SR Ca^{2+}-pump activity is inhibited by the regulatory protein **phospholamban**. When phospholamban is phosphorylated by cyclic adenosine monophosphate (cAMP)-dependent protein kinase (PKA), its ability to inhibit the SR Ca^{2+} pump is lost. Thus, activators of PKA, such as the neurotransmitter epinephrine, may enhance the rate of cardiac myocyte relaxation (p. 525).

SR Ca^{2+}-pump activity is also inhibited by high $[Ca^{2+}]$ within the SR lumen. This inhibition of SR Ca^{2+}-pump activity is delayed by Ca^{2+}-binding proteins within the SR lumen. These Ca^{2+}-binding proteins buffer the $[Ca^{2+}]$ increase in the SR during Ca^{2+} re-uptake and thus markedly increase the Ca^{2+} capacity of the SR. The principal Ca^{2+}-binding protein in skeletal muscle, **calsequestrin**, is also present in cardiac and some smooth muscle. **Calre-**

ticulin** is a ubiquitous Ca^{2+}-binding protein that is found in particularly high concentrations within the SR of smooth muscle. These proteins have a tremendous capacity to bind Ca^{2+}, with up to 50 binding sites per protein molecule.

Ca^{2+}-binding proteins are not located diffusely within the SR. Rather, calsequestrin is highly localized to the region of the SR immediately beneath the triad junction. Calsequestrin appears to bind directly at the triad, where it forms a complex with the Ca^{2+}-release channel and with two other triad proteins, junctin and triadin. Here, calsequestrin is poised not only to aid muscle relaxation by buffering Ca^{2+} within the SR lumen but also to unload its Ca^{2+} in the vicinity of the Ca^{2+}-release channel and thus facilitate EC coupling. It has been hypothesized that EC coupling promotes Ca^{2+} release from calsequestrin, making Ca^{2+} available for exit from the SR.

In Smooth Muscle, Terminating Contraction Also Requires Dephosphorylation of the Myosin Light Chain

Because Ca^{2+} triggers smooth muscle contraction by inducing phosphorylation of the myosin regulatory light chain, merely restoring $[Ca^{2+}]_i$ to its low resting value may not allow muscle relaxation. Rather, relaxation of smooth muscle requires MLC dephosphorylation, which is accomplished by **myosin light chain phosphatase**. This phosphatase is a heterotrimer consisting of subunits with molecular masses of 130, 20, and 37 kDa. The 130-kDa subunit confers specificity by binding to myosin, whereas the 37-kDa protein is the catalytic subunit responsible for the dephosphorylating activity.

REGULATING MUSCLE CONTRACTION

Muscle Contractions Produce Force and/or Shortening and, in the Extreme, Can Be Studied Under Either Isometric or Isotonic Conditions

The total force generated by a muscle is the sum of the forces generated by many independently cycling actin-myosin cross-bridges. The number of simultaneously cycling cross-bridges depends substantially on the initial length of the muscle fiber and on the pattern or frequency of muscle-cell stimulation. When muscle is stimulated to contract, it exerts a force tending to pull the attachment points at either end toward each other. This force is referred to as the **tension** developed by the muscle.

Two mechanical—and artificial—arrangements can be used to study muscle contraction. In one, the attachment points are immobile, thereby fixing the muscle *length*. Here, stimulation causes an increase in tension, but no shortening. Because these contractions occur at constant length, they are referred to as **isometric contractions** (Fig. 9–12A). In the second arrangement, one of the two attachment points is mobile, and a force—or load—

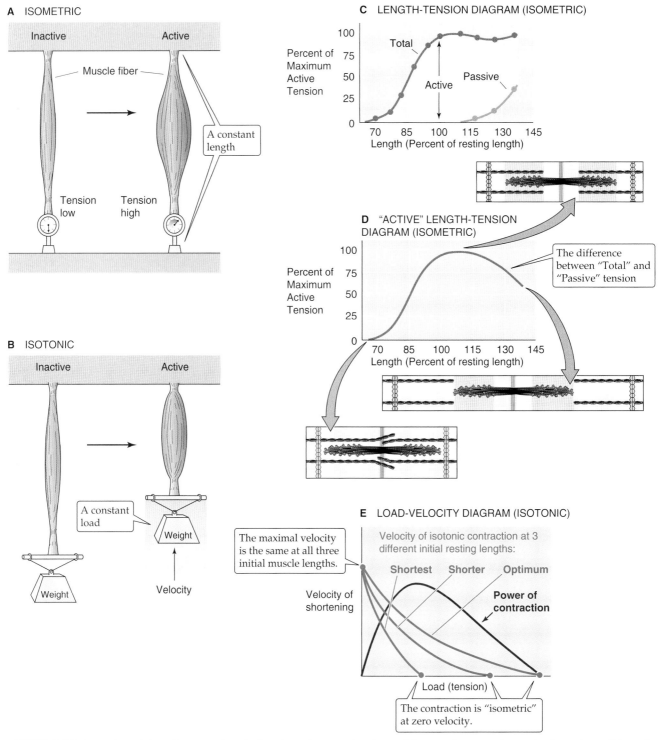

FIGURE 9–12. Isometric and isotonic contraction. *A*, Experimental preparation for studying muscle contraction under *isometric* conditions. *B*, Experimental preparation for studying muscle contraction under *isotonic* conditions. *C*, The *"passive"* curve represents the tension that is measured at various muscle lengths prior to muscle contraction. The *"total"* curve represents the tension that is measured at various muscle lengths during muscle contraction. *D*, The "active" tension is the difference between the "total" and the "passive" tensions in *C*. *E*, Each of the *three blue curves* shows that the velocity of muscle shortening is faster if the muscle lifts a lighter weight—it is easier to lift a feather (left side of each curve/low load) than to lift a barbell (right side of each curve/high load). The *three blue curves* also show that, for any given velocity of shortening, a longer muscle can develop a greater tension than can a shorter muscle.

MEASURING THE FORCE OF A SINGLE CROSS-BRIDGE CYCLE

The force of a single cross-bridge cycle has been measured directly. Finer, Simmons, and Spudich used **optical tweezers** to manipulate a single actin filament and place it in proximity to a myosin molecule immobilized on a bead (Fig. 9–13). With the use of video-enhanced microscopy these investigators were able to detect movements of the actin filament as small as 1 nm. The optical tweezers could also exert an adjustable force opposing movement of the actin filament. When the tweezers applied only a small opposing force and the experiment was conducted in the presence of adenosine triphosphate (ATP), they observed that the actin moved over the myosin bead in step-like displacements of 11 nm. This observation, made under "microscopically isotonic" conditions, suggests that the quantal displacement of a single cross-bridge cycle is approximately 11 nm. When the tweezers applied a force sufficiently large to immobilize the actin filament, the investigators observed step-like impulses of force that averaged around 5 pN. This observation, made under "microscopically isometric" conditions, suggests that the quantal force developed during a single cross-bridge cycle is about 5 pN. Interestingly, these isometric force impulses lasted longer when the ATP concentration was lower. This last finding is consistent with the notion that ATP binding to myosin must occur to allow detachment of the cross-bridges (*step 1* in the cycle in Fig. 9–7).

tends to pull this mobile point away from the fixed one. Here, stimulation causes shortening, provided that the tension developed by the muscle is greater than the opposing load. Because these shortenings occur at constant load, they are referred to as **isotonic contractions** (see Fig. 9–12B). Both isometric and isotonic contractions can be examined at different initial muscle lengths. Moreover, they can be measured during individual muscle twitches that are evoked by single muscle action potentials, as well as during other patterns of stimulation.

Muscle Length Influences Tension Development By Determining the Degree of Overlap Between Actin and Myosin Filaments

The iso*metric* force of contractions depends on the initial length of the muscle fiber. Unstimulated muscle may be elongated somewhat by applying tension and stretching it. The tension measured before muscle contraction is referred to as **passive tension** (see Fig. 9–12C). Because muscle gets stiffer as it is distended, it takes increasing amounts of "passive" tension to progressively elongate the muscle cell. If at any fixed length (i.e., isometric conditions) the muscle is stimulated to contract, an additional **active tension** develops because of cross-bridge cycling. The total measured tension is thus the sum of the passive and active tension. This incremental or *active* tension— the difference between total tension and passive tension—is quite small when the muscle is less than approximately 70% of its normal resting length (see Fig. 9–12D). As muscle length increases toward its normal length, active tension increases. Active tension is maximal at a length—usually called L_0—that is near the normal muscle length. Active tension decreases with further lengthening; thus, active tension is again small when the muscle is stretched beyond 150% of its normal resting length. Although the relationship between muscle length and tension has been best characterized for skeletal muscle, the tension of cardiac and smooth muscle also appears to depend on length in a similar manner.

This length-tension relationship is a direct result of the anatomy of the thick and thin filaments within individual sarcomeres (see Fig. 9–12D). As muscle length increases, the ends of the actin filaments arising from neighboring Z disks are pulled away from each other. When length is increased beyond 150% of its resting sarcomere length, the ends of the actin filaments are pulled beyond the ends of the myosin filaments. Under this condition, no interaction occurs between actin and myosin filaments and hence no development of active tension. As muscle length shortens from this point, actin and myosin filaments begin to overlap and tension can develop; the amount of tension developed corresponds to the degree of overlap between the actin and the myosin filaments. As the muscle shortens further, opposing actin filaments slide over one another and the ends of the myosin filaments and—with extreme degrees of shortening—eventually butt up against the opposing Z disks. Under these conditions, the spatial relationship between actin and myosin is distorted and active tension falls. The maximal degree of overlap between actin and myosin filaments, and hence maximal active tension, corresponds to a sarcomere length that is near its normal resting length.

At Higher Loads, the Velocity of Shortening Is Lower Because More Cross-Bridges Are Simultaneously Active

Under iso*tonic* conditions, the velocity of shortening decreases as the applied load opposing contraction of the muscle fiber increases. This point is obvious; anyone can lift a single French fry much faster than a sack of potatoes. As shown for any of the three *blue curves* in Figure 9–12E—each of which represents a different initial length of muscle—the relationship between velocity and load is hyperbolic. Thus, the smaller the load applied to the muscle, the greater its velocity of shortening. Conversely, the greater the load, the lower the velocity of shortening.

A EXPERIMENTAL PREPARATION

FIGURE 9–13. Microscopic measurements of cross-bridge force and displacement. *A,* An actin filament is attached at each end to a polystyrene bead. The "optical tweezers," a finely focused beam of laser light, can "trap" the bead at its focal point and physically move it. By adjusting the laser intensity, the experimenter can alter the strength of the trap (i.e., the force with which the bead is held). In this experiment, two optical tweezers were used to suspend the actin filament above a coverglass. Attached to this coverslip is a silica bead, and myosin molecules are bound to the bead. *B,* In an "isotonic" experiment, the force between the actin filament and the fixed myosin/silica bead is kept constant by using a stable laser intensity. The experimenter measures, as a function of time, the displacement of the polystyrene bead (*blue*) away from the center of the trap. Thus, in one cross-bridge cycle, the myosin-actin interaction pulls the polystyrene bead approximately 11 nm away from the center of the trap. *C,* In an "isometric" experiment, the experimenter measures, as a function of time, the extra force that needs to be applied (i.e., increase in laser intensity) to keep the polystyrene bead (*blue*) at a fixed position near the center of the trap. Thus, in one cross-bridge cycle, the myosin-actin interaction exerts a force of approximately 5 pN. (Data from Finer JT, Mehta AD, Spudich JA: Characterization of single actin-myosin interactions. Biophys J 68:291s–296s, 1995.)

The load (or tension)-velocity relationship is perhaps best understood by considering the situation at maximum load for a resting muscle length (i.e., *isometric* conditions). This situation is represented by the *upper blue curve* in Figure 9–12E. At any time, all the available cross-bridges are engaged in resisting the opposing force. None are left over to make the muscle shorten. If the number of engaged cross-bridges were decreased, the muscle would lengthen. At a slightly smaller load but at the same isotonic muscle length, fewer cross-bridges need to be engaged to resist the opposing load. Thus, extra cross-bridges are available to ratchet the thick myosin filaments over the thin actin filaments, but at a very low velocity. At a still lower load, even more cross-bridges are available for ratcheting the myosin over the actin, and the velocity increases further. At very low loads, it is reasonable to expect that as the myosin filament slides along the actin filament, only a tiny fraction of the actin monomers need

to interact with myosin heads to overcome the load. Under these conditions of vanishingly small loads, the speed with which the thick and thin filaments slide over each other is limited only by the time that it takes for the ATP-consuming cross-bridge cycle to occur. With increasing velocity, the probability of actin-myosin interactions decreases. Thus, fewer cross-bridges are simultaneously active at higher shortening velocities, and less tension develops.

Note that the *upper blue curve* in Figure 9–12E applies to a particular initial length of the muscle, that is, the *resting* length. We already saw in Figure 9–12C that the total isometric tension (i.e., the maximal load that the muscle can sustain at zero velocity) increases with initial muscle length. This principle is confirmed in Figure 9–12E: the longer the initial length, the larger the maximal load under zero-velocity conditions (i.e., the three different intercepts with the abscissa). In contrast to this maxi-

FIGURE 9–14. Frequency summation of skeletal muscle twitches.

mal *load*, which depends very much on length, maximal *velocity* is independent of length, as shown by the common intercept of the family of curves with the ordinate. The explanation for this effect—as we have already noted—is that maximal velocity (at no load) depends on the maximal rate of cross-bridge turnover, not on the initial overlap of the thin and thick filaments.

The velocity-tension curve reveals an interesting relationship between muscle power and applied load. Muscle does measurable mechanical work only when it displaces a load. This mechanical **work** (*W*) is the product of load (*F*) and displacement (Δx). **Power** (*P*) is the rate at which work is performed, or work per unit time (Δt):

Equation 9–1

$$P = W/\Delta t = F \times \Delta x/\Delta t$$

Because velocity (*v*) is $\Delta x/\Delta t$, it follows that

Equation 9–2

$$P = F \times v$$

For a given load (*F*), we can calculate the power by reading the velocity (*v*) from the uppermost of the three blue load-velocity relationships in Figure 9–12E. Power is maximal at intermediate loads (where both *F* and *v* are moderate) and falls to zero at maximum load (where *v* = 0) and at zero load (where *F* = 0).

In a Single Skeletal Muscle Fiber, the Force Developed May Be Increased By Summing Multiple Twitches In Time

At sufficiently low stimulation frequencies, the tension developed falls to the resting level between individual twitches (Fig. 9–14A). Single skeletal-muscle twitches last between 25 and 200 msec, depending on the type of muscle. Although each twitch is elicited by a single muscle action potential, the duration of contraction is long when compared with the duration of the exciting action potential, which lasts only several milliseconds. Because the muscle twitch far exceeds the duration of the action potential, it is possible to initiate a second *action potential* before a first *contraction* has fully subsided. When this

situation occurs, the second action potential stimulates a twitch that is superimposed on the residual tension of the first twitch, thereby achieving greater isometric tension than the first (compare Fig. 9–14A and B). This effect is known as **summation**.

If multiple action potentials occur closely enough in time, the multiple twitches can summate and thus greatly increase the tension developed. Summation is more effective at increasing tension when the action potentials are grouped more closely in time, as in Figure 9–14C. In other words, tension is higher when action potentials are evoked at higher frequency. Because this type of tension enhancement depends on the frequency of muscle stimulation, it is referred to as **frequency summation**.

When the stimulation frequency is increased sufficiently, the individual twitches occur so closely together in time that they fuse (see Fig. 9–14D) and cause the muscle tension to remain at a steady plateau. The state in which the individual twitches are no longer distinguishable from each other is referred to as **tetanus**. Tetanus arises when the time between successive action potentials is insufficient to return enough Ca^{2+} back to the SR to lower $[Ca^{2+}]_i$ below a level that initiates relaxation. In fact, a sustained increase in $[Ca^{2+}]_i$ persists until the tetanic stimulus ceases. At stimulation frequencies above the **fusion frequency** that causes tetanus, muscle fiber tension increases very little.

In a Whole Skeletal Muscle, the Force Developed May Be Increased By Summing the Contractions of Multiple Fibers

In addition to determining the frequency with which it stimulates a single muscle fiber, the central nervous system (CNS) can control muscle force by determining the number of individual muscle fibers that it stimulates at a given time. As each additional motor-neuron cell body within the spinal cord is excited, those muscle fibers that are part of the *motor unit* of that motor neuron are added to the contracting pool of fibers (Fig. 9–15). This effect is known as **multiple-fiber summation**. Generally, smaller motor neurons serve motor units consisting of fewer individual muscle fibers. Because a given excitatory stimulus will generate a larger excitatory postsynaptic potential (p.

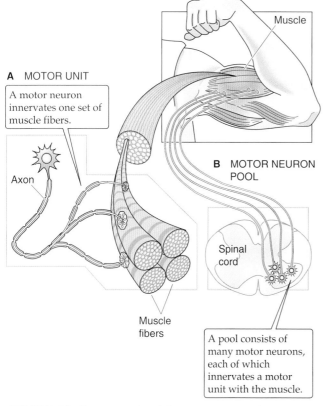

A MOTOR UNIT

A motor neuron innervates one set of muscle fibers.

Axon

Muscle

B MOTOR NEURON POOL

Spinal cord

Muscle fibers

A pool consists of many motor neurons, each of which innervates a motor unit with the muscle.

FIGURE 9–15. The motor unit and the motor-neuron pool.

212) in motor neurons with smaller cell bodies, the small motor units are recruited even with minimal neuronal stimulation. As neuronal stimulation intensifies, larger motor neurons innervating larger motor units are also recruited. The progressive recruitment of first small and then larger and larger motor units is referred to as the **size principle**. The group of all motor neurons innervating a single muscle is called a **motor-neuron pool**.

Multiple-fiber summation, sometimes referred to as **spatial summation**, is an important mechanism that allows the force developed by a whole muscle to be relatively constant in time. It is true that the CNS could direct the force to be relatively constant over time merely by driving a fixed number of motor units within the muscle to tetanus, where the force fluctuations are very small (see Fig. 9–14D). However, adding tetanic motor units would increase total muscle force by rather large individual increments. Instead, the CNS can activate individual motor units asynchronously so that some units are developing tension while others are relaxing. Thus, whole-muscle force can be relatively constant with time, even when individual fibers are not stimulated to tetanus. Smooth, nontetanic contraction is essential for fine motor control.

In Cardiac Muscle, Increasing the Entry of Ca²⁺ Enhances the Contractile Force

Whereas frequency summation and multiple-fiber summation are important mechanisms for regulating the strength of skeletal-muscle contractions, these mechanisms would

not be consistent with the physiological demands of cardiac muscle. Because cardiac muscle must contract only once with each heartbeat and must fully relax between each contraction, frequency summation is precluded. Furthermore, the extensive electrical coupling between cardiac myocytes, as well as the requirement that cardiac muscle contract homogeneously, eliminates the potential for multiple-fiber summation. Therefore, the strength of cardiac muscle contraction must be regulated by modulating the contractile force generated during each individual muscle twitch. This type of regulation is an important part of the adaptive response to exercise and is mediated by norepinephrine, a neurotransmitter released by the sympathetic nervous system.

Because an increase in $[Ca^{2+}]_i$ activates contraction by removing the inhibitory influence of the regulatory proteins, it is reasonable to consider that contractile function may be regulated either by modulating the magnitude of the rise in $[Ca^{2+}]_i$ or by altering the Ca^{2+} sensitivity of the regulatory proteins. In fact, both these mechanisms are important in controlling the force of cardiac muscle contraction.

In cardiac muscle, a significant proportion of the activator Ca^{2+} enters the cell via voltage-gated Ca^{2+} channels that open during the cardiac action potential. Most of this Ca^{2+} influx occurs via L-type Ca^{2+} channels. How does norepinephrine increase the contractile force of the heart? This hormone acts through the β-type adrenergic receptor to increase the generation of cAMP, activate PKA (p. 97), and in turn phosphorylate the L-type Ca^{2+} channels, thereby increasing the passive influx of Ca^{2+}. An increased $[Ca^{2+}]_i$ leads to an increase in contractile force. The cAMP pathway also appears to increase the Ca^{2+} sensitivity of the contractile apparatus by phosphorylating one or more of the regulatory proteins. Thus, cAMP causes an increase in the force generated for any given $[Ca^{2+}]_i$.

Reciprocal control over Ca^{2+} entry is provided by cyclic guanosine monophosphate (cGMP)-dependent phosphorylation of the L-type Ca^{2+} channels. Acetylcholine, acting through muscarinic ACh receptors, raises intracellular cGMP concentrations. In turn, the cGMP-dependent phosphorylation of L-type Ca^{2+} channels, at sites distinct from those phosphorylated by the cAMP-dependent kinase, causes a decrease in Ca^{2+} influx during the cardiac action potential and thus a decrease in the force of contraction.

Ca^{2+} entry may also be regulated indirectly by modulating other ion channels so that they either change their Ca^{2+} permeability or alter the duration of the action potential. Norepinephrine, for example, may increase the Ca^{2+} permeability of voltage-gated Na^+ channels. Receptor transduction mechanisms that inhibit voltage-gated K^+ currents may prolong the cardiac action potential and thereby increase net Ca^{2+} influx through L-type Ca^{2+} channels without modulating the Ca^{2+} channels themselves.

In Smooth Muscle, Contractile Force Is Enhanced By Increasing the Entry of Ca²⁺, As Well As By Increasing the Ca²⁺ Sensitivity of the Contractile Apparatus

Unlike skeletal muscle, in which force development results from the summation of individual muscle *twitches*, individual smooth muscle cells can maintain a sustained contraction that can be graded in strength over a wide range. Contractile force in smooth muscle largely depends on the relative balance between the phosphorylation and dephosphorylation of MLCs. The rate of MLC phosphorylation is regulated by the Ca^{2+}-CaM complex, which in turn depends on *levels of intracellular Ca^{2+}*. Smooth muscle cells can regulate $[Ca^{2+}]_i$ over a wider range than skeletal and cardiac muscle can for several reasons. First, some smooth muscle cells do not generate action potentials. Rather, their membrane potential varies slowly in response to neurotransmitters or hormones. This graded response of V_m allows finer regulation of Ca^{2+} influx through voltage-gated channels. Second, release of Ca^{2+} from intracellular stores may be modulated through neurotransmitter-induced generation of intracellular second messengers such as IP_3. This modulation allows finer control of Ca^{2+} release than occurs in the SR Ca^{2+} release channel by L-type Ca^{2+} channels in skeletal and cardiac muscle.

A second level of control over contractile force occurs by regulating the *Ca^{2+} sensitivity* of proteins that regulate contraction. For example, inhibiting *myosin light chain phosphatase* alters the balance between phosphorylation and dephosphorylation, in effect allowing a greater contraction at a lower $[Ca^{2+}]_i$. Some neurotransmitters act by inhibiting the phosphatase, which appears to occur through activation of G-protein–coupled receptors. Another mechanism for governing the Ca^{2+} sensitivity of proteins that regulate contraction is alteration of the Ca^{2+} sensitivity of the *myosin light chain kinase*. For example, MLCK itself is phosphorylated at specific sites by several protein kinases, including PKA, protein kinase C, and Ca^{2+}-CaM–dependent kinases. Phosphorylation by any of these kinases decreases the sensitivity of MLCK to activation by the Ca^{2+}-CaM complex.

Smooth Muscle Maintains High Force at Low Energy Consumption

Smooth muscle is often called upon to maintain high force for long periods. If smooth muscle consumed ATP at rates similar to striated muscle, metabolic demands would be considerable and the muscle would be prone to fatigue. Unlike striated muscle, however, smooth muscle is able to maintain high force at a low rate of ATP hydrolysis. This low–energy consumption/high-tension state is referred to as the **latch state**. The latch state in smooth muscle is unique because high tension can be maintained despite a decrease in the degree of muscle activation by excitatory stimuli. As a result, force is maintained at a lower level of MLCK phosphorylation.

The mechanism underlying the latch state is not entirely known, although it appears to be due in large part to changes in the kinetics of actin-myosin cross-bridge formation and detachment. These changes may be a direct result of a decrease in the rate at which dephosphorylated cross-bridges detach. Tension is directly related to the number of attached cross-bridges. Furthermore, the proportion of myosin heads cross-bridged to actin is related to the ratio of attachment rates to detachment rates.

Therefore, it is reasonable to expect that a decrease in the detachment rate would allow a greater number of cross-bridges to be maintained and would result in a lower rate of cross-bridge cycling and ATP hydrolysis. Thus, smooth muscle appears to be able to slow down cross-bridge cycling just before detachment, a feat that can be accomplished in skeletal muscle (see Fig. 9–7) only at low ATP levels (as in *rigor mortis*).

DIVERSITY AMONG MUSCLES

Each muscle type (i.e., skeletal, cardiac, and smooth) is distinguishable on the basis of its unique histology, EC-coupling mechanisms, and regulation of contractile function. However, even within each of the three categories, muscle in different locations must serve markedly different purposes, with different demands for strength, speed, and fatigability. This diversity is possible because of differences in the expression of specific isoforms for various contractile and regulatory proteins (Table 9–1).

Skeletal Muscle Is Composed of Slow-Twitch and Fast-Twitch Fibers

Some skeletal muscles must be resistant to fatigue and be able to maintain tension for relatively long periods, although they need not contract rapidly. Examples are muscles that maintain body posture, such as the soleus muscle of the lower part of the leg. In contrast, some muscles need to contract rapidly, yet infrequently. Examples are the extraocular muscles, which must contract rapidly to redirect the eye as an object of visual interest moves about.

Individual muscle fibers are classified as *slow twitch* (*type I*) or *fast twitch* (*type II*), depending on their rate of force development. These fiber types are also distinguished by their histologic appearance and their ability to resist fatigue.

Slow-twitch fibers (Table 9–2) are generally thinner and have a more dense capillary network surrounding them. Slow-twitch fibers also appear red because of a large amount of the oxygen-binding protein **myoglobin** (p. 656) within the cytoplasm. This rich capillary network together with myoglobin facilitates oxygen transport to the slow-twitch fibers, which mostly rely on oxidative metabolism for energy. The metabolic machinery of the slow-twitch fiber also favors oxidative metabolism because it has low glycogen content and glycolytic-enzyme activity but a rich mitochondrial and oxidative-enzyme content.

Fast-twitch fibers differ among themselves with respect to fatigability. Some fast-twitch fibers are fatigue resistant; they rely on oxidative metabolism (**type IIa**) and are quite similar to slow-twitch fibers with respect to myoglobin content (indeed, they are red) and metabolic machinery. One important difference is that fast-twitch oxidative fibers contain abundant glycogen and have a greater number of mitochondria than slow-twitch fibers do. These features ensure adequate ATP generation to compensate for the increased rate of ATP hydrolysis in fast-twitch fibers.

TABLE 9–1

ISOFORM EXPRESSION OF CONTRACTILE AND REGULATORY PROTEINS

	SKELETAL SLOW (I)	SKELETAL FAST OXIDATIVE (IIa)	SKELETAL FAST FATIGABLE (IIb)	CARDIAC	SMOOTH
Myosin heavy chain	MHC-I	MHC-IIa	MHC-IIb, -IIx	MHC-α and -β	MHC-SM1, 2 (multiple isoforms)
Myosin light chain	MLC-1aS, -1bS	MLC-1f, -3f	MLC-1f, -3f	MLC-1v, -1a	MLC-17a, -17b
SR Ca ATPase	SERCA2a	SERCA1	SERCA1	SERCA2a	SERCA2a, 2b (b > > > a)
Phospholamban	Present	Absent	Absent	Present	Present
Calsequestrin	"Fast" and "cardiac"	"Fast"	"Fast"	"Cardiac"	? "Cardiac" ? "Fast"
Ca^{2+} release mechanisms	RyR1 (Ca^{2+} release channel or "ryanodine" receptor)	RyR1	RyR1	RyR2	IP_3R (3 isoforms) RyR3
Ca^{2+} sensor	Troponin C_1	Troponin C_2	Troponin C_2	Troponin C_1	Calmodulin (multiple isoforms)

IP_3R, inositol 1,4,5-triphosphate receptor; SR, sarcoplasmic reticulum.

Other fast-twitch fibers are not capable of sufficient oxidative metabolism to sustain contraction. Because these fibers must rely on the energy that is stored within glycogen (and phosphocreatine), they are more easily fatigable. Fatigable fast-twitch fibers (**type IIb**) have fewer mitochondria and lower concentrations of myoglobin and oxidative enzymes. Because of their low myoglobin content, type IIb muscle fibers are white. They are, however, richer in glycolytic enzyme activity than other fiber types are.

In reality, slow- and fast-twitch fibers represent the extremes of a continuum of muscle fiber characteristics. Moreover, each whole muscle is composed of fibers of each twitch type, although in any given muscle one of the fiber types predominates. The differences between fiber types derive in large part from differences in isoform expression of the various contractile and regulatory proteins (see Table 9–1).

Differences in the rate of contraction, for example, may be directly correlated with the maximal rate of myosin ATPase activity. As many as 10 different **myosin heavy chain** isoforms have been identified. Individual isoform expression varies among muscle types and is developmentally regulated. At least four isoforms of the MHC protein are expressed in skeletal muscle (MHC-I, MHC-IIa, MHC-IIb, MHC-IIx/d). For the most part, a muscle fiber type expresses a single MHC isoform, the ATPase activity of which appears to correspond to the rate of contraction in that fiber type. Whereas most fibers express one of these isoforms, some fibers express a combination of two different isoforms. These hybrid cells have rates of contraction that are intermediate between the two pure fiber types.

Differences in the rates and strength of contraction may also result from differences in **myosin light chain** isoform expression or from isoform differences among other components of the EC coupling process. Three skeletal muscle isoforms have been identified. MLC-1as and MLC-1bs are expressed in slow-twitch fibers, whereas MLC-1f and MLC-3f are expressed in fast-twitch fibers.

Isoform differences also exist for the **SR Ca^{2+} pump** (i.e., the SERCA), calsequestrin, the Ca^{2+}-release channel,

TABLE 9–2

PROPERTIES OF FAST- AND SLOW-TWITCH MUSCLE FIBERS

	SLOW TWITCH	FAST TWITCH	FAST TWITCH
Synonym	Type I	Type IIa	Type IIb
Fatigue	Resistant	Resistant	Fatigable
Color	Red (myoglobin)	Red (myoglobin)	White (low myoglobin)
Metabolism	Oxidative	Oxidative	Glycolytic
Mitochondria	High	Higher	Fewer
Glycogen	Low	Abundant	High

and troponin C. Furthermore, some proteins, such as phospholamban, are expressed in one fiber type (slow twitch) and not the other.

One particularly interesting feature of muscle differentiation is that fiber-type determination is not static. Through exercise training or changes in patterns of neuronal stimulation, alterations in contractile and regulatory protein isoform expression may occur. For example, it is possible for a greater proportion of fast-twitch fibers to develop in a specific muscle with repetitive training. It is even possible to induce cardiac-specific isoforms in skeletal muscle, given appropriate stimulation patterns.

The Properties of Cardiac Cells Vary with Location in the Heart

Just as skeletal muscle consists of multiple fiber types, so too does heart muscle. The electrophysiological and mechanical properties of cardiac muscle vary with their location (i.e., atria versus conducting system versus ventricle). Moreover, even among cells within one anatomic location, functional differences may exist between muscle cells near the surface of the heart (*epicardial cells*) and those lining the interior of the same chambers (*endocardial cells*). As in skeletal muscle, many of these differences reflect differences in isoform expression of the various contractile and regulatory proteins. Although some of the protein isoforms expressed in cardiac tissue are identical to those

expressed in skeletal muscle, many of the proteins have cardiac-specific isoforms (see Table 9–1). The MHC in heart, for example, exists in two isoforms, α and β, which may be expressed alone or in combination.

Smooth Muscle Cells May Differ Markedly Among Tissues and May Adapt Their Properties with Time Even in a Single Tissue

When one considers that smooth muscle has a broad range of functions, including regulating the diameter of blood vessels, propelling food through the gastrointestinal tract, regulating the diameter of airways, and delivering a newborn infant from the uterus, it is not surprising that smooth muscle is a particularly diverse type of muscle. In addition to being distinguished as unitary or multiunit muscle (p. 231), smooth muscle in different organs diverges with respect to nerve and hormonal control, electrical activity, and characteristics of contraction.

Even among smooth muscle cells within the same sort of tissue, important functional differences may exist. For example, vascular smooth muscle cells within the walls of two arterioles that perfuse different organs may vary in their contractile response to various stimuli. Differences may even exist between vascular smooth muscle cells at two different points along one arterial pathway.

The phenotype of smooth muscle within a given organ may change with shifting demands. The uterus, for exam-

TABLE 9–3

SUMMARY OF COMPARISONS BETWEEN MUSCLE TYPES			
	SKELETAL	**CARDIAC**	**SMOOTH**
Mechanism of excitation	Neuromuscular transmission	Pacemaker potentials Electrotonic depolarization via gap junctions	Synaptic transmission Hormone-activated receptors Electrical coupling Pacemaker potentials
Electrical activity of muscle cell	Action potential spikes	Action potential plateaus	Action potential spikes, plateaus Graded membrane potential changes Slow waves
Ca^{2+} sensor	Troponin	Troponin	Calmodulin
Excitation-contraction coupling	L-type Ca^{2+} channel (DHP receptor) in T-tubule membrane coupling to Ca^{2+} release channel (ryanodine receptor) in SR	Ca^{2+} entry via L-type Ca^{2+} channel (DHP receptor) triggers Ca^{2+}-induced Ca^{2+} release from SR	Ca^{2+} entry via voltage-gated Ca^{2+} channels Ca^{2+}- and IP_3-mediated Ca^{2+} release from SR Ca^{2+} entry through store-operated Ca^{2+} channels
Terminates contraction	Breakdown of ACh by acetylcholinesterase	Action potential repolarization	Myosin light chain phosphatase
Twitch duration	20–200 msec	200–400 msec	200 msec—sustained
Regulation of force	Frequency and multifiber summation	Regulation of calcium entry	Balance between MLCK phosphorylation and dephosphorylation Latch state
Metabolism	Oxidative, glycolytic	Oxidative	Oxidative

ACh, acetylcholine; DHP, dihydropyridine; IP_3, inositol 1,4,5-triphosphate receptor; MLCK, myosin light chain kinase; SR, sarcoplasmic reticulum.

ple, is composed of smooth muscle—the myometrium—that undergoes remarkable transformation during gestation as it prepares for parturition (see Chapter 55). In addition to hypertrophy, greater coupling develops between smooth muscle cells through the increased formation of gap junctions. The cells also undergo changes in their expression of contractile protein isoforms. Changes in the expression of ion channels and hormone receptors facilitate rhythmic electrical activity. This activity is coordinated across the myometrium by propagation of action potentials and increases in $[Ca^{2+}]_i$ through the gap junctions. These rhythmic, coordinated contractions develop spontaneously, but they are strongly influenced by the hormone oxytocin, levels of which increase just before and during labor and just after parturition.

These differences in smooth muscle function among various tissues or even over the lifetime of a single cell probably reflect differences in protein composition. Indeed, in comparison to striated muscle, smooth muscle cells express a wider variety of isoforms of contractile and regulatory proteins (see Table 9–1). This variety is a result of both multiple genes and alternative splicing (p. 139). This richness in diversity is likely to have important consequences for smooth muscle cell function, although the precise relationship between the structure and function of these protein isoforms is not yet clear.

Smooth Muscle Cells Express a Wide Variety of Neurotransmitter and Hormone Receptors

Perhaps one of the most impressive sources of diversity among smooth muscle relates to differences in response to neurotransmitters, environmental factors, and circulating hormones. Smooth muscle cells differ widely with respect to the types of cell-surface receptors that mediate the effects of these various mediators. In general, smooth muscle cells each express a variety of such receptors, and receptor stimulation may lead to either contraction or relaxation. Many substances act through different receptor subtypes in different cells, and these receptor subtypes may act through different mechanisms. For example, whereas some neurotransmitter/hormone receptors may be ligand-gated ion channels, others act through heterotri-

meric G proteins that either act directly on targets or act through intracellular second messengers such as cAMP, cGMP, or IP_3 and DAG.

The list of neurotransmitters, hormones, and environmental factors regulating the function of vascular smooth muscle cells alone is vast (see Chapter 22). A few of these vasoactive substances include epinephrine, norepinephrine, serotonin, angiotensin, vasopressin, neuropeptide Y, nitric oxide, endothelin, and oxygen. Identical stimuli, however, may result in remarkably different physiologic responses by smooth muscle in different locations. For example, systemic arterial smooth muscle cells relax when the oxygen concentration around them decreases, whereas pulmonary arterial smooth muscle contracts when local oxygen decreases (p. 699).

See Table 9–3 for a comparison of muscle types.

REFERENCES

Books and Reviews

Farah CS, Reinach FC: The troponin complex and regulation of muscle contraction. FASEB J 9:755–767, 1995.

Franzini-Armstrong C, Protasi F: Ryanodine receptors of striated muscles: A complex channel capable of multiple interactions. Physiol Rev 77:699–729, 1997.

Holda J, Klishin A, Sedova M, et al: Capacitative calcium entry. News Physiol Sci 13:157–163, 1998.

Horowitz A, Menice CB, Laporte R, Morgan KG: Mechanisms of smooth muscle contraction. Physiol Rev 76:967–1003, 1996.

Parekh AB, Penner R: Store depletion and calcium influx. Physiol Rev 77:901–930, 1997.

Striggow F, Ehrlich BE: Ligand-gated calcium channels inside and out. Curr Opin Cell Biol 8:490–495, 1996.

Journal Articles

Cannell MB, Cheng H, Lederer WJ: The control of calcium release in heart muscle. Science 268:1045–1049, 1995.

Finer JT, Simmons RM, Spudich JA: Single myosin molecule mechanics: Piconewton forces and nanometer steps. Nature 368:113–119, 1994.

Gordon AM, Huxley AF, Julian FJ: The variation in isometric tension with sarcomere length in vertebrate muscle. J Physiol 184:170–192, 1966.

Mickelson JR, Louis CF: Malignant hyperthermia: Excitation-contraction coupling, Ca^{2+} release channel, and cell Ca^{2+} regulation defects. Physiol Rev 76:537–592, 1996.

Cellular Physiology of the Nervous System

CHAPTER 10

Organization of the Nervous System

Bruce R. Ransom

The human brain is the most complex tissue in the body. It mediates behavior ranging from simple movements and sensory perception to learning and memory. It is the organ of the mind. Many of the brain's functions are poorly understood. In fact, the most prominent function of the human brain, its capacity to think, is hardly understood at all. Our lack of knowledge about fundamental aspects of brain function stands in marked contrast to the level of comprehension that we have about the primary functions of other organ systems such as the heart, lungs, or kidneys. Nevertheless, tremendous strides have been made in the past few decades. While philosophers ponder the paradox of a person thinking about thinking, physiologists are trying to learn about learning.

In this part of the book, we present the physiology of the nervous system in a manner that is intended to be complementary to texts on neurobiology and neuroanatomy. In this chapter, we review the basic cellular, developmental, and gross anatomy of the nervous system. Chapters 11 through 14 focus on the broad physiological principles that underlie how the brain's cellular elements operate. The second major goal of this section is to provide more detailed information on those parts of the nervous system that play key roles in the physiology of other systems in the body. Thus, in Chapter 15, we discuss the autonomic nervous system (ANS), which controls "viscera" such as the heart, lungs, and gastrointestinal tract. Finally, in Chapter 16, we discuss the fluid environment of the neurons in the brain and how this environment interacts with the rest of the extracellular fluid of the body.

The Nervous System Can Be Divided Into Central, Peripheral, and Autonomic Nervous Systems

The manner in which the nervous system is subdivided is somewhat arbitrary. All elements of the nervous system work closely together in a way that has no clear boundaries. Nevertheless, the traditional definitions of the subdivisions provide a useful framework for talking about the brain and its connections and are important if only for that reason.

The **central nervous system** (CNS) consists of the brain and spinal cord (Table 10–1). It is covered by three "membranes"—the meninges. The outer membrane is the dura mater; the middle is the arachnoid; and the delicate inner membrane is called the pia mater. Within the CNS, some neurons that share similar functions are grouped into aggregations called **nuclei**.

TABLE 10-1

SUBDIVISIONS OF THE NERVOUS SYSTEM		
SUBDIVISION	**COMPONENTS**	**SPECIAL FEATURES**
Central	Brain (including CN II and retina) and spinal cord	Oligodendrocytes provide myelin Axons cannot regenerate
Peripheral	Peripheral ganglia (including cell bodies); sensory receptors; peripheral portions of spinal and cranial nerves (except CN II), both afferent and efferent	Schwann cells provide myelin Axons can regenerate
Autonomic	Selected portions of the CNS and PNS	Functionally distinct system

CN, cranial nerve; CNS, central nervous system; PNS, peripheral nervous system.

The **peripheral nervous system** (PNS) consists of those parts of the nervous system that lie outside the dura mater (see Table 10–1). These elements include sensory receptors for various kinds of stimuli, the peripheral portions of spinal and cranial nerves, as well as all the peripheral portions of the ANS (see the next paragraph). The **sensory** nerves that carry messages from the periphery to the CNS are termed **afferent nerves** (Latin, *ad + ferens*, or carrying toward). Conversely, the peripheral **motor** nerves that carry messages from the CNS to peripheral tissues are called **efferent nerves** (Latin, *ex + ferens*, or carrying away). **Peripheral ganglia** are groups of nerve cells concentrated into small knots or clumps that are located outside the CNS.

The **autonomic nervous system** is that portion of the nervous system that regulates and controls visceral functions, including heart rate, blood pressure, digestion, temperature regulation, and reproductive function. Although the ANS is a functionally distinct system, it is anatomically composed of parts of the CNS and PNS (see Table 10–1). The ANS was originally defined to include only efferent (i.e., motor) neurons that send messages from the CNS to peripheral tissues, but this practice is no longer suitable. Visceral control is achieved by reflex arcs that consist of visceral afferent (i.e., sensory) neurons that send messages from the periphery to the CNS, control centers in the CNS that receive this input, and visceral motor output. Moreover, visceral afferent fibers typically travel together with visceral efferent fibers.

Each Area of the Nervous System Has Unique Nerve Cells and a Different Function

Nervous tissue is composed of neurons and neuroglial cells. **Neurons** vary greatly in their morphology throughout the nervous system, but they all share certain features that tailor them for the unique purpose of electrical communication (see Chapter 11). Neuroglial cells, often simply called **glia**, are not primary signalling cells and have variable structures that are suited for their diverse functions (see Chapter 16).

The human brain contains about 10^{11} neurons and 10 times as many glial cells. Each of these neurons may interact with thousands of other neurons, which helps explain the awesome complexity of the nervous system.

No evidence suggests that the human brain contains receptors, ion channels, or cells that are unique to humans and not seen in other mammals. The unparalleled capabilities of the human brain are presumed to result from its unique patterns of connectivity and its large size.

The brain's diverse functions are the result of tremendous regional specialization. Different brain areas are composed of neurons that have special shapes, physiological properties, and connections. One part of the brain, therefore, cannot substitute functionally for another part that has failed. Any compensation of neural function by a patient with a brain lesion—e.g., a stroke—reflects enhancement of existing circuits or recruitment of latent circuits. A corollary is that damage to a specific part of the brain causes predictable symptoms that can enable a clinician to establish the anatomic location of the problem, a key step in diagnosing neurologic diseases.

CELLS OF THE NERVOUS SYSTEM

The "Neuron Doctrine" First Asserted That the Nervous System Is Composed of Many Individual Signaling Units—The Neurons

In 1838, Schleiden and Schwann proposed that the nucleated cell is the fundamental unit of structure and function in both plants and animals. They reached this conclusion by microscopic observation of plant and animal tissues that had been stained to reveal their cellular composition. However, the brain proved to be more difficult to stain than other tissues, and until 1885, when Camillo Golgi introduced his silver impregnation method—"the black reaction"—there was no clear indication that the brain was composed of individual cells. The histologist Santiago Ramon y Cajal worked relentlessly with the silver-staining method and eventually concluded that not only was nervous tissue composed of individual cells, but the anatomy of these cells also conferred a functional polarization to the passage of nervous signals; the tapering branches near the cell body were the receptive end of the cell, and the long-axis cylinder conveyed signals away from the cell. In the absence of any reliable physiological evidence, Cajal was nevertheless able to correctly anticipate how complex cell aggregates in the brain would communicate with each other.

The pathologist Heinrich von Waldeyer referred to the individual cells in the brain as "neurons." He wrote a monograph in 1891 that assembled the evidence in favor of the cellular composition of nervous tissue, a theory that became known as the "neuron doctrine." It is ironic that Golgi, whose staining technique made these advances possible, never accepted the neuron doctrine, and he argued vehemently against it when he received his Nobel Prize along with Cajal in 1906. The ultimate proof of the neuron doctrine was established by electron microscopic observations that definitively demonstrated that neurons are entirely separate from one another, even though their processes come into very close contact.

Nerve Cells Have Four Specialized Regions: The Cell Body, the Dendrites, the Axon, and the Presynaptic Terminals

Neurons are specialized for sending and receiving signals, a purpose reflected in their unique shapes and physiological adaptations. The structure of a typical neuron can generally be divided into four distinct domains: (1) the cell body, also called the soma or perikaryon; (2) the dendrites; (3) the axon; and (4) the presynaptic terminals (Fig. 10–1).

CELL BODY. As the name *perikaryon* implies, the cell body is the portion of the cell surrounding the nucleus. It contains much of the cell's complement of endoplasmic reticular membranes, as well as the Golgi complex. The cell body appears to be responsible for many of the neuronal housekeeping functions, including the synthesis and processing of proteins.

DENDRITES. Dendrites are tapering processes of variable complexity that arise from the cell body. The dendrites and cell body are the main areas for receiving information. Thus, their membranes are endowed with **receptors** that bind and respond to the neurotransmitters released by neighboring cells. The chemical message is translated by membrane receptors into an electrical or a biochemical event that influences the state of excitability of the receiving neuron. The cytoplasm of the dendrites contains dense networks of microtubules, as well as extensions of the endoplasmic reticulum.

THE AXON. Perhaps the most remarkable feature of the neuron, the axon, like the dendrites, is a projection that arises from the cell body. Its point of origin is a tapered region known as the **axon hillock**. Just distal to the cone-shaped hillock is an untapered, unmyelinated region known as the **initial segment**. This latter area is also called the "spike-initiation zone" because it is where an action potential (p. 172) normally arises as the result of the electrical events that have occurred in the cell body and dendrites. In contrast to the dendrites, the axon is thin, does not taper, and can extend for more than a meter. Because of its length, the typical axon contains much more cytoplasm than does the cell body, up to 1000 times as much. The neuron uses special metabolic mechanisms to sustain this unique structural component. The cytoplasm of the axon, the axoplasm, is packed with parallel arrays of microtubules and microfilaments that provide structural stability and a means to rapidly convey materials back and forth between the cell body and the axon terminus.

Axons are the message-sending portion of the neuron.

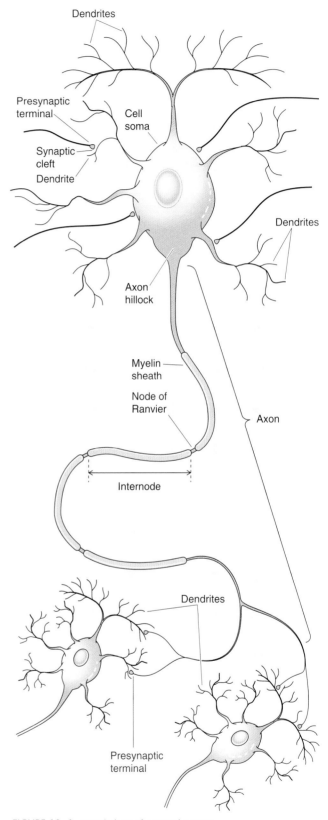

FIGURE 10–1. Morphology of a typical neuron.

The axon carries the neuron's signal, the action potential, to a specific target such as another neuron or a muscle. Some axons have a special electrical insulation, called **myelin**, that consists of the coiled cell membranes of glial cells that wrap themselves around the nerve axon (p. 417). If the axon is *not* covered with myelin, the action potential travels down the axon by continuous propagation. On the other hand, if the axon is myelinated, the action potential jumps from one node of Ranvier (the space between adjacent myelin segments) to another in a process called saltatory conduction (p. 200). This adaptation greatly speeds impulse conduction.

PRESYNAPTIC TERMINALS. At its target, the axon terminates in multiple endings—the presynaptic terminals— usually designed for rapid conversion of the neuron's electrical signal into a chemical signal. When the action potential reaches the presynaptic terminal, it causes the release of chemical signalling molecules in a complex process called synaptic transmission (see Chapters 8 and 12).

The junction formed between the presynaptic terminal and its target is called a chemical synapse. "**Synapse**" is derived from the Greek for "joining together" or "junction"; this word and concept were introduced in 1897 by the neurophysiologist Charles Sherrington. A synapse comprises the presynaptic terminal, the membrane of the target cell ("postsynaptic membrane"), and the space between the two ("synaptic cleft"). The width of the synaptic cleft is determined and maintained by components of the extracellular matrix. In synapses between two neurons, the presynaptic terminals primarily contact dendrites and the cell body. The area of the postsynaptic membrane is frequently amplified to increase the surface that is available for receptors. This amplification can occur either through infolding of the plasma membrane or through the formation of small projections called **dendritic spines**.

The molecules released by the presynaptic terminals diffuse across the synaptic cleft and bind to receptors on the postsynaptic membrane. The receptors then convert the chemical signal of the transmitter molecules—either directly or indirectly—back into an electrical signal.

In many ways, neurons can be thought of as highly specialized *endocrine cells*. They package and store hormones and hormone-like molecules, which they release rapidly into the extracellular space by exocytosis (p. 36) in response to an external stimulus, in this case a nerve action potential. However, instead of entering the bloodstream to exert *systemic* effects, the substances secreted by neurons act over the very short distance of a synapse to communicate *locally* with a single neighboring cell (p. 88).

In a different sense, neurons can be thought of as *polarized cells* with some of the properties of epithelial cells. Like epithelial cells, neurons have different populations of membrane proteins at each of the distinct domains of the neuronal plasma membrane, an arrangement that reflects the individual physiological responsibilities of these domains. Thus, the design of the nervous system permits information transfer across synapses in a selective and coordinated way that serves the needs of the organism and summates to produce complex behavior.

The Cytoskeleton Helps Compartmentalize the Neuron and Also Provides the Tracks Along Which Material Travels Between Different Parts of the Neuron

Neurons are very compartmentalized in both structure and function. *Dendrites* are tapered, have limited length, and contain neurotransmitter receptor proteins in their membranes. *Axons* can be very long and have a high density of Na^+ channels. *Dendrites* and the *cell body* contain mRNA, ribosomes, and a Golgi apparatus. These structures are absent in axons.

How does this compartmentalization come about? The answer is not certain, but **microtubule-associated proteins** (MAPs) appear to play an important role. (Note that these MAPs are totally unrelated to the mitogen-activated protein [MAP] kinase introduced on p. 134.) Two major classes of MAPs are found in the brain: high-molecular-weight proteins such as MAP-1 and MAP-2 and lower-molecular-weight tau proteins. Both classes of MAPs associate with microtubules and help link them to other cell components. MAP-2 is found only in cell bodies and dendrites. Dephosphorylated tau proteins are confined entirely to axons. In cultured neurons, suppressing the expression of tau protein prevents formation of the axon without altering formation of the dendrites.

Microtubules may also help create the remarkable morphologic and functional divisions in neurons. In axons, microtubules assemble with their plus ends pointed away from the cell body; this orientation polarizes the flow of material into and out of the axon. The cytoskeletal "order" provided in part by the microtubules and the MAPs helps define what should or should not be in the axonal cytoplasm. In dendrites, the microtubules do not have a consistent orientation, which gives the dendrites a greater structural and functional similarity to the cell body.

The neuron cell body is the main manufacturing site for the membrane proteins and membranous organelles that are necessary for the structural integrity and function of its processes. Axons have no protein synthetic ability, whereas dendrites have some free ribosomes and may be able to engage in limited protein production. The transport of proteins from the cell body all the way to the end of long axons is a challenging task. The neuron also has a second task: moving various material in the opposite direction, from presynaptic terminals at the end of the axon to the cell body. The neuron solves these problems by using two distinct mechanisms for moving material to the presynaptic terminals in an "anterograde" direction and a third mechanism for transport in the opposite or "retrograde" direction (Table 10–2).

FAST AXOPLASMIC TRANSPORT. Vesicles carrying newly synthesized membrane proteins and lipids that are destined for insertion in the axonal membrane must travel down the length of the axon before delivering their cargo. Similarly, the peptide and protein contents of "dense-core secretory granules," which are found in the presynaptic axonal terminals, are synthesized as standard "secretory proteins" (p. 36). Thus, they are cotranslationally inserted across the membranes of the rough endoplasmic reticulum and subsequently processed in the cisternae of

TABLE 10–2

FEATURES OF AXOPLASMIC TRANSPORT

TRANSPORT TYPE	SPEED (mm/day)	MECHANISM	MATERIAL TRANSPORTED
Fast anterograde	~400	Saltatory movement along microtubules via the motor molecule kinesin (ATP dependent)	Mitochondria Vesicles containing peptide and other neurotransmitters, some degradative enzymes
Fast retrograde	~1–5	Saltatory movement along microtubules via the motor molecule dynein (ATP dependent)	Degraded vesicular membrane Absorbed exogenous material (toxins, viruses, growth factors)
Slow anterograde	~200–300	Not clear; possibly via molecular motors	Cytoskeletal elements (e.g., neurofilament and microtubule subunits) Soluble proteins of intermediary metabolism Actin

ATP, adenosine triphosphate.

the Golgi complex. They are shipped to the axon in the lumens of Golgi-derived carrier vesicles. If the flow of these membrane vesicles to the distant axon terminus were left to the whims of simple diffusion, their delivery would be far too slow to be of practical use. It could take months for needed proteins to diffuse to the end of an axon, and the presynaptic terminals are high-volume consumers of these molecules. To overcome this difficulty, neurons exploit a rapid, pony express–style system of conveyance known as fast axoplasmic transport (see Table 10–2). Protein-containing vesicles move along **microtubules** (p. 25) with the help of a microtubule-dependent motor protein called **kinesin** (Fig. 10–2A). The kinesin motor (p. 26) is itself an adenosine triphosphatase (ATPase) that produces vectorial movement of its payload along the microtubule. This system can move vesicles down the axon at rates of up to 1 m/day. Kinesins always move toward the plus end of microtubules (i.e., away from the cell body), and transport function is lost if the microtubules are disrupted. The nervous system has many forms of kinesin that recognize and transport different cargo. Other membranous organelles, such as mitochondria, are also shipped to the axon by this mechanism.

FAST RETROGRADE TRANSPORT. Axons move material back toward the cell body with a different motor protein called **dynein** (see Fig. 10–2B). Like kinesin, dynein (p. 26) also moves along microtubule tracks and is an ATPase (see Table 10–2). However, dynein moves along microtubules in the opposite direction of kinesin (see Fig. 10–2C). It is not known how the motor proteins recognize and attach to their intended payloads. The loss of ATP production, as occurs with blockade of oxidative metabolism, causes fast axonal transport in both the anterograde and retrograde directions to fail.

SLOW AXOPLASMIC TRANSPORT. Axons also have a need for cytoskeletal proteins and soluble proteins that are used as enzymes for intermediary metabolism. These proteins are delivered by a slow anterograde axoplasmic transport mechanism that moves material at a mere 1 to 5 mm/day—the nervous system's equivalent of snail mail. The cytoskeletal proteins that travel by this route are neurofilament and microtubule subunits. The mechanism of slow axoplasmic transport is not understood, but motor molecules may be involved.

Neurons Can Be Classified on the Basis of Their Axonal Projection, Their Dendritic Geometry, and the Number of Processes Emanating from the Cell Body

The trillions of nerve cells in the CNS have great structural diversity. Typically, neurons are classified on the basis of where their axons go (i.e., where they "project"), the geometry of their dendrites, and the number of processes that emanate from the cell body (Fig. 10–3). The real significance of these schemes is that they have functional implications.

AXONAL PROJECTION. Neurons with long axons that connect with other parts of the nervous system are called **projection neurons** (or principal neurons or Golgi type I cells). Each of these cells has a clearly defined axon that arises from the axon hillock located on the cell body or proximal dendrite and extends away from the cell body, sometimes for remarkable distances. A motor neuron in the cortex, for example, may project to the distal part of the spinal cord, a stretch of nearly a meter. All the other processes that a projection neuron has are dendrites. The other type of neuron that is defined in this way has all of its processes confined to one region of the brain. These neurons are called **interneurons** (or intrinsic neurons or Golgi type II cells). Some of these cells have very short axons, whereas others seem to lack a conventional axon altogether and may be referred to as *anaxonal*. The anax-

A ANTEROGRADE MOVEMENT

Proteins synthesized in the "secretory pathway" are packaged by budding off in membrane-enclosed vesicles from the Golgi.

The vesicles and mitochondria are carried down the axon on microtubule "tracks" by kinesin motors that are energized by ATP.

B RETROGRADE MOVEMENT

Vesicles now move in reverse, carried by dynein motors, which also split ATP and move along microtubule "tracks."

C MICROTUBULE

FIGURE 10–2. Fast axoplasmic transport.

onal neuron in the retina is called an amacrine (from the Greek for "no large/long fiber") cell.

DENDRITIC GEOMETRY. A roughly pyramid-shaped set of dendritic branches characterizes **pyramidal cells**, whereas a radial pattern of dendritic branches defines **stellate cells**. This classification often includes mention of the presence or absence of dendritic spines, those small, protuberant projections that are sites for synaptic contact. All

pyramidal cells appear to have spines, but stellate cells may have them ("spiny") or not ("aspiny").

NUMBER OF PROCESSES. Neurons can also be classified by the number of processes that extend from their cell bodies. The dorsal root ganglion cell is the classic **unipolar** neuron. The naming of the processes of primary sensory neurons, like the dorsal root ganglion cell, is often ambiguous. The process that extends into the CNS from

Basis for classification	Example	Functional implication	Structure
1. Axonal projection			
Goes to a distant brain area	Projection neuron or Principal neuron or Golgi type I cell (cortical motor neuron)	Affects different brain areas	Dorsal root ganglion cell
Stays in a local brain area	Intrinsic neuron or Interneuron or Golgi type II cell (cortical inhibitory neuron)	Affects only nearby neurons	Retinal bipolar cell
2. Dendritic pattern			Pyramidal cell
Pyramid-shaped spread of dendrites	Pyramidal cell (hippocampal pyramidal neuron)	Large area for receiving synaptic input; determines the pattern of incoming axons that can interact with the cell (i.e., pyramid-shaped)	
Radial-shaped spread of dendrites	Stellate cell (cortical stellate cell)	Large area for receiving synaptic input; determines pattern of incoming axons that can interact with the cell (i.e., star-shaped)	Stellate cell Spine
3. Number of processes			
One process exits the cell body	Unipolar neuron (dorsal root ganglion cell)	Small area for receiving synaptic input: highly specialized function	Unipolar Soma
Two processes exit the cell body	Bipolar neuron (retinal bipolar cell)	Small area for receiving synaptic input: highly specialized function	Bipolar
Many processes exit the cell body	Multipolar neuron (spinal motor neuron)	Large area for receiving synaptic input; determines the pattern of incoming axons that can interact with the cell	Multipolar

FIGURE 10–3. Classification of neurons based on their structure.

this unipolar neuron is easily recognized as an "axon" because it carries information *away* from the cell body. On the other hand, the process that extends to sensory receptors in the skin and elsewhere is less easily defined. It is a typical "axon" in the sense that it can conduct an action potential, has myelin, and is characterized by an axonal cytoskeleton. However, it conveys information *toward* the cell body, which is usually the function of a "dendrite." **Bipolar** neurons, such as the retinal bipolar cell, have two processes extending from opposite sides of the cell body. Most neurons in the brain are **multipolar**. Cells with many dendritic processes are designed to receive large numbers of synapses.

Most neurons in the brain can be categorized by two or more of these schemes. For example, the typical motor neuron in the cortex is a "multipolar," "pyramidal," "projection" neuron. Similarly, a retinal bipolar cell is both an "interneuron" and a "bipolar" cell.

Glial Cells Provide a Physiological Environment for Neurons

Glial cells are defined in part by what they lack: axons, action potentials, and synaptic potentials. They are much more numerous than neurons and are diverse in structure and function. The main types of CNS glial cells are oligodendrocytes, astrocytes, and microglial cells. In the PNS, the main types of glial cells are satellite cells in autonomic and sensory ganglia, Schwann cells, and enteric glial cells. Glial function is discussed in Chapter 16. Oligodendrocytes form the myelin sheaths of CNS axons, and Schwann cells myelinate peripheral nerves. Glial cells are involved in nearly every function of the brain and are far more than simply "nerve glue," a literal translation of the name neuroglia (from the Greek *neuron* for nerve and *glia* for glue).

In depictions of the nervous system, the presence of glial cells is sometimes minimized or neglected altogether. Glia fills in almost all the space around neurons, with a narrow extracellular space left between neurons and glial cells that has an average width of only approximately 0.02 μm. The composition of the extracellular fluid, which has a major impact on brain function, as well as the function of glial cells, is taken up in detail in Chapter 16.

DEVELOPMENT OF NEURONS AND GLIAL CELLS

Neurons Differentiate from the Neuroectoderm

Although the embryology of the nervous system may seem like an odd place to begin studying the physiology of the brain, there are a number of reasons to start here. Knowledge of the embryology of the nervous system greatly facilitates comprehension of its complex organization. Events in the development of the nervous system highlight how different neuronal cell types evolve from a single type of precursor cell and how these neurons establish astonishingly specific connections. Finally, the

characteristics of brain cell proliferation, as well as the growth of neuronal processes during development, provide insight into the consequences of brain injury.

The vertebrate embryo consists of three primitive tissue layers at the stage of gastrulation: the endoderm, mesoderm, and ectoderm (Fig. 10–4). The entire nervous system arises from ectoderm, which also gives rise to the skin. Underlying the ectoderm is a specialized cord of mesodermal cells called the notochord. Cells of the notochord somehow direct or "induce" the overlying ectoderm, or **neuroectoderm**, to form the neural tube in a complex process called neurulation.

The first step in neurulation is formation of the neural plate at about the beginning of the third fetal week. Initially, the neural plate is only a single layer of neuroectoderm cells. Rapid proliferation of these cells, especially at the lateral margins, creates a neural groove bordered by neural folds. Continued cell division enlarges the neural folds, and they eventually fuse dorsally to form the neural tube. The neural tube is open at both ends, the anterior and posterior neuropores. The neural tube ultimately gives rise to the brain and spinal cord. The lumen of the neural tube, the neural canal, becomes the four **ventricles** of the brain and the central canal of the spinal cord. Congenital malformations of the brain commonly arise from developmental defects in the neural tube.

The **neural crest** derives from symmetric lateral portions of the neural plate. Neural crest cells migrate to sites in the body where they form the vast majority of the PNS and most of the peripheral cells of the ANS, including the sympathetic ganglia and the chromaffin cells of the adrenal medulla. On the sensory side, these neural crest derivatives include unipolar neurons whose cell bodies are in the dorsal root ganglia, as well as the equivalent sensory cells of cranial nerves V, VII, IX, and X. Neural crest cells also give rise to several non-neuronal structures, including Schwann cells, satellite glial cells in spinal and cranial ganglia, and pigment cells of the skin.

The human brain begins to exhibit some regional specialization around the fourth gestational week (Fig. 10–6A, B). By then, it is possible to discern an anterior part called the **prosencephalon**, a midsection called the **mesencephalon**, and a posterior part called the **rhombencephalon**. Rapid brain growth ensues, and important new regions emerge in just another week (see Fig. 10–6C). Distinct regions called *brain vesicles*, which are destined to become separate parts of the adult brain are set apart as swellings in the rostral-caudal plane (see Fig. 10–6B, C). The prosencephalon is now divisible into the **telencephalon**, which will give rise to the basal ganglia and cerebral cortex, and the **diencephalon**, which becomes the thalamus, subthalamus, hypothalamus, and neurohypophysis (the posterior or neural portion of the pituitary). Similarly, the rhombencephalon can now be divided into the **metencephalon**, which will give rise to the pons and cerebellum, and the **myelencephalon**, which becomes the medulla. Robust development of the cerebral cortex becomes apparent in mammals, especially humans, after the seventh week. This structure gradually expands so that it enwraps the rostral structures.

As the neural tube thickens with cell proliferation, a groove called the **sulcus limitans** forms on the inner,

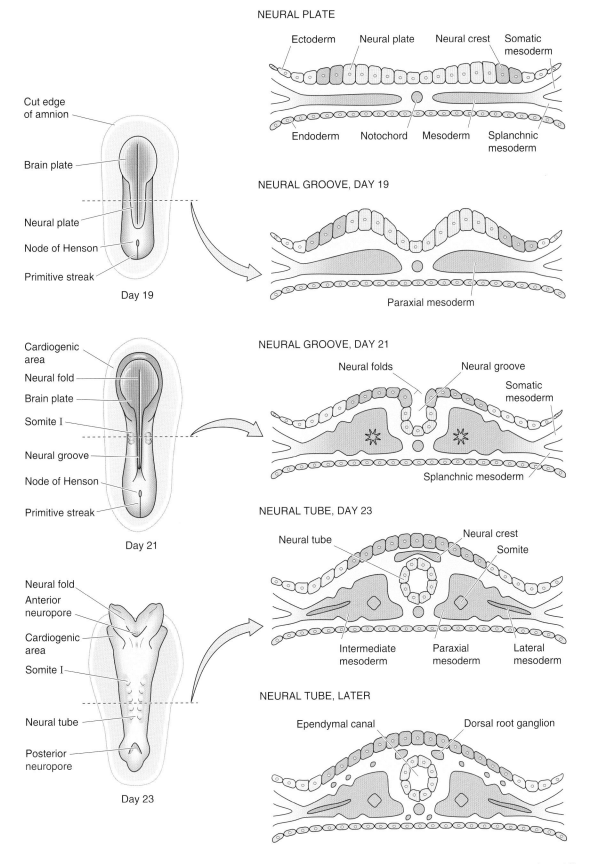

NEURAL PLATE

Ectoderm   Neural plate   Neural crest   Somatic mesoderm

Endoderm   Notochord   Mesoderm   Splanchnic mesoderm

NEURAL GROOVE, DAY 19

Paraxial mesoderm

NEURAL GROOVE, DAY 21

Neural folds   Neural groove   Somatic mesoderm

Splanchnic mesoderm

NEURAL TUBE, DAY 23

Neural tube   Neural crest   Somite

Intermediate mesoderm   Paraxial mesoderm   Lateral mesoderm

NEURAL TUBE, LATER

Ependymal canal   Dorsal root ganglion

Cut edge of amnion

Brain plate

Neural plate

Node of Henson

Primitive streak

Day 19

Cardiogenic area

Neural fold

Brain plate

Somite I

Neural groove

Node of Henson

Primitive streak

Day 21

Neural fold

Anterior neuropore

Cardiogenic area

Somite I

Neural tube

Posterior neuropore

Day 23

FIGURE 10–4. Development of the nervous system. The *left column* provides a dorsal view of the developing nervous system at three different time points. The *right column* shows cross sections of the dorsal portion of the embryo at five different stages, three of which correspond to the dorsal views shown at the left.

ABNORMALITIES OF NEURAL TUBE CLOSURE

Closure of the neural tube in humans normally occurs between 26 and 28 days of gestation. A disturbance in this process results in a midline congenital abnormality called a **dysraphism** (from the Greek *dys,* abnormal, + *raphe,* seam or suture). The defect can be so devastating that it is incompatible with life or, alternatively, have so little consequence that it goes unnoticed throughout life. These midline embryonic abnormalities also involve the primitive mesoderm and ectoderm associated with the neural tube. Therefore, the vertebral bodies or skull (derived from mesoderm) and the overlying skin (derived from ectoderm) may be affected along with the nervous system.

The most serious neural tube defect is **anencephaly,** in which the cerebral hemispheres are absent and the rest of the brain is severely malformed. Overlying malformations of the skull, brain coverings, and scalp are present (Table 10–3). Affected fetuses are often spontaneously aborted.

The most common dysraphisms affect formation of the spinal vertebral bodies and are called **spina bifida.** The problem may be very slight and cause only a minor problem in closure of the vertebral arch, called spina bifida occulta (Fig. 10–5*A*). This malformation affects about 10% of the population, usually at the fifth lumbar or first sacral vertebra, and generally causes no significant sequelae. If the dura and arachnoid membranes herniate (i.e., protrude) through the vertebral defect, the malformation is called spina bifida cystica (Fig. 10–5*B*); if the spinal cord also herniates through the defect, it is called myelomeningocele (Fig. 10–5*C*). These latter problems are often more significant and may cause severe neurologic disability.

Genetic and nongenetic factors can cause dysraphism. Some severe forms of this condition appear to be inherited, although the genetic pattern suggests that multiple genes are involved. Nongenetic factors may also play a role, as in the case of folic acid deficiency. Mothers taking folic acid (p. 1182) before and during the periconceptional period have a decreased risk of having a fetus with a neural tube closure defect. Current medical recommendations are that women *contemplating* becoming pregnant receive folic acid supplementation, and it has been suggested that bread products should be enriched with folic acid to ensure that women will have the protective advantage of this vitamin if they become pregnant. Other factors that increase the risk of these defects are maternal heat exposure (e.g., from a hot tub) and certain drugs such as the anticonvulsant valproate. Neural tube disorders can be detected during pregnancy by measuring the concentration of α-fetoprotein in maternal blood or amniotic fluid. α-Fetoprotein is synthesized by the fetal liver and, for unclear reasons, increases in concentration abnormally with failure of neural tube closure.

A   SPINA BIFIDA OCCULTA

B   SPINA BIFIDA CYSTICA OR MENINGOCELE

C   MYELOMENINGOCELE

FIGURE 10–5. Variations of spina bifida. *A,* An incomplete vertebral arch with no herniation. *B,* The dura and arachnoid membranes herniate through the vertebral defect. *C,* The spinal cord and meninges herniate through the vertebral defect.

TABLE 10–3

DEFECTS OF NEURAL TUBE CLOSURE

MALFORMATION	CHARACTERISTICS
Brain Defects	
Anencephaly	Absence of the brain, with massive defects in the skull, meninges, and scalp. Frequency: 1/1000 deliveries
Cephalocele	Partial brain herniation through a skull defect (cranium bifidum)
Meningocele	Skull or spine defect associated with herniation of the meninges
Spina Bifida Defects	
Spina bifida occulta	Vertebral arch defect only
Spina bifida cystica	Herniation of the dura and arachnoid through a vertebral defect
Myelomeningocele	Herniation of the spinal cord and meninges through a vertebral defect

lateral wall of the neural tube (Fig. 10–7A). This anatomic landmark extends throughout the neural tube except in the farthest rostral area that will become the diencephalon and cortex. The sulcus limitans divides the neural tube into a ventral area called the basal plate and a dorsal area called the alar plate.

Structures that derive from the **basal plate** mediate efferent functions, and structures that arise from the **alar plate** mediate afferent and associative functions. Efferent neurons are mainly motor neurons that convey information from the CNS to outside effectors (i.e., muscles or secretory cells). In a strict sense, the only true *afferent* neurons are those that derive from neural crest cells and that convey sensory information from various kinds of receptors to the CNS. In the CNS, these afferent neurons synapse on other neurons derived from the alar plate; these alar plate neurons may be referred to as "afferent" because they receive sensory information and pass it along to other parts of the CNS. However, it is also appropriate to call these alar plate–derived neurons "associative."

The development of the spinal cord and medulla illustrates how this early anatomic division into alar and basal plates helps make sense of the final organization of these complex regions. Neurons of the alar and basal plates proliferate, migrate, and aggregate into discrete groups that have functional specificity. In the spinal cord (see Fig. 10–7B, C), the basal plate develops into the ventral horn, which contains the cell bodies of somatic motor neurons, and the intermediolateral column, which contains the cell bodies of autonomic motor neurons. Both regions contain interneurons. The alar plate in the spinal cord develops into the dorsal horn, which contains the cell bodies onto which sensory neurons synapse.

In the medulla (see Fig. 10–7D, E), as well as in the rest of the brain, aggregates of neurons are called **nuclei**. Nuclei that develop from the alar plate are generally afferent, such as the nucleus tractus solitarius, which plays an important sensory role in the ANS. Nuclei that develop from the basal plate are generally efferent, such as the dorsal motor nucleus of the vagus nerve, which plays an important *motor* role in the ANS. The choroid plexus that invaginates into the lumen of the central canal is responsible for secreting cerebrospinal fluid (p. 400).

Neurons and Glial Cells Originate from Cells in the Proliferating Germinal Matrix Near the Ventricles

The trillions of neurons and glial cells that populate the brain arise from rapidly dividing **stem cells** located near the ventricles (which derive from the neural canal) of the embryonic CNS. This area is called the germinal matrix or **ventricular zone** (Fig. 10–8A). Most of the neurons in the human brain are generated during the first 100 days of embryogenesis. Growth factors such as epidermal growth factor and platelet-derived growth factor and hormones such as growth hormone influence the rate of cell division of the **neuroepithelial germinal cells**, as these stem cells are called. The signals that direct one immature neuron to become a cortical pyramidal cell and another to become a retinal ganglion cell are not understood. It is believed, however, that neurons are probably not fully differentiated when first created and that their mature characteristics depend on their interactions with the chemical environment or other cells in a specific anatomic region of the nervous system.

The ventricular zone appears to produce separate **progenitor cells** that produce only neurons, astrocytes, or oligodendrocytes. It also appears likely that different progenitor cells provide white matter or fibrous astrocytes and gray matter or protoplasmic astrocytes. The ventricular zone does not contribute to the population of Schwann cells, which derive from neural crest tissue and myelinate peripheral nerves, nor to microglial cells, which arise from the mesoderm.

Of the various progenitor cells of the ventricular zone, the neuronal progenitor cells appear earliest and produce the entire complement of adult neurons during early embryonic life. Glial cells are created later in development. Neurons are confined to specific locations of the brain, whereas glial cells are more evenly distributed. For example, astrocytes and oligodendrocytes are found everywhere in the brain, although their characteristics may vary from region to region. Regional variability is particularly true for oligodendrocytes. In white matter, most oligodendrocytes produce myelin sheaths that enwrap nearby axons, whereas in gray matter, oligodendrocytes do not produce myelin and exist as perineuronal satellite cells.

Many more neurons are created during fetal development than are present in the adult brain. Most neurons, having migrated to a final location in the brain and differentiated, are lost through a process called programmed cell death, or **apoptosis**. Apoptosis (Greek for "falling off") is a unique form of cell death that requires protein synthesis and can be triggered by removal of specific

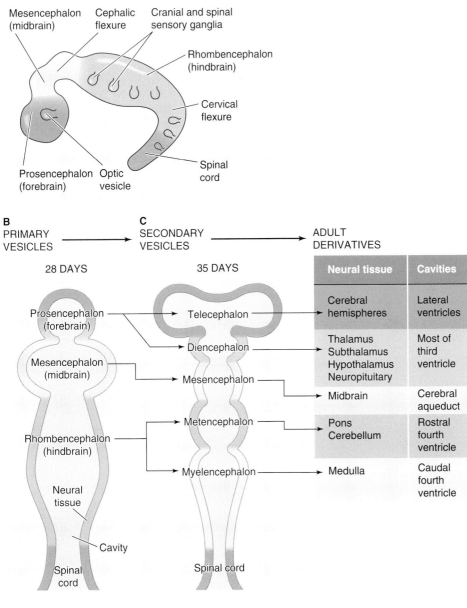

FIGURE 10–6. Embryonic development of the brain.

trophic influences, such as the action of a growth factor. In contrast to necrotic cell death, which rapidly leads to loss of cell membrane integrity after some insult causes a toxic increase in $[Ca^{2+}]_i$, apoptosis evolves more slowly. For example, in the retina, approximately 60% of the ganglion cells and thus about 60% of the retinal axons are lost in the first 2 weeks of extrauterine life as a result of programmed retinal ganglion cell death. This process of sculpting the final form of a neuronal system by discarding neurons through programmed death is a common theme in developmental biology.

The number of glial cells in different areas of the brain appears to be determined by signals from nearby neurons or axons. For example, in the optic nerve, the final number of glia in the nerve is closely determined by the number of axons. When programmed cell death is prevented by expression of the *bcl-2* gene in transgenic animals, the number of axons in the optic nerve is dramatically increased, as well as the number of astrocytes and oligodendrocytes. Thus, glial cell–to–axon ratios remain relatively constant. The axon-dependent signal or signals responsible for these adjustments in glial cell number are not known, but the process appears to operate by influencing both glial cell survival and proliferation.

Neurons Migrate to their Correct Anatomic Position in the Brain with the Help of Cell-Cell Adhesion Molecules, As Well As Radial Glial Cells

The navigation mechanisms used by migrating cells in the nervous system and elsewhere in the body are only partially understood. Proteins that promote selective cellular aggregation are called cell-cell adhesion molecules (CAMs; p. 19) and include the Ca^{2+}-dependent cadherins and

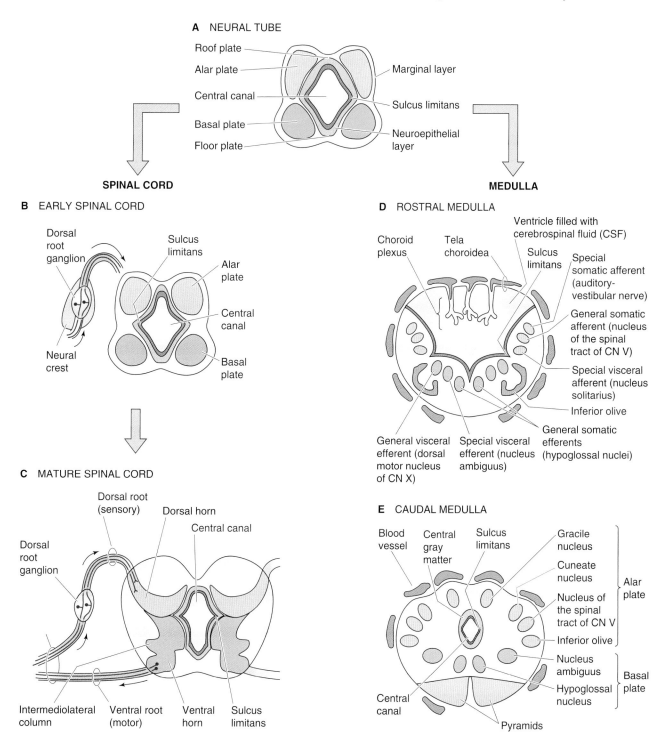

FIGURE 10–7. Development of the spinal cord and medulla. *A,* In this cross section through the neural tube, the sulcus limitans is the landmark that separates the ventral basal plate from the dorsal alar plate. The basal plate will form efferent (or motor-type) structures, whereas the alar plate will form afferent and associative (or sensory-type) functions. *B,* The true afferent neurons are those in the dorsal root ganglion, which derive from neural crest cells. These afferents will contact the neurons in the alar plate, which will become associative. *C,* The basal plate has developed into the ventral horn and intermediolateral column (motor), whereas the alar plate has developed into the dorsal horn (associative). *D,* The basal plate has developed into nuclei with motor functions, whereas the alar plate has developed into nuclei with sensory functions. The roof of the rostral medulla becomes the fourth ventricle. *E,* This cross section shows the same gross separation between motor and associative/sensory functions as is seen with the rostral medulla and the spinal cord. CN V, cranial nerve V; CN X, cranial nerve X.

DEFINITIONS OF NEURAL MODALITIES

The type of information, or neural **modality,** that a neuron transmits is classically categorized by three terms that refer to different attributes of the neuron.

1. The first category defines the *direction* of information flow.

   Afferent (sensory): Neurons that transmit information into the central nervous system (CNS) from sensory cells or sensory receptors outside the nervous system. Examples are the dorsal root ganglion cell and neurons in the sensory nucleus of the fifth cranial nerve.

   Efferent (motor): Neurons that transmit information out of the CNS to muscles or secretory cells. Examples are spinal motor neurons and motor neurons in the autonomic nervous system.

2. The second category defines the *anatomic distribution* of the information flow.

   Visceral: Neurons that transmit information to or from internal organs or regions that arise embryologically from the branchial arch (e.g., chemoreceptors of the carotid body).

   Somatic: Neurons that transmit information to or from all nonvisceral parts of the body, including skin and muscle.

3. The third category, which is somewhat arbitrary, defines the information flow on the basis of the *embryologic origin* of the structure being innervated.

   Special: Neurons that transmit information to or from a "special" subset of visceral or somatic structures. For example, in the case of **special visceral** neurons, information travels to or from structures derived from the branchial arch region of the embryo (e.g., pharyngeal muscles). In the case of **special somatic** neurons, which handle only sensory information, the neurons arise from the organs of special sense (e.g., retina, taste receptors, cochlea).

   General: Neurons that transmit information to or from visceral or somatic structures that are not in the "special" group.

Each axon in the body conveys information of only a single modality. In this classification scheme, a motor neuron in the spinal cord would be described as a "general somatic efferent" neuron. A motor neuron in the brain stem that innervates branchial arch–derived chewing muscles would be described as a "special visceral efferent" neuron. Because each of these three categories defines two options, you might expect a total of eight distinct neural modalities. In practice, however, only seven neural modalities exist. The term "special somatic efferent" neuron is not used.

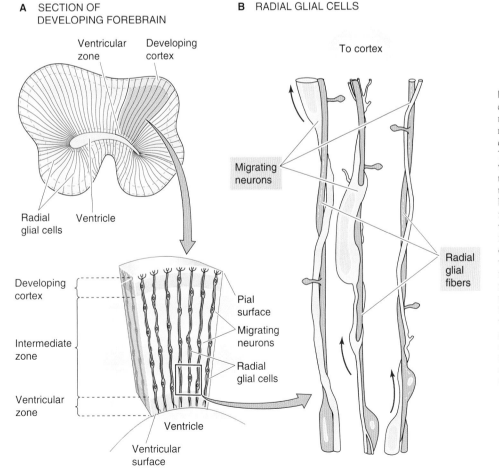

A SECTION OF DEVELOPING FOREBRAIN

Ventricular zone
Developing cortex
Radial glial cells
Ventricle

Developing cortex
Intermediate zone
Ventricular zone
Pial surface
Migrating neurons
Radial glial cells
Ventricle
Ventricular surface

B RADIAL GLIAL CELLS

To cortex
Migrating neurons
Radial glial fibers

FIGURE 10–8. Arrangement of radial glial cells and migrating neurons. *A,* The *upper portion* is a coronal section of developing occipital cerebral lobe of fetal monkey brain. The *lower portion* is a magnified view. The ventricular zone contains the germinal cells that give rise to the neurons as well as to the cell bodies of the radial glial cells. These radial glial cells extend from the ventricular surface to the pial surface, which overlies the developing cortex. *B,* This is a more magnified view and shows the cell bodies of three radial glial cells as well as their processes that extend upward toward the cortex. Also shown are three neurons migrating from the ventricular zone toward the cortex along the fibers of the radial glial cells. (Data from Rakic P: Mode of cell migration to the superficial layers of fetal monkey neocortex. J Comp Neurol 145:61–84, 1972.)

AXONAL DEGENERATION AND REGENERATION

Axons have their own mitochondria and produce the adenosine triphosphate that they need to maintain the steep ion gradients necessary for excitability and survival. In this sense, they are metabolically independent of the cell body. However, they cannot make proteins and are unable to sustain themselves if separated from the cell body (see Fig. 10–2). If an axon is cut, either in the peripheral nervous system (PNS) or the central nervous system (CNS), a characteristic series of changes take place (Fig. 10–9):

Step 1: **Degeneration of the synaptic terminals distal to the lesion.** Synaptic transmission occurring at the axon terminal fails within hours because this complex process is very dependent on material provided by axonal transport. Visible changes in the degenerating terminal are seen a few days after the lesion. The terminal retracts from the postsynaptic target.

Step 2: **Wallerian degeneration.** The lesion divides the axon into proximal and distal segments. The distal segment degenerates slowly over a period of several weeks in a process named after its discoverer, Augustus Waller. Eventually, the entire distal segment is destroyed and removed.

Step 3: **Myelin degeneration.** If the affected axon is myelinated, the myelin degenerates. The myelinating cell (i.e., the Schwann cell in the PNS and the oligodendrocyte in the CNS) usually survives this process. Schwann cells are immediately induced to divide, and they begin to synthesize

trophic factors that may be important for regeneration.

Step 4: **Scavenging of debris.** Microglia in the CNS and macrophages and Schwann cells in the PNS scavenge the debris created by the breakdown of the axon and its myelin. This step is more rapid in the PNS than the CNS.

Step 5: **Chromatolysis.** After axonal injury, most neuron cell bodies swell and undergo a characteristic rearrangement of organelles called chromatolysis. The nucleus also swells and moves to an eccentric position. The endoplasmic reticulum, normally close to the nucleus, reassembles around the periphery of the cell body. Chromatolysis is reversible if the neuron survives and is able to reestablish its distal process and contact the appropriate target.

Step 6: **Retrograde transneuronal degeneration.** Neurons that are synaptically connected to injured neurons may themselves be injured, a condition called transneuronal or trans-synaptic degeneration. If the neuron that synapses on the injured cell undergoes degeneration, it is called retrograde degeneration.

Step 7: **Anterograde transneuronal degeneration.** If a neuron that received synaptic contacts from an injured cell degenerates, it is called anterograde degeneration. The magnitude of these transneuronal effects (retrograde and anterograde degeneration) is quite variable.

Ca^{2+}-independent neural cell-adhesion molecules (N-CAMs). These molecules are expressed by developing cells in an organized, sequential manner. Cells that express the appropriate adhesion molecules have a strong tendency to adhere to one another. These "Velcro-like" molecules can assemble cells in a highly ordered fashion; experimentally, disrupted germ cells can properly reorganize themselves into a three-layered structure that replicates the normal embryonic pattern.

Another mechanism that assists migrating cells is the presence of **extracellular matrix** molecules such as laminin and fibronectin (p. 19). These molecules are selectively secreted by both neurons and astrocytes and form a kind of extracellular roadway with which migrating cells can interact. Perhaps the least well understood mechanism related to cell migration is chemotaxis, the ability of a cell to follow a chemical signal emitted from a target cell. The tips of developing axons, called growth cones, appear to follow such chemical cues as they grow toward their specific targets.

Unlike most glial cells, which appear developmentally *after* neurons, one type of glial cell is present when neurons first appear. These glial cells, a special type of astrocyte, are called **radial glia**. The cell bodies of radial glia are located in the ventricular zone, and their processes project to the outer edges of the developing brain (see Fig. 10–8A). The processes of radial glial cells create an

organized, cellular scaffolding on which neurons can migrate to their final position in the brain shortly after they appear. Migrating neurons contact radial glial cells (see Fig. 10–8B) and move along the glial processes toward their final positions in the developing cortex. Thus, the prearranged positions of these radial glial processes determine the direction of neuronal migration. The importance of the radial glial framework for assisting neuronal migration is illustrated by the failure of neurons to populate the cortex normally when the radial glial processes are interrupted by hemorrhage in the fetal brain.

Neurons Do Not Regenerate If Lost

NEURONS. Most human neurons arise in about the first 3 months of intrauterine life. After birth, neurons do not divide, and if a neuron is lost for any reason, it is not replaced, which is the main reason for the relatively limited recovery from serious brain and spinal cord injuries. It has been argued that this lack of regenerative ability is a design principle to ensure that learned behavior and memories are preserved in stable populations of neurons throughout life. A notable exception to this rule is olfactory bulb neurons, which are continually renewed throughout adult life by a population of stem cells or neuronal progenitor cells.

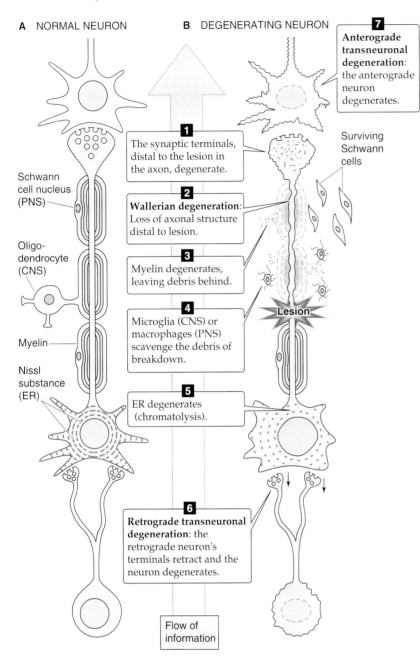

A NORMAL NEURON   **B** DEGENERATING NEURON

Schwann cell nucleus (PNS)

Oligo-dendrocyte (CNS)

Myelin

Nissl substance (ER)

7 **Anterograde transneuronal degeneration**: the anterograde neuron degenerates.

Surviving Schwann cells

1 The synaptic terminals, distal to the lesion in the axon, degenerate.

2 **Wallerian degeneration**: Loss of axonal structure distal to lesion.

3 Myelin degenerates, leaving debris behind.

Lesion

4 Microglia (CNS) or macrophages (PNS) scavenge the debris of breakdown.

5 ER degenerates (chromatolysis).

6 **Retrograde transneuronal degeneration**: the retrograde neuron's terminals retract and the neuron degenerates.

Flow of information

FIGURE 10–9. Nerve degeneration. *A*, Normal neuron. *B*, Degenerating neuron. ER, endoplasmic reticulum; PNS, peripheral nervous system.

GLIA. Unlike neurons, glial cells can be replaced if lost or injured in an adult. Such repopulation depends on progenitor cells committed to the glial cell lineage. Either the progenitor cells reside in a latent state (or are slowly turning over) in adult brains, or true multipotential stem cells are activated by specific conditions, such as brain injury, to produce de novo glial progenitors. The most typical reaction of mammalian brains to a wide range of injuries is the formation of an **astrocytic glial scar**. This scar is produced primarily by an enlargement of individual astrocytes, a process called *hypertrophy*, and increased expression of a particular cytoskeleton protein, glial acidic fibrillary protein. Only a small degree of astrocytic *proliferation* (i.e., an increase in cell number) accompanies this reaction. **Microglial cells**, which derive from cells related to the monocyte/macrophage lineage in blood and not

from neuroepithelium, also react strongly to brain injury and are the main cells that proliferate at the injury site.

AXONS. Another reason that relatively little recovery follows severe brain and spinal cord injury is that axons within the CNS do not regenerate effectively. This lack of axon regeneration in the CNS is in sharp contrast to the behavior of axons in the PNS, which can regrow and reconnect to appropriate end organs, either muscle or sensory receptors. For example, if the median nerve of the forearm was crushed by blunt trauma, the distal axon segments would die off in a process called Wallerian degeneration (see the box titled Axonal Degeneration and Regeneration) because the sustaining relationship with their proximal cell bodies is lost. These PNS axons can slowly regenerate and connect to muscles and sensory receptors in the hand. It is believed that the inability of

CNS axons to regenerate is more the fault of the local environment than it is an intrinsic property of these axons. For example, oligodendrocytes and myelin carry on their surface molecules, such as myelin-associated glycoprotein, that inhibit axon growth. Experiments have shown that if severed CNS axons are given the opportunity to regrow in the same environment that surrounds axons in the PNS, they are capable of regrowth and can make functional connections with CNS targets. The remarkable ability of damaged peripheral nerves to regenerate, even in mammals, has encouraged hope that CNS axons might, under the right conditions, be able to perform this same feat. It would mean that victims of spinal cord injury might walk again. Learning how to induce the regeneration of CNS neurons is the holy grail of regeneration research.

SUBDIVISIONS OF THE NERVOUS SYSTEM

A rudimentary knowledge of the anatomy of the nervous system is a prerequisite to discussing its physiology. This section provides an overview of nervous system anatomy that builds on what has already been discussed about its embryologic development. We, in turn, consider the CNS, PNS, and ANS (see Table 10−1).

The directional terms used to describe brain structures can be somewhat confusing because the human nervous system, unlike that of lower vertebrates, bends during development. Thus, the "dorsal" surface of the cerebral cortex is also "superior," whereas the "dorsal" surface of the spinal cord is also "posterior" (Fig. 10−10*A*).

The CNS Consists of the Telencephalon, Cerebellum, Diencephalon, Midbrain, Pons, Medulla, and Spinal Cord

The CNS can be conveniently divided into four major areas: (1) the telencephalon, (2) cerebellum, (3) brainstem (consisting of the diencephalon, midbrain, pons, and medulla), and (4) spinal cord (see Fig. 10−10*B*). Each of these areas has symmetric right and left sides.

TELENCEPHALON. One of the crowning glories of evolution is the human **cerebral cortex**, the most conspicuous part of the paired cerebral hemispheres. The human cerebral cortex has a surface area of approximately 2200 cm^2 and is estimated to contain 1.5 to 2×10^{10} neurons. The number of synaptic contacts between these cells is roughly 3×10^{14}. The capacity for information processing by this neuronal machine is staggering and includes a remarkable range of functions: thinking, learning, memory, and consciousness.

The cortex is topographically organized in two ways. First, certain areas of the cortex mediate specific functions. For example, the area that mediates motor control is a well-defined strip of cortex located in the frontal lobe (see Fig. 10−10*C*). Second, within a portion of cortex that manages a specific function (e.g., motor control, somatic sensation, hearing, or vision), the parts of the body spatially map onto this cortex in an orderly way. We discuss this principle of **somatotopy** on p. 370.

The other parts of the telencephalon are the basal ganglia and the great mass of axons that stream into and out of the cerebral cortex and connect it with other regions. The **basal ganglia** consist of the striatum (caudate nucleus and putamen) and globus pallidus. These structures have indirect connections with motor portions of the cerebral cortex and are involved in motor control.

The **cerebellum** lies immediately dorsal to the brainstem. Although it represents only about 10% of the CNS by volume, it contains roughly 50% of all CNS neurons. The exceedingly large number of input connections to the cerebellum conveys information from nearly every type of receptor in the nervous system, including visual and auditory input. Combined, these afferent fibers outnumber the efferent projections by an estimated ratio of 40:1.

Functionally and by virtue of its connections, the cerebellum can be divided into three parts. Phylogenetically, the vestibulocerebellum (also called the archicerebellum) is the oldest of these three parts, followed by the spinocerebellum (also called the paleocerebellum) and then by the cerebrocerebellum (also called the neocerebellum).

The **vestibulocerebellum** is closely related to the vestibular system, whose sensors are located in the inner ear and whose way stations are located in the pons and medulla. It helps maintain the body's balance. The **spinocerebellum** receives strong input from muscle stretch receptors via connections in the spinal cord and brainstem. It helps regulate muscle tone. The **cerebrocerebellum**, the largest part of the human cerebellum, receives a massive number of projections from sensorimotor portions of the cerebral cortex via neurons in the pons. It coordinates motor behavior. Much of the cerebellum's output reaches the contralateral (i.e., on the opposite side of the body) motor cortex by way of the thalamus. Other efferent projections reach neurons in all three parts of the brainstem.

DIENCEPHALON. This rostral portion of the brainstem consists of the thalamus, the subthalamus, and the hypothalamus. Each of these areas has very different functions. The **thalamus** is the main integrating station for sensory information that is bound for the cerebral cortex, where it will reach the level of conscious perception. Along with the **subthalamus**, the thalamus also receives projections from the basal ganglia that are important for motor function. Input to the thalamus from the cerebellum (specifically, the cerebrocerebellum) is important for normal motor control. Patients with **Parkinson disease**, a severe movement disorder, gradually lose the ability to make voluntary movements; in some of these patients, it is possible to improve movement by stimulating certain areas of the thalamus or subthalamus. Control of arousal and certain aspects of memory function also reside in discrete areas of the thalamus.

The **hypothalamus** is the CNS structure that most affects the ANS. It performs this function through strong, direct connections with autonomic nuclei in the brainstem and spinal cord. It also acts as part of the endocrine system in two major ways. First, specialized neurons located within specific nuclei in the hypothalamus synthesize certain hormones (e.g., arginine vasopressin and oxytocin) and transport them down their axons to the posterior pituitary gland, where the hormones are se-

A AXES OF THE CNS

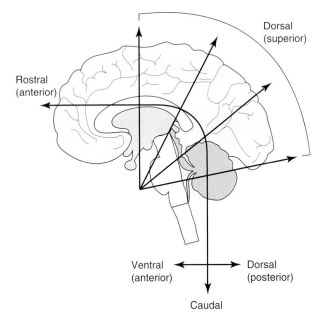

B MAJOR COMPONENTS OF THE CNS

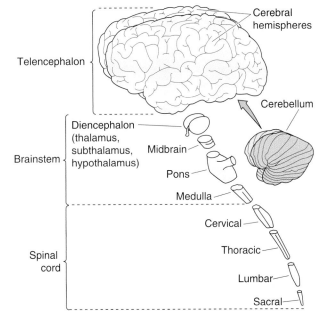

C SURFACE ANATOMY OF THE CEREBRAL CORTEX

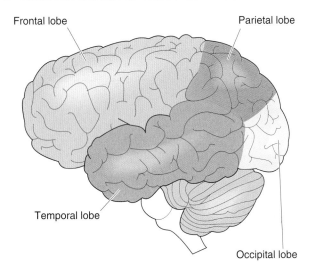

FIGURE 10–10. Gross anatomy of the central nervous system (CNS).

creted into the blood. Second, other specialized neurons in other nuclei synthesize "releasing hormones" (e.g., gonadotropin-releasing hormone) and release them into a plexus of veins, called a "portal system," that carries the releasing hormones to cells in the anterior pituitary. There, the releasing hormones stimulate certain cells (e.g., gonadotrophs) to secrete hormones (e.g., follicle-stimulating hormone or luteinizing hormone) into the bloodstream. We discuss these principles. The hypothalamus also has specialized centers that play important roles in controlling body temperature (p. 1236), hunger (p. 1227), thirst (p. 871), and the cardiovascular system. It is the main control center of the ANS.

MIDBRAIN, PONS, AND MEDULLA. This caudal portion of the brainstem lies immediately above, or rostral to, the spinal cord. Like the spinal cord, the midbrain, pons, and

medulla have a segmental organization, receive sensory (afferent) information, and send out motor (efferent) signals via paired nerves that are called **cranial nerves**. The midbrain, pons, and medulla also contain important control centers for the ANS (see Chapter 15). In addition to motor neurons, autonomic neurons, and sensory neurons present at each level, the caudal brainstem serves as a conduit for a large volume of axons traveling from higher CNS centers to the spinal cord (descending pathways) and vice versa (ascending pathways). Additionally, this portion of the brainstem contains a loosely organized interconnected collection of neurons and fibers called the **reticular formation**. This neuronal network has diffuse connections with the cortex and other brain regions and affects the level of consciousness or arousal.

The **midbrain** has somatic motor neurons that control eye movement. These neurons reside in the nuclei for cranial nerve III (CN III) and CN IV. Other midbrain neurons are part of a system, along with the cerebellum and cortex, for motor control. The midbrain also contains groups of neurons that are involved in relaying signals related to hearing and vision.

Just caudal to the midbrain is the **pons**, which contains the somatic motor neurons that control mastication (nucleus for CN V), eye movement (nucleus for CN VI), and facial muscles (nucleus for CN VII). The pons also receives somatic sensory information from the face, scalp, mouth, and nose (portion of the nucleus for CN V). It is also involved in processing information that is related to hearing and equilibrium (nucleus for CN VIII). Neurons in the ventral pons receive input from the cortex, and these neurons in turn form a massive direct connection with the cerebellum (see earlier) that is crucial for coordinating motor movements.

The most caudal portion of the brainstem is the **medulla**. The organization of the medulla is most similar to that of the spinal cord. The medulla contains somatic motor neurons that innervate the muscles of the neck (nucleus of CN XI) and tongue (nucleus of CN XII). Along with the pons, the medulla is involved in controlling blood pressure, heart rate, respiration, and digestion (nuclei of CN IX and X). The medulla is the first CNS way station for information traveling from the special senses of hearing and equilibrium.

SPINAL CORD. Continuous with the caudal portion of the medulla is the spinal cord. The spinal cord runs from the base of the skull to the body of the first lumbar vertebra. Thus, it does not run the full length of the vertebral column in adults.

The spinal cord consists of 31 segments that each have a motor and sensory nerve root. (The sensory nerve root of the first cervical segment is very small and can be missing.) These nerve roots combine to form 31 bilaterally symmetrical pairs of spinal nerves. The spinal roots, nerves, and ganglia are part of the PNS (see later).

Sensory information from the skin, muscle, and visceral organs enters the spinal cord via fascicles of axons called dorsal roots (Fig. 10–11A). The point of entry is called the dorsal root entry zone. Dorsal root axons have their cell bodies of origin in the spinal ganglia (i.e., **dorsal root ganglia**) associated with that spinal segment.

Ventral roots contain strictly efferent fibers (see Fig. 10–11B). These fibers arise from motor neurons (i.e., general somatic efferent neurons) whose cell bodies are located in the ventral (or anterior) *gray* horns of the spinal cord (gray because they contain mainly cell bodies without myelin) and from preganglionic autonomic neurons (i.e., general visceral efferent neurons) whose cell bodies are located in the intermediolateral gray horns (i.e., between the dorsal and ventral gray horns) of the cord. Most of the efferent fibers are somatic efferents that innervate skeletal muscle to mediate voluntary movement. The other fibers are visceral efferents that synapse with postganglionic autonomic neurons, which in turn innervate visceral smooth muscle or glandular tissue.

Each segment of the spinal cord contains groups of "associative" neurons in its dorsal gray horns. Some, but not all, incoming sensory fibers synapse on these associative neurons, which in turn contribute axons to fiber paths that both mediate synaptic interactions within the spinal cord and convey information to more rostral areas of the CNS by way of several conspicuous **ascending tracts** of axons (see Fig. 10–11C). Similarly, **descending tracts** of axons from the cerebral cortex and brainstem control the motor neurons whose cell bodies are in the ventral horn, thus leading to coordinated voluntary or posture-stabilizing movements. The most important of these descending tracts is called the lateral **corticospinal tract**; about 90% of its cell bodies of origin are in the contralateral cerebral cortex. These ascending and descending tracts are located in the *white* portion of the spinal cord (white because it contains mostly myelinated axons). The spatial organization of spinal cord neurons and fiber tracts is complex but orderly and varies somewhat among the 31 segments.

If sensory fibers enter the spinal cord and synapse directly on motor neurons in that same segment, this connection underlies a simple **segmental reflex** or interaction. If the incoming fibers synapse with neurons in other spinal segments, they can participate in an **intersegmental reflex** or interaction. Finally, if the incoming signals travel rostrally to the brainstem before they synapse, they constitute a **suprasegmental interaction**.

The Peripheral Nervous System Comprises the Cranial and Spinal Nerves, Their Associated Sensory Ganglia, and Various Sensory Receptors

The PNS serves four main purposes: (1) it transduces physical or chemical stimuli both from the external environment and from within the body into raw sensory information via receptors; (2) it conveys sensory information to the CNS along axon pathways; (3) it conveys motor signals from the CNS along axon pathways to target organs, primarily skeletal and smooth muscle; and (4) it converts the motor signals to chemical signals at synapses on target tissues in the periphery. Figure 10–11B summarizes these four functions for a simple reflex arc in which a painful stimulus to the foot results in retraction of the foot from the source of the pain.

Like the CNS, the PNS can be divided into *somatic* and *autonomic* parts. The somatic division includes the sensory neurons and axons that innervate the skin, joints, and muscle, as well as the motor axons that innervate skeletal muscle. The somatic division of the PNS primarily deals with the body's *external environment*, either to gather information about this environment or to interact with it through voluntary motor behavior. The ANS, discussed in the next section and in Chapter 15, is a functionally distinct part of both the CNS and PNS (see Table 10–1). The autonomic portion of the PNS consists of the motor and sensory axons that innervate smooth muscle, the exocrine glands, and other viscera. This division mainly deals with the body's *internal environment*.

Three important aspects of the PNS are discussed in other chapters. Sensory transduction is reviewed in Chapter 13, synaptic transmission in Chapters 8 and 12, and peripheral neuronal circuits in Chapter 14. Here, we fo-

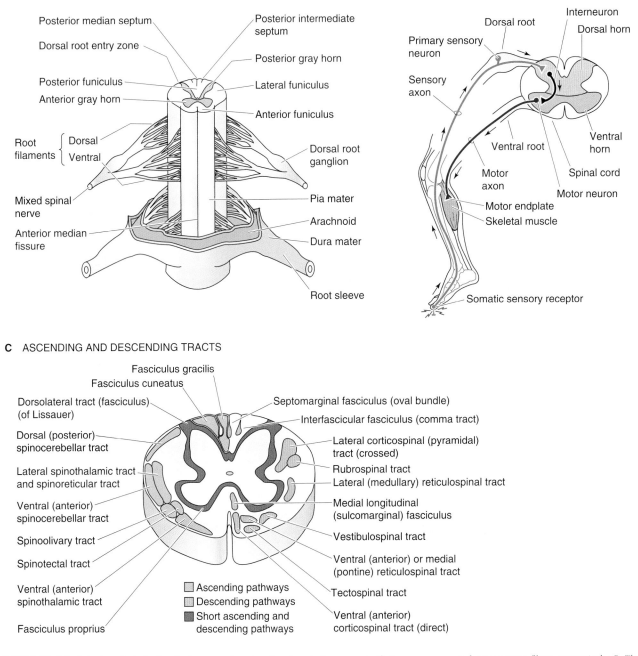

A SPINAL CORD AND NERVE ROOTS

Posterior median septum

Dorsal root entry zone

Posterior funiculus

Anterior gray horn

Root filaments { Dorsal / Ventral }

Mixed spinal nerve

Anterior median fissure

Posterior intermediate septum

Posterior gray horn

Lateral funiculus

Anterior funiculus

Dorsal root ganglion

Pia mater

Arachnoid

Dura mater

Root sleeve

B A SPINAL REFLEX ARC

Dorsal root

Primary sensory neuron

Sensory axon

Motor axon

Motor endplate

Skeletal muscle

Somatic sensory receptor

Interneuron

Dorsal horn

Ventral horn

Spinal cord

Motor neuron

Ventral root

C ASCENDING AND DESCENDING TRACTS

Fasciculus gracilis

Fasciculus cuneatus

Dorsolateral tract (fasciculus) (of Lissauer)

Dorsal (posterior) spinocerebellar tract

Lateral spinothalamic tract and spinoreticular tract

Ventral (anterior) spinocerebellar tract

Spinoolivary tract

Spinotectal tract

Ventral (anterior) spinothalamic tract

Fasciculus proprius

Septomarginal fasciculus (oval bundle)

Interfascicular fasciculus (comma tract)

Lateral corticospinal (pyramidal) tract (crossed)

Rubrospinal tract

Lateral (medullary) reticulospinal tract

Medial longitudinal (sulcomarginal) fasciculus

Vestibulospinal tract

Ventral (anterior) or medial (pontine) reticulospinal tract

Tectospinal tract

Ventral (anterior) corticospinal tract (direct)

☐ Ascending pathways
☐ Descending pathways
☐ Short ascending and descending pathways

FIGURE 10–11. Spinal cord. *A*, Each spinal segment has dorsal and ventral nerve roots that carry sensory and motor nerve fibers, respectively. *B*, The simple "flexor" reflex arc is an illustration of the four functions of the peripheral nervous system: (1) a receptor transduces a painful stimulus into an action potential, (2) a primary sensory neuron conveys the information to the central nervous system (CNS), (3) the CNS conveys information to the target organ via a motor neuron, and (4) the electrical signals are converted to signals at the motor endplate. *C*, Ascending pathways, which carry information to more rostral areas of the CNS, are shown on the *left*. Descending pathways, which carry information in the opposite direction, are shown on the *right*.

cus primarily on the system of axons that is such a prominent feature of the PNS.

Axons in the PNS are organized into bundles called **peripheral nerves** (Fig. 10–12). These nerves contain, in a large nerve such as the sciatic nerve, tens of thousands of axons. Individual axons are surrounded by loose connective tissue called the **endoneurium**. Within the nerve, axons are bundled together in small groups called fascicles, each one covered by a connective tissue sheath known as the **perineurium**. The perineurium contributes structural stability to the nerve. Fascicles are grouped together and surrounded by a matrix of connective tissue called the **epineurium**. Fascicles within a nerve anastomose with neighboring fascicles. Axons shift from one fascicle to another along the length of the nerve, but they tend to remain in roughly the same general area

FIGURE 10–12. Peripheral nerve.

within the nerve over long distances. The interlocking meshwork of fascicles adds further mechanical strength to the nerve. Axons range in diameter from less than 1 to 20 μm. Because axons are extremely fragile, adaptations that enhance mechanical stability are very important. The PNS is designed to be much tougher, physically, than nervous tissue in the CNS. The PNS must be mechanically flexible, tolerant of minor physical trauma, and sustainable by a blood supply that is less dependable than the one providing for the CNS. A spinal cord transplanted to the lower part of the leg would not survive the running of a 100-meter dash.

Axons in peripheral nerves are closely associated with Schwann cells. In the case of a myelinated axon, a Schwann cell forms a myelinated wrap around a single adjacent axon, a single internodal myelin segment between 250 and 1000 μm in length. Many such internodal myelin segments, and thus many Schwann cells, are necessary to myelinate the entire length of the axon. In an unmyelinated nerve, the cytoplasm of a Schwann cell envelops but does not wrap around axons. Unmyelinated axons outnumber myelinated axons by about 2:1 in typical human nerves. Diseases that affect the PNS can disrupt nerve function by causing either loss of myelin or axonal injury.

The functional organization of a peripheral nerve is best illustrated by a typical thoracic spinal nerve and its branches. Every spinal nerve is formed by the dorsal and ventral roots joining together and emerging from the spinal cord at that segmental level (see Fig. 10–11). The dorsal roots coalesce and display a spindle-shaped swell-

ing called the spinal or dorsal root ganglion, which contains the cell bodies of the sensory axons in the dorsal roots. Individual neurons are called dorsal root ganglion cells or spinal ganglion cells and are typical unipolar neurons that give rise to a single process that bifurcates in a "T-like" manner into a peripheral and central branch (see Fig. 10–3). The central branch carries sensory information into the CNS and the peripheral branch terminates as a sensory ending. The peripheral process, which brings information toward the cell body, meets one definition of a dendrite; however, it has all the physiological and morphologic features of a peripheral axon.

Spinal nerves divide into several branches that distribute motor and sensory axons to the parts of the body associated with that segment. Axons conveying autonomic motor or autonomic sensory signals also travel in these branches. These branches are said to be "mixed," because they contain both efferent and afferent axons. Further nerve division occurs as axons travel to supply their targets, such as the skin, muscle, or blood vessels. In the case of thoracic spinal nerves, the subdivision is orderly and has a similar pattern for most of the nerves. In the cervical and lumbosacral areas, however, the spinal nerves from different segments of the spinal cord intermingle to form a **nerve plexus**. The subsequent course of the nerves in the upper and lower extremities is complex. The pattern of cutaneous innervation of the body is shown in Figure 10–13. The area of cutaneous innervation provided by a single dorsal root and its ganglion is called a **dermatome**. Severing a single dorsal root does not produce anesthesia in that dermatome because of

PERIPHERAL NERVE DISEASE

The symptoms of peripheral nerve disease, or **"neuropathy,"** are numbness (i.e., a sensory deficit) and/or weakness (i.e., a motor deficit). Such symptoms may arise from disturbances in many parts of the nervous system. How, then, can one tell whether a problem is the result of disease in the peripheral nervous system (PNS)?

Motor axons directly innervate and have "trophic" effects on skeletal muscle. If the axon is cut or dies, this trophic influence is lost and the muscle undergoes denervation atrophy. In addition, individual muscle fibers may twitch spontaneously **("fibrillation").** The cause of fibrillation is still debated, but it may be related to the observation that acetylcholine receptors spread beyond the neuromuscular junction and become "supersensitive" to their agonist. If true, these observations imply continuing exposure to acetylcholine, even if in smaller quantities. Schwann cells at denervated junctions may be the source of acetylcholine. When a motor axon is first damaged but has not yet lost continuity with the muscle fibers that it innervates, these muscle cells may twitch in unison. These small twitches can be seen under the skin and are called **fasciculations.** They are probably due to spontaneous action potentials in dying or injured motor neurons or their axons.

When the PNS is affected by a diffuse or generalized disease (e.g., the result of a metabolic problem or toxin), all peripheral nerves are involved, but symptoms arise first in the longest nerves of the body (i.e., those traveling from the spinal cord to the feet). This predilection for affecting the longest nerves often causes a "stocking pattern" defect in sensation and sometimes in strength. If both the feet and hands are affected, the process is called a "stocking and glove" defect. With progression of the disease, the level of involvement moves centripetally (i.e., up the leg, toward the trunk), and the sensory or motor dysfunction comes to involve more proximal portions of the legs and arms. One of the most common causes of this diffuse pattern of PNS involvement is the sensorimotor polyneuropathy associated with diabetes. Other causes include chronic renal failure (uremia), thiamine deficiency (often seen with alcohol abuse), and heavy-metal poisoning.

If a patient exhibits weakness or sensory loss that is associated with muscle fibrillation and atrophy and a "stocking" or "stocking and glove" pattern of sensory disturbance, a PNS problem is likely. Patients with peripheral neuropathy may also complain of tingling sensations **("paresthesias")** or pain in areas of the body supplied by the diseased nerves.

overlap between the cutaneous innervation provided by adjacent dorsal roots. The sole exception to this rule is the C2 root, sectioning of which causes a patch of analgesia on the back of the head; neither C3 nor the trigeminal nerve innervates skin in this area. Also note that no dermatomes are shown for the first cervical and the coccygeal segments because they are small or may be missing (in the case of the first cervical segment).

The Autonomic Nervous System Innervates Effectors That Are Not Under Voluntary Control

The nervous system regulates some physiological mechanisms in a way that is independent or *autonomous* of voluntary control. Control of body temperature is an example of a fundamental process that most individuals

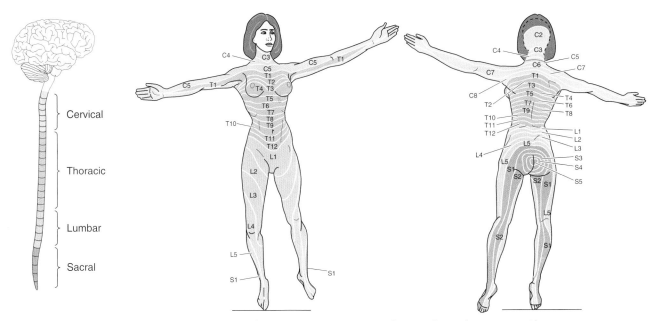

FIGURE 10–13. Dermatomes. A dermatome is the area of cutaneous sensory innervation that a single spinal segment provides.

cannot consciously regulate. Other examples include blood pressure and heart rate. The absence of voluntary control means that the ANS has little cortical representation.

The ANS has three divisions: sympathetic, parasympathetic, and enteric. The sympathetic and parasympathetic divisions have both CNS and PNS parts. The enteric is entirely in the PNS. The **parasympathetic** and **sympathetic** efferent systems are composed of two neurons. The cell body of the first neuron is located in the CNS, and that of the second in the PNS. The sympathetic and parasympathetic divisions innervate most visceral organs and have a yin-yang functional relationship. The **enteric** division regulates the rhythmic contraction of intestinal smooth muscle and also regulates the secretory functions of intestinal epithelial cells. It receives afferent input from the gut wall and is subject to modulation by the two other divisions of the ANS.

All the divisions have both efferent and afferent connections, although the efferent actions of the ANS are usually emphasized. We consider the ANS in detail in Chapter 15.

REFERENCES

Books and Reviews

Gage FH: Stem cells of the central nervous system. Curr Opin Neurobiol 8:671–676, 1998.

Hirokawa N: Kinesin and dynein superfamily proteins and the mechanism of organelle transport. Science 279:519–526, 1998.

Kandel ER, Schwartz JH, Jessell TM: Principles of Neural Science, 4th ed. New York, McGraw-Hill, 2000.

Weiss S, Reynolds BA, Vescovi AL, et al: Is there a neural stem cell in the mammalian forebrain? Trends Neurosci 19:387–393, 1996.

Journal Articles

Burne JF, Staple JK, Raff MC: Glial cells are increased proportionally in transgenic optic nerves with increased numbers of axons. J Neurosci 16:2064–2073, 1996.

Chiasson BJ, Tropepe V, Morshead CM, van der Kooy D: Adult mammalian forebrain ependymal and subependymal cells demonstrate proliferative potential, but only subependymal cells have neural stem cell characteristics. J Neurosci 19:4462–4471, 1999.

Colbert CM, Johnston D: Axonal action-potential initiation and Na^+ channel densities in the soma and axon initial segment of subicular pyramidal neurons. J Neurosci 16:6676–6686, 1996.

CHAPTER 11

Physiology of Neurons

Barry W. Connors

Neurons Receive, Combine, Transform, Store, and Send Information

Neurons have arguably the most complex job of any cell in the body. Consequently, they have an elaborate morphology and physiology. Each neuron is an intricate computing device. A single neuron may receive chemical input from tens of thousands of other neurons. It then combines these myriad signals into a much simpler set of electrical changes across its cellular membrane. The neuron subsequently transforms these ionic transmembrane changes according to rules determined by its particular shape and electrical properties and transmits a *single new message* through its axon, which itself may contact and inform hundreds of other neurons. Under the right circumstances, neurons also possess the property of *memory*; some of the information coursing its synapses may be stored for periods as long as years.

This general scheme of neuronal function applies to most neurons in the vertebrate nervous system. However, the scheme is endlessly variable. For example, each region of the brain has several major classes of neurons, and each of these classes has a physiology adapted to perform specific and unique functions. In this chapter, the general principles of neuronal function are outlined, and the almost unlimited variability contained within the general schema is discussed.

Neural Information Flows from Dendrite to Soma to Axon to Synapse

Numerous dendrites converge on a central soma, or cell body, from which a single axon emerges and branches multiple times (see Fig. 10–1). Each branch culminates at a presynaptic terminal that contacts another cell. In most neurons, dendrites are the principal synaptic input sites, although synapses may also be found on the soma, on the axon hillock (the region of the soma neighboring the axon), or even directly on the axons. In some primary sensory neurons, the dendrites themselves are transducers of environmental energy. Regardless of their source, signals—in the form of voltage changes across the membrane—typically flow from dendrites to soma to axon and finally to synapses on the next set of cells.

Excitatory input to a neuron usually generates an inward flow of positive charge (i.e., an "inward current") across the dendritic membrane (p. 281). Because the interior of a resting neuron is polarized negatively with respect to the external environment, this inward current, which makes the mem-

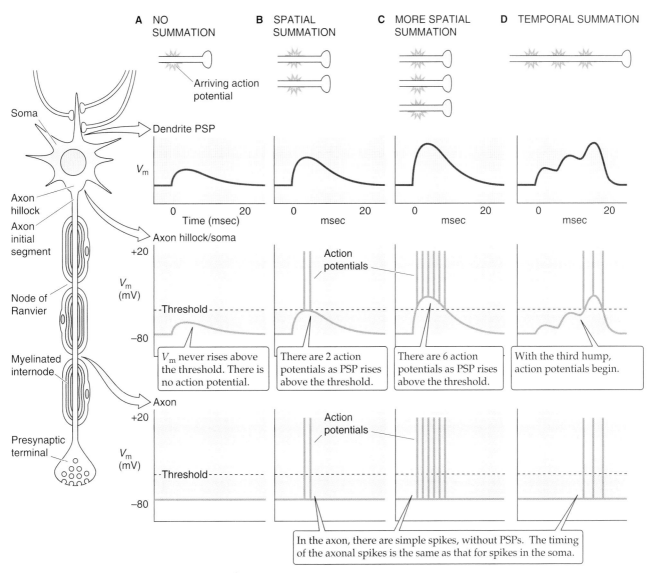

A NO SUMMATION

B SPATIAL SUMMATION

C MORE SPATIAL SUMMATION

D TEMPORAL SUMMATION

Arriving action potential

Dendrite PSP

V_m

Time (msec)

msec

msec

msec

Axon hillock/soma

+20

Action potentials

V_m (mV)

Threshold

−80

V_m never rises above the threshold. There is no action potential.

There are 2 action potentials as PSP rises above the threshold.

There are 6 action potentials as PSP rises above the threshold.

With the third hump, action potentials begin.

Axon

+20

Action potentials

V_m (mV)

Threshold

−80

In the axon, there are simple spikes, without PSPs. The timing of the axonal spikes is the same as that for spikes in the soma.

Soma

Axon hillock

Axon initial segment

Node of Ranvier

Myelinated internode

Presynaptic terminal

FIGURE 11–1. Spatial versus temporal summation of EPSPs.

brane voltage more positive (i.e., less negative), is said to **depolarize** the cell. Conversely, inhibitory input to a neuron usually generates an outward current and, thus, hyperpolarization.

If the neuron receives its input from a neighboring cell via a chemical synapse, neurotransmitters trigger currents by activating ion channels. If the cell is a sensory neuron, environmental stimuli (e.g., chemicals, light, mechanical deformation) activate ion channels and produce a flow of current. The change in membrane potential (V_m) caused by the flow of charge is called a **postsynaptic potential** (PSP) if it is generated at the postsynaptic membrane by a neurotransmitter and a **receptor potential** if it is generated at a sensory nerve ending by an external stimulus. In the case of synaptic transmission, the postsynaptic V_m changes may be either positive or negative. If the neurotransmitter is excitatory and produces a *depolarizing* PSP, we refer to the PSP as an **excitatory postsynaptic potential** (EPSP; p. 212). On the other hand, if the neurotransmitter is inhibitory and produces a *hyperpolarizing* PSP,

the PSP is an **inhibitory postsynaptic potential** (IPSP). In all cases, the stimulus produces a V_m change that may be *graded* from small to large depending on the strength or quantity of input stimuli (p. 173). Stronger sensory stimuli generate larger receptor potentials; similarly, more synapses activated together generate larger PSPs. A graded response is one form of neural coding whereby the size and duration of the input are encoded as the size and duration of the change in the dendritic V_m.

The synaptic (or receptor) potentials generated at the ends of a dendrite are communicated to the soma, but not usually without substantial attenuation of the signal (Fig. 11–1A). Extended cellular processes such as dendrites behave like leaky electrical cables (p. 200). As a consequence, dendritic potentials usually decline in amplitude before reaching the soma. As an EPSP reaches the soma, it may also combine with EPSPs arriving via other dendrites on the cell; this behavior is a type of **spatial summation** and can lead to EPSPs that are substantially larger than those generated by any single synapse (see

Fig. 11–1B, C). **Temporal summation** occurs when EPSPs arrive rapidly in succession; when the first EPSP has not yet dissipated, a subsequent EPSP tends to add its amplitude to the residual of the preceding EPSP (see Fig. 11–1D).

The tendency for synaptic and receptor potentials to diminish with distance along a dendrite puts significant limitations on their signalling abilities. If nothing else happened, these depolarizing potentials would simply dwindle back to the resting membrane potential as they spread through the soma and down into the axon. At best, this passive signal might be carried a few millimeters, clearly inadequate for wiggling a toe when the axon of the motor neuron stretching from the spinal cord to the foot might be 1000 mm long. Some amplification is, therefore, necessary for certain inputs to generate effective signals to and from the central nervous system (CNS). Amplification is provided in the form of regenerating **action potentials**. If the V_m change in the soma is large enough to reach the threshold voltage (p. 172), the depolarization may trigger one or more action potentials between the soma and axon, as shown in Figure 11–1B to D. Action potentials are large, rapid fluctuations in V_m. As described in Chapter 7, an action potential is an efficient, rapid, and reliable way to carry a signal over long distances. However, notice that generating action potentials entails another transformation of neuronal information: the neuron converts the graded-voltage code of the dendrites (i.e., the PSPs) to a temporal code of action potentials in the axon.

Action potentials are fixed in amplitude, not graded, and have uniform shape. So how is information encoded by action potentials? This question has no simple answer and is still hotly debated. Because one axonal spike looks like another (with slight exceptions), neurons can vary only their timing. For a single axon, information may be encoded by the average rate of action potential firing, the total number of action potentials, their temporal pattern, or some combination of these mechanisms. Figure 11–1 illustrates that as the synaptic potential in the soma increases in size, the resultant action potentials occur more frequently, and the burst of action potentials in the axon lasts longer. Notice also that by the time the signal has propagated well down the axon, the transformation has become complete—the graded potential has waned and vanished, whereas the action potentials have retained their size, number, and temporal pattern. The final output of the neuron is entirely encoded in these action potentials. When action potentials reach axonal terminals, they may trigger the release of a neurotransmitter at the next set of synapses, and the cycle begins again.

SIGNAL CONDUCTION IN DENDRITES

The word "dendrite" is derived from the Greek word *dendron* for "tree," and indeed some dendritic trees resemble the branches or roots of an oak tree. Inspired by trees, no doubt, the anatomist Camillo Golgi suggested in 1886 that the function of dendrites is to collect nutrients for the neuron. The truth is analogous but more interesting: dendrites arborize through a volume of brain tissue

so that they can collect *information* in the form of synaptic input. The dendrites of different types of neurons exhibit a great diversity of shapes. Dendrites are often very extensive, accounting for up to 99% of a neuron's membrane. The dendrites of a single neuron may receive as many as 200,000 synaptic inputs. The electrical and biochemical properties of dendrites are quite variable from cell to cell, and they have a profound influence on the transfer of information from synapse to soma.

Dendrites Attenuate Synaptic Potentials

Dendrites tend to be long and thin. Their cytoplasm has relatively low electrical resistivity, and their membrane has relatively high resistivity. These are the properties of a *leaky electrical cable*, which is the premise for **cable theory** (p. 200). Leaky cables are like leaky garden hoses; if ionic current (or water) enters at one end, the fraction of it that exits at the other end depends on the number of channels (or holes) in the cable (hose). A good hose has no holes and all the water makes it through, but most dendrites have a considerable number of channels that serve as leaks for ionic current (see Fig. 7–22).

Cable theory predicts how much current flows down the length of the dendrite via the cytoplasm and how much of it leaks out of the dendrite across the membrane. As summarized in Table 7–3, we can express the leakiness of the membrane by the resistance per unit area of dendritic membrane (**specific membrane resistance,** R_m), which can vary widely among neurons. The intracellular resistance per cross-sectional area of dendrite (**specific resistivity of the cytoplasm,** R_i) is also important in determining current flow inasmuch as a very resistive cytoplasm forces more current to flow out across the membrane rather than down the axis of the dendrite. Another important factor is cable diameter; thick dendrites let more current flow toward the soma than thin dendrites do. Figure 7–22C illustrates the consequences of a point source of steady current flowing into a leaky, uniform, infinitely long cable made of purely passive membrane. The transmembrane voltage generated by the current falls off exponentially with distance from the site of current injection. The steepness with which the voltage falls off is defined by the length constant (λ; p. 201), which is the distance over which a steady voltage decays by a factor of $1/e$ (about 37%). Estimates of the parameter values vary widely, but for brain neurons at rest, reasonable numbers are approximately 50,000 $\Omega \cdot cm^2$ for R_m and 200 $\Omega \cdot cm$ for R_i. If the radius of the dendrite (a) is 1 μm (10^{-4} cm), we can estimate the length constant of a dendrite by applying Equation 7–8.

Equation 11–1

$$\lambda = \sqrt{\frac{aR_m}{2R_i}} = \sqrt{\frac{(10^{-4}\ cm)(5 \times 10^4\ \Omega\ cm^2)}{2(200\ \Omega\ cm)}}$$
$$= 0.1118\ cm = 1118\ \mu m$$

Because dendrite diameters vary greatly, λ should also vary greatly. For example, assuming the same cellular properties, a thin dendrite with a radius of 0.1 μm would have a λ of only 354 μm, whereas a thick one with a

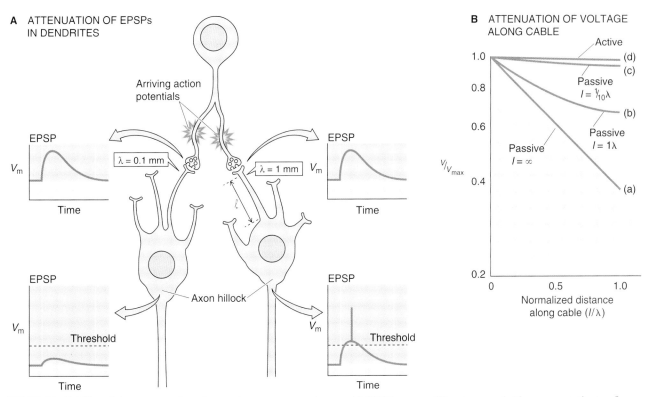

A ATTENUATION OF EPSPs IN DENDRITES

Arriving action potentials

EPSP

V_m

Time

$\lambda = 0.1$ mm

$\lambda = 1$ mm

V_m

EPSP

Time

ℓ

EPSP

V_m

Threshold

Time

Axon hillock

EPSP

V_m

Threshold

Time

B ATTENUATION OF VOLTAGE ALONG CABLE

Active

Passive $l = \frac{1}{10}\lambda$

Passive $l = \infty$

Passive $l = 1\lambda$

(d)
(c)
(b)
(a)

V/V_{max}

1.0
0.8
0.6
0.4
0.2

0   0.5   1.0

Normalized distance along cable (l/λ)

FIGURE 11–2. Effect of λ on propagation of an excitatory postsynaptic potential (EPSP) to two different axons. *A,* The neuron at the top fires an action potential that reaches the left and right neurons below, each at a single synapse. The EPSPs are identical. However, the left neuron has a thin dendrite, and therefore a small length constant ($\lambda = 0.1$ mm). As a result, the signal is almost completely attenuated by the time it reaches the axon hillock and there is no action potential. In the *right* neuron, the dendrite is thicker and, therefore, has a larger length constant ($\lambda = 1$ mm). As a result, the signal that reaches the axon hillock is large enough to trigger an action potential. *B,* The graph shows four theoretical plots of the decay of voltage (logarithmic plot) along a dendritic cable. The voltage is expressed as a fraction of maximal voltage. The length along the cable is normalized for the length constant (λ). Thus, an l/λ of 1.0 corresponds to one length constant along the dendrite. *Curve* (a): If the cable is infinitely long and passive, the voltage decays exponentially with increasing length, so that the semilog plot is linear. *Curve* (b): If the cable is terminated at a length that is equal to one length constant, then voltage decays less steeply. *Curve* (c): If the cable is terminated at a length that is equal to 10% of the length constant, the voltage decays even less steeply. *Curve* (d): If the membrane is not passive, but has a slow voltage-gated conductance, the dendritic attenuation will be much smaller. (Data from Jack JJB, Noble D, Tsien RW: Electrical Current Flow in Excitable Cells. Oxford, Oxford University Press, 1975.)

radius of 5 μm would have a λ of 2500 μm. Thus, the graded signal spreads farther in a thick dendrite.

Real dendrites are certainly not infinitely long, uniform, and unbranched, nor do they have passive membranes. Thus, quantitative analysis of realistic dendrites is complex. Sharp termination of a dendrite *decreases* attenuation because current cannot escape farther down the cable. Branching *increases* attenuation because current has more paths to follow. Gradually expanding to an increased diameter progressively increases λ and thus *decreases* attenuation. Real membranes are never completely passive because all have voltage-gated channels; and, therefore, their R_m values can change as a function of voltage. Finally, in the working brain, cable properties are not constant but may vary dynamically with ongoing brain activity. For example, as the general level of synaptic input to a neuron rises (which might happen when a brain region is actively engaged in a task), more membrane channels will open and thus R_m will drop as a function of time, with consequent shortening of dendritic length constants. However, all these caveats do not alter the fundamental *qualitative* conclusion: *voltage signals are attenuated as they travel down a dendrite.*

So far, we have described only how a dendrite might

attenuate a *sustained* voltage change. Indeed, the usual definition of length constant applies only to a *steady-state* voltage shift. An important complication is that the signal attenuation along a cable depends on the *frequency* components of that signal—how rapidly voltage changes over time. When V_m varies over time, some current is lost to membrane capacitance (p. 157), and less current is carried along the dendrite downstream from the source of the current. Because action potentials and EPSPs entail rapid changes in V_m, with the fastest of them rising and falling within a few milliseconds, they are attenuated much more strongly than the steady-state λ implies. If V_m varies in time, we can define a λ that depends on signal frequency ("λ_{AC}," where the "AC" stands for "alternating current"). When signal frequency is zero (i.e., V_m is steady), $\lambda = \lambda_{AC}$. However, as frequency increases, λ_{AC} may fall sharply. Thus, *dendrites attenuate high-frequency (i.e., rapidly changing) signals more than low-frequency or steady signals.* Another way to express this concept is that most dendrites tend to be **low-pass filters** in that they let slowly changing signals pass more easily than rapidly changing ones.

Figure 11–2*A* shows how an EPSP propagates along two different dendrites with very different length constants: when the dendrites have a longer λ, a larger signal arrives at the axon hillock. How do leaky dendrites manage to communicate a useful synaptic signal to the soma? The problem is solved in two ways. The first solution deals with the passive properties of the dendrite membrane. The length (l) of dendrites tends to be relatively small in comparison to their λ; thus, none extend more than one or two steady-state length constants (i.e., the l/λ ratio is smaller than 1). One way that dendrites achieve a small l/λ ratio is to have a combination of diameter and R_{m} that gives them a large λ. Another way is that dendrites are not infinitely long cables, but "terminated cables." Figure 11–2*B* shows that a signal is attenuated more in an infinitely long cable (*curve a*) than in a "terminated cable" whose length (l) is equal to λ (*curve b*). The attenuation of a purely passive cable would be even less if the terminated cable had a λ 10-fold greater than l (*curve c*). Recall that in our example in Figure 11–2*A*, such a 10-fold difference in λ underlies the difference in the amplitudes of the EPSPs arriving at the axon hillock.

The second solution to the attenuation problem is to endow dendrites with voltage-gated ion channels (p. 182) that enhance the signal more than would be expected in a purely "passive" system (*curve d*). We discuss the properties of such "active cables" in the next section.

Dendritic Membranes Have Voltage-Gated Ion Channels

All mammalian dendrites have voltage-gated ion channels that influence their signalling properties. Dendritic characteristics vary from cell to cell, and the principles of dendritic signalling are studied intensively. Most dendrites have a relatively low density of voltage-gated channels (p. 182) that may amplify, or boost, synaptic signals by adding additional inward current as the signals propagate from distal dendrites toward the soma. We have already introduced the principle of an **active cable** in *curve d* of Figure 11–2*B*. If the membrane has voltage-gated channels that are able to carry more inward current (usually Na^+ or Ca^{2+}) under depolarized conditions, a sufficiently strong EPSP would drive V_{m} into the activation range of the voltage-gated channels. These voltage-gated channels would open, and their additional inward current would add to that generated initially by the synaptic channels. Thus, the synaptic signal would fall off much less steeply than in a passive dendrite. Voltage-gated channels can be distributed all along the dendrite, and thus amplify the signal along the entire dendritic length, or they can be clustered at particular sites. In either case, voltage-gated channels can boost the synaptic signal considerably, even if the densities of channels are far too low to generate action potentials.

An even more dramatic solution, used by a few dendrites, is to have such a high density of voltage-gated ion channels that they can produce *action potentials*, just as in the case of an axon. One of the best documented examples is the Purkinje cell, which is the large output neuron of the cerebellum. As Rodolfo Llinás and colleagues have shown, when the dendrites of Purkinje cells are stimulated strongly, they can generate large, sharp action po-

tentials that are mediated by voltage-gated Ca^{2+} channels (Fig. 11–3). Such Ca^{2+} spikes can sometimes propagate toward—or even into—the soma, but these Ca^{2+} action potentials do not continue down the axon. Instead, they may trigger fast Na^+-dependent action potentials that are generated by voltage-gated Na^+ channels in the soma and initial segment. The Na^+ spikes carry the signal along the axon in the conventional way, and those in the soma are considerably quicker and larger than the dendritic Ca^{2+} spikes. The faster Na^+ spikes do not propagate very far backward into the dendritic tree because the rapid time course of the Na^+ spike is strongly attenuated by the inherent filtering properties of the dendrites (i.e., the λ_{AC} is smaller for the rapid frequencies of the Na^+ action potentials than for the slower Ca^{2+} action potentials). The dendrites of certain other neurons of the CNS, including some pyramidal cells of the cerebral cortex, can also generate spikes that are dependent on Ca^{2+}, Na^+, or both.

Dendritic action potentials, when they exist at all, tend to be slower and weaker than those in axons. The reason is probably that one of the functions of dendrites is to collect and integrate information from a large number of synapses (often tens of thousands). If each synapse were capable of triggering an action potential, there would be little opportunity for most of the input to have a meaningful influence on a neuron's output. The cell's dynamic range would be truncated; that is, a very small number of active synapses would bring the neuron to its maximum firing rate. However, if dendrites are only weakly excitable, the problem of signal attenuation along dendritic cables can be solved while still allowing the cell to generate an output (i.e., the axonal firing rate) that is indicative of the proportion of its synapses that are active.

Another advantage of voltage-gated channels in dendrites may be the selective boosting of high-frequency synaptic input. Recall that passive dendrites attenuate signals of high frequency more than those of low frequency. However, if dendrites possess the appropriate voltage-gated channels, they will be better able to communicate high-frequency synaptic input.

CONTROL OF SPIKING PATTERNS IN THE SOMA

Electrical signals from dendrites converge and summate at the soma. Although action potentials themselves often appear first at the nearby axon hillock and initial segment of the axon, the large variety of ion channels in the soma and proximal dendritic membranes is critically important in determining and modulating the temporal patterns of action potentials that ultimately course down the axon.

Neurons Can Transform a Simple Input into a Variety of Output Patterns

Neurophysiologists have sampled the electrical properties of many different types of neurons in the nervous system, and one general conclusion seems safe: no two types behave the same. The variability begins with the **shape and height** of individual action potentials. Most neurons

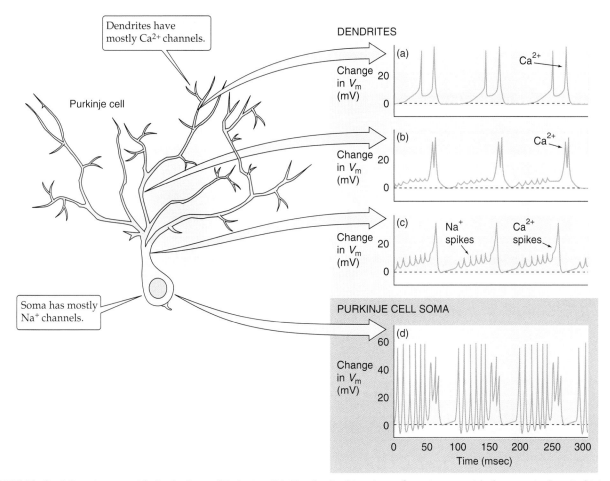

Dendrites have mostly Ca^{2+} channels.

Purkinje cell

Soma has mostly Na$^+$ channels.

DENDRITES

(a)

Change in V_m (mV)   20   0   Ca^{2+}

(b)

Change in V_m (mV)   20   0   Ca^{2+}

(c)

Change in V_m (mV)   20   0   Na$^+$ spikes   Ca^{2+} spikes

PURKINJE CELL SOMA

(d)

Change in V_m (mV)   60   40   20   0

0   50   100   150   200   250   300
Time (msec)

FIGURE 11–3. Ca^{2+} action potentials (in dendrites of Purkinje cells). Usually, dendrites do not fire action potentials; however, in these Purkinje cells of the cerebellum (*left panel*), the high density of voltage-gated Ca^{2+} channels in the dendrites allows the generation of *slow* dendritic Ca^{2+} spikes (*records a, b, c on right*), which propagate all the way to the axon soma. In the axon soma, these Ca^{2+} action potentials trigger fast Na$^+$ action potentials (*record d on right*). Moreover, the fast Na$^+$ spikes back propagate into the dendritic tree but are attenuated. Thus, these fast Na$^+$ spikes appear as small spikes in the proximal dendrites (*record c*), and even smaller blips in the midlevel dendrites (*record b*). (Data from Llinás R, Sugimori M: Electrophysiological properties of *in vitro* Purkinje cell dendrites in mammalian cerebellar slices. J Physiol 305:197–213, 1981.)

within the CNS generate action potentials in the conventional way, as described in Chapter 7 (see Fig. 7–4). Fast, voltage-gated Na$^+$ channels (p. 186) generate a strong inward current that depolarizes the membrane from rest, usually in the range of −60 to −80 mV, to a peak that is usually between +10 and +40 mV. This depolarization represents the upstroke of the action potential. The Na$^+$ channels then very quickly inactivate and close, and certain K$^+$ channels (often voltage-gated "delayed outward rectifier" channels; p. 194) open and thus cause V_m to fall and terminate the spike. However, many neurons have somewhat different spike-generating mechanisms and produce spikes with a range of shapes (Fig. 11–4). Although a fast Na$^+$ current invariably drives the fast upstroke of neuronal action potentials, frequently, an additional fast Ca^{2+} current (p. 189) can occur and, if large enough, broaden the spike duration. The greatest variability occurs in the repolarization phase. Many neurons are repolarized by other voltage-gated K$^+$ currents in addition to the delayed outward rectifier K$^+$ current, and some also have a K$^+$ current carried by channels that are rapidly activated by the combination of membrane depolarization and a rise in [Ca^{2+}]$_i$ (p. 194).

More dramatic variations occur in the **repetitive spiking patterns** of neurons, observed when the stimulus is of long duration. One way to illustrate this principle is to apply a simple, continuous stimulus (a current pulse, for example) to each neuron and measure its output (the number and pattern of action potentials fired at its soma). The current pulse is the equivalent of a steady, strong input of excitatory synaptic currents. The transformation from stimulus input to spiking output can take many different forms. Some examples are shown in Figure 11–5, which illustrates recordings from three types of neurons in the cerebral cortex. In response to a sustained current stimulus, some cells generate a rapid train of action potentials that *do not adapt* (see Fig. 11–5A); that is, the spikes occur at a regular interval throughout the current pulse. Other cells fire rapidly at first but then *adapt strongly* (see Fig. 11–5B); that is, the spikes gradually become less frequent during the current pulse. Some cells fire a burst of action potentials and then stop firing altogether, and still others generate very *rhythmic bursts* of action potentials that continue as long as the stimulus (see Fig. 11–5C). These varied behaviors are not arbitrary but are characteristic of each neuron type, and they are as

FIGURE 11–4. Shapes of action potentials in various neurons.

distinctive as each cell's morphology. They are also an intrinsic property of each neuron; that is, a neuron's fundamental firing pattern is determined by the membrane properties of the cell and does not require fluctuations in synaptic input. Of course, synaptic input may also impose particular firing patterns on a neuron. When a neuron is operating in situ, its firing patterns are determined by the interaction of its intrinsic membrane properties and synaptic input.

Rhythmically bursting cells are particularly interesting and occur in a variety of places in the brain. As described on p. 367, they may participate in the central circuits that generate rhythmic motor output for behavior such as locomotion and respiration. Cells that secrete peptide neurohormones, such as the magnocellular neurons of the hypothalamus, are also often characterized by rhythmic bursting behavior. These cells release either arginine vasopressin or oxytocin and help to control water retention (p. 871) and lactation (p. 1189), respectively. Rhythmic bursting is a more effective stimulus for the synaptic release of peptides than are tonic patterns of action potential. It may be that the bursting patterns and the Ca^{2+} currents that help drive them can elicit the relatively high $[Ca^{2+}]_i$ necessary to trigger the exocytosis of peptide-containing vesicles (p. 222). One additional role of rhythmically bursting neurons is to help drive the synchronous oscillations of neural activity in forebrain circuits (i.e., thalamus and cortex) during certain behavioral states, particularly sleep.

Although it has been difficult to prove, the diverse electrical properties of neurons are probably adapted to each cell's particular functions. For example, in the first stage of auditory processing in the brain, cranial nerve VIII axons from the cochlea innervate several types of neurons in the cochlear nucleus of the brainstem. The axons provide similar synaptic drive to each type of neuron, yet the output from each neuron type is distinctly different. Some are tuned to precise timing and respond only to the *onset* of the stimulus and ignore anything else; some respond, pause, and respond again; others chop the ongoing stimulus into a more rhythmic output; and still other cells transform the input very little. The mechanisms for this range of transformations include both synaptic circuitry and the diverse membrane properties of each cell type. The different properties allow some cells to be particularly well tuned to specific features of the stimulus—its onset, duration, or amplitude modulation—and they can then communicate this signal to the appropriate auditory nuclei for more complex processing.

Intrinsic Firing Patterns Are Determined by a Variety of Ion Currents with Relatively Slow Kinetics

What determines the variety of spiking patterns in each type of neuron, and why do neurons differ in their intrinsic patterns? The key is a large set of ion channel types that have variable and often relatively *slow* kinetics compared with the *quick* Na^+ and K^+ channels that shape the spike. For a discussion of the properties of such channels, see Chapter 7. Each neuron expresses a different complement of these slow channels and has a unique spatial arrangement of them on its dendrites, soma, and axon initial segment. The channels are gated primarily by membrane voltage and $[Ca^{2+}]_i$, and a neuron's ultimate spiking pattern is determined by the net effects of the slow currents that it generates. We illustrate three examples of systems that have been studied in detail:

1. A neuron with only fast, voltage-gated Na^+ channels and delayed rectifier K^+ channels will generate repetitive spikes when presented with a long stimulus. The pattern of those spikes will be quite regular over time, as for the cerebral cortical interneuron that we have already seen in Figure 11–5A.
2. If the neuron also has another set of K^+ channels that activate only very slowly, the spiking pattern becomes more time dependent: the spiking frequency may initially be very high, but it adapts to progressively lower rates as a slow K^+ current turns on to counteract the stimulus, as shown for the small pyramidal cell in Figure 11–5B. The strength and rate of adaptation depend strongly on the number and properties of the fast and slow K^+ channels.
3. A neuron, by exploiting the interplay between two voltage-gated currents, can generate spontaneous rhythmic bursting—as in the case of the large pyramidal neuron in Figure 11–5C—even without ongoing synaptic activity to drive it.

Another example of a bursting neuron comes from the thalamus; in this case the neuron produces a rhythmic bursting activity during certain sleep states (Fig. 11–6A). Each burst consists of a cluster of standard Na^+-dependent action potentials and is driven by a slower and smaller wave of depolarization. Bursts recur at a rate of about 2 Hz. It is easy to show that the fast Na^+ spikes have no role in generating the underlying slow waves that establish the burst rhythm because abolishing them with tetrodotoxin, an Na^+ channel blocker (p. 178), leaves the slow waves intact (see Fig. 11–6B). Underlying the slow depolarizing waves are two inward currents (see Fig. 11–6C), a low-threshold Ca^{2+} current (I_{Ca}) and a cation current (I_{cation}) carried by a relatively nonselective cation channel. The rhythm depends on a repeating cycle of interaction between these two slow currents: activation of I_{Ca} drives the more rapid phase of the depolarizing waves, but the same depolarization causes both I_{Ca} and I_{cation} to inactivate; as a result, the wave terminates and the membrane then hyperpolarizes. Stimulated by the hyperpolarization, I_{cation} then reactivates and slowly begins to depolarize the membrane again. At a critical threshold V_m, activation of I_{Ca} again drives the more rapid phase of the depolarizing wave. Small changes in the properties of the intrinsic thalamic currents alter the cell's behavior. During waking behavioral states, thalamic neurons tend to have a more positive resting potential because levels of certain neurotransmitters affect the cell's various channel properties. Rhythmic bursting does not occur then because both I_{Ca} and I_{cation} remain inactivated. Thalamic neurons are a dramatic example of the important role of transmitters in modulating the electrical behavior of neurons, a theme that we will examine in Chapter 12.

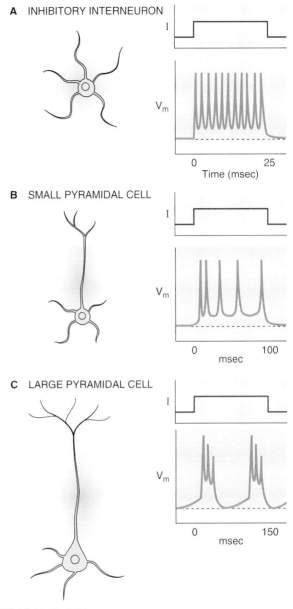

FIGURE 11–5. Spiking patterns.

AXONAL CONDUCTION

Axons Are Specialized for Rapid, Reliable, and Efficient Transmission of Electrical Signals

At first glance, the job of the axon seems mundane when compared with the complex computational functions of synapses, dendrites, and somata. After all, the axon has the relatively simple job of carrying the computed signal—a sequence of action potentials—from one place in the brain to another without changing it significantly. Some axons are thin, unmyelinated, and slow; these properties are sufficient to achieve their functions. However, the axon can be exquisitely optimized, with myelin and nodes of Ranvier, for fast and reliable saltatory conduction of action potentials over very long distances (p. 200). Consider the sensory endings in the skin of your foot,

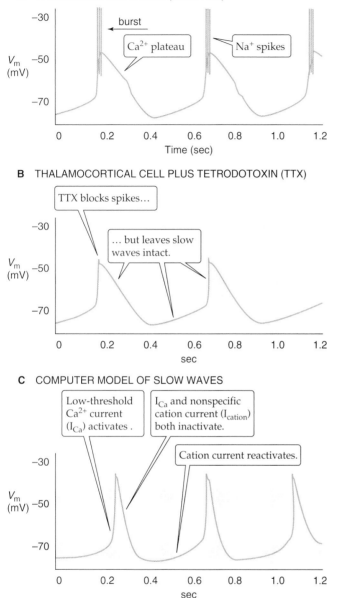

A THALAMOCORTICAL CELL (CONTROL)

burst

Ca²⁺ plateau

Na⁺ spikes

V_m (mV)

B THALAMOCORTICAL CELL PLUS TETRODOTOXIN (TTX)

TTX blocks spikes...

... but leaves slow waves intact.

V_m (mV)

C COMPUTER MODEL OF SLOW WAVES

Low-threshold Ca²⁺ current (I_{Ca}) activates .

I_{Ca} and nonspecific cation current (I_{cation}) both inactivate.

Cation current reactivates.

V_m (mV)

FIGURE 11–6. Spontaneous rhythmic bursting in single neurons. *A*, The *record* shows the spontaneous rhythmic bursting of a thalamic relay neuron. Bursts recur at a rate of about 2 Hz. The fast bursts are Na⁺ spikes; the slow waves are due to Ca²⁺ currents. *B*, This is a *record* from the same neuron as that in *A*, after treatment with tetrodotoxin (TTX). The Na⁺ channel blocker TTX abolishes fast spikes but does not affect the underlying rhythmic, Ca²⁺-dependent slow waves. Thus, the fast Na⁺ spikes in *A* have no role in generating the underlying burst rhythm. *C*, The basis for the slow thalamic rhythm is the interaction between two voltage-dependent currents. (Data from Huguenard JR, McCormick DA: Simulation of the currents involved in rhythmic oscillations in thalamic relay neurons. J Neurophysiol 68:1373–1383, 1992.)

which must send their signals to your lumbar spinal cord 1 m away (see Fig. 10–11B). The axon of such a sensory cell transmits its message in just a few tens of milliseconds! As we see in our discussion of spinal reflexes on p. 362, axons of similar length carry signals in the opposite direction, from your spinal cord to the muscles within your feet, and they do it even faster than the sensory axons. Axons within the CNS can also be very long; examples include the corticospinal axons that originate in the cerebral cortex and terminate in the lumbar spinal cord. Alternatively, many central axons are quite short, only tens of micrometers in length, and they transmit their messages locally between neurons. The spinal interneuron between a sensory neuron and a motor neuron (see Fig. 10–11B) is an example. Some axons target their signal precisely, from one soma to only a few other cells, whereas others may branch profusely to target thousands of postsynaptic cells.

Different parts of the brain have different signalling needs, and their axons are adapted to the local requirements. Nevertheless, the primary function of all axons is to carry electrical signals, in the form of action potentials, from one place to other places and to do so rapidly, efficiently, and reliably. Without myelinated axons, the large, complex brains necessary to control warm, fast mammalian bodies could not exist. For *un*myelinated axons to conduct action potentials sufficiently fast for many purposes, their diameters would have to be so large that the axons alone would take up far too much space and use impossibly large amounts of energy.

Action Potentials Are Usually Initiated at the Initial Segment

The soma, axon hillock, and initial segment of the axon together serve as a kind of focal point in most neurons.

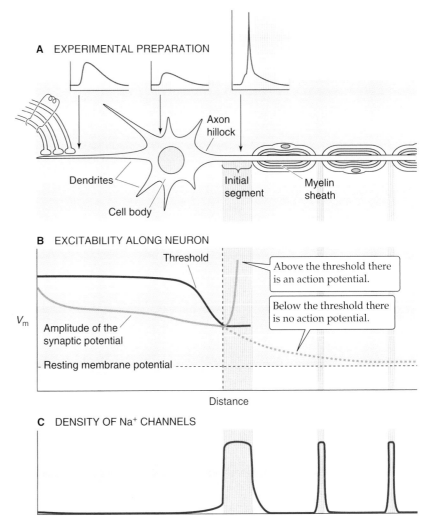

FIGURE 11–7. Simultaneous recording of action potentials from different parts of a neuron. *A,* In this hypothetical experiment, an excitatory synapse on a dendrite is stimulated and the response near that dendrite is recorded in the soma and at the initial segment. The excitatory postsynaptic potential (EPSP) attenuates in the soma and the initial segment, but the EPSP is large enough to trigger an action potential at the initial segment. *B,* The threshold is high (-35 mV) in regions of the neuron that have few Na^+ channels, but starts to fall rather steeply in the hillock and initial segment. Typically, a stimulus of sufficient strength triggers an action potential at the initial segment. *C,* The density of Na^+ channels is high only at the initial segment and at each node of Ranvier.

The many graded synaptic potentials carried by numerous dendrites converge at the soma and generate one electrical signal. During the 1950s, Sir John Eccles and colleagues used glass microelectrodes to probe the details of this process in spinal motor neurons. Because it appeared that the threshold for action potentials in the initial segment was only about 10 mV above the resting potential whereas the threshold in the soma was closer to 30 mV above resting potential, they concluded that the neuron's action potentials would be first triggered at the initial segment. Direct evidence now indicates that spikes may begin at the initial segment, at least for some neurons. EPSPs evoked in the dendrites propagate down to and through the soma and trigger an action potential in the initial segment (Fig. 11–7A). The action potential then propagates in two directions: forward ("**orthodromically**") into the axon, with no loss of amplitude, and backward into the soma and dendrites, with strong attenuation, as we saw earlier in Figure 11–3. Orthodromic propagation carries the signal to the next set of neurons. The function of backward propagation, if indeed such a role exists, is not known. It is possible that backwardly propagating spikes trigger biochemical changes in the neuron's dendrites and synapses and they may have a role in synaptic plasticity.

The axon achieves a uniquely *low threshold* in its initial segment (see Fig. 11–7B) by packing voltage-gated Na^+ *channels at a remarkably high density* (in comparison to the soma and dendrites) *in the initial segment* (see Fig. 11–7C). The Na^+ channel density in the axon initial segment is about 2000 channels/μm^2, about 1000-fold higher than in the membrane of the soma and dendrites.

Conduction Velocity of a Myelinated Axon Increases Linearly with Diameter

The larger the diameter of an axon, the faster its conduction velocity, other things remaining equal. However, conduction velocity is usually far greater in myelinated axons than it is in unmyelinated axons (p. 199). Thus, a myelinated axon 10 μm in diameter conducts impulses at about the same velocity as an unmyelinated axon about 500 μm in diameter. Not only does myelination confer substantial speed advantages but also advantages in efficiency. Almost 2500 of the 10-μm myelinated axons can pack into the volume occupied by one 500-μm axon!

It should be stressed that unmyelinated axons still have a role in vertebrates. At diameters below approximately 1 μm, unmyelinated axons in the peripheral nervous system

TABLE 11–1

CLASSES OF PERIPHERAL SENSORY AND MOTOR AXONS, BY SIZE AND CONDUCTION VELOCITY

Erlanger and Gasser's Classification*	Aα	Aβ	Aγ	Aδ	B	C
Function	Sensory afferents from proprio-ceptors of skeletal mus-cle Motor neurons to skeletal muscle	Sensory afferents from mecha-noreceptors of skin	Motor fibers to intra-fusal fi-bers of muscle spindles	Sensory afferents from pain and temperature receptors	Preganglionic neurons of the ANS	Sensory afferents from pain, temperature and itch re-ceptors
Diameter (μm)	13–20	6–12	3–6	1–5	<3	0.2–1.5
Conduction ve-locity of action potential (m/s)	80–120	35–75	12–30	5–30	3–15	0.5–2
Alternative classi-fication of sen-sory axons from muscle and tendon†	Ia (sensory from muscle spin-dle fibers) Ib (sensory from Golgi tendon organs)	II		III		IV

*This A–C classification was introduced by Joseph Erlanger and Herbert Gasser, who shared the 1944 Nobel Prize in Medicine or Physiology for describing the relationship among axon diameter, conduction velocity, and function in a complex peripheral nerve.

†This I–IV classification was introduced by other investigators. It applies only to sensory axons and only to those from muscle and tendon.

Modified from Bear MF, Connors BW, Paradiso MP: Neuroscience: Exploring the Brain. Baltimore, Williams & Wilkins, 1996.

conduct more rapidly than myelinated ones do. In a testament to evolutionary frugality, the thinnest axons of the peripheral sensory nerves, called **C fibers**, are about 1 μm wide or less, and all are unmyelinated. Axons larger than about 1 μm in diameter are all myelinated (Table 11–1). Every axon has its biologic price: the largest axons obviously take up the most room and are the most expensive to synthesize and maintain metabolically. The largest, swiftest axons are therefore used sparingly. They are only used to carry sensory information about the most rapidly changing stimuli over the longest distances (e.g., stretch receptors in muscle, mechanoreceptors in tendons and skin), or they are used to control finely coordinated contractions of muscles. The thinnest, slowest C fibers are mainly sensory axons related to chronic pain and temperature, for which the speed of the message is not as critical.

The relationship between form and function for axons in the CNS is less obvious than it is in the periphery, in part because it is harder to identify each axon's function. Interestingly, in the brain and spinal cord, the critical diameter for the myelination transition may be smaller than in the periphery. Many central myelinated axons are as thin as 0.2 μm. At the other extreme, very few myelinated central axons are larger than 4 μm in diameter.

FIGURE 11–8. Demyelination in the CNS. *A,* A cross section of a spinal root from a dystrophic mouse that shows amyelinated bundles of axons (*thin borders*) that are surrounded by myelinated fibers (*thick borders*). (From Rosenbluth J: In Waxman SG, Kocsis JD, Stys PK (eds): The Axon: Structure, Function, and Pathophysiology. New York, Oxford University Press, 1995.) *B,* This is a transverse section stained so that myelinated axons are *black.* Note the large, light plaques (regions of demyelination) around the midline and at the *center, right,* and *left.* (From Ludwin SK: In Waxman SG, Kocsis JD, Stys PK (eds): The Axon: Structure, Function, and Pathophysiology. New York, Oxford University Press, 1995.)

A NORMAL CONDUCTION

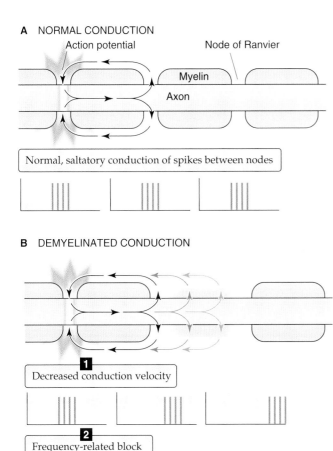

B DEMYELINATED CONDUCTION

C CROSSTALK BETWEEN DEMYELINATED AXONS

FIGURE 11–9. Demyelination. *A*, Four action potentials at the *leftmost* node of Ranvier are conducted—unchanged in amplitude and frequency—to the nodes that are farther to the *right. B,* Action potentials propagate from a normally myelinated region into a demyelinated area. The axial action current that was generated at the last healthy node is distributed across a long region of bare or partially myelinated axonal membrane, with its decreased resistivity and increased capacitance. Thus, the current density at the two affected nodes is greatly reduced. This panel shows five consequences of demyelination: (1) decreased velocity, which is manifest as longer delays for the arrival of the train of spikes; (2) frequency-related block, which does not pass high-frequency trains—as a result, some of the spikes are missing distally; (3) total blockade; (4) ectopic impulse generation—even though there is no input in the proximal portion of the axon, action potentials arise spontaneously beyond the lesion; and (5) increased mechanosensitivity—ectopic action potentials arise due to mechanical stimulation. *C,* If the demyelination affects two adjacent axons, action potentials in one (the *top axon* in this case) cause action potentials to propagate in both directions in the adjacent axon.

The myelinated axon membrane has a variety of ion channels that may contribute to its normal and pathologic function. Of primary importance is the *voltage-gated Na⁺ channel*, which provides the rapidly activating and inactivating inward current that yields the action potential. Na⁺ channels are packed into the nodal membrane at a density of 1000 to 2000 channels/μm^2 (see Fig. 11–7). The same axonal membrane in the internodal regions, under the myelin, has fewer than 25 channels/μm^2 (versus between 2 and 200 channels/μm^2 in unmyelinated axons). The dramatically different distribution of channels between nodal and internodal membrane has important implications for conduction along pathologically demyelinated

axons (see later). *K⁺ channels* are relatively less important in myelinated axons than they are in most other excitable membranes. Very few of these channels are present in the nodal membrane, and fast K⁺ currents contribute little to repolarization of the action potential in mature myelinated axons. This diminished role for K⁺ channels may be a cost-cutting adaptation because the absence of K⁺ currents decreases the metabolic expense of a single action potential by about 40%. However, some K⁺ channels are located in the axonal membrane *under* the myelin, particularly in the paranodal region. The function of these K⁺ channels is unclear; they may set the resting V_m of the internodes and help stabilize the firing properties of the axon.

Demyelinated Axons Conduct Action Potentials Slowly, Unreliably, or Not at All

Numerous clinical disorders selectively damage or destroy myelin sheaths and leave the axonal membranes intact but bare. These **demyelinating diseases** may affect either peripheral or central axons and can lead to severely impaired conduction (Fig. 11–8). The most common demyelinating disease of the CNS is **multiple sclerosis** (see the box titled Demyelinating Diseases), a progressive disorder that is characterized by distributed zones of demyelination in the brain and spinal cord. Among the demyelinating diseases of peripheral nerves is *Landry-Guillain-Barré syndrome*, which is an inflammatory disorder that may rapidly incapacitate but often ends in substantial recovery. The specific clinical signs of these disorders vary and depend on the particular sets of axons affected.

In a normal, myelinated axon, the action currents generated at a node can effectively charge the adjacent node and bring it to threshold within about 20 μsec (Fig. 11–9A), because myelin serves to increase the resistance and reduce the capacitance of the pathways between the axoplasm and the extracellular fluid (p. 200). The current flowing across each node is actually 5- to 7-fold higher than necessary to initiate an action potential at the adjacent node. Removing the insulating myelin, however, means that the same nodal action current is distributed across a much longer, leakier, higher-capacitance stretch of axonal membrane (see Fig. 11–9B). Several consequences are possible. When compared with normal conduction, conduction in a demyelinated axon may continue, but at a *lower velocity*, if the demyelination is not too severe (see Fig. 11–9B, *record 1*). In experimental studies, the internodal conduction time through demyelinated fibers can be as slow as 500 μsec, 25 times longer than normal. The ability of axons to transmit *high-frequency* trains of impulses may also be impaired (*record 2*). Extensive demyelination of an axon causes *total blockade* of conduction (*record 3*). Clinical studies indicate that the

DEMYELINATING DISEASES

Multiple sclerosis (MS), the most common demyelinating disease of the central nervous system (CNS), affects more than 200,000 Americans alone. MS is an autoimmune disease directed against the myelin or oligodendrocytes (p. 417) and is thus a purely CNS disease. The trigger is unclear. Some have proposed a viral antigen (including canine distemper virus), but many other theories abound, none of which has been clearly proven. The viral antigen theory is based at least in part on classic studies that concluded that MS has a greater incidence in temperate regions than in the tropics and that one's risk depends on where one spent one's childhood, not adulthood. According to this view, the "incubation" period, or the delay between exposure to an as yet unspecified environmental factor and onset of the first attack, is 10 to 25 years. However, some contemporary neurologists doubt the statistical significance of the temperate/tropic data. No good evidence has been presented for a viral etiology yet. MS is more common in women than in men. Susceptibility to MS has also been linked to a number of genetic alleles of the HLA system.

The signs and symptoms of MS are protean, but common features include the following: (1) An optic neuritis may cause decreased visual acuity. (2) An internuclear ophthalmoplegia results in an inability of the eyes to adduct on lateral conjugate gaze, reflecting a lesion in the medial longitudinal fasciculus, a white matter tract. The result is double vision. (3) The Lhermitte sign is an electrical sensation that shoots down the back and into the legs when flexing the neck. Elevated IgG levels are typically found in the cerebrospinal fluid (CSF), and electrophoresis reveals oligoclonal bands in the IgG region. Magnetic resonance imaging can demonstrate the lesions in MS. Evoked potential studies, which measure nerve fiber conduction in various sensory pathways, are abnormal in almost all established cases and in about two thirds of suspected cases of MS.

MS is defined clinically as a disease that involves demyelination of the CNS with episodes separated in both time and space—at least two episodes of demyelination

involving at least two separated regions of the CNS. A characteristic of many patients with MS is remissions and relapses. Thus, episodes of demyelination may be separated by intervals during which the symptoms and signs improve or even completely resolve. It is only the minority of patients who inexorably progress to the point of disability.

An exacerbation is due to the occurrence of active inflammation of a white matter tract in the CNS. A remission then occurs when the inflammation subsides and the axons that have now been demyelinated recover some of their function and are able to conduct action potentials through the area of myelin damage. However, the pathologically demyelinated fibers are not normal. Conduction is often barely adequate under normal circumstances and may become inadequate under stressful situations, such as illness, emotional stress, and exhaustion. Under these circumstances, symptoms will reappear. Such reappearance of symptoms must be distinguished clinically from a new exacerbation. In the former case, it is an old area of damage that has become dysfunctional. In the latter case, it is a new area of damage caused by new inflammation. The treatments for these two causes of symptoms are very different.

The reasons for remissions and exacerbations are not entirely clear. One explanation focuses on the impaired conduction in the pathologically demyelinated fibers. If conduction is just barely adequate under normal circumstances, it may become inadequate under certain stressful situations, such as illness, emotional stress, and exhaustion; only then will symptoms become evident. A change in **temperature** is a classic example of circumstances changing conduction. Conduction through demyelinated axons is exquisitely sensitive to temperature, but the direction of the effect is counterintuitive: conduction is "safer" at low temperature. *Lower* temperatures slow the gating kinetics of Na^+ channels, thereby lengthening the duration of the action potentials and slowing conduction velocity. A decrease of just 2°C increases the duration of an action potential by about 20%. The augmented cur-

DEMYELINATING DISEASES *Continued*

rents of the broader spike are better able to charge the increased capacitance of the axonal membrane of a demyelinated region, thus making it more likely that the threshold for continued conduction will be reached (Fig. 11–10). When the body temperature of a patient with MS is elevated, for example, by fever or immersion in a hot bath, conduction is compromised and neurologic deficits may appear. Conversely, the slightly increased impulse duration gained by cooling the body may be sufficient to restore conduction through a demyelinated region. Thus, MS patients may experience improved nerve function in cold versus hot environments. These temperature effects on symptoms are explained nicely by the physiology of neural conduction, and probably account for evanescent changes in symptoms in many patients. However, the temperature effects do not explain exacerbations and remissions, which are due to appearance and disappearance of inflammation.

Certain drugs can also prolong the duration of action potentials and facilitate conduction through demyelinated axons. Demyelination may expose the voltage-gated K⁺ channels, which are normally hidden under the myelin. Activation of outwardly rectifying K⁺ channels can further impair spike production in demyelinated axons. However, the K⁺ channels also become accessible to pharmacologic agents, such as the class of K⁺ channel blockers called **aminopyridines.** Because fast K⁺ channels may contribute to the repolarization phase of an action potential, blocking these K⁺ channels can prolong the spike and facilitate its propagation through demyelinated regions. Aminopyridines are being tested in clinical trials and show some promise for symptomatic relief in patients with MS.

At present, standard treatment for MS exacerbations includes immunosuppressive agents. The most common is interferon-β, which is one of the class of interferons that have antiviral, antiproliferative, and immune-modulating activity. This drug reduces the number and severity of exacerbations in patients with mild or moderate relap-

sing and remitting MS and may also help patients with chronic progressive MS. Many new drugs are currently under investigation for helping to prevent the autoimmune attack, to reduce the damage during an attack, and/or to improve function in already demyelinated regions.

Other demyelinating diseases of the CNS include **progressive multifocal leukoencephalopathy,** a fatal illness common in patients with acquired immunodeficiency disease and caused by opportunistic infection of the oligodendroglia (myelin-producing cells) by a strain of human papovavirus. Another disorder, **central pontine myelinolysis,** is caused by too rapid correction of hyponatremia; the sudden osmotic fluctuations appear to produce demyelination.

The most common demyelinating disease of the peripheral nervous system is **Landry-Guillain-Barré syndrome.** After a respiratory or other viral infection, an ascending neurologic syndrome develops that is characterized by the onset of weakness, leading to paralysis of the legs and subsequent involvement of the hands and arms. In severe cases, the paralysis involves the nerves feeding the brain stem, and patients may lose the ability to swallow or even breathe. The latter requires mechanical ventilation for a time. This initial stage of Landry-Guillain-Barré syndrome reaches a plateau in several weeks and then gradually resolves. Most patients recover completely as long as the physician recognizes the syndrome and initiates supportive treatment. Untreated, this syndrome is often fatal.

The pathologic lesions of Landry-Guillain-Barré syndrome consist of lymphocytic infiltration of the myelin sheath produced by Schwann cells in the peripheral nervous system (p. 418). The result is segmental demyelination. These patients generally recover fully because the peripheral nervous system has the ability to remyelinate itself. Axons of the CNS do not remyelinate to any significant extent, which explains why complete recovery in patients with MS is not as common as in these patients.

FIGURE 11–10. Temperature dependence of axonal conduction. (Data from Sears TA, Bostock H: Conduction failure in demyelination: Is it inevitable? Adv Neurol 31:357–375, 1981.)

blockade of action potentials is more closely related to symptoms than is the simple *slowing* of conduction. Demyelinated axons can also become the source of spontaneous, **ectopically generated action potentials** because of changes in their intrinsic excitability (*record 4*) or *mechanosensitivity* (*record 5*). Moreover, the signal from one demyelinated axon can excite an adjacent demyelinated axon and induce "**crosstalk**" (see Fig. 11–9C), which may cause action potentials to be conducted in both directions in the adjacent axon.

REFERENCES

Books and Reviews

Bear MF, Connors BW, Paradiso MP: Neuroscience: Exploring the Brain, 2nd ed. Baltimore, Lippincott Williams & Wilkins, 2001.
Connors BW, Gutnick MJ: Intrinsic firing patterns of diverse neocortical neurons. Trends Neurosci 13:99–104, 1990.

Johnston D, Magre JC, Colbert CM, Christie BR: Active properties of neuronal dendrites. Annu Rev Neurosci 19:165–186, 1996.

Rall W: Core conductor theory and cable properties of neurons. In Kandel ER (ed): Handbook of Physiology, Section 1. The Nervous System, Vol 1. Bethesda, MD, American Physiological Society, 1970, pp 39–98.

Journal Articles

Connor JA, Stevens CF: Prediction of repetitive firing behavior from voltage clamp data on an isolated neurone soma. J Physiol (Lond) 213:31–53, 1971.

Coombs JS, Curtis DR, Eccles JC: The interpretation of spike potentials of motoneurones. J Physiol (Lond) 139:198–231, 1957.

Häusser M, Stuart G, Racca C, Sakmann B: Axonal initiation and active dendritic propagation of action potentials in substantia nigra neurons. Neuron 15:637–647, 1995.

Huguenard JR, Hamill OP, Prince DA: Sodium channels in dendrites of rat cortical pyramidal neurons. Proc Natl Acad Sci U S A 86:2473–2477, 1989.

Llinás R, Nicholson C: Electrophysiological properties of dendrites and somata in alligator Purkinje cells. J Neurophysiol 34:534–551, 1971.

Magee JC, Johnston D: Synaptic activation of voltage-gated channels in the dendrites of hippocampal pyramidal neurons. Science 268:301–304, 1995.

Stuart G, Sakmann B: Active propagation of somatic action potentials into neocortical pyramidal cell dendrites. Nature 367:69–72, 1994.

CHAPTER 12

Synaptic Transmission in the Nervous System

Barry W. Connors

After meticulous study of spinal reflexes, Charles Sherrington deduced that neurons somehow communicate information, one to the next, by a mechanism that is fundamentally different from the way that they conduct signals along their axons. Sherrington had merged his physiologic conclusions with the anatomic observations (Fig. 12–1) of his contemporary, the preeminent neuroanatomist Santiago Ramón y Cajal. Cajal had proposed that neurons were distinct entities, fundamental units of the nervous system, that were *discontinuous* with each other. Discontinuous neurons must nevertheless communicate, and Sherrington in 1897 proposed that the **synapse**, a specialized apposition between cells, mediated the signals. The word "synapse" implies "contiguity, not continuity" between neurons, as Cajal himself explained it. When the fine structure of synapses was finally revealed with the electron microscope in the 1950s, the vision of Cajal and Sherrington was amply sustained. Neurons come very close together at chemical synapses (p. 206), but their membranes and cytoplasm remain distinct (Fig. 12–2). At electrical synapses (p. 206), which are far less common than chemical synapses, the membranes remain distinct, but ions and other small solutes can diffuse through the gap junctions, a form of "continuity."

NEURONAL SYNAPSES

The Molecular Mechanisms of Neuronal Synapses Are Similar, But Not Identical, to Those of the Neuromuscular Junction

Chemical synapses use diffusible **transmitter molecules** to communicate messages between two cells. The first chemical synapse to be understood in detail was the neuromuscular junction (the nerve-muscle synapse) in vertebrate skeletal muscle, which is described in Chapter 8. In this chapter, we are concerned with the properties of the synapses that occur *between* neurons. We now know that all synapses share certain basic biochemical and physiologic mechanisms, and thus many basic insights gained from the neuromuscular junction are also applicable to synapses in the brain. However, neuronal synapses differ from neuromuscular junctions in many important ways; they also differ widely among themselves, and it is the diverse properties of synapses that help make each part of the brain unique.

It is useful to begin by reviewing some of the mechanisms that are

FIGURE 12–1. Synapses of the mammalian brain. Drawings by Ramón y Cajal taken from Golgi-stained cortex of the cerebellum. *A,* Basket cell (B) from the mouse, making synaptic contacts onto the somata of numerous postsynaptic Purkinje cells (A). The axon (c) of the basket cell branches several times to make baskets (a and b) that synapse onto the somata of Purkinje cells (axosomatic synapse). Ramón y Cajal used the osmic method to stain the Purkinje cell and the Golgi method to stain the basket cell. *B,* A single climbing fiber (a) from a human, making numerous synaptic contacts onto the dendrites of a single Purkinje cell (b). This is an example of axodendritic synapses. Ramón y Cajal used the Golgi method to stain the climbing fiber. (From Ramón y Cajal S: Histology of the Nervous System of Man and Vertebrates, Vol 1. New York, Oxford University Press, 1995 [*Histologie du Système Nerveux de l'Homme et des Vertebrés,* 1909–1911—translated by Swanson N and Swanson LW].)

common to all chemical synapses (see Fig. 12–2). Synaptic transmission at chemical synapses occurs in seven steps:

Step 1: Neurotransmitter molecules are packaged into membranous vesicles, and the vesicles are concentrated and docked at the presynaptic terminal.

Step 2: The presynaptic membrane depolarizes, usually as the result of an action potential.

Step 3: The depolarization causes voltage-gated Ca^{2+} channels to open and allows Ca^{2+} ions to flow into the terminal.

Step 4: The resulting increase in intracellular $[Ca^{2+}]$ triggers fusion of vesicles with the presynaptic membrane (p. 222). The Ca^{2+} dependence of fusion may be conferred by a neuron-specific protein component of the fusion apparatus called synaptotagmin. The actual fu-

sion events are incredibly fast, with each individual exocytosis requiring only a fraction of a millisecond to complete.

Step 5: The transmitter is released into the extracellular space in quantized amounts and diffuses passively across the synaptic cleft.

Step 6: Some of the transmitter molecules bind to receptors in the postsynaptic membrane, and the activated receptors trigger some postsynaptic event, usually the opening of an ion channel or the activation of a G-protein–coupled signal cascade.

Step 7: Transmitter molecules diffuse away from postsynaptic receptors and are eventually cleared away by continued diffusion, enzymatic degradation, or active uptake into cells. In addition, the presynaptic machinery retrieves the membrane of the exocytosed synaptic vesicle, perhaps via endocytosis from the cell surface.

A RESTING STATE   **B** ACTIVATED STATE

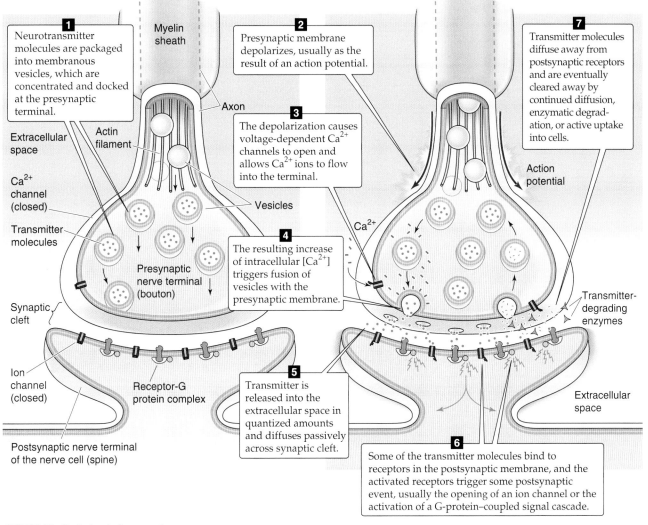

1 Neurotransmitter molecules are packaged into membranous vesicles, which are concentrated and docked at the presynaptic terminal.

Myelin sheath

Axon

2 Presynaptic membrane depolarizes, usually as the result of an action potential.

7 Transmitter molecules diffuse away from postsynaptic receptors and are eventually cleared away by continued diffusion, enzymatic degradation, or active uptake into cells.

Extracellular space

Actin filament

3 The depolarization causes voltage-dependent Ca^{2+} channels to open and allows Ca^{2+} ions to flow into the terminal.

Ca^{2+} channel (closed)

Vesicles

Action potential

Transmitter molecules

Ca^{2+}

4 The resulting increase of intracellular $[Ca^{2+}]$ triggers fusion of vesicles with the presynaptic membrane.

Presynaptic nerve terminal (bouton)

Synaptic cleft

Transmitter-degrading enzymes

Ion channel (closed)

Receptor-G protein complex

5 Transmitter is released into the extracellular space in quantized amounts and diffuses passively across synaptic cleft.

Extracellular space

Postsynaptic nerve terminal of the nerve cell (spine)

6 Some of the transmitter molecules bind to receptors in the postsynaptic membrane, and the activated receptors trigger some postsynaptic event, usually the opening of an ion channel or the activation of a G-protein–coupled signal cascade.

FIGURE 12–2. A chemical synapse between neurons.

The molecular machinery of synapses is closely related to components that are universal in eukaryotic cells (p. 39). A large set of proteins is involved in the docking and fusion of vesicles, and the proteins present in nerve terminals are amazingly similar to the ones mediating fusion and secretion in yeast. Docking and fusion of synaptic vesicles are discussed on p. 222. Ligand-gated ion channels and G-protein–coupled receptors, the receptors on the postsynaptic membrane, are also present in all eukaryotic cells and mediate processes as disparate as the recognition of nutrients and poisons as well as the identification of other members of the species. Even most of the neurotransmitters themselves are simple molecules, identical or very similar to those used in general cellular metabolism. Clearly, the evolutionary roots of synaptic transmission are much older than nervous systems themselves.

Within nervous systems, however, myriad variations on the basic molecular building blocks yield synapses with wide-ranging properties. Neuronal synapses vary widely in the size of the synaptic contact, the identity of the neurotransmitter, the nature of the postsynaptic receptors, the efficiency of synaptic transmission, the mechanism used for terminating transmitter action, and the degree and modes of synaptic plasticity. Thus, the properties of neuronal synapses can be tuned to achieve the diverse functions of the brain.

A major difference between the neuromuscular junction and most neuronal synapses is the type of neurotransmitter used. All skeletal neuromuscular junctions use acetylcholine (ACh). In contrast, neuronal synapses use many transmitters. The most ubiquitous are amino acids: glutamate and aspartate excite, whereas γ-aminobutyric acid (GABA) and glycine inhibit. Other transmitters include simple amines, such as ACh, norepinephrine, serotonin, and histamine, as well as a wide array of peptides.

Even more varied than the neuronal transmitters are their receptors. Whereas skeletal muscle manufactures a few slight variants of its ACh receptors, the nervous system typically has several major receptor variants for each neurotransmitter. Knowledge about the wide range of transmitters and receptors is essential to understanding the chemical activity of the brain, as well as the drugs that influence brain activity. For one thing, the many transmitter systems in the brain generate responses with

FIGURE 12–3. Time courses of synaptic events in the nervous system. Different transmitter systems in the brain generate responses that vary widely in how long they last in the postsynaptic cell. Note that the time axis is logarithmic. (Data from Shepherd GM: Neurobiology, 3rd ed. New York, Oxford University Press, 1994.)

widely varying durations that range from a few milliseconds to days (Fig. 12–3).

Presynaptic Terminals May Contact Neurons at the Dendrite, Soma, or Axon and May Contain Both Clear Vesicles and Dense-Core Granules

Chemical synapses between neurons are generally small, often less than 1 μm in diameter, which means that their detailed structure can be seen only with an electron microscope (Fig. 12–4); under the light microscope, brain synapses are usually visible only as swellings along or at the termination of the axons (see Fig. 12–1). These swellings are actually the silhouettes of the **bouton terminals**—the presynaptic terminals. Most presynaptic terminals arise from axons, and they can form synapses on virtually any part of a neuron. The contact site and direction of communication determine the way in which a synapse is named: **axodendritic**, **axosomatic**, and **axoaxonic** synapses (Fig. 12–5). These synapses are the most common types in the nervous system. In many cases, synapses occur on small outpockets of the dendritic membrane called **spines** and are termed **axospinous** synapses. However, not all synapses arise from axons, and **dendrodendritic**, **somatosomatic**, and even **somatodendritic** synapses may be found in the mammalian brain.

Despite their differences in size, site, and shape, all synapses share one basic function: they *deliver a small amount of chemical transmitter onto a circumscribed patch of postsynaptic membrane*. To accomplish this task, they use certain common anatomic features, most of them familiar from discussions of the neuromuscular junction (see Chapter 8).

Synapses are polarized, which means that their two apposed sides have different structures. This polarity reflects the fact that most synapses transmit information in one direction but not in the other (we will see that some rare exceptions do exist). The presynaptic side contains numerous clear **vesicles**, 40 to 50 nm in diameter, that

appear empty when viewed by transmission electron microscopy. Synaptic termini may also contain large (100 to 200 nm in diameter), **dense-core secretory granules** that are morphologically quite similar to the secretory granules of endocrine cells. These granules contain neuropeptides, that is, peptides or small proteins that act as neurotransmitters and for which receptors exist in the postsynaptic membranes. Many of these neuropeptides are identical to substances secreted by "traditional" endocrine cells. Endocrine hormones such as adrenocorticotropic hormone (ACTH), vasoactive intestinal polypeptide (VIP), and cholecystokinin (CCK) are all found in dense-core secretory granules present in the terminals of certain central and peripheral neurons.

The clear synaptic vesicles (i.e., not the dense-core granules) are anchored and shifted about by a dense network of cytoskeletal proteins. Some vesicles are clustered close to the part of the presynaptic membrane that apposes the synaptic contact; these vesicle attachment sites are called **active zones**. Synaptic vesicles are lined up several deep along the active zones, which are probably the regions of actual exocytosis. The number of active zones per synapse varies greatly (active zones are marked with *arrows* in the synapses of Fig. 12–4). Most synapses in the central nervous system (CNS) have relatively few active zones, often only 1 but occasionally as many as 10 or 20 (versus the hundreds in the neuromuscular junction). If we could view the presynaptic face of an active zone from the perspective of a synaptic vesicle, we would see filaments and particles projecting from the presynaptic membrane, often forming a regular hexagonal arrangement called a **presynaptic grid**. Specific points along the grid are thought to be the vesicle release sites.

Unlike the clear synaptic vesicles containing nonpeptide transmitters, dense-core secretory granules are distributed randomly throughout the cytoplasm of the synaptic terminus. They are not concentrated at the presynaptic density, and they do not appear to release their contents at the active zone. Although the molecular pathways that control exocytosis of the neuronal dense-core granules are still being elucidated, it appears that a rise in $[Ca^{2+}]_i$ is a primary stimulus.

FIGURE 12–4. Electron micrograph of synapses in the cochlear nucleus. Three presynaptic terminals are filled with vesicles and make contact with the same postsynaptic dendrite. Postsynaptic densities (marking active zones) are indicated by *arrows*. (From Peters A, Palay SL, Webster HD: The Fine Structure of the Nervous System: The Neurons and Supporting Cells. Philadelphia, WB Saunders, 1976.)

The Postsynaptic Membrane Contains Transmitter Receptors and Numerous Proteins Clustered in the "Postsynaptic Density"

The postsynaptic membrane lies parallel to the presynaptic membrane, and they are separated by a narrow **synaptic cleft** (about 30-nm thick) that is filled with extracellular fluid. Transmitter molecules released from the presynaptic terminal must diffuse across the cleft to reach postsynaptic receptors. The most characteristic anatomic feature of the postsynaptic side is the **postsynaptic density**, a strip of granular material visible under the electron microscope on the cytoplasmic face of the membrane (see Fig. 12–4). The most important molecular feature of the postsynaptic side is the cluster of transmitter receptors

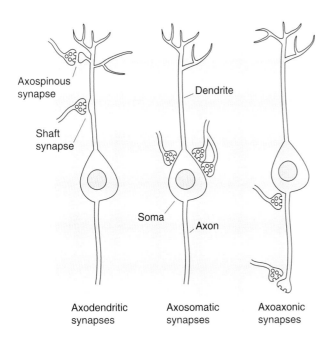

FIGURE 12–5. The most common synaptic arrangements in the central nervous system.

embedded within the postsynaptic membrane. The positions of the receptors are revealed by staining methods that use specific antibodies, toxins, or ligands coupled to some visible tag molecule.

In over 90% of all excitatory synapses in the CNS the postsynaptic site is a **dendritic spine**. The ubiquity of spines implies that they serve prominent functions, but their small size (usually less than 1 μm long) makes their function extremely difficult to study. Spines come in a variety of shapes, and their density varies from one dendrite to another (Fig. 12–6); indeed, many central neurons have no spines. The postsynaptic density of spines (as for all central synapses) contains over 30 proteins in high concentration, including transmitter receptors, protein kinases, a host of structural proteins, and proteins that are involved in endocytosis and glycolysis.

Numerous functions for spines have been proposed. It may be that spines increase the opportunity for a dendrite to form synapses with nearby axons. Many hypotheses have focused on the possibility that spines isolate individual synapses from the rest of a cell. This isolation may be electrical or chemical; the narrow spine neck may reduce current flow or the diffusion of chemicals from the spine head into the dendritic shaft. Recently, the idea that the electrical resistance of the spine neck is important has fallen into disfavor; with the small conductance that is generated by single synapses, neck diameter has a minimal effect on current flow. However, activation of some excitatory synapses allows substantial amounts of Ca^{2+} to enter the postsynaptic cell. Spines may compartmentalize this Ca^{2+}, thus allowing it to rise to higher levels or preventing it from influencing other synapses on the cell. Because increases in postsynaptic $[Ca^{2+}]_i$ are an essential trigger for many forms of long-term synaptic plasticity, an

attractive but unproven possibility is that dendritic spines play an important role in learning mechanisms.

Some Transmitters Are Used by Diffusely Distributed Systems of Neurons to Modulate the General Excitability of the Brain

The brain carries out many sensory, motor, and cognitive functions that require fast, specific, spatially organized neural connections and operations. Consider the detailed neural mapping that allows you to read this sentence or the precise timing required to play the piano. These functions require *spatially focused* networks (Fig. 12–7A).

Other functions, such as falling asleep, waking up, becoming attentive, or changing mood, involve more general alterations of the brain. Several systems of neurons regulate the general excitability of the CNS. Each of these **modulatory systems** uses a different neurotransmitter, and the axons of each make widely dispersed, diffuse, almost meandering synaptic connections to carry a simple message to vast regions of the brain. This arrangement can be achieved by a *widely divergent* network (Fig. 12–7B). The functions of the different systems are not well understood, but each appears to be essential for certain aspects of arousal, motor control, memory, mood, motivation, and metabolic state. The modulatory systems are of central importance to clinical medicine. Both the activity of psychoactive drugs and the pathology of most psychiatric disorders seem to involve alterations in one or more of the modulatory systems.

The brain has several modulatory systems with very diffuse central connections. Although they differ in structure and function, they have certain similarities:

1. Typically, a small set of neurons (several thousand) forms the center of the system.
2. Neurons of the diffuse systems arise from the central core of the brain, most of them from the brain stem.
3. Each neuron can influence many others because each one has an axon that may contact more than 100,000 postsynaptic neurons spread widely across the brain.
4. The synapses made by some of these systems seem designed to release transmitter molecules into the extracellular fluid so that they can diffuse to many neurons rather than be confined to the vicinity of a single synaptic cleft.

The main modulatory systems of the brain are distinct anatomically and biochemically. Separate systems use norepinephrine, serotonin (5-hydroxytryptamine [5-HT]), dopamine, ACh, or histamine as their neurotransmitter. They all tend to involve numerous **metabotropic transmitter receptors**. Unlike ionotropic receptors, which are themselves channels, metabotropic receptors are coupled to enzymes such as adenylyl cyclase or phospholipase C via G proteins (p. 207). For example, the brain has 10 to 100 times more metabotropic (i.e., muscarinic) ACh receptors than ionotropic (i.e., nicotinic) ACh receptors. We will briefly describe the anatomy and possible functions of each major system (Fig. 12–8).

Norepinephrine is used by neurons of the tiny **locus coeruleus** (from the Latin for "blue spot" because of the

FIGURE 12–6. Dendritic spines. *A,* Drawings of various dendrites in the neocortex, taken from Golgi-stained material. The numerous protrusions are "spines." *B,* Electron micrograph of an axospinous synapse in the neocortex. Note that the dendritic spine protrudes from the dendritic shaft, making contact with a presynaptic terminal. (From Feldman ML: In Peters A, Jones EG (eds): Cerebral Cortex: Cellular Components of the Cerebral Cortex, Vol 1. New York, Plenum, 1984, pp 123–200.)

pigment in its cells), located bilaterally in the brain stem (see Fig. 12–8*A*). Each human locus coeruleus has about 12,000 neurons. Axons from the locus coeruleus innervate just about every part of the brain: the entire cerebral cortex, the thalamus and hypothalamus, the olfactory bulb, the cerebellum, the midbrain, and the spinal cord. Just one of its neurons can make more than 250,000 synapses, and that cell can have one axon branch in the *cerebral* cortex and another in the *cerebellar* cortex! Locus coeruleus cells seem to be involved in the regulation of attention, arousal, and sleep-wake cycles, as well as in learning and memory, anxiety and pain, mood, and brain metabolism. Recordings from awake rats and monkeys in behavioral studies show that locus coeruleus neurons are best activated by new, unexpected, nonpainful sensory stimuli in the animal's environment. They are least active when the animals are not vigilant, just sitting around quietly digesting a meal. The locus coeruleus may participate in general arousal of the brain during interesting events in the outside world.

Serotonin-containing neurons are mostly clustered within the nine **raphe nuclei** (see Fig. 12–8*B*). Raphe means "ridge" or "seam" in Greek, and indeed, the raphe nuclei lie to either side of the midline of the brain stem. Each nucleus projects to different regions of the brain, and together they innervate most of the CNS in the same diffuse way as the locus coeruleus neurons. Similar to neurons of the locus coeruleus, cells of the raphe nuclei fire most rapidly during wakefulness, when an animal is aroused and active. Raphe neurons are quietest during certain stages of sleep. The locus coeruleus and the raphe nuclei are part of a venerable concept called the **ascending reticular activating system**, which implicates the reticular "core" of the brain stem in processes that arouse and awaken the forebrain. Raphe neurons seem to be intimately involved in the control of sleep-wake cycles, as well as the different stages of sleep. Serotonergic raphe neurons have also been implicated in the control of mood and certain types of emotional behavior. Many hallucinogenic drugs, such as LSD, apparently exert their effects through interaction with serotonergic systems. Serotonin may also be involved in clinical depression; some of the

A   SPATIALLY FOCUSED   **B**   WIDELY DIVERGENT

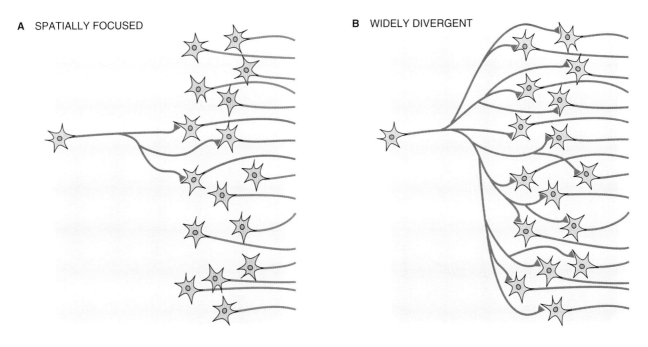

FIGURE 12–7. Synaptic connections.

most effective drugs now used to treat depression (e.g., fluoxetine [Prozac]) are potent blockers of serotonin reuptake and thus prolong its action in the brain.

Although **dopamine**-containing neurons are scattered throughout the CNS, two closely related groups of dopaminergic cells have characteristics of the diffuse modulatory systems (see Fig. 12–8C). One of these groups is the **substantia nigra** in the midbrain. Its cells project axons to the striatum, a part of the basal ganglia, and they somehow facilitate the initiation of voluntary movement. Degeneration of the dopamine-containing cells in the substantia nigra produces the progressively worsening motor disorders of Parkinson's disease. Another set of dopaminergic neurons lies in the **ventral tegmental area** of the midbrain; these neurons innervate the part of the forebrain that includes the prefrontal cortex and parts of the limbic system. They have been implicated in neural systems that mediate reinforcement or reward, as well as in aspects of drug addiction and psychiatric disorders, most notably schizophrenia. Members of the class of antipsychotic drugs called neuroleptics are antagonists of certain dopamine receptors.

Acetylcholine is the familiar transmitter of the neuromuscular junction and the autonomic nervous system. Within the brain are two major diffuse modulatory cholinergic systems: the **basal forebrain complex** (which innervates the hippocampus and all of the neocortex) and the **pontomesencephalotegmental cholinergic complex** (which innervates the dorsal thalamus and parts of the forebrain) (see Fig. 12–8D). The functions of these systems are obscure, but interest has been fueled by evidence that they are involved in the regulation of general brain excitability during arousal and sleep-wake cycles, as well as perhaps learning and memory formation.

Collectively, the diffuse modulatory systems may be viewed as general regulators of brain function, much as

the autonomic nervous system (see Chapter 15) regulates the organ systems of the body. Because their axons spread so widely within the CNS, the few modulatory neurons can have an inordinately strong influence on behavior.

Electrical Synapses Serve Specialized Functions in the Mammalian Nervous System

Many cells are coupled to one another through gap junctions. The large and unselective gap-junction channels (p. 164) allow ion currents to flow in both directions (in most types of gap junctions) or unidirectionally (in rare types). It follows from Ohm's law that if two cells are coupled by gap junctions and they have different membrane voltages, current will flow from one cell into the other (see Fig. 6–18C). If the first cell generates an action potential, current will flow through the gap junction channels and depolarize the second cell; this type of current flow, for example, is the basis for conduction of excitation across cardiac muscle. Such an arrangement has all the earmarks of a synapse, and indeed, when gap junctions interconnect neurons, we describe them as electrical synapses.

Electrical synapses would seem to have many advantages over chemical synapses: they are extremely fast and limited only by the time constants of the systems involved, they use relatively little metabolic energy or molecular machinery, they are highly reliable, and they can be bidirectional. In certain species, electrical synapses have been identified occasionally in the cerebral cortex, at scattered sites in the brain stem and hypothalamus, between certain motor neurons controlling eye movements, and in a few other places. However, in all these areas, they are vastly outnumbered by chemical synapses. Gap

FIGURE 12–8. Four diffusely connected systems of central neurons using modulatory transmitters. *A,* Neurons containing norepinephrine are located in the locus coeruleus and innervate nearly every part of the central nervous system. *B,* Neurons containing serotonin are located in two groups of raphe nuclei and project to most of the brain. *C,* Neurons containing dopamine are located in the substantia nigra (and these project to the striatum) and the ventral tegmental area of the midbrain (and these project to the prefrontal cortex the limbic system). *D,* Neurons containing acetylcholine are located in the basal forebrain complex, which includes the septal nuclei and nucleus basalis. The neurons project to the hippocampus and the neocortex. Other acetylcholine-containing neurons originate in the pontomesencephalotegmental cholinergic complex and project to the dorsal thalamus and part of the forebrain.

junctions universally interconnect the photoreceptors of the retina, the astrocytic glia (p. 414) of all parts of the CNS, and most cells early in development.

Why are chemical synapses, as complex and relatively slow as they are, so much more prevalent than electrical synapses in the mature brain? Comparative studies suggest several reasons for the predominance of chemical synapses among mammalian neurons. The first is **amplification**. Electrical synapses do not amplify the signal passed from one cell to the next; they can only degrade it. Therefore, if a presynaptic cell is small relative to its coupled postsynaptic cell, the current that it can generate through an electrical synapse will also be small, and thus

"synaptic strength" will be low. By contrast, a small bolus of neurotransmitter from a chemical synapse can trigger an amplifying cascade of molecular events that can cause a relatively large postsynaptic change.

A second advantage of chemical synapses is their ability to generate inhibition. **Inhibition** is difficult (although not impossible in specialized cases) to achieve in electrical synapses. Chemical synapses perform this function with ease, by simply opening channels that are selective for ions with relatively negative equilibrium potential.

A third advantage of chemical synapses is that they can transmit information over a **broad time domain**. By using different transmitters, receptors, second messengers, and effectors, chemical synapses can produce a wide array of postsynaptic effects with time courses ranging from a few milliseconds to minutes and even hours. The effects of electrical synapses are generally limited to the time course of the presynaptic event.

A fourth advantage of chemical synapses is that they are champions of **plasticity**; their strength can be a strong function of recent neural activity, and they can therefore play a role in learning and memory, which are essential to the success of vertebrate species.

It might also be noted that the few perceived advantages of electrical synapses may be more apparent than real. Bidirectionality is clearly not useful in many neural circuits, and the difference in speed of transmission may be too small to matter in most cases. Electrical synapses serve important, but specialized functions in the nervous system. They seem to be most prevalent in neural circuits in which speed or high degrees of synchrony are at a premium: quick-escape systems in invertebrates or the fine coordination of rapid eye movements in vertebrates. They are also very effective in diffusely spreading current through large networks of cells, which appears to be their function in photoreceptors and glia.

NEUROTRANSMITTER SYSTEMS OF THE BRAIN

The mammalian nervous system uses dozens of different neurotransmitters that act on more than 100 types of receptors; these receptors stimulate numerous second-messenger systems, which in turn regulate several dozen ion channels and enzymes. We call these pathways of synaptic signalling the *transmitter systems*. It is not enough to know the identity of a transmitter to predict its effect—you also need to know the nature of the components that it interacts with, and these components may vary from one part of the brain to another and even between parts of a single neuron. The components of the transmitter systems are extremely complex. This subchapter introduces the intricate and vital web of neurotransmitters. The clinical importance of the subject is hard to overstate. It is likely that most drugs that alter mental function do so by interacting with neurotransmitter systems in the brain. Disorders of neurotransmitter systems are also implicated in many devastating brain disorders, such as schizophrenia, depression, epilepsy, Parkinson disease, the damage of stroke, and drug addiction.

Most of the Brain's Transmitters Are Common Biochemicals

Most neurotransmitters are similar or identical to the standard chemicals of life, the same substances that all cells use for metabolism. Transmitter molecules can be large or small. The small ones, such as the **amino acids** glutamate, aspartate, GABA, and glycine, are also simple foods (Fig. 12–9A). Cells use amino acids as an energy source and to build essential proteins, but they have co-opted these common molecules for essential and widespread messenger functions in the brain. Another impor-

tant class of small neurotransmitters is the amines, including the **monoamines** (e.g., ACh, serotonin, and histamine) listed in Figure 12–9B and the **catecholamines** (e.g., dopamine, norepinephrine, and epinephrine) listed in Figure 12–9C. Neurons synthesize these small transmitters by adding only a few chemical steps to the glucose and amino acid pathways that are present in every cell. **Purine derivatives** can also be important transmitters. For example, a key molecule of cell metabolism that has recently achieved neurotransmitter status is adenosine triphosphate (ATP). ATP is the major chemical intermediate of energy metabolism and is present in many synaptic vesicles. It is also released from various synapses in the central and peripheral nervous systems. ATP appears to be the transmitter responsible for sympathetic vasoconstriction in small arteries and arterioles, for example. ATP acts on a variety of nucleotide receptors, both ionotropic and metabotropic. Adenosine is also a transmitter in the CNS.

The large-molecule transmitters, which constitute a much more numerous group, are proteins or small bits of protein called **neuroactive peptides**. A few of the better-studied neuropeptides are shown in Figure 12–10. Many were originally identified in non-neural tissues such as the gut or endocrine glands, and were only later found in nerve terminals of the brain or peripheral nervous system. They vary in size from two–amino acid peptides to large polypeptides. Among the neuroactive peptides are the endorphins (*endogenous* substances with m*orphine*-like actions), which include small peptides called enkephalins. The term "opioids" includes all substances with a morphine-like pharmacology—the endorphins (endogenous), as well as morphine and heroin (exogenous).

The synthesis of most neuropeptides begins like any other secretory protein (p. 36), with the ribosome-directed assembly of a large **prehormone**. The prehormone is then cleaved to form a smaller **prohormone** in the Golgi apparatus and further reduced into small active neuropeptides that are packaged into vesicles. Thus, the synthesis of neuropeptides differs significantly from that of the small transmitters.

In summary, then, the neurotransmitters consist of a dozen or so small molecules, plus 50 to 100 peptides of various size. The small transmitters are, as a rule, each stored and released by separate sets of neurons. The peptides, however, are usually stored and released from the same neurons as one of the small transmitters (Table 12–1), an arrangement called **co-localization** of neurotransmitters. Thus, GABA may be paired with somatostatin in some synapses, serotonin and enkephalin in others, and so on. The colocalized transmitters may be released together, but of course each acts on its own receptors.

One of the most unique of the substances proposed as a transmitter is a gaseous molecule, the labile free radical **nitric oxide** (NO). **Carbon monoxide** has also been suggested to be a transmitter, although evidence thus far is meager. NO is synthesized from L-arginine by many cells of the body (p. 110), and it has powerful biologic effects. As a neurotransmitter, NO may have unique functions. It seems to be released from both presynaptic and what we normally think of as *post*synaptic neurons. Because NO is *not* packaged into vesicles, its release does not require an

A AMINO ACIDS

C CATECHOLAMINES

B MONOAMINES

FIGURE 12–9. Biosynthesis of some common small transmitter molecules.

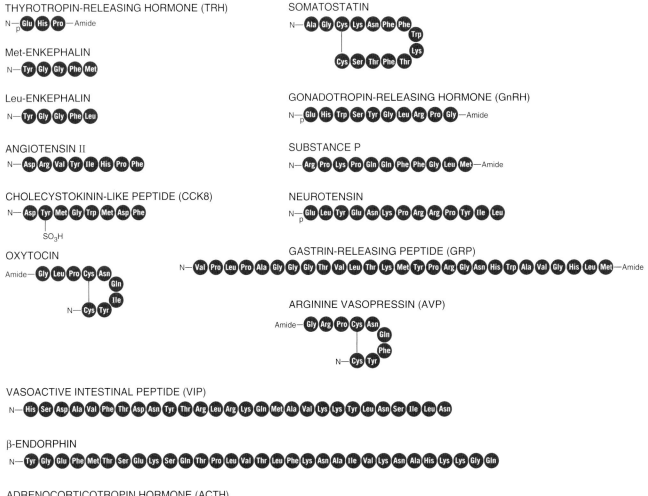

FIGURE 12–10. Structure of some neuroactive peptides. All peptides are presented with their NH_2 termini (i.e., the first to be synthesized) to the left, as is now customary for proteins in general. However, note that for many of the peptide hormones, the amino-acid residues were numbered before this convention was established. The *p* on the amino-terminal glutamate on some of these peptides stands for "pyroglutamate."

increase in $[Ca^{2+}]_i$, although its synthesis does (Fig. 12–11). NO may sometimes act as a retrograde messenger, that is, from postsynaptic to presynaptic structures. Because NO is small and membrane permeable, it can diffuse about much more freely than other transmitter molecules, even penetrating through one cell to affect another beyond it. On the other hand, NO is evanescent, and it breaks down very rapidly. The functions of gaseous transmitters are now being vigorously studied and hotly debated.

Obviously, most of the chemicals we call "neurotransmitters" also exist in non-neural parts of the body. Each chemical may serve dual purposes in that it can mediate communication in the nervous system but do something similar or even entirely different elsewhere. Amino acids, of course, are used to make protein everywhere. NO is a local hormone that relaxes the smooth muscle in blood vessels (p. 478). Surprisingly, the cells with the highest ACh levels are in the cornea of the eye, although corneal cells lack specific receptors for ACh. It is not clear what ACh does for corneal cells, but it almost certainly is not

acting as a "transmitter." One of the most interesting nonmessenger functions of transmitter molecules is their role in the development of the brain, even before synapses have appeared. At these early stages of development, transmitters may regulate cell proliferation, migration, and differentiation, somehow helping to form the brain before they help operate it.

Synaptic Transmitters Can Stimulate, Inhibit, or Modulate the Postsynaptic Neuron

Each neuromuscular junction has a simple and stereotyped job: when an action potential fires in the motor neuron, the junction must reliably excite its muscle cell to fire an action potential and contract. Decisions about muscle contractions (where, when, and how much) are made within the CNS, and the neuromuscular junction exists simply to communicate that decision to the muscle unambiguously. To perform this function, neuromuscular transmission has evolved to be very strong so that it is

TABLE 12–1

EXAMPLES OF NEUROACTIVE PEPTIDES THAT COLOCALIZE WITH SMALL-MOLECULE NEUROTRANSMITTERS*

SMALL MOLECULE	PEPTIDE
ACh	Enkephalin VIP CGRP Substance P Somatostatin and enkephalin GnRH Neurotensin Galanin
Dopamine	CCK Enkephalin Neurotensin
Epinephrine	Enkephalin Neuropeptide Y Neurotensin Substance P
GABA	CCK Enkephalin Somatostatin Neuropeptide Y Substance P VIP
Glutamate	Substance P
Glycine	Neurotensin
Norepinephrine	Enkephalin Neuropeptide Y Neurotensin Somatostatin Vasopressin
Serotonin	CCK Enkephalin Substance P and TRH TRH

*Each row on the right gives a peptide or combination of peptides that co-localize with the small molecule in the row on the left.

ACh, acetylcholine; CCK, cholecystokinin; CGRP, calcitonin-gene–related peptide; GABA, gamma-aminobutyric acid; GnRH, gonadotropin-releasing hormone. TRH, thyrotropin-releasing hormone; VIP, vasoactive intestinal polypeptide.

Data from Hall ZW: An Introduction to Molecular Neurobiology. Sunderland, Mass, Sinauer, 1992.

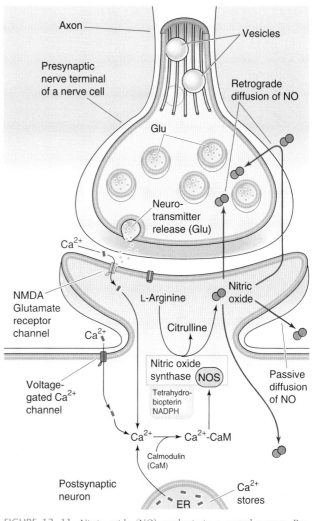

FIGURE 12–11. Nitric oxide (NO) synthesis in a central neuron. Presynaptic glutamate release triggers the entry of Ca^{2+} through NMDA glutamate receptor channels or voltage-gated Ca^{2+} channels. Via calmodulin (CaM), Ca^{2+} stimulates nitric oxide synthase (NOS; p. 110). NO diffuses out and through cells to affect presynaptic and postsynaptic elements of the same synapse or of nearby synapses. NADPH, nicotinamide adenine dinucleotide phosphate; NMDA, N-methyl-D-aspartate.

fail-safe under even the most extreme of physiological conditions.

Synapses between neurons usually have a more subtle role in communication, and they use a variety of mechanisms to accomplish their more complex tasks. Like neuromuscular junctions, some neuron-neuron synapses (**excitatory**) can rapidly excite. However, other synapses (**inhibitory**) can cause profound inhibition by decreasing postsynaptic excitability directly (postsynaptic inhibition). In a third broad class of synapse (**modulatory**), the synapse often has little or no direct effect of its own but, instead, regulates or modifies the effect of other excitatory or inhibitory synapses by acting on either presynaptic or postsynaptic membranes. These three basic types of neural synapses are exemplified by their input to the *pyramidal neuron* of the cerebral cortex. In the example shown in Figure 12–12, a pyramidal neuron in the visual cortex receives an excitatory synaptic input from the thalamus (using glutamate as the neurotransmitter), an inhibitory synaptic input from an interneuron (using GABA as the neurotransmitter), and a modulatory input from the locus coeruleus (using norepinephrine as the neurotransmitter).

EXCITATORY SYNAPSES. Pyramidal cells receive excitatory synapses from many sources, including the axons of the thalamus. Most fast *excitatory synapses* in the brain use **glutamate** or **aspartate** as their transmitter, and the thalamus-to-cortex synapses are no exception (see Fig. 12–12). Both amino acids have similar effects on the postsynaptic excitatory amino acid receptors, and it has

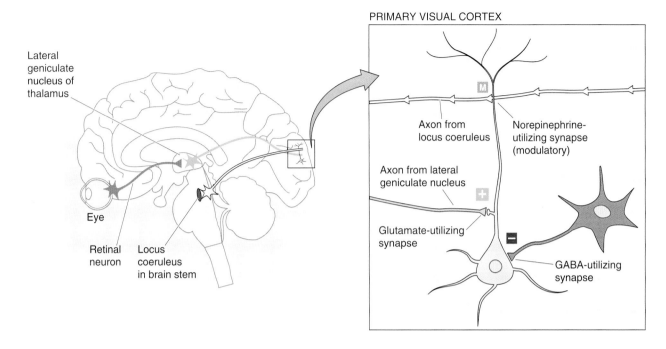

FIGURE 12–12. Synaptic circuitry of the visual cortex. Visual pathways that originate in the retina activate neurons in the lateral geniculate nucleus of the thalamus. These glutamate-containing neurons in turn synapse on cortical pyramidal neurons and produce some *excitation*. Also within the primary visual cortex, a GABA-containing neuron mediates localized *inhibition*. Small cells in the locus coeruleus, a brainstem nucleus, make widely divergent connections onto cortical neurons and release norepinephrine and thus produce *modulation*. GABA, γ-aminobutyric acid.

proved difficult to determine which excitatory amino acid is used in which synapse. For convenience, these types of synapses are often presumptuously referred to as "**glutamatergic**." These excitatory amino acids bind to a group of fast, ligand-gated cation channels. When activated by synaptic glutamate, glutamate-gated channels generate an **excitatory postsynaptic potential** (EPSP) that is very similar to the one produced by ACh at the neuromuscular junction (p. 212), except that it is much smaller than the EPSP in muscle. In the example shown in Figure 12–13 (*left side*), glutamate produces the EPSP by activating a nonselective cation channel that has about the same conductance for Na^+ and K^+. Thus, the **reversal potential** (p. 153) of the EPSP is 0 mV, about midway between the equilibrium potential for Na^+ (E_{Na}) and that for K^+ (E_K). An EPSP from the activation of a *single* glutaminergic synapse peaks at 0.01 to 1 mV (depending on many factors, including the size of the postsynaptic cell and the size of the synapse), whereas one neuromuscular EPSP reaches a peak of about 40 mV—a difference of 40- to 4000-fold. Obviously, most glutaminergic synapses are not designed to be fail-safe. It takes the summation of EPSPs from many such synapses to depolarize a postsynaptic neuron to the threshold for triggering an action potential.

INHIBITORY SYNAPSES. Skeletal muscle cells in vertebrates have only excitatory synapses. On the other hand, virtually all central neurons have numerous excitatory *and* inhibitory synapses. Thus, the excitability of most neurons is governed by the dynamic balance of excitation and inhibition at any moment. The inhibitory transmitters

GABA and **glycine** are the transmitters at the large majority of inhibitory synapses. Indeed, the inhibitory synapse between the interneuron and the pyramidal cell in Figure 12–12 uses GABA. Both GABA and glycine bind to receptors that gate Cl^--selective channels (p. 215). Cl^- conductance usually has an inhibitory influence because the equilibrium potential for Cl^- (E_{Cl}) in neurons is near or slightly negative to the resting potential of the neuron. Thus, the reversal potential for the Cl^--mediated **inhibitory postsynaptic potential** (IPSP) is the same as the E_{Cl}. If Cl^- conductance increases, the membrane potential (V_m) has a tendency to move toward E_{Cl} (see Fig. 12–13, *right side*). The effect is inhibitory because it tends to oppose other factors (mainly EPSPs) that might otherwise move the V_m to the threshold for an action potential.

MODULATORY SYNAPSES. The nervous system is influenced by many forms of *synaptic modulation*, and their mechanisms will be covered in more detail later. As an example, consider the axons arising from the *locus coeruleus*, which synapse widely on pyramidal cells in the cerebral cortex (see Figs. 12–8A and 12–12). These axons release the transmitter **norepinephrine**, a classic modulator with multiple effects. Norepinephrine acts on β-adrenergic receptors in the pyramidal cell membrane (it may also act on α receptors at the same time). Unlike the actions of the fast amino acid forms of synaptic transmission, this effect of norepinephrine by itself has little or no obvious influence on the activity of a resting neuron. However, a cell exposed to norepinephrine will react more powerfully when it is stimulated by a strong excitatory input (usually by glutaminergic synapses), as shown

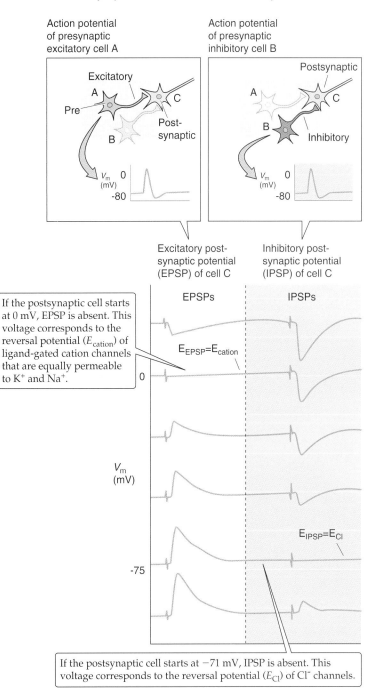

FIGURE 12–13. Voltage dependence of EPSPs and IPSPs of the nervous system. An excitatory presynaptic neuron (cell A) and an inhibitory presynaptic neuron (cell B) both synapse on a third neuron (cell C). In this experiment, the investigators injected enough constant current into cell C to initially set the V_m to each of the six values shown in the figure. For each record, the experimenter first stimulated the stimulatory presynaptic neuron to produce an EPSP in the postsynaptic neuron and then stimulated the inhibitory presynaptic neuron to produce an IPSP. These EPSPs and IPSPs reflect the activities of multiple synapses onto cell C. The reversal potential for the EPSP is about 0 mV (i.e., stimulating the stimulatory presynaptic neuron has no effect) because Na^+ and K^+ conduct through the channel equally well. The reversal potential for the IPSP is at about −71 mV (i.e., stimulating the inhibitory presynaptic neuron has no effect). This value is E_{Cl}, indicating that the IPSP is mediated by a Cl^- channel.

in Figure 12–14. Thus, norepinephrine *modulates* the cell's response to other inputs.

The molecular mechanisms of **neuromodulators** are complex and diverse, but all begin with a G-protein–coupled membrane receptor that activates an intracellular signal cascade (p. 92). Binding of norepinephrine to the β-adrenergic receptor stimulates the intracellular enzyme adenylyl cyclase, which increases intracellular levels of cyclic adenosine monophosphate (cAMP, the second messenger), which in turn stimulates other enzymes to increase their rates of phosphorylation. Within the cortical neuron, phosphorylation of one or more types of K^+ channel decreases the probability of the channels being open (p. 162). Fewer open K^+ channels mean higher membrane resistance, greater excitability, and less adaptation of spike firing rates during prolonged stimuli. This K^+ channel pathway is but one of the many mechanisms by which norepinephrine can affect cells. Other effects are generated when norepinephrine activates other subtypes of adrenergic receptors and thus different second-messenger systems coupled to different channels or enzymes. Modulatory transmitters allow the nervous system tremendous potential and flexibility to vary its state of excitability.

FIGURE 12–14. Modulatory effect of norepinephrine. *A,* Injecting a neuron from the hippocampus with a sustained depolarizing current pulse leads to a "phasic" action-potential response: frequent spiking at the beginning but adaptation as the depolarizing current pulse is maintained. *B,* The application of norepinephrine causes the spiking that is elicited by the depolarizing current pulse to be sustained longer ("tonic"). *C,* The cell returns to its control state as in *A.* (Data from Madison DV, Nicholl RA: Actions of noradrenaline recorded intracellularly in rat hippocampal CA1 pyramidal neurones, in vitro. J Physiol 372:221–244, 1986.)

G Proteins May Affect Ion Channels Directly, or Indirectly Through Second Messengers

G-protein–coupled receptors exist in every cell (p. 92). In the preceding section we described one example, the receptor for norepinephrine and its second-messenger–mediated effect on certain K+ channels. However, norepinephrine alone has at least five major receptor types—two α receptors and three β receptors—that act on numerous effectors. In fact, each transmitter has multiple G-protein–coupled receptors, and their effects are complex and interactive and engage almost all aspects of cell function via several intracellular messenger systems. The various G-protein–coupled receptors can recognize a wide range of transmitter types, from small molecules to peptides.

Activated G proteins can trigger a wide array of responses at synapses by either of the two general pathways introduced in Chapter 4: (1) the G protein may modulate the gating of an ion channel directly or by a very short second-messenger pathway, and (2) the G protein may activate one of several enzyme systems that involve second messengers and subsequent signal cascades.

The first—and simplest—G-protein cascade involves a very direct receptor G-protein–channel linkage and is sometimes called the **membrane-delimited pathway**. In this case the G protein may be the only messenger between the receptor and the effector. A variety of neurotransmitter–G-protein–channel systems use this pathway. For example, in heart muscle ACh binds to a certain type of muscarinic ACh receptor (M2) that activates a G protein, the βγ subunits of which in turn cause a K+ channel to open. (We discuss this example later in Figure 12–15B.) Other receptors in various cells can modulate other K+ and Ca2+ channels in a similar way.

One advantage of the membrane-delimited pathway is that it is relatively fast, beginning within 30 to 100 msec—not quite as fast as a ligand-gated channel, which uses no intermediary between receptor and channel, but faster than the many-messenger cascades described next. The membrane-delimited pathway is also very localized in comparison to the other cascades. Because the G protein cannot diffuse very far within the membrane, only chan-

nels nearby can be affected. This type of coupling also allows flexibility because many types of receptors can be coupled to a variety of channels by using the appropriate G-protein intermediate.

The other general type of G-protein signalling involves enzyme systems and second messengers, often diffusing through the cytoplasm, to influence an ion channel. The terminology deserves some clarification. Traditionally, the small, diffusible intracellular chemicals (e.g., cAMP, inositol 1,4,5-triphosphate [IP3]) that help carry the message between a transmitter receptor and a channel are called *second messengers.* The transmitter itself is counted as the first messenger, but notice that by this logic the receptor is not a messenger at all, even though it transfers a signal from the neurotransmitter to a G protein. The G protein is also not counted as a messenger, nor are the various enzymes that may come before and after the traditional "second messenger" in any signal cascade. Different cascades involve different numbers of messengers, but obviously, most have many more than two! Alas, the terminology is entrenched, although when we speak of "second messengers," one should remember that a multiple-messenger cascade is almost always involved. As an added complication, two or more cascades, each with different types of messengers, may sometimes be activated by one type of receptor (an example of *divergence,* see later).

In Chapter 4, we discussed three of these longer, and slower, G-protein signal cascades: (1) the adenylyl cyclase pathway, (2) the phospholipase C pathway, and (3) the phospholipase A2 pathway. Each is activated by a different set of receptors, each uses a different G protein, and each generates different intracellular messengers. Some of these messengers dissolve in the watery cytoplasm, whereas others diffuse within the fatty lipid bilayer. The final link in most of the messenger cascades is a **kinase**.

In a well-known example, cAMP binds to cAMP-dependent protein kinase (protein kinase A [PKA]), which then phosphorylates amino acids on K+ or Ca2+ channels in the membrane. The addition of phosphate groups to the channel protein changes its conformation slightly, which may strongly influence its probability of being open (p.

162). In Chapter 20 we discuss the stimulation of the *β*-adrenergic receptor by norepinephrine, which ultimately results in a stronger heartbeat through phosphorylation and opening of myocardial voltage-gated Ca²⁺ channels. By contrast, in the pyramidal cell of the hippocampus, stimulation of *β*-adrenergic receptors also results in an increase in cAMP, but it has no influence on the cell's Ca²⁺ channels. Instead, it inhibits some of its K⁺ channels. As a result, the cell can fire more action potentials during prolonged stimuli (see Fig. 12–14).

If transmitter-stimulated kinases were allowed to madly phosphorylate without some method of reversing the process, all proteins would quickly become saturated with phosphates and further regulation would become impossible. Protein phosphatases save the day. They act rapidly to remove phosphate groups (p. 98), and thus the degree of channel phosphorylation at any moment depends on the dynamic balance of phosphorylation and dephosphorylation.

Signalling Cascades Allow Amplification, Regulation, and a Long Duration of Transmitter Responses

At this point you may be wondering about the perversity of such complex, interconnected, indirect messenger cascades. Do these long chains of command have any bene-fit? Why not use simple, fast ligand-gated channels (Fig. 12–15A) for all transmitter purposes? In fact, complex messenger cascades seem to have advantages.

One important advantage is *amplification*. When activated, one ligand-gated channel is just that: one ion channel in one place. However, activate one G-protein–coupled receptor and you potentially influence many channels. Signal amplification can occur at several places in the cascade (p. 91), and a few transmitter molecules can generate a sizable cellular effect. One stimulated receptor can activate perhaps 10 to 20 G proteins, each of which can activate a channel by a membrane-delimited pathway such as the *βγ* pathway (Fig. 12–15B). Alternatively, the *α* subunit of one G protein can activate an adenylyl cyclase, which can make many cAMP molecules, and the cAMP molecules can spread to activate many kinases; each kinase can then phosphorylate many channels (see Figure 12–15C). If all cascade components were tied together in a clump, signalling would be severely limited. The use of small messengers that can diffuse quickly (e.g., cAMP) also allows signalling at a distance, over a wide stretch of cell membrane. Signalling cascades also provide many sites for further *regulation*, as well as interaction between cascades. Finally, signal cascades can generate very *long-lasting chemical changes* in cells, which may form the basis for, among other things, a lifetime of memories.

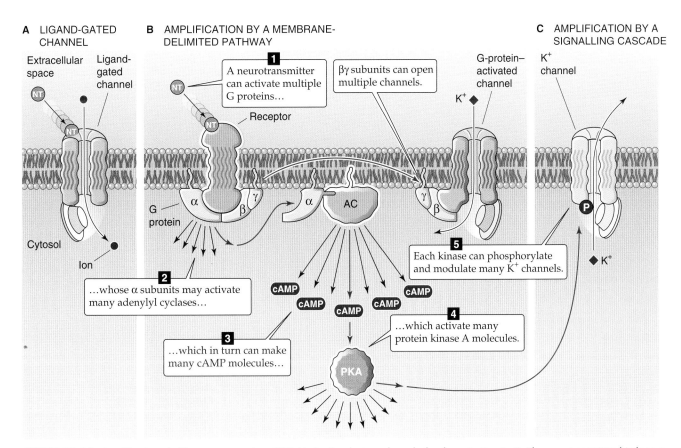

FIGURE 12–15. Amplification. *A*, The neurotransmitter (NT) binds directly to a channel, thereby activating it. *B*, The neurotransmitter binds to a receptor that in turn activates 10 to 20 G proteins. In this example, the *βγ* subunits directly activate K⁺ channels. In addition, the activated *α* subunits each activate an adenylyl cyclase molecule, each of which produces many cAMP molecules that activate protein kinase A (PKA). *C*, Each activated PKA can phosphorylate and thereby modulate many channels. AC, adenylyl cyclase; cAMP, cyclic adenosine monophosphate.

Neurotransmitters May Have Both Convergent and Divergent Effects

Two of the most common neurotransmitters in the brain are glutamate and GABA. Either molecule can bind to any of several kinds of receptors, and each of these receptors can mediate a different effect. This ability of one transmitter to activate more than one type of receptor is sometimes called divergence.

Divergence is the rule among neurotransmitters. Every well-studied transmitter can activate multiple receptor subtypes, and recent experience indicates that the number of receptors will continue to escalate as the powerful methods of molecular biology continue to be applied to each system. Divergence means that one transmitter can affect different neurons (or even different parts of the same neuron) in very different ways. It also means that *if* a transmitter affects different neurons in different ways, it *could* be because each neuron has a different type of receptor. However, among transmitter systems that use second messengers, divergence may also occur at points beyond the level of the receptor. For example, norepi-

nephrine can turn on or turn off a variety of ion channels in different cells (Fig. 12–16A). Some of these effects occur because norepinephrine activates different receptors, but some of these receptors may each activate more than one second messenger, *or* a single second messenger (e.g., cAMP) may activate a kinase that influences numerous different channels. Divergence may occur at any stage in the cascade of transmitter effects.

Neurotransmitters can also exhibit **convergence** of effects. This property means that multiple transmitters, each activating their own receptor type, converge on a single type of ion channel in a single cell. For example, some pyramidal cells of the hippocampus have GABA$_B$, 5-HT$_{1A}$, A1 (specific for adenosine), and SS (specific for somatostatin) receptors, all of which activate the same K$^+$ channel (see Fig. 12–16B). Furthermore, in the same cells, norepinephrine, ACh, 5-HT, corticotropin-releasing hormone, and histamine all converge on and depress the slow Ca^{2+}-activated K$^+$ channels. Analogous to divergence, the molecular site of convergence may occur at a common second-messenger system, or different second messengers may converge on the same ion channel.

A   DIVERGENT TRANSMITTER ACTIONS

FIGURE 12–16. Divergence and convergence of transmitter effects on channels. *A,* One transmitter, norepinephrine in this case, can activate multiple receptors, which stimulate different G-protein/second messengers, which in turn either stimulate or depress the gating of many types of ion channels. I$_{AHP}$ stands for afterhyperpolarization current, which is mediated by a Ca^{2+}-activated K$^+$ channel. I$_h$ stands for hyperpolarization-activated cation current. *B,* Multiple transmitters bind to their specific receptors and, via the same or different second-messenger systems, influence the same set of ion channels. ACh, acetylcholine; DA, dopamine; Enk, enkephalin; GABA, γ-aminobutyric acid; 5-HT, 5-hydroxytryptamine (serotonin); NE, norepinephrine; SS, somatostatin; SSTR, somatostatin receptor.

B   CONVERGENT TRANSMITTER ACTIONS

Divergence and convergence can occur simultaneously within neurotransmitter systems, and many of them have chemical feedback regulation built in as well.

FAST, AMINO ACID–MEDIATED SYNAPSES IN THE CENTRAL NERVOUS SYSTEM

Fast, amino acid–mediated synapses account for most of the neural activity that we associate with specific information processing in the brain: events directly responsible for sensory perception, motor control, and cognition, for example. Glutamate-mediated excitation and GABA-mediated inhibition have been intensively studied. In physiological terms, these are also the best understood of the brain's synapses, and this section describes their function.

As a rule, postsynaptic events are more easily measured than presynaptic events, thus we know more about them. Of course, by measuring postsynaptic events we also have a window onto the functions of the presynaptic terminal, and in fact this is usually the best view we can get of presynaptic functions. For this reason, we begin our description with the downstream, postsynaptic side of the synapse and then work backward to the presynaptic side.

Most Excitatory Postsynaptic Potentials in the Brain Are Mediated by Two Types of Glutamate-Gated Channels

Most glutamate-mediated synapses generate an EPSP with two distinct components, one much faster than the other. Both are triggered by the same presynaptic terminal releasing a single bolus of transmitter, but the two EPSP components are generated by different types of ion channels that are gated by distinct postsynaptic receptors—a case of transmitter divergence. The behavior of these channels helps understand the characteristics of the EPSP.

Glutamate can act on four major classes of receptors: one is a G-protein–coupled or *metabotropic* receptor, and three of them are ion channels or *ionotropic* receptors. As noted earlier, **metabotropic receptors** (mGluRs—the "m" stands for "metabotropic") have seven membrane-spanning segments and are linked to heterotrimeric G proteins (Fig. 12–17A). At least eight metabotropic receptors have been identified, and comparisons of their primary structure have been used to infer the evolutionary relationships among receptor subunits (see Fig. 12–17B). The mGluRs form three groups that differ in their sequence similarity, pharmacology and associated signal-transduction systems.

The three classes of **ionotropic glutamate receptors** are the AMPA, NMDA, and kainate receptors (Table 12–2). By definition, each is activated by binding glutamate, but their pharmacology differs. The receptor names are derived from their relatively specific agonists: **AMPA** stands for α-amino-3-hydroxy-5-methyl-4-isoxazole propionic acid. The AMPA receptor is sometimes called the

"quisqualate" receptor, after another of its agonists, or even the "quisqualate/AMPA" receptor. **NMDA** stands for N-methyl-D-aspartate. The **kainate** receptor is named for one of its agonists, kainic acid, and can also be activated by domoic acid. The three ionotropic glutamate receptors can also be distinguished by their selective antagonists: *AMPA* and kainate receptors but not NMDA receptors are blocked by drugs such as **CNQX** (6-cyano-7-nitroquinoxaline-2,3-dione). Moreover, AMPA receptors can be specifically antagonized by 2,3-benzodiazepine derivatives such as GYKI53655. No specific antagonists for *kainate* receptors are known. Finally, *NMDA* receptors, but not AMPA and kainate receptors, are blocked by **APV** (2-amino-5-phosphonovaleric acid).

At least 22 ionotropic glutamate receptor cDNAs—plus a variety of splice variants—have been cloned, and more are likely to come. Each of these cDNAs represents a monomer with a large extracellular glutamate-binding domain, followed by a transmembrane segment, a loop that partially enters the membrane from the cytosolic side, and then two more transmembrane segments (see Fig. 12–17C). The loop appears to line the channel pore. Based on kinetic studies, the channel appears to consist of a tetramer of four subunits. Comparisons of primary structures can be used to infer evolutionary relationships among receptor monomeric subunits. Figure 12–17D shows the hypothesized phylogenetic tree for the three classes of ionotropic glutamate receptors, with the major subtypes clustered together. Note that the various NMDA receptor subunits (e.g., NMDAR1, NMDAR2A to NMDAR2D) that combine to make the NMDA receptors are more closely related to each other than to the subunits (e.g., KA1, KA2, GluR5 to GluR7) that combine to make the kainate receptors or to the subunits (e.g., GluR1 to GluR4) that combine to make the AMPA receptors. The *metabotropic* and *ionotropic* glutamate receptors have separate family trees because although both receptor types bind glutamate, they are so different in structure that it is highly probable that they evolved from different ancestral protein lines.

As noted earlier, most glutamate-mediated synapses generate an EPSP with two temporal components (Fig. 12–18A, C). The two phases of the glutamate-mediated EPSP have different pharmacologic profiles, kinetics, voltage dependencies, ion dependencies, and permeabilities, and most importantly, they serve distinct functions in the brain. Pharmacologic analysis reveals that the faster phase is mediated by an AMPA-type glutamate receptor and the slower phase by an NMDA-type glutamate receptor. These glutamate-gated channels have been extensively studied with single-channel recording methods. Both AMPA and NMDA receptors have nearly equal permeability to Na^+ and K^+, but they differ in several ways.

AMPA-gated channels are found in most excitatory synapses in the brain, and they mediate fast excitation, with most receptor channels normally letting very little Ca^{2+} into cells. Their single-channel conductance is relatively low, about 15 pS, and they show little voltage dependence.

NMDA-gated channels have more complex behavior. They have higher conductance, around 50 pS, and much slower kinetics. The ion selectivity of NMDA channels is

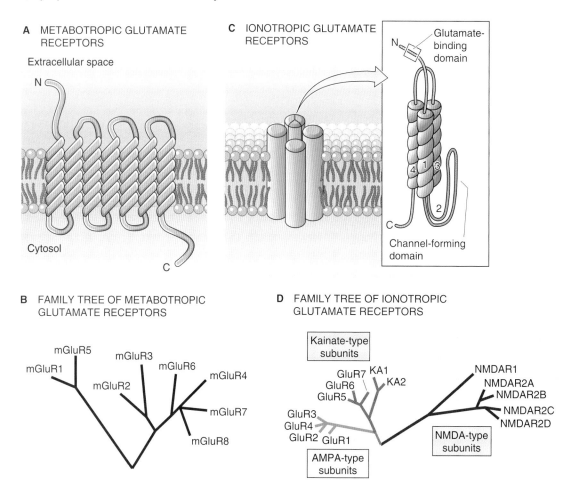

FIGURE 12–17. Comparison of ionotropic and metabotropic glutamate receptors. In *C*, the *inset* shows a prototypical subunit, with a large extracellular glutamate-binding domain, a membrane-spanning segment, a short loop that partially re-enters the membrane from the cytosolic side, and two more membrane-spanning segments. Four of these subunits appear to come together to form a single channel/receptor with a central pore. AMPA, α-amino-3-hydroxy-5-methyl-4-isoxazole propionic acid; NMDA, N-methyl-D-aspartate.

the key to their functions: permeability to Na^+ and K^+ causes depolarization and thus excitation of a cell, but their high permeability to Ca^{2+} allows them to influence $[Ca^{2+}]_i$ significantly. It is hard to overstate the importance of intracellular $[Ca^{2+}]$. Ca^{2+} can activate many enzymes, regulate the opening of a variety of channels, and affect the expression of genes. Excess Ca^{2+} can even precipitate the death of a cell.

The gating of NMDA channels is unusual: at normal resting voltage (about -70 mV), the channel is clogged by Mg^{2+}, and few ions pass through it; the Mg^{2+} pops out only when the membrane is depolarized above about

TABLE 12–2

IONOTROPIC GLUTAMATE RECEPTORS				
CLASS OF RECEPTOR	**AGONIST**	**ANTAGONIST**	**KINETICS**	**PERMEABILITY**
AMPA	α-Amino-3-hydroxy-5-methyl-4-isoxazole propionic acid	CNQX (6-cyano-7-nitroquinoxaline-2,3-dione) GYKI53655 (2,3-benzodiazepine derivatives)	Fast	Na^+, K^+ (Ca^{2+} in a few cases)
NMDA	N-methyl-D-aspartate	APV (2-amino-5-phosphonovaleric acid)	Slow	Na^+, K^+, Ca^{2+}
Kainate	Kainic acid Domoic acid	CNQX	Fast	Na^+, K^+

FIGURE 12–18. Glutamate-gated channels A, At most glutamate-mediated synapses, the EPSP (*red curve*) is the sum of two components: (1) a rapid component that is mediated by an AMPA receptor channel (*green curve*) and (2) a slow component that is mediated by an NMDA receptor channel (*orange curve*). In this example, in which the postsynaptic V_m is relatively negative, the contribution of the NMDA receptor channel is very small. B, At a relatively negative initial V_m in the postsynaptic cell, as in A, the NMDA receptor channel does not open. The AMPA receptor channel, which is independent of postsynaptic V_m, opens. The result is a fast depolarization. C, In this example, in which the postsynaptic V_m is relatively positive, the contribution of the NMDA receptor channel is fairly large. D, At a relatively positive initial V_m in the postsynaptic cell, as in C, glutamate activates both the AMPA- and the NMDA-receptor channels. The recruitment of the NMDA-receptor channels is important, because, unlike most AMPA-receptor channels, they allow the entry of Ca^{2+} and have slower kinetics. AMPA, α-amino-3-hydroxy-5-methyl-4-isoxazole propionic acid; NMDA, N-methyl-D-aspartate.

−60 mV. Thus, the NMDA channel is **voltage dependent**, in addition to being ligand gated; both glutamate and a relatively positive V_m are necessary for the channel to open. How do the NMDA-gated channels open? NMDA-gated channels coexist with AMPA-gated channels in many synapses of the brain. When the postsynaptic cell is at a relatively negative resting potential (Fig. 12–18A, B), the glutamate released from a synaptic terminal can open the AMPA-gated channel, which is voltage independent, but not the NMDA-gated channel. However,

when the postsynaptic cell is more depolarized because of the action of other synapses (Fig. 12–18C, D), the larger depolarization of the postsynaptic membrane now allows the NMDA-gated channel to open by relieving its Mg^{2+} block. Indeed, under natural conditions, the slower NMDA channels open only after the membrane has been sufficiently depolarized by the action of the faster AMPA channels from many simultaneously active synapses.

The physiological function of **kainate-gated channels** is still a mystery, although recent evidence suggests that they may contribute in a small way to some glutamate-mediated EPSPs. The kainate receptor channels may also exist on *presynaptic* GABAergic terminals, where they regulate release of the inhibitory transmitter (i.e., GABA).

Most Inhibitory Postsynaptic Potentials in the Brain Are Mediated by the GABA$_A$ Receptor, Which Is Activated by Several Classes of Drugs

GABA mediates the large majority of synaptic inhibition in the CNS, and glycine mediates most of the rest. Both the GABA$_A$ receptor and the glycine receptor are ionotropic receptors that are, in fact, Cl$^-$-selective channels. Note that GABA can also activate the relatively common GABA$_B$ receptor, which is a G-protein–coupled or *metabotropic* receptor that is linked to either the opening of K$^+$ channels or the suppression of Ca^{2+} channels. Finally, GABA can activate the ionotropic GABA$_C$ receptor, which is rare in the brain.

Synaptic inhibition must be tightly regulated in the brain. Too much inhibition causes loss of consciousness and coma, whereas too little leads to a seizure. The need to control inhibition may explain why the GABA$_A$ receptor channel has, in addition to its GABA binding site, several other sites where chemicals can bind and thus dramatically modulate the function of the GABA$_A$ receptor channel. For example, two classes of drugs, **benzodiazepines** (one of which is the tranquilizer diazepam [Valium]) and **barbiturates** (e.g., the sedative phenobarbital), each binds to its own specific site on the outside face of the GABA$_A$ receptor channel. By themselves, these drugs do very little to the channel's activity. However, when GABA is around, benzodiazepines increase the *frequency* of channel opening, whereas barbiturates increase the *duration* of channel opening. In addition, the benzodiazepines can increase Cl$^-$ conductance of the GABA$_A$ receptor channel. Figure 12–19A to D shows the effects of barbiturates on both the IPSP and the single-channel currents. The result, both for the benzodiazepines and the barbiturates, is more inhibitory Cl$^-$ current, stronger IPSPs, and the behavioral consequences of enhanced inhibition.

Surely, however, the GABA$_A$ receptor did not evolve specialized binding sites just for the benefit of our modern drugs. This sort of logic has motivated research to find endogenous ligands, or natural chemicals that bind to the benzodiazepine and barbiturate sites and serve as regulators of inhibition. Figure 12–19E shows some of the binding sites on the GABA$_A$ receptor. Among the potential natural modulators of the GABA$_A$ receptor may be various metabolites of the steroid hormones progesterone, corticosterone, and testosterone. Some of these hormones increase the lifetime or opening frequency of GABA-activated single-channel currents and may thus enhance inhibition. The steroid effect is unlike the usual genomic mechanisms of steroid hormones (p. 131). Instead, steroids modulate the GABA$_A$ receptor in a manner similar to barbiturates—directly, via binding sites that are distinct from the other drug-binding sites on the GABA$_A$

FIGURE 12–19. Physiology and structure of the GABA$_A$-receptor channel. *A,* When a pulse of GABA is released from a synapse, it elicits a small IPSP. *B,* In the presence of a low dose of pentobarbital, the pulse of synaptic GABA elicits a much larger IPSP. Thus, the barbiturate enhances inhibition. *C,* At the single-channel level, GABA by itself elicits brief channel openings. *D,* A barbiturate (50 μM pentobarbital, in this case) does not by itself activate the GABA$_A$ receptor channel, but increases the channel open time when GABA is present. *E,* The channel receptor is a heteropentamer. It not only has a pore for Cl$^-$, but also separate binding sites for GABA and several classes of channel modulators. The *inset* shows the presumed structure of one of the five monomers. The M2 domain of each of the five subunits presumably lines the central channel pore. GABA, γ-aminobutyric acid; IPSP, inhibitory postsynaptic potential. (Data in *C* and *D* from Puia G, Santi MR, Vicini S, et al: Neurosteroids act on recombinant human GABA$_A$ receptors. Neuron 4:759–765, 1990.)

receptor. Thus, these steroids are not the natural agonists of the benzodiazepine and barbiturate-binding sites. The GABA$_A$ receptor is also subject to modulation by the effects of phosphorylation triggered by second-messenger signalling pathways within neurons.

The Ionotropic Receptors for Acetylcholine, Serotonin, GABA, and Glycine Belong to the Superfamily of Ligand-Gated/Pentameric Channels

We now know the amino acid sequences of many ligand-gated ion channels in the brain, including the receptors for ACh, serotonin, GABA, and glycine. Even though they are gated by such different ligands and have such different permeabilities, virtually all have the same overall structure: five protein subunits, with each subunit being made up of four membrane-spanning segments (as shown for the GABA$_A$ receptor channel in Fig. 12–19E and *inset*). For example, inhibitory GABA$_A$ and glycine receptors have structures very similar to those of excitatory nicotinic ACh receptors, even though the first two are selective for anions whereas the last is selective for cations. For both the glycine and nicotinic ACh receptors, the transmitters bind only to the α subunits, whereas for the GABA$_A$ receptor, the transmitter can bind to either the α or the β subunit.

The primary structures of the many subunit types are remarkably similar, particularly within the amino acid sequences of the hydrophobic membrane-spanning segments. One such stretch, called the **M2 domain**, tends to have repeating sequences of the polar amino acids threonine and serine. Each of the five subunits that constitute a channel contributes one such polar M2 domain, and the set of five combine to form the water-lined pore through which ions can flow (see Fig. 12–19E). For the channels gated by GABA and glycine, selectivity for Cl$^-$ may be determined by positively charged arginines and lysines near the mouth of the pore.

Not quite *all* ligand-gated channels belong to the same superfamily. We have already seen that the family of ionotropic glutamate receptors is distinct from the family of ligand-gated/pentameric channels. Extensive evidence also indicates that ATP is a synaptic transmitter between certain neurons and at neuron–smooth muscle cell synapses, with rapid actions similar to those of glutamate and ACh. One of the "purinoceptors," called P$_{2X}$, is an ATP-gated cation channel with relatively high Ca^{2+} permeability. The sequence of this receptor bears little resemblance to either the ionotropic glutamate receptor family or the ligand-gated/pentameric channel superfamily. Instead, each subunit appears to have only two membrane-spanning segments. Functionally, the ATP-gated channel closely resembles the nicotinic ACh receptor; structurally, it is much more akin to the channel family that includes voltage-gated Na$^+$ and K$^+$ channels (p. 182) and to mechanosensitive channels. This similarity appears to be a case of convergent evolution among ion channels.

Most Neuronal Synapses Release a Very Small Number of Transmitter Quanta with Each Action Potential

A single neuromuscular junction has about 1000 active zones (p. 209). A single presynaptic impulse releases 100 to 200 quanta of transmitter molecules (i.e., ACh), which generates an EPSP of over 40 mV in the muscle cell. This is excitation with a vengeance because the total number of quanta is far more than necessary to cause the muscle cell to fire an action potential and generate a brief contraction. Evolution has designed a neuromuscular junction that works every time, with a large margin of excess for safety. Synapses in the brain are quite different. A typical glutamatergic synapse, which has as few as one active zone, generates EPSPs of only 10 to 1000 μV. In most neurons, one EPSP is rarely enough to cause a postsynaptic cell to fire an action potential.

The basis for the small effect of central synapses has been explored by quantal analysis, with refinements of methods originally applied to the neuromuscular junction. In this approach, a single presynaptic axon is stimulated repeatedly while the postsynaptic response is recorded under voltage-clamp conditions. The frequency distribution of amplitudes of excitatory postsynaptic currents (EPSCs) is analyzed, as described for the neuromuscular junction (see Fig. 8–12B). Recall that according to standard quantal theory:

$$m = np$$

Here, *m* is the total number of quanta released, *n* is the maximal number of releasable quanta (perhaps equivalent to the number of active zones), and *p* is the average probability of release. Measuring these parameters is very difficult. Only in rare cases in central neurons is it possible to find amplitude distributions of EPSCs with clearly separate peaks that may correspond to quantal increments of transmitter. In most cases, EPSC distributions are smooth and broad, which makes quantal analysis hard to interpret. The analysis is hampered because EPSCs are small, it is extremely difficult to identify each small synapse, the dendrites electrically filter the recorded synaptic signals, noise arises from numerous sources (including the ion channels themselves), and synapses exhibit considerable variability. Nevertheless, what is clear is that most synaptic terminals in the CNS release only a small number of transmitter molecules per impulse, often just those contained in a single quantum (i.e., 1000 to 5000 glutamate molecules). Furthermore, the probability of release of that single quantum is usually substantially less than 1; in other words, a presynaptic action potential often results in the release of no transmitter at all. When a quantum of transmitter molecules is released, only a very limited number of postsynaptic receptors is available for the transmitter to bind to, usually not more than 100. In addition, because not all the receptors open their channels during each response, only 10 to 40 channels contribute current to each postsynaptic response, as compared with the thousands of channels opening in concert during each neuromuscular EPSP.

Because most glutamatergic synapses in the brain contribute such a weak excitatory effect, it may require the nearly simultaneous action of many synapses (and the summation of their EPSPs) to bring the postsynaptic membrane potential above the threshold for an action potential. *The threshold number of synapses varies greatly among neurons, but it is roughly in the range of 10 to 100.*

Some exceptions to the rule of small synaptic strengths

B LOW-FREQUENCY STIMULATION

Localized [Ca²⁺]
increases

A PRESYNAPTIC TERMINAL AT REST

Presynaptic
terminal

Large,
peptide-filled
vesicles

Small
vesicles
filled with
small transmitters

Ca²⁺
channels

C HIGH-FREQUENCY STIMULATION

Widespread [Ca²⁺]
increases

FIGURE 12–20. Selective release of co-localized small transmitters and neuroactive peptides. *A*, The presynaptic terminal at rest is filled with small vesicles (containing small transmitter molecules) and large, dense-core vesicles (containing neuroactive peptides). *B*, Fusion of small vesicles containing small transmitters. *C*, Fusion of large, dense-core vesicles.

in the CNS may be noted. One of the strongest connections in the CNS is the one between the climbing fibers and Purkinje cells of the cerebellum (see Fig. 12–1*B*). **Climbing fibers** are glutaminergic axons arising from cells in the inferior olivary nucleus, and they are a critical input to the cerebellum. Climbing fibers and Purkinje cells have a dedicated, one-to-one relationship. The

climbing fiber branches extensively and winds intimately around each **Purkinje cell**, making numerous synaptic contacts. When the climbing fiber fires, it generates a massive EPSP (about 40 mV, similar to the neuromuscular EPSP) that evokes a burst of spikes in the Purkinje cell. Like the neuromuscular junction, the climbing fiber–Purkinje cell relationship seems to be designed to deliver a suprathreshold response every time it is activated. It achieves this strength in the standard way: each climbing fiber makes about 200 synaptic contacts with each Purkinje cell.

When Multiple Transmitters Co-Localize to the Same Synapse, the Exocytosis of Large Vesicles Requires High-Frequency Stimulation

As we mentioned previously, some presynaptic terminals have two or more transmitters co-localized within them. In these cases the small transmitters are packaged into relatively small vesicles (~40 nm in diameter), whereas neuropeptides are in larger dense-core vesicles (100 to 200 nm in diameter), as noted earlier. This dual-packaging scheme allows the neuron some control over the relative release of its two types of transmitters (Fig. 12–20*A*). In general, **low-frequency stimulation** of the presynaptic terminal triggers the release of only the small transmitter (see Fig. 12–20*B*); corelease of both transmitters requires bursts of **high-frequency stimulation** (see Fig. 12–20*C*). This frequency sensitivity may result from the size and spatial profile of presynaptic [Ca²⁺]ᵢ levels achieved by the different patterns of stimulation. Presynaptic Ca²⁺ channels are located very close to the vesicle fusion sites. Low frequencies of activation yield only very localized elevations of [Ca²⁺]ᵢ, an amount sufficient to trigger the exocytosis of small vesicles near active zones. Larger peptide-filled vesicles are farther from active zones, and high-frequency stimulation may be necessary to achieve higher, more distributed elevations of [Ca²⁺]ᵢ. With this arrangement, it is obvious that the synaptic effect (resulting from the mixture of transmitters released) depends strongly on the way that the synapse is activated.

PLASTICITY OF CENTRAL SYNAPSES

Use-Dependent Changes in Synaptic Strength Underlie Many Forms of Learning

Arguably, the greatest achievement of a brain is its ability to learn and store the experience and events of the past so that it is better adapted to deal with the future. Memory is the ability to store and recall learned changes, and nervous systems without memory are extremely handicapped. Studies of the biologic bases for learning and memory have been intense. Although far from understood, certain principles have become clear. First, no single mechanism can explain all forms of memory. Even within a single organism a variety of types of memory exist—and undoubtedly a variety of mechanisms underlie them. Second, evidence is strong that synapses are the physical site of many, if not all forms of memory storage in the brain. As the major points of interaction

A   RESPONSE TO HIGH-FREQUENCY STIMULATION

FIGURE 12–21. Facilitation, potentiation, depression, and habituation. (Data from Levitan IB, Kaczmarek LK: The Neuron. Cell and Molecular Biology, 2nd ed. New York, Oxford University Press, 1997.

between neurons, synapses are well placed to alter the processing capabilities of a neural circuit in interesting and useful ways. Third, the **synaptic strength** (i.e., the mean amplitude of the postsynaptic response) of many synapses may depend on their previous activity. The sensitivity of a synapse to its past activity can lead to a long-term change in its future effectiveness, which is all we need to build memory into a neural circuit.

Some forms of memory last just a few seconds or minutes, only to be lost or replaced by new memories. **Working memory** is an example. It is the continual series of fleeting memories that we use during the course of a day to remember facts and events, what was just spoken to us, where we put the phone down, whether we are coming or going—things that are useful for the moment but need not be stored longer. Other forms of memory may last for hours to decades and strongly resist disruption and replacement. Such **long-term memory** allows the accumulation of knowledge over a lifetime. Some memories may be formed after only a single trial (recall a particularly dramatic, but unique event in your life), whereas others form only with repeated practice

(examples include speaking a language or playing the piano). Detailed descriptions of the many types of memory are beyond the scope of this chapter, but it seems obvious that no single synaptic mechanism would suffice to generate all of them. Neurophysiologists have identified many types of **synaptic plasticity**, the term for activity-dependent changes in the effectiveness of synapses, and some of their mechanisms are well understood. However, it has been very difficult to demonstrate that specific forms of memory use particular types of synaptic plasticity, and correlating memory with synaptic plasticity remains a coveted goal of current research.

Short-Term Synaptic Plasticity Usually Reflects Presynaptic Changes

Repetitive stimulation of neuronal synapses often yields brief periods of increased or decreased synaptic strength (Fig. 12–21). The usual nomenclature for the short-term increases in strength is **facilitation** (which lasts tens to hundreds of milliseconds), **augmentation** (lasting several seconds), and **potentiation** (lasting tens of seconds to several minutes and outlasting the period of high-frequency stimulation). They are not all expressed at every type of synapse. In general, the longer-lasting modifications require longer periods of conditioning stimuli. Short-term *decreases* in synaptic strength include **depression**, which can occur during high-frequency stimulation, and **habituation**, which is a slowly progressing decrease that occurs during relatively low-frequency activation.

Three potential explanations may be offered for short-term *increases* in synaptic strength. First, the presynaptic terminal may release more transmitter for each action potential. Second, the postsynaptic receptors may be more responsive to transmitter because of a change in their number or sensitivity. Third, both of these explanations may occur simultaneously. Studies involving a variety of synapses suggest that the first explanation is most often true. In these cases, quantal analysis usually shows that synapses become stronger because more neurotransmitter is released during each presynaptic action potential; postsynaptic mechanisms generally do not play a role. This form of plasticity seems to depend on the influx of presynaptic Ca^{2+} during the conditioning tetanus. Katz and Miledi first proposed that synaptic strength is increased because of residual Ca^{2+} left in the terminal after a conditioning train of stimuli at the neuromuscular junction. Recent work supports this hypothesis. The idea is that: (1) a tetanic stimulus leads to a substantial increase in presynaptic $[Ca^{2+}]_i$; (2) it takes a relatively long time for presynaptic $[Ca^{2+}]_i$ to decline to baseline, and prolonged stimulation requires prolonged recovery times; and (3) presynaptic action potentials arriving after the conditioning tetanus generate a Ca^{2+} influx that sums with the residual $[Ca^{2+}]_i$ from the preceding tetanus to yield a larger than normal peak $[Ca^{2+}]_i$. Because the dependence of transmitter release on presynaptic $[Ca^{2+}]_i$ is highly nonlinear, the increase in release after conditioning stimuli can be large. It also seems likely that several types of Ca^{2+}-sensitive proteins are present in the presynaptic terminal; the Ca^{2+} binding site that triggers exocytosis is distinct from Ca^{2+} binding sites that regulate short-term increases in transmitter release.

The physiology of a short-term *decrease* in synaptic strength, namely, habituation, has been studied in the marine invertebrate *Aplysia*. The animal reflexively withdraws its gill in response to a stimulus to its skin. Vincent Castellucci and Eric Kandel found that withdrawal becomes less vigorous—that is, the animal habituates—when the stimulus is presented repeatedly. The basis for this behavioral habituation is a decrease in the strength of synapses made by skin sensory neurons onto gill withdrawal motor neurons. Using quantal analysis, Castellucci and Kandel showed that synaptic habituation is due to fewer transmitter quanta being released per action potential. Thus, as with the short-term enhancements of synaptic strength, this example of habituation is due to presynaptic modifications.

Long-Term Potentiation in the Hippocampus May Last for Days or Weeks

In 1973, Timothy Bliss and Terje Lømo described a form of synaptic enhancement that lasted for days or even weeks. This phenomenon, now called **long-term potentiation** (LTP), occurred in excitatory synapses of the mammalian cerebral cortex. LTP was generated by trains of high-frequency stimulation applied to the presynaptic axons, and it was expressed as an increase in the size of EPSPs. Several properties of LTP, including its longevity and its location in cortical synapses, made it immediately attractive as a candidate for the cellular basis of certain forms of vertebrate learning. Years of intensive research have revealed many details of the molecular mechanisms of LTP. They have also provided some evidence, albeit still indirect, that LTP is involved in learning. Several types of LTP have been discovered; here we will discuss only the best-studied example.

LTP is easily demonstrated in several synaptic relays within the **hippocampus**, a part of the cerebral cortex that has often been considered essential for the formation of certain long-term memories. The best studied of these synapses is between the Schaffer collateral axons of CA3 pyramidal neurons (forming the presynaptic terminals) and CA1 pyramidal neurons (the postsynaptic neurons). In a typical experiment, the strength of synapses to the CA1 neuron is tested by giving a single shock about once every 10 seconds. Stimuli are applied separately to two sets of Schaffer collateral fibers that form two different sets of synapses (Fig. 12–22A). If we stimulate a "control" Schaffer collateral once every 10 seconds, the amplitude of the EPSPs recorded in the postsynaptic CA1 neuron remain rather constant over many tens of minutes (see Fig. 12–22B). However, if we *pair* the presynaptic test shocks occurring once every 10 seconds to the "test" pathway with simultaneous postsynaptic depolarization of the CA1 neuron, the amplitude of the EPSP gradually increases several-fold (see Fig. 12–22C), indicative of LTP. In this case, the trigger for LTP was the *pairing* of a low-frequency presynaptic input and a strong postsynaptic depolarization. We already saw that Bliss and Lømo originally induced LTP by pairing the low-frequency presynaptic input with brief bursts of tetanic stimulation (50 to 100 stimuli at a frequency of ~100 Hz).

The induction of LTP has several interesting features that enhance its candidacy as a memory mechanism. First, it is **input specific**, which means that only the activated set of synapses onto a particular cell will be potentiated whereas unactivated synapses to that same neuron remain unpotentiated. Second, induction of LTP requires coincident activity of the presynaptic terminals plus significant depolarization of the postsynaptic membrane. We saw this effect in Figure 12–22C, which showed that inducing LTP required coincident synaptic input and depolarization. Because single hippocampal synapses are quite weak, the requirement for substantial postsynaptic activation means that LTP is best induced in an in vivo situation by **cooperativity**—enough presynaptic axons must cooperate, or fire coincidently, to strongly activate the postsynaptic cell. The cooperative property of LTP can be used to form associations between synaptic inputs. Imagine that two sets of weak inputs onto one cell are, by themselves, too weak to induce LTP. Perhaps each encodes some sensory feature of an object: the sight (input 1) and sound (input 2) of your pet cat. If the two firing together are strong enough to induce LTP,

FIGURE 12–22. Causing LTP by pairing presynaptic and postsynaptic stimuli. *A,* Pyramidal CA3 neurons in the hippocampus send axons (Schaffer collaterals) to synapse on pyramidal CA1 neurons. In the case of the "control" stimulus, the stimulating electrode stimulates collaterals that activate one set of synapses on the postsynaptic CA1 neuron. In this case, the CA1 neuron receives only *presynaptic* stimuli. In the case of the "test" stimulus, a second electrode stimulates a different set of collaterals that activate a different set of synapses on that *same* CA1 neuron. However, in this case, the presynaptic stimuli will be paired with a *postsynaptic* depolarization that is delivered by a third microelectrode. Aside from pairing or not pairing the presynaptic stimuli with a postsynaptic stimulus, the "test" and "control" pathways are equivalent. The third microelectrode records the EPSPs from the CA1 neuron in both the "test" and "control" experiments. *B,* In this case, the "control" Schaffer collaterals are stimulated. Each test pulse is represented by a point on the graph. However, because the CA1 neuron is not depolarized, the amplitude of the EPSPs remains constant (i.e., there is no LTP). *C,* In this case, the "test" Schaffer collaterals are stimulated. When the CA1 neuron is also depolarized, the amplitude of the EPSPs greatly increases (i.e., LTP has been induced). EPSP, excitatory postsynaptic potential; LTP, long-term potentiation. (Data from Gustafsson B, Wigstrom H, Abraham WC, Huang YY: Long-term potentiation in the hippocampus using depolarizing current pulses as the conditioning stimulus to single-volley synaptic potentials. J Neurosci 7: 774–780, 1987.)

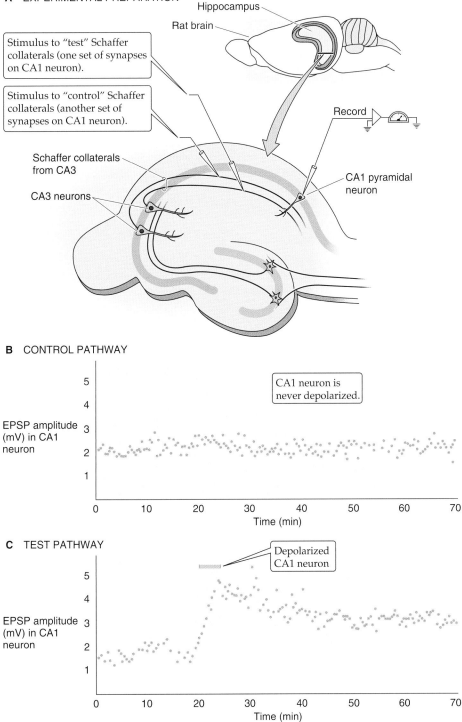

both sets of synaptic input will tend to strengthen, and the features that they encode (the sight and sound of the cat) will become associated in their enhanced ability to fire the postsynaptic cell. In contrast, for example, the sight of your cat and the sound of your telephone will rarely occur together, and their neural equivalents will not become associated.

The molecular mechanisms of one form of LTP in the CA1 region of hippocampus have been partially eluci-

dated. The synapse uses glutamate as its transmitter, and both AMPA and NMDA receptors are activated to generate an EPSP. Induction of LTP depends absolutely on an increase in *post*synaptic $[Ca^{2+}]_i$ levels beyond a critical level and lasting for about 1 to 2 seconds. (Recall that the *short*-term forms of enhancement required a *pre*synaptic increase in $[Ca^{2+}]_i$—see the previous section.) Under most conditions, postsynaptic $[Ca^{2+}]_i$ levels rise during a tetanic stimulus because of the activation of NMDA receptors, the only type of glutamate-activated channel that is usually permeable to Ca^{2+} (see Fig. 12–18). Recall also that the NMDA-type glutamate receptor channel is voltage dependent: it requires V_m to be relatively positive in order to open. The cooperativity requirement of LTP is really a requirement for the activation of NMDA receptors so that Ca^{2+} can enter—if the postsynaptic V_m is too negative (as it is when synaptic activation is weak), NMDA channels remain mostly closed. If activation is strong (as it is when multiple inputs cooperate or when tetanus occurs), V_m becomes positive enough to allow NMDA channels to open. The stimulus-induced rise in postsynaptic $[Ca^{2+}]_i$ is thought to activate two essential kinases: **protein kinase C** and **calcium-calmodulin–dependent protein kinase II**. Blocking either of these kinases with drugs prevents induction of LTP.

The molecular pathway toward the maintenance of LTP is more obscure after the Ca^{2+}-induced activation of kinases. Evidence has been presented both for and against postsynaptic and presynaptic changes explaining the increase in synaptic strength. Postsynaptically, there may be an increased number or effectiveness of AMPA receptors; presynaptically, there may be an enhancement of transmitter release. Sometimes, postsynaptic AMPA receptors appear to be functionally "silent" until LTP mechanisms activate them or insert them into the membrane. Note that the presynaptic hypothesis requires the presence of some rapidly diffusing retrograde messenger that can carry a signal from the postsynaptic side (where rising $[Ca^{2+}]_i$ is clearly a trigger for LTP) back to the presynaptic terminal. Even proponents of the presynaptic hypothesis are not in agreement about the identity of this messenger, although NO and CO are among the candidates.

Long-Term Depression and Long-Term Potentiation in the Hippocampus May Depend on the Same Phosphoproteins

It is theoretically very reasonable to suspect that memory systems have mechanisms to not only increase synaptic strength but decrease it as well. In fact, **long-term depression** (LTD) can be induced in the same synapses within the hippocampus that generate the $[Ca^{2+}]_i$-dependent LTP described in the previous section. The critical feature that determines whether the synapses will strengthen or weaken is simply the frequency of stimulation that they receive. For example, several hundred stimuli delivered at 50 Hz produce LTP, the same number delivered at 10 Hz has little effect, and at 1 Hz they produce LTD. One set of synapses can be strengthened or weakened repeatedly, which suggests that each process (LTP and LTD) acts on the same molecular component of the synapses. LTD induced in this way shows the same input specificity as LTP—only the stimulated synapses onto a cell are depressed.

The induction requirements of hippocampal LTD are paradoxically similar to those of LTP: LTD induced by low-frequency stimulation depends on the activation of NMDA receptors, and it requires an increase in postsynaptic $[Ca^{2+}]_i$. The key determinant for whether a tetanic stimulus induces LTP or LTD may be the level to which

postsynaptic $[Ca^{2+}]_i$ rises. A simple model that integrates the induction mechanisms of LTD and LTP is shown in Figure 12–23. Synaptic activation releases glutamate, which activates NMDA receptors, which in turn allow Ca^{2+} to enter the postsynaptic cell. In the case of high-frequency stimulation, postsynaptic $[Ca^{2+}]_i$ rises to very high levels; if stimulation is of low frequency, the rise in postsynaptic $[Ca^{2+}]_i$ is more modest. High levels of $[Ca^{2+}]_i$ lead to a net activation of protein *kinases*, whereas modest levels of $[Ca^{2+}]_i$ preferentially activate protein *phosphatases*. Kinase and phosphatase in turn act on a common synaptic phosphoprotein (or proteins) that somehow regulates synaptic strength. Note that the simple scheme shown in Figure 12–23 leaves unidentified many of the steps between the rise in postsynaptic $[Ca^{2+}]_i$ and the change in synaptic strength; most of the molecular details remain to be determined. However, if the model is correct, it means that synaptic strength (and by implication, some memory) is under the dynamic control of cellular processes that determine postsynaptic $[Ca^{2+}]_i$. Once again in physiology, $[Ca^{2+}]_i$ has been assigned a pivotal role in a vital process.

Long-Term Depression in the Cerebellum May Be Important for Motor Learning

It is important to note that a variety of other types of LTP and LTD have been described in other synapses and even within the same synapses of the CA1 region in the hippocampus. Clearly, multiple means and mechanisms may be used to strengthen and weaken synapses in the brain over a range of time courses. We will briefly describe one other well-studied type of synaptic modification in the mammalian brain, LTD in the cerebellum.

The cerebellum is a large brain structure that is important in motor control and strongly implicated in motor learning. The cortex of the cerebellum is a thin, multiply folded sheet of cells with an intricate, but highly repetitious neural structure. The principal cell of the cerebellum is the **Purkinje cell**, a large neuron that uses GABA as its transmitter and whose axon forms the sole output of the cerebellar cortex. Purkinje cells receive two types of excitatory synaptic input: (1) each Purkinje cell receives powerful synaptic contact from just a single climbing fiber, which comes from a cell in the inferior olivary nucleus (see Fig. 12–1B), and (2) each Purkinje cell also

---

FIGURE 2–23. Proposed molecular mechanism for LTP and LTD. Glutamate release from the presynaptic terminal activates NMDA receptor channels, which allow Ca^{2+} to enter the postsynaptic cell. The glutamate also activates AMPA receptor channels. Whether the ultimate effect is LTP or LTD appears to depend on the extent to which $[Ca^{2+}]_i$ rises. High levels of $[Ca^{2+}]_i$—produced by high-frequency stimulation—lead to a net activation of protein kinases and thus phosphorylation of one or more synaptic proteins that regulate synaptic strength. One hypothetical pathway has the phosphorylated/dephosphorylated synaptic proteins modulating the AMPA receptor channel. The result is LTP. The postsynaptic neuron also seems to be able to stimulate the presynaptic terminal. A moderate increase in $[Ca^{2+}]_i$—produced by low-frequency stimulation—preferentially activates protein phosphatases, which presumably dephosphorylate the same synaptic proteins as in the previous example. The result is LTD. AMPA, α-amino-3-hydroxy-5-methyl-4-isoxazole propionic acid; LTD, long-term depression; LTP, long-term potentiation.

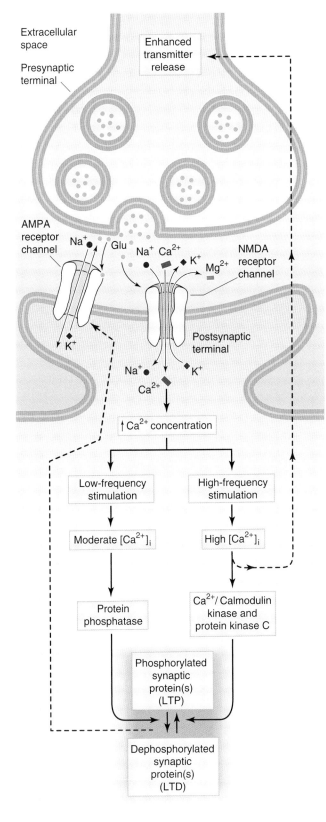

Extracellular space

Presynaptic terminal

Enhanced transmitter release

AMPA receptor channel

Na⁺   Glu   Na⁺ Ca²⁺   K⁺   Mg²⁺   NMDA receptor channel

K⁺

Postsynaptic terminal

Na⁺   K⁺

Ca²⁺

↑Ca²⁺ concentration

Low-frequency stimulation

High-frequency stimulation

Moderate [Ca²⁺]ᵢ

High [Ca²⁺]ᵢ

Protein phosphatase

Ca²⁺/ Calmodulin kinase and protein kinase C

Phosphorylated synaptic protein(s) (LTP)

Dephosphorylated synaptic protein(s) (LTD)

FIGURE 2–23. *See legend on opposite page.*

receives a synapse from about 150,000 **parallel fibers**, which originate from the tiny granule cells of the cerebellum itself. This remarkable conjunction of synaptic inputs is the basis for a theory of motor learning that was proposed by David Marr and James Albus in 1970. They predicted that the parallel-fiber synapses should change their strength only if they are active at the same time as the climbing fiber onto the same cell. This idea received important experimental support from the laboratory of Masao Ito.

Ito and colleagues monitored EPSPs in a Purkinje cell while stimulating some of its inputs from parallel fibers and its one climbing fiber input. They found that the EPSPs generated by the parallel fibers became smaller when both the parallel fibers *and* the cell's climbing fiber were coactivated at low frequencies. Stimulating either input alone did not cause any change. Cerebellar LTD can last at least several hours. As with the hippocampal LTP and LTD described before, cerebellar LTD showed input specificity: only those parallel fibers coactivated with the climbing fiber were depressed, whereas other synapses onto the cell were unchanged.

The mechanism of cerebellar LTD has some similarities to that of LTD in the hippocampus, but it is also distinctly different. Parallel-fiber synapses weaken because of reduced effectiveness—either a reduction in the number or sensitivity—of *postsynaptic* AMPA-type glutamate receptors. As in the hippocampus, induction of cerebellar LTD requires an increase in postsynaptic [Ca²⁺]ᵢ. However, unlike the hippocampus, no NMDA-type glutamate receptors are present in the mature cerebellum to mediate Ca²⁺ flux. Instead, Ca²⁺ can enter Purkinje cells via voltage-gated Ca²⁺ channels that are opened during the exceptionally powerful EPSP that the climbing fiber generates. In addition to a rise in postsynaptic [Ca²⁺]ᵢ, cerebellar LTD induction seems to require the activation of metabotropic glutamate receptors and protein kinase C by the parallel fibers. Increases in postsynaptic [Na⁺]ᵢ and NO have also been implicated in LTD induction. At present, the relationships between these putative induction factors and the molecular pathways leading to the expression of cerebellar LTD are obscure.

As we pointed out for the hippocampus, most efficient memory systems need mechanisms for both weakening and strengthening their synapses. It turns out that parallel-fiber synapses of the cerebellum can be induced to generate LTP as well as LTD by stimulating them at relatively low (2 to 8 Hz) frequencies. Cerebellar LTP, unlike hippocampal LTP, requires presynaptic but not postsynaptic increases in [Ca²⁺]ᵢ. Potentiation seems to occur as a result of increased transmitter release from the presynaptic terminal.

REFERENCES

Books and Reviews

Brenman JE, Bredt DS: Synaptic signaling by nitric oxide. Curr Opin Neurobiol 7:374–378, 1997.

Clapham DE: Direct G protein activation of ion channels? Annu Rev Neurosci 17:441–464, 1994.

Hanson PI, Heuser JE, Jahn R: Neurotransmitter release—four years of SNARE complexes. Curr Opin Neurobiol 7:310–315, 1997.

Hollmann M, Heinemann S: Cloned glutamate receptors. Annu Rev Neurosci 17:31–108, 1994.

Linden DJ, Connor JA: Long-term synaptic depression. Annu Rev Neurosci 18:319–357, 1995.

MacDonald RL, Olsen RW: GABA_A receptor channels. Annu Rev Neurosci 17:569–602, 1994.

Südhof TC: RAB3 and synaptotagmin: The yin and yang of synaptic membrane fusion. Annu Rev Neurosci 21:75–95, 1998.

Journal Articles

Kamiya H, Zucker RS: Residual Ca^{2+} and short-term synaptic plasticity. Nature 371:603–606, 1994.

Katz B, Miledi R: The role of calcium in neuromuscular facilitation. J Physiol (Lond) 195:481–492, 1968.

Rosenmund C, Stern-Bach Y, Stevens CF: The tetrameric structure of a glutamate receptor channel. Science 280:1596–1599, 1998.

Valera S, Hussy N, Evans RJ, et al: A new class of ligand-gated ion channel defined by P2x receptor for extracellular ATP. Nature 371:516–519, 1994.

Vignes M, Collingridge GL: The synaptic activation of kainate receptors. Nature 388:179–182, 1997.

CHAPTER 13

Sensory Transduction

Barry W. Connors

Sensory Receptors Convert Environmental Energy into Neural Signals

Sensation is a cognitive process that requires the full powers of the central nervous system (CNS). Sensation begins with the sensory receptors that actually interface with the world, and these receptors use energy from the environment to trigger electrochemical signals that can be transmitted to the brain—a process called **sensory transduction**. Understanding transduction processes is crucial for several reasons. Without these processes, sensation fails. Moreover, a variety of diseases that specifically affect sensory receptors can impair or abolish sensation without damaging the brain. Transduction also sets the basic limits of perception. It determines the sensitivity, range, speed, versatility, and vigor of a sensory system.

We have a variety of senses, each tuned to particular types of environmental energy. These **sensory modalities** include the familiar ones of seeing, hearing, touching, smelling, and tasting, as well as our senses of pain, balance, body position, and movement. In addition, other intricate sensory systems of which we are not conscious monitor the internal milieu and report on the body's chemical and metabolic state. Early in the 19th century, the physiologist Johannes Müller recognized that neurons that are specialized to evaluate a particular type of stimulus energy will produce the appropriate sensation regardless of how they were activated. For example, banging your eye can produce perceptions of light even in the dark, and seizure activity in a region of the cortex devoted to olfaction can evoke repulsive smells even in a rose garden. This property has been called **univariance**; in other words, the sensory receptor and its subsequent neural circuits do not know what stimulated them—they give the same type of response regardless. Specificity for each modality is ensured by the structure and position of the sensory receptor.

Sensory Transduction Uses Adaptations of Common Molecular Signalling Mechanisms

Evolution is a conservative enterprise. Good ideas are retained, and with slight modification they are adapted to new purposes. Sensory transduction is a prime example of this principle. The sensory processes that are now understood at the molecular level use systems that are closely related to the ubiquitous signalling molecules in eukaryotic cells. Some modalities (vision, olfaction, some types of taste and other chemoreception) begin with integral membrane proteins that belong to the superfamily of G-protein–coupled receptors (p. 92). The second-messenger pathways use the same substances that are used for so many nonsensory tasks in cells, such as cyclic nucleotides, inositol phosphates, and kinases. Other sensory systems (mechanoreceptors, including the hair cells of audition and the vestibular organs, as well some taste cells) use modified membrane ion channels in the primary transduction process. Although the structures of these channels have not yet been deduced, their biophysical properties are mostly unremarkable, and they are likely related to other, nonsensory ion channels. Indeed, the gating of many ion channels (p. 161) from "nonsensory" cells is sensitive to the physical distortion of the membrane that they lie in, which implies that mechanosensitivity is a widespread (although perhaps epiphenomenal) feature of integral membrane proteins.

To achieve a specificity for certain stimulus energies, many sensory receptors must use specialized cellular structures. These, too, are usually adapted from familiar components. Various receptors are slightly modified epithelial cells. Some situate their transduction sites on modified cilia, whereas others use muscle cells or collagen fibers to channel the appropriate forces to the sensory axon. Many are neurons alone, often just bare axons with no specialization visible by microscopy. Most sensory transduction cells (e.g., oxygen and taste sensors, but not olfactory receptors) lack their own axon to communicate with the CNS. For these cells, the communication system of choice is a relatively standard, Ca^{2+}-dependent system of synaptic transmission onto a primary sensory neuron.

Sensory Transduction Requires Detection and Amplification, Usually Followed by a Local Receptor Potential

Functionally, sensory transducers follow certain general steps. Obviously, they must detect stimulus energy, but they must do so with enough selectivity and speed that stimuli of different types, from different locations, or with different timing are not confused. In most cases, transduction also involves one or more steps of signal amplification so that the sensory cell can reliably communicate small stimuli (e.g., a few stray photons or a smattering of drifting molecules) to a large brain in an environment with much sensory noise. The sensory cell must then convert the amplified signal into an electrical change by altering the gating of some ion channel. This channel gating leads to alterations of the membrane potential (V_m) in the receptor cell—otherwise known as a **receptor potential**. The receptor potential is not an action potential, but a graded electrotonic event (p. 173) that can either modulate the activity of other channels (e.g., voltage-gated Na^+ or Ca^{2+} channels) or trigger action potentials in a different portion of the same cell. Very often, the receptor potential regulates the flux of Ca^{2+} into the cell and thus controls the release of some synaptic-transmitter molecule onto the sensory afferent neuron.

Ultimately, receptor potentials determine the rate and pattern with which action potentials fire in a sensory neuron. This firing pattern is the signal that is actually communicated to the CNS. Useful information may be encoded in many features of the firing, including its rate, its temporal patterns, its periodicity, its consistency, and its patterns when compared when other sensory neurons of the same, or even different modalities.

CHEMORECEPTION

Chemoreceptors Are Ubiquitous, Diverse, and Evolutionarily Ancient

Every cell is bathed in chemicals. Molecules can be food or poison, or they may serve as signals of communication between cells, organs, or individuals. The ability to recognize and respond to environmental chemicals can allow cells to find nutrients, avoid harm, attract a mate, navigate, or regulate a physiologic process. Chemoreception has basic and universal advantages. It is the oldest form of sensory transduction, and it exists in many forms. Chemoreception does not even require a nervous system. Single-celled organisms such as bacteria can recognize and respond to substances in their environment. In the broadest sense, every cell in the human body is chemosensitive, and chemical signalling between cells is the basis for internal communication through endocrine systems and neurotransmission. In this chapter we restrict ourselves to chemoreception as a sensory system, the interface between the nervous system and the external and internal chemical milieu.

Chemicals reach the human body by oral or nasal ingestion, contact with the skin, or inhalation, and, once there, they diffuse or are carried to the surface membranes of receptor cells through the various aqueous fluids of the body (e.g., mucus, saliva, tears, cerebrospinal fluid, blood plasma). The nervous system constantly monitors these chemical comings and goings with a diverse array of chemosensory receptors. The most familiar of these receptors are the sensory organs of taste (**gustation**) and smell (**olfaction**). However, chemoreception is widespread throughout the body. Chemoreceptors in the skin, mucous membranes, and gut warn against irritating substances, and chemoreceptors in the carotid bodies (p. 723) measure blood levels of O_2, CO_2, and $[H^+]$.

Taste Receptors Are Modified Epithelial Cells, Whereas Olfactory Receptors Are Neurons

The tasks of gustatory and olfactory receptors appear similar at first glance: Both recognize the concentration and identity of dissolved molecules, and they communicate this information to the CNS. In fact, the two systems operate in parallel during eating, and the flavors of most foods are strongly dependent on both taste *and* smell. However, the receptor cells of the two systems are quite different. Olfactory receptors are neurons. Each olfactory cell has small dendrites at one end that are specialized to identify chemical stimuli, and at the other end an axon projects directly into the brain. Taste receptor cells are not neurons but rather collections of modified epithelial cells that synapse onto the axons of sensory neurons that communicate with the CNS.

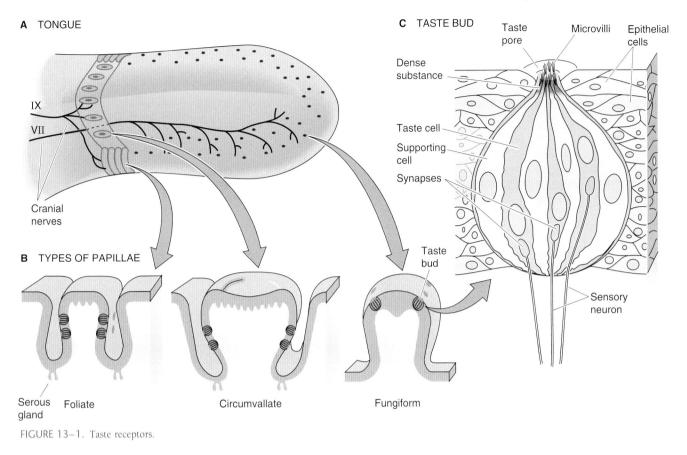

A TONGUE

IX

VII

Cranial
nerves

B TYPES OF PAPILLAE

Serous
gland   Foliate

Circumvallate

Fungiform

C TASTE BUD

Taste
pore   Microvilli   Epithelial
cells

Dense
substance

Taste cell

Supporting
cell

Synapses

Taste
bud

Sensory
neuron

FIGURE 13–1. Taste receptors.

TASTE RECEPTOR CELLS. Taste receptors are located mainly on the dorsal surface of the tongue (Fig. 13–1A), concentrated within small, but visible projections called **papillae** (see Fig. 13–1B). Papillae are shaped like ridges, pimples, or mushrooms, and each is a few millimeters in diameter. Each papilla in turn has numerous **taste buds** (see Fig. 13–1C). One taste bud contains 50 to 150 taste receptor cells, numerous basal and supporting cells that surround the taste cells, plus a set of sensory afferent axons. Most people have 2000 to 5000 taste buds, although exceptional cases range from 500 to 20,000.

The chemically sensitive part of a taste receptor cell is a small apical-membrane region near the surface of the tongue. The apical ends have thin extensions called **microvilli** that project into the **taste pore**, a small opening on the surface of the tongue where the taste cells are exposed to the contents of the mouth. Taste cells form synapses with the primary sensory axons near the bottom of the taste bud. However, processing may be more complicated than a simple receptor-to-axon relay. Receptor cells also make both electrical and chemical synapses onto some of the basal cells, some basal cells synapse onto the sensory axons, and some type of information-processing circuit may be present within each taste bud itself.

Cells of the taste bud undergo a constant cycle of growth, death, and regeneration. This process depends on the influence of the sensory nerve because if the nerve is cut, taste buds degenerate.

OLFACTORY RECEPTOR CELLS. We smell with receptor cells in the thin **olfactory epithelium**, which is placed high in the nasal cavity (Fig. 13–2A). The olfactory epithelium has three main cell types: **olfactory receptor cells** are the site of transduction; **support cells** are similar to glia and, among other things, help produce mucus; and **basal cells** are the source of new receptor cells (see Fig. 13–2B). Olfactory receptors (similar to taste receptors) continually die, regenerate, and grow in a cycle that lasts about 4 to 8 weeks. Olfactory receptor cells are one of the very few types of neurons in the mammalian nervous system that are regularly replaced throughout life.

As we breathe or sniff, chemical odorants waft through the many folds of the nasal passages. However, to contact the receptor cells, odorants must first dissolve in and diffuse through a thin mucous layer, which has both a viscous and a watery portion. The normal olfactory epithelium exudes a mucous layer 20 to 50 μm thick. Mucus flows constantly and is normally replaced about every 10 minutes. Mucus is a complex, water-based substance containing dissolved glycosaminoglycans (p. 40); a variety of proteins, including antibodies, odorant-binding proteins, and enzymes; and various salts. The antibodies are critical because olfactory cells offer a direct route for viruses (e.g., rabies) or bacteria to enter the brain. **Odorant-binding proteins** in the mucus probably facilitate the diffusion of odorants toward and away from the receptors. Enzymes may help clear the mucus of odorants and thus speed recovery of the receptors from transient odors.

Both the absolute size and the receptor density of the olfactory epithelium vary greatly among species, and they help determine olfactory acuity. The surface area of the human olfactory epithelium is only about 10 cm², but

A   NASAL CAVITY AND OLFACTORY BULB

B   OLFACTORY EPITHELIUM

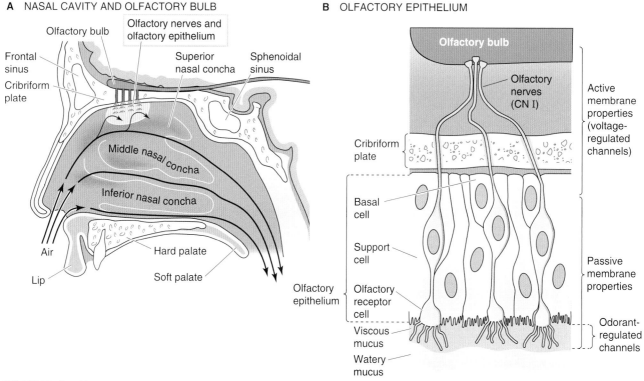

FIGURE 13–2. Olfactory reception.

this limited area is enough to detect some odorants at concentrations as low as a few parts per trillion. The olfactory epithelia of some dogs may be over 170 cm², and dogs have more than 100 times as many receptors in each square centimeter as humans do. The olfactory acuity of some breeds of dog is legendary and far surpasses that of humans. By sniffing the aromatic air above the ground, they can often detect the few molecules left by someone walking there hours before.

Complex Flavors Are Derived from a Few Basic Types of Taste Receptors, with Contributions from Sensory Receptors of Smell, Temperature, Texture, and Pain

Studies of taste discrimination in humans imply that we can distinguish among 4000 to 10,000 different chemicals with our taste buds. However, behavioral evidence suggests that these discriminations represent only four or five primary taste qualities: **bitter**, **salt**, **sweet**, and **sour**. Many taste researchers also define a fifth primary quality, often called **umami** ("delicious" in Japanese), which is epitomized by the taste of the amino acid glutamate (monosodium glutamate [MSG] is the familiar culinary form). Unlike the olfactory receptor cells, which contain only one receptor type (see later), taste receptor cells may have several.

In many cases, there is an obvious correlation between the chemistry of **tastants** (i.e., chemicals being tasted) and the quality of their taste. Most acids taste sour and most salts taste salty. However, for many other tastants, the linkage between taste and chemical structure is not clear. The familiar sugars (e.g., sucrose and fructose) are satisfyingly sweet, but certain proteins (e.g., monellin) and artificial sweeteners (e.g., saccharin and aspartame, the latter of which is made from two amino acids: L-aspartyl-L-phenylalanine methyl ester) are 10,000 to 100,000 times sweeter by weight than these sugars. Bitter substances are also chemically diverse. They include simple ions such as K^+ (KCl actually simultaneously evokes both bitter and salty tastes), larger metal ions such as Mg^{2+}, and complex organic molecules such as quinine.

If the tongue has only four or five primary taste qualities available to it, how does it discriminate among the myriad complex flavors that embellish our lives? First, the tongue's response to each tastant reflects distinct proportions of each of the primary taste qualities. In this sense, the taste cells are similar to the photoreceptors of our eyes; with only three different types of color-selective photoreceptive cone cells, we can distinguish a huge palette of colors (see later). Second, the flavor of a tastant is determined not only by its taste but also by its smell. Taste and smell operate in parallel, with information converging in the CNS to aid the important discrimination of foods and poisons. For example, without the aid of olfaction, an onion tastes much like an apple—and both are quite bland. Third, the mouth is filled with other types of sensory receptors that are sensitive to texture, temperature, and pain, and these modalities enhance both the identification and enjoyment of foods. A striking example is the experience of spicy food, which is enjoyable to some but painful to others. The spiciness of hot peppers is generated by the chemical **capsaicin**, not because of its activation of taste receptor cells, but because of its stimulation of pain receptors in the mouth.

Taste Transduction Involves Many Types of Molecular Signalling Systems

The chemicals that we taste have very diverse structures, and taste receptors have evolved a variety of mechanisms for transduction. The taste system has adapted virtually all known types of membrane-signalling systems to its purposes. Tastants may pass directly through ion channels (salt and sour), bind to and block ion channels (sour and bitter), bind to and open ion channels (some sweet amino acids), or bind to membrane receptors that activate second-messenger systems, which in turn open or close ion channels (sweet and bitter). Taste cells have simply used specialized variations of these processes to initiate meaningful signals to the brain.

The receptor potentials of taste cells are usually depolarizing. At least some taste receptor cells can fire action potentials, similar to those of neurons, but if the membrane is sufficiently depolarized by whatever means, voltage-gated Ca^{2+} channels open, and Ca^{2+} enters the cytoplasm and triggers the release of transmitter molecules. The identity of the taste receptor's transmitter or transmitters is unknown.

More than 90% of receptor cells respond to two or more of the basic taste groups, and many respond to all. What varies is the relative sensitivity of taste cells to the spectrum of basic tastes. Some cells are salt lovers only; others prefer salt and sour; still others have a preference for sweet and sour; and a few respond eagerly to everything. Presumably, single taste cells can express one, some, or all of the various taste transduction mechanisms that are outlined in the following sections.

The complex diversities of taste transduction are not yet fully understood. Many of the details have come from research on the taste cells of catfish, mudpuppies, mice, and rats. Each animal has certain experimental advantages (e.g., very large taste cells), but the differences among species suggest that we may be surprised when it becomes possible to study human mechanisms directly. The following is a summary of the best-understood transduction processes for the five primary taste qualities (Fig. 13–3).

SALT. The most common salty tasting chemical is NaCl, or table salt. The taste of salt is mainly the taste of the cation Na^+, and transduction of $[Na^+]$ in taste cells is relatively simple. Salt-sensitive taste cells have an Na^+-selective channel called ENaC (see Fig. 13–3A), common to many epithelial cells, that is blocked by the drug amiloride (p. 779). Unlike the Na^+ channel that generates action potentials in excitable cells, the taste channel is relatively insensitive to voltage and stays open at rest. However, transduction of the $[Na^+]$ in a mouthful of food is somewhat analogous to the behavior of a neuron during the upstroke of an action potential. When $[Na^+]$ rises outside the receptor cell, the gradient for Na^+ across the membrane becomes steeper, Na^+ diffuses down its electrochemical gradient (i.e., it flows into the cell), and the resultant inward current causes the membrane to depolarize to a new voltage. Neurons depolarize during their action potential by increasing Na^+ conductance at a fixed Na^+ gradient (see Fig. 7–4). In contrast, Na^+-sensitive taste cells depolarize by increasing the Na^+ gradient at a fixed Na^+ permeability. The resultant graded depolarization of the taste cell is defined as its receptor potential.

Anions may affect the taste of salts by modulating the saltiness of the cation or by adding a taste of their own. NaCl tastes saltier than Na acetate, perhaps because the larger an anion is, the more it *inhibits* the salty taste of the cation. Na saccharin is sweet because the anion saccharin activates sweetness receptors; it is not salty because Na^+ is present at a very low concentration.

SOUR. Sourness is evoked by protons (H^+ ions). Acidity affects taste receptors in two ways (see Fig. 13–3A). First, H^+ can permeate the ENaC Na^+ channel, the same channel that mediates the taste of salt. This H^+ influx is an inward current and could depolarize the cell. Second, H^+ ions can bind to and *block* a K^+-selective channel. The fall in K^+ permeability causes the membrane to depolarize. In addition, because pH can affect virtually all cellular processes, it is possible that other less specific influences of low pH are involved in sour transduction.

SWEET. Sweetness is sensed when molecules bind to specific receptor sites on the taste-cell membrane and activate a cascade of second messengers (see Fig. 13–3B). This mechanism is also quite familiar and resembles the response of many cells to the modulator norepinephrine (p. 97). A tastant (e.g., a sugar molecule) binds to the receptor, activates a G protein that stimulates the formation of cyclic adenosine monophosphate (cAMP) within the cytoplasm, and ultimately blocks a K^+-selective channel (apparently a different one from that involved in sourness). As a result, the cell membrane depolarizes. Recent studies suggest that some sweet stimuli can activate a second-messenger pathway that involves inositol 1,4,5-triphosphate (IP_3), similar to one of the bitter mechanisms described next. Finally, sugars may also directly gate cation channels without second-messenger intermediaries.

BITTER. Bitterness usually warns of poison. Perhaps because poisons are so chemically diverse, several mechanisms have evolved for the transduction of bitterness. Similar to the sourness mechanism, some bitter compounds (e.g., calcium and quinine) bind directly to K^+-selective channels and block them (see Fig. 13–3C). In addition, at least two types of membrane receptor proteins are specific for bitter substances, both of which activate G-protein–mediated second-messenger cascades that are different from those of the sweet system. In one, the bitter tastant binds to a member of the T2R class of receptors. These couple to a G protein called **gustducin,** which triggers a *decrease in cAMP.* Gustducin is very similar to the G-protein transducin, which is important in the transduction of light in photoreceptors (see later). The effect of the lowered $[cAMP]_i$ is not entirely clear, but it may affect certain channels that are gated by cyclic nucleotide monophosphates in the taste-cell membrane. The other class of bitter receptors triggers increased production of the intracellular messenger IP_3. IP_3 releases Ca^{2+} from intracellular stores (p. 100), and Ca^{2+} then triggers transmitter release onto the primary sensory axon.

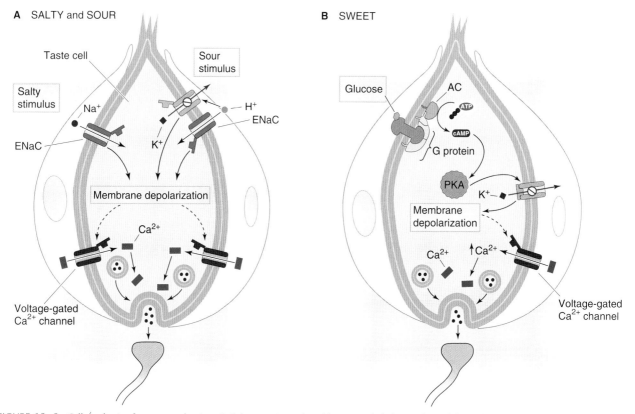

FIGURE 13–3. Cellular basis of taste transduction. *A*, Salty taste is mediated by an epithelial Na$^+$ channel (ENaC) that is sensitive to amiloride. Sour is mediated by H$^+$ entering through the same ENaC channel or by the effect of low pH inhibiting a K$^+$ channel. The resulting depolarization opens voltage-gated Ca^{2+} channels, increasing [Ca^{2+}]$_i$ and leading to transmitter release. *B*, Sugar binds to a 7-transmembrane receptor that activates heterotrimeric G protein, stimulating AC, increasing cAMP, and activating PKA, which then closes a K$^+$ channel. The resulting depolarization opens voltage-gated Ca^{2+} channels, increasing [Ca^{2+}]$_i$ and leading to transmitter release.

AMINO ACIDS. Amino acids are critical nutrients that are vital as an energy source and for constructing proteins. Probably as a consequence, many amino acids taste good, although some taste bitter. The **umami** taste, which we know well from Chinese restaurants, may be generated when glutamate (and perhaps certain other amino acids) binds to and activates a cation channel that is permeable to Na$^+$ and Ca^{2+} and subsequently causes depolarization (see Fig. 13–3*D*). This mechanism is very similar to the one mediating most synaptic excitation between CNS neurons; in that case, glutamate opens an *ionotropic* glutamate receptor that is a nonselective cation channel (p. 313). Glutamate may also activate a particular subtype of *metabotropic* glutamate receptor and thus lead to a decrease in [cAMP]$_i$ and unknown subsequent effects. Other amino acids taste bitter (leucine, for example), and they may trigger either cAMP- or IP$_3$-mediated messenger systems.

Olfactory Transduction Involves Specific Receptors, G-Protein–Coupled Signalling, and a Cyclic-Nucleotide–Gated Ion Channel

Our ability to smell chemicals is better developed than our ability to taste them. By one estimate, we can smell more than 400,000 different substances. Interestingly, about 80% of them smell unpleasant. As with taste, it seems likely that smell evolved to serve important protec-

tive functions, such as warning us away from harmful substances. With the ability to discriminate so many different smells, you might also expect many different types of transduction mechanisms, as in the taste system. In fact, olfactory receptors probably use only one second-messenger mechanism. Figure 13–4 summarizes the chain of events that leads to an action potential in the olfactory nerve (i.e., cranial nerve I [CN I]):

Step 1: The odorant binds to a specific **olfactory receptor protein** in the cell membrane of a cilium of an olfactory receptor cell.

Step 2: Receptor activation stimulates a heterotrimeric G protein called G$_{olf}$ (p. 92).

Step 3: The α subunit of G$_{olf}$ in turn activates adenylyl cyclase, which produces cAMP.

Step 4: The cAMP binds to a cAMP-gated cation channel.

Step 5: Opening of this channel increases permeability to Na$^+$, K$^+$, and Ca^{2+}.

Step 6: The net inward current leads to membrane depolarization and increased [Ca^{2+}]$_i$.

Step 7: The increased [Ca^{2+}]$_i$ opens Ca^{2+}-activated Cl$^-$ channels. Opening of these channels produces more depolarization because of the relatively high [Cl$^-$]$_i$ of olfactory receptor neurons.

Step 8: If the receptor potential exceeds the threshold, it triggers action potentials in the soma that travel down the axon and into the brain.

C BITTER

D UMAMI

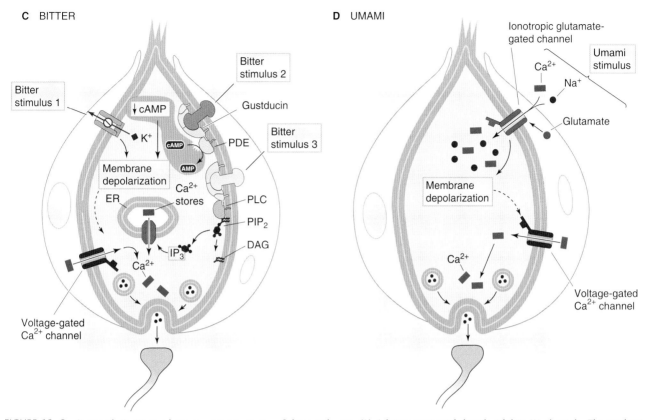

FIGURE 13-3. *Continued. C,* Bitter substances can act via any of three pathways. (1) A bitter compound directly inhibits K^+ channels. The resulting depolarization opens voltage-gated Ca^{2+} channels, increasing $[Ca^{2+}]_i$ and leading to transmitter release. (2) A ligand binds to a 7-transmembrane receptor and activates a G protein called gustducin that stimulates phosphodiesterase. The resultant *decrease* in $[cAMP]_i$ somehow leads to depolarization. (3) Ligand binds to a receptor that is linked to a G protein, which activates phospholipase C. The resultant increase in $[IP_3]$ releases Ca^{2+} from stores, raises $[Ca^{2+}]_i$, and leads to transmitter release. *D,* Glutamate binds to a glutamate-gated, nonselective cation channel and opens it. The resultant depolarization opens voltage-gated Ca^{2+} channels, increases $[Ca^{2+}]_i$, and leads to transmitter release. AC, adenylyl cyclase; AMP, adenosine monophosphate; cAMP, cyclic adenosine monophosphate; DAG, diacylglycerol; ER, endoplasmic reticulum; IP_3, inositol 1,4,5-triphosphate; PDE, phosphodiesterase; PIP_2, phosphatidyl inositol 4,5-biphosphate; PLC, phospholipase C.

All this molecular machinery, with the exception of the action-potential mechanism, is squeezed into the thin cilia of olfactory receptor cells. Moreover, additional modulatory schemes also branch from this basic pathway.

Olfactory receptor cells express a huge family of perhaps 1000 different olfactory receptor proteins, which means that they belong to the largest family of genes yet discovered! This family of olfactory receptor proteins belongs to the superfamily of G-protein–coupled receptors (p. 92) that also includes the phototransduction protein rhodopsin, as well as the receptors for a wide variety of ligands. The extracellular surfaces of olfactory receptor proteins have odorant-binding sites, each slightly different from the others. Presumably, each receptor protein can bind only certain types of odorants, therefore some degree of selectivity is conferred to different olfactory receptor cells. Each receptor cell expresses only a single gene of the 1000 different odorant-receptor genes. Thus, 1000 different types of olfactory receptor cells are present, each identified by the one receptor gene that it expresses. Because each odorant may activate a large proportion of the different receptor types, the central olfactory system's task is to decode the patterns of receptor-cell activity that signals the identity of each smell.

The structure of the olfactory cAMP-gated channel is closely related to the light-activated channel in photoreceptors of the retina, which is normally gated by an increase in intracellular cyclic guanosine monophosphate ($[cGMP]_i$). The olfactory channel and the photoreceptor channel almost certainly evolved from one ancestral cyclic nucleotide–gated channel, just as the olfactory receptor and photoreceptor proteins probably evolved from an ancestral receptor with seven membrane-spanning segments.

Termination of the olfactory response occurs when odorants diffuse away, scavenger enzymes in the mucous layer break them down, or cAMP in the receptor cell activates other signalling pathways that end the transduction process.

VISUAL TRANSDUCTION

The environment of most species is enveloped by light (Fig. 13–5). Animals have evolved a variety of mechanisms to transduce and detect light. Their brains analyze visual information to help them locate food, avoid becoming food, find a mate, navigate, and generally recognize distant objects. Light is an exceptionally useful source of information about the world because it is nearly ubiquitous and it can travel far and fast and in straight lines

FIGURE 13–4. Cellular mechanism of odor sensation. ATP, adenosine triphosphate; cAMP, cyclic adenosine monophosphate.

with relatively little dispersion of its energy. The vertebrate eye, which we describe here, has two major components: an **optical** part to gather and focus light and form an image and a **neural** part (the retina) to convert the optical image into a neural code.

The Optical Components of the Eye Collect Light and Focus It onto the Retina

The optical structures of the eye are among the most sophisticated of the specialized non-neural sensory endings, and they are often compared with a camera. As cameras have become more technologically sophisticated, the analogy has improved because the eye has systems to focus automatically, adjust its sensitivity for widely different light levels, move to track and stabilize a target, and even keep its surface washed and clear (obviously, cameras still have room for improvement). The similarity to a camera breaks down when we consider the retina, which is decidedly not like standard photographic film.

Figure 13–6A shows a cross section through the human eye. A ray of light entering the eye passes through

FIGURE 13–5. The electromagnetic spectrum. AC, alternating current.

A ANATOMY

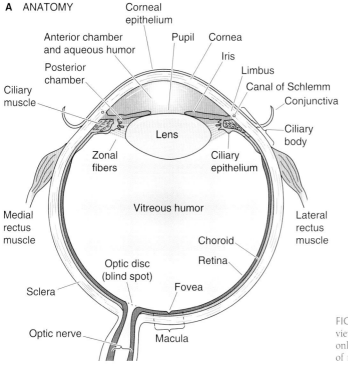

B REFRACTIVE INDEX OF
EYE COMPONENTS

FIGURE 13–6. The eye. *A,* A cross section of the right human eye, viewed from the top. *B,* The bending of light by a structure depends not only on the radius of curvature but also on the difference in the indices of refraction of the two adjoining media.

several relatively transparent elements to reach the retina: these elements include a thin film of tears and then the cornea, the aqueous humor, the lens, and finally the vitreous humor. **Tears** are a surprisingly complex liquid, based on a plasma ultrafiltrate. They bathe the cornea in a layer that is less than 10 μm thick, keep it wet, and allow oxygen to diffuse from the air to the corneal cells. Tears also contain lysozymes and antibodies to counter infection, a superficial oily layer that greatly slows evaporation and prevents spillage at the lid margins, and a thin mucoid layer to wet the surface of the cornea and allow the tears to spread smoothly. Tears also help flush away foreign substances. The **cornea** is a thin, transporting epithelium that is devoid of blood vessels and has a cell structure that is specialized to maintain its high transparency. The ciliary epithelium constantly secretes the **aqueous humor**, a protein-free ultrafiltrate of blood plasma, into the posterior chamber of the eye. The aqueous humor then flows between the iris and the anterior surface of the lens and reaches the **anterior chamber** via the pupil. This aqueous humor keeps the anterior portion of the eye slightly pressurized ($\sim$20 mm Hg), which helps maintain the eye's shape. The canals of Schlemm drain the aqueous humor. Excess pressure in the anterior chamber produces a disease called glaucoma. The **lens** is an onion-like structure with closely packed columnar cells that are arranged in concentric shells and encased by a thin, tough, transparent capsule that is composed of epithelial cells. The cells of the lens have a high concentration of proteins called α-crystallins, which help increase the density of the lens and enhance its focusing power. The **posterior chamber**, which is filled with a gelatinous substance called **vitreous humor**, is also kept pressurized by the production of aqueous humor.

The light must be focused to generate a clear optical image on the retina. This is accomplished by the cornea and, to a lesser extent, the lens. Focusing requires that the path of the light is bent, or refracted. Refraction can occur when light passes from a medium in which it travels relatively fast into a medium in which it travels relatively slowly, or vice versa. The **index of refraction** for a substance is essentially a measure of the speed of light within it; for example, light travels faster through air (index of refraction, 1.0003) than through the denser substance of the cornea (index of refraction, 1.376). Two things determine how much a light ray is refracted: the difference in the refractive indices of the two media and the angle between the incident light and the interface between the two media. Simple convex lenses use curved surfaces to control the refraction of light rays so that they converge (or focus) on a distant surface. The focal power (D) of one surface of a spherical lens is

Equation 13–1

$$\text{Focal power} = \frac{n_2 - n_1}{r}$$

Here, n_1 and n_2 are the refractive indices of the first and second medium and r is the radius of curvature of the lens in meters. The unit of focal power is a *diopter* (1 D = 1 m^{-1}). Focal power is the reciprocal of focal length. Thus, parallel light rays entering a 1 D lens are focused at 1 m and those entering a 2 D lens are focused at 0.5 m.

In the case of the eye, most of the focusing takes place at the interface between the air and the tear-covered anterior surface of the cornea because this region is where light encounters the greatest disparity in refractive index on its path to the retina (see Fig. 13–6B). With a change of 0.376 in refractive index and a radius of outer curvature of 7.8 mm in a typical human cornea, the focal power is 48.2 D. The curvature on the inner surface of the cornea is reversed, so some focal power is lost as light passes into the aqueous humor. However, the change in refractive index at this surface is only 0.040, so the change is only −5.9 D. The lens of the eye, with convex curvature on both sides, has a potentially greater focal power than the cornea. However, because of the small difference in refractive index between the substance of the lens and the aqueous and vitreous humor surrounding it, the effective focal power of the lens is lower. The summed focal power of the optics of the relaxed eye is about 60 D, which allows it to focus light from distant objects onto the retina, the center of which is about 24 mm behind the surface of the cornea. The position of the retinal image is, of course, upside down relative to the object that produced it.

A normal *resting* eye is focused on distant objects, beyond about 7 m. If it were fixed in this position, it would be impossible to see objects that are close up. To focus objects that are closer than 7 m away, the eye needs to increase its focal power, a process called **accommodation**. The eye achieves this goal by changing the shape of the lens. At rest, the lens is suspended around its edge by elastic **zonal fibers** that keep its capsule stretched and relatively flattened. To accommodate, the ciliary muscle fibers contract and release some of the tension in the zonal fibers. Relieved of the radial pull of its fibers, the lens becomes rounder. This increased curvature means increased focal power and a shift of the focal point closer to the eye (Equation 13–1). There are limits to accommodation, of course, and they are strongly age dependent. Young children have the most pliable lenses and can increase their focal power up to 12 to 14 D. Their **near point**, the closest distance that they are able to focus, is about at the end of their nose. With age, the lens becomes stiffer and less able to round up and accommodate. By age 30 the near point is about 10 cm, and by the mid-40s it stretches beyond arm's length. The loss of accommodation with age is called **presbyopia**; it is the reason that glasses for reading are unavoidable for almost everyone past middle age. Additional refractive flaws may be caused by an eye that is too long or short for its focusing power or by aberrations in the refracting surfaces of the eye. **Astigmatism**, for example, results from uneven curvature of the refractive surfaces of the eye. As a result, a point source of light cannot be brought to a precise focus on the retina. The resultant diffuse focusing leads to blurring of the image.

The **iris** is the colored structure that is visible through the window of the cornea. The iris's hue comes from pigments in its cells, but its function is to create and adjust the round opening that it encircles—the **pupil**. The pupil is like the aperture of the camera, and the iris is the diaphragm that regulates the amount of light allowed to enter the eye. The iris has sphincter muscles that allow it to constrict (**miosis**), as well as radially oriented muscles for dilatation (**mydriasis**). Regulating pupillary size is the job of nuclei in the brainstem, which receive information about light levels directly from the retina. Control of the pupils in the two eyes is yoked: An increase in light to only one eye causes its pupil to constrict (the **direct light response**), but it also causes an identical constriction in the other eye, even if that eye saw only constant light levels (the **consensual light response**). Pupillary responses serve two functions: (1) they regulate the total amount of light that enters the eye (over a range of about 16-fold), and (2) they affect the quality of the retinal image in the same way that aperture affects the depth of focus of a camera (a smaller pupil diameter gives a greater depth of focus).

Other peripheral structures are also essential to proper visual function. The most important are the extraocular muscles that control eye movements and thus the direction of gaze, the tracking of objects, and the coordination of the two eyes to keep their retinal images aligned as the eye, head, and visual world move about. Nuclei in the brainstem also control these tracking functions.

The Retina Is a Small, Displaced Part of the Central Nervous System

The retina is a very thin (~200 μm thick in humans) sheet of tissue that lines the back of the eye and contains the light-sensitive cells, the **photoreceptors**. Photoreceptors capture photons, convert their light energy into chemical free energy, and ultimately generate a synaptic signal for relay to other visual neurons in the retina.

The retina is, histologically and embryologically, a part of the CNS. Not only does it transduce light into neural signals, but it also does some remarkably complex processing of visual information before passing it on to other regions of the brain. In addition to the photoreceptor cells, the retina has four additional types of neurons that form an orderly, but intricate neural circuit (Fig. 13–7). One type, the **ganglion cell**, generates the sole output of the retina by sending its axons to the thalamus via the optic nerve (CN II).

The retina is a highly laminated structure. Through a quirk of evolution, the photoreceptors of the vertebrate eye are on the *outer* surface of the retina, that is, the side facing *away* from the vitreous humor and incoming light. Thus, to reach the transducing cells, light has to first pass through all the retinal neurons. This path causes only minor distortion of image quality because of the thinness and transparency of the neural layers. This seemingly inverted arrangement may actually be an advantage for housekeeping of the eye. Photoreceptors undergo a continuous process of renewal, sloughing off membrane from their outer segments and rebuilding them. They also demand a relatively high energy supply. Because they face the back of the eye, photoreceptors are close to the **pigment epithelium**, which aids the renewal process, and to the blood vessels that supply the retina. These poorly transparent structures (i.e., pigment epithelium and blood vessels) are thus isolated from the light path. In fact, the pigment epithelium also *absorbs* photons that are not first captured by photoreceptors, before they can be reflected and degrade the visual image.

Each human eye has over 100×10^6 photoreceptors, but only 1×10^6 ganglion cells, which implies a high

FIGURE 13–7. The retina. The neural circuits in the retina of a primate. Notice that the incoming light reaches the photoreceptor cells (*rods* and *cones*) only after passing through several thin, transparent layers of other neurons. The pigment epithelium absorbs the light that is not absorbed by the photoreceptor cells and thus minimizes reflections of stray light. The ganglion cells communicate to the thalamus by sending action potentials down their axons. However, the photoreceptor cells and other neurons communicate by graded synaptic potentials that are conducted electrotonically.

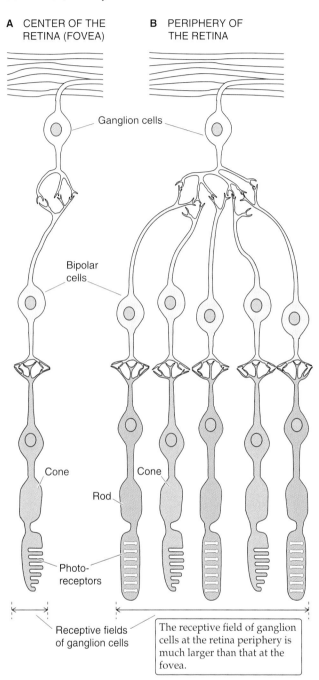

A CENTER OF THE RETINA (FOVEA)

B PERIPHERY OF THE RETINA

Ganglion cells

Bipolar cells

Cone

Cone

Rod

Photo-receptors

Receptive fields of ganglion cells

The receptive field of ganglion cells at the retina periphery is much larger than that at the fovea.

FIGURE 13–8. Comparison of receptive fields in the fovea and periphery of the retina.

retina. **Amacrine cells** synapse within the inner layer of the retina and interconnect both bipolar cells and ganglion cells. The circuitry of the retina is much more complex than this picture implies. One hint of this complexity is that its four primary types of neurons are in turn divided into at least 10 to 20 distinct subtypes, each with different physiology and morphology.

The thinness of the mammalian retina has an interesting biophysical consequence. Because signalling distances are so short, synaptic potentials can spread effectively within its neurons without the help of conventional action potentials. Electrotonic spread of potentials along the dendrites is generally enough. The main exceptions are the ganglion cells, which use action potentials to speed visual information along their axons to the thalamus.

There Are Two Types of Photoreceptors: Rods and Cones

The two types of photoreceptors, rods and cones, are named for their characteristic shapes (see Fig. 13–7). The human retina has only one type of rod, which is responsible for our monochromatic dark-adapted vision, and three subtypes of cones, which are responsible for the color-sensitive vision that we experience in brighter environments. Rods outnumber cones by at least 16:1, and each is spread in a distinct pattern across the retina.

In the central area of the primate retina is a small pit 300 to 700 μm in diameter (which accounts for 1 to 2.3 degrees of visual angle) called the **fovea**, which collects light from the center of our gaze (see Fig. 13–6). Several adaptations of the fovea allow it to mediate the highest visual acuity in the retina. Neurons of the inner layer of retina are actually displaced laterally to the side of the fovea to minimize light scattering on the way to the receptors. In addition, within the fovea the ratio of photoreceptors to ganglion cells falls dramatically. Most foveal receptors synapse on only one bipolar cell, which synapses on only one ganglion cell (Fig. 13–8A). Because each ganglion cell is devoted to a very small portion of the visual field, central vision has high resolution. In other words, the receptive field of a foveal ganglion cell is small. At the periphery, the ratio of receptors to ganglion cells is high (see Fig. 13–8B); thus, each ganglion cell has a large receptive field. The large receptive field reduces the spatial resolution of the peripheral portion of the retina but increases its sensitivity because more photoreceptors collect light for a ganglion cell. Foveal vision is purely cone mediated, and the sheet of foveal photoreceptors consists of only the smallest cones packed at the highest density (about 0.3 μm from the center of one cone to another). Cone density falls to very low levels outside the fovea, and rod density rises. Peripheral vision (i.e., nonfoveal vision, or vision at visual angles >10 degrees away from the center of the fovea and thus the center of gaze) is mediated by both rods and cones.

Photoreceptors are elongated cells with synaptic terminals, an inner segment, and an outer segment (see Fig. 13–7). The **synaptic terminals** connect to the inner segment via a short axon. The **inner segment** contains the nucleus and metabolic machinery; it synthesizes the pho-

degree of convergence of information as it flows from the transducing cells to the output cells. Some of this convergence is mediated by a set of interneurons (i.e., cells that make synaptic connections only within the retina) called **bipolar** cells, which directly connect photoreceptors and ganglion cells in a mainly radial direction (see Fig. 13–7). The two remaining types of retinal neurons, horizontal cells and amacrine cells, are interneurons that mainly spread horizontally. **Horizontal cells** synapse within the outer layer of the retina and interconnect photoreceptors and bipolar cells to themselves and to each other. Horizontal cells often mediate interactions over a wide area of topigments and has a high density of mitochondria. The inner segment also serves an optical function—its high density funnels photons into the outer segment. A thin ciliary stalk connects the inner segment to the outer segment. The **outer segment** is the transduction site, although it is the last part of the cell to see the light. Structurally, the outer segment is a highly modified cilium. Each rod outer segment has about 1000 tightly packed stacks of *disk membranes*, which are flattened, membrane-bound intracellular organelles that have pinched off from the outer membrane. Cone outer segments have similarly stacked membranes, except that they are infolded and remain continuous with the outer membrane. The disk membranes contain the photopigments—**rhodopsin** in rods and molecules related to rhodopsin in cones. Rhodopsin moves from its synthesis site in the inner segment through the stalk and into the outer segment via small vesicles whose membranes are packed with rhodopsin to be incorporated into the disks.

Photoreceptors Hyperpolarize in Response to Light

The remarkable psychophysical experiments of Hecht and colleagues in 1942 demonstrated that five to seven photons, each acting on only a single rod, are sufficient to evoke a sensation of light in humans. Thus, the rod is performing at the edge of its physical limits because there is no light level smaller than one photon. To detect a single photon requires a prodigious feat of signal amplification. As Denis Baylor has pointed out, "the sensitivity of rod vision is so great that the energy needed to lift a sugar cube one centimeter, if converted to a blue-green light, would suffice to give an intense sensation of a flash to every human who ever existed."

Phototransduction involves a cascade of chemical and electrical events to detect, amplify, and signal a response to light. As in many other sensory receptors, photoreceptors use electrical events (receptor potentials) to carry the visual signal from the outer segment to their synapses. Chemical messengers diffusing over such a distance would simply be too slow. The surprising fact about the receptor potential of rods and cones is that it is *hyperpolarizing*. Light causes the cell's V_m to become *more negative* than the resting potential that it maintains in the dark (Fig. 13–9A). At low light intensities, the size of the receptor potential rises linearly with light intensity, but at higher intensities the response saturates.

Hyperpolarization is an essential step in relaying the visual signal because it directly modulates the rate of transmitter release from the photoreceptor onto its postsynaptic neurons. This synapse is conventional in that it releases more transmitter—in this case glutamate—when its presynaptic terminal is depolarized and less when it is hyperpolarized. Thus, a flash of light causes a *decrease* in transmitter secretion. The upshot is that the vertebrate photoreceptor is most active in the dark.

How is the light-induced hyperpolarization generated? In the dark, each photoreceptor produces an ionic current that flows steadily into the outer segment and out of the inner segment. This **dark current** is carried mainly by inwardly directed Na^+ ions in the outer segment and by outwardly directed K^+ ions from the inner segment (see Fig. 13–9B). Na^+ flows through a nonselective cation channel of the outer segment, which light indirectly regulates, and K^+ flows through a K^+ channel in the inner segment, which light does not regulate. Na^+ carries approximately 90% of the dark current in the outer segment, and Ca^{2+}, approximately 10%. In the dark, V_m is about -40 mV. Na-K pumps, primarily located within the inner segments, remove the Na^+ and import K^+. A Na-Ca exchanger removes Ca^{2+} from the outer segment.

Absorption of photons leads to closure of the nonselective cation channels in the outer segment. The total conductance of the cell membrane decreases. Because the K^+ channels of the inner segment remain open, K^+ continues to flow out of the cell, and this outward current causes the cell to hyperpolarize (see Fig. 13–9C). The number of cation channels that close depends on the number of photons that are absorbed. The range of one rod's sensitivity is from 1 to approximately 1000 photons. Cones are less sensitive, but they are faster than rods; moreover, cone responses do not saturate even at the brightest levels of natural light.

Using the clever method shown in Figure 13–10, in which they sucked up a single rod outer segment into a recording pipette, Baylor and colleagues in 1979 measured the minimum amount of light required to produce a change in receptor current. They found that absorption of one photon suppresses a surprisingly large current, equivalent to the entry of more than 10^6 Na^+ ions, and thus represents an enormous amplification of energy. At the peak of the response, this decrease in Na^+ influx represents about 3% of the cell's entire dark current. The single-photon response is also much larger than the background electrical noise in the rod, as it must be to produce the rod's high sensitivity to dim light. Cones respond similarly to single photons, but they are inherently noisier and their response is only about 1/50th the size of that in the rod.

Rhodopsin Is a G-Protein–Coupled "Receptor" for Light

How can a single photon stop the flow of 1 million Na^+ ions across the membrane of a rod cell? The process begins when the photon is absorbed by rhodopsin, the light receptor molecule. Rhodopsin is one of the most tightly packed proteins in the body, with a density of about 30,000 molecules per square micrometer in the disk membranes. Thus, the packing ratio is 1 protein molecule for every 60 lipid molecules! One rod contains about 10^9 rhodopsin molecules. This staggering density ensures an optimized capture rate for photons passing through a photoreceptor. Even so, only about 10% of the light entering the eye is used by the receptors. The rest is either absorbed by the optical components of the eye or passes between or through the receptors. Rhodopsin has two key components: retinal (vitamin A aldehyde, $\sim$500 Da) and the protein opsin ($\sim$41 kDa). **Opsin** is a single polypeptide with seven membrane-spanning segments (Fig. 13–11A). It is a member of the superfamily of

A LIGHT-EVOKED HYPERPOLARIZATIONS

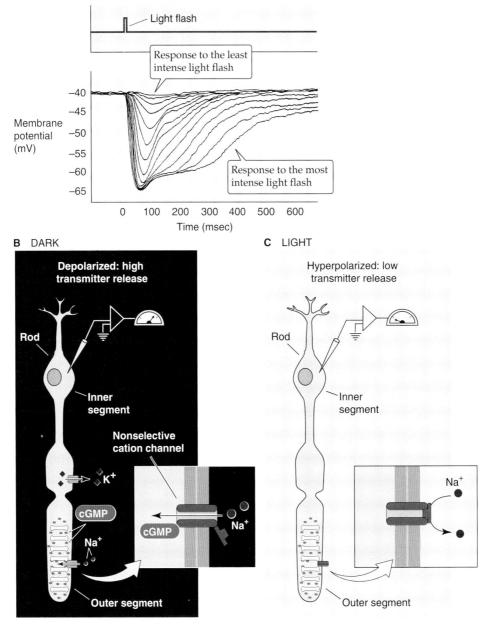

FIGURE 13–9. Phototransduction. *A,* The experiment summarized here was performed on a red-sensitive cone from a turtle. A brief flash of light causes a hyperpolarization of the photoreceptor cell. The size of the peak and the duration of the receptor potential increase with the increasing intensity of the flash. At low light intensities, the magnitude of the peak increases linearly with light intensity. At high intensities, the peak response saturates, but the plateau becomes longer. (Data from Baylor DA, Hodgkin AL, Lamb TD: The electrical response of turtle cones to flashes and steps of light. J Physiol 242:685–727, 1974.) *B,* In the absence of light, Na^+ enters the outer segment of the rod through cGMP-gated channels and depolarizes the cell. The electrical circuit for this dark current is completed by K^+ leaving the inner segment. The dark current, which depolarizes the cell, leads to constant transmitter release. *C,* In the presence of light, Na^+ can no longer enter the cell because cGMP levels are low, and the cGMP-gated channel closes. The photoreceptor cell thus hyperpolarizes, and transmitter release decreases. cGMP, cyclic guanosine monophosphate.

Figure 13-10. Use of a suction pipette to record the current through the outer segment of a single rod. *A,* A suction pipette is positioned just above a group of rods from a toad retina. *B,* One of these rods has been sucked into the pipette, allowing the investigators to monitor the current in a single photoreceptor cell. The *horizontal white band* is the light used to stimulate the rod. (Reproduced from Baylor DA, Lamb TD, Yau K-W: Responses of retinal rods to single photons. J Physiol (Lond) 288:613–634, 1979.)

G-protein–coupled membrane receptors (p. 92) that includes many neurotransmitter receptors as well as the odor receptor molecules (see earlier).

To be transduced, photons are actually absorbed by **retinal**, which is responsible for rhodopsin's color. The tail of retinal can twist into a variety of geometric configurations, one of which is a kinked and unstable version called **11-*cis* retinal** (see Fig. 13–11*B*). The *cis* form sits within a pocket (comparable to the ligand-binding site of other G-protein–linked receptors) of the opsin and is covalently bound to it. However, because of its instability, the *cis* form can exist only in the dark. If 11-*cis* retinal absorbs a photon, it isomerizes within one picosecond to a straighter and more stable version called **all-*trans* retinal**. This isomerization in turn triggers a series of conformational changes in the opsin that lead to a form called **metarhodopsin II**, which can activate an attached molecule called transducin. Transducin carries the signal forward in the cascade and causes a reduction in Na⁺ conductance. Soon after isomerization, all-*trans* retinal and opsin separate in a process called **bleaching**; this separa-

tion causes the color to change from the rosy red (*rhodon* is Greek for the color "rose") of rhodopsin to the pale yellow of opsin. The photoreceptor cell converts all-*trans* retinal to retinol (vitamin A), which then translocates to the pigment epithelium and becomes 11-*cis* retinal. This compound makes its way back to the outer segment, where it recombines with opsin. This cycle of rhodopsin regeneration takes a few minutes.

Transducin is so named because it transduces the light-activated signal from rhodopsin into the photoreceptor membrane's response (see Fig. 13–11*C*). Transducin was the first of the large family of guanosine triphosphate (GTP)-binding proteins (G proteins) to be identified, and its amino acid sequence is very similar to that of other G-protein–coupled receptors (p. 92). When activated by metarhodopsin, the α subunit of transducin exchanges a bound guanosine diphosphate (GDP) for a GTP and then diffuses within the plane of the membrane to stimulate a **phosphodiesterase** that hydrolyzes cGMP to 5′-guanylate monophosphate (GMP).

cGMP is the diffusible second messenger that links the light-activated events of the disk membranes to the electrical events of the outer membrane. A key discovery by Fesenko and colleagues in 1985 showed that the "light-sensitive" cation channel of rods is actually a cGMP-gated cation channel (p. 170). This cyclic-nucleotide–gated channel was the first of its kind to be discovered (we have already discussed a similar channel in olfactory receptors). In the dark, a **constitutively active guanylyl cyclase** that synthesizes cGMP from GTP keeps cGMP levels high within the photoreceptor cytoplasm. This high [cGMP]$_i$ causes the cGMP-gated cation channels to spend much of their time open and accounts for the dark current (see Fig. 13–9*B*). Because light stimulates the phosphodiesterase and thus decreases [cGMP]$_i$, light reduces the number of open cGMP-gated cation channels and thus reduces the dark current. The photoreceptor then hyperpolarizes, transmitter release falls, and a visual signal is passed to retinal neurons.

Strong amplification occurs along the phototransduction pathway. The absorption of 1 photon activates 1 metarhodopsin molecule, which can activate about 700 transducin molecules within approximately 100 msec. These transducin molecules activate phosphodiesterase, which increases the rate of cGMP hydrolysis by approximately 100-fold. One photon leads to the hydrolysis of about 1400 cGMP molecules by the peak of the response, thus reducing [cGMP] by about 8% in the cytoplasm around the activated disk. This decrease in [cGMP]$_i$ closes approximately 230 of the 11,000 cGMP-gated channels that are open in the dark. As a result, the dark current falls by about 2%.

The cGMP-gated channel has additional interesting properties. It responds within milliseconds when [cGMP]$_i$ rises, and it does not desensitize in response to cGMP. The concentration-response curve is very steep at low [cGMP]$_i$ because opening requires the simultaneous binding of three cGMP molecules. Thus, the channel has switch-like behavior at physiological levels of cGMP. Ion conductance through the channel also has steep voltage dependence, because Ca²⁺ and Mg²⁺ strongly block the

A   OPSIN

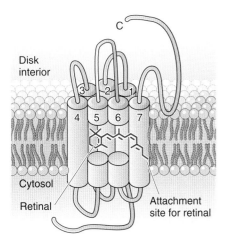

Disk interior

Cytosol

Retinal

Attachment site for retinal

B   RETINAL

11-*cis* retinal

Light

All-*trans* retinal

C   VISUAL TRANSDUCTION

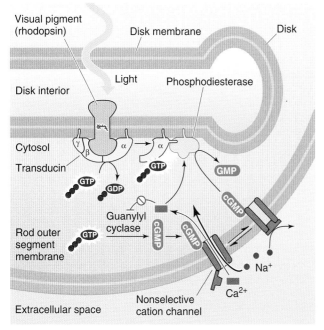

channel (as well as permeate it) within its physiologic voltage range. This open-channel block (see Fig. 7–20D in Chapter 7) makes the normal single-channel conductance very small, among the smallest of any ion channel; the open channel normally carries a current of only 3 × 10^{-15} amperes (3 fA)! The current of ion channels is inherently "noisy" as they flicker open and closed. However, the 11,000 channels—each with currents of 3 fA—summate to a rather noise-free dark current of 11,000 channels × 3 fA per channel = 33 pA. In contrast, if 11 channels—each with currents of 3 pA—carried the dark current of 33 pA, the 2% change in this signal (0.66 pA) would be smaller than the noise produced by the opening and closing of a single channel (3 pA). Thus, the small channels give the photoreceptor a high signal-to-noise ratio.

The [cGMP]$_i$ in the photoreceptor cell represents a dynamic balance between the synthesis of cGMP by guanylyl cyclase and the breakdown of cGMP by phosphodiesterase. Ca^{2+}, which enters through the relatively nonselective cGMP-gated channel, synergistically inhibits the guanylyl cyclase and stimulates the phosphodiesterase. These Ca^{2+} sensitivities set up a negative feedback system. In the dark, the incoming Ca^{2+} prevents runaway increases in [cGMP]$_i$. In the light, the ensuing decrease in [Ca^{2+}]$_i$ relieves the inhibition on guanylyl cyclase, inhibits the phosphodiesterase, increases [cGMP]$_i$, and thus poises the system for channel reopening.

The process of terminating the light-activated state of the photoreceptor cell has not been as well defined as is the activation process. One mechanism appears to involve the channels themselves. As described in the preceding paragraph, closure of the cGMP-gated channels in the light leads to a fall in [Ca^{2+}]$_i$, which helps replenish cGMP and facilitates channel reopening. Two additional mechanisms involve the proteins rhodopsin kinase and arrestin. **Rhodopsin kinase** phosphorylates light-activated rhodopsin and allows it to be recognized by arrestin. **Arrestin**, an abundant cytosolic protein, binds to the phosphorylated light-activated rhodopsin and helps terminate the activated state of the receptor, probably by competing with transducin.

Figure 13–11. Rhodopsin, transducin, and signal transduction at the molecular level. *A,* The opsin molecule is a classic 7-transmembrane receptor that couples to transducin, a G protein. The attachment site of the retinal is amino-acid residue 296 in the seventh (i.e., most C-terminal) membrane-spanning segment. *B,* The absorption of a photon by 11-*cis* retinal causes the molecule to isomerize to all-*trans* retinal. *C,* After rhodopsin absorbs a photon of light, it activates many transducins. The activated α subunit of transducin (Gα$_t$) in turn activates phosphodiesterase, which hydrolyzes cGMP. The resultant decrease in [cGMP]$_i$ closes cGMP-gated channels and produces a hyperpolarization (receptor potential). cGMP, cyclic guanosine monophosphate; GDP, guanosine diphosphate; GTP, guanosine triphosphate.

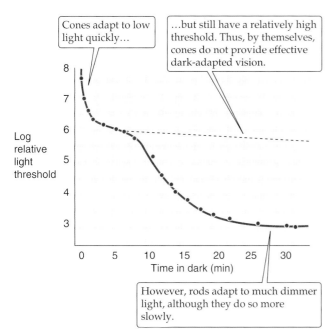

Cones adapt to low light quickly...

...but still have a relatively high threshold. Thus, by themselves, cones do not provide effective dark-adapted vision.

However, rods adapt to much dimmer light, although they do so more slowly.

Figure 13–12. The effect of dark adaptation on the visual threshold. The subject was exposed to light at a level of 1600 millilumens and then switched to the dark. The graph is a plot of the time course of the subject's relative threshold (on a log scale) for detecting a light stimulus. (Data from Hecht S, Shlaer S, Smith EL, et al.: The visual functions of the complete color blind. J Gen Physiol 31:459–472, 1948.)

photoreceptor mechanisms. The *neural* mechanisms are relatively fast, operate at relatively low ambient light levels, and involve multiple mechanisms within the neuronal network of the retina. The *photoreceptor* mechanisms involve some of the processes that are described in the previous section. Thus, in bright sunlight, rods become ineffective because most of their rhodopsin remains inactivated, or bleached. After returning to darkness, the rods slowly regenerate rhodopsin and become sensitive once again. However, a component of the cGMP system also regulates photoreceptor sensitivity. In the dark, when baseline $[cGMP]_i$ is relatively high, substantial amounts of Ca^{2+} enter via cGMP-gated channels. The resultant high $[Ca^{2+}]_i$ inhibits guanylyl cyclase and stimulates phosphodiesterase, thereby preventing $[cGMP]_i$ from rising too high. Conversely, when background light levels are high, this same feedback system causes baseline $[cGMP]_i$ to remain high so that $[cGMP]_i$ can fall in response to further increases in light levels. Otherwise, the signal-transduction system would become saturated. In other words, the photoreceptor adapts to the increased background light intensity and remains responsive to small changes. Additional adaptation mechanisms regulate the sensitivity of rhodopsin, guanylyl cyclase, and the cGMP-gated channel. Clearly, adaptation involves an intricate network of molecular interaction.

The Eye Uses a Variety of Mechanisms to Adapt to a Wide Range of Light Levels

The human eye can operate effectively over a 10^{10}-fold range of light intensities, which is the equivalent of going from almost total darkness to bright sunlight on snow. However, moving from a bright to a dark environment, or vice versa, requires time for adaptation before the eye can respond optimally. Adaptation is mediated by several mechanisms. One mechanism mentioned earlier is regulating the size of the pupil by the iris, which can change light sensitivity by about 16-fold. That still leaves the vast majority of the range to account for. During **dark adaptation,** two additional mechanisms with very different time courses are evident, as we can see from a test of the detection threshold for the human eye (Fig. 13–12). The first phase of adaptation is finished within approximately 10 minutes and is a property of the cones; the second takes at least 30 minutes and is attributed to the rods. A fully dark-adapted retina, relying on rods, can have a light threshold that is as much as 15,000 times lower than a retina relying on cones. In essence, then, the human eye has two retinas in one, a rod retina for low light levels and a cone retina for high light levels. These two systems can operate at the same time; when dark-adapted, the rods can respond to the lowest light levels, but cones are available to respond when brighter stimuli appear.

The rapid and slow phases of adaptation that are discussed in the previous paragraph have both neural and

Color Vision Depends on the Different Spectral Sensitivities of the Three Types of Cones

The human eye responds only to a small region of the electromagnetic spectrum (see Fig. 13–5), but within it we are exquisitely sensitive to the light's wavelength. We see assorted colors in a daytime panorama because objects absorb some wavelengths while reflecting, refracting, or transmitting others. Different sources of light may also affect the colors of a scene; the light from tungsten bulbs is reddish, whereas that of fluorescent bulbs is bluish.

Research on color vision has a long history. In 1801, Thomas Young first outlined the trichromatic theory of color vision, which was championed later in the 19th century by Hermann von Helmholtz. These investigators found that they could reproduce a particular sample hue by mixing the correct intensities of three lights with the primary hues blue, green, and red. They proposed that color vision, with its wide range of distinct, perceived hues, was based on only three different pigments in the eye, each absorbing a different range of wavelengths. Microspectrophotometry of single cones in 1964 amply confirmed this scheme. Thus, although analysis of color by the human brain is sophisticated and complex, it all derives from the responses of only three types of photopigments in cones.

Our sensitivity to the wavelength of light depends on the retina's state of adaptation. When dark-adapted (also called **scotopic** conditions), the spectral sensitivity curve for human vision is shifted toward shorter wavelengths

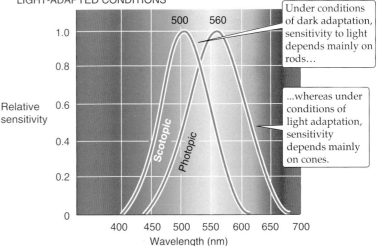

A SPECTRAL SENSITIVITY UNDER DARK- AND LIGHT-ADAPTED CONDITIONS

> Under conditions of dark adaptation, sensitivity to light depends mainly on rods…

> …whereas under conditions of light adaptation, sensitivity depends mainly on cones.

Figure 13–13. Sensitivity of vision and photoreceptors at different wavelengths of light. *A*, The figure shows the results of a psychophysical experiment. Under dark-adapted ("scotopic") conditions, the eye is maximally sensitive at approximately 500 nanometers (nm). Under light-adapted ("photopic") conditions, the human eye is maximally sensitive at approximately 560 nm. (Data from Knowles A: The biochemical aspects of vision. In Barlow HB, Mollon JD [eds]: The Senses. Cambridge, Cambridge University Press, 1982, pp 82–101.) *B*, The spectral sensitivity of rods—obtained with a spectro-photometer—peaks at approximately 500 nm, whereas that of the three types of cones peak at approximately 420 nm for the S (*blue*), approximately 530 nm for the M (*green*) and approximately 560 nm for L (*red*). (Data from Dartnell HJ, Bowmaker JK, Mollon JD: Microspec-trophotometry of human photoreceptors. In Mollon JD, Sharpe LT [eds]: Colour Vision. London, Academic Press, 1983, pp 69–80.)

B ABSORBANCE SPECTRA OF THE HUMAN ROD AND CONE RHODOPSINS

when compared with the curve obtained after light adaptation (**photopic** conditions; Fig. 13–13*A*). The absolute sensitivity to light can also be several orders of magnitude higher under scotopic conditions (see Fig. 13–12). The primary reason for the difference in these curves is that rods are doing the transduction of dim light under dark-adapted conditions whereas cones transduce in the light-adapted eye. As we would predict, the spectral sensitivity curve for scotopic vision is quite similar to the absorption spectrum of the rods' rhodopsin, with a peak at 500 nm.

The spectral sensitivity of the light-adapted eye depends on the photopigments in the cones. Humans have three different kinds of cones, and each expresses a photopigment with a different absorbance spectrum. The peaks of their absorbance curves fall at about 420, 530, and 560 nm, which correspond to the violet, yellow-green, and yellow-red regions of the spectrum (see Fig. 13–13*B*). The three cones and their pigments were historically called blue, green, and red, respectively. They are now more commonly called S, M, and L (for short, medium, and long wavelengths); we use the latter terminology. Because the absolute sensitivity of the short-wavelength cone is only one tenth that of the other two, the

spectral sensitivity of photopic human vision is dominated by the two longer-wavelength cones (compare the spectral sensitivity functions in Fig. 13–13*A* with the absorbance spectra of the cones in Fig. 13–13*B*).

It is important to recognize that *single* cones do not encode the wavelength of a light stimulus. If a cone responds to a photon, it generates the same response regardless of the wavelength of that photon. A glance at Figure 13–13*B* shows that each type of cone pigment can absorb a wide range of wavelengths. The pigment in a cone is more likely to absorb photons when their wavelength is at its peak absorbance, but light hitting the cone on the fringe of its absorbance range can still generate a large response if the light's intensity is sufficiently high. This property of response **univariance** is the reason that vision in an eye with only one functioning pigment (e.g., scotopic vision using only rods) can only be monochromatic. With a single pigment system, the distinction between different colors and between differences in intensity is confounded. Two different cones (as in most New World monkeys), each with a different but overlapping range of wavelength sensitivity, remove much of the ambiguity in encoding the wavelength of light stimuli. With

INHERITED DEFECTS IN COLOR VISION

Inherited defects in color vision are relatively common, and many are caused by mutations in visual pigment genes. For example, 8% of white males and 1% of white females have some defect in their L or M pigments caused by X-linked recessive mutations. A single abnormal pigment can lead to either **dichromacy** (the absence of one functional pigment) or **anomalous trichromacy** (the absorption spectrum of one pigment shifted relative to normal), often with a consequent inability to distinguish certain colors. Jeremy Nathans and colleagues found that men have only one copy of the L pigment gene, but located right next to it on the X chromosome they may have from one to three copies of the M pigment gene. He proposed that homologous recombination could account for the gene duplication, loss of a gene, or production of the hybrid L-M genes that occur in red-green color blindness. Hybrid L-M pigments have spectral properties intermediate between those of the two normal pigments, probably because their opsins consist of a combination of the traits of the two normal pigments.

Lack of two of the three functional cone pigments leads to **monochromacy.** The number of people who have such true color blindness is very small, less than 0.001% of the population. For example, S-cone monochromacy is a rare X-linked disorder in which both L and M photopigments are missing because of mutations on the X chromosome. The S pigment is on chromosome 7.

three overlapping pigments (as in Old World monkeys and humans), light of a single wavelength stimulates each of the three cones to different degrees, and light of any other wavelength stimulates these cones with a distinctly different pattern. Because the nervous system can compare the *relative* stimulation of the three cone types to decode the wavelength, it can also distinguish changes in the intensity (luminance) of the light from changes in its wavelength.

Color capabilities are not constant across the retina. The use of multiple cones is not compatible with fine spatial discrimination because of wavelength-dependent differences in the eye's ability to focus light (**chromatic aberration**) and because very small objects may stimulate only single cones. The fovea has only M and L cones, which limits its color discrimination in comparison to the peripheral portions of the retina but leaves it best adapted to discriminate fine spatial detail.

The four different human visual pigments have a similar structure. The presence of retinal and the mechanisms of its photoisomerization are essentially identical in each. The main difference is the primary structure of the attached protein, the opsin. M and L opsins share 96% of their amino acids. Pairwise comparisons among the other opsins show only 44% or lower sequence similarity, however. Apparently, the different amino-acid structures of the opsins affect their charge distributions in the region of the 11-*cis* retinal and shift its absorption spectrum to give the different pigments their specific spectral sensitivities.

AUDITORY AND VESTIBULAR TRANSDUCTION: HAIR CELLS

Listening to music and balancing on one foot both involve sensory systems that have similar transduction mechanisms. Sensation in both the auditory and vestibular systems begins with the inner ear, and both use a highly specialized kind of receptor called the **hair cell**. Common structure and function often suggest a common origin, and indeed, the organs of mammalian hearing and balance both evolved from the **lateral line organs** present in all aquatic vertebrates. The lateral line consists of a series of pits or tubes along the flanks of an animal. Within each indentation are clusters of sensory cells that are similar to hair cells. These cells have cilia projecting into a gelatinous material that is in contact with the water in which the animal swims. In many animals, the lateral line is exquisitely sensitive to vibrations or pressure changes in the water, although in some species they are also sensitive to temperature or electric fields. Reptiles abandoned the lateral line during their evolution, but they retained the hair-cell–centered sensory structures of the inner ear that evolved from the lateral line.

The **auditory system** provides our senses of hearing, and the **vestibular system** generates our sense of balance. Auditory stimuli are often at the forefront of our conscious experience, whereas vestibular information is rarely noticed unless something goes wrong. Hearing is an exceptionally versatile process that allows us to detect things in our environment, precisely identify their nature, localize them well at a distance, and, through language, communicate with speed, complexity, nuance, and emotion. Vestibular sensation has a more focused task. It operates constantly while we are awake and informs the brain how our head and body are oriented and which way and how fast they are moving. Such information is essential for generating muscular contractions that will put our body where we want it to be, to reorient the body when something pushes us aside, and to move our eyes continually so that the visual world stays fixed on our retinas even though our head may be nodding about. Vestibular dysfunction can make it impossible to stabilize an image on our moving retinas, and it causes the disconcerting feeling that the world is uncontrollably moving around. Walking and standing can be difficult or impossible. With time, compensatory adjustments are made as the brain learns to substitute more visual and proprioceptive cues to help guide smooth and accurate movements.

Bending the Stereocilia of Hair Cells Along One Axis Causes Cation Channels to Open or Close

Hair cells (Fig. 13–14) are mechanoreceptors that are specialized to detect minuscule movement along one particular axis. The cells are polarized, with their hair bundle projecting from the apical end and synaptic contacts made at their basal end (Fig. 13–15A). The hair bundle consists of one large **kinocilium**, which is a true cilium with nine pairs of microtubules around a core (see Fig. 2–12A), and 50 to 150 **stereocilia**, which are filled with

Figure 13–14. Structure of a hair cell. This is a scanning electron micrograph of bullfrog hair cells from the sensory epithelium of the saccule. (Reproduced from Corey DP, Assad JA: In Corey DP, Roper SD [eds]: Sensory Transduction. New York, Rockefeller University Press, 1992.)

actin and are more akin to microvilli. Hair cells of the mammalian cochlea lose their kinocilium with maturity, whereas vestibular hair cells retain them. The stereocilia are 0.2 to 0.8 μm in diameter and are generally 4 to 10 μm in height. These "hairs" are arranged in a neat array, with the kinocilium standing tallest along one side of the bundle and the stereocilia falling away in height to the opposite side. Cilia are narrower at their base and insert into the apical membrane of the hair cell, where they make a sort of hinge before connecting to a cuticular plate. Within the bundle, stereocilia are connected one to the next, but they can slide with respect to each other as the bundle is deflected side to side. The ends of the cilia are interconnected with very fine strands called **tip links**, which can be seen with the electron microscope.

The appropriate stimulus for a hair cell is the bending of its hairs, but not just any deflection will do. Bending the hair bundle toward the kinocilium (see Fig. 13–15B) excites the cell and causes a depolarizing receptor potential. Bending the hair bundle away from the kinocilium (see Fig. 13–15C) hyperpolarizes the cell. Only tiny movements are needed; as little as 0.5 nm (which is the diameter of a large atom) gives a detectable response, and the response is saturated at less than 0.5 μm, about the diameter of one cilium (see Fig. 13–15D)! In fact, the sensitivity of hair cells is limited only by noise from brownian motion of surrounding molecules. The cell is also exquisitely selective to direction. If the hairs are bent along the axis 90 degrees to their preferred direction, they are less than one tenth as responsive.

Hair cells are part of an epithelium that separates perilymph from endolymph. The **perilymph** that bathes the basolateral side of the hair cells is similar to cerebrospinal fluid and has a relatively low [K$^+$]. Its voltage is zero— close to that of most other extracellular fluids in the body. The basolateral resting potential of the hair cell is about -60 mV and is dominated by its K$^+$ conductance and the large in-to-out K$^+$ gradient across its basolateral

membrane. The **endolymph** bathing the stereocilium is singular in both composition and voltage. It has a very high [K$^+$] (150 mM) and a very low [Na$^+$] (1 mM), more like cytoplasm than extracellular fluid. The voltage of the endolymph is about $+80$ mV relative to perilymph. Across the apical membrane, the *chemical* gradient for K$^+$ is small. However, the *electrical* gradient is extraordinarily large (higher in the auditory than the vestibular system). Indeed, the sum of the endolymph potential ($+80$ mV relative to perilymph) and the basolateral membrane potential (-60 mV relative to perilymph) creates a very large voltage difference (140 mV) across the apical membrane of the hair cells. An unidentified electrogenic pump presumably maintains this large apical voltage gradient.

Mechanotransduction in hair cells seems to be accomplished by directly linking ciliary movement to the gating of apical mechanosensitive cation channels. Electrical measurements, as well as the imaging of intracellular Ca^{2+}, imply that the transduction channels are located near the tips of the cilia. How is channel gating connected to movement of the hairs? The latency of channel opening is extremely short, less than 40 μsec. If one deflects the hairs more rapidly, the channels are activated more quickly. This observation suggests a direct, physical coupling inasmuch as diffusion of a second messenger would take much longer. Corey and Hudspeth have suggested a spring-like molecular linkage between ciliary movement and channel gating. Indirect evidence suggests that the "tip links" may be the tethers between cilia and the channels. Brief exposure to low-Ca^{2+} solutions abolishes transduction, and it also destroys the "tip links" without otherwise causing obvious harm to the cells.

The mechanosensitive channels at the tips of the stereocilia are relatively large (about 100 pS each) and unselective in that they allow all alkali cations and some divalent cations, including Ca^{2+}, to pass easily. Each hair cell has fewer than 100 channels. Under physiologic conditions, K$^+$ carries most of the transduction current. Opening the apical channels leads to *influx* of K$^+$ and thus *depolarization*. K$^+$ leaves the cell through mechano*in*sensitive K$^+$ channels on the basolateral side (see Fig. 13–15B), along a favorable electrochemical gradient.

A hair cell is not a neuron. Hair cells do not project an axon of their own, and most do not generate action potentials. Instead, the membrane near the presynaptic (i.e., basolateral) face of the cell has voltage-gated Ca^{2+} channels that are somewhat active at rest but more active during mechanically induced depolarization (i.e., the receptor potential) of the hair cell. The Ca^{2+} that flows through these channels triggers the release of an excitatory transmitter, probably glutamate, that stimulates the postsynaptic terminal of the sensory neuron. The rate of action-potential firing in the postsynaptic axon is a function of the transmitter output of the presynaptic hair cell.

When the cell is at rest (i.e., with its hairs straight up), a small but steady leak of depolarizing K$^+$ current flows through the cell. This leak allows the hair cell to respond to both positive deflections of its cilia, which cause *depolarization* by increasing cation (K$^+$) conductance, and negative deflections, which cause *hyperpolarization* by decreasing conductance (see Fig. 13–15C).

In mammals, all hair cells—whether part of the audi-

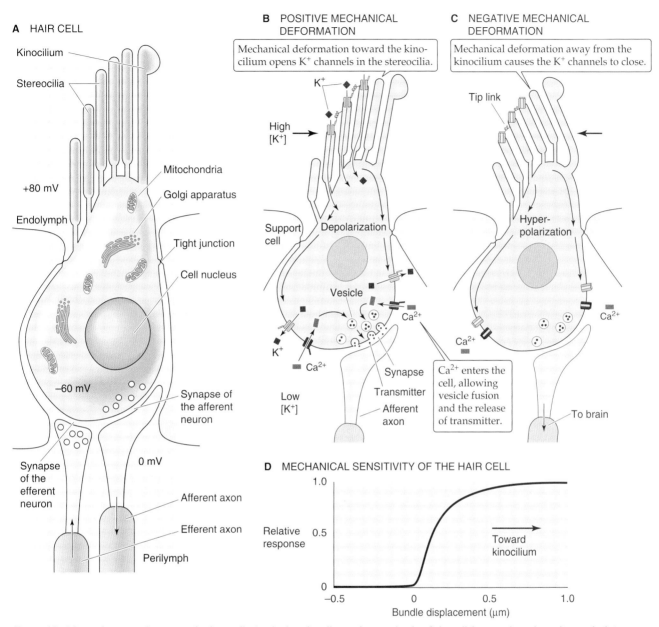

Figure 13–15. Mechanotransduction in the hair cell. *A,* The hair bundle on the apical side of the cell has one large kinocilium, which is a true cilium with a 9 + 2 arrangement of microtubules, as well as 50 − 150 stereocilia, which contain actin and are similar to microvilli. Endolymph, which has a very high [K+], bathes the apical surface. Perilymph, with a much lower [K+], bathes the basolateral surface. Each cell contacts an afferent and efferent axon. *B,* At rest, a small amount of K+ leaks into the cells, driven by the negative membrane potential and high apical [K+]. Mechanical deformation of the hair bundle *towards* the kinocilium increases the opening of non-selective cation channels at the tips of the stereocilia, allowing K+ influx, depolarizing the cell, activating voltage-sensitive Ca++ channels on the basal membrane, causing release of synaptic vesicles, and stimulating the postsynaptic membrane of the accompanying sensory neuron. *C,* Mechanical deformation of the hair bundle *away* from the kinocilium causes the non-selective cation channels to close, leading to hyperpolarization and reduced transmitter release. *D,* The graph shows the relative conductance of a hair cell on the y axis, and the displacement of the hair bundle on the x axis. A displacement of only 0.5 μm, roughly the diameter of a single stereocilium, nearly saturates the conductance change. (*D,* Data from Crawford AC, Fettiplace R: Auditory nerve responses to imposed displacements of the turtle basilar membrane. Hearing Res 12:199–208, 1983.)

tory or vestibular system—are contained within bilateral sets of interconnected tubes and chambers called, appropriately enough, the **membranous labyrinth** (Fig. 13–16A, B). The labyrinth is filled with endolymph and is encased in the temporal bone. The **auditory** portion of the labyrinth is the spiraling **cochlea**, which detects rapid vibrations (sound) transmitted to it from the surrounding air. The **vestibular** portion contains two structures: the **otolith organs**, which detect gravity and head tilt, and the **semicircular canals**, which are sensitive to head rotation. The ultimate function of each of these structures is to transmit mechanical energy to their hair cells. In each case, transduction occurs in the manner described earlier. The specificity of the transduction process comes much less from the hair cells than from the structure of the labyrinth organs around them.

A EAR

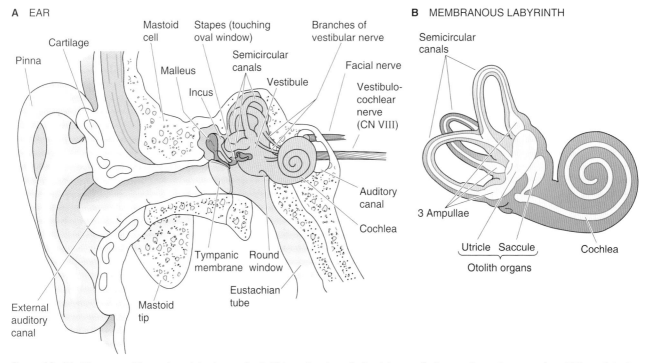

B MEMBRANOUS LABYRINTH

Figure 13–16. The ear, cochlea, and semicircular canals. *A,* This section through the right ear of a human shows the outer, the middle, and the inner ear. *B,* The labyrinth consists of an auditory and a vestibular portion. The auditory portion is the cochlea. The vestibular portion includes the two otolith organs (the utricle and saccule) and the three semicircular canals.

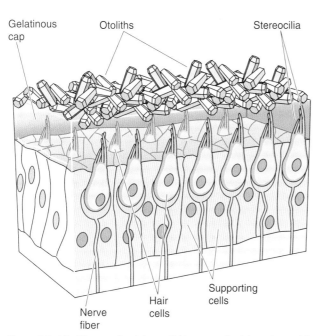

Figure 13–17. The macula of the otolithic organs (utricle and saccule). The macula is a sensory epithelium that contains hair cells and supporting cells. The hair bundles project into the gelatinous cap. Crystals of calcium carbonate, called otoliths, are embedded on the surface of this cap. The hair cells synapse on the ending of a primary sensory axon, which is part of the vestibular nerve (CN VIII).

The Otolithic Organs (Saccule and Utricle) Transduce the Steady Tilt of the Head

The **otolithic organs** are a pair of relatively large chambers near the center of the labyrinth (see Fig. 13–16B). Each contains a sensory epithelium called the **macula**, which is vertically oriented (in the sagittal plane) within the **saccule** and horizontally oriented within the **utricle** when the head is upright. The macula contains the hair cells, which lie among a bed of supporting cells with their cilia projecting into a gelatinous cap (Fig. 13–17). Each hair cell synapses on the ending of a primary sensory axon that is part of the **vestibular nerve**, which in turn is a branch of the vestibulocochlear nerve (CN VIII). **Otoliths** are particles of calcium carbonate, 1 to 5 μm in diameter, that encrust the surface of the gelatinous cap. The otoliths have a higher density than the endolymph that surrounds them, and this difference is the basis for the tilt sensitivity of the otolithic organs. When the angle of the head changes, the otoliths are pulled by gravity and a force is exerted in the same direction on the gelatinous cap; the cap moves slightly, and the cilia of the hair cells are deflected.

The saccule and utricle are specialized for detecting changes in linear acceleration. They respond well to changes in head angle and to acceleration of the sort that you experience as a car or an elevator starts or stops. Of course, the head can tilt in many directions, but the hair cells of the utricle and saccule are oriented to effectively transduce all of them. Single hair cells are polarized and respond best to ciliary bending along one particular axis. The hair cells of each macula are organized so that their polarities cover a full range of directions. Any tilt of the

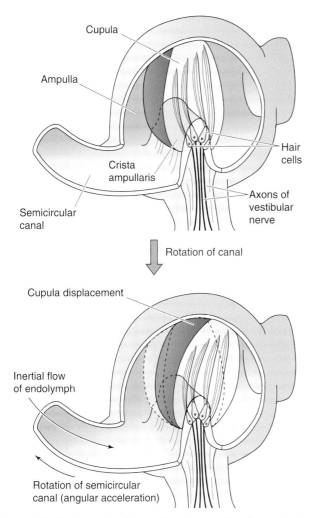

Figure 13–18. Activation of hair cells in the ampulla of a semicircular canal. The *top panel* shows the head at rest. The hair bundles (cilia) of the hair cells project into the cupula, which is a gelatinous mass suspended within the ampulla. When the head rotates in the plane of the canal, as in the *bottom panel*, the rotation of the canal causes an inertial movement of endolymph in the opposite direction. The force of this movement of endolymph bends the deformable cupula and thus bends the cilia of the hair cells. This bending (*shown*) stimulates transmitter release by the hair cells onto axons of the vestibular nerve (CN VIII). Head rotation in the opposite direction would inhibit transmitter release.

nals. Shake your head side to side or nod it up and down, and some of your canals will become very excited.

The semicircular canals stimulate their hair cells differently than do the otolith organs. Hair cells of the canals are clustered within a sensory epithelium (the **crista ampullaris**), which is located in a bulge along the canal called the **ampulla** (Fig. 13–18). The hair bundles project into the gelatinous **cupula**, which spans the lumen of the ampulla. No otoliths are present in the canals, and all the hair cells are oriented in the same direction. Bending of the hairs occurs when the canal is rotated; as the canal moves, endolymph tends to stay behind because of its inertia. The relatively stagnant endolymph exerts a force on the movable cupula, much like wind on a sail. This force bows the cupula, which bends the hairs and (depending on the direction of rotation) either excites or suppresses the release of transmitter from the hair cells onto the sensory axons of the vestibular nerve. This arrangement makes the semicircular canals very sensitive to angular acceleration of the head. If head rotation is maintained at a constant velocity, the friction of endolymph with the canal walls eventually makes the two move together, and bending of the cupula is reduced and then eliminated in about 15 seconds. When rotation is then stopped, the inertia of the endolymph causes bending of the cupula in the other direction and thus gives a temporary sensation of counter-rotation.

Each side of the head has three semicircular canals that lie in approximately orthogonal planes. The **anterior** canal is tilted about 41 degrees anterolaterally from the sagittal plane, the **posterior** canal is tilted about 56 degrees posterolaterally from the sagittal plane, and the **lateral** canal is tipped about 25 degrees back from the horizontal plane. Because each canal best senses rotation about a particular axis, the three together give a good representation of all possible angles of head rotation. This complete representation is further ensured because each canal is paired with another on the opposite side of the head. Each member of a pair sits within the same plane and responds to rotation about the same axis. However, whereas rotation excites the hair cells of one canal, it inhibits the canals of its contralateral axis mate. This push-pull arrangement presumably increases the sensitivity of detection.

head will excite some, reduce the excitability of others, and have no effect on the rest. Because the saccule and utricle are paired structures (one on each side of the head) oriented at right angles to one another, all possible head tilts are well represented by their hair-cell responses. The CNS, by simultaneously using the information encoded by the full population of otolithic hair cells, can unambiguously interpret any angle of movement.

Semicircular Canals Transduce the Angular Acceleration of the Head

Semicircular canals (Fig. 13–16B) also sense acceleration, but not the linear acceleration that the otolith organs prefer. Angular acceleration generated by sudden head rotations is the primary stimulus for the semicircular ca-

Outer and Middle Ears Collect and Condition Air Pressure Waves for Transduction Within the Inner Ear

Sound is a perceptual phenomenon that is produced by periodic waves of pressure through air or water. These waves vary in frequency, amplitude, and direction; our auditory systems are specialized to discriminate all three. We can also interpret the rapid and intricate temporal patterns of sound frequency and amplitude that constitute words and music. Encoding of sound frequency and amplitude begins with mechanisms in the cochlea, followed by further analysis in the CNS. To distinguish the direction of a sound along the horizontal plane, the brain compares signals from the two ears.

All mammalian ears are strikingly similar in structure.

The ear is traditionally divided into outer, middle, and inner components (see Fig. 13–16A). Proceeding from outside to inside, the part most visible is the **pinna**, a skin-covered flap of cartilage, and its small extension the **tragus**. Together, they collect and focus sound waves into the **external auditory canal**. Many animals (e.g., cats) can turn each pinna independently to facilitate hearing without changing head position. The shape of the pinna/tragus tends to emphasize certain sound frequencies over others, depending on their angle of incidence. The external ear parts in humans are essential for localizing sounds in the vertical plane. Sound enters the auditory canal both directly and after being reflected; the sound that we hear is a combination of the two. Depending on a sound's angle of elevation, it is reflected differently off the pinna and tragus. Thus, we hear a sound coming from above our head slightly differently than a sound coming from straight in front of us.

The external auditory canal is also skin lined, and it penetrates approximately 2.5 cm into the temporal bone and ends blindly at the eardrum (or **tympanic membrane**). Sound causes the tympanic membrane to vibrate, much like the head of drum.

The middle ear is an air-filled chamber that is bounded by the tympanic membrane on one side and the **oval window** on the other (see Fig. 13–16). The **eustachian tube** connects the middle ear to the nasopharynx and makes it possible to equalize the air pressure on opposite sides of the tympanic membrane. The primary function of the middle ear is to transfer the vibrations of the tympanic membrane to the oval window. It accomplishes this task with a chain of three delicate bones called **ossicles**: the **malleus** (or hammer), **incus** (anvil), and **stapes** (stirrup). The ossicles are the smallest bones in the body.

Vibration transfer is not as simple as it might seem because sound starts as a set of pressure waves in the air (within the ear canal) and ends up as pressure waves in a watery fluid (within the inner ear). Air and water have a very different **acoustic impedance**, which is the tendency of each medium to oppose movement brought about by a pressure wave. This impedance mismatch means that sound traveling directly from air to water has insufficient pressure to move the dense water molecules. Instead, without some system of compensation, more than 97% of a sound's energy would be reflected when it met a surface of water. The middle ear serves as an *impedance-matching device* that saves most of the aforementioned energy by two primary methods. First, the tympanic membrane has an area that is approximately 20-fold larger than that of the oval window, so a given pressure at the air side (the tympanic membrane) is amplified as it is transferred to the water side (the footplate of the stapes). Second, the malleus and incus act as a lever system, again amplifying the pressure of the wave. Rather than being reflected, most of the energy is successfully transferred to the liquids of the inner ear.

Two tiny muscles of the middle ear, the **tensor tympani** and the **stapedius**, insert onto the malleus and the stapes, respectively. These muscles exert some control over the stiffness of the ossicular chain, and their contraction serves to dampen the transfer of sound to the inner ear. They are reflexively activated when ambient sound levels become high. It is possible that this property has a protective function, but more likely it is a device for suppressing self-produced sounds, such as the roar you produce in your head when you speak or chew.

The Frequency Sensitivity of Auditory Hair Cells Depends on Their Position Along the Basilar Membrane of the Cochlea

The subjective experience of tonal discrimination is called **pitch**. Young humans can hear sounds with frequencies from about 20 to 20,000 Hz. This range is modest by the standards of most mammals because many hear up to 50,000 Hz and some, notably whales and bats, can hear sounds with frequencies greater than 100,000 Hz.

The auditory portion of the inner ear is mainly the **cochlea**, a tube that is approximately 35 mm long and coiled 2.5 times into a snail shape about the size of a large pea (Fig. 13–19A). The cochlea has a million moving parts (mostly the stereocilia of the hair cells), which makes it the most complex mechanical apparatus in the body. The cochlea is innervated by the **auditory or cochlear nerve**, a branch of CN VIII. This nerve provides the primary auditory nerve axons, which contact cochlear hair cells at one end and enter the brain stem at the other. Cell bodies of the sensory or *afferent* neurons of the cochlear nerve lie alongside the spiral ganglion and run along the interior of the cochlear spiral. The cochlea also receives motor or *efferent* innervation, the olivocochlear axons arising in the brain stem (from the superior olivary complex) and synapsing mainly on the outer hair cells and, sparsely, on the afferent axons that innervate the inner hair cells.

The inner structure of the cochlea is complex, but in essence it consists of several long, narrow membranes that vibrate along with sound pressure waves. Hair cells cover one of these membranes. Movement of the membranes wiggles the cilia of the hair cells. The frequency of the sound determines which part of the membranes vibrates most—high frequencies at one end and low at the other—and thus which hair cells are stimulated. This selectivity is the basis for the idea of **place coding** in the auditory system: the longitudinal *position* of a hair cell along the cochlear membranes is the primary determinant of its frequency selectivity. The cochlea is essentially a spectral analyzer in which a complex sound is analyzed according to its pure tonal components, with each pure tone stimulating a specific region of the cochlea. The process is more complicated than that, but place coding is a general principle of auditory coding both within the ear and in the CNS.

If we view a cross section of the cochlea anywhere along its length, we see that two membranes divide it into three fluid-filled compartments (see Fig. 13–19A). On one side is the compartment called the **scala vestibuli**, which connects at its large end with the space that is adjacent to the oval window—where vibrations enter the inner ear. *Reissner's membrane* separates the scala vestibuli from the middle compartment, the **scala media**. The other boundary of the scala media is the *basilar membrane*, on which rides the organ of Corti and its hair cells.

A CROSS SECTION OF COCHLEA

B ORGAN OF CORTI

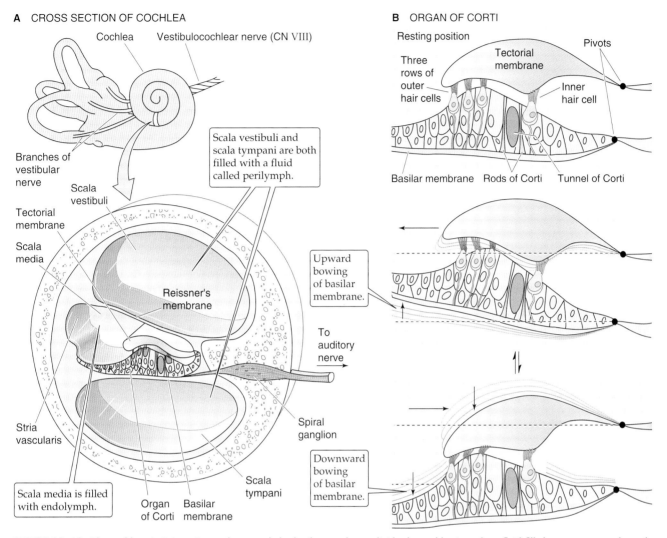

FIGURE 13–19. The cochlea. *A,* Reissner's membrane and the basilar membrane divide the cochlea into three fluid-filled compartments: the scala vestibuli, the scala media, and the scala tympani. *B,* The *top panel* shows the relationship between the gelatinous tectorial membrane and the three rows of outer hair cells and the single row of inner hair cells in the organ of Corti. The *middle* and *lower panels* show how the movement of the stapes against the oval window, which causes a cyclic increase and decrease in the pressure of the scala vestibuli, results in a downward and upward bowing of the basilar membrane.

Below the basilar membrane is the **scala tympani**, which connects at its basal or large end to the round window. These three compartments are filled with two different fluids: **perilymph** (in the scala vestibuli and scala tympani) and **endolymph** (in the scala media). In fact, the space and fluids of the scala vestibuli and scala tympani are continuous and interconnect through a small opening at the apex of the cochlea called the **helicotrema**.

The business end of the cochlea is the **organ of Corti**, which stretches the length of the basilar membrane. It has four rows of hair cells: one row of about 3500 inner hair cells and three rows with a total of approximately 20,000 outer hair cells (Fig. 13–20). The hair cells lie within a matrix of supporting cells, with their apical ends facing the endolymph of the scala media and their cilia projecting into the gelatinous, collagen-containing **tectorial membrane**. The tectorial membrane is firmly attached only along one edge, with a sort of hinge, so that it is free to tilt up and down. Hair cells transmit their infor-

mation by synapsing on auditory nerve axons, but the connections are not made in a simple one-to-one ratio. Instead, about 95% of the roughly 30,000 axons of each cochlear nerve innervate the relatively few inner hair cells, and only a few thousand axons innervate the abundant outer hair cells. The reason for this puzzling arrangement is, as discussed later, that the inner hair cells are the primary source of sound transduction; outer hair cells serve a very different role.

How are the auditory hair cells actually stimulated? Pressure waves are created within the cochlear fluids by movement of the stapes against the oval window. As the stapes moves inward, pressure in the scala vestibuli increases. Because the perilymph that fills the scala vestibuli and scala tympani is incompressible and the cochlea is encased in rigid bone, the inward displacement of the oval window is matched by an opposite, outward movement of the round window. During this process, the pressure in the scala vestibuli exceeds that in the scala tym-

FIGURE 13–20. Hair cells of the cochlea. A scanning electron microscopic image of outer and inner hair cells of the organ of Corti of a chinchilla after removal of the tectorial membrane. The three rows of outer hair cells are on the bottom, and the single row of inner hair cells is along the top. (Courtesy of I. Hunter-Duvar, M.D., and R. Harrison, Ph.D., D.Sc., The Hospital for Sick Children, Toronto, Canada.)

pani. Because Reissner's membrane is very thin and flexible, the bulging scala vestibuli pushes down on the incompressible scala media, which in turn causes the **basilar membrane** (and the organ of Corti) to bow downward into the scala tympani. When the stapes reverses direction and moves outward, the pressure gradients reverse and the basilar membrane tends to move upward. The bowing movements of the basilar membrane create a shear force relative to the parallel sheet of the tectorial membrane. Because the two membranes are connected by the cilia of the hair cells and because the tectorial membrane is hinged along one edge only, this sheer results in bending of the cilia. Transduction ensues! As discussed earlier, the molecular mechanisms of transduction in auditory hair cells are similar to those in vestibular hair cells.

What is the origin of the auditory place code? A continuous, pure tone produces a wave that travels along the basilar membrane and has different amplitudes at different points along the base-apex axis (Fig. 13–21A). Georg von Békésy used optical methods and cadaver ears to show that sounds of a particular frequency generate relatively localized waves in the basilar membrane, and that the envelope of these waves changes position according to the frequency of the sound (see Fig. 13–21B). Low frequencies generate their maximal amplitudes near the apex. As sound frequency increases, the envelope shifts progressively toward the basal end. The mechanical basis for the low-apical, high-basal pattern on the basilar membrane derives from two factors: its taper and its stiffness

yield a gradient of resonance (see Fig. 13–21C). If the cochlea is unwound and stretched straight, we see that it tapers from base to apex. The basilar membrane tapers in the opposite direction—wider at the apex, narrower at the base. More important, the basal end is about 100-fold stiffer than its apical end. The basilar membrane resembles a harp. At one end it has short, taut strings that vibrate at high frequencies, and at the other end it has longer, looser strings that vibrate at low frequencies. As described in the next section, active processes further sharpen the tuning of the basilar membrane.

Inner Hair Cells Transduce Sound, Whereas the Movement of Outer Hair Cells Sharpens Tuning

von Békésy's experiments on movements of the basilar membrane were illuminating, but paradoxic. A variety of experimental data suggested that the tuning of auditory cells was considerably sharper than the broad envelopes of von Békésy's traveling waves on the basilar membrane could possibly produce. Recordings from primary auditory nerve cells were also very sharp, which implied that this tuning must occur within the cochlea, not in the CNS. Some enhancement of tuning comes from the structure of the inner hair cells themselves. Those near the base have shorter, stiffer cilia, which makes them resonate to higher frequencies than possible with the longer, less stiff cilia on cells near the apex.

The *blue curve* in Figure 13–22 approximates von Békésy's envelope of traveling waves for a passive basilar membrane (recall that von Békésy worked with *cadavers*!). von Békésy had also used unnaturally loud sounds, but with reasonable sound levels, maximum displacement of the basilar membrane would be slightly more than 0.1 nm. This distance is less than the pore diameter of an ion channel and also less than the threshold (0.3 to 0.4 nm) for an electrical response from a hair cell. However, measurements from the basilar membrane in *living* animals (*orange curve* in Fig. 13–22) by very sensitive methods show that movements of the basilar membrane are much more localized and much larger than predicted by von Békésy. The maximal physiologic displacement is about 20-fold greater than threshold and about 40-fold greater than that predicted by the passive von Békésy model. Moreover, the physiological displacement decays sharply on either side of the peak, over 100-fold within approximately 0.5 mm (recall that the human basilar membrane has a total length greater than 30 mm).

Sharp tuning of the cochlea depends on active, energy-dependent processes inasmuch as such tuning disappears quickly during anoxia; the elements responsible for this cochlear tuning have come to be known as the **"cochlear amplifier."** A fascinating clue to the existence of the amplifier was the early observation that not only does the ear receive sounds, it also generates them! Short click sounds trigger an "echo," a brief vibration of the tympanic membrane that far outlasts the click. The echo can be heard with a microphone in the auditory canal. Occasionally, damaged ears may produce spontaneous "otoacoustic

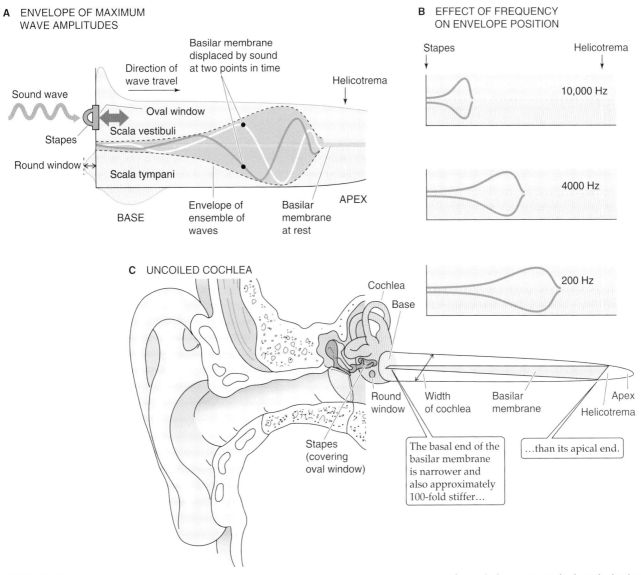

A ENVELOPE OF MAXIMUM WAVE AMPLITUDES

Direction of wave travel

Basilar membrane displaced by sound at two points in time

Sound wave

Helicotrema

Oval window

Stapes

Scala vestibuli

Round window

Scala tympani

APEX

Envelope of ensemble of waves

Basilar membrane at rest

BASE

B EFFECT OF FREQUENCY ON ENVELOPE POSITION

Stapes

Helicotrema

10,000 Hz

4000 Hz

200 Hz

C UNCOILED COCHLEA

Cochlea

Base

Round window

Width of cochlea

Basilar membrane

Apex

Helicotrema

Stapes (covering oval window)

The basal end of the basilar membrane is narrower and also approximately 100-fold stiffer...

...than its apical end.

FIGURE 13–21. Waves along the basilar membrane of the cochlea. *A*, As a wave generated by a sound of a single frequency travels along the basilar membrane, its amplitude changes with distance. The *green* and *yellow curves* represent a sample wave at two different points in time. The *upper* and *lower broken lines* (i.e,. the envelope) encompass all the maximum amplitudes that are achieved by all waves, at all points in time. Thus, a wave can never escape the envelope. Note that the amplitudes of the traveling waves have been exaggerated about 1 million-fold in these diagrams. *B*, For a pure tone of 10,000 Hz, the envelope is confined to a short region of the basilar membrane near the stapes. For a pure tone of 4000 Hz, the widest part of the envelope is further along the basilar membrane. Finally, for a pure tone of 200 Hz, the widest part of the envelope is near the helicotrema. *C*, Note that the cochlea narrows in diameter from base to apex, whereas the basilar membrane widens from stapes to helicotrema. The basilar membrane is also stiffer at the basal end. These differences in size and stiffness create a gradient of resonating frequencies along the basilar membrane, explaining the effect of frequency on envelope position.

emissions" that can even be loud enough to be heard by a nearby listener.

Several lines of evidence strongly suggest that the cochlear amplifier is in the organ of Corti and that the outer hair cells are the motor for that amplifier. First, if outer hair cells are selectively damaged—by large doses of certain antibiotics, for example—the sharpness of cochlear tuning is considerably dulled. Second, outer hair cells respond to sound with both an electrical response and a change in their shape. Sound causes receptor potentials in outer hair cells that are similar to those of inner hair cells. However, outer hair cells are so poorly innervated by auditory axons that they must contribute very little

direct information about sound to the brain. Observations of isolated cells have shown that imposed changes in their V_m cause changes in the length of the cell, up to a maximum of about 5%. The change in shape is fast, beginning within 100 μsec. The mechanism of the mechanical response of the outer hair cell is not yet understood and the molecules involved have not been identified, but the mechanism does not depend on adenosine triphosphate (ATP), microtubule or actin systems, extracellular Ca^{2+}, or changes in cell volume.

Putting the data together, a current hypothesis is that the outer hair cells provide positive feedback to sound-stimulated regions of the basilar membrane: (1) Sound vibrates the basilar membrane through the purely mechanical mechanisms just described. (2) Outer hair cells respond to sound when their hair bundles bend, triggering mechanical-to-electrical transduction typical of all hair cells. (3) Outer hair cells, through an electrical-to-mechanical mechanism, then generate a force by shortening their soma when the membrane depolarizes and lengthening their soma when the membrane hyperpolarizes. The current guess is that large numbers of intramembranous proteins in the hair cell soma produce this movement. (4) The movements of outer hair cells somehow enhance local movement of the basilar/tectorial membranes. The amplified movement of the membranes facilitates the local stimulation of the inner hair cells, which relay auditory signals to the brain stem.

Tuning of hair cells is also under efferent control by the olivocochlear nerve fibers, which release acetylcholine onto both the outer hair cells and the afferent axons connected to the inner hair cells. Stimulation of the efferent fibers suppresses the responsiveness of the cochlea to sound. The efferent axons hyperpolarize the outer hair cells—effectively an inhibitory postsynaptic potential (IPSP)—thereby reducing their electrical response to sound. Presumably, the IPSP also reduces the mechanical contributions of the outer hair cells to the cochlear amplifier. The efferent axons allow the brain to actively control the gain of the inner ear, perhaps to protect it from too much stimulation or to regulate its responsiveness in noisy environments.

SOMATIC SENSORY RECEPTORS, PROPRIOCEPTION, AND PAIN

Somatic sensation is the most widespread and diverse of the body's sensory systems (*soma* means "body" in Greek). Its receptors are distributed throughout the body instead of being condensed into small and specialized sensory surfaces, as most other sensory systems are arranged. Somatosensory receptors cover the skin, subcutaneous tissue, skeletal muscles, bones and joints, major internal organs, epithelia, and the cardiovascular system. These receptors also vary widely in their specificity. The body has mechanoreceptors to transduce pressure, stretch, vibration, and tissue damage; thermoreceptors to gauge temperature; and chemoreceptors to sense a variety of substances. Somatic sensation (or **somesthesia**) is usually considered to be a combination of at least four sensory modalities: the senses of touch, temperature, body position (proprioception), and pain (nociception).

A Variety of Sensory Endings in the Skin Transduce Mechanical, Thermal, and Chemical Stimuli

To meet a wide array of sensory demands, many kinds of specialized receptors are required. Somatic sensory receptors range from simple, bare nerve endings to complex combinations of nerve, muscle, connective tissue, and supporting cells. As we have seen, the other major sensory systems have only one type of sensory receptor or a set of very similar subtypes.

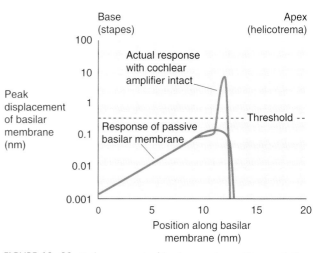

FIGURE 13–22. Peak movement of basilar membrane. The graph illustrates the displacement of the basilar membrane—in response to a pure tone—as a function of distance along the base-to-apex axis of the basilar membrane. The *blue curve* represents the *passive* response of the basilar membrane (recorded, for example, during anoxia). The *orange curve* represents the *actual* response of the living cochlea and includes the contribution of active amplification (the cochlear amplifier) by the outer hair cells. The *dotted line* indicates the displacement threshold for triggering an electrical response. (Data from Ashmore JF: Mammalian hearing and the cellular mechanisms of the cochlear amplifier. In Corey DP, Roper SD [eds]: Sensory Transduction. New York, Rockefeller University Press, 1992, pp 396–412.)

Mechanoreceptors, which are sensitive to physical distortion such as bending or stretching, account for many of the somatic sensory receptors. They exist throughout our bodies and monitor the following: physical contact with the skin, blood pressure in the heart and vessels, stretching of the gut and bladder, and pressure on the teeth. The transduction site of these mechanoreceptors is one or more unmyelinated axon branches. Our progress in understanding the molecular nature of mechanosensory transduction has been relatively slow. Similar to the transduction process in hair cells, cutaneous mechanoreceptive nerve endings probably involve the gating of ion channels. These ion channels can be physically coupled to either extracellular structures (e.g., collagen fibers) or cytoskeletal components (e.g., microtubules) that transfer energy from deformation of the cell to the gating mechanism of the channel. Studies of mechanosensation in nematodes and *Drosophila* suggest that multiple molecular mechanisms have evolved. These specialized structures that surround the mechanically sensitive axons give them much of their specific sensitivity to different stimuli. **Thermoreceptors** respond best to changes in temperature, whereas **chemoreceptors** are sensitive to various kinds of chemical alterations. In the next three sections, we discuss mechano-, thermo-, and chemoreceptors that are located in the skin.

Mechanoreceptors in the Skin Provide Sensitivity to Specific Stimuli Such as Vibration and Steady Pressure

Skin protects us from our environment by preventing evaporation of body fluids, invasion by microbes, abra-

A GLABROUS (HAIRLESS) SKIN

B PACINI'S CORPUSCLE

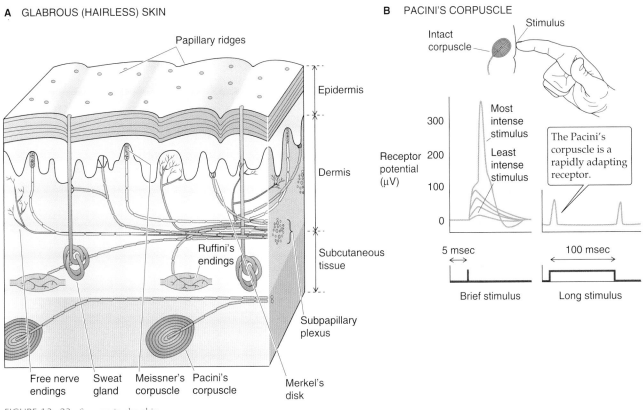

FIGURE 13–23. Sensors in the skin.

sion, and damage from sunlight. However, skin also provides our most direct contact with the world. The two major types of mammalian skin are *hairy* and *glabrous*. **Glabrous skin** (or hairless) is found on the palms of our hands and fingertips and on the soles of our feet and pads of our toes (Fig. 13–23A). **Hairy skin** makes up most of the rest and differs widely in its hairiness. Both types of skin have an outer layer, the **epidermis**, and an inner layer, the **dermis**, and sensory receptors innervate both. The receptors in the skin are sensitive to many types of stimuli and respond when the skin is vibrated, pressed, pricked, and stroked or when its hairs are bent or pulled. These are quite different kinds of mechanical energy, yet we can feel them all and easily tell them apart. Skin also has exquisite sensitivity; for example, we can reliably feel a dot only 0.006 mm high and 0.04 mm across when stroked across a fingertip. The standard Braille dot is 167 times higher!

The sensory endings in the skin take many shapes, and most of them are named after the 19th century European histologists who observed them and made them popular. The largest and best studied mechanoreceptor is the **Pacini's corpuscle**, which is up to 2 mm long and almost 1 mm in diameter (see Fig. 13–23B). The Pacini's corpuscle is located in the subcutaneous tissue of both glabrous and hairy skin. It has an ovoid capsule with 20 to 70 onion-like, concentric layers of connective tissue and a nerve terminal in the middle. The capsule is responsible for the rapidly adapting nature of the Pacini's corpuscle's responses. When the capsule is compressed, energy is transferred to the nerve terminal, its membrane is de-

formed, and mechanosensitive channels open. Current flowing through the channels generates a depolarizing receptor potential that, if large enough, causes the axon to fire an action potential (see Fig. 13–23B, *left panel*). However, the capsule layers are slick, with viscous fluid between them. If the stimulus pressure is maintained, the layers slip past one another and transfer the stimulus energy away so that the underlying axon terminal is no longer deformed and the receptor potential dissipates (Figure 13–23B, *right panel*). When pressure is released, the events reverse themselves and the terminal is depolarized again. In this way, the non-neural covering of the Pacini's corpuscle specializes the corpuscle for sensing vibrations and makes it almost unresponsive to steady pressure. The Pacini's corpuscle is most sensitive to vibrations of 200 to 300 Hz, and its threshold increases dramatically below 50 Hz and above about 500 Hz. The sensation evoked by stimulating a Pacini's corpuscle is a poorly localized humming feeling.

Werner Lowenstein and colleagues in the 1960s showed the importance of the Pacini's corpuscle's capsule to its frequency sensitivity. With fine microdissection, they were able to strip away the capsule from single corpuscles. They found that the resultant naked nerve terminal is much less sensitive to vibrating stimuli and much more sensitive to steady pressure. Clearly, the capsule modifies the sensitivity of the bare mechanoreceptive axon. The encapsulated Pacini's corpuscle is an example of a **rapidly adapting** sensor, whereas the decapsulated nerve ending is an example of a **slowly adapting** sensor.

Several other types of encapsulated mechanoreceptors

A RECEPTIVE FIELD OF   **B** RECEPTIVE FIELD OF   **C** TWO-POINT DISCRIMINATION ACROSS THE SKIN
       PACINI'S CORPUSCLES   MEISSNER'S CORPUSCLES

Pacinian corpuscles   Meissner's corpuscles

FIGURE 13–24. Receptive fields and spatial discrimination of skin mechanoreceptors. *A,* Each of the two *black dots* indicates an area of maximal sensitivity of a single corpuscle. The *green area* is the receptive field of a corpuscle; the corpuscle responds when the stimulus strength increases sufficiently anywhere within that area. *B,* Each *dot* represents the entire receptive field of a single Meissner's corpuscle. Note that the fields are much smaller than in *A. C,* The *horizontal bars* represent the minimum distance at which two points can be perceived as distinct at various locations over the body. Spatial discrimination depends on both the receptive-field size of the receptors and the density of the receptors. (*A, B,* Data from Vallbo AB, Johansson RS: Properties of cutaneous mechanoreceptors in the human hand related to touch sensation. Human Neurobiology 3:3–14, 1984. *C,* Data from Weinstein S: Intensive and extensive aspects of tactile sensitivity as a function of body part, sex and laterality. In Kenshalo DR [ed]: The Skin Senses. Springfield, IL, Charles C Thomas, 1968.)

are located in the dermis, but none have been studied as well as the Pacini's corpuscle. **Meissner's corpuscles** (see Fig. 13–23A) are located in the ridges of glabrous skin and are about one tenth the size of a Pacini's corpuscle. They are rapidly adapting, although less so than Pacini's corpuscles. **Ruffini's corpuscles** resemble diminutive Pacini's corpuscles and, like their Pacini's corpuscles counterparts, occur in the subcutaneous tissue of both hairy and glabrous skin. Their preferred stimuli might be called "fluttering" vibrations. As relatively *slowly* adapting receptors, they respond best to low frequencies. **Merkel's disks** are also slowly adapting receptors made from a flattened, non-neural epithelial cell that synapses on a nerve terminal. They lie at the border of the dermis and epidermis of glabrous skin. It is not clear whether it is the nerve terminal or epithelial cell that is mechanosensitive. The nerve terminals of **Krause end bulbs** appear knotted. They innervate the border areas of dry skin and mucous membranes (e.g., around the lips and external genitalia) and are probably rapidly adapting mechanoreceptors.

The **receptive fields** of different types of skin receptors vary greatly in size. Pacini's corpuscles have extremely broad receptive fields (Fig. 13–24A), whereas those of

Meissner's corpuscles (see Fig. 13–24B) and Merkel's disks are very small. The latter two seem to be responsible for the ability of the fingertips to make very fine tactile discriminations. Small receptive fields are an important factor in achieving high spatial resolution. Resolution varies widely, a fact easily demonstrated by measuring the skin's two-point discrimination. Bend a paper clip into a U shape. Vary the distance between the tips, and test how easily you can distinguish the touch of one tip versus two on your palm, your fingertips, your lips, your back, and your foot. To avoid bias, a colleague—rather than you—should apply the stimulus. Compare the results with standardized data (see Fig. 13–24C).

Two things determine the sensitivity of spatial discrimination in an area of skin. The first is the size of the receptors' receptive fields—if they are small, the two tips of your paper clip are more likely to stimulate different sets of receptors. The second parameter that determines spatial discrimination is the density of the receptors in the skin. Indeed, two-point discrimination of the fingertips is better than that of the palm, even though their receptive fields are the same size. The key to finer discrimination in the fingertips is their higher *density* of receptors. Crowd-

A   STEADY (TONIC) RESPONSES

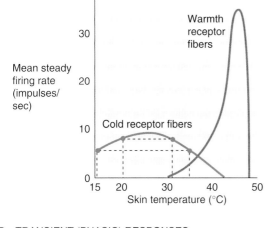

B   TRANSIENT (PHASIC) RESPONSES OF "COLD" FIBERS

FIGURE 13–25. Temperature sensitivity of cutaneous thermoreceptors. *A,* The *orange curve* represents the mean, steady firing rate of neurons from warmth receptors as a function of temperature. The *blue curve* represents the mean, steady firing rate of neurons from cold receptors. *B,* These two experiments on cold receptors show the effects of two cooling steps of nearly identical magnitude starting from different temperatures (20.5°C and 35°C). In both instances, the transient ("phasic") responses are the same: an increase in the firing rate. When the starting temperature is 20.5°C (to the *left* of the *peak* of the *blue curve* in *A*), the final firing rate is less than the initial one. However, when the initial temperature is 35°C (to the *right* of the *peak* of the *blue curve* in *A*), the final rate is greater than the initial one. (Data from Somjen GG: Sensory Coding in the Mammalian Nervous System. New York, Appleton-Century-Crofts, 1972.)

ing more receptors into each square millimeter of fingertip has a second advantage: because the CNS receives more information per stimulus, it has a better chance of transducing very small stimuli.

Although we rarely think about it, **hair** is a sensitive part of our somatic sensory system. For some animals, hairs are a major sensory system. Rodents whisk long facial vibrissae (hairs) and feel the texture, distance, and shape of their local environment. Hairs grow from **follicles** embedded in the skin, and each follicle is richly innervated by free, mechanoreceptive nerve endings that either wrap around it or run parallel to it. Bending of the hair causes deformation of the follicle and surrounding tissue, which stretches, bends, or flattens the nerve endings and increases or decreases their firing frequency. Various mechanoreceptors innervate hair follicles, and they may be either slowly or rapidly adapting.

Separate Thermoreceptors Detect Warm and Cold

Neurons are sensitive to changes in temperature, as are all of life's chemical reactions. This temperature sensitivity has two consequences: first, neurons can measure temperature, but second, to work properly, most neural circuits need to be kept at a relatively stable temperature. Neurons of the mammalian CNS are especially vulnerable to temperature changes. Whereas skin tissue temperatures can range from 20°C to 40°C without harm or discomfort, brain temperature must be near 37°C to avoid serious dysfunction. The body has complex systems to control brain (i.e. body core) temperature tightly (p. 1236).

Even though all neurons are sensitive to temperature, not all neurons are thermoreceptors. Because of specific (but poorly understood) membrane mechanisms, some neurons are extremely sensitive to temperature and seem to be adapted to the job of sensing it. We can perceive changes in our average skin temperature of as little as 0.01°C. Within the skin are separate types of thermoreceptors that are sensitive to a range of relatively hot or cold temperatures. Figure 13–25A shows how the steady discharge rate of both types of receptors varies with temperature. **Warmth receptors** begin firing above about 30°C and increase their firing rate until 44°C to 46°C, beyond which the rate falls off steeply and a sensation of pain begins, presumably mediated by nociceptive endings (see the next section). **Cold receptors** have a much broader temperature response. They are relatively quiet at skin temperatures of about 40°C, but their steady discharge rate increases as the temperature falls to 24°C to 28°C. Further decreases in temperature cause the steady discharge rate of the cold receptors to decrease until the temperature falls to around 10°C. Below that temperature, firing ceases and cold becomes a very effective local anesthetic.

In addition to the *tonic* response just described (i.e., the steady discharge rate), cold receptors also have a *phasic* response that enables them to report *changes* in temperature. As shown in Figure 13–25B, when the temperature suddenly shifts from 20.5°C to 15.2°C (both points are to the left of the peak in Fig. 13–25A), the firing rate transiently increases (i.e., the "phasic" response). However, the new steady-state level is lower, as suggested by the "left" pair of points in Figure 13–25A. When the temperature suddenly shifts from 35°C to 31.5°C (both points are to the right of the peak in Fig. 13–25A), the firing rate transiently increases, and the new steady-state level is higher, as suggested by the "right" pair of points in Figure 13–25A.

Perceptions of temperature apparently reflect warmth and cold receptors located in the skin. Thermoreceptors, like mechanoreceptors, are not spread uniformly across the skin. When you map the skin's sensitivity to temperature with a small cold or warm probe, you find spots about 1 mm across that are especially sensitive to *either* hot or cold, but not both. In addition, some areas of skin in between are relatively insensitive. The spatial dissociation of the hot and cold maps shows that they are separate submodalities, with separate receptors to encode each. Recordings from single sensory fibers have con-

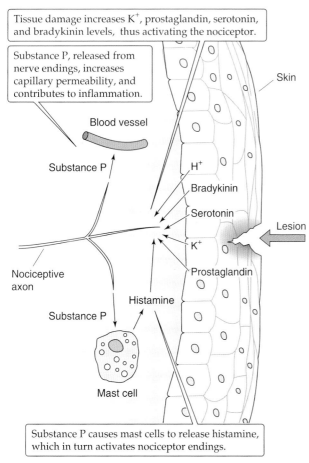

Tissue damage increases K⁺, prostaglandin, serotonin, and bradykinin levels, thus activating the nociceptor.

Substance P, released from nerve endings, increases capillary permeability, and contributes to inflammation.

Blood vessel

Substance P

Nociceptive axon

Substance P

Histamine

Mast cell

Skin

H⁺

Bradykinin

Serotonin

Lesion

K⁺

Prostaglandin

Substance P causes mast cells to release histamine, which in turn activates nociceptor endings.

FIGURE 13–26. Hyperalgesia of inflammation.

firmed this conclusion. The responses of thermoreceptors adapt during long stimuli (see Fig. 13–25*B*), as many sensory receptors commonly do. Most cutaneous thermoreceptors are probably free nerve endings, without obvious specialization. Their axons are small, either unmyelinated *C fibers* or the smallest-diameter myelinated *Aδ fibers* (Table 11–1).

Temperature-sensitive neurons are also clustered in the hypothalamus and the spinal cord (p. 1236). The hypothalamic temperature sensors, like their cutaneous counterparts, are important for regulating the physiological responses that maintain stable body temperature.

Nociceptors Are Specialized Sensory Endings That Transduce Painful Stimuli

Physical energy that is informative at low and moderate levels can be destructive at higher intensity. Sensations of pain motivate us to avoid such situations. Nociceptors are the receptors that mediate painful feelings that warn us that body tissue is being damaged or is at risk of being damaged (as their Latin roots imply; i.e., *nocere* means to hurt, and *recipere*, to receive). The pain-sensing system is entirely separate from the other modalities we have discussed; it has its own peripheral receptors and a complex, dispersed, chemically unique set of central circuits.

Nociceptors vary in their selectivity. **Mechanical** noci-

ceptors respond to strong pressure, in particular, pressure from sharp objects. **Thermal** nociceptors signal either burning heat (above about 45°C, when tissues begin to be destroyed) or unhealthy cold. **Chemically sensitive**, mechanically insensitive nociceptors respond to a variety of agents, including K⁺, extremes of pH, neuroactive substances such as histamine and bradykinin from the body itself, and various irritants from the environment. Finally, **polymodal** nociceptors are single nerve endings that are sensitive to combinations of mechanical, thermal, and chemical stimuli. Nociceptive axons include both fast Aδ fibers and slow, unmyelinated C fibers. Aδ axons mediate sensations of sharp, intense pain, whereas C fibers elicit more persistent feelings of dull, burning pain.

Nociceptors are free nerve endings that are widely distributed throughout the body. They innervate the skin, bone, muscle, most internal organs, blood vessels, and the heart. Ironically, they are generally absent from the brain substance itself, although they are in the meninges.

Sensations of pain can be modulated in a variety of ways. Skin, joints, or muscles that have been damaged or inflamed are unusually sensitive to further stimuli. This phenomenon is called **hyperalgesia**, and it can be manifested as a reduced threshold for pain, an increased intensity of painful stimuli, or spontaneous pain. **Primary hyperalgesia** occurs within the area of damaged tissue, but within about 20 minutes after an injury, tissues surrounding a damaged area may become supersensitive by a process called **secondary hyperalgesia**. Hyperalgesia seems to involve processes near peripheral receptors (Fig. 13–26), as well as mechanisms in the CNS. Damaged skin releases a variety of chemical substances from itself, blood cells, and nerve endings. These substances include bradykinin, prostaglandins, serotonin, substance P, K⁺, H⁺, and others; they trigger the set of local responses that we know as **inflammation**. As a result, blood vessels become more leaky and cause tissue swelling (or edema) and redness (see box on p. 473). Nearby mast cells release the chemical histamine, which directly excites nociceptors. Finally, the spreading axon branches of the nociceptors themselves may release substances that sensitize nociceptive terminals and make them responsive to previously nonpainful stimuli. Such "silent" nociceptors among our small Aδ and C fibers are normally unresponsive to stimuli—even destructive ones. Only after sensitization do they become responsive to mechanical or chemical stimuli and contribute greatly to hyperalgesia.

The cognitive sensations of pain are under remarkably potent control by the brain, more so than other sensory systems. In some cases, nociceptors may fire wildly, although perceptions of pain are absent; on the other hand, pain may be crippling, although nociceptors are silent. Pain can be modified both by nonpainful sensory input and by neural activity from various nuclei within the brain. For example, pain evoked by activity in nociceptors (Aδ and C fibers) can be reduced by simultaneous activity in low-threshold mechanoreceptors (Aα and Aβ fibers). This phenomenon is a familiar experience—some of the discomfort of a burn, cut, or bruise can be relieved by gentle massage or rubbing (stimulating mechanoreceptors) around the injured area. In 1965, Melzack and Wall proposed that this phenomenon involves a circuit in the spinal cord that can "gate" the transmission of nociceptive information to the brain; control of the gate could be provided by other sensory information (e.g., tactile stimulation) or by descending control from the brain itself.

A second mechanism for modifying the sensation of pain involves the relatively small peptides called endorphins. In the 1970s, it was discovered that a class of drugs called opioids (including morphine, heroin, and codeine) act by binding tightly and specifically to **opioid receptors** in the brain and, furthermore, that the brain itself manufactures "endogenous morphine-like substances", collectively called endorphins (p. 304).

Muscle Spindles Sense Changes in the Length of Skeletal Muscle Fibers, Whereas Golgi Tendon Organs Gauge the Muscle's Force

The somatic sensory receptors described thus far provide information about the *external* environment. However, the

body also needs detailed information about itself to know where each of its parts is in space, whether it is moving, and if so, in which direction and how fast. **Proprioception** provides this sense of self and serves two main purposes. First, knowledge of the positions of our limbs as they move helps us judge the identity of external objects. It is much easier to recognize an object if you can actively palpate it than if it is placed passively into your hand so that your skin is stimulated but you are not allowed to personally guide your fingers around it. Second, proprioceptive information is essential for accurately guiding many movements, especially while they are being learned.

Skeletal muscles, which mediate voluntary movement, have two mechanosensitive proprioceptors: the muscle spindles (or stretch receptors) and Golgi tendon organs (Fig. 13–27). Muscle spindles measure the length and rate of stretch of the muscles, whereas the Golgi tendon organs gauge the force generated by a muscle by measur-

FIGURE 13–27. Golgi tendon organ and muscle spindle fibers. A muscle contains two kinds of muscle fibers, "extrafusal" fibers (ordinary muscle fibers that cause contraction) and "intrafusal" fibers (in parallel with the extrafusal fibers). Some of the extrafusal fibers have Golgi tendon organs located in series between the end of the muscle fiber and the macroscopic tendon. The intrafusal fibers contain muscle spindles, which receive both afferent (sensory) and efferent (motor) innervation. The spindle (*inset*) contains both bag fibers, with nuclei bunched together, and chain fibers, with nuclei in row.

ing the tension in its tendon. Together, they provide a full description of the dynamic state of each muscle. The different sensitivities of the spindle and the tendon organ are partly due to their structures, but also to their placement: spindles are located in modified muscle fibers called *intrafusal* muscle fibers, which are aligned in *parallel* with the "ordinary" force-generating or *extrafusal* skeletal muscle fibers. On the other hand, Golgi tendon organs are aligned in *series* with the extrafusal fibers.

The **Golgi tendon organ** consists of bare nerve endings of group Ib axons (see Table 11–1). These endings intimately invest an encapsulated collagen matrix and usually sit at the junction between skeletal muscle fibers and the tendon. When tension develops in the muscle as a result of either passive stretch or active contraction, the collagen fibers tend to squeeze and distort the mechanosensitive nerve endings, triggering them to fire action potentials.

The mammalian **muscle spindle** is a complex of modified skeletal muscle fibers (**intrafusal fibers**) combined with both afferent and efferent innervation. The spindle does not contribute significant force generation to the muscle, but serves a purely sensory function. A simplified summary of the muscle spindle is that it contains two kinds of intrafusal muscle fibers ("bag" and "chain"), with two kinds of sensory endings entwined about them (the "primary" and "secondary" endings). The different viscoelastic properties of the muscle fibers make them differentially sensitive to the consequences of muscle stretch. Because the primary sensory endings of group Ia axons coil around and strongly innervate individual bag muscle fibers (in addition to chain fibers), they are very sensitive to the dynamics of muscle length (i.e., *changes* in its length). The secondary sensory endings of group II axons mainly innervate the chain fibers and most accurately transduce the static length of the muscle; in other words, they are slowly adapting receptors. The discharge rate of afferent neurons increases when the whole muscle—and therefore the spindle—is stretched.

What is the function of the motor innervation of the muscle spindle? Consider what happens when the α motor neurons stimulate the force-generating extrafusal fibers and the muscle contracts. The spindle, connected in parallel to the extrafusal fibers, quickly tends to go slack, which makes it insensitive to further changes in length. To avoid this situation and to continue to maintain control over the sensitivity of the spindle, γ motor neurons cause the intrafusal muscle fibers to contract in parallel with the extrafusal fibers. This ability of the spindle's intrafusal fibers to change their length as necessary greatly increases the range of lengths over which the spindle can work. It also means that the sensory responses of the spindle depend not only on the *length* of the whole muscle in which the spindle sits but also on the *contractile state* of its own intrafusal muscle fibers. Presumably, the ambiguity in this code is sorted out centrally by circuits that simultaneously keep track of the spindle's sensory output and the activity of its motor nerve supply.

In addition to the muscle receptors, various mechanoreceptors are found in the connective tissues of **joints**, especially within the capsules and ligaments. Many resemble Ruffini's, Golgi, and Pacini's end organs; others are free nerve endings. They respond to changes in the angle, direction, and velocity of movement in a joint. Most are rapidly adapting, which means that sensory information about a *moving* joint is rich. Nerves encoding the resting *position* of a joint are few. We are, nevertheless, quite good at judging the position of a joint, even with our eyes closed. It seems that information from joint receptors is combined with that from muscle spindles and Golgi tendon organs, and probably from cutaneous receptors as well, to estimate joint angle. Removing one source of information can be compensated by use of the other sources. When an arthritic hip is replaced with a steel and plastic one, patients are still able to tell the angle between their thigh and their pelvis, even though all hip joint mechanoreceptors are long gone.

REFERENCES

Books and Reviews

Bowmaker JK: Visual pigments and molecular genetics of color blindness. News Physiol Sci 13:63–69, 1998.

Hudspeth AJ: How hearing happens. Neuron 19:947–950, 1997.

Hunt CC: Mammalian muscle spindle: Peripheral mechanisms. Physiol Rev 70:643–663, 1990.

Kinnamon SC, Margolskee RF: Mechanisms of taste transduction. Curr Opin Neurobiol 6:506–513, 1996.

Nathans J: In the eye of the beholder: Visual pigments and inherited variation in human vision. Cell 78:357–360, 1994.

Nobili R, Mammano F, Ashmore J: How well do we understand the cochlea? Trends Neurosci 21:159–167, 1998.

Journal Articles

Buck L, Axel R: A novel multigene family may encode odorant receptors: A molecular basis for odor recognition. Cell 65:175–187, 1991.

Crawford AC, Fettiplace R: Auditory nerve responses to imposed displacements of the turtle basilar membrane. Hear Res 12:199–208, 1983.

Fesenko EE, Kolesnikov SS, Lyubarsky AL: Induction by cyclic GMP of cationic conductance in plasma membrane of retinal rod outer segment. Nature 313:310–313, 1985.

Hecht S, Shlaer S, Pirenne MH: Energy, quanta, and vision. J Gen Physiol 25:819–840, 1942.

Nakamura T, Gold GH: A cyclic nucleotide–gated conductance in olfactory receptor cilia. Nature 325:442–444, 1987.

Zhao H, Ivic L, Otaki JM, et al: Functional expression of a mammalian odorant receptor. Science 279:237–242, 1998.

CHAPTER 14

Circuits of the Central Nervous System

Barry W. Connors

ELEMENTS OF NEURAL CIRCUITS

Neural Circuits Process Sensory Information, Generate Motor Output, and Create Spontaneous Activity

A neuron never works alone. Even in the most primitive nervous systems, all neurons participate in synaptically interconnected networks called **circuits**. In some hydrozoans (small jellyfish), the major neurons lack specialization and are multifunctional. They serve simultaneously as photodetectors, pattern generators for swimming rhythms, and motor neurons. Groups of these cells are monotonously interconnected by two-way electrical synapses into simple ring-like arrangements, and these networks coordinate the rhythmic contraction of the animal's muscles during swimming. This simple neural network also has the flexibility to command defensive changes in swimming patterns when a shadow passes over the animal. Thus, neuronal circuits have profound advantages over unconnected neurons.

In more complex animals, each neuron within a circuit may have very *specialized properties*. By interconnecting various specialized neurons, even a simple neuronal circuit may accomplish astonishingly intricate functions. Some neural circuits may be primarily sensory (e.g., the retina) or motor (e.g., the ventral horns of the spinal cord). Many circuits combine features of both, with some neurons dedicated to providing and processing **sensory input**, others to commanding **motor output**, and many neurons (perhaps most!) doing both. Neural circuits may also generate their own intrinsic signals, with no need for any sensory or central input to activate them. The brain does more than just respond reflexively to sensory input, as a moment's introspection will amply demonstrate. Some neural functions—such as walking, running, breathing, chewing, talking, and piano playing—require precise timing, with coordination of rhythmic temporal patterns across hundreds of outputs. These basic rhythms may be generated by neurons and neural circuits called **pacemakers** because of their clock-like capabilities. The patterns and rhythms generated by a pacemaking circuit can almost always be modulated—stopped, started, or altered—by input from sensory or central pathways. Neuronal circuits that produce rhythmic motor output are sometimes called **central pattern generators**; we discuss these in a later section.

This chapter introduces the basic principles of neural circuits in the mammalian central nervous system (CNS). We describe a few examples of specific systems in detail to illuminate general principles, as well as the

A BEHAVIOR

B SYSTEMS AND PATHWAYS

C LOCAL CIRCUITS

D NEURON

Action potential

H GENES

G MEMBRANES, MOLECULES, IONS

Channel protein   Ion

Channel activity

Neurotransmitter or neuromodulator

Second messenger

F SYNAPSE

E MICROCIRCUITS

FIGURE 14−1. Levels of organization of the nervous system. (Data from Shepherd GM: Neurobiology, 3rd ed. New York, Oxford University Press, 1994.)

diversity of neural solutions to life's complex problems. However, this topic is enormous, and we have necessarily been selective and somewhat arbitrary in our presentation.

Nervous Systems Have Several Levels of Organization

The function of a nervous system is to generate behavior. Because different species face unique problems, we expect brains to differ in their organization and mechanisms. Nevertheless, certain principles apply to most nervous systems. It is useful to define various levels of organization. In Figure 14−1, we analyze a complex **behavior**—reading the words on this page (see Fig. 14−1A)—in progressively finer detail, down to the level of ion channels, receptors, messengers, and the genes that control them. At the highest level, we recognize neural **subsystems and pathways**, which in this case include the sensory input leading to the visual cortex, the central processing regions that make sense of the visual information, and the motor systems that coordinate movement of the eyes and head (see Fig. 14−1B). Many of these systems can be recognized in the gross anatomy of the brain. Figure 14−1B is, of course, highly oversimplified; the brain is not a simple chain of neurons. Rather, each brain

region is extensively interconnected with other regions that serve different primary functions. These regions tend to have profuse connections that send information *in both directions* along most sensory/central motor pathways. The advantages of this complexity are obvious: while interpreting visual information, for example, it can be very useful to simultaneously analyze sound and to know where your eyes are pointing and how your body is oriented.

The systems of the brain can be more deeply understood by studying their organization at the cellular level. Within a local brain region, the arrangement of neurons and their synaptic connections is called a **local circuit** (see Fig. 14−1C). A local circuit typically includes the set of inputs, outputs, and all the interconnected neurons that are essential to functions of the local brain region. Many regions of the brain are composed of a large number of stereotyped local circuits, almost modular in their interchangeability, that are themselves interconnected. Within the local circuits are finer arrangements of neurons (see Fig. 14−1D) and synapses sometimes called **microcircuits** (see Fig. 14−1E). Microcircuits may be repeated numerous times within a local circuit, and they determine the transformations of information that occur within small areas of dendrites and the collection of syn-

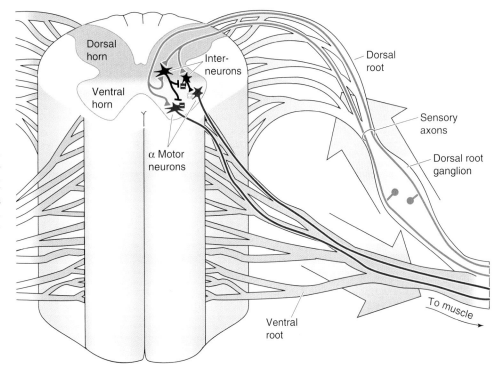

FIGURE 14–2. Local circuits in the spinal cord. A basic local circuit in the spinal cord consists of inputs (e.g., sensory axons of the dorsal roots), interneurons (both excitatory and inhibitory), and output neurons (e.g., α motor neurons that send their axons through the ventral roots).

apses impinging on them. At even finer resolution, neural systems can be understood by the properties of their **synapses** (Fig. 14–1F), membranes, **molecules** (e.g., neurotransmitters and neuromodulators), and ions, as well as the **genes** that encode and control the system's molecular biology (see Fig. 14–1G and H).

Most Local Circuits Have Three Elements: Input Axons, Interneurons, and Projection (Output) Neurons

One of the most fascinating things about the nervous system is the wide array of different local circuits that have evolved for different behavioral functions. Despite this diversity, we can define a few general components of local circuits, which we will illustrate with two examples from very different parts of the CNS: the ventral horn of the spinal cord and the cerebral neocortex. Some of the functions of these circuits are described in subsequent sections; here, we examine their cellular anatomy.

All local circuits have some form of **input**, which is usually a set of axons that originate elsewhere and terminate in synapses within the local circuit. A major input to the spinal cord (Fig. 14–2) is the afferent sensory axons in the dorsal roots. These axons carry information from somatic sensory receptors in the skin, connective tissue, and muscles (p. 352). However, local circuits in the spinal cord also have many other sources of input, including descending input from the brain and input from the spinal cord itself, both from the contralateral side and from spinal segments above and below. Input to the local circuits of the neocortex (Fig. 14–3) is also easily identified; relay neurons of the thalamus send axons into particular layers of the cortex to bring a range of information about sensation, motor systems, and the body's internal state. By

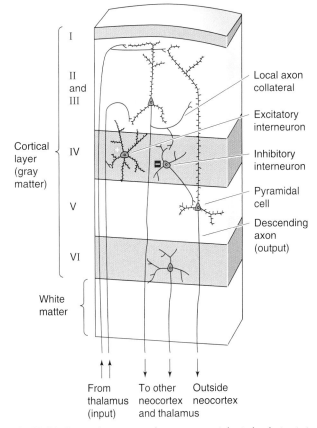

FIGURE 14–3. Local circuits in the neocortex. A basic local circuit in the neocortex consists of inputs (e.g., afferent axons from the thalamus), excitatory and inhibitory interneurons, and output neurons (e.g., pyramidal cells).

far, the most numerous input to the local circuits of the neocortex comes from the neocortex itself—from adjacent local circuits, distant areas of cortex, and the contralateral hemisphere. These two systems illustrate a basic principle: local circuits receive multiple types of input.

Output is usually achieved with a subset of cells known as *projection neurons*, or *principal neurons*, which send axons to one or more targets. The most obvious spinal output comes from the α motor neurons, which send their axons out through the ventral roots to innervate skeletal muscle fibers. Output axons from the neocortex come mainly from large pyramidal cells in layer V, which innervate many targets in the brainstem and spinal cord, and from cells in layer VI, which make their synapses back onto the cells of the thalamus. However, as was true with input, most local circuits have multiple output. Thus, spinal neurons innervate other regions of the spinal cord and the brain, whereas neocortical circuits make most of their connections to other neocortical circuits.

Rare, indeed, is the neural circuit that has only input and output cells. **Local processing** is achieved by additional neurons whose axonal connections remain within the local circuit. These neurons are usually called *interneurons*, or *intrinsic neurons*. Interneurons vary widely in structure and function, and a single local circuit may have many different types. Both the spinal cord and neocortex have excitatory and inhibitory interneurons, interneurons that make very specific or widely divergent connections, and interneurons that either receive direct contact from input axons or process only information from other interneurons. In many parts of the brain, interneurons vastly outnumber output neurons. To take an extreme example, the cerebellum has as many as 10^{11} granule cells—a type of excitatory interneuron—which is more than the total number of all types of neurons in the rest of the brain!

Numerous variations on the "principles" of local circuits outlined here may be mentioned. For example, a projection cell may have some of the characteristics of an interneuron, as when a branch of its output axon stays within the local circuit and makes synaptic connections. This branching is the case for the projection cells of both the neocortex (pyramidal cells) and the spinal cord (α motor neurons). On the other hand, some interneurons may entirely lack an axon and instead make their local synaptic connections via very short neurites or even dendrites. In some rare cases, the source of the input to a local circuit may not be purely synaptic, but chemical (as with CO_2-sensitive neurons in the medulla; p. 729) or physical (as with temperature-sensitive neurons in the hypothalamus; p. 1236). It is important to emphasize that although the neurons within a generic local circuit are wired in *series* (see Figs. 14–2 and 14–3), local circuits, often in massive numbers, operate in *parallel* with one another. Furthermore, these circuits usually demonstrate a tremendous amount of *crosstalk*; information from each circuit is shared mutually, and each circuit continually influences its neighbors. Indeed, one of the things that makes analysis of local neural circuits so exceptionally difficult is that they operate in highly interactive, simultaneously interdependent, and expansive networks.

SIMPLE, STEREOTYPED RESPONSES: SPINAL REFLEX CIRCUITS

Passively Stretching a Skeletal Muscle Causes a Reflexive Contraction of That Same Muscle and Relaxation of the Antagonist Muscles

Reflexes are among the most basic of neural functions and involve some of the simplest neuronal circuits. A motor *reflex* is a rapid, stereotyped motor response to a particular sensory stimulus. Although the existence of reflexes was long appreciated, it was Sir Charles Sherrington who, beginning in the 1890s, first defined the anatomic and physiological bases for some simple spinal reflexes. So meticulous were Sherrington's observations of reflexes and their timing that they offered him compelling evidence for the existence of synapses, a term he originated.

Reflexes are essential, if rudimentary, elements of behavior. Because of their relative simplicity, more than a century of research has taught us a lot about their biologic basis. However, reflexes are also important for understanding more complex behaviors. Intricate behaviors may sometimes be built up from sequences of simple reflexive responses. In addition, neural circuits that generate reflexes almost always mediate or participate in much more complex behaviors. Here we examine a relatively well-understood example of reflex-mediating circuitry.

The CNS commands the body to move about by activating motor neurons, which excite skeletal muscles (Sherrington called motor neurons the "final common path"). Motor neurons receive synaptic input from many sources within the brain and spinal cord, and the output of large numbers of motor neurons must be closely coordinated to achieve even uncomplicated actions such as walking. However, in some circumstances, motor neurons can be commanded directly by a simple sensory stimulus—muscle stretch—with only the minimum of neural machinery intervening between the sensory cell and motor neuron: one synapse. Understanding this simplest of reflexes, the **stretch reflex**, first requires knowing some anatomy.

Each motor neuron, with its soma in the spinal cord or brain stem, commands a group of skeletal muscle cells; a single motor neuron and the muscle cells that it synapses on are collectively called a **motor unit** (p. 249). Each muscle cell belongs to only one motor unit. The size of motor units varies dramatically and depends on muscle function. In small muscles that generate very finely controlled movements, such as the extraocular muscles of the eye, motor units tend to be small and may contain just a few muscle fibers. Large muscles that generate strong forces, such as the gastrocnemius muscle of the leg, tend to have large motor units with more than several thousand muscle fibers. There are two types of motor neurons (see Table 11–1): α **motor neurons** innervate the main force-generating muscle fibers (the "extrafusal" fibers), whereas γ **motor neurons** innervate only the fibers of the muscle spindles. The group of all motor neurons innervating a single muscle is called a **motor neuron pool** (p. 250).

When a skeletal muscle is abruptly stretched, often a

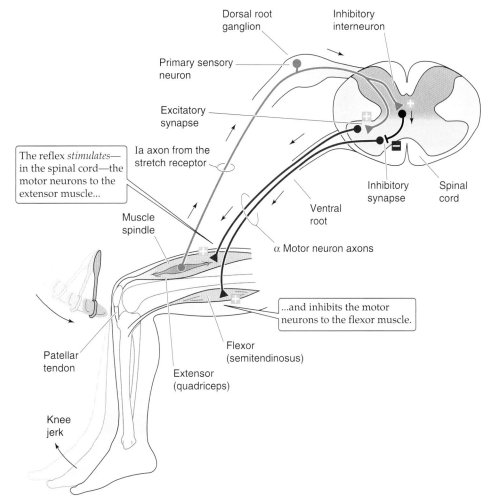

FIGURE 14–4. Knee-jerk (myotatic) reflex. Tapping the patellar tendon with a percussion hammer elicits a reflexive knee-jerk caused by contraction of the quadriceps muscle: the *stretch reflex*. Stretching the tendon pulls on the muscle spindle, exciting the primary sensory afferents, which convey their information via group Ia axons. These axons make monosynaptic connections to the α motor neurons that innervate the quadriceps, resulting in the contraction of this muscle. The Ia axons also excite inhibitory interneurons that reciprocally innervate the motor neurons of the antagonist muscle of the quadriceps (the flexor), resulting in relaxation of the semitendinosus muscle. Thus, the reflex relaxation of the antagonistic muscle is polysynaptic.

Labels in figure:
Dorsal root ganglion
Inhibitory interneuron
Primary sensory neuron
Excitatory synapse
Inhibitory synapse
Spinal cord
Ia axon from the stretch receptor
The reflex *stimulates*—in the spinal cord—the motor neurons to the extensor muscle...
Ventral root
Muscle spindle
α Motor neuron axons
...and inhibits the motor neurons to the flexor muscle.
Flexor (semitendinosus)
Patellar tendon
Extensor (quadriceps)
Knee jerk

rapid, reflexive contraction of the same muscle occurs. The contraction increases muscle tension and opposes the stretch. This stretch reflex is particularly strong in physiological extensor muscles—those that resist gravity—and is sometimes called the **myotatic reflex** because it is specific for the same muscle that is stretched. The most familiar version is the "knee jerk," which is elicited by a light tap on the patellar tendon. The tap deflects the tendon, which then pulls on and briefly stretches the quadriceps femoris muscle. A reflexive contraction of the quadriceps quickly follows (Fig. 14–4). Stretch reflexes are also easily demonstrated in the biceps of the arm and the muscles that close the jaw. Sherrington showed that the stretch reflex depends on the nervous system and requires sensory feedback from the muscle. For example, cutting the dorsal (sensory) roots to the lumbar spinal cord abolishes the stretch reflex in the quadriceps muscle. The basic circuit for the stretch reflex begins with the primary sensory axons from the **muscle spindles** (p. 358) in the muscle itself. Increasing the length of the muscle stimulates the spindle afferents, particularly the large group Ia axons from the primary sensory endings. In the spinal cord, these group Ia sensory axons terminate monosynaptically onto the α motor neurons that innervate the same (i.e., the "homonymous") muscle from which the group Ia axons originated. Thus, stretching a

muscle causes rapid feedback excitation of the same muscle through the minimum possible circuit: one sensory neuron, one synapse, and one motor neuron.

Monosynaptic connections account for much of the rapid component of the stretch reflex, but they are only the beginning of the story. At the same time the stretched muscle is being stimulated to contract, parallel circuits are inhibiting the α motor neurons of its *antagonist* muscles, those muscles that move a joint in the opposite direction. Thus, as the knee-jerk reflex causes contraction of the quadriceps muscle, it simultaneously causes relaxation of its antagonist, the semitendinosus muscle (see Fig. 14–4). To achieve inhibition, branches of the group Ia sensory axons excite specific interneurons that *inhibit* the α motor neurons of the antagonists. This **reciprocal innervation** increases the effectiveness of the stretch reflex by minimizing the antagonistic forces of the antagonist muscles.

Force Applied to the Golgi Tendon Organ During Active Muscle Contraction Causes Relaxation of the Same Muscle and Contraction of the Antagonistic Muscles

Skeletal muscle contains another sensory transducer in addition to the stretch receptor: the **Golgi tendon organ**

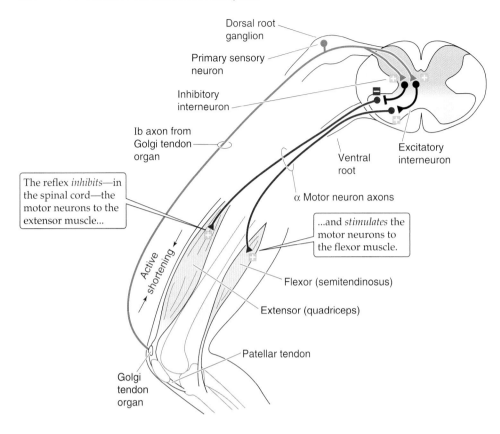

Dorsal root ganglion

Primary sensory neuron

Inhibitory interneuron

Ib axon from Golgi tendon organ

The reflex *inhibits*—in the spinal cord—the motor neurons to the extensor muscle...

Ventral root

Excitatory interneuron

α Motor neuron axons

...and *stimulates* the motor neurons to the flexor muscle.

Active shortening

Flexor (semitendinosus)

Extensor (quadriceps)

Patellar tendon

Golgi tendon organ

FIGURE 14–5. Golgi tendon organ (inverse myotatic) reflex. Active contraction of the quadriceps muscle elicits a reflexive relaxation of this muscle and contraction of the antagonistic semitendinosus muscle: the *inverse mytotatic reflex*. Contraction of the muscle pulls on the tendon, which squeezes and excites the sensory endings of the Golgi tendon organ, which convey their information via group Ib axons. These axons synapse on both inhibitory and excitatory interneurons in the spinal cord. The inhibitory interneurons innervate α motor neurons to the quadriceps, relaxing this muscle. The excitatory interneurons innervate α motor neurons to the antagonistic semitendinosus muscle, contracting it. Thus, both limbs of the reflex are polysynaptic.

(p. 358). Tendon organs are aligned in series with the muscle; they are exquisitely sensitive to the *tension* within a tendon and thus respond to the force generated by the muscle rather than to muscle length. Tendon organs may respond during passive muscle stretch, but they are stimulated particularly well during active contractions of a muscle. The group Ib sensory axons of the tendon organs excite both excitatory and inhibitory interneurons within the spinal cord (Fig. 14–5). However, this interneuron circuitry *inhibits* the muscle in which tension has increased and *excites* the antagonistic muscle; therefore, activity in the tendon organs yields effects that are almost the opposite of the stretch reflex. This response has been called the **inverse myotatic reflex**, and it may serve to control the force within muscles and the stiffness of particular joints.

Noxious Stimuli Can Evoke Complex Reflexive Movements

Sensations from the skin and connective tissue can also evoke strong spinal reflexes. Imagine walking on a beach and stepping on a sharp piece of shell (Fig. 14–6). Your response is swift and coordinated and does not require thoughtful reflection: you rapidly withdraw the wounded foot by activating the leg flexors and inhibiting the extensors. To keep from falling, you also extend your opposite leg by activating its extensors and inhibiting its flexors. This response is an example of a **flexor reflex**. The original stimulus for the reflex came from fast pain afferent neurons in the skin, primarily the group Aδ axons.

The above bilateral flexor reflex response is coordinated by sets of inhibitory and excitatory interneurons within

the spinal gray matter. Note that this coordination requires circuitry not only on the side of the cord ipsilateral to the wounded side but also on the contralateral side. Flexor reflexes can be activated by most of the various sensory afferents that detect noxious stimuli. Motor output spreads widely up and down the spinal cord, as it must to orchestrate so much of the body's musculature into an effective response. A remarkable feature of flexor reflexes is their specificity. Touching a hot surface, for example, elicits reflexive withdrawal of the hand in the direction opposite the side of the stimulus, and the strength of the reflex is related to the intensity of the stimulus. Unlike simple stretch reflexes, flexor reflexes coordinate the movement of entire limbs and even pairs of limbs. Such coordination requires precise and widespread wiring of the spinal interneurons.

Spinal Reflexes Are Strongly Influenced by Control Centers Within the Brain

Axons descend from numerous centers within the brainstem and the cerebral cortex and terminate primarily onto the spinal interneurons, with some direct input to the motor neurons. This descending control is essential for all conscious (and much unconscious) command of movement, a topic beyond the scope of this chapter. Less obvious is that the descending pathways can alter the strength of reflexes. For example, to heighten an anxious patient's stretch reflexes, a neurologist will sometimes ask the patient to perform the **Jendrassik maneuver**. The patient clasps his or her hands together and pulls; while the patient is distracted with that task, the examiner tests the stretch reflexes of the leg. Another example of the

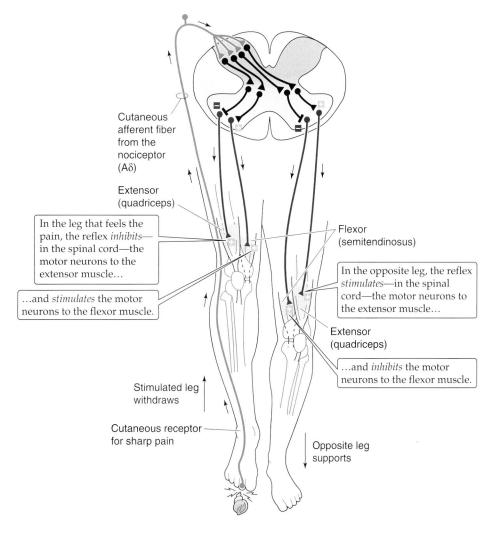

FIGURE 14–6. The flexor reflex. A painful stimulus to the right foot elicits a reflexive flexion of the right knee and an extension of the left knee: the *flexor reflex*. The noxious stimulus activates nociceptor afferents, which convey their information via group Aδ axons. These axons synapse on both inhibitory and excitatory interneurons. The inhibitory interneurons that project to the *right side* of the spinal cord innervate α motor neurons to the quadriceps and relax this muscle. The excitatory interneurons that project to the *right* side of the spinal cord innervate α motor neurons to the antagonistic semitendinosus muscle and contract it. The net effect is a coordinated *flexion* of the right knee. Similarly, the inhibitory interneurons that project to the *left* side of the spinal cord innervate α motor neurons to the left semitendinosus muscle and relax this muscle. The excitatory interneurons that project to the *left* side of the spinal cord innervate α motor neurons to the left quadriceps and contract it. The net effect is a coordinated *extension* of the left knee.

Cutaneous afferent fiber from the nociceptor (Aδ)

Extensor (quadriceps)

In the leg that feels the pain, the reflex *inhibits*—in the spinal cord—the motor neurons to the extensor muscle...

...and *stimulates* the motor neurons to the flexor muscle.

Flexor (semitendinosus)

In the opposite leg, the reflex *stimulates*—in the spinal cord—the motor neurons to the extensor muscle...

Extensor (quadriceps)

...and *inhibits* the motor neurons to the flexor muscle.

Stimulated leg withdraws

Cutaneous receptor for sharp pain

Opposite leg supports

brain's modulation of a stretch reflex occurs when catching a falling ball. If a ball were to fall unexpectedly from the sky and hit your outstretched hand, the force applied to your arm would cause a rapid *stretch reflex*—contraction in the *stretched* muscles and reciprocal inhibition in the *antagonist* muscles. The result would be that your hand would slap the ball back up into the air. However, if you *anticipate* catching the falling ball, for a short period around the time of impact (about ±60 msec), both your stretched muscles *and* the antagonist muscles contract! This maneuver stiffens your arm just when you need to squeeze that ball in order to not drop it. Stretch reflexes of the leg also vary dramatically during each step as we walk, thereby facilitating movement of the legs.

Like stretch reflexes, flexor reflexes can also be strongly affected by descending pathways. With mental effort, painful stimuli can be tolerated and withdrawal reflexes suppressed. On the other hand, anticipation of a painful stimulus may heighten the vigor of a withdrawal reflex when the stimulus actually arrives. Most of the brain's influence on spinal circuitry is achieved by control of the many spinal interneurons.

Spinal reflexes are frequently studied in isolation from one another, and textbooks often describe them this way. However, under realistic conditions, many reflex systems operate simultaneously, and motor output from the spinal cord depends on interactions among them, as well as on the state of controlling influences descending from the brain. It is now well accepted that reflexes do not simply correct for external perturbations of the body; in addition, they play a key role in the control of all movements.

The neurons involved in reflexes are the same neurons that generate other behaviors. Think again of the flexor response to the sharp shell—the pricked foot is withdrawn while the opposite leg extends. Now imagine that a crab pinches that opposite foot—you respond with the opposite pattern of withdrawal and extension. Repeat this a few times, crabs pinching you left and right, and you have achieved the basic pattern necessary for walking! Indeed, rhythmic locomotor patterns use components of these same spinal reflex circuits, as discussed next.

RHYTHMIC ACTIVITY: CENTRAL PATTERN GENERATORS

Central Pattern Generators in the Spinal Cord Can Create a Complex Motor Program Even Without Sensory Feedback

A common feature of motor control is the **motor program**, a set of structured muscle commands that are de-

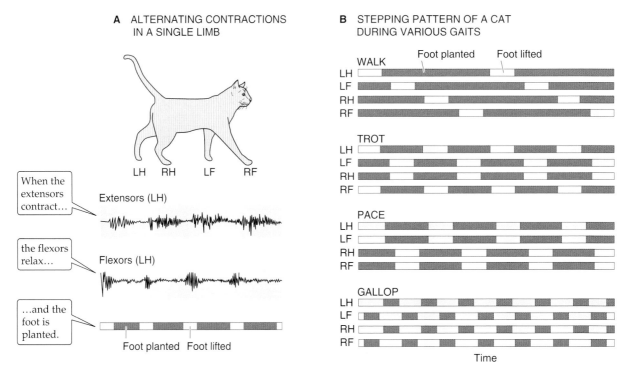

A   ALTERNATING CONTRACTIONS IN A SINGLE LIMB

When the extensors contract...

Extensors (LH)

the flexors relax...

Flexors (LH)

...and the foot is planted.

Foot planted   Foot lifted

B   STEPPING PATTERN OF A CAT DURING VARIOUS GAITS

Foot planted   Foot lifted

WALK
LH
LF
RH
RF

TROT
LH
LF
RH
RF

PACE
LH
LF
RH
RF

GALLOP
LH
LF
RH
RF

Time

FIGURE 14–7. Rhythmic patterns during locomotion. *A*, The experimental tracings are electromyograms (EMGs)—extracellular recordings of the electrical activity of muscles—from the extensor and flexor muscles of the left hind limb of a walking cat. The *pink bars* indicate that the foot is lifted; *purple bars* indicate that the foot is planted. *B*, The *walk, trot, pace,* and *gallop* not only represent different patterns and frequencies of planting and lifting for a single leg but also different patterns of coordination among the legs. LF, left front; LH, left hind; RF, right front; RH, right hind. (Data from Pearson K: The control of walking. Sci Am 2:72–86, 1976.)

termined by the nervous system before a movement begins and that can be sent to the muscles with the appropriate timing so that a sequence of movements occurs without any need for sensory feedback. The best evidence for the existence of motor programs is that the brain or spinal cord can command a variety of voluntary and automatic movements, such as walking and breathing (p. 719), even in the complete absence of sensory feedback from the periphery. The existence of motor programs certainly does not mean that sensory information is unimportant; on the contrary, motor behavior without sensory feedback is always different from that with normal feedback. The neural circuits responsible for various motor programs have been defined in a wide range of species. Although the details vary endlessly, certain broad principles emerge, even when comparing vertebrates and invertebrates. Here we focus on **central pattern generators**, well-studied circuits that underlie many of the rhythmic motor activities that are central to animal behavior.

Rhythmic behavior includes walking, running, swimming, breathing, chewing, certain eye movements, shivering, and even scratching. The central pattern generators driving each of these activities share certain basic properties. At their core is a set of cyclic, coordinated timing signals that are generated by a cluster of interconnected neurons. These basic signals are used to command as many as several hundred muscles, each precisely contracting or relaxing during a particular phase of the cycle—for example, with each walking step, the knee must first be flexed and then extended. Figure 14–7A shows how

the extensor and flexor muscles of the left hind limb of a cat contract rhythmically—and out of phase with one another—while the animal walks. Rhythms must also be coordinated with other rhythms—in order for humans to walk, one leg must move forward while the other thrusts backward, then vice versa, and the arms must swing in time with the legs, but with the opposite phase. For four-footed animals, the rhythms are even more complicated and must be able to accommodate changes in gait (see Fig. 14–7B). To achieve coordination among the various limbs, sets of central pattern generators must be interconnected. The motor patterns must also have great flexibility so that they can be altered on a moment's notice—consider the adjustments necessary when one foot strikes an obstacle while walking, or the changing motor patterns necessary to go from walking, to trotting, to running, to jumping. Finally, reliable methods must be available for turning the patterns on and off.

The central pattern generators for some rhythmic functions, such as breathing, are in the brain stem. Surprisingly, those responsible for locomotion reside in the spinal cord itself. Even with the spinal cord transected so that the lumbar segments are isolated from all higher centers, cats on a treadmill can generate well-coordinated stepping movements. Furthermore, stimulation of sensory afferents or descending tracts can induce the spinal pattern generators in four-footed animals to switch rapidly from walking, to trotting, to galloping patterns by altering not only the frequency of motor commands but also their pattern and coordination. During walking and trotting and pacing, the hind legs *alternate* their movements, but

FIGURE 14–8. Half-center model for alternating rhythm generation in flexor and extensor motor neurons. Stimulating the upper excitatory interneuron has two effects. First, the stimulated excitatory interneuron excites the motor neuron to the flexor muscle. Second, the stimulated excitatory interneuron excites an inhibitory interneuron, which inhibits the lower pathway. Stimulating the lower excitatory interneuron has the opposite effects. Thus, when one motor neuron is active, the opposite one is inhibited.

during galloping, they both flex and extend *simultaneously* (compare the leg patterns in Fig. 14–7B). Grillner and colleagues showed that each limb has at least one central pattern generator. If one leg is prevented from stepping, the other continues stepping normally. Under most circumstances, the various spinal pattern generators are coupled to one another, although the nature of the coupling must change to explain, for example, the switch from trotting to galloping patterns.

Pacemaker Cells and Synaptic Interconnections Both Contribute to Central Pattern Generation

How do neural circuits generate rhythmic patterns of activity? There is no single answer, and different circuits use different mechanisms. The simplest pattern generators are single neurons whose membrane properties endow them with pacemaker properties that are analogous to those of cardiac muscle cells (p. 489) and smooth muscle cells (p. 234). Even when experimentally isolated from other neurons, pacemaker neurons may be able to generate rhythmic activity by relying only on their intrinsic membrane conductance (see Fig. 11–6A). It is easy to imagine how intrinsic pacemaker neurons might act as the primary rhythmic driving force for sets of motor neurons that in turn command cyclic behavior. However, within vertebrates, although pacemaker neurons may contribute to some central pattern generators, they do not appear to be solely responsible for generating rhythms. Instead, they are embedded within interconnected circuits, and it is the combination of intrinsic pacemaker properties and synaptic interconnections that generates rhythm.

Neural circuits without pacemaker neurons can also generate rhythmic output. In 1911 Graham Brown proposed a pattern-generating circuit for locomotion. The essence of Brown's "half-center" model is a set of excitatory and inhibitory interneurons arranged to inhibit one another reciprocally (Fig. 14–8). The half-centers are the two halves of the circuit, each commanding one of a pair of antagonist muscles. For the circuit to work, a tonic drive must be applied to the excitatory interneurons; this drive could come from axons originating outside the circuit or from the intrinsic excitability of the neurons themselves. Furthermore, some built-in mechanism must limit the duration of the inhibitory activity so that excitability

can cyclically switch from one half-center to the other. Note that feedback from the muscles is not needed for the rhythms to proceed indefinitely. In fact, studies of more than 50 vertebrate and invertebrate motor circuits have confirmed that rhythm generation can continue in the absence of sensory information.

Central Pattern Generators in the Spinal Cord Take Advantage of Sensory Feedback, Interconnections Among Spinal Segments, and Interactions with Brainstem Control Centers

The half-center model can produce rhythmic, alternating neural activity, but it is clearly too simplistic to account for all features of locomotor pattern generation. Analysis of vertebrate pattern generators is a daunting task, made difficult by the complexity of the circuits and the behaviors they control. In the most detailed and successful investigation, Grillner and colleagues studied a very simple model of vertebrate locomotion circuits: the spinal cord of the sea lamprey. Lampreys swim with undulating motions of their body by using precisely coordinated waves of body-muscle contractions. At each spinal segment, muscle activity alternates—one side contracts as the other relaxes. As in mammals, the rhythmic pattern is generated within the spinal cord, and neurons in the brainstem control the initiation and speed of the patterns. The basic pattern-generating circuit for the lamprey spinal cord is repeated in each of the animal's 100 or so spinal segments.

The lamprey pattern-generating circuit improves on the half-center model in three ways. The first is **sensory feedback**. The lamprey has two kinds of stretch receptor neurons in the lateral margin of the spinal cord itself. These neurons sense stretching of the cord and body, which occurs as the animal bends during swimming. One type of stretch receptor excites the pattern generator interneurons on that same side and facilitates contraction, whereas the other type inhibits the pattern generator on the contralateral side and suppresses contraction. Because stretching occurs on the side of the cord that is currently relaxed, the effect of both stretch receptors is to terminate activity on the contracted side of the body and initiate contraction on the relaxed side.

The second improvement of the lamprey circuit over

the half-center model is the **interconnection of spinal segments**, which ensures the smooth progression of contractions down the length of the body, so that swimming can be efficient. Specifically, each segment must command its muscles to contract slightly later than the one anterior to it, with a lag of about 1% of a full activity cycle for normal forward swimming. Under some circumstances, the animal can also reverse the sequence of intersegment coordination to allow it to swim backward!

A third improvement over the half-center model is the **reciprocal communication** between the lamprey spinal pattern generators and control centers in the brainstem. Not only does the brainstem use numerous pathways and transmitters to modulate the generators, but the spinal generators also inform the brainstem of their activity.

The features outlined for swimming lampreys are relevant to walking cats and humans. All use spinal pattern generators to produce rhythms. All use sensory feedback to modulate locomotor rhythms (in mammals, feedback from muscle, joint, and cutaneous receptors is all important). All coordinate the spinal pattern generators across segments, and all maintain reciprocal communication between spinal generators and brainstem control centers.

SPATIAL REPRESENTATIONS: SENSORY AND MOTOR MAPS IN THE BRAIN

We have already seen that the spinal cord can receive sensory input, integrate it, and produce motor output that is totally independent of the brain. The brain also receives this sensory information and uses it to control the motor activity of the spinal reflexes and central pattern generators. How does the brain organize this sensory input and motor output? In many cases, it organizes these functions spatially by using maps.

In everyday life, we use maps to represent spatial locations. You may use endless ways to construct a map, depending on which features of an area you want to highlight and what sort of transformation you make as you take measurements from the source (the thing being mapped) and place them on the target (the map). Maps of the earth may emphasize topography, the road system, political boundaries, the distributions of air temperature and wind direction, population density, or vegetation. A map is a model of a part of the world—and a very limited model at that. The brain also builds maps, most of which represent very selected aspects of our sensory information about the environment or the motor systems controlling our body. These maps can be spatial, or they can express nonspatial qualities of various sensory modalities (e.g., smell).

The Nervous System Contains Maps of Sensory and Motor Information

Almost all sensory receptors are laid out in planar sheets. In some cases these receptor sheets are straightforward **spatial maps** of the sensory environment that they encode. For example, the somatic sensory receptors of the skin literally form a map of the body surface. Similarly, a tiny version of the visual scene is projected onto the mosaic of retinal photoreceptors. The topographies of other sensory receptor sheets represent qualities other than spatial features of the sensory stimuli. For example, the position of a hair cell along the basilar membrane in the cochlea determines the range of sound frequencies to which it will respond. Thus, the sheet of hair cells is a **frequency map** of sound rather than a map of the location of sounds in space. Olfactory and taste receptors also do not encode stimulus position; instead, because the receptor specificity varies topographically, the receptor sheets may be **chemical maps** of the types of stimuli. The most interesting thing about sensory receptor maps is that they often project onto many different regions of the CNS. In fact, each sensory surface may be mapped and remapped many times within the brain, the characteristics of each map being unique. In some cases the brain constructs maps of stimulus features even when these features are not mapped at the level of the receptors themselves. Sound localization is a good example of this property (see the next section). Some neural maps may also combine the features of other neural maps, for example, overlaying visual information with auditory information.

The Cerebral Cortex Has Multiple Visuotopic Maps

Some of the best examples of brain maps are those of the visual fields. Figure 14–9A shows the basic anatomic pathway extending from the retina to the lateral geniculate nucleus of the thalamus and on to the **primary visual cortex** (area V1). Note that area V1 actually maps the visual thalamus, which in turn maps the retina, the first visuotopic map in the brain. Thus, the V1 map is sometimes referred to as a *retinotopic map*. Figure 14–9B shows how the visual fields are mapped onto cortical area V1. The first thing to notice is that the *left* half of the visual field is represented on the *right* cortex and the *upper* half of the visual field is represented on the *lower* portions of the cortex. This orientation is strictly determined by the system's anatomy. For example, all the retinal axons from the *left*most halves of both eyes (which are stimulated by light from the *right* visual hemifield) project to the *left* half of the brain. Compare the *red* and *blue pathways* in Figure 14–9A. During development, each axon must therefore make an unerring decision about which side of the brain to innervate when it reaches the optic chiasm!

The second thing to notice is that scaling of the visual fields onto visual cortex—often called the **magnification factor**—is not constant. In particular, the central region of the visual fields—the fovea—is greatly magnified on the cortical surface. Behavioral importance ultimately determines mapping in the brain. Primates require particularly high-resolution vision in the center of their gaze; photoreceptors and ganglion cells are thus packed as densely as possible into the central retinal region (p. 336). About half of the primary visual cortex is devoted to input from the relatively small fovea and the retinal area just surrounding it.

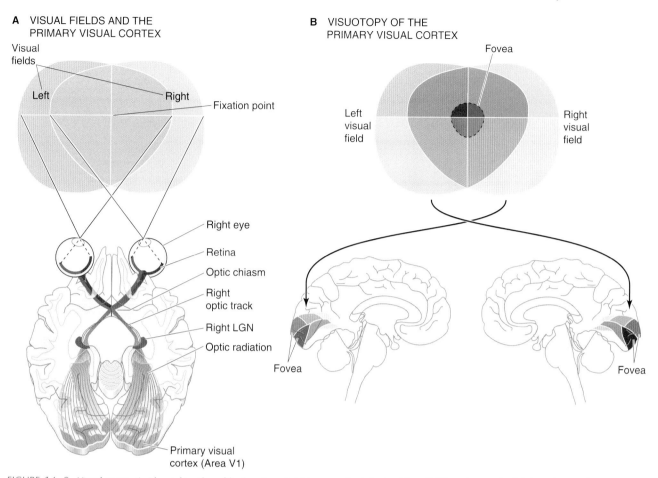

A VISUAL FIELDS AND THE
  PRIMARY VISUAL CORTEX

Visual
fields

Left   Right

                    Fixation point

                    Right eye

                    Retina

                    Optic chiasm

                    Right
                    optic track

Right LGN

                    Optic radiation

                    Primary visual
                    cortex (Area V1)

B VISUOTOPY OF THE
  PRIMARY VISUAL CORTEX

                    Fovea

Left   Right
visual   visual
field   field

Fovea   Fovea

FIGURE 14–9. Visual maps. *A*, The right sides of both retinas (which sense the left visual hemifield) project to the left lateral geniculate, which in turn projects to the left primary visual cortex (*area V1*). *B*, The upper parts of the visual fields project to lower parts of the contralateral visual cortex, and vice versa. Although the fovea represents only a small part of the visual field, its representation is greatly magnified in the primary visual cortex, reflecting the large number of retinal ganglion cells that are devoted to the fovea. LGN, lateral geniculate nucleus.

Understanding a visual scene requires us to analyze many of its features simultaneously. An object may have shape, color, motion, location, and context, and the brain can usually organize these features to present a seamless interpretation, or image. The details of this process are only now being worked out, but it appears that the task is accomplished with the help of *numerous* visual areas within the cerebral cortex. Studies of monkey cortex by a variety of electrophysiologic and anatomic methods have identified more than 25 areas, most of which are in the vicinity of area V1, that are mainly visual in function. According to recent estimates, humans devote almost half of their neocortex primarily to the processing of visual information. Several features of a visual scene, such as motion, form, and color, are processed in parallel and, to some extent, in separate stages of processing. The neural mechanisms by which these separate features are somehow melded into one image or concept of an object remain unknown, but they depend on strong and reciprocal interconnections between the visual maps in various areas of the brain.

The apparently simple topography of a sensory map looks much more complex and discontinuous when examined in detail. Many cortical areas can be described as maps upon maps. Such an arrangement is especially strik-

ing in the visual system. For example, within area V1 of Old World monkeys and humans, the visuotopic maps of the two eyes remain segregated. In layer IV of the primary visual cortex, this segregation is accomplished by having visual input derived from the left eye alternate every 0.25 to 0.5 mm with visual input from the right. Thus, two sets of information, one from the left and one from the right eye, remain separated but adjacent. When viewed edge on, these left-right alternations look like columns (Fig. 14–10*A*); hence their name: **ocular dominance columns**. When viewed from the surface of the brain, this alternating left-right array of input looks like bands or zebra stripes (Fig. 14–10*B*).

Superimposed on the zebra-stripe ocular dominance pattern in layer IV of the primary visual cortex, but quite distinct from these zebra stripes, layers II and III have structures called **blobs**. These blobs are visible when the cortex is stained for the mitochondrial enzyme cytochrome oxidase. When viewed edge on, these blobs look like round pegs (see Fig. 14–10*A*). When viewed from the surface of the brain (see Fig. 14–10*A*, *B*), the blobs appear as a polka-dot pattern of small dots that are approximately 0.2 mm in diameter.

Adjacent to the primary visual cortex (V1) is the secondary visual cortex (V2), which has, instead of blobs, a

A LAYERS OF AREA V1

B SPLIT-OPEN VIEW

FIGURE 14–10. Ocular dominance columns and blobs in the primary visual cortex (*area V1*). *A*, Ocular dominance columns are shown as *alternating black* (right eye) and *gray* (left eye) structures in layer IV. The *alternating light* and *dark bands* are the result of an autoradiograph taken 2 weeks after injecting one eye with ³H-labeled proline and fucose. The ³H label moved from the optic nerve to neurons in the lateral geniculate and then to the axon terminals in the V1 cortex that are represented in this figure. The blobs are shown as *teal-colored pegs* in layers II and III. They represent the regular distribution of cytochrome oxidase–rich neurons and are organized in pillar-shaped clusters. *B*, Cutting the brain parallel to its surface, but between layers III and IV, reveals a *polka-dot pattern of blobs* in layer II/III and *zebra-like stripes* in layer IV. (Data from Hubel D: Eye, Brain and Vision. New York, WH Freeman, 1988.)

series of thick and thin **stripes** that are separated by pale interstripes. Some other higher-order visual areas also have striped patterns. Whereas ocular dominance columns demarcate the left and right eyes, blobs and stripes seem to demarcate clusters of neurons that process and channel different types of visual information between areas V1 and V2 and pass them on to other visual regions of the cortex. For example, neurons within the blobs of area V1 seem to be especially attuned to information about color, and project to neurons in the thin stripes of V2. Other neurons throughout area V1 are very sensitive to motion but are insensitive to color. They channel their information mainly to neurons of the thick stripes in V2.

Maps of Somatic Sensory Information Magnify Some Parts of the Body More Than Others

One of the most famous depictions of a neural map came from studies of the human somatosensory cortex by Penfield and colleagues. Penfield stimulated small sites on the cortical surface of locally anesthetized, but conscious patients during neurosurgical procedures, and from their verbal descriptions of the position of their sensations he drew a "homunculus," a little person representing the **somatotopy**—mapping of the body surface—of the primary somatic sensory cortex (Fig. 14–11A). The basic features of Penfield's map have been confirmed with other methods, including recording from neurons while stimulating the body surface and modern brain imaging methods, such as positron emission tomography and functional magnetic resonance imaging. The human somatotopic

map resembles a trapeze artist hanging upside down, the legs hooked over the top of the postcentral gyrus and dangling into the medial cortex between the hemispheres, and the trunk, upper limbs and head draped over the lateral aspect of the postcentral gyrus.

Two interesting features should be noticed about the somatotopic map in Figure 14–11A. First, mapping of the body surface is not always continuous. For example, the representation of the hand separates those of the head and face, whereas the genitals map onto the most hidden part of the cortex, somewhere below the toes. Second, the map is not scaled like the human body. Instead, it looks like a cartoon character: the mouth, tongue, and fingers are very large, whereas the trunk, arms, and legs are tiny. As was the case for mapping of the visual fields onto the visual cortex, it is clear in Penfield's map that the magnification factor for the body surface is not a constant but varies for different parts of the body. Fingertips are magnified on the cortex much more than the tips of the toes. The relative size of cortex that is devoted to each body part is correlated with the *density* of sensory input received from that part, and 1 mm² of fingertip skin has many more sensory endings than a similar patch on the buttocks. Size on the map is also related to the *importance* of the sensory input from that part of the body; information from the tip of the tongue is more useful than that from the elbow. The mouth representation is probably large because tactile sensations are important in the production of speech, and the lips and tongue are one of the last lines of defense when deciding whether a morsel is a potential piece of food or poison.

The importance of each body part differs among spe-

A SOMATOSENSORY

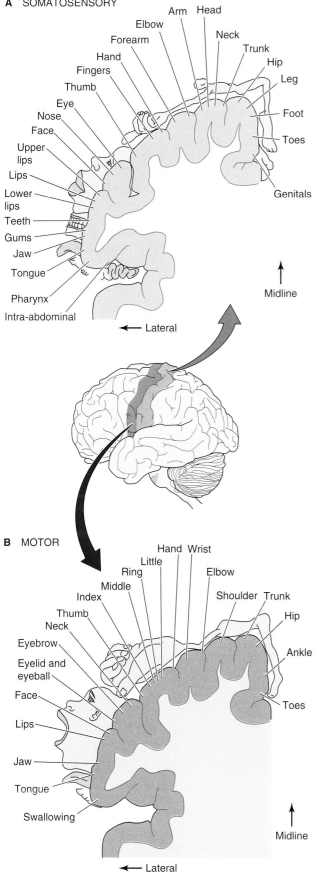

cies, and indeed, some species have body parts that others do not. For example, the whiskers of rodents have a huge representation on the cortex, whereas the digits of the paws receive relatively little. Rodent behavior explains this paradox. Most are nocturnal, and to navigate they actively sweep their whiskers about as they move. By touching their local environment they can sense shapes, textures, and movement with remarkable acuity. For a rat or mouse, seeing things with their eyes is usually less important than "seeing" things with their whiskers.

As we have already seen for the visual system, other sensory systems usually map their information numerous times. Maps may be carried through many anatomic levels. The somatotopic maps in the cortex begin with the primary somatic sensory axons (see Table 11–1) that enter the spinal cord or the brainstem, each at the spinal segment appropriate to the site of the information that it carries. The sensory axons synapse on second-order neurons, and these cells project their axons into various nuclei of the thalamus and form synapses. Thalamic relay neurons in turn send their axons into the neocortex. The topographic order of the body surface (i.e., *somatotopy*) is maintained at each anatomic stage, and somatotopic maps are located within the spinal cord, brainstem, and the thalamus, as well as in the somatosensory cortex. Within the cortex, the somatic sensory system has several maps of the body, each unique and each concerned with different types of somatotopic information. Multiple maps are the rule in the brain.

The Cerebral Cortex Has a Motor Map That Is Adjacent to and Well Aligned with the Somatosensory Map

Neural maps are not limited to sensory systems; they also appear regularly in brain structures that are considered to be primarily motor. Studies done in the 1860s by Fritsch and Hitzig showed that stimulating particular parts of the cerebral cortex evokes specific muscle contractions in dogs. Penfield and colleagues generated maps of the primary motor cortex in humans (see Fig. 14–11B) by microstimulating and observing the evoked movements. They noted an orderly relationship between the site of cortical stimulation and the body part that moved. Penfield's motor maps look remarkably similar to his somatosensory maps, which lie in the adjacent cortical gyrus (see Fig. 14–11A). Note that the *sensory and motor maps are adjacent and similar* in basic layout (legs represented medially and head laterally) and both have a striking magnification of the head and hand regions. Not surprisingly, there are myriad axonal interconnections between the primary motor and primary somatosensory areas. Functional magnetic resonance imaging of the human motor cortex shows that the motor map for hand movements is not nearly as simple and somatotopic as Penfield's drawings might imply. Movements of individual fingers or the wrist, initiated by the individual, activate specific and widely distributed regions of motor cortex, but these regions also overlap one another. Rather than following an obvious somatotopic progression, it instead appears that neurons in the arm area of the motor cortex form

B MOTOR

FIGURE 14–11. Somatosensory and motor maps. *A,* The plane of section runs through the postcentral gyrus of the cerebral cortex, shown as a *blue band* on the image of the brain. *B,* The plane of section runs through the precentral gyrus of the cerebral cortex, shown as a *violet band* on the image of the brain. (Data from Penfield W, Rasmussen T: The Cerebral Cortex of Man. New York, Macmillan, 1952.)

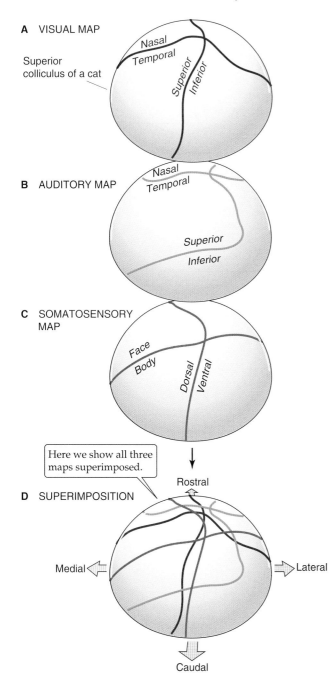

A VISUAL MAP

Superior colliculus of a cat

Nasal
Temporal
Superior
Inferior

B AUDITORY MAP

Nasal
Temporal
Superior
Inferior

C SOMATOSENSORY MAP

Face
Body
Dorsal
Ventral

Here we show all three maps superimposed.

D SUPERIMPOSITION

Rostral
Medial
Lateral
Caudal

FIGURE 14–12. Polysensory space in the superior colliculus. In *A*, the illustration shows the representation of visual space that is projected onto the right superior colliculus of a cat. Note that visual space is divided into nasal versus temporal space and superior versus inferior space. In *B* and *C*, the illustrations show comparable auditory and somatosensory maps, respectively. In *D*, which shows the superimposition, note the approximate correspondence among the visual (*red*), auditory (*green*), and somatosensory (*blue*) maps, which are superimposed on one another. The motor map for orienting the eyes (not shown) is in almost perfect register with the visual map in *A*. (Data from Stein BE, Wallace MT, Meredith MA: Neural mechanisms mediating attention and orientation to multisensory cues. In Gazzaniga M [ed]: The Cognitive Neurosciences. Cambridge, MA, MIT Press, 1995.)

distributed and cooperative networks that control collections of arm muscles. Other regions of the motor cortex also have a distributed organization when examined on a fine scale, although Penfield's somatotopic maps still suffice to describe the gross organization of the motor cortex.

In other parts of the brain, *motor and sensory functions may even occupy the same tissue,* and precise alignment of the motor and sensory maps is usually the case. For example, a paired midbrain structure called the *superior colliculus* receives direct, retinotopic connections from the retina, as well as input from the visual cortex. Accordingly, a spot of light in the visual field activates a particular patch of neurons in the colliculus. The same patch of collicular neurons can also command, via other brainstem connections, eye and head movements that bring the image of the light spot into the center of the *visual* field so that it is imaged onto the fovea. The *motor map* for orientation of the eyes is in precise register with the visual response map. In addition, the superior colliculus has maps of both *auditory* and *somatosensory* information superimposed on its visual and motor maps; the four aligned maps work in concert to represent points in polysensory space and help control an animal's orienting responses to prominent stimuli (Fig. 14–12).

Sensory and Motor Maps Are Fuzzy and Plastic

We have described a sample of the sensory and motor maps in the brain, but we are left to wonder just why neural maps are so ubiquitous, elaborate, and varied. What is the advantage of mapping neural functions in an orderly way? You could imagine other arrangements: spatial information might be widely scattered about on a neural structure, such as on the hard disk of a computer. Various explanations may be proposed for the phenomenon of orderly mapping in the nervous system, although most remain speculations. Maps may be the most efficient way of generating **nearest-neighbor relationships** between neurons that must be interconnected for proper function. For example, the collicular neurons that participate in sensing stimuli 10 degrees up and 20 degrees to the left and other collicular neurons that command eye movements toward that point undoubtedly need to be strongly interconnected. Orderly collicular mapping enforces togetherness for those cells and minimizes the length of axons necessary to interconnect them. In addition, if brain structures are arranged topographically, neighboring neurons will be most likely to become activated synchronously. Neighboring neurons are very likely to be interconnected in structures such as the cortex, and their synchronous activity serves to reinforce the strength of their interconnections because of the inherent rules governing synaptic plasticity (p. 318).

An additional advantage of mapping is that it may simplify establishment of the proper connections between neurons during **development**. For example, it is easier for an axon from neuron A to find neuron B if distances are short. Maps may thus make it easier to establish interconnections precisely among the neurons that represent the three sensory and one motor map in the superior colliculus. Another advantage of maps may be to facilitate the effectiveness of **inhibitory connections**. Perception of the edge of a stimulus (edge detection) is heightened by lateral connections that suppress the activity of neurons representing the space slightly away from the edge. If sen-

A SOMATOSENSORY REORGANIZATION

B MOTOR-SYSTEM REORGANIZATION

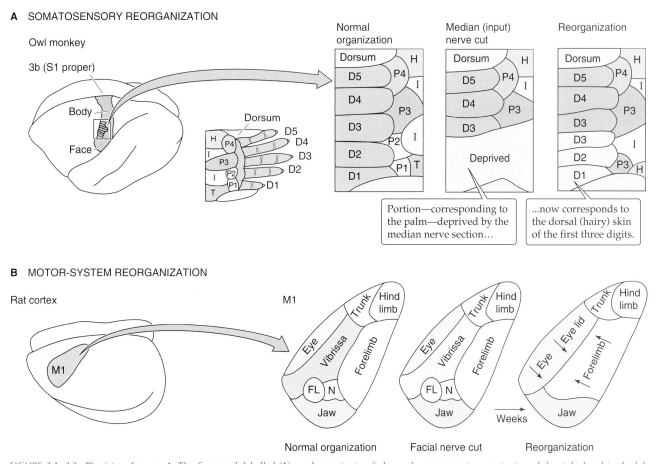

FIGURE 14–13. Plasticity of maps. *A, The first panel,* labelled "Normal organization," shows the somatotopic organization of the right hand in the left somatosensory cortex of the monkey brain. The colors correspond to different regions of the hand (viewed from the palm side, except for portions labelled "dorsum"). The *second panel* shows (*in gray*) the territory that is deprived of input by sectioning the median nerve. The *third panel* shows that the cortical map is greatly changed several months after nerve section. The nerve was not allowed to regrow, but the previously deprived cortical region now responds to the dorsal skin of D3, D2, and D1. Notice that responses to regions P1, P2, and T have disappeared; *region I* has encroached; and *regions H* and *P3* have suddenly appeared at a second location. (Data from Kaas JH: The reorganization of sensory and motor maps in adult mammals. In Gazzaniga M [ed]: The Cognitive Neurosciences. Cambridge, MA, MIT Press, 1995.) *B, The first panel,* labelled "Normal organization," shows the somatotopic organization of the left motor cortex (*M1*) of the rat brain. The colors correspond to the muscles that control different regions of the body. The *second panel* shows (*in gray*) the territory that normally provides motor output to the facial nerve, which has been severed. The *third panel* shows that, after several weeks, the deprived cortical territory is now remapped. Notice that the deprived territory that once evoked whisker movements now evokes eye, eyelid, and forelimb movements. (Data from Sanes J, Suner S, Donoghue JP: Dynamic organization of primary motor cortex output to target muscles in adult rats: Long-term patterns of reorganization following motor or mixed peripheral nerve lesions. Exp Brain Res 79:479–491, 1990.)

sory areas are mapped, it is a simple matter to arrange the inhibitory connections onto nearby neurons and thereby construct an edge-detector circuit.

It is worth clarifying several general points about neural maps. "The map is not the territory, the word is not the thing it describes."* In other words, all maps, including neural maps, are abstract representations of particular experimental measurements. A problem with neural maps is that different experimenters, using different methods, may sometimes generate quite different maps of the same part of the brain. As more and better refined methods become available, our understanding of these maps is evolving. Moreover, the brain itself muddies its maps. Maps of sensory space onto a brain area are not point-to-point representations. On the contrary, a point in sensory space (e.g., a spot of light) activates a relatively large group of

neurons in a sensory region of the brain. However, such activation of many neurons is not due to errors of connectivity; the spatial dissemination of activity is part of the mechanism used to encode and process information. The *strength* of activation is most intense within the center of the activated neuronal group, but the population of more weakly activated neurons may encompass a large portion of an entire brain. This diversity in strength of activation means that a point in sensory space is unlikely to be encoded by the activity of a single neuron, but instead it is represented by the distributed activity in a large population of neurons. Such a distributed code has computational advantages, and some redundancy also guards against errors, damage, and loss of information.

Finally, maps may change with time. All sensory and motor maps are clearly dynamic and can be reorganized rapidly and substantially as a function of development, behavioral state, training, or damage to the brain or periphery. Such changes are referred to as **plasticity**. Figure 14–13 illustrates two examples of dramatic changes in

---

*From Van Vogt AE: The Players of Null-A. London, Dobson, 1970, p 158, as quoted by Dykes and Ruest.

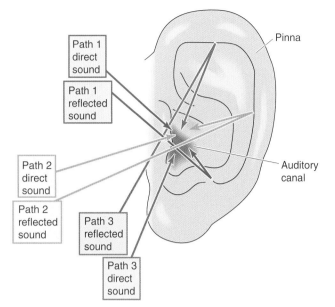

FIGURE 14–14. Detection of sound in the vertical plane. The detection of sound in the vertical plane requires only one ear. Regardless of the source of a sound, the sound reaches the auditory canal by both direct and reflected pathways. The brain localizes the source of the sound in the vertical plane by detecting differences in the combined sounds from the direct and reflected pathways.

neocortical mapping, one sensory and one motor, after damage to peripheral nerves. In both cases, severing a peripheral nerve causes the part of the map that normally relates to the body part served by this severed nerve to become remapped to another body part. Although the mechanisms of these reorganizations are not yet known, they probably reflect the same types of processes that underly our ability to learn sensorimotor skills with practice, and to adjust and improve after neural damage from trauma or stroke.

TEMPORAL REPRESENTATIONS: TIME-MEASURING CIRCUITS

To Localize Sound, the Brain Compares the Timing and Intensity of Input to the Ears

Neural circuits are very good at resolving time intervals down to microseconds. One of the most demanding tasks of timing is performed by the auditory system as it localizes the source of certain sounds. Sound localization is an important skill, whether you are prey, predator, or pedestrian. Vertebrates use several different strategies for localization of sound, depending on the species, the frequency of the sound, and whether the task is to localize the source in the horizontal (left-right) or vertical (up-down) plane. In this subchapter we briefly review general strategies of sound localization and then explain the mechanism by which a brainstem circuit measures the relative timing of low-frequency sounds so that the source of the sounds can be localized with precision.

Sound localization along the **vertical plane** (the degree of elevation) depends, in humans at least, on the distinctive shape of the external ear, the *pinna*. Much of the sound that we hear enters the auditory canal directly, and its energy is transferred to the cochlea. However, some sound reflects off the curves and folds of the pinna and tragus before it enters the canal and thus takes slightly longer to reach the cochlea. Notice what happens when the vertical direction of the sound changes. Because of the arcing shape of the pinna, the reflected path of sounds coming from above is shorter than that of sounds from below (Fig. 14–14). The two sets of sounds (the *direct* and, slightly delayed, the *reflected*) combine to create sounds that are slightly different on entering the auditory canal. Because of the interference patterns created by the direct and reflected sounds, the combined sound has spectral properties that are characteristic of the elevation of the sound source. This mechanism of vertical sound localization works well even with one ear at a time, although its precise neural mechanisms are not very clear.

Accurately determining the direction of a sound along the **horizontal plane** (the "azimuth") necessitates two working ears. Sounds must first be processed by the

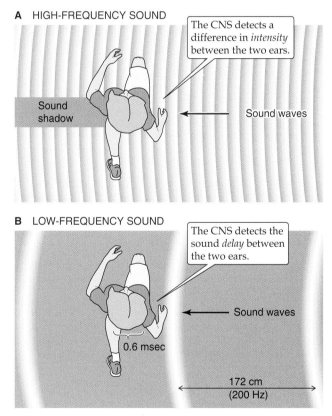

FIGURE 14–15. Sound detection in a horizontal plane. *A,* Two ears are necessary for the detection of sound in a horizontal plane. For frequencies between 2 kHz and 20 kHz, the CNS detects the ear-to-ear *intensity* difference. In this example, the sound comes from the right. The left ear hears a weaker sound because it is in the shadow of the head. *B,* For frequencies below 2 kHz, the CNS detects the ear-to-ear *delay*. In this example, the width of the head is 20 cm, and sound with a frequency of 200 Hz (wavelength of 172 cm) comes from the right. The peak of each sound wave reaches the left ear approximately 0.6 msec after it reaches the right. CNS, central nervous system.

cochlea in each ear and then compared by neurons within the CNS to estimate horizontal direction. But what exactly is compared? For sounds that are relatively high in frequency (about 2 to 20 kHz), the important measure is the *interaural* (i.e., ear-to-ear) *intensity difference*. Stated simply, the ear facing the sound hears it louder than the ear facing away because the head casts a "sound shadow" (Fig. 14–15A). If the sound is directly to the right or left of the listener, this difference is maximal; if the sound is straight ahead, no difference is heard; and if the sound comes from an oblique direction, intensity differences are intermediate. Note that this system can be fooled. A sound straight ahead gives the same intensity difference (i.e., none) as a sound directly behind.

The interaural intensity difference is not helpful at lower frequencies. Sounds below about 2 kHz have a wavelength that is longer than the width of the head itself. Longer sound waves are diffracted around the head, and differences in *interaural intensity* no longer occur. At low frequencies, the nervous system uses another strategy—it measures *interaural delay* (see Fig. 14–15B). Consider a 200-Hz sound coming directly from the right. Its peak-to-peak distance (i.e., the wavelength) is about 172 cm, which is considerably more than the 20-cm width of the head. Each sound wave peak will reach the right ear about 0.6 msec before it reaches the left ear. If the sound comes from a 45-degree angle ahead, the interaural delay is about 0.3 msec; if it comes from straight ahead (or directly behind), the delay is 0 msec. Delays of small fractions of a millisecond are well within the capabilities of certain brainstem auditory neurons to detect. Sounds need not be continuous for the interaural delay to be detected. Sound onset or offset, clicks, or any abrupt changes in the sound give opportunities for interaural time comparisons. Obviously, measurement of interaural delay is subject to the same front-back ambiguity as interaural intensity, and indeed, it is sometimes difficult to distinguish whether a sound is in front of or behind your head.

The Brain Measures Interaural Timing by a Combination of Neural Delay Lines and Coincidence Detectors

How does the auditory system measure interaural timing? Surprisingly, to detect very small *time* differences, the nervous system uses a precise arrangement of neurons in *space*. Figure 14–16A summarizes the neuroanatomy of the first stages of central auditory processing within the brainstem. Notice that neurons in each of the cochlear nuclei receive information from only the ear on that one side whereas neurons from the medial superior olivary (MSO) nucleus—and higher CNS centers—receive abundant input from both ears. Because horizontal sound localization requires input from both ears, we may guess that "direction-sensitive neurons" will probably be found somewhere central to the cochlear nuclei. When cochlear-nucleus neurons are activated by auditory stimuli, their action potentials tend to fire with a particular phase relationship to the sound stimulus. For example, such a neu-

ron might fire at the peak of every sound wave or at the peak of every fifth sound wave. That is, its firing is *phase-locked* to the sound waves, at least for relatively low frequencies. Hence cochlear neurons preserve the timing information of sound stimuli. Neurons in the MSO receive synaptic input from axons originating in both cochlear nuclei, so they are well placed to compare the timing (the phase) of sounds arriving at the two ears. Recordings from MSO neurons demonstrate that they are exquisitely sensitive to interaural time delay, and the optimal delay for olivary neurons varies systematically across the nucleus. In other words, the MSO has a spatial map of *interaural delay*. The olive also has a systematic map of sound *frequency*, so it simultaneously maps two qualities of sound stimuli.

The tuning of MSO neurons to interaural delay seems to depend on neural circuitry that combines "delay lines" with "coincidence detection," an idea first proposed by Jeffress in 1948. **Delay lines** are the axons from each cochlear nucleus; their length and conduction velocity determine how long it takes sound-activated action potentials to go from a cochlear nucleus to the axon's presynaptic terminals onto MSO neurons (see Fig. 14–16B). Axons from both the right and left cochlear nuclei converge and synapse onto a series of neurons in the MSO. However, each axon (each delay line) may take a different time to conduct its action potential to the same olivary neuron. The difference in conduction delay between the axon from the right side and that from the left side determines the optimal interaural delay for that particular olivary neuron. It is the olivary neuron that acts as the **coincidence detector:** only when action potentials from *both* the left and right ear axons reach the postsynaptic olivary neuron simultaneously (meaning that sound has reached the two ears at a particular interaural delay) is that neuron likely to fire an action potential. If input from the two ears arrives at the neuron out of phase, without coincidence in time, the neuron will not fire. All these postsynaptic superior olivary neurons are fundamentally the same: they fire when there is coincidence between input from the left and right. However, because neurons arrayed across the olive are mapped so that the axons connecting them have different delays, they display coincidence for different interaural delays. Thus, each is **tuned** to a different interaural delay and a different sound locale along the horizontal axis. The orderly arrangement of delay lines across the olive determines each of the neurons' preferred delays (and thus sound location preferences) and leads to the orderly spatial mapping of sound direction.

Neural maps of sound localization are an interesting example of a sensory map that the brain must *compute*. This computed map contrasts with many other sensory maps that are derived more simply, such as by an orderly set of connections between the sensory receptor sheet (e.g., the retinal photoreceptors) and a central brain structure (e.g., the superior colliculus), as described in the previous subchapter (see Fig. 14–9). The cochlea does not have any map for sound location. Instead, the CNS localizes low-frequency sounds by calculating an interaural *time-delay* map, using information from both ears

A SOME MAJOR AUDITORY PATHWAYS

FIGURE 14–16. CNS processing of sounds. *A*, The figure shows a cross section of the medulla. After a sound stimulus to the cochlea, the cochlear nerve carries an action potential to the cochlear nucleus, which receives information only from the ear on the same side. However, higher auditory centers receive input from both ears. *B*, Neurons in the medial superior olivary (MSO) nucleus are each tuned to a different interaural delay. Only when action potentials from the right and left sides arrive at the MSO neuron simultaneously does the neuron fire an action potential (coincidence detection). In this example, the two action potentials are coincident at MSO neuron D because the brief acoustic delay to the left ear is followed by a long neuronal-conduction delay, whereas the long acoustic delay to the right ear is followed by a brief neuronal-conduction delay.

B CALCULATION OF INTERAURAL DELAY BY COINCIDENCE DETECTION

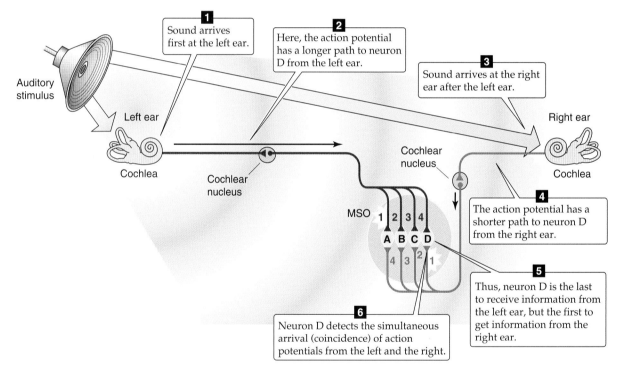

1 Sound arrives first at the left ear.

2 Here, the action potential has a longer path to neuron D from the left ear.

3 Sound arrives at the right ear after the left ear.

4 The action potential has a shorter path to neuron D from the right ear.

5 Thus, neuron D is the last to receive information from the left ear, but the first to get information from the right ear.

6 Neuron D detects the simultaneous arrival (coincidence) of action potentials from the left and the right.

together. Other circuits can build a computed map of interaural *intensity differences*, which can be used for localization of high-frequency sounds (see Fig. 14–15*A*). Once these two orderly sensory maps have been computed, they can be remapped onto another part of the brain by a simple system of orderly connections. For instance, the inferior colliculus receives parallel information on both timing delay and intensity difference; it transforms these two sets of information, combines them, and produces a complete map of sound direction. This combination of hierarchic (lower to high centers) and parallel information processing is probably ubiquitous in the CNS and is a general strategy for the analysis of much more complex sensory problems than those described here.

REFERENCES

Books and Reviews

Bear MF, Connors BW, Paradiso MA: Neuroscience: Exploring the Brain, 2nd ed. Baltimore, Lippincott Williams & Wilkins, 2001.

Carr CE: Processing of temporal information in the brain. Annu Rev Neurosci 16:223–243, 1993.

Middlebrooks JC, Green DM: Sound localization by human listeners. Annu Rev Psychol 42:135–159, 1991.

Journal Articles

Barlow HB: Why have so many cortical areas? Vis Res 26:81–90, 1986.

Carr CE, Konishi M: A circuit for detection of interaural time differences in the brainstem of the barn owl. J Neurosci 10:3227–3246, 1990.

Delcomyn F: Neural basis of rhythmic behavior in animals. Science 210: 492–498, 1980.

Donoghue JP, Sanes JN: Motor areas of the cerebral cortex. J Clin Neurophysiol 11:382–396, 1994.

Lacquaniti F, Borghese NA, Carrozzo M: Transient reversal of the stretch reflex in human arm muscles. J Neurophysiol 49:16–27, 1991.

Sanes J, Suner S, Donoghue JP: Dynamic organization of primary motor cortex output to target muscles in adult rats. I. Long-term patterns of reorganization following motor or mixed peripheral nerve lesions. Exp Brain Res 79:479–491, 1990.

CHAPTER 15

The Autonomic Nervous System

George B. Richerson

When we are awake, we are constantly aware of sensory input from our external environment, and we consciously plan how to react to it. When we are asleep, the nervous system has a variety of mechanisms for dissociating cortical function from sensory input and somatic motor output. Among these mechanisms are closing the eyes, blocking the transmission of sensory impulses to the cortex as they pass through the thalamus, and effecting a nearly complete paralysis of skeletal muscles during rapid eye movement (REM) sleep to keep us from physically acting out our dreams.

The conscious and discontinuous nature of cortical brain function stands in sharp contrast with those parts of the nervous system that are responsible for controlling our internal environment. These "autonomic" processes never stop attending to the wide range of metabolic, cardiopulmonary, and other visceral requirements of our body. Autonomic control continues whether we are awake and attentive, preoccupied with other activities, or asleep. While we are awake, we are unaware of most visceral sensory input, and we avoid any conscious effort to act on it unless it induces distress. In most cases we have no awareness of motor commands to the viscera, and most individuals can exert voluntary control over motor output to the viscera only in minor ways. Consciousness and memory are frequently considered the most important functions of the human nervous system, but it is the visceral control system—the **autonomic nervous system** (ANS)—that makes life and higher cortical function possible.

We have a greater understanding of the physiology of the ANS than of many other parts of the nervous system, largely because it is reasonably easy to isolate peripheral neurons and study them. As a result of its accessibility, the ANS has served as a key model system for the elucidation of many principles of neuronal and synaptic function.

ORGANIZATION OF THE VISCERAL CONTROL SYSTEM

The Autonomic Nervous System Has Sympathetic, Parasympathetic, and Enteric Divisions

Output from the central nervous system (CNS) travels along two anatomically and functionally distinct pathways: the **somatic motor neurons**, which innervate striated skeletal muscle, and the **autonomic motor neurons**, which innervate smooth muscle, cardiac muscle, secretory epithelia, and glands. All viscera are richly supplied by efferent axons from the ANS that constantly adjust organ function.

The autonomic (from the Greek for "self-governing," functioning independently of the will) nervous system was first defined by Langley in 1898 as including the local nervous system of the gut and the efferent neurons innervating glands and involuntary muscle. Thus, the original definition of the ANS included only *efferent* neurons and *enteric* neurons. Since that time, it has become clear that it is impossible to separate the efferent ANS from accompanying *afferents*, as well as from those parts of the CNS that control the viscera and other autonomic functions. This *CNS portion* of the ANS monitors autonomic afferents from the viscera and the rest of the body, compares this input with current and anticipated needs, and controls output to the body's organ systems.

The ANS has three divisions: sympathetic, parasympathetic, and enteric. The **sympathetic** and **parasympathetic divisions** of the ANS are the two major efferent pathways controlling targets other than skeletal muscle (Fig. 15–1). Each arises in the CNS, and each innervates target tissue by a two-synapse pathway. The cell bodies of the first neurons lie within the CNS. These **preganglionic neurons** are found in columns of cells in the brain stem and spinal cord and send axons out of the CNS to make synapses with **postganglionic neurons** in peripheral ganglia interposed between the CNS and their target cells. Axons from these postganglionic neurons then project to their targets. The sympathetic and parasympathetic divisions can act independently of each other. However, in general they work synergistically to control visceral activity and often act in opposite ways, like an accelerator and brake to regulate visceral function. An increase in output of the sympathetic division occurs under conditions of stress, anxiety, physical activity, fear, or excitement, whereas parasympathetic output increases during sedentary activity, eating, or other "vegetative" behavior.

The **enteric division** of the ANS is a system of afferent neurons, interneurons, and motor neurons that form networks of neurons called **plexuses** (from the Latin "to braid") that surround the gastrointestinal (GI) tract. It can function as a separate and independent nervous system, but it is normally controlled by the CNS via sympathetic and parasympathetic fibers.

Sympathetic Preganglionic Neurons Originate Between Spinal Cord Segments T1 and L3 and Synapse with Long Postganglionic Neurons in Paravertebral or Prevertebral Ganglia

PREGANGLIONIC NEURONS. The cell bodies of preganglionic sympathetic motor neurons are located in the thoracic and upper lumbar spinal cord between levels T1 and L3. At these spinal levels, autonomic neurons lie in the **intermediolateral cell column**, or lateral horn, between the dorsal and ventral horns (Fig. 15–2). Axons from preganglionic sympathetic neurons exit the spinal cord through the ventral roots, along with axons from *somatic* motor neurons. After entering the spinal nerves, sympathetic efferents diverge from somatic motor axons

FIGURE 15–1. Organization of the sympathetic and parasympathetic divisions of the autonomic nervous system.

to enter the white **rami communicantes**. These rami, or branches, are white because most preganglionic sympathetic axons are myelinated.

PARAVERTEBRAL GANGLIA. Axons from preganglionic neurons enter the nearest sympathetic paravertebral ganglion via a white ramus. These ganglia lie adjacent to the vertebral column. Although preganglionic sympathetic fibers emerge only from levels T1 through L3, the chain of sympathetic ganglia extends all the way from the upper part of the neck to the coccyx, where the left and right sympathetic chains merge in the midline and form the coccygeal ganglion. In general, one ganglion is positioned at the level of each spinal root, but in some cases adjacent ganglia are fused. The most rostral ganglion, the **superior cervical ganglion**, arises from fusion of C1 through C4 and supplies the head and neck. The next two ganglia are the **middle cervical ganglion**, which arises from fusion of C5 and C6, and the **inferior cervical ganglion** (C7 and C8), which is usually fused with the first thoracic ganglion to form the **stellate ganglion**. Together, the middle cervical and stellate ganglia, along with the upper thoracic ganglia, innervate the heart, lungs, and bronchi. The remaining paravertebral ganglia supply organs and portions of the body wall in a segmental fashion.

After entering a paravertebral ganglion, a preganglionic sympathetic axon has one or more of three fates. It may (1) synapse within that segmental paravertebral ganglion, (2) travel up or down the sympathetic chain to synapse within a neighboring paravertebral ganglion, and/or (3) exit its segmental paravertebral ganglion without synapsing and then enter the greater or lesser splanchnic nerve to synapse within one of the ganglia of the *pre*vertebral plexus.

PREVERTEBRAL GANGLIA. The **prevertebral plexus** lies in front of the aorta and along its major arterial branches and includes the prevertebral ganglia and interconnected fibers (Fig. 15–3). The major prevertebral ganglia are named according to the arteries that they are adjacent to and include the celiac, superior mesenteric, aorticorenal, and inferior mesenteric ganglia. Portions of the prevertebral plexus extend down the major arteries and contain other named and unnamed ganglia and plexuses of nerve fibers, altogether making up a dense and extensive network of sympathetic neuron cell bodies and nerve fibers.

Each *pre*ganglionic sympathetic fiber synapses on many

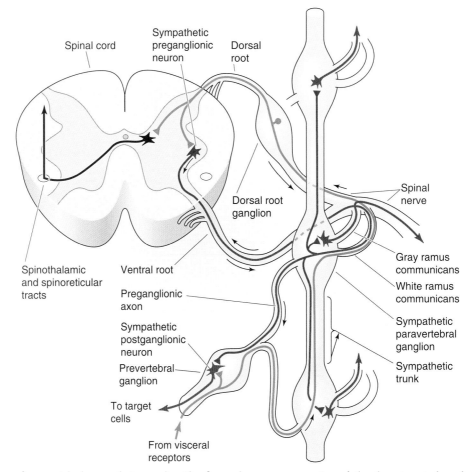

FIGURE 15–2. Anatomy of *paravertebral* sympathetic ganglia. The figure shows a cross section of the thoracic spinal cord and the nearby paravertebral ganglia, as well as a prevertebral ganglion. Sympathetic preganglionic neurons are shown in *red*, and postganglionic neurons in dark *blue-violet*. Afferent (sensory) pathways are in *blue*. Interneurons are shown in *black*.

*post*ganglionic sympathetic neurons that are located within one or several nearby paravertebral or prevertebral ganglia. It has been estimated that each preganglionic sympathetic neuron branches and synapses on as many as 200 postganglionic neurons, thus enabling the sympathetic output to have more widespread effects. However, any impulse arriving at its target end organ has only crossed a single synapse between the preganglionic and postganglionic sympathetic neurons.

POSTGANGLIONIC NEURONS. The cell bodies of postganglionic sympathetic neurons that are located within *para*vertebral ganglia send out their axons via the nearest **gray rami communicantes**, which rejoin the spinal nerves (see Fig. 15–2). These rami are gray because most postganglionic axons are unmyelinated. Because preganglionic sympathetic neurons are located only in the thoracic and upper lumbar spinal segments (T1 through L3), *white* rami are found only at these levels (Fig. 15–4, *left*). However, because *each* sympathetic ganglion sends out postganglionic axons, *gray* rami are present at all spinal levels from C2 or C3 to the coccyx. Postganglionic sympathetic axons from paravertebral and prevertebral ganglia travel to their target organs within other nerves or by traveling along blood vessels to reach their target organ. Because the paravertebral and prevertebral sympathetic

ganglia lie near the spinal cord and thus relatively far from their target organs, the postganglionic axons of the sympathetic division tend to be long. On their way to reach their targets, some postganglionic sympathetic axons travel through *para*sympathetic terminal ganglia or cranial nerve ganglia without synapsing.

Parasympathetic Preganglionic Neurons Originate from the Brain Stem and Sacral Spinal Cord and Synapse with Short Postganglionic Neurons in "Terminal" Ganglia That Are Located Near Target Organs

The cell bodies of preganglionic parasympathetic neurons are located in specific nuclei of the medulla, pons, and midbrain and in the S2 through S4 level of the spinal cord (see Fig. 15–4, *right*). Thus, unlike the sympathetic—or **thoracolumbar**—division, whose preganglionic cell bodies are in the thoracic and lumbar spinal cord, the parasympathetic—or **craniosacral**—division's preganglionic cell bodies are cranial and sacral. The preganglionic parasympathetic fibers originating in the brain distribute with four cranial nerves: the oculomotor nerve (CN III), the facial nerve (CN VII), the glossopharyngeal nerve (CN IX), and the vagus nerve (CN X). The pregan-

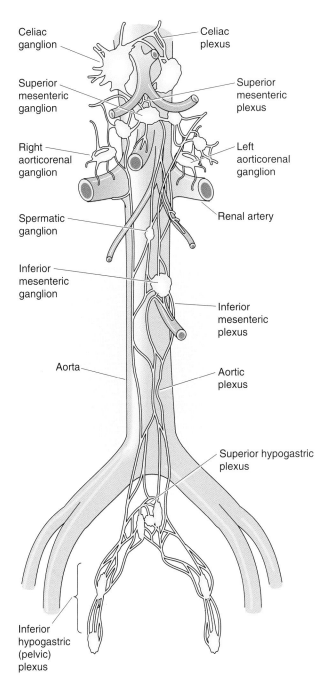

FIGURE 15–3. Anatomy of the *prevertebral* plexus. The ganglia and each associated plexus are named after the artery with which they are associated.

glionic parasympathetic fibers originating in S2 through S4 distribute with the pelvic splanchnic nerves.

Postganglionic parasympathetic neurons are located in **terminal ganglia** that are more peripherally located and more widely distributed than are the sympathetic ganglia. Terminal ganglia often lie within the walls of their target organs. Thus, in contrast to the sympathetic division, postganglionic fibers of the parasympathetic division are short. In some cases, individual postganglionic parasym-

pathetic neurons are found in isolation or in scattered cell groups rather than in encapsulated ganglia.

CRANIAL NERVES III, VII, AND IX. The preganglionic parasympathetic neurons that are distributed with CN III, VII, and IX originate in three groups of nuclei: (1) the **Edinger-Westphal nucleus** is a subnucleus of the oculomotor complex in the mesencephalon (Fig. 15–5). Parasympathetic neurons in this nucleus project to the eye via the **oculomotor nerve** (CN III) and synapse onto postganglionic neurons in the ciliary ganglion (see Fig. 15–4, *right*). The postganglionic fibers supply the pupillary constrictor smooth muscle, as well as the smooth muscle of the ciliary body, which controls the shape of the lens. (2) The *superior* salivary nucleus is in the rostral medulla (see Fig. 15–5) and contains parasympathetic neurons that project, via a branch of the **facial nerve** (CN VII), to the pterygopalatine ganglion (see Fig. 15–4, *right*). The postganglionic fibers supply the lacrimal glands, which produce tears. Another branch of the facial nerve carries preganglionic fibers to the submandibular ganglion. The postganglionic fibers supply two salivary glands, the submandibular and sublingual glands. (3) The *inferior* salivatory nucleus and the rostral part of the **nucleus ambiguus** in the rostral medulla (see Fig. 15–5) contain parasympathetic neurons that project via the **glossopharyngeal nerve** (CN IX) to the otic ganglion (see Fig. 15–4, *right*). The postganglionic fibers supply a third salivary gland, the parotid gland.

CRANIAL NERVE X. Most parasympathetic output occurs via the **vagus nerve** (CN X). Cell bodies of vagal preganglionic parasympathetic neurons are found in the medulla within the **nucleus ambiguus** and the **dorsal motor nucleus of the vagus** (see Fig. 15–5). This nerve supplies parasympathetic innervation to all the viscera of the thorax and abdomen, including the GI tract between the pharynx and distal end of the colon (see Fig. 15–4, *right*). Among other effects, electrical stimulation of the nucleus ambiguus results in activation of striated muscle in the pharynx, larynx, and esophagus and slows the heart. Stimulation of the dorsal motor nucleus of the vagus initiates secretion of gastric acid, insulin, and glucagon. Preganglionic parasympathetic fibers of the vagus nerve join the esophageal, pulmonary, and cardiac plexuses and travel to terminal ganglia that are located within their target organs.

SACRAL NERVES. The cell bodies of preganglionic parasympathetic neurons in the sacral spinal cord (S2 through S4) are located in a position that is similar to that of the preganglionic *sympathetic* neurons—although they do not form a distinct intermediolateral column. Their axons leave via ventral roots and travel with the pelvic splanchnic nerves to their terminal ganglia in the descending colon and rectum (p. 888), as well as the bladder (p. 754) and reproductive organs (pp. 1136 & 1162).

The Visceral Control System Also Has an Important Afferent Limb

All internal organs are densely innervated by visceral afferents. Some of these receptors monitor nociceptive

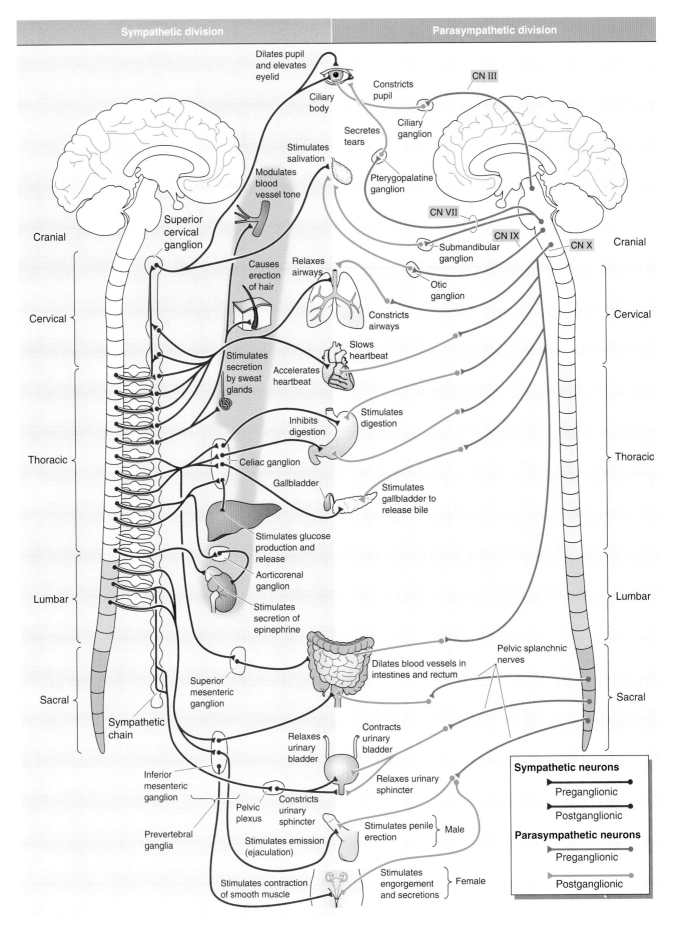

Sympathetic division

Parasympathetic division

Dilates pupil and elevates eyelid

Ciliary body

Constricts pupil

CN III

Ciliary ganglion

Secretes tears

Stimulates salivation

Modulates blood vessel tone

Superior cervical ganglion

Cranial

Pterygopalatine ganglion

CN VII

Submandibular ganglion

CN IX

CN X

Cranial

Causes erection of hair

Relaxes airways

Otic ganglion

Cervical

Cervical

Constricts airways

Stimulates secretion by sweat glands

Slows heartbeat

Accelerates heartbeat

Inhibits digestion

Stimulates digestion

Thoracic

Celiac ganglion

Thoracic

Gallbladder

Stimulates gallbladder to release bile

Stimulates glucose production and release

Aorticorenal ganglion

Stimulates secretion of epinephrine

Lumbar

Lumbar

Sacral

Superior mesenteric ganglion

Sympathetic chain

Dilates blood vessels in intestines and rectum

Pelvic splanchnic nerves

Sacral

Inferior mesenteric ganglion

Relaxes urinary bladder

Contracts urinary bladder

Relaxes urinary sphincter

Prevertebral ganglia

Pelvic plexus

Constricts urinary sphincter

Stimulates penile erection } Male

Stimulates emission (ejaculation)

Stimulates contraction of smooth muscle

Stimulates engorgement and secretions } Female

Sympathetic neurons
Preganglionic
Postganglionic
Parasympathetic neurons
Preganglionic
Postganglionic

FIGURE 15–5. Supraspinal nuclei involved in the autonomic nervous system. Several nuclei in the brain stem participate in the control of the autonomic nervous system (*bold labels*). Some of these nuclei contain the cell bodies of the preganglionic parasympathetic neurons (i.e., efferent). The Edinger-Westphal nucleus contains cell bodies of preganglionic fibers that travel with cranial nerve (CN) III to the ciliary ganglion. The superior salivatory nucleus contains cell bodies of preganglionic fibers that travel with CN VII to the pterygopalatine and submandibular ganglia. The inferior salivatory nucleus contains cell bodies of preganglionic fibers that travel with CN IX to the otic ganglion. The rostral portion of the nucleus ambiguus contains preganglionic cell bodies that distribute with CN IX, whereas the rest of the nucleus ambiguus, as well as the dorsal motor nucleus of the vagus, contain cell bodies of preganglionic fibers that travel with CN X to a host of terminal ganglia in the viscera of the thorax and abdomen. For the sake of completeness, the figure also illustrates other cranial nerves that are not involved in controlling the autonomic nervous system (*gray labels*).

(painful) input. Others are sensitive to a variety of mechanical and chemical ("physiological") stimuli, including stretch of the heart, blood vessels, and hollow viscera, as well as P_{CO_2}, P_{O_2}, pH, blood glucose, and temperature of the skin and internal organs. Many visceral nociceptive fibers travel in sympathetic nerves (*blue* projections in Fig. 15–2). Most axons from physiological receptors travel with parasympathetic fibers. As is the case with somatic afferents (p. 276), the cell bodies of visceral afferent fibers are located within the dorsal root ganglia or cranial nerve ganglia (e.g., nodose and petrosal ganglia). Ninety percent of these visceral afferents are unmyelinated.

The largest concentration of visceral afferent axons can be found in the **vagus nerve**, which carries non-nociceptive afferent input to the CNS from all viscera of the

thorax and abdomen. Most fibers in the vagus nerve are *afferents*, even though all parasympathetic preganglionic output (i.e., *efferents*) to the abdominal and thoracic viscera also travels in the vagus nerve. Vagal afferents, whose cell bodies are located in the nodose ganglion, carry information about the distention of hollow organs (e.g., blood vessels, cardiac chambers, stomach, bronchioles), blood gases (e.g., P_{O_2}, P_{CO_2}, pH), and body chemistry (e.g., glucose concentration) to the medulla.

Internal organs also have nociceptive receptors that are sensitive to excessive stretch and noxious chemical irritants. In the CNS, this visceral pain input is mapped (p. 368) *viscerotopically* at the level of the spinal cord because most visceral nociceptive fibers travel with the sympathetic fibers and enter the spinal cord at a specific segmental level along with a spinal nerve (see Fig. 15–2). This viscerotopic mapping is also present in the brain stem, but not at the level of the cerebral cortex. Thus, awareness of visceral pain is not usually localized to a specific organ but is instead "referred" to the dermatome (p. 277) that is innervated by the same spinal nerve. This **referred pain** results from lack of precision in the central organization of visceral pain pathways. Thus, you know that the pain is associated with a particular spinal nerve, but you do not know where the pain is coming from (i.e., from the skin or a visceral organ). For example, nociceptive input from the left ventricle of the heart is referred to the left T1 to T5 dermatomes and leads to discomfort in the left arm and left side of the chest,

FIGURE 15–4. Organization of the sympathetic and parasympathetic divisions of the autonomic nervous system (ANS). The *left panel* shows the sympathetic division. The cell bodies of sympathetic preganglionic neurons (*red*) are in the intermediolateral column of the thoracic and lumbar spinal cord (T1-L3). Their axons project to paravertebral ganglia (the sympathetic chain) and prevertebral ganglia. Postganglionic neurons (*blue-violet*) therefore have long projections to their targets.

The *right panel* shows the parasympathetic division. The cell bodies of parasympathetic preganglionic neurons (*orange*) are either in the brain (midbrain, pons, medulla) or in the sacral spinal cord (S2-S4). Their axons project to ganglia very near (or even inside) the end organs. Postganglionic neurons (*green*) therefore have short projections to their targets.

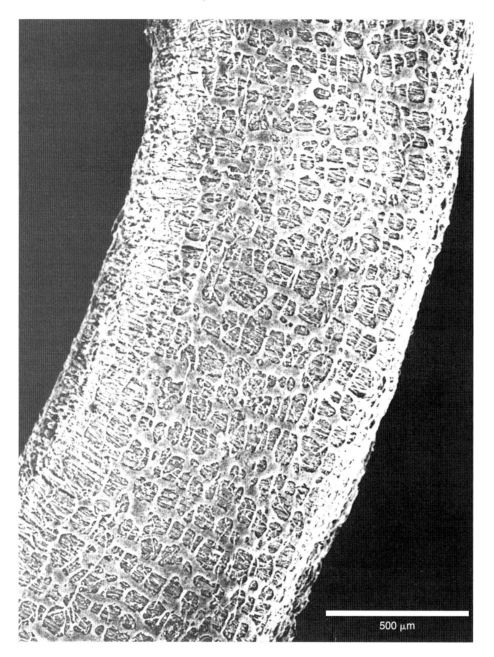

FIGURE 15–6. The myenteric or Auerbach's plexus. The photograph is a scanning electron micrograph of the myenteric plexus of the mouse large intestine. The external longitudinal muscle of the intestine was removed, so that the view is of the plexus (the highly interconnected meshwork on the surface) spreading over the deeper circular layer of muscle. (From Burnstock G: Autonomic neuromuscular junctions: Current developments and future directions. J. Anat 146: 1–30, 1986.)

500 μm

whereas nociceptive input from the diaphragm is referred to the C3 through C5 dermatomes and is interpreted as pain in the shoulder. This visceral pain is often felt as a vague burning or pressure sensation.

The Enteric Division Is a Self-Contained Nervous System That Surrounds the Gastrointestinal Tract and Receives Sympathetic and Parasympathetic Input

The enteric nervous system (ENS) is a collection of nerve plexuses that surround the GI tract, including the pancreas and biliary system. Although it is entirely peripheral, the ENS receives input from the sympathetic and parasympathetic divisions of the ANS. The ENS is estimated to contain over 100 million neurons, including afferent neurons, interneurons, and efferent postganglionic

parasympathetic neurons. Enteric neurons contain many different neurotransmitters and neuromodulators. Thus, not only does the total number of neurons in the enteric division exceed that of the spinal cord, but the neurochemical complexity of the ENS also approaches that of the CNS. The anatomy of the ENS, as well as its role in controlling GI function, is discussed in Chapter 40.

The plexuses of the ENS are a system of ganglia that is sandwiched between the layers of the gut and are connected to each other by a dense meshwork of nerve fibers. The **myenteric,** or Auerbach's, plexus (Fig. 15–6) lies between the external longitudinal and the deeper circular smooth-muscle layers, whereas the **submucosal,** or Meissner's, plexus lies between the circular muscle and the most internal layer of smooth muscle, the muscularis mucosae (see Fig. 40–3A). In the intestinal wall, the myenteric plexus is involved primarily in the control of motility, whereas the submucosal plexus is involved in the control of ion and fluid transport. Both the myenteric and the submucosal plexuses receive *preganglionic parasympathetic* innervation from the vagus nerve (or sacral nerve in the case of the distal portion of colon and rectum). Thus, in one sense, the enteric division is homologous to a large and complex parasympathetic terminal ganglion. The other major input to the ENS is from *postganglionic sympathetic* neurons. Thus, the ENS can be thought of as "postganglionic" with respect to the parasympathetic division and "postpostganglionic" with respect to the sympathetic division. Input from both the sympathetic and parasympathetic divisions modulates the activity of the ENS, but the ENS can by and large function normally without extrinsic input. The isolated ENS can respond appropriately to local stimuli and control many aspects of gut function, including initiating peristaltic activity in response to gastric distention, controlling secretory and absorptive functions, and triggering biliary contractions.

SYNAPTIC PHYSIOLOGY OF THE AUTONOMIC NERVOUS SYSTEM

The Sympathetic and Parasympathetic Divisions Have Opposite Effects on Most Visceral Targets

All innervation of skeletal muscle in humans is excitatory. In contrast, many visceral targets receive both inhibitory and excitatory synapses. These antagonistic synapses arise from the two opposing divisions of the ANS, the sympathetic and the parasympathetic.

In organs that are stimulated during physical activity, the sympathetic division is excitatory and the parasympathetic division is inhibitory. For example, sympathetic input increases the heart rate, whereas parasympathetic input decreases it. In organs whose activity increases while the body is at rest, the opposite is true. For example, the parasympathetic division stimulates peristalsis of the gut, whereas the sympathetic division inhibits it.

Although antagonistic effects of the sympathetic and parasympathetic divisions of the ANS are the general rule for most end organs, exceptions exist. For example, the salivary glands are stimulated by both divisions, although stimulation by the sympathetic division has different characteristics than does parasympathetic stimulation (p. 929).

In addition, some organs receive innervation from only one of these two divisions of the ANS. For example, sweat glands, piloerector muscles, and most peripheral blood vessels receive input from only the sympathetic division.

Synapses of the ANS are specialized for their function. Rather than possessing synaptic terminals that are typical of somatic motor axons, many postganglionic autonomic neurons have bulbous expansions, or **varicosities**, that are distributed along their axons within their target organ (Fig. 15–7). It was once believed that these varicosities indicated that neurotransmitter release sites of the ANS did not form close contact with end organs and that neurotransmitters needed to diffuse long distances across the extracellular space to reach their targets. However, we now recognize that many varicosities form synapses with their targets, with a synaptic cleft extending approximately 50 nm across. At each varicosity, autonomic axons form an "en passant" synapse with their end-organ target. This arrangement results in an increase in the number of targets that a single axonal branch can influence, with wider distribution of autonomic output.

All Preganglionic Neurons—Both Sympathetic and Parasympathetic—Release Acetylcholine and Stimulate N_2 Nicotinic Receptors on Postganglionic Neurons

At their synapses between their postganglionic neurons and target cells, the two major divisions of the ANS use different neurotransmitters and receptors (Table 15–1). However, in both the sympathetic and parasympathetic divisions, synaptic transmission between preganglionic and postganglionic neurons (termed "ganglionic transmission" because the synapse is located in a ganglion) is mediated by **acetylcholine** (ACh) acting on nicotinic receptors (Fig. 15–8). Nicotinic receptors are ligand-gated channels (i.e., ionotropic receptors) with a pentameric structure (p. 213). Table 15–2 summarizes some of the properties of nicotinic receptors. The nicotinic receptors on postganglionic autonomic neurons are a different molecular subtype (N_2) than are those found at the neuromuscular junction (N_1). Both are ligand-gated ion channels that are activated by ACh or nicotine. However, whereas the N_1 receptors at the neuromuscular junction (p. 212) are stimulated by decamethonium and preferentially blocked by D-tubocurarine, the autonomic N_2 recep-

FIGURE 15–7. Synapses of autonomic neurons with their target organs. Varicosities in the axon make multiple points of contact with their targets. Shown is a scanning electron micrograph of the axon of a postganglionic sympathetic neuron from a guinea pig, grown in tissue culture. (From Burnstock G: Autonomic neuromuscular junctions: Current developments and future directions. J. Anat 146: 1–30, 1986.)

TABLE 15–1

PROPERTIES OF THE SYMPATHETIC AND PARASYMPATHETIC DIVISIONS

	SYMPATHETIC PREGANGLIONIC	SYMPATHETIC POSTGANGLIONIC	PARASYMPATHETIC PREGANGLIONIC	PARASYMPATHETIC POSTGANGLIONIC
Location of neuron cell bodies	Intermediolateral cell column in the spinal cord (T1–L3)	Prevertebral and paravertebral ganglia	Brain stem and sacral spinal cord (S2–S4)	Terminal ganglia in or near target organ
Myelination	Yes	No	Yes	No
Primary neurotransmitter	Acetylcholine	Norepinephrine	Acetylcholine	Acetylcholine
Primary postsynaptic receptor	Nicotinic	Adrenergic	Nicotinic	Muscarinic

tors are stimulated by tetramethylammonium, but resistant to D-tubocurarine. When activated, N_1 and N_2 receptors are both permeable to Na^+ and K^+, with entry of Na^+ dominating. Thus, nicotinic transmission triggered by stimulating preganglionic neurons leads to rapid depolarization of postganglionic neurons.

All Postganglionic Parasympathetic Neurons Release Acetylcholine and Stimulate Muscarinic Receptors on Visceral Targets

All postganglionic *para*sympathetic neurons act through muscarinic ACh receptors on the postsynaptic membrane

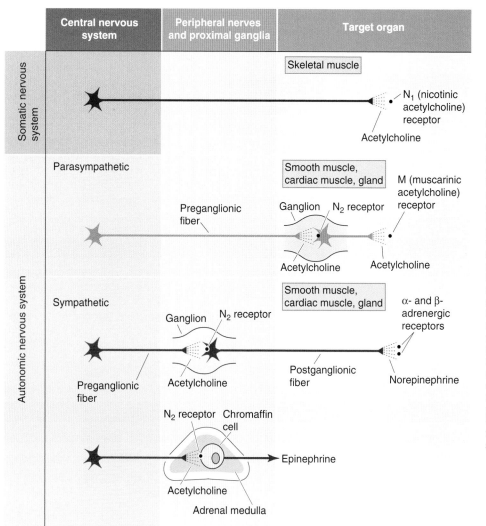

FIGURE 15–8. Major neurotransmitters of the autonomic nervous system. In the case of the **somatic** neuron, the pathway between the central nervous system and effector cell is monosynaptic. The neuron releases acetylcholine (ACh), which binds to N_1-type nicotinic receptors on the postsynaptic membrane (i.e., skeletal muscle cell). In the case of both the parasympathetic and sympathetic divisions, the **preganglionic** neuron releases ACh, which acts at N_2-type nicotinic receptors on the postsynaptic membrane of the postganglionic neuron. In the case of the **postganglionic parasympathetic** neuron, the neurotransmitter is ACh, but the postsynaptic receptor is a muscarinic receptor, which is a metabotropic (i.e., G-protein–linked) receptor of one of five subtypes (M_1–M_5). In the case of most **postganglionic sympathetic** neurons, the neurotransmitter is norepinephrine. The postsynaptic receptor is a metabotropic (i.e., G-protein–linked) adrenergic receptor of one of two major subtypes (α and β).

TABLE 15–2

SIGNALLING PATHWAYS FOR NICOTINIC, MUSCARINIC, AND ADRENERGIC RECEPTORS

RECEPTOR TYPE	AGONISTS*	ANTAGONISTS	G PROTEIN	LINKED ENZYME	2ND MESSENGER
N_1 nicotinic ACh	ACh (nicotine, decamethonium)	D-Tubocurarine, α-Bungaro-toxin	—	—	—
N_2 nicotinic ACh	ACh (nicotine, TMA)	Hexamethonium	—	—	—
$M_1/M_3/M_5$ muscarinic ACh	ACh (muscarine)	Atropine, pirenzepine (M_1)	$G\alpha_q$	PLC	IP_3 and DAG
M_2/M_4 muscarinic ACh	ACh (muscarine)	Atropine, methoctra-mine (M_2)	$G\alpha_i$ and $G\alpha_o$	Adenylyl cyclase	↓ $[cAMP]_i$
α_1-Adrenergic	NE ≥ Epi (phenylephrine)	Phentolamine	$G\alpha_q$	PLC	IP_3 and DAG
α_2-Adrenergic	NE ≥ Epi (clonidine)	Yohimbine	$G\alpha_i$	Adenylyl cylase	↓ $[cAMP]_i$
β_1-Adrenergic	Epi > NE (dobutamine, isoproterenol)	Metoprolol	$G\alpha_s$	Adenylyl cyclase	↑ $[cAMP]_i$
β_2-Adrenergic	Epi > NE (terbutaline, isoproterenol)	Butoxamine	$G\alpha_s$	Adenylyl cyclase	↑ $[cAMP]_i$
β_3-Adrenergic	Epi > NE (isoproterenol)	SR-59230A	$G\alpha_s$	Adenylyl cyclase	↑ $[cAMP]_i$

* Selective agonists are in parentheses.
ACh, acetylcholine; cAMP, cyclic adenosine monophosphate; DAG, diacylglycerol; Epi, epinephrine; IP_3, inositol 1,4,5-triphosphate; NE, norepinephrine; PLC, phospholipase C; TMA, tetramethylammonium.

of the target cell (see Fig. 15–8). Activation of this receptor can either stimulate or inhibit function of the target cell. Cellular responses induced by muscarinic receptor stimulation are more varied than are those induced via nicotinic receptors. Muscarinic receptors are metabotropic receptors that interact with heterotrimeric G proteins (p. 92) to (1) stimulate the hydrolysis of phosphoinositide and thus increase $[Ca^{2+}]_i$ and activate protein kinase C, (2) inhibit adenylyl cyclase and thus decrease cyclic adenosine monophosphate (cAMP) levels, or (3) directly modulate K^+ channels via the G-protein $\beta\gamma$ complex (see Table 15–2). Because they are mediated by second messengers, muscarinic responses, unlike the rapid responses evoked by nicotine receptors, are slow and prolonged.

Muscarinic receptors exist in five different pharmacologic subtypes (M_1 through M_5) that are encoded by five different genes. All five subtypes are highly homologous to each other, but very different from the nicotinic receptors, which are ligand-gated ion channels. Subtypes M_1 through M_5 are each stimulated by ACh and muscarine and are blocked by atropine. Although a wide variety of *antagonists* inhibit the muscarinic receptors, none is completely selective for a specific subtype. However, it is possible to classify a receptor on the basis of its affinity profile for a battery of antagonists. Selective *agonists* for the different isoforms have not been available.

A molecular characteristic of the muscarinic receptors is

that the third cytoplasmic loop (i.e., between the fifth and sixth membrane-spanning segments) is different in M_1, M_3, and M_5 on the one hand and M_2 and M_4 on the other. This loop appears to play a role in coupling of the receptor to the G protein downstream in the signal-transduction cascade. In general M_1, M_3, and M_5 preferentially couple to $G\alpha_q$ and then to phospholipase C, with release of inositol 1,4,5-triphosphate (IP_3) and diacylglycerol (p. 100). On the other hand M_2 and M_4 preferentially couple to $G\alpha_i$ or $G\alpha_o$ to inhibit adenylyl cyclase and thus decrease $[cAMP]_i$ (p. 95).

The five muscarinic subtypes have a heterogeneous distribution among tissues, and this heterogeneity varies among species. Muscarinic receptors are found both presynaptically and postsynaptically throughout the ANS. Many smooth muscles coexpress multiple muscarinic subtypes, each of which may play different roles in neurotransmission. Thus, it is sometimes difficult to predict the effects of applying ACh to a particular tissue.

Most Postganglionic Sympathetic Neurons Release Norepinephrine onto Visceral Targets

Postganglionic sympathetic neurons release **norepinephrine** (see Fig. 15–8), which acts on target cells via adre-

FIGURE 15–9. Muscarinic neurotransmission at ganglionic synapses. *A,* In this experiment, stimulation of the preganglionic sympathetic neuron of a frog releases acetylcholine, which triggers a fast EPSP (due to activation of *nicotinic* receptors on the postganglionic sympathetic neuron), followed by a slow EPSP (due to activation of *muscarinic* receptors on the postsynaptic neuron). EPSP, excitatory postsynaptic potential. (*A,* Data from Adams PR, Brown DA: Synaptic inhibition of the M-current: Slow excitatory post-synaptic potential mechanism in bullfrog sympathetic neurones. J Physiol 332: 263–272, 1982.) *B,* In this experiment on a rat sympathetic postganglionic neuron, the M current (mediated by a K^+ channel) normally hyperpolarizes the neuron, thereby inhibiting the generation of action potentials. Thus, injecting current elicits only a single action potential. *C,* In the same experiment as that in *B,* adding muscarine stimulates a G-protein–linked muscarinic receptor and triggers a signal-transduction cascade that blocks the M current. One result is a steady-state depolarization of the cell. In addition, injecting current now elicits a train of action potentials. (*B* and *C,* Data from Brown DA, Constanti A: Intracellular observations on the effects of muscarinic agonists on rat sympathetic neurones. Br J Pharmacol 70:593–608, 1980.)

nergic receptors. The sympathetic innervation of sweat glands is an exception to this rule. Sweat glands are innervated by sympathetic neurons that release ACh and act via muscarinic receptors (p. 573). The adrenergic receptors are all G-protein–coupled (i.e., metabotropic) receptors and are highly homologous to the muscarinic receptors. Two major types of adrenergic receptor are recognized, α and β, each of which exists in multiple subtypes (e.g., α_1, α_2, β_1, β_2, and β_3). Additionally, there are heterogeneous α_1 and α_2 receptors, with three cloned subtypes of each. Table 15–2 lists the signalling pathways that are generally linked to these receptors. For example, β_1 receptors in the heart activate the G_s heterotrimeric G protein and stimulate adenylyl cyclase, which antagonizes the effects of muscarinic receptors.

Adrenergic receptor subtypes have a tissue-specific distribution. α_1 Receptors predominate on blood vessels, α_2 on presynaptic terminals, β_1 in the heart, β_2 in high concentration in the bronchial muscle of the lungs, and β_3 in fat cells. This distribution has permitted the development of many clinically useful agents that are selective for different subtypes and tissues. For example, α_1 agonists are effective as nasal decongestants, and α_2 antagonists have been used to treat impotence. β_1 Agonists increase cardiac output in congestive heart failure, whereas β_1 antagonists are useful antihypertensive agents. β_2 Agonists are used as bronchodilators in patients with asthma and chronic lung disease.

The adrenal medulla (p. 1061) is a special adaptation of the sympathetic division, homologous to a sympathetic ganglion (see Fig. 15–8). It is innervated by preganglionic sympathetic neurons, and the postsynaptic target cells, which are called **chromaffin cells**, are analogous to postganglionic sympathetic neurons. Thus, chromaffin cells have nicotinic ACh receptors. However, rather than possessing axons that release norepinephrine onto a specific target organ, the chromaffin cells reside near blood vessels and release **epinephrine** into the bloodstream. This neuroendocrine component of sympathetic output enhances the ability of the sympathetic division to broadcast its output throughout the body. Norepinephrine and epinephrine both activate all five subtypes of adrenergic receptor, but with different affinities (see Table 15–2). In general, the α receptors have a greater affinity for norepinephrine, whereas the β receptors have a greater affinity for epinephrine.

Postganglionic Sympathetic and Parasympathetic Neurons Often Have Muscarinic As Well As Nicotinic Receptors

Two additional superimposed layers of complexity are also present in the ANS. First, some postganglionic neurons, both sympathetic and parasympathetic, have *muscarinic* in addition to nicotinic receptors. Second, at all levels of the ANS, certain neurotransmitters and postsynaptic receptors are neither cholinergic nor adrenergic. We will discuss the first exception in this section and the second in the following section.

If we stimulate the release of ACh from preganglionic neurons or apply ACh to the ganglionic synapse, many postganglionic neurons exhibit both nicotinic and muscarinic responses. Because *nicotinic receptors* (N_2) are ligand-gated ion channels, nicotinic neurotransmission causes a fast, monophasic excitatory postsynaptic potential (EPSP). In contrast, because *muscarinic receptors* are G-protein linked, neurotransmission by this route leads to a slower electrical response. Thus, the result is a multiphasic postsynaptic response that, depending on the ganglion, can be a combination of a fast EPSP via a nicotinic receptor plus either a slow EPSP or a slow inhibitory postsynaptic potential (IPSP) via a muscarinic receptor. Figure 15–9*A* is an example of a fast EPSP followed by a slow EPSP.

A well-characterized effect of muscarinic neurotransmission in autonomic ganglia is inhibition of a specific K^+ current called the **M current**. The M current is widely distributed in visceral end organs, autonomic ganglia, and the CNS. In the baseline state, the K^+ channel that underlies the M current is active, thereby producing slight hyperpolarization. In the example shown in Figure 15–9*B*, with the stabilizing M current present, electrical stimulation of the neuron causes only a single spike. If we now add muscarine to the neuron, the stimulated muscarinic receptor turns off the hyperpolarizing M current and thus leads to a small depolarization. If we repeat the electrical stimulation in the continued presence of muscarine (Fig. 15–9*C*), repetitive spikes appear because the absence of the stabilizing influence of the M current increases the excitability of the neuron. Thus, muscarinic receptor activation modulates the repetitive firing properties of this neuron. The slow, modulatory effects of muscarinic responses greatly enhance the ability of the ANS to control visceral activity.

Nonclassic Transmitters Can Be Released at Each Level of the ANS

In the 1930s, Sir Henry Dale first proposed that sympathetic nerves release a transmitter that is similar to epinephrine (now known to be norepinephrine) and parasympathetic nerves release ACh. For many years, attention was focused on these two neurotransmitters, primarily because they mediate large and fast postsynaptic responses that can be easily studied. In addition, a variety of antagonists are available to block cholinergic and adrenergic receptors and thereby permit clear characterization of the roles of these receptors in the control of visceral function. More recently, it has become evident that some neurotransmission in the ANS involves neither adrenergic nor cholinergic pathways. Table 15–3 lists some of the multitude of neurotransmitters used in the ENS. Moreover, many neuronal synapses use more than a single neurotransmitter. Such **cotransmission** is now known to be common in the ANS. As many as eight different neurotransmitters may be found within some neurons, a phenomenon known as **colocalization** (see Table 12–1). Thus, ACh and norepinephrine play important but not exclusive roles in autonomic control.

The distribution and function of nonadrenergic, non-

TABLE 15–3

NEUROTRANSMITTERS AND NEUROMODULATORS PRESENT IN THE ENTERIC NERVOUS SYSTEM

Acetylcholine (ACh)

Norepinephrine (NE)

Serotonin (5-HT)

Dopamine

Tachykinins (substance P, neurokinin A, neuropeptide K, neuropeptide γ)

Nitric oxide (NO)

Adenosine triphosphate (ATP)

Vasoactive intestinal polypeptide (VIP)

γ-Aminobutyric acid (GABA)

Cholecystokinin (CCK)

Galanin

Neuropeptide Y

Somatostatin

Gastrin-releasing peptide (GRP)

Enkephalins

Dynorphin

Calcitonin gene–related peptide (CGRP)

Neurotensin

TABLE 15–4

NEUROTRANSMITTERS PRESENT WITHIN THE AUTONOMIC NERVOUS SYSTEM

SYNAPSE		TRANSMITTERS RELEASED
Presynaptic	**Postsynaptic**	
CNS neurons	Preganglionic autonomic neurons	Glutamate Glycine Substance P Serotonin Norepinephrine TRH Enkephalins Neuropeptide Y Neurotensin Neurophysin II Oxytocin Somatostatin
Preganglionic autonomic neurons	Postganglionic autonomic neurons	Acetylcholine Substance P CGRP
Postganglionic autonomic neurons	Target cell	Norepinephrine Acetylcholine NO ATP Neuropeptide Y Galanin Somatostatin VIP Opioid peptides
Visceral afferents	Neurons in autonomic ganglia or spinal cord	Substance P CGRP
Interneurons	Peripheral autonomic ganglia and ENS	Dopamine Enkephalins

ATP, adenosine triphosphate; CGRP, calcitonin gene–related peptide; CNS, central nervous system; ENS, enteric nervous system; NO, nitric oxide; TRH, thyrotropin-releasing hormone; VIP, vasoactive intestinal peptide.

cholinergic transmitters are only partially understood. However, these transmitters are found at every level of autonomic control (Table 15–4), where they can cause a wide range of postsynaptic responses. These nonclassic transmitters may cause slow synaptic potentials or may modify repetitive firing properties (as in the case of the M current) without having obvious direct effects. In other cases, nonclassic transmitters have no known effects and may be acting in ways that have not been determined.

Although colocalization of neurotransmitters is recognized as a common property of neurons, it is not clear what controls the release of each of the many neurotransmitters. In some cases, the proportion of neurotransmitters released depends on the level of neuronal activity (p. 318). For example, medullary raphe neurons project to the intermediolateral cell column in the spinal cord, where they corelease serotonin, thyrotropin-releasing hormone (TRH), and substance P onto sympathetic preganglionic neurons. The proportions of released neurotransmitters are controlled by neuronal firing frequency; as the firing rate increases, TRH release makes up a higher percentage of the total release. Frequency-dependent modulation of synaptic transmission provides a mechanism for enhancing the versatility of the ANS.

Two of the Most Unusual "Nonclassic" Neurotransmitters, Adenosine Triphosphate and Nitric Oxide, Were First Identified in the Autonomic Nervous System

It was not until the 1970s that a nonadrenergic, noncholinergic class of *sympathetic* or *parasympathetic* neurons was first proposed by Geoffrey Burnstock and colleagues, who suggested that adenosine triphosphate (ATP) might act as the neurotransmitter. This idea, that a molecule used as an intracellular energy substrate could also be a synaptic transmitter, was initially difficult to prove. However, it is now clear that neurons use a variety of classes of molecules for intercellular communication (p. 304). Two of the most surprising examples of nonclassic transmitters, nitric oxide (NO) and ATP, were first identified and studied as neurotransmitters in the ANS, but they are now known to be more widely used throughout the nervous system.

ADENOSINE TRIPHOSPHATE. ATP is colocalized with norepinephrine in postganglionic sympathetic vasoconstrictor neurons. It is contained in synaptic vesicles, is released on electrical stimulation, and induces vascular constriction when applied directly to vascular smooth

Varicosity of sympathetic axon

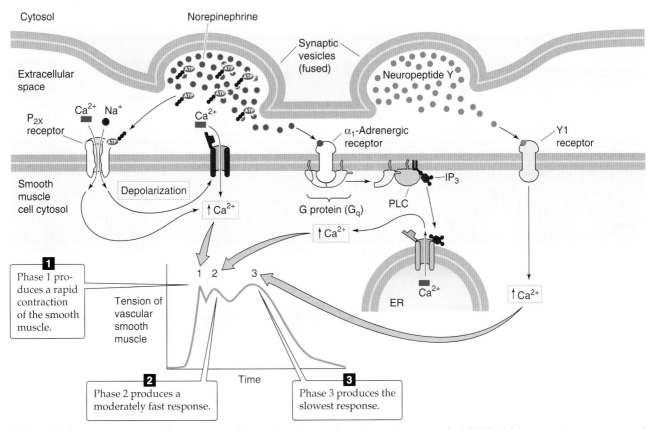

FIGURE 15–10. Cotransmission with adenosine triphosphate (ATP), norepinephrine, and neuropeptide Y (NPY) in the autonomic nervous system. In this example, stimulation of a postganglionic sympathetic neuron causes three phases of contraction of a vascular smooth muscle cell. Each phase corresponds to the release of a different neurotransmitter or group of transmitters. In *phase 1*, ATP binds to a P_{2X} purinoceptor (a ligand-gated cation channel) on the smooth muscle cell, leading to depolarization, activation of voltage-gated Ca^{2+} channels, increased $[Ca^{2+}]_i$, and the rapid phase of contraction. In *phase 2*, norepinephrine binds to an α_1-adrenergic receptor, which—via a G_q/PLC/IP_3 cascade, leads to Ca^{2+} release from internal stores and the second phase of contraction. In *phase 3*, when present, NPY binds to a Y_1 receptor and somehow causes an increase in $[Ca^{2+}]_i$ and thus produces the slowest phase of contraction. ER, endoplasmic reticulum; IP_3 inositol 1,4,5-triphosphate; PLC, phospolipase C.

muscle. The effect of ATP results from activation of P_2 **purinoceptors** on smooth muscle, which include ligand-gated ion channels (P_{2X}) and G-protein–coupled receptors (P_{2Y} and P_{2U}). P_{2X} receptors are present on autonomic neurons and smooth-muscle cells of blood vessels, the urinary bladder, and other visceral targets. P_{2X} receptor channels have a relatively high Ca^{2+} permeability (p. 317). In smooth muscle, depolarization can also activate voltage-gated Ca^{2+} channels (p. 189) and thus lead to an elevation in $[Ca^{2+}]_i$ and a rapid phase of contraction (Fig. 15–10). Norepinephrine, by binding to α_1-adrenergic receptors, acts through a heterotrimeric G protein (p. 92) to facilitate the release of Ca^{2+} from intracellular stores and thereby produce a slower phase of contraction. Finally, the release of neuropeptide Y may, after prolonged and intense stimulation, elicit a third component of contraction.

NITRIC OXIDE. In the 1970s, it was also discovered that the vascular endothelium produces a substance that induces relaxation of vascular smooth muscle. First called endothelium-derived relaxation factor (EDRF), in 1987 it was identified as the free radical NO. **Nitric oxide** is an unusual molecule for intercellular communication because it is a short-lived gas that is produced locally from

L-arginine by the enzyme nitric oxide synthase (NOS; p. 110). Inhibition of NO signalling blocks long-term potentiation in hippocampal brain slices, which has led to speculation that NO acts as a retrograde messenger from postsynaptic neurons to presynaptic terminals during this cellular correlate of learning (p. 324). Similar effects of NO on synaptic strength have also been observed in autonomic neurons, even though learning has not typically been considered an important property of the ANS.

NOS is found in the preganglionic and postganglionic neurons of both the sympathetic and parasympathetic divisions, as well as in vascular endothelial cells. It is not specific for any type of neuron inasmuch as it is found in both norepinephrine- and ACh-containing cells, as well as neurons containing a variety of neuropeptides. Figure 15–11 shows how a parasympathetic neuron may simultaneously release NO, ACh, and vasoactive intestinal peptide, each acting in concert to lower $[Ca^{2+}]_i$ and relax vascular smooth muscle. Why NO is so ubiquitous and when its release is important are not known. However, evidence now indicates that abnormalities of the NO system are involved in the pathophysiology of adult respiratory distress syndrome, high-altitude pulmonary edema, stroke, and other diseases. Understanding its physiological and pathophysiological roles has led to the introduction

FIGURE 15–11. Action of nitric oxide in the autonomic nervous system. Stimulation of a postganglionic parasympathetic neuron can cause more than one phase of relaxation of a vascular smooth muscle cell, corresponding to the release of a different neurotransmitter or group of transmitters. The first phase in this example is mediated by both nitric oxide (NO) and acetylcholine. The neuron releases NO, which diffuses to the smooth muscle cell. In addition, acetylcholine (ACh) binds to M_3 muscarinic receptors (G-protein linked) on endothelial cells, leading to production of NO, which also diffuses to the smooth muscle cell. Both sources of NO raise $[cGMP]_i$ in the smooth muscle cell and contribute to the first phase of relaxation. In the second phase, which tends to occur more with prolonged or intense stimulation, the neuropeptide VIP (or a related peptide) binds to receptors on the smooth muscle cell and causes a delayed relaxation via an increase in $[cAMP]_i$ or a decrease in $[Ca^{2+}]_i$. cGMP, cyclic guanosine monophosphate.

of clinical treatments that modulate the NO system. Examples include the use of NO generators such as nitroglycerin for treating angina, use of the cyclic guanosine monophosphate (cGMP) phosphodiesterase inhibitor sildenafil (Viagra) for treating penile erectile dysfunction, and gaseous NO for treating pulmonary edema.

CNS CONTROL OF THE VISCERA

Sympathetic Output Can Be Massive and Nonspecific, As in the "Fight-or-Flight" Response, or Can Be Selective for Specific Target Organs

In 1915, Walter Cannon proposed that the entire sympathetic division is activated together and has a uniform

effect on all target organs. This effect is in contrast to that of the parasympathetic division, which typically functions in a more discrete, organ-specific, and reflexive manner. In response to fear, exercise, and other types of stress, the sympathetic division produces a massive and coordinated output to all end organs simultaneously, and parasympathetic output ceases. This type of sympathetic output is used to ready the body for life-threatening situations—the so-called "fight-or-flight" response. Thus, when a person is presented a fearful or menacing stimulus, the sympathetic division coordinates all body functions to respond appropriately to the stressful situation. This response includes increases in heart rate, cardiac contractility, blood pressure, and ventilation of the lungs; bronchial dilatation; sweating; piloerection; liberation of glucose into the blood; inhibition of insulin secretion; reduction in blood clotting time; mobilization of blood cells via contraction of the spleen; and decreased GI activity. This mass response is a primitive mechanism for survival. In some people, such a response can be triggered spontaneously or with minimal provocation; each individual episode is then called a "panic attack."

The fight-or-flight response is an important mechanism for survival, but under normal nonstressful conditions, output of the sympathetic division can also be more discrete and organ specific. In contrast to Cannon's original proposal, the sympathetic division does not actually produce uniform effects on all visceral targets. Different postganglionic sympathetic neurons have different electrophysiologic properties and, in addition to norepinephrine, release other neurotransmitters. This specific distribution of neuroactive chemicals among neurons is called "chemical coding." For example, depolarization of guinea pig postganglionic sympathetic neurons in the *lumbar* sympathetic chain ganglia causes a *brief* burst of action potentials in 95% of the neurons and release of norepinephrine together with neuropeptide Y. These neurons are thought to innervate arteries and induce vasoconstriction (see Fig. 15–10). In contrast, depolarization of postganglionic sympathetic neurons in the *inferior mesenteric ganglion* causes sustained firing in 80% of the neurons and release of norepinephrine together with somatostatin. These neurons appear to control gut motility and secretion. Thus, sympathetic neurons have cellular properties that are substantially variable. This variability permits the sympathetic division to produce different effects on targets with different functions, rather than what was originally conceived: that all sympathetic pathways produce uniform output.

A Variety of Brainstem Nuclei, in Addition to Those That Contain Parasympathetic Preganglionic Neurons, Provide Basic Control of the Autonomic Nervous System

In addition to nuclei that contain parasympathetic preganglionic neurons, a variety of other brainstem structures are also involved in visceral control (see Fig. 15–5). These structures include the nucleus tractus solitarius (NTS), ventrolateral medulla, medullary raphe, reticular formation, locus coeruleus, and parabrachial nucleus. These autonomic nuclei within the lower part of the brain stem mediate autonomic reflexes, control specific autonomic functions, or modulate the general level of autonomic tone. In some cases, these nuclei play a well-defined role in one specific autonomic function. For example, stimulation of a group of neurons in the rostral portion of the ventrolateral medulla increases sympathetic output to the cardiovascular system—without affecting respiration or sympathetic output to other targets. In other cases, these nuclei are linked to more than one autonomic function. For example, the medullary raphe contains serotonergic neurons that project to cardiovascular, respiratory, and GI neurons; the reticular activating system; and pain pathways. Therefore, these neurons can affect the background level of autonomic tone. The specific functions of some nuclei are not known, and their involvement in autonomic control is inferred from their anatomic connections, a correlation between spike activity and activity in autonomic nerves, or the effect of lesions.

One of the most important lower brainstem structures is the **nucleus tractus solitarius** in the medulla. The NTS contains second-order sensory neurons that receive all peripheral chemoreceptor (p. 723) and baroreceptor input (p. 535), as well as non-nociceptive afferent input from every organ of the thorax and abdomen. Visceral afferents from the vagus nerve make their first synapse within the NTS, where they combine with other afferent impulses that are derived from the glossopharyngeal (CN IX), facial (CN VII), and trigeminal (CN V) nerves. These visceral afferents form a large bundle of nerve fibers—the *tractus solitarius*—that the NTS surrounds. Afferent input is distributed to the NTS in a viscerotopic manner, with major subnuclei devoted to respiratory, cardiovascular, gustatory, and GI input. The NTS also receives input and sends output to many other CNS regions (Table 15–5), including the brainstem nuclei described earlier, as well as the hypothalamus and the forebrain. These widespread interconnections allow the NTS to influence and be influenced by a wide variety of CNS functions. Thus, the NTS is the major lower brainstem command center for visceral control. It integrates multiple inputs from visceral afferents and exerts control over autonomic output, thereby participating in autonomic reflexes that maintain the homeostasis of many basic visceral functions.

The Forebrain Can Modulate Brainstem Autonomic Nuclei, and Reciprocally, Visceral Afferents Integrated in the Brain Stem Can Influence or Even Overwhelm the Forebrain

Only a subset of the nervous system is necessary for maintaining "autonomic" body homeostasis under most conditions. The necessary structures include: (1) the brainstem nuclei discussed in the previous section, (2) the brainstem nuclei that contain the parasympathetic preganglionic neurons, (3) the spinal cord, and (4) the peripheral ANS. These components are capable of acting autonomously, even without input from higher (i.e., rostral) brain regions. However, such forebrain regions do play a role in coordinating and modulating activity in the lower centers. Many rostral CNS centers project to autonomic nuclei; these centers include the hypothalamus, amygdala, prefrontal cortex, entorhinal cortex, insula, and other forebrain nuclei.

The **hypothalamus**, especially the paraventricular nucleus, is the most important brain region for coordinating autonomic output. The hypothalamus projects to the parabrachial nucleus, medullary raphe, NTS, central gray matter, locus coeruleus, dorsal motor nucleus of the vagus, nucleus ambiguus, and intermediolateral cell column of the spinal cord. Thus, the hypothalamus can initiate and coordinate an integrated response to the body's needs, including modulation of autonomic output, as well as control of neuroendocrine function via the pituitary gland (p. 1010). The hypothalamus coordinates autonomic function with feeding, thermoregulation, circadian rhythms, water balance, emotions, sexual drive, reproduction, motivation, and other brain functions and thus plays a dominant role in the integration of higher cortical and limbic systems with autonomic control.

The hypothalamus often mediates interactions between

TABLE 15–5

CONNECTIONS TO/FROM THE NUCLEUS TRACTUS SOLITARIUS

Receives Input from

Vagus n. (peripheral chemoreceptor/aortic bodies and aortic baroreceptor, as well as non-nociceptive afferent input from every organ of the thorax and abdomen)

Glossopharyngeal n. (taste and peripheral chemoreceptors/carotid bodies, carotid baroreceptor)

Facial n. (taste)

Trigeminal n. (teeth, sinuses)

Ventrolateral medulla

Medullary raphe

Area postrema

Periaqueductal gray

Parabrachial nucleus

Hypothalamus

Cerebral cortex

Sends Output to

Intermediolateral cell column (preganglionic sympathetic neurons) and sacral parasympathetic neurons

Phrenic motor nucleus and other respiratory output pathways

Dorsal motor nucleus of the vagus (preganglionic parasympathetic neurons from the vagus nerve)

Nucleus ambiguus (preganglionic parasympathetic neurons from the vagus nerve)

Ventrolateral medulla

Medullary raphe

Area postrema

Parabrachial nuclei

Reticular formation

Forebrain nuclei

Hypothalamus

the forebrain and the brain stem. However, a number of forebrain regions also have direct connections to brainstem autonomic nuclei. Most of these forebrain regions are part of the **limbic system** rather than the neocortex. The paucity of direct neocortical connections probably explains why individuals trained to control autonomic output by biofeedback can generally produce only relatively minor effects on overall autonomic activity rather than regulate output to specific organs. Most individuals are incapable of even limited cortical control over the ANS. However, even though we may have only minimal *conscious* control of autonomic output, cortical processes can strongly modulate the ANS. Emotions, mood, anxiety, stress, and fear can all alter autonomic output (Table 15–6A). The pathways for these effects are unknown, but they could be mediated by direct connections or via the hypothalamus.

Not only does forebrain function influence the ANS, autonomic activity also influences forebrain function. Visceral afferents reach the neocortex. However, because these afferents are not well represented viscerotopically, they cannot be well localized. Nevertheless, visceral afferents can have profound effects on cortical function. Visceral input can modulate the excitability of cortical neurons (see the box titled Vagus Nerve Stimulation in the Treatment of Epilepsy) and, in some cases, can result in such overpowering sensory stimuli that it is not possible to focus cortical activity on any other purpose (see Table 15–6B).

CNS Control Centers Oversee Visceral Feedback Loops and Orchestrate a Feedforward Response to Meet Anticipated Needs

The ANS maintains physiological parameters within an optimal range by means of **feedback loops** made up of sensors, afferent fibers, central autonomic control centers (discussed in the previous section), and effector systems.

TABLE 15–6

INTERACTIONS BETWEEN CORTICAL AND AUTONOMIC FUNCTION

A. Examples of Descending Cortical Control of Autonomic Output

Fear—initiates fight-or-flight response

Panic attacks—initiate spontaneous fight-or-flight response

Emotional stress (e.g., first day in gross anatomy lab) or painful stimuli—lead to massive vasodilation and hypotension, i.e., vasovagal syncope (fainting)

Cortical seizures—can induce sudden cardiac death from massive sympathetic output and arrhythmias

Chronic stress—can lead to peptic ulcers from increased gastric acid secretion

Sleep deprivation—in rats leads to death from loss of thermoregulation and cardiovascular control

Cognitive activity—can initiate sexual arousal

Nervousness, such as before an exam—can lead to diarrhea

B. Examples in Which Visceral Afferents Overwhelm Cortical Function (i.e., Nothing Else Seems to Matter)

Hunger

Nausea

Dyspnea

Visceral pain

Bladder and bowel distention

Hypothermia/hyperthermia

VAGUS NERVE STIMULATION IN THE TREATMENT OF EPILEPSY

It is often not appreciated just how much effect the autonomic nervous system can have on cortical function. Table 15–6B lists several examples in which strong input from visceral afferents can overwhelm cortical function, to the point that concentrating on anything else is nearly impossible. As we have already noted, not only does the vagus nerve contain parasympathetic preganglionic *motor* fibers, it also contains a wide variety of *sensory* fibers from viscera in the thorax and abdomen. Discovery of the influence of vagal afferent input on seizures has led to development of the vagus nerve stimulator, which is used clinically. The surgically implanted stimulator electrically triggers the vagus nerve for 30 seconds every 5 minutes, 24 hours per day. Additionally, when patients feel a seizure coming on (an aura), they can activate the device with a hand-held magnet to deliver extra pulses. Clinical studies have shown that this treatment reduces the number of seizures by about half in about one in four patients. It remains to be determined whether a subgroup of patients may be particularly responsive to this treatment. Side effects include hoarseness, coughing, and breathlessness. That this approach works at all indicates how important visceral input is to cortical function. Vagal input to the nucleus tractus solitarius can influence many rostral brain structures, but is not yet clear whether stimulation of peripheral chemoreceptor afferents, pulmonary afferents, or other visceral afferent pathways is important for the anticonvulsant effect. If the specific pathways could be identified, it might be possible to selectively stimulate these pathways or activate them pharmacologically to produce an anticonvulsant effect with fewer side effects.

These feedback loops achieve homeostasis by monitoring input from visceral receptors and adjusting the output of both the sympathetic and parasympathetic divisions to specific organs so that they maintain activity at a set-point that is determined by involuntary CNS control centers. As we have already noted, the sympathetic and parasympathetic divisions usually act in opposite ways to make these adjustments. Blood pressure control is an example of a visceral feedback loop in which the CNS monitors current blood pressure via afferents from baroreceptors, compares it with an internally determined set-point, and appropriately adjusts output to the heart, blood vessels, adrenal gland and other targets. An increase in blood pressure (p. 536) causes a reflex decrease in sympathetic output to the heart and an increase in parasympathetic output.

Instead of merely responding via feedback loops, the ANS also anticipates the future needs of the individual. For example, when a person begins to exercise, sympathetic output increases before the increase in metabolic need to prevent an exercise debt from occurring (p. 1249). Because of this anticipatory response, alveolar ventilation rises to such an extent that blood levels of CO_2 (a

byproduct of exercise) can actually drop at the onset of exercise. This response is the opposite of what would be expected if the ANS worked purely via feedback loops because one would then predict that an increase in respiratory output would be driven by an obligatory increase in CO_2 levels (p. 723). Similarly, a trained athlete's heart rate begins to increase several seconds before the starting gun fires to signal the beginning of a 100-m dash. This anticipation of future activity, or **feedforward** stimulation during exercise, is a key component of the regulation of homeostasis during stress because it prevents large changes in physiological parameters that could be detrimental to optimal function. This type of response probably resulted in an evolutionary advantage that permitted the body to respond rapidly and more efficiently to a threat of danger. A system relying solely on feedback could produce a response that is delayed or out of phase with respect to the stimulus. The central neuronal pathways responsible for this anticipatory or feedforward response are not known.

The Autonomic Nervous System Has Multiple Levels of Reflex Loops

The human nervous system is built in a hierarchy that mirrors phylogenetic evolution (p. 273). Each of the successively more primitive components is capable of independent, organized, and adaptive behavior. In turn, the activity of each of the more primitive levels is modulated by more rostral, more phylogenetically advanced components (Fig. 15–12).

The **enteric nervous system** of humans is homologous to the most primitive nervous system, the neural net of jellyfish. In both cases, the component neurons control motility and nutrient absorption and respond appropriately to external stimuli.

The **autonomic ganglia** are homologous to ganglionic nervous systems, such as those of annelid worms. Autonomic ganglia were previously considered a simple relay station for signals from the CNS to the periphery, but it is now clear that they integrate afferent input from the viscera and have substantial independent control mechanisms. The largest of the sympathetic ganglia, the superior cervical ganglion, contains about 1 million neurons. In addition to postganglionic cell bodies, autonomic ganglia also contain interneurons. Axons from interneurons, sensory receptors located in the end organs, and preganglionic neurons converge with postganglionic neuron dendrites to form a dense network of nerve fibers, or a **neuropil**, within the ganglion. This neuropil confers considerable computational capability on the ganglia. As opposed to feedback from skeletal muscle, which only occurs in the CNS, the peripheral synapses of visceral afferents result in substantial integration of autonomic activity at peripheral sites. This integration is enhanced by the variety of neurotransmitters present. Thus, although fast neurotransmission from preganglionic neurons to postganglionic neurons is an important role of the autonomic ganglia, the ganglia are not simply relays.

The **spinal cord,** which coordinates activity among different root levels, first appeared with the evolution of chordates. The CNS of *Amphioxus*, a primitive chordate, is

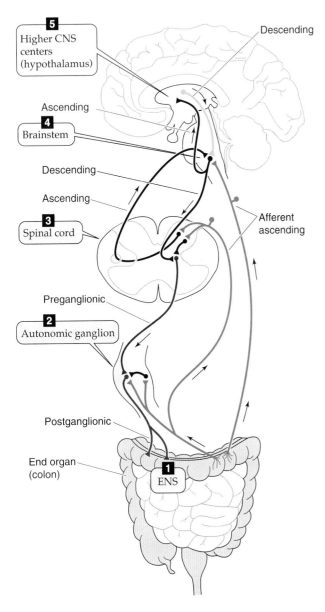

FIGURE 15–12. Hierarchical reflex loops in the autonomic nervous system. CNS, central nervous system; ENS, enteric nervous system.

CROSSTALK BETWEEN AUTONOMIC FUNCTIONS CAN BE PATHOLOGIC

Visceral control of each of the body's organs occurs relatively independently of the others. However, some overlap in control systems can be noted for different components of the ANS. For example, stimulating the baroreceptors causes inhibition of respiration. Conversely, the decrease in thoracic pressure that occurs during inspiration normally triggers a reflex decrease in heart rate. Many neurons in the brain stem and spinal cord have a firing pattern that is modulated in time with both the heartbeat and respiratory activity. This spillover may be responsible for the frequent observation of **sinus arrhythmia** on electrocardiograms of normal patients, whereby the heart rate is irregular because of an exaggeration of the normal influence of respiration on heart rate. These phenomena have no clear evolutionary advantage. Instead, they may simply be due to an error in separating closely related physiological control mechanisms.

In some cases, overlap between physiological control mechanisms can have serious consequences. For example, control of micturition overlaps with cardiorespiratory control. An increase in bladder pressure can lead to apnea and hypertension. Conversely, each breath is accompanied by an increase in neural outflow to the bladder. In patients with obstruction of urinary outflow, as can be seen in men with enlarged prostates, the bladder can become severely distended. If this obstruction is relieved suddenly by inserting a catheter and the bladder is drained too rapidly, blood pressure can drop precipitously. In extreme cases, the hypotension causes syncope (fainting) or a stroke. A similar phenomenon can occur in some people with less provocation. While emptying a relatively full bladder, blood pressure can drop precipitously and lead to **postmicturition syncope,** with the patient suddenly falling unconscious on the bathroom floor.

---

essentially just a spinal cord. In humans who suffer transsection of the low cervical spinal cord—and in whom the outflow of the respiratory system is spared (see Chapter 31)—the caudal spinal cord and lower autonomic ganglia can still continue to maintain homeostasis. However, these individuals are incapable of more complex responses that require reflexes that are mediated by the cranial nerve afferents and cranial parasympathetic outflow. In many patients, this situation can lead to maladaptive reflexes such as autonomic hyper-reflexia, where a full bladder results in hypertension and sweating (see the box on pathologic crosstalk).

All vertebrates have a brain that is segmented into three parts (p. 264), the prosencephalon, mesencephalon, and rhombencephalon. With evolution, the more rostral parts took on a more dominant role. The brain of the ammocoete larva of the lamprey is dominated by the **medulla,** which is also the most vital part of the human brain—in contrast to more rostral structures, destroying the medulla leads to instant death. The medulla coordinates all visceral control and optimizes it for survival. In humans, normal body homeostasis can continue indefinitely with only a medulla, spinal cord, and peripheral ANS.

In fish, the **midbrain** became the dominant CNS structure in response to the increasing importance of vision. The brain of primitive reptiles is only a brain stem and paleocortex, without a neocortex; the corpus striatum is the dominant structure. Thus, the brain stem is sometimes referred to as the "reptilian brain." Finally, the **neocortex** appeared in mammals and became dominant. The phylogenetically advanced portions of the CNS rostral to the medulla—including the hypothalamus, limbic system, and cortex—coordinate activity of the ANS with complex behaviors, motivations, and desires, but they are not required for normal homeostasis.

As a result of this hierarchy, impulses from most vis-

HORNER SYNDROME

One of the keys to neurologic diagnosis has always been neuroanatomic localization (Fig. 15–13). A classic condition in which defining neuroanatomy is important is **Horner syndrome:** the combination of unilateral **ptosis** (drooping eyelid), **miosis** (small pupil), and **anhidrosis** (lack of sweating). Sympathetic neurons innervate the smooth muscle that elevates the eyelid, the pupillary dilator muscle, and the sweat glands of the face. Horner syndrome results from loss of the normal sympathetic innervation on one side of the face. The differential diagnosis of this syndrome is large, but it can be narrowed if the site of involvement of the sympathetic pathways can be identified. Involvement of *first-order sympathetic neurons* can occur at their cell bodies in the hypothalamus or along their axons traveling down to the ipsilateral intermediolateral column of the spinal cord. Thus a first-order Horner syndrome can be due to ischemia of the lateral medulla (e.g., occlusion of the posterior inferior cerebellar artery, the so-called Wallenberg syndrome). In this case, other brainstem abnormalities will also be present. The *second-order sympathetic neurons,* or *pre*ganglionic neurons, can be affected at their origin in the intermediolateral column or along their axons. Those that supply the eye synapse in the superior cervical ganglion. A second-order Horner syndrome can be the first sign that a Pancoast tumor exists in the apex of the lung and is encroaching on the sympathetic nerves as they travel to the superior cervical ganglion. Finally, *third-order sympathetic neurons,* or *post*ganglionic neurons, can be involved at the ganglion or along their course to the eye. Because they travel within the wall of the carotid artery, these sympathetic nerves can be damaged during a carotid artery "dissection". Dissection is damage to the wall of the artery, often caused by a neck injury. In time, the damage to the vessel can lead to a blood clot that will obstruct blood flow. Thus a Horner syndrome can be a warning that without treatment, a stroke may be imminent. The key to proper diagnosis is to determine what nearby structures may be involved (the company that it keeps). Two pharmacologic tests can also be administered. A dilute 2% to 10% cocaine solution blocks norepinephrine re-uptake into the synaptic terminals so that the buildup of norepinephrine near the pupil dilator muscle will dilate the pupil in a healthy person. Cocaine treatment will have no effect on the pupil if the lesion involves the postganglionic neurons because the presynaptic terminals are absent. A sufficiently dilute (1 : 1000) norepinephrine solution will not affect a normal pupil, but it will dilate a pupil that has lost its postganglionic innervation because denervation causes supersensitivity of the pupillary dilator muscle. A combination of a careful neurologic examination with these tests will usually allow one to determine where in the sympathetic pathways damage has occurred, thus narrowing the differential diagnosis.

FIGURE 15–13. Anatomy of the innervation to the pupil—Horner syndrome. Cartoon showing pathways from (1) the hypothalamus to the intermediolateral (IML) column in the spinal cord (first-order neuron). (2) A preganglionic sympathetic neuron with the cell body in the intermediolateral column gets a synapse from (1) and sends an axon to the superior cervical ganglion (SCG). (3) A postganglionic sympathetic neuron with the cell body in the SCG sends axons to pupillary dilator (smooth) muscles.

ceral afferents never reach the cortex, and we are not usually conscious of them. Instead, they make synapses within the enteric plexuses, autonomic ganglia, spinal cord, and brain stem, and they close reflex loops that regulate visceral output at each of these levels.

REFERENCES

Books and Reviews

Andresen MC, Kunze DL: Nucleus tractus solitarius—gateway to neural circulatory control. Annu Rev Physiol 56:93–116, 1994.

Bennett MR: Transmission at sympathetic varicosities. News Physiol Sci 13:79–84, 1998.

Caulfield MP, Birdsall NJ: International Union of Pharmacology. XVII. Classification of muscarinic acetylcholine receptors. Pharmacol Rev 50: 279–290, 1998.

Janig W, McLachlan E: Characteristics of function-specific pathways in the sympathetic nervous system. Trends Neurosci 15:475–481, 1992.

Lundberg JM: Pharmacology of cotransmission in the autonomic nervous system: Integrative aspects on amines, neuropeptides, adenosine triphosphate, amino acids and nitric oxide. Pharmacol Rev 48:113–178, 1996.

Journal Articles

Evans RJ, Derkach V, Surprenant A: ATP mediates fast synaptic transmission in mammalian neurons. Nature 357:503–505, 1992.

Furchgott RF, Zawadzki JV: The obligatory role of endothelial cells in the relaxation of arterial smooth muscle by acetylcholine. Nature 288:373–376, 1980.

Jansen ASP, van Nguyen X, Karpitskiy V, et al: Central command neurons of the sympathetic nervous system: Basis of the fight-or-flight response. Science 270:644–646, 1995.

Kawasaki J, Kobayashi S, Miyagi Y, et al: The mechanisms of the relaxation induced by vasoactive intestinal peptide in the porcine coronary artery. Br J Pharmacol 121:977–985, 1997.

Palmer RMJ, Ferrige AG, Moncada S: Nitric oxide release accounts for the biological activity of endothelium-derived relaxing factor. Nature 327:524–526, 1987.

CHAPTER 16

The Neuronal Microenvironment

Bruce R. Ransom

Extracellular Fluid in the Brain Provides a Highly Regulated Environment for Central Nervous System Neurons

Everything that surrounds individual neurons can be considered part of the **neuronal microenvironment**. Technically, therefore, the neuronal microenvironment includes the extracellular fluid (ECF), capillaries, glial cells, and adjacent neurons. Although the term often is restricted to just the immediate ECF, the ECF cannot be meaningfully discussed in isolation because of its extensive interaction with brain capillaries, glial cells, and cerebrospinal fluid (CSF). How the microenvironment interacts with neurons and how the brain (used here synonomously with CNS) stabilizes it to provide constancy for neuronal function are the subjects of this discussion.

The concentrations of solutes in **brain extracellular fluid** (BECF) fluctuate with neural activity, and conversely, changes in extracellular fluid composition can influence nerve cell behavior. Not surprisingly, therefore, the brain carefully controls the composition of this important compartment. It does so in three major ways. First, the brain uses the blood-brain barrier (BBB) to protect the BECF from fluctuations in blood composition. Second, the CSF, which is synthesized by choroid-plexus epithelial cells, strongly influences the composition of the BECF. Third, the surrounding glial cells "condition" the BECF.

The Brain Is Physically and Metabolically Fragile and Must Be Protected

The ratio of brain weight to body weight in humans is the highest in the animal kingdom. The average adult male brain weighs approximately 1400 g; the average woman's brain weighs approximately 1300 g. This large and vital structure, which has the consistency of thick pudding, is protected from mechanical injury by a surrounding layer of bone and by the CSF in which it floats.

The brain is also *metabolically* fragile. This fragility arises from its high rate of energy consumption, absence of significant stored fuel in the form of glycogen (~10% of the amount in the liver), and the rapid development of cellular damage when adenosine triphosphate (ATP) is depleted. However, the brain is not the greediest of the body's organs; both the heart and kidney cortex have higher metabolic rates. Nevertheless, although it constitutes only 2% of the body by weight, the brain receives approximately 15% of resting blood flow and accounts for about 20% and 50%, respectively, of total resting O_2 and glucose utilization. The brain's high metabolic demands arise from the need of its neurons to maintain the steep ion gradients on which neuronal excitability depends. Neuroglial cells, the other major cells in the brain, also maintain steep transmembrane ion gradients. More than half of the energy consumed by the brain is directed to maintain ion gradients, primarily through operation of the Na-K pump (p. 61). An interruption of the continuous supply of oxygen or glucose to the brain results in rapid depletion of energy stores and disruption of ion gradients. Because of falling ATP levels in the brain, consciousness is lost within 10 seconds of a blockade in cerebral blood flow. Irreversible nerve cell injury can occur after only 5 minutes of interrupted blood flow.

CEREBROSPINAL FLUID

CSF is a colorless, watery liquid. It fills the ventricles of the brain and forms a thin layer around the outside of the brain and spinal cord in the subarachnoid space. CSF is secreted within the brain by a highly vascularized epithelial structure called the **choroid plexus** and circulates to sites in the subarachnoid space where it enters the venous blood system. The composition of CSF is highly regulated and, because CSF is in slow diffusional equilibrium with BECF, helps regulate the composition of BECF. The choroid plexus can be thought of as the brain's "kidney" in that it stabilizes the composition of CSF, just as the kidney stabilizes the composition of blood plasma.

CSF Fills the Ventricles and Subarachnoid Space

The **ventricles** of the brain are four small compartments located within the brain (Fig. 16–1A). Each ventricle contains a choroid plexus and is filled with CSF. The ventricles are linked together by channels, or foramina, that allow CSF to move easily between them. The two **lateral ventricles** are the largest and are symmetrically located within the cerebral hemispheres. The choroid plexus of each lateral ventricle is located along the inner radius of this horseshoe-shaped structure (see Fig. 16–1B). The two lateral ventricles each communicate with the **third ventricle**, which is located in the midline between the thalami, via the two interventricular **foramina of Monro**. The choroid plexus of the third ventricle lies along the ventricle roof. The third ventricle communicates with the fourth ventricle by the **cerebral aqueduct of Sylvius**. The **fourth ventricle** is the most caudal ventricle and is located in the brain stem. It is bounded by the cerebellum superiorly and by the pons and medulla inferiorly. The choroid plexus of the fourth ventricle lies along only a portion of this ventricle's tent-shaped roof. The fourth ventricle is continuous with the central canal of the spinal cord. CSF escapes from the fourth ventricle and flows into the subarachnoid space via three foramina: the two laterally placed **foramina of Luschka** and the midline opening in the roof of the fourth ventricle, called the **foramen of Magendie**. We shall see later how CSF circulates throughout the subarachnoid space of the brain and spinal cord.

The brain and spinal cord are covered by two membra-

nous tissue layers called the **leptomeninges**, which are in turn surrounded by a third, tougher layer. The innermost of these three layers is the pia mater; the middle is the arachnoid mater (or arachnoid membrane); and the outermost layer is the dura mater (Fig. 16–2). Between the arachnoid mater and pia mater (i.e., the leptomeninges) is the **subarachnoid space**, which is filled with CSF that escaped from the fourth ventricle. The CSF in the subarachnoid space completely surrounds the brain and spinal cord. In adults, the subarachnoid space plus the ventricles with which they are continuous contain approximately 150 ml of CSF, 30 ml in the ventricles and 120 ml in the subarachnoid spaces of the brain and spinal cord.

The **pia mater** (Latin for "tender mother") is a thin layer of connective tissue cells that is very closely applied to the surface of the brain and covers blood vessels as they plunge through the arachnoid into the brain. A nearly complete layer of astrocytic endfeet—the *glia limitans*—abuts the pia from the brain side and is separated from the pia by a basement membrane. The pia adheres so tightly to the associated glia limitans in some areas that they seem to be continuous with each other; this combined structure is sometimes called the pial-glial membrane or layer. This layer does *not* restrict diffusion of substances between the BECF and the CSF.

The **arachnoid membrane** (Greek for "cobweb-like") is composed of layers of cells, resembling those that make up the pia, that are linked together by *tight junctions*. The arachnoid isolates the CSF in the subarachnoid space from blood in the overlying vessels of the dura mater. The cells that constitute the arachnoid and the pia are continuous in the trabeculae that span the subarachnoid space. These arachnoid and pial layers are relatively avascular; thus, the leptomeningeal cells that form them probably derive nutrition from the CSF that they enclose, as well as the extracellular fluid that surrounds them. The leptomeningeal cells can phagocytize foreign material in the subarachnoid space.

The **dura mater** is a thick, inelastic membrane that forms an outer protective envelope around the brain. The dura has two layers that split to form the intracranial venous sinuses. Blood vessels in the dura mater are outside the BBB (see later), and substances could easily diffuse from dural capillaries into the nearby CSF if it were not for the blood-CSF barrier created by the arachnoid.

The Brain Floats in CSF, Which Acts As a Shock Absorber

An important function of CSF is to buffer the brain from mechanical injury. The CSF that surrounds the brain reduces the practical weight of the brain to less than 50 g (normal weight, ~1400 g). This buoyancy is a consequence of the difference in the specific gravities of brain tissue (1.040) and CSF (1.007). The mechanical buffering that the CSF provides greatly diminishes the risk of acceleration-deceleration injuries in the same way that wearing a bicycle helmet reduces the risk of head injury. As you strike a tree, the foam insulation of the helmet gradually compresses and reduces the velocity of your head. Thus, the deceleration of your head is not nearly as severe as

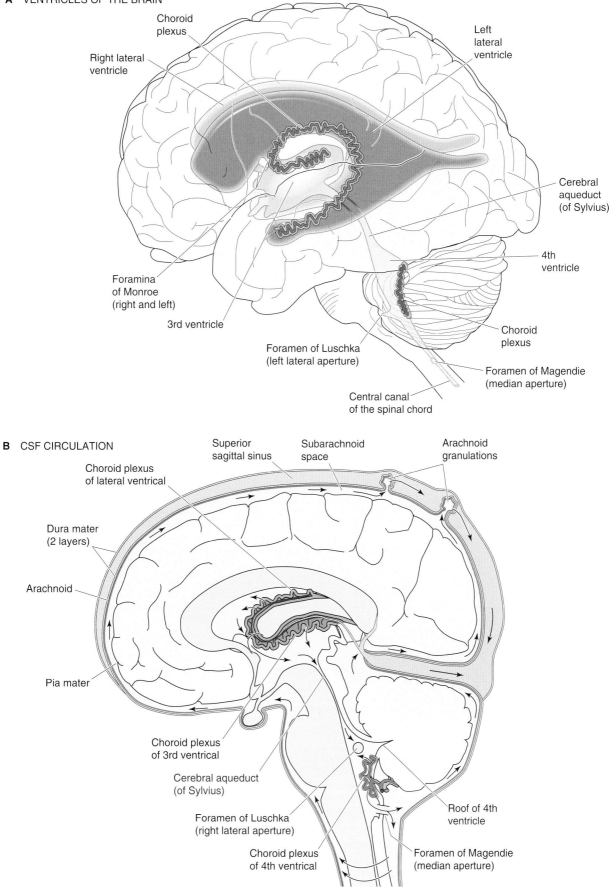

A VENTRICLES OF THE BRAIN

Choroid plexus

Right lateral ventricle

Left lateral ventricle

Cerebral aqueduct (of Sylvius)

4th ventricle

Choroid plexus

Foramina of Monroe (right and left)

3rd ventricle

Foramen of Luschka (left lateral aperture)

Foramen of Magendie (median aperture)

Central canal of the spinal chord

B CSF CIRCULATION

Superior sagittal sinus

Subarachnoid space

Arachnoid granulations

Choroid plexus of lateral ventrical

Dura mater (2 layers)

Arachnoid

Pia mater

Choroid plexus of 3rd ventrical

Cerebral aqueduct (of Sylvius)

Foramen of Luschka (right lateral aperture)

Choroid plexus of 4th ventrical

Roof of 4th ventricle

Foramen of Magendie (median aperture)

FIGURE 16–1. The brain ventricles and the cerebrospinal fluid. *A,* This is a transparent view, looking from the left side of the brain. The two lateral ventricles communicate with the third ventricle, which in turn communicates with the fourth ventricle. *B,* Each ventricle contains a choroid plexus, which secretes cerebrospinal fluid (CSF). The CSF escapes from the fourth ventricle and into the subarachnoid space via the two lateral foramina of Luschka and the single foramen of Magendie.

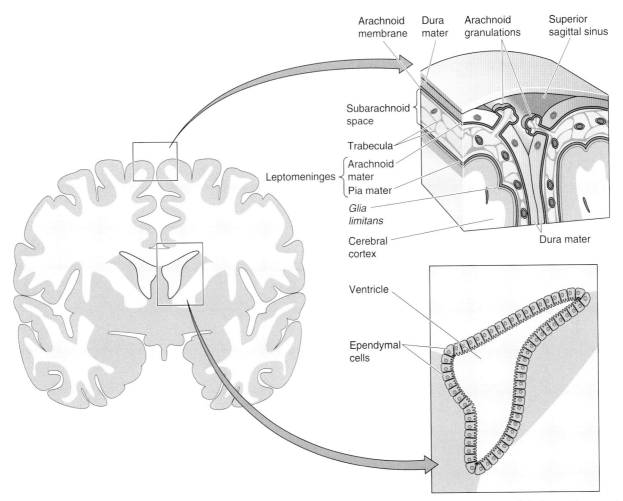

FIGURE 16–2. The meninges and ependymal cells. The figure represents a coronal section through the anterior portion of the brain. The *upper inset* shows the three layers of meninges: (1) the dura mater, which here is split into two layers to accommodate the superior sagittal sinus (filled with venous blood); (2) the arachnoid mater, which is formed by cells that are interconnected by tight junctions; and (3) the pia mater, which closely adheres to a layer that is composed of astrocyte endfeet that are covered by a basement membrane (*glia limitans*). The *lower inset* shows ependymal cells lining the interior of the frontal horn of the left ventricle. Both the subarachnoid space and the cavities of the ventricles are filled with cerebrospinal fluid.

the deceleration of the outer shell of your helmet. The importance of this fluid suspension system is underscored by the consequences of reduced CSF pressure, which sometimes happens transiently after the diagnostic procedure of removing CSF from the spinal subarachnoid space (see the box titled Lumbar Puncture). Patients with reduced CSF pressure experience severe pain when they try to sit up or stand, because the brain is no longer cushioned by shock-absorbing fluid and small gravity-induced movements put strain on pain-sensitive structures. Fortunately, the CSF leak that can result from lumbar puncture is only temporary; the puncture hole easily heals itself, with prompt resolution of all symptoms.

The Choroid Plexuses Secrete CSF into the Ventricles

Most of the CSF is produced by the **choroid plexuses**, which are present in four locations (see Fig. 16–1): the two lateral ventricles, the third ventricle, and the fourth

ventricle. The capillaries within the brain appear to form a small amount of CSF. Total CSF production is about 500 ml/day. Therefore, the entire volume of CSF, about 150 ml, is replaced or "turns over" about three times each day.

Secretion of new CSF creates a slight pressure gradient, which drives the circulation of CSF from its ventricular sites of origin into the subarachnoid space via three openings in the fourth ventricle, as discussed earlier. CSF percolates throughout the subarachnoid space and is finally absorbed into venous blood in the superior sagittal sinus, which lies between the two cerebral hemispheres (see Fig. 16–2). The sites of absorption are specialized evaginations of the arachnoid membrane into the venous sinus (Fig. 16–3A). These absorptive sites are called pacchionian granulations or simply **arachnoid granulations** when they are large (up to 1 cm in diameter) and called **arachnoid villi** if their size is microscopic. These structures act as pressure-sensitive, one-way valves for bulk CSF clearance: CSF can cross into venous blood but ve-

LUMBAR PUNCTURE

One of the most important diagnostic tests in neurology is the sampling of cerebrospinal fluid (CSF) by lumbar puncture. Critical information about the composition of CSF and about intracranial pressure can be obtained from this procedure. The anatomist Vesalius noted in 1543 that the ventricles are filled with a clear fluid, but the diagnostic technique of placing a needle into the lumbar subarachnoid space to obtain CSF was not introduced until 1891 by the neurologist Heinrich Quincke. The method of lumbar puncture is dictated by spine anatomy. In adults, the spinal cord ends at the interspace between L1 and L2 (p. 275). A hollow needle for sampling CSF can be safely inserted into the subarachnoid space at the level of the L3-4 interspace, well below the end of the spinal cord.

Once it is in the subarachnoid space, the physician attaches the needle to a manometer for measuring pressure. With the patient lying on the side, normal pressure varies from 100 to 180 mm H_2O, or 7 to 13 mm Hg. With the subject in this position and in the absence of a block to the free circulation of CSF, lumbar CSF pressure roughly corresponds to intracranial pressure. The physician can demonstrate direct communication of the pressure in the intracranial compartment to the lumbar subarachnoid space by gently compressing the external jugular veins in the neck for 10 seconds. This maneuver, called the **Queckenstedt test,** rapidly increases intracranial pressure because it increases the volume of intracranial venous blood. It quickly leads to an increase in lumbar pressure, which just as rapidly dissipates when the jugular pressure is removed.

CSF pressure can become elevated because of a pathologic mass within the cranium, such as a tumor or collection of blood, or because the brain is swollen as a result of injury or infection (see the later Box titled Cerebral Edema). If a "mass lesion" (i.e., any pathologic process that occupies intracranial space) is large or critically placed, it can displace the brain and cause interference with the free circulation of CSF. For example, an expanding mass in the cerebellum can force the inferior part of the cerebellum into the foramen magnum and block flow of CSF into the spinal subarachnoid space. Under these conditions, performing a lumbar puncture can precipitate a neurologic catastrophe. If a needle is placed in the lumbar subarachnoid space and fluid is removed for diagnostic examination or leaks out after the needle is removed, the ensuing decrease in pressure in the lumbar space creates a pressure gradient across the foramen magnum and potentially forces the brain down into the spinal canal. This disaster is called *herniation.* For this reason, a computed tomographic scan or magnetic resonance image of the head is usually obtained before attempting a lumbar puncture; the imaging study can rule out the possibility of a large intracranial lesion that might raise intracranial pressure and increase the risk of herniation when the subarachnoid space is punctured and CSF withdrawn. The Queckenstedt test must also be avoided when an intracranial mass is suspected because it could enhance the pressure gradient and hasten herniation.

A MECHANISM OF CSF ABSORPTION

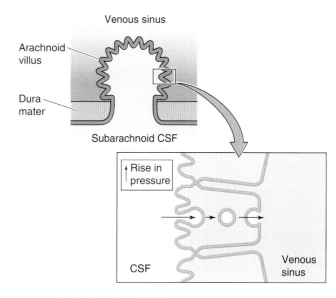

B RATE OF CSF ABSORPTION

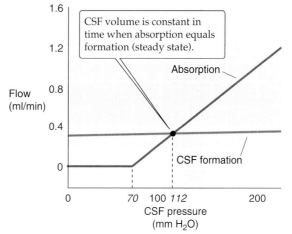

FIGURE 16–3. Absorption of cerebrospinal fluid. *A,* Arachnoid villi—or the larger arachnoid granulations (not shown)—are specialized evaginations of the arachnoid membrane through the dura mater and into the lumen of the venous sinus. The absorption of cerebrospinal fluid (CSF) may involve transcytosis. Note that arachnoid villi and granulations serve as one-way valves; fluid cannot move from the vein to the subarachnoid space. *B,* The rate of CSF formation is virtually insensitive to changes in the pressure of the CSF. On the other hand, the absorption of CSF increases steeply at CSF pressures that are above approximately 70 mm H_2O.

nous blood cannot enter CSF. The actual mechanism of CSF absorption may involve transcytosis (p. 464), or the formation of giant fluid-containing vacuoles that cross from the CSF side of the arachnoid epithelial cells to the blood side (see Fig. 16–3*A*). CSF may also be absorbed into spinal veins from herniations of arachnoid cells into these venous structures. Net CSF movement into venous blood is promoted by the pressure of the CSF, which is higher than that of the venous blood. When intracranial pressure (equivalent to CSF pressure) exceeds approximately 70 mm H_2O, absorption commences and increases with intracranial pressure (see Fig. 16–3*B*). In contrast to

"NORMAL-PRESSURE" HYDROCEPHALUS

Impaired cerebrospinal fluid (CSF) absorption is one mechanism proposed to explain a clinical form of ventricular enlargement called **"normal-pressure" hydrocephalus.** This condition is somewhat misnamed because the intracranial pressure is often intermittently elevated. Damage to the arachnoid villi can occur most commonly from infection or inflammation of the meninges, or from the presence of an irritating substance, such as blood in the CSF after a subarachnoid hemorrhage. Patients with normal-pressure hydrocephalus typically have progressive dementia, urinary incontinence, and gait disturbance. A spinal tap reveals normal pressure readings, but computed tomography, or magnetic resonance imaging of the head shows enlargement of all four ventricles. A flexible plastic tube can be placed in one of the lateral ventricles to shunt CSF to venous blood or to the peritoneal cavity, thereby reducing CSF pressure. This procedure may reduce ventricular size and decrease neurologic symptoms. The "shunting" procedure is also used for patients with obstructive hydrocephalus. In this condition, CSF outflow from the ventricles is blocked, typically at the aqueduct of Sylvius.

CSF absorption, CSF formation is not sensitive to intracranial pressure. This arrangement helps stabilize intracranial pressure.

If intracranial pressure increases, CSF absorption selectively increases as well so that absorption exceeds formation (see Fig. 16–3B). This response results in a lower CSF volume and a tendency to counteract the increased intracranial pressure. However, if absorption of CSF is impaired even at an initially normal intracranial pressure, CSF volume increases and causes an increase in intracranial pressure. Such an increase in intracranial pressure can lead to a decrease in brain function, as described in the box titled "Normal-Pressure" Hydrocephalus.

CSF Communicates Freely with the Extracellular Fluid Surrounding Neurons and Stabilizes the Composition of the Neuronal Microenvironment

CSF in the ventricles and the subarachnoid space can exchange freely with BECF across two borders, the pia mater and ependymal cells. The **pial-glial membrane** (see Fig. 16–2, upper *inset*) has paracellular gaps (p. 46) through which substances can equilibrate between the subarachnoid space and BECF. **Ependymal cells** (see Fig. 16–2, lower *inset*) are special glial cells that line the walls of the ventricles and form the cellular boundary between the CSF and the BECF. These cells form gap junctions between themselves that mediate intercellular communication, but they do not create a tight epithelium (p. 82). Thus, macromolecules and ions can also easily pass through this cellular layer via paracellular openings (some

notable exceptions to this rule are considered later) and equilibrate between the CSF in the ventricle and the BECF. Because CSF and BECF can readily exchange with one another, it is not surprising that they have a similar chemical composition (see later).

CSF is an efficient waste-management system because of its high rate of production, its circulation over the surface of the brain, and the free exchange between CSF and BECF. Products of metabolism and other substances released by cells, perhaps for signalling purposes, can diffuse into the chemically stable CSF and ultimately be removed on a continuous basis either by bulk resorption into the venous sinuses or by active transport across the choroid plexus into the blood. For example, choroid plexus actively absorbs the breakdown products of the neurotransmitters serotonin and dopamine, 5-hydroxyindoleacetic acid and homovanillic acid, respectively.

Transport by the Epithelial Cells of the Choroid Plexus Determines the Composition of the CSF

Each of the four choroid plexuses is formed during embryologic development by invagination of the tela choroidea into the ventricular cavity (Fig. 16–4). The tela choroidea consists of a layer of ependymal cells covered by the pia mater and its associated blood vessels. The choroid epithelial cells are specialized ependymal cells and therefore contiguous with the ependymal lining of the ventricles at the margins of the choroid plexus. Choroid epithelial cells are cuboidal in shape and have an apical border with microvilli and cilia that project into the ventricle (i.e., into the CSF). The plexus receives its blood supply from the anterior and posterior choroidal arteries; blood flow to the plexuses—per unit mass of tissue—is about 10-fold greater than the average cerebral blood flow. Sympathetic and parasympathetic nerves innervate each plexus, and sympathetic input appears to inhibit CSF formation. A high density of relatively leaky capillaries is present within each plexus; as discussed later, these capillaries are outside the BBB. The choroid epithelial cells are bound to one another by tight junctions that completely encircle each cell, an arrangement that makes the epithelium an effective barrier to free diffusion. Thus, although the choroid capillaries are outside the BBB, the choroid epithelium insulates the ECF around these capillaries (which has a composition that is more similar to that of arterial blood) from the CSF. Moreover, the thin neck that connects the choroid plexus to the rest of the brain isolates the ECF near the leaky choroidal capillaries from the highly protected BECF in the rest of the brain.

The composition of CSF differs considerably from that of plasma; thus, CSF is not just an ultrafiltrate of plasma (Table 16–1). For example, CSF contains lower concentrations of K^+ and amino acids than plasma does, and it contains almost no protein. Moreover, the choroid plexuses rigidly maintain the concentration of ions in CSF in the face of large swings in ion concentration in plasma. This ion homeostasis includes K^+, H^+/HCO_3^-, Mg^{2+},

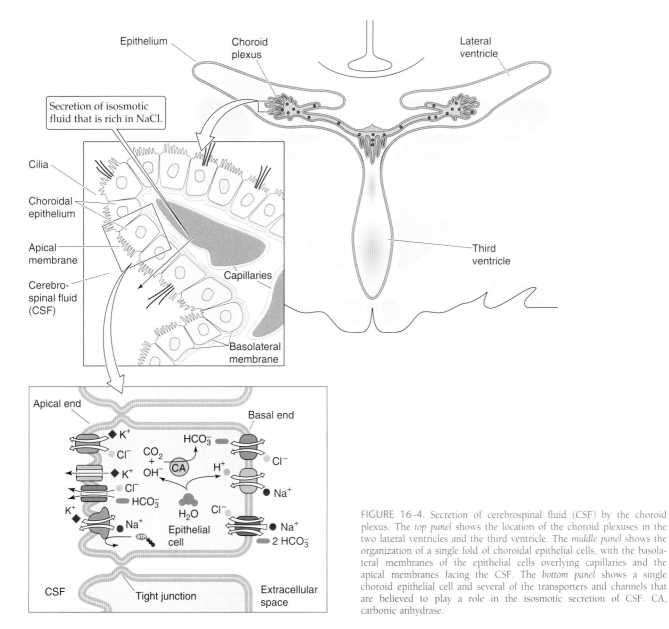

FIGURE 16–4. Secretion of cerebrospinal fluid (CSF) by the choroid plexus. The *top panel* shows the location of the choroid plexuses in the two lateral ventricles and the third ventricle. The *middle panel* shows the organization of a single fold of choroidal epithelial cells, with the basolateral membranes of the epithelial cells overlying capillaries and the apical membranes facing the CSF. The *bottom panel* shows a single choroid epithelial cell and several of the transporters and channels that are believed to play a role in the isosmotic secretion of CSF. CA, carbonic anhydrase.

Ca^{2+}, and to a lesser extent, Na^+ and Cl^-. All these ions can affect neural function, hence the need for tight homeostatic control. The neuronal microenvironment is so well protected from the blood by the choroid plexuses and the rest of the BBB that essential **micronutrients**, such as vitamins and trace elements that are needed in very small amounts, must be selectively transported into the brain. Some of these micronutrients are transported into the brain primarily by the choroid plexus and others primarily by the endothelial cells of the blood vessels. In comparison, the brain continuously metabolizes relatively large amounts of "macronutrients" such as glucose and some amino acids.

Evidence indicates that CSF forms in two sequential steps: first, ultrafiltration of plasma occurs across the fenestrated capillary wall (p. 464) into the ECF beneath the basolateral membrane of the choroid epithelial cell. Sec-

ond, choroid epithelial cells secrete fluid into the ventricle. CSF production occurs with a net transfer of NaCl that drives water movement isosmotically. Isosmotic *absorption* of fluid occurs in the renal proximal tubule (p. 781) and small intestine (p. 85). The most striking difference between these epithelia and choroidal epithelium is that the choroid *secretes* an isosmotic fluid. As we have already seen, the choroid plexus also conditions CSF by absorbing certain substances (e.g., a metabolite of serotonin: 5-hydroxyindoleacetic acid).

The ion transport processes that are mediated by the choroid epithelial cells are shown schematically in Figure 16–4. As in the case of other epithelial cells, the asymmetric distribution of transport mechanisms within the choroid epithelial cells is responsible for net transepithelial transport (p. 84). The Na-K pump, which is unusual in being located on the *apical* membrane, moves Na^+ out

TABLE 16–1

COMPOSITION OF CEREBROSPINAL FLUID

SOLUTE	PLASMA (mM OF PROTEIN-FREE PLASMA)	CSF (mM)	CSF/PLASMA RATIO
Na^+	153	147	0.96
K^+	4.7	2.9	0.62
Ca^{2+}	1.3 (ionized)	1.1 (ionized)	0.85
Mg^{2+}	0.6 (ionized)	1.1 (ionized)	1.8
Cl^-	110	113	1.03
HCO_3^-	24	22	0.92
$H_2PO_4^-$ and HPO_4^{2-}	0.75 (ionized)	0.9	1.2
pH	7.40	7.33	
Amino acids	2.6	0.7	0.27
Proteins	7 g/dl	0.03 g/dl	0.004
Osmolality (mOsm)	290	290	1.00

of the cell into the CSF. The Na-K pump is directly responsible for CSF secretion; blocking it with ouabain blocks CSF formation. Active movement of Na^+ out of the cell generates an Na^+ gradient across the basolateral (plasma-facing) membrane, which sets up the entry of Na^+ across the basolateral membrane via Na-H exchange and Na^+-coupled HCO_3^- transport. In the case of Na-H exchange, the limiting factor is the availability of intracellular H^+, which carbonic anhydrase generates, along with HCO_3^-, from CO_2 and H_2O. Indeed, blockade of carbonic anhydrase by the drug acetazolamide inhibits CSF formation.

The net movement of Cl^- from plasma to CSF is also a two-step process. The first step is the intracellular accumulation of Cl^- via the basolateral Cl-HCO_3 exchanger. Note that the net effect of parallel Cl–HCO_3 exchange and Na-H exchange is NaCl uptake. The second step is efflux of Cl^- across the apical border into the CSF via either a Cl^- channel or a K/Cl cotransporter.

The net movement of HCO_3^- into CSF is important for neutralizing acid produced by central nervous system (CNS) cells. However, the precise steps by which the choroid plexus secretes HCO_3^- are unclear. The basolateral step of HCO_3^- secretion may involve direct uptake of HCO_3^- from the plasma filtrate into the cell via a transporter such as the Na^+-driven Cl-HCO_3 exchanger (see Fig. 3–12, #17). Alternatively, CO_2 may simply enter the cell and form HCO_3^- and H^+, catalyzed by intracellular carbonic anhydrase. The apical step, movement of intracellular HCO_3^- into the CSF, could occur through Cl^- channels (which are generally permeable to HCO_3^-) or a transporter such as an electrogenic Na/HCO_3 cotransporter (see Fig. 3–12, #19).

The concentration of K^+ in freshly secreted CSF is about 3.3 mM. Even with very large changes in plasma $[K^+]$, the $[K^+]$ in CSF changes very little. The value of $[K^+]$ in CSF is significantly lower in the subarachnoid space than in choroid secretions, which suggests that

brain capillary endothelial cells remove extracellular K^+ from the brain (see later).

BRAIN EXTRACELLULAR SPACE

Neurons, Glia, and Capillaries Are Packed Tightly Together in the CNS and Share a Common Extracellular Space That Plays a Role in Cell-Cell Communication

The average width of the space between brain cells is about 20 nm, which is about three orders of magnitude smaller than the diameter of either a neuron or glial cell body (Fig. 16–5). However, because the surface membranes of neurons and glial cells are highly folded (i.e., have a large surface-to-volume ratio), the BECF in toto has a sizable volume fraction, approximately 20%, of the total brain volume. The fraction of the brain that is occupied by BECF varies somewhat in different areas of the CNS. Moreover, because brain cells can increase volume rapidly during intense neural activity, the BECF fraction can reversibly decrease within seconds by as much as 15%.

Even though the space between brain cells is extremely small, diffusion of ions and other solutes within this thin BECF space is reasonably high. However, a particle that diffuses through the BECF from one side of a neuron to the other must take a very circuitous route that is described by a parameter called **tortuosity**. For a normal width of the cell-to-cell spacing, this tortuosity reduces the rate of diffusion by approximately 60% when compared with movement in free solution. Decreases in cell-to-cell spacing can further slow diffusion. For example, brain cells, especially glial cells, swell under certain pathologic conditions and sometimes with intense neural activity. Cell swelling is associated with a reduction in BECF because water moves from the BECF into cells. The

FIGURE 16–5. The brain extracellular space. This is an electron micrograph of a section of the spinal cord from an adult rat showing the intermingling and close apposition of neurons and glial cells. Neurons and glial cells are separated by narrow clefts that are approximately 20 nm wide. The brain extracellular fluid (BECF) in this space creates a tortuous path for the extracellular diffusion of solutes. Astrocyte processes are *colored. As,* astrocytes; *At, en passant* synapses; *Ax,* unmyelinated axons, *Ax$_1$* and *Ax$_2$,* myelinated axons; *Den,* dendrites; *f,* astrocytic fibrils; *nf,* neurofilaments; *S,* synapses; *SR,* smooth endoplasmic reticulum. (Modified from Peters A, Palay SL, Webster H: The Fine Structure of the Nervous System. WB Saunders, Philadelphia, 1976.)

intense cell swelling associated with acute anoxia, for example, can reduce BECF volume to 5% of total brain volume. By definition, this reduced extracellular volume translates to reduced cell-to-cell spacing, further slowing the extracellular movement of solutes between the blood and brain cells (see the box titled Cerebral Edema).

The BECF is the route by which important molecules such as oxygen, glucose, and amino acids reach brain cells and by which the products of metabolism, including CO_2 and catabolized neurotransmitters, leave the brain. The BECF also permits molecules that are released by brain cells to diffuse to adjacent cells. Neurotransmitter molecules released at synaptic sites, for example, can spill over from the synaptic cleft and contact nearby glial cells and neurons, in addition to their target postsynaptic cell. Glial cells express neurotransmitter receptors, and neurons have **extrajunctional receptors**; therefore, these cells are capable of receiving "messages" sent via the BECF. Numerous trophic molecules secreted by brain cells diffuse in the BECF to their targets; these factors include brain-derived neurotrophic factor (BDNF), ciliary neuro-

CEREBRAL EDEMA

Almost any type of insult to the brain causes cell swelling. Frequently, this swelling is accompanied by a *net accumulation of water* within the brain that is referred to as **cerebral edema.** It is important to emphasize that cell swelling in the absence of net water accumulation in the brain does *not* constitute cerebral edema. For example, intense neural activity causes a rapid shift of fluid from the brain extracellular fluid (BECF) to the intracellular space, with no net change in brain water content. In cerebral edema, the extra water comes from the blood, as shown in Figure 16–6.

The mechanisms by which glial cells and neurons swell are not completely understood. Neuron cell bodies and dendrites, but not axons, swell when exposed to high concentrations of the neurotransmitter **glutamate.** This transmitter, along with others, is released to the BECF in an uncontrolled fashion with brain injury. Activation of ionotropic glutamate receptors (p. 313) allows Na$^+$ to enter neurons, and water and Cl$^-$ follow passively. Glial cells, both astrocytes and oligodendrocytes, swell vigorously under pathologic conditions. One mechanism of glial swelling in an increase in [K$^+$]$_o$, which is a common ionic disturbance in a variety of brain pathologies. This elevated [K$^+$]$_o$ causes a net uptake of K$^+$, accompanied by the passive influx of Cl$^-$ and water.

Cerebral edema can be life threatening when severe. The problem is a mechanical one. The skull is an inelastic container housing three relatively noncompressible substances: brain, CSF, and blood. A significant increase in the volume of CSF, blood, or brain rapidly causes increased pressure within the skull (see Fig. 16–3). If the cerebral edema is *generalized,* it can be tolerated until intracerebral pressure exceeds arterial blood pressure, at which point blood flow to the brain stops, with disastrous consequences. Fortunately, sensors in the medulla detect the increased intracerebral pressure and can partially compensate ("Cushing reflex"), to a point, by increasing arterial pressure (p. 562). *Focal* cerebral edema (i.e., edema involving an isolated portion of the brain) causes problems by displacing nearby brain tissue. This abnormality may result in distortion of normal anatomic relationships, with selective pressure on critical structures such as the brain stem.

Clinical evidence of cerebral edema results directly from the increased intracranial pressure and includes headache, vomiting, altered consciousness, and focal neurologic problems such as stretching and dysfunction of the sixth cranial nerve.

Hyperventilation is the most effective means of combating the acute increase in intracranial pressure associated with severe cerebral edema. Hyperventilation causes a prompt respiratory alkalosis (p. 641) that is rapidly translated to an increase in the pH surrounding vascular smooth muscle, thereby triggering vasoconstriction and reduced cerebral blood flow (p. 561). Thus, total intracranial blood content falls, with a rapid subsequent drop in intracranial pressure. Alternatively, the brain can be partially dehydrated by adding osmoles to the blood in the form of intravenously administered mannitol (p. 76).

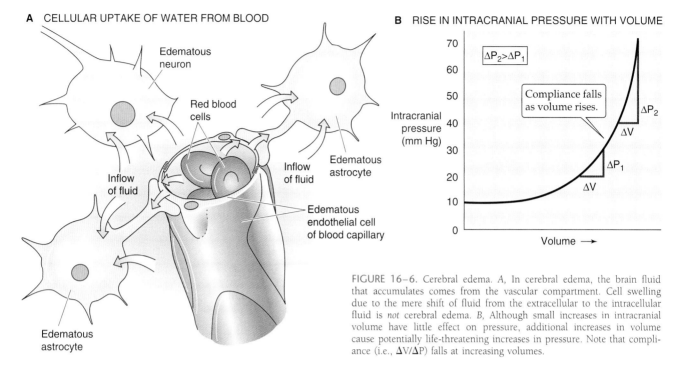

FIGURE 16–6. Cerebral edema. *A*, In cerebral edema, the brain fluid that accumulates comes from the vascular compartment. Cell swelling due to the mere shift of fluid from the extracellular to the intracellular fluid is *not* cerebral edema. *B*, Although small increases in intracranial volume have little effect on pressure, additional increases in volume cause potentially life-threatening increases in pressure. Note that compliance (i.e., $\Delta V/\Delta P$) falls at increasing volumes.

trophic factor (CNTF), and neurotrophin 3. Intercellular communication by way of the BECF is especially well suited for the transmission of tonic signals that are ideal for longer-term modulation of the behavior of aggregates of neurons and glial cells. The chronic presence of variable amounts of neurotransmitters in the BECF supports this idea.

Because the Extracellular Volume Between Adjacent Cell Membranes Is Exceedingly Small, the Ion Fluxes Accompanying Neural Activity Cause Large Changes in Extracellular Ion Concentration

As discussed in Chapter 7, ionic currents through cell membranes underlie the synaptic and action potentials by which neurons communicate. These currents lead to changes in the ion concentrations of the BECF. It is estimated that even a single action potential can transiently lower $[Na^+]_o$ by about 0.75 mM and increase $[K^+]_o$ by a similar amount. Repetitive neuronal activity causes larger perturbations in these extracellular ion concentrations. Because ambient $[K^+]_o$ is much lower than $[Na^+]_o$, activity-induced changes in $[K^+]_o$ are proportionately larger and are of special interest because of the important effect that $[K^+]_o$ has on membrane potential (V_m). For example, K^+ accumulation in the vicinity of active neurons depolarizes nearby glial cells. In this way, neurons signal to glial cells the pattern and extent of their activity. Even small changes in $[K^+]_o$ can alter metabolism and ionic transport in glial cells and may be used for signalling. Changes in the extracellular concentrations of certain common amino acids, such as glutamate and glycine, can also affect neuronal V_m and synaptic function by acting at specific receptor sites. If the nervous system is to function reliably, its signalling elements must have a

regulated environment. Glial cells and neurons both function to prevent excessive extracellular accumulation of K^+ and neurotransmitters.

Brain Extracellular Fluid Resembles CSF, but Both Differ from Blood Plasma

The conccentrations of ions and other molecules in BECF closely resemble those seen in CSF. For example, $[K^+]$ is approximately 3.3 mM in freshly secreted CSF and approximately 3 mM in both the CSF of the subarachnoid space (see Table 16–1) and BECF. The $[K^+]$ of blood, however, is approximately 4.5 mM. However, because of the extent and vast complexity of the extracellular space, changes in the composition of CSF are reflected slowly in the BECF and probably incompletely. As noted earlier, this equilibration takes place across the pia mater and across the ependymal cells that line the ventricles. Blood is not a suitable environment for neurons because its composition is highly changeable. For example, marked fluctuations occur in blood composition during strenuous exercise; the drop in pH and rise in $[K^+]$ can be substantial. If these changes were communicated to the BECF, they could affect brain function; running a foot race might temporarily lower your IQ. Fortunately, as we shall see later, BECF is protected from blood by the BBB.

THE BLOOD-BRAIN BARRIER

Because of the Blood-Brain Barrier, Not All Blood Constituents Can Pass Freely into the Brain Extracellular Space

The unique protective mechanism called the BBB was first demonstrated by Ehrlich in 1885. He injected aniline

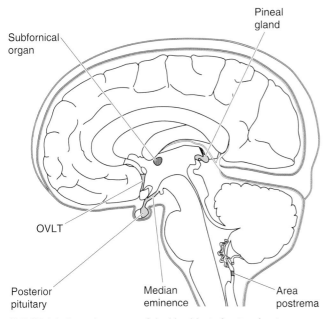

FIGURE 16–7. Leaky regions of the blood-brain barrier: the circumventricular organs. The capillaries of the brain are leaky in several areas: the area postrema, the posterior pituitary, the subfornical organ, the median eminence, the pineal gland, and the organum vasculosum laminae terminalis (OVLT). In these regions, the neurons are directly exposed to the solutes of the blood plasma. A midline sagittal section is shown.

dyes intravenously and discovered that the soft tissues of the body, except for the brain, were uniformly stained. Even though aniline dyes, such as trypan blue, extensively bind to serum albumin, the dye-albumin complex passes across capillaries in most areas of the body, but not the brain. This special property of CNS blood vessels to exclude certain substances from brain tissue is called the **blood-brain barrier**. We now recognize that a BBB is present in all vertebrates and many invertebrates as well.

The need for a BBB can be understood by considering the nature of blood. Blood is a complex medium that contains a large variety of solutes, some of which can vary greatly in concentration, depending on factors such as diet, metabolism, illness, and age. For example, the concentration of many amino acids increases significantly after a protein-rich meal. Some of these amino acids act as neurotransmitters within the brain, and if these molecules could move freely from the blood into the neuronal microenvironment, they would nonselectively activate receptors and disturb normal neurotransmission. Similarly, athletic activity can increase concentrations of K^+ and H^+ within blood. If these ionic changes were communicated directly to the microenvironment of neurons, they could disrupt ongoing activity. Increases in $[K^+]_o$ would depolarize neurons and thus increase their likelihood of firing and releasing transmitter. H^+ can nonspecifically modulate neuronal excitability and influence the action of certain neurotransmitters. A broad range of blood constituents—including hormones, other ions, and inflammatory mediators such as cytokines—can influence the behavior of neurons or glial cells, which can express receptors for

these molecules. For the brain to function efficiently, it must be spared such influences.

First, it should be stressed that the choroid plexus and several restricted areas of the brain lack a BBB; that is, they are supplied by leaky capillaries. Intra-arterially injected dyes can pass into the brain ECS at these sites through gaps between endothelial cells. The small brain areas that lack a BBB are called the **circumventricular organs** because they surround the ventricular system; these areas include the *area postrema, posterior pituitary, subfornical organ, median eminence, pineal gland,* and *organum vasculosum laminae terminalis* (OVLT) (Fig. 16–7). The ependymal cells that overlie the leaky capillaries in some of these regions (e.g., the choroid plexus) are linked together by tight junctions. Thus, these specialized ependymal cells form a barrier between the local BECF—which is more similar to blood plasma than are other areas of the BECF—and the CSF, which must be insulated from the blood. Whereas dyes with molecular weights up to 5000 can normally pass from CSF across the ependymal cell layer into the BECF, they do not pass across the specialized ependymal layer at the median eminence, area postrema, and infundibular recess. At these points, the localized BECF-CSF barrier is similar to the one in the choroid plexus. Their specialized ependymal cells often have long processes that extend to capillaries within the portal circulation of the pituitary. Although the function of these cells is not known, it has been suggested that they may form a special route for neurohumoral signalling; molecules secreted by hypothalamic cells into the third ventricle could be taken up by these cells and transmitted to the general circulation or to cells in the pituitary.

Neurons within the circumventricular organs are directly exposed to blood solutes and macromolecules; this arrangement is believed to be part of a neuroendocrine control system for maintaining such parameters as osmolality (p. 871) and appropriate hormone levels, among other things. Humoral signals are integrated by connections of circumventricular organ neurons to endocrine, autonomic, and behavioral centers within the CNS. In the median eminence, leaky capillaries pick up releasing hormones for carriage via the pituitary portal system to the anterior pituitary (p. 1010). The lack of a BBB in the posterior pituitary is necessary to allow hormones that are released there to enter the general circulation (p. 1013). In the OVLT, leakiness is important in the action of cytokines from the periphery, which act as signals to temperature control centers that are involved in fever (p. 1240).

Brain Capillary Endothelial Cells Are Linked Together by Continuous Tight Junctions That Prevent Free Diffusion into the Brain

The BBB should be thought of as a physical barrier to diffusion from blood to brain and as a selective set of regulatory transport mechanisms that determine how certain organic solutes move between the blood and brain.

FIGURE 16–8. The blood-brain barrier function of brain capillaries. *A,* Capillaries from most other organs often have interendothelial clefts or fenestrae, which makes them relatively leaky. *B,* Brain capillaries are not leaky and have reduced transcytosis. *C,* Continuous tight junctions connect the endothelial cells in the brain, making the capillaries relatively tight.

Thus, the BBB contributes to stabilization and protection of the neuronal microenvironment by facilitating the entry of needed substances, removing waste metabolites, and excluding toxic or disruptive substances.

The structure of brain capillaries differs from that of capillaries in other organs (Fig. 16–8A). Capillaries from other organs generally have small, simple openings—or clefts—between their endothelial cells. In some of these other organs, windows, or fenestrae, provide a pathway that bypasses the cytoplasm of capillary endothelial cells. Thus, in most capillaries outside the CNS, solutes can easily diffuse through the clefts and fenestrae. The physical barrier to solute diffusion in *brain* capillaries (see Fig. 16–8B) is provided by the capillary endothelial cells, which are fused to each other by continuous **tight junctions** (or *zonula occludens*; p. 46). The tight junctions prevent water-soluble ions and molecules from passing from the blood into the brain via the paracellular route. Not surprisingly, the electrical resistance of the cerebral capillaries is 100 to 200 times higher than that of most other systemic capillaries.

Elsewhere in the systemic circulation, molecules may traverse the endothelial cell by the process of **transcytosis** (p. 464). In cerebral capillaries, transcytosis is uncommon. Indeed, brain endothelial cells have fewer endocytic vesicles than systemic capillaries do. However, brain endothelial cells have many more **mitochondria** than systemic endothelial cells do, which may reflect the high metabolic demands imposed on brain endothelial cells by active transport.

Other interesting features of brain capillaries are the thick **basement membrane** that underlies the endothelial cells, the presence of occasional **pericytes** within the basement membrane sheath, and the **astrocytic end-feet** (or processes) that provide a nearly continuous covering of the capillaries. Astrocytes may play a crucial role in forming tight junctions between endothelial cells; experiments have shown that these glial cells can induce the formation of tight junctions between endothelial cells derived from capillaries outside the CNS. The close apposition of the astrocyte endfoot to the capillary also could facilitate transport of substances between these cells and blood.

Molecules That Are Uncharged and Lipid Soluble More Readily Pass the Blood-Brain Barrier

The capacity of the brain capillaries to exclude large molecules is strongly related to the molecular weight of the molecule and its hydrated diameter (Table 16–2). With a weight of 61 kDa, prealbumin is 14 times as concentrated in blood as in CSF (essentially equivalent to BECF for purposes of this comparison), whereas fibrinogen, which has a molecular weight of 340 kDa, is approximately 5000 times more concentrated in blood than in CSF. Diffusion of a solute is also generally limited by ionization at physiological pH, by low lipid solubility, and by binding to plasma proteins. For example, highly lipid-soluble gases such as CO_2 and O_2 and drugs such as ethanol, caffeine, nicotine, heroin, and methadone readily cross the BBB. However, ions such as K^+ or Mg^{2+} and protein-bound metabolites such as bilirubin have very restricted access to the brain. Finally, the BBB is very permeable to water because of the presence of water channels in the endothelial cells. Thus, water moves across the BBB in response to changes in plasma osmolarity. When dehydration raises the osmolality of blood plasma (see box titled Disorders of Extracellular Osmolality on p. 77), the increased osmolality of the CSF and BECF can affect the behavior of brain cells.

Cerebral capillaries also express enzymes that can affect the movement of substances from blood to brain and vice versa. Peptidases, acid hydrolases, monoamine oxidase,

TABLE 16–2

COMPARSON OF PROTEINS IN BLOOD PLASMA VERSUS CEREBROSPINAL FLUID

PROTEIN	MOLECULAR WEIGHT (kDa)	HYDRODYNAMIC RADIUS (nm)	PLASMA/CSF RATIO*
Prealbumin	61	3.3	14
Albumin	69	3.6	240
Transferrin	81	3.7	140
Ceruloplasmin	152	4.7	370
IgG	150	5.3	800
IgA	150	5.7	1350
α_2-Macroglobulin	798	9.4	1100
Fibrinogen	340	11.0	4940
IgM	800	12.1	1170
β-Lipoprotein	2240	12.4	6210

*The greater the plasma/CSF ratio, the more the blood-brain barrier excludes the protein from the CSF.
CSF, cerebrospinal fluid.

and other enzymes are present in CNS endothelial cells and can degrade a range of biologically active molecules, including enkephalins, substance P, proteins, and norepinephrine. Orally administered dopamine is not an effective treatment for Parkinson's disease (p. 302), a condition in which CNS dopamine is depleted, because dopamine is rapidly broken down by monoamine oxidase in the capillaries. Fortunately, the dopamine precursor compound L-dopa is effective for this condition. Neutral amino-acid transporters in capillary endothelial cells move L-dopa to the BECF, where presynaptic terminals take up the L-dopa and convert it to dopamine in a reaction that is catalyzed by dopa decarboxylase.

Capillary Endothelial Cells Have Transport Mechanisms That Contribute to the Blood-Brain Barrier

Two classes of substances can pass readily from blood into the brain. The first consists of the small, highly lipid soluble molecules discussed in the previous section. The second group consists of compounds that are not extremely lipid soluble, but that enter via specific transporters. Some examples include glucose, several amino acids, nucleic acid precursors, and several organic acids. The transporters are bidirectional and exhibit saturation kinetics and stereospecificity. These mechanisms have evolved to provide pathways both for the entry of critical, water-soluble nutrients into the brain and for the exit of water-soluble metabolites.

Capillary endothelial cells appear to express certain functional membrane proteins selectively on either the luminal or basal surface. The Na-K pump and Na-H exchanger are located exclusively on the basolateral membrane, whereas amiloride-sensitive Na^+ channels and Na/K/Cl transporters are located on the luminal surface (see Fig. 16–8C). This arrangement permits the endothe-

lial cells of the brain to control $[K^+]$ and pH in the BECF by removing excess K^+ or H^+.

Although most CSF is secreted by the choroid plexuses, CNS endothelial cells produce some interstitial fluid with a composition similar to that of CSF.

GLIAL CELLS

Glial Cells Constitute Half the Volume of the Brain and Outnumber Neurons Approximately 10:1

The three major types of glial cells in the CNS are astrocytes, oligodendrocytes, and microglial cells (Fig. 16–9; Table 16–3). As discussed in Chapter 10, the peripheral nervous system (PNS) contains other, distinctive types of glial cells, including satellite cells, Schwann cells, and enteric glia. Glial cells represent about half the volume of the brain and are about 10-fold more numerous than neurons. Unlike neurons, which have little capacity to replace themselves when lost, neuroglial (or simply glial) cells can proliferate throughout life. An injury to the nervous system is the usual stimulus for proliferation.

Historically, glial cells were viewed as a type of CNS connective tissue whose main function was to provide support for the true functional cells of the brain, the neurons. This firmly entrenched concept remained virtually unquestioned for the better part of a century after the early description of these cells by Virchow in 1858. Knowledge about glial cells has accumulated slowly because these cells have proved far more difficult to study than neurons. Because glial cells do not exhibit easily recorded action potentials or synaptic potentials, these cells were sometimes referred to as "silent cells." However, glial cells are now recognized as intimate partners with neurons in virtually every function of the brain.

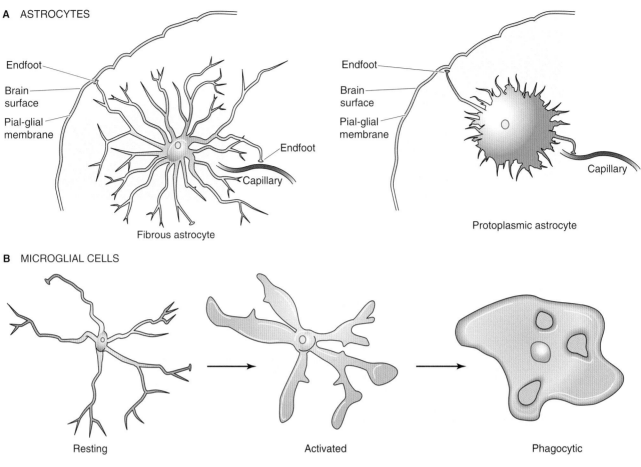

FIGURE 16–9. Astrocytes and microglial cells. *A,* The endfeet of both fibrous and protoplasmic astrocytes abut the pia mater and the capillaries. See Figure 16–2. *B,* Resting microglial cells become activated by injury to the brain, which causes them to proliferate and become phagocytic.

TABLE 16–3

GLIAL TYPES

GLIAL CELL TYPE	SYSTEM	LOCATION	GFAP
Astrocytes			
Fibrous	CNS	White matter	Positive
Protoplasmic	CNS	Gray matter	Weakly positive
Radial glial cells	CNS	Throughout brain during development	Positive
Müller cells	CNS	Retina	Positive
Bergmann glia	CNS	Cerebellum	Positive
Ependymal cells	CNS	Ventricular lining	Positive
Oligodendrocytes	CNS	Mainly white matter	Negative
Microglial cells	CNS	Throughout the brain	Negative
Satellite cells	PNS	Sensory and autonomic ganglia	Weakly positive
Schwann cells	PNS	Peripheral axons	Negative
Enteric glial cells	ENS	Gut wall	Positive

CNS, central nervous system; ENS, enteric nervous system; GFAP, glial fibrillary acidic protein; PNS, peripheral nervous system.

Different Varieties of Astrocytes Are Present Throughout the CNS and Supply Fuel to the Neurons in the Form of Lactic Acid

Astrocytes have great numbers of extremely elaborate processes that closely approach both blood vessels and neurons. This arrangement led to the idea that astrocytes transport substances between the blood and neurons. This notion may be true, but it has not been proved. Astrocytes envelop neurons, and both cells bathe in a common BECF. Therefore, astrocytes are ideally positioned to modify and control the immediate environment of neurons. Most astrocytes in the brain are traditionally subdivided into fibrous and protoplasmic types (see Table 16–3). **Fibrous astrocytes** (found mainly in white matter) have long, thin, and well-defined processes, whereas **protoplasmic astrocytes** (found mainly in gray matter) have shorter, frilly processes. The cytoskeleton of these and other types of astrocytes contains an identifying intermediate filament (p. 24) that is composed of a unique protein called **glial fibrillar acidic protein** (GFAP). The basic physiological properties of both types of astrocyte are similar, but specialized features, such as the expression of neurotransmitter receptors, varies among astrocytes from different brain regions.

During development, another type of astrocyte called the **radial glial cell** (p. 271) is also present. As discussed in Chapter 10, these cells create an organized "scaffolding" by spanning the developing forebrain from the ventricle to the pial surface. Astrocytes in the retina and cerebellum are similar in appearance to radial glial cells. Like astrocytes elsewhere, these cells contain the intermediate filament GFAP. Retinal astrocytes, called **Müller cells**, are oriented so that they span the entire width of the retina. **Bergmann glial cells** in the cerebellum have processes that run parallel to the processes of Purkinje cells.

Astrocytes store virtually all the **glycogen** present in the adult brain. They also contain all the enzymes needed for metabolizing glycogen. The brain's high metabolic needs are primarily met by glucose transferred from blood because the brain's glucose supply in the form of glycogen is very limited. In the absence of glucose from blood, astrocytic glycogen could sustain the brain for only about 5 minutes. As implied, astrocytes can share with neurons the energy stored in glycogen, but *not* by the direct release of glucose into the BECF. Instead, astrocytes break glycogen down to glucose and even further to lactate, which is transferred to nearby neurons where it can be aerobically metabolized (Fig. 16–10). The extent to which this metabolic interaction takes place under normal conditions is not known, but it may be important during periods of intense neuronal activity, when the demand for glucose exceeds the supply from blood.

Astrocytes can also provide fuel to neurons in the form of lactate derived directly from glucose, independent of glycogen. Glucose entering the brain from blood first encounters the astrocytic end-foot. Although it can diffuse past this point to neurons, glucose is preferentially taken up by astrocytes and shuttled through astrocytic glycolysis to lactic acid, a significant portion of which is excreted into the BECF surrounding neurons. Several observations support the notion that astrocytes provide lactate to neu-

rons. First, astrocytes have higher *anaerobic* metabolic rates and export much more lactate than do neurons. Second, neurons and their axons function normally when glucose is replaced by lactate, and some neurons seem to prefer lactate to glucose as fuel. Note that the two molecules of lactate derived from the breakdown of one molecule of glucose provide 28 molecules of ATP when aerobically metabolized, compared with the 30 ATP provided by the complete oxidation of glucose itself (see Table 57–2). The advantage of this scheme for neuronal function is that it provides a form of **substrate buffering**, a second energy reservoir that is available to neurons. The availability of *glucose* in the neuronal microenvironment depends on moment-to-moment supply from the blood and probably also varies as a result of changes in neural activity. The concentration of extracellular *lactate*, however, is buffered against such variability by the surrounding astrocytes, which continuously shuttle lactate to the BECF through the metabolism of glucose or by breaking down glycogen.

Astrocytes Are Predominantly Permeable to K^+ and Also Help Regulate $[K^+]_o$

The membrane potential of glial cells is more negative than that of neurons. For example, astrocytes have a V_m of about −85 mV, whereas the resting neuronal V_m is about −65 mV. Because the equilibrium potential for K^+ is about −90 mV in both neurons and glia, the more negative V_m in astrocytes indicates that glial membranes have higher K^+ selectivity than neuronal membranes do (p. 155). Although glial cells express a variety of K^+ channels, inwardly rectifying K^+ channels seem to be important in setting the resting potential. These channels are voltage gated and are open at membrane potentials that are more negative than about −80 mV, close to the observed resting potential of astrocytes. Astrocytes express many other voltage-gated ion channels that were once thought to be restricted to neurons. The significance of voltage-gated Na^+ and Ca^{2+} channels in glial cells is unknown. Because the ratio of Na^+ to K^+ channels is low in adult astrocytes, these cells are not capable of regenerative electrical responses such as the action potential.

One consequence of the higher K^+ selectivity of astrocytes is that the V_m of astrocytes is far more sensitive than neurons to changes in $[K^+]_o$. For example, when $[K^+]_o$ is raised from 4 to 20 mM, astrocytes depolarize by approximately 25 mV, versus only about 5 mV for neurons. This relative insensitivity of neuronal resting potential to changes in $[K^+]_o$ in the "physiological" range may have emerged as an adaptive feature that stabilizes the resting potential of *neurons* in the face of the transient increases in $[K^+]_o$ that accompany neuronal activity. In contrast, natural stimulation, such as viewing visual targets of different shapes or orientations, can cause depolarizations of up to 10 mV in *astrocytes* of the visual cortex. The accumulation of extracellular K^+ that is secondary to neural activity may serve as a signal—to glial cells—that is proportional to the extent of the activity. For example, small increases in $[K^+]_o$ cause astrocytes to increase their glucose metabolism and provide more lactate for active

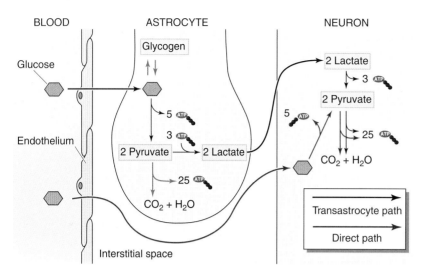

FIGURE 16–10. Role of astrocytes in providing lactate as fuel for neurons. Neurons have two fuel sources. They can obtain glucose directly from the blood plasma or lactate from astrocytes. In the neuron, the conversion of glucose to pyruvate yields five ATP molecules, two directly, plus three from the oxidation of two NADH (we assume that the glycerol 3-phosphate shuttle moves the reducing equivalents into the mitochondrion; see Table 57–2). The oxidation of two pyruvates to CO_2 and H_2O yields an additional 25 ATP. Thus, the total is 30 ATP/glucose. The astrocyte, which has a very high rate of anaerobic glycolysis, can take up glucose and generate two pyruvates; this process would create five ATP under anaerobic conditions. The conversion of two pyruvates to two lactates consumes two NADH, which is equivalent to losing three ATP. The lactate then moves from the astrocyte to the neuron. The conversion of two lactates to two pyruvates generates three ATP from the oxidation of two NADH. Thus, the complete oxidation of two molecules of lactate in the neuron yields 28 ATP.

neurons. In addition, the depolarization that is triggered by the increased $[K^+]_o$ leads to the influx of HCO_3^- into astrocytes via the electrogenic Na/HCO_3 cotransporter (p. 67); this influx of bicarbonate in turn causes a fall in extracellular pH that may diminish neuronal excitability.

Not only do astrocytes respond to changes in $[K^+]_o$, they also help regulate it (Fig. 16–11A). The need for homeostatic control of $[K^+]_o$ is clear because changes in brain $[K^+]_o$ can influence transmitter release, cerebral blood flow, cell volume, glucose metabolism, and neuronal activity. Active neurons lose K^+ into the BECF, and the resulting increased $[K^+]_o$ tends to act as a positive feedback signal that increases excitability by further depolarizing neurons. This potentially unstable situation is combatted by efficient mechanisms that expedite K^+ removal and limit its accumulation to a maximum level of 10 to 12 mM, the so-called ceiling level. $[K^+]_o$ would rise far above this ceiling with intense neural activity if K^+ clearance depended solely on passive redistribution of K^+ in the BECF. Neurons and blood vessels can contribute to K^+ homeostasis, but glial mechanisms are probably most important. Astrocytes can take up K^+ in response to elevated $[K^+]_o$ by three major mechanisms: the Na-K pump, the Na/K/Cl cotransporter, and uptake of K^+ and Cl^- via channels. Conversely, when neural activity decreases, K^+ and Cl^- leave the astrocytes via ion channels.

Astrocytes Couple to One Another via Gap Junctions That Permit the Passage of Small Molecules and Ions

The anatomic substrate for cell-cell coupling among astrocytes is the **gap junction,** which is composed of membrane proteins called connexins that form aqueous pores connecting the cytoplasm of two adjacent cells (p. 164). Coupling between astrocytes is strong because hundreds of gap junction channels may be present between two astrocytes. Astrocytes may also be weakly coupled to oligodendrocytes. Ions and organic molecules that are up to 1 kDa in size, regardless of charge, can diffuse from one cell into another via these large channels. Thus, a

broad range of biologically important molecules, including nucleotides, sugars, amino acids, small peptides, cyclic adenosine monophosphate (cAMP), Ca^{2+}, and inositol 1,4,5-triphosphate (IP_3), have access to this pathway.

Gap junctions may coordinate the metabolic and electrical activities of cell populations, amplify the consequences of signal transduction, and control intrinsic proliferative capacity. The strong coupling among astrocytes ensures that all cells in the aggregate have similar intracellular concentrations of ions and small molecules and similar membrane potentials. Thus, the network of astrocytes functionally behaves as a **syncytium,** much like the myocytes in the heart (p. 483). In ways that are not yet clear, gap junctional communication can be important for the control of cellular proliferation. The most common braincell–derived tumors in the CNS arise from astrocytes. Malignant astrocyte tumors, like malignancies derived from other cells that are normally coupled (e.g., liver cells), lack gap junctions.

The coupling among astrocytes may also play an important role in controlling $[K^+]_o$ via a mechanism known as **spatial buffering.** The selective K^+ permeability of glia, together with their low-resistance cell-cell connections, permits them to transport K^+ from focal areas of high $[K^+]_o$, where a portion of the glial syncytium would be depolarized, to areas of normal $[K^+]_o$, where the glial syncytium would be more normally polarized (see Fig. 16–11B). Redistribution of K^+ proceeds by way of a current loop in which K^+ enters glial cells at the point of high $[K^+]_o$ and leaves them at sites of normal $[K^+]_o$, with the extracellular flow of Na^+ completing this circuit. At a site of high neuronal activity, $[K^+]_o$ might rise to 12 mM, which would produce a very large depolarization of an isolated, uncoupled astrocyte. However, because of the electrical coupling among astrocytes, the V_m of the affected astrocyte remains more negative than the E_K predicted for a $[K^+]_o$ of 12 mM. Thus, K^+ would tend to passively enter coupled astrocytes through channels at sites of high $[K^+]_o$. As discussed in the previous section, K^+ may also enter the astrocyte via transporters.

An additional specialization that contributes to spatial

A MECHANISMS OF K⁺ UPTAKE BY ASTROCYTES

B SPATIAL BUFFERING

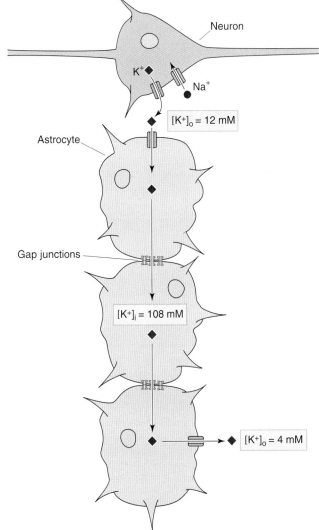

FIGURE 16–11. K⁺ handling by astrocytes. *A,* Each action potential is accompanied by a net movement of K⁺ from the neuron into the extracellular space. Astrocytes can take up this K⁺, and store it briefly, via K⁺ channels, the Na-K pump, or the Na/K/Cl cotransporter. *B,* The K⁺ taken up by an astrocyte in a region of high $[K^+]_o$ can move from astrocyte to astrocyte via gap junctions and finally exit into a region of low $[K^+]_o$.

buffering is a nonuniform distribution of K⁺ channels on a single cell. The density of K⁺ channels on the cell membrane of retinal Müller cells (Fig. 16–12*A*), which are specialized astrocytes, is highest on the cell's endfoot. Thus, focal increases in $[K^+]_o$ at the endfoot cause greater depolarization than if they occur elsewhere along the cell's membrane (see Fig. 16–12*B*). Because the endfoot of the Müller cell, which abuts the vitreous humor of the eye, has the highest density of K⁺ channels, excess extracellular K⁺ is preferentially transported to the vitreous, which acts as a disposal site. It is not known whether nonuniform K⁺ channel distribution is a general feature of astrocytes.

Astrocytes Synthesize Neurotransmitters, Take Them Up from the Extracellular Space, and Have Neurotransmitter Receptors

Astrocytes synthesize at least 20 neuroactive compounds, including both glutamate and γ-aminobutyric acid

(GABA). Neurons can manufacture glutamate from glucose or from the immediate precursor molecule glutamine (Fig. 16–13). The glutamine pathway appears to be the primary one in the synthesis of synaptically released glutamate. Glutamine, however, is manufactured only in astrocytes by using the astrocyte-specific enzyme **glutamine synthetase** to convert glutamate to glutamine. This glutamine is then released to the BECF to be taken up by neurons. Consistent with its apparent role in the synthesis of glutamate for neurotransmission, glutamine synthetase is localized to astrocytic processes surrounding glutamatergic synapses. In the presynaptic terminals of neurons, glutaminase converts the glutamine to glutamate, for release into the synaptic cleft by the presynaptic terminal. Finally, some of the glutamate is taken back up into astrocytes (see later) to complete this **glutamate-glutamine cycle**. Disrupting this metabolic interaction between astrocytes and neurons can depress glutamate-dependent synaptic transmission.

Glutamine derived from astrocytes is also important for

A CROSS SECTION OF RETINA

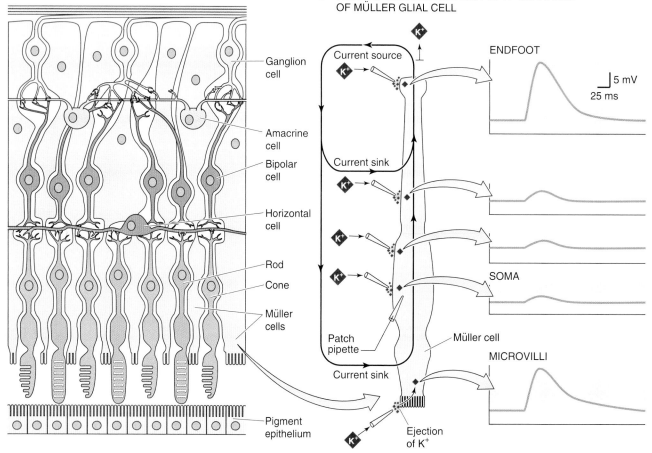

B NONUNIFORM DISTRIBUTION OF K$^+$ CHANNELS
OF MÜLLER GLIAL CELL

FIGURE 16–12. Role of Müller cells in spatial buffering. *A*, The Müller cells are the predominant glial cell of the retina. *B*, In this experiment on an isolated Müller cell from a salamander retina, the investigator monitored membrane potential from the soma of the cell while ejecting K$^+$ from a second pipette at different points along the Müller cell. These ejections, which raise local [K$^+$]$_o$, produced the largest depolarizations when K$^+$ was ejected at the endfoot and microvilli.

FIGURE 16–13. Role of astrocytes in the glutamate-glutamine cycle. Most of the glutamate of glutamatergic neurons is generated from glutamine, which the neurons themselves cannot make. However, astrocytes take up some of the glutamate that is released at synapses (or produced by metabolism) and convert it into glutamine. The glutamine then enters the neuron, where it is converted back to glutamate. This glutamate also serves as the source for γ-aminobutyric acid in inhibitory neurons.

The dicarboxylic amino acid glutamate is the most prevalent excitatory neurotransmitter in the brain (p. 307). Although glutamate is present at millimolar levels inside neurons, the brain extracellular fluid (BECF) has only micromolar levels of glutamate, except at sites of synaptic release (see Fig. 16–13). Excessive accumulation of glutamate in the BECF—induced by ischemia, anoxia, hypoglycemia, or trauma—can lead to neuronal injury. Astrocytes are intimately involved in the metabolism of glutamate and its safe disposition after synaptic release.

In anoxia and ischemia, the sharp drop in cellular levels of adenosine triphosphate (ATP) inhibits the Na-K pump, thereby rapidly leading to large increases in $[K^+]_o$ and $[Na^+]_i$. These changes result in membrane depolarization, with an initial burst of glutamate release from vesicles in presynaptic terminals. This release, however, requires cytoplasmic ATP and probably halts rapidly. The ability of astrocytes to remove glutamate from the BECF is impeded by the elevated $[K^+]_o$, elevated $[Na^+]_i$, and membrane depolarization. In fact, the unfavorable gradients can cause the transporter to run in reverse and dump glutamate into the BECF. The action of rising levels of extracellular glutamate on *postsynaptic* and astrocytic receptors reinforces the developing ionic derangements by opening channels permeable to Na^+ and K^+. This vicious cycle at the level of the astrocyte can rapidly cause extracellular glutamate to reach levels that are toxic to neurons.

synthesis of the brain's most prevalent inhibitory neurotransmitter, GABA. In the neuron, the enzyme **glutamic acid decarboxylase** converts glutamate (generated from glutamine) to GABA (see Fig. 12–9A). Because astrocytes play such an important role in the synthesis of synaptic transmitters, these glial cells are in a position to modulate synaptic efficacy.

Astrocytes have **high-affinity uptake systems** for a large number of neural transmitter molecules, including the excitatory transmitter glutamate and the inhibitory transmitter GABA. In the case of glutamate uptake via the EAAT family (p. 996), astrocytes appear to play the dominant role. The Na^+ gradient provides the energy to move glutamate into cells, accompanied by two Na^+ and an H^+; at the same time, K^+ moves in the opposite direction (Fig. 16–13). Uptake of glutamate by this transport mechanism is associated with movement of a net positive charge into the cell. For this reason, glutamate uptake causes membrane depolarization. The presynaptic cytoplasm may contain glutamate at a concentration as high as 10 mM, and vesicles may contain as much as 100 mM glutamate. Nevertheless, the glutamate uptake systems can maintain extracellular glutamate at concentrations as low as approximately 1 μM.

Neurotransmitter uptake systems are important because they help terminate the action of synaptically released neurotransmitters. Astrocyte processes frequently surround synaptic junctions and are, therefore, ideally placed for this function. Under pathologic conditions in which transmembrane ion gradients break down, high-affinity uptake systems may work in reverse and release transmitters, such as glutamate, into the BECF (see the box titled Excitatory Amino Acids and Neurotoxicity).

Astrocytes also have a variety of **release mechanisms** for the neurotransmitters they take up or synthesize. The mechanism of release is variable, but certain neurotransmitters and elevated $[K^+]_o$ can trigger neurotransmitter release. Astrocytes may also function as a source for neurons of trophic factors, including BDNF, glial-derived neurotrophic factor (GDNF), basic fibroblast growth factor (bFGF), and CNTF.

Astrocytes express a wide variety of inotropic and metabotropic **neurotransmitter receptors** that are similar or identical to those present on neuronal membranes. As in neurons, activation of these receptors can open ion channels or generate second messengers. In most astrocytes, glutamate produces depolarization by increasing Na^+ permeability, whereas GABA hyperpolarizes cells by opening Cl^- channels, similar to the situation in neurons (p. 308). Transmitter substances released at synapses can diffuse in the BECF to activate nearby receptors on astrocytes, thus providing, at least theoretically, a form of neuronal-glial signalling. Applying glutamate to cultured astrocytes causes an increase in $[Ca^{2+}]_i$, which may oscillate. Moreover, these increases in $[Ca^{2+}]_i$ can travel in waves across adjacent astrocytes via gap junctions. Most provocative of all is the observation that waves of increased $[Ca^{2+}]_i$ in astrocytes can lead to changes in the activity of nearby neurons, which may be mediated by a neurotransmitter released from astrocytes. This interaction represents another form of glial-neuronal communication.

Oligodendrocytes and Schwann Cells Make and Sustain Myelin

The primary function of oligodendrocytes, as well as their PNS equivalent, the Schwann cell, is to provide and maintain myelin sheaths on axons of the central and peripheral nervous systems, respectively. As discussed in Chapter 7, myelin is the insulating electrical tape of the nervous system (see Fig. 7–21B) **Oligodendrocytes** are present in all areas of the CNS, although their morphology is highly variable and depends on their location within the brain. In regions of the brain that are dominated by myelinated nerve tracts, called "white matter," the oligodendrocytes responsible for myelination have a distinctive appearance (Fig. 16–14A). Such an oligodendrocyte has 15 to 30 processes, each of which connects a myelin sheath to the oligodendrocyte's cell body. Each myelin sheath, which is up to 250 μm wide, wraps many times around the long axis of one axon in the nerve fiber. The small exposed area of axon between adjacent myelin sheaths is called the **node of Ranvier** (p. 260).

During the myelination process, the leading edge of one of the processes of the oligodendrocyte cytoplasm wraps around the axon many times (Fig. 16–14A, upper axon). The cytoplasm is then squeezed out of the many

A OLIGODENDROCYTE

B SCHWANN CELL

FIGURE 16–14. Myelination of axons by oligodendrocytes and Schwann cells.

different (Table 16–4). For example, proteolipid protein is the most common protein in CNS myelin (~50% of total protein) but is absent in PNS myelin. Conversely, P0 is found almost exclusively in PNS myelin.

Myelination greatly enhances conduction of the action potential down the axon because it allows the regenerative electrical event to skip from one node to the next rather than gradually spreading down the whole extent of the axon. This process is called **saltatory conduction** (p. 200). Besides being responsible for CNS myelin, oligodendrocytes play another key role in saltatory conduction: they induce the clustering of Na^+ channels at the nodes (see Fig. 11–7C), which is essential for saltatory conduction.

FIGURE 16–15. Ensheathed versus myelinated axons. *A*, Ensheathed axons. This transmission electron micrograph shows a Schwann cell surrounding several *unmyelinated* peripheral axons, some of which are marked with an *asterisk*. The *arrows* point to the basal lamina. The *arrowhead* points to collagen fibrils. *B*, Myelinated axons. This transmission electron micrograph shows a Schwann cell (nucleus on right side of picture) surrounding a peripheral axon with several layers of myelin. The *lower star* shows the beginning of the spiraling myelin sheath, whereas the *upper star* indicates the termination of the spiral and a small region of noncompacted cytosol. The final magnification is about 14,000 in both panels. (Reproduced from Bunge RP, Fernandez-Valle C: In Kettemann H, Ransom RR [eds]: Neuroglia. New York, Oxford University Press, 1995, pp. 44–57; courtesy of Mary Bartlett Bunge.)

cell layers surrounding the axon in a process called **compaction**. This process creates layer upon layer of tightly compressed membranes that is called **myelin**. The myelin sheaths remain continuous with their parent glial cells.

In the PNS, a single **Schwann cell** provides a single myelin segment to a single axon of a myelinated nerve (see Fig. 16–14B). This situation stands in contrast to that in the CNS, where one oligodendrocyte myelinates many axons. The process of myelination that occurs in the PNS is analogous to that outlined earlier for oligodendrocytes. Axons of unmyelinated nerves are also associated with Schwann cells. In this case, the axons indent the surface of the Schwann cell and are completely surrounded by Schwann cell cytoplasm (Fig. 16–15).

Myelin has a different biochemical composition than the oligodendrocyte or Schwann cell plasma membrane from which it arose. Although PNS myelin and CNS myelin look similar, some of the constituent proteins are

TABLE 16-4

	CNS (% OF TOTAL MYELIN PROTEINS)	PNS (% OF TOTAL MYELIN PROTEINS)
PROTEIN		
MBP	30	18
PLP	50	<0.01
MAG	1	0.1
CNP	4	0.4
P0	<0.01	>50
P2	<1	1-15
PMP22	<0.01	5-10
MOG	0.05	<0.01

CNP, cyclic nucleotide phosphodiesterase; CNS, central nervous system; MAG, myelin-associated glycoprotein; MBP, myelin basic protein; MOG, myelin/oligodendrocyte glycoprotein; PLP, proteolipid protein; PMP22, peripheral myelin protein-22; PNS, peripheral nervous system.

It is well known that severed axons in the PNS can regenerate with restoration of lost function. Regrowth of these damaged axons is coordinated by the Schwann cells in the distal portion of the cut nerve. Severed axons in the CNS do not show functional regrowth, in part because of the growth-retarding nature of CNS myelin (p. 273).

Oligodendrocytes Are Involved in pH Regulation and Iron Metabolism in the Brain

Oligodendrocytes and myelin contain most of the enzyme carbonic anhydrase within the brain. The appearance of this enzyme during development closely parallels the maturation of these cells and the formation of myelin. Carbonic anhydrase rapidly catalyzes the reversible hydration of CO_2 (Box on p. 637) and may thus allow the CO_2/HCO_3^- buffer system to be maximally effective in buffering acid-base disturbances in the brain. pH regulation in the brain is important because it influences neuronal excitability. The classic example of the brain's sensitivity to pH is the reduced seizure threshold caused by the respiratory alkalosis secondary to hyperventilation (p. 641).

Oligodendrocytes are the cells in the brain most involved with iron metabolism. They contain the iron storage protein ferritin and the iron transport protein transferrin. Iron is necessary as a cofactor for certain enzymes and may catalyze the formation of free radicals under pathologic circumstances such as disruption of blood flow to the brain.

Microglial Cells Are the Macrophages of the CNS and Mediate Immune Responses Within the Brain

Microglial cells are of mesodermal origin and derive from cells related to the monocyte/macrophage lineage. Microglia represent about 20% of the total glial cells within the mature CNS. These cells are rapidly activated by injury to the brain, which causes them to proliferate, change shape, and become phagocytic (see Fig. 16-9B). When activated, they are capable of releasing substances that are toxic to neurons, including free radicals and nitric oxide. It is believed that microglia are involved in most brain diseases, not as initiators but as highly reactive cells that shape the brain's response to any insult.

Microglia are also the most effective antigen-presenting cells within the brain. Activated T lymphocytes are able to breech the BBB and enter the brain. To become mediators of tissue-specific disease or to destroy an invading infectious agent, T lymphocytes must recognize specific antigenic targets. Such recognition is accomplished through the process of antigen presentation, which is a function of the microglia.

REFERENCES

Books and Reviews

Abbott NJ (ed): Glial-neuronal interaction. Ann N Y Acad Sci 633:1–639, 1991.
Bunge RP: Glial cells and the central myelin sheath. Physiol Rev 48:197–251, 1968.
Kettenmann H, Ransom BR (eds): Neuroglia. New York, Oxford University Press, 1995.
Ransom BR, Sontheimer H: The neurophysiology of glial cells. J Clin Neurophysiol 9:224–251, 1992.

Journal Articles

Connors BW, Ransom BR, Kunis DM, Gutnick MJ: Activity-dependent K+ accumulation in the developing rat optic nerve. Science 216:1341–1343, 1982.
Hertz L, Dringen R, Schousboe A, Robinson SR: Astrocytes: Glutamate producers for neurons. J Neurosci Res 57:417–428, 1999.
Kaplan MR, Meyer-Franke A, Lambert S, et al: Induction of sodium channel clustering by oligodendrocytes. Nature 386:724–728, 1997.
Karwoski CJ, Lu HK, Newman EA: Spatial buffering of light-evoked potassium increases by retinal Müller (glial) cells. Science 244:578–580, 1989.
Newman EA, Zahs KR: Modulation of neuronal activity by glial cells in the retina. J Neurosci 18:4022–4028, 1998.
Ransom BR, Fern R: Does astrocytic glycogen benefit axon function and survival in CNS white matter during glucose deprivation? Glia 21:134–141, 1997.

IV

The Cardiovascular System

CHAPTER 17

Organization of the Cardiovascular System

Emile L. Boulpaep

ELEMENTS OF THE CARDIOVASCULAR SYSTEM

The Circulation Is an Evolutionary Consequence of Body Size

Isolated single cells and small organisms do not have a circulatory system. They can meet their metabolic needs by the simple processes of diffusion and convection of solutes from the *external* to the *internal milieu* (Fig. 17–1A). The requirement for a circulatory system is an evolutionary consequence of the increasing size and complexity of multicellular organisms. Simple diffusion (p. 56) is not adequate to supply nutrients to centrally located cells, nor to eliminate waste products; in large organisms, the distances separating the central cells from the *external milieu* are too long. A simple closed-end tube (see Fig. 17–1B), penetrating from the extracellular compartment and feeding a central cell deep in the core of the organism, would not be sufficient. The concentration of nutrients inside the tube would become very low at its closed end, because of both the uptake of these nutrients by the cell and the long path for re-supply leading to the cell. Conversely, the concentration of waste products inside the tube would become very high at the closed end. Such a tube represents a long **unstirred layer**; as a result, the concentration gradients for both nutrients and wastes across the membrane of the central cell are very small.

In complex organisms, a **circulatory system** provides a steep concentration gradient from the blood to the central cells for nutrients, and in the opposite direction for waste products. Maintaining such steep intracellular-to-extracellular concentration gradients requires a fast convection system that rapidly circulates fluid between surfaces that equilibrate with the *external milieu* (e.g., the lung, gut, and kidney epithelia) and individual central cells deep inside the organism (see Fig. 17–1C). In mammals and birds, the exchange of gases with the external milieu is so important that they have evolved a two-pump, dual circulatory system (see Fig. 17–1D) that delivers the full output of the "heart" to the lungs (p. 695).

The primary role of the circulatory system is the distribution of dissolved gases and other molecules for nutrition, growth, and repair. Secondary roles have also evolved: (1) fast chemical signalling to cells by means of circulating hormones or neurotransmitters, (2) dissipating heat by delivering heat from the core to the surface of the body, and (3) mediating inflammatory and host defense responses against invading microorganisms.

A UNICELLULAR ORGANISM

B MULTICELLULAR ORGANISM

The concentration of waste gradually decreases in its path from left (central cell) towards the right (stirred external milieu).

The concentration of nutrients gradually decreases in its path from right (stirred external milieu) to left (central cell).

C CIRCULATION WITH ONE PUMP

D CIRCULATION WITH TWO PUMPS / TWO CIRCUITS

The circulatory system of humans integrates three basic functional parts, or organs: a pump (the **heart**) that circulates a liquid (the **blood**) through a set of containers (the **vessels**). This integrated system is able to adapt to the changing circumstances of normal life. Demand on the circulation fluctuates widely between sleep and wakefulness, between rest and exercise, with acceleration/deceleration, during changes in body position or intrathoracic pressure, during digestion, and under emotional or thermal stress. To meet these variable demands, the entire system requires sophisticated and integrated regulation.

The Heart Is a Dual Pump That Drives the Blood in Two Serial Circuits: The Systemic and the Pulmonary Circulations

A remarkable pump, weighing approximately 300 g, drives the human circulation. The heart really consists of two pumps, the **left heart** or main pump, and the **right heart** or boost pump (see Fig. 17–1D). These operate in series and require a delicate equalization of their outputs. The output of each pump is approximately 5 liters/min, but this can easily increase fivefold during exercise.

Over a 75-year lifetime, the two ventricles combined pump 400 million liters of blood (enough to fill a lake 1 km long, 40 m wide, and 10 m deep). The circulating fluid itself is an organ, kept in a liquid state by mechanisms that actively prevent cell-cell adhesion and coagulation. With each heartbeat, the ventricles impart the energy necessary to circulate the blood by generating the pressure head that drives the flow of blood through the **vascular system**. On the basis of its anatomy, we can divide this system of tubes into two main circuits: the **systemic** and the **pulmonary** circulations (see Fig. 17–1D). We could also divide the vascular system into a **high-pressure** part (extending from the contracting left ventricle to the systemic capillaries) and a **low-pressure** part (extending from the systemic capillaries, through the right heart, across the pulmonary circulation and left atrium, and into the left ventricle in its relaxed state). The vessels also respond to the changing metabolic demands of the tissues they supply by directing blood flow to (or away from) tissues as demands change. The circulatory system is also self-repairing/self-expanding. Endothelial cells lining vessels mend the surfaces of existing blood vessels and generate new vessels (**angiogenesis**).

Some of the most important life-threatening human diseases are caused by failure of the heart as a pump (e.g., congestive heart failure), failure of the blood as an effective liquid organ (e.g., thrombosis and embolism), or failure of the vasculature either as a competent container (e.g., hemorrhage) or as an efficient distribution system (e.g., atherosclerosis). Moreover, failure of the normal interactions among these three organs can by itself elicit or aggravate many human pathologies.

Blood Is a Suspension of Cellular Elements in Plasma

Blood is a complex fluid. If you spin down a sample of blood containing an anticoagulant, the bottom fraction contains formed elements—red blood cells (RBCs), white blood cells (i.e., granulocytes, lymphocytes, and monocytes), and platelets—whereas the top fraction is blood plasma. The hematocrit (p. 51) is the fraction of the total column occupied by RBCs.

Plasma is a pale-white watery solution of electrolytes, plasma proteins, carbohydrates, and lipids (Table 2–02). The electrolyte composition of plasma differs only slightly from that of interstitial fluid. The principal plasma proteins (p. 472) are albumin, globulins, fibrinogen, and other coagulation factors. The electrophoretic mobility of plasma proteins in decreasing order comprises albumins (lowest molecular weight), α_1-globulins, α_2-globulins, β-globulins, fibrinogen, and γ-globulins. The γ-globulins include the circulating antibodies (i.e., immunoglobulins). The liver produces albumin and most of the globulins and coagulation factors. The remaining globulins are the immunoglobulins synthesized by B lymphocytes.

Many proteins are involved in blood coagulation through a "coagulation cascade" in which serine proteases cleave inactive coagulation factors into active factors, which are themselves serine proteases. This cascade can begin via either the intrinsic or the extrinsic pathway, which converge. The end point of the cascade is the cleavage of fibrinogen into fibrin monomers, which assemble into a fibrin polymer. Cross-linked fibrin polymers form strands that trap red and white cells, platelets, and plasma inside the thrombus (i.e., blood clot). Subsequent interaction of myosin and actin in the platelets of the clot allows the clot to shrink to a plug that expels a slightly yellow-tinged fluid. This residual fluid is **serum**, which differs principally from plasma by the absence of fibrinogen and other coagulation factors; however, serum still contains antibodies. Note that *plasma* can also form a clot, but a plasma clot does not retract because it lacks platelets.

Blood is normally in a liquid state inside blood vessels because it does not come into contact with negatively charged surfaces (e.g., the collagen beneath endothelial cells) that activate the *intrinsic* coagulation pathway, nor does it contact tissue factors (e.g., thromboplastin released from damaged tissue) that activate the *extrinsic* pathway. Furthermore, thrombolytic pathways keep the coagulation pathways in check. Indeed, plasma contains plasminogen,

---

FIGURE 17–1. Role of circulatory system in promoting diffusion In *C*, nutrients and wastes exchange across two barriers: a "surface for equilibration" between external milieu and blood, and another surface between blood and the "central cell." As shown in the *inset*, blood is the conduit that connects the external milieu (e.g., lumina of lung, gut, and kidney) to the internal milieu (i.e., extracellular fluid bathing central cells). In *D*, the system is far more efficient because it uses one circuit for exchanging gases with the stirred external milieu, and another circuit for exchanging nutrients and nongaseous wastes.

FIGURE 17–2. Flow through a straight tube The flow (F) between a high-pressure point (P_1) and low-pressure point (P_2) is proportional to pressure difference (ΔP). A_1 and A_2 are cross-sectional areas at these two points. A cylindrical bolus of fluid—between the disks at points 1 and 2—moves down tube with a linear velocity, v.

which tissue plasminogen activator (t-PA) can convert to **plasmin**, a protease that digests fibrin and thereby lyses blood clots.

HEMODYNAMICS

Blood Flow Is Driven by a Constant Pressure Head Across Variable Resistances

To keep concepts simple, first think of the left heart as a constant pressure generator that maintains a steady mean arterial pressure at its exit (i.e., the aorta). In other words, assume that blood flow throughout the circulation is steady or nonpulsatile (later in the chapter, see discussion of the consequences of normal cyclic variations in flow and pressure that occur as the result of the heartbeat). As a further simplification, assume that the entire systemic circulation is a single, straight tube.

To understand the *steady flow* of blood, driven by a *constant pressure* head, we can apply classical hydrodynamic laws. The most important is analogous to Ohm's law of electricity:

Equation 17–1

$$\Delta V = I \cdot R \qquad \text{for electricity}$$

$$\Delta P = F \cdot R \qquad \text{for liquids}$$

That is, the pressure difference (ΔP) between an upstream point (pressure P_1) and a downstream site (pressure P_2) is equal to the product of the flow (F) and the resistance (R) between those two points (Fig. 17–2). Ohm's law of hydrodynamics holds at any instant in time, regardless of how simple or how complicated the circuit. This equation also does not require any assumptions about whether the vessels are rigid or compliant, as long as R is constant.

In reality, the **pressure difference (ΔP)** between the beginning and end points of the human systemic circulation—that is, between the high-pressure side (aorta) and the low-pressure side (vena cava)—turns out to be fairly constant over time. Thus, the heart behaves more as a generator of a constant pressure head than as a generator of constant flow, at least within physiologic limits. Indeed, **flow (F)**—the output of the left heart—is quite variable in time and depends greatly on the physiologic

circumstances (e.g., whether one is active or at rest). Like flow, **resistance (R)** varies with time; in addition, it varies with location within the body. The overall resistance of the circulation reflects the contributions of a complex network of vessels in both the systemic and pulmonary circuits.

Blood can take many different pathways *from the left heart to the right heart* (Fig. 17–3): (1) a single capillary bed (e.g., coronary capillaries), (2) two capillary beds in series (e.g., glomerular and peritubular capillaries in the kidney), or (3) two capillary beds in parallel that subsequently merge and feed into a single capillary bed in series (e.g., the parallel splenic and mesenteric circulations, which merge on entering the portal hepatic circulation). In contrast, blood flow *from the right heart to the left heart* can take only a single pathway, across a single capillary bed in the pulmonary circulation. Finally, some blood also courses *from the left heart directly back to the left heart* across shunt pathways, the most important of which is the bronchial circulation.

The overall resistance (R_{Total}) across a circulatory bed results from parallel and serial arrangements of branches, and is governed by laws similar to those for the electrical resistance of DC circuits. For multiple resistance elements (R_1, R_2, $R_3 \cdots$) arranged in series:

Equation 17–2

$$R_{Total} = R_1 + R_2 + R_3 + \cdots$$

For multiple elements arranged in parallel:

Equation 17–3

$$\frac{1}{R_{Total}} = \frac{1}{R_1} + \frac{1}{R_2} + \frac{1}{R_3} + \cdots$$

Blood Pressure Is Always Measured as a Pressure Difference Between Two Points

Physicists measure pressure in the units of Pascals, g/cm^2, or $dynes/cm^2$. However, physiologists most often gauge blood pressure by the height it can drive a column of liquid. This pressure is:

Equation 17–4

$$P = \rho \, g \, h$$

where ρ is the density of the liquid in the column, g is the gravitational constant, and h is the height of the column.

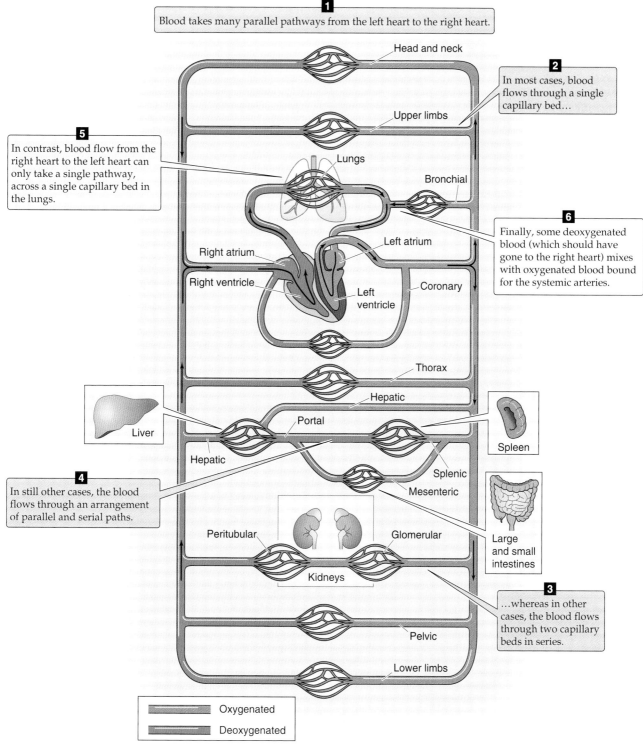

1
Blood takes many parallel pathways from the left heart to the right heart.

Head and neck

2
In most cases, blood flows through a single capillary bed…

Upper limbs

5
In contrast, blood flow from the right heart to the left heart can only take a single pathway, across a single capillary bed in the lungs.

Lungs

Bronchial

Left atrium

6
Finally, some deoxygenated blood (which should have gone to the right heart) mixes with oxygenated blood bound for the systemic arteries.

Right atrium

Right ventricle

Left ventricle

Coronary

Thorax

Hepatic

Liver

Portal

Spleen

Hepatic

Splenic

4
In still other cases, the blood flows through an arrangement of parallel and serial paths.

Mesenteric

Large and small intestines

Peritubular

Glomerular

Kidneys

3
…whereas in other cases, the blood flows through two capillary beds in series.

Pelvic

Lower limbs

Oxygenated
Deoxygenated

FIGURE 17–3. Circulatory beds.

Therefore, if we neglect variations in g, and know ρ for the fluid in the column (usually water or mercury), we can take the height of the liquid column as a measure of blood pressure. Physiologists usually express this pressure in mm Hg or cm H_2O. Clinicians use the classical blood pressure gauge (sphygmomanometer) to report arterial blood pressure in mm Hg.

Pressure is never expressed in absolute terms, but as a **pressure difference** ΔP, relative to some "reference" pressure. We can make this concept intuitively clear by considering pressure as a force $\mathscr{F}$ applied to a surface area A.

Equation 17–5

$$P = \mathscr{F}/A$$

If we apply a force to one side of a free-swinging door, we cannot predict the direction the door will move unless we know what force a colleague may be applying on the opposite side. In other words, we can define a movement or distortion of a mechanical system only by the *difference* between two forces. In electricity, we compare the difference between two voltages. In hemodynamics, we compare the difference between two pressures. When not explicitly stated, the reference pressure in human physiology is the atmospheric or barometric pressure (P_B). Because P_B on earth is never zero, a pressure reading obtained at some site within the circulation, and referred to P_B, actually does not express the absolute pressure in that blood vessel, but rather the difference between the pressure inside the vessel and P_B.

Because a pressure difference is always between two points—and these two points are separated by some **distance** (Δx), and have a **spatial orientation** to one another—we can define a **pressure gradient** ($\Delta P/\Delta x$) with a spatial orientation. Considering orientation, we can define three different kinds of pressure differences in the circulation:

1. **Driving pressure.** In Figure 17–4, the ΔP between points x_1 and x_2 inside the vessel—along the axis of the vessel—is the **axial pressure difference**. Because this ΔP causes blood to flow from x_1 to x_2, it is also known as the driving pressure. In the circulation, the driving pressure is the ΔP between the arterial and venous ends of the systemic (or pulmonary) circulation, and it governs blood flow. Indeed, this is the only ΔP we need to consider to understand flow in horizontal rigid tubes (see Fig. 17–2).
2. **Transmural pressure.** The ΔP in Figure 17–4 between point r_1 (inside the vessel) and r_2 (just outside the vessel)—along the radial axis—is an example of a **radial pressure difference**. Although there is normally no pressure difference through the blood along the radial axis, the pressure drops steeply across the vessel

wall itself. The ΔP between r_1 and r_2 is the transmural pressure, that is, the difference between the intravascular pressure and the tissue pressure. Because blood vessels are distensible, transmural pressure governs vessel diameter, which is in turn the major determinant of resistance.
3. **Hydrostatic pressure.** Because of the density of blood and gravitational forces, a third pressure difference arises if the vessel does not lie in a horizontal plane, as was the case in Figure 17–2. The ΔP in Figure 17–4 between point h_1 (*top of a liquid column*) and h_2 (*bottom of column*)—along the height axis—is the hydrostatic pressure difference. This ΔP is similar to the P in Equation 17-4 (here, ρ is the density of blood) and it exists even in the absence of any blood flow.

Total Blood Flow, or Cardiac Output, Is the Product (Heart Rate) × (Stroke Volume)

The flow of blood delivered by the heart, or the total mean flow in the circulation, is the **cardiac output** (CO). The output during a single heartbeat, from either the left or the right ventricle, is the **stroke volume** (SV). For a given **heart rate** (HR):

Equation 17–6

$$CO = F = HR \cdot SV$$

The cardiac output is usually expressed in liters/min; at rest, it is approximately 5 liters/min. The **principle of continuity** of flow requires that two sets of vessels in series have the same flow, assuming that between them no fluid has been added or subtracted. Therefore, the cardiac outputs of the right and left hearts must be equal in the steady state.

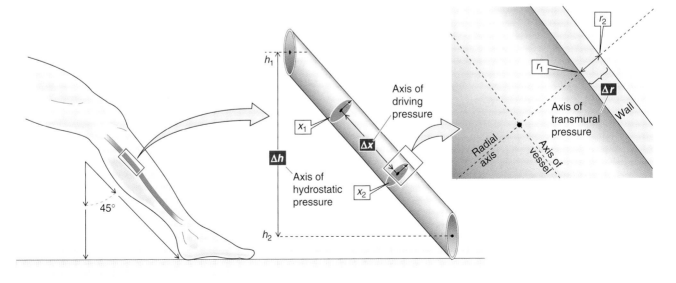

FIGURE 17–4. Three kinds of pressure differences—and their axes—in a blood vessel.

Flow in an Idealized Vessel Increases with the Fourth Power of Radius (Poiseuille's Equation)

Flow (F) is the displacement of volume (ΔV) per unit time (Δt):

Equation 17–7

$$F = \frac{\Delta V}{\Delta t}$$

In Figure 17–2, we could be watching a bolus (*the blue cylinder*)—with an area A and a length L—move along the tube with a mean velocity $\bar{v}$. During a time interval Δt, the cylinder advances by Δx, so that the volume passing some checkpoint (e.g., at P_2) is (A · Δx). Thus,

Equation 17–8

$$F = \frac{\overbrace{A \cdot \Delta x}^{\frac{\Delta V}{\Delta t}}}{\Delta t} = A \cdot \overbrace{\frac{\Delta x}{\Delta t}}^{\bar{v}} = A \cdot \bar{v}$$

This equation holds at any point along the circulation, regardless of how complicated the circulation is, or how irregular the cross-sectional area.

In a physically well-defined system, it is also possible to *predict* the flow from the geometry of the vessel and the properties of the fluid. In 1840 and 1841, Jean Poiseuille observed the flow of liquids in tubes of small diameter, and derived the law associated with his name. In a straight, rigid, cylindrical tube:

Equation 17–9

$$F = \Delta P \cdot \underbrace{\frac{\pi r^4}{8 \eta \ell}}_{1/R}$$

This is the Poiseuille-Hagen equation, where *F* is the flow, ΔP is the driving pressure, *r* is the inner radius of the tube, ℓ is its length, and η is the viscosity. The Poiseuille equation requires that both driving pressure and the resulting flow be constant.

Three implications of Poiseuille's law are that flow is:

1. Directly proportional to the axial pressure difference, ΔP. The proportionality constant—(π r⁴)/(8 η ℓ)—is the reciprocal of resistance (R), as is presented later.
2. Directly proportional to the fourth power of vessel radius.
3. Inversely proportional to both the length of the vessel and the viscosity of the fluid.

Unlike Ohm's law of hydrodynamics (F = ΔP/R), which applies to *all* vessels, no matter how complicated, Poiseuille's equation applies only to rigid, cylindrical tubes. Moreover, later discussion in this chapter reveals that the fluid flowing through the tube must satisfy certain conditions.

Viscous Resistance to Flow Is Proportional to the Viscosity of Blood, but Does Not Depend on Properties of the Blood-Vessel Walls

The simplest approach for expressing vascular resistance is to rearrange Ohm's law of hydrodynamics (see Equation 17–1):

Equation 17–10

$$R = \frac{\Delta P}{F}$$

This approach is independent of geometry, and is even applicable to very complex circuits, such as the entire peripheral circulation. Moreover, we can conveniently express resistance in units used by physicians for pressure (mm Hg) and flow (ml/sec). Thus, the units of total peripheral resistance are mm Hg/(ml/sec)—also known as **peripheral resistance units** (PRUs).

Alternatively, if the flow through the tube fulfills Poiseuille's requirements, we can express "viscous" resistance in terms of the dimensions of the vessel and the *viscous* properties of the circulating fluid. Combining Equation 17–9 and Equation 17–10:

Equation 17–11

$$R = \frac{8}{\pi} \cdot \frac{\eta \ell}{r^4}$$

Thus, *viscous* resistance is proportional to the *viscosity* of the fluid and the length of the tube, but inversely proportional to the fourth power of the radius of the blood vessel. Note that this equation makes no statement regarding the properties of the vessel wall per se. The resistance to flow results from the geometry of the fluid—as described by ℓ and *r*—and the internal friction of the fluid, the **viscosity** (η). Viscosity is a property of the content (i.e., the fluid), unrelated to any property of the container (i.e., the vessel).

The Viscosity of Blood Is a Measure of the Internal Slipperiness between Layers of Fluid

Viscosity is an expression of the degree of slipperiness between two layers of fluid. Isaac Newton described the interaction as illustrated in Figure 17–5A. Imagine that two parallel planes of fluid, each with an area A, are moving past one another. The velocity of the first is v, and the velocity of the slightly faster moving second plane is v + Δv. The separation between the two planes is Δx. The *velocity gradient* between the moving planes, Δv/Δx (units: (cm/sec)/cm = sec⁻¹), is the **shear rate**. The *force* that we must apply to the second sheet to make it move faster than the first is the **shear stress**. The greater the area of the sheets, the greater is the force needed to overcome the friction between them. Thus, shear stress is expressed as force per unit area (F/A). The *shear stress* required to produce a particular *shear rate* Newton defined as the viscosity:

Equation 17–12

$$\eta = \frac{\text{shear stress}}{\text{shear rate}} = \frac{F/A}{\Delta v/\Delta x}$$

A   DEFINITION OF VISCOSITY

B   VISCOUS FLOW IN A CYLINDER

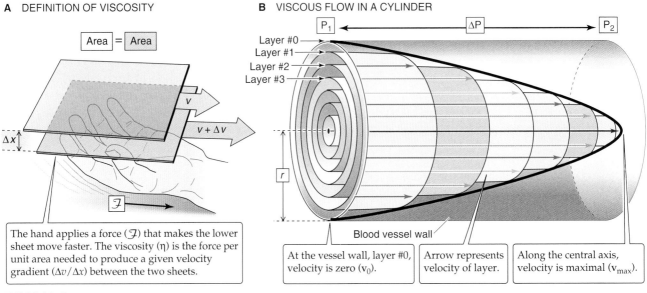

The hand applies a force ($\mathcal{F}$) that makes the lower sheet move faster. The viscosity (η) is the force per unit area needed to produce a given velocity gradient ($\Delta v / \Delta x$) between the two sheets.

At the vessel wall, layer #0, velocity is zero (v_0).

Arrow represents velocity of layer.

Along the central axis, velocity is maximal (v_{max}).

Blood vessel wall

FIGURE 17–5. Viscosity.

Viscosity measures the resistance to sliding when layers of fluid are shearing against each other. The unit of viscosity is a **poise** (P). Whole blood has a viscosity of approximately 3 centipoise (cP).

If one applies Newton's definition of viscosity to a cylindrical blood vessel, the shearing laminae of the blood are not planar, but concentric cylinders (see Fig. 17–5B). If we apply a pressure head to the blood in the vessel, each lamina will move parallel to the long axis of the tube. Because of cohesive forces between the inner surface of the vessel wall and the blood, we can assume that an infinitesimally thin layer of blood (Fig. 17–5B, *layer #0*) close to the wall of the tube cannot move. However, the next concentric cylindrical layer, *layer #1*, moves in relation to the stationary outer layer #0, but slower than the next inner concentric cylinder, *layer #2*, and so on. Thus, the velocities increase from the wall to the center of the cylinder. The resulting velocity profile is a parabola with a maximum velocity, v_{max}, at the central axis. The lower the viscosity, the sharper the point of the bullet-shaped velocity profile.

HOW BLOOD FLOWS

As discussed, Poiseuille's relationship (Equation 17–9) is based on solid empirical and theoretical grounds. However, the equation requires the following assumptions:

1. The fluid must be incompressible.
2. The tube must be straight, rigid, cylindrical, and unbranched, and have a constant radius.
3. The velocity of the thin fluid layer at the wall must be zero (i.e., no "slippage"). This assumption holds for aqueous solutions, but not for some "plastic" fluids.
4. The flow must be laminar. That is, the fluid must move in concentric undisturbed laminae, without the gross exchange of fluid from one concentric shell to another.

5. The viscosity of the fluid must be constant. First, it must be constant throughout the cross section of the cylinder. Second, it must be constant in the "Newtonian" sense; that is, the viscosity must be independent of the magnitude of the shear stress (i.e., force applied) and the shear rate (i.e., velocity gradient produced).
6. The flow must be steady (i.e., not pulsatile).

To what extent does the circulatory system fulfill the conditions of Poiseuille's equation? The first condition (i.e., incompressible fluid) is well satisfied by blood. If we consider only flow in a vessel segment that is of fairly fixed size (e.g., thoracic aorta), the second assumption (i.e., simple geometry) is also reasonably satisfied. The third requirement (i.e., no "slippage") is true for blood in blood vessels. Indeed, if one forms a reservoir out of a piece of vessel (e.g., aorta) and fills it with blood, a meniscus forms with the concave surface facing upward, indicating adherence of blood to the vessel wall.

The last three assumptions, which are more complex, are the subject of the next three sections.

Blood Flow Is Laminar

From Ohm's law of hydrodynamics ($\Delta P = F \cdot R$), flow should increase linearly with driving pressure if resistance is constant. In cylindrical vessels, flow does indeed increase linearly with ΔP *up to a certain point* (Fig. 17–6A). However, at high flow rates—beyond a critical velocity—flow rises less steeply and is no longer proportional to ΔP, but to roughly the square root of ΔP, because R apparently increases. Here, blood flow is no longer laminar, but **turbulent**. Because turbulence causes substantial kinetic energy losses, it is energetically wasteful.

The critical parameter that determines when flow becomes turbulent is a dimensionless quantity called **Reynolds number (Re)**, named after Osborne Reynolds:

A PRESSURE-FLOW RELATIONSHIP

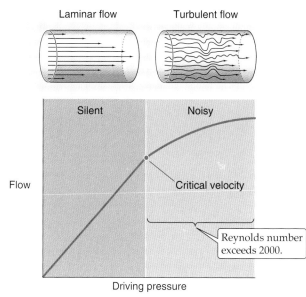

Laminar flow   Turbulent flow

Silent   Noisy

Flow

Critical velocity

Reynolds number
exceeds 2000.

Driving pressure

FIGURE 17–6. Laminar versus turbulent flow.

B VELOCITY PROFILES

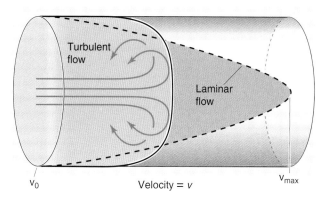

Turbulent
flow

Laminar
flow

v_0 Velocity = v v_{max}

Equation 17–13

$$Re = \frac{2r\bar{v}\rho}{\eta}$$

Blood flow is laminar when Re is below approximately 2000, and is mostly turbulent when Re exceeds approximately 3000. The terms in the numerator reflect disruptive forces produced by the *inertial momentum* in the fluid. Thus, turbulent blood flow occurs where r is large (e.g., aorta) or when $\bar{v}$ is large (e.g., high cardiac output). Turbulent flow can also occur when a local decrease in vessel diameter (e.g., arterial stenosis) causes a local increase in $\bar{v}$. The term in the denominator of Equation 17–13, viscosity, reflects the cohesive forces that tend to keep the layers well organized. Therefore, a low viscosity (e.g., anemia—a low red blood cell count) predisposes to turbulence. When turbulence arises, the parabolic profile of the linear velocity across the radius of a cylinder becomes blunted (see Fig. 17–6B).

The distinction between laminar and turbulent flow is clinically very significant. Laminar flow is silent, whereas vortex formation during turbulence sets up **murmurs.** These "Korotkoff sounds" are useful in assessing arterial blood flow in the traditional auscultatory method for determining blood pressure. These murmurs are also important for diagnosing vessel stenosis, vessel shunts, and cardiac valvular lesions (see the box on Heart Murmurs and Arterial Bruits). Intense forms of turbulence may be detected not only as loud acoustic murmurs, but also as mechanical vibrations or **thrills** that can be felt by touch.

Whole Blood Has an Anomalous Viscosity

Water and saline solutions are homogenous or Newtonian liquids. For these, the relationship between shear stress (force needed to move one lamina faster than its neighbor) and shear rate (velocity gradient between laminae) is linear and passes through the origin (Fig. 17–7, *blue*

HEART MURMURS AND ARTERIAL BRUITS

Turbulence as blood flows across diseased heart valves creates murmurs that can be readily detected by auscultation with a stethoscope. The factors causing turbulence are the ones that increase Reynolds number: increases in vessel diameter or blood velocity and decreases in viscosity. Before the advent of sophisticated technology, such as cardiac ultrasound, clinicians made a fine art of detecting these murmurs in an attempt to diagnose cardiac valvular disease. In general, it was appreciated that normal blood flow across normal heart valves is silent, although murmurs can occur with increased blood flow (e.g., exercise) and are not infrequently heard in young, thin individuals with dynamic circulations. The grading of heart murmurs helps to standardize the cardiac examination from observer to observer. Thus, a grade 1 heart murmur is barely audible, grade 2 is one that is slightly more easily heard, and grades 3 and 4 are progressively louder. A grade 5 murmur is the loudest murmur that still requires a stethoscope to hear. A grade 6 murmur is so loud it can be heard with the stethoscope off the chest, and is often accompanied by a thrill. The location, duration, pitch, and quality of a murmur aid in identifying the underlying valvular disorder.

Blood flowing through diseased arteries can also create a murmur or a thrill. By far the most common cause is atherosclerosis, which narrows the vessel lumen and thus increases velocity. In patients with advanced disease, these murmurs can be heard in virtually every major artery, most easily in the carotid and femoral arteries. Arterial murmurs are usually referred to as bruits.

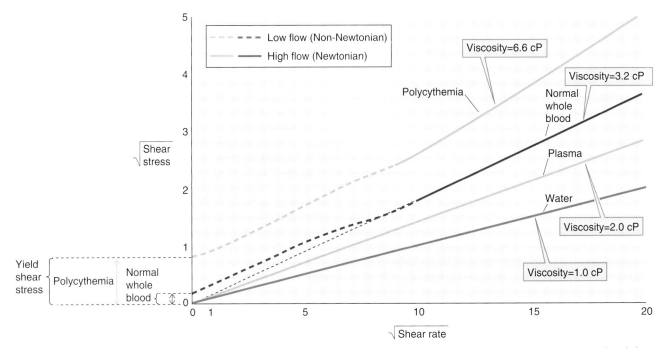

FIGURE 17–7. Anomalous viscosity of blood. To emphasize deviations from linearity, we plot the square roots of shear stress (Force/Area) and shear rate ($\Delta v/\Delta x$). cP, centipoise.

line). Viscosity (see Equation 17–12) is the slope of this line. The shear-stress to shear-rate relationship for a non-Newtonian fluid, such as latex house paint, is nonlinear. Blood plasma (see Fig. 17–7, *yellow line*) and serum are very nearly Newtonian. However, normal *whole blood is non-Newtonian*: it has a nonlinear shear-stress to shear-rate relationship that intersects the y-axis above the origin (see Fig. 17–7, *red curve*). In other words, one has to apply some threshold force (i.e., the "*yield shear stress*") before the fluid will move at all. At lower forces, the fluid is immobile. However, at higher shear rates (such as those achieved physiologically after the velocity of blood flow has increased sufficiently), the relationship between shear stress and shear rate assumes the Newtonian ideal, with a slope that corresponds to a viscosity of approximately 3.2 cP.

The concept of "yield shear stress" can best be understood by comparing two familiar viscous solutions: honey and mayonnaise. By estimating the effort needed to stir a pot of honey or a jar of mayonnaise with a spoon, one might assume that their apparent viscosity is the same because each solution offers about the same resistance to deformation. However, using a more modest deforming force, such as gravity, a striking difference between the two fluids emerges. As one removes the spoon from the pot of honey, gravity causes the honey to drip from the spoon in a continuous stream. In contrast, a glob of mayonnaise stays attached to the spoon. The velocity of the mayonnaise is zero because its "yield shear stress" is greater than the force of gravity. Honey is a Newtonian fluid that behaves similarly at low and high forces of deformation. Mayonnaise is similar to blood in that its viscosity appears to be infinite at low forces of deformation.

In practice, the effective viscosity of whole blood depends on several physiologic factors: (1) fibrinogen concentration, (2) hematocrit, (3) vessel radius, (4) linear velocity, and (5) temperature. As noted previously, the viscosity of whole blood in the linear (or Newtonian) region of Figure 17–7 is approximately 3.2 cP, assuming a typical fibrinogen concentration of 260 mg/dl, a hematocrit of 40%, and a temperature of 37°C. We will now see how each of these five factors influences the viscosity of blood.

FIBRINOGEN. Fibrinogen is a major protein component of human blood and a key element in the coagulation cascade responsible for clotting. The main reason for the non-Newtonian behavior of blood is the interaction of this fibrinogen with red blood cells. Thus, plasma (which contains fibrinogen, but not RBCs) is Newtonian, as is a suspension of washed RBCs in saline (without fibrinogen). However, the simultaneous presence of fibrinogen and blood cells causes the nonlinear behavior illustrated by the red curve in Figure 17–7. At normal hematocrits, fibrinogen, and, perhaps, the β-lipoproteins are the only plasma proteins capable of creating a "yield shear stress."

At normal hematocrits, the absence of fibrinogen (afibrinogenemia) eliminates the "yield shear stress" altogether. Conversely, hyperfibrinogenemia elevates "yield shear stress" and, in the extreme, leads to a clustering of RBCs that increases their "effective density." This increased effective density, in turn, causes the RBCs to settle toward the bottom of a vertical tube—easily measured as an increased **erythrocyte sedimentation rate** (see the box on Erythrocyte Sedimentation Rate).

HEMATOCRIT. Increases in hematocrit elevate blood viscosity by two mechanisms (Fig. 17–8). One prevails at physiological hematocrits, and the other at higher hematocrits. Starting from values of 30%, raising the hematocrit

ERYTHROCYTE SEDIMENTATION RATE

Almost any acute stress to the body (e.g., trauma, infection, disease) induces a reaction called the **acute phase response**. Over the course of several hours, the liver rapidly synthesizes and secretes into the circulatory system a number of proteins that aid in the host response to the threat. Among these proteins is fibrinogen, which causes RBCs to cluster and increases their effective density. When anticoagulated blood from a patient with hyperfibrinogenemia is placed in a glass tube, the RBCs fall more quickly under the influence of gravity than when the blood is from a healthy subject. After 1 hour, this sedimentation leaves a layer of clear plasma on the top of the tube, 15 mm thick for normal blood, and often greater than 40 mm in certain inflammatory disorders. This rate of fall is called the erythrocyte sedimentation rate (ESR). Although very nonspecific because so many different conditions can cause it to increase, the ESR is still widely used by clinicians to assess the presence and severity of inflammation. It is a simple technique, easily performed in a physician's office. As an example of its utility, a patient with an inflammatory process that naturally waxes and wanes, such as lupus erythematosus, may present with nonspecific complaints such as fatigue, weakness, and achiness. An elevated ESR would suggest that these complaints are due to the reactivation of the disease, and not just to a poor night's sleep or depression.

increases the interactions among RBCs—both directly and via proteins such as fibrinogen—and thereby increases viscosity. The reason is that forcing two RBCs more closely together at higher hematocrits makes them more likely to stick to each other. At hematocrits above 60%, the cells are so tightly packed that further increases lead to cell-cell interactions that increasingly deform the RBCs, thereby increasing viscosity. In patients with polycythemia, not only is viscosity high, but the yield stress

can be more than 4-fold higher than normal (see Fig. 17–7, *green curve*). Obviously, the combination of a high hematocrit and a high fibrinogen level can be expected to lead to extremely high viscosities.

VESSEL RADIUS. In reasonably large vessels (radius > approximately 1 mm), blood viscosity is independent of vessel radius (Fig. 17–9A). However, the viscosity decreases steeply at lower radii. This Fahraeus-Lindqvist phenomenon has four major causes:

1. Poiseuille observed not only that red blood cells move faster in the center of an arteriole or venule than at the periphery, but also that the *concentration* of RBCs is greater at the center. Indeed, very near the wall, he observed a "transparent space" occupied only by plasma (see Fig. 17–9B). This **axial accumulation** of RBCs occurs because the plasma imparts a spin to an erythrocyte caught between two layers of plasma sliding past one another at different velocities (see Fig. 17–5B). This spin causes the cell to move toward the center of the vessel, much as a billiard ball curves when struck off center (see Fig. 17–9B, *inset of upper panel*). One consequence of axial accumulation is that local viscosity is lowest in the cell-poor region near the vessel wall, and greatest in the cell-enriched core. The net effect in smaller vessels is that the overall viscosity of the blood is *decreased* because the cell-poor plasma (low intrinsic viscosity) moves to the periphery where the shearing forces are the greatest, whereas the cell-enriched blood (high intrinsic viscosity) is left along the central axis where the shearing forces are least. A second consequence of axial accumulation is that branch vessels preferentially skim the plasma ("plasma skimming") from the main stream of the parent vessel, leading to a lower hematocrit in branch vessels. However, some anatomic sites prevent skimming by means of an arterial cushion (see Fig. 17–9B, *lower panel*).

2. Poiseuille's equation does not hold in vessels small enough to hold only a few RBCs in their cross section. Hagen's derivation of the equation assumes an infinite number of concentric laminae inside the vessel. In reality, a lamina can be no smaller than the thickness

FIGURE 17–8. Dependence of viscosity on hematocrit. cP, centipoise.

A   DEPENDENCE OF RELATIVE
VISCOSITY ON VESSEL RADIUS

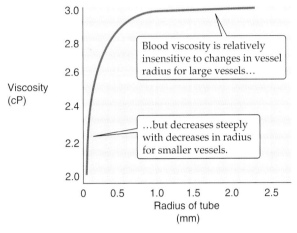

Viscosity
(cP)

Blood viscosity is relatively
insensitive to changes in vessel
radius for large vessels…

…but decreases steeply
with decreases in radius
for smaller vessels.

B   AXIAL ACCUMULATION

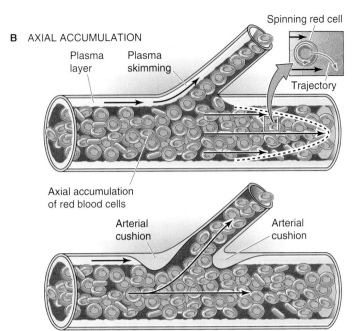

Plasma
layer

Plasma
skimming

Spinning red cell

Trajectory

Axial accumulation
of red blood cells

Arterial
cushion

Arterial
cushion

C   LIMITED NUMBER OF LAMINAE IN SMALL VESSEL

D   TANK TREADING OF RED BLOOD CELLS

Spinning plasma

E   DEFORMATION OF RED BLOOD CELLS

FIGURE 17–9. Dependence of viscosity of vessel radius. cP, centipoise.

of an erythrocyte, thus severely limiting the number of laminae in small vessels (see Fig. 17–9C). If we were to re-derive a Poiseuille-like equation to model a small vessel, it would predict a viscosity that is *lower* than that predicted by Poiseuille's equation for a large vessel.

3. In vessels (e.g., capillaries) so small that their diameter is about the size of a single erythrocyte, we can no longer speak of the friction between concentric laminae. Instead, in small capillaries, the membrane of the RBC rolls around the cytoplasm in a movement called "tank treading," similar to that of the track of a bulldozer (see Fig. 17–9D). As two treading erythrocytes shoot down a capillary, they spin the bolus of plasma trapped between them ("bolus flow").

4. In vessels smaller than an erythrocyte, highly deformed—literally bullet-shaped—RBCs squeeze through the capillaries, making the effective viscosity fall even further below that of the bulk solution (see Fig. 17–9E). Under these conditions, a layer of plasma separates the erythrocytes from the capillary wall. The cells automatically "focus" themselves to the centerline of the capillary, and maintain a fixed distance between two successive cells.

VELOCITY OF FLOW. As for an ideal fluid (see Fig. 17–6A), the dependence of flow on pressure is linear for blood *plasma* (Fig. 17–10). However, for *whole blood,* the pressure-flow relationship deviates slightly from linearity at velocities close to zero, and the situation is

even worse for polycythemia. These deviations at very low flows have two explanations. First, at low flows, the shear rate is also low, causing the whole blood (like mayonnaise) to behave in a non-Newtonian manner (see Fig. 17–7) and to have a high apparent viscosity. In fact, as was already seen, one must apply a threshold force to get the blood to move at all. Thus, the *red* and *green curves* in Figure 17–10 have shallower slopes at low flows than at high flows. The second reason for the nonlinear pressure-flow relationship is that the tendency for RBCs to move to the center of the stream—thereby lowering viscosity—requires a modest flow. After this axial accumulation "saturates," however, the relationship becomes linear.

TEMPERATURE. Cooling normal whole blood from 37°C to 0°C increases its viscosity approximately 2.5-fold. However, physiologically, this effect is negligible in humans except during intense cooling of the extremities. On the other hand, in some patients, the presence of **cryoglobulins** in the blood can cause an abnormal rise in viscosity even with less intense cooling of limbs. Cryoglobulins are immunoglobulins that precipitate at a temperature that is less than 37°C, but can partially resolubilize upon warming. Different cryoglobulins are associated with infections, particularly hepatitis C, as well as with several autoimmune and lymphoproliferative disorders. High blood viscosity from the precipitated cryoglobulins can lead to vessel obstruction and local thrombosis.

Pressure and Flow Oscillate with Each Heartbeat Between Maximum Systolic and Minimum Diastolic Values

Thus far we have considered blood flow to be steady and driven by a constant pressure generator. That is, we have been working with a *mean* blood flow and a *mean* driving pressure (i.e., the difference between the mean arterial and venous pressures). However, we are all aware that the heart is a pump of the "two-stroke" variety, with a filling and an emptying phase. Because both the left and right hearts perform their work in a cyclic fashion, flow is pulsatile in both the systemic and pulmonary circulations.

The mean blood pressure in the large systemic arteries is approximately 95 mm Hg. This is a single, time-averaged value. In reality, the blood pressure cycles between a maximal **systolic** arterial pressure (approximately 120 mm Hg) that corresponds to the contraction of the ventricle, and a minimal **diastolic** arterial pressure (approximately 80 mm Hg) that corresponds to the relaxation of the ventricle (Fig. 17–11). The difference between the systolic and the diastolic pressure is **pulse pressure**. Note that the mean arterial pressure is not the arithmetic mean of systolic and diastolic values, which would be (120 + 80)/2 = 100 mm Hg in our example, but rather the area beneath the curve, which describes the pressure in a single cardiac cycle (see Fig. 17–11, *blue area*) divided by the duration of the cycle. A reasonable value for the mean arterial pressure is 95 mm Hg.

Like arterial pressure, flow through arteries also oscillates with each heartbeat. Because both pressure and flow are pulsatile, and because the pressure and flow waves are not perfectly matched in time, we cannot describe the relationship between these two parameters by a simple

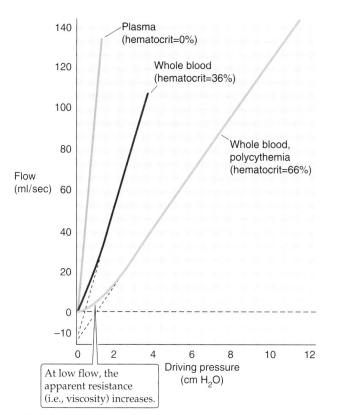

FIGURE 17–10. Pressure-flow relationships over a range of hematocrits. The slope of the linear portion of each curve is 1/resistance; resistance (or viscosity) increases from plasma to normal whole blood to polycythemic blood.

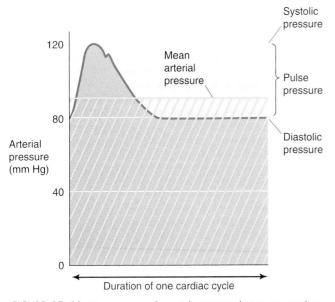

FIGURE 17–11. Time course of arterial pressure during one cardiac cycle. The area beneath the *blue pressure curve,* divided by the time of one cardiac cycle, is mean arterial pressure (*horizontal yellow line*). The *yellow cross-hatched area* is the same as blue area.

Ohm's Law–like relationship ($\Delta P = F \cdot R$), which is analogous to a simple DC circuit in electricity. Rather, if we were to model pressure and flow in the circulatory system, we would have to use a more complicated approach, analogous to that used for understanding AC electrical circuits.

ORIGINS OF PRESSURE IN THE CIRCULATION

Four factors help generate pressure in the circulation: gravity, compliance of the vessels, viscous resistance, and inertia.

Gravity Causes a Hydrostatic Pressure Difference When There Is a Difference in Height

Because gravity produces a hydrostatic pressure difference between two points whenever there is a *difference in height* (Δh; Equation 17–4), one must always express pressures relative to some reference "h" level. In cardiovascular physiology, this reference—zero height—is the level of the heart.

Whether the body is recumbent (i.e., horizontal) or upright (i.e., erect) has a tremendous effect on the intravascular pressure. In the horizontal position (Fig. 17–12A), where we assume that the entire body is at the level of the heart, we do not need to add a hydrostatic pressure component to the various intravascular pressures. Thus, the mean pressure in the aorta is 95 mm Hg and—because it takes a driving pressure of approximately 5 mm Hg to pump blood into the end of the large arteries—the mean pressure at the end of the large arteries in the foot and head is 90 mm Hg. Similarly, the

mean pressure in the large veins draining the foot and head is 5 mm Hg and—because it takes a driving pressure of approximately 3 mm Hg to pump blood to the right atrium—the mean pressure in the right atrium is 2 mm Hg.

When a 180-cm tall person is standing (see Fig. 17–12B), we must *add* a 130-cm column of blood (the Δh between the heart and large vessels in the foot) to the pressure prevailing in the large arteries and veins of the foot. Because a water column of 130 cm is equivalent to 95 mm Hg, the mean pressure for a large artery in the foot will be 90 + 95 = 185 mm Hg, and the mean pressure for a large vein in the foot will be 5 + 95 = 100 mm Hg. On the other hand, we must *subtract* a 50-cm column of blood from the pressure prevailing in the head. Because a water column of 50 cm is equivalent to 37 mm Hg, the mean pressure for a large artery in the head will be 90 − 37 = 53 mm Hg, and for a large vein in the head, 5 − 37 = −32 mm Hg. Of course, this "negative" value really means that the pressure in a large vein in the head is 32 mm Hg lower than the reference pressure at the level of the heart.

In this example, we have simplified things somewhat by ignoring the valves that interrupt the blood column. In reality, the veins of the limbs have a series of one-way valves that allow blood to flow only toward the heart. These valves act like a series of relay stations, so that the contraction of skeletal muscle around the veins pushes blood from one valve to another (p. 519). Thus, veins in the foot do not "see" the full hydrostatic column of 95 mm Hg when the leg muscles pump blood away from the foot veins.

Although the absolute arterial and venous pressures are much higher in the foot than in the head, the ΔP that *drives* blood flow is the same in the vascular beds of the foot and head. Thus, in the horizontal position, the ΔP across the vascular beds in the foot or head is 90 − 5 = 85 mm Hg. In the upright position, the ΔP for the foot is 185 − 100 = 85 mm Hg, and for the head, 53 − (−32) = 85 mm Hg. Thus, gravity does not affect the driving pressure that governs flow. On the other hand, in "dependent" areas of the body (i.e., vessels "below" the heart in a gravitational sense), the hydrostatic pressure does tend to increase the *transmural* pressure (intravascular versus extravascular "tissue" pressure), and thus the diameter of distensible vessels. Because various anatomic barriers separate different "tissue" compartments, it is assumed that gravity does not appreciably affect this tissue pressure.

Low Compliance of a Vessel Causes the Transmural Pressure to Increase When the Vessel Blood Volume Is Increased

Until now, we have considered blood vessels to be rigid tubes, which, by definition, have fixed volumes. If we were to try to inject a volume of fluid into a truly rigid tube with closed ends, we could in principle increase the pressure to infinity without increasing the volume of the tube (Fig. 17–13A). At the other extreme, if the wall of the tube were to offer no resistance to deformation (i.e., infinite compliance), we could inject an infinite volume of fluid without increasing the pressure at all (see Fig. 17–

A RECUMBENT   **B** UPRIGHT

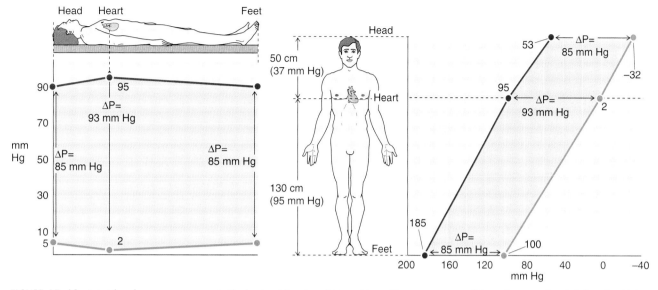

FIGURE 17–12. Arterial and venous pressures in the horizontal and upright positions. The pressures are different between *A* and *B*, but the driving pressures (ΔP) between arteries and veins (*separation between red and blue lines, violet background*) are the same.

13*B*). Blood vessels lie between these two extremes: They are distensible, but have a finite compliance (p. 455). Thus, if we were to inject a volume of blood into the vessel, the volume of the vessel would increase by the same amount (ΔV), and the intravascular pressure would also increase (see Fig. 17–13*C*). The ΔP accompanying a given ΔV is greater if the compliance of the vessel is lower. The relationship between ΔP and ΔV is a *static* property of the vessel wall, and holds whether or not there is flow in the vessel. Thus, if we were to infuse blood into a patient's blood vessels, the intravascular pressure would rise throughout the circulation, even if the heart were stopped.

The Viscous Resistance of Blood Causes an Axial Pressure Difference When There Is Flow

As we saw in Ohm's law of hydrodynamics (see Equation 17–1), during steady flow down the axis of a tube (see Fig. 17–2), the driving pressure (ΔP) is proportional to both flow and resistance. Viewed differently, if we want to achieve a constant flow, then the greater the resistance, the greater the ΔP that we must apply along the axis of flow. Of the four sources of pressure in the circulatory system, this ΔP due to viscous resistance is the only one that appears in Poiseuille's law (see Equation 17–9).

The Inertia of the Blood and Vessels Causes Pressure to Decrease When the Velocity of Blood Flow Increases

For the most part, we have been assuming that the flow of blood, as well as its mean linear velocity, is steady. However, as we have already noted, blood flow in the circulation is not steady: The heart imparts its energy in a *pulsatile* manner, with each heartbeat. Therefore, $\bar{v}$ in the aorta increases and reaches a maximum during systole, and falls off during diastole. As we shall shortly see, these

A ZERO COMPLIANCE   **B** INFINITE COMPLIANCE   **C** FINITE COMPLIANCE

FIGURE 17–13. Compliance: Changes in pressure with vessels of different compliances.

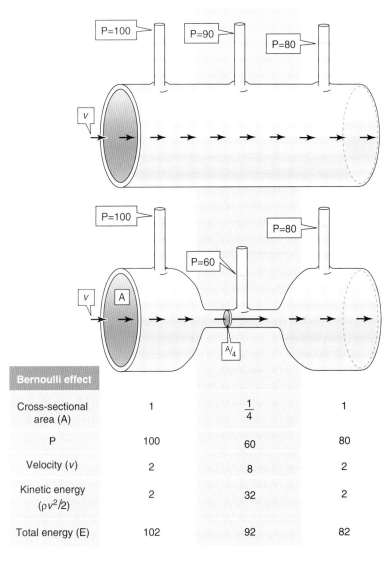

FIGURE 17–14. Bernoulli effect. For *top tube*, which has a uniformly high radius, velocity (v) is uniform and transmural pressure (P) falls linearly with length. The bottom tube has the same upstream and downstream pressures, but a constriction in the middle with a cross-sectional area that is only one fourth that of the two ends. Thus, velocity in the *narrow portion* must be fourfold higher than it is at the *ends*. Although the *total energy* of fluid falls linearly along tube, *pressure* is lower in the middle than at the distal end.

Bernoulli effect

Cross-sectional area (A)	1	$\frac{1}{4}$	1
P	100	60	80
Velocity (v)	2	8	2
Kinetic energy ($\rho v^2/2$)	2	32	2
Total energy (E)	102	92	82

changes in velocity lead to compensatory changes in intravascular *pressure*.

The trade-off between velocity and pressure reflects the conversion between two forms of energy. Although we generally state that fluids flow from a higher to a lower *pressure*, it is more accurate to say that fluids flow from a higher to a lower *total energy*. This energy is made up of both the pressure or **potential energy** and the **kinetic energy** (KE = ½ mv²). The impact of the interconversion between these two forms of energy is manifested by the familiar **Bernoulli effect**. As fluid flows along a horizontal tube with a narrow central region, which has half the diameter of the two ends, the pressure in the central region is actually lower than the pressure at the distal end of the tube (Fig. 17–14). How can the fluid paradoxically flow against the *pressure gradient* from the lower-pressure central to the higher-pressure distal region of the tube? We saw earlier that flow is the product of cross-sectional area and velocity (see Equation 17–8). Because the flow is the same in both portions of the tube, but the cross-sectional area in the center is lower by a factor of 4, the

velocity in the central region must be fourfold higher (see Fig. 17–14, *table at bottom*). Although the blood in the central region has a lower potential energy (pressure = 60) than the blood at the distal end of the tube (pressure = 80), it has a 16-fold higher kinetic energy. Thus, the total energy of the fluid in the center exceeds that in the distal region, so that the fluid does indeed flow down the *energy gradient*.

The previous example illustrates an interconversion between potential energy (pressure) and kinetic energy (velocity) in *space*, because velocity changes along the length of a tube even though flow is constant. We will see on p. 513 that during ejection of blood from the left ventricle into the aorta, the flow and velocity of blood change with *time* at any point within the aorta. These changes in velocity contribute to the changes in pressure inside the aorta.

The Bernoulli effect has important practical implications for measurement of blood pressure with an open-tipped catheter. The pressure recorded with the open tip facing the flow is higher than the actual pressure by an amount corresponding to the kinetic energy of the oncoming fluid

FIGURE 17–15. Effects of kinetic energy on the measurement of blood pressure with catheters.

(Fig. 17–15). Conversely, the pressure recorded with the open tip facing away from the flow is lower than the actual pressure by an equal amount. The measured pressure is correct only when the opening is on the side of the catheter, perpendicular to the flow of blood.

HOW TO MEASURE BLOOD PRESSURE, BLOOD FLOW, AND CARDIAC VOLUMES

Blood Pressure Can Be Measured Directly by Puncturing the Vessel

One can record blood pressure anywhere along the circulation—inside a heart chamber, inside an artery, within a capillary, or within a vein. Clinicians generally are concerned with the intravascular pressure at a particular site (e.g., in a systemic artery) in reference to the barometric pressure outside the body, and generally not with pressure *differences* between two sites.

FIGURE 17–16. Direct method for determining blood pressure.

The most direct approach for measuring pressure is to introduce a needle or a catheter into a vessel and position the open tip at a particular site. In the first measurements of blood pressure ever performed, Stephen Hales in 1733 found that a column of blood from a presumably agitated horse rose to fill a brass pipe to a height of 3 m. It was Poiseuille who measured blood pressure for the first time by connecting a mercury-filled U-tube to arteries via a tube containing a solution of saturated $NaHCO_3$. In modern times, a saline-filled transmission or conduit system connects the blood vessel to a pressure transducer. In its most primitive form, a catheter was connected to a closed chamber, one wall of which was a deformable diaphragm. Nowadays, the pressure transducer is a stiff diaphragm bonded to a strain gauge that converts mechanical strain into a change in electrical resistance, capacitance, or inductance (Fig. 17–16). The opposite face of the diaphragm is open to the atmosphere, so that the blood pressure is referenced to barometric pressure. The overall performance of the system depends largely on the properties of the catheter and the strain gauge. The presence of air bubbles and a long or narrow catheter can decrease the displacement, velocity, and acceleration of the fluid in the catheter. Together, these properties determine overall performance characteristics such as sensitivity, linearity, damping of the pressure wave, and frequency response. To avoid problems with fluid transmission in the catheter, some high-fidelity devices employ a solid-state pressure transducer at the catheter tip.

In catheterizations of the **right heart**, the clinician begins by sliding a fluid-filled catheter into an antecubital vein and, while continuously recording pressure, advances the catheter tip into the superior vena cava, through the right atrium and the right ventricle, and past the pulmonary valve into the pulmonary artery. Eventually, the tip reaches and snugly fits into a smaller branch of the pulmonary artery, recording the **pulmonary wedge pressure** (p. 522). The wedge pressure effectively measures the pressure downstream from the catheter tip, that is, the left atrial pressure.

In catheterizations of the **left heart**, the clinician slides a catheter into the brachial artery or femoral artery, obtaining the **systemic arterial blood pressure**. From there, the catheter is advanced into the aorta, the left ventricle, and finally the left atrium.

Clinical measurements of **venous pressure** are typically made by inserting a catheter into the jugular vein. Because of the low pressures, these venous measurements require very sensitive pressure transducers or water manometers.

In the research laboratory, one can measure **capillary pressure** in exposed capillary beds by inserting a micropipette that is pressurized just enough (with a known pressure) to keep fluid from entering or leaving the pipette.

Blood Pressure Can Be Measured Indirectly Using a Sphygmomanometer

In clinical practice, one may measure arterial pressure indirectly using a manual sphygmomanometer (Fig. 17–

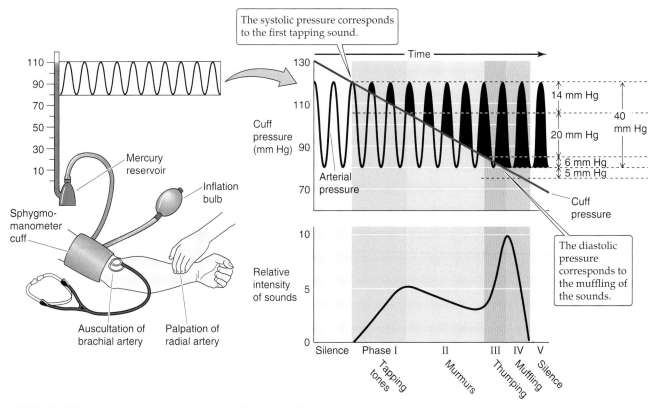

FIGURE 17–17. Sphygmomanometry. The clinician inflates the cuff to a pressure that is higher than the anticipated systolic pressure, and then slowly releases the pressure in the cuff.

17). An inextensible cuff containing an inflatable bag is wrapped around the arm (or occasionally, the thigh). Inflating the bag by means of a rubber squeeze-bulb to a pressure level above the expected systolic pressure occludes the underlying brachial artery and halts blood flow downstream. The pressure in the cuff, measured by means of a mercury or aneroid manometer, is then allowed to slowly decline (see Fig. 17–17, *diagonal red line*). The physician can use either of two methods to monitor the blood flow downstream of the slowly deflating cuff. In the **palpatory method**, one detects the pulse as an indicator of flow by feeling the radial artery at the wrist. In the **auscultatory method**, the physician detects flow by using a stethoscope to detect the changing character of Korotkoff sounds over the brachial artery in the antecubital space.

The palpatory method permits determination of the systolic pressure, that is, the pressure in the cuff below which it is just possible to detect a radial pulse. Because of limited sensitivity of the finger, palpation probably slightly underestimates systolic pressure. The auscultatory method permits the detection of both systolic and diastolic pressure. The sounds heard during the slow deflation of the cuff can be divided into five phases (see Fig. 17–17). During Phase I, there is a sharp tapping sound, indicating that a spurt of blood is escaping under the cuff when cuff pressure is just below systolic pressure. The pressure at which these taps are first heard closely represents systolic pressure. In Phase II, the sound becomes a

blowing or swishing murmur. During Phase III, the sound becomes a louder thumping. In Phase IV, as the cuff pressure falls toward the diastolic level, the sound becomes muffled and softer. Finally, in Phase V, the sound disappears. Although some debate persists about whether the point of muffling or the point of silence is the correct diastolic pressure, most favor the point of muffling as being more consistent. Actual diastolic pressure may be somewhat overestimated by the point of muffling, but underestimated by the point of silence.

Practical problems arise when a sphygmomanometer is used with children or obese adults, or when it is used to obtain a measurement on a thigh. Ideally, one would like to use a pressure cuff that is wide enough to ensure that the pressure inside the cuff is the same as that in the tissue surrounding the artery. In 1967, the American Heart Association recommended that the pneumatic bag within the cuff be 20% wider than the diameter of the limb, extend at least halfway around the limb, and be centered over the artery. More recent studies indicate that accuracy and reliability improve when the pneumatic bag completely encircles the limb, as long as the width of the pneumatic bag is at least the limb diameter.

Blood Flow Can Be Measured Directly by Electromagnetic and Ultrasound Flowmeters

The spectrum of blood-flow measurements in the circulation ranges from determinations of total blood flow (car-

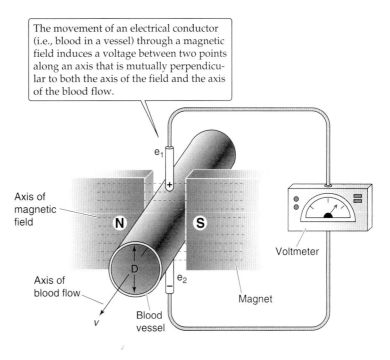

The movement of an electrical conductor (i.e., blood in a vessel) through a magnetic field induces a voltage between two points along an axis that is mutually perpendicular to both the axis of the field and the axis of the blood flow.

FIGURE 17–18. Electromagnetic flowmeter.

diac output) to assessment of flow within an organ or a particular tissue within an organ. Moreover, one can average blood-flow measurements over time, or record continuously. Examples of the latter include recordings of the phasic blood flow that occurs during the cardiac cycle or any other periodic event (e.g., breathing). We will discuss both invasive and noninvasive approaches.

INVASIVE METHODS. These approaches require direct access to the vessel under study, and are thus useful only in research laboratories. The earliest measurements of blood flow involved collecting venous outflow into a graduated cylinder and timing the collection with a stopwatch. This direct approach was limited to short time intervals to minimize blood loss and the resulting changes in hemodynamics. Blood loss could be avoided by ingenious, but now antiquated, devices that returned the blood to the circulation, in either a manual or a semiautomated fashion.

The most frequently used modern instruments for measuring blood flow in the research laboratory are **electromagnetic flowmeters** based on the electromagnetic induction principle (Fig. 17–18). The vessel is placed in a magnetic field. According to Faraday's induction law, moving any conductor (including an electrolyte solution, such as blood) at right angles to lines of the magnetic field generates a voltage difference between two points along an axis perpendicular to both the axis of the movement and the axis of the magnetic field. The induced voltage is

Equation 17–14

$$E = B \, \bar{v} \, D$$

where B is the density of magnetic flux, $\bar{v}$ is the average linear velocity, and D is the diameter of the moving column of blood.

Ultrasound flowmeters employ a pair of probes,

placed at two sites along a vessel. One probe emits an ultrasound signal, and the other records it. The linear velocity of blood in the vessel either induces a change in the frequency of the ultrasound signal (Doppler effect) or alters the transit time of the ultrasound signal. Both the electromagnetic and ultrasound methods measure linear velocity, not flow per se.

NONINVASIVE METHODS. The electromagnetic or ultrasonic flowmeters discussed earlier require the surgical isolation of a vessel. However, **ultrasonic methods** are also widely used transcutaneously on surface vessels in humans. This method is based on recording the backscattering of the ultrasound signal from moving red blood cells. To the extent that the RBCs move, the reflected sound has a different frequency than the emitted sound (Doppler effect). This frequency difference may thus be calibrated to measure flow. **Plethysmographic methods** are noninvasive approaches for measuring changes in the volume of a limb, or even of a whole person (p. 610). Inflating a pressure cuff enough to occlude veins but not arteries allows blood to continue to flow *into* (but not out of) a limb or an organ, so that the volume increases with time. The record of this rise in volume, as recorded by the plethysmograph, is a measure of blood flow.

With the exception of transcutaneous ultrasound, the direct methods discussed earlier for measuring blood flow are largely confined to research laboratories. The next two sections include discussions of two indirect methods that clinicians use to measure mean blood flow.

Cardiac Output Can Be Measured Indirectly by the Fick Method, Which Is Based on the Conservation of Mass

The Fick method requires that a substance be removed from or added to the blood during its flow through an

A THE FICK PRINCIPLE

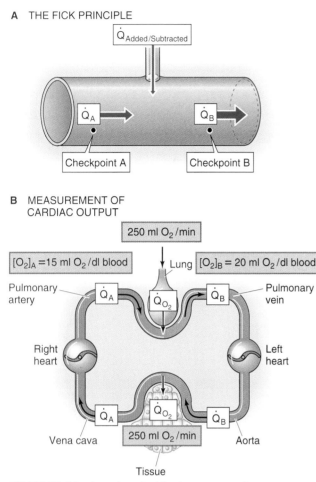

B MEASUREMENT OF CARDIAC OUTPUT

FIUGRE 17–19. The Fick method for determining cardiac output.

organ. The rate at which X passes a checkpoint in the circulation ($\dot{Q}$) is simply the product of the rate at which blood volume passes the checkpoint (F) and the concentration of X in that blood:

$$\dot{Q} = F \cdot [X]$$

Equation 17–15

$$\text{Units:} \quad \frac{\text{moles}}{\text{s}} = \frac{\text{liter}}{\text{s}} \cdot \frac{\text{moles}}{\text{liter}}$$

The **Fick principle** is a restatement of the law of conservation of mass. The amount of X per unit time that passes a downstream checkpoint ($\dot{Q}_B$) minus the amount of X that passes an upstream checkpoint ($\dot{Q}_A$) must equal the amount of X added or subtracted per unit time ($\dot{Q}_{Added/Subtracted}$) between these two checkpoints (Fig. 17–19A):

$$\dot{Q}_{Added/Subtracted} = \dot{Q}_B - \dot{Q}_A$$

Equation 17–16

$\dot{Q}_{Added/Subtracted}$ is positive for the addition of X. If the volume flow is identical at both checkpoints, combining Equation 17–15 and Equation 17–16 yields:

$$\dot{Q}_{Added/Subtracted} = F ([X]_B - [X]_A)$$

Equation 17–17

We can calculate flow from the amount of X added or subtracted, and the concentrations of X at the two checkpoints:

$$F = \frac{\dot{Q}_{Added/Subtracted}}{[X]_B - [X]_A} = \frac{\text{moles/min}}{\text{moles/liter}} = \frac{\text{liter}}{\text{min}}$$

Equation 17–18

It is easiest to apply the Fick principle to the blood flow through the lungs, which is the cardiac output (see Fig. 17–19B). The quantity added to the bloodstream is the O_2 uptake ($\dot{Q}_{O_2}$) by the lungs, which we obtain by measuring the subject's O_2 consumption. This value is typically 250 ml of O_2 gas per minute. The upstream checkpoint is the pulmonary artery (*point A*), where the O_2 content ($[O_2]_A$) is typically 15 ml O_2 per dl blood. The sample for this checkpoint must reflect the O_2 content of mixed-venous blood, obtained by means of a catheter within the right atrium, or the right ventricle or pulmonary artery. The downstream checkpoint is a pulmonary vein (*point B*), where the O_2 content ($[O_2]_B$) is typically 20 ml O_2/dl blood. We can obtain the sample for this checkpoint from any systemic artery. Using these particular values, we calculate a cardiac output of 5 liters/min:

$$F = \frac{\dot{Q}_{O_2}}{[O_2]_B - [O_2]_A} = \frac{250 \text{ ml } O_2/\text{min}}{(20 - 15) \text{ ml } O_2/\text{dl blood}}$$

$$= 5 \text{ liters blood/min}$$

Equation 17–19

Cardiac Output Can Be Measured Indirectly by Dilution Methods

The dye-dilution method, inaugurated by G.N. Stewart in 1897 and extended by W.F. Hamilton in 1932, is a variation on the Fick procedure. One injects a known quantity of a substance (X) into a systemic vein (e.g., antecubital vein) at site A while simultaneously monitoring the concentration downstream at site B (Fig. 17–20A). It is important that the substance not leave the vascular circuit and that it is easy to follow the concentration, by either successive sampling or continuous monitoring. If we inject a single known amount (Q_X) of the indicator, an observer downstream at checkpoint B will see a rising concentration of X, which after reaching its peak, falls off exponentially. Concentration measurements provide the interval (Δt) between the time the dye makes its first appearance at site B and the time the dye finally disappears there.

If site B is in the *pulmonary artery,* then *the entire amount Q_X* that we injected into the peripheral vein must pass site B during the interval Δt, carried by the entire cardiac output. We can deduce the average concentration $[\overline{X}]$ during the interval Δt from the concentration-versus-time curve in Figure 17–20B. From the conservation of mass, we know that

$$Q_X = V \cdot [\overline{X}]$$

Equation 17–20

$$\text{Units:} \quad \text{moles} = \text{liter} \cdot \frac{\text{moles}}{\text{liter}}$$

A PRINCIPLE OF DYE DILUTION

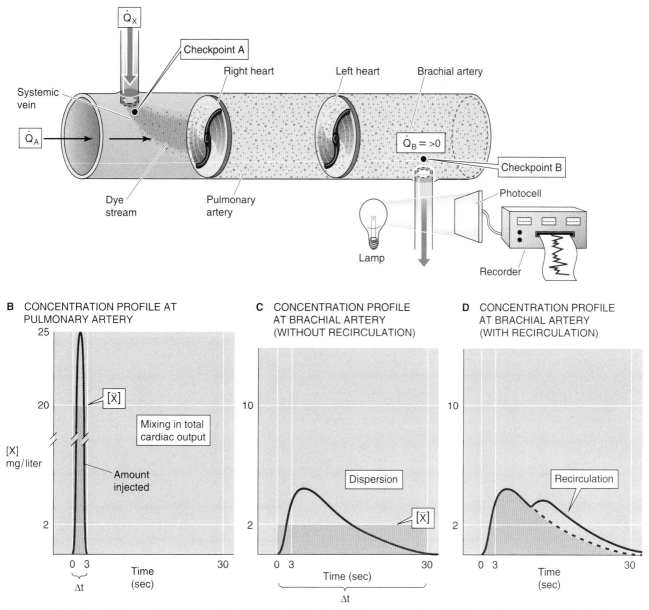

FIGURE 17-20. Dye dilution method for determining blood flow. In B, C, and D, the *areas underneath the three red curves*—as well as the *three green areas*—are all the same.

Because the volume of blood (V) that flowed through the pulmonary artery during the interval Δt is, by definition, the product of cardiac output and the time interval (CO · Δt),

Equation 17-21

$$Q_X = CO \cdot \Delta t \cdot [\overline{X}]$$

Units: $\text{moles} = \dfrac{\text{liter}}{\text{s}} \cdot \text{s} \cdot \dfrac{\text{moles}}{\text{liter}}$

Note that the product $\Delta t \cdot [\overline{X}]$ is the area under the concentration-versus-time curve in Figure 17-20B. Solving for CO, we have

Equation 17-22

$$CO = \frac{Q_X}{[\overline{X}] \times \Delta t} = \frac{Q_X}{\text{Area}}$$

In practice, cardiologists monitor [X] in the *brachial artery*. Obviously, only a fraction of the cardiac output passes through a brachial artery; however, this fraction is the same as the fraction of Q_X that passes through the brachial artery. If we were to re-derive Equation 17-22 for the brachial artery, we would end up multiplying both the CO and Q_X terms by this same fraction. Therefore, even though only a small portion of both cardiac output and injected dye passes through any single systemic artery, we can still use Equation 17-22 to compute cardiac output using data from that artery.

THALLIUM SCANNING FOR ASSESSING CORONARY BLOOD FLOW

Thallium (Th) is an ion that acts as a potassium analog and enters cells via the same channels or transporters as K+. Active cardiac muscle takes up injected thallium, provided there is adequate blood flow. Therefore, the rate of uptake of the [201]Th isotope by the heart is a useful qualitative measure of coronary blood flow. Complete [201]Th myocardial imaging is possible by two-dimensional scanning of the emitted γ rays or by computed tomography for a three-dimensional image. Thus, in those portions of myocardial tissue supplied by stenotic coronary vessels, the uptake is slower, and these areas appear as defects on a thallium scan. Thallium scans are used for detecting coronary artery disease during exercise stress tests.

Compared to the [X] profile in the pulmonary artery, the [X] profile in the brachial artery is not as tall and is more spread out, so that [X] is smaller and Δt is longer. However, the product $[\overline{X}] \cdot \Delta t$ in the brachial artery—or any other systemic artery—is the same as in the pulmonary artery. Indocyanine green dye (cardiogreen) is the most common dye employed. Because the liver removes this dye from the circulation, it is possible to repeat the injections, after a sufficient wait, without progressive accumulation of dye in the plasma. Imagine that, after we inject 5 mg of the dye, $[\overline{X}]$ under the curve is 2 mg/liter, and Δt is 0.5 min. Thus,

Equation 17–23

$$CO = \frac{5 \text{ mg}}{2 \text{ mg/liter} \times 0.5 \text{ min}} = 5 \text{ liters/min}$$

A practical problem is that, after we inject a marker into a systemic vein, blood moves more quickly through some pulmonary beds than others, so that the marker arrives at checkpoint B at different times. This process, known as dispersion, is the main cause of the flattening of the [X] profile in the brachial artery (see Fig. 17–20C) versus the pulmonary artery (see Fig. 17–20B). If we injected the dye into the *left atrium* and monitored it in the *systemic veins*, the dispersion would be far worse because of longer and more varied path lengths in the systemic as compared with the pulmonary circulation. In fact, the concentration curve would be so flattened that it would be difficult to resolve the area underneath the [X] profile.

A second practical problem with a closed circulatory system is that, before the initial [X] wave has waned, recirculation causes the injected indicator to reappear for a second time in front of the sensor at checkpoint B (see Fig. 17–20D). Extrapolating the exponential decay of the first wave can correct for this problem.

An alternative approach to the dye technique is to inject a bolus of cold saline and use an indwelling thermistor to follow the dilution of these "negative calories"

as a change of temperature at the downstream site. In this thermodilution technique, a temperature-versus-time profile replaces the concentration-versus-time profile. During cardiac catheterization, the cardiologist injects a bolus of cold saline into the right atrium, and records the temperature change in the pulmonary artery. The distance between upstream injection and downstream recording site is kept short to avoid heat exchange in the pulmonary capillary bed. The advantages of this method are that: (1) the injection of cold saline can be repeated without harm, (2) a single venous (versus venous and arterial) puncture allows access to both the upstream and the downstream sites, (3) less dispersion occurs because no capillary beds are involved, and (4) less recirculation occurs because of adequate temperature equilibration in the pulmonary and systemic capillary beds. A potential drawback is incomplete mixing, which may result from the proximity between injection and detection sites.

Regional Blood Flow Can Be Measured Indirectly by "Clearance" Methods

The methods used for measuring regional blood flow are often called "clearance" methods, although the term here has a somewhat different meaning than it does in kidney physiology. They are another application of the Fick principle, using the rate of uptake or elimination of a substance by an organ, together with a determination of the difference in concentration of the indicator between the arterial inflow and venous outflow (i.e., the **a–v difference**). By analogy with Equation 17–18, we can compute the blood flow through an organ (F) from the rate at which the organ removes the test substance X from the blood $(\dot{Q}_X)$ and the concentrations of the substance in arterial blood $([X]_a)$ and venous blood $([X]_v)$:

Equation 17–24

$$F = \frac{\dot{Q}_X}{[X]_a - [X]_v} = \frac{\text{moles/min}}{\text{moles/liter}} = \text{liter/min}$$

One can determine **hepatic blood flow** using BSP (Bromosulphthalein), a dye that the liver almost completely clears and excretes into the bile (p. 983). Here, $\dot{Q}_X$ is the rate of removal of BSP from the blood, estimated as the rate at which BSP appears in the bile. $[X]_a$ is the concentration of BSP in a systemic artery, and $[X]_v$ is the concentration of BSP in the hepatic vein.

In a similar manner, one can determine **renal blood flow** using PAH (para-aminohippurate). The kidneys almost completely remove this compound from the blood and secrete it into the urine (p. 767).

It is possible to determine **coronary blood flow** or **regional blood flow through skeletal muscle** from the tissue clearance of rapidly diffusing inert gases, such as the radioisotopes ^{133}Xe and [85]Kr.

Finally, one can use the rate of disappearance of nitrous oxide (N_2O), a gas that is historically important as the first anesthetic, to compute cerebral blood flow.

A similar, though qualitative, approach is the use of thallium scanning to assess coronary blood flow. Here one measures the uptake of an isotope by the heart muscle, rather than its clearance (see the box on Thallium Scanning for Assessing Coronary Blood Flow).

Ventricular Dimensions, Ventricular Volumes, and Volume Changes Can Be Measured by Angiography and Echocardiography

Clinicians can use a variety of approaches to examine the cardiac chambers. **Gated radionuclide imaging** employs compounds of the γ-emitting isotope technetium-99m (^{99m}Tc), which has a half-life of 6 hours. After ^{99m}Tc is injected, a gamma camera provides imaging of the cardiac chambers. ECG gating (i.e., synchronization to a particular spot on the electrocardiogram) allows the apparatus to snap a picture at a specific part of the cardiac cycle, and to sum these pictures up over many cycles. Because this method does not provide a high-resolution image, it yields only a *relative* ventricular volume. From the difference between the count at the maximally filled state (end-diastolic volume) and at its minimally filled state (end-systolic volume), the cardiologist can estimate the fraction of ventricular blood that is ejected during systole—**the ejection fraction**—which is an important measure of cardiac function.

Angiography can accurately provide the linear dimensions of the ventricle, allowing the cardiologist to calculate *absolute* ventricular volumes. A catheter is threaded into either the left or the right ventricle, and saline containing a contrast substance (i.e., a chemical opaque to x-rays) is injected into the ventricle. This approach provides a two-dimensional projection of the ventricular volume as a function of time. In **magnetic resonance imaging** (MRI), one obtains a nuclear magnetic resonance (NMR) image of the protons in the water of the heart muscle and blood. However, because standard NMR requires long data-acquisition times, it does not provide very good time resolution.

Echocardiography, which exploits ultrasonic waves to visualize the heart and great vessels, can be used in two modes. In *M-mode echocardiography* ("M" is for motion), the technician places a single transducer in a fixed position on the chest wall and obtains a one-dimensional view of heart components. In the upper portion of Figure 17–21A, the ultrasonic beam transects the anterior wall of the right ventricle, the right ventricle, the septum, the left ventricle, the leaflets of the mitral valve, and the posterior wall of the left ventricle. The lower portion of Figure 17–21A shows the positions of the borders between these structures (x-axis) during a single cardiac cycle (y-axis), and thus how the size of the left ventricle—along the axis of the beam—changes with time. Of course, the technician can obtain other views by changing the orientation of the beam.

In *two-dimensional echocardiography*, the probe automatically and rapidly pivots, scanning the heart in a single anatomic slice or plane (Fig. 17–21A, *area between the two broken lines*) and providing a true cross section. This approach is therefore superior to angiography, which provides only a two-dimensional projection. Because cardiac

A PRINCIPLE OF ECHOCARDIOGRAPHY

B ASSUMED VENTRICULAR GEOMETRY

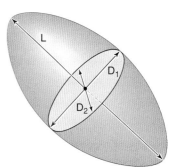

FIGURE 17–21. M-mode and two-dimensional echocardiography. In *A*, the tracing on the *bottom* shows the result of an M-mode echocardiogram (i.e., transducer in single position) during one cardiac cycle. The waves represent motion ("M") of heart boundaries transected by stationary ultrasonic beam. In two-dimensional echocardiography (*upper panel*), the probe rapidly rotates between the two extremes (*broken lines*), producing an image of a slice through the heart at one instant in time.

FIGURE 17–22. The colors, which encode the velocity of blood flow, are superimposed on a two-dimensional echocardiogram, which is shown in a gray scale. In A, blood moves through the mitral valve and into the left ventricle during diastole. Because blood is flowing toward the transducer, its velocity is encoded as red. In B, blood moves out of the ventricle and toward the aortic valve during systole. Because blood is flowing away from the transducer, its velocity is encoded as blue. (From Feigenbaum H: Echocardiography. In Braunwald E (ed): Heart Disease: A Textbook of Cardiovascular Medicine, 5th ed. Philadelphia, WB Saunders, 1997.)

output is the product of heart rate and stroke volume, one can calculate cardiac output from echocardiographic measurements of ventricular end-diastolic and end-systolic volume.

A problem common to angiography and M-mode echocardiography is that it is impossible to compute ventricular volume from a single dimension because the ventricle is not a simple sphere. As is shown in Figure 17–21B, the left ventricle is often assumed to be a *prolate ellipse*, with a long axis L and two short axes D_1 and D_2. To simplify the calculation, and to allow ventricular volume to be computed from a single measurement, it is sometimes assumed that D_1 and D_2 are identical, and that D_1 is half of L. Unfortunately, using this algorithm and just a single dimension, as provided by M-mode echocardiography, often yields grossly erroneous volumes. Using two-dimensional echocardiography to sum information from several parallel slices through the ventricle, or from planes that are at a known angle to one another, can yield more accurate volumes.

In contrast to standard echocardiography, **Doppler echocardiography** provides information on the velocity, direction, and character of blood flow, just as police radar monitors traffic. In Doppler echocardiography (as with police radar), most information is obtained with the beam parallel to the flow of blood. In the simplest application of Doppler flow measurements, one can continuously monitor the velocity of flowing blood in a blood vessel or part of the heart. On such a record, the x-axis represents time, and the y-axis represents the spectrum of *velocities* of the moving red blood cells (i.e., different cells can be moving at different velocities). Flow toward the transducer appears above baseline, whereas flow away from the transducer appears below baseline. The intensity of the record at a single point on the y-axis (encoded by a gray scale or false color) represents the strength of the returning signal, which depends on the *number* of red blood cells moving at that velocity. Thus, Doppler echo-

cardiography is able to distinguish the character of flow: laminar versus turbulent. Alternatively, at one instant in time, the Doppler technician can scan a region of a vessel or the heart, obtaining a two-dimensional, color-encoded map of blood velocities. If we overlay such two-dimensional Doppler data on a two-dimensional echocardiogram, which shows the positions of the vessel or cardiac structures, the result is a color, flow-imaging Doppler echocardiogram (see Fig. 17–22B).

HEMOSTASIS AND FIBRINOLYSIS

We have already noted that two essential requirements of the circulatory system are that the blood must be a liquid and that it cannot leak through the walls of the blood vessels. Meeting these two requirements is the job of the fibrinolytic and hemostatic machinery.

Hemostasis (from the Greek *hemos* [blood] + *stasis* [standing]), or the prevention of hemorrhage, can be achieved by four methods: (1) vasoconstriction, (2) increased tissue pressure, (3) the formation of a platelet plug in the case of capillary bleeding, and (4) coagulation or clot formation.

Vasoconstriction contributes to hemostasis because it raises the critical closing pressure—as we discuss on page 455—and thus collapses vessels that have an intravascular pressure below the critical closing pressure. Vessel constriction is also promoted by chemical byproducts of platelet-plug formation and of coagulation. For example, activated platelets release the vasoconstrictors thromboxane A_2 (TXA_2) (p. 106) and serotonin (5-HT) (p. 305). Moreover, thrombin, a major product of the clotting machinery, triggers the endothelium to generate endothelin-1 (ET-1) (p. 480), the most powerful physiological vasoconstrictor.

Increased tissue pressure contributes to hemostasis

because it decreases transmural pressure (p. 428), which is the difference between intravascular pressure and tissue pressure. Transmural pressure is the main determinant of blood-vessel radius. Given the fourth-power relationship between flow and blood-vessel radius (p. 429), an increase in tissue pressure that causes radius to decrease by a factor of 2 would diminish flow by a factor of 16. We all take advantage of this principle when we press a finger against a small cut to stop the bleeding. A tourniquet increases extravascular pressure and can thus halt an arterial hemorrhage in a limb. Finally, surgeons routinely make use of this principle when applying hemostatic clamps to close off "bleeders."

In this section, we discuss the third and fourth methods of hemostasis, platelet-plug formation and coagulation.

Platelets Can Plug Holes in Small Vessels

Platelets form in the bone marrow by budding off from large cells called **megakaryocytes**, each of which can produce up to a few thousand platelets. In their unactivated state, these nucleus-free fragments are disk shaped and 2 to 3 μm in diameter. Normal blood contains 150,000 to 450,000 platelets per microliter. The lifespan of these platelets is about ten days.

In a highly controlled fashion, platelets plug small breaches in the vascular endothelium. Plug formation is a process that includes adhesion, activation, and aggregation.

ADHESION. Normally platelets do not adhere to themselves, to other blood cells, or to endothelial membranes. One preventive factor may be the negative surface charge on both platelets and endothelial cells. In the case of endothelial cells, the negative surface charge reflects the presence of proteoglycans, mainly heparan sulfate. Platelet adhesion occurs in response to an increase in the shearing force (p. 429) at the surface of platelets or endothelial cells and in response to vessel injury or humoral signals.

Platelet adhesion—the binding of platelets to themselves or to other components—is mediated by "**platelet receptors**," which are glycoproteins in the platelet membrane. These platelet receptors are integral membrane proteins belonging to a class of matrix receptors known as **integrins** (p. 19). They are usually heterodimers linked by disulfide bonds. One ligand naturally present in the blood plasma is **von Willebrand factor** (vWf), a glycoprotein made by endothelial cells and megakaryocytes (and carried by the product of megakaryoctyes—platelets). High shear, certain cytokines, and hypoxia all trigger the release of vWf from endothelial cells. vWf binds to the platelet receptor known as glycoprotein Ib/Ia (Gp Ib/Ia), which is a dimer of Gp Ib linked to Gp Ia.

A breach of the endothelium exposes platelet receptors to ligands that are components of the subendothelial matrix. These ligands include **collagen**, which binds to Gp Ia/IIa, and **fibronectin** and **laminin** (p. 19), both of which bind to Gp Ic/IIa.

ACTIVATION. The binding of the above ligands—or of certain other agents (e.g., thrombin) that we will discuss

later—triggers a conformational change in the platelet receptors that initiates an intracellular signaling cascade that leads to an exocytotic event known as the "release reaction" or platelet activation. The signal transduction cascade involves the activation of phospholipase C (p. 100) and an influx of Ca^{2+}. Activated platelets exocytose the contents of their **dense storage granules**, which include ADP, serotonin, and Ca^{2+}. Activated platelets also exocytose the contents of their **α granules**, which contain several proteins, including a host of growth factors and three hemostatic factors: von Willebrand factor (see above) and two clotting factors that we will discuss below, clotting factor V and fibrinogen. Activated platelets also use cyclooxygenase (p. 104) to initiate the breakdown of arachidonic acid to thromboxane A_2, which they release. Platelet activation is also associated with marked cytoskeletal and morphological changes as the platelet extends first a broad lamellipodium and then many fingerlike filopodia.

AGGREGATION. Signaling molecules released by activated platelets amplify the platelet-activation response. ADP (which binds to $P2Y_{12}$ receptors on platelets), serotonin, and TXA_2 all activate additional platelets, and this recruitment promotes platelet aggregation. Aspirin, an inhibitor of cyclooxygenase, inhibits clotting by reducing the release of TXA_2. As noted above, the von Willebrand factor released by activated platelets binds to the platelet receptor Gp Ib/Ia, thereby activating even more platelets and forming molecular bridges between platelets. Platelet activation also induces a conformational change in Gp IIb/IIIa, another platelet receptor, endowing it with the capacity to bind fibrinogen. Thus, as a result of the conformational change in Gp IIb/IIIa, the fibrinogen that is always present in blood forms bridges between platelets and thus participates in the formation of a platelet plug. As we will see later, when cleaved by thrombin, fibrinogen also plays a critical role in clotting.

A Controlled Cascade of Proteolysis Creates a Blood Clot

A **blood clot** is a semisolid mass composed of both platelets, fibrin, and —entrapped in the mesh of fibrin— erythrocytes, leukocytes, and serum. A **thrombus** is also a blood clot, but the term is usually reserved for an *intravascular* clot. Thus, the blood clot formed at the site of a skin wound would usually not be called a thrombus. The relative composition of thrombi varies with the site of **thrombosis** (i.e., thrombus formation). A higher proportion of platelets is present in clots of the arterial circulation, whereas a higher proportion of fibrin is present in clots of the venous circulation.

Platelet-plug formation and blood clotting are related but distinct events that may occur in parallel or in the absence of the other. As we will see later, activated platelets can release small amounts of some of the factors (e.g., Ca^{2+}) that play a role in blood clotting. Conversely, as we have already noted, some clotting factors (e.g., thrombin and fibrinogen) play a role in platelet-plug formation. Thus, molecular crosstalk between the machinery involved in platelet-plug formation and clot formation helps coordinate hemostasis.

The cardiovascular system normally maintains a precarious balance between two pathological states. On the one hand, inadequate clotting would lead to the leakage of blood from the vascular system and, ultimately, to hypovolemia. On the other hand, overactive clotting would lead to thrombosis and, ultimately, to cessation of blood flow. The cardiovascular system achieves this balance between an **antithrombotic** (anticoagulant) and a **prothrombotic** (procoagulant) state by a variety of components of the vascular wall and blood. Promoting an "antithrombotic" state is a normal layer of endothelial cells, which line all luminal surfaces of the vascular system. Promoting a "prothrombotic" state are events associated with vascular damage: (1) the failure of endothelial cells to produce the proper antithrombotic factors or (2) the physical removal or injury of endothelial cells, which permits the blood to come into contact with thrombogenic factors that lie beneath the endothelium. Also promoting a "prothrombotic" state is the activation of platelets by any of the ligands that bind to platelet receptors, as discussed earlier. For instance, as platelets flow past artificial mechanical heart valves, the shearing forces can activate the platelets.

According to the classical view, two distinct sequences can precipitate coagulation: the intrinsic pathway and the extrinsic pathway. It is the **intrinsic pathway** that becomes activated when blood comes into contact with a negatively charged surface—in the laboratory we can mimic this process by putting blood into a glass test tube. The **extrinsic pathway** is activated when blood comes in contact with material from damaged cell membranes. In both cases, the precipitating event triggers a chain reaction that converts precursors into activated factors, which in turn catalyze the conversion of other precursors into other activated factors, and so on. Most of these "precursors" are zymogens that give rise to "activated factors" that are serine proteases. Thus, *controlled proteolysis* plays a central role in amplifying the clotting signals. However, the cascades do not occur in the fluid phase of the blood, where the concentration of each of these factors is low. In the case of the intrinsic pathway, the chain reaction

TABLE 17–1

PROCOAGULANT AND ANTICOAGULANT FACTORS

NAME	ALTERNATE NAMES	PROPERTIES
Procoagulant Factors		
Factor I	Fibrinogen	A plasma globulin
Factor Ia	Fibrin	
Factor II	Prothrombin	A plasma α_2 globulin Synthesis in liver requires Vitamin K*
Factor IIa	Thrombin	A serine protease
Factor III (cofactor)	Tissue factor Tissue thromboplastin	An integral membrane glycoprotein; member of Type II cytokine receptor family Receptor for Factor VIIa Must be present in a phospholipid membrane for procoagulant activity
Factor IV	Ca²⁺	
Factor V	Labile factor Proaccelerin Accelerator globulin	A plasma protein synthesized by liver and stored in platelets Single-chain protein
Factor Va (cofactor)		Heterodimer held together by a single Ca²⁺ ion Highly homologous to Factor VIIIa
Factor VII	Stable factor Serum prothrombin conversion accelerator (SPCA) Proconvertin	A plasma protein Synthesis in liver requires Vitamin K*
Factor VIIa		A serine protease
Factor VIII	Antihemophilic factor (AHF) Factor VIII procoagulant component (FVIII:C)	A plasma protein with phospholipid binding domain
Factor VIIIa (cofactor)		Highly homologous to Factor Va
Factor IX	Christmas factor Plasma thromboplastin component (PTC)	A plasma protein Synthesis in liver requires Vitamin K*
Factor IXa		A protease A disulfide-linked heterodimer
Factor X	Stuart factor	A plasma glycoprotein Synthesis in liver requires Vitamin K*
Factor Xa		A protease

TABLE 17–1

PROCOAGULANT AND ANTICOAGULANT FACTORS *Continued*

NAME	ALTERNATE NAMES	PROPERTIES
Factor XI	Plasma thromboplastin anteced-ent (PTA)	A plasma protein produced by megakaryocytes and stored in platelets
Factor XIa		A protease A disulfide-linked homodimer
Factor XII	Hageman factor (HAF)	A plasma glycoprotein
Factor XIIa		A protease
Factor XIII	Fibrin stabilizing factor (FSF)	A plasma protein stored in platelets
Factor XIIIa		A transglutaminase A tetramer of two A chains and two B chains
HMWK	High molecular weight kininogen Fitzgerald factor	A plasma protein stored in platelets Kallikrein clips bradykinin from HMWK
Plasma prekallikrein	Fletcher factor Plasma kallikrein precursor	A plasma protein
Plasma kallikrein		A serine protease Kallikrein clips bradykinin from HMWK
von Willebrand factor	vWf	A plasma glycoprotein made by endothelial cells and mega-karyocytes Stabilizes Factor VIIIa Promotes platelet adhesion and aggregation

Anticoagulant Factors

NAME	ALTERNATE NAMES	PROPERTIES
TFPI	Tissue factor pathway inhibitor	Protease inhibitor produced by endothelial cells GPI-linked to the cell membrane
Antithrombin III	AT III	A plasma protein Serine protease inhibitor, member of serpin family Inhibits Factor Xa and thrombin, and probably also Factors XIIa, XIa, and IXa Heparan and heparin enhance the inhibitory action
Thrombomodulin (cofactor)		Glycosaminoglycan on surface of endothelial cell Binds thrombin and promotes activation of protein C
Protein C	Anticoagulant protein C Autoprothrombin IIA	A plasma protein Synthesis in liver requires Vitamin K*
Protein Ca		A serine protease Disulfide-linked heterodimer
Protein S (cofactor)		A plasma protein Synthesis in liver requires Vitamin K* Cofactor for protein C

*See page 1226 for a discussion of vitamin K.

occurs mainly at the membrane of activated platelets. In the case of the extrinsic pathway, the reactions occur mainly at a "tissue factor" that is membrane bound. Both pathways converge on a **common pathway** that culminates in generating thrombin and, ultimately, "stable" fibrin. Table 17–1 summarizes the names, synonyms, and properties of the procoagulant and anticoagulant factors in various parts of the clotting scheme.

INTRINSIC PATHWAY (SURFACE CONTACT-ACTIVA-TION). The left branch of Figure 17–23 shows the intrinsic pathway, a cascade of protease reactions initiated by factors that are all present within blood. When in contact with a negatively charged surface such as glass or the membrane of an activated platelet, a plasma protein called Factor XII (Hageman factor) can become **Factor XIIa**—

the suffix "a" indicates that this is the *activated* form of Factor XII. A molecule called **high molecular weight kininogen** (HMWK), a product of platelets that may in fact be attached to the platelet membrane, helps to anchor Factor XII to the charged surface, and thus serves as a cofactor. However, this HMWK-assisted conversion of Factor XII to Factor XIIa is limited in speed. Once a small amount of Factor XIIa accumulates, this protease converts prekallikrein to kallikrein, with HMWK as an anchor. In turn, the newly produced **kallikrein** accelerates the conversion of Factor XII to Factor XIIa—an example of positive feedback. On page 555, we see another example of an interaction between kallikreins and kininogens (e.g., HMWK), in which the proteolytic activity of kallikreins on kininogens leads to the release of small vasodilatory peptides called kinins.

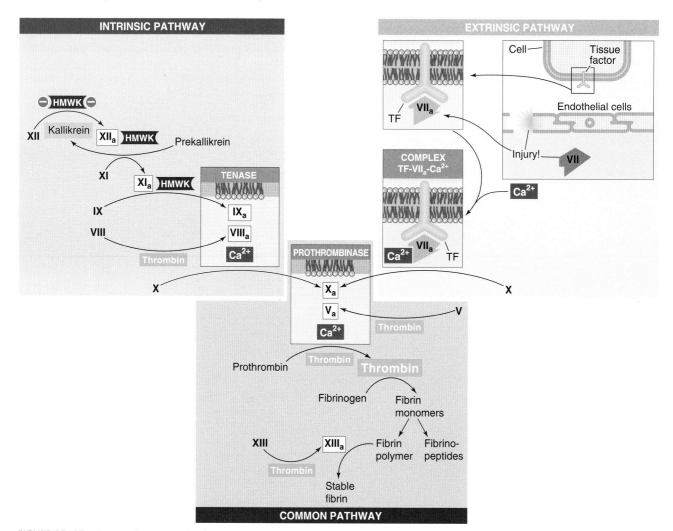

FIGURE 17–23. The coagulation cascade, showing only the procoagulant factors. The abbreviations are listed in Table 17–1.

In addition to amplifying its own generation by forming kallikrein, Factor XIIa (together with HMWK) also proteolytically cleaves Factor XI to Factor XIa. In turn, Factor XIa (also bound to the charged surface by HMWK) proteolytically cleaves Factor IX (Christmas factor) to Factor IXa, which is a protease. Factor IXa and two downstream products of the cascade—Factors Xa and, most importantly, thrombin—proteolytically cleave Factor VIII to Factor VIIIa, a cofactor in the next reaction. Finally, Factors IXa and VIIIa, together with Ca^{2+} (which may come largely from activated platelets) and negatively charged phospholipids form a trimolecular complex called "tenase." **Tenase** then converts Factor X (Stuart factor) to Factor Xa, yet another protease.

EXTRINSIC PATHWAY (TISSUE FACTOR ACTIVATION). The right branch of Figure 17–23 shows the extrinsic pathway, a cascade of protease reactions initiated by factors that are outside the vascular system. Nonvascular cells constitutively express an integral membrane protein called **tissue factor** (tissue thromboplastin, or Factor III), which is a receptor for a plasma protein called Factor VII. When an injury to the endothelium allows Factor VII

to come into contact with tissue factor, the tissue factor nonproteolytically activates Factor VII to Factor VIIa. Subsequently, tissue factor, Factor VIIa, and Ca^{2+} form a trimolecular complex analogous to tenase. Like tenase, the trimolecular complex of [tissue factor + Factor VIIa + Ca^{2+}] proteolytically cleaves the proenzyme Factor X to Factor Xa. An interesting feature is that when Factor X binds to the trimolecular complex, Factor VIIa undergoes a conformational change that prevents it from dissociating from tissue factor.

Regardless of whether Factor Xa arises by the intrinsic or extrinsic pathway, the cascade proceeds along the "common pathway."

COMMON PATHWAY. Factor Xa from either the intrinsic or extrinsic pathway is the first protease of the common pathway (*center* of Figure 17–23). Reminiscent of the conversion of Factor VIII to the cofactor VIIIa in the intrinsic pathway, the downstream product thrombin clips Factor V to form the cofactor Va. Factor V is highly homologous to Factor VIII, and in both cases the proteolytic activation clips a single protein into two peptides that remain attached to one another. Factors Xa and Va,

FIGURE 17–24. An abbreviated version of the coagulation cascade, showing the anticoagulant factors. The anticoagulant pathways are indicated in red. The abbreviations are listed in Table 17–1.

together with Ca^{2+} and phospholipids, form yet another trimolecular complex called **prothrombinase**. Prothrombinase acts on a plasma protein called prothrombin to form thrombin.

Thrombin is the central protease of the coagulation cascade, responsible for three major kinds of actions:

1. **Activation of downstream components in the clotting cascade.** The main action of thrombin is to catalyze the proteolysis of a soluble plasma protein called fibrinogen (p. 432) to form **fibrin monomers** that are still soluble. Fibrin monomers then polymerize to form a *gel* of **fibrin polymers** that traps blood cells. Thrombin also activates Factor XIII to Factor XIIIa, which mediates the covalent crosslinking of the fibrin polymers to form a *mesh* called **stable fibrin** that is even less soluble than fibrin polymers.
2. **Positive feedback at several upstream levels of the cascade.** Thrombin can catalyze the formation of new thrombin from prothrombin and can also catalyze the formation of the co-factors Va and VIIIa.
3. **Paracrine actions that influence hemostasis.** First, thrombin causes endothelial cells to release NO, PGI_2, ADP, von Willebrand factor, and tissue plasminogen activator (see below). Second, thrombin can activate platelets through PAR-1, a protease-activated receptor

that belongs to the family of G-protein–coupled receptors (p. 92). Thus, thrombin is a key part of the molecular crosstalk introduced earlier between platelet activation and blood clotting, both of which are required for optimal clot formation. On the one hand, thrombin is a strong catalyst for platelet activation, and on the other hand, activated platelets offer the optimal surface for the intrinsic pathway leading to additional thrombin generation.

COAGULATION AS A CONNECTED DIAGRAM. The concept of independent intrinsic and extrinsic branches converging on a common pathway is becoming obsolete. In such a "branching tree" (see p. 574), multiple branches converge to form larger downstream branches, eventually converging on a single "trunk"—with no crosstalk between branches. However, coagulation is best conceptualized as a "connected diagram" (p. 574) in which the branches may interconnect in both the upstream and downstream directions. One example of interconnections is thrombin's multiple actions just discussed. Another example is the trimolecular complex of [tissue factor + Factor VIIa + Ca^{2+}] of the extrinsic pathway, which activates Factors IX and XI of the intrinsic pathway. In the other direction, Factors IXa and Xa of the intrinsic pathway can activate Factor VII of the extrinsic pathway.

Thus, the intrinsic pathway and extrinsic pathway are strongly interconnected to form a *network*.

What parts of this network are most important for coagulation in vivo? Clinical evidence suggests that coagulation depends largely on the extrinsic pathway. Although tissue factor is normally absent from intravascular cells, inflammation can trigger peripheral blood monocytes and endothelial cells to express tissue factor, increasing the risk of coagulation. Indeed, during sepsis, the tissue factor produced by circulating monocytes initiates intravascular thrombosis.

Anticoagulants Keep the Clotting Network in Check

Thus far, our discussion has focused on the coagulation cascade and attendant positive feedback. Just as important are the mechanisms that prevent hemostasis from running out of control. Endothelial cells are the main sources of the agents that help maintain normal blood fluidity. These agents are of two general types, paracrine factors and anticoagulant factors.

PARACRINE FACTORS. Endothelial cells generate prostacyclin (PGI_2; see p. 106), which promotes vasodilation (p. 479) and thus blood flow, and also inhibits platelet activation and thus clotting. Stimulated by thrombin, endothelial cells also produce nitric oxide (NO; see p. 110). Via cGMP, NO inhibits platelet adhesion and aggregation.

ANTICOAGULANT FACTORS. As summarized in Figure 17–24, endothelial cells also generate anticoagulant factors that interfere with the clotting cascade that generates fibrin. Table 17–1 lists these factors:

1. **Tissue factor pathway inhibitor (TFPI).** TFPI is a plasma protein that binds to the tri-molecular complex [tissue factor + Factor VIIa + Ca^{2+}] in the extrinsic pathway and blocks the protease activity of Factor VIIa. TFPI is GPI linked (p. 34) to the endothelial cell membrane, where it maintains an antithrombotic surface.
2. **Antithrombin III (AT III).** AT III binds to and inhibits Factor Xa and thrombin. The sulfated glycosaminoglycans (p. 40) **heparan sulfate** and **heparin** enhance the binding of AT III to Factor Xa or to thrombin, thus inhibiting coagulation. Heparan sulfate is present on the external surface of most cells, including endothelial surfaces. Mast cells and basophils release heparin.
3. **Thrombomodulin.** A glycosaminoglycan product of endothelial cells, thrombomodulin can form a complex with thrombin, thereby removing thrombin from the circulation and inhibiting coagulation. In addition, thrombomodulin also binds protein C.
4. **Protein C.** After protein C binds to the thrombomodulin portion of the thrombin-thrombomodulin complex, the thrombin activates protein C. Activated protein C (Ca) is a protease. Together with its cofactor protein S, Ca inactivates the cofactors Va and VIIIa, thus inhibiting coagulation.
5. **Protein S.** This is the cofactor of protein C and is thus an anticoagulant.

Fibrinolysis Breaks Up Clots

As noted on page 425, cross-linked stable fibrin traps red and white blood cells as well as platelets in a freshly formed thrombus. Through the interaction of actin and myosin in the platelets, the clot shrinks to a plug and thereby expels serum. After plug formation, **fibrinolysis**—the breakdown of stable fibrin—breaks up the clot in a more general process known as **thrombolysis**. As shown in Figure 17–25, the process of fibrinolysis begins with the conversion of plasminogen to plasmin, catalyzed by one of two activators: tissue-type plasminogen activator or urokinase-type plasminogen activator. Table 17–2 summarizes the properties of fibrinolytic factors.

The source of **tissue plasminogen activator** (t-PA), a serine protease, is endothelial cells. t-PA consists of a single peptide chain with two "kringles" at the N-terminal portion of the molecule and a protease motif in the C-terminal portion. Kringles are loop structures created by three disulfide bonds and serve to anchor the molecule to its substrate. t-PA converts the plasma zymogen plasminogen to the active fibrinolytic protease plasmin. The presence of fibrin greatly accelerates the conversion of plasminogen to plasmin.

Besides t-PA, the other plasminogen activator, **urokinase-type plasminogen activator** (u-PA), is present in plasma either as a single-chain protein or as the two-chain product of a proteolytic cleavage. Like t-PA, u-PA converts plasminogen to the active protease plasmin. However, this proteolysis requires that u-PA attaches to a receptor on the cell surface called urokinase plasminogen activator receptor (u-PAR).

Plasminogen is a large, single-chain glycoprotein that is composed of an N-terminal heavy chain (A chain) and a C-terminal light chain (B chain). The N-terminal heavy chain contains five kringles, and the C-terminal light chain contains the protease domain. t-PA cleaves plasminogen at the junction between the heavy and light chains, yielding plasmin. However, the two chains in plasmin remain connected by disulfide bonds.

Plasmin is a serine protease that can break down both fibrin and fibrinogen. The five kringles of the heavy chain of plasminogen are still present in plasmin. These anchors attach to lysine residues on fibrin, holding the protease portion of the molecule in place to promote hydrolysis. Plasmin proteolytically cleaves stable fibrin to fibrin breakdown products. Plasmin can also cleave t-PA between the kringle and protease motifs of t-PA. The C terminus of single-chain t-PA nonetheless retains its protease activity.

FIGURE 17–25. The fibrinolytic cascade. The abbreviations are listed in Table 17–2 on the following page.

TABLE 17–2

FIBRINOLYTIC FACTORS

NAME	ALTERNATE NAMES	PROPERTIES
Tissue-type plasminogen activator	t-PA	A serine protease that catalyzes hydrolysis of plasminogen at the junction between the N-terminal heavy chain and C-terminal light chain N terminus contains two loop structures called kringles
Urokinase-type plasminogen activator	u-PA	A serine protease
Urokinase-type plasminogen activator receptor	u-PAR	Binds to and required for the activity of u-PA
Plasminogen		Single-chain plasma glycoprotein with large N-terminal and small C-terminal domain. N terminus contains five kringles
Plasmin	Fibrinolysin	A serine protease
Plasminogen activator inhibitor-1	PAI-1	A serpin (serine protease inhibitor) In plasma and platelets Forms 1:1 complex with t-PA in blood
Plasminogen activator inhibitor-2	PAI-2	A serpin (serine protease inhibitor) Detected only in pregnancy
α_2-Antiplasmin	α_2-AP	A serpin (serine protease inhibitor) Forms 1:1 complex with plasmin in blood

The cardiovascular system regulates fibrinolysis at several levels, using both enhancing and inhibitory mechanisms. Catecholamines and bradykinin increase the levels of circulating t-PA. Two *serine protease inhibitors* ("serpins") reduce the activity of the plasminogen activators: plasminogen activator inhibitor-1 (PAI-1) and plasminogen activator inhibitor-2 (PAI-2). **PAI-1** complexes with and inhibits both single-chain and two-chain t-PA. **PAI-2** mainly inhibits u-PA. It is of interest that activated protein C, which inhibits coagulation as shown in Figure 17–24, also inhibits PAI-1 and PAI-2, thereby facilitating fibrinolysis. Only one serpin targets plasmin, α_2-**antiplasmin** (α_2-AP). When plasmin is not bound to fibrin (i.e., when the plasmin is in free solution), α_2-AP complexes with and thereby readily inactivates plasmin. However, when plasmin is attached to lysine residues on fibrin, this inhibition is greatly reduced. In other words, the very presence of a clot (i.e., fibrin) promotes the breakdown of the clot (i.e., fibrinolysis).

REFERENCES

Books and Reviews

Caro CG, Pedley TJ, Schroter RC, Seed WA: The Mechanics of the Circulation. Oxford, Oxford University Press, 1978.

Haynes RH: Physical basis of the dependence of blood viscosity on tube radius. Am J Physiol 198:1193–1200, 1960.

Lassen NA, Henriksen O, Sejrsen P: Indicator methods for measurement of organ and tissue blood flow. In Handbook of Physiology, Section 2: The Cardiovascular System, Vol III. Bethesda, MD, American Physiological Society, 1979, pp. 21–63.

Levine RA, Gillam LD, Weyman AE: Echocardiography in cardiac research. In Fozzard HA, Haber E, Jennings RB, et al (eds): The Heart and Cardiovascular System. New York, Raven Press, 1986, pp 369–452.

Maeda N, Shiga T: Velocity of oxygen transfer and erythrocyte rheology. News Physiol Sci 9:22–27, 1994.

Journal Articles

Coulter NA Jr, Pappenheimer JR: Development of turbulence in flowing blood. Am J Physiol 159:401–408, 1949.

Cournand A, Ranges HA: Catheterization of the right auricle. Proc Soc Exp Biol Med 46:462–466, 1941.

Fåhraeus R, Lindqvist T: The viscosity of the blood in narrow capillary tubes. Am J Physiol 96:562–568, 1931.

Hamilton WF, Moore JW, Kinsman JM, Spurling RG: Studies on the circulation. IV. Further analysis of the injection method and of changes in hemodynamics under physiological and pathological conditions. Am J Physiol 99:534–551, 1932.

Poiseuille JLM: Recherches expérimentales sur le mouvement des liquides dans les tubes de très petits diamètres. Mém Savant Etrangers Paris 9:433–544, 1846.

Reynolds O: An experimental investigation of the circumstances which determine whether the motion of water shall be direct or sinuosid, and of the law of resistance in parallel channels. Philos Trans R Soc Lond B Biol Sci 174:935–982, 1883.

CHAPTER 18

Arteries and Veins

Emile L. Boulpaep

THE ARTERIAL-DISTRIBUTION AND VENOUS-COLLECTION SYSTEMS

Hemodynamics is the study of the physical laws of blood circulation. It therefore addresses the properties of both the "content" (i.e., blood) and the "container" (i.e., blood vessels). In Chapter 17, we discussed the properties of the blood. This chapter is primarily concerned with the properties of the blood vessels. The circulation is not a system of rigid tubes. Moreover, the anatomy and functions of the various segments of the vasculature differ greatly from one to another. Because the function of the circulation is to carry substances all over the body, the circulatory system branches out into a network of billions of tiny capillaries. We can think of the **arteries** as a *distribution system*, the **microcirculation** as a *diffusion and filtration system*, and the **veins** as a *collection system*.

Physical Properties of Vessels Follow Closely the Level of Branching in the Circuit

The aorta branches out into billions of capillaries that ultimately regroup into a single vena cava (Fig. 18–1, *panel 1*). At each level of arborization of the peripheral circulation, the values of several key parameters vary dramatically:

1. Number of vessels at each level of arborization
2. Radius of a typical individual vessel
3. Aggregate cross-sectional area of all vessels at that level
4. Mean linear velocity of blood flow within an individual vessel
5. Flow (i.e., volume/second) through a single vessel
6. Relative blood volume (i.e., the fraction of the body's total blood volume present in all vessels of a given level)
7. Circulation (i.e., transit) time between two points of the circuit
8. Pressure profile along that portion of the circuit
9. Structure of the vascular walls
10. Elastic properties of the vascular walls

We discuss items 1 through 5 in this section, and items 6 through 8 in the following two sections. Items 9 and 10 are the subject of the second subchapter.

The **number of vessels** at a particular level of arborization (Table 18–1)

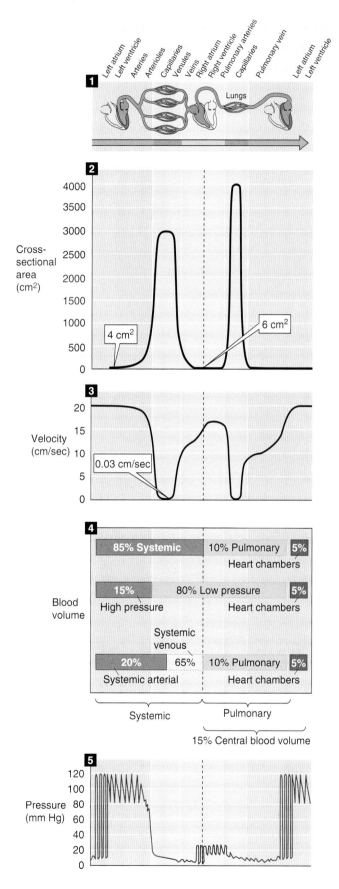

FIGURE 18–1. Profile of key parameters along the cardiovascular system. *Panel 1 (top)* shows branching of the cardiovascular system, from left heart to right heart, and back to left. *Panel 2* shows the variation of aggregate cross-sectional area of all vessels at any level of branching. *Panel 3* shows how mean linear velocity of blood varies in typical vessels. *Panel 4* shows ways of grouping blood volume in various compartments. *Panel 5* shows profile of blood pressure, with superimposed oscillations that represent variations in time.

TABLE 18–1

KEY SYSTEMIC VASCULAR PARAMETERS THAT VARY WITH ARBORIZATION

PARAMETER	AORTA	SMALL ARTERIES*	ARTERIOLES*	CAPILLARIES†	VENA CAVA
Number of units (N)	1	8000	2×10^7	1×10^{10} open (4×10^{10} total)	1
Internal radius (r_i)	1.13 cm	0.5 mm	15 μm	3 μm	1.38 cm
Cross-sectional area ($A_i = \pi r_i^2$)	4 cm²	7.9×10^{-3} cm²	7.1×10^{-7} cm²	2.8×10^{-7} cm²	6 cm²
Aggregate cross-sectional area ($A_{Total} = N\pi r_i^2$)	4 cm²	63 cm²	141 cm²	2827 cm²‡	6 cm²
Aggregate flow (F_{Total})	83 cm³/s (ml/s)	83 cm³/s	83 cm³/s	83 cm³/s	83 cm³/s
Mean linear velocity ($\bar{v} = F_{Total}/A_{Total}$)	21 cm/s	1.3 cm/s	0.6 cm/s	0.03 cm/s‡	14 cm/s
Single-unit flow ($F_i = F_{Total}/N = A_i \cdot \bar{v}$)	83 cm³/s (ml/s)	0.01 cm³/s	4×10^{-6} cm³/s	8×10^{-9} cm³/s‡	83 cm³/s

*The statistics for this column are for a representative generation.
†The values in this column are for the smallest capillaries, at the highest level of branching.
‡Assuming that only 25% of the capillaries are open.

increases enormously from a single aorta, to approximately 10^4 small arteries, approximately 10^7 arterioles, and finally approximately 4×10^{10} capillaries. However, only about one fourth of all capillaries are normally open to flow at any particular time. Finally, all of the blood returns to a single vessel where the superior and inferior venae cavae join.

The **radius of an individual vessel** (r_i, see Table 18–1) declines as a result of the arborization, decreasing from 1.1 cm in the aorta to a minimum of approximately 3 μm in the smallest capillaries. Because the **cross-sectional area** of an individual vessel is proportional to the square of the radius, this parameter decreases even more precipitously.

The **aggregate cross-sectional area** (see Table 18–1)

at any level of branching is the sum of the single cross-sectional areas of all parallel vessels at that level of branching. That is, it is the area that you would see if you sliced through all of the vessels at the same level of branching in *Panel 1* of Figure 18–1.

A fundamental law of vessel branching is that, at each branch point, the combined cross-sectional area of daughter vessels exceeds the cross-sectional area of the parent vessel. In this process of bifurcation, the steepest increase in total cross-sectional area occurs in the microcirculation (see Fig. 18–1, *Panel 2*). A typical **microcirculation** in the smooth muscle and submucosa of the intestine (Fig. 18–2) encompasses a first-order arteriole, several orders of progressively smaller arterioles, capillaries, several orders of venules into which the capillaries empty, and

FIGURE 18–2. Branching in a typical microcirculation, that of the smooth muscle and submucosa of the intestine. r, radius.

eventually a first-order venule. In humans, the maximum cross-sectional area occurs not at the level of the capillaries, but at the "postcapillary" (i.e., fourth-order) venules. Because of anastomoses among capillaries, capillaries only slightly outnumber fourth-order venules, whereas the cross-sectional unit area of each venule is appreciably greater than the area of a capillary. Assuming that only a quarter of the capillaries are usually open, the peak aggregate cross-sectional area of these postcapillary venules can be approximately 1000-fold greater than the cross section of the parent artery (e.g., aorta), as is shown in *Panel 2* of Figure 18–1.

The profile of the **mean linear velocity** of flow ($\bar{v}$) along a vascular circuit (see Fig. 18–1, *Panel 3*) is roughly a mirror image of the profile of the total cross-sectional area. According to the principle of continuity, **total volume flow** must be the same at any level of arborization. Indeed, as we make multiple vertical slices along the abscissa of *Panel 1* in Figure 18–1, the aggregate flow for each slice is the same:

Equation 18–1

$$F_{Total} = \underbrace{A_1 \cdot \bar{v}_1}_{Level\ \#1} = \underbrace{A_2 \cdot \bar{v}_2}_{Level\ \#2} = \underbrace{A_3 \cdot \bar{v}_3}_{Level\ \#3} = \ \ldots$$

As a consequence, $\bar{v}$ must be minimal in the postcapillary venules (~0.03 cm/sec), where A_{Total} is maximal. Conversely, $\bar{v}$ is maximal in the aorta (~20–50 cm/sec). Thus, A_{Total} and $\bar{v}$ values range approximately 1000-fold from the aorta to the capillaries, but are mirror images of one another. The vena cava, with a cross-sectional area approximately 50% larger than that of the aorta, has a mean linear velocity that is approximately 1/3 less.

Single-vessel flow, in contrast to total flow, ranges by approximately 10 orders of magnitude. In the aorta, the flow is approximately 83 ml/sec, the same as the cardiac output (~5 liters/min). When approximately 25% of the capillaries are open, a *typical* capillary has a mean linear velocity of 0.03 cm/sec, and a flow of 8×10^{-9} ml/sec (8 pl/sec)—10 orders of magnitude less than the flow in the aorta. Within the microcirculation, single-vessel flow has considerable range. At one extreme, a first-order arteriole (r_i ~30 μm) may have a flow of 20×10^{-6} ml/sec. At the other, the capillaries that are closed at any given time have zero flow.

Most of the Blood Volume Resides in the Systemic Veins

The body's **total blood volume** (V) of approximately 5 liters is not uniformly distributed along the x-axis of *Panel 1* in Figure 18–1. At any level of branching, the total blood volume is the sum of the volumes of all parallel branches. Table 18–2 summarizes—for a hypothetical 70-kg woman—the distribution of total blood volume expressed as both absolute blood volumes and **relative blood volumes** (% of total blood volume). *Panel 4* in Figure 18–1 summarizes four useful ways of grouping these volumes.

First, we can divide the blood volume into the *systemic* circulation (where ~85% of blood resides), the *pulmonary* circulation (~10%), and the *heart* chambers (~5%). The

pulmonary blood volume is quite adjustable (i.e., it can be much higher than 10%) and is carefully regulated.

Second, as can be seen in the next section, we can divide blood volume into what is contained in the *high-pressure* system (~15%), the *low-pressure* system (~80%), and the heart chambers (~5%).

Third, we can group the blood volumes into those in the *systemic venous system* versus the remainder of the circulation. Of the 85% of the total blood volume that resides in the systemic circulation, approximately ¾—or 65% of the total—is on the venous side, particularly in the smaller veins. Thus, the venous system acts as a volume reservoir. Changes in the diameters of veins have a major impact on the amount of blood they contain. For example, an abrupt increase in venous capacity causes pooling of blood in venous segments, and may lead to **syncope** (i.e., fainting).

We can also use a fourth approach for grouping blood volumes—dividing the blood into the **central blood volume** (volumes of the right heart + pulmonary circulation) versus the rest of the circulation. This central blood volume is very adjustable, and it constitutes the filling reservoir for the left heart. Left heart failure can cause the normally careful regulation of the central blood volume to break down.

The **circulation time** is the time required for a bolus of blood to travel either across the entire length of the circulation, or across a particular vascular bed. Total circulation time (the time to go from left to right across *Panel 1* in Figure 18–1) is approximately 1 minute. Circulation time across a single vascular bed (e.g., coronary circulation) may be as short as 10 sec. Circulation times may be obtained in humans by injecting a substance such as ether into an antecubital vein and measuring the time to its appearance in the lung (4–8 sec), or by injecting a bitter or sweet substance and measuring the time to the

TABLE 18–2

DISTRIBUTION OF BLOOD VOLUME*				
REGION	**ABSOLUTE VOLUME (ml)**		**RELATIVE VOLUME (%)**	
Systemic Circulation		4200		84
Aorta and Large Arteries	300		6.0	
Small Arteries	400		8.0	
Capillaries	300		6.0	
Small Veins	2300		46.0	
Large Veins	900		18	
Pulmonary Circulation		440		8.8
Arteries	130		2.6	
Capillaries	110		2.2	
Veins	200		4.0	
Heart (End-Diastole)	360	360	7.2	7.2
Total	5000	5000	100	100

*Values are for a 70-kg woman. For a 70-kg man, scale up the absolute values by 10%.

TABLE 18–3

MEAN PRESSURES IN THE SYSTEMIC AND PULMONARY CIRCULATIONS	
LOCATION	**MEAN PRESSURE (mm Hg)**
Systemic large arteries	95
Systemic arterioles	60
Systemic capillaries	25 (range, 35–15)
Systemic venules	15
Systemic veins	15–3
Pulmonary artery	15
Pulmonary capillaries	10
Pulmonary veins	5

perception of taste in the tongue (10–18 sec). Although, in the past, circulation time was used clinically as an index of cardiac output, the measurement has little physiological significance. The rationale for determining circulation time was that a shortening of circulation time could signify an improvement of cardiac output. However, the interpretation is more complicated because circulation time is actually the ratio of blood volume to blood flow:

Equation 18–2

$$t = \frac{V}{F}$$

Units: $\sec = \dfrac{ml}{ml/sec}$

Circulation time may thus reflect changes in volume as well as flow. For instance, a patient in heart failure may have a decreased cardiac output (i.e., F) and/or an increased blood volume (i.e., V), both of which would contribute to an elevation of transit time.

The Intravascular Pressures Along the Systemic Circuit Are Higher Than Those Along the Pulmonary Circuit

Panel 5 in Figure 18–1 shows the profile of pressure along the systemic and pulmonary circulations. Pressures are far higher in the systemic than in the pulmonary circulation. Although the cardiac outputs of the left and right hearts are the same, the total resistance of the systemic circulation is far higher than that of the pulmonary circulation (p. 695). This difference explains why the upstream driving pressure averages approximately 95 mm Hg in the *systemic circulation*, but only approximately 15 mm Hg in the *pulmonary circulation*. Table 18–3 summarizes typical mean values at key locations in the circulation. In both the systemic and pulmonary circulations, the systolic and diastolic pressures decay downstream from the ventricles (Fig. 18–3). The instantaneous pressures vary throughout each cardiac cycle for much of the circulatory system (see Fig. 18–1, *Panel 5*). In addition, the *systemic venous* and pulmonary pressures vary with the respiratory cycle, and venous pressure in the lower limbs varies with the contraction of skeletal muscle.

As has been noted earlier, the circulation can be divided into a high-pressure and a low-pressure system. The **high-pressure system** extends from the left ventricle *during* contraction all the way to the systemic arterioles.

FIGURE 18–3. Pressure profiles along systemic and pulmonary circulations, In *A* and *B*, the oscillations represent variations in time, not distance. *Boxed numbers* indicate mean pressures.

The **low-pressure system** extends from the systemic capillaries, through the rest of the systemic circuit, into the right heart, and then through the pulmonary circuit into the left heart in the *relaxed state*. The pulmonary circuit, unlike the systemic circuit, is entirely a low-pressure system; mean arterial pressures normally do not exceed 15 mm Hg and the capillary pressures do not rise above 10 mm Hg.

Under Normal Conditions, the Steepest Pressure Drop in the Systemic Circulation Occurs in Arterioles, the Site of Greatest Vascular Resistance

If we assume for simplicity's sake that the left heart behaves as a constant pressure generator of 95 mm Hg, and the right heart as a constant pressure generator of 15 mm Hg, it is the resistance of each vascular segment that determines the profile of pressure fall between the upstream arterial and downstream venous ends of the circulation. In particular, the pressure difference between two points along the axis of the vessel (i.e., the driving pressure difference, ΔP) depends on flow and resistance: $\Delta P = F \cdot R$ (p. 426). According to Poiseuille's law (p. 429), the resistance (R_i) of an individual, unbranched vascular segment is inversely proportional to the fourth power of the radius. Thus, the *pressure drop between any two points along the circuit depends critically* on the *diameter of the vessels* between these two points. However, the steepest pressure drop ($\Delta P/\Delta x$) does *not* occur along the capillaries, where vessel diameters are smallest, but rather, along the *precapillary arterioles*. Why? The **aggregate resistance** contributed by vessels of a particular order of arborization depends not only on their average radius, but also on the *number* of vessels in parallel. The more vessels in parallel, the smaller the aggregate resistance (see Equation 17–3). Although the resistance of a single capillary exceeds that of a single arteriole, capillaries far outnumber arterioles (Table 18–4). The result is that the aggregate resistance is larger in the arterioles, and this is where the steepest ΔP occurs.

TABLE 18–4

ESTIMATES OF TOTAL ARTERIOLAR AND CAPILLARY RESISTANCES*		
	ARTERIOLES	**CAPILLARIES**
Internal radius (r_i)	15 μm	4 μm†
Individual resistance (R_i) (units: dyne · s/cm^5)	~15 × 10^7	~3000 × 10^7
Number of units (N)	1 × 10^7	1 × 10^{10}
Total resistance ($R_{total} = R_i/N$) (units: dyne · s/cm^5)	15	3

*Assuming a blood viscosity of 3 cP and a vessel length of 100 μm.
†The value of 4 μm is near the average radius of capillaries.

A   NORMAL

Capillary pressure (P_c) is less than the arithmetic mean between arteriolar (P_a) and venular pressure (P_v) because $R_{pre} > R_{post}$.

$\dfrac{R_{post}}{R_{pre}}<1$

| Arteriole | Capillary | Venule |
| 60 mm Hg | 25 mm Hg | 15 mm Hg |

R_{pre} R_{post}

B   ARTERIOLAR DILATION OR VENULAR CONSTRICTION

P_c rises, tending to track P_a

$\dfrac{R_{post}}{R_{pre}}>1$

| Arteriole | Capillary | Venule |
| 60 mm Hg | 40 mm Hg | 15 mm Hg |

↓R_{pre} ↑R_{post}

C   ARTERIOLAR CONSTRICTION OR VENULAR DILATION

P_c falls, tending to track P_v

$\dfrac{R_{post}}{R_{pre}}\ll 1$

| Arteriole | Capillary | Venule |
| 60 mm Hg | 20 mm Hg | 15 mm Hg |

↑R_{pre} ↓R_{post}

FIGURE 18–4. Effect of precapillary and postcapillary resistances on capillary pressure.

Local Intravascular Pressure Depends on the Distribution of Vascular Resistance

We have just seen that the ΔP between an upstream checkpoint and a downstream checkpoint depends on the resistance between these points. What determines the absolute pressure at some location *between* the two checkpoints? To answer this question, we need to know not only the upstream arterial and downstream venous pressures, but also the *distribution of resistance* between the two checkpoints. A good example for explaining this concept is the distribution of resistance and pressure in the systemic microvasculature. Just how the upstream pressure in the arteriole and the downstream pressure in the venule affect the pressure at the midpoint of the capillary (P_c) depends on the relative size of the upstream and downstream resistances. For the simple circuit illustrated in Figure 18–4A:

Equation 18–3

$$P_c = \frac{(R_{post}/R_{pre}) \cdot P_a + P_v}{1 + (R_{post}/R_{pre})}$$

P_a is arteriolar pressure, P_v is venular pressure, R_{pre} is precapillary resistance upstream of the capillary bed, and R_{post} is postcapillary resistance downstream of the capillary.

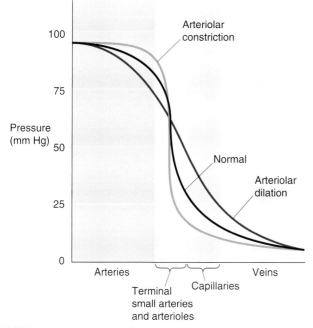

FIGURE 18–5. Pressure profiles during vasomotion. In this example, we assume that constriction or dilatation of terminal arteries and arterioles does not affect the overall driving pressure (ΔP) between aorta and vena cava. This assumption is reasonable in two cases: (1) Vasoconstriction or vasodilatation is confined to a single parallel vascular bed (e.g., one limb) and does not substantially change total peripheral resistance. (2) Even if total peripheral resistance *does* change, the cardiac pump could still maintain constant systemic arterial and venous pressures.

From this equation, we can draw three conclusions regarding local microvascular pressure. First, even though the arteriolar pressure is 60 and the venular pressure is 15 mm Hg in our example (see Table 18–3), capillary pressure is not necessarily 37.5 mm Hg, the arithmetic mean. According to Equation 18–3, P_c would be the arithmetic mean only if the precapillary and postcapillary resistances were identical (i.e., $R_{post}/R_{pre} = 1$). The finding that P_c is approximately 25 mm Hg in most vascular beds (see Figure 18–4A) implies that R_{pre} exceeds R_{post} (i.e., $R_{post}/R_{pre} < 1$). Under normal conditions in most microvascular beds, R_{post}/R_{pre} ranges from 0.2 to 0.4.

The second implication of Equation 18–3 is that, as long as the *sum* ($R_{pre} + R_{post}$) is constant, reciprocal changes in R_{pre} and R_{post} would not alter the total resistance of the circuit and would therefore leave both P_a and P_v constant. However, as R_{post}/R_{pre} increases, P_c would increase, thereby approaching P_a (see Fig. 18–4B). Conversely, as R_{post}/R_{pre} decreases, P_c would decrease, approaching P_v (see Fig. 18–4C). This conclusion is also intuitive: If we reduced R_{pre} to zero (but increased R_{post} to keep $R_{post} + R_{pre}$ constant), no pressure drop would occur along the precapillary vessels, and P_c would be the same as P_a. Conversely, if R_{post} were zero, P_c would be the same as P_v.

The third conclusion from Equation 18–3 is that, depending on the value of R_{post}/R_{pre}, P_c may be more sensitive to changes in arteriolar than venular pressure, or vice versa. For example, when the ratio R_{post}/R_{pre} is low (i.e., $R_{pre} > R_{post}$, as in Fig. 18–4A or 4C), capillary pressure tends to follow the downstream pressure in large veins.

This phenomenon explains why standing may cause the ankles to swell: The elevated pressure in large leg veins translates to an increased P_c, which, as is discussed later, leads to increased transudation of fluid from the capillaries into the interstitial spaces (p. 469). It also explains why elevating the feet, which lowers the pressure in the large veins, reverses ankle edema.

Vascular resistance varies in time and depends critically on the action of vascular smooth-muscle cells. The *major site of control* of vascular resistance in the systemic circulation is the *terminal small arteries (or "feed arteries") and arterioles.* Figure 18–5 illustrates the effect of vasoconstriction or vasodilation on the pressure profile. Whereas the overall ΔP between source and end point may not vary appreciably during a change in vascular resistance, the *shape* of the local pressure profile may change appreciably. Thus, during arteriolar constriction, the pressure drop between two points along the circuit (i.e., axial pressure gradient, $\Delta P/\Delta x$) is steep and concentrated at the arteriolar site (see Fig. 18–5, *green curve*). During arteriolar dilation, the gradient is shallow and more spread out (see Fig. 18–5, *violet curve*).

Although the effects of vasoconstriction and vasodilation are greatest in the local arterioles (*lighter red band* in Fig. 18–5), the effects extend both upstream (*darker red band*) and downstream (*purple and blue bands*) from the site of vasomotion because the pressure profile along the vessel depends on the resistance profile. Thus, if one vascular element contributes a greater fraction of the total resistance, a greater fraction of the pressure drop will occur along that element.

ELASTIC PROPERTIES OF BLOOD VESSELS

Blood Vessels Are Elastic Tubes

The wall of blood vessels consists of three layers: the intima, the media, and the adventitia. Capillaries, which have only an intimal layer of endothelial cells resting on a basal lamina, are the exception. Regardless of the organization of layers, one can distinguish four building blocks that make up the vascular wall: endothelial cells, elastic fibers, collagen fibers, and smooth muscle cells. Figure 18–6 shows how the relative abundance of these components varies throughout the vascular circuit. In addition to these principal components, fibroblasts, nerve endings, and blood cells invade the intima; other extracellular components (e.g., proteoglycans) may also be present.

Endothelial cells form a single, continuous layer that lines all vascular segments. Junctional complexes keep the endothelial cells together in arteries, but are less numerous in veins. The organization of the endothelial cell layer in capillaries varies greatly depending on the organ (p. 464). The glomus bodies in the skin and elsewhere are unusual in that their "endothelial cells" exist in multiple layers of cells called **myoepithelioid cells**. These glomus bodies control small arteriovenous shunts or anastomoses (p. 572).

Elastic fibers are a rubber-like material that accounts for most of the stretch of vessels at normal pressures, as well as the stretch of other tissues (e.g., lungs). Elastic

	Aorta	Medium artery	Arteriole	Precapillary sphincter	True capillary	Venule	Vein	Vena cava
Internal radius:	12 mm	2 mm	15 μm	15 μm	3 μm	10 μm	2.5 mm	15 mm
Wall thickness:	2 mm	1 mm	20 μm	30 μm	1 μm	2 μm	0.5 mm	1.5 mm

FIGURE 18–6. Structure of blood vessels. Medium arteries, arterioles, venules, and veins can have a wide range of dimensions. The values here are merely illustrative.

fibers have two components: a core of elastin and a covering of microfibrils. The elastin core consists of a highly insoluble polymer of **elastin**, a protein rich in nonpolar amino acids (i.e., glycine, alanine, valine, proline). After being secreted into the extracellular space, the elastin molecules remain in a random-coil configuration. They covalently cross-link and assemble into a highly elastic network of fibers, capable of stretching more than 100% under physiological conditions. The **microfibrils**, which are composed of glycoproteins and have a diameter of approximately 10 nm, are similar to those found in the extracellular matrix in other tissues. In arteries, elastic fibers are arranged as concentric, cylindrical lamellae. A network of elastic fibers is abundant everywhere except in the true capillaries, venules, and in the aforementioned arteriovenous anastomoses.

Collagen fibers constitute a jacket of far less extensible material than the elastic fibers, like the fabric woven inside the wall of a rubber hose. Collagen can be stretched only 3% to 4% under physiological conditions. The basic unit of the collagen fibers in blood vessels is type I and III collagen molecules, which are two of the fibrillar collagens. After being secreted, these triple-helical molecules assemble into fibrils that may be 10 to 300 nm in diameter; these in turn aggregate into collagen fibers that may be several microns in diameter, and are visible with a light microscope. Collagen fibers are present throughout the circulation except in the capillaries. Collagen and elastic fibers form a network that is more loosely arranged toward the inner surface of the vessel than at the outer surface. Collagen fibers are usually attached to the other components of the vascular wall with some slack, so that they are normally not under tension. Stretching these other components may take up the slack on the collagen fibers, which may then contribute to the overall tension.

Vascular smooth-muscle cells (VSMCs) are also present in all vascular segments except the capillaries. In *elastic* arteries, VSMCs are arranged in spirals with pitch varying from near-longitudinal to near transverse-circular, whereas in *muscular* arteries, they are arranged either in concentric rings or as helices with a low pitch. Relaxed VSMCs do not contribute appreciably to the elastic tension of the vascular wall, which is mainly determined by the elastin and collagen fibers. VSMCs exert tension primarily by means of active contraction (pp. 247 & 460).

Because of the Elastic Properties of Vessels, the Pressure-Flow Relationship of Passive Vascular Beds Is Nonlinear

Because blood vessels are elastic, we must revise our concept of blood flow, which was based on Poiseuille's law for rigid tubes (p. 429). Poiseuille's law predicts a linear pressure-flow relationship (Fig. 18–7A, *broken line*). However, in reality, the *pressure-flow relationship is markedly nonlinear* in an *in vivo* preparation of a vascular bed (see Fig. 18–7A, *red curve*). Starting at the foot of the red curve at a driving pressure of approximately 6 mm Hg, we see that the curve rises more steeply as the driving pressure increases. The reason is that increasing the driving pressure (i.e., axial pressure gradient) also increases the transmural pressure, causing the vessel to distend. Because radius increases, resistance falls and flow rises more than it would in a rigid tube. Thus, the plot curves upward. The *elastic properties* of vessels are the major cause of such nonlinear pressure-flow relationships in vascular beds exhibiting little or no "active tension."

As driving pressure—and thus transmural pressure—increases, vessel radius increases as well, causing resistance (p. 429) to fall (see Fig. 18–7B, *red curve*). Con-

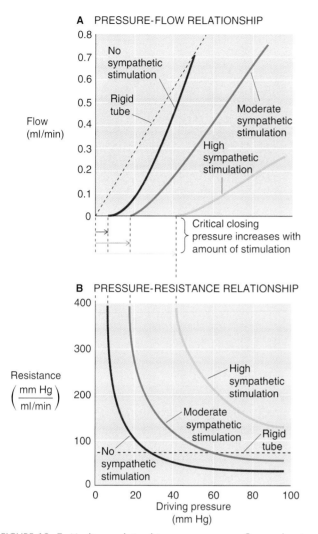

A PRESSURE-FLOW RELATIONSHIP

B PRESSURE-RESISTANCE RELATIONSHIP

FIGURE 18–7. Nonlinear relationships among pressure, flow, and resistance.

versely, resistance increases toward infinity when driving pressure falls. In Poiseuille's case, of course, resistance would be constant (see Fig. 18–7B, *broken line*), regardless of the driving pressure. Although many vascular beds behave as do the *red curves* in Figures 18–7A and *B*, we will see in Chapter 23 that some are highly regulated (i.e., active tension varies with pressure). These special circulations therefore exhibit a pressure-flow relationship that differs substantially from that of a system of elastic tubes.

Contraction of Smooth Muscle Halts Blood Flow When Driving Pressure Falls Below the Critical Closing Pressure

As we have already seen, at low values of driving pressure, resistance rises abruptly toward infinity (see Fig. 18–7B, *red curve*). Viewed differently, flow totally ceases when the pressure falls below approximately 6 mm Hg, the **critical closing pressure** (see Fig. 18–7A, *red curve*). The stoppage of flow occurs because of the combined action of elastic fibers and *active tension* from vascular smooth-muscle cells. Graded increases in active tension—produced, for example by sympathetic stimulation—shift

the pressure-flow relationship to the right and decrease the slope (see Fig. 18–7A, *blue and green curves*), reflecting an increase in resistance over the entire pressure range (see Fig. 18–7B, *blue and green curves*). The critical closing pressure also shifts upward with increasing degrees of vasomotor tone. This phenomenon is important in *hypotensive shock*, where massive vasoconstriction occurs—in an attempt to raise arterial pressure—and critical closing pressures rise to 40 mm Hg or more. As a result, blood flow can stop completely in the limb of a patient in hypotensive shock, despite the persistence of a finite, albeit small, pressure difference between the main artery and vein.

Elastic and Collagen Fibers Determine the Distensibility and Compliance of Vessels

Arteries and veins must withstand very different transmural pressures in vivo (see Table 18–3). Moreover, their relative blood volumes respond in strikingly different ways to increases in transmural pressure (Fig. 18–8). Arteries have a low volume capacity, but can withstand large transmural pressure differences. In contrast, veins have a large volume capacity (and are thus able to act as blood reservoirs), but can withstand only small transmural pressure differences.

The abundance of structural elements in the vascular walls also differs between arteries and veins (see Fig. 18–6). These disparities contribute to differences in the elastic behavior of arteries and veins. We can study the elastic properties of an isolated blood vessel either by recording the "static" volume change produced by pressurizing the vessel to different levels, or, conversely, by recording the "static" pressure change produced by filling the vessel with liquid to different volumes. After experimentally altering the pressure or volume, it is important to wait until the vessel has finished responding (i.e., it becomes static) before recording the measurements.

The **volume distensibility** expresses the elastic properties of blood vessels. Three measurements are useful for assessing distensibility. First, the **absolute distensibility** is the change in volume for a *macroscopic* step change in pressure, $\Delta V/\Delta P$. Second, because the unstretched size varies among vessels, it is preferable to normalize the volume change to the initial, unstretched volume (V_0) and thus to use a **normalized distensibility** instead:

$$\text{Equation 18–4}$$

$$\text{Normalized Distensibility} = \frac{(\Delta V/V_0)}{\Delta P}$$

This ratio is a measurement of the fractional change in volume with a given step in pressure. Third, the most useful index of distensibility is **compliance** (C), which is the slope of the tangent to any point along the pressure-volume diagram in Figure 18–8:

$$\text{Equation 18–5}$$

$$C = \frac{\Delta V}{\Delta P}$$

Here, the ΔV and ΔP values are *minute* displacements. The steeper the slope of a pressure-volume diagram, the

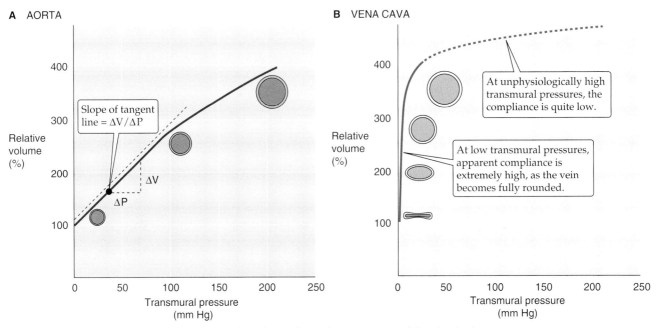

FIGURE 18-8. Compliance of blood vessels. In *A* and *B*, relative volume of 100% represents fully relaxed volume.

greater the compliance (i.e., the easier it is to increase volume). In Figure 18-8, the slope—and thus the compliance—decreases with increasing volumes. For such a nonlinear relationship, this variable compliance is the slope of the tangent to the curve at any point. Thus, a compliance reading should always include the transmural pressure or the volume at which it was made. Similar principles apply to the compliance of airways in the lung (p. 615).

Differences in Compliance Cause Arteries to Act as Resistors, and Veins to Act as Capacitors

As we increase transmural pressure, **arteries** increase in volume. As they accommodate the volume of blood ejected with every heartbeat, large, muscular systemic arteries (e.g., femoral artery) increase in radius by approximately 10%. This change for a typical *muscular* artery is much smaller than the distention that one would observe for *elastic* arteries (e.g., aorta), which have fewer layers of smooth muscle and are not under nervous control. The higher compliance of elastic arteries is evident in the pressure-volume diagram in Figure 18-8*A*—obtained after relaxing the smooth muscle. The compliance of a relaxed elastic artery is substantial: Increasing the transmural pressure from 0 to 100 mm Hg (near the normal, mean arterial pressure) increases relative volume by approximately 180%. With further increases in pressure and diameter, compliance decreases only modestly. For example, increasing transmural pressure from 100 to 200 mm Hg increases relative volume by a further approximately 100 percentage points. Thus, arteries are properly constituted for developing and withstanding high transmural pressures. Because an increase in pressure raises the radius only modestly under physiological conditions, particularly in muscular arteries, the resistance of the artery (inversely proportional to r⁴) does not fall markedly. Be-

cause muscular arteries have a rather stable resistance, they are sometimes referred to as **resistance vessels**.

Veins behave very differently. The pressure-volume diagram of a vein (see Fig. 18-8*B*) shows that compliance is extremely high—far higher than for "elastic arteries"—at least in the low-pressure range. For a relaxed vein, a relatively small increase of transmural pressure from 0 to 10 mm Hg increases volume by approximately 200%. This high compliance in the low-pressure range is not due to a property of the elastic fibers. Rather, it reflects a change in geometry. At pressures below 6 to 9 mm Hg, the vein's cross section is ellipsoidal. A small rise in pressure causes the vein to become circular, without an increase in perimeter, but with a greatly increased cross-sectional area. Thus, in their normal pressure range (see Table 18-3), veins can accept relatively large volumes of blood with little buildup of pressure. Because they act as *volume reservoirs*, veins are sometimes referred to as **capacitance vessels**. The true distensibility or compliance of the venous wall—related to the increase in *perimeter* produced by pressures above 10 mm Hg—is rather poor, as shown by the flat slope at higher pressures in Figure 18-8*B*.

How do veins and elastic arteries compare in response to a sudden increase in volume (ΔV)? When the heart ejects its stroke volume into the aorta, the intravascular pressure increases modestly, from 80 to 120 mm Hg. This change in intravascular pressure—also known as the pulse pressure (p. 435)—is the same as the change in transmural pressure. We have already seen that venous compliance is low in this "arterial" pressure range. Thus, if we were to challenge a vein with a sudden increase in volume (ΔV) in the arterial pressure range, the increase in transmural pressure (ΔP) would be much higher than an artery of equal size. This is indeed the case when a surgeon uses a saphenous vein segment in a coronary artery bypass graft, and anastomoses the vein between

A EXPERIMENTAL PREPARATION

B STRESS-STRAIN RELATIONSHIP

FIGURE 18–9. Elastic properties of a spring.

two sites on a coronary artery, forming a bypass around an obstructed site.

Changes in the volume of vessels during the cardiac cycle are due to changes in radius, rather than in length. During ejection of blood during systole, the length of the thoracic aorta may increase by only approximately 1%.

Laplace's Law Describes How Tension in the Vessel Wall Increases with Transmural Pressure

Because compliance depends on the elastic properties of the vessel wall, the discussion here focuses on how an external force deforms elastic materials. When the force vanishes, the deformation vanishes, and the material returns to its original state. The simplest mechanical model of a linearly elastic solid is a spring (Fig. 18–9A). The elongation ΔL is proportional to the **force** ($\mathcal{F}$), according to **Hooke's law**:

Equation 18–6

$$\mathcal{F} = k \cdot \Delta L$$

k is a constant. If an elastic body requires a larger force to achieve a certain deformation, it is stiffer or less compliant. The largest stress that the material can withstand while remaining elastic is the **elastic limit**. If deformed beyond this limit, the material reaches its yield point and, eventually, its breaking point.

Stress is the force per unit cross-sectional area ($\mathcal{F}/A$). Thus, if we pull on an elastic band—stretching it from an initial length L_0 to a final length L—the stress is the

TABLE 18–5

ELASTIC MODULI (i.e., STIFFNESS) OF VARIOUS MATERIALS	
MATERIAL	**ELASTIC MODULUS (dyne/cm²)***
Smooth muscle	10^4 or 10^5
Elastin	4×10^6
Rubber	4×10^7
Collagen	1×10^{10}
Wood	10^{10} to 10^{12}

*1 mm Hg = 1334 dynes/cm²

force we apply, divided by the area of the band in cross section. **Strain** is the fractional increase in length, that is, $\Delta L/L_0$ or $(L-L_0)/L_0$ (see Fig. 18–9B). An equation analogous to Hooke's law describes the relationship between stress and strain:

Equation 18–7

$$\underbrace{\frac{\mathcal{F}}{A}}_{\text{Stress}} = Y \underbrace{\left(\frac{L - L_0}{L_0} \right)}_{\text{Strain}}$$

The proportionality factor, Young's **elastic modulus** (Y), is the force per cross-sectional area required to stretch the material to twice its initial length, and also the slope of the strain-stress diagram in Figure 18–9B. Thus, the stiffer a material is, the steeper the slope, and the greater the elastic modulus. For example, collagen is more than 1000-fold stiffer than elastin (Table 18–5).

Because the elastic and collagen fibers in blood vessels are not arranged as simple linear springs, the stresses and strains that arise during the pressurization or filling of a vessel occur, at least in principle, along three axes (Fig. 18–10): (1) an elongation of the circumference (θ), (2) an elongation of the axial length (x), and (3) a compression of the thickness of the vessel wall in the direction of the radius (r). In fact, blood vessels actually change little in length during distention, and the thinning of the wall is usually not a major factor. Thus, we can describe the elastic properties of a vessel by considering only what happens along the circumference.

The transmural pressure (ΔP) is the distending force that tends to increase the circumference of the vessel. Opposing this elongation is a force inside the vessel wall. It is convenient to express this wall **tension** (T) as the force that must be applied to bring together the two edges of an imaginary slit, of unit length L, cut in the wall along the longitudinal axis of the vessel (Fig. 18–11). Note that in using tension (units: dynes/cm) rather than stress (units: dynes/cm²), we assume that the thickness of the vessel wall is constant.

The equilibrium between ΔP and T depends on the vessel radius, and is expressed by a law derived independently by Thomas Young and Marquis de Laplace in the early 1800s. For a cylinder,

Equation 18–8

$$T = \Delta P \cdot r$$

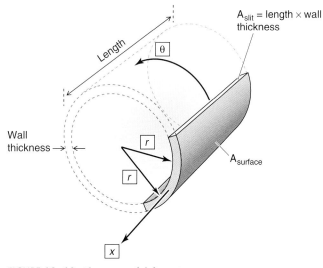

FIGURE 18–10. Three axes of deformation.

Thus, for a given transmural pressure, the wall tension in the vessel gets larger as the radius increases.

The Vascular Wall Is Adapted to Withstand Wall Tension, Not Transmural Pressure

In Figure 18–8, we plotted the volume of a vessel against transmural pressure, finding that the slope of this relationship is compliance. However, this sort of analysis does not provide us with direct information on the spring-like properties of the materials that make up the vessel wall. With Laplace's law ($T = \Delta P \cdot r$), we can transform the pressure-volume relationship into the same kind of "elastic diagram" that we used in Figure 18–9B to understand the properties of a rubber band.

Figure 18–12A is a replot of the pressure-volume diagrams in Figure 18–8A and B. In Figure 18–12B, we

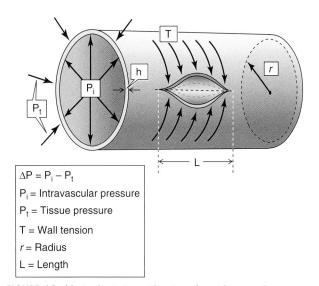

$$\Delta P = P_i - P_t$$

P_i = Intravascular pressure

P_t = Tissue pressure

T = Wall tension

r = Radius

L = Length

FIGURE 18–11. Laplace's Law. The *circumferential arrows* that attempt to bring together the edges of an imaginary slit along the length of the vessel represent the constricting force of the tension in the wall. The *radial arrows* that push the wall outward represent the distending force. At equilibrium, the two sets of forces balance.

reverse the coordinate system so that volume is now on the x-axis and pressure on the y-axis. Finally, in Figure 18–12C, we convert volume to radius on the x-axis, and use Laplace's law to convert pressure into wall tension on the y-axis. The plots in Figure 18–12C are analogous to a stress-strain diagram for a rubber band (see Fig. 18–9B). Thus, stretching the radius of the aorta (*solid red curve*) causes a considerable rise in wall tension, reflecting the aorta's moderate compliance. The vena cava, on the other hand, fills over a wide range of radii before developing any wall tension, reflecting the shape change that makes it *appear* to be very compliant at the low pressures that are physiological for a vein. However, further stretching the vein's radius results in a steep rise in wall tension, reflecting the inherently limited compliance of veins.

What does Laplace's law (see Equation 18–8) tell us about the wall tension necessary to withstand the pressure inside a blood vessel? On the plot of tension versus radius for the aorta in Figure 18–12C, we have chosen a single point at a radius of 6 mm; because the aorta is relatively stiff, stretching it to this radius produces a wall tension of 120,000 dynes/cm. According to Laplace's law, exactly one *pressure*—200,000 dynes/cm² or 150 mm Hg—satisfies this combination of r and T. In Figure 18–12C, this pressure is indicated by the *slope* of the *red broken line* that connects the origin with our point. In a similar exercise for the vena cava, we assume a radius of approximately 6.7 mm, which is similar to the one we chose for the aorta; because the vena cava is readily deformed in this range, expanding it to this radius produces a wall tension of only 12,000 dynes/cm (*blue broken line*). This combination of r and T yields a much lower pressure—18,000 dynes/cm², or 13.5 mm Hg. Thus, comparing vessels of *similar size*, Laplace's law tells us that a high wall tension is required to withstand a high pressure.

Comparing two vessels of very *different size* reveals a disparity between wall tension and pressure. A large vein, such as the vena cava, must resist only 10 mm Hg in transmural pressure, but is equipped with a fair amount of elastic tissue. A capillary, on the other hand, which must resist a transmural pressure of 25 mm Hg, does not have any elastic tissue at all. Why? The key concept is that what the vessel really has to withstand is not pressure, but *wall tension*. According to Laplace's law (see Equation 18–8), wall tension is the product of transmural pressure and radius ($\Delta P \cdot r$). Hence, wall tension in a capillary (10 dynes/cm) is much smaller than that in the vena cava (18,000 dynes/cm), even though the capillary is at a higher pressure. Table 18–6 shows that the amount of elastic tissue correlates extremely well with wall tension, but very poorly with transmural pressure. The higher the tension that the vessel wall must bear, the greater is its complement of elastic tissue.

Elastin and Collagen Separately Contribute to the Wall Tension of Vessels

The *solid red and blue curves* in Figure 18–12C are quite different from the linear behavior predicted by Hooke's law (see Fig. 18–9B). With increasing stretch, the vessel wall resists additional deformation more; that is, the slope of the relationship becomes steeper. The increasing slope

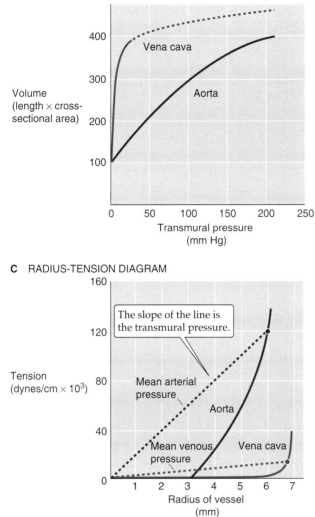

A PRESSURE-VOLUME DIAGRAM

Volume (length × cross-sectional area)

Vena cava

Aorta

Transmural pressure (mm Hg)

B VOLUME-PRESSURE DIAGRAM

Transmural pressure (P = T/r)

Aorta

Vena cava

Volume (V = length × πr^2)

C RADIUS-TENSION DIAGRAM

Tension (dynes/cm × 10^3)

The slope of the line is the transmural pressure.

Mean arterial pressure

Aorta

Mean venous pressure

Vena cava

Radius of vessel (mm)

FIGURE 18–12. Elastic diagram (tension versus radius) of blood vessels. In *A*, the *curves* are re-plots of the curves in Figure 18–8, *A* and *B*. In *B*, the plot is the result of reversing the two axes in *A*. In *C*, the *solid red and blue curves* are transformations of the curves in *B*. If we solve for r, the *x-axis* of *B* (volume) becomes radius in *C*; if we use Laplace's law (T = P · r) to solve for T, the *y-axis* of *B* (transmural pressure) becomes tension in *C*.

(i.e., increasing elastic modulus) of the radius-tension diagram of a blood vessel is due to the heterogeneity of the elastic material of the vascular wall. Elastic and collagen fibers have different elastic moduli (see Table 18–5). We can quantitate the separate contributions of elastic and collagen fibers by "chemical dissection." After selective digestion of the elastic fibers with elastase, which un-

masks the behavior of collagen fibers, the length-tension relationship is very steep and closer to the linear relationship expected from Hooke's law (Fig. 18–13, *orange curve*). After selective digestion of collagen fibers with formic acid, which unmasks the behavior of elastic fibers, the length-tension relationship is fairly flat (see Fig. 18–13, *blue curve*). The *orange curve* (collagen) is steeper than

TABLE 18–6

COMPARISON OF WALL TENSIONS AND ELASTIC-TISSUE CONTENT IN VARIOUS VESSELS

	MEAN TRANSMURAL PRESSURE ΔP (mm Hg)	RADIUS (r)	WALL TENSION T (dynes/cm)	ELASTIC TISSUE*
Aorta	95	1.13 cm	140,000	++++
Small arteries	90	0.5 cm	60,000	+++
Arterioles	60	15 μm	1200	+
Capillaries	25	3 μm	10	0
Venules	15	10 μm	20	0
Veins	12	>0.02 cm	320	+
Vena cava	10	1.38 cm	18,000	++

*The number of plus signs is a relative index of the amount of elastic tissue.

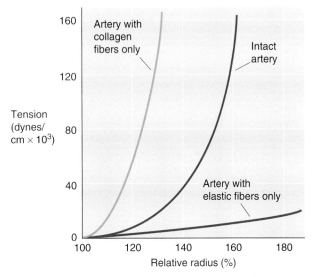

FIGURE 18–13. Chemical dissection of elastic moduli of collagen and elastin.

the *blue curve* (elastin) because collagen is stiffer than elastin (see Table 18–5). In a normal vessel (see Fig. 18–13, *red curve*), modest degrees of stretch elongate primarily the elastin fibers along a relatively flat slope. Progressively greater degrees of stretch recruit collagen fibers, resulting in a steeper slope.

Aging Reduces the Distensibility of Arteries

With aging, important changes occur in the elastic properties of blood vessels, primarily arteries. We can look at these age relationships for arteries from two perspectives, the pressure-volume curve and the radius-tension curve.

The most obvious difference in aortic pressure-volume curves with increasing age is that the curves shift to progressively higher volumes (Fig. 18–14A), reflecting an increase in diameter. In addition, the compliance of the aorta first rises during growth and development to early adulthood, and then falls during later life. After early adulthood, two unfavorable changes occur. First, arteriosclerotic changes reduce the vessel's compliance per se. Thus, during ventricular ejection, a normal-sized increase in aortic volume (ΔV) in a young adult produces a relatively small pulse pressure (ΔP) in the aorta. In contrast, the same change in aortic volume in an elderly individual produces a much larger pulse pressure. Second, because blood pressure frequently rises with age, the older person operates on a flatter portion of the pressure-volume curve, where the compliance is even lower than at lower pressures. Thus, a normal-sized increase in aortic volume produces an even larger pulse pressure.

The second approach for assessing the effects of age on the elastic properties of blood vessels is to examine the radius-tension diagram (see Fig. 18–14B). Because of the progressive, diffuse fibrosis of vessel walls with age, and because of an increase in the amount of collagen, the maximal slope of the radius-tension diagram increases with age. In addition, with age, these curves start to bend upward at lower radii, as the same degree of stretch recruits a larger number of collagen fibers. Underlying this phenomenon is an increased cross-linking among collagen fibers, and thus less slack in their connections to other elements in the arterial wall. Thus, even modest elongations challenge the stiffer collagen fibers to stretch.

Active Tension from Smooth-Muscle Activity Adds to the Elastic Tension of Vessels

Although we have been treating blood vessels as though their walls were purely elastic, the **active tension** (p. 247)

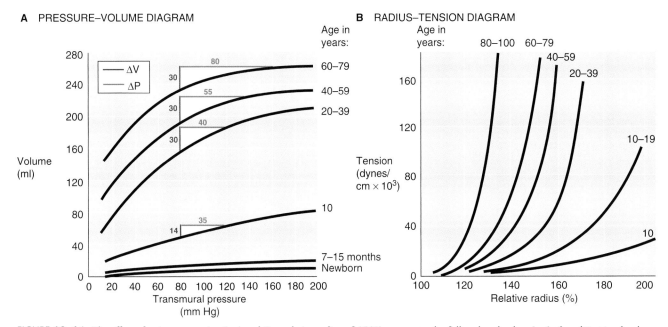

FIGURE 18–14. The effect of aging on arteries. In *A* and *B*, a relative radius of 100% represents the fully relaxed value. In *A*, the *white triangles* show the expected change in transmural pressure (*blue line*) for increase in aortic blood volume (*red line*) produced by each heartbeat—assuming a diastolic pressure of 80 mm Hg.

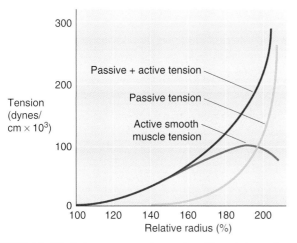

FIGURE 18–15. Active versus passive tension. The relative radius of 100% is that of an excised vessel maximally stimulated by norepinephrine (*red curve*, total tension), but not "stressed" (i.e., transmural pressure is 0). When the vessel is maximally poisoned with potassium cyanide, the baseline radius is approximately 150% (*green curve*, passive tension), reflecting its relaxed state. The *blue curve* is just the active (i.e., smooth-muscle) component of tension.

from vascular smooth-muscle cells also contributes to wall tension. Stimulation of VSMCs can reduce the internal radius of muscular feed arteries by 20% to 50%. Laplace's law (T = ΔP · r) tells us that, as the VSMC shortens—thereby reducing vessel radius against a constant transmural pressure—there is a decrease in the tension that the muscle must exert to maintain that new, smaller radius.

For a blood vessel in which both passive elastic components and active smooth-muscle components contribute to the total tension, the radius-tension relationship reflects the contributions of each. The red curve in Figure 18–15 shows such a compounded ("passive" + "active") radius-tension diagram for an artery in which the sympathetic neurotransmitter norepinephrine (p. 387) has maximally stimulated the VSMCs. The *green curve* shows a "passive" radius-tension relationship for just the elastic component of the tension (after the active component is eliminated by poisoning of the VSMCs with potassium cyanide). Of course, the *green curve* is the radius-tension diagram on

which we have focused the previous figures (e.g., see Fig. 18–12C). Subtracting the *green* from the *red curve* in Fig. 18–15 yields the *active* length-tension diagram (*blue curve*) for the vascular smooth muscle.

Elastic Tension Helps Stabilize Vessels Under Vasomotor Control

Consider a vessel initially stretched to a radius that is 80% greater than the unstressed radius (i.e., 180 vs 100 on the x-axis of Fig. 18–15). As we inject more fluid into the vessel, the radius increases (i.e., the vessel is more "stressed"). As a result, total wall tension must increase (see Fig. 18–15, *red curve*). The opposite, of course, would happen if we were to withdraw some fluid from the vessel. During such changes in total wall tension, what are the individual contributions of vascular smooth-muscle tension and the passive connective-tissue tension? In Figure 18–16, we consider two extreme examples, one in which the vessel has only elastic elements, and another in which it has only a fixed (i.e., isotonic) active tension.

First, consider a vessel lacking smooth muscle, so that only elastic elements contribute to total wall tension (see Fig. 18–16A). If we increase transmural pressure from P (*Panel 1*) to P+ΔP (*Panel 2*), thereby increasing the radius from r to r+Δr, wall tension will automatically increase from T to T+ΔT. This increase in tension allows the vessel to reach a new equilibrium, according to Laplace's law:

Equation 18–9
$$T + \Delta T = (P + \Delta P) \cdot (r + \Delta r)$$

Conversely, a decrease in pressure must lead to a decrease in radius and a decrease in tension (*Panel 3*). To achieve either the stable inflation of *Panel 2* or the stable deflation of *Panel 3*, ΔT cannot be zero. In other words, the passive radius-tension diagram (see Fig. 18–15, *green curve*) cannot have a slope of zero. The vessel wall must have some elasticity.

Second, consider a hypothetical case in which *no elastic fibers* are present, and in which the total tension T is kept constant by active elements (i.e., VSMCs) alone. For example, this would be approximately the case for the *blue curve* in Figure 8–15, between relative radii of 180% to

A STABILITY OF VESSEL WITH ELASTIC WALL TENSION

Start	+ΔP $\rightarrow$ +Δr	−ΔP $\rightarrow$ −Δr
T = P × r	T + ΔT = (P + ΔP)(r + Δr)	T − ΔT = (P − ΔP)(r − Δr)
Stable equilibrium	Stable inflation	Stable deflation

B INSTABILITY OF VESSEL WITH ONLY A FIXED, ACTIVE WALL TENSION

Start	+ΔP $\rightarrow$ +Δr	−ΔP $\rightarrow$ −Δr
T = P × r	T < (P + ΔP)(r + Δr)	T > (P − ΔP)(r − Δr)
Unstable equilibrium	Pressure wins to blowout	Tension wins to collapse

FIGURE 18–16. Mechanical stability of vessels.

200%. At the start (see Fig. 18–16B, *Panel 1*), we will assume that the smooth-muscle tension exactly balances the P · r product. However, when we now increase pressure *(Panel 2)*, the automatic adaptation of tension that we saw in the previous example would *not* occur. Indeed any increase in pressure would make the product $(P + \Delta P) \cdot (r + \Delta r)$ exceed the fixed T of the VSMCs. As a result, the vessel would blow out. Conversely, any decrease in pressure would make the product $(P - \Delta P) \cdot (r - \Delta r)$ fall below the fixed T and lead to full collapse of the vessel *(Panel 3)*. This type of instability does in fact occur in **arteriovenous anastomoses**, which are characterized by poor elastic tissue and abundant myoepithelioid cells.

A real vessel, whose wall contains both elastic and smooth-muscle elements, can be stable (i.e., neither blown out nor collapsed) over a wide range of radii. The role of elastic tissue in vessels is, therefore, not only to withstand high transmural pressures, but also to stabilize the vessel. Thus, elastic tissue ensures a graded response when smooth-muscle tone changes. If vessels had only smooth muscle—and no elastic fibers—they would be like those in *Panels 2* and *3* of Figure 18–16B, and tend to be either completely open or completely closed.

An imbalance between passive and active elastic components in blood vessels can be important in disease. For example, when the passive, elastic fibers of a blood vessel are reduced or damaged, vessels tend to become larger (e.g., **aneurysms** or **varicosities**). If the radius exceeds the value compatible with the physical equilibrium governed by Laplace's law, a blowout may occur.

A second pathologic example is seen when smooth muscle has undergone maximal stimulation and, conversely, passive elastic elements have regressed. This is the case in **Raynaud's disease**, in which exposure to cold leads to extreme constriction of arterioles in the extremities, particularly the fingers. Vessel closure occurs because active smooth-muscle tension dominates the radius tension diagram.

REFERENCES

Books and Reviews

Burton AC: Relation of structure to function of the tissues of the wall of blood vessels. Physiol Rev 34:619–642, 1954.

Dobrin PB: Vascular mechanics. In Shepherd JT, Abboud FM (eds): Handbook of Physiology, Sect 2. The Cardiovascular System, Vol III, Part 1. Bethesda, MD, American Physiological Society, 1979, pp 65–102.

Monos E, Bérczi V, Nádasy G: Local control of veins: Biomechanical, metabolic, and humoral aspects. Physiol Rev 75:611–666, 1995.

Mulvany MJ, Aalkjær C: Structure and function of small arteries. Physiol Rev 70:921–961, 1990.

Rother CF: Venous system: Physiology of the capacitance vessels. In Shepherd JT, Abboud FM (eds): Handbook of Physiology, Sect 2. The Cardiovascular System, Vol III, Part 1. Bethesda, MD, American Physiological Society, 1979, pp 397–452.

Journal Articles

Bayliss WM: On the local reactions of the arterial wall to changes in internal pressure. J Physiol London 28:220–231, 1902.

Bowditch N: *Mécanique Céleste by the marquis de La Place* (translated and with a commentary by Nathaniel Bowditch). Boston, Little, Brown, 1829–1839, 4 volumes.

Burton AC: On the physical equilibrium of small blood vessels. Am J Physiol 164: 319–329, 1947.

McDonald DA, Taylor MG: The hydrodynamics of the arterial circulation. Progr Biophys 9:105–173, 1959.

Young T: Hydraulic investigations subservient to an intended Croonian lecture on the motion of the blood. Philos Trans R Soc London 98: 164–186, 1808.

CHAPTER 19

The Microcirculation

Emile L. Boulpaep

The Microcirculation Serves Both Nutritional and Non-Nutritional Roles

The primary function of the cardiovascular system is to maintain a suitable environment for the tissues. The microcirculation is the "business end" of the system. The capillary is the principal site for the exchange of gases, water, nutrients, and waste products. In most tissues, capillary flow exclusively serves these **nutritional** needs. In a few tissues, however, a large portion of capillary flow is **non-nutritional**. For example, in the glomeruli of the kidneys, capillary flow forms the glomerular filtrate (p. 757). Blood flow through the skin, some of which may shunt through arteriovenous anastomoses, plays a key role in temperature regulation (p. 1237). Capillaries also serve other non-nutritional roles, such as signalling (e.g., delivery of hormones) and host-defense (e.g., delivery of platelets). In the first part of this chapter, we discuss the nutritional role of capillaries, and we examine how gases, small water-soluble substances, macromolecules, and water pass across the endothelium. In the last two subchapters, we will discuss lymphatics, as well as the regulation of the microcirculation.

The morphology and local regulatory mechanisms of the microcirculation are designed to meet the particular needs of each tissue. Because these needs may be quite different, the structure and function of the microcirculation may be quite different from one tissue to the next.

The Microcirculation Extends from the Arterioles to the Venules

The microcirculation is defined as the blood vessels from the first-order arteriole to the first-order venule. Although the details vary from organ to organ, the principal components of an idealized microcirculation include a single arteriole and venule, between which extends a network of true capillaries (Fig. 19–1). Sometimes a metarteriole—somewhat larger than a capillary—provides a shortcut through the network. Both the arteriole and the venule have vascular smooth-muscle cells (VSMCs). Precapillary sphincters—at the transition between a capillary and either an arteriole or a metarteriole—control the access of blood to particular segments of the network. Sphincter closure/opening creates small local pressure differences that may reverse the direction of blood flow in some segments of the network.

Arteries consist of an inner layer of endothelium, an internal elastic lamina, and a surrounding sheath of at least two continuous layers of

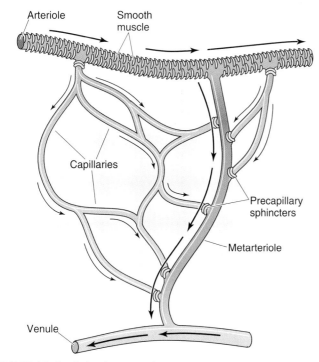

FIGURE 19-1. Idealized microcirculatory circuit.

innervated VSMCs (p. 453). The inner radius of **terminal arteries** (called "feed" arteries in muscle) may be as small as 25 μm. **Arterioles** (inner radius: 5–25 μm) are similar to arteries, but have only a *single* continuous layer of VSMCs, which are innervated. **Metarterioles** are similar to arterioles, but of shorter length. Moreover, their VSMCs are discontinuous and are not usually innervated. The **precapillary sphincter** is a small cuff of smooth muscle that usually is not innervated, but is very responsive to local tissue conditions. Relaxation or contraction of the precapillary sphincter may modulate tissue blood flow by an order of magnitude or more. Metarterioles and precapillary sphincters are not found in all tissues.

True capillaries (inner radius: 2–5 μm) consist of a single layer of endothelial cells surrounded by a basement membrane, a fine network of reticular collagen fibers, and—in some tissues—pericytes. The endothelial cells have a smooth surface and are extremely thin (as little as 200–300 nm in height), except at the nucleus. The thickness and density of the capillary **basement membrane** vary among organs. Where large transcapillary pressures occur or other large mechanical forces exist, the basement membrane is thickest. Some endothelial cells have, on both their luminal and basal surfaces, numerous **coated pits** and **coated vesicles** that are involved in fluid-phase and receptor-mediated endocytosis (p. 42). Indeed, the cytoplasm of capillary endothelial cells is rich in endocytotic (pinocytotic) **vesicles** (<100 nm in diameter). These vesicles contribute to the **transcytosis** of water and water-soluble compounds across the wall of the endothelial cells. In some cases, the endocytotic vesicles are lined up in a string and even appear linked together to form a **transendothelial channel.**

Linking endothelial cells together are **inter-endothelial junctions** (Fig. 19–2); here, the two cell membranes are approximately 10 nm apart, although there may be constricted regions where the space or **cleft** between the two cells is only 4 nm wide. Endothelial cells may also have **tight junctions** (p. 46), in which the apposed cell membranes actually fuse and claudins are present. Some endothelial cells have membrane-lined, cylindrical conduits—**fenestrations**—that run completely through the cell, from the capillary lumen to the interstitial space. These fenestrations are 50 to 80 nm in diameter, and are seen primarily in tissues with large fluid and solute fluxes across the capillary walls (e.g., intestine, choroid plexus, exocrine glands, and renal glomeruli). The perforations of the fenestrae are often closed by a thin diaphragm (e.g., in intestinal capillaries).

The endothelia of the sinusoidal capillaries in the liver, bone marrow, and spleen have very large fenestrations, as well as **gaps** 100 nm to 1000 nm wide *between* adjacent cells. Vesicles, transendothelial channels, fenestrae, and gaps—as well as structures of intermediate appearance—are probably part of a spectrum of regulated permeation across the endothelial cells.

Capillaries fall into three groups, based on their degree of leakiness (Fig. 19–3).

1. **Continuous capillary.** This is the most common form of capillary. It has inter-endothelial junctions 10 to 15 nm wide. These clefts are absent in the blood-brain barrier (p. 408), whose capillaries have narrow tight junctions.
2. **Fenestrated capillary.** In these capillaries, the endothelial cells are thin and perforated with fenestrations. These capillaries most often surround epithelia (e.g., small intestine, exocrine glands).
3. **Discontinuous capillary.** In addition to fenestrae, these capillaries have large gaps. Discontinuous capillaries are found in sinusoids (e.g., liver).

At their distal ends, true capillaries merge into **venules** (inner radius: 5–25 μm), which carry blood back into low-pressure veins that return blood to the heart. Venules have a discontinuous layer of VSMCs and, therefore, can control local blood flow. Venules may also exchange some solutes across their walls.

FIGURE 19–2. Capillary endothelial junctions. This electron micrograph shows the interendothelial junction between two endothelial cells in a muscle capillary. *Arrows* point to tight junctions. (From Fawcett DW: Bloom and Fawcett. A textbook of histology, 12th ed. New York, Chapman & Hall, 1994, p 964.)

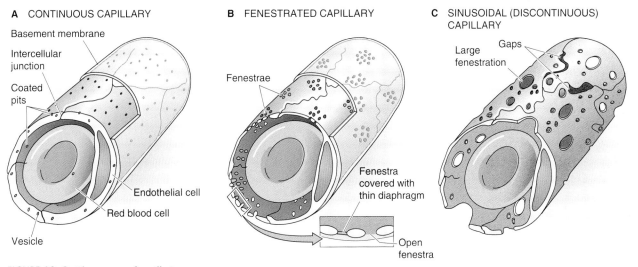

A CONTINUOUS CAPILLARY

Basement membrane
Intercellular junction
Coated pits
Endothelial cell
Red blood cell
Vesicle

B FENESTRATED CAPILLARY

Fenestrae
Fenestra covered with thin diaphragm
Open fenestra

C SINUSOIDAL (DISCONTINUOUS) CAPILLARY

Large fenestration
Gaps

FIGURE 19–3. Three types of capillaries.

CAPILLARY EXCHANGE OF SOLUTES

The Exchange of Oxygen and Carbon Dioxide Across Capillaries Depends on the Diffusional Properties of the Surrounding Tissue

Gases diffuse by a **transcellular route** across the two cell membranes and cytosol of the endothelial cells of the capillary with the same ease that they diffuse through the surrounding tissue. In this section, we focus primarily on the exchange of oxygen. Very similar mechanisms exist for the exchange of carbon dioxide, but they run in the opposite direction. Arterial blood has a relatively high O_2 level. As blood traverses a systemic capillary, the principal site of gas exchange, O_2 diffuses across the capillary wall and into the tissue space, which includes the interstitial fluid and the neighboring cells.

The most frequently used model of gas exchange is August Krogh's **tissue cylinder**, a volume of tissue that a single capillary supplies with O_2 (Fig. 19–4A). The cylinder of tissue surrounds a single capillary. According to this model, the properties of the tissue cylinder govern the rate of diffusion of both O_2 and CO_2. The radius of a tissue cylinder in an organ is typically half the average spacing from one capillary to the next, that is, half the mean intercapillary distance. Capillary density and, therefore, mean intercapillary distance vary greatly among tissues. Among systemic tissues, capillary density is highest in tissues with high O_2 consumption (e.g., myocardium), and lowest in tissues consuming little O_2 (e.g., joint cartilage). Capillary density is extraordinarily high in the lungs (p. 696).

The Krogh model predicts how the concentration or partial pressure of oxygen (PO_2) within the capillary lumen falls along the length of the capillary as O_2 exits for the surrounding tissues (see Fig. 19–4A). The PO_2 within the capillary at any site along the length of the capillary depends on several factors:

1. The concentration of **free O_2** in the arteriolar blood that feeds the capillary. This dissolved [O_2], which is

the same in the plasma and the cytoplasm of the erythrocytes (red blood cells [RBCs]), is proportional to the partial pressure of O_2 (p. 654) in the arterioles.

2. The **O_2 content** of the blood. Less than 2% of the total O_2 in arterial blood is dissolved; the rest is bound to hemoglobin inside the RBCs. Each 100 ml of arterial blood contains approximately 20 ml of O_2 gas, or 20 volume%—the **O_2 content** (see Table 28–3).

3. The **capillary blood flow** (F).

4. The **radial diffusion coefficient** (D_r), which governs the diffusion of O_2 out of the capillary lumen. For simplicity, we assume that D_r is the same within the blood, the capillary wall, and the surrounding tissue, and that it is the same along the entire length of the capillary.

5. The **capillary radius** (r_c).

6. The **radius of tissue cylinder** (r_t) that the capillary is supplying with O_2.

7. The **O_2 consumption** by the surrounding tissues ($\dot{Q}O_2$).

8. The **axial distance** (x) along the capillary.

The combination of all these factors accounts for the shape of the concentration profiles within the vessel and the tissue. Although this model appears complicated, it is actually based on many simplifying assumptions.

The O_2 Extraction Ratio of a Whole Organ Depends Primarily on Blood Flow and Metabolic Demand

In principle, beginning with a model like Krogh's but more complete, one could sum up the predictions for a single capillary segment, and then predict gas exchange in an entire tissue. However, it is more convenient to pool all the capillaries in an organ and focus on a single arterial inflow and single venous outflow. The difference in the concentration of a substance in the arterial inflow and venous outflow of that organ is the **arteriovenous (a–v) difference** of that substance. For example, if the

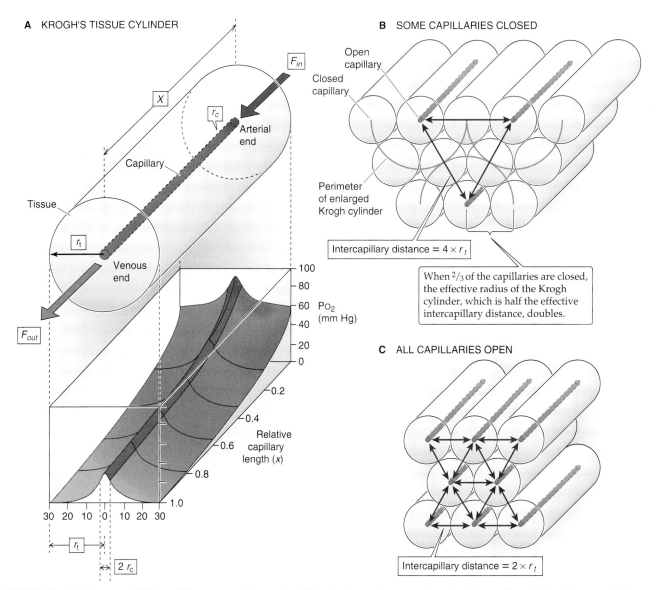

A KROGH'S TISSUE CYLINDER

B SOME CAPILLARIES CLOSED

Open capillary

Closed capillary

Perimeter of enlarged Krogh cylinder

Intercapillary distance = $4 \times r_t$

When $2/3$ of the capillaries are closed, the effective radius of the Krogh cylinder, which is half the effective intercapillary distance, doubles.

C ALL CAPILLARIES OPEN

Intercapillary distance = $2 \times r_t$

FIGURE 19–4. Delivery and diffusion of O_2 to systemic tissues. In A, Krogh's tissue cylinder consists of a single capillary (radius r_c), surrounded by a concentric cylinder of tissue (radius r_t) that the capillary supplies with O_2 and other nutrients. Blood flow into the capillary is F_{in}, and blood flow out of the capillary is F_{out}. The *lower panel* of A shows how profile of partial pressure of O_2 (P_{O_2}) along the longitudinal axis of the capillary and the radial axis of the tissue cylinder.

arterial O_2 *content* ($[O_2]_a$) entering the tissue is 20 ml O_2/dl blood, and the venous O_2 content leaving it ($[O_2]_v$) is 15 ml O_2/dl blood, then the O_2 a–v difference for that tissue is 5 ml O_2 gas/dl blood.

For a substance like O_2, which *exits* the capillaries, another way of expressing the amount that the tissues remove is the **extraction ratio**. This parameter is merely the a–v difference *normalized* to the arterial content of the substance. Thus, the extraction ratio of oxygen (E_{O_2}) is:

Equation 19–1

$$E_{O_2} = \frac{[O_2]_a - [O_2]_v}{[O_2]_a}$$

Thus, in our example:

Equation 19–2

$$E_{O_2} = \frac{20 \text{ ml } O_2/dl - 15 \text{ ml } O_2/dl}{20 \text{ ml } O_2/dl} = \frac{5}{20} = 25\%$$

In other words, the muscle in this example removes (and burns) 25% of the O_2 presented to it by the arterial blood.

What are the factors that determine O_2 extraction? To answer this question, we return to the hypothetical Krogh cylinder. The same eight factors that influence the P_{O_2} profiles in Figure 19–4A also determine the whole-organ O_2 extraction. Of these factors, the two most important are capillary flow (*item #3* in the list) and metabolic demand (*item #7*). The O_2 extraction ratio decreases with increased flow, but increases with increased O_2 consumption. These conclusions make intuitive sense. Greater flow supplies more O_2, so the tissue needs to extract a smaller fraction of the incoming O_2 in order to satisfy its fixed needs. Conversely, increased metabolic demands require that the tissue extract more of the incoming O_2. These conclusions are merely a restatement of the Fick principle (p. 442), which we can rewrite as:

Equation 19–3

$$\underbrace{[O_2]_a - [O_2]_v}_{\text{Related to Extraction Ratio}} = \frac{\dot{Q}O_2}{F}$$

The term on the left is the a–v difference. The extraction ratio is merely the a–v difference normalized to $[O_2]_a$. Thus, the Fick principle confirms our intuition that the extraction ratio should increase with increasing metabolic demand, but decrease with increasing flow.

Another important factor that we have so far ignored is that not all of the capillaries in a tissue may be active at any one time. For example, skeletal muscle contains roughly a half million capillaries per gram of tissue. However, only approximately 20% are perfused at rest (see Fig. 19–4B). During exercise, when the O_2 consumption of the muscle increases, the resistance vessels and precapillary sphincters dilate to meet the increased demand. This vasodilation increases muscle blood flow and the density of perfused capillaries (see Fig. 19–4C). This response is equivalent to decreasing the tissue radius of Krogh's cylinder because each perfused capillary now supplies a smaller region. Other things being equal, the reduced diffusion distances will cause the PO_2 in the tissue to increase.

The velocity of blood flow in the capillaries also increases during exercise. All things being equal, this increased velocity would cause PO_2 to fall *less steeply* along the capillary lumen. For example, if the velocity were infinite, PO_2 would not fall at all! In fact, because O_2 consumption rises during exercise, PO_2 actually falls *more steeply* along the capillary.

According to Fick's Law, the Diffusion of Small, Water-Soluble Solutes Across a Capillary Wall Depends on Both the Permeability and the Concentration Gradient

Although the endothelial cell is freely permeable to O_2 and CO_2, it offers a significant barrier to the exchange of lipid-insoluble substances. Hydrophilic solutes that are smaller than albumin can traverse the capillary wall by **diffusion** via a paracellular route (i.e., through the clefts and inter-endothelial junctions, as well as gaps and fenestrae, if these are present).

The amount of solute that crosses a particular surface area of a capillary per unit time is called a **flux**. It seems intuitive that the flux ought to be proportional to the magnitude of the concentration difference across the capillary wall, and that it ought to be bigger in leakier capillaries (Fig. 19–5). These ideas are embodied in a form of Fick's law:

Equation 19–4

$$J_X = P_X \cdot ([X]_c - [X]_{if})$$

In Figure 19–5, J_X is the flux of the solute X (units: moles/(cm²/s)), assuming a positive J_X with flow out of the capillary, into the interstitial fluid. $[X]_c$ and $[X]_{if}$ are the dissolved concentrations of the solute in the capillary and interstitial fluid, respectively. Because the capillary wall thickness, a (units: cm), is difficult to determine, we combined the diffusion coefficient, D_X (units: cm²/s), and wall thickness into a single term (D_X/a) called P_X, the **permeability coefficient** (units: cm/s). Thus, P_X expresses the ease with which the solute crosses a capillary by diffusion.

Because, in practice, the surface area (S) of the capillary is often unknown, it is impossible to compute the *flux* of a solute, which is expressed per unit area. Rather, it is more common to compute the *mass flow* ($\dot{Q}$), which is simply the amount of solute transferred per unit time (units: moles/s):

Equation 19–5

$$\dot{Q} = S \cdot J_X = S \cdot P_X \cdot ([X]_c - [X]_{if})$$

The Whole-Organ Extraction Ratio for Small, Hydrophilic Solutes Provides an Estimate of the Solute Permeability of Capillaries

How could we estimate the permeability coefficient for a solute in different capillaries, or for different solutes in the same capillary? Unfortunately, it is difficult to determine permeability coefficients in single capillaries. Therefore, investigators use an indirect approach that begins with measuring the *whole-organ* extraction ratio for the solute X. As we have already seen for O_2 (see Equation 19–1), the extraction ratio (E_X) is a normalized arteriovenous difference for X:

Equation 19–6

$$E_X = \frac{[X]_a - [X]_v}{[X]_a}$$

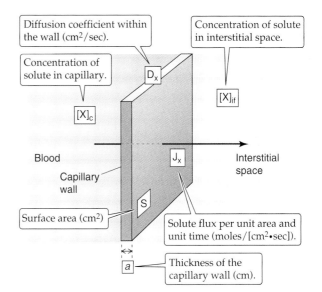

FIGURE 19–5. Diffusion of a solute across a capillary wall.

TABLE 19–1

$P_X \cdot S$ PRODUCTS FOR VARIOUS CAPILLARY BEDS

TISSUE	$P_X S$ FOR INULIN* (10^{-3} cm³/s) (measured)	S, CAPILLARY SURFACE AREA* (cm²) (measured)	P_X, PERMEABILITY TO INULIN ($\times 10^{-6}$ cm/s) (calculated)
Heart	4.08	800	5.1
Lung	3.80	950	4.0
Small intestine	1.79	460	3.9
Diaphragm	0.76	400	1.9
Ear	0.34	58	5.9
Skeletal muscle at rest	0.09	75	1.2

*All calculations are normalized for 1 g of tissue from rabbits. (Adapted from Wittmers LE, Barlett M, Johnson JA: Estimation of the capillary permeability coefficients of inulin in various tissues of the rabbit. Microvasc Res 11:67–78, 1976.)

Thus, E_X describes the degree to which an organ removes a solute from the circulation. Unlike the situation for O_2, the extraction ratio for small hydrophilic solutes depends not only on total organ blood flow (F) but also on the overall "exchange properties" of all of its capillaries, expressed by the product of permeability and total capillary area ($P_X \cdot S$). The dependence of E_X on the $P_X \cdot S$ product and F is described by the following equation:

Equation 19–7

$$E_X = 1 - e^{-(P_X S/F)}$$

Therefore, by knowing the whole-organ extraction ratio for a solute and blood flow through the organ, we can calculate the product $P_X \cdot S$. The first column of Table 19–1 lists the $P_X \cdot S$ products for a single solute (inulin), determined from Equation 19–7, for a number of different organs. Armed with independent estimates of the capillary surface area (see Table 19–1, *column 2*), we can compute P_X (*column 3*). P_X increases by a factor of approximately 4 from resting skeletal muscle to heart, reflecting a difference in the density of fluid-filled transendothelial clefts. Because a much greater fraction of the capillaries in the heart are open to blood flow (i.e., S is ~10-fold larger), the $P_X \cdot S$ product for heart is approximately 40-fold higher than for resting skeletal muscle.

The **cerebral vessels** have very unique characteristics that constitute the basis of the blood-brain barrier (p. 408). The tight junctions of most brain capillaries do not permit any paracellular flow of hydrophilic solutes; therefore, they exhibit a very low permeability to sucrose or inulin due to the presence of claudin-5. In contrast, the *water* permeability of cerebral vessels is similar to that of other organs. Hydrophilic solutes in other tissues move largely by the paracellular route. On the other hand, a large fraction of water exchange in cerebral vessels must occur through the endothelial cells.

"Whole-organ" $P_X \cdot S$ values are not constant. First, arterioles and precapillary sphincters control the number of capillaries being perfused, and thus the available surface area (S). Second, in response to a variety of signalling molecules (e.g., cytokines), endothelial cells can reorganize their cytoskeleton, thereby changing their shape. This deformation widens inter-endothelial clefts and increases P_X. One example is the increased leakiness that develops during inflammation in response to the secretion of histamine by mast cells and basophilic granulocytes.

Small Polar Molecules Have a Relatively Low Permeability Because They Can Traverse the Capillary Wall Only by Diffusing Through Clefts or Through Water-Filled Pores

Having compared the permeabilities of a single hydrophilic solute (inulin) in several capillary beds, we may address the selectivity of a single capillary wall to several solutes. Table 19–2 shows that the permeability coefficient falls as molecular radius increases. These small, water-soluble, polar molecules have a relatively low permeability because they can traverse the capillary wall only by diffusing through inter-endothelial clefts or other water-filled pathways, which constitute only a fraction of the total capillary area. For *lipid-soluble* substances such as CO_2 and O_2, which can diffuse through the *entire* capillary endothelial cell and not just the water-filled pathways, the permeability is much larger than for the solutes in Table 19–2.

TABLE 19–2

PERMEABILITY COEFFICIENTS FOR LIPID-INSOLUBLE SOLUTES*

SUBSTANCE	RADIUS OF EQUIVALENT SPHERE† (nm)	PERMEABILITY (cm/s)
NaCl	0.14	310×10^{-6}
Urea	0.16	230×10^{-6}
Glucose	0.36	90×10^{-6}
Sucrose	0.44	50×10^{-6}
Raffinose	0.56	40×10^{-6}
Inulin	1.52	5×10^{-6}

*Permeability data are from skeletal muscle of the cat, assuming that the capillary surface area is 70 cm²/gram wet tissue.
† Stokes-Einstein radius.
Data from Pappenheimer JR: Passage of molecules through capillary walls. Physiol Rev 33:387–423, 1953.

The inter-endothelial clefts are wider—and fenestrae are more common—at the venular end of the capillary than at its arteriolar end, so that P_X increases along the capillary. Therefore, if the transcapillary concentration difference ($[X]_c - [X]_{if}$) were the same, the solute flux would actually be larger at the venous end of the microcirculation.

Small proteins can also diffuse across inter-endothelial clefts or through fenestrae. In addition to molecular size, the *electrical charge* of proteins and other macromolecules is a major determinant of their apparent permeability coefficient. In general, the flux of negatively charged proteins is much smaller than that of neutral macromolecules of equivalent size, whereas positively charged macromolecules have the highest apparent permeability coefficient. Fixed negative charges in the diffusion path across the endothelium exclude macromolecules with negative charge and favor the transit of macromolecules with positive charge. Selective permeability based on the electrical charge of the solute is a striking feature of the filtration of proteins across the glomerular barrier of the nephron (p. 760).

The diffusive movement of solutes is the dominant mode of transcapillary exchange. However, the convective movement of water can also carry solutes. This **solvent drag** is the flux of a dissolved solute that is swept along by the bulk movement of the solvent. Compared with the diffusive flux of a small solute with a high permeability coefficient (e.g., glucose), the contribution of solvent drag is minor.

The Exchange of Macromolecules Across Capillaries Can Occur by Transcytosis

Macromolecules with a radius exceeding 1 nm (e.g., plasma proteins) can cross the capillary, at a low rate, through intercellular clefts and fenestrations, when they are present. A second mechanism of macromolecular translocation is **transcytosis**. Ultrastructural images of endothelial cells show pinocytotic or transport vesicles (diameter 50–100 nm) free in the cytoplasm or opening with a short neck onto either the luminal or the basal membrane. The transcytosis of very large macromolecules by vesicular transport involves: (1) equilibration of dissolved macromolecules in the capillary lumen with the

fluid phase inside the open vesicle; (2) pinching off of the vesicle; (3) vesicle shuttling to the cytoplasm and probably transient fusion with other vesicles within the cytoplasm, allowing intermixing of the vesicular content; (4) fusion of vesicles with the opposite plasma membrane; and (5) equilibration with the opposite extracellular fluid phase.

Although one can express the transcytotic movement of macromolecules as a *flux*, the laws of diffusion (see Equation 19–4) do not govern transcytosis. Nevertheless, investigators have calculated the "apparent permeability" of typical capillaries to macromolecules (Table 19–3). The resulting "permeability"—which reflects the total movement of the macromolecule, regardless of the pathway— falls off steeply with increases in molecular radius, a feature called **sieving**. This sieving may be the result of steric hindrance when large macromolecules equilibrate across the neck of nascent vesicles, or when a network of glycoproteins on the surface of the vesicle excludes the large macromolecules. In addition, sieving of macromolecules according to molecular size could occur as macromolecules diffuse through infrequent chains of fused vesicles that span the full width of the endothelial cell.

Transcytosis is not as simple as the luminal loading and basal unloading of "ferry-boats"—the cell may process some of the cargo. Although the luminal surface of endothelial cells avidly takes up ferritin (750 kDa), only a tiny portion of endocytosed ferritin translocates to the opposite side of the cell (see Table 19–3). The remainder stays for a time in intracellular compartments, where it is finally broken down.

Both transcytosis and chains of fused vesicles are less prominent in brain capillaries. The presence of continuous tight junctions and the low level of transcytosis account for the blood-brain barrier's much lower apparent permeability to macromolecules.

CAPILLARY EXCHANGE OF WATER

Fluid Transfer Across Capillaries Is Convective and Depends on Net Hydrostatic and Osmotic Forces (i.e., Starling Forces)

The pathway for fluid movement across the capillary wall is a combination of transcellular and paracellular pathways. Endothelial cell membranes express constitutively active **aquaporin 1** (AQP 1) water channels (p. 58). It is likely that AQP 1 constitutes the principal *transcellular* pathway for water movement. The inter-endothelial clefts, fenestrae, or gaps may be the anatomic substrate of the *paracellular* pathway.

Whereas the main mechanism for the transfer of gases and other solutes is *diffusion*, the main mechanism for the net transfer of fluid across the capillary membrane is **convection**. As first outlined in 1896 by Ernest Starling, the two driving forces for the convection of fluid—or bulk water movement—across the capillary wall are the transcapillary hydrostatic pressure difference and *effective* osmotic pressure difference, also known as the colloid osmotic pressure or oncotic pressure difference (p. 72).

The **hydrostatic pressure difference** (ΔP) across the

TABLE 19–3

CAPILLARY PERMEABILITY TO MACROMOLECULES		
MACROMOLECULE	**RADIUS OF EQUIVALENT SPHERE (nm)***	**APPARENT PERMEABILITY (cm/s)**
Myoglobin	1.9	0.5×10^{-6}
Plasma albumin[†]	3.5	0.01×10^{-6}
Ferritin	6.1	~ 0

* Stokes-Einstein radius.
[†] Representative value for skeletal muscle.
 Data from Pappenheimer JR: Passage of molecules through capillary walls. Physiol Rev 33:387–423, 1953.

capillary wall is the difference between the intravascular pressure (i.e., capillary hydrostatic pressure, P_c) and the extravascular pressure (i.e., interstitial fluid hydrostatic pressure, P_{if}).

The **colloid osmotic pressure difference** ($\Delta\pi$) across the capillary wall is the difference between the intravascular colloid osmotic pressure caused by plasma proteins (π_c) and the extravascular colloid osmotic pressure caused by interstitial proteins and proteoglycans (π_{if}). A positive ΔP tends to drive water *out of* the capillary lumen, whereas a positive $\Delta\pi$ attracts water *into* the capillary lumen.

Starling's hypothesis for describing the volume flow (J_V) of fluid across the capillary wall is embodied in the following equation, which is similar to Equation 3–24 (p. 73):

Equation 19–8

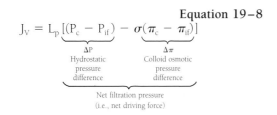

$$J_V = L_p [(P_c - P_{if}) - \sigma(\pi_c - \pi_{if})]$$

Table 19–4 summarizes the terms in this equation. The equation is written so that the flux of water leaving the capillary is positive and that of fluid entering the capillary is negative.

The **hydraulic conductivity** (L_p) is the proportionality constant that relates the net driving force to J_V and expresses the total permeability provided by the ensemble of AQP 1 channels and the paracellular pathway.

According to van't Hoff's law, the theoretical colloid osmotic pressure difference ($\Delta\pi_{Theory}$) is proportional to the protein concentration difference ($\Delta[X]$):

Equation 19–9

$$\Delta\pi_{Theory} = RT\,\Delta[X]$$

However, because capillary walls exclude proteins *imperfectly*, the observed colloid osmotic pressure difference ($\Delta\pi_{Obs}$) is less than the ideal. The ratio $\Delta\pi_{Obs}/\Delta\pi_{Theory}$ is the **reflection coefficient** (σ) that describes how a semipermeable barrier excludes or "reflects" solute X as water moves across the barrier, driven by hydrostatic or osmotic pressure gradients.

The value of σ can range from 0 to 1. When σ is zero, the moving water perfectly "entrains" the solute, which moves with the water and exerts no osmotic pressure across the barrier. When σ is 1, the barrier completely excludes the solute as the water passes through, and the solute exerts its full or ideal osmotic pressure. To the extent that σ exceeds zero, the membrane sieves out the solute. The σ for plasma proteins is nearly 1.

Because small solutes such as Na^+ and Cl^- freely cross the endothelium, their σ is zero, and they are not included in the Starling equation for the capillary wall (Equation 19–8). Thus, changing the intravascular or interstitial concentrations of such "crystalloids" does *not* create a net effective osmotic driving force across the capillary wall. (Conversely, because plasma membranes have an effective $\sigma_{NaCl} = 1$, NaCl gradients *do* shift water between the *intracellular and interstitial* compartments.)

The net driving force in the Starling equation (see Equation 19–8), $[(P_c - P_{if}) - \sigma(\pi_c - \pi_{if})]$, has a special name, the **net filtration pressure**. **Filtration** of fluid from the capillary into the tissue space occurs when the net filtration pressure is positive. In the special case when σ for proteins is 1, the fluid leaving the capillary is protein free; this process is called ultrafiltration. Conversely, **reabsorption** of fluid from the tissue space into the vascular space occurs when the net filtration pressure is negative. At the arterial end of the capillary, the net filtration pressure is generally positive, so that filtration occurs. At the venous end, the net filtration pressure is generally negative, so that absorption occurs. However, as is discussed later, some organs do not adhere to this general rule.

TABLE 19–4

TERMS IN STARLING EQUATION		
J_v	Volume flux across the capillary wall	$cm^3\ cm^{-2}\ s^{-1}$ [$cm^3/(cm^2 \times s)$]
L_p	Hydraulic conductivity*	$cm\ s^{-1}\ (mm\ Hg)^{-1}$ [$cm/(s \times mm\ Hg)$]
P_c	Capillary hydrostatic pressure	mm Hg
P_{if}	Tissue (interstitial fluid) hydrostatic pressure	mm Hg
π_c	Capillary colloid osmotic pressure caused by plasma proteins	mm Hg
π_{if}	Tissue (interstitial fluid) colloid osmotic pressure caused by interstitial proteins and proteoglycans	mm Hg
σ	Average colloid osmotic reflection coefficient	(dimensionless, varies between 0 and 1)
F	Flow of fluid across the capillary wall	cm^3/s
S_f	Functional surface area	cm^2

*Alternatively, the leakiness of the capillary wall to water may be expressed in terms of water permeability (P_f; units: cm/s). In this case, the hydrostatic and osmotic forces are given in the units of osmolality.

In the next four sections, we will examine each of the four "Starling forces" that constitute the net filtration pressure: P_c, P_{if}, π_c, and π_{if}.

Capillary Blood Pressure (P_C) Falls from Approximately 35 mm Hg at the Arteriolar End to Approximately 15 mm Hg at the Venular End

Capillary blood pressure is also loosely called the capillary *hydrostatic* pressure, to distinguish it from capillary *colloid osmotic* pressure. It is only possible to record P_c in an exposed organ, ideally in a thin tissue (e.g., a mesentery) that allows for good transillumination. One impales the lumen of the capillary with a fine micropipette (tip diameter < 5 μm) filled with saline and heparin. The micropipette lumen connects to a manometer, which has a side-arm to a syringe. Immediately after the impalement, blood begins to rise slowly up the pipette. A pressure reading at this time would underestimate the actual P_c because pipette pressure is less than P_c. The syringe makes it possible to apply just enough pressure to the pipette lumen to reach true pressure equilibrium—when fluid flows neither from nor to the pipette. Using this **null-point** approach, the recorded pressure is the true P_c. In the human skin, P_c is approximately 35 mm Hg at the arteriolar end and approximately 15 mm Hg at the venular end.

When the arteriolar pressure is 60 mm Hg and the venous pressure is 15 mm Hg, the midcapillary pressure is not the mean value of 37.5 mm Hg, but only 25 mm Hg (Table 19–5, *top row*). The explanation for the difference is that normally the precapillary upstream resistance exceeds the postcapillary downstream resistance (R_{post}/R_{pre} is typically 0.3) (p. 453). However, the midcapillary pressure is not a constant and uniform value. In the previous chapter, we saw that P_c varies with changes in R_{pre} and R_{post} (Fig. 18–4). P_c also varies with changes in four other parameters: (1) upstream and downstream pressure, (2) location, (3) time, and (4) gravity.

ARTERIOLAR (P_a) AND VENULAR (P_v) PRESSURE. Because R_{post} is less than R_{pre}, P_c follows P_v more closely than P_a (p. 452). Thus, increasing P_a by 10 mm Hg—at a constant R_{post}/R_{pre} of 0.3—causes P_c to rise by only 2 mm Hg (see Table 19–5, *middle row*). On the other hand, increasing P_v by 10 mm Hg causes P_c to rise by 8 mm Hg (see Table 19–5, *bottom row*).

LOCATION. Capillary pressure differs markedly among tissues. For example, the high P_c of glomerular capillaries in the kidney, approximately 50 mm Hg (p. 762), is required for ultrafiltration. The retinal capillaries in the eye must also have a high P_c because they bathe in a vitreous humor that is under a pressure of approximately 20 mm Hg (p. 333). A higher P_c is needed to keep the capillaries patent in the face of the external compressing force. The pulmonary capillaries have unusually *low* P_c values, 5 to 15 mm Hg, minimizing the ultrafiltration that otherwise would lead to the accumulation of edema fluid in the alveolar air spaces (p. 695).

TIME. Capillary blood pressure varies considerably from moment to moment at any given site, depending on the arteriolar diameter and tone of the precapillary sphincter (i.e., R_{pre}). In individual capillaries, these fluctuations lead to times of net filtration and other times of net fluid absorption.

GRAVITY. Finally, the effect of gravity on P_c is the same as that discussed for arterial and venous pressure. Thus, a capillary bed below the level of the heart has a higher P_c than a capillary bed at the level of the heart.

Interstitial-Fluid Pressure (P_{if}) Is Slightly Negative, Except in Encapsulated Organs

The interstitium consists of both a solid and a liquid phase. The solid phase is made up of collagen fibers and proteoglycans. In the liquid phase, only a small fraction of interstitial water is totally "free" and capable of moving under the influence of convective forces. Most of the water is trapped in gels (e.g., proteoglycans), in which both water and small solutes move by diffusion. It was once thought that P_{if} in the liquid phase is slightly above barometric pressure throughout the interstitium, but more recent measurements indicate that P_{if} is sub-atmospheric in many tissues.

Estimating P_{if} is very difficult because the probe used to make the measurement is far larger than the interstitial space; thus, the measurement itself can alter P_{if}. If one inserts a probe percutaneously, and immediately uses a null-point method to measure P_{if} (as outlined earlier for capillary pressure), the values are +1 to +2 mm Hg. However, during the next 4 to 5 hours, the measured value drops to −1 to −2 mm Hg. Arthur Guyton implanted a perforated, hollow plastic sphere under the skin to provide a chronic record of P_{if} (Fig. 19–6). After the wound has healed, the pressure inside the sphere may be as low as −2 to −10 mm Hg after 1 or 2 weeks.

A value of −2 mm Hg is a reasonable average in *loose tissues*, such as the lung and subcutaneous tissue. P_{if} is slightly negative because of fluid removal by the lymphatics (see later). Inside *rigid enclosed compartments*, such as the bone marrow or brain, P_{if} is positive. It is also positive in *encapsulated organs* such as the kidney, where P_{if} is +1 to +3 mm Hg within the parenchyma. Expansion of high-pressure vessels in the kidney pushes the interstitial fluid against an unyielding fibrous capsule, raising P_{if}. The same principle applies to skeletal muscle, which is surrounded by layers of fascia. In some cases, it is not the interstitial fluid but another specialized compartment that provides the pressure around the capillaries. For renal

TABLE 19–5

EFFECT OF UPSTREAM AND DOWNSTREAM PRESSURE CHANGES ON CAPILLARY PRESSURE*			
	P_a (mm Hg)	P_c (mm Hg)	P_v (mm Hg)
Control	60	25	15
Increased arteriolar pressure	70	27	15
Increased venular pressure	60	33	25

* Constant R_{post}/R_{pre} = 0.3.

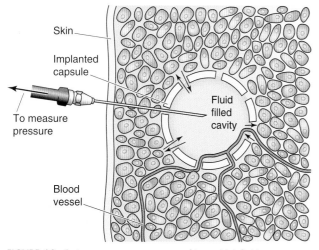

FIGURE 19–6. Long-term measurement of interstitial fluid pressure using an implanted capsule.

glomerular capillaries, it is Bowman's space (p. 761)—filled with glomerular filtrate to a pressure of about +10 mm Hg—that is the relevant outside compartment. For pulmonary capillaries, the relevant outside compartment is the alveolus, the pressure of which varies during the respiratory cycle (p. 626).

P_{if} is also sensitive to the addition of fluid to the interstitial compartment. When small amounts of fluid are added to the interstitial compartment, the interstitium behaves as a "low-compliance" system, so that P_{if} rises steeply for the small amount of added fluid. Adding more fluid disrupts the solid phase of collagen fibers and the gel of proteoglycans, so that large volumes can now accumulate with only small additional pressure increases. In this high-volume range, the interstitial compartment thus behaves as a "high-compliance" system. This high compliance is especially high in loose subcutaneous tissues, which can accommodate more edema fluid (see clinical box on interstitial edema) than can muscle.

Capillary Colloid Osmotic Pressure (π_c), Which Reflects the Presence of Plasma Proteins, Is Approximately 25 mm Hg

The colloid osmotic pressure difference across the capillary endothelium is due solely to the plasma proteins, such as albumin, globulins, and fibrinogen. Total plasma protein concentration is approximately 7.0 g/dl, which corresponds to approximately 1.5 mM of protein. According to van't Hoff's law (see Equation 19–9), these proteins would exert an osmotic pressure of approximately 28 mm Hg if perfectly reflected by the capillary wall ($\sigma = 1$). The σ is indeed close to 1 for the principal plasma proteins—albumin (3.5–5.5 g/dl) and the globulins (2.0–3.5 g/dl)—so that the actual colloid osmotic pressure ($\sigma\pi_c$) in capillaries is approximately 25 mm Hg. This value is the same as if osmotically active solutes were present at approximately 1.3 mM. Note that because of the very definition of colloid osmotic pressure, we have ignored the osmotic effects of the small solutes in plasma, which have an *osmolality* of 290 mOsm (p. 53).

π_c does vary appreciably along the length of the capillary. Indeed, most capillary beds filter less than 1% of the fluid entering at the arteriolar end. Thus, the loss of protein-free fluid does not measurably concentrate plasma proteins along the capillary, and does not appreciably raise π_c.

Because clinical laboratories report plasma protein concentrations in g/dl, and not all proteins have the same molecular weight, a plasma protein concentration of 7 g/dl can produce different π_c values, depending on the protein *composition* of the plasma. Because albumin has a much lower molecular weight than γ-globulin, replacing 1 g of the heavier γ-globulin with 1 g of the lighter albumin raises π_c. Whereas van't Hoff's law (see Equation 19–9) predicts a *linear* relationship between osmotic pressure and concentration, colloid osmotic pressure actually increases more steeply, even when the albumin/globulin ratio is held constant at 1.8 (Fig. 19–7, *orange curve*). Obviously, the steepness of the curve varies from one plasma protein to the next because all have different molecular weights.

Not only does π_c vary markedly with protein composition and concentration, the reflection coefficient for colloids also varies widely among organs. The lowest values for σ (i.e., greatest leakiness) are in discontinuous capillary beds (e.g., liver), intermediate values are in muscle capillaries, and the highest values ($\sigma = 1$) are in the tight, continuous capillary beds of the brain.

The plasma proteins do more than just act as osmotic agents. Because these proteins also carry negative charges, the Donnan effect causes an increase in both the concentrations of cations (p. 53) and the colloid osmotic pressure (see Fig. 3–13) in the capillary lumen.

FIGURE 19–7. Dependence of colloid osmotic pressure on the concentration of plasma proteins. The point on the *orange curve* indicates that normal plasma, a mixture of proteins at a concentration of 7 g/dl, has a colloid osmotic pressure (π_c) of 25 mm Hg.

INTERSTITIAL EDEMA

Edema (from the Greek oidema, for "swelling") is characterized by an excess of salt and water in the extracellular space, particularly in the interstitium. Edema may be associated with any disease leading to salt retention and expansion of the extracellular fluid volume, in particular, renal, cardiac, and hepatic disease (p. 864). However, interstitial edema can also occur without overall salt and water retention because of microcirculatory alterations that affect the Starling forces. Regardless of the cause, the resulting edema can be either generalized (e.g., widespread swelling of subcutaneous tissue, often first evident in facial puffiness) or localized (e.g., limited to the dependent parts of the body). In this box, we focus on how edema can result from changes in terms that make up the Starling equation.

HYDROSTATIC FORCES

When a person is **standing** for a sustained period of time, venous pressure and thus capillary pressure (P_c) in the legs increase because of gravity. The result is movement of fluid into the tissue space. In most cases, the lymphatic system can take up the extra interstitial fluid and return it to the vascular space, maintaining proper fluid balance. The return of fluid requires contractions of the leg muscles to compress the veins and lymphatics, and to propel the fluid upward through the valves in these vessels and toward the heart (p. 475). If the standing person does not contract these muscles, the transudation of fluid can exceed the lymphatic return, causing interstitial edema.

An organ that is particularly sensitive to proper fluid balance is the lung. Slight increases in the hydrostatic pressure of the pulmonary capillaries (pulmonary hypertension) can lead to **pulmonary edema**. This condition decreases lung compliance (making lung inflation more difficult; p. 615) and also may severely compromise gas exchange across the pulmonary capillary bed (p. 671). Left heart failure causes blood to back up into the vessels of the lung, raising pulmonary vascular pressures and causing pulmonary edema.

In right heart failure, blood backs up into the systemic veins. As a result, central venous pressure (i.e., the pressure inside the large systemic veins leading to the right heart) rises, causing an increase in the P_c in the lower extremities and abdominal viscera. Fluid transudated from the hepatic and intestinal capillaries may leave the interstitial space and enter the peritoneal cavity, a condition called **ascites**.

COLLOID OSMOTIC FORCES

In **nephrotic syndrome**, a manifestation of a number of renal diseases, protein is lost in the urine. The result is a fall in plasma colloid osmotic pressure, a decrease in the ability of the capillaries to retain fluid, and generalized peripheral edema.

In **pregnancy**, synthesis of plasma proteins by the mother does not keep pace with the expanding plasma volume and nutritional demands of the fetus. As a result, maternal plasma protein levels fall. The same occurs in **protein malnutrition**. Although less severe than in nephrotic syndrome, the lower capillary colloid osmotic pressure nevertheless leads to edema in the extremities.

The opposite effect is seen in dehydration. A deficit of salt and water causes an *increase* in the plasma-protein concentration, increasing the capillary colloid osmotic pressure and thus pulling fluid out of the interstitial space. The result is reduced turgor of the interstitial space. This effect is easily noticed by pinching the skin, which is unable to spring back to its usual firm position.

PROPERTIES OF THE CAPILLARY WALL

Inflammation causes the release of vasodilators, such as histamine and cytokines, into the surrounding tissue. Vasodilation increases the number of open capillaries and therefore the functional surface area (S_f). Cytokines also cause widening of inter-endothelial clefts and a fall in the reflection coefficient (σ) for proteins. The net effect is enhanced filtration of fluid from capillary lumen to interstitium, so that tissue swelling is one of the hallmarks of inflammation.

Severe head injuries can result in **cerebral edema**, a result of the breakdown of the normally tight endothelial barrier of the cerebral vessels (p. 408). Because the rigid skull prevents expansion of the brain, cerebral edema can lead to occlusion of the cerebral microcirculation.

During ischemia—when blood flow to a tissue is severely reduced or completely stopped—blood vessels deteriorate, causing hydraulic conductivity (L_p) to increase and reflection coefficient to decrease. Once blood flow is reestablished (**reperfusion**), these changes lead to local edema. If the increased leakiness is substantial, large quantities of plasma proteins freely move into the interstitial space, dissipating the colloid osmotic gradient across the capillary wall and aggravating the edema.

LYMPHATIC DRAINAGE

Lymphatic drainage may become impaired after removal of lymph nodes for cancer surgery, or when lymph nodes are obstructed by malignancies. The reduction in the lymphatic drainage leads to local edema, upstream from the affected nodes.

TABLE 19–6

				EFFECTIVE INTERSTITIAL-	
	CAPILLARY BLOOD PRESSURE (P_c)	**INTERSTITIAL FLUID PRESSURE (P_{if})**	**EFFECTIVE CAPILLARY COLLOID OSMOTIC PRESSURE ($\sigma \pi_c$)**	**FLUID COLLOID OSMOTIC PRESSURE ($\sigma \pi_{if}$)**	**NET FORCE**
Anteriolar end	+35 mm Hg	−2 mm Hg	+25 mm Hg	+0.1 mm Hg	+12 mm Hg
Venular end	+15 mm Hg	−2 mm Hg	+25 mm Hg	+3 mm Hg	−5 mm Hg

TYPICAL VALUES OF TRANSCAPILLARY DRIVING FORCES FOR FLUID MOVEMENT IN LOOSE, NON-ENCAPSULATED TISSUE

Interstitial Fluid Colloid Osmotic Pressure (π_{if}) Varies Between 0 and 10 mm Hg Among Different Organs

It is difficult to measure the interstitial fluid colloid osmotic pressure because it is practically impossible to obtain uncontaminated samples. As a first approximation, we generally assume that π_{if} is the same as the colloid osmotic pressure of *lymph*. The protein content of lymph varies greatly from region to region; for example, it is 1 to 3 g/dl in the legs, 3 to 4 g/dl in the intestine, and 4 to 6 g/dl in the liver. Such lymph data predict that π_{if} ranges from 0.1 to 10 mm Hg. However, the protein concentration in the interstitial fluid is probably somewhat higher than in the lymph. A total-body average value for π_{if} is approximately 3 mm Hg, substantially less than the value of 25 mm Hg for π_c in the capillary lumen.

The π_{if} appears to increase along the axis of the capillary (Table 19–6). The lowest values are near the arteriolar end, where the interstitium receives protein-free fluid from the

A   INDIVIDUAL HYDROSTATIC AND OSMOTIC PRESSURES

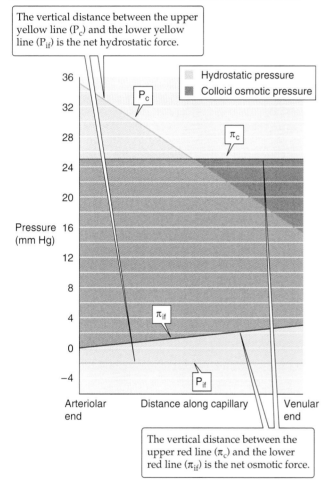

The vertical distance between the upper yellow line (P_c) and the lower yellow line (P_{if}) is the net hydrostatic force.

The vertical distance between the upper red line (π_c) and the lower red line (π_{if}) is the net osmotic force.

FIGURE 19–8. Starling forces along a capillary. In *A*, the *yellow lines* are idealized profiles of capillary (P_c) and interstitial (P_{if}) hydrostatic pressures. Red lines are idealized capillary (π_c) and interstitial (π_{if}) colloid osmotic pressures. In *B*, the net filtration pressure is $(P_c - P_{if}) - \sigma(\pi_c - \pi_{if})$.

B   NET FILTRATION PRESSURE

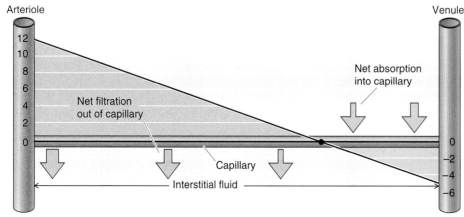

capillary as the result of filtration. The highest values are near the venular end, where the interstitium loses protein-free fluid to the capillary as the result of reabsorption.

The Capillary Beds of Most Organs Perform Ultrafiltration at the Arteriolar End and Reabsorption at the Venular End

The idealized forces acting on fluid movement across a capillary are shown in Figure 19–8A. Using the Starling equation and the values in Table 19–6, we can calculate the net transfer of fluid (J_V) at both the arteriolar and venular ends of a typical capillary:

$$\text{Equation } 19-10$$
$$J_V = L_p[(P_c - P_{if}) - (\sigma\pi_c - \sigma\pi_{if})]$$

Arteriolar end: $J_V = L_p[(35 - (-2)) - (25 - 0.1)]$
$$= L_p(+12 \text{ mm Hg})$$

Venular end: $J_V = L_p[(15 - (-2)) - (25 - 3)]$
$$= L_p(-5 \text{ mm Hg})$$

The net filtration pressure is thus positive (favoring filtration) at the arteriolar end, and it gradually makes the transition to negative (favoring reabsorption) at the venular end (see Fig. 19–8B). At the point where the filtration and reabsorptive forces balance each other, an equilibrium exists, and no net movement of water occurs across the capillary wall.

Net filtration pressure varies—sometimes considerably—among tissues. For example, in the intestinal mucosa, P_c is so much lower than π_c that reabsorption occurs continually along the entire length of the capillary. On the other hand, in glomerular capillaries, P_c exceeds π_c throughout most of the network, so that filtration may occur along the entire capillary (p. 763). Hydraulic conductivity also can affect the filtration/reabsorption profile along the capillary. Because the inter-endothelial clefts become larger toward the venular end of the capillary, L_p increases along the capillary, from the arteriolar to the venular end.

Ignoring glomerular filtration in the kidney, the net effect of filtration at the arteriolar end of the capillary, and reabsorption at the venular end, is a net *filtration* of approximately 2 to 4 liters/day from blood to interstitial fluid. This 2 to 4 liters of net filtration does not occur uniformly in all capillary beds. The *flow* of fluid across a group of capillaries (F) is the product of the *flux* (J_v) and the functional surface area (S_f): $F = J_v \cdot S_f$. Thus, net filtration of fluid in an organ depends not only on the net filtration pressure and the hydraulic conductivity of the capillary wall (terms that contribute to J_V), but also on the surface area of the perfused capillaries. Thus, as exercise recruits additional open capillaries in muscle and raises S_f, it increases filtration.

LYMPHATICS

Lymphatics Return Excess Interstitial Fluid to the Blood, Thus Completing Local Fluid Balance

Lymphatics arise in the interstitium as small thin-walled channels that then join together to form increasingly larger vessels (Fig. 19–9). Some authors view the **terminal lymphatics** as being open at their ends, and thus continuous with the liquid phase of the interstitial space. Others describe the terminal lymphatics as closed-ended vessels similar to capillaries, but with many open inter-endothelial junctions, gaps, and fenestrations. Terminal lymphatics are tethered, to some degree, to surrounding connective tissue. Although small lymphatics may appear collapsed, muscle contraction can deform them so that the openings become more patent. The walls of the larger lymphatics are similar to those of small veins, consisting of endothelium and sparse smooth muscle.

Lymphatics are absent from some tissues (e.g., myocardium, brain). They are most prevalent in the skin and the genitourinary, respiratory, and gastrointestinal tracts. The large lymphatic vessels, like the veins, have valves, which restrict the movement of lymph in the retrograde direction. The large lymphatics ultimately drain into the left and right subclavian veins.

As we have already seen, filtration at the arteriolar end of capillaries exceeds reabsorption at the venular end by 2 to 4 liters/day. However, fluid does not normally accumulate in the interstitium because this excess fluid and protein move into the lymphatics. Thus, each day, the lymphatics return to the circulation 2 to 4 liters of interstitial fluid, maintaining a steady state.

Hydrostatic pressure in the small lymphatics (P_{Lymph}) ranges from −1 mm Hg to +1 mm Hg. Inasmuch as the mean interstitial fluid pressure is somewhat more *negative* than these values, what provides the driving force for interstitial fluid to move into the terminal lymphatics? Transient increases in P_{if} temporarily raise P_{if} above P_{Lymph}. Indeed, increases in mean P_{if} cause an increase in lymph flow (Fig. 19–10).

Because the interstitium exhibits a variable compliance (p. 472), fluid added to the interstitium in its low-compliance range raises the P_{if} substantially, providing the driving force for fluid to enter the lymphatics. In this same range of P_{if} values, lymphatic flow is especially sensitive to increases in P_{if} (*steep portion* of Fig. 19–10). Thus, lymphatic efflux nicely matches the excess capillary filtration, so that the interstitial fluid volume changes very little. The situation is very different if the interstitium is already expanded and in its high-compliance range. In this case, fluid added to the interstitium raises the already elevated P_{if} only moderately (e.g., from +2 to +4 mm Hg).

FIGURE 19–9. Lymph vessels.

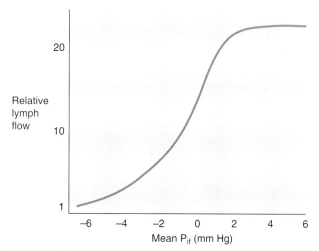

FIGURE 19–10. Dependence of lymph flow on interstitial pressure.

In this range of P_{if} values, lymphatic uptake is not very responsive to increases in P_{if} (*flat portion* of Fig. 19–10). Thus, in this case, lymphatic return does not compensate well for the excess capillary filtration, so that interstitial fluid volume increases further (i.e., edema begets more edema).

As pressure rises in the larger lymphatic vessels, smooth muscle in the lymphatic walls actively contracts by an intrinsic "myogenic" mechanism that, as discussed later, also plays a role in blood vessels. Thus, downstream occlusion of a lymphatic vessel increases P_{Lymph} and hence the frequency of smooth-muscle contractions, whereas an upstream occlusion does the opposite. Because these larger lymphatic vessels contain one-way valves, smooth-muscle contraction drives lymph toward the veins. In addition, passive processes also propel lymph toward the blood. Extravascular pressure changes elicited by skeletal muscle contraction, respiratory movements, and intestinal contractions all passively compress the lymphatics. Pressures in the large lymphatics range from +1 to +10 mm Hg, and they increase progressively with each valve along the vessel. This intermittent pumping action moves lymph from the interstitium to the veins, and may be largely responsible for the sub-atmospheric values of the P_{if} observed in many tissues.

Macromolecules filtered at the arteriolar end of a capillary cannot return to the circulation at the venular end because of the adverse chemical gradient across the capillary endothelial wall. The buildup of these macromolecules in the interstitium creates a diffusional gradient from the interstitium to the lymph that complements the convective movement of these macromolecules (along with fluid) into the lymphatic system. In an average person, the lymphatics return 100 to 200 g of proteins to the circulation per day.

The Circulation of Extracellular Fluids Involves Three Convective Loops: Blood, Interstitial Fluid, and Lymph

Extracellular fluid moves in *three convective loops* (Fig. 19–11). The first is the **cardiovascular loop**. Assuming a

cardiac output of 5 liters/min, the convective flow of blood through the circulation at rest is 7200 liters/day. The second is the **transvascular loop**, in which fluid moves out of the capillaries at their arteriolar end, and into the capillaries at their venular end. Not counting the kidney, whose glomeruli filter a vast amount of fluid (p. 757), all the other tissues of the body filter approximately 20 liters/day at the arteriolar end of their capillaries. Of this 20 liters, the venular end of the capillary network reabsorbs 16 to 18 liters. The third is the **lymphatic loop**, which returns to the venous vascular system the 2 to 4 liters/day that represents the difference between transvascular filtration and reabsorption.

In addition to convective exchange, a *diffusional exchange* of water and solutes also occurs across the capillaries. The diffusional exchange of **water** occurs at a much higher rate than does convective movement. Using deuterium oxide as a marker, investigators have found that this diffusional exchange is approximately 80,000 liters/day across all of the body's systemic capillaries. This value is about an order of magnitude greater than blood flow in the cardiovascular loop, and three orders of magnitude larger than the convective flow in the transvascular filtration/reabsorption loop of the microcirculation. However, the diffusion of water molecules is an *exchange* process that does not contribute appreciably to the *net* movement of water. In other words, every day 80,000 liters of water diffuse out of the capillaries, and 80,000 liters diffuse back.

With regard to **small solutes** that can diffuse across the capillary endothelium, the traffic is quite different from the convective loops for water. Take glucose as an example. The plasma contains approximately 100 mg/dl glucose, RBCs have little glucose, and the cardiac output of *plasma* is approximately 2.75 liters/min (assuming a hematocrit of 45%). Therefore, each day the heart pumps approximately 4000 g of glucose. This glucose can enter the interstitium by two mechanisms. First, glucose is dissolved in the water filtered from the arteriolar end of the capillaries. Each day, this filtration process carries 20 liters × 100 mg/dl = 20 g of glucose into the interstitium. Second, each day approximately 20,000 g of glucose enters the interstitium by diffusion. Convection can supply only a small fraction of the approximately 400 g of glucose that the body consumes each day. Instead, diffusion supplies the majority of the glucose. Nevertheless, the 400 g/day of metabolized glucose is a minuscule fraction of the amount that enters the interstitium by diffusion. Thus, the vast majority of the glucose that diffuses into the interstitium diffuses back out again.

Protein traffic provides yet another pattern of circulatory loops. Plasma contains 7 g/dl of proteins. Given a cardiac *plasma* output of 2.75 liters/min, the heart pumps approximately 277,000 g of protein through the circulation every day. Of this protein, 100 to 200 g/day moves by convection across the capillary walls, dissolved in the filtered fluid (i.e., solvent drag). Because only very small amounts of filtered protein return to the circulation by solvent drag at the venular end of capillaries (~5 g/day), nearly all of the filtered protein (95–195 g/day) depends on the convective lymphatic loop for its ultimate recovery. The vital importance of lymphatic recovery is readily

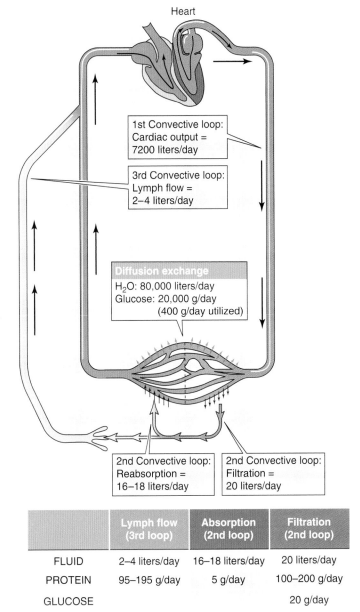

FIGURE 19–11. Convective loops of extracellular fluid and protein.

Heart

1st Convective loop:
Cardiac output =
7200 liters/day

3rd Convective loop:
Lymph flow =
2–4 liters/day

Diffusion exchange
H_2O: 80,000 liters/day
Glucose: 20,000 g/day
(400 g/day utilized)

2nd Convective loop:
Reabsorption =
16–18 liters/day

2nd Convective loop:
Filtration =
20 liters/day

	Lymph flow (3rd loop)	Absorption (2nd loop)	Filtration (2nd loop)
FLUID	2–4 liters/day	16–18 liters/day	20 liters/day
PROTEIN	95–195 g/day	5 g/day	100–200 g/day
GLUCOSE			20 g/day

apparent if one considers that the total protein content of plasma in a 70-kg human is only 200 to 250 g.

REGULATION OF THE MICROCIRCULATION

The Active Contraction of Vascular Smooth Muscle Regulates Precapillary Resistance, Which Controls Capillary Blood Flow

Smooth-muscle tone in arterioles, metarterioles, and precapillary sphincters (p. 460) determines the access resistance to the capillary beds. This resistance upstream of the capillary bed is also known as the afferent or **precapillary** resistance (R_{pre}). The overall resistance of a microcirculatory bed is the sum of R_{pre}, the resistance of the capillary bed itself (R_{cap}), and the efferent or postcapillary resistance (R_{post}).

How do these resistances influence the flow of blood (F_{cap}) through a capillary bed? We can answer this question by rearranging the Ohm's Law–like expression that we introduced as Equation 17–1:

Equation 19–11

$$F_{cap} = \frac{\Delta P}{R_{total}} = \frac{P_a - P_v}{R_{pre} + R_{cap} + R_{post}}$$

P_a is the pressure just before the beginning of the precapillary resistance, and P_v is the pressure just after the end of the postcapillary resistance. Because the aggregate R_{cap} is small, and R_{post}/R_{pre} is usually approximately 0.3, R_{pre} is usually much greater than $R_{cap} + R_{post}$. Because R_{pre} is the principal determinant of total resistance, capillary flow is roughly inversely proportional to R_{pre}.

Modulating the contractility of vascular smooth muscle cells in *precapillary* vessels is the main mechanism for adjusting perfusion of a particular tissue. VSMCs rely on a different molecular mechanism of contraction than skeletal muscle, although an increase in $[Ca^{2+}]_i$ is the principal trigger of contraction in both cases. Whereas an increase in $[Ca^{2+}]_i$ in skeletal muscle elicits contraction by interacting with troponin C, an increase in $[Ca^{2+}]_i$ in VSMCs elicits contraction by activating calmodulin (p. 102). The Ca^{2+}-calmodulin complex (Ca^{2+}-CaM) activates myosin light chain kinase (MLCK), which in turn phosphorylates the regulatory myosin light chain (MLC) on each myosin head (p. 238). Phosphorylation of MLC allows the myosin to interact with actin, producing contraction. Relaxation occurs when myosin light chain phosphatase dephosphorylates the MLC. In addition to changes in $[Ca^{2+}]_i$, changes in the activity of MLCK itself can modulate the contraction of VSMCs. Phosphorylation of MLCK by cAMP-dependent protein kinase (PKA) or cGMP-dependent protein kinase (PKG) inactivates the enzyme and thus *prevents* contraction.

Smooth-muscle cells can function as a syncytium when they are coupled through gap junctions ("unitary" smooth muscle), or they can function independently of one another as do skeletal muscle fibers ("multi-unit" smooth muscle; p. 231). Most vascular smooth muscle has a multi-unit organization. In contrast to skeletal muscle, VSMCs receive multiple excitatory as well as inhibitory inputs (p. 254). Moreover, these inputs come not only from chemical synapses (i.e., neural control), but also from circulating chemicals (i.e., humoral control). The actual contraction of VSMCs may follow smooth-muscle electrical activity in the form of action potentials, slow waves of depolarization, or graded depolarizations without spikes. However, humoral agents can also trigger contraction of VSMCs via increases in $[Ca^{2+}]_i$, without measurable fluctuations in membrane potential (pharmacomechanical coupling; p. 244).

Table 19–7 summarizes the roles that various membrane proteins (channels, receptors, and transporters) play in controlling the tone of VSMCs. Together with their associated signal transduction pathways, these membrane proteins lead to either contraction (i.e., vasoconstriction) or relaxation (i.e., vasodilation). Although different neural and humoral agents act on smooth muscle through different membrane proteins and transduction pathways, their effects converge on regulating the activity of MLCK.

Tissue Metabolites Regulate Local Blood Flow in Specific Vascular Beds, Independently of the Systemic Regulation

Vascular smooth-muscle cells not only control the resistance of arterioles (i.e., R_{pre}), and thus local blood flow, they also control the resistance of small terminal arteries and thereby play an important role in regulating systemic arterial blood pressure. In Chapter 22, we discuss this control of arterial blood pressure (a whole-body function) via VSMCs of small arteries and arterioles, both of which are under the control of *central* mechanisms—the autonomic nervous system and systemic humoral agents (e.g., angiotensin II). However, the subject of the present discussion is *local regulatory mechanisms* that use the arteri-

oles to regulate blood flow through specific vascular beds. These local control mechanisms can override any of the aforementioned neural or systemic humoral influences.

Mechanisms of local control involve (1) myogenic activity and (2) local chemical and humoral factors. **Myogenic regulation** refers to an *intrinsic* mode of control of activity, in which stretch of the VSMC membrane activates stretch-sensitive channels (see Table 19–7). The result is a depolarization that affects pacemaker activity, thereby increasing contractility of the VSMC.

The most prominent **chemical factors** are interstitial P_{O_2}, P_{CO_2}, and pH, as well as local concentrations of K^+, lactic acid, ATP, ADP, and adenosine (Table 19–8). Total osmolality may also make a contribution. The local regulation of VSMCs by *interstitial* P_{O_2}, P_{CO_2}, and pH is distinct from the regulation of systemic blood pressure by the peripheral chemoreceptors, which respond to changes in *arterial* P_{O_2}, P_{CO_2}, and pH (p. 723) and initiate a complex neural reflex that modulates VSMC activity (p. 546). In the case of *local* control, chemical changes in interstitial fluid act *directly* on the VSMCs through one of the mechanisms listed in Table 19–7. Changes that typically accompany increased metabolism (e.g., low P_{O_2}, high P_{CO_2}, and low pH) vasodilate vessels in the systemic circulation. Such local changes in P_{O_2}, P_{CO_2}, and pH have opposite effects in the pulmonary circulation (p. 699).

Because blood flow itself can influence the local concentration of the metabolic intermediates listed previously, blood flow in capillary beds tends to oscillate spontaneously over time in a process known as **vasomotion**. The timing of the components of the local feedback system may set the periodicity of vasomotion in the microcirculation. For example, if interstitial P_{O_2} falls as a result of increased local O_2 consumption, the ensuing vasodilation will increase O_2 delivery to the metabolizing cells, and in turn, will tend to cause the local interstitial P_{O_2} to increase. As the P_{O_2} now increases, vascular tone will increase. Spontaneous fluctuations in metabolism contribute to the periodicity of vasomotion. The interstitial volume around the active cells—the volume in which vasoactive metabolites are distributed—also affects this periodicity, because it affects the time lag for the concentration of vasoactive substances to rise or fall.

The Endothelium of Capillary Beds Is the Source of Several Vasoactive Compounds, Including NO, EDHF, and Endothelin

The capillary endothelium is the source of several important vasoactive compounds (Table 19–9).

Nitric oxide (NO), originally called endothelium-derived relaxing factor (EDRF), is a potent vasodilator. NO also inhibits platelet aggregation, induces platelet disaggregation, and inhibits platelet adhesion. Bradykinin and acetylcholine both stimulate the NOS III isoform of NO synthase (p. 110) that is constitutively present in endothelial cells. Increases in shear stress—the force acting on the endothelial cell along the axis of blood flow—can also stimulate the enzyme. NOS III, which depends on both Ca^{2+} and calmodulin for its activity, catalyzes the

TABLE 19–7

MOLECULAR MECHANISMS UNDERLYING THE CONTRACTION AND RELAXATION OF VASCULAR SMOOTH MUSCLE

CONTRACTION (VASOCONSTRICTION)	RELAXATION (VASODILATION)
Voltage-gated Ca^{2+} channels Depolarization $\rightarrow$ voltage-gated Ca^{2+} channels open $\rightarrow$ Ca^{2+} entry $\rightarrow$ $\uparrow [Ca^{2+}]_i$	**Voltage-gated K^+ channels** Depolarization $\rightarrow$ voltage-gated K^+ channels open $\rightarrow$ hyperpolarization $\rightarrow$ Ca^{2+} channels close $\rightarrow$ $\downarrow [Ca^{2+}]_i$
Voltage-gated Na^+ channels Depolarization $\rightarrow$ voltage-gated Na^+ channels open $\rightarrow$ more depolarization $\rightarrow$ voltage-gated Ca^{2+} channels open $\rightarrow$ Ca^{2+} entry $\rightarrow$ $\uparrow [Ca^{2+}]_i$	**Ca^{2+}-dependent K^+ channels** Hyperpolarization $\rightarrow$ voltage-gated Ca^{2+} channels close $\rightarrow$ $\downarrow [Ca^{2+}]_i$
Stretch-activated (SA) nonselective cation channels Stretch $\rightarrow$ SA channels open $\rightarrow$ depolarization $\rightarrow$ voltage-gated Ca^{2+} channels open $\rightarrow$ Ca^{2+} entry $\rightarrow$ $\uparrow [Ca^{2+}]_i$	**ATP-sensitive K^+ channels (K_{ATP})** $\downarrow [ATP]_i \rightarrow K_{ATP}$ channels open $\rightarrow$ hyperpolarization $\rightarrow$ Ca^{2+} channels close $\rightarrow$ $\downarrow [Ca^{2+}]_i$
Receptor-operated Ca^{2+} channels (ROCs) Agonist (e.g., adenosine) $\rightarrow$ ROC Ca^{2+} channels open $\rightarrow$ Ca^{2+} entry $\rightarrow$ $\uparrow [Ca^{2+}]_i$ (pharmacomechanical coupling)	**NO receptor (a soluble guanylyl cyclase)** NO $\rightarrow$ $\uparrow GC$ activity $\rightarrow$ $\uparrow [cGMP]_i \rightarrow$ $\uparrow PKG$ activity $\rightarrow$ • Phosphorylation of MLCK $\rightarrow$ $\downarrow$ MLCK activity $\rightarrow$ $\downarrow$ phosphorylation of MLC • Activation of Ca^{2+}-H pump (Ca^{2+} ATPase) in the SR $\rightarrow$ $\downarrow [Ca^{2+}]_i$
Adrenergic receptor α_1 Agonist (e.g., norepinephrine) $\rightarrow$ Adrenoreceptor $\alpha_1 \rightarrow$ activation of $G\alpha_q \rightarrow$ $\uparrow PLC$ activity $\rightarrow$ $\uparrow [IP_3]_i$ and $[DAG]_i \rightarrow$ IP_3 receptor in SR opens Ca^{2+} channels $\rightarrow$ $\uparrow [Ca^{2+}]_i$	**Adrenergic receptor β_2** Agonist (e.g., epinephrine) $\rightarrow$ adrenoreceptor $\beta_2 \rightarrow$ activation of $G\alpha_s \rightarrow$ $\uparrow AC$ activity $\rightarrow$ $\uparrow [cAMP]_i \rightarrow$ $\uparrow PKA$ activity $\rightarrow$ phosphorylation of MLCK $\rightarrow$ $\downarrow$ MLCK activity $\rightarrow$ $\downarrow$ phosphorylation of MLC
Muscarinic receptor M_2 Agonist (e.g., acetylcholine) $\rightarrow$ Muscarinic receptor $M_2 \rightarrow$ activation of $G\alpha_i \rightarrow$ $\downarrow AC$ activity $\rightarrow$ $\downarrow [cAMP]_i \rightarrow$ $\downarrow PKA$ activity $\rightarrow$ $\downarrow$ phosphorylation of MLCK $\rightarrow$ $\uparrow$ MLCK activity $\rightarrow$ $\uparrow$ phosphorylation of MLC	**VIP receptor** Vasoactive peptide $\rightarrow$ VIP receptor $\rightarrow$ activation of $G\alpha_s \rightarrow$ $\uparrow AC$ activity $\rightarrow$ $\uparrow [cAMP]_i \rightarrow$ $\uparrow PKA$ activity $\rightarrow$ • $\uparrow$ Phosphorylation of MLCK $\rightarrow$ $\downarrow$ MLCK activity $\rightarrow$ $\downarrow$ phosphorylation of MLC • Both Ca^{2+}-dependent and voltage-gated K^+ channels open $\rightarrow$ hyperpolarization $\rightarrow$ Ca^{2+} channels close $\rightarrow$ $\downarrow [Ca^{2+}]_i$
Endothelin receptor ET_A ET $\rightarrow$ Endothelin receptor $ET_A \rightarrow$ activation of $G\alpha_q \rightarrow$ $\uparrow PLC$ activity $\rightarrow$ $\uparrow [IP_3]_i$ and $[DAG]_i \rightarrow IP_3$ receptor in SR opens Ca^{2+} channels $\rightarrow$ $\uparrow [Ca^{2+}]_i$	**Prostacyclin (PGI_2)** $PGI_2 \rightarrow$ $\uparrow AC$ activity $\rightarrow$ $\uparrow [cAMP]_i \rightarrow$ $\uparrow PKA$ activity $\rightarrow$ $\uparrow$ phosphorylation of MLCK $\rightarrow$ $\downarrow$ MLCK activity $\rightarrow$ $\downarrow$ phosphorylation of MLC
Angiotensin receptor AT_{1A} ANGII $\rightarrow$ Angiotensin receptor $AT_{1A} \rightarrow$ activation of $G\alpha_q \rightarrow$ $\uparrow PLC$ activity $\rightarrow$ $\uparrow [IP_3]_i$ and $[DAG]_i \rightarrow IP_3$ receptor in SR opens Ca^{++} channels $\rightarrow$ $\uparrow [Ca^{++}]_i$	**Histamine receptor H_2** Histamine $\rightarrow$ H_2 receptor $\rightarrow$ activates $G\alpha_s \rightarrow$ $\uparrow AC$ activity $\rightarrow$ $\uparrow [cAMP]_i \rightarrow$ $\uparrow PKA$ activity $\rightarrow$ phosphorylation of MLCK $\rightarrow$ $\downarrow$ MLCK activity $\rightarrow$ $\downarrow$ phosphorylation of MLC
Purinergic receptor ATP $\rightarrow$ P_{2X} receptor (ligand-gated Ca^{2+} channel, an example of an ROC) $\rightarrow$ Ca^{2+} entry $\rightarrow$ $\uparrow [Ca^{2+}]_i$	**Purinergic receptor** • Adenosine $\rightarrow$ A_1, A_{2A}, and A_{2B} adenosine receptors $\rightarrow$ K_{ATP} channels open $\rightarrow$ hyperpolarization $\rightarrow$ voltage-gated Ca^{2+} channels close $\rightarrow$ $\downarrow [Ca^{2+}]_i$ • ATP $\rightarrow$ P_{2Y} receptors $\rightarrow$ activation of $G\alpha_{q/11} \rightarrow$ $\uparrow PLC$ activity $\rightarrow$ $\uparrow [Ca^{2+}]_i \rightarrow$ $\uparrow NOS \rightarrow$ NO release
Na-Ca exchanger Depolarization $\rightarrow$ voltage-gated Na^+ channels open $\rightarrow$ Na^+ entry $\rightarrow$ $\uparrow [Na^+]_i \rightarrow$ slows Na-Ca^{2+} exchange $\rightarrow$ $\uparrow [Ca^{2+}]_i$	**SR Ca^{2+} pump (SERCA)** Activation of Ca^{2+} pump (Ca^{2+}-ATPase) in the SR $\rightarrow$ $\downarrow [Ca^{2+}]_i$
	Na-K pump Activation of Na-K pump in plasma membrane $\rightarrow$ $\downarrow [Na^+]_i \rightarrow$ activation of Na-Ca^{2+} exchange $\rightarrow$ $\downarrow [Ca^{2+}]_i$

AC, adenylyl cyclase; DAG, diacylglycerol; GC, guanylyl cyclase; IP_3, inositol trisphosphate; MLC, myosin light chain; MLCK, myosin light-chain kinase; NOS, nitric oxide synthase; PKA, cAMP-stimulated protein kinase (protein kinase A); PKG, cGMP-stimulated protein kinase (protein kinase G); PLC, phospholipase C; SR, sarcoplasmic reticulum; VIP, vasoactive intestinal peptide.

TABLE 19–8

LOCAL METABOLIC CHANGES THAT CAUSE VASODILATION IN THE SYSTEMIC CIRCULATION

CHANGE	MECHANISM*
↓ P_{O_2}	↓ $[ATP]_i$, adenosine release
↑ P_{CO_2}	↓ pH_o
↓ pH	↓ pH_o
↑ $[K^+]_o$	Transient hyperpolarization → closes voltage-gated Ca^{2+} channels
↑ [lactic acid]$_o$	Probably ↓ pH_o
↓ $[ATP]_i$	Opens K_{ATP} channels
↑ $[ATP]_o$	Activates purinergic receptors
↑ $[ADP]_o$	Activates purinergic receptors
↑ $[Adenosine]_o$	Activates purinergic receptors

*The subscript "i" refers to intracellular levels, and the subscript "o" refers to interstitial levels.

formation of NO from arginine. NO, a lipophilic gas with a short half-life, diffuses locally outside the endothelial cell. Inside the VSMC is the "receptor" for NO, a soluble guanylyl cyclase that converts guanosine triphosphate (GTP) to cyclic guanosine monophosphate (cGMP). cGMP-dependent protein kinase (i.e., PKG) then phosphorylates MLCK and SERCA. Phosphorylation *inhibits* the MLCK, thus leading to a net decrease in the phosphorylation of MLC, and a decrease in the interaction between myosin and actin. Phosphorylation *activates* SERCA, thereby decreasing $[Ca^{2+}]_i$. The net result is that NO released by endothelial cells relaxes VSMCs, producing vasodilation.

Physicians have used exogenous organic nitrates (e.g., nitroglycerin) for decades to dilate peripheral vessels in order to relieve the pain of angina pectoris. These powerful vasodilators exert their activity by breaking down chemically, thereby releasing NO near VSMCs.

In addition to releasing NO, endothelial cells release another relaxing factor in response to acetylcholine, called **EDHF** (i.e., endothelium-derived hyperpolarizing factor). EDHF causes VSMC relaxation by making the membrane potential more negative.

TABLE 19–9

VASOACTIVE AGENTS PRODUCED BY ENDOTHELIAL CELLS

VASODILATORS	VASOCONSTRICTORS
Nitric oxide (NO)	Endothelin (ET)
Endothelium-derived hyperpolarizing factor (EDHF)	Endothelium-derived constricting factor-1 ($EDCF_1$)
Prostacyclin (PGI_2)	Endothelium-derived constricting factor-2 ($EDCF_2$)

Prostacyclin (PGI_2) is derived from arachidonic acid through the action of prostacyclin synthase (see Fig. 4–11). Prostacyclin is a vasodilator that acts by increasing $[cAMP]_i$ and promoting the phosphorylation of MLCK, ultimately decreasing the phosphorylation of myosin light chains. PGI_2 is especially important for dilating pulmonary vessels at birth (p. 1202).

The **endothelins (ETs)** are 21-residue peptides produced by endothelial cells; they cause an extremely potent and long-lasting **vasoconstriction** in most VSMCs. Many acute and chronic pathologic conditions, including hypoxia, promote the release of endothelin, which exists as three isopeptides: ET-1, ET-2, and ET-3. The precursor of ET-1 is *preproendothelin*, which the endothelial cell converts first to *proendothelin* and then to the mature *endothelin*, which it releases. The ET receptor subtype for vasoconstriction is ET_A. Other endothelin receptors also exist: ET_{B1} mediates vasodilation, ET_{B2} mediates vasoconstriction, and ET_C has as yet no clearly defined function. ET_A receptors predominate in high-pressure parts of the circulation, whereas ET_B receptors predominate in low-pressure parts of the circulation.

The binding of an endothelin to any endothelin receptor subtype ultimately results in an increase in $[Ca^{2+}]_i$. In the *vasoconstriction* response, ET-1 binding to ET_A receptors acts through the phospholipase C pathway to generate inositol triphosphate, release Ca^{2+} from intracellular stores, and raise $[Ca^{2+}]_i$ (p. 100). In a second, delayed phase, which is not well understood, Ca^{2+} entering from the outside contributes to the increase in $[Ca^{2+}]_i$. The increased $[Ca^{2+}]_i$ activates Ca^{2+}-CaM, stimulating MLCK to phosphorylate myosin light chains, and culminating in contraction.

Investigators have also described other **endothelial factors of unknown chemical composition**. In some arteries of the dog, *anoxia* produces an unexpected effect: an endothelium-dependent *increase* in tension mediated by a putative factor, $EDCF_1$ (endothelium-derived constricting factor). In some dog arteries, rapid *stretch* evokes a contraction that is also endothelium dependent. This putative factor, $EDCF_2$, could be a superoxide anion because superoxide dismutase prevents the contractions.

FIGURE 19–12. Autoregulation of blood flow. The *gray and red curves* are also shown in Figure 18–7A.

Autoregulation Stabilizes Blood Flow Despite Large Fluctuations in Systemic Arterial Pressure

As we saw in Chapter 17, the pressure-flow relationship of an idealized, rigid vessel is linear (Fig. 19–12, *gray line*). In most real (i.e., elastic) vessels, however, increases in pressure cause a dilation that reduces resistance and leads to a steeper-than-linear flow (see Fig. 19–12, *red curve*). However, some vascular beds behave very differently: Despite large changes in the systemic arterial pressure—and thus large changes in the driving pressure—these special vascular beds maintain local blood flow within a narrow range. This phenomenon is called **autoregulation**. These vascular beds behave more or less as rigid tubes at very low and at very high perfusion pressures (see Fig. 19–12, *blue curve*). However, in the physiological pressure range over which autoregulation occurs, changes in perfusion pressure have little effect on flow. Instead, increases in *pressure* lead to increases in *resistance* that keep blood flow within a carefully controlled range.

Autoregulatory behavior takes time to develop and is due to an active process. If the perfusion pressure were to increase abruptly, we would see that—immediately after the pressure increase—the pressure-flow diagram would look much like the one for the rigid tube in Figure 19–12. However, the vascular arteriolar tone then slowly adjusts itself to produce the characteristic autoregulatory pressure-flow diagram. The contraction of VSMCs that underlies autoregulation is *autonomous*, that is, it is entirely local and independent of neural and endocrine mechanisms. Both myogenic and metabolic mechanisms play an important role in the adjustments of smooth-muscle tone during autoregulation. For example, the stretch of VSMCs that accompanies the increased perfusion pressure triggers a "myogenic" contraction that reduces blood flow. Also, the increase in PO_2 (or decrease in PCO_2 or increase in pH) that accompanies increased perfusion pressure triggers a "metabolic" vasoconstriction that reduces blood flow (see Table 19–8).

Autoregulation is useful for at least two reasons. First, with an increase in perfusion pressure, autoregulation avoids a waste of perfusion in organs in which the flow was already sufficient. Second, with a decrease in perfusion pressure, autoregulation maintains capillary flow and capillary pressure. Autoregulation is very important under these conditions for organs—particularly the heart, brain, and kidneys—that are very sensitive to ischemia or hypoxia, or for organs (again, the kidney) whose job it is to filter the blood.

New Blood Vessels Proliferate in Response to Growth Factors By a Process Known as Angiogenesis

In adults, the anatomy of the microcirculation remains rather constant. Notable exceptions are the growth of new vessels during wound healing, inflammation, tumor growth, and in the endometrium during the menstrual cycle. Increased capillary density is important in physical training (p. 1253) and in acclimatization to altitude (p. 1264).

The development of new vessels is called **angiogenesis**. The first step is dissolution of the venular basement

membrane at a specific site, followed by activation and proliferation of previously quiescent endothelial cells. The new cells, attracted by growth factors, migrate to form a tube. Eventually, the budding tubes connect with each other, allowing the flow of blood and the development of vascular smooth muscle as the new microvascular network establishes itself. Angiogenesis relies on a balance between positive and negative regulation. The body normally produces some factors that promote angiogenesis and others that inhibit it (Table 19–10).

PROMOTERS OF VESSEL GROWTH. The principal peptides that induce angiogenesis are two polypeptides: vascular endothelial growth factor (VEGF) and fibroblast growth factor (FGF). Both interact with endothelium-specific receptor tyrosine kinases (p. 110). **VEGF**, which is related to platelet-derived growth factor (PDGF), is produced by fibroblasts and is frequently expressed in cancers. Activated coagulation factor VII (FVIIa) promotes VEGF production. **FGF** mediates many cellular responses during embryonic, fetal, and postnatal development. At least 16 different fibroblast growth factors (FGF-1 to FGF-16) exist.

The targeted delivery of these growth factors is a major obstacle in their therapeutic use. One approach has been to link the growth factor to small beads delivered into the coronary circulation. Cardiologists have successfully used FGF-1 (also known as basic fibroblast growth factor or bFGF) to promote the growth of vessels in the myocardium of patients with ischemic heart disease. NO, which is also a vasodilator, may play a role in terminating proliferation of endothelial cells and promoting the differentiation of vascular tubes.

Other growth factors have indirect angiogenic effects that are distinct from those of VEGF or FGF. **Angiopoietin-1** (ANGPT1) acts through a receptor tyrosine kinase (TIE2) that is expressed almost exclusively in endothelial cells. The tyrosine phosphorylation of TIE2 does not promote the growth of endothelial cells directly, but is required for critical interactions between endothelial cells and the surrounding matrix. ANGPT1 appears to play a major role in the angiogenesis of wound healing. **Angiogenin**, a 14-kDa protein, is one of the most potent angiogenic factors in experimental models; its plasma levels rise in cancer patients.

INHIBITORS OF VESSEL GROWTH. The concept of anti-angiogenesis was first advanced by Judah Folkman as a strategy to stop the growth of tumors. He and his colleagues have described two peptides, angiostatin and endostatin, that are inhibitors of angiogenesis.

Angiostatin is a 38-kDa internal fragment of plasminogen, a key fibrinolytic protein (p. 425). Angiostatin arises

TABLE 19–10

AGENTS THAT AFFECT VASCULAR GROWTH

PROMOTERS	INHIBITORS
Vascular endothelial growth factor (VEGF)	Endostatin
Fibroblast growth factors (FGFs)	Angiostatin
Angiopoietin-1 (ANGPT1)	Angiopoietin-2 (ANGPT2)

by proteolytic cleavage of plasminogen by connective tissue enzymes, such as matrix metalloproteinases and elastase. Angiostatin inhibits angiogenesis by enhancing apoptosis of endothelial cells and inhibiting migration and tube formation, rather than by affecting proliferation.

Endostatin is a peptide breakdown product of collagen XVIII. It is produced by the extracellular matrix of tumors.

Angiopoietin-2 (ANGPT2) is a relative of ANGPT1 that was identified by homology screening of cDNAs. However, ANGPT2 turns out to be a naturally occurring *antagonist* of angiopoietin-1, acting at the TIE2 receptor.

We can illustrate the importance of angiogenesis by highlighting three clinical situations in which angiogenesis plays an important role. First, enhancing vessel growth is important during coronary artery disease, when chronic ischemia of the heart leads to the development of new vessels and thus collateral circulation. Second, angiogenesis enhances the blood supply to a tumor, thereby promoting its growth and opening the principal route by which tumor cells exit the primary tumor during metastasis. Oncologists are exploring the use of angiogenesis inhibitors to treat cancer. Third, angiogenesis may also be important in diabetic retinopathy, where blood vessel proliferation can cause blindness.

REFERENCES

Books and Reviews

Aukland K, Reed RK: Interstitial-lymphatic mechanism in the control of extracellular fluid volume. Physiol Rev 73:1–78, 1993.

Davies PF: Flow-mediated endothelial mechanotransduction. Physiol Rev 75:519–560, 1995.
Grossman JD, Morgan JP: Cardiovascular effects of endothelin. News Physiol Sci 12:113–117, 1997.
Hudlicka O, Brown M, Egginton S: Angiogenesis in skeletal and cardiac muscle. Physiol Rev 72:369–417, 1992.
Schmid-Schönbein GW, Zweifach BW: Fluid pump mechanisms in initial lymphatics. News Physiol Sci 9:67–71, 1994.

Journal Articles

Buga GM, Gold ME, Fukuto JM, Ignarro LJ: Shear-stress induced release of nitric oxide from endothelial cells grown on beads. Hypertension 17:187–193, 1991.
Furchgott RF, Zawadzki V: The obligatory role of endothelial cells in the relaxation of arterial smooth muscle by acetylcholine. Nature 336:385–388, 1988.
Krogh A: The number and distribution of capillaries in muscles with calculation of the oxygen pressure head necessary for supplying the tissue. J Physiol London 52:409–415, 1919.
Landis EM: The capillary pressure in frog mesentery as determined by micro-injection methods. Am J Physiol 75:548–570, 1925–1926.
O'Reilly MS, Holmgren L, Shing Y, et al: Angiostatin: A novel angiogenesis inhibitor that mediates the suppression of metastases by a Lewis lung carcinoma. Cell 79:315–328, 1994.
Rees DD, Palmer RMJ, Moncada S: Role of endothelium-derived nitric oxide in the regulation of blood pressure. Proc Natl Acad Sci U S A 86:3375–3378, 1989.
Starling EH: On the absorption of fluids from connective tissue spaces. J Physiol 19:312–326, 1896.

CHAPTER 20

Cardiac Electrophysiology and the Electrocardiogram

W. Jonathan Lederer

Different cardiac cells serve different and very specialized functions, but all are electrically active. The heart's electrical signal normally originates in a group of cells high in the right atrium that depolarize spontaneously; it then spreads throughout the heart from cell to cell (Fig. 20–1A). As this action potential propagates through the heart—sometimes carried by cells that form specialized conducting pathways and sometimes by the very cells that generate the force of contraction—it assumes different appearances within the different cardiac cells (Fig. 20–1). Based on the speed of the upstroke, we can characterize action potentials as either **slow** (SA and AV nodes) or **fast** (atrial myocytes, Purkinje fibers, and ventricular myocytes).

Because the excitation of cardiac myocytes triggers contraction—a process called *excitation-contraction coupling* (p. 242)—the propagation of action potentials must be carefully timed to coordinate the complex mechanics of contraction. This chapter focuses on the membrane currents responsible for the generation and transmission of action potentials in heart tissue. We also examine how to record the heart's electrical flow by placing electrodes on the surface of the body, creating one of the simplest and yet one of the most useful diagnostic tools available to the clinician—the electrocardiogram, or ECG.

ELECTROPHYSIOLOGY OF CARDIAC CELLS

The Cardiac Action Potential Starts in Specialized Muscle Cells of the Sinoatrial Node, and Then Propagates in an Orderly Fashion Throughout the Heart

The cardiac action potential originates in a group of cells called the **sinoatrial (SA) node** (see Fig. 20–1), located in the right atrium. These cells depolarize spontaneously and fire off action potentials at a regular rate, usually between 60 and 100 times per minute. This intrinsic **pacemaker** activity, or *automaticity* (p. 367) is influenced by both parasympathetic and sympathetic neural input.

Because cardiac cells are electrically coupled through gap junctions (Fig. 20–2A), the action potential propagates from cell to cell in the same way that an action potential in nerve conducts along a single, long axon. A spontaneous action potential originating in the SA node will conduct from cell to cell throughout the right atrial muscle and spread to the left atrium. The existence of discrete conducting pathways in the atria is still disputed. About one tenth of a second after its origination, the signal arrives at the **atrioventricular (AV) node** (see Fig. 20–1). The impulse does not spread directly from the atria to the ventricles because of the presence of a fibrous

A CONDUCTION PATHWAYS THROUGH HEART

B CARDIAC ACTION POTENTIALS

FIGURE 20–1. Electrical activity in heart tissue. *A*, Conduction pathways through the heart. A section through the long axis of the heart is shown. *B*, Cardiac action potentials. The distinctive shapes of action potentials at five sites along the spread of excitation are shown. AV, atrioventricular; SA, sinoatrial.

atrioventricular ring. Instead, the only available pathway is for the impulse to travel from the AV node to the **His-Purkinje fiber system**, a network of specialized conducting cells that carries the signal to the muscle of both ventricles.

The Cardiac Action Potential Conducts from Cell to Cell via Gap Junctions

The electrical influence of one cardiac cell on another depends on the voltage difference between the cells and on the resistance of the gap-junction connection between them. A gap junction (p. 206) is an **electrical synapse** (see Fig. 20–2*A*) that permits electrical current to flow between neighboring cells. According to Ohm's law, the current flowing between cell A and the adjacent cell B (I_{AB}) is proportional to the voltage difference between the

two cells (ΔV_{AB}), but inversely proportional to the electrical resistance between them (R_{AB}):

Equation 20–1

$$I_{AB} = \frac{V_A - V_B}{R_{AB}} = \frac{\Delta V_{AB}}{R_{AB}}$$

When R_{AB} is very small (i.e., when the cells are tightly coupled), the gap junctions are minimal barriers to the flow of depolarizing current.

Imagine that several interconnected cells are initially all at their normal resting potentials (see Fig. 20–2*B*). An action potential propagating from the left of cell A now injects depolarizing current into cell A. As a result, the cell depolarizes to V_A, which is now somewhat positive compared to V_B. Thus, a small depolarizing current (i.e., positive charges) will also move from cell A to cell B and

A   CURRENT FLOW THROUGH GAP JUNCTIONS

B   ELECTROTONIC SPREAD OF CURRENT

C   THRESHOLD AND RATE OF PROPAGATION OF ACTION POTENTIAL

FIGURE 20–2. Conduction in the heart. *A*, An action potential conducting from left to right causes intracellular current to flow from fully depolarized cells on the left, through gap junctions, and into cell A. Depolarization of cell A causes current to flow from cell A to cell B (I_{AB}). Part of I_{AB} discharges the capacitance of cell B (depolarizing cell B), and part flows downstream to cell C. *B*, Subthreshold depolarization of cell A decays with distance. *C*, The speed of conduction increases with greater depolarization of cell A (*blue vs. red curves*) and/or with a more negative threshold.

depolarize cell B. In turn, current flowing from cell B will then depolarize cell C. By this process, the cells closest to the current source undergo the greatest depolarization.

Imagine that the injected current, coming from the active region of the heart to the left, depolarizes cell A just to its threshold (see Fig. 20–2C, *red curve*)—but that cell A has not yet fired an action potential. At this instant, the current passing from cell A to cell B cannot bring cell B to its threshold. Of course, cell A will eventually fire an action potential and, in the process, depolarize enough to inject enough current into cell B to raise cell B to its threshold. Thus, the action potential propagates down the chain of cells, but relatively slowly. On the other hand, if the active region to the left injects *more* current into cell A (see Fig. 20–2C, *blue curve*)—producing a larger depolarization in cell A—the current passing from cell A to cell B will be greater, and sufficient to depolarize cell B beyond its voltage threshold for a regenerative action potential. However, at this instant, the current passing from cell B to cell C is still not sufficient to trigger an action potential in cell C. That will have to wait until the active region moves closer to cell C, but the wait is not as long as in the first example *(red curve)*. Thus, the action potential propagates more rapidly in this second example *(blue curve)*.

In principle, we could make the action potential propagate more rapidly down the chain of cells in two ways. First, we could allow more ion channels to open in the active region of the heart, so that depolarizing current is larger (*blue curve* in Fig. 20–2C). Second, we could lower the threshold for the regenerative action potential ("more negative threshold" in Fig. 20–2C), so that even the small current represented by the *red curve* is now sufficient to trigger cell B.

Just as in a nerve axon conducting an action potential, the intracellular and extracellular currents in heart muscle must be equal and opposite. In the active region of the heart (to the left of cell A in Fig. 20–2B), cells have reached threshold and their action potentials provide the *source* of current that depolarizes cells that are approaching threshold (e.g., cells A and B). As cell A itself is depolarizing to and beyond threshold, its Na^+ and Ca^{2+} channels are opening, enabling these cations (i.e., positive charge) to enter. The positive charge that enters cell A not only depolarizes cell A, but also produces a flow of positive charge to cell B—**intracellular current**. This flow of positive charge discharges the membrane capacitance of cell B, thereby depolarizing cell B and releasing extracellular positive charges that had been associated with the membrane. The movement of this extracellular positive charge from around cell B toward the extracellular region around cell A constitutes the **extracellular current**. The flow of intracellular current from cell A to cell B and the flow of extracellular current from around cell B to around cell A are equal and opposite. It is the flow of this *extracellular* current in the heart that gives rise to the electrocardiogram (ECG).

Cardiac Action Potentials Have as Many as Five Distinctive Phases

The initiation time, shape, and duration of the action potential are distinctive for different parts of the heart, reflecting their different functions. These important differences arise because the myocytes in different regions of the heart have different sets of channels and different anatomy. Underlying cardiac action potentials are four major time-dependent and voltage-gated membrane currents (Table 20–1):

1. The **Na^+ current** (I_{Na}) is responsible for the rapid **depolarizing** phase of the action potential in atrial and ventricular muscle and in Purkinje fibers.

TABLE 20–1

MAJOR CARDIAC MEMBRANE CURRENTS THAT ARE TIME DEPENDENT AND VOLTAGE GATED					
CURRENT	NAME	CHANNEL	IONS THAT CARRY CURRENT	REVERSAL POTENTIAL OF CURRENT (mV)	INHIBITORS
I_{Na}	Na^+ current	Voltage-gated Na^+ channel	Na^+	+60	TTX Local anesthetics
I_{Ca}	Ca^{2+} current	L-type Ca^{2+} channel	Ca^{2+}	+120	nifedipine verapamil
I_K	Repolarizing I_{K_R}	HERG + miRP1*	K^+	−100	Ba^{2+} Cs^+ TEA
	Repolarizing I_{K_S} I_{to} G protein activated ATP-sensitive	KvLQT1 + minK* Kv4.3 GIRK* K_{ATP}*			
I_f	Pacemaker current	HCN	Na^+, K^+	−35	Cs^+

*These are heteromultimeric channels.

TTX, tetrodotoxin; TEA, tetraethylammonium; HERG, *h*uman *e*ther-a-go-go *r*elated *g*ene (related to Kv family of K^+-channel genes); GIRK, G protein–activated inwardly rectifying K^+ channel; HCN, Hyperpolarization-activated cyclic nucleotide gated.

FIGURE 20–3. Phases of cardiac action potentials. The records in this figure are idealized. I_K, I_{Na}, I_{Ca}, and I_f are currents through K^+, Na^+, Ca^{2+}, and nonselective cation channels, respectively.

2. The **Ca^{2+} current** (I_{Ca}) is responsible for the rapid **depolarizing** phase of the action potential in the SA node and AV node; it also triggers contraction in all cardiomyocytes.
3. The **K^+ current** (I_K) is responsible for the **repolarizing** phase of the action potential in all cardiomyocytes.
4. The "**pacemaker current**" (I_f) is responsible, in part, for pacemaker activity in SA nodal cells, AV nodal cells, and Purkinje fibers.

In addition to these four currents, channels carry numerous other currents in heart muscle. In addition, two *electrogenic* transporters carry current across plasma membranes: the Na-Ca exchanger and the Na-K pump.

Traditionally, the changes in membrane potential (V_m) during the cardiac action potential are divided into separate "phases," as illustrated in Figure 20–3A for cardiac action potentials from the SA node, and in Figure 20–3B for those from ventricular muscle.

Phase 0 is the upstroke of the action potential. If upstroke is due only to I_{Ca} (see Fig. 20–3A), it will be slow. If the upstroke is due to both I_{Ca} and I_{Na} (see Fig. 20–3B), it will be fast.

Phase 1 is the rapid repolarization component of the action potential (when it exists). This phase is due to almost total inactivation of I_{Na} or I_{Ca}, and may also depend on the activation of a minor K^+ current not listed previously, called I_{to} (for transient outward current).

Phase 2 is the plateau phase of the action potential, which is prominent in ventricular muscle. It depends on the continued entry of Ca^{2+} or Na^+ ions through their major channels, and on a minor membrane current due to the Na-Ca exchanger (see later).

Phase 3 is the repolarization component of the action potential. It depends on I_K.

Phase 4 constitutes the electrical diastolic phase of the action potential. V_m during phase 4 is termed the **diastolic potential**; the most *negative* V_m during phase 4 is the **maximum diastolic potential**. In SA and AV nodal cells, changes in I_K, I_{Ca}, and I_f produce pacemaker activity during phase 4. Purkinje fibers also exhibit pacemaker activity, but use only I_f. Atrial and ventricular muscle have no time-dependent currents during phase 4.

The Na^+ Current Is the Largest Current in the Heart

The sodium current (I_{Na}; see Table 20–1) is the largest current in heart muscle, which may have as many as 200 Na^+ channels per square micron of membrane. These channels are abundant in ventricular and atrial muscle, in Purkinje fibers, and in specialized conduction pathways of the atria. This current is not present in SA or AV nodal cells.

The channel that underlies I_{Na} is a classic voltage-gated Na^+ channel, with both an α and a β_1 subunit (p. 185). The unique cardiac α subunit has several phosphorylation sites that make it sensitive to stimulation by cAMP-dependent protein kinase (p. 97).

At the negative resting potentials of the ventricular muscle cells, the Na^+ channels are closed. However, these channels rapidly activate (in 0.1–0.2 ms) in response to local depolarization produced by conducted action potentials, and produce a massive inward current that underlies most of the rapid upstroke of the cardiac action potential (phase 0 in Fig. 20–3B). If V_m remains at a positive level, these channels close gradually—in a process known as **inactivation**. This process, which is slower than activation but is still fairly rapid (half-time, ~1 ms), is partly responsible for the rapid repolarization of the action potential (phase 1). At the potentials maintained during the plateau of the cardiac action potential—slightly positive to 0 mV during phase 2—a very small but important component of this current remains. This sustained level of I_{Na} helps prolong phase 2.

In cardiac tissues other than the SA and AV nodes, the regenerative spread of the conducted action potential depends in large part on the *magnitude* of I_{Na} (see Fig. 20–

2*C*). The depolarization produced by the Na$^+$ current not only activates I$_{Na}$ in neighboring cells, but also activates other membrane currents in the same cell, including I$_{Ca}$ and I$_K$. Local anesthetic **antiarrhythmic drugs**, such as lidocaine, work by partially blocking I$_{Na}$.

The Ca²⁺ Current in the Heart Passes Primarily Through L-Type Ca²⁺ Channels

The calcium current (I$_{Ca}$; see Table 20–1) is present in all cardiac myocytes. The "L-type" Ca^{2+} channel (p. 190) is the dominant one in the heart. T-type Ca^{2+} channels, with different biophysical and pharmacologic properties, are also present, but in smaller amounts.

In the SA node, the role of I$_{Ca}$, like that of the other time- and voltage-dependent membrane currents, is to contribute to pacemaker activity. In both the SA and AV nodes, I$_{Ca}$ is the inward current source that is responsible for the upstrokes (phase 0) of the SA and AV nodal action potentials. Because the nodal cells lack the larger I$_{Na}$, their upstrokes are slower than those in atrial and ventricular muscle (compare Fig. 30–3*A* and *B*). Therefore, the smaller I$_{Ca}$ discharges the membrane capacitance of neighboring cells in the SA and AV nodes less rapidly, so that the speed of the conducted action potential is much slower than that of any other cardiac tissue. This feature in the AV node leads to an **electrical delay** between atrial contraction and ventricular contraction that permits more time for the atria to empty blood into the ventricles.

Although it is smaller, I$_{Ca}$ sums with I$_{Na}$ during the upstroke of the action potentials of the ventricular and atrial muscle and the Purkinje fibers. In this way, it increases the velocity of the conducted action potential in these tissues. Like I$_{Na}$, I$_{Ca}$ produces virtually no current at very negative potentials because the channels are closed. At more positive values of V$_m$, the Ca^{2+} channels rapidly *activate* (in ~1 ms) and, by a completely separate and time-dependent process, *inactivate* (half-time, 10–20 ms). A small I$_{Ca}$ remains during the phase 2 of the action potential, helping to prolong the plateau. In atrial and ventricular muscle cells, the Ca^{2+} entering via L-type Ca^{2+} channels activates the release of Ca^{2+} from the sarcoplasmic reticulum (SR) by calcium-induced Ca^{2+} release (p. 242). **Blockers of L-type Ca²⁺ channels**—therapeutic agents such as verapamil, diltiazem, and nifedipine—act by inhibiting I$_{Ca}$.

The Repolarizing K⁺ Current Turns On Slowly

Cardiac action potentials last two orders of magnitude longer than action potentials in skeletal muscle because the repolarizing potassium current turns on very slowly and—in the case of atrial myocytes, Purkinje fibers, and ventricular myocytes—with a considerable delay. The **repolarizing potassium current** (I$_K$; see Table 20–1) is found in all cardiac myocytes and is responsible for repolarizing the membrane at the end of the action potential (phase 3 in Fig. 20–3*A* and *B*). Two currents underlie I$_K$—a relatively rapid component (I$_{K_r}$) and a relatively slow component (I$_{K_s}$; see the box on p. 196). The I$_K$ membrane current is very small at negative potentials. With depolarization, it slowly activates (20 to 100 msec)

but does not inactivate. In SA and AV nodal cells, it contributes to pacemaker activity by deactivating at the diastolic voltage.

In addition to I$_K$, several other K$^+$ currents are present in cardiac tissue:

EARLY OUTWARD K⁺ CURRENT (A-TYPE CURRENT). Atrial and ventricular muscle cells have some early *transient* outward current (I$_{to}$). This current is activated by depolarization but rapidly inactivates. It contributes to phase 1 repolarization and is analogous to the "A-type" currents (p. 194) seen in nerves. A Kv4.3 channel mediates the A-type current in heart and certain other cells.

G PROTEIN–ACTIVATED K⁺ CURRENT. Acetylcholine activates muscarinic receptors and, through the $\beta\gamma$ subunits of a G protein, activates an outward K$^+$ current mediated by GIRK K$^+$ channels (see p. 197). This current is prominent in SA and AV nodal cells, where it decreases pacemaker rate when activated by cell hyperpolarization. It also slows the conduction of the action potential through the AV node.

K$_{ATP}$ CURRENT. ATP-sensitive K$^+$ channels (K$_{ATP}$; p. 198) are present in abundance and may play a role in electrically regulating contractile behavior.

The I$_f$ Current Is Mediated by a Nonselective Cation Channel

The "pacemaker current" (I$_f$) is found in SA and AV nodal cells and in Purkinje fibers (see Fig. 20–3*A*, *blue curve*). The channel underlying this current is a nonspecific cation channel called HCN (for *Hyperpolarization-activated Cyclic Nucleotide-gated*), which is related to the cyclic nucleotide–gated channels (p. 170). Because the HCN channels conduct both K$^+$ and Na$^+$, the reversal potential of I$_f$ is around −20 mV, between the Nernst potentials for K$^+$ (about −90 mV) and Na$^+$ (about +50 mV). The HCN channels have the unusual property (hence the subscript "f," for "funny" current) that they do not conduct at positive potentials, but are activated by *hyperpolarization* at the end of phase 3. The activation is slow (100 ms), and the current does not inactivate. Thus, I$_f$ produces an inward, *depolarizing* current as it slowly activates at the end of phase 3. Despite its name, the I$_f$ current is not the only current that contributes to pacemaker activity; in SA and AV nodal cells, I$_{Ca}$ and I$_K$ also contribute significantly to the phase 4 depolarization.

Different Cardiac Tissues Uniquely Combine Ionic Currents to Produce Distinctive Action Potentials

The shape of the action potential differs among different cardiac cells because of the unique combination of various currents—both the voltage-gated/time-dependent currents discussed in the previous four sections and the "background" currents—present in each cell type. In Chapter 6, we introduced Equation 6–12, which describes V$_m$ in terms of the conductances for the different ions (G$_{Na}$, G$_K$, G$_{Ca}$, G$_{Cl}$) relative to the total membrane conductance (G$_m$), and the equilibrium potentials (E$_{Na}$, E$_K$, E$_{Ca}$, E$_{Cl}$):

TABLE 20–2

EQUILIBRIUM POTENTIALS

ION	INTRACELLULAR CONCENTRATION (mM)	EXTRACELLULAR CONCENTRATION (mM)	EQUILIBRIUM POTENTIAL (mV)
Na^+	10	145	+72
K^+	120	4.5	−88
Cl^-	35	116	−32
H^+	pH = 7.1	pH = 7.4	−19
Ca^{2+}	0.0001	1.0	+123

Equation 20–2

$$V_m = \frac{G_K}{G_m} E_K + \frac{G_{Na}}{G_m} E_{Na} + \frac{G_{Ca}}{G_m} E_{Ca} + \frac{G_{Cl}}{G_m} E_{Cl} \cdots$$

Therefore, as the relative contribution of a particular membrane current becomes dominant, V_m approaches the equilibrium potential for that membrane current (Table 20–2). How fast V_m changes during the action potential depends on the magnitude of each of the currents (see Equation 6–12). Not only does each current *independently* affect the shape of the action potential, but the voltage- and time-dependent currents interact with one another because they affect—and are affected by—V_m. Other important influences on the shape of the cardiac action potential are the membrane capacitance of each cell and the geometry of the conduction pathway (e.g., AV node, bundle of His, ventricular muscle) as the action potential propagates from cell to cell via gap junctions. Therefore, it is easy to understand, at a conceptual level, how a particular cell's unique complement of ion channels, the properties of these channels at a particular instant in time, intracellular ion concentrations, and the cell's geometry can all contribute to the shape of an action potential.

The Sinoatrial Node Is the Primary Pacemaker of the Heart

THE CONCEPT OF PACEMAKER ACTIVITY. The normal heart has three intrinsic pacemaking tissues: the SA node, the AV node, and the Purkinje fibers. The term **pacemaker activity** refers to the spontaneous time-dependent depolarization of the cell membrane that leads to an action potential in an otherwise quiescent cell. Any cardiac cell with pacemaker activity can initiate the heartbeat. The pacemaker with the highest frequency will be the one to trigger an action potential that will propagate throughout the heart. In other words, the fastest pacemaker sets the heart rate and overrides all slower pacemakers. Thus, cardiac pacemakers have a hierarchy among themselves, based on their intrinsic frequency. Under normal conditions, the SA node is the fastest pacemaker.

Two fundamental principles underlie pacemaker activity. The first is that inward or depolarizing membrane currents interact with outward or hyperpolarizing membrane currents to establish regular cycles of spontaneous depolarization and repolarization. The second is that, in a particular cell, these currents interact during phase 4 within a narrow range of diastolic potentials: between −70 and −50 mV in SA and AV nodal cells, and between −90 and −65 mV in Purkinje fibers.

SINOATRIAL NODE. The sinoatrial (SA) node is found in the right atrium and is the primary site of origin of the electrical signal in the mammalian heart (Table 20–3). It is the smallest electrical region of the heart and constitutes the fastest normal pacemaker, with an intrinsic rate of 60 beats/min or faster. SA cells are stable oscillators whose currents are always varying with time. The interactions among three time-dependent and voltage-gated membrane currents control the intrinsic rhythmicity of the SA node: (1) I_{Ca}, (2) I_K, and (3) I_f. The sum of a *decreasing outward* current (I_K; *green curve* in Fig. 20–3A) and two *increasing inward* currents (I_{Ca} and I_f; *red and blue curves* in Fig. 20–3A) produces the slow pacemaker depolarization (phase 4) associated with the SA node. The maximum diastolic potential (i.e., the most negative V_m) of the SA nodal cells, which occurs during phase 4 of the action potential, is between −60 and −70 mV. As V_m rises toward the threshold of about −55 mV, I_{Ca} becomes increasingly activated and eventually becomes regenerative, producing the upstroke of the action potential. This depolarization rapidly turns off (i.e., deactivates) I_f, and the whole process begins again.

These membrane currents discussed in the previous paragraph are under the control of local and circulating agents (e.g., acetylcholine, epinephrine, and norepinephrine), and are also targets for therapeutic agents designed to modulate the heart's rhythm (e.g., Ca^{2+}-channel blockers and β-adrenergic blockers).

ATRIOVENTRICULAR NODE. The atrioventricular (AV) node, located just above the atrioventricular ring, is the secondary site of origin of the electrical signal in the mammalian heart. Normally, the AV node may be excited by an impulse reaching it by way of the specialized atrial conduction pathways (see later). Like the SA node, the intrinsic rhythmicity of the AV node depends on the interaction of three time-dependent and voltage-gated currents: (1) I_K, (2) I_{Ca}, and (3) I_f. Electrically, the SA and AV nodes share many properties: They have similar action potentials, pacemaker mechanisms, and drug sensitivities, and a similarly slow conduction of action potentials. Because the intrinsic pacemaker rate of the AV node is

TABLE 20–3

ELECTRICAL PROPERTIES OF DIFFERENT CARDIAC TISSUES

TISSUE NAME	FUNCTION	PRINCIPAL TIME-DEPENDENT & VOLTAGE-DEPENDENT CURRENTS	β-ADRENERGIC EFFECT (e.g., epinephrine)	CHOLINERGIC EFFECT (e.g., acetylcholine)
SA node	Primary pacemaker	I_{Ca}, I_K, I_f	↑ Conduction velocity ↑ Pacemaker rate	↓ Pacemaker rate ↓ Conduction velocity
Atrial muscle	Expel blood from atria	I_{Na}, I_{Ca}, I_K	↑ Strength of contraction	Little effect
AV node	Secondary pacemaker	I_{Ca}, I_K, I_f	↑ Conduction velocity ↑ Pacemaker rate	↓ Pacemaker rate ↓ Conduction velocity
Purkinje fibers	Rapid conduction of action potential Tertiary pacemaker	I_{Na}, I_{Ca}, I_K, I_f	↑ Pacemaker rate	↓ Pacemaker rate
Ventricular muscle	Expel blood from ventricles	I_{Na}, I_{Ca}, I_K	↑ Contractility	Little effect

AV, atrioventricular; SA, sinoatrial.

slower (around 40 beats/min) than that of the SA node, it does not set the heart rate; its pacemaker activity is thus considered "secondary." However, if the SA node should fail, the AV node can assume control of the heart and drive it successfully.

PURKINJE FIBERS. The His-Purkinje fiber system originates at the AV node with the "bundle of His," and splits to form the left and right bundle branches (see Fig. 20–1). The right bundle conducts the electrical signal to the right ventricle, and the left bundle conducts the signal to the left ventricle. The anatomy of the left bundle is variable, but this bundle frequently divides into two main branches—the left anterosuperior fascicle (or hemibundle) and the left posteroinferior fascicle.

Purkinje fiber cells have the slowest intrinsic pacemaker rate (20 beats/min or less). Thus, Purkinje fiber cells become functional pacemakers only if the SA and AV pacemakers fail, and are considered "tertiary" pacemakers. On the other hand, the bundle of His and the Purkinje fibers are an effective conduction system within the ventricles because they conduct action potentials more quickly than any other tissue within the heart (Table 20–4).

The action potential of the Purkinje fibers depends on four time- and voltage-dependent membrane currents: (1) I_{Na} (not present in the SA and AV nodal cells), (2) I_{Ca}, (3) I_K, and (4) I_f. The maximum diastolic potential is −80 mV. From that negative V_m, these cells produce a very slow pacemaker depolarization (phase 4) that depends on I_f. Because of their low rate of pacemaker depolarization and therefore the uncertainty of reaching the threshold for triggering an action potential, Purkinje fiber cells are very unreliable as pacemakers. Normally, the action potential passing through the AV node activates the Purkinje fiber cells, resulting in a very rapid upstroke (phase 0), mediated by I_{Na} and I_{Ca}. Because I_{Na} is large, Purkinje fibers conduct action potentials rapidly.

Atrial and Ventricular Myocytes Fire Action Potentials but Do Not Have Pacemaker Activity

The resting potential of atrial and ventricular myocytes is substantially more negative (about −80 mV) than the maximum diastolic potential of pacemaker cells (see Fig. 20–1).

ATRIAL MUSCLE. Within each atrium, the action potential spreads among cardiac myocytes via a direct cell-to-cell pathway. The atrial action potential depends on three primary time- and voltage-dependent membrane currents: (1) I_{Na}, (2) I_K, and (3) I_{Ca}. There is no normal spontaneous (i.e., pacemaker) activity in atrial muscle. It has been proposed that atrial muscle has four special conducting bundles (see Fig. 20–1). One, **Bachman's bundle** (anterior interatrial myocardial band), is interatrial, and conducts the cardiac action potential from the SA node to the left atrium. Three other internodal pathways—the anterior, middle, and posterior internodal pathways—ap-

TABLE 20–4

CONDUCTION VELOCITY IN DIFFERENT CARDIAC TISSUES

TISSUE	CONDUCTION VELOCITY (m/s)
SA node	0.05
Atrial pathways	1
AV node	0.05
Bundle of His	1
Purkinje system	4
Ventricular muscle	1

AV, atrioventricular; SA, sinoatrial.

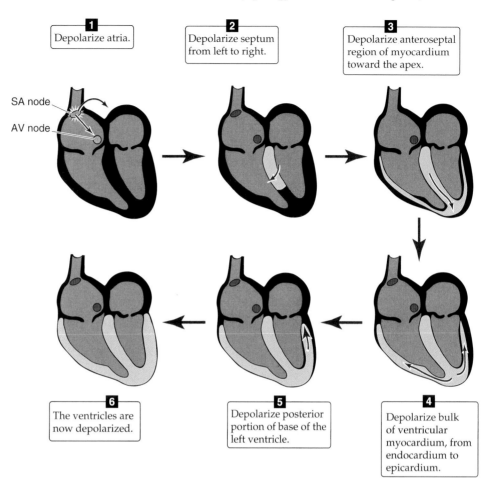

FIGURE 20-4. Sequence of depolarization in cardiac tissue. AV, atrioventricular; SA, sinoatrial.

1 Depolarize atria.

2 Depolarize septum from left to right.

3 Depolarize anteroseptal region of myocardium toward the apex.

4 Depolarize bulk of ventricular myocardium, from endocardium to epicardium.

5 Depolarize posterior portion of base of the left ventricle.

6 The ventricles are now depolarized.

pear to conduct the action potential from the SA node to the AV node. Therefore, the first step in propagation of the cardiac action potential is the depolarization of the atria, following a general axis from right to left and downward (Fig. 20–4, *step 1*).

If the conduction path through the AV node is blocked, the ventricles will not be activated electrically and will not contract. The spontaneous activity that can arise in the Purkinje fiber cells may provide the necessary electrical signal to activate the ventricles, but this activation occurs normally only at a very low rate, and Purkinje fiber pacemaker activity is fairly unreliable.

VENTRICULAR MUSCLE. After the action potential reaches the AV node, it travels to the His-Purkinje fiber network and out into the ventricular muscle. The only electrical access between the atrial muscle and the ventricles is the AV node. Because of this single electrical connection between the atria and the ventricles, there is a well-defined and orderly sequence of electrical activity through the rapidly conducting His-Purkinje network to the ventricles. Within the ventricular muscle, the action potential conducts from cell to cell. Steps 2 through 6 in Figure 20–4 summarize the sequence of events in ventricular activation, which is completed in approximately 100 ms:

Step 2: The septum depolarizes from left to right.
Step 3: The anteroseptal region depolarizes.

Step 4: The myocardium always depolarizes from the endocardium (the cells lining the ventricles) toward the epicardium (cells on the outer surface of the heart). The left ventricle depolarizes at the apex, while the Purkinje fibers are still in the process of conducting the action potential toward the base of the left ventricle.
Step 5: Depolarization spreads from the apex toward the base, carried by the Purkinje fibers. This spread to the base begins even as the signal in the "apex" is still spreading from the endocardium to the epicardium. The last region to depolarize is the posterobasal region of the left ventrical.
Step 6: The ventricles are fully depolarized.

Ventricular muscle has three major time- and voltage-gated membrane currents. (1) I_{Na}, (2) I_{Ca}, and (3) I_K (see Fig. 20–3B). Ventricular muscle has no I_f, and healthy ventricular muscle cells show no pacemaker activity. Starting from a resting potential of −80 mV, the rapid upstroke of the ventricular action potential results from the activation of I_{Na} by an external stimulus (e.g., an impulse conducted to the muscle by a Purkinje fiber, or conducted to it by a neighboring ventricular muscle cell). The Ca^{2+} current is of particular importance to ventricular muscle because it provides the Ca^{2+} influx that activates the release of Ca^{2+} from the sarcoplasmic reticulum. The rapid repolarization (phase 1), the plateau (phase 2), and the repolarization (phase 3) all appear to be governed by mechanisms similar to those found in the Purkinje fibers. However, the plateau phase is prolonged in ventricular muscle because inward and outward currents are rather stable during that time (*green, orange, and red curves* in Fig. 20–3B).

Once a ventricular muscle cell is activated electrically, it is refractory to additional activation. This **effective refractory period** (ERP) arises because the inward currents (I_{Na} and I_{Ca}) that are responsible for activation are largely inactivated by the membrane depolarization (see Fig. 20–3B). The ERP is the same as the *absolute* refractory period in nerve and skeletal muscle. During the ERP, an additional electrical stimulus has no effect on the action potential. At the end of the plateau, the cell begins to repolarize as I_K increases in magnitude. As I_{Ca} and I_{Na} begin to recover from inactivation, the **relative refractory period** (RRP) begins. During this period, an additional electrical stimulus can produce an action potential, but a smaller one than usual. Refractoriness provides the heart with a measure of electrical safety because it prevents extraneous pacemakers (which may arise pathologically)

from triggering **ectopic beats**. An extrasystolic contraction would make the heart a less efficient pump. Refractoriness also prevents tetanus (p. 249), a feature observed in skeletal muscle. Tetanus of the heart would mean perpetual systole, and no further contractions.

Acetylcholine and Catecholamines Modulate Pacemaker Activity, Conduction Velocity, and Contractility

In principle, the SA node can slow the firing rate of its pacemaker by three mechanisms. First, the steepness of the depolarization during phase 4 can decrease, thereby lengthening the time necessary for V_m to reach threshold (Fig. 20–5A, *blue curve*). In this way, diastole is longer and the heart rate falls. Second, the maximum diastolic potential can become more negative (see Fig. 20–5B, *green curve*). In this case, beginning at a lower value, V_m requires a longer time to reach the threshold, assuming no change in the steepness of the phase 4 depolarization.

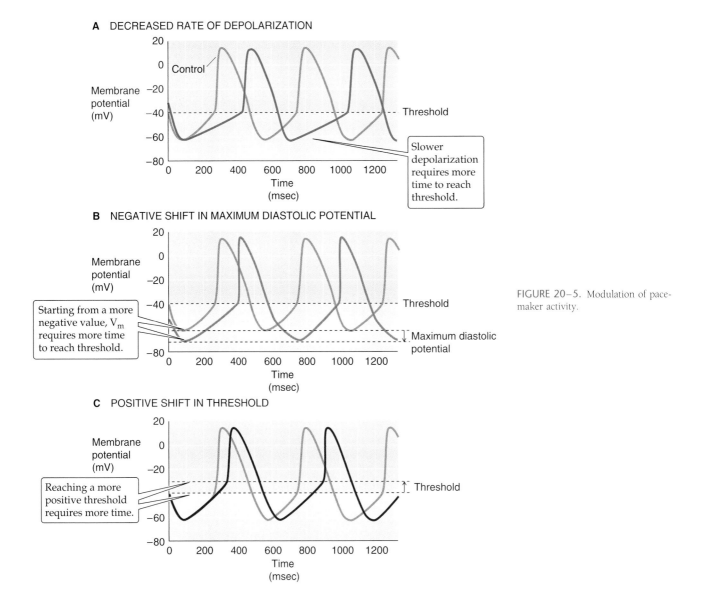

FIGURE 20–5. Modulation of pacemaker activity.

Third, the threshold for the action potential can become more positive (see Fig. 20–5C, *purple curve*). Assuming no change in either the maximum diastolic potential (i.e., starting point) or the steepness of the phase 4 depolarization, V_m requires a longer time to reach a more positive threshold. Obviously, a combination of these three mechanisms would have an enhanced effect. Conversely, the SA node cells can use each of these three mechanisms in the opposite sense to increase their firing rate.

ACETYLCHOLINE. The vagus nerve, which is parasympathetic (p. 380), releases acetylcholine (ACh) onto the SA and AV nodes and slows the intrinsic pacemaker activity by all three mechanisms discussed in the previous paragraph. First, ACh decreases I_f in the SA node (see Table 20–1), reducing the steepness of the phase 4 depolarization (see Fig. 20–5A). Second, ACh opens GIRK channels, increasing relative K^+ conductance and making the maximum diastolic potential of SA nodal cells more negative (see Fig. 20–5B). Third, ACh reduces I_{Ca} in the SA node, thereby reducing the steepness of the phase 4 depolarization (see Fig. 20–5A) and also moving the threshold to more positive values (see Fig. 20–5C). All three effects cooperate to lengthen the time for the SA node to depolarize to threshold; the net effect is to lower the heart rate.

Acetylcholine has similar effects on currents in the AV node as it does in the SA node. However, because the pacemaker normally does not reside in the AV node, the physiological effect of ACh on the AV node is to slow **conduction velocity**. The mechanism is an inhibition of I_{Ca} that also makes the threshold more positive for AV nodal cells. Because it is more difficult for one cell to depolarize its neighbors to threshold, conduction velocity falls.

CATECHOLAMINES. Sympathetic innervation to the heart is plentiful, releasing mostly norepinephrine. In addition, the adrenal medulla releases epinephrine into the circulation. Catecholamines, which act through β_1-adrenergic receptors, produce an increase in heart rate by two mechanisms. First, catecholamines increase I_f in the nodal cells, thereby increasing the steepness of the phase 4 depolarization (i.e., opposite to the effect in Fig. 20–5A). Second, catecholamines increase I_{Ca} in all myocardial cells. The increase in I_{Ca} in the SA and AV nodal cells steepens the phase 4 depolarization (i.e., opposite to the effect in Fig. 20–5A), and also makes the threshold more negative (i.e., opposite to the effect in Fig. 20–5C). Note that catecholamines do not appear to change the maximum diastolic potential.

In atrial and ventricular muscle, catecholamines cause an increase in the strength of contraction (**positive inotropic effect**) for four reasons. First, the increased I_{Ca} (i.e., Ca^{2+} influx) leads to a greater local increase in $[Ca^{2+}]_i$, and also a greater Ca^{2+}-induced Ca^{2+} release (p. 242) from the SR. Second, the catecholamines increase the sensitivity of the SR Ca^{2+}-release channel to cytoplasmic Ca^{2+} (p. 241). Third, catecholamines also enhance Ca^{2+} pumping into the SR by stimulating the SERCA Ca^{2+} pump (p. 64), thereby increasing Ca^{2+} stores for later release. Fourth, the increased I_{Ca} presents more Ca^{2+} to SERCA, so that SR Ca^{2+} stores increase over time. The

four mechanisms make more Ca^{2+} available to troponin C, enabling a more forceful contraction.

THE ELECTROCARDIOGRAM

An Electrocardiogram Generally Includes Five Waves

The electrocardiogram (ECG or EKG) is the standard clinical tool used to measure the electrical activity of the heart. It is a recording of the small *extracellular* signals produced by the movement of action potentials through cardiac myocytes. In order to obtain a standard 12-lead ECG, one places two **electrodes** on the upper extremities, two on the lower extremities, and six on standard locations across the chest. In various combinations, the electrodes on the extremities generate the six limb leads (three standard and three augmented), and the chest electrodes produce the six precordial leads. In a **lead**, one electrode is treated as the positive side of a voltmeter, and one or more electrodes as the negative side. Therefore, a lead records the fluctuation in voltage difference between positive and negative electrodes. By varying which elec-

FIGURE 20–6. Components of the electrocardiogram (ECG) recording. AV, atrioventricular; SA, sinoatrial.

trodes are positive and which are negative, the ECG machine records a standard 12-lead ECG. Each lead looks at the heart from a unique angle and plane, that is, from what is essentially its own unique point of view.

The fluctuations in extracellular voltage recorded by each lead vary from fractions of a millivolt to several millivolts. These fluctuations are called **waves**, and are named with the letters of the alphabet (Fig. 20–6). The **P** wave reflects depolarization of the right and left atrial muscle. The **QRS** complex represents depolarization of ventricular muscle. The **T** wave represents repolarization of both ventricles. Finally, the rarely seen **U** wave may reflect repolarization of the papillary muscle. The shape and magnitude of these waves are different in each lead, because each lead views the electrical activity of the heart from a unique position in space. For his discovery of the mechanism of the electrocardiogram, Willem Einthoven was awarded the 1924 Nobel Prize in Physiology or Medicine.

Because the ECG machine uses electrodes attached to the skin to measure the sum of the heart's electrical activity, it requires special amplifiers. The ECG machine also has electrical filters that reduce the electrical noise. Moving limbs, breathing, coughing, shivering, or faulty contact between the skin and an electrode produces artifacts on the recorded ECG.

Because the movement of charge (i.e., the spreading wave of electrical activity in the heart) has both a three-dimensional **direction** and a **magnitude**, the signal measured on an ECG is a **vector**. The system that clinicians use to measure the heart's three-dimensional, time-dependent electrical vector is simple to understand and easy to implement, but it can be challenging to interpret.

A Pair of Electrocardiogram Electrodes Defines a "Lead"

In order to record the complicated time-dependent electrical vector of the heart, the physician or ECG technician constructs a system of leads in two planes that are perpendicular to each other. One plane, the **frontal plane**, is defined by the six **limb leads** (Fig. 20–7A). A perpendicular **transverse plane** is defined by the six **precordial leads** (see Fig. 20–7B). Each lead is an axis in one of the two planes, onto which the heart projects its electrical activity. The ECG recording from a single lead shows how that lead views the time-dependent changes in voltage of the heart.

Older ECG machines recorded data from the 12 leads one at a time, sequentially. Thus, relatively rare events captured by the recording in one lead might not be reflected in any of the others, which were obtained at different times. Modern ECG machines obtain leads synchronously in groups of 3 or 12. Because the real electrical vector of the heart consists of just one time-dependent vector signal, you might think that a three-lead recording would suffice to localize the vector signal in space. In principle, this is true: Only two leads in one plane and one lead in another plane are needed to fully define the original electrical vector of the heart at all moments. However, recording from all 12 leads is extremely useful because a signal of interest may be easier to see in one lead than another. For example, an acute myocardial infarction involving the inferior (diaphragmatic) portion of the heart might be easily visualized in leads II, III, and aVF, but go completely undetected (or produce so-called reciprocal changes) in the other leads.

THE LIMB LEADS. One obtains a 12-lead ECG by having the patient relax in a supine position, and connecting four electrodes to the limbs (see Fig. 20–7A). Electrically, the torso and limbs are viewed as an equilateral triangle (Einthoven's triangle) with one vertex on the groin and the other two on the shoulder joints (Fig. 20–8A). Because the body is an electrical "volume conductor," an electrical attachment to an arm is electrically equivalent to a connection at the shoulder joint, and an attachment to

A FRONTAL PLANE LEADS

B TRANSVERSE PLANE–PRECORDIAL LEADS

FIGURE 20–7. The ECG leads.

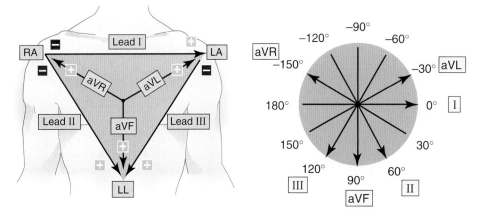

A EINTHOVEN'S TRIANGLE

B CIRCLE OF AXES

FIGURE 20–8. Axes of the limb leads. *A,* The frontal plane limb leads behave as if located at the shoulders (RA, right arm; LA, left arm) and groin (LL, left leg). Leads I, II, and III are separated from one another by 60 degrees. The augmented leads, referenced to the center of the heart, bisect each of the 60-degree angles formed by leads I, II, and III. *B,* Translating each of the six frontal leads so that they pass through a common point defines a polar coordinate system, providing views of the heart at 30-degree intervals.

either leg is equivalent to a connection at the groin. By convention, the left leg represents the groin. The fourth electrode, connected to the right leg, is used for electrical grounding. The three initial limb leads represent the difference between two of the limb electrodes:

▷ I (positive connection to left arm, negative connection to right arm). This lead defines an axis in the frontal plane at 0 degrees (see Fig. 20–8*A* and *B*).
▷ II (positive to left leg, negative to right arm). This lead defines an axis in the frontal plane at 60 degrees.
▷ III (positive to left leg, negative to left arm). This lead defines an axis in the frontal plane at 120 degrees.

An electronic reconstruction of the three limb leads defines an electrical reference point in the middle of the heart (see Fig. 20–8*A*) that constitutes the "negative" connection for the augmented "unipolar" limb leads and for the chest leads. The three augmented "unipolar" limb leads compare one limb electrode to the average of the other two:

▷ **aVR** (positive connection to *Right* arm, negative connection is electronically defined in the middle of the heart). The axis defined by this limb lead in the frontal plane is −150 degrees (see Fig. 20–8*B*). The "a" stands for augmented, and the "V" represents unipolar.
▷ **aVL** (positive to *Left* arm, negative is middle of the heart). The axis defined by this limb lead in the frontal plane is −30 degrees.
▷ **aVF** (positive to left leg [*Foot*], negative is middle of the heart). The axis defined by this limb lead in the frontal plane is +90 degrees.

Thus, the positive and negative ends of these six leads define axes every 30 degrees in the frontal plane (see Fig. 20–8*B*).

THE PRECORDIAL LEADS. These leads lie in the transverse plane, perpendicular to the plane of the frontal leads. The "positive" connection is one of six different locations on the chest wall (see Fig. 20–7*B*), and the "negative" connection is electronically defined in the middle of the heart by averaging the three limb electrodes. The resultant leads are named V_1 through V_6, where the "V" stands for unipolar:

▷ V_1: fourth intercostal space to the right of the sternum
▷ V_2: fourth intercostal space to the left of the sternum
▷ V_4: fifth intercostal space at the midclavicular line
▷ V_3: halfway between V_2 and V_4
▷ V_6: fifth intercostal space at the midaxillary line
▷ V_5: halfway between V_4 and V_6.

It is also possible, on rare occasions, to obtain **special leads** by employing the same negative connection used for the unipolar limb and precordial leads and a positive "probe" lead. Special leads that are used include esophageal leads and an intracardiac lead (e.g., that used to obtain a recording from the His-bundle).

A Simple Two-Cell Model Can Explain How a Simple Electrocardiogram Can Arise

We can illustrate how the ECG arises from the propagated action potentials of myocytes by examining the electrical activity in two neighboring cardiac cells, A and B, connected by gap junctions (Fig. 20–9*A*). The depolarization and action potential begin first in cell A (V_A in Fig. 20–9*A*, *green record*). The current from cell A then depolarizes cell B through the gap junctions, and a brief time later triggers an action potential in cell B (V_B). If we subtract the V_B record from the V_A record, we obtain a record of the intracellular voltage *difference* $V_A - V_B$ (see Fig. 20–9*B*).

We have already seen that, according to Ohm's law (see Equation 20–1), the *intracellular* current from cell A to cell B (I_{AB}) is proportional to ($V_A - V_B$). The *extracellular* current flowing from the region of cell B to the region of cell A is equal, but opposite in direction, to the intracellular current flowing from cell A to cell B. Imagine that an extracellular voltmeter has its negative electrode placed to the left of cell A, and its positive electrode to the right of cell B (forming a lead with an axis of 0 degrees). During the upswing in the action potential of cell A, while cell B is still at rest, ($V_A - V_B$) and I_{AB} are both positive, and the voltmeter detects a *positive* difference in voltage (see Fig. 20–9*C*)—analogous to the QRS complex in a real ECG. Later, during the recovery from the action potential in cell A, while cell B is still depolarized, ($V_A - V_B$) and I_{AB} are both negative, and the voltmeter

A ACTION POTENTIALS OF TWO SEPARATE CELLS

Two intracellular electrodes record normal action potentials displaced in time.

V_A V_B

Gap junction

R_{AB} is resistance of gap junctions.

B SUBTRACTED ACTION POTENTIALS

Subtracted intracellular voltage records show the equivalent of a QRS complex and T wave.

$$I_{AB} = \frac{V_A - V_B}{R_{AB}}$$

C DEPOLARIZATION MOVING TOWARD POSITIVE ELECTRODE

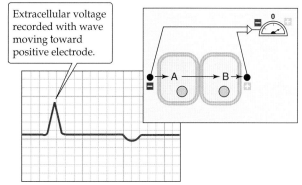

Extracellular voltage recorded with wave moving toward positive electrode.

D DEPOLARIZATION MOVING PERPENDICULAR TO ELECTRODE AXIS

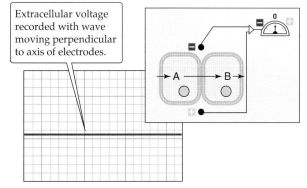

Extracellular voltage recorded with wave moving perpendicular to axis of electrodes.

E DEPOLARIZATION MOVING AWAY FROM POSITIVE ELECTRODE

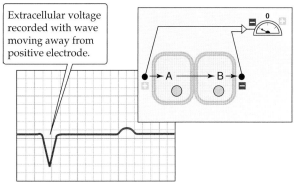

Extracellular voltage recorded with wave moving away from positive electrode.

FIGURE 20–9. Two-cell model of the ECG.

would detect a *negative* difference in voltage. From the extracellular voltage difference in Figure 20–9C, we can conclude that when the wave of depolarization moves *toward* the positive lead, there is a positive deflection in the *extracellular* voltage difference.

If we place the two electrodes at the junction between the two cells, with the positive connection on the bottom and the negative connection on the top, we create a lead with an axis of 90 degrees to the direction of current flow (see Fig. 20–9D). Under these conditions, we observe no voltage difference because both extracellular electrodes sense the same voltage at each instant in time. Thus, when a lead is perpendicular to the wave of depolarization, the measured deflection on that lead is **isoelectric**.

If we put our extracellular electrodes in yet a third configuration—with the positive electrode on the left and the negative electrode on the right—we observe a *negative* deflection during the depolarization of cell A because the wave of depolarization is moving *away from* the positive electrode (see Fig. 20–9E).

This simple two-cell model demonstrates that the wave of depolarization behaves as a vector, with both magnitude and direction. The box on p. 498 presents two practical methods for determining the direction (or axis) of the vector.

The "QRS equivalent" in the extracellular voltage record of our simplistic two-cell analysis is due to a spreading wave of *depolarization*. The T-wave equivalent is negative

BASIC INTERPRETATION OF THE ELECTROCARDIOGRAM

An electrocardiogram provides a direct measurement of the rate, rhythm, and time-dependent electrical vector of the heart. It also provides fundamental information about the origin and conduction of the cardiac action potential within the heart. Because the different parts of the heart activate sequentially, we can attribute the time-dependent changes in the electrical vector of the heart to different regions of the heart. The P wave reflects the atrial depolarization. The QRS complex corresponds to ventricular depolarization. The T wave reflects ventricular repolarization.

ECG paper has a grid of small 1-mm square boxes, and larger 5-mm square boxes. The vertical axis is calibrated at 0.1 mV/mm, and the horizontal (time) axis, at 0.04 s/mm *(small box)*—or 0.2 s/5 mm *(large box)*. Thus, five large boxes correspond to 1.0 second (Fig. 20–10). Table 20–5 summarizes the steps for interpreting an ECG.

Rate. We can measure rate in two ways. The direct method is to measure the number of seconds between waves of the same type, for example, the R-R interval. The quotient of 60 divided by the interval in seconds is the heart rate in beats per minute:

$$\text{Rate (beats/min)} = \frac{60 \text{ s/min}}{\text{R-R interval (s/beat)}}$$

A quick, alternative method is quite popular (Table 20–6). Measure the number of large boxes that form the R-R interval and remember the series: 300, 150, 100, 75, 60, 50—which corresponds to an interval of 1, 2, 3, 4, 5, or 6 large boxes. Thus, if 4 large boxes separate the R waves, the heart rate is 75 beats/min.

Rhythm. The determination of rhythm is more complex. One must answer the following questions: Where is the heart's pacemaker? What is the conduction path from the pacemaker to the last cell in the ventricles? Is the pacemaker functioning regularly and at the correct speed? The normal pacemaker is the SA node; the signal then propagates through the AV node, and activates the ventricles. When the heart follows this pathway at a normal rate and in this sequence, the rhythm is called a **"normal sinus rhythm."**

Careful examination of the intervals, durations, and segments in the ECG tracing can reveal a great deal about the conducted action potential (see Fig. 20–6). The **P-wave** duration indicates how long atrial depolarization takes. The **PR interval** indicates how long it takes the action potential to conduct through the AV node before activating the ventricles. The **QRS duration** reveals how long it takes for the wave of depolarization to spread throughout the ventricles. The **QT interval** indicates how long the ventricles remain depolarized, and is thus a rough measure of the duration of the overall "ventricular" action potential. The QT segment gets shorter as the heart rate increases, reflecting the shorter action potentials that are observed at high rates. In addition, many other alterations in these waves—and the segments separating them—reflect important physiological and pathophysiological changes in the heart.

Vector (or axis) of a wave in the frontal plane. Determining the vector of current flow through the heart is not just an intellectual exercise, but can be of great clinical importance. The normal axis of ventricular depolarization in the frontal plane lies between −30 and +90 degrees. However, this axis can change in a number of pathologic situations, including hypertrophy of one or both ventricular walls (a common sequela of severe or prolonged hypertension) and conduction blocks in one or several of the ventricular conducting pathways.

We can use two approaches for measuring the axis of a wave within the frontal plane (i.e., using limb leads). The first is more accurate, but the second is quicker and easier, and is usually sufficient for clinical purposes.

The first approach is a **geometric method**. It uses our knowledge of the axes of the different leads and the measured magnitude of the wave projected onto at least two leads in the frontal plane, and involves five steps:

Step 1. **Measure** the height of the wave on the ECG records in two leads, using any arbitrary unit (e.g., number of boxes). A *positive deflection* is one that rises above the baseline, and a *negative deflection* is one that falls below the baseline. In the example in Figure 20–11A, we are estimating the axis of the R wave of the QRS complex. The R wave is +2 units in lead II, and −1 unit in lead aVR.

Step 2. **Mark** the height of the measured deflections on the corresponding "lead" lines on a "circle of axes." Any unit of measure will suffice, as long as you use the same unit for both markings. Starting at the center of the circle, mark a *positive deflection* toward the *arrowhead*, and a *negative deflection* toward the *tail of the arrow.*

Step 3. **Draw** lines, perpendicular to the lead axes, through each of your two marks.

Step 4. **Connect** the center of the circle of axes (tail of vector) to the intersection of the two perpendicular lines (head of vector). In our example, the intersection is close to the aVF axis.

Step 5. **Estimate** the axis of the vector that corresponds to the R wave, using the "angle" scale of the circle of axes. In this case, the vector is at approximately 95 degrees, just clockwise to the aVF lead (i.e., 90 degrees).

The second approach is a qualitative **inspection method**. It exploits the varying magnitudes of the wave of interest in recordings from different leads. When the wave is isoelectric (i.e., no deflection, or equal positive and negative deflections), then the electrical vector responsible for that projection must be perpendicular to the isoelectric lead, as we already saw for the two-cell model in Figure 20–9D. The inspection approach requires two steps:

Step 1. **Identify a lead in which the wave of interest is isoelectric** (or nearly isoelectric). In the example in Figure 20–11B, the QRS complex is isoelectric in aVL (−30 degrees). The vector must be perpendicular (or nearly perpendicular) to that lead (i.e., aVL). In our example, the vector must point 90 degrees from −30 degrees, and therefore is at either +60 degrees or −120 degrees. Because the leads in the frontal plane define axes every 30 degrees, every lead has another lead to which it is perpendicular.

Step 2. **Identify a lead in which the wave is largely positive**. In Figure 20–11B, this would be lead II. The vector must lie roughly in the same direction as the orientation of that lead. Because lead II is at +60 degrees, the axis of the vector of the QRS wave must be approximately +60 degrees, and not −120 degrees.

If the wave of interest is not isoelectric in any lead, then find two leads onto which the projections are of similar magnitude and sign. The vector has an axis halfway between those two leads.

FIGURE 20–10. A normal 12-lead ECG recording. The recordings were obtained synchronously, three leads at a time (I, II, and III simultaneously; aVR, aVL, and aVF simultaneously; V_1, V_2, and V_3 simultaneously; and V_4, V_5, and V_6 simultaneously). A 1-mV, 200-msec calibration pulse is visible in the three top recordings.

compared with the QRS equivalent, and it reflects the wave of *repolarization*. If cell A has an action potential that is much longer than cell B (so that positive current again propagates from A to B after the action potential in B is completed), then the T-wave equivalent will be upright, as it is in most ECGs. Thus, on average, the ventricular myocytes that depolarize last are the first to repolarize. In other words, the B cells have shorter action potentials than the A cells.

What happened to the P wave that we see in a real ECG? The P wave reflects the depolarization of the *atrial* myocytes. In our model, we could represent the P wave by introducing a second pair of myocytes (i.e., the atrial cells), and allowing them to fire their action potentials much earlier than the two ventricular myocytes. We do not see an atrial equivalent of the T wave on the ECG because the small atrial T wave is buried within the QRS complex.

CARDIAC ARRHYTHMIAS

Any change in cardiac rhythm from the "normal sinus rhythm" is defined as an **arrhythmia**. Although some arrhythmias are pathologic and even life-threatening, others are normal and appropriately adaptive, including sinus tachycardia and sinus arrhythmia.

Sinus tachycardia is a heart rate faster than normal, driven by the sinus node. This arrhythmia is seen in frightened or startled individuals, or during normal exercise. Rarely, sinus tachycardia can be pathologic, for example, in patients with acute hyperthyroidism (p. 1042).

Sinus arrhythmia, a normal phenomenon, is a subtle change in heart rate with each respiratory cycle. Inspiration accelerates the heart rate (p. 549); expiration slows it. Deepening the respirations exaggerates these cyclic changes. The magnitude of the effect can vary signifi-

TABLE 20–5

EIGHTFOLD APPROACH FOR READING ELECTROCARDIOGRAMS

1	Search for P waves.
2	Determine the relationship of P waves and QRS complexes.
3	Identify pacemaker.
4	Measure the heart rates from different waves (e.g., P-P interval, R-R interval).
5	Characterize QRS shape (i.e., narrow vs wide).
6	Examine features of ST segment.
7	Estimate the mean QRS axis (and the axes of the other waves of interest).
8	Examine the cardiac rhythm (e.g., look at a 20- to 30-s ECG record from lead II).

ECG, electrocardiogram.

TABLE 20–6

DETERMINATION OF HEART RATE FROM THE ECG

R-R INTERVAL (in number of "large boxes" of 0.2 s)	HEART RATE (beats per minute)
1	300
2	150
3	100
4	75
5	60
6	50

Note that, on each row, the product of column 1 and column 2 is always 300.

cantly among individuals. The heart rate is still under the control of the SA node, but cyclic variations in sympathetic and parasympathetic tone modulate the SA node's pacemaker rate. The loss of sinus arrhythmia can be a sign of autonomic system dysfunction, as may be seen in patients with diabetes.

Although the list of pathologic arrhythmias is long, two

FIGURE 20–11. Estimation of the ECG axis in the frontal plane.

MYOCARDIAL INFARCTION

An acute myocardial infarction, or "heart attack," begins with the occlusion of a coronary artery. The region of myocardium subserved by that coronary artery is deprived of oxygen and, unless blood flow resumes shortly, will die. During the initial stages, the myocardial cells are electrically active but their function is impaired, producing characteristic changes in the ECG. Complete but transient blockade of blood flow to the myocardium—even though it does not lead to cell death—may lead to a pattern of ECG changes similar to that seen during the acute phase of myocardial infarction. Because blood flow is regional, the areas of infarction are also regional. Thus, the physician can best observe the changes in electrical activity by examining the specific ECG leads that provide the best view of the involved region of myocardium.

The first electrical change associated with an acute myocardial infarction is **peaking of the T waves**, followed soon after by **T-wave inversion**. These T-wave changes are not specific for infarction, and are reversible if blood flow is restored.

The next change, and one that is more characteristic of an acute myocardial infarction, is **elevation of the ST segment**. This change occurs because the myocytes closest to the epicardium become depolarized by the cellular anoxic injury, but they are still electrically coupled. Returning to the two-cell model (Fig. 20–12A), consider the cell on the left (cell A) to be normal, and the cell on the right (cell B) to be damaged. Figure 20–12B shows the extracellular current, which is proportional to the differences in the action potentials of the two cells shown in Figure 20–12A. Because cell B has a more positive resting potential than cell A, but has the same plateau during the action potential, the difference in voltage between cell A and cell B is depressed everywhere but at the ST segment—making the ST segment appear elevated. This is also the ECG change that one views with an acute myocardial infarction.

Brief periods of **coronary artery spasm** can also produce ST elevation, presumably by the same mecha-

nism. Rapid reperfusion of coronary arteries after acute blockage may lead to rapid and complete recovery of the myocardial cells, as indicated by the evanescent nature of the ECG changes.

Ischemia without cell death due to a "fixed" degree of occlusion (e.g., that caused by a thrombus or atherosclerosis) is often associated with changes in the ECG, typically ST-segment and T-wave changes. However, these changes are quite variable, presumably brought about by altered action potential duration in the affected regions. Patients experiencing exertional chest pain (angina) due to diminished coronary blood flow frequently have ECG changes during the anginal episode that include **ST-segment depression** and T-wave inversion.

With irreversible cell death, the ECG typically shows the evolution of **deep Q waves** (a large negative deflection at the beginning of the QRS complex). Q waves develop only in those leads overlying or near the region of the infarction. The Q waves signify an area of myocardium that has become electrically silent. Because action potentials cannot propagate into the infarcted area, the net vector of the remaining areas of ventricular depolarization—by default—points *away* from this area. The result is a deep *negative* deflection on the ECG in the appropriate leads. Thus, an inferior wall infarction inscribes deep Q waves in leads II, III, and aVF. An infarction affecting the large, muscular anterior wall of the heart will inscribe deep Q waves in some of the precordial leads (V_1 through V_6).

Not all infarctions create deep Q waves; the only visible changes may be T-wave inversion and ST-segment depression. Clinically, these infarctions behave like incomplete infarctions, and patients are at risk of a second, "completing" event. Therefore, these patients are investigated and treated aggressively to prevent further infarction.

A   ACTION POTENTIALS OF TWO SEPARATE CELLS

B   SUBTRACTED ACTION POTENTIALS

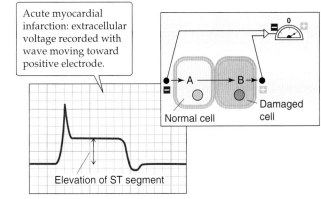

FIGURE 20–12. Two-cell model of a myocardial infarction. A, The damaged cell B *(blue record)* has a lower resting potential, but the plateau of its action potential is at same level as the normal cell A *(green record)*. B, After subtracting the records in A, the elevation of ST segment is the same as the difference in resting potentials.

basic problems are responsible for nearly all arrhythmias: altered conduction and altered automaticity.

Conduction Abnormalities Are a Major Cause of Arrhythmias

Disturbances of conduction make up the first major category of cardiac arrhythmias. Conduction disturbances can have multiple causes and can occur at any point in the conduction pathway. Conduction disturbances can be partial or complete. The two major causes of conduction disturbances are depolarization and abnormal anatomy.

If a tissue is injured (e.g., by stretch or anoxia), an altered balance of ionic currents can lead to a **depolarization**. The depolarization, in turn, partially inactivates I_{Na} and I_{Ca}, slowing the spread of current (i.e., slowing conduction). As a result, the tissue may become less excitable (partial conduction block) or completely inexcitable (complete conduction block).

Another type of conduction disturbance is the presence of an aberrant conduction pathway, reflecting **abnormal anatomy**. One such example is an accessory conduction pathway that rapidly transmits the action potential from the atria to the ventricles, bypassing the AV node, which normally imposes a conduction delay. Patients with the common Wolff-Parkinson-White syndrome have a bypass pathway called the bundle of Kent. The existence of a second pathway between the atria and ventricles predisposes affected individuals to supraventricular arrhythmias (see Accessory Conduction Pathways on p. 505).

PARTIAL (OR INCOMPLETE) CONDUCTION BLOCK. Three major types of partial conduction block exist: slowed conduction, intermittent block, and unidirectional block. We will defer the discussion of unidirectional block until we consider re-entry phenomena.

In **slowed conduction**, the tissue conducts all the impulses, but more slowly than normal. **First-degree AV block** reflects a *slowing* of conduction through the AV node. On an ECG, first-degree AV block appears as an unusually long PR interval (compare Fig. 20–13A and B).

A second example of partial conduction block is **intermittent block**, in which the tissue conducts some impulses but not others. In the AV node, intermittent block leads to **second-degree AV block**, of which there are two types. Both reflect incomplete (i.e., intermittent) coupling of the atria to the ventricles. In a **Möbitz type I block** (or Wenckebach block), the PR interval gradually lengthens from one cycle to the next until the AV node fails completely, skipping a ventricular depolarization (see Fig. 20–13C). With Möbitz type I block, it is most common to see every third or fourth atrial beat fail to conduct to the ventricles. In a **Möbitz type II block**, the P-R interval is constant from beat to beat, but every n^{th} ventricular depolarization is missing. In Figure 20–13D, the first cardiac cycle is normal. However, the second P wave is not followed by a QRS or T. Instead, the ECG record is flat until the third P wave arrives at the expected time, followed by a QRS and a T. Thus, we say that every second QRS is dropped (2:1 block).

Another form of intermittent conduction block, called **rate-dependent block**, reflects pathology often seen in the large branches of the His-Purkinje fiber system (i.e., the "bundle branches"). When the heart rate exceeds a critical level, the ventricular conduction system fails, presumably because a part of the conducting system lacks sufficient time to repolarize. With intermittent failure of the His-Purkinje fiber system, the impulse is left to spread slowly and inefficiently through the ventricles by conducting from one myocyte to the next. Such a failure, whether intermittent or continuous, is known as a **bundle branch block** and appears in the ECG as an intermittently wide QRS complex (see Fig. 20–13E). Because this block impairs the coordinated spread of the action potential throughout the ventricles, the resulting contraction loses some efficiency.

COMPLETE CONDUCTION BLOCK. In complete block, or **third-degree AV block**, no impulses conduct through the affected area, in either direction. For example, **complete block** at the AV node stops any supraventricular electrical impulse from triggering a ventricular contraction. Thus, AV nodal block electrically severs the atria and ventricles, each of which beats under control of its own pacemakers. This situation is called **AV dissociation**. The only ventricular pacemakers that are available to initiate cardiac contraction are the Purkinje fiber cells, which are notoriously unreliable and slow. Thus, cardiac output may fall, and blood pressure along with it. AV dissociation can therefore constitute a medical emergency, and placement of an artificial ventricular pacemaker can prove lifesaving. On an ECG, complete block appears as regularly spaced P waves (i.e., the SA node properly triggers the atria), and as irregularly spaced QRS and T waves that have a low frequency and no fixed relationship to the P waves (see Fig. 20–13F).

RE-ENTRY. An independent focus of pacemaker activity can develop as a consequence of a conduction disturbance. This class of conduction disturbance is called re-entry (or "re-entrant excitation" or "circus movement"). It occurs when a wave of depolarization travels in an endless circle. Re-entry has three requirements: (1) a closed conduction loop, (2) a region of unidirectional block (at least briefly), and (3) a sufficiently slow conduction of action potentials around the loop.

Before further considering re-entry, we need to discuss a conduction defect that is essential for re-entry—unidirectional block. **Unidirectional block** is a type of partial conduction block in which impulses travel in one direction, but not in the opposite one. Unidirectional block may arise as a result of a local depolarization or may be due to pathologic changes in functional anatomy. Normal cardiac tissue can conduct impulses in both directions (Fig. 20–14A). However, after an asymmetric anatomic lesion develops, many more healthy cells may remain on one side of the lesion than on the other. When conduction proceeds in the direction from the many healthy cells to the few healthy cells, the current from the "many" may be sufficient to excite the "few" (right to left in Fig. 20–14B). On the other hand, when conduction proceeds in the opposite direction, the few healthy cells cannot generate enough current to excite the region of many healthy

FIGURE 20–13. Pathological ECGs. In *F*, right bundle branch block is visible in the V₁ or V₂ precordial leads, whereas left bundle branch block is visible in the V₅ or V₆ leads. (Data from Chernoff HM: Workbook in Clinical Electrocardiography. New York, Medcom, 1972.)

cells (left to right in Fig. 20–14*B*). The result is a unidirectional block.

We return now to the problem of re-entry. Imagine that an impulse is traveling down a bifurcating Purkinje fiber and is about to reach a group of ventricular myocytes—a *closed conduction loop* (see Fig. 20–14*C*). However, the refractory zones prevent impulses from the right to re-enter the left, and vice versa. We now introduce a lesion that causes a *unidirectional conduction block* in the left branch of the Purkinje fiber. When the impulse reaches the fork in the road, it spreads in both directions (see Fig. 20–14*D, step 1*). However, the impulse cannot

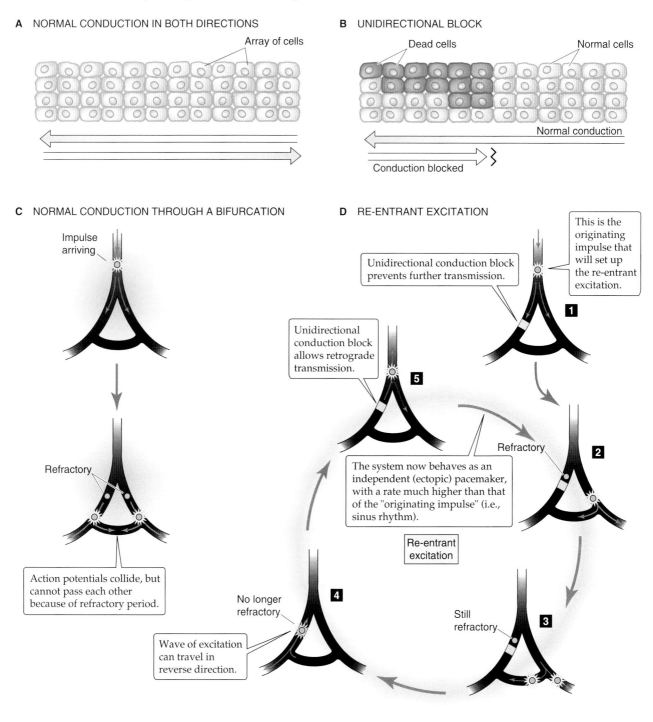

A NORMAL CONDUCTION IN BOTH DIRECTIONS

Array of cells

B UNIDIRECTIONAL BLOCK

Dead cells   Normal cells

Normal conduction

Conduction blocked

C NORMAL CONDUCTION THROUGH A BIFURCATION

Impulse arriving

Refractory

Action potentials collide, but cannot pass each other because of refractory period.

D RE-ENTRANT EXCITATION

This is the originating impulse that will set up the re-entrant excitation.

Unidirectional conduction block prevents further transmission.

1

Unidirectional conduction block allows retrograde transmission.

5

The system now behaves as an independent (ectopic) pacemaker, with a rate much higher than that of the "originating impulse" (i.e., sinus rhythm).

Refractory

2

Re-entrant excitation

No longer refractory

4

Wave of excitation can travel in reverse direction.

Still refractory

3

FIGURE 20–14. Abnormal conduction.

continue past the unidirectional block in the left branch. The impulse traveling down the right branch stimulates the distal conducting cells (see Fig. 20–14D, *step 2*), leaving them in an effective refractory period (p. 492). When the impulse reaches the ventricular muscle, it begins to travel back toward the damaged left branch (*step 3*). At this point, the cells in the normal right branch may still be refractory to excitation. The impulse finally

reaches the damaged left branch and travels in a retrograde fashion up this branch, reaching and passing through the region of the unidirectional conduction block (*step 4*). Finally, the impulse again reaches the bifurcation (*step 5*). Because enough time has elapsed for the cells at the bifurcation, as well as in the right branch, to recover from their refractory period, the impulse can now travel retrograde up the main part of the Purkinje fiber, as well as orthograde down the right branch—for a second time.

If this re-entrant movement (steps $2 \rightarrow 5 \rightarrow 2$, etc.) continues, the frequency of re-entry will generally outpace the SA nodal pacemaker (frequency of *step 1*) and is often responsible for diverse tachyarrhythmias because the fastest pacemaker sets the heart rate. Re-entry excitation may be responsible for atrial and ventricular tachycardia, atrial and ventricular fibrillation, and many other arrhythmias. Re-entry can occur in big loops (see Fig. 20–14*D*), or in small loops consisting entirely of myocardial cells.

ACCESSORY CONDUCTION PATHWAYS. The **Wolff-Parkinson-White syndrome** (WPW), briefly mentioned earlier in the chapter, is a common example of an accessory conduction pathway, which in this case provides a short circuit (i.e., bundle of Kent) around the delay in the AV node. The fast accessory pathway conducts the action potential directly from the atria to the ventricular septum, depolarizing some of the septal muscle earlier than if the depolarization had reached it via the slower, normal AV nodal pathway. As a result, ventricular depolarization is more spread out in time than is normal, giving rise to a broader-than-normal QRS complex. The general direction of ventricular depolarization is reversed, so that the events normally underlying the Q wave of the QRS complex have an axis opposite to that normally seen. This early depolarization, or **pre-excitation**, appears as a small, positive **delta wave** at the beginning of the QRS complex (see Fig. 20–13*G*). In addition, because the time between atrial depolarization and ventricular depolarization (i.e., beginning of delta wave) is shortened, the interval between the P wave and the QRS complex is shortened.

The aberrant conduction pathway in WPW syndrome also establishes a loop that may meet the requirements for re-entry, and may therefore be associated with a **supraventricular tachycardia**. Although in general a benign condition, WPW syndrome is associated with at least one attack of supraventricular tachycardia in at least 50% of affected individuals. The two most common supraventricular tachycardias seen in this population are atrial fibrillation (described later) and paroxysmal supraventricular tachycardia. **Paroxysmal supraventricular tachycardia** (PSVT) is a regular tachycardia with a ventricular rate usually exceeding 150 beats per minute. Because ventricular depolarization still occurs via the normal conducting pathways, the QRS complex appears normal.

Less commonly, the re-entry loop may run in the reverse direction—down the accessory pathway and back up through the AV node. This arrangement produces a PSVT with wide and bizarre QRS complexes because ventricular depolarization does not occur along the normal bundle branches. A small number of people with WPW syndrome have more than one accessory pathway, so that multiple re-entry loops are possible.

FIBRILLATION. In fibrillation, many regions of re-entrant electrical activity are present, creating electrical chaos that is not associated with useful contraction. **Atrial fibrillation** (see Fig. 20–13*H*) is commonly found in elderly patients, sometimes with mitral valve or coronary artery disease, but often without any evidence of underlying cardiac disease. The re-entry loop within the atria moves wildly and rapidly, generating a very rapid succession of action potentials—as many as 500 per minute. This wandering re-entry circuit easily becomes the fastest pacemaker in the heart, outpacing the SA node and bombarding the AV node. Fortunately, the AV node cannot repolarize fast enough to pass along all of these impulses. Only some make it through to the ventricles, resulting in the irregular appearance of QRS complexes without any detectable P waves. The baseline between QRS complexes may appear straight or may show small, rapid fluctuations. Although only some atrial impulses reach the ventricles, the ventricular rate can still be quite high.

Because the atria function mainly as a booster pump (see box on Atrial Contraction on p. 511), many patients tolerate atrial fibrillation without harm, and may even be unaware that they have it. Others may suffer greatly from the loss of a coordinated atrial contraction, particularly the elderly or those with coexisting cardiac disease. If possible, attempts should be made to convert most individuals back to normal sinus rhythm by either electrical or chemical means. If this is not possible, then attempts can be made to at least slow conduction through the AV node. For example, digitalis compounds increase parasympathetic and decrease sympathetic stimulation to the AV node, decreasing the speed of AV conduction and thus reducing the ventricular rate (see box on Vagal Maneuvers, earlier in this chapter).

Ventricular fibrillation (see Fig. 20–13*I*) is a life-threatening medical emergency. The heart cannot generate cardiac output because the ventricles are not able to pump blood without a coordinated ventricular depolarization.

Altered Automaticity Can Originate from the Sinus Node or from an Ectopic Locus

The automaticity of any cardiac tissue can change. Pacemaker cells can experience an alteration or even a complete absence of automaticity. Conversely, other cells that normally have no automaticity (e.g., ventricular muscle) can become "ectopic" pacemakers. These disturbances of automaticity make up the second major category of cardiac arrhythmias.

DEPOLARIZATION-DEPENDENT TRIGGERED ACTIVITY. A positive shift in the maximum diastolic potential brings V_m closer to the threshold for an action potential, and can induce automaticity in cardiac tissue that otherwise has no pacemaker activity. The development of such depolarization-induced triggered activity depends on the interaction of the Ca^{2+} current (I_{Ca}) and the repolarizing K^+ current, I_K. This mechanism can produce a more rapid pacemaker depolarization in the SA or AV nodal cells, causing them to accelerate their pacemakers. It can also increase the intrinsic pacemaker rate in Purkinje fiber cells, which normally have a very slow pacemaker.

Depolarization-induced triggered activity is particularly dramatic in nonpacemaker tissues (e.g., ventricular muscle), which normally exhibit no diastolic depolarization. Fac-

A PROLONGED ACTION POTENTIAL LEADS
TO EARLY AFTER-DEPOLARIZATION

B PROLONGED ACTION POTENTIAL LEADS
TO A "RUN" OF SPONTANEOUS ACTIVITY

FIGURE 20–15. Abnormal automaticity in ventricular muscle. The records in this figure are idealized. *A*, The prolonged action potential keeps I_{Na} inactivated but permits I_{Ca} and I_K to interact and thereby produce a spontaneous depolarization—the "early after-depolarization." *B*, The after-depolarization reaches threshold, triggering a sequence of several slow pacemaker-like action potentials that generate extrasystoles.

tors that significantly prolong action potential duration can cause depolarization-dependent triggered activity. During the repolarization phase, I_{Na} remains inactivated because the cell is so depolarized (Fig. 20–15A). On the other hand, I_{Ca} has had enough time to recover from inactivation and—because the cell is still depolarized—triggers a slow, positive deflection in V_m known as an "**early afterdepolarization.**" Eventually, I_K increases and returns V_m toward the resting potential. Such early after-depolarizations, if larger than the one shown in Figure 20–15A, may trigger an extrasystole. Isolated ventricular extrasystoles (known by many names, including premature ventricular contractions, or PVCs) may occur in normal individuals. Alterations in cellular Ca^{2+} metabolism (discussed in the next section) may increase the tendency of a prolonged action potential to produce an extrasystole. Ironically, a class of drugs used to treat arrhythmias can become *arrhythmogenic* by producing early afterdepolarizations. For example, quinidine can produce this dangerous adverse effect, presumably by inhibiting Na^+ channels and some K^+ channels and thus prolonging the ventricular muscle action potential.

More than one extrasystole—a **"run" of extrasystoles** (see Fig. 20–15B)—is pathologic. A run of three or more ventricular extrasystoles is the minimal requirement for diagnosing **ventricular tachycardia**. This arrhythmia is life threatening, because it can degenerate into ventricular fibrillation (see Fig. 20–13I), which is associated with no meaningful cardiac output. The heart rate in ventricular tachycardia is much faster than normal, usually between 120 and 150 beats/min (or faster), and the pacemaker driving the heartbeat is located in the ventricle itself. The heart rate in ventricular tachycardia may be so fast that the heart cannot pump blood effectively.

LONG QT SYNDROME (LQTS). Patients with LQTS have a prolonged ventricular action potential, and are prone to

ventricular arrhythmias. In particular, these patients are susceptible to a form of ventricular tachycardia called **torsades de pointes**, or "twisting of the points," in which the QRS complexes appear to spiral around the baseline, constantly changing their axes and amplitude. LQTS can be congenital or acquired. The congenital form can involve mutations of cardiac Na^+ channels (see box on p. 189) or K^+ channels (see box on p. 196). The acquired form of LQTS, which is much more common, can result from various electrolyte disturbances (especially hypokalemia and hypocalcemia) or from prescribed or over-the-counter medications (e.g., several antiarrhythmic drugs, tricyclic antidepressants, and some nonsedating antihistamines when taken together with certain antibiotics, notably erythromycin).

Ca^{2+} Overload and Metabolic Changes Can Also Cause Arrhythmias

Ca^{2+} OVERLOAD. Ca^{2+} overload in the heart has many potential causes. One frequent factor is digitalis intoxication. Another is injury-related cellular depolarization. Ca^{2+} overload occurs when $[Ca^{2+}]_i$ increases, causing the sarcoplasmic reticulum to sequester too much Ca^{2+}. Thus overloaded, the SR begins to cyclically—and spontaneously—dump Ca^{2+} and then take it back up. The Ca^{2+} release may be large enough to stimulate a Ca^{2+}-activated nonselective cation channel and the Na-Ca exchanger (p. 68). These current sources combine to produce I_{ti}, a **transient inward current** that produces a **delayed afterdepolarization**. When large enough, I_{ti} can depolarize the cell beyond threshold and produce a spontaneous action potential.

METABOLISM-DEPENDENT CONDUCTION CHANGES. During ischemia and anoxia, many cellular events take place, including a fall in intracellular ATP levels. This fall in

[ATP]$_i$ activates the ATP-sensitive K$^+$ channel (K$_{ATP}$), which is plentiful in cardiac myocytes. Thus, when [ATP]$_i$ falls sufficiently, K$_{ATP}$ is less inhibited and the cells tend to become less excitable (i.e., K$_{ATP}$ helps to keep V$_m$ close to E$_K$). The activation of this channel may explain, in part, the slowing or blocking of conduction that may occur during ischemia or in the peri-infarction period.

ELECTROMECHANICAL DISSOCIATION. Rarely, patients being resuscitated from cardiac arrest exhibit a phenomenon called electromechanical dissociation, in which the heart's ECG activity is not accompanied by the pumping of blood. In many cases, the basis of electromechanical dissociation is not understood. However, in other cases, the cause is obvious. For example, the heart of a patient with a large pericardial effusion may manifest normal electrical activity, but the fluid between the heart and the pericardium may press in on the heart (cardiac tamponade) and prevent effective pumping.

REFERENCES

Chernoff HM: Workbook in Clinical Electrocardiography. New York, Medcom Press, 1972.

Deal KK, England SK, Tamkun MM: Molecular physiology of cardiac potassium channels. Physiol Rev 76:49–67, 1996.

Einthoven W: The string galvanometer and the measurement of action currents of the heart. In Nobel Lecture in Physiology or Medicine, Vol. 2. Amsterdam, Elsevier, 1964.

Hiraoka M, Furukawa T: Functional modulation of cardiac ATP-sensitive K$^+$ channels. News Physiol Sci 13:131–137, 1998.

Irisawa H, Brown HF, Giles W: Cardiac pacemaking in the sinoatrial node. Physiol Rev 73:197–227, 1993.

Levick JR: An Introduction to Cardiovascular Physiology, 2nd ed. Oxford, Butterworth Heinemann, 1995.

Sanguinetti MC, Keating MT: Role of delayed rectifier potassium channels in cardiac repolarization and arrhythmias. News Physiol Sci 12: 152–157, 1997.

Weidmann S: Effect of current flow on the membrane potential of cardiac muscle. J Physiol 115:227–236, 1951.

Winsor T: The electrocardiogram in myocardial infarction. Clinical Symposia, 29:1–29, 1977.

CHAPTER 21

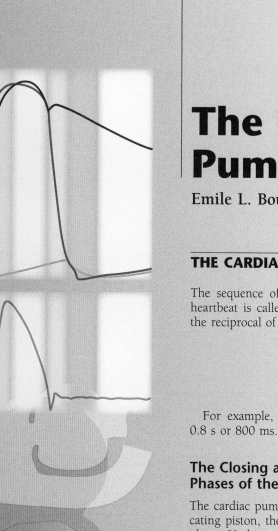

The Heart as a Pump

Emile L. Boulpaep

THE CARDIAC CYCLE

The sequence of mechanical and electrical events that repeats with every heartbeat is called the **cardiac cycle**. The **duration** of the cardiac cycle is the reciprocal of heart rate:

Equation 21–1

$$\text{Duration (s/beat)} = \frac{60 \text{ (s/min)}}{\text{Heart Rate (beats/min)}}$$

For example, for a heart rate of 75 beats/min, the cardiac cycle lasts 0.8 s or 800 ms.

The Closing and Opening of the Cardiac Valves Define Four Phases of the Cardiac Cycle

The cardiac pump is of the two-stroke variety. Like a pump with a reciprocating piston, the heart alternates between a filling phase and an emptying phase. Under normal circumstances, the electrical pacemaker in the sinoatrial node (p. 489) determines the duration of the cardiac cycle, and the electrical properties of the cardiac conduction system and cardiac myocytes determine the relative duration of contraction and relaxation. As long as the heart rate remains unchanged, this pattern remains steady.

The cardiac **atria** are small chambers. The right atrium receives deoxygenated systemic venous return from the inferior and superior vena cava. The left atrium receives oxygenated blood from the lungs via the pulmonary circulation. Both atria operate more as passive reservoirs than as mechanical pumps. However, they do contract, and this contraction does enhance ventricular filling and cardiac output to a small degree (see box on p. 511).

The inlet valves of the ventricles are called the **AV (atrioventricular) valves**. They permit blood to flow in one direction only, from the atria to the ventricles. The valve located between the *right* atrium and the right ventricle is called the **tricuspid valve** because it has three flaps, or cusps. The valve located between the *left* atrium and the left ventricle is called the **mitral valve** because it has only two cusps, which resemble a bishop's miter.

The outlet valves of the ventricles are called **semilunar valves**. They also allow blood to flow in just a single direction, from each ventricle into a large outflow-tract vessel. Both the **pulmonary valve**, located between the right ventricle and pulmonary artery, and the **aortic valve**, located between the left ventricle and aorta, have three cusps.

Cardiac valves open passively when upstream pressure exceeds downstream pressure. They close passively when downstream pressure exceeds upstream pressure. The movement of the valve leaflets can be detected by echo-cardiography (p. 445); their closure makes **heart sounds** that can be heard with a stethoscope. The stethoscope can also detect leaks in the valves that permit jets of blood to flow backward across the valvular orifice (i.e., regurgitation), as well as stenotic lesions that narrow the valve opening, forcing the blood to pass through a narrower space (i.e., stenosis). During certain parts of the cardiac cycle, blood passing through either **regurgitant** or **stenotic** lesions makes characteristic sounds that are called **murmurs** (see box on p. 431).

The cardiac cycle can be artificially divided into phases in any number of ways. However, from the point of view of the ventricles and the positions of their valves, we must consider a minimum of four distinct **phases**:

1. **Inflow phase**. The inlet valve is open and the outlet valve is closed.
2. **Isovolumetric contraction**. Both valves are closed, with no blood flow.
3. **Outflow phase**. The outlet valve is open and the inlet valve is closed.
4. **Isovolumetric relaxation**. Both valves are closed, with no blood flow.

Table 21–1 summarizes these four phases and the key events of the cardiac cycle. Note that the same events occur on the right side of the heart as on the left side.

It is common to separate these phases into two parts. **Systole** includes phases 2 and 3, when the ventricles are contracting, whereas **diastole** includes phases 4 and 1, when the ventricles are relaxing. For a heart rate of 75 (cycle duration = 800 ms), systole occupies approximately 300 ms, and diastole approximately 500 ms. With increasing heart rate—and thus decreasing cycle length—diastole shortens relatively more than systole.

For convenience, the events in Table 21–1 start a short time after the beginning of diastole, with the opening of the AV valves and the start of ventricular filling (phase 1).

Changes in Ventricular Volume, Pressure, and Flow Accompany the Four Phases of the Cardiac Cycle

Figure 21–1 illustrates the changes in pressure and volume that occur during the cardiac cycle. The four vertical lines indicate the timing of the four *valvular events*, which terminate each of the four phases defined previously:

▷ AV valve closure terminates phase 1
▷ Semilunar valve opening terminates phase 2
▷ Semilunar valve closing terminates phase 3
▷ AV valve opening terminates phase 4

The shapes of pressure tracings for the right heart (see Fig. 21–1A) and the left heart (see Fig. 21–1B) are quite similar except that the pressures on the right are a scaled-down version of those on the left. In both cases, the tracings begin in the *middle* of phase 1—that is, toward the end of diastole or the **diastasis** (i.e., period of decreased filling). Note that the volume changes in the left ventricle are exactly the same as those in the right ventricle because the cardiac outputs of the right and left sides

TABLE 21–1

EVENTS IN THE CARDIAC CYCLE

VALVULAR EVENTS	CARDIAC CHAMBER EVENTS	PHASE	
Opening of AV valves (tricuspid and mitral)			
	Rapid ventricular filling	1	Diastole
	Decreased ventricular filling. Diastasis	1	Diastole
	Atrial contraction (additional ventricular filling)	1	Diastole
Closing of AV valves (tricuspid and mitral)			
	Isovolumetric ventricular contraction (with all valves closed)	2	Systole
Opening of semilunar valves (pulmonary and aortic)			
	Rapid ventricular ejection (fast muscle shortening)	3	Systole
	Decreased ventricular ejection (slower muscle shortening)	3	Systole
Closing of semilunar valves (pulmonary and aortic)			
	Isovolumetric ventricular relaxation (with all valves closed)	4	Diastole
Opening of AV valves (tricuspid and mitral)			

AV, atrioventricular.

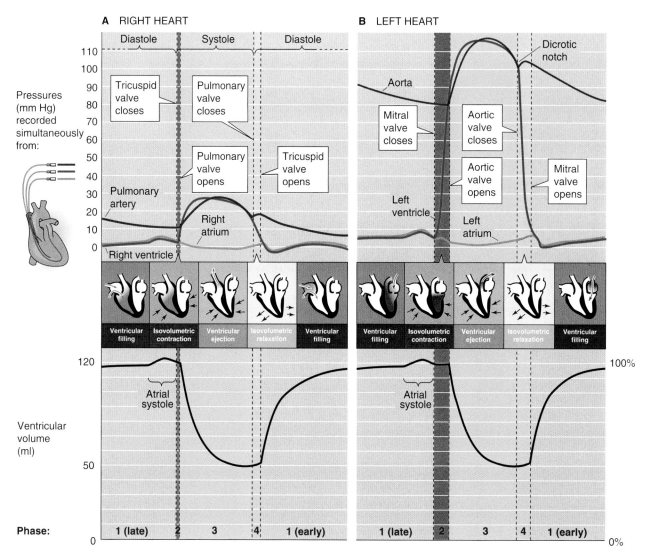

FIGURE 21–1. Pressures and ventricular volumes during the cardiac cycle. *A*, Right heart. *B*, Left heart. The inset shows the placement of catheters used for pressure measurements in the right heart.

of the heart are virtually identical (p. 428). For purposes of illustration, we now focus on the records for the *left* heart (see Fig. 21–1*B*).

DIASTASIS PERIOD (MIDDLE OF PHASE 1). During the diastasis, the mitral valve is open, but little blood flows from the left atrium to the left ventricle; ventricular volume slowly rises and approaches a plateau. The pressures in both the left atrium and the left ventricle rise slowly, driven by the pressure in the pulmonary veins, which is only slightly higher. The atrial pressure parallels—and is only slightly above—the ventricular pressure because the mitral valve is wide open, and the flow between the two chambers is minimal. The P wave of the electrocardiogram (ECG; p. 494), which corresponds to atrial excitation, occurs at the end of this phase.

ATRIAL CONTRACTION (END OF PHASE 1). Immediately following the ECG's P wave is the atrial contraction, which causes a variable amount of blood to enter the left ventricle. In a person at rest, the atrial contraction transfers into the left ventricle a volume of blood that repre-

sents less than 20% of the subsequent stroke volume and often only a few percent. During heavy exercise, this figure can rise to 40% (see box on p. 511). Atrial contraction causes a slight rise in intra-atrial pressure, and a comparable rise in ventricular pressure and volume. All during this period, the aortic pressure decreases as blood flows out to the periphery.

ISOVOLUMETRIC CONTRACTION (PHASE 2). When the ventricles begin to depolarize, as evidenced by the QRS complex on the ECG, systole commences. The ventricles contract, and very soon the pressure in the left ventricle exceeds that in the left atrium (*first crossover of blue and orange pressure tracings in Fig. 21–1B, top panel*). As a result, the *mitral valve closes*. The aortic valve has been closed this entire time. Thus, the left ventricle contracts with both mitral and aortic valves closed. Because the blood has no place to go, the result is an isovolumetric contraction that causes the pressure in the left ventricle to rise rapidly, eventually exceeding the pressure in the aorta (*first crossover of blue and red tracings*) and causing the aortic valve to open.

IMPORTANCE (AND UNIMPORTANCE) OF ATRIAL CONTRACTION

The relative importance of atrial contraction to overall cardiac function is evident in patients who develop *atrial fibrillation* (see Fig. 20–13H), an arrhythmia associated with loss of this atrial "kick." In atrial fibrillation, chaotic electrical activity, bombarding the atria with as many as 500 impulses per minute from all directions, prevents the concerted action of atrial cardiac muscle fibers that is necessary for coordinated atrial contraction. As a result, the atria fibrillate—they look like a wriggling bag of worms. In healthy persons with otherwise normal hearts, the loss of atrial contraction usually causes no symptoms at rest, or perhaps only a sensation of an irregular or rapid heartbeat (i.e., the result of atrial fibrillation). However, if the patient already has a compromised myocardium (e.g., from ischemic heart disease, prolonged hypertension, or mitral stenosis), or if the patient is debilitated by dysfunction of other organs (e.g., chronic emphysema), the loss of the atrial contraction may further reduce cardiac output just enough to send the patient into florid congestive heart failure (see box on Cardiac Hypertrophy on p. 533) or even shock (i.e., arterial pressure so low that it compromises perfusion of peripheral tissues). The physician may treat a patient from the former group in a leisurely fashion, or perhaps not at all. In the latter group, emergency chemical or electrical cardioversion may be necessary.

EJECTION OR OUTFLOW (PHASE 3). As the *aortic valve opens*, the ejection phase begins. During the first part of phase 3—**rapid ejection**—ventricular pressure (*blue tracing* in Fig. 21–1B, *top*) continues to rise, closely followed by a rapid elevation of aortic pressure, which, at first, is slightly less (*red tracing*). Accompanying these rapid pressure increases is a precipitous reduction in ventricular volume (see Fig. 21–1B, *bottom*), as blood flows into the aorta. Aortic pressure continues to rise and eventually exceeds ventricular pressure (*second crossover of blue and red tracings* in Fig. 21–2, *top*) just before both the aortic and ventricular pressures begin to fall. Despite the reversal of the pressure gradient across the aortic valve, the cusps of the aortic valve do not immediately snap shut because of the inertia of blood flow, which imparts considerable kinetic energy to the blood. During the latter part of phase 3—**decreased ejection**—the decrease in ventricular volume becomes less rapid, and both the ventricular and aortic pressures fall off. During the entire ejection phase, approximately 70 ml of blood flows into the aorta, leaving approximately 50 ml behind in the ventricle.

ISOVOLUMETRIC RELAXATION (PHASE 4). Late in the ejection phase, blood flow across the aortic valve falls to extremely low values, until it actually reverses direction (i.e., retrograde or negative flow). At this point, the *aortic valve closes*, defining the onset of diastole. As blood flow in the aorta again becomes briefly positive (i.e., forward), causing a small upward deflection in the aortic pressure trace. The result is the **dicrotic notch** (from the Greek

dikrotos, "double-beating"), or **incisura**, and the subsequent dicrotic wave, which interrupts the generally downward trend of aortic pressure. Because both the aortic and mitral valves are closed, and no blood can enter the left ventricle, this is the period of isovolumetric relaxation. Pressure falls rapidly in the left ventricle.

RAPID VENTRICULAR FILLING PERIOD (BEGINNING OF PHASE 1). When ventricular pressure falls below that in the left atrium (*second crossover of blue and orange tracings* in Fig. 21–1B), the *mitral valve opens*. Immediately following mitral valve opening, left ventricular volume begins to increase rapidly (see Fig. 21–1B, *bottom*). During this period of rapid ventricular filling, the left atrial and ventricular pressures evolve in parallel because the mitral valve is wide open. A period of relatively decreased filling follows, the period of diastasis with which we began our discussion. Thus, diastole includes both the rapid ventricular filling period and diastasis. As already noted, the length of diastole decreases with elevations in heart rate. This decreased diastolic period comes first at the expense of the period of slower ventricular filling (i.e., diastasis).

During rapid ventricular filling, the aortic valve remains closed. Because blood continues to flow out to the periphery, owing to the recoil of the aorta's elastic wall (see Box on p. 516), the aortic pressure falls. This fall continues during diastasis.

The Electrocardiogram, Phonocardiogram, and Echocardiogram All Follow the Cyclic Pattern of the Cardiac Cycle

Accompanying the basic cyclic pattern of cardiac pressure and volume changes are characteristic mechanical, electrical, acoustic, and echocardiographic changes. Figure 21–2 illustrates these events for the left side of the heart and the systemic circulation. Notice that the pressure records in the *top panel* of Figure 21–2 start with the atrial contraction—that is, slightly later than in Figure 21–1.

AORTIC BLOOD FLOW (see Fig. 21–2, *second panel*). Blood flow from the left ventricle to the ascending aorta rises most rapidly during the rapid ejection phase of the left ventricle. The peaking of aortic flow defines the beginning of the decreased ejection phase.

JUGULAR VENOUS PULSE. The *third panel* of Figure 21–2 includes the jugular venous pulse, for comparison with the timing of other events. We will discuss the jugular venous pulse later in the chapter.

THE ELECTROCARDIOGRAM (see Fig. 21–2, *fourth panel*). The ECG, discussed in the previous chapter (p. 493), begins with the middle of the P wave (atrial depolarization). The QRS complex (ventricular depolarization) is the prelude to the upswing in ventricular pressure. The T wave (ventricular repolarization) occurs in the decreased-ejection phase.

PHONOCARDIOGRAM AND HEART SOUNDS (See Fig. 21–2, *fifth panel*). The opening and closing of the valves are accompanied by **heart sounds**, easily heard through a stethoscope or recorded on a phonocardiogram (Table 21–2). Each of the vertical dotted lines in

FIGURE 21–2. Mechanical, electrical, acoustic and echocardiographic events in the cardiac cycle. *Top*, A repeat of Figure 21–1B, with three modifications: (1) The cardiac cycle begins with atrial contraction; (2) phase 1 of the cardiac cycle has three subparts: rapid ventricular filling, decreased ventricular filling, and atrial systole; (3) phase 3 has two subparts: rapid and decreased ventricular ejection.

TABLE 21-2

THE HEART SOUNDS

SOUND		ASSOCIATED EVENTS
S_1	▷ First heart sound (sounds like "lub") ▷ Two bursts, a mitral M_1 and a tricuspid T_1 component	Closure of mitral and tricuspid valves
S_2	▷ Second heart sound (sounds like "dub") ▷ An aortic A_2 and a pulmonary P_2 component	Closure of aortic and pulmonary valves
OS	Opening snap	Opening of a stenotic mitral valve
S_3	Third heart sound	Diastolic filling gallop or ventricular or protodiastolic gallop
S_4	Fourth heart sound	Atrial sound that creates an atrial or presystolic gallop

Figure 21–2 indicates the movement of two valves, one on the right side of the heart and one on the left. Thus, two valves can contribute to a single heart sound, although the two components can often be separated by the ear. The phonocardiogram in Figure 21–2 shows the timing of the two major, or physiological, heart sounds (S_1 and S_2), as well as two other sounds (S_3 and S_4) that are occasionally heard.

The physiological heart sounds **S_1** and **S_2** are heard following the closure of the cardiac valves: the mitral and tricuspid valves for S_1, and the aortic and pulmonary valves for S_2. However, the actual apposition of the valve leaflets (i.e., "slamming the door") does not produce the sound. Instead, vibrations resulting from sudden tension in the AV valves and the adjacent ventricular walls produce S_1. Similarly, vibrations of the large vessel walls and columns of blood produce S_2 following closure of the semilunar valves. These vibrations propagate through adjacent tissues to the chest wall, where one can normally hear the first and second heart sounds through a stethoscope. S_1 is usually stronger, longer, and of lower frequency than S_2.

Although the four vertical lines that define the four phases of the cardiac cycle are very similar for the right and left hearts, they do not line up perfectly with one another, as can be seen by comparing Figure 21–1A and B. For example, the aortic valve usually closes just before the pulmonary valve. This timing difference produces the **physiological splitting** of the A_2 (i.e., aortic) and P_2 (i.e., pulmonary) components of the second heart sound. As we shall see later in the chapter, inspiration accentuates the splitting of S_2. Pathology that accentuates the asyn-

chrony between left and right hearts may also lead to splitting of the first heart sound.

With stiffening of the mitral valve, seen in mitral stenosis, the opening of the mitral valve may produce an additional sound, an opening snap (**OS**), just after S_2.

A physiological **S_3** is present in some normal individuals, particularly children. S_3 occurs in early diastole when rapid filling of the ventricles results in recoil of the ventricular walls, which have a limited distensibility. An S_3 also can be heard in adults when the ventricle is so overfilled at the end of systole that adding 70 ml more blood during diastole brings the ventricle into a volume range where ventricular compliance is very low. The result is an accentuated recoil, heard as an S_3. If heart rate is increased above normal, the addition of an S_3 to the physiological S_1 and S_2 creates an S_1-S_2-S_3 sequence that is termed a **protodiastolic gallop** rhythm. A "gallop rhythm" is a grouping of three heart sounds that, together, sound like hoofs of a galloping horse.

When present, a fourth sound (**S_4**) coincides with atrial contraction. It is usually heard in pathologic conditions in which an unusually strong atrial contraction occurs in combination with low compliance of the left ventricle. The presence of S_4 produces the sequence S_4 S_1 S_2, which is also a gallop rhythm, a **presystolic gallop**.

ECHOCARDIOGRAM. We discussed echocardiography on p. 445. The echocardiogram in the *bottom panel* of Figure 21–2 shows that the separation between the anterior and posterior leaflets of the mitral valve increases during atrial contraction. The leaflets meet at the beginning of phase 2 and remain together until rapid ventricular filling occurs in the beginning of phase 1, when the separation between leaflets becomes maximal. During the decreased phase of ventricular filling, the leaflets once again move closer together, until the next atrial contraction.

The Cardiac Cycle Causes Flow Waves in the Aorta and Peripheral Vessels

With the closing and opening of the heart's exit valves (i.e., pulmonary and aortic valves), blood flow and blood velocity across these valves oscillate from near zero, when the valves are closed, to high values, when the valves are open. *Blood flow* in the aortic arch actually oscillates between slightly negative to highly positive values (Fig. 21–3A, panel #1). *Pressure* in the aortic arch typically oscillates between approximately 80 and approximately 120 mm Hg (see Fig. 21–3B, panel #1), but varies greatly among individuals. Phasic changes in pressure and flow also occur in the peripheral arteries. Arterial pressure is usually measured in a large artery, such as the brachial artery (p. 440). Because very little pressure drop occurs between the aorta and such a large, proximate artery, the measured **systolic** and **diastolic** arterial pressures, as well as the pulse pressure and mean arterial pressure (p. 435), closely approximate the corresponding aortic pressures.

If blood vessels were rigid tubes, so that the resistance (R) were constant, and if the driving pressure (ΔP) were also constant throughout the cardiac cycle, we could describe blood flow (F) using a simple Ohm's law–like relationship, as we did in Chapter 17 (see Equation 17–

A FLOWS

B PRESSURES

FIGURE 21–3. Flow (*A*) and pressure (*B*) profiles in the aorta and smaller vessels.

A STEADY INPUT PRESSURE (CONTINUOUS FLOW)

B SQUARE-PULSE PRESSURE (PULSATILE FLOW)

C "WINDKESSEL" MODEL OF AORTA

FIGURE 21–4. Effect of pulsatile pressure on flow through a compliant vessel.

1). However, because blood vessels are compliant (so that R varies with pressure, as in Fig. 18–7B) and because both aortic pressure and flow vary during the cardiac cycle, we cannot describe real arteries in this way. In the field of hydraulics, oscillating flows and pressures have not only an **amplitude**, but also a **phase**. As a result, the ratio $\Delta P/F$ is no longer resistance—a simple, time-independent quantity—but a *complex* quantity called the **mechanical impedance** that depends on the classical "resistance," as well as the compliance and inertial properties of the vessels and blood.

Because of these resistive, compliant, and inertial properties, the pressure and flow waves in vessels distal to the aorta are not quite the same as in the aorta. Instead, the farther the vessels are from the aorta, the more different the pressure and flow waves become.

AORTIC ARCH. During the rapid-ejection phase, peak *flow* through the aortic arch is remarkably high, approximately 30 liters/min (*dark beige band* in Fig. 21–3A, panel #1). The peak linear velocity is approximately 100 cm/s, which makes it more likely that the blood will reach the

critical Reynolds number value for turbulence (p. 430). The rapid ejection of blood also causes a rapid rise of the *pressure* in the aorta to above that in the ventricle (see Fig. 21–3B, panel #1). Even though the pressure gradient across the valve reverses, the valve does not close, as is evidenced by the continuous flow of blood from the ventricle into the aorta. The reason that flow continues in the forward direction is the *inertial* component of the blood flow, which represents considerable kinetic energy. Eventually, blood in the aortic arch decelerates sufficiently that the flow becomes zero and eventually negative (producing reflux through the valve). As the aortic valve closes, it produces the dicrotic notch in the aortic pressure trace.

THORACIC/ABDOMINAL AORTA AND LARGE ARTERIES. Just distal to the aortic arch, a transformation of the flow and pressure curves begins to occur. The records in panels #2 through #4 in Figure 21–3A show the *flow* curves for the abdominal aorta and some of its large branches. Peak systolic flow becomes smaller as one moves from the aorta toward the periphery (i.e., iliac and femoral ar-

EFFECT OF AORTIC COMPLIANCE ON BLOOD FLOW

There is a large diastolic component to total blood flow in the large arteries that lie close to the aorta, such as the carotid and renal arteries (*panels #5 and #6 in Fig. 21–3A*). This large diastolic component is largely the result of the **compliance** of the blood vessel wall and the **radial expansion** of the vessels that occurs during ventricular ejection. We can reach at least an intuitive understanding of the radial contribution to flow in the aorta and large arteries by examining the ability of the aorta to store and give up energy during the acceleration and deceleration of flow.

Figure 21–4 compares two branches of a hydraulic system that are identical in radius and length. One branch (branch #1) is rigid and made of glass, the other (branch #2) is elastic and made of rubber. Both branches terminate in a spout with an outflow resistance that is analogous to the resistance of arterioles. We assume that the resistance of the spout is much greater than that of the glass or rubber tube, so that we can ignore small changes in the diameter of the rubber tube on overall resistance. If we apply a *steady pressure* to both branches, the flows through the two branches are continuous and identical (see Fig. 21–4A).

However, if we apply the *pressure in square pulses*, the flows in the two branches are quite different (see Fig. 21–4B). The flow through the glass tubing instantly rises to a maximum value with the onset of the pressure wave, and then instantly falls to zero when the driving pressure falls to zero. Thus, the plot of flow through the glass tube perfectly mirrors the plot of the applied square wave pressure. The flow through the rubber tube has a very different profile. During the interval of peak pressure, the rubber vessel gradually dilates, storing a volume of fluid. Therefore, the flow rises slowly to its maximum value. During the interval of the cycle when the driving pressure falls to zero, the expanded rubber vessel delivers its stored volume downstream, resulting in some forward flow despite the absence of any pressure head. The time-averaged outflow from the rubber tube exceeds that from the glass tube.

The aorta and large vessels behave like the rubber tube in Figure 21–4B. The oscillating pressure head in our model (i.e., between zero and a peak value) represents ventricular pressure. The maintenance of flow during interruption of the pressure head is equivalent to the continuing flow from the aorta during diastole.

Figure 21–4C shows an alternative mechanical model, that of a Windkessel (German for "air chamber"), in which the distensible rubber tube is replaced with a compressible air chamber.

The two models illustrated in Figure 21–4B and C show how compliant blood vessels can convert discontinuous flow into a more continuous flow. The so-called Windkessel action of the arterial system considerably improves the efficiency of the pump (i.e., the heart) because the vessels are able to convert the phasic flow peaks of the pump into a more continuous flow.

teries), as would be predicted because of the branching of the vessels. However, in the abdominal aorta, a new phenomenon is seen: As the elastic aorta—which stored blood during systole—releases it during diastole, a second peak of flow appears. Note that this *diastolic component* of flow is larger in the abdominal aorta than in the more distal iliac artery, and is almost absent in the femoral artery. Of particular importance is the sizable diastolic flow in the carotid and renal arteries (*panels #5 and #6*). The basis for the diastolic component of flow is the subject of the box titled Effect of Aortic Compliance on Blood Flow.

The Cardiac Cycle Also Causes Pressure Waves in the Aorta and Peripheral Vessels

The *pressure* curves in Figure 21–3B show that, with increasing distance from the heart (*panels #1–#4*), the rising portion of the wave becomes steeper and the peak is narrower. Because the peak gradually increases in height and the minimum pressure gradually decreases, the pulse pressure becomes greater. With increasing distance from the heart, an important secondary pressure oscillation appears during diastole (Fig. 21–4B, *fourth panel*). Thus, although the pressure waves are distorted, they are not damped. Although it might seem counterintuitive that the peak arterial pressure should increase as we get farther from the heart (i.e., Is the blood flowing against a pressure gradient?), it turns out that the *mean* arterial pressure does fall very slightly with increasing distance from the heart.

TERMINAL ARTERIES AND ARTERIOLES. In the smallest arteries, the flows must be small. Here, the trend toward an increased peak pressure reverses. Instead, the pulse wave gets damped out for two reasons. First, because we are dealing with many parallel vessels with a large aggregate wall area, the aggregate compliance increases, damping the pressure wave. Second, because these smaller arteries have a smaller radius and thus a far greater resistance, the mean arterial pressure must fall in proportion to the much higher resistance. Thus, in contrast to the situation in the larger arteries, damping predominates over distortion.

CAPILLARIES. By the time the blood reaches the capillaries, the damping is so severe that pulsations (i.e., pressure oscillations) do not normally occur—blood flow is continuous. The pulmonary capillaries are an exception: Their upstream vessels are short, and they have low resistance and high compliance. The pulsation of systemic capillaries occurs only in cases of markedly increased pulse pressure, such as in patients with aortic regurgitation or hyperthyroidism, or in cases of generalized peripheral vasodilation (e.g., certain forms of shock).

Distortion of Pressure Waves Is the Result of Their Propagation Along the Arterial Tree

Imagine that you are listening to a patient's heart with a stethoscope, while simultaneously feeling the pulse of the radial artery near the wrist. For each heartbeat that you

A ARTERIAL PRESSURE WAVES

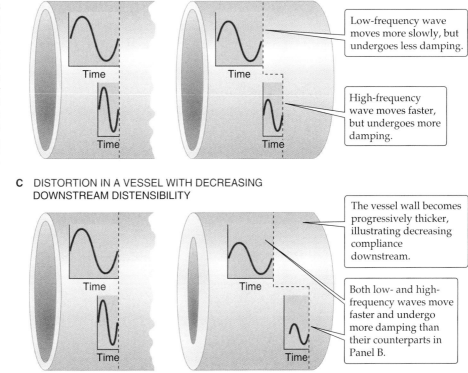

B DISTORTION IN A VESSEL WITH UNIFORM DISTENSIBILITY

Low-frequency wave moves more slowly, but undergoes less damping.

High-frequency wave moves faster, but undergoes more damping.

C DISTORTION IN A VESSEL WITH DECREASING DOWNSTREAM DISTENSIBILITY

The vessel wall becomes progressively thicker, illustrating decreasing compliance downstream.

Both low- and high-frequency waves move faster and undergo more damping than their counterparts in Panel B.

FIGURE 21–5. Propagation of pressure waves. *A*, These simultaneous pressure records are from a dog, with catheters placed at 0, 10, 20, and 30 cm from the aortic arch. As the wave moves down the vessel, the upstroke is delayed, but the peak is higher. In *B* and *C*, the flow is from left to right. The left pair of pressure waves is at the same early time, whereas the right pair of pressure waves is at the same late time. If on the right (i.e., end of the vessel) we summate waves of different frequency at the same instant in time, then the composite wave is distorted (like the more distal curves—e.g., femoral artery—in *A*).

hear, you feel a radial pulse. You know that the peak pressure in the left ventricle occurs about midway between the first and second heart sounds, but the delay between the midpoint of the two heart sounds and the peak of the radial pulse is only approximately 0.1 s. Red blood cells (RBCs) take several seconds to flow from the heart to the wrist. Why, then, are you able to feel the pulse so soon after the heartbeat?

The answer is that the blood vessels conduct the palpable pulse as a **pressure wave**. The linear velocity of RBCs—carried in the blood by convection—ranges from approximately 1 m/s in the aorta to vanishingly small values in the capillaries (p. 450). However, the pressure wave travels at a velocity of 5 to 6 m/s in the aorta, increasing to 10 to 15 m/s in the small arteries.

The following example illustrates the difference between a pressure wave and convection: Imagine that two people are submerged in a river, floating downstream (convection). Now the upstream person makes a sound under water. The sound waves (an example of a pressure wave) travel to the downstream person with a velocity that is far greater than the velocity of the river.

We could illustrate how pressure waves propagate along arteries by replotting the arterial pressure profiles from Figure 21–3B, and stacking them one on top of the other. The four pressure waves in Figure 21–5A actually represent data obtained simultaneously in a dog with four catheters, the first placed in the aortic arch, and the last three placed precisely 10 cm downstream from the previous one. The downstream propagation of the wave through the larger arteries is accompanied by a serious *distortion* of the pressure profile: It gets narrower and taller as we move downstream.

EFFECT OF FREQUENCY ON WAVE VELOCITY AND DAMP-ING. The pressure wave moving from the aorta to the periphery is actually an ensemble of many individual waves, each with its own frequency. Higher-frequency

A JUGULAR VENOUS PRESSURE CHANGES
CAUSED BY CARDIAC CYCLE

Pressure
(mm Hg)

B JUGULAR VENOUS PRESSURE CHANGES
CAUSED BY RESPIRATORY CYCLE

Intrathoracic
pressure
(cm H$_2$O)

Mean
jugular
venous
pressure
(cm H$_2$O)

FIGURE 21–6. Venous pressure changes. In *A*, the time scale is a single cardiac cycle. The relative heights of the peaks and valleys are variable. In *B* and *C*, the time scale surrounds one protracted inspiration (i.e., several heartbeats); the y-axis shows the *mean* jugular venous pressure. (*B*, Data from Brecher GA: Venous Return. New York, Grune and Stratton, 1956. *C*, Data from Pollack AA, Wood EH: Venous pressure in the saphenous vein at the ankle in man during exercise and changes in posture. J Appl Physiol 1:649–662, 1949.)

C VENOUS PRESSURE CHANGES IN FOOT
CAUSED BY MUSCLE CONTRACTION

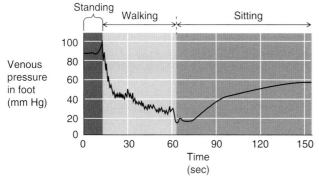

Venous
pressure
in foot
(mm Hg)

waves travel faster and undergo more damping than low-frequency waves (see Fig. 21–5*B*). Recombining these waves at a more peripheral site thus produces a new wave with a shape that is a distorted version of the original aortic wave.

EFFECT OF WALL STIFFNESS ON WAVE VELOCITY. As the pressure wave reaches vessels that have a stiffer wall (e.g., greater ratio of wall thickness to vessel diameter), the velocity of the wave increases (see Fig. 21–5*C*). Conversely, with a more compliant vessel, some of the energy of the pressure pulse goes into dilating the vessel, so that the pressure wave spreads out and slows down. Because aging causes a decrease in vessel compliance (i.e., distensibility), the velocity of propagation actually increases.

Pressure Waves in Veins Do Not Originate From Arterial Waves

We have seen earlier in this chapter that flow in *capillaries* is usually not pulsatile. Nevertheless, blood flow in systemic capillaries can exhibit slow oscillations, unrelated to the cardiac cycle. The action of upstream vasomotor control elements in arterioles and precapillary sphincters can cause fluctuations. In addition, changes in tissue pressure (e.g., caused by muscle contraction) can compress capillaries and cause further fluctuations in capillary flow. Pulmonary capillaries are especially susceptible to changes in the surrounding alveolar pressure (p. 700).

Although systemic *veins* have pressure waves, these waves do not originate from arterial waves propagating through the capillary beds, which are nonpulsatile. Three mechanisms can contribute to the **venous pulse**: (1) retrograde action of the heartbeat during the cardiac cycle, (2) the respiratory cycle, and (3) the contraction of skeletal muscles.

EFFECT OF THE CARDIAC CYCLE. A large vein close to the heart, such as the **jugular vein**, has a complex pulse wave (Fig. 21–6*A*) synchronized to the cardiac cycle. The three maxima, or peaks, in the jugular pulse wave are labeled *a*, *c*, and *v*. The three minima, or dips, are labeled *av, x,* and *y.* These pressure transients reflect events in the cardiac cycle:

▷ The *a* **peak** is caused by the contraction of the right atrium.

▷ The *av* **minimum** is due to relaxation of the right atrium and closure of the tricuspid valve.

▷ The *c* **peak** reflects the pressure rise in the right ventricle early during systole, and the resultant bulging of the tricuspid valve—which has just closed—into the right atrium.

▷ The *x* **minimum** occurs as the ventricle contracts and shortens during the ejection phase, later in systole. The shortening heart—with tricuspid valve still closed—pulls on and therefore elongates the veins, lowering their pressure.

▷ The *v* **peak** is related to filling of the right atrium against a closed tricuspid valve, which causes right atrial pressure to rise. As the tricuspid valve opens, the *v* peak begins to wane.

▷ The *y* **minimum** reflects a fall in right atrial pressure during rapid ventricular filling, as blood leaves the right atrium through an open tricuspid valve and enters the right ventricle. The increase in venous pressure after the *y* minimum occurs as venous return continues in the face of reduced ventricular filling.

EFFECT OF THE RESPIRATORY CYCLE. Poiseuille was the first to observe that the pressure in the jugular vein becomes negative during inspiration (see Fig. 21–6B). During inspiration, the diaphragm descends, causing intrathoracic pressure (and therefore the pressure inside the thoracic vessels) to decrease and intra-abdominal pressure to increase (p. 612). Consequently, the venous return from the head and upper extremities transiently increases, as low-pressure vessels literally suck blood into the thoracic cavity. Simultaneously, the venous flow decreases from the lower extremities because of the relatively high pressure of the abdominal veins during inspiration. Therefore, during inspiration, pressure in the jugular vein falls while pressure in the femoral vein rises.

EFFECT OF SKELETAL MUSCLE CONTRACTION ("MUSCLE PUMP"). The contraction of skeletal muscle can also affect pressure and flow in veins. Large veins in the lower limbs are equipped with valves that prevent retrograde movement of blood (p. 436). When a person is at rest and in the recumbent position, all venous valves are open and venous blood flow toward the heart is continuous. Standing causes the venous pressure in the foot to rise gradually to the hydrostatic pressure dictated by the vertical blood column from the foot to the heart (see Fig. 21–6C). If the person begins to walk, the combination of the pumping action of the leg muscles on the leg veins, and the action of the venous valves as hydrostatic relay stations, causes the venous pressure in the foot to decrease. Each step causes both a small oscillation and a small net decrease in foot vein pressure. Once foot vein pressure has bottomed out, each step simply causes a small pressure oscillation. Walking causes a net decrease in pressure in both the superficial and deep foot veins, as well as in the corresponding capillaries. When the exercise ceases, the venous pressure again rises.

CARDIAC DYNAMICS

The heart is a system of two pumps linked in series. The muscular wall of the left ventricle is thicker and more powerful than that of the right. The interventricular septum welding the two pumps together is even thicker. The thick muscular walls of the ventricles are mainly responsible for exerting the heart's pumping action.

The heart does not depend on a rhythm generator in the brain, like the central pattern generators (p. 367) that drive other rhythmic behaviors, such as respiration, locomotion, chewing, and shivering. Instead, pacemaker cells within the heart itself initiate cardiac excitation. When the heart is in a normal sinus rhythm, the pacemaker cells setting the rate are located in the sinoatrial (SA) node of the right atrium (p. 489). The action potential then spreads through atrial myocytes and specialized tracts or bundles. The impulse cannot cross from the atria to the ventricles except through the atrioventricular (AV) node. The AV node inserts a time delay into the conduction that is essential for allowing the ventricles to finish filling with blood before contraction and ejection occur. From the AV node, the impulse spreads through the bundle of His, the right and left bundle branches, and the Purkinje system. It finally excites the ventricular myocytes from cell to cell via gap junctions.

The Right Ventricle Contracts Like a Bellows, Whereas the Left Ventricle Contracts Like a Hand Squeezing a Tube of Toothpaste

The two ventricles share a common envelope of spiral and circular muscle layers. The arrangement of the spiral bundles ensures that ventricular contraction virtually wrings the blood out of the heart, although incompletely. The apex contracts before some of the basal portions of the ventricle, a sequence that propels blood upward to the aortic and pulmonary valves.

The mechanical action of the **right ventricle** resembles that of a bellows used for fanning a fire (Fig. 21–7A). Although the distance between the free wall and the septum is small, the free wall has such a large surface area that a small movement of the free wall toward the septum ejects a large volume.

The mechanism of emptying the right ventricle involves three motions: First, the longitudinal axis of the right ventricle shortens when spiral muscles pull the tricuspid valve ring toward the apex. Second, the free wall of the right ventricle moves toward the septum in a bellows-like motion. Third, the contraction of the deep circular fibers of the *left* ventricle forces the septum into a convex shape, so that the septum bulges into the right ventricle. This bulging of the septum stretches the free wall of the right ventricle over the septum. These three motions are well suited for ejecting a large volume, but not for developing a high pressure. The right ventricle ejects the same blood volume as the left ventricle, but it does so at much lower intraventricular pressures.

The mechanical action of the **left ventricle** occurs by a dual motion (see Fig. 21–7B): First, constriction of the *circular muscle layers* reduces the diameter of the cham-

A RIGHT VENTRICULAR CONTRACTION

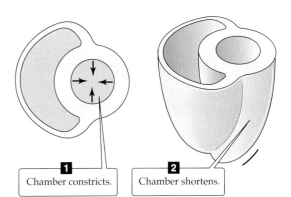

2 The free wall moves toward septum.

1 The free wall shortens.

3 The septum moves toward free wall.

B LEFT VENTRICULAR CONTRACTION

1 Chamber constricts.

2 Chamber shortens.

C TIMING OF EVENTS IN CARDIAC CYCLE

D RIGHT VENTRICULAR PRESSURE AND FLOW   **E** LEFT VENTRICULAR PRESSURE AND FLOW

FIGURE 21–7. Comparison of the dynamics of the left and right ventricles.

ber, progressing from the apex to the base, akin to squeezing a tube of toothpaste. Second, contraction of the *spiral muscles* pulls the mitral valve ring toward the apex, thereby shortening the long axis. The first mechanism is the more powerful and is responsible for the high pressures developed by the left ventricle. The conical shape of the lumen gives the left ventricle a smaller surface-to-volume ratio than the right ventricle, and contributes to the ability of the left ventricle to generate high pressures.

Atrial contraction normally makes only a minor contribution to the filling of the two ventricles when the subject is at rest (see box on p. 511). However, the contraction of the atria is a useful safety factor in at least two circumstances. During tachycardia, when the diastolic interval—and thus the time for passive filling—is short, the atrial contraction can provide a much-needed boost. Atrial contraction is also useful in certain pathologic conditions. For example, when a narrowed (i.e., stenotic) AV valve offers substantial resistance to the flow of blood from atrium to ventricle, the atrial pump can make an important contribution to ventricular filling.

The Right Atrium Contracts Before the Left, But the Left Ventricle Contracts Before the Right

When introducing the cardiac cycle earlier in the chapter, we assumed that the events on the right and left sides of the heart happen simultaneously. However, as we have already noted in our discussion of the splitting of heart sounds, the timing of the two sides of the heart is slightly different (see Fig. 21–7C).

ATRIAL CONTRACTION. Because the SA node is located in the right atrium, atrial contraction begins and ends earlier in the right atrium than in the left (see Fig. 21–7C, *Contraction*).

INITIATION OF VENTRICULAR CONTRACTION. Ventricular contraction starts slightly earlier on the *left* side, and the mitral valve closes before the tricuspid valve. However, this timing difference in the closure of the AV valves (see Fig. 21–7C, *Valve movements*) is so small that it is unusual to hear a split S_1. On the other hand, the right ventricle has a briefer period of isovolumetric contraction because it does not need to build up as much pressure to open its semilunar (i.e., outflow) valve and initiate ejection. Thus, the pulmonary valve opens slightly ahead of the aortic valve.

VENTRICULAR EJECTION. Ejection from the right ventricle lasts longer than that from the left. The semilunar valves do not close simultaneously: The aortic valve, with its higher downstream pressure, closes before the pulmonary valve. Therefore, the pulmonary valve—with its lower downstream pressure—opens first and closes last. This timing difference in the closure of the semilunar valves explains the normal physiological splitting of S_2 (see Fig. 21–7C, *Sounds*). During inspiration, the relatively negative intrathoracic pressure enhances filling of the right heart, causing it to have a larger end-diastolic volume and therefore more blood to eject. The additional time required for right ventricular ejection postpones the

closure of the pulmonary valve, broadening the splitting of S_2.

VENTRICULAR RELAXATION. Isovolumetric relaxation is briefer in the right heart than in the left: The pulmonary valve closes *after* the aortic valve, and the tricuspid valve opens *before* the mitral valve. Therefore, the right ventricle begins filling before the left.

Measurements of Ventricular Volumes, Pressures, and Flows Allow Clinicians to Judge Cardiac Performance

DEFINITIONS OF CARDIAC VOLUMES. The cardiac output is the product of heart rate and stroke volume (p. 428). The **stroke volume** (SV) is the difference between ventricular **end-diastolic volume** (EDV) and ventricular **end-systolic volume** (ESV), that is, the difference between the maximal and minimal ventricular volumes. EDV is typically 120 ml, and the ESV is 50 ml, so that

$$\text{Equation } 21-2$$
$$
\begin{aligned}
SV &= EDV - ESV \\
&= 120 \text{ ml} - 50 \text{ ml} \\
&= 70 \text{ ml}
\end{aligned}
$$

The **ejection fraction** (EF) is a dimensionless value, defined as the stroke volume normalized to the end-diastolic volume:

$$\text{Equation } 21-3$$
$$
EF = \frac{SV}{EDV}
$$

In our example, the ejection fraction is (70 ml)/(120 ml) or approximately 0.6; it should exceed 55% in a healthy person.

MEASUREMENTS OF CARDIAC VOLUMES. Clinicians routinely measure the volume of the cardiac chambers by means of angiography or echocardiography (p. 445). **One-dimensional (or M-mode) echocardiography** allows one to assess left ventricular performance in terms of linear dimensions and velocities by providing measurements of: (1) velocity of the posterior left ventricular wall, (2) fractional shortening of the left ventricular circumference, and (3) rate of fractional circumferential shortening. **Two-dimensional echocardiography** makes it possible to determine several ventricular volumes:

▷ Left-ventricular end-diastolic volume (LVEDV)
▷ Left-ventricular end-systolic volume (LVESV)
▷ Stroke volume (SV = LVEDV–LVESV)
▷ Left ventricular ejection fraction (LVEF = SV/LVEDV)

MEASUREMENT OF VENTRICULAR PRESSURES. Clinicians use a Swan-Ganz catheter to monitor intraventricular pressures. This catheter consists of three parallel tubes of different length; the longest is an end-hole catheter with a balloon flotation device, whereas the other two tubes are side-hole catheters. The physician advances the catheter percutaneously through a large systemic vein, into the right heart, and then into the pulmonary circulation where the tip of the longest tube literally *wedges* in a small pulmonary artery. Because a continuous and presumably closed column of blood connects the probe's end and the left atrium, the **wedge pressure** is often taken as an index of left atrial pressure. Table 21–3 lists some of the most important pressure values for the right and left heart.

MEASUREMENT OF FLOWS. The cardiologist can calculate flow from changes in ventricular volume, as measured by echocardiography and the Doppler ultrasound technique (p. 446), both of which measure the flow of blood in the outflow tract (i.e., aorta). Figure 21–7D and E illustrates the profiles of outflow pressure and velocity for the two ventricles. Although the two ventricles expel on average the same *amount* of blood in a single cardiac cycle, the peak *velocity* is much higher in the left ventricle. In addition, the velocity rises far more rapidly in the left ventricle, indicating greater acceleration of the blood during ejection. The *pressure* wave is about five times larger in the left ventricle than in the right, and the rate at which the pressure rises ($\Delta P/\Delta t$) is more rapid in the left ventricle.

The Pressure-Volume Loop of a Ventricle Illustrates the Ejection Work of the Ventricle

In Figure 21–1, we saw separate plots of ventricular *pressure* against time, and *volume* against time. If, at each point in time, we now plot pressure against volume, the result is a **pressure-volume loop**, as is shown in Figure 21–8A for the left ventricle. This loop is a "phase plot" that describes the relationship between left ventricular pressure and left ventricular volume during the cardiac cycle. Notice that, although *time* does not explicitly appear in this plot, as we make one complete cycle around the loop, we sequentially plot all of the time points of the cardiac cycle. However, the distance between two points on the loop is not proportional to elapsed time.

In examining this pressure-volume loop, we will arbitrarily start at point A in Figure 21–8A, and then consider each of the segments of the loop (e.g., AB, BC, etc.) before again returning to point A. Although we use the left ventricle as an example, a similar analysis applies to the right ventricle.

SEGMENT AB. Point A represents the instant at which the *mitral valve opens*. At this point, left ventricular volume is at its minimal value of approximately 50 ml, and left ventricular pressure is at the fairly low value of approximately 7 mm Hg. As the mitral valve opens, the ventricle begins to fill passively, because atrial pressure is higher than ventricular pressure. During interval AB, ventricular pressure falls slightly to approximately 5 mm Hg because the ventricular muscle is continuing to relax during diastole. Thus, despite the rapid entry of blood, ventricular pressure falls to its lowest value in the cardiac cycle.

SEGMENT BC. During a second phase of ventricular filling, volume rises markedly from approximately 70 to approximately 120 ml, accompanied by a rather modest increase in pressure from approximately 5 to approximately 10 mm Hg. The modest rise in pressure, despite a doubling of ventricular volume, reflects the high compliance ($C = \Delta V/\Delta P$) of the ventricular wall during late diastole. The relationship between pressure and volume during segment BC is similar to that in blood vessels (p. 455).

SEGMENT CD. Point C represents the *closure of the mitral valve*. At this point, ventricular filling has ended and **isovolumetric contraction**—represented by the vertical line CD—is about to begin. Thus, by the definition of "isovolumetric," ventricular volume remains at 120 ml while left ventricular pressure rises to approximately 80 mm Hg, about equal to the aortic end-diastolic pressure.

SEGMENT DE. Point D represents the *opening of the aortic valve*. With the outlet to the aorta now open, the ventricular muscle can begin to shorten and eject blood. During this period of rapid ejection, ventricular volume decreases from approximately 120 to approximately 75 ml. Notice that as contraction continues during interval DE, the ventricular pressure rises even farther, reaching a peak systolic value of approximately 130 mm Hg at point E.

SEGMENT EF. Point E represents the instant at which the ventricular muscle starts to relax. During this period of decreased ejection, ventricular pressure falls from approximately 130 to approximately 100 mm Hg. Nevertheless, blood continues to leave the ventricle, and ventricular volume falls from approximately 75 ml at point E to approximately 50 ml at point F. Point F represents end-systolic volume and pressure. Notice that the ventricle does not shrink to zero volume at the end of systole. In total, 120 − 50, or 70 ml of blood has left the ventricle during systole (i.e., between points D and F). Therefore, the stroke volume is substantially less than the maximum ventricular volume (i.e., EDV). The ejection fraction in

TABLE 21–3

COMPARISON OF PRESSURES IN THE RIGHT AND LEFT CIRCULATIONS

PRESSURES (in mm Hg)

Right Atrium		Left Atrium		
Mean	2	Mean		8
		a wave	13	
		c wave	12	
		v wave	15	
Right Ventricle		**Left Ventricle**		
Peak systolic	30	Peak systolic	130	
End diastolic	6	End diastolic	10	
Pulmonary Artery		**Aorta**		
Mean	15	Mean		95
Peak systolic	25	Peak systolic	130	
End diastolic	8	End diastolic	80	
Pulmonary Capillaries		**Systemic Capillaries**		
Mean	10	Mean		25

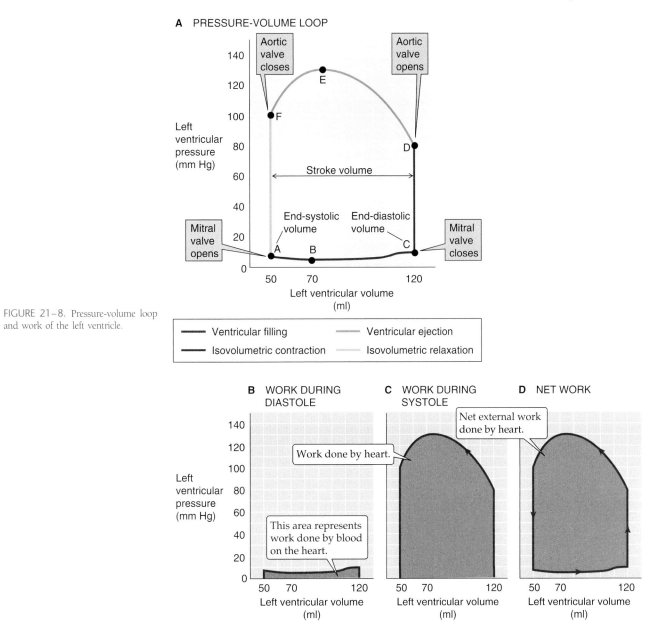

FIGURE 21–8. Pressure-volume loop and work of the left ventricle.

this example is approximately 60%, which is in the normal range. Ejection occurs against aortic pressures ranging between 80 and 130 mm Hg. Therefore, ejection is not "isotonic" (p. 247).

SEGMENT FA. Point F represents the *closing of the aortic valve*. At this point, ejection has ended and **isovolumetric relaxation** is about to begin. The ventricular volume remains at 50 ml, while left ventricular pressure falls from approximately 100 mm Hg at point F to approximately 7 mm Hg at point A. At the end of isovolumetric relaxation, the mitral valve opens and the cardiac cycle starts all over again with ventricular filling.

The six segments of the pressure-volume loop correspond to different phases of the cardiac cycle:

▷ Phase 1, the inflow phase, includes segments AB and BC
▷ Phase 2, isovolumetric contraction, includes segment CD

▷ Phase 3, the outflow phase, includes segments DE and EF
▷ Phase 4, isovolumetric relaxation, includes segment FA

Segments CDEF represent systole, whereas segments FABC represent diastole.

The "Pumping Work" Done by the Heart Is a Small Fraction of the Total Energy the Heart Consumes

The heart does its useful work as a pump by imparting momentum to the blood and propelling it against the resistance of the periphery.

Work, in its simplest definition, is the product of the force applied to an object and the distance the object moves (W = force × distance). When considering **pressure-volume work**, we must revise this definition. Imagine that we have a volume of blood in a syringe. If we apply a *constant* force to the plunger, that is, if we apply a *constant* pressure to the blood, the plunger moves a certain distance as we eject the blood through a needle, thereby reducing blood volume by an amount ΔV. How much work have we done? For pressure moving a fluid, the external work is:

Equation 21–4

$$W = P \cdot \Delta V$$

If the aortic pressure were constant, the work done with each heartbeat would be simply the product of the aortic pressure (P) and the stroke volume ($\Delta V = SV = EDV − ESV$).

The pressure-volume relationships in Figure 21–8*B*, *C*, and *D* illustrate the pressure-volume work of the heart. The surface below the *segment ABC* (i.e., filling phase) is the work done *by the blood* (previously contained in the venous reservoirs and atria) on the ventricle (see Fig. 21–8*B*). The surface below DEF (i.e., ejection phase) is the work done *by the heart* on the blood during the ejection (see Fig. 21–8*C*). The difference between the areas in Figure 8*B* and *C*—that is, the area within the single-cycle loop—is the *net* external work done by the heart (see Fig. 21–8*D*).

The pressure-volume diagram for the **right ventricle** has the same general shape. However, the area (i.e., *net* external work) is only about one fifth as large because the pressures are so much lower.

The area of the loop in Figure 21–8*D*—that is, the pressure-volume work (P · V)—ignores the speed at which the ventricle pumps the blood (i.e., acceleration that the heart imparts to the blood, or the time it takes to complete one cardiac cycle). Thus, the work per beat should also include the **kinetic energy** ($\frac{1}{2}$ mv²) that the heart imparts to the ejected blood:

Equation 21–5

$$\underbrace{W}_{\substack{\text{Total} \\ \text{external} \\ \text{work}}} = \underbrace{P \cdot V}_{\substack{\text{Pressure-} \\ \text{Volume} \\ \text{work}}} + \underbrace{\frac{1}{2} \, mv^2}_{\substack{\text{Kinetic} \\ \text{energy}}}$$

Of its total external work, the heart delivers only a relatively small fraction as kinetic energy. Moreover, the total external work is itself only a small portion of the total energy that the heart actually expends. Like other muscles, the heart not only shortens and performs *classical* work (e.g., isotonic contraction), but it can also maintain active tension without shortening (i.e., isometric contraction; p. 245). During the isovolumetric contraction, the ventricle develops and maintains a high pressure without performing any total external work—just as we perform no useful work when we hold a weight without lifting it. However, in both isometric exercises, the muscle breaks down adenosine triphosphate (ATP) as long as it maintains isometric tension; the energy ends up as heat. This type of energy cost in heart muscle is called **tension heat**, which is proportional to the product of the tension of the ventricular wall (T) and the length of time (Δt) that the ventricle maintains this tension (i.e., tension-time integral). In the case of the heart, the pressure against which the ventricle must pump is a major determinant of the wall tension.

The total energy transformed in one cardiac cycle is the sum of the total external work done on the blood and the tension heat:

Equation 21–6

$$E = \underbrace{\underbrace{P \cdot V}_{\substack{\text{Pressure-} \\ \text{Volume} \\ \text{work}}} + \underbrace{\frac{1}{2} \, mv^2}_{\substack{\text{Kinetic} \\ \text{energy}}}}_{\text{Total External Work}} + \underbrace{k \cdot T \cdot \Delta t}_{\substack{\text{Tension} \\ \text{heat}}}$$

k is a proportionality constant that converts $T \cdot \Delta t$ into units of energy. The tension heat is the *major* determinant of the total energy requirements of the heart. The total external work represents a relatively small fraction (3%) of the total energy needs of the heart at rest, rising to as much as 10% during exercise. The heat developed as part of the tension-time integral remains the major component of the total energy consumption, even during exercise.

The tension heat is not only far more costly for the heart than the pressure-volume work, but is also of considerable practical interest for the patient with coronary artery disease who wishes to step up cardiac output during increased physical activity. The major burden for such an individual may be not so much the total external work expended in driving additional blood through the circulation (i.e., increasing the cardiac output), but rather an increase in *tension heat* ($k \cdot T \cdot \Delta t$). Thus, it is advantageous to the patient to have a low wall tension (T)—that is, a low blood pressure. It is also advantageous for the patient not to spend too much time (Δt) in systole. The heart spends a greater fraction of its time in systole when the heart rate is high. Thus, the cardiac patient is better off to increase cardiac output at low pressure and low heart rate (i.e., a low $T \cdot \Delta t$ product). The only option left is to increase stroke volume.

The ratio of the ventricle's total external work (P · V + $\frac{1}{2}$ mv²) to the total energy cost (i.e., W/E) is the heart's **mechanical efficiency**. Note that the mechanical efficiency has nothing to do with how effective the ventricle is at expelling blood (i.e., ejection fraction).

FROM CONTRACTILE FILAMENTS TO A REGULATED PUMP

In Chapter 9, we examined the general features of muscle contraction, and compared the properties of skeletal, cardiac, and smooth muscle. In this chapter, we examine how some of the features of cardiac muscle underlie cardiac performance.

The Entry of Ca²⁺ from the Outside Triggers Ca²⁺-Induced Ca²⁺ Release from the SR, Initiating Contraction of Cardiac Myocytes

Excitation-contraction (EC) coupling in cardiac ventricular myocytes (p. 242) is similar to EC coupling in skeletal muscle (p. 241). One major difference is that, in the case of skeletal muscle, the initiating event is the arrival of an action potential at the neuromuscular junction, the release of acetylcholine, and the initiation of an end-plate potential. In the ventricular myocyte, action potentials in adjacent myocytes depolarize the target cell via gap junctions (p. 484), and thereby generate an action potential.

As in a skeletal muscle fiber (p. 241), the depolarization of the plasma membrane in the ventricular myocyte invades T tubules that run radially to the long axis of the myocyte. Unlike skeletal muscle cells, cardiac myocytes also have *axial* T tubules that run parallel to the long axis of the cell and interconnect adjacent radial T tubules.

Another major difference in EC coupling between cardiac and skeletal muscle is in the way that the L-type Ca^{2+} channels (i.e., dihydropyridine receptors) in the T-tubule membrane activate the Ca^{2+}-release channels (CRCs, or ryanodine receptors) in the sarcoplasmic reticulum (SR) membrane. In skeletal muscle, the linkage is mechanical, and does not require Ca^{2+} entry per se. In cardiac muscle, Ca^{2+} entry through the L-type Ca^{2+} channel is essential for raising $[Ca^{2+}]_i$ in the vicinity of the CRCs on the SR. This trigger Ca^{2+} activates an adjacent cluster of CRCs, causing them to release Ca^{2+} into the cytoplasm (**Ca^{2+}-induced Ca^{2+} release**). Thus, if you place a heart in a Ca^{2+}-free solution, it will quickly stop beating, whereas a skeletal muscle can continue contracting until its intracellular Ca^{2+} stores become depleted. A single episode of Ca^{2+}-induced Ca^{2+} release causes a large but localized increase in $[Ca^{2+}]_i$ that appears as a **Ca^{2+} spark** when monitored with a Ca^{2+}-sensitive dye using confocal microscopy. If many L-type Ca^{2+} channels open simultaneously, the cardiac myocyte exhibits multiple foci or Ca^{2+} sparks, leading to a global increase in $[Ca^{2+}]_i$.

The basic structure of the thin and thick filaments is the same as for skeletal muscle (see Fig. 9–5). After $[Ca^{2+}]_i$ increases, Ca^{2+} binds to troponin C (TnC), and the Ca^{2+}/TnC complex releases the inhibition of troponin I on actin. As a result, the tropomyosin filaments on the actin shift out of the way (see Fig. 9–6A), allowing myosin to interact with active sites on the actin. The cross-bridge cycling (see Fig. 9–7) is fueled by ATP. Because the heart can never rest, cardiac myocytes have a very high density of mitochondria, and thus are capable of sustaining very high rates of oxidative phosphorylation (i.e., ATP synthesis).

The cross-bridge cycling causes thick filaments to slide past thin filaments, generating tension. When we discussed the mechanics of skeletal muscle in Chapter 9, we introduced the concept of a length-tension diagram (see Fig. 9–12), which is a plot of muscle tension as a function of muscle length. The length parameter in such a plot can be either the length of the whole skeletal muscle or the length of a single sarcomere. For heart muscle, which wraps around the ventricle, the length parameter can be either the ventricular volume, which is analogous to whole-muscle length, or the sarcomere length. The sarcomere, stretching from one Z line to another, is the functional unit in both skeletal and cardiac muscle.

Phosphorylation of Phospholamban and of Troponin I Speeds Cardiac Muscle Relaxation

With the waning of the phase 2 plateau of the cardiac action potential (see Fig. 20–3B), the influx of Ca^{2+}

through L-type Ca^{2+} channels decreases, lessening the release of Ca^{2+} by the SR. By itself, halting Ca^{2+} entry and release can only prevent a further increase in $[Ca^{2+}]_i$. The actual relaxation of the contractile proteins depends on three processes: (1) extrusion of Ca^{2+} into the extracellular fluid (ECF); (2) re-uptake of Ca^{2+} from the cytosol by the SR; and (3) dissociation of Ca^{2+} from TnC. The last two of these processes are highly regulated.

EXTRUSION OF Ca^{2+} INTO THE EXTRACELLULAR FLUID. As in most other cells (p. 70), the extrusion of Ca^{2+} into the ECF occurs by two pathways: (1) a sarcolemmal Na-Ca exchanger (NCX), which operates at relatively high levels of $[Ca^{2+}]_i$; and (2) a sarcolemmal Ca^{2+} pump (PMCA), which functions at even low levels of $[Ca^{2+}]_i$. Even during the plateau of the action potential, the myocyte extrudes some Ca^{2+}. After the membrane potential returns to more negative values, the extrusion processes gain the upper hand and lower $[Ca^{2+}]_i$. In the steady state (i.e., over the course of several action potentials), all the Ca^{2+} that enters the cytosol from the extracellular fluid through L-type Ca^{2+} channels must be extruded.

RE-UPTAKE OF Ca^{2+} BY THE SR. Even during the plateau of the action potential, some of the Ca^{2+} accumulating in the cytoplasm is sequestered into the SR by a Ca^{2+} pump known as SERCA2 in the case of the heart (p. 64). **Phospholamban**, an integral SR membrane protein with a single transmembrane segment, is an important regulator of the SERCA2 in cardiac muscle. In SR membranes of cardiac, smooth, and slow-twitch skeletal muscle, phospholamban can exist as a pentamer that may function as an ion channel or as a regulator of Cl^- channels in the SR. The dissociation of the pentamer allows the hydrophilic cytoplasmic domain of phospholamban monomers to inhibit SERCA2. However, phosphorylation of phospholamban by any of several kinases relieves phospholamban's inhibition of SERCA2, allowing Ca^{2+} resequestration to accelerate. The net effect is an increase in the rate of cardiac muscle relaxation. Therefore, it is not surprising that knockout mice deficient in phospholamban have uninhibited SERCA2 Ca^{2+} pumps, and thus an increased velocity of muscle relaxation.

Phosphorylation of phospholamban by protein kinase A (PKA) explains why β_1-adrenergic agonists (e.g., epinephrine), which act via the PKA pathway (p. 97), speed up the relaxation of cardiac muscle.

DISSOCIATION OF Ca^{2+} FROM TROPONIN C. As $[Ca^{2+}]_i$ falls, Ca^{2+} dissociates from TnC (p. 236), blocking actin-myosin interactions, and causing relaxation. β_1-Adrenergic agonists accelerate relaxation by promoting phosphorylation of troponin I (TnI), which in turn enhances the dissociation of Ca^{2+} from troponin C.

The Overlap of Thick and Thin Filaments Cannot Explain the Unusual Shape of the Cardiac Length-Tension Diagram

We discussed passive and active length-tension diagrams for skeletal muscle in Chapter 9 (see Fig. 9–12C and D). We obtain a passive length-tension diagram by holding a piece of resting skeletal or cardiac muscle at several predefined lengths, and measuring the tension at each length

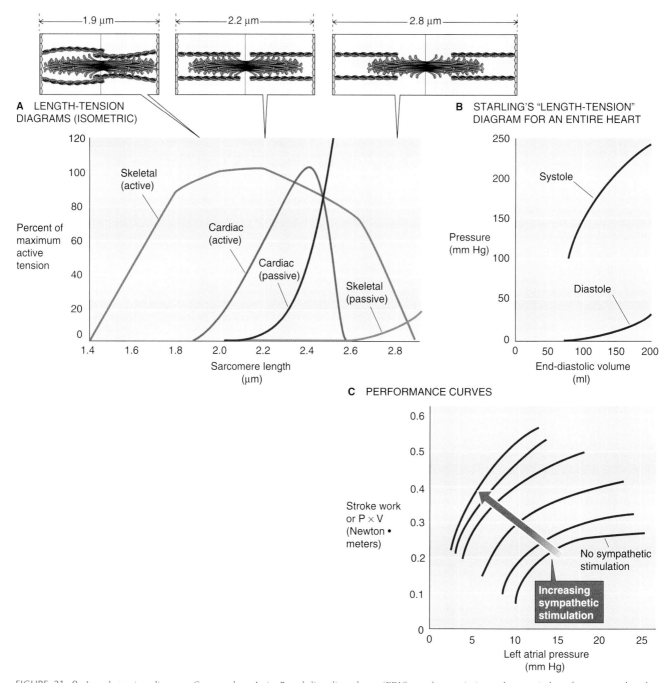

FIGURE 21–9. Length-tension diagram. Compared to *A*, in *B* end-diastolic volume (EDV) on the x-axis is used as an index of sarcomere length. (Because EDV was difficult to measure before the days of echocardiography, Starling actually used left atrial pressure as an index of the degree of filling.) Starling measured pressure on the y-axis as an index of tension. Thus, systolic pressure replaces active tension, and diastolic pressure replaces passive tension. In *C*, left atrial pressure on the x-axis is used as an index of sarcomere length, and stroke work (systolic pressure × ejected volume) on the y-axis is used instead of tension.

(Fig. 21–9*A*, *green and violet curves*). We obtain the *active* length-tension diagram by stimulating the muscle at each predefined length (i.e., isometric conditions) and measuring the *increment* in tension from its resting or passive value (*turquoise and brown curves*).

The **passive length-tension diagrams** for skeletal and cardiac muscle are quite different. The passive tension of a skeletal muscle (see Fig. 21–9*A*, *green curve*) is practically nil until the length of the sarcomere exceeds 2.6 μm. Beyond this length, passive tension rises slowly. On the other hand, the passive tension of cardiac muscle

(*violet curve*) begins to rise at much lower sarcomere lengths, and rises much more steeply. The reason for this difference is that the noncontractile (i.e., elastic) components of cardiac muscle are less distensible. The most important of these elastic components is the giant protein **titin** (~2500 kDa), which runs from the Z line to the M line of a sarcomere (see Fig. 9–4*B*). As a result, cardiac muscle will break if stretched beyond a sarcomere length of 2.6 μm, whereas it is possible to stretch skeletal muscle to a sarcomere length of 3.6 μm.

The **active length-tension diagrams** also differ between skeletal and cardiac muscle. The active tension of skeletal muscle (*turquoise curve*) is high and varies only modestly between sarcomere lengths of 1.8 and 2.6 μm (see Fig. 21–9A). In Chapter 9, we accounted for the shape of this curve as caused by the degree of myofilament overlap (p. 247). In cardiac muscle (*brown curve*), active tension has a relatively sharp peak. For example, as cardiac sarcomere length decreases from 2.4 to 1.8 μm, active tension falls steeply. We cannot account for this fall by a decrease in the overlap of thick and thin filaments because the filament dimensions of cardiac and skeletal muscle are similar. Rather, the fall in tension at lower sarcomere lengths in cardiac muscle probably has two causes: (1) Short sarcomere lengths somehow reduce the Ca^{2+} affinity of TnC, thereby reducing the Ca^{2+} sensitivity of the myofilaments; and (2) for reasons that are unclear, reducing the cardiac sarcomere length reduces Ca^{2+} entry from the extracellular fluid or Ca^{2+}-induced Ca^{2+} release. As cardiac sarcomere length increases above 2.4, active tension declines precipitously, compared with the gradual fall in skeletal muscle. Once again, this fall-off does not reflect a problem in the overlap of thin and thick filaments. Instead, the same noncontractile components that increase the passive *stiffness* of cardiac muscle may also impede development of *active tension* at high sarcomere lengths.

Starling's Law States that a Greater Fiber Length (i.e., Greater Ventricular Volume) Causes the Heart to Deliver More Mechanical Energy

Long before the development of the sliding filament hypothesis and our understanding that active tension should depend on sarcomere length, Ernest Starling in 1914 anticipated the results of Figure 21–9A, using an isolated heart-lung preparation. **Starling's law** states that, "the mechanical energy set free in the passage from the resting to the active state is a function of the length of the fiber." Therefore, the initial length of myocardial fibers determines the work done during the cardiac cycle. Figure 21–9B shows the results of experiments that Starling performed on the intact heart. Starling assumed that the initial *length* of the myocardial fibers is proportional to the end-diastolic volume (EDV). Further, he assumed that

tension in the myocardial fibers is proportional to the systolic pressure. Therefore, starting from a volume-pressure diagram, Starling was able to reconstruct an equivalent length-tension diagram (Table 21–4).

His diagram for *diastole* (see Fig. 21–9B, *purple curve*), which shows a rising pressure (tension) with increased EDV (fiber length), is very similar to the early part of the *passive* length-tension diagram for cardiac muscle (see Fig. 21–9A, *violet curve*). His diagram for *systole* (see Fig. 21–9B, *red curve*) is more or less equivalent to the ascending phase of the *active* length-tension diagram for cardiac muscle (see Fig. 21–9A, *brown curve*). Therefore, Starling's systole curve shows that the heart is able to generate more pressure (i.e., deliver more blood) when more is presented to it.

A **ventricular performance curve** (see Fig. 21–9C) is another representation of Starling's length-tension diagram, but it is one a clinician can obtain on a patient. A ventricular performance curve is a plot of stroke work (P · ΔV, see Equation 21–4), which is the equivalent of Starling's systolic pressure (which itself is an estimate of muscle tension), against left atrial pressure, which corresponds to Starling's end-diastolic volume (which itself is an estimate of muscle length). What we learn from performance curves obtained on living subjects is that Starling's law *is not a fixed relationship*. For instance, the norepinephrine released during sympathetic stimulation—which increases myocardial contractility (as we will see later in this chapter)—shifts the performance curve upward and to the left (see Fig. 21–9C). Similar shifts occur with other **positive inotropic** agents (e.g., cardiac glycosides)—that is, drugs that increase myocardial contractility. Note also that ventricular performance curves show no descending component because sarcomere length does not increase beyond 2.2 to 2.4 μm in healthy hearts.

The Velocity of Cardiac Muscle Shortening Falls when the Contraction Occurs against a Greater Opposing Force (or Pressure) or at a Shorter Muscle Length (or Lower Volume)

The functional properties of cardiac muscle—how much tension it can develop, how rapidly it can contract—depend on many factors, but especially on two properties intrinsic to the cardiac myocyte:

TABLE 21–4

EQUIVALENT UNITS FOR CONVERTING BETWEEN A THREE-DIMENSIONAL HEART AND A LINEAR MUSCLE FIBER

ISOLATED MUSCLE = LINEAR		CARDIAC VENTRICLE = HOLLOW ORGAN	
Parameter	Units	Parameter	Units
Length	mm	Volume	ml
Extent of shortening	mm	Stroke volume	ml
Velocity of shortening	mm/s	Velocity of ejection	ml/s
Load or Force or Tension	gram dyne dyne/cm^2	Pressure	mm Hg

This table shows the equivalence between dimensions when converting from the contraction of a hollow organ, such as a cardiac ventricle, to a linear model of a single muscle contraction.

1. **Initial sarcomere length**. For the beating heart, a convenient index of initial sarcomere length is *end-diastolic volume*. Both initial sarcomere length and EDV are measures of the **preload** imposed on the cardiac muscle *just before* it ejects blood from the ventricle during systole. *Starling's law*, in which the independent variable is EDV, focuses on preload.

2. **Force that the contracting myocytes must overcome**. In the beating heart, a convenient index of opposing force is the *arterial pressure* that opposes the outflow of blood from the ventricle. Both opposing force and arterial pressure are measures of the **after-load** the ventricular muscle must overcome *as it ejects blood during systole*. Experiments on *isotonic contractions* focus on the after-load, factors that the ventricle can sense only *after* the contraction has begun.

Figure 21–10 shows how one might measure the *velocity of shortening* in a way that is relevant for a cardiac muscle facing both a preload and an after-load. In Figure 21–10A, the muscle starts off at rest, stretched between a fixed support *(bottom of the muscle)* and the left end of a lever *(top of the muscle)*. A weight attached to the other end of the lever, but resting on a table, applies stretch to the muscle—to the extent allowed by the screw, which adjusts the "stop" of the lever's left end. Thus, the combination of the weight and the screw determines initial sarcomere length (i.e., preload). At this time, the muscle cannot sense the full extent of the weight. The more we stretch the muscle by retracting the screw, the greater the preload. When we begin to stimulate the muscle, it develops a gradually increasing tension (see Fig. 21–10C, *lower blue curve*), but the length between the fixed point and the left end of the lever (see Fig. 21–10A) remains constant. That is, the muscle cannot shorten. Therefore, in the first phase of the experiment, the muscle exerts increasing *isometric tension*.

When the muscle has built up enough tension, it can now begin lifting the weight off the table (see Fig. 21–10B). This phase of the contraction is termed "after-loaded" shortening. The tension now remains at a fixed after-load value *(flat portion of lower curve in Fig. 21–10C)* but the muscle gradually shortens *(rising portion of upper blue curve)*. Therefore, in the second phase of the experiment, the muscle exerts *isotonic contraction*. From the slope of the upper curve in Figure 21–10C, we can compute the velocity of shortening at a particular after-load.

This experiment roughly mimics the actions of ventricular muscle during systole. Initially, during its iso*metric* contraction, our hypothetical muscle increases its tension at constant length, as during the iso*volumetric* contraction in segment CD of Figure 21–8A. The initial length corresponds to EDV, the preload. Later, the muscle shortens while overcoming a constant force (i.e., generating a constant tension), as during the ejection phase in segment DEF of Figure 21–8A. The tension corresponds to arterial pressure, the after-load.

What happens if we vary the after-load (i.e., change the weight)? As we already observed in our discussion of skeletal muscle, it is easier to lift a feather than a barbell. Thus, with a heavier weight, the muscle develops a lot of

tension, but shortens slowly (see Fig. 21–10D, *red tracings*). Conversely, with a lighter weight, the muscle develops only a little bit of tension, but shortens rapidly *(purple curves)*.

If we plot the velocities of shortening in Figure 21–10D as a function of the three different after-loads being lifted, we obtain the purple, blue, and red points on the load-velocity curve in Figure 21–10E. This curve applies to a muscle that we stretched only slightly in the preload phase (i.e., low preload in Fig. 21–10A). The red curve in Figure 21–10E shows a similar load-velocity relationship for a muscle that was stretched greatly in the preload phase (i.e., high preload). In both cases, the velocity of shortening increases as the tension (i.e., after-load) falls.

When the after-load is so large that no shortening ever occurs, that after-load is the **isometric tension**, shown as the point of zero velocity on the x-axis of Figure 21–10E. As expected from Starling's law, the greater the initial stretch (i.e., preload), the greater the isometric tension. In fact, at *any* velocity (see Fig. 21–10E, *dashed horizontal line*), the tension is greater in the muscle that was stretched more in the preload phase *(red curve)*—a restatement of Starling's law.

In summary, at a given preload (i.e., walking up the black curve in Fig. 21–10E), the velocity of shortening for cardiac muscle becomes greater with lower after-loads (i.e., opposing pressure). Conversely, at a given after-load—that is, comparing the *black and red curves* for any common x value (see Fig. 21–10E, *dashed vertical line*)—the velocity of shortening for cardiac muscle becomes greater with a greater preload (i.e., sarcomere length).

Finally, the curves in Figure 21–10E do not represent a fixed set of relationships. Positive inotropic agents shift all curves up and to the right. Thus, a positive inotropic agent allows the heart to achieve a given velocity against a greater load, or to push a given load with a greater velocity.

Another way of representing how velocity of shortening depends on the initial muscle length (i.e., preload) is to monitor velocity of shortening during a single isotonic contraction. If we first apply a large preload to stretch a piece of muscle to an initial length of 9.0 mm (see Fig. 21–10F), and then stimulate it, the velocity instantly rises to a peak value of approximately 8.5 mm/s; it then gradually falls to zero as the muscle shortens to 7.5 mm. If we start by applying a smaller preload, thereby stretching the muscle to an initial length of 8.5 or 8.0 mm, the peak velocity falls. Thus, initial length determines not only the tension that cardiac muscle can generate, but also the speed with which the muscle can shorten.

Increases in Heart Rate Enhance Myocardial Tension

Heart muscle tension has a special dependence on the frequency of contraction. If we stimulate isolated heart muscle only a few times per minute, the tension developed is much smaller than if we stimulate it at a physiological rate of 70/min. The progressive rise of tension

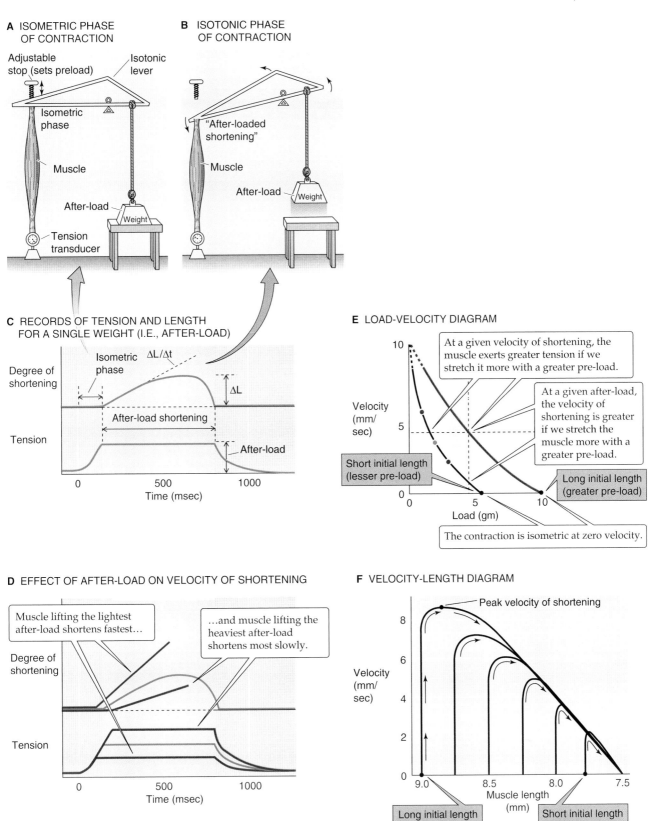

A   ISOMETRIC PHASE OF CONTRACTION

Adjustable stop (sets preload)

Isotonic lever

Isometric phase

Muscle

After-load

Weight

Tension transducer

B   ISOTONIC PHASE OF CONTRACTION

"After-loaded shortening"

Muscle

After-load

Weight

C   RECORDS OF TENSION AND LENGTH FOR A SINGLE WEIGHT (I.E., AFTER-LOAD)

Degree of shortening

Isometric phase

$\Delta L/\Delta t$

ΔL

After-load shortening

Tension

After-load

0   500   1000
Time (msec)

E   LOAD-VELOCITY DIAGRAM

At a given velocity of shortening, the muscle exerts greater tension if we stretch it more with a greater pre-load.

At a given after-load, the velocity of shortening is greater if we stretch the muscle more with a greater pre-load.

Velocity (mm/ sec)

10

5

0

Short initial length (lesser pre-load)

Long initial length (greater pre-load)

0   5   10
Load (gm)

The contraction is isometric at zero velocity.

D   EFFECT OF AFTER-LOAD ON VELOCITY OF SHORTENING

Muscle lifting the lightest after-load shortens fastest...

...and muscle lifting the heaviest after-load shortens most slowly.

Degree of shortening

Tension

0   500   1000
Time (msec)

F   VELOCITY-LENGTH DIAGRAM

Peak velocity of shortening

Velocity (mm/ sec)

8

6

4

2

0

9.0   8.5   8.0   7.5
Muscle length (mm)

Long initial length (greater pre-load)

Short initial length (lesser pre-load)

FIGURE 21–10. Effect of preload and after-load on velocity of shortening. In *A*, the developed tension is not yet sufficient to lift the weight (i.e., after-load). In *B*, the muscle, which has now developed sufficient tension to lift the weight, shortens against a constant after-load. In *C*, the slope of the *blue curve* (dL/dt) is the velocity of shortening. The velocities of shortening for three different after-loads (tensions) in *D* are plotted as the three colored points of the lower curve in *E*. In *F*, the x-axis has the longest lengths on the left, so that "time" runs from left to right (*arrows*). Note that the family of curves is enclosed by the envelope created by the curve for the greatest initial length.

following an increase in rate—the "**staircase phenomenon**"—was first observed by Henry Bowditch in 1871. Underlying the staircase phenomenon is an increase in Ca^{2+} availability, which has two causes. First, the larger number of action potentials per minute provides a longer aggregate period of Ca^{2+} entry into the cell, which loads up SR Ca^{2+} stores. Second, it appears that during each action potential plateau, more Ca^{2+} enters the cell.

Contractility Is an Intrinsic Measure of Cardiac Performance

Now that we know that the performance of the heart depends on such factors as degree of filling (i.e., preload), arterial pressure (i.e., after-load), and heart rate, it would be useful to have a measure of the heart's *intrinsic* contractile performance, independent of these *extrinsic* factors. **Contractility** is such a measure.

Contractility is a somewhat vague but clinically useful term that distinguishes a better-performing heart from a poorly performing one. In a patient, it is difficult to assess cardiac performance by using the approaches in Figures 21–9 and 21–10. One clinically useful measurement of contractility is the ejection fraction (p. 521). However, according to Starling's law, ejection depends on end-diastolic volume (i.e., preload), which is *external* to the heart. Two somewhat better gauges of contractility are the **rate of pressure development** during ejection ($\Delta P/\Delta t$) and the velocity of ejection. Both correlate well with the velocity of shortening in Figure 21–10E and F, and they are very sensitive guides to the effect of inotropic interventions.

A third assessment of contractility focuses on the physiological relationship between pressure and volume during the cardiac cycle. In the era of echocardiography, these volume data are now reasonably easy to obtain. We return to the ventricular **pressure-volume loop** that we introduced in Figure 21–8A, and redraw it as the purple loop in Figure 21–11A. In this example, the end-diastolic volume is 120 ml. Point D′ on the loop represents the relationship between pressure and volume at the end of the isovolumetric contraction, when the aortic valve opens. If we had prevented the aortic valve from opening, ventricular pressure would have continued to rise until the ventricle could generate no additional tension. In this case, the pressure would rise to point G′, the theoretical maximum isovolumetric pressure. We could repeat the measurement at very different EDVs by decreasing or increasing the venous return. Point G represents the maximum isovolumetric pressure for an EDV below 120 ml (*red loop*), and point G″ for an EDV above 120 ml (*green loop*). A line through points G, G′, and G″ would describe the relationship between pressure and EDV under isometric (i.e., aortic valve closed) conditions—the equivalent of an isometric *Starling curve* (e.g., *brown curve* in Fig. 21–9A). The steeper this line, the greater the contractility.

It is impossible to measure maximum isovolumetric pressures in a patient because it is hardly advisable to prevent the aortic valve from opening. However, we can use the **end-systolic pressure** at point F′, on the normal pressure-volume loop with an EDV of 120 ml (*purple loop*). For an EDV below 120 ml (*red loop*), the corner point would slide down and to the left (F). Conversely,

for an EDV above 120 ml (*green loop*), the corner point would slide upward and to the right (F″). The corner points of many such pressure-volume loops fall along a line—the **end-systolic pressure-volume relation** (ESPVR)—that is very similar to that generated by the points G, G′, and G″.

EFFECT OF CHANGES IN CONTRACTILITY. The ESPVR is a clinically useful measure of contractility. Increasing contractility increases the slope of the ESPVR line, as in the shifts in the ventricular performance curves seen earlier (see Fig. 21–9C). For example, imagine that—with the same EDV and aortic pressure as in the control situation (see Fig. 21–11B, *violet area*)—we increase contractility. We represent increased contractility by steepening the ESPVR line (see Fig. 21–11B, *red dotted line*). The result is that ejection continues from point D′ to a new point F on the red loop until the left ventricular volume reaches a much lower value than normal. In other words, increased contractility increases *stroke volume*. Decreasing contractility would flatten the slope of the ESPVR and decrease stroke volume.

EFFECT OF CHANGES IN PRELOAD (i.e., INITIAL SARCOMERE LENGTH). A pressure-volume loop nicely illustrates the effect of an increased preload (i.e., increased filling or EDV) without changing contractility. Starting from the control situation (see Fig. 21–11C, *purple area*), increasing the EDV shifts the isovolumetric segment to the right (*CD on the red loop*). Because the volume change along segment DEF is larger than for the control situation, stroke volume increases—as predicted by Starling's law.

EFFECT OF CHANGES IN AFTER-LOAD. A pressure-volume loop also illustrates the effect of an increased after-load (i.e., increase in aortic pressure). Starting from the control situation (see Fig. 21–11D, *purple area*), increasing the aortic pressure shifts the upper right corner of the loop from point D′ to D (*red curve*) because the ventricle cannot open the aortic valve until ventricular pressure reaches the higher aortic pressure. During the ejection phase—assuming that contractility (i.e., slope of the ESPVR) does not change—the ventricle necessarily ejects less blood until segment DEF intersects the ESPVR line. Therefore, an increase in after-load (at constant contractility) causes the loop to be taller and narrower, so that stroke volume and ejection fraction both decrease. However, if we were to increase contractility (i.e., increase the slope of the ESPVR), we could return the stroke volume to normal.

Positive Inotropic Agents Increase Myocardial Contractility by Raising $[Ca^{2+}]_i$

Modifiers of contractility can affect the dynamics of cardiac muscle contraction, independent of preload or afterload. These factors have in common their ability to change $[Ca^{2+}]_i$. When these factors increase myocardial contractility, they are called positive inotropic agents. When they decrease myocardial contractility, they are called negative inotropic agents.

POSITIVE INOTROPIC AGENTS. Factors that increase myocardial contractility increase $[Ca^{2+}]_i$, either by opening

A STANDARD CONTRACTILITY CONDITIONS

B INCREASED CONTRACTILITY

C INCREASED PRELOAD (FILLING)

D INCREASED AFTER-LOAD (AORTIC PRESSURE)

FIGURE 21–11. Assessment of contractility using a ventricular pressure-volume loop. The *purple* pressure-volume loop is the normal curve in Figure 21–8*A*. In *A*, at the same normal state of cardiac contractility, the *red* loop is generated by decreasing end-diastolic volume (EDV), and the *green* loop is generated by increasing EDV. The slope of the line through the points at the end of systole (F, F′, and F″) represents the end-systolic pressure-volume relation (ESPVR).

CARDIAC HYPERTROPHY

Either volume overload or pressure overload can mechanically compromise the heart. A **volume overload** is an excessive EDV (i.e., preload). For example, a large arteriovenous shunt would volume overload both the left and right heart. The increased EDV leads to an increase in stroke volume (see Fig. 21–11 C), which elevates cardiac output. Systemic arterial pressure usually remains normal. A **pressure overload** is an excessive pressure in the ventricle's outflow tract (i.e., after-load). For the left heart, the problem would be an increase in systemic arterial pressure (i.e., hypertension). The increased aortic pressure leads to a decrease in stroke volume (see Fig. 21–11 D). However, because of a compensatory increase in heart rate, cardiac output usually remains normal.

Because cells of the adult heart are terminally differentiated, stimuli that might be mitogenic in other cells cannot elicit cell division in the heart, but rather cause the cardiac myocytes to hypertrophy and increase muscle mass. When, over time, this adaptive process becomes inadequate to cope with demand, the result is mechanical dysfunction and, ultimately, heart failure (see box titled Cellular Basis of Heart Failure). A host of events may trigger hypertrophy, including various hypertrophic factors, increases in $[Ca^{2+}]_i$, and mechanical forces.

Hypertrophic factors. Agents implicated in cardiac hypertrophy include the cardiac peptides **myotrophin** and **cardiotrophin**, as well as catecholamines, angiotensin II (ANG II), endothelin-1, insulin-like growth factor-II, transforming growth factor-β (TGF-β), and interleukin-1. Catecholamines and ANG II both activate the MAP kinase cascade (p. 134). Farther downstream the signal transduction pathway, the transcriptional response to hypertrophic stimuli includes the zinc finger transcription factor, GATA4 (p. 121), and perhaps also the transcription factors SRF and Sp1, as well as the TEF-1 family.

Calcium. Elevated $[Ca^{2+}]_i$ may be both a trigger for hypertrophy and part of signal transduction pathways that lead to hypertrophy. $[Ca^{2+}]_i$ in heart cells is probably elevated initially during chronic volume or pressure overloads, just as $[Ca^{2+}]_i$ would be elevated in a normal heart that is working hard. Elevated $[Ca^{2+}]_i$ may activate calcineurin, a Ca^{2+}-dependent phosphatase (p. 98). After being dephosphorylated by calcineurin, the transcription factor NF-AT3 can enter the nucleus and bind to GATA4 (see earlier), which transcriptionally activates genes responsible for hypertrophy. Mice that express constitutively activated forms of calcineurin develop cardiac hypertrophy and heart failure.

Mechanical factors. Mechanical stretch induces the expression of specific genes. The mechanical sensor that triggers cardiac hypertrophy may be MLP (muscle LIM protein), part of the myocardial cytoskeleton. Stretch activates a phosphorylation cascade of protein kinases: Raf-1 kinase, extracellular signal–regulated kinase (ERK), and a separate subfamily of the MAP kinases called SAPKs (for stretch-activated protein kinases). These various kinases regulate gene expression by activating the transcription factor AP-1 (p. 124).

The pathways we have just discussed lead to several changes in gene expression within cardiac myocytes during hypertrophy. In addition to synthesizing many housekeeping proteins, hypertrophic cardiac myocytes undergo other changes that are more specific for contraction. Some of the most striking changes include *reduced* levels of the mRNA encoding three critical proteins in the membrane of the sarcoplasmic reticulum: (1) the Ca^{2+} release channel, (2) phospholamban, and (3) the SR Ca^{2+} pump (SERCA2). In addition, cardiac hypertrophy is associated with increased levels of mRNA for the skeletal α actin, which is normally expressed in fetal, but not adult heart. Hypertrophic hearts also have increased expression of the angiogenic factor VEGF (p. 481).

Although a hypertrophied myocardial cell may be able to do more work than a nonhypertrophied cell, it has a lower "contractility" when normalized to its cross-sectional area. Why should hypertrophied cardiac muscle not be as good as normal muscle? Possibilities include alterations in the transient increases in $[Ca^{2+}]_i$ during the cardiac action potential and alterations in the expression of the contractile filaments, particularly the myosin isoenzymes.

Ca^{2+} channels, inhibiting Na-Ca exchange, or inhibiting the Ca^{2+} pump—all at the plasma membrane.

1. **Adrenergic agonists**. Catecholamines (e.g., epinephrine, norepinephrine) act on β_1 adrenoceptors to activate the α subunit of G_s-type heterotrimeric G proteins. The activated α_s subunits produce effects by two pathways. First, α_s raises intracellular levels of cyclic adenosine monophosphate (cAMP) and stimulates protein kinase A (p. 97), which can then act by the mechanisms summarized in Table 22–2 to increase contractility and speed relaxation. Second, α_s can directly open L-type Ca^{2+} channels in the plasma membrane, leading to an increased Ca^{2+} influx during action potentials, increased $[Ca^{2+}]_i$, and enhanced contractility.

2. **Cardiac glycosides**. Digitalis derivatives inhibit the Na-K pump on the plasma membrane (p. 63), and therefore raise $[Na^+]_i$. We would expect the increased $[Na^+]_i$ to slow down Na-Ca exchange, raise steady-state $[Ca^{2+}]_i$, and enhance contractility. Recent evidence suggests that cardiac glycosides may also increase $[Ca^{2+}]_i$ by a novel pathway—increasing the Ca^{2+} permeability of Na^+ channels in the plasma membrane.

3. **High extracellular $[Ca^{2+}]$**. Acting in two ways, elevated $[Ca^{2+}]_o$ increases $[Ca^{2+}]_i$ and thereby enhances contractility. First, it decreases the exchange of external Na^+ for internal Ca^{2+}. Secondly, more Ca^{2+} enters the myocardial cell through L-type Ca^{2+} channels during the action potential.

4. **Low extracellular $[Na^+]$**. Reducing the Na^+ gradient decreases Na-Ca exchange, raising $[Ca^{2+}]_i$ and enhancing contractility.

5. **Increased heart rate**. As we noted when introducing the staircase phenomenon (p. 530), an increased heart rate increases SR stores of Ca^{2+}, and also increases Ca^{2+} influx during the action potential.

CELLULAR BASIS OF HEART FAILURE

Heart failure is among the most common causes of hospitalization in developed countries for people aged 65 or older, and is a leading cause of death. People whose hearts cannot sustain an adequate cardiac output become breathless (because blood backs up from the left heart into the lungs) and have swollen feet and ankles (because blood backs up from the right heart and promotes net filtration in systemic capillaries—see box on edema on p. 473). On the cellular level, decreased contractility in heart failure could be a result of cardiac hypertrophy (see box titled Cardiac Hypertrophy), reflecting alterations in the transient increases of $[Ca^{2+}]_i$, the expression of the contractile filaments, or both.

Changes in $[Ca^{2+}]_i$ physiology could reflect altered properties of the L-type Ca^{2+} channel in the plasma membrane or the Ca^{2+} release channel (CRC) in the SR membrane. In an animal model of hypertension-induced cardiac hypertrophy that leads to heart failure, the L-type Ca^{2+} channels exhibit an impaired ability to activate the CRC via Ca^{2+}-induced Ca^{2+} release. A distortion of the microarchitecture in hypertrophic cells, and thus a distortion of the spacing between L-type Ca^{2+} channels and CRCs, could be responsible for impaired coupling.

Changes in the expression of contractile proteins can reduce contractility. Two isoforms of myosin heavy chain, αMHC and βMHC, are present in heart (see Table 9–1). The speed of muscle shortening increases with the relative expression of αMHC. In human heart failure, the amount of αMHC mRNA, relative to total MHC mRNA, falls from approximately 35% to approximately 2%.

An interesting animal model of heart failure is the knockout mouse that lacks the gene encoding MLP, the muscle LIM protein. MLP-deficient mice have the same disrupted cytoskeletal architecture seen in failing hearts. In addition, these mice have a dilated cardiomyopathy. Although humans with failing hearts are generally not deficient in MLP, the evidence from these knockout mice suggests that the MLP system could play a role in certain forms of cardiomyopathy.

NEGATIVE INOTROPIC AGENTS. Factors that decrease myocardial contractility all decrease $[Ca^{2+}]_i$.

1. **Ca^{2+}-channel blockers.** Inhibitors of L-type Ca^{2+} channels (p. 190)—such as verapamil, diltiazem, and nifedipine—reduce Ca^{2+} entry during the plateau of the cardiac action potential. By reducing $[Ca^{2+}]_i$, they decrease contractility.

2. **Low extracellular $[Ca^{2+}]$.** Depressed $[Ca^{2+}]_o$ lowers $[Ca^{2+}]_i$, both by increasing Ca^{2+} extrusion via Na-Ca exchange and by reducing Ca^{2+} entry through L-type Ca^{2+} channels during the plateau of the cardiac action potential.

3. **High extracellular $[Na^+]$.** Elevated $[Na^+]_o$ increases Na-Ca exchange, thereby decreasing $[Ca^{2+}]_i$.

REFERENCES

Books and Reviews

Cooper G IV: Load and length regulation of cardiac energetics. Annu Rev Physiol 52:505–522, 1990.

Sadoshima J, Izumo S: The cellular and molecular response of cardiac myocytes to mechanical stress. Annu Rev Physiol 59:551–571, 1997.

Simmerman HKB, Jones LR: Phospholamban: Protein structure, mechanism of action, and role in cardiac function. Physiol Rev 78:921–947, 1998.

Sonnenblick EH: Determinants of active state in heart muscle: Force, velocity, instantaneous muscle length, time. Federation Proc 24:1396–1409, 1965.

Wier WG: Cytoplasmic $[Ca^{2+}]$ in mammalian ventricle: Dynamic control by cellular processes. Annu Rev Physiol 52:467–485, 1990.

Zimmer H-G: The isolated perfused heart and its pioneers. News Physiol Sci 13:203–210, 1998.

Journal Articles

Frank O: Zur Dynamik des Herzmuskels. Zeitschr Biol 32:370–437, 1895.

Gómez AM, Valdivia HH, Cheng H, et al: Defective excitation-contraction coupling in experimental cardiac hypertrophy and heart failure. Science 276:800–806, 1997.

Patterson SW, Piper H, Starling EH: The regulation of the heart beat. J Physiol 48:465–513, 1914.

Sarnoff JS, Berglund E: Ventricular function. I. Starling's law of the heart studied by means of simultaneous right and left ventricular function curves in the dog. Circulation 9:706–718, 1954.

Wiggers CJ, Katz LN: The contours of ventricular volume curves under different conditions. Am J Physiol 58:439–475, 1922.

CHAPTER 22

Regulation of Arterial Pressure and Cardiac Output

Emile L. Boulpaep

When faced with a patient who appears seriously ill, clinicians focus their immediate attention on the patient's vital signs: temperature, respiratory rate, pulse, and blood pressure. These parameters are aptly named "vital" because they reflect the most fundamental aspects of health and even survival; a significant abnormality in any of these components indicates that emergent care is required.

In this chapter, we focus on blood pressure, a critical hemodynamic factor and one that is easily measured. An adequate blood pressure is necessary for proper organ perfusion. Too low, and we say that the patient is in shock. Too high, and we say that the patient is hypertensive; an acute and profound elevation of the blood pressure can be just as dangerous as one that suddenly plummets. Here, we examine both the short- and long-term mechanisms that the body uses to regulate arterial blood pressure.

Because the arterial blood pressure depends to a large degree on the cardiac output, we also examine the regulation of this critical parameter. Finally, because cardiac output also depends on the venous return of blood to the heart, we discuss the matching between input (i.e., venous return) and cardiac output.

SHORT-TERM REGULATION OF ARTERIAL PRESSURE

Systemic Mean Arterial Blood Pressure Is the Principal Variable That the Cardiovascular System Controls

Imagine that we must distribute city water to 1000 houses. We could decide in advance that each house uses 500 liters/day, and then pump this amount to each house at a constant rate. In other words, we would deliver approximately 20 liters/hr, regardless of actual water usage. The cardiovascular equivalent of such a system would be a circulation in which the cardiac output and the delivery of blood to each tissue remain constant.

Alternatively, we could connect all the houses to a single, large water tower that provides a constant pressure head. Because the height of the water level in the tower is fairly stable, all faucets in all houses see the same pressure at all times. This system offers several advantages. First, each house can regulate its water usage by opening faucets according to need. Second, heavy water usage in one house with all faucets open does not affect the pressure head in the other houses with only one faucet open. Third, the pressure head in the water tower guarantees that each house will receive sufficiently high pressure to send water to houses with upper floors.

This water tower system is analogous to our own circulatory system, which provides the same flexibility for distributing blood flow by, first and foremost, *controlling the systemic mean arterial blood pressure.*

The priority given to arterial pressure control is necessary because of the anatomy of the circulatory system: A network of branched arteries delivers to each organ a mean arterial pressure that approximates the mean aortic pressure. Thus, all organs, whether close to or distant from the heart, receive the same mean arterial pressure. Each organ, in turn, controls local blood flow by increasing or decreasing local arteriolar resistance. In Chapter 19, we described these local control mechanisms in a general way, and in Chapter 23, we will discuss specific vascular beds.

The system that we just introduced works because a change in blood flow in one vascular bed does not affect blood flow in other beds—as long as the heart can maintain the mean arterial pressure. However, the circulatory system must keep mean arterial pressure not only *constant*, but also *high enough* for glomerular filtration to occur in the kidneys or to overcome high tissue pressures in organs such as the eye.

Since Chapter 17, we have regarded the heart as the generator of a constant driving pressure. The principles of the feedback loops that the body uses to control the circulation are similar to those involved in the regulation of many other physiological systems. The short-term regulation of arterial pressure—on a time scale of seconds to minutes—occurs via neural pathways, and targets the heart, vessels, and adrenal medulla. This short-term regulation is the topic of the present discussion. The long-term regulation of arterial pressure—on a time scale of hours or days—occurs via pathways that target the blood vessels, as well as the kidneys, in their control of extracellular fluid volume. This long-term regulation is the topic of the final portion of the chapter.

Neural Reflexes Mediate the Short-Term Regulation of Mean Arterial Blood Pressure

The neural reflex systems that regulate mean arterial pressure operate as a series of **negative feedback loops**. All such loops are composed of the following elements:

1. A **detector**. A sensor or receptor quantitates the controlled variable and transduces it into an electrical signal that is a measure of the controlled variable.
2. **Afferent neural pathways**. These convey the message away from the detector, to the central nervous system (CNS).
3. A **coordinating center**. A control center in the CNS compares the signal detected in the periphery to a set point, generates an error signal, processes the information, and generates an appropriate response.
4. **Efferent neural pathways**. These convey the response from the coordinating center to the periphery.
5. **Effectors**. These elements act on the controlled variable and correct its deviation from the set point.

A dual system of sensors and neural reflexes controls mean arterial pressure. The primary sensors are baroreceptors, which are actually stretch receptors or mechano-

receptors that detect distention of the vascular walls. The secondary sensors are chemoreceptors that detect changes in blood PO_2, PCO_2, and pH. The control centers are located within the CNS, mostly in the medulla, but sites within the cerebral cortex and hypothalamus also exert control. The effectors include pacemaker and muscle cells in the heart, vascular smooth-muscle cells (VSMCs) in arteries and veins, and the adrenal medulla.

We all know from common experience that the CNS influences the circulation. Emotional stress can cause blushing of the skin or an increase in heart rate. Pain—or the stress of your first day in a gross anatomy laboratory—can elicit fainting because of a profound, generalized vasodilation and a decrease in heart rate (i.e., bradycardia).

Early physiologists, such as Claude Bernard, observed that stimulating peripheral sympathetic nerves causes vasoconstriction, and that interrupting the spinal cord in the lower cervical region drastically reduces blood pressure (i.e., produces hypotension). However, the first idea that a *reflex* might be involved in regulating the cardiovascular system came from experiments in which stimulating a particular sensory (i.e., afferent) nerve caused a change in heart rate and blood pressure. In 1866, E. de Cyon and Carl Ludwig studied the depressor nerve, a branch of the vagus nerve. After they transected this nerve, they found that stimulating the central (i.e., cranial) end of the cut nerve slows down the heart and produces hypotension. Hering showed that stimulating the central end of another cut nerve—the sinus nerve (nerve of Hering), which innervates the carotid sinus—also causes bradycardia and hypotension. These two experiments strongly suggested that the depressor and sinus nerves carry sensory information to the brain, and that the brain in some fashion uses this information to control cardiovascular function.

High-Pressure Baroreceptors at the Carotid Sinus and Aortic Arch Are Stretch Receptors That Sense Changes in Mean Arterial Blood Pressure

Corneille Heymans was the first to demonstrate that pressure receptors—called **baroreceptors**—are located in arteries, and that they are part of a neural feedback mechanism that regulates mean arterial pressure. He found that injecting epinephrine—also known as adrenaline—into a dog raises blood pressure and, later, lowers heart rate. Heymans hypothesized that increased blood pressure stimulates arterial sensors, which send a neural signal to the brain, and that the brain in turn transmits a neural signal to the heart, resulting in bradycardia.

In order to demonstrate that the posited feedback loop did not depend on the blood-borne traffic of chemicals between the periphery and the CNS, Heymans cross-perfused two dogs, so that only nerves connected the head of the dog to the rest of the animal's body. The dog's head received its blood flow from a second animal. (Today, one would use a heart-lung machine to perfuse the head of the first dog.) Heymans found that the vagus nerve carried both the upward and the downward traffic

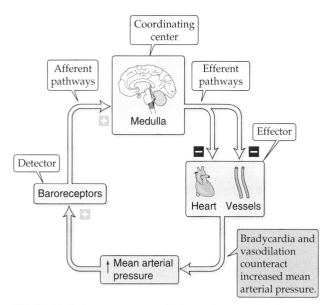

FIGURE 22–1. Baroreceptor control of arterial pressure. In this example, we assume that an increase in mean arterial pressure *(violet box)* is the primary insult.

for the reflex arc, and that agents carried in the blood played no role. He used a similar approach to demonstrate the role of the peripheral chemoreceptors in the control of respiration (p. 723). For his work on the neural control of respiration, Heymans received the Nobel Prize in Physiology or Medicine for 1938.

The entire control process, known as the **baroreceptor control of arterial pressure** (Fig. 22–1), consists of baroreceptors (i.e., the detectors), afferent neuronal pathways, control centers in the medulla, efferent neuronal pathways, and the heart and blood vessels (i.e., the effectors). The negative feedback loop is designed so that *increased mean arterial pressure causes vasodilation and bradycardia, whereas decreased mean arterial pressure causes vasoconstriction and tachycardia* (i.e., increased heart rate).

The sensor component consists of a set of mechanoreceptors located at strategic *high-pressure sites* within the cardiovascular system. As discussed later, the cardiovascular system also has *low-pressure* sensors that detect changes in venous pressure. The two most important high-pressure loci are the carotid sinus and the aortic arch. Stretching the vessel walls at either of these sites causes vasodilation and bradycardia. The **carotid sinus** (Fig. 22–2A) is a very distensible portion of the wall of the internal carotid artery, located just above the branching of the common carotid artery into the external and internal carotid arteries. The arterial wall at the carotid sinus contains thin lamellae of elastic fibers, but very little collagen or smooth muscle. The **aortic arch** (see Fig. 22–2B) is also a highly compliant portion of the arterial tree that distends during each left ventricular ejection.

The baroreceptors in both the carotid sinus and the aortic arch are the branched and coiled bare ends of myelinated sensory nerve fibers, which are intermeshed within the elastic layers. The cell bodies of these *bipolar neurons* are located in ganglia near the brain stem, and

the other end of the neuron projects to the medulla. An increase in the transmural pressure difference enlarges the vessel, and thereby deforms these receptors. Therefore, the baroreceptors are not really pressure sensitive, but *stretch sensitive*. Directly stretching the receptors results in increased firing of the baroreceptor's sensory nerve. The difference between stretch sensitivity and pressure sensitivity becomes apparent when one prevents the expansion of the vessel by surrounding the arterial wall with a plaster cast. When this is done, increasing the transmural pressure fails to increase the firing rate of the baroreceptor nerve. Removing the cast restores the response. Other tissues surrounding the receptors act as a sort of mechanical filter, although much less so than the plaster cast.

As shown by the *red records* in the upper two panels of Figure 22–3A, a step increase in transmural pressure (i.e., stretch) produces an inward current that depolarizes the receptor, generating a **receptor potential** (p. 326). The pressure increase actually causes a biphasic response in the receptor voltage. Following a large initial depolarization (the *dynamic* component) is a more modest but steady depolarization (the *static* component). This receptor potential, unlike a regenerative action potential, is a graded response, whose amplitude is proportional to the degree of stretch (compare *red and purple records*). Patch-clamp experiments on the cell bodies of the aortic baroreceptor neurons, which are located in the nodose ganglion (a sensory ganglion of the vagus nerve), have identified nonselective cation channels that are stretch sensitive and blocked by Gd^{3+}. These channels may be the mechano-electrical transducers in baroreceptor nerve endings, although other channels may help to set the sensitivity of the baroreceptor.

Increased Arterial Pressure Increases the Firing Rate of Afferent Baroreceptor Pathways

If, in the absence of a pressure step, we depolarize the baroreceptor nerve ending, the result is an increase in the frequency of action potentials in the sensory nerve. Therefore, it is not surprising that graded increases in pressure produce graded increases in the spike frequency (see Fig. 22–3A, lower two panels). Graded *decreases* in pressure gradually diminish receptor activity until the firing falls to vanishingly low frequencies at pressures around 40 to 60 mm Hg. Therefore, the baroreceptor encodes the mechanical response as a **frequency-modulated signal**.

The large initial depolarization produced by a step increase in pressure is accompanied by a transiently high frequency of discharge. The smaller, steady depolarization is accompanied by a steady but lower spike frequency. Because baroreceptors have both a static and a dynamic component, they are sensitive to the *waveform* as well as the *amplitude* of a pressure oscillation. Therefore, it is not surprising that bursts of action potentials may occur in phase with the cardiac cycle; they encode information on the pulse pressure (i.e., difference between the peak systolic and lowest diastolic pressures). The **static** pressure-activity curve in Figure 22–3B—obtained on single units

A INNERVATION OF CAROTID SINUS AND BODY

B INNERVATION OF AORTIC ARCH AND BODIES

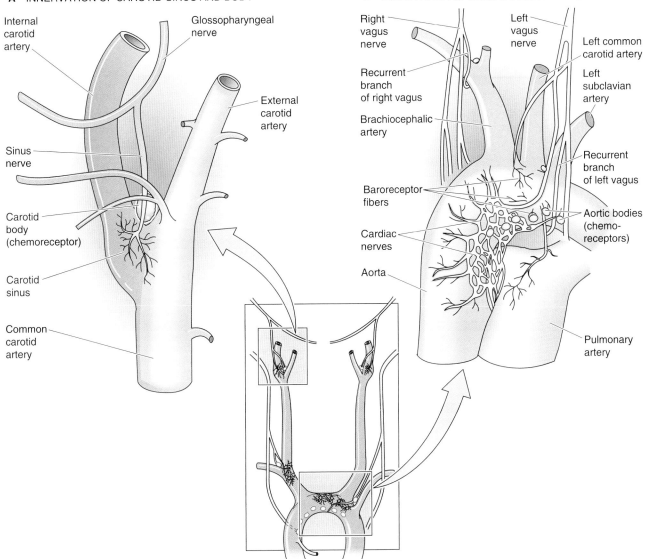

FIGURE 22–2. Afferent pathways of the high-pressure baroreceptors. In B, the chemoreceptors (i.e., aortic bodies) are located on the underside of the aortic arch, as well as at the bifurcation of the right brachiocephalic artery. On the *left*, aortic bodies, if present, are in a notch between the common carotid and the left subclavian arteries.

of the sinus nerve—shows that the spike frequency rises sigmoidally with increases in *steady* blood pressure. The **pulsatile** pressure-activity curve in Figure 22–3B shows that, when the pressure is *oscillating*, the mean discharge frequency at low mean pressures is higher than when pressure is steady.

Not all receptors within an arterial site have the same properties. As we gradually increase intravascular pressure, different single units in the isolated carotid sinus begin to fire at different static pressures. Thus, the overall baroreceptor response to a pressure increase includes both an increased firing rate of active units and the **recruitment** of more units, until a saturation level is reached at approximately 200 mm Hg. The carotid sinus in some individuals is unusually sensitive. When wearing a tight collar, such a person may faint just from turning

the head because compressing or stretching the carotid sinus orders the medulla to lower blood pressure.

The responses of the receptors in the carotid sinus and the aortic arch are different. In a given individual, a change in the carotid sinus pressure has a greater effect on the systemic arterial pressure than does a change in the aortic pressure. Compared with the carotid sinus receptor, the **aortic arch receptor**

▷ Has a higher threshold for activating the static response (~110 mm Hg vs ~50 mm Hg),
▷ Has a higher threshold, likewise, for the dynamic response,
▷ Continues responding to pressure increases at pressures at which the carotid baroreceptor has already saturated,

A RESPONSE TO INCREASED PRESSURE

B PRESSURE-ACTIVITY RELATIONSHIPS

FIGURE 22–3. Afferent pathways of the high-pressure baroreceptors.

▷ Is less sensitive to the rate of pressure change, and
▷ Responds less effectively to a decrease in pressure than to an increase in pressure (over the same pressure range).

Once a change in the arterial pressure has produced a change in the firing rate of the sensory nerve, the signal travels to the medulla. The afferent pathway for the carotid sinus reflex is the **sinus nerve**, which then joins the **glossopharyngeal** trunk (CN IX; see Fig. 22–2A). The cell bodies of the carotid baroreceptors are located in the petrosal (or inferior) ganglion of the glossopharyngeal nerve (Fig. 22–4A). The afferent pathways for the aortic arch reflex are sensory fibers in the **depressor branch** of the **vagus nerve** (CN X; see Fig. 22–2B). After joining the superior laryngeal nerves, the sensory fibers run cranially to their cell bodies in the nodose (or inferior) ganglion of the vagus (see Fig. 22–4A).

The Medulla Coordinates Afferent Baroreceptor Signals

The entire complex of medullary nuclei involved in cardiovascular regulation is called the **medullary cardiovascular center**. Within this center, broad subdivisions can be distinguished, such as a vasomotor area and a cardioinhibitory area. The medullary cardiovascular center receives all important information from the baroreceptors and is the major coordinating center for cardiovascular homeostasis.

Most afferent fibers from the two high-pressure baroreceptors project to the **nucleus tractus solitarius** (NTS; p. 393), one of which is located on each side of the medulla (see Fig. 22–4A and B). The neurotransmitter released by the baroreceptor afferents onto the NTS neurons is probably glutamate or substance P. Some neurons in the NTS (and also in the dorsal motor nucleus of the vagus, see later) have P_{2x} purinoceptors that are activated by extracellular ATP.

Inhibitory interneurons project from the NTS onto the **vasomotor area** in the ventrolateral medulla (see Fig. 22–4B). This "vasomotor area" includes the A1 and C1 areas in the rostral ventrolateral medulla, as well as the inferior olivary complex and other nuclei. Stimulating the neurons in the **C1 area** produces a vasoconstrictor response. Unless inhibited by output from the NTS interneurons, neurons within the C1 area produce a tonic output that promotes vasoconstriction. Therefore, an increase in pressure stimulates baroreceptor firing, which, in turn, causes NTS interneurons to inhibit C1 neurons, resulting in va*sodilation*. This C1 pathway largely accounts for the *vascular* component of the baroreceptor reflex. The bursting pattern of C1 neurons is locked to the cardiac cycle.

Other *excitatory* interneurons project from the NTS onto a **cardioinhibitory area**, which includes the nucleus ambiguus and the dorsal motor nucleus of the vagus (p. 389). Neurons in the dorsal motor nucleus of the vagus largely account for the *cardiac* component of the baroreceptor reflex (i.e., bradycardia). Also located in the dorsal medulla is a **cardioacceleratory** area. Stimulating neurons

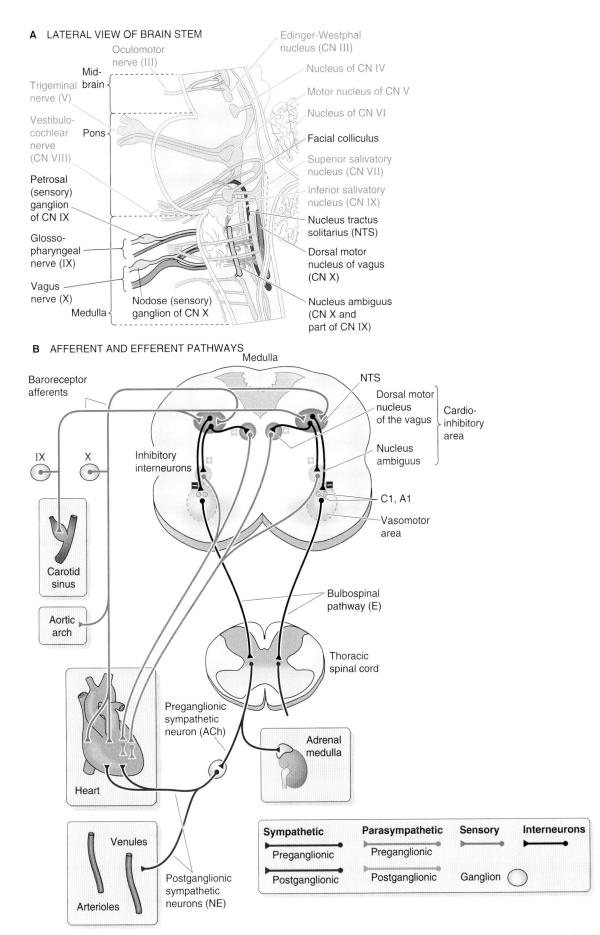

A LATERAL VIEW OF BRAIN STEM

Oculomotor nerve (III)

Edinger-Westphal nucleus (CN III)

Mid-brain

Trigeminal nerve (V)

Nucleus of CN IV

Motor nucleus of CN V

Vestibulo-cochlear nerve (CN VIII)

Pons

Nucleus of CN VI

Facial colliculus

Superior salivatory nucleus (CN VII)

Petrosal (sensory) ganglion of CN IX

Inferior salivatory nucleus (CN IX)

Nucleus tractus solitarius (NTS)

Glosso-pharyngeal nerve (IX)

Dorsal motor nucleus of vagus (CN X)

Vagus nerve (X)

Medulla

Nodose (sensory) ganglion of CN X

Nucleus ambiguus (CN X and part of CN IX)

B AFFERENT AND EFFERENT PATHWAYS

Medulla

Baroreceptor afferents

NTS

Dorsal motor nucleus of the vagus

Cardio-inhibitory area

IX   X

Inhibitory interneurons

Nucleus ambiguus

C1, A1

Vasomotor area

Carotid sinus

Aortic arch

Bulbospinal pathway (E)

Thoracic spinal cord

Preganglionic sympathetic neuron (ACh)

Adrenal medulla

Heart

Venules

Arterioles

Postganglionic sympathetic neurons (NE)

Sympathetic	Parasympathetic	Sensory	Interneurons
Preganglionic	Preganglionic		
Postganglionic	Postganglionic	Ganglion	

FIGURE 22–4. Medullary control centers for the cardiovascular system. In *A*, the relevant nuclei and cranial nerves are colorized and labeled in dark type. *B* is a hypothetical section through the medulla, showing projections of structures that do not necessarily co-exist in a single cross section. ACh, acetylcholine; CN, cranial nerve; NTS, nucleus tractus solitarius.

in this area causes heart rate and cardiac contractility to increase. NTS interneurons probably inhibit the cardioacceleratory area, resulting in decreased heart rate and contractility.

The Efferent Pathways of the Baroreceptor Response Include Both Sympathetic and Parasympathetic Divisions of the Autonomic Nervous System

After the medullary cardiovascular center has processed the information from the afferent baroreceptor pathways, and has integrated it with data coming from other pathways, this center must send signals back to the periphery via efferent (i.e., motor) pathways. The baroreceptor response has two major efferent pathways: the sympathetic and parasympathetic divisions of the autonomic nervous system (ANS).

SYMPATHETIC EFFERENTS. As was discussed earlier, increased baroreceptor activity instructs the NTS to *inhibit* the C1 (i.e., vasomotor) and cardioacceleratory areas of the medulla. "Bulbospinal" neurons in both areas send axons down the spinal cord to synapse directly with preganglionic sympathetic neurons in the spinal cord. The excitatory neurotransmitter at this synapse is not known, which is unfortunate, because this synapse could be a target for the pharmacologic control of blood pressure.

The cell bodies of the preganglionic sympathetic neurons are located in the intermediolateral gray matter of the spinal cord, between levels T1 and L3 (see Fig. 15–4). After considerable convergence and divergence, most of the axons from these preganglionic neurons synapse with postganglionic sympathetic neurons located within ganglia of the paravertebral sympathetic chain, as well as within prevertebral ganglia (see Fig. 15–2). The neurotransmitter between the preganglionic and postganglionic sympathetic neurons is acetylcholine (ACh), which acts at N_2 nicotinic acetylcholine receptors (p. 385). Because of the convergence and divergence, sympathetic output does not distribute according to dermatomes (p. 383). Postganglionic sympathetic fibers control a wide range of functions (see Fig. 15–4). Those that control blood pressure run with the large blood vessels and innervate both *arteries/arterioles and veins*.

Increased sympathetic activity produces vasoconstriction. Indeed, the baroreceptor reflex produces *vasodilation* because it *inhibits* the tonic stimulatory output of the vasomotor C1 neurons. Because the bulbospinal C1 neurons synapse with preganglionic sympathetic neurons between T1 and L3, severing the spinal cord above T1 causes a severe fall in blood pressure. Sectioning the cord below L3 produces no fall in blood pressure.

Another important target of postganglionic neurons with a cardiovascular mission is the heart. Output from the middle cervical and stellate ganglia, along with that from several upper thoracic ganglia (see Fig. 15–4), ramifies and, after extensive convergence and divergence, forms the cardiac nerves. Thus, severing the spinal cord above T1 would block the input to the preganglionic sympathetic fibers to the heart. In addition, some preganglionic fibers do not synapse in sympathetic ganglia at all, but directly innervate the chromaffin cells of the *adrenal*

medulla via the splanchnic nerve. These cells release epinephrine, which acts on the heart and blood vessels (see later in chapter).

PARASYMPATHETIC EFFERENTS. As was noted earlier, increased baroreceptor activity instructs the NTS to stimulate neurons in the nucleus ambiguus and the dorsal motor nucleus of the vagus (cardioinhibitory area). The target neurons in these two nuclei are preganglionic parasympathetic fibers of the vagus nerve (CN X) that project to the heart. These efferent vagal fibers follow the common carotid arteries, ultimately synapsing in small ganglia in the walls of the atria. There, they release acetylcholine onto the N_2 nicotinic receptors of the postganglionic parasympathetic neurons. The short postganglionic fibers then innervate the *sinoatrial (SA) node, the atria, and the ventricles*, where they act primarily to slow conduction through the heart (see below).

The Principal Effectors in the Neural Control of Arterial Pressure Are the Heart, the Arteries, the Veins, and the Adrenal Medulla

The cardiovascular system uses several effector organs to control systemic arterial pressure: the heart, arteries, veins, and adrenal medulla (Fig. 22–5).

SYMPATHETIC INPUT TO THE HEART (CARDIAC NERVES). The sympathetic division of the ANS influences the heart through the cardiac nerves, which form a plexus near the heart (see Fig. 22–2). The postganglionic fibers, which release **norepinephrine**, innervate the SA node, atria, and ventricles. Their effect is to increase both heart rate and contractility (Table 22–1). Because it dominates the innervation of the SA node (which is in the right atrium), sympathetic input from the *right* cardiac nerve has more effect on the *heart rate* than input from the left cardiac nerve. On the other hand, sympathetic input from the *left* cardiac nerve has more effect on *contractility*. In general, the cardiac nerves do not exert a strong tonic cardioacceleratory activity on the heart. At rest, their firing rate is less than that of the vagus nerve.

PARASYMPATHETIC INPUT TO THE HEART (VAGUS NERVE). The vagus normally exerts an intense tonic, parasympathetic activity on the heart via **acetylcholine** released by the postganglionic fibers. Severing the vagus nerve or administering atropine (which blocks the action of acetylcholine) increases heart rate. Indeed, experiments on the effects of the vagus on the heart led to the discovery of the first neurohumoral transmitter, acetylcholine (p. 205). Vagal stimulation decreases heart rate by its effect on pacemaker activity (p. 493). Just as the actions of the right and left cardiac nerves are somewhat different, the right vagus is a more effective inhibitor of the SA node than the left. The left vagus is a more effective inhibitor of conduction through the AV node. Vagal stimulation, to some extent, also reduces cardiac contractility.

SYMPATHETIC INPUT TO BLOOD VESSELS (VASOCONSTRICTOR RESPONSE). The vasoconstrictor sympathetic fibers are disseminated widely throughout the blood vessels of the body. These fibers are most abundant in the kidney and the skin, relatively sparse in the coronary and

FIGURE 22–5. Autonomic control of cardiovascular end organs.

TABLE 22-1

EFFECTS OF SYMPATHETIC AND PARASYMPATHETIC PATHWAYS ON THE CARDIOVASCULAR SYSTEM

EFFECTOR RESPONSE	ANATOMIC PATHWAY	NEUROTRANSMITTER RELEASED AT EFFECTOR	RECEPTOR	G PROTEIN	ENZYME OR PROTEIN	2nd MESSAGE
Tachycardia	Sympathetic	Norepinephrine	β_1 on cardiac pacemaker	$G\alpha_s$	Activates AC	↑ $[cAMP]_i$
Bradycardia	Parasympathetic	Acetylcholine	M_2 on cardiac pacemaker	Direct action of dimeric $G_i\beta\gamma$	GIRK K^+ channels	ΔV_m
Increase cardiac contractility	Sympathetic	Norepinephrine	β_1 on cardiac myocyte	$G\alpha_s$ Direct action of $G\alpha_s$ on L-type Ca^{2+} channels	Activates AC	↑ $[cAMP]_i$
Decrease cardiac contractility	Parasympathetic	Acetylcholine	M_2 on cardiac myocyte	$G\alpha_i$	↓ AC	↓ [cAMP]
			Presynaptic M_2 receptor on noradrenergic neuron	$G\alpha_i$	↓ AC	↓ $[cAMP]_i$ in neuron
Vasoconstriction in most blood vessels (e.g., skin)	Sympathetic	Norepinephrine	α_1 on VSMC	$G\alpha_q$	Activates PLC	↑ $[Ca^{2+}]_i$
Vasoconstriction some blood vessels	Sympathetic	Norepinephrine	α_2 on VSMC	$G\alpha_{i/o}$	↓ AC	↓ $[cAMP]_i$
Vasodilation in most blood vessels (e.g., muscle)	Adrenal medulla	Epinephrine	β_2 on VSMC	$G\alpha_s$	Activates AC	↑ $[cAMP]_i$
Vasodilation in erectile blood vessels	Parasympathetic	Acetylcholine	Presynaptic M_2 receptor on noradrenergic neurons	$G\alpha_i$	Inhibits AC	↓ $[cAMP]_i$ in neuron
		Acetylcholine	M_3 on endothelial cell	$G\alpha_q$	Activates PLC, Ca^{2+} release, activates NOS	NO diffuses to VSMC
		NO	NO receptor (i.e., GC) inside VSMC	—	Stimulates GC	↑ $[cGMP]_i$
		VIP	VIP receptor on VSMC	$G\alpha_s$	Stimulates AC	↑ $[cAMP]_i$
Vasodilation in blood vessels of salivary gland	Parasympathetic	Acetylcholine	M_3 receptor on gland cell	$G\alpha_q$	Activates kallikrein	Kinins
Vasodilation in blood vessels of muscle in "fight or flight" response	Sympathetic	Acetylcholine	Presynaptic M_2 receptor on noradrenergic neurons	$G\alpha_i$	Inhibits AC	↓ $[cAMP]_i$ in neuron
		NANC	Receptor on VSMC			

AC, adenylyl cyclase; cAMP, cyclic adenosine monophosphate; GC, guanylyl cyclase; GIRK, G-protein–activated/inwardly rectifying K^+ channel; NANC, non-adrenergic/non-cholinergic; NO, nitric oxide; NOS, nitric oxide synthase; PLC, phospholipase C; VIP, vasoactive intestinal peptide; VSMC, vascular smooth-muscle cell.

cerebral vessels, and absent in the placenta. They release norepinephrine, which binds to adrenoceptors on the membrane of vascular smooth-muscle cells. In most vascular beds, *vasodilation* is the result of a decrease in the tonic discharge of the vasoconstrictor sympathetic nerves.

PARASYMPATHETIC INPUT TO BLOOD VESSELS (VASO*DI-LATOR* **RESPONSE).** Parasympathetic vaso*dilator* fibers are far less common than sympathetic vaso*constrictor* fibers. The parasympathetic vasodilator fibers supply the salivary and some gastrointestinal glands, and are also crucial for vasodilating erectile tissue in the external genitalia (p. 1136 and 1162). Postganglionic parasympathetic fibers release acetylcholine, which, as we shall see, *indirectly* causes vasodilation. In addition, these fibers may produce vasodilation by releasing nitric oxide (NO) (p. 391) or other cotransmitters.

SYMPATHETIC INPUT TO BLOOD VESSELS IN SKELETAL MUSCLE (VASO*DILATOR* **RESPONSE).** In addition to the more widespread sympathetic vasoconstrictor fibers, skeletal muscle in nonprimates has a special system of sympathetic fibers that produce *vasodilation* (p. 388). These special fibers innervate the large precapillary vessels in skeletal muscle. The origin of the sympathetic vasodilator pathway is very different from that of the vasoconstrictor pathway, which receives its instructions—ultimately—from the vasomotor area of the medulla. Instead, the sympathetic vasodilator fibers receive their instructions—ultimately—from neurons in the cerebral cortex, which synapse on other neurons in the hypothalamus or in the mesencephalon. The fibers from these second neurons (analogous to the bulbospinal neurons discussed earlier) transit through the medulla without interruption, and reach the spinal cord. There, these fibers synapse on preganglionic sympathetic neurons in the intermediolateral column, just as do other descending neurons. The vasodilatory preganglionic fibers synapse in the sympathetic ganglia on postganglionic neurons that terminate on VSMCs surrounding skeletal-muscle blood vessels. These postganglionic vasodilatory fibers release acetylcholine and perhaps other transmitters.

Therefore, blood vessels within skeletal muscle receive both sympathetic adrenergic and sympathetic cholinergic innervation. The cholinergic system, acting directly via muscarinic receptors (p. 387), relaxes VSMCs and causes rapid vasodilation. This vasodilation in skeletal muscle occurs in the "fight or flight" response, as well as perhaps during the anticipatory response in exercise (p. 394). In both cases, mobilization of the sympathetic vasodilator system is accompanied by extensive activation of the sympathetic division, including cardiac effects (i.e., increased heart rate and contractility) and generalized vasoconstriction of all vascular beds *except those in skeletal muscle.* (Little vasoconstriction occurs in cerebral and coronary beds, which have sparse sympathetic vasoconstrictor innervation.)

ADRENAL MEDULLA. We have already mentioned that some preganglionic sympathetic fibers in the sympathetic splanchnic nerves also innervate the chromaffin cells in the adrenal medulla. Therefore, the adrenal medulla is the equivalent of a sympathetic ganglion. The synaptic terminals of the preganglionic fibers release ACh, which acts

on nicotinic receptors of the **chromaffin cells** of the adrenal medulla (p. 1061). Chromaffin cells are thus modified postganglionic neurons that release their transmitters—**epinephrine** and, to a far lesser degree, norepinephrine—into the bloodstream rather than onto a specific end organ. Thus, the adrenal medulla participates as a global effector that, through its release of epinephrine, causes generalized effects on the circulation. As we will see in the next section, the epinephrine released by the adrenal medulla acts on both the heart and the blood vessels, and thereby contributes to the control of the systemic arterial pressure.

The Unique Combination of Agonists and Complement of Receptors Determine the End Response in the Cardiac and Vascular Effector Cells

ADRENERGIC RECEPTORS IN THE HEART. The *sympathetic* output to the heart affects both heart rate and contractility. Norepinephrine, released by the postganglionic sympathetic neurons, acts on postsynaptic β_1-adrenergic receptors of pacemaker cells in the SA node, as well as on similar receptors of myocardial cells in the atria and ventricles. The β_1 adrenoceptor, via the G-protein G_s, acts via the cyclic adenosine monophosphate (cAMP)–protein kinase A (PKA) pathway (p. 97) to phosphorylate multiple effector molecules in both pacemaker cells and cardiac myocytes (see Table 22–1).

In **pacemaker cells**, β_1 and L-type agonists stimulate (1) I_{Ca}, a Ca^{2+} current through T-type Ca^{2+} channels (p. 488); and (2) I_f, the diastolic Na^+ current through nonselective cation channels (p. 488). The net effect of these two changes is an increased rate of diastolic depolarization (i.e., "phase 4" of action potential; see Fig. 20–3A) and a negative shift in the threshold for the action potential (p. 493). Because diastole shortens, the *heart rate* increases.

In **myocardial cells**, β_1 agonists exert several parallel effects via PKA (Table 22–2). In addition, the activated α_s subunit of the G protein can directly activate L-type Ca^{2+} channels. The net effect of these pathways are contractions that are both stronger (p. 493) and briefer (p. 525).

CHOLINERGIC RECEPTORS IN THE HEART. Parasympathetic output to the heart affects heart rate and, to a much lesser extent, contractility. Acetylcholine released by postsynaptic parasympathetic neurons binds to M_2 muscarinic (i.e., G protein–coupled) receptors on pacemaker cells of the SA node and on ventricular myocytes (see Table 22–1).

In **pacemaker cells**, ACh triggers a membrane-delimited signalling pathway mediated not by the G-protein α subunits, but rather by the $\beta\gamma$ heterodimers (p. 95). The newly released $\beta\gamma$ subunits directly open inward-rectifier K^+ channels (GIRK) in pacemaker cells (p. 488). The resulting elevation of the K^+ conductance makes the maximum diastolic potential more negative during phase 4 of the action potential. ACh also reduces I_f and I_{Ca} (p. 493), thereby reducing the rate of diastolic depolarization, and making the threshold more positive. The net effect is a reduction in heart rate.

In **myocardial cells**, M_2 receptor occupancy has a mi-

TABLE 22-2

EFFECTS OF ACTIVATING THE β_1 ADRENERGIC RECEPTOR IN VENTRICULAR MUSCLE

β_1 adrenoceptor
↓
Activated α_s
↓
↑ Adenylyl cyclase
↓
↑ cAMP
↓
↑ PKA
↓

Phosphorylation of L-type Ca^{2+} channels	Phosphorylation of phospholamban	Phosphorylation of troponin I	Interaction of α_s with L-type Ca^{2+} channels
↑ Open probability of L-type Ca^{2+} channels	↑ SR Ca^{2+} pump	↑ Off-rate of Ca^{2+} from Ca^{2+}/troponin C complex	↑ Open probability of L-type Ca^{2+} channels
↑ Ca^{2+} influx	↑ Ca^{2+} re-uptake into SR ↑ Ca^{2+} stores	↑ Speed of relaxation (lusitropic)	↑ Ca^{2+} influx
↑ $[Ca^{2+}]_i$	↑ Speed of relaxation (lusitropic effect)	↓ Duration of contraction	↑ $[Ca^{2+}]_i$
↑ Ca^{2+}-induced Ca^{2+} release from the SR (CICR)	↓ Duration of contraction		↑ Ca^{2+}-induced Ca^{2+} release from the SR (CICR)
↑ Contractility			↑ Contractility

nor negative inotropic effect. The sequence of events appears to be sequential activation of G proteins, phospholipase C (PLC), and then nitric oxide synthase (NOS) (p. 110), which forms NO. The NO stimulates guanylyl cyclase, and thereby increases levels of cyclic guanosine monophosphate (cGMP), which somehow inhibits L-type Ca^{2+} channels and decreases Ca^{2+} influx. Hence, the cholinergic increase in $[cGMP]_i$ counteracts the increased Ca^{2+} influx triggered by an adrenergic increase in $[cAMP]_i$. Thus, cGMP reduces contractile strength, while keeping the contractions rather long.

ADRENERGIC RECEPTORS IN BLOOD VESSELS. The sympathetic division of the ANS can modulate the tone of vascular smooth muscle in arteries, arterioles, and veins via two distinct routes—postganglionic sympathetic neurons and the adrenal medulla. Whether the net effect of sympathetic stimulation in a particular vessel is vasoconstriction (increased VSMC tone) or vasodilation (decreased VSMC tone) depends on four factors: (1) which agonist is released, (2) which adrenoceptors that agonist binds to, (3) whether receptor occupancy tends to cause vasoconstriction or vasodilation, and (4) which receptor subtypes happen to be present on a particular VSMC.

Which agonist is released is the most straightforward of the factors—postganglionic sympathetic neurons release norepinephrine, and the adrenal medulla releases primarily epinephrine.

Which receptors the agonist binds to is more complex. Norepinephrine and epinephrine do not have exclusive affinity for a single type of adrenoceptor. The original α and β designations followed from the observation that

norepinephrine appeared to have its greatest activity on α receptors, and epinephrine, on β receptors. However, although norepinephrine binds with a greater affinity to α receptors than to β receptors, it also can activate β receptors. Similarly, although epinephrine binds with a greater affinity to β receptors than to α receptors, it can also activate α receptors. Of course, synthetic agonists may be more specific and potent than either norepinephrine or epinephrine (e.g., the α agonist phenylephrine and β agonist isoproterenol). A finer pharmacologic and molecular dissection reveals that both α and β receptors have subgroups (e.g., β_1 and β_2), and even the subgroups have subgroups (p. 388). Each of these many adrenoceptor types has a unique pharmacology. Thus, the β_1 receptor has about the same affinity for epinephrine and norepinephrine, but the β_2 receptor has a higher affinity for epinephrine than for norepinephrine.

Whether receptor occupancy tends to cause vasoconstriction or vasodilation is straightforward (see Table 22–1). The *vasoconstriction* elicited by catecholamines is an α effect, in particular, an α_1 effect. Thus, norepinephrine released from nerve terminals acts on the α_1 adrenoceptor, which is coupled to the G protein G_q. The resulting activation of phospholipase C (p. 100) and formation of inositol-1,4,5-triphosphate (IP_3) lead to a rise in $[Ca^{2+}]_i$ and smooth-muscle contraction. In contrast, *vasodilation*, elicited by epinephrine released from the adrenal medulla, is a β_2 effect. Occupancy of the β_2 adrenoceptor triggers the cAMP-PKA pathway, leading to phosphorylation of myosin light chain kinase (MLCK; see p. 238), which reduces the sensitivity of MLCK to the Ca^{2+}-calmodulin complex, resulting by default in smooth-muscle relaxation (p. 478).

Which receptor subtypes happen to be present on a particular VSMC is a complex issue. Many blood vessels are populated with a mixture of α-receptor or β-receptor subtypes, each stimulated to varying degrees by norepinephrine and epinephrine. Therefore, the response of the cell depends on the relative dominance of the subtype of receptor present on the cell surface. Fortunately, the only two subtypes in blood vessels that matter clinically are α_1 and β_2.

The ultimate outcome in the target tissue (vasoconstriction vs. vasodilation) depends on both the heterogeneous mixture of agonists (norepinephrine vs. epinephrine) applied and the heterogeneous mixture of receptors (α_1 and β_2) present in the VSMC. As an example, consider blood vessels in the skin and heart. Because cutaneous blood vessels have *only* α_1 receptors, they can only vasoconstrict, regardless of whether the agonist is norepinephrine or epinephrine. On the other hand, epinephrine causes coronary blood vessels to dilate because they have a greater number of β_2 receptors than α_1 receptors.

CHOLINERGIC RECEPTORS IN OR NEAR BLOOD VESSELS. Adding ACh to an isolated VSMC causes contraction. Thus, in an artificial situation in which the nerve terminals release only ACh, and in which no other tissues are present, ACh would lead to vasoconstriction (see Table 19–9). In real life, however, ACh dilates blood vessels by binding to muscarinic receptors on neighboring cells, and generating *other* messengers that indirectly cause vasodilation (see Table 22–1). For example, in erectile tissue and skeletal muscle, ACh may bind to M_2 receptors on the presynaptic membranes of postganglionic sympathetic neurons, decreasing $[cAMP]_i$ and inhibiting the release of norepinephrine. Thus, inhibiting vasoconstriction produces vasodilation.

In erectile tissue, ACh also binds to M_3 receptors on vascular *endothelial cells*, and acts through the PLC pathway to release IP_3 and raise $[Ca^{2+}]_i$ (see Fig. 15–11). The Ca^{2+} stimulates nitric oxide synthase to produce nitric oxide (p. 110), which diffuses from the endothelial to the vascular smooth-muscle cell. Inside the VSMC, the NO activates soluble guanylyl cyclase, resulting in the production of cGMP and activation of protein kinase G (PKG). The subsequent phosphorylation of MLCK causes relaxation (p. 478).

In **salivary glands**, postganglionic parasympathetic neurons release ACh, which may stimulate gland cells to secrete kallikrein, an enzyme that cleaves kininogens to vasodilating kinins (e.g., bradykinin). A similar paracrine sequence of events may occur in the **sweat glands** of non-apical skin, where postganglionic sympathetic fibers release ACh, indirectly leading to local vasodilation (p. 573).

NON-ADRENERGIC, NONCHOLINERGIC (NANC) RECEPTORS IN BLOOD VESSELS. Postganglionic parasympathetic nerve terminals may cause vasodilation by co-releasing neurotransmitters other than ACh (see Table 22–1), such as NO, vasoactive intestinal peptide (VIP), and calcitonin gene-related peptide (CGRP). This neural NO acts in the same way as endothelium-derived NO. VIP and, presumably, CGRP act by raising $[cAMP]_i$ and phosphorylating MLCK (see Table 19–9).

The Medullary Cardiovascular Center Tonically Maintains Blood Pressure, and Is Also Under the Control of Higher Brain Centers

The medullary cardiovascular center normally exerts its tonic activity on the sympathetic preganglionic neurons, whose cell bodies lie in the thoracolumbar segments of the spinal cord. However, a variety of somatic and visceral afferents also make connections with this efferent pathway in the spinal cord, and these afferents are responsible for several reflexes that occur at the spinal level. The sympathetic preganglionic neurons are normally so dependent on medullary input that they are not very sensitive to local afferents. Rather, these somatic and visceral afferents exert their major effect by ascending to the medulla and synapsing in the NTS. Nevertheless, some spinal (i.e., segmental) cardiovascular reflexes do exist. For example, the skin blanches in response to both pain and inflammation. These spinal reflexes become most powerful after a spinal transverse lesion.

Neurons of the C1 area of the medulla (see Fig. 22–4) are responsible for maintaining a normal mean arterial pressure. In general, C1 neurons are tonically active and excite sympathetic preganglionic neurons to produce vasoconstriction (p. 531). The presence of tonically active neurons in the C1 area raises the possibility that these neurons play a role in some forms of hypertension. Interestingly, clonidine, an antihypertensive agent, acts by binding to imidazole receptors on C1 area neurons.

Besides the afferents from the baroreceptors, the medullary cardiovascular center receives afferents from respiratory centers and from higher CNS centers, such as the hypothalamus and forebrain areas (see Fig. 22–5). The hypothalamus is an important area for integrating many cardiovascular responses (e.g., during exercise). Indeed, using a microelectrode to stimulate particular sites in the hypothalamus can reproduce a variety of physiological responses. Cortical areas influence the hypothalamic integration areas along both excitatory and inhibitory pathways. Thus, a strong emotion can lead to precipitous hypotension with syncope (i.e., fainting). Conditioned reflexes can also elicit cardiovascular responses. For example, it is possible, by reward conditioning, to train an animal to increase or decrease its heart rate.

Secondary Neural Regulation of Arterial Blood Pressure Depends on Chemoreceptors

Although baroreceptors are the primary sensors for blood pressure control, a second set of receptors, the peripheral chemoreceptors, also play a role. Whereas input from baroreceptors exerts a *negative* drive on the medullary *vasomotor center*, causing vasodilation, the peripheral chemoreceptors exert a *positive* drive on the vasomotor center, causing vasoconstriction (Fig. 22–6A). As far as the heart is concerned, input from *both* the baroreceptors and the peripheral chemoreceptors exerts a positive drive on the *cardioinhibitory center*; that is, they both decrease heart rate (compare Figs. 22–1 and 22–6A).

The medullary *respiratory* centers—which include the areas that integrate the input from the peripheral chemo-

A INTRINSIC CARDIOVASCULAR RESPONSE

B INTEGRATED RESPONSE

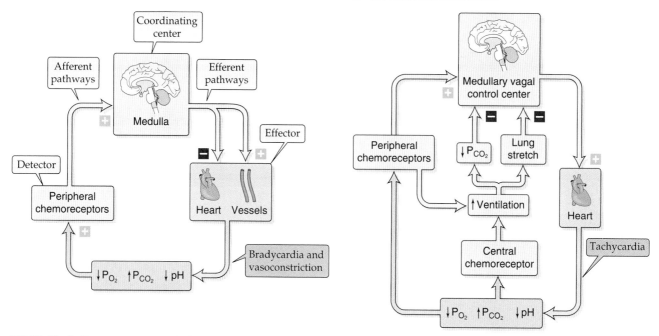

FIGURE 22–6. Chemoreceptor control of the cardiovascular system. In this example, we assume that a decrease in P_{O_2}, an increase in P_{CO_2}, or a decrease in pH is the primary insult (*violet box*). In *A*, the bradycardia occurs only when ventilation is fixed or prevented (e.g., breath-holding). In *B*, the effects of breathing overcome the intrinsic cardiovascular response, producing tachycardia.

receptors—strongly influence medullary *cardiovascular* centers. A fall in arterial P_{O_2}, a rise in P_{CO_2}, or a fall in pH stimulates the peripheral chemoreceptors to increase the firing frequency of the afferent nerves to the medulla. In the absence of conflicting input, which we discuss next, the intrinsic response of the medulla to this peripheral chemoreceptor input is to direct efferent pathways to cause *vasoconstriction* and *bradycardia* (see Fig. 22–6A). Opposite changes in the P_{O_2}, P_{CO_2}, and pH have the opposite effects.

The **peripheral chemoreceptors**—whose primary role is to regulate ventilation (p. 723)—lie close to the baroreceptors. Just as there are two types of high-pressure baroreceptors (i.e., carotid sinus and aortic arch), there are also two types of peripheral chemoreceptors: the carotid bodies and the aortic bodies (compare the location of the baroreceptor and chemoreceptor systems in Fig. 22–2A and B).

CAROTID BODIES. The carotid body—or glomus caroticum—is located between the external and internal carotid artery. Although the human carotid body is small (i.e., ~1 mm³ in size), it has an extraordinarily high blood flow per unit mass and a minuscule arteriovenous difference for P_{O_2}, P_{CO_2}, and pH—putting it in an excellent position to monitor the composition of the *arterial blood*. The chemosensitive cell in the carotid body is the **glomus cell**, which synapses with nerve fibers that join the glossopharyngeal nerve (CN IX). A fall in arterial P_{O_2}, a rise in arterial P_{CO_2}, or a fall in the pH increases the spike frequency in the sensory fibers of the afferent sinus nerve.

AORTIC BODIES. The aortic bodies are situated immediately under the concavity of the aortic arch, and in the

angle between the *right* subclavian and carotid arteries. Aortic bodies may also be present at the angle between the *left* subclavian and common carotid arteries. The aortic glomus cells synapse with nerve fibers that are afferent pathways in the vagus nerve (CN X).

AFFERENT FIBER INPUT TO THE MEDULLA. The most important signal affecting the glomus cells is a low P_{O_2}, which triggers an increase in the firing rate of the sensory fibers. We will discuss ways in which this signal triggers neuronal firing on p. 725. Like the afferent fibers from the baroreceptors, the afferent fibers from both the carotid body (CN IX) and the aortic bodies (CN X) project to the NTS in the medulla. Indeed, the responses to input from the peripheral chemoreceptors overlap with those to input from the baroreceptors.

PHYSIOLOGICAL ROLE OF THE PERIPHERAL CHEMORECEPTORS IN CARDIOVASCULAR CONTROL. The fluctuations in P_{O_2} that normally occur in humans are not large enough to affect the blood pressure or heart rate. For the cardiovascular system, the peripheral chemoreceptors play a role only during severe hypoxia (e.g., hemorrhagic hypotension). As was already noted, the *intrinsic* cardiovascular effects of hypoxia on the peripheral chemoreceptors include vasoconstriction and bradycardia (see Fig. 22–6A). However, it is not easy to demonstrate this primary reflex bradycardia; indeed, it is observed only during forced apnea. Under real-life conditions, *hypoxia causes tachycardia.* Why? Hypoxia—via the peripheral chemoreceptors—normally stimulates the medullary respiratory centers, which in turn stimulate ventilation (see Fig. 22–6B). As discussed later, the high P_{CO_2} that may accompany hypoxia stimulates the central chemoreceptors, which independently stimulates ventilation. This increased ventilation has two effects. First, it stretches the lungs, which in turn stimulates pulmonary stretch receptors. Afferent impulses from these pulmonary stretch receptors ultimately inhibit the cardioinhibitory center, causing reflex tachycardia. Second, as is discussed on p. 691, increased alveolar ventilation caused by hypoxia lowers systemic P_{CO_2}, raising the pH of the brain extracellular fluid and inhibiting the cardioinhibitory center. Again, the net effect is tachycardia. Thus, the physiological response to hypoxia is tachycardia.

CENTRAL CHEMORECEPTORS. In addition to peripheral chemoreceptors, *central* chemoreceptors are present in the medulla (p. 728). However, in contrast to the peripheral chemoreceptors, which primarily sense a low P_{O_2}, the central chemoreceptors mainly sense a low brain pH, which generally reflects a high arterial P_{CO_2}.

As already noted (see Fig. 22–4B), tonic baroreceptor input to the NTS in the medulla stimulates inhibitory interneurons that project onto the vasomotor area. This pathway exerts a considerable restraining influence on sympathetic output, which would otherwise cause vasoconstriction. Thus, cutting these baroreceptor afferents causes vasoconstriction. The central chemoreceptor also influences the vasomotor area. Indeed, a high arterial P_{CO_2} (i.e., low brain pH), which stimulates the central chemoreceptor, dis-inhibits the vasomotor area—just as cutting baroreceptor afferents dis-inhibits the vasomotor area. The result is also the same: an increase in the sympathetic output and vasoconstriction.

In summary, a low P_{O_2} acting on the peripheral chemoreceptor and a high P_{CO_2} acting on the central chemoreceptor act in concert to enhance vasoconstriction.

REGULATION OF CARDIAC OUTPUT

Other things being unchanged, an increased cardiac output raises mean arterial pressure. Therefore, it is not surprising that as we have just seen, the heart is an important effector organ in the feedback loops that regulate mean arterial pressure. Cardiac output is the product of the heart rate and stroke volume (see Equation 17–6), and both factors are under the dual control of (1) regulatory mechanisms intrinsic to the heart, and (2) neural and hormonal pathways that are extrinsic to the heart.

Mechanisms Intrinsic to the Heart Modulate Both Heart Rate and Stroke Volume

INTRINSIC CONTROL OF HEART RATE. As the length of diastole increases, the heart rate necessarily decreases. The diastolic interval is determined by the nature of the action potential fired off by the SA node. Such factors as the maximum diastolic potential, the slope of the diastolic depolarization (phase 4), and the threshold potential all influence the period between one SA node action potential and the next (see Fig. 20–5). Intrinsic modifiers of the SA node pacemaker, such as $[K^+]_o$ and $[Ca^{2+}]_o$, greatly influence the ionic currents responsible for SA node pacemaker activity, but are not part of any cardiovascular feedback loops.

INTRINSIC CONTROL OF STROKE VOLUME. Stroke volume is simply the difference between end-diastolic volume and end-systolic volume (see Equation 21–2). Various processes intrinsic to the heart affect both of these variables.

The **end-*diastolic* volume** (EDV) depends on:

1. **Filling pressure**. Ventricular filling pressure depends to a large degree on *atrial* filling pressure. When increased venous return causes atrial filling pressure to rise, EDV rises as well.
2. **Filling time**. The longer the filling time, the greater the EDV. As heart rate rises, diastole shortens to a greater extent than does systole, thereby decreasing EDV.
3. **Ventricular compliance** (reciprocal of the slope of the "Diastole" curve in Fig. 21–9B). As ventricular compliance increases, a given filling pressure will produce a greater increase in ventricular volume, thus resulting in a greater EDV.

The **end-*systolic* volume** (ESV) depends on:

1. **Preload** (i.e., end-*diastolic* volume). According to the Starling principle, increasing the EDV increases the stretch on the cardiac muscle and the force of the contraction (see the "Systole" curve in Fig. 21–9B), and thus the stroke volume. Only at a very large EDV does contraction begin to weaken as the muscle fibers are stretched too far to generate maximal power.
2. **After-load** (force against which the ventricle must eject its contents). For the left ventricle, the after-load is the mean systemic arterial pressure; for the right ventricle, it is the mean pulmonary arterial pressure. Increased after-load impedes the heart's ability to empty, and thereby increases ESV.
3. **Heart rate**. An increased heart rate leads to greater Ca^{2+} entry into myocardial cells, thereby increasing contractility and reducing ESV (p. 530).
4. **Contractility**. Positive inotropic agents act by increasing $[Ca^{2+}]_i$ within the myocardial cells (p. 530), thereby enhancing the force of contraction and decreasing ESV.

Note that a particular variable may affect both end-diastolic and end-systolic volumes. For example, an increased heart rate decreases EDV and decreases ESV. Therefore, its effect on stroke volume—the *difference* between these two volumes—may be difficult to predict.

Mechanisms Extrinsic to the Heart (e.g., Baroreceptors and Chemoreceptors) Also Modulate Both Heart Rate and Stroke Volume

We have already seen that the sympathetic and parasympathetic pathways are the efferent limbs of the feedback loops that control mean arterial pressure (see Fig. 22–5). These efferent limbs also control cardiac output via heart rate and stroke volume. Because we have already described the anatomy, neurotransmitters, and transduction mechanisms involved in these pathways, we focus here on how these pathways specifically affect the heart rate and stroke volume.

BARORECEPTOR REGULATION. Baroreceptor responses affect both heart rate and stroke volume, the *product of*

A ANATOMICAL DISTRIBUTION

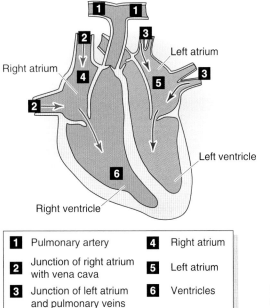

1 Pulmonary artery
2 Junction of right atrium with vena cava
3 Junction of left atrium and pulmonary veins
4 Right atrium
5 Left atrium
6 Ventricles

B RESPONSE OF ATRIAL A– AND B–TYPE RECEPTORS

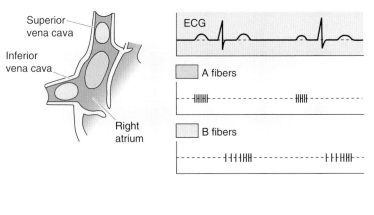

FIGURE 22–7. Low-pressure receptors. In *B*, A-type receptors (*orange*), located mainly in the body of right atrium; B-type receptors, located mainly in superior and inferior vena cava. ECG, electrocardiogram.

which is *cardiac output.* However, baroreceptors do not monitor cardiac output per se, but rather, arterial pressure. Thus, the baroreceptor response does *not* correct spontaneous alterations in cardiac output unless they happen to change mean arterial pressure. For example, when an increase in the cardiac output matches a commensurate decrease in the peripheral resistance, leaving the mean arterial pressure unchanged, the baroreceptors do not respond. On the other hand, even if cardiac output is unchanged, it will be the target of the baroreceptor response if other factors (e.g., changes in peripheral resistance) alter arterial pressure.

CHEMORECEPTOR REGULATION. In Figure 22–6B, we saw that the integrated response to hypoxia and respiratory acidosis is *tachycardia.* This tachycardia response turns out to be a very helpful feedback mechanism for maintaining cardiac output. For example, a reduced cardiac output lowers arterial P_{O_2}, raises P_{CO_2}, and lowers pH. These changes stimulate the peripheral chemoreceptors, indirectly producing tachycardia and thereby increasing cardiac output. Thus, the chemoreceptor response corrects changes in blood chemistry that are likely to result from reduced cardiac output. Once again, the detector (i.e., the peripheral chemoreceptors) does not sense changes in the cardiac output per se, but rather in the metabolic consequences of altered cardiac output. Changes in cardiac output go unnoticed by the chemoreceptors if they do not affect arterial P_{O_2}, P_{CO_2}, or pH.

It is fortunate that a high P_{CO_2} increases the heart rate (see Fig. 22–6B) because a high P_{CO_2} has a direct effect on the heart, *decreasing* myocardial contractility. An increased P_{CO_2} leads to intracellular acidosis of the myocardial cells (p. 653). The fall in myocardial pH decreases the Ca^{2+} sensitivity of the myofilaments, so that they develop *less* force. In the absence of reflex tachycardia, this decreased force would lower cardiac output.

Low-Pressure Baroreceptors in the Atria Respond to Increased "Fullness" of the Vascular System, Triggering Tachycardia, Renal Vasodilation, and Diuresis

The baroreceptors located at *high*-pressure sites (i.e., the carotid sinus and aortic arch) are not the only stretch receptors involved in feedback regulation of the circulation. **Low-pressure baroreceptors**—bare ends of myelinated nerve fibers—are located at strategic *low*-pressure sites, including the pulmonary artery, the junction of the atria with their corresponding veins, the atria themselves, and the ventricles (Fig. 22–7A). Distention of these receptors depends largely on venous return to the heart. Therefore, these mechanoreceptors detect the "fullness" of the circulation, and are part of a larger system of volume sensors that control the effective circulating volume of blood (p. 864). These low-pressure receptors also help to control cardiac output. By regulating both effective circulating volume and cardiac output, these receptors also *indirectly* regulate mean arterial blood pressure.

ATRIAL RECEPTORS. The most extensively studied low-pressure receptors are the atrial receptors. These are located at the ends of afferent axons—either A or B fibers—that join the vagus nerve (CN X). The A fibers fire in synchrony with atrial systole, and therefore monitor heart rate (see Fig. 22–7B). The B fibers fire in a burst during ventricular systole, and gradually increase their firing rate as the atria fill. Thus, the B fibers monitor the rising atrial volume. Because the **central venous pressure** (CVP)—the pressure inside large systemic veins leading to the right heart—is the main determinant of right atrial filling, the B fibers also detect changes in CVP. Therefore, the B-type low-pressure stretch receptors primarily monitor effective circulating volume and venous return.

The afferent pathways for the low-pressure receptors are similar to those for high-pressure baroreceptors and peripheral chemoreceptors traveling along the vagus nerve and projecting to the NTS (p. 538) and other nuclei of the medullary cardiovascular center. To some extent, the efferent pathways and effector organs (i.e., heart and blood vessels) also are similar. However, whereas increased stretch of the high-pressure receptors *lowers* heart rate, increased stretch of the atrial B-type receptors *raises* heart rate (the "Bainbridge reflex," which we discuss in the next section). Moreover, whereas increased stretch of the high-pressure receptors causes *generalized* vasodilation, increased stretch of the atrial B-type receptors decreases sympathetic vasoconstrictor output *only to the kidney.* The net effect of increased atrial stretch (i.e., tachycardia and renal vasodilation) is an increase in renal blood flow, and—as is seen in Chapter 33—an increase in urine output (i.e., diuresis). Decreased atrial stretch has little effect on heart rate, but increases sympathetic output to the kidney. Therefore, as far as their direct cardiovascular effects are concerned, the high-pressure baroreceptors respond to stretch (i.e., increased blood pressure) by attempting to decrease blood pressure. The low-pressure baroreceptors respond to stretch (i.e., increased fullness) by attempting to eliminate fluid.

The afferent fibers of the atrial receptors project not only to the medulla, but also to the hypothalamus, which contains neurons that synthesize **arginine vasopressin** (AVP)—also known as antidiuretic hormone (p. 840)—and then transport it down their axons to the posterior pituitary for release into the blood (p. 1012). Increased atrial stretch lowers AVP secretion, producing a water diuresis and thus decreasing total body water (p. 872).

In addition to stimulating bare nerve endings, atrial stretch causes a *non*-neural response by stretching the atrial myocytes themselves. When stretched, atrial myocytes release **atrial natriuretic peptide** (ANP) or factor (ANF). ANP is a powerful vasodilator. It also causes diuresis (p. 867) and thus enhances the renal excretion of Na^+ (i.e., it causes natriuresis). In these ways, it lowers effective circulating volume blood pressure.

Thus, enhanced atrial filling with consequent stretching of the atrial mechanoreceptors promotes diuresis by at least three efferent mechanisms. The first two are neurally mediated responses—tachycardia in combination with a reduced sympathetic vasoconstrictor output to the kidney and a decreased secretion of AVP. The third response is the enhanced release of ANP by the atrial myocytes themselves.

VENTRICULAR RECEPTORS. Stretching the ventricular *low*-pressure stretch receptors causes bradycardia and vasodilation, responses similar to those associated with stretching of the arterial *high*-pressure receptors. However, these ventricular receptors do not contribute appreciably to homeostasis of the cardiac output.

Cardiac Output Is Roughly Proportional to Effective Circulating Blood Volume

The **Bainbridge reflex** is the name given to the tachycardia caused by an increase in venous return. An increase in blood volume leads to increased firing of low-pressure B fibers (see Fig. 22–7B) during atrial filling. The efferent limb of this Bainbridge reflex is limited to instructions carried by both parasympathetic and sympathetic pathways to the SA node, which determines heart rate. Effects on cardiac contractility and stroke volume are insignificant. Because the Bainbridge reflex saturates, the increase in heart rate is greatest at low baseline heart rates.

The *orange curve* on the right half of Figure 22–8 illustrates the Bainbridge reflex: Increasing the effective circulating volume (i.e., increasing venous return and stimulating *low-pressure* receptors) increases heart rate. On the other hand, we have already noted that decreased atrial stretch has little effect on heart rate. Indeed, a decrease in blood volume does not cause a fall in heart rate, but rather an increase (*orange curve*, left half of Fig.

FIGURE 22–8. Effect of blood volume on cardiac output. The investigators changed effective circulating volume (*x axis*) by altering blood volume.

22–8). The tachycardia caused by volume depletion is due to the intervention of the *high-pressure* baroreceptors. That is, a significant reduction in blood volume leads to a fall in mean arterial pressure, reduced baroreceptor firing, and—via the cardioinhibitory and cardioacceleratory areas in the medulla (see Fig. 22–4B)—stimulation of the SA node. Therefore, heart rate exhibits a biphasic response to changes in blood volume or venous return. By different mechanisms, volume loading and volume depletion *both* increase heart rate. In general, during volume loading, the Bainbridge reflex prevails, whereas during volume depletion, the high-pressure baroreceptor reflex dominates. *Heart rate is at its minimum when effective circulating volume is normal.*

In contrast to heart rate, which has a biphasic response to changes in effective circulating volume, cardiac output rises monotonically (see Fig. 22–8, *red curve*). The reason for this smooth increase is that cardiac output is the product of heart rate *and* stroke volume, and stroke volume has a peculiar dependence on effective circulating volume (see Fig. 22–8, *blue curve*). Starting from very low blood volumes, increasing the blood volume causes a gradual rise in stroke volume, until blood volume and stroke volume reach normal levels. Further increases in blood volume have no effect on stroke volume.

Like the biphasic response of the heart rate (see Fig. 22–8, *orange curve*), the biphasic response of stroke volume is the result of two competing effects—in this case, Starling's law and the baroreceptor reflex. According to Starling's law, as venous blood volume increases, enhanced ventricular filling increases EDV, thereby improving cardiac performance and thus stroke volume (p. 527). The Starling relationship reflects the *intrinsic* properties of the heart muscle. However, in a real person, the baroreceptor reflex has a major influence on the dependence of stroke volume on blood volume. At low blood volumes, the baroreceptor reflex produces high sympathetic output, increasing contractility and steepening the *blue curve* on the left half of Figure 22–8. At high blood volumes, the Starling relationship would tend to be less steep. Moreover, the baroreceptor reflex reduces sympathetic output, thus decreasing contractility and further flattening the *blue curve* on the right half of Figure 22–8.

Therefore, the dependence of cardiac output on effective circulating volume is the result of the complex interplay among three factors: (1) the Bainbridge reflex, (2) the baroreceptor reflex, and (3) Starling's law.

MATCHING OF VENOUS RETURN AND CARDIAC OUTPUT

Venous return is the blood flow returning to the heart. Most often, the term is used to mean the *systemic* venous return, that is, return of blood to the right heart. Because the right heart's input must equal its output in the steady state, and because the cardiac outputs of the right and left hearts are almost exactly the same, the input to the right heart must equal the output of the left heart. Thus, the systemic venous return must match the systemic cardiac output.

Increases in Cardiac Output Cause Right Atrial Pressure to Fall

The right atrial pressure (RAP) determines the extent of ventricular filling, and indeed was the first of the three determinants of end-diastolic volume discussed on p. 547. In turn, RAP depends on the venous return of blood to the heart. Imagine that we replace the heart and lungs with a simple pump—with adjustable flow—that delivers blood into the aorta and simultaneously takes it back up from the vena cava (Fig. 22–9A). Using this simple pump, we can study the factors that govern venous return from the peripheral systemic circulation to the right heart by varying flow (the *independent* variable) while recording right atrial pressure (the *dependent* variable).

We start our experiment with the pump generating a normal cardiac output of 5 liters/min; the right atrial pressure is 2 mm Hg. This situation is represented by point A in Figure 22–9B, which is a plot of right atrial pressure versus venous return (i.e., our pump rate). When we reverse the axes, the plot is known as a **vascular function curve**. Note that we express venous return (i.e., cardiac *input*) in the same units as cardiac *output*. We now turn off the pump, a situation analogous to cardiac arrest. For several seconds, blood continues to flow from the arteries and capillaries into the veins because the arterial pressure continues to exceed the venous pressure. Remember that the aortic pressure does not fall to zero during diastole because of the potential energy stored in the elastic recoil of the arterial walls (see Box on p. 516). Similarly, after a cardiac arrest, this potential energy continues to push blood to the venous side until all pressures are equal throughout the vascular tree, and flow stops everywhere.

When blood flow finally ceases after a cardiac arrest, the pressures in the arteries, capillaries, veins, and right atrium are all uniform. This pressure is called the **mean systemic filling pressure** (MSFP), and is approximately 7 mm Hg (*point B* in Fig. 22–9B). Why is the MSFP not zero? When you fill an elastic container (e.g., a balloon) with fluid, the pressure inside depends on how much fluid you put in, as well as the compliance of the container (see Equation 18–5). In the case of the cardiovascular system, MSFP depends on the blood volume and the overall compliance of the entire vascular system. Now that blood flow has ceased, there is obviously no longer any force (i.e., no ΔP) driving the blood from the veins to the pump. Therefore, RAP equals MSFP.

Now, starting with the system at a standstill (*point B* in Fig. 22–9B), we will increase the pump rate and measure the steady-state RAP, repeating this procedure several times. As the pump rate increases, RAP falls (see Fig. 22–9B) because the inflow to the pump draws blood out of the right atrium, the site closest to the inlet of the pump. As the pump rate rises to 5 liters/min, the right atrial pressure falls to about +2 mm Hg, its original value. As

A MODEL OF SYSTEMIC CIRCULATION

B VASCULAR FUNCTION CURVE WITH REVERSED AXES

FIGURE 22–9. Vascular function. In *A*, a heart-lung machine replaces the right heart, pulmonary circulation, and the left heart. We can set the pump flow to predetermined values and examine how cardiac output determines central venous pressure (CVP) and right atrial pressure (RAP). C_V and C_A are vascular compliances. *B* shows dependent variable (RAP) on the *y axis*, whereas *C* shows RAP on *x axis*.

the pump rate increases even farther, RAP eventually falls to negative values.

Cardiovascular physiologists usually work with the vascular function curve with the axes reversed from those shown in Figure 22–9*B*, treating RAP as the independent variable, and plotting it on the abscissa (see Fig. 22–9*C*). As RAP becomes less positive, it provides a greater ΔP for increasing the return of blood from the periphery to the right atrium, as it must in order for cardiac output to increase. Therefore, the cardiac output steadily rises as RAP falls. However, as RAP becomes increasingly negative, the transmural pressure of the large veins becomes negative, so that the large veins feeding blood to the right atrium collapse. No further increment in venous return can occur, even though the driving pressure, ΔP, is increasing. Therefore, the vascular function curve plateaus at negative values of RAP, around −1 mm Hg (see Fig. 22–9*C*).

Two different theories attempt to explain the shape of the vascular function curve in Figure 22–9*C*. One explanation for the curve's steepness emphasizes the high compliance of the venous capacitance vessels; the other focuses on their small viscous resistance. In reality, both compliance and resistance are responsible for the steepness of the vascular function curve.

Changes in Blood Volume Shift the Vascular Function Curve to Different Right Atrial Pressures, Whereas Changes in Arteriolar Tone Alter the Slope of the Curve

Because the vascular function curve depends on how full the capacitance vessels are, *changing the blood volume* affects the vascular function curve. An increase in blood volume (e.g., a transfusion) shifts the curve to the right. In the example in Figure 22–10*A*, the intercept with the x-axis (i.e., mean systemic filling pressure, MSFP) moves from 7 to 9 mm Hg, as would be expected if more blood were put into a distensible container, whether a balloon or the circulatory system. A decrease in blood volume (e.g., hemorrhage) shifts the curve and the x-intercept to the left. Thus, MSFP increases with transfusion and decreases with hemorrhage. However, changes in blood volume do *not* affect the *slope* of the linear portion of the vascular function curve as long as there is no change in either vessel compliance or resistance.

Changing the venomotor tone, by constricting or dilating *only the veins*, is equivalent to changing the blood volume. Returning to our balloon analogy, even if we hold the amount of blood constant, we can increase pressure inside the balloon by increasing the tension in the wall.

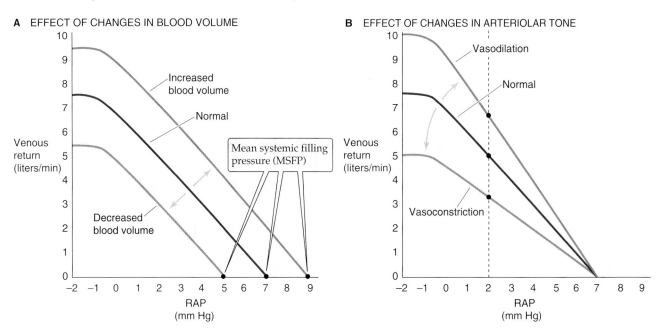

FIGURE 22–10. Effect of changes in blood volume and vasomotor tone on the vascular function curve. The *purple curves* are the same as the *vascular function curve* in Figure 22–9C. In *B*, dilating the arterioles increases central venous pressure (CVP), and thus raises the driving force (CVP-RAP) for venous return. Constricting arterioles has the opposite effects. RAP, right atrial pressure.

Thus, a pure increase in venomotor tone would be equivalent to a blood transfusion (see Fig. 22–10A). Conversely, a pure decrease in venomotor tone would reduce the tension in the wall of the container, shifting the curve to the left, just as in a hemorrhage.

Changing the tone of the arterioles has a very different effect on the vascular function curve. Because the arterioles contain only a minor fraction of the blood volume, changes in the arteriolar tone have little effect on MSFP, and thus on the x-intercept. However, changes in the arteriolar tone can have a marked effect on the central venous pressure, which, along with the right atrial pressure, determines the driving force for the venous return. Arteriolar constriction flattens the vascular function curve; arteriolar dilation has the opposite effect (see Fig. 22–10B). We can understand this effect by examining the vertical line through the three curves at an RAP of 2 mm Hg. For the middle or "normal" curve, the difference between a CVP of, say, 5 mm Hg and a RAP of 2 mm Hg ($\Delta P = 3$ mm Hg) produces a venous return of 5 liters/min. Arteriolar constriction might lower the CVP from 5 to 4 mm Hg, thereby reducing ΔP from 3 to 2 mm Hg. Because the driving pressure (ΔP) drops to $\frac{2}{3}$ of normal, venous return also falls to $\frac{2}{3}$ of normal. Thus, arteriolar constriction flattens the vascular function curve. Similarly, arteriolar dilation might raise CVP from 5 to 6 mm Hg, so that the ΔP increases from 3 to 4 mm Hg, producing a venous return that is $\frac{4}{3}$ of normal. Thus, arteriolar dilation steepens the vascular function curve.

In the preceding analysis, we assumed "pure" changes in blood volume or vessel tone. In real life, things can be more complicated. For example, hemorrhage is typically followed by arteriolar constriction for maintenance of the systemic arterial pressure. Thus, real situations may both shift the x-intercept and change the slope of the vascular function curve.

Because Vascular Function and Cardiac Function Depend on Each Other, Cardiac Output and Venous Return Match at Exactly One Value of Right Atrial Pressure

Just as there is a vascular function curve, there is also a **cardiac function curve** that, in effect, is Starling's law. The classical Starling's law relationship (see Figure 21–9B, *red curve*) which is valid for both ventricles, is a plot of developed pressure versus EDV. However, we already expressed Starling's law as a cardiac performance curve in Figure 21–9C, plotting stroke work on the y-axis and atrial pressure on the x-axis. Because stroke work—at a fixed arterial pressure and heart rate—is proportional to cardiac output, we can replace stroke work with *cardiac output* on the y-axis of the cardiac performance curve. The result is the *red cardiac function curve* in Figure 22–11A. Note that the *cardiac function curve* is a plot of cardiac output versus right atrial pressure, and it has the same *units* as the *vascular function curve*. We can plot the two relationships on the same graph (see Fig. 22–11A). However, the y-axis for the cardiac function curve is *cardiac output*, whereas the y-axis for the vascular function curve is *venous return*. Of course, cardiac output and venous return (i.e., cardiac input) must be the same in the steady state.

We can now ask, Do the cardiac output and venous return depend on RAP? Or, does RAP depend on the cardiac output and venous return? The answer to both questions is an emphatic "yes"! They all depend on each

A MATCHING OF A SINGLE CARDIAC FUNCTION CURVE
WITH A SINGLE VASCULAR FUNCTION CURVE

B SHIFT OF VASCULAR FUNCTION CURVE

C SHIFT OF CARDIAC FUNCTION CURVE

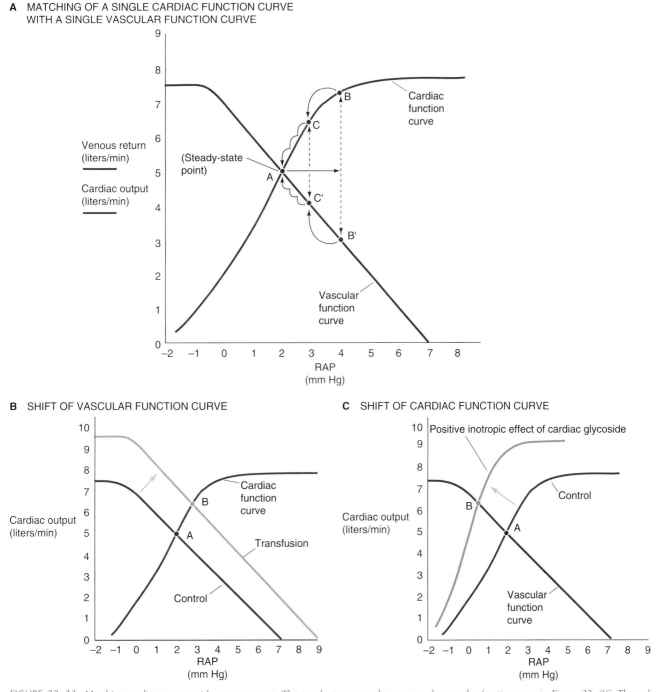

FIGURE 22–11. Matching cardiac output with venous return. The *purple curves* are the same as the *vascular function curve* in Figure 22–9C. The *red cardiac function curves* represent Starling's law. In *A*, point A is the single right atrial pressure at which venous return and cardiac output match. A transient increase in RAP from 2 to 4 mm Hg causes an initial mismatch between cardiac output (*point B*) and venous return (*point B'*), which eventually resolves (B'C'A and BCA). In *B*, permanently increasing blood volume ("transfusion") shifts the *vascular function curve* to the right (as in Fig. 22–10A), so that a match between the cardiac output and venous return now occurs at a higher RAP (*point B*). In *C*, permanently increasing cardiac contractility shifts the *cardiac function curve* upward, so that a match between the cardiac output and the venous return now occurs at a lower RAP (*point B*). RAP, right atrial pressure.

other. There is no absolute dependent or independent variable in this closed circuit because, in the steady state, venous return and cardiac output must be equal. Venous return (from the vascular function curve) and cardiac output (from the cardiac function curve) can be equal only at the single point where the two curves intersect

(*point A* in Fig. 22–11A). Only transient and small deviations in these two curves are possible unless either or both of the function curves change in shape.

Imagine what would happen if RAP transiently increased from 2 to 4 mm Hg (see Fig. 22–11A). Starling's law states that the increased ventricular filling initially increases cardiac output from starting point A (5 liters/min) to point B (7.3 liters/min). Simultaneously, the increase in RAP causes a decrease in the driving pressure for venous return, that is, the difference CVP − RAP. Thus, the increase in RAP would initially reduce the venous return from point A (5 liters/min) to point B′ (3 liters/min). This imbalance between cardiac output and venous return cannot last very long. The transiently elevated cardiac output will have two effects. First, by sucking the right atrium dry, it will tend to lower RAP. Second, by pumping blood toward the veins, it will raise CVP. As a result, the difference CVP − RAP increases, and venous return moves from point B′ to C′. Because RAP at point C′ is lower than at B′, the cardiac output must also be less at point C than at point B. The imbalance between C and C′ (6.5 vs 4 liters/min) is now less than that between B and B′ (7.3 vs 3 liters/min). In this way, venous return gradually increases, cardiac output gradually decreases, and RAP gradually decreases until once again they all come into balance at point A. Thus, the cardiovascular system has an intrinsic mechanism for counteracting small, transient imbalances between cardiac input and output.

The only way to produce a *permanent change* in cardiac output, venous return, and RAP is to change at least one of the two function curves. The vascular function curve may be any one of a large family of such curves (see Fig. 22–10A and B), depending on the precise blood volume and arteriolar tone. Thus, a transfusion of blood shifts the vascular function curve to the right, establishing a new steady-state operating point at a higher RAP (point A → point B in Fig. 22–11B). Similarly, vasodilation would rotate the vascular function curve to a steeper slope, also establishing a new steady-state operating point at a higher RAP.

The cardiac function curve also may be any one of a large family (see Fig. 21–9C), depending on afterload, heart rate, and, above all, the heart's contractile state. Therefore, increasing contractility by adding a cardiac glycoside such as digitalis (p. 532) shifts the cardiac function curve upward and to the left, establishing another steady-state operating point (point A → point B in Fig. 22–11C). Both physiological and pathologic conditions can reset the vascular and cardiac function curves, resulting in a wide range of operating points for the match between venous return and cardiac output.

INTERMEDIATE AND LONG-TERM CONTROL OF THE CIRCULATION

In addition to the rapidly acting neural mechanisms that control the total peripheral resistance and cardiac output, humoral controls contribute to the homeostasis of the circulation. In most instances, these control systems operate on a time scale of hours or days, far more slowly than the neurotransmitter-mediated reflex control by the CNS.

Two classes of humoral controls influence the circulation: (1) Vasoactive substances released in the blood, or in the proximity of vascular smooth muscle, modulate the vasomotor tone of arteries and veins, affecting blood pressure and the distribution of blood flow and (2) Nonvasoactive substances, which act on targets other than the cardiovascular system, control the effective circulating volume by modulating extracellular fluid volume. By determining the filling of the blood vessels, these nonvasoactive agents also modulate the mean arterial pressure and cardiac output.

Endocrine and Paracrine Vasoactive Compounds Control the Circulatory System on an Intermediate to Long-Term Basis

Vasoactive substances, both endocrine and paracrine, cause blood vessels to contract or relax (Table 22–3). In many instances, paracrine control dominates over endocrine control. The chemical messengers controlling the blood vessels can be amines, peptides, or proteins; derivatives of arachidonic acid; or gases such as nitric oxide.

BIOGENIC AMINES. Monoamines may be either vasoconstrictors (epinephrine and serotonin) or vasodilators (histamine).

1. **Epinephrine.** The source of this hormone is the adrenal medulla (p. 1061). In blood vessels, as we already noted (see p. 544), epinephrine binds to α_1 receptors, causing *vasoconstriction*, and to β_2 receptors, causing *vasodilation*. Because β_2 receptors are largely confined to the blood vessels of skeletal muscle, the heart, the liver, and the adrenal medulla itself, epinephrine is not a systemic vasodilator. Epinephrine also binds to β_1 receptors in the heart, thereby *increasing the heart rate and contractility* (p. 543). For the cardiovascular system, the effects of catecholamines originating from the adrenal medulla are usually minor compared with those of the norepinephrine released from the sympathetic nerve endings.

2. **Serotonin.** Also known as 5-hydroxytryptamine (see Fig. 12–9B), this monoamine may be present in nerve terminals, and is also present in platelets and mast cells. Serotonin is a *vasoconstrictor*. Circulating serotonin is generally not involved in systemic control of the circulation, but rather in local control. Serotonin is

TABLE 22–3

VASOACTIVE COMPOUNDS	
VASOCONSTRICTORS	**VASODILATORS**
Epinephrine (via α_1 receptors)	Epinephrine (via β_2 receptors)
Serotonin	Histamine
ANG II	ANP
AVP	Bradykinins
Endothelin	PGE_2, PGI_2
	NO

ANG II, angiotensin II; ANP, atrial natriuretic peptide; AVP, arginine vasopressin; NO, nitric oxide; PGE_2, prostaglandin E_2; PGI_2, prostacyclin.

particularly important with vessel damage, where it contributes to hemostasis.

3. **Histamine**. Like serotonin, histamine (see Fig. 12–9*B*) may also be present in nerve terminals. In addition, mast cells release histamine in response to tissue injury and inflammation. Histamine is a *vasodilator*. Although histamine causes vascular smooth muscle to relax, it causes visceral smooth muscle (e.g., bronchial smooth muscle in asthma) to contract.

PEPTIDES. Vasoactive peptides may be either vasoconstrictors or vasodilators (see Table 22–3).

1. **Angiotensin II** (ANG II). Part of the renin-angiotensin-aldosterone cascade (p. 866), ANG II, as its name implies, is a powerful *vasoconstrictor*. The liver secretes angiotensinogen into the blood. The enzyme renin, released into the blood by the kidney, then converts angiotensinogen to the decapeptide ANG I. Finally, angiotensin-converting enzyme (ACE), which is present primarily on endothelial cells, particularly those of the lung, cleaves ANG I to the octapeptide ANG II. Aminopeptidases further cleave it to the heptapeptide ANG III, which is somewhat less vasoactive than ANG II.

In VSMCs, ANG II binds to G protein–coupled **AT$_{1A}$ receptors**, activating phospholipase C, raising $[Ca^{2+}]_i$ (p. 100), and leading to contraction. However, ANG II is *normally* not present in plasma concentrations high enough to produce systemic vasoconstriction. In contrast, ANG II plays a major role in cardiovascular control during blood loss (p. 588), exercise, and similar circumstances that reduce renal blood flow. Reduced perfusion pressure in the kidney causes the release of renin (p. 866). Plasma ANG II levels rise, leading to an intense vasoconstriction in the splanchnic and renal circulations. The resulting reduced renal blood flow leads to even more renin release and higher ANG II levels, a dangerous positive feedback system that can lead to acute renal failure. A widely studied model of hypertension that demonstrates the importance of this mechanism is the Goldblatt model for hypertension (see box on hypertension).

ANG II has a range of other effects—besides direct vasoactive effects—that indirectly increase mean arterial pressure: (1) ANG II increases cardiac contractility; (2) it reduces renal plasma flow, thereby enhancing Na$^+$ reabsorption in the kidney; (3) as is discussed in the next section, ANG II and ANG III also stimulate the adrenal cortex to release aldosterone; (4) in the CNS, ANG II stimulates thirst and leads to the release of another vasoconstrictor—AVP; (5) ANG II facilitates the release of norepinephrine by postganglionic sympathetic nerve terminals; and (6) finally, ANG II also acts as a cardiac growth factor (see box on cardiac hypertrophy).

2. **Arginine vasopressin** (AVP). The posterior pituitary releases AVP, also known as antidiuretic hormone. AVP has a *vasoconstrictor* effect, but only at concentrations that are higher than those that are strongly antidiuretic (p. 840). Hemorrhagic shock causes enhanced AVP release and a vasoconstriction that contributes to a transient restoration of arterial pressure (p. 586).

3. **Endothelins** (ETs). Endothelial cells produce ETs (p. 480). Although, on a molar basis, ETs are the most powerful *vasoconstrictors*, it is not clear whether these paracrine agents play a dominant role in overall blood pressure homeostasis.

4. **Atrial natriuretic peptide** (ANP or ANF). Released from atrial myocytes in response to stretch (p. 549), this 28-amino-acid peptide is a potent *vasodilator*. Although ANP lowers blood pressure, its role in the overall regulation of mean arterial pressure is doubtful. Because ANP also has powerful diuretic and natriuretic actions, it ultimately reduces plasma volume and therefore blood pressure.

5. **Kinins**. At least three different *vasodilator* kinins exist: (1) the nonapeptide **bradykinin**, which is formed in plasma; (2) the decapeptide **lysyl-bradykinin**, which is liberated from tissues; and (3) **methionyl-lysyl-bradykinin**, which is present in the urine. These kinins are breakdown products of **kininogens**, catalyzed by **kallikreins**—enzymes that are present in plasma and in tissues such as the salivary glands, pancreas, sweat glands, intestine, and kidney. Kallikreins form in the blood from the following cascade: Plasmin acts on clotting factor XII, releasing fragments with proteolytic activity. These factor XII fragments convert an inactive precursor, prekallikrein, to kallikreins. The kinins formed by the action of these kallikreins are eliminated by the **kininases** (kininase I and II). Kininase II is the same as angiotensin-converting enzyme. Thus, the same enzyme (ACE) that generates a vasoconstrictor (ANG II) also disposes of vasodilators (bradykinin). Like histamine, the kinins *relax* vascular smooth muscle, but *contract* visceral smooth muscle.

PROSTAGLANDINS. Many tissues synthesize these derivatives of arachidonic acid (p. 103). PGI$_2$ (prostacyclin) and prostaglandin E$_2$ (PGE$_2$) are particularly strong *vasodilators*. It is doubtful that prostaglandins play a role in systemic vascular control. In veins, and also in some arteries, arachidonic acid or Ca^{2+} ionophores cause endothelium-dependent contractions. Because cyclooxygenase inhibitors prevent this vasoconstrictor response, venous endothelial cells probably metabolize arachidonic acid into a vasoconstrictive cyclooxygenase product, presumably thromboxane A$_2$.

NITRIC OXIDE (NO). Nitric oxide synthase (NOS) produces NO from arginine in endothelial cells (p. 478). Although NO is a powerful, paracrine *vasodilator*, it is not clear that it plays an important role in overall blood pressure homeostasis.

Pathways That Target the Renal Control of Extracellular Fluid Volume Are the Primary Long-Term Regulators of Mean Arterial Pressure

The *volume of the extracellular fluid* (ECF) includes both the blood plasma and the interstitial fluid. The small solutes in the plasma and interstitial fluid exchange freely across the capillary wall, so that the entire ECF constitutes a single osmotic compartment. Because the plasma volume is a more-or-less constant fraction ($\sim$20%) of the ECF volume, changes in the ECF volume produce proportional changes in plasma volume. Thus, assuming that the compliance of the vasculature is constant (see Equation 18–5), such an increase in plasma volume will lead to an increase in transmural blood pressure.

We saw in Chapter 19 that the *Starling forces* across a capillary (i.e., the hydrostatic and colloid osmotic pressure differences) determine the traffic of fluid between the plasma and the interstitial fluid (see box on p. 473). Thus, alterations in the Starling forces acting across the capillary wall can affect the plasma volume, and therefore blood pressure.

Because of the importance of the ECF volume and Starling forces in determining the plasma volume, one might expect that the body would have specific sensors for ECF volume, interstitial fluid volume, and blood volume. However, the parameter that the body controls in the intermediate and long-term regulation of the mean arterial pressure is none of these, but rather a more vague parameter termed the **"effective circulating volume."** The effective circulating volume is not an anatomic volume, but the *functional* blood volume that reflects the extent of tissue perfusion, as sensed by the fullness or pressure in the vessels. The control mechanisms that defend effective circulating volume include the two classes of stretch receptors described in this chapter. First, the high-pressure receptors in the carotid sinus and aorta (p. 535) do double duty. In the short term, these baroreceptors regulate blood pressure via their direct cardiovascular effects, as was already discussed. In the longer term, they regulate effective circulating volume. Second, the low-pressure receptors—located in the pulmonary artery, the junction of the atria with their corresponding veins, the atria themselves, and the ventricles (p. 548)—regulate effective circulating volume by direct and indirect effects on the cardiovascular system. In addition to these already familiar receptors involved in neural control of the circulation, other sensors monitor effective circulating volume (see Table 39–2): the baroreceptors in the renal artery, the stretch receptors in the liver, and the atrial myocytes themselves, as well as—to some extent—osmoreceptors in the CNS.

As we will see in Chapter 39, these sensors of effective circulating volume send signals to the dominant effector organ—the kidney—to change the rate of Na^+ excretion in the urine. These signals to the kidney follow four parallel effector pathways (p. 864): (1) the renin-ANG II-aldosterone axis, (2) the autonomic nervous system, (3) the posterior pituitary that releases AVP, and (4) atrial myocytes that release ANP. Among these four parallel pathways, the most important is the **renin-angiotensin-aldosterone** system. By regulating total-body Na^+ content, the kidney determines ECF volume. Therefore, the kidney ultimately governs the blood volume and is thus the principal agent in the long-term control of mean arterial pressure.

HYPERTENSION

Hypertension is found in approximately 20% of the adult population. It can damage endothelial cells, producing a number of proliferative responses, including arteriosclerosis. In the long term, hypertension can lead to coronary artery disease, myocardial infarction, heart failure, stroke, and renal failure. In the great majority of cases, hypertension is the result of dysfunction of the mechanisms used by the circulation for the long-term, rather than short-term, control of arterial pressure. In fact, chronically hypertensive patients may have diminished sensitivity of their arterial baroreceptors.

Most people with an elevated blood pressure have **"primary hypertension,"** in which it is not possible to identify a specific cause. Renal artery stenosis, which compromises renal blood flow, is the most common cause of *secondary* hypertension. An experimental equivalent of renal artery stenosis is the "one-clip two-kidney" model of hypertension first described by Goldblatt (see box on p. 868). This model does not explain the vast majority of cases of hypertension, but it does give us our best description of the pathophysiology involved in at least some patients with elevated blood pressure. The most common cause of renal artery stenosis is the narrowing of the renal artery by atherosclerotic plaque. Fibromuscular disease of the renal arterial wall can also be responsible, usually in young women, as can any space-occupying lesion (e.g., metastatic cancer or benign cysts). If the stenosis is removed by angioplasty or surgery, and if preliminary tests show that the stenosis is the likely cause of the elevation in blood pressure, then a significant percentage of patients will experience resolution of their hypertension.

The cumulative obstruction of smaller arteries and arterioles may also produce hypertension, as is often seen in diseases of the renal parenchyma or any end-stage renal disease. Conversely, constriction of larger vessels proximal to the kidneys can also cause hypertension, as is the case with coarctation of the aorta, a congenital malformation that constricts flow through the aorta to the lower parts of the body. Other causes of secondary hypertension include chronic volume overload, primary aldosteronism (caused by either a benign adenoma or bilateral hyperplasia), and pheochromocytoma (a tumor of the adrenal medulla that releases excessive amounts of catecholamines into the circulation).

REFERENCES

Books and Reviews

Andresen MC, Kunze DL: Nucleus tractus solitarius: Gateway to neural circulatory control. Annu Rev Physiol 56:93–116, 1994.

Cowley AW Jr: Long-term control of arterial blood pressure. Physiol Rev 72:231–300, 1992.

Hainsworth R: Reflexes from the heart. Physiol Rev 71:617–658, 1991.

Marshall JM: Peripheral chemoreceptors and cardiovascular regulation. Physiol Rev 74:543–594, 1994.

Navar LG, Zou L, Von Thun A, et al: Unraveling the mystery of Goldblatt hypertension. News Physiol Sci 13:170–176, 1998.

Sved AF, Gordon FJ: Amino acids as central neurotransmitters in the baroreceptor reflex pathway. News Physiol Sci 9:243–246, 1994.

Journal Articles

Barger G, Dale HH: Chemical structure and sympathomimetic action of amines. J Physiol London 41:19–59, 1910.

Bronk DW, Stella G: Afferent impulses in the carotid sinus nerve. I. The relation of the discharge from single end organs to arterial blood pressure. J Cell Comp Physiol 1:113–130, 1932.

Chapleau MW, Abboud FM: Contrasting effects of static and pulsatile pressure on carotid baroreceptor activity in dogs. Circ Res 61:648–658, 1987.

Loewi O: Über humorale Übertragbarkeit der Herznervenwirkung. Pflügers Arch 189:239–242, 1921.

CHAPTER 23

Special Circulations

Steven S. Segal

In the preceding chapters, we considered blood flow to peripheral capillary beds as if the "periphery" were a single entity. In this chapter, we break that entity down into some of its component parts. Because each organ in the body has its own unique set of requirements, special circulations within each organ have evolved with their own particular features and regulatory mechanisms. Especially for times of great stress to the body, each organ possesses circulatory adaptations that allow it to make the changes appropriate for causing minimal harm to the overall organism. Here, we focus on the circulations of the brain, heart, skeletal muscle, abdominal viscera, and skin. We discuss other special circulations in the context of particular organs—the lungs in Chapter 30, the kidneys in Chapter 33, the placenta in Chapter 55, and the fetal circulation in Chapter 56.

The Blood Flow to Individual Organs Must Vary to Meet the Needs of the Particular Organ, As Well As of the Whole Body

The blood flow to each tissue must meet the nutritional needs of that tissue's parenchymal cells, while at the same time allowing those cells to play their role in the homeostasis of the whole individual. The way in which the circulatory system distributes blood flow must be flexible so that changing demands can be met. In the process of meeting these demands, the body makes compromises. Consider the circulatory changes that accompany exercise. Blood flow to active skeletal muscle increases tremendously through both an increase and a redistribution of cardiac output. Blood flow to the coronary circulation must also rise to meet the demands of exercise. Furthermore, in order to dispose of the heat generated during exercise, the vessels in the skin dilate, thereby promoting heat transfer to the environment. As cardiac output is increasingly directed to active muscle and skin, circulation to the splanchnic and renal circulations decreases, while blood flow to the brain is preserved.

This chapter focuses on the perfusion of select *systemic* vascular beds, but keep in mind that the lungs receive the entire cardiac output, and therefore must also be able to accommodate any changes in total blood flow.

Neural, Myogenic, Metabolic, and Endothelial Mechanisms Control Regional Blood Flow

Several mechanisms govern vascular resistance, and thus the distribution of blood circulating throughout the body. The extent to which a particular bed depends on a particular blood flow control mechanism varies from organ to organ. We have discussed these mechanisms in the preceding chapters, and briefly review them here.

NEURAL MECHANISMS. The resistance vessels of nearly every organ are invested with fibers of the autonomic nervous system (ANS), particularly those of the sympathetic division (p. 540). In addition to its critical role in controlling blood pressure and cardiac output, the ANS modulates local blood flow to meet the needs of particular tissues.

MYOGENIC MECHANISMS. Many vessels, particularly the muscular arteries and arterioles that govern vascular resistance, are inherently responsive to changes in transmural pressure. Increased pressure and the accompanying stretch of vascular smooth muscle cells (VSMCs) elicit vasoconstriction (p. 478), whereas decreased pressure elicits vasodilation. This myogenic response plays an important role in the autoregulation (p. 480) that occurs in the vessels of the brain, heart, skeletal muscle, and kidneys.

METABOLIC MECHANISMS. Throughout the body, the vessels that govern blood flow are sensitive to the local metabolic needs of parenchymal cells. Table 19–8 lists several changes that act synergistically to increase local blood flow. For example, a decrease in PO_2 or pH causes vasodilation. Tissues with high energy demands—such as the brain, heart, and skeletal muscle during exercise—rely heavily on such local control mechanisms.

ENDOTHELIAL MECHANISMS. Endothelial cells release a variety of vasoactive substances (Table 19–9). For example, the shear stress exerted by the movement of blood through the vessel lumen stimulates the release of nitric oxide, which relaxes VSMCs and prevents leukocyte adhesion.

The interplay among the previous four mechanisms establishes a resting level of vasomotor tone. VSMCs and endothelial cells also use gap junctions for electrical and chemical signalling between themselves, thereby coordinating their activity during vasomotor control.

In addition to the previous mechanisms, which are part of a sophisticated feedback control system, other factors—which are *not* regulatory in nature—can affect the local circulation. These *other* factors are all mechanical forces that are external to the blood vessels and that tend to either collapse or open them (p. 519). For example, in the heart and skeletal muscle, muscular contraction transiently halts blood flow by compressing blood vessels within the tissue.

THE BRAIN

Anastomoses at the Circle of Willis and Among the Branches of Distributing Arteries Protect the Blood Supply to the Brain, Which Is Approximately 15% of Cardiac Output

The brain accounts for only about 2% of the body's weight, yet it receives approximately 15% of the resting cardiac output. Of all the tissues in the body, the brain is the least tolerant of ischemia. It depends entirely on oxidative sources of energy production. Each day, the human brain oxidizes approximately 100 g of glucose, which is roughly equivalent to the amount stored as glycogen in the liver. Interruption of cerebral blood flow for just a few seconds causes unconsciousness. If ischemia persists for even a few minutes, irreversible cellular damage is likely.

ARTERIES. Blood reaches the brain through four *source arteries*—the two internal carotid arteries and the two vertebral arteries (Fig. 23–1). The vertebral arteries join to form the basilar artery, which then splits to form the two posterior cerebral arteries, which in turn, are part of the **circle of Willis** at the base of the brain. The internal carotid arteries are the major source of blood to the circle. Three bilateral pairs of *distributing arteries* (anterior, middle, and posterior cerebral arteries) arise from the circle of Willis to envelop the cerebral hemispheres. Smaller branches from the vertebral and basilar arteries distribute blood to the brain stem and cerebellum. The distributing arteries give rise to branches that course over the surface of the brain, forming anastomoses, and then branch again to penetrate the tissue at right angles to the brain surface. These penetrating vessels branch centripetally to give rise to capillaries. The anastomoses on the cortical surface provide the collateral circulation that is so important should a distributing artery or one of its branches become occluded. Each of the four source arteries tends to supply the brain region closest to where the source artery joins the circle of Willis. If a stenosis develops in one source artery, other source arteries to the circle of Willis can provide alternative flow. Nevertheless, if flow through a carotid artery becomes severely restricted (e.g., with atherosclerotic plaque), ischemia may occur in the ipsilateral hemisphere, with impairment of function.

VEINS. The veins of the brain are wide, thin-walled structures that are nearly devoid of smooth muscle and have no valves. In general, the veins drain the brain radially, in a centrifugal direction. The intracerebral veins converge into a superficial pial plexus lying under the arteries. The plexus drains into collecting veins, which course over the distributing arteries and empty into the **dural sinuses** (see Fig. 16–1B). The exception to this radial pattern is the deep white matter of the cerebral hemispheres and basal ganglia; these regions drain centrally into veins that course along the walls of the lateral ventricles to form a deep venous system, which also empties into the dural sinuses. Nearly all of the venous blood from the brain leaves the cranium by way of the **internal jugular vein.**

A   MAJOR ARTERIAL SUPPLY AND CIRCLE OF WILLIS

B   DISTRIBUTING ARTERIES

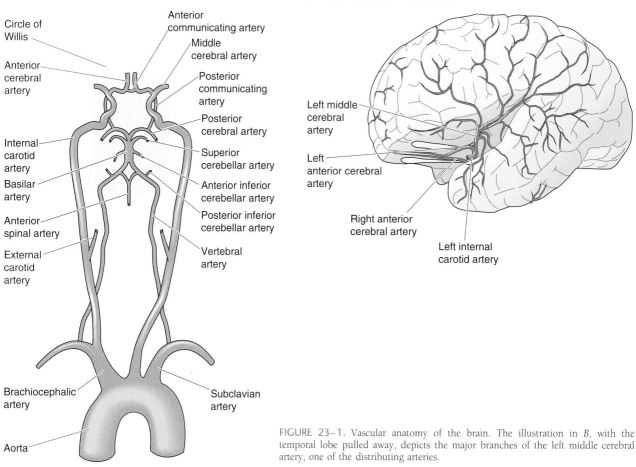

FIGURE 23–1. Vascular anatomy of the brain. The illustration in *B*, with the temporal lobe pulled away, depicts the major branches of the left middle cerebral artery, one of the distributing arteries.

CAPILLARIES. One of the most characteristic features of the brain vasculature is the **blood-brain barrier** (p. 408), which prevents the solutes in the lumen of the capillaries from having direct access to the brain extracellular fluid (BECF). For this reason, many drugs that act on other organs or vascular beds have no effect on the brain. Polar and water-soluble compounds cross the blood-brain barrier slowly, and the ability of proteins to cross the barrier is extremely limited. Only water, O_2, and CO_2 (or other gases) can readily diffuse across the cerebral capillaries. Glucose crosses more slowly via facilitated diffusion. No substance is *entirely* excluded from the brain; the critical variable is the rate of transfer. The blood-brain barrier protects the brain from abrupt changes in the composition of arterial blood. In a similar manner, a blood-testis barrier protects the germinal epithelia in males. The blood-brain barrier may become damaged in regions of the brain that are injured, infected, or occupied by tumors. Such damage can be helpful in identifying the location of tumors because tracers that are excluded from healthy CNS tissue can enter the tumor. In specialized areas of the brain—the **circumventricular organs** (p. 409)—the capillaries are fenestrated and have permeability characteristics similar to those of capillaries in the intestinal circulation.

LYMPHATICS. The brain lacks lymphatic vessels.

VASCULAR VOLUME. The skull encloses all of the cerebral vasculature, along with the brain and the cerebrospinal fluid compartments. Because the rigid cranium has a fixed total volume, vasodilation and an increase in vascular volume in one region of the brain must be met by reciprocal volume changes elsewhere within the cranium. Tight control of the cerebral blood volume is essential for preventing elevation of the intracranial pressure. With cerebral edema or hemorrhage, or with the growth of a brain tumor, neurologic dysfunction can result from the restriction of blood flow due to vascular compression. An analogous situation can occur in the eyes of patients with glaucoma (p. 333). Pressure buildup within the eye compresses the optic nerve and retinal artery, and blindness can result from the damage caused by diminished blood flow to the retinal cells.

Neural, Metabolic, and Myogenic Mechanisms Control Blood Flow to the Brain

Cerebral blood flow averages 50 ml/min for each 100 g of brain tissue and, because of autoregulation, is relatively constant. Nevertheless, regional changes in blood distribution occur in response to changing patterns of neuronal activity (Fig. 23–2).

NEURAL CONTROL. *Sympathetic* nerve fibers supplying the brain vasculature originate from postganglionic neurons in the superior cervical ganglia, and travel with the internal carotid and vertebral arteries into the skull, branching with the arterial supply. The sympathetic nerve terminals release norepinephrine, which causes contraction of VSMCs. *Parasympathetic* innervation of the cerebral vessels arises from branches of the facial nerve; they elicit a modest vasodilation when activated. The cerebral vessels are also supplied with sensory nerves, whose cell bodies are located in the trigeminal ganglia and whose sensory processes contain substance P and CGRP, both of which are vasodilatory neurotransmitters. Local perturbations (e.g., changes in pressure or chemistry) may stimulate the sensory nerve endings to release these vasodilators, an example of an "axon reflex."

Despite this innervation, neural control of the cerebral vasculature is relatively weak. Instead, it is the local metabolic requirements of the brain cells that primarily govern vasomotor activity in the brain.

METABOLIC CONTROL. A local increase in brain metabolism lowers P_{O_2} in the nearby BECF, and also raises P_{CO_2} and lowers pH. These changes trigger vasodilation and thus a compensatory increase in blood flow. Cerebral VSMCs relax mainly in response to low *extra*cellular pH; these cells are insensitive to increased P_{CO_2} per se, and decreased intracellular pH actually causes a weak vasoconstriction.

How does brain blood flow respond to systemic changes in pH? Lowering *arterial* pH at a constant P_{CO_2} (metabolic acidosis; p. 642) has little effect on cerebral blood flow because arterial H^+ cannot easily penetrate the blood-brain barrier, and therefore does not readily reach cerebral VSMCs. On the other hand, lowering arterial pH by increasing P_{CO_2} (respiratory acidosis) (p. 640) rapidly leads to a fall in the pH around VSMCs because CO_2 readily crosses the blood-brain barrier. This fall in pH of the BECF evokes pronounced dilation of the cerebral vasculature, with an increase in blood flow that occurs within seconds. The rise in arterial P_{CO_2} caused by inhaling 7% CO_2 can cause cerebral blood flow to double. Conversely, the fall in arterial P_{CO_2} caused by hyperventilation raises the pH of the BECF, producing cerebral vasoconstriction, decreased blood flow, and dizziness.

A fall in the blood and tissue P_{O_2}—from hypoxemia or impaired cardiac output—may also contribute to cerebral vasodilation, although the effects are less dramatic than those produced by arterial hypercapnia. The vasodilatory effects of hypoxia may be direct or may be mediated by release of adenosine, K^+, or nitric oxide into the BECF.

MYOGENIC CONTROL. Cerebral resistance vessels are inherently responsive to changes in their transmural pressure, with increases in diameter leading to vasoconstriction.

Autoregulation Maintains a Fairly Constant Cerebral Blood Flow Across a Broad Range of Perfusion Pressures

The perfusion pressure to the brain is the difference between the systemic arterial pressure (mean pressure, ~95 mm Hg) and intracranial venous pressure, which is nearly equal to the intracranial pressure (<10 mm Hg). A decrease in cerebral blood flow could thus result from a fall in arterial pressure or a rise in intracranial (or venous)

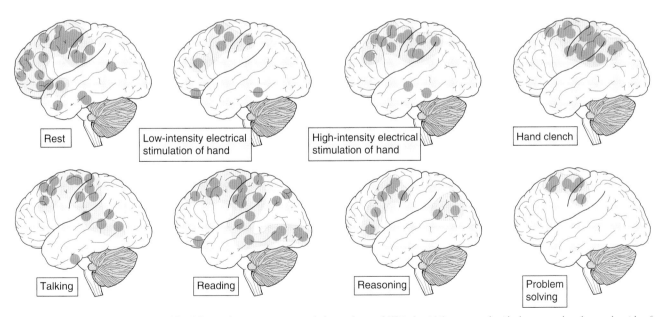

FIGURE 23–2. Changes in regional blood flow. The investigators used the washout of ^{133}Xe (p. 444), measured with detectors placed over the side of the patient's head, as an index of regional blood flow in the dominant cerebral hemisphere. The *turquoise* "hot spots" represent regions where blood flow was more than 20% above mean blood flow for the entire brain. At rest, blood flow is greatest in the frontal and premotor regions. The patterns of blood flow change in characteristic ways with the other seven forms of cerebral activity. (Data from Ingvar DH: Functional landscapes of the dominant hemisphere. Brain Res 107:181–197, 1976.)

pressure. However, the local control of cerebral blood flow maintains a nearly constant blood flow through perfusion pressures ranging from approximately 70 to 150 mm Hg. This constancy of blood flow—**autoregulation** (p. 480)—maintains a continuous supply of O_2 and nutrients. In patients with hypertension, the cerebral blood flow remains normal because cerebral vascular resistance increases. Conversely, vascular resistance falls with hypotension. This autoregulation of blood flow has both myogenic and metabolic components.

Increases in intracranial pressure compress the brain vasculature and tend to reduce blood flow despite autoregulatory vasodilation. In such cases, the brain regulates its blood flow by inducing reflexive changes in *systemic arterial pressure*. This principle is exemplified by the **Cushing reflex**, an increase in arterial pressure that occurs in response to an increase in intracranial pressure. It appears that intracranial compression causes a local ischemia that stimulates vasomotor centers in the medulla. Increased sympathetic activity then triggers a rise in total peripheral resistance. The Cushing reflex may occur acutely with the swelling following a head injury, or more gradually with growth of a brain tumor. Over a considerable pressure range, the Cushing reflex ensures that the perfusion pressure can offset the effects of vascular compression, and thereby maintain the cerebral blood flow.

THE HEART

The Coronary Circulation Receives 5% of the Resting Cardiac Output from the Left Heart, and Mostly Returns It to the Right Heart

The heart receives approximately 5% of the resting cardiac output, although it represents less than 0.5% of total body weight. The heart normally uses oxidative phosphorylation to generate the adenosine triphosphate (ATP) required for pumping blood. However, of all the O_2 that the heart consumes, no more than 40% reflects the oxidation of carbohydrate. More than 60% of myocardial O_2 consumption in the fasting state is due to the oxidation of fatty acids. The myocardium readily oxidizes ketone bodies (p. 1083), which can provide considerable energy during starvation or during diabetic ketoacidosis. When the O_2 supply is adequate, the heart takes up and oxidizes both lactate and pyruvate, as do red (i.e., oxidative) skeletal muscle fibers, although the arterial concentration of pyruvate is usually low. When the energetic demand for ATP exceeds the supply of O_2, the heart can no longer take up lactate, but instead releases lactate by breaking down its own glycogen stores. In this manner, the heart can continue to function for a short time when deprived of O_2. If hypoxia develops in the myocardium, nociceptive fibers trigger the sensation of referred pain, known as **angina pectoris**. More severe or prolonged insults damage the myocardial tissue, which eventually becomes necrotic (**myocardial infarction**).

The entire blood supply to the myocardium derives from the right and left coronary arteries, which originate at the root of the aorta behind the cusps of the aortic valves (Fig. 23–3). Although anatomy is subject to individual variation, the **right coronary artery** generally supplies the right ventricle and atrium, and the left coronary artery supplies the left ventricle and atrium. The **left coronary artery** divides near its origin into two principal branches: The **left circumflex artery** sends branches to the left atria and ventricle, and the **left anterior descending artery** descends to the apex of the heart and branches to supply the interventricular septum and a portion of the right as well as the left ventricle. These arteries course over the heart, branching into segments that penetrate into the tissue, and dividing into capillary networks. Capillary density in histologic sections of the human heart exceeds 3000/mm² (skeletal muscle has only ~400/mm²). The small diameter of cardiac muscle fibers (<20 μm), less than half that of skeletal muscle (~50 μm), facilitates O_2 diffusion into the cardiac cells, which have a high energetic demand.

Once blood passes through the capillaries, it collects in venules, which drain outward from the myocardium to

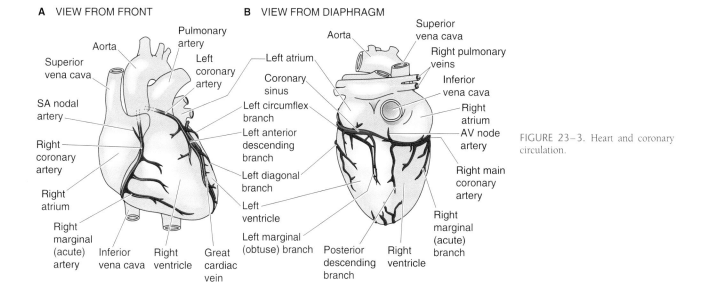

A VIEW FROM FRONT

Aorta, Pulmonary artery, Left coronary artery, Superior vena cava, SA nodal artery, Right coronary artery, Right atrium, Right marginal (acute) artery, Inferior vena cava, Right ventricle, Great cardiac vein

B VIEW FROM DIAPHRAGM

Left atrium, Coronary sinus, Left circumflex branch, Left anterior descending branch, Left diagonal branch, Left ventricle, Left marginal (obtuse) branch, Posterior descending branch, Right ventricle, Aorta, Superior vena cava, Right pulmonary veins, Inferior vena cava, Right atrium, AV node artery, Right main coronary artery, Right marginal (acute) branch

FIGURE 23–3. Heart and coronary circulation.

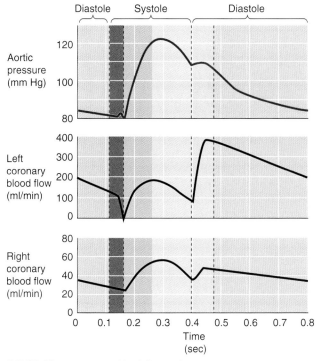

FIGURE 23–4. Coronary blood flow cycle.

converge into the epicardial veins. These veins empty into the right atrium via the **coronary sinus**. Other vascular channels drain directly into the cardiac chambers. These include the **thebesian veins**, which drain capillary beds within the ventricular wall. Because the deoxygenated blood carried by the thebesian veins exits predominantly into the ventricles, this blood flow bypasses the pulmonary circulation. Numerous *collateral* vessels among branches of the arterial vessels and throughout the venous system act as anastomoses; these provide alternative routes for blood flow should a primary vessel become occluded.

Extravascular Compression Impairs Coronary Blood Flow During Systole

In other systemic vascular beds, blood flow roughly parallels the pressure profile in the aorta, rising in systole and falling in diastole (see Fig. 21–3A). However, in the coronary circulation, flow is somewhat paradoxical: Although the heart is the source of its own perfusion pressure, myocardial contraction effectively compresses its own vascular supply. Therefore, the profile of blood flow through the coronary arteries depends on both the perfusion pressure in the aorta (Fig. 23–4, *top panel*) and the extravascular compression provided by the contracting ventricles, particularly the left ventricle.

Blood flow in the *left coronary artery* may actually reverse transiently in early systole (see Fig. 23–4, *middle panel*), as the force of the left ventricle's isovolumetric contraction compresses the left coronary vessels, while the aortic pressure has not yet begun to rise (i.e., aortic valve is still closed). As aortic pressure increases later during systole, coronary blood flow increases, but never reaches

very high values. However, early during diastole, when the relaxed ventricles no longer compress the left coronary vessels and aortic pressure is still high, left coronary flow rises rapidly to extremely high levels. All told, approximately 80% of total left coronary blood flow occurs during diastole.

In contrast, the profile of flow through the *right coronary artery* (see Fig. 23–4, *lower panel*) is very similar to the pressure profile of its feed vessel, the aorta. Here, systole contributes a greater proportion of the total flow, and systolic reversal does not occur. The reason for this difference is the lower wall tension developed by the right heart, which pumps against the low resistance of the pulmonary circulation.

The impact of systolic contraction on the perfusion of the left coronary vessels is highlighted by the effect of ventricular fibrillation (see Fig. 20–13I). At the onset of this lethal arrhythmia, left coronary perfusion transiently *increases*, reflecting the loss of mechanical compression of the vasculature.

Changes in heart rate, because they affect the duration of diastole more than that of systole, also affect coronary flow. During tachycardia, the fraction of the cardiac cycle spent in diastole decreases, minimizing the time available for maximal left coronary perfusion. If the heart is healthy, the coronary vessels can adequately dilate in response to the metabolic signals generated by increased cardiac work, which offsets the negative effects of the shorter diastole. On the other hand, a high heart rate can be dangerous when severe coronary artery disease restricts blood flow.

Coronary blood flow not only varies in *time* during the cardiac cycle, it also varies with *depth* in the wall of the heart. Blood flows to cardiac myocytes through arteries that penetrate from the epicardium toward the endocardium. During systole, the intramuscular pressure is greatest near the endocardium and least near the epicardium. All things being equal, the perfusion of the endocardium would therefore be less than that of the epicardium. However, total blood flows to the endocardial and epicardial halves are approximately equal because the endocardium has a lower intrinsic vascular resistance, and thus a greater blood flow during *diastole*. When the diastolic pressure at the root of the aorta is pathologically low (e.g., aortic regurgitation) or coronary arterial resistance is high (e.g., coronary artery occlusion), endocardial blood flow falls below the epicardial flow. Thus, the inner wall of the left ventricle often experiences the greatest damage with atherosclerotic heart disease.

Myocardial Blood Flow Parallels Myocardial Metabolism

A striking feature of the coronary circulation is the nearly linear correspondence between myocardial O_2 consumption and myocardial blood flow. This relationship persists in isolated heart preparations, emphasizing that metabolic signals are the principal determinants of O_2 delivery to the myocardium. In a resting individual, each 100 g of heart tissue receives 60 to 70 ml/min of blood flow. Normally, the heart extracts 70% to 80% of the O_2 content of arterial blood (normally ~20 ml/dl blood), thereby producing an extremely low venous O_2 content (~5 ml/dl). Therefore, the myocardium cannot respond to increased metabolic demands by extracting much more O_2 than it already does when the individual is at rest. The heart can meet large increases in O_2 demand only by increasing coronary blood flow, which can exceed 250 ml/min per 100 g with exercise.

Because blood pressure normally varies within fairly narrow limits, the only way to substantially increase blood flow through the coronary circulation during exercise is by vasodilation. The heart relies primarily on metabolic mechanisms to increase the caliber of its coronary vessels. **Adenosine** has received particular emphasis in this regard. An increased metabolic activity of the heart, an insufficient coronary blood flow, or a fall in myocardial PO_2 results in adenosine release. Adenosine then diffuses to the vascular smooth-muscle cells, activating purinoceptors to induce vasodilation by lowering $[Ca^{2+}]_i$ (see Table 19–7). Thus, inadequate perfusion to a region of tissue would elevate interstitial adenosine levels, causing vasodilation and restoration of flow to the affected region.

When cardiac demand outstrips the blood supply, a transient rise in $[K^+]_o$ may also contribute to the initial increase in coronary perfusion (see Table 19–8). However, it is unlikely that K^+ mediates sustained elevations in blood flow. An elevation of the PCO_2 and a fall in the PO_2 may also lower coronary vascular resistance.

Coronary blood flow is relatively stable between perfusion pressures of approximately 70 mm Hg and more than 150 mm Hg. Thus, like the brain, the blood flow to the heart exhibits autoregulation. In addition to the myogenic response, metabolites such as adenosine and O_2 contribute to coronary autoregulation.

Although Sympathetic Stimulation Directly Constricts Coronary Vessels, Accompanying Metabolic Effects Predominate, Producing an Overall Vasodilation

Sympathetic nerves course throughout the heart, following the arterial supply. Stimulating these nerves causes the heart to beat more frequently and more forcefully. β_1 adrenoceptors on the cardiac myocytes mediate these chronotropic and inotropic responses. As discussed in the previous section, the increased metabolic work of the myocardium leads to coronary vasodilation via metabolic pathways. However, during pharmacologic inhibition of the β_1 receptors on the cardiac myocytes, which prevents the increase in metabolism, sympathetic nerve stimulation causes a coronary *vasoconstriction*. This response is the direct effect of sympathetic nerve activity on α adrenoceptors on the VSMCs of the coronary resistance vessels. Thus, blocking β_1 receptors "unmasks" adrenergic constriction. However, under normal circumstances (i.e., no β blockade), the tendency of the *metabolic* pathways to vasodilate far overwhelms the tendency of the *sympathetic* pathways to vasoconstrict.

Activation of the **vagus nerve** has only a mild vasodilatory effect on the coronary resistance vessels. This muted response is not due to insensitivity of the resistance vessels to acetylcholine, which elicits a pronounced vasodilation when administered directly. Rather, the release of acetylcholine from the vagus nerve is restricted to the vicinity of the sinoatrial node. Thus, the vagus nerve has a much greater effect on heart rate than on coronary resistance.

Collateral Vessel Growth Can Provide Blood Flow to Ischemic Regions

When a coronary artery or one of its primary branches becomes abruptly occluded, ischemia can produce necrosis (i.e., a myocardial infarct) in the region deprived of blood flow. However, if a coronary artery narrows *gradually* over time, collateral blood vessels may develop and at least partially ameliorate the reduced delivery of O_2 and nutrients to the compromised area, preventing or at least diminishing tissue damage. Collateral vessels originate from existing branches that undergo remodeling with the proliferation of endothelial and smooth-muscle cells. Stimuli for collateral development include angiogenic molecules (p. 481) released from the ischemic tissue and changes in mechanical stress in the walls of vessels supplying the affected region.

Vasodilator Drugs May Compromise Myocardial Flow Through "Coronary Steal"

A variety of drugs can promote vasodilation of the coronary arteries. These are typically prescribed for patients suffering from angina pectoris, the chest pain associated with inadequate blood flow to the heart (see box titled Treating Coronary Artery Disease). If the buildup of atherosclerotic plaque—which underlies angina pectoris—occurs in the large epicardial arteries, the increased resistance lowers the pressure in the downstream microvessels. Under such conditions, the physician should be cautious in using pharmacologic agents to dilate the coronary vessels: In an ischemic area of the myocardium, downstream from a stenosis, metabolic stimuli may have already maximally dilated the arterioles. Administering a vasodilator can then only increase the diameter of blood vessels in *nonischemic* vascular beds that are parallel to the ischemic ones. The result is **coronary steal**, a further reduction in the pressure downstream from the site of stenosis, and further compromise of the blood flow to the ischemic region. When vasodilator therapy relieves angina, the favorable result is more likely attributable to the vasodilation of the *noncoronary* systemic vessels, which reduces the work of the heart.

THE SKELETAL MUSCLE

Perhaps the most impressive characteristic of the blood flow to skeletal muscle is its extreme range. Muscle blood flow at rest is 5 to 10 ml/min for each 100 g of tissue. With maximal aerobic exercise, it may increase 50-fold, reaching 250 ml/min or more for each 100 g of active muscle. The linear correspondence among work rate, O_2 consumption, and muscle blood flow implies a "coupling" between muscle fiber activity and O_2 delivery to capillaries. Muscle blood flow during exercise is the subject of Chapter 59. Here we discuss the key features of the

TREATING CORONARY ARTERY DISEASE

For many patients with gradual narrowing of their coronary arteries by atherosclerotic plaque, the first sign of disease may be the development of **angina pectoris**. Pain results when the metabolic demands of a region of myocardium exceed the ability of the compromised blood supply to satisfy those needs. Attacks of angina are often accompanied by characteristic changes on the electrocardiogram. If the diagnosis is in doubt—the chest pain of angina can sometimes be mimicked by gastroesophageal reflux, hyperventilation, costochondritis, and other clinical entities—an exercise test may stress the heart sufficiently to bring on the pain, induce ECG changes, or alter coronary blood flow as monitored by a thallium scan (see box on p. 444). Some patients with significant coronary artery narrowing never experience angina, and are said to have silent *ischemia*. In these patients, only an astute clinician may detect the coronary disease.

Many patients with a stable anginal pattern respond well to medication. *Nitrates* induce vasodilation by releasing nitric oxide (p. 110). The nitrates dilate peripheral veins, reducing venous return and thus the preload to the heart (p. 528); they also dilate the arteries and arterioles, reducing blood pressure and therefore the afterload. Finally, nitrates may increase coronary collateral flow to the involved region of myocardium (however, see discussion of "coronary steal" on p. 564). *Beta blockers* prevent the sympathetic nervous system from stimulating myocardial β_1 receptors, thereby reducing both heart rate and contractility, and thus metabolic demand. *Calcium channel blockers* lessen the contractility of the heart muscle and the vascular smooth muscle. These interventions all reduce the metabolic demands of the heart.

In patients for whom medication cannot control the angina, or who develop a pattern of unstable angina with an increasing frequency and severity of anginal attacks, mechanical revascularization may be required. For a long time, the only option was coronary artery bypass grafting, but nowadays **percutaneous transluminal coronary angioplasty** may often be successful. A cardiologist can perform this procedure at the same time as a diagnostic coronary artery catheterization. The physician advances a balloon-tipped catheter through a peripheral artery into the left ventricle, and then loops the catheter back out the left ventricle to have a favorable angle for entering the coronary vessels from the aorta. Inflating the balloon at the site of the obstruction flattens the plaque into the wall of the vessel and restores blood flow. Recurrence of the obstruction may be due to proliferation of VSMCs. Refinements in the technique, the placing of stents at the treated site, and the use of aggressive anticoagulation have all contributed to the technique's growing success. Variants of this technique, in which lasers are used, are coming under study increasingly.

Given the continued prevalence of coronary artery disease, a great deal of research has been aimed at developing alternatives to medication and mechanical revascularization. Among the most promising of these is the use of angiogenesis promoters that promote the growth of new blood vessels (p. 481).

organization of the skeletal muscle vasculature, and the integration of its blood flow control mechanisms.

A Microvascular Unit Is the Capillary Bed Supplied by a Single Terminal Arteriole

The vascular supply to skeletal muscle begins externally to the tissue in the **feed arteries**. These muscular vessels are the last branches of the arterial supply, located just before entry into the tissue. As much as 30% to 50% of the total resistance to blood flow through skeletal muscle resides in these feed arteries. Therefore, an important site of blood flow control is located *proximally* to the microvessels that are in direct contact with skeletal muscle fibers.

The arteriolar network originates from the site at which a feed artery enters the muscle. Within the muscle, arterioles branch through several orders (Fig. 23–5A) until reaching the **terminal arterioles** (see Fig. 23–5B), which are the last branches to contain smooth muscle and, therefore, the last branches still able to control blood flow. Thus, the terminal arteriole is the functional equivalent of the precapillary sphincter (p. 464). The group of capillaries supplied by a terminal arteriole represents one **microvascular unit**, which is the smallest functional unit of blood flow control in skeletal muscle. Each unit consists of 15 to 20 capillaries that run parallel to the muscle fibers in each direction, for a distance of 1 mm or less, ending in a **collecting venule**.

Owing to the profound differences in length between capillaries (≤ 1 mm) and muscle fibers (centimeters), many such microvascular units are required to span the distance of each muscle fiber. When a muscle fiber contracts, blood flow must increase throughout all of the microvascular units that supply that fiber.

Metabolites Released by Active Muscle Trigger Vasodilation and an Increase in Blood Flow

When skeletal muscle is at rest, its vascular resistance is high, blood flow is low, and the venous O_2 content is only a few milliliters per deciliter lower than the arterial O_2 content. As exercise begins, the terminal arterioles (those closest to the capillaries) dilate first. This vasodilation increases blood flow through capillaries that are already conducting blood, and also opens up quiescent capillaries, thus increasing the number of perfused capillaries and decreasing the effective intercapillary distance (p. 465). If total blood flow has not yet increased very much, the increased muscle demand for O_2 produces a large increase in the O_2 extraction ratio (p. 465). As metabolic demand later increases, additional O_2 delivery is required. The vasculature meets this demand by progressively dilating the terminal arterioles, then the more proximal arteriolar branches and feed arteries. Thus, vasodilation "ascends" the resistance network.

A coordinated vasodilation throughout the resistance network is essential when segments having substantial resistance are organized *in series* with each other. Dilating the downstream arterioles, without dilating the proximal

A   SKELETAL-MUSCLE CIRCULATION

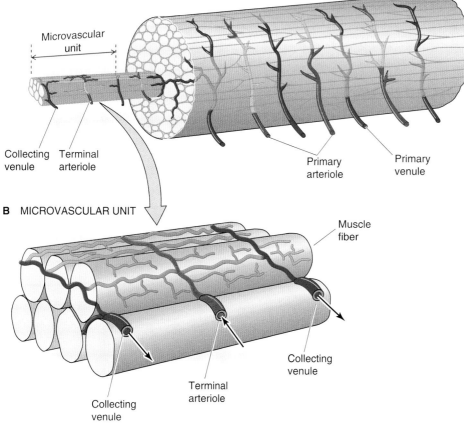

B   MICROVASCULAR UNIT

FIGURE 23–5. Microvascular units in skeletal muscle. *A*, A feed artery (not shown) branches into primary arterioles, which undergo several more orders of branching before reaching the level of a terminal arteriole. *B*, The terminal arteriole supplies a "microvascular unit" (<1 mm in length).

arterioles and feed arteries, would result in only a limited ability to increase muscle blood flow because of the high resistance of upstream vessels. Thus, when feed arteries dilate in concert with arterioles, the increase in muscle blood flow is profound.

The primary stimulus triggering vasodilation is the release of vasodilator substances (e.g., adenosine, CO_2, K^+) from active muscle fibers in proportion to the energy expenditure. These metabolites diffuse locally and relax the VSMCs of resistance vessels, thereby increasing blood flow in proportion to local demand. Although a variety of substances released by muscle fibers can contribute to the hyperemia, no single stimulus yet explains the integrated response of blood flow control to muscle contraction. Furthermore, the hyperemic response to increased muscle activity occurs within a second or two of the onset of exercise. In contrast, it would take several seconds for these substances to be produced by the skeletal muscle fibers, reach the interstitium, and diffuse to the arteriolar VSMCs in sufficient concentration to elicit vasodilation.

The initiation of muscle fiber contraction leads to a release of K^+ that may hyperpolarize the nearby VSMCs (see Table 19–8). Once triggered, this hyperpolarization causes the small proximal arterioles to dilate, and the electrical signal spreads from cell to cell, conducting upstream to the larger vessels and causing them to dilate in concert. This mechanism of conducted vasodilation, together with the action of the muscle pump, likely contributes to the rapid onset of hyperemia (discussed later). In

the steady state, changes in the levels of other metabolites (e.g., increases in adenosine and CO_2 levels, or decreases in PO_2 levels) sustain the hyperemic response.

Sympathetic Innervation Increases the Intrinsic Tone of Resistance Vessels

Sympathetic nerve fibers invest the entire resistance network, from feed arteries to terminal arterioles. The release of norepinephrine by these nerve terminals leads to vasoconstriction. Increased transmural pressure results in increased myogenic tone, also producing vasoconstriction. On the other hand, the shear stress of blood flowing past the endothelial cells produces vasodilators such as nitric oxide (NO). The interactions among these vasoconstrictor and vasodilatory mechanisms maintain the intrinsic basal tone of the VSMCs. Venules also constrict in response to sympathetic nerve stimulation, but are not directly innervated, and instead respond to norepinephrine that diffuses from the nearby arterioles.

With nearly half of the body mass composed of muscle, the sympathetic control of vasomotor tone to skeletal muscle is an integral component of the regulation of both systemic arterial pressure (via total peripheral resistance) and cardiac filling (via venous capacitance and return). This principle is particularly true during maximal aerobic exercise, when more than 80% of the cardiac output flows to the active skeletal muscles.

The basal firing rate of the sympathetic nerves to skeletal muscle is 1 to 2 Hz, which contributes only modestly to the resting vasomotor tone. However, when high-pressure baroreceptors detect a fall in blood pressure (p. 535), sympathetic firing to skeletal muscle may increase to 8 to 16 Hz. This degree of sympathetic activity can close the lumens of arterioles in skeletal muscle.

During exercise, the proportion of cardiac output flowing through skeletal muscle increases. This redistribution of systemic blood flow occurs for two reasons. First, an increase in sympathetic tone constricts splanchnic circulation (see later), renal circulation (p. 771), and the vessels of *inactive* skeletal muscle. Indeed, only the brain and heart are spared. Second, the metabolites released by *active* skeletal muscle overcome the vasoconstriction that sympathetic activity would otherwise produce. In addition, substances released during muscle fiber contraction (e.g., NO and adenosine) may inhibit norepinephrine release from sympathetic neurons.

The vasodilatory effects of the metabolites notwithstanding, sympathetic vasoconstrictor activity can be overwhelming, particularly when another large mass of muscle is active simultaneously and requires a substantial portion of cardiac output. Thus, during "whole body" exercise, each muscle group may receive only a fraction of the blood flow it would otherwise get if it were the *only* active group in the body. It is at the level of the feed arteries—which are external to the muscle and thus physically removed from the direct influence of the vasoactive products of muscular activity—that sympathetic

vasoconstriction puts an upper limit on blood flow during intense aerobic exercise. Dilation of arterioles *within* the muscle maximizes O_2 extraction by promoting capillary perfusion.

Rhythmic Contraction Promotes Blood Flow Through the "Muscle Pump"

During exercise, skeletal muscle undergoes rhythmic changes in length and tension, giving rise to mechanical forces within the tissue analogous to those of the beating heart. The contraction of muscle forces venous blood out of the muscle and impedes arterial inflow (Fig. 23–6). Because valves in the veins prevent backflow of blood, each muscle contraction squeezes and empties the veins, driving blood toward the heart (see also p. 519). During the subsequent relaxation, the reduction in venous pressure increases the driving force for capillary perfusion. In addition, peak arterial inflow occurs during relaxation between contractions. This pumping action of skeletal muscle on the vasculature imparts substantial kinetic energy to the blood, thereby reducing the work of the heart. Remarkably, the skeletal muscle pump may generate up to half of the energy required to circulate blood, an essential contribution for achieving the high blood flows experienced during maximal aerobic exercise. By contrast, using drugs to pharmacologically dilate blood vessels in inactive muscle can increase blood flow to a lesser extent than is observed with rhythmic contractions.

THE SPLANCHNIC CIRCULATION

The splanchnic circulation includes the blood flow through the stomach, small intestine, large intestine, pancreas, spleen, and liver (Fig. 23–7A). The majority of flow to the liver occurs through the portal vein, which carries the venous blood draining from all of these organs except the liver itself.

The Vascular Supply to the Gut Is Highly Interconnected

The **celiac artery** is the primary blood supply to the stomach, pancreas, and spleen. The **superior and inferior mesenteric arteries** supply the large and small intestines, as well as parts of the stomach and pancreas. The superior mesenteric artery is the largest of all the splanchnic branches from the aorta, carrying over 10% of the cardiac output. The extensive interconnections between the arcading arterial branches (see Fig. 23–7B) provide multiple collateral pathways through which blood can reach each portion of the intestines. This arrangement lessens the risk that the intestines may become ischemic should one of the arteries become occluded.

The microvascular network in the small intestine (see Fig. 23–7C) is representative of that throughout the gastrointestinal tract. After penetrating the wall of the intestine, small arteries course through the various muscle layers and reach the submucosa, where they branch into arterioles. Some arterioles remain in the submucosa to

1 Before muscle contraction, blood enters vein.

2 When the muscle contracts, upper valve opens further, but lower valve closes, so that contracting muscle pushes blood up.

3 After muscle relaxes, upper valve closes, preventing backflow...

A

B

Open valve

Closed valve

C

...and lower valve opens, allowing veins to fill.

FIGURE 23–6. Muscle pump.

A MAJOR VESSELS

Liver

Hepatic vein

Portal vein

Hepatic artery

Spleen

Stomach

Celiac artery

Superior mesenteric artery

Inferior mesenteric artery

Pancreas

Intestines

Abdominal aorta

Inferior vena cava

B MESENTERIC ARTERIES

Superior mesenteric artery

Inferior mesenteric artery

Large intestine

Abdominal aorta

C BLOOD SUPPLY TO LAYERS OF INTESTINAL WALL

Artery

Villus

Muscularis

Sub mucosa

Mucosa

Muscularis mucosae

Vein

D MICROVASCULATURE OF THE VILLUS

Blood capillaries

Central lacteal

Arteriole

Venule

FIGURE 23–7. Splanchnic circulation.

form a submucosal vascular plexus. Others project toward the intestinal lumen and into the mucosa, including the villi. Still others project away from the mucosa, and course along the smooth-muscle bundles. Venules emerging from the villi and mucosal and muscularis layers converge into veins. These exit the intestinal wall, paralleling the arterial supply.

The arrangement of microvessels within a villus is like a fountain (see Fig. 23–7D). The incoming arteriole courses up the center of the villus, branching into many capillaries along the way to the tip of the villus. Capillaries converge into venules and carry blood back to the base of the villus. Capillaries also interconnect the arteriole and the venule all along the villus. These microvessels are permeable to solutes of low molecular weight or high lipid solubility.

The arrangement just described creates a **countercurrent flow** system that enables permeable solutes to move from the arteriole to the venule without having to traverse the entire length of the villus. For example, much of the bloodborne O_2 short circuits from the arteriole to the venule before reaching the tip of the villus, which therefore is particularly susceptible to anoxic damage. The situation is just the opposite for solutes (e.g., Na^+) that the villus epithelium absorbs during digestion. These solutes enter capillaries and then pass into venules. As the venous blood travels toward the base of the villus, the solute can diffuse out of the venules, into the interstitium, and then into the arterioles. In this way, the solute concentration in the arterial blood increases as the blood flows to the tip of the villus. This process increases the interstitial osmolarity near the tip of the villus, in a manner analogous to the mechanism that maintains high osmolality at the tip of the renal medulla (p. 831).

Because the capillaries in the villi are fenestrated (i.e., they have large pores) and have a large surface area, they are well suited for absorbing nutrients from the intestinal lumen. The venous blood carries away the majority of **water-soluble nutrients** absorbed from the gut, eventually delivering them to the portal vein. **Lipophilic nutrients** absorbed from the intestinal lumen enter the central lacteal of the villus (see Fig. 23–7D), which merges with the intestinal lymphatics. The lymph then delivers these substances into the bloodstream via the thoracic duct.

Blood Flow to the Gastrointestinal Tract Increases up to Eight-Fold Following a Meal ("Postprandial Hyperemia")

Throughout the gastrointestinal tract, blood flow in each layer of the gut wall closely correlates with the local metabolism (which reflects digestive and absorptive activity). Intestinal blood flow at rest, in the fasting state, is typically 30 ml/min for each 100 g of tissue. However, flow can reach 250 ml/min for each 100 g during peak hyperemia following a meal. The increase in blood flow with the ingestion and digestion of a meal reflects a complex interplay of several factors.

First, the central nervous system (CNS) initiates an "anticipatory" response that increases splanchnic blood flow with the mere thought of food—corresponding to the "cephalic phase" of gastric (p. 900) and pancreatic secretion (p. 921).

Second, mucosal metabolic activity during digestion and absorption primarily depends on the rate of active transport of substances across the epithelium. These activities consume O_2 and produce **vasodilator metabolites** (e.g., adenosine and CO_2) that increase blood flow locally.

Third, the absorption of nutrients generates hyperosmolality in both the blood and the lymphatic vessels of the villus. Hyperosmolality itself stimulates an increase in blood flow.

Fourth, during digestion, the gastrointestinal tract releases several hormones, some of which are vasoactive. Of these, **cholecystokinin** and **neurotensin** (see Table 40–1) may reach high enough concentrations in the local circulation to promote intestinal blood flow. The intestinal epithelium also releases various kinins (e.g., bradykinin and kallidin), which are powerful vasodilators. The magnitude of the postprandial hyperemia further depends on the nature of the luminal content. Bile acids and partially digested fats are particularly effective in promoting hyperemia by acting on chemoreceptors in the intestinal mucosa.

The circulatory system does not distribute the increased splanchnic blood flow equally to all digestive organs, nor does it distribute the flow equally throughout the wall of even one segment of bowel. During and following a meal, blood flow increases sequentially along the gastrointestinal tract, first in the stomach and then, sequentially, in more distal segments of the intestine as digestion proceeds. In all segments, blood flow through the muscularis layers primarily provides nutrition for the smooth-muscle cells. However, flow through the villi and submucosal vessels supports the absorption of foodstuffs, as well as the secretion of electrolytes, fluids, and enzymes. After a meal, splanchnic blood flow is elevated for 2 to 4 hours, primarily reflecting the vasodilation in the *mucosal* layer.

As in the heart and skeletal muscle, muscle contraction in the intestine (i.e., peristalsis) decreases blood flow, probably as a result of the compression applied by the muscularis in conjunction with the distending pressure of the luminal contents.

Sympathetic Activity Directly Constricts Splanchnic Vessels, Whereas Parasympathetic Activity Indirectly Dilates Them

The gastrointestinal tract is endowed with its own division of the autonomic nervous system, the **enteric nervous system** (ENS; pp. 384 and 883). At one level, the ENS is its own independent nervous system, with sensory neurons, the capacity to integrate and process sensory data, and motor neurons. One of the components of the ENS, the myenteric (or Auerbach) plexus, releases vasoactive neurotransmitters. However, this plexus probably achieves its major influence on blood flow by controlling the peristaltic activity of the intestinal smooth muscle.

The enteric division sends sensory information upstream to the peripheral ganglia and to the CNS. The ENS also receives important input from the sympathetic and parasympathetic divisions of the ANS. Postganglionic **sympathetic neurons** originate in the celiac, superior mesenteric, and inferior mesenteric ganglia and send nerve fibers that travel along the corresponding major arteries to all splanchnic organs. Except for the capillaries, all splanchnic blood vessels receive sympathetic innervation. The predominant neural influence is *sympathetic vasoconstriction*, mediated by norepinephrine acting on α adrenoceptors on VSMCs. The vasoconstriction occurs to a similar extent in both the muscularis and mucosal layers, without redistribution of flow between the layers. Vasoconstriction elicited by sympathetic activity can reduce blood flow to less than 10 ml/min per 100 g of tissue (i.e., ~25% of resting values).

Parasympathetic preganglionic fibers travel to the intestine via vagal or pelvic nerves, which contact postganglionic parasympathetic neurons in the intestinal wall. The effect of parasympathetic activity on blood flow is indirect. Parasympathetic activity stimulates intestinal motility and glandular secretion, which in turn, increases intestinal metabolism, thereby enhancing blood flow to the gut.

Changes in the Splanchnic Circulation Regulate Total Peripheral Resistance and the Distribution of Blood Volume

The splanchnic circulation serves both as a site of adjustable resistance and as a major reservoir of blood. During exercise, when blood flow increases to active skeletal muscle, sympathetic constriction of the splanchnic resistance vessels decreases the proportion of cardiac output directed to the viscera. Therefore, abdominal cramping can result from attempts to exercise too soon after eating, when the gastrointestinal tract still demands blood flow to support its digestive and absorptive activities.

The splanchnic circulation contains approximately 15% of the total blood volume, with the majority contained in the liver; sympathetic constriction of the capacitance vessels can rapidly mobilize about half of this blood volume. During increases in sympathetic tone, splanchnic arteriolar constriction reduces perfusion, resulting in the passive collapse of the splanchnic veins. Blood contained in these veins moves into the inferior vena cava, thus increasing the circulating blood volume. With a greater increase in sympathetic activity, as would occur with intense exercise or severe hemorrhage, active venoconstriction mobilizes even more venous blood, thereby helping to maintain arterial pressure.

Exercise and Hemorrhage Can Substantially Reduce Splanchnic Blood Flow

A reduction in blood flow leads to the production of vasodilator metabolites (e.g., adenosine and CO_2), which stimulate arteriolar dilation and increase O_2 delivery. Nevertheless, during maximal exercise or severe hemorrhage, blood flow through the gut may fall to less than 25% of its resting value. Fortunately, temporary reductions in splanchnic flow can occur without serious O_2 deprivation; at rest, the viscera normally extract only about 20% of the O_2 carried in the blood, so that extraction can increase several-fold. However, extended periods of compromised splanchnic blood flow can irreversibly damage the intestinal parenchyma.

Following a severe hemorrhage and sustained splanchnic vasoconstriction, the ischemic mucosal epithelia slough off, even after repletion of the blood volume and restoration of blood flow. Sloughing occurs particularly at the tips of the villi, where the epithelial cells are particularly susceptible to ischemia because of countercurrent flow (see p. 559). As these cells slough, it appears that pancreatic enzymes generate "activators" that enter the circulation and produce multiple organ failure. For example, such factors can lead to an irreversible decline in cardiovascular function. In an experimental setting, one can avoid damage to the heart by collecting the blood draining from the gut during the first several minutes of reperfusion, thereby preventing access of these as yet unidentified substances to the heart. Another major consequence of damaging the epithelium is **endotoxic shock**, which results from disruption of the barrier that normally prevents bacteria and toxins from escaping the intestinal lumen and entering the systemic circulation and peritoneal cavity.

The Liver Receives Its Blood Flow from Both the Systemic and the Portal Circulation

The liver receives nearly one fourth of resting cardiac output. Of this blood flow, approximately 25% is arterial blood that arrives via the hepatic artery. The remaining 75% of the hepatic blood flow comes from the portal vein, which drains the stomach, intestines, pancreas, and spleen (see Fig. 23–7A). Because the portal venous blood has already given up much of its O_2 to the gut, the hepatic artery is left to supply approximately 75% of the O_2 used by the liver.

We discuss the anatomy of the hepatic circulation in more detail on p. 977. Small branches of the portal vein give rise to terminal portal venules, and branches of the hepatic artery give rise to hepatic arterioles. These two independent sources of blood flow enter the liver lobule at its periphery. Blood flows from these terminal vessels into the sinusoids, which form the capillary network of the liver. The sinusoids converge at the center of the lobule to form terminal hepatic venules (i.e., central veins), which drain into progressively larger branches of the hepatic veins and finally into the inferior vena cava. Within the sinusoids, rapid exchange occurs between the blood and the hepatocytes because the vascular endothelial cells have large fenestrations and gaps, and thus do not meet to form interendothelial junctions as in other capillaries. Thus, the liver sinusoids are more permeable to protein than are capillaries elsewhere in the body. The passage of blood from the gastrointestinal tract past the reticuloendothelial cells of the liver (p. 975) also removes bacteria and particulate matter, thereby preventing the access of potentially harmful material to the general circulation.

The mean blood pressure in the portal vein is normally 10 to 12 mm Hg. In contrast, the pressure in the hepatic

PORTAL HYPERTENSION

The cirrhotic liver is hard, shrunken, scarred, and laced with thick bands of fibrotic tissue. The most common cause of this in the United States is chronic alcoholism, but worldwide, hepatitis B and hepatitis C are also leading causes. Less commonly, inherited diseases, such as hemochromatosis (iron overload) and Wilson disease (altered copper metabolism), can be responsible, as can diseases of unclear etiology, such as biliary cirrhosis and sclerosing cholangitis.

When damage to the liver becomes severe, the clinical consequences of cirrhosis can become life threatening. The 5-year survival rate is the same as that for primary lung cancer—less than 10%. The three major complications of cirrhosis are metabolic abnormalities, portal hypertension, and hepatic encephalopathy.

Metabolic abnormalities. The liver's inability to maintain its normal synthetic activities (p. 995) results in a range of metabolic problems. Both albumin and cholesterol levels fall, and the prothrombin time rises, indicating failure of the liver to manufacture proteins in the coagulation cascade. Decreased plasma levels of K^+ and Na^+ often herald the onset of renal failure, a consequence of the *hepatorenal syndrome*.

Portal hypertension. The scarring that accompanies cirrhosis causes increased resistance to blood flow through the liver. When the portal venous pressure rises, the signs and symptoms of portal hypertension can appear. The increased portal venous pressure leads to increased pressure in the splanchnic capillaries. The Starling forces (p. 469) thus promote the filtration and extravasation of fluid. The result is abdominal edema (i.e., fluid accumulation in the interstitium), which can progress to frank **ascites** (i.e., fluid in the peritoneal cavity). As the portal pressure rises farther, a portion of the portal blood begins to flow through and dilate the portal anastomoses with systemic veins. These anastomoses are present in the lower esophagus, around the umbilicus, at the rectum, and in the retroperitoneum.

Dilation of the vessels in the lower esophagus can lead to the development of *esophageal varices*. These veins, and similar veins in the stomach, can burst and cause life-threatening hemorrhage. When varices are associated with persistent or recurrent bleeding, the physician can inject sclerosing agents directly into the varices, a procedure called sclerotherapy. However, even after sclerotherapy, recurrent bleeding is not uncommon, and complications include perforation, stricture formation, infection, and aspiration. It is possible to prevent rupture of the varices in some patients by placing an intrahepatic portosystemic shunt. One introduces a catheter through the jugular vein and into the liver, and then places a stent between a branch of the hepatic vein and a branch of the portal vein, allowing portal blood to shunt directly into the vena cava.

In some cases of portal hypertension, surgical intervention is necessary. Portacaval shunts (i.e., those linking the portal vein and inferior vena cava) can stop rebleeding and reduce portal hypertension, but hepatic encephalopathy (see later) can occur and overall mortality is not improved. The distal splenorenal shunt is now the more popular choice of treatment. It is very effective in preventing rebleeding and, because it diverts only a portion of the blood flow away from the liver (i.e., just the blood exiting the spleen; see Fig. 23–7A), it is associated with a much lower incidence of encephalopathy.

Hepatic encephalopathy. Even as hepatic scarring increases vascular resistance through the liver, hepatic perfusion continues for a while. However, as we have just seen, eventually some of the portal blood flow shunts around the damaged liver into systemic veins, through pre-existing anastomoses. Because the liver is critical for removing and inactivating naturally occurring toxic metabolites (p. 985), as well as pharmacologic agents, toxins that bypass the liver directly enter the systemic veins and can build up in the plasma. If these toxins (e.g., NH_3) (see Fig. 38–6) cross the blood-brain barrier, they can cause acute delirium.

artery averages 90 mm Hg. These two systems, with very different pressures, feed into the sinusoids (8–9 mm Hg). The sinusoids drain into the hepatic veins ($\sim$5 mm Hg), and these in turn drain into the vena cava (2–5 mm Hg). These remarkable values lead us to three conclusions. First, there must be a very high "precapillary" resistance between the hepatic artery (90 mm Hg) and the sinusoids (8–9 mm Hg), causing the arterial pressure to step down to sinusoidal values. If the sinusoidal pressure were as high as in typical capillaries (e.g., 25 mm Hg), blood would flow from the hepatic artery to the sinusoids and then backward into the portal vein. Second, because the pressure in the portal vein (10–12 mm Hg) is only slightly higher than that in the sinusoids (8–9 mm Hg), the precapillary resistance of the portal inflow (75% of the total flow) must be very low. Third, because the pressure in the sinusoids is only slightly higher than that in the hepatic vein ($\sim$5 mm Hg), the resistance of the sinusoids must also be extremely low.

As a result of the unique hemodynamics of the liver,

changes in pressure within the hepatic vein have profound effects on fluid exchange across the wall of sinusoids. For example, in right-sided congestive heart failure, an elevated vena cava pressure can result in transudation of fluid from the liver into the peritoneal cavity, a condition known as **ascites**.

A change in the blood flow through one of the inputs to the liver (e.g., portal vein) leads to a reciprocal change in flow through the other input (i.e., hepatic artery). However, these adjustments do not fully stabilize total hepatic blood flow. For example, if the inflow through the hepatic artery decreases, the pressure inside the sinusoids falls slightly, leading to an increase in flow from the portal vein into the sinusoids. When the inflow through the portal vein decreases, metabolic factors (e.g., decreases in metabolites carried by the portal blood) trigger an increase in flow from the hepatic arteriolar system. The hepatic arterial supply displays autoregulation (p. 480), which is absent in the portal venous system. With changes in O_2 delivery, the liver compensates with corresponding changes in O_2 extraction ratio. Hence, the liver tends to maintain constant O_2 consumption.

THE SKIN

The Skin Is the Largest Organ of the Body

The skin is the major barrier between the internal milieu of the body and the unregulated environment of the outside world. Changes in blood flow to the skin also play a central role in the body's temperature regulation (p. 1237).

In terms of blood flow, we can divide the skin into "apical" skin (Fig. 23–8*A*—which is present on the nose, lips, ears, hands, and feet—and "nonapical" skin (see Fig. 23–8*B*). As in other vascular beds, arterioles break up into capillaries, which reunite to form venules. The capillaries reach only as superficially as the dermis; the epidermis does not have a blood supply. The venules that are part of a plexus of vessels near the dermal-epidermal border (i.e., the most superficial vessels) may contain an appreciable volume of blood, thereby imparting a pinkish hue to individuals with light-colored skin. When cutaneous blood flow decreases, this volume of blood also decreases, lessening the reddish component of skin color

(i.e., pallor). Local nutritional flow through the precapillary sphincters and capillaries is under the control of local vasodilator metabolites and sensory stimuli (e.g., temperature, touch, pain). For example, the vascular beds can respond to local thermal changes, largely independent of sympathetic nerve activity: The blood vessels dilate when the skin is directly heated, and constrict when cooled.

In addition to the effects of local metabolites and local warming and cooling, the blood flow to the skin is under sympathetic neural control. Increases in body core temperature increase blood flow to the skin, leading to a loss of heat. Decreases in core temperature result in the opposite effect of conserving heat. In contrast to other vascular beds, this neural control is far more important than local metabolic control in the overall regulation of skin blood flow.

Specialized Arteriovenous Anastomoses in Apical Skin Help Control Heat Loss

APICAL SKIN. The apical skin at the extremities of the body has a very high surface-to-volume ratio that favors heat loss. Circulation to these apical regions has an unusual feature—*arteriovenous (a–v) anastomoses* called **glomus bodies.** (These glomus bodies are unrelated to the

FIGURE 23–8. Blood flow to the skin. *A*, The density of glomus bodies (arteriovenous anastomoses) is ~500 per cm² in the nail beds. *B*, The nonapical skin lacks glomus bodies. Postganglionic sympathetic fibers release norepinephrine (NE), causing the usual vasoconstriction. Preganglionic sympathetic fibers release acetylcholine (ACh) and cause vasodilation, perhaps mediated by formation of bradykinin.

glomus cells of the peripheral chemoreceptors.) Glomus bodies are tiny nodules found in many parts of the body, including the ears, the pads of the fingers and toes, and the nail beds. As the afferent arteriole enters the connective tissue capsule of the glomus body, it becomes a vessel with a small lumen and a thick, muscular wall comprising multiple layers of myoepithelioid cells. These vessels—which have a rich sympathetic innervation—connect with short, thin-walled veins that eventually drain into larger skin veins. The a–v anastomoses, which are involved in heat exchange, are in parallel with the capillaries of the skin, which are involved in nutrient exchange (see Fig. 23–8A).

The anastomotic vessels are under neural control, rather than the control of local metabolites, and play a critical role in temperature regulation. In these apical regions, blood flow is under the control of sympathetic fibers that release norepinephrine and thereby constrict the arterioles, anastomotic vessels, and venules. Therefore, the increase in sympathetic tone that occurs in response to decreases in core temperature elicits vasoconstriction in the a–v anastomoses, a fall in blood flow, and a reduction in heat loss. Maximal sympathetic stimulation can completely obliterate the lumen of an anastomotic vessel, thus greatly reducing total blood flow to the skin. On the other hand, when the core temperature rises, the withdrawal of sympathetic tone leads to passive vasodilation; there is no active vasodilation. Indeed, blocking the sympathetic input to a hand in a neutral thermal environment can increase blood flow 4-fold above basal levels—as much as heat stress can produce. Thus, sympathetic tone is substantial at rest.

NONAPICAL SKIN. The body uses a very different approach for regulating blood flow in nonapical skin. One important difference is that the vasculature of this skin almost completely lacks a–v anastomoses. A second important difference is that there are two types of sympathetic neurons innervating the vessels of the skin: Some release *norepinephrine* and some release *acetylcholine*.

Vasoconstriction occurs in response to the release of norepinephrine. In contrast to the situation in *apical* skin, blockade of sympathetic innervation to *nonapical* skin in a thermoneutral environment produces little change in skin blood flow, demonstrating little vasoconstrictor activity at rest.

Vasodilation in nonapical skin occurs in response to sympathetic neurons that release acetylcholine (p. 388).

Indeed, blockade of sympathetic innervation to the nonapical skin in a warm environment produces vasoconstriction and a decrease in skin blood flow, demonstrating neurally directed vasodilation before the blockade. The precise mechanism of this vasodilation is obscure. One proposal is that the acetylcholine stimulates eccrine sweat glands, causing the secretion of sweat as well as enzymes that lead to the local formation of vasoactive molecules. For instance, gland cells release kallikrein, a protease that converts kininogens to kinins, one of which is bradykinin (p. 555). These kinins may act in a paracrine fashion on nearby blood vessels to relax VSMCs and thereby increase local perfusion. Cholinergic sympathetic neurons may cause vasodilation by means of a second pathway involving the co-release of vasodilatory neurotransmitters (e.g., CGRP, vasoactive intestinal polypeptide) that act directly on VSMCs, independent of sweat gland activity.

REFERENCES

Books and Reviews

Bohr DF, Somlyo AP, Sparks HV (eds): Handbook of Physiology. The Cardiovascular System. Vol. 2: Vascular Smooth Muscle. Bethesda, MD, American Physiological Society, 1980.

Faraci FM, Heistad DD: Regulation of the cerebral circulation: Role of endothelium and potassium channels. Physiol Rev 78:53–97, 1998.

Heistad DD, Kontos HA: Cerebral circulation. In Shepherd JT, Abboud FM (eds): Handbook of Physiology. The Cardiovascular System. Peripheral Circulation and Organ Blood Flow, Part 1, pp. 137–182. Bethesda, MD, American Physiological Society, 1983.

Hoffman JIE, Spaan JAE: Pressure-flow relations in coronary circulation. Physiol Rev 70:331–390, 1990.

Shepherd JT, Abboud FM (eds): Handbook of Physiology. The Cardiovascular System. Vol. 3, Part 1: Peripheral Circulation and Organ Blood Flow. Bethesda, MD, American Physiological Society, 1983.

Journal Articles

Apkon M, Boron WF: Extracellular but not intracellular alkalinization constricts rat cerebral arterioles. J Physiol 484:743–753, 1995.

Berne RM: Role of adenosine in the regulation of coronary blood flow. Circ Res 47:807–813, 1980.

Emerson GG, Segal SS: Alignment of microvascular units along skeletal muscle fibers of hamster retractor. J Appl Physiol 82:42–48, 1997.

Laughlin MH: Skeletal muscle blood flow capacity: Role of muscle pump in exercise hyperemia. Am J Physiol 253:H993–H1004, 1987.

Mitsuoka H, Kistler EB, Schmid-Schönbein GW: Generation of in vivo activating factors in the ischemic intestine by pancreatic enzymes. Proc Natl Acad Sci USA 97:1772–1777, 2000.

Segal SS, Duling BR: Flow control among microvessels coordinated by intercellular conduction. Science 234:868–870, 1986.

CHAPTER 24

Integrated Control of the Cardiovascular System

Emile L. Boulpaep

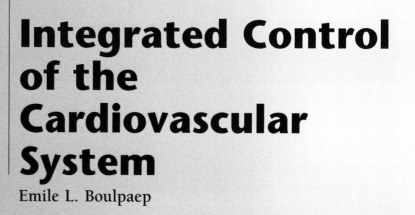

In the preceding chapters, we examined cardiovascular regulation at several different levels. Powerful *systemic* mechanisms operate over both the short term and the long term to control mean arterial pressure and cardiac output. Operating independently of these are *local* mechanisms of control that regulate blood flow at the microcirculatory level. In addition, individual organs have their own, unique tools for managing specific circulatory requirements. In this chapter, we put it all together, and learn how the cardiovascular system integrates the complex systemic, local, and individualized regulatory mechanisms in response to the demands of everyday life.

INTERACTION AMONG THE DIFFERENT CARDIOVASCULAR CONTROL SYSTEMS

The Control of the Cardiovascular System Involves "Linear," "Branched," and "Connected" Interactions

In the previous chapters, we often presented physiological responses in a linear sequence, or on a **linear chart**. For instance, we might represent the carotid-baroreceptor feedback loop (p. 536) as a linear sequence of events (Fig. 24–1A). However, cardiovascular parameters and associated physiological responses are often related by multiple factors, requiring a more complex diagram called a **branching tree** (or an algorithmic tree). For example, in our discussion of the control of cardiac output (p. 547), we started with the knowledge that cardiac output (CO) depends on *two* parameters—stroke volume (SV) and heart rate (HR). Therefore, with our very first step, we come to a fork in the road—an example of a branching tree (see Fig. 24–1B). At the next level, we encounter a pair of forks because SV and HR both depend on two parameters. Finally, at the third level, we see that each of the determinants of SV and HR depends on multiple factors (i.e., multiple forks).

The control of some cardiovascular parameters is even more complex, requiring that we graft branches from smaller trees. For example, we know from Ohm's law that *mean arterial pressure* depends on both *cardiac output* (and all the elements in its "branching tree" in Fig. 24–1B) and *total peripheral resistance*, which requires a branching tree of its own (see Fig. 24–1C). Moreover, sometimes an element in one part of the "forest" interacts with another element that is far away. A physiological system with such complex interactions is best represented by a **connected diagram**, which may include feedback loops (Fig. 24–1C, *red arrows*), parameters

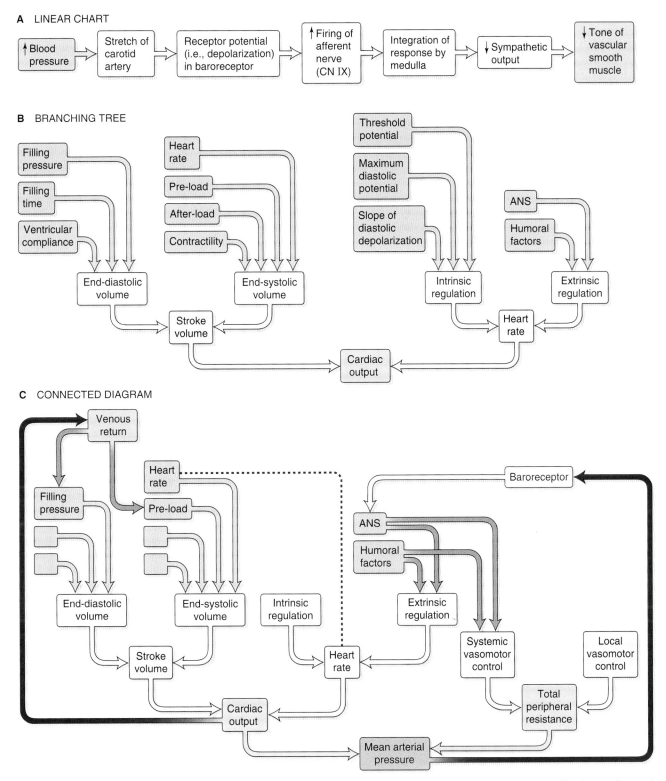

FIGURE 24–1. Patterns of cardiovascular control. *A,* The baroreceptor reflex is depicted as if increased blood pressure affected a single stretch receptor, which ultimately would influence a single effector (i.e., vascular smooth muscle). *B,* Cardiac output depends on multiple parameters, which in turn depend on multiple parameters, and so on. However, we ignore potential interactions among parameters. *C,* A branching tree represents the control of mean arterial pressure. The left limb repeats *B.* Superimposed on this simple tree are three more complex interactions: (1) feedback loops (*red arrows*), (2) two occurrences of the same parameter (connected by the *red dashed line*), and (3) examples of parameters exerting effects on two different branches of the tree (*brown arrows*). ANS, autonomic nervous system.

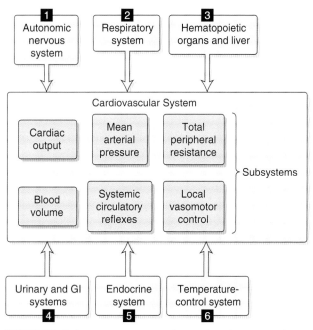

FIGURE 24–2. Interaction among cardiovascular subsystems and noncirculatory systems. GI, gastrointestinal.

that appear more than once in the tree (*connected by a red dashed line*), or factors that modulate parameters in two different branches of the tree (*connected by brown arrows*). Although not shown in Figure 24–1C, several feedback loops may impinge on a single element, and some loops are more dominant than others. The complex interactions among parameters make it difficult for one to distinguish factors of primary importance from those of lesser weight. In previous chapters, we have chosen situations that artificially isolate one portion of the cardiovascular system (e.g., heart, microcirculation) in order to explain in a simple way the homeostatic control mechanisms that govern that subsystem. However, conditions isolating subsystems rarely apply to a real person.

How can we evaluate which parameters are important? As an example, consider one subsystem, the heart. Let us assume that we can rigorously analyze all determinants of cardiac function—such as Starling's law, force-velocity relationships, effect of heart rate on contractility, and so forth. These analyses take the form of mathematical expressions, which we can combine using "systems analysis" to create a **model** that describes the behavior of the entire heart—at least theoretically. How can we test whether our model is reasonable? We can compare the physiological response of the heart in vivo with the response predicted by a computer simulation of the model. Using this approach, we may be able to establish whether we have used the correct feedback loops, whether we have assigned proper values to various elements, and whether we have assigned the proper importance to each interaction. In this way, we can use any agreement between the experimental data and the performance of the model as evidence—but not proof—that the concepts contained in the model are reasonable.

Regulation of the Entire Cardiovascular System Depends on the Integrated Action of Multiple Subsystem Controls As Well As Noncardiovascular Controls

In performing a "systems analysis" of the entire cardiovascular system, we must consider the interrelationships among the various "subsystems" summarized in the central, yellow block of Figure 24–2. Not surprisingly, we cannot fully understand how a particular disturbance affects the overall circulation unless we consider all subsystems in an integrated fashion. For instance, consider the effects of administering norepinephrine, which has a high affinity for α_1 adrenoceptors, less for β_1 adrenoreceptors, and far less for β_2 adrenoceptors. These receptors are present, in varying degrees, in both the blood vessels and the heart. A *branching tree* would predict the following: Because α_1 adrenoceptors (high affinity) are present in most vascular beds, we expect widespread vasoconstriction. Because β_2 adrenoceptors (low affinity) are present in only a few vascular beds, we predict little vasodilation. Because β_1 adrenoceptors (intermediate affinity) are present in pacemaker and myocardial cells of the heart, we would anticipate an increase in both heart rate and contractility, and, therefore, an increase in cardiac output.

Although our analysis predicts that the *heart rate* should increase, in most cases, the dominant effect of norepinephrine is to slow down the heart. The explanation, which relies on a *connected diagram*, is that the increased peripheral resistance (caused by stimulation of α_1 receptors) and increased cardiac output (caused by stimulation of β_1 receptors) combine to cause a substantial rise in mean arterial pressure. The baroreceptor reflex (see *red arrow* on right in Fig. 24–1C) then intervenes to instruct the heart to slow down (p. 536). However, bradycardia may not occur if many vascular beds were dilated before the administration of norepinephrine; in this case, the rise in blood pressure would be modest. Bradycardia might also not occur if the baroreceptor reflex were less sensitive, as would be the case in a chronically hypertensive patient (see the box on p. 556). Therefore, the effect of norepinephrine on heart rate depends on the pre-existing state of various subsystems.

In trying to understand the integrated response of the cardiovascular system to an insult, we must include in our analysis not only all the subsystems of the cardiovascular system, but also the pertinent control systems outside the circulation (see *blue boxes* in Fig. 24–2):

1. **Autonomic nervous system**. Part of the autonomic nervous system (ANS) is intimately involved in cardiovascular control (e.g., high-pressure baroreceptor response). On the other hand, a generalized activation of the ANS—such as occurs with the fight-or-flight response (p. 392) also can affect the circulation.
2. **Respiratory system**. We have already seen that ventilatory activity converts the intrinsic bradycardia response to tachycardia during stimulation of the peripheral chemoreceptors (p. 546). In addition, the action of the respiratory muscles during inspiration causes intrathoracic pressure to become more negative (p. 612), thereby increasing venous return. A third exam-

ple is that the evaporative loss of water during breathing reduces total body water and, ultimately, blood volume.

3. **Hematopoietic organs and liver.** These systems control blood composition in terms of cell constituents and plasma proteins. The hematocrit and large proteins (e.g., fibrinogen) are major determinants of blood viscosity (p. 432) and therefore of blood flow. Because the plasma proteins also determine colloid osmotic pressure (p. 472), they are a major component of the Starling forces (p. 469), which determine the distribution of extracellular fluid (ECF) between the interstitium and the blood plasma.

4. **Gastrointestinal and urinary systems.** Because the gastrointestinal (GI) tract and kidneys are the principal organs determining the input and output of electrolytes and water, they are mainly responsible for controlling the volume and electrolyte composition of ECF. Extracellular fluid volume plays a central role in the long-term control of blood pressure (p. 864).

5. **Endocrine system.** Part of the endocrine system is intimately involved in cardiovascular control (e.g., epinephrine release by the adrenal medulla). Other hormones influence the cardiovascular system either because they are vasoactive agents (p. 554) or because they regulate fluid volume and electrolyte composition by acting on the kidney and GI system.

6. **Temperature control system.** The cardiovascular system is a major effector organ for thermoregulation, carrying blood from the body core to the skin, where heat loss then occurs (p. 1237). In part, this heat loss occurs as sweat glands secrete fluid that then evaporates. However, the loss of extracellular fluid volume reduces the effective circulating volume (p. 556).

Inclusion of control elements outside the circulation (see Fig. 24–2) in our connected diagram of the cardiovascular system (see Fig. 24–1C) would expand the computer model to include hundreds of independent and dependent variables. Rather than trying to grasp such an exhaustive model, we work here through the integrated cardiovascular responses to four important circulatory "stresses": (1) orthostasis (i.e,. standing up), (2) emotional stress, (3) exercise, and (4) hemorrhage.

RESPONSE TO ERECT POSTURE

Because of Gravity, Standing Up ("Orthostasis") Tends to Shift Blood from the Head and Heart to Veins in the Legs

About two thirds of the total blood volume resides in the systemic veins (p. 450). When a recumbent subject assumes an upright position, the blood shifts from the central blood volume reservoirs and other veins to large veins in the dependent limbs. In discussing Figure 17–12B, we assumed that the cardiovascular system somehow made the adjustments necessary to keep right atrial pressure constant at approximately 2 mm Hg. Indeed, unless compensatory mechanisms intervene, blood redistribution will lower not only arterial blood pressure, but also venous return, and thus cardiac output.

To illustrate the effect of blood redistribution on venous return, we will represent the entire circulatory system by a horizontal, distensible cylinder 180 cm in length (the height of our person) and 3 cm in radius (Fig. 24–3A). This cylinder holds approximately 5000 ml of blood (the normal blood volume). We know that immediately following a cardiac arrest, the entire vascular system will have a mean systemic filling pressure (MSFP) of approximately 7 mm Hg (p. 550). The MSFP is the pressure in the circulation that would remain in the absence of any pumping or any gravity effects. Thus, if a subject is re-

FIGURE 24–3. Model of the orthostatic redistribution of blood. *A,* A horizontal tube (3 cm radius, 180 cm long) contains the entire blood volume (5 liters). With no blood flow, pressure inside tube is uniform and corresponds to a mean systemic filling pressure of 7 mm Hg. *B,* With the cylinder upright ("orthostasis"), pressure gradually increases toward the bottom, causing increasingly greater distention of this compliant tube. Because blood volume has shifted to the bottom, the upper level of the blood column is 30 cm below the level of the heart, preventing venous return. *C,* Reducing compliance of the tube by half also causes distention to fall by half. With the reduced shift of blood volume, the upper level of the blood column now just reaches the heart.

cumbent and has no heartbeat, and if the cardiovascular system is filled with a normal blood volume of 5000 ml, the overall compliance of the system will produce a uniform pressure of approximately 7 mm Hg. If we were to transfuse an additional 100 ml of blood into our cylinder, the MSFP would rise by approximately 1 mm Hg. We can conclude that the compliance, expressed as a normalized distensibility (p. 455), is:

Equation 24–1

$$\text{Relative Distensibility} = \frac{(\Delta V/V_o)}{\Delta P}$$
$$= \frac{(100 \text{ ml}/5000 \text{ ml})}{1 \text{ mm Hg}}$$
$$= 0.02 \frac{\text{ml}}{\text{ml} \times \text{mm Hg}} = 0.02/(\text{mm Hg})$$

Thus, for every 2% increase in blood volume, the MSFP of the cylinder increases by 1 mm Hg.

What will happen to our cylinder if we now turn it upright ("orthostasis," from the Greek *orthos* = upright + *stasis* = standing)? Because we have a vertical column of blood 180 cm tall, we must now consider gravity (see Fig. 24–3B). The highest pressures will be at the bottom of the cylinder. (Figure 17–12B shows that orthostasis causes venous pressure at the ankle to rise from 5 to 100 mm Hg). Therefore, our cylinder will distend maximally at the bottom, and this distention represents a shift in blood volume. The bottom of the cylinder (corresponding to the "dependent areas" of a person) gains volume, whereas the top (i.e., corresponding to the cranial portion of a person) loses blood volume. In fact, there would be no blood at all at the top of the cylinder.

By just how much would the column of blood fall in our upright, 180-cm-tall cylinder? If the overall vascular volume distensibility were 0.02/(mm Hg), then the actual height of the blood column inside the cylinder would be only about 100 cm. If the heart were 50 cm below the top of the cylinder, then the top of the column would now be approximately 30 cm below the level of the heart. Therefore, there would be no blood to return to the heart. Moreover, the right atrial pressure (RAP) would be negative (−30 cm H_2O, or about −22 mm Hg). Because the heart cannot create a vacuum this large at its input by "sucking" blood—in fact, the heart must be filled by a positive RAP—cardiac output would fall to zero.

The Autonomic Nervous System Mediates an "Orthostatic Response" That Raises Heart Rate and Peripheral Vascular Resistance, and, Thus, Tends to Restore Mean Arterial Pressure

If our model predicts that orthostasis should cause right atrial pressure to fall to −22 mm Hg, how is it that the body manages to maintain RAP at approximately 2 mm Hg in the upright position? The answer is that pooling of blood in the dependent vessels is much less pronounced during orthostasis than would be predicted by Figure 24–

3B, where approximately 2.2 liters disappeared from the top of the cylinder. The actual amount of pooling in both legs of a real person is only about 500 ml. Four major factors help to reduce pooling and maintain RAP.

NONUNIFORM INITIAL DISTRIBUTION OF BLOOD. In our "cylinder" example, the blood was initially distributed evenly throughout the length of the cylinder. In a recumbent human, however, most of the blood in large veins is located in the "central blood volume" (p. 450), that is, the vessels near the heart. If a large fraction of the blood had started off in the head, the orthostatic shift of blood would have been more dramatic, as in Figure 24–3B. The majority of the 500 ml of blood that pools in the legs during orthostasis comes from the intrathoracic vascular compartments. What is the sequence of events by which blood volume redistributes during orthostasis? As one stands, the output from the heart for a number of beats exceeds the venous return into the thoracic pool. This excess blood ends up filling the vessels in the dependent regions of the body. The result is a net transfer of blood—by way of the heart—from the intrathoracic vascular compartments to the dependent vessels.

NONUNIFORM DISTENSIBILITY OF THE VESSELS. In Figure 24–3B, we assumed a relative distensibility of 0.02/(mm Hg). If we had instead used a value of 0.01/(mm Hg)—that is, if the vessels were *less* distensible—standing would cause a less dramatic shift of blood to the dependent vessels, approximately 1.4 liters (see Fig. 24–3C) instead of approximately 2.2 liters (see Fig. 24–3B). As a result, the height of the blood column would fall from 180 to only 130 cm (see Fig. 24–3C) in the upright position, rather than to 100 cm (see Fig. 24–3B). Assuming a lower distensibility for the leg veins is reasonable because small vessels are far stiffer than larger ones, such as the aorta and vena cava. With the lower relative distensibility of 0.01/(mm Hg), the column of blood would just reach the heart. Indeed, when a subject stands quietly, the zero effective pressure level—the height in the body where vascular pressure equals atmospheric pressure—is about at the level of the right atrium. Obviously, if the circulatory system reduces its distensibility even further through the regulated contraction of vascular smooth muscle (discussed later), the height of the column of blood will increase and improve venous return.

"MUSCLE PUMPS." An important compensation for blood pooling during orthostasis comes from skeletal muscle contraction. When a person stands, the muscles of the legs and abdomen tighten. The presence of valves in the veins, as well as intermittent muscular movement, contributes to the flow of blood upward along the veins (see Fig. 23–6). Vessels of the abdominal region remain nearly unaffected by orthostasis because the abdominal viscera are contained in a water-filled jacket that is maintained by the tone of the abdominal muscles.

AUTONOMIC REFLEXES. Because of decreased venous return, cardiac output tends to fall by approximately 20% soon after one assumes an erect position. However, the fall in cardiac output would be even greater in the absence of autonomic reflexes. The decreased venous return

TABLE 24–1

FACTORS INFLUENCING THE DEGREE OF ORTHOSTATIC RESPONSE*

Total blood volume

Distribution of blood volume

Size of vessels in dependent regions of the body

Vascular distensibility

Mean systemic filling pressure (pressure in the absence of cardiac output)

Level at which zero effective pressure is normally located in a particular individual

Degree of tilt

Skeletal muscle tone; strength and rate of intermittent contraction of skeletal muscles

Vascular sufficiency

Abdominal muscle tone

Temperature

Response of low-pressure receptors

Response of high-pressure baroreceptors

Activity of the sympathetic system

Initial heart rate

Initial myocardial contractility

Sensitivity of vascular smooth muscle to sympathetic stimulation

*That is, by how much does standing up increase heart rate and peripheral vascular resistance?

leads to a fall in RAP, which in turn, leads to a decrease in stroke volume, and thus arterial pressure. High-pressure baroreceptors (p. 536) sense this decrease in arterial pressure, which leads to an increased sympathetic output that raises vascular tone throughout the body and increases heart rate and contractility. Together, the constriction of arterioles (which raises total peripheral resistance) and the increased heart rate restore the systemic mean arterial pressure, despite a small decrease in stroke volume. In the dependent regions of the body, the sympathetic response also increases the tone of the veins, thereby decreasing their diameter and their capacity (compare Fig. 24–3B and C).

In summary, of the four factors that contribute to the stability of RAP during orthostasis, two are anatomic (i.e., nonuniformities of initial blood volume distribution and distensibility) and two are physiological (i.e., muscle pumps and autonomic reflexes). The two physiological mechanisms are both important. Indeed, following a lumbar sympathectomy, patients tend to faint when standing. However, after some months, they are able to compensate, perhaps by using the muscle pumps more effectively, or by enhancing the sympathetic response of the heart.

The extent of the **orthostatic response**—how much the heart rate or peripheral vascular resistance increases

under the control of the ANS—depends on a variety of factors (Table 24–1), which involve nearly the entire cardiovascular system. Because these factors may differ from person to person, or may differ within any one individual according to the circumstances, the orthostatic response is highly variable. We will now discuss an example of each type of variability.

POSTURAL HYPOTENSION. In very sensitive subjects lying on a tilt table, a sudden orthostatic tilt can cause such a large fall in arterial pressure that the individual becomes dizzy or even faints. **Fainting** is caused by a transient fall in arterial pressure that causes cerebral perfusion to become inadequate.

TEMPERATURE EFFECTS. In a *cool environment*, where the arterioles in the lower extremities are constricted, the initial dip in arterial pressure can be small, despite the decrease in stroke volume. The explanation is that the high arteriolar resistance delays the transfer of blood from the thoracic pool to the legs. As a result, the sympathetic response to the small drop in mean arterial pressure may already be in effect before further pooling can occur. In a *warm environment*, where the arterioles in the skin are more dilated, orthostasis leads to faster transfer of blood from the thoracic pool to the legs so that—before the sympathetic response can develop—the initial decreases in stroke volume, mean arterial pressure, and pulse pressure can be large. Thus, soldiers standing quietly at attention in hot weather are more likely to faint than soldiers marching in a cold environment because of differences in muscle pump activity and vasoconstriction.

RESPONSES TO ACUTE EMOTIONAL STRESS

The Fight-or-Flight Reaction Is a Sympathetic Response That Is Centrally Controlled in the Cortex and Hypothalamus

Emotional situations vary greatly among people. A severe emotional reaction can resemble the **fight-or-flight response** in animals (p. 392). This defense reaction causes a generalized increase in skeletal muscle tone and increased sensory attention.

Fight-or-flight behavior is an extreme example of an integrated response that originates entirely within the central nervous system (CNS), without involvement of peripheral sensors or reflexes. The response is due to the activation of cortical and hypothalamic brain centers, and is quite variable among individuals and according to the degree of stress. Under the overarching control of the cortex, the hypothalamus acts through two pathways—the **medullary cardiovascular center** (p. 538) and the **postganglionic sympathetic *cholinergic* neurons** (p. 388).

The overall fight-or-flight response involves (Fig. 24–4):

1. **Skeletal muscle blood flow.** In animals—but perhaps not humans—activation of sympathetic cholinergic vasodilator fibers *directly* causes a rapid and massive increase in blood flow to skeletal muscle (p. 543).

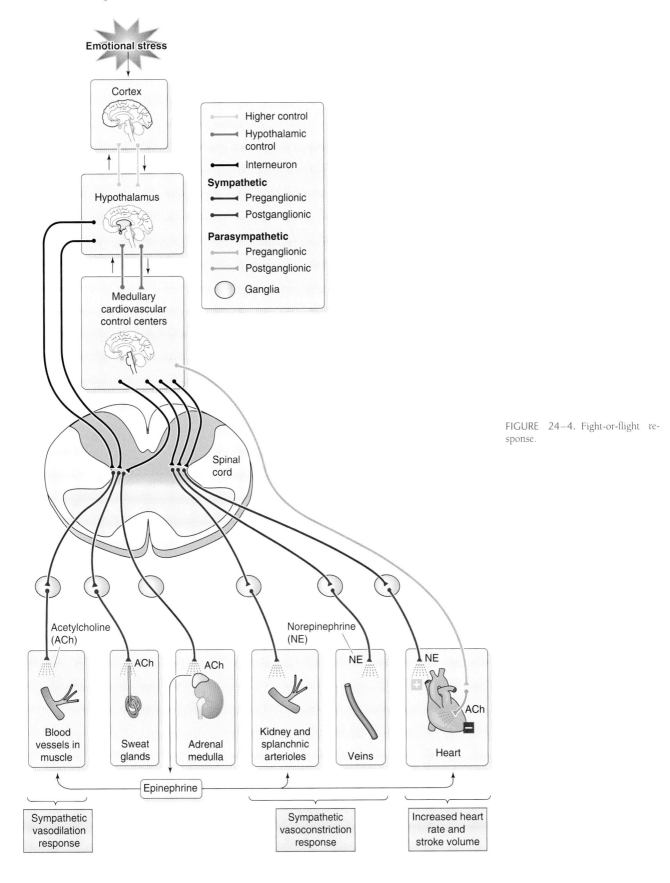

FIGURE 24–4. Fight-or-flight response.

In humans as well as other mammals, flow also increases *secondarily* more slowly and less dramatically because the adrenal medulla releases epinephrine, which acts on β_2 adrenoceptors on skeletal muscle blood vessels. The result is dilation and an increase in blood flow. In a full-blown fight-or-flight reaction, muscle exercise generates metabolites that further increase skeletal muscle blood flow (p. 565). Of course, humans may not exercise skeletal muscle when responding to internal stress (e.g., anxiety or panic).

2. **Cutaneous blood flow**. The sympathetic response causes little change in blood flow to skin unless it stimulates sweating. The neural pathway involves sympathetic cholinergic neurons (p. 388), which release acetylcholine and perhaps vasodilatory neurotransmitters (e.g., calcitonin gene–related peptide [CGRP], vasoactive intestinal peptide [VIP]). The acetylcholine causes the secretion of sweat and possibly also the local formation of kinins (p. 555). These kinins increase capillary permeability, and presumably also dilate arterioles but constrict venules (i.e., increasing the midcapillary pressure). The result would be an increased filtration of fluid from the skin capillaries into the interstitium, causing dermal swelling.

3. **Adrenal medulla**. Preganglionic sympathetic neurons stimulate the chromaffin cells to release epinephrine, which causes vasodilation in muscle (via β_2 adrenoceptors) and vasoconstriction in the kidney and splanchnic beds (via α_1 adrenoceptors).

4. **Renal and splanchnic blood flow**. In virtually all vascular beds, increased sympathetic output causes vasoconstriction and thereby decreases blood flow. The systemic release of epinephrine also vasoconstricts these vascular beds rich in α_1 adrenoceptors.

5. **Veins**. Most veins constrict in response to sympathetic output.

6. **The heart**. Increased sympathetic output and decreased vagal output cause a rise in heart rate and contractility, so that cardiac output increases.

7. **Mean arterial pressure**. Depending on the balance of vasodilation and vasoconstriction, the overall result of vascular resistance changes may be either a decrease or an increase in total peripheral resistance. Nevertheless, because cardiac output increases, the net result of an increased cardiac output and a resistance change is an increase in arterial pressure.

The Common Faint Reflects Mainly a Parasympathetic Response Caused by Sudden Emotional Stress

About one fifth of humans experience one or more episodes of fainting during adolescence. This type of fainting is known as vasodepressor syncope, or **vasovagal syncope**. It can occur in response to a sudden emotional stress, phlebotomy, the sight of blood, or acute pain. Fainting starts usually when the individual is standing or sitting, rarely when the individual is recumbent. The loss of consciousness is due to a transient fall in perfusion pressure to the brain. The "playing dead" reaction in animals is the equivalent of vasovagal syncope in humans.

Vasovagal syncope originates with activation of specific areas in the cerebral cortex; stimulating areas in the anterior cingulate gyrus can trigger a faint. The events associated with vasovagal syncope have in common a massive stimulation of the parasympathetic system and the removal of sympathetic tone.

Vasovagal syncope involves changes in several parameters (Fig. 24–5):

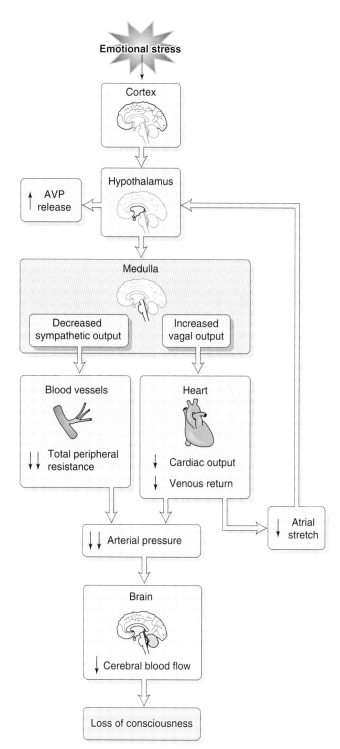

FIGURE 24–5. Vagovagal syncope. AVP, arginine vasopressin.

1. **Total peripheral resistance**. A massive vasodilation occurs, resulting from the removal of sympathetic tone from the resistance vessels of the skeletal muscle, splanchnic, renal, and cerebral circulations. The resulting fall in blood pressure is not corrected by a baroreceptor response, which would normally increase cardiac output.
2. **Cardiac output**. Intense vagal output to the heart causes bradycardia and decreased stroke volume, resulting in a marked decrease in cardiac output. Because atropine, a muscarinic receptor blocker, does not reliably prevent syncope, decreased sympathetic tone to the heart may also play a role in causing bradycardia.
3. **Arterial pressure**. The combination of a sudden decrease in total peripheral resistance and decreased cardiac output causes a profound fall in mean arterial pressure.
4. **Cerebral blood flow**. The fall in mean arterial pressure causes global cerebral ischemia to develop. If the decreased cerebral blood flow persists for only a few seconds, the result is dizziness or faintness. If it lasts for approximately 10 seconds, the subject loses consciousness. The stress underlying the common faint also may provoke hyperventilation, which lowers arterial P_{CO_2} (p. 691). The resulting constriction of cerebral blood vessels (p. 561) further impairs cerebral blood flow, which increases the likelihood of a faint.
5. **Other manifestations of altered ANS activity**. Pallor of the skin and sweating (beads of perspiration) are signs that often appear before the loss of consciousness. Intense vagal stimulation of the GI tract may cause epigastric pain that is interpreted as nausea. Mydriasis (pupillary dilation), as well as visual blurring, can also result from parasympathetic stimulation.

Fainting is more likely to occur in a warm room (see earlier), after a volume loss (e.g., dehydration or hemorrhage), or after standing up or other maneuvers that tend to lower mean arterial pressure. You might think that these stresses would trigger the usual responses that increase cardiac output and vascular resistance, thereby making fainting less likely. However, the same integrated pattern of brain activity that orchestrates vasovagal syncope also appears to suppress the expected reflexes that would otherwise counteract the syncope.

After regaining consciousness, the patient often notices oliguria (reduced urine output), caused by high plasma levels of arginine vasopressin (AVP, also known as antidiuretic hormone; p. 840). Elevated levels of AVP can result in part from the reduced atrial stretch that occurs during periods of decreased venous return (p. 549). The pallor and nausea that persist after fainting may also result from the high levels of circulating AVP.

RESPONSE TO EXERCISE

Adaptation to exercise probably places the greatest demands on circulatory function. The main feature of the cardiovascular response to exercise is an increased cardiac output, up to 4 or 5 times the resting cardiac output. The increase in cardiac output during exercise is more the result of increased heart rate (~3 times control) than of increased stroke volume (~1.3 times control). The cardiovascular response to exercise has both early and late components, and originates from higher centers in the CNS ("early"), from mechanical and chemical changes triggered by contracting skeletal muscle ("delayed"), and from various reflexes ("delayed").

Early Physiologists Suggested That Muscle Contraction Leads to Mechanical and Chemical Changes That Trigger an Increase in Cardiac Output

Contracting skeletal muscle produces cardiovascular changes that mimic many of those that occur during exercise. In fact, early physiologists believed that these skeletal muscle effects triggered *all* of the cardiovascular changes associated with exercise. We now know that these skeletal muscle effects are important only for the *delayed* cardiovascular responses in exercise. Muscle contraction directly affects the cardiovascular system in two ways (Fig. 24–6)—a mechanical response that increases venous return and a chemical response that dilates blood vessels in active muscle.

MECHANICAL RESPONSE: INCREASED VENOUS RETURN. The pumping action of contracting skeletal muscle improves venous return (pp. 519 and 567). As a result, right atrial pressure, ventricular end-diastolic pressure, and end-diastolic volume (EDV) should all increase. According to the Starling mechanism (p. 527), the result should be an increase in stroke volume.

CHEMICAL RESPONSE: LOCAL VASODILATION IN ACTIVE MUSCLE. Enhanced skeletal muscle metabolism produces multiple changes in the chemistry of the interstitial fluid. The P_{O_2} and pH fall, whereas other metabolites (CO_2, lactic acid, K^+, and adenosine) accumulate. Moreover, the accumulation of metabolites causes interstitial osmolarity to increase. After a small delay following the onset of muscle contraction, the developing chemical changes cause the arterioles to dilate (pp. 478 and 565), which may lead to an initial fall in arterial pressure. However, this fall is transient because of the intervening baroreceptor response (p. 536), which increases heart rate and stroke volume, both of which enhance cardiac output. At the same time, the baroreceptor reflex vasoconstricts inactive muscle regions, as well the splanchnic, renal, and cutaneous circulations.

Cardiovascular physiologists believed for a long time that the mechanical and chemical limbs in Figure 24–6, both of which originate in active muscle, are responsible for the overall effect of exercise on cardiac output. However, Figure 24–6 is not only incomplete, some of its predictions are incorrect, and others do not occur in the predicted order. As far as the *mechanical effect* on venous return is concerned, the model predicts a rise in ventricular end-diastolic pressure and thus EDV. As far as the *chemical effect* is concerned, the model predicts that it

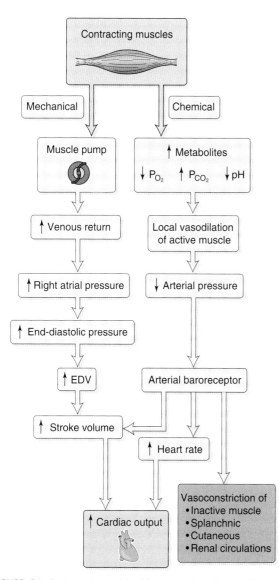

FIGURE 24–6. An early model of how exercise affects cardiovascular function. EDV, end-diastolic volume.

The explanation for the discrepancies between the predicted and actual findings is the presence of an overriding control mechanism that rapidly activates the sympathetic division of the ANS. The ventricular changes that occur in response to exercise are the result of the increased firing of sympathetic nerves, which increases both heart rate and contractility (i.e., stroke volume).

The Early Integrated Response to Exercise Originates in the Hypothalamus

An increased sympathetic output from the medullary cardiovascular center would explain the immediate *ventricular response* during exercise. Increased sympathetic output from medullary centers would also explain the immediate vasoconstriction in inactive muscles, and in the splanchnic, renal, and cutaneous circulations. However, sympathetic signals originating in the medulla *cannot* account for yet another immediate exercise response that occurs in dogs (though not humans and other primates)—a rapid vasodilation that occurs only in *active* skeletal muscle. On the contrary, experimental stimulation of medullary centers would constrict *all* muscle beds. Because the hypothalamus is an important center of integration for the ANS, Rushmer and his colleagues explored various sites in the diencephalon to determine if stimulating any of them might mimic the integrated sympathetic response to exercise. In the 1950s, Rushmer found that stimulating the H_2 fields of Forel in the hypothalamus, or neurons in the preventricular gray matter, reproduced all the details of the cardiac response to exercise, even though the muscles were completely quiescent.

The **early response** to exercise is orchestrated by the hypothalamus, under the general control of the cerebral cortex, which initiates the motor activity (Fig. 24–7). The early response consists of at least three major components:

1. **Increased cardiac output.** The hypothalamus instructs the medulla to increase sympathetic output to the heart. The ensuing tachycardia and increased contractility account for the rapid upsurge of cardiac output that Rushmer observed with the initiation of exercise.
2. **Vasoconstriction.** When one decides to exercise, the cerebral cortex stimulates hypothalamic centers, which in turn activate the medullary cardiovascular centers. Sympathetic output from the medulla causes vasoconstriction in inactive muscle regions, as well as in the renal, splanchnic, and cutaneous circulations. The net effect is to make more blood available for diversion to the contracting muscles. Except during maximal exercise, the increase in splanchnic and renal resistance does not result in a fall in local blood flow to the abdominal viscera and kidneys. Rather, because the arterial pressure increases along with the renal and splanchnic vascular resistance, the *absolute* blood flow remains close to resting levels in these tissues, even as the flow to the skeletal muscle increases markedly. However, *fractional* blood flow (i.e., local blood flow normalized to cardiac output) does fall in these regions. In the early phase of exercise, skin blood flow also decreases. However, cutaneous blood flow eventu-

should take time for chemical changes in active skeletal muscle to produce local vasodilation. Therefore, there ought to be a time lag between the initiation of exercise and the fall in mean arterial pressure that triggers the baroreceptor response (e.g., increased heart rate).

In the 1950s, Rushmer tested these predictions on trained unanesthetized dogs. Recording the *mechanical limb* of Figure 24–6, he found that, at the onset of exercise, left ventricular end-diastolic pressure does *not* rise and that left ventricular EDV diminishes rather than increases. These findings cast doubt on the primary role of the Starling mechanism in raising stroke volume during exercise. Recording the *chemical limb* of Figure 24–6, Rushmer found *no* transient fall in mean arterial pressure, thus casting doubt on the importance of the baroreceptor reflex. Furthermore, he saw *no* delay between the onset of exercise and the increase of heart rate, thus calling into question the idea that the chemically induced vasodilation is at the root of the tachycardia.

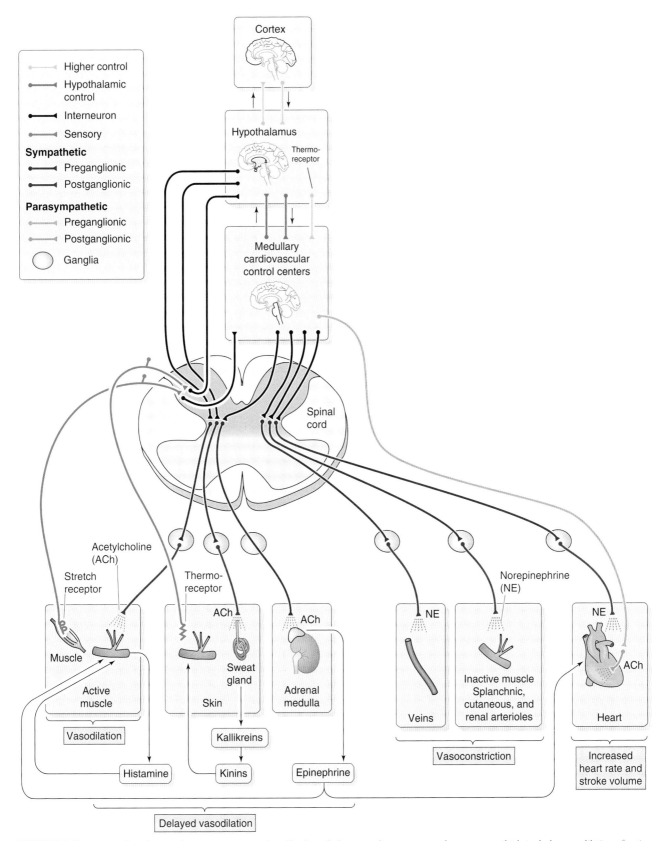

FIGURE 24–7. Integrated cardiovascular response to exercise. The hypothalamus orchestrates an *early* response, which includes vasodilation of active muscle (the mechanism of which is controversial in humans), vasoconstriction of certain inactive tissues, and increased cardiac output. In addition to those responses shown in Figure 24–6, the *delayed* responses (highlighted in *yellow*) include release of histamine, kallikreins, and epinephrine, leading to delayed vasodilation. Delayed local chemical responses from contracting muscles sustain early cardiovascular responses. Cutaneous thermoreceptors trigger delayed vasodilation in the skin.

ally rises, reflecting the attempt of the temperature regulatory system to prevent body temperature from rising too much (p. 1237).

3. **Early vasodilation in active muscle.** In dogs—although not in humans or other primates—at the initiation of exercise, the cerebral cortex stimulates hypothalamic neurons whose axons bypass the medullary cardiovascular centers and synapse on preganglionic sympathetic neurons in the spinal cord (p. 543). The postganglionic neurons synapse on cholinergic sympathetic vasodilator fibers that innervate the vascular smooth muscle of skeletal muscle and trigger early peripheral vasodilation in active skeletal muscle. As discussed in the next section, the delayed local "chemical" response later reinforces this vasodilation.

The increased alertness that accompanies the anticipation of exercise can elicit all the components of the early response to exercise. The early response resembles the fight-or-flight reaction. In humans, the anticipatory cardiovascular adjustments prepare the body for the increased metabolism of the exercising skeletal muscle. For sprinters at the start of a 100-m dash, the anticipatory response prepares them to deliver an increased cardiac output, and simultaneously to divert the increased blood flow away from tissues that do not require increased blood flow.

In Addition to Mechanical and Chemical Events, Histamine and Epinephrine Release, Muscle Reflexes, and Increases in Temperature Reinforce the Delayed Cardiovascular Response to Exercise

The integrated response to exercise includes a delayed component that consists of two key elements:

VASODILATION TRIGGERED BY METABOLITES IN SKELETAL MUSCLE. *Metabolites* released locally (see Fig. 24–7) dilate the resistance vessels and recruit capillaries that had received no blood flow at rest (p. 565). As a result of this decrease in resistance, in concert with the increase in cardiac output, blood flow to active skeletal muscle can be as much as 20 times that to resting skeletal muscle. This vasodilator effect of metabolites thus more than overcomes any vasoconstrictive tendency produced by norepinephrine.

CARDIAC OUTPUT. The neural pathways discussed in the previous section are responsible for the *early* increase in cardiac output during exercise. The sustained increase of cardiac output depends on both the mechanical and the chemical limbs in Figure 24–6. The vasodilation of active muscle beds results in the rapid mobilization of blood from the central blood volume to exercising muscle. The early increase in cardiac output could not be sustained if the *muscle pump* did not also increase venous return, and if the *Starling mechanism* did not respond by increasing stroke volume. In addition, because vasodilation in exercising skeletal muscle would reduce total peripheral resistance, mean arterial pressure would fall if the *baroreceptor reflex* did not sustain the generalized sympathetic outflow.

Other factors also contribute to the delayed component of the response to exercise.

HISTAMINE RELEASE. Cells near the arterioles may release their intracellular stores of **histamine**, a potent vasodilator (see Table 19-7 on p. 479). Although these histamine-containing cells are quiescent when sympathetic nerves release *norepinephrine*, they release histamine when sympathetic tone wanes. Because of relaxation of the arterioles and precapillary sphincters, the pressure in the muscle capillaries rises, leading to increased extravasation of fluid and enhanced lymph flow.

EPINEPHRINE RELEASE. During severe exercise, preganglionic sympathetic fibers to the adrenal medulla stimulate epinephrine release. The systemic effects of circulating epinephrine on cardiac β_1 adrenoceptors enhance the neural effects on the heart, thus increasing cardiac output. Circulating epinephrine also acts on vascular β_2 adrenoceptors, augmenting vasodilation mainly in skeletal muscle and heart.

REFLEXES ORIGINATING FROM CONTRACTING MUSCLE. Within the exercising muscle itself, contraction activates stretch receptors that sense muscle tension and may also activate chemoreceptors that sense metabolites. Signals from these receptors travel through small myelinated and unmyelinated sensory fibers to the spinal cord, and then on to the medullary cardiovascular control centers. This sensory input reinforces the central input to the cardiovascular control center and thus sustains the sympathetic activation.

REGULATION OF BODY CORE TEMPERATURE. As exercise continues, increased metabolism causes body core temperature to rise, activating **temperature-sensitive cells** in the hypothalamus (p. 1236). This activation has two effects, both of which promote heat loss via the skin as part of a temperature regulatory response (p. 1237). First, the hypothalamus signals the medulla to inhibit its sympathetic vasoconstrictor outflow to the skin, thereby increasing cutaneous blood flow. Recall that vasoconstriction is part of the early response to exercise (see earlier). Second, the hypothalamus activates sympathetic cholinergic fibers to sweat glands, causing an increase in sweat production as well as an indirect cutaneous vasodilation that may involve kinin formation. In addition, these neurons may co-release neurotransmitters that directly dilate cutaneous vessels (p. 573).

RESPONSE TO HEMORRHAGE

If a person rapidly loses more than 10% or 20% of total blood volume from a large *vein*, the inadequate intravascular volume causes sequential decreases in central blood volume, venous return, ventricular filling, stroke volume, cardiac output, and thus mean arterial pressure. However, if the blood loss comes from a large peripheral *artery*, the mean arterial pressure in central arteries does not fall until cardiac output falls secondary to decreased venous return. Of course, if the blood loss occurs as a blown aortic aneurysm, mean arterial pressure falls immediately.

Large hemorrhages, in which one loses 30% or more of total blood volume, produce **hypovolemic shock**. Shock is a state of peripheral circulatory failure that is characterized by inadequate perfusion of the peripheral tissues. During shock, the *systolic* arterial pressure is usually below 90 mm Hg, and the *mean* arterial pressure is below 70 mm Hg. For reasons that will become clear, by the time one records a significant fall in mean arterial pressure, other signs of shock are evident. The first signs may be narrowing of the pulse pressure, as well as a sensation of faintness when sitting or standing. The subject in hypovolemic shock has cold and moist (i.e., "clammy") skin, as well as a rapid and weak pulse. Moreover, urine output drops to less than 25 ml/hr, even though fluid intake had been normal.

Following its abrupt initial fall, arterial pressure tends to return to normal (Fig. 24–8A, red curve), although in some cases, blood pressure falls irreversibly (blue dashed curve). Under favorable circumstances, the body restores blood pressure toward normal values by mobilizing two lines of defense. First, circulatory control mechanisms act on the heart and blood vessels to restore cardiac output and increase peripheral resistance. Second, mechanisms of capillary exchange and fluid conservation restore the intravascular volume.

Following Hemorrhage, Cardiovascular Reflexes Restore Mean Arterial Pressure

Several cardiovascular reflexes cooperate to compensate for the fall in mean arterial pressure. These reflexes originate from four major groups of receptors (numbered 1–4 in Fig. 24–8B):

1. **High-pressure baroreceptors.** The fall in arterial pressure leads to a decrease in the firing rate of afferents from the carotid and aortic baroreceptors (p. 535). The resulting enhanced sympathetic output and diminished vagal output increase heart rate and cardiac contractility, and also produce venoconstriction and selective arteriolar constriction. These responses cooperate to re-establish the arterial pressure.
2. **Low-pressure baroreceptors.** Reduced blood volume directly decreases effective circulating volume, which, in turn, lessens the activity of low-pressure stretch receptors (p. 548). The resulting increased sympathetic outflow causes vasoconstriction in a number of vascular beds, particularly the kidney, reducing glomerular filtration rate and urine output. In response to decreased stretch, low-pressure receptors at various sites in the circulation ultimately have divergent effects on heart rate. The afferents of the atrial stretch receptors also project to the hypothalamus, enhancing the release of AVP, which reduces water excretion by the kidneys (p. 840). During shock, the vasoconstrictor effects of AVP appear to be important for maintaining peripheral vascular resistance. Reduced atrial stretch also lowers the level of circulating atrial natriuretic peptide (p. 549), thereby reducing salt and water loss by the kidneys (p. 867).
3. **Peripheral chemoreceptors.** As blood pressure drops, perfusion of the carotid and aortic bodies declines, causing local hypoxia near the glomus cells and an increase in the firing rate of the chemoreceptor afferents (p. 723), a response enhanced by increased sympathetic tone to the peripheral chemoreceptor vessels (p. 725). Increased *chemoreceptor* discharge leads to increased firing of the sympathetic vasoconstrictor fibers and ventilatory changes that indirectly increase heart rate (p. 546).
4. **Central chemoreceptors.** Severe hypotension results in brain ischemia, which leads to a fall in the P_{O_2} of brain extracellular fluid, as well as a rise in P_{CO_2} and a fall in pH. The acidosis has a profound effect on the central chemoreceptors in the medulla, leading to a greatly enhanced sympathetic vasoconstrictor output (p. 547).

These four reflex pathways have in common the activation of a massive sympathetic response that results in the release of norepinephrine from postganglionic sympathetic neurons. In addition, the sympathetic response triggers the **adrenal medulla** to release epinephrine and norepinephrine roughly in proportion to the severity of the hemorrhage. Lowering the mean arterial pressure to 40 mm Hg causes circulating levels of epinephrine to rise 50-fold, and norepinephrine, 10-fold. The consequences of the four combined reflex actions are the following responses (see Fig. 24–8B).

TACHYCARDIA AND INCREASED CONTRACTILITY. Increased sympathetic activity increases heart rate roughly in proportion to the volume of shed blood. Thus, the degree of tachycardia is an index of the severity of the hemorrhage. Increased sympathetic tone increases myocardial contractility but can increase stroke volume only after venous return also improves.

ARTERIOLAR CONSTRICTION. Sympathetic constriction of the resistance vessels is most pronounced in the blood vessels of the *extremities, skin, skeletal muscle, and abdominal viscera.* Although both precapillary and postcapillary resistance vessels constrict, the *precapillary* response initially dominates. As a result, capillary pressure falls precipitously, leading to the transcapillary refill discussed in the next section. *Renal* blood flow falls rapidly after hemorrhage as a result of the fall in blood pressure, but recovers after a few minutes because of autoregulation (p. 769). The responses of both high- and low-pressure stretch receptors lead to enhanced sympathetic vasoconstrictor traffic to the kidney. Although renal blood flow has a high threshold for this sympathetic traffic, the sympathetic vasoconstriction eventually overrides renal autoregulation if arterial pressure remains low or continues to fall. In hypovolemic shock, renal blood flow falls to a proportionately greater extent than does cardiac output, which explains why severe hemorrhage often results in renal failure. Blood flow in the medulla of the kidney is less compromised than in the cortex, leading to "medullary washout" of the hypertonic interstitial fluid in the renal medulla (p. 837), and an inability to produce a concentrated urine. Both *coronary blood flow and cerebral blood flow* initially fall after hemorrhage, but autoregulation can largely restore blood flow to normal.

VENOUS CONSTRICTION. The fall in blood volume with hemorrhage occurs primarily in the large capacitance ves-

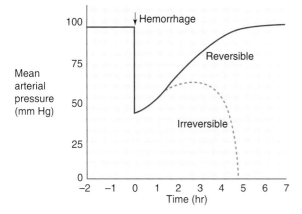

A CHANGES IN BLOOD PRESSURE WITH HEMORRHAGE

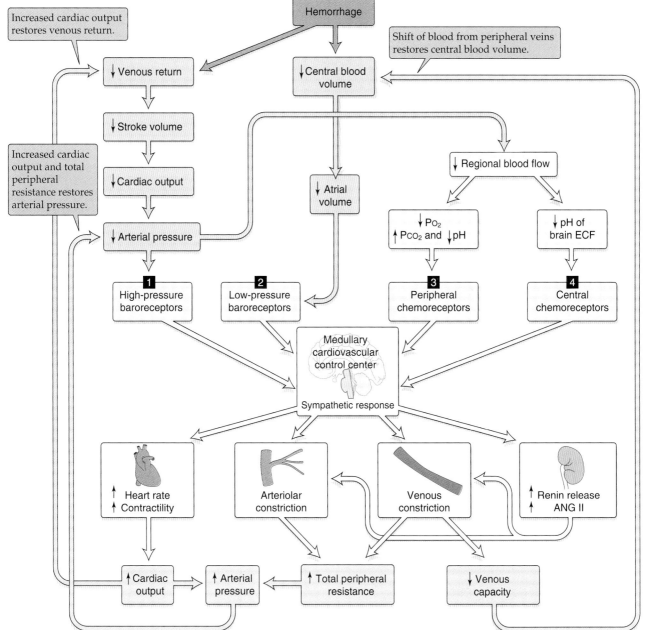

B INTEGRATED RESPONSE TO HEMMORRHAGE

FIGURE 24–8. Effect of hemorrhage on cardiovascular function. *A,* At time zero, the investigator removes enough blood from the experimental animal to lower mean arterial pressure to 45 mm Hg. *B,* Blood loss triggers four kinds of receptors (numbered 1 to 4) to produce an integrated response orchestrated by the medulla. ANG, angiotensin; ECF, extracellular fluid.

sels, especially those that contain the central blood volume. These vessels are very sensitive to sympathetic stimulation (which causes constriction), and less so to local metabolites (which causes dilation). The sympathetic venous constriction decreases both the *capacity* and the compliance of the large veins, thereby tending to restore central venous pressure. In addition, sympathetic venous constriction increases *postcapillary resistance*, which is important for transcapillary refill (see later).

OTHER EFFECTS. Sympathetic stimulation of the granular cells in the juxtaglomerular apparatus of the kidney leads to an increased release of renin and, ultimately, increased plasma levels of angiotensin II (ANG II) (p. 555). In hemorrhagic shock, ANG II rises to concentrations that are vasoconstrictive. Activation of the sympathetic system also triggers sympathetic cholinergic stimulation of the sweat glands (p. 573), causing the patient's extremities to become clammy.

With moderate blood losses (10% to 20%), these four responses can increase total peripheral resistance sufficiently to keep arterial pressure at about normal levels. However, cardiac output remains depressed.

Following Hemorrhage, Transcapillary Refill, Fluid Conservation, and Thirst Restore the Blood Volume

The reflexes discussed in the previous section compensate for the principal *consequences* of blood loss—decreased blood pressure and reduced cardiac output. The responses discussed here compensate for the *primary disturbance*, the loss of blood volume.

TRANSCAPILLARY REFILL. The movement of fluid from the interstitium to the blood plasma is the major defense against reduced blood volume. Starling forces (p. 469) are critically important during hemorrhage and hypovolemic shock. Immediately following hemorrhage, a phase of **hemodilution** develops, as was first observed during World War I, when medics noted that injured soldiers arrived at the first aid station with diluted blood (i.e., low hematocrit). Within an hour, interstitial fluid replaces approximately 75% of the shed blood volume. Studies performed around World War II showed that the dilution of *hemoglobin* is more pronounced than the dilution of *plasma proteins* following hemorrhage. Therefore, not only do fluid and electrolytes move from the interstitium to the blood, but proteins also enter the vascular compartment.

Transcapillary refill involves two steps. The first is *fluid movement* from the interstitium to the vasculature. Capillary hydrostatic pressure (P_c) (Fig. 24–9A) depends on arteriolar and venular pressures, as well as on the relation of the precapillary to the postcapillary resistance (p. 452). Immediately after the hemorrhage, the upstream arteriolar pressure and the downstream venular pressure both fall, causing P_c to fall (see Fig. 24–9B). The Starling forces thus produce a large net movement of fluid and small electrolytes from the interstitium into the capillaries. As compensation occurs, total peripheral resistance increases, in part restoring arteriolar pressure (see Fig. 24–9C). However, because precapillary resistance increases more

than does postcapillary resistance, P_c remains relatively low, sustaining the net movement of fluid into the capillaries. Normally, little protein would enter with the fluid because most capillary walls reflect proteins very effectively (p. 470). The entry of protein-free fluid into the capillary gradually modifies the three other Starling forces. First, the interstitial fluid volume decreases, lowering interstitial hydrostatic pressure (P_{if}). Second, the plasma proteins become diluted, so that capillary colloid osmotic pressure (π_c) falls. Finally, the removal of a protein-free solution from the interstitium raises interstitial colloid osmotic pressure (π_{if}). The result of these dissipating Star-

A   NORMAL

B   UNCOMPENSATED HEMORRHAGE

C   COMPENSATED HEMORRHAGE

D   DECOMPENSATED HEMORRHAGE

FIGURE 24–9. Effect of hemorrhage on capillary hydrostatic pressure. *A,* In this figure (which is similar to Fig. 18–4A), R_{pre} and R_{post} are the precapillary and postcapillary resistances, respectively. Here, the ratio $R_{post}/R_{pre} = 0.35$. *B,* The fall in capillary hydrostatic pressure reverses the Starling forces, causing net movement of fluid from the interstitium to the capillary lumen. *C,* Sympathetic stimulation increases total peripheral resistance ($R_{post}/R_{pre} = 0.25$ in this example). *D,* Capillary pressure rises sufficiently to favor filtration ($R_{post}/R_{pre} = 0.45$ in this example).

ling forces is that transcapillary refill gradually wanes and eventually ceases.

The second step in transcapillary refill is the appearance of *plasma proteins* in the blood. These proteins probably enter the blood across fenestrae of the mesenteric and hepatic capillaries, two regions in which the interstitium has a very high interstitial colloid osmotic pressure. In addition, hemorrhage rapidly stimulates albumin synthesis by the liver. Plasmapheresis, the artificial removal of plasma proteins from the blood, has the same effect on albumin synthesis, suggesting that a reduction in the concentration of plasma proteins per se stimulates the liver to make albumin.

Water from the *intracellular* compartments ultimately replaces the lost *interstitial* fluid. What the driving force is for water to leave the cells and enter the interstitium is somewhat controversial. The blood osmolality often rises after hemorrhage, presumably reflecting interstitial hyperosmolality. The additional interstitial osmoles come from ischemic tissues that release the products of proteolysis, glycolysis, and lipolysis. Therefore, interstitial hyperosmolality may provide the **osmotic** drive for the movement of water from the intracellular to the interstitial compartment.

RENAL CONSERVATION OF SALT AND WATER. Arterial hypotension and lowered renal blood flow reduce the glomerular filtration rate (p. 757), and therefore diminish the urinary excretion of salt and water. In addition to the direct hemodynamic effects, the reduced effective circulating volume promotes the renal retention of Na^+ by four mechanisms, which are discussed more fully in Chapter 39. First, reduced effective circulating volume activates the renin-angiotensin cascade (p. 866), increasing aldosterone release, and thus enhancing salt and water reabsorption by the distal nephron. Second, increased sympathetic nerve activity (p. 867) promotes Na^+ retention by altering renal hemodynamics, enhancing renin release, and stimulating Na^+ reabsorption by renal tubule cells. Third, the release of AVP reduces water excretion (p. 867). Finally, reduced effective circulating volume inhibits release of atrial natriuretic peptide (ANP) (see p. 867) and thus promotes renal Na^+ retention. Therefore, the overall response of the kidney to blood loss is to reduce the excretion of water and salt, thereby contributing to the conservation of extracellular fluid. However, the renal response only *conserves* fluid; by itself, it does not *add* any water to the extracellular fluid.

THIRST. Reduced effective circulating volume produced by severe hemorrhage is one of the most potent stimuli for thirst (p. 876); it also stimulates the Na^+ appetite. These urges, if fulfilled, actually provide some of the raw materials for replacing the blood lost in hemorrhage.

Positive Feedback Mechanisms Cause Irreversible Hemorrhagic Shock

In some cases, hemorrhagic shock can be irreversible. Following an initial fall in arterial pressure and perhaps some recovery, arterial pressure and the perfusion of pe-

ripheral tissues may inexorably deteriorate (see Fig. 24-8A, *blue dashed curve*). Moreover, in these cases, the fall in arterial pressure does not reverse even if the physician intervenes at this time and replaces the volume of blood lost as the result of hemorrhage.

The best experimental model for irreversible hemorrhagic shock is **prolonged hypotension**. Typically, the researcher acutely removes blood from an experimental animal—thereby reducing blood pressure to some low target value—and then *clamps* the mean arterial pressure at this low target by either removing or infusing blood as the normal physiological responses evolve. Studies of this kind reveal that hemorrhagic shock can become irreversible as a result of the failure of multiple response components: (1) the vascular response, (2) the cardiac response, and (3) the response of the CNS.

FAILURE OF THE VASCULAR RESPONSE. With prolonged hemorrhagic hypotension, the total peripheral resistance—which first increases in response to sympathetic stimulation—tends to return to prehemorrhage levels. This failure may have many causes, including desensitization of the vascular adrenoceptors or depletion of neurotransmitters in the nerve terminals close to the blood vessels. In addition, the ischemic tissues release metabolites and other vasodilator compounds that act on local blood vessels, thereby counteracting the vasoconstricting stimuli. In the late phases of irreversible shock, humans may become completely unresponsive to a range of vasoconstrictor drugs. At the same time, plasma AVP levels may have fallen substantially from the peak value during the early phase of hemorrhage—perhaps reflecting a decreased ability of the low-pressure baroreceptor reflex to trigger hypothalamic neurons to release AVP, or a depletion of AVP stores. Under these conditions, restoring AVP levels to their initial peak can markedly increase blood pressure.

Some blood vessels are able to sustain the initial increase in resistance better than others. Over time, precapillary sphincters fail first, followed by the precapillary resistance vessels (i.e., arterioles), the postcapillary resistance vessels, and the capacitance vessels. Figure 24-9D shows an example in which, after prolonged hypotension, the precapillary constrictor response has fully faded, whereas the postcapillary response is partially maintained. Because the ratio R_{post}/R_{pre} has risen, the midcapillary pressure (p. 452) increases from 16 mm Hg (see Fig. 24-9C) to 21 mm Hg (see Fig. 24-9D). You will recall that, early during hemorrhage, the net Starling forces reverse, favoring the movement of fluid from the interstitium to the blood. The gradual increase of R_{post}/R_{pre} (see Fig. 24-9D) reverses this reversal, so that fluid once again leaves the capillary, even though the blood volume has not yet been restored. Thus, following the initial large influx of water and electrolytes into the capillary lumen, not only does transcapillary refill decline, but a net loss occurs. This phenomenon contributes to the hemoconcentration that occasionally occurs in prolonged hemorrhagic states.

FAILURE OF THE HEART. Several factors may contribute to the weakening of the heart. Acidosis reduces $[Ca^{2+}]_i$ in the myocardium, and thus reduces contractility. In severe cases, subendocardial hemorrhage and necrosis of the heart muscle render the myocardium nonfunctional. Various organs may also release cardiotoxic shock factors, which exert a negative inotropic effect on the heart (p. 533).

CENTRAL NERVOUS SYSTEM DEPRESSION. Moderate ischemia, via effects on the central chemoreceptors, stimulates the cardiovascular control centers in the brain (p. 586). However, prolonged cerebral ischemia depresses neural activity throughout the brain. This general decrease in neuronal activity also depresses the sympathetic output, which may be responsible for the decay in both vascular and cardiac responses. A progressive fall in the circulating levels of catecholamines of adrenal origin further worsens the outcome.

REFERENCES

Books and Reviews

Butler PJ, Jones DR: Physiology of diving of birds and mammals. Physiol Rev 77:837–899, 1997.

Kunze DL: Role of baroreceptor resetting in cardiovascular regulation: Acute resetting. Fed Proc 44:2408–2411, 1985.

Persson PB: Modulation of cardiovascular control mechanisms and their interaction. Physiol Rev 76:193–244, 1996.

Uvnäs B: Sympathetic vasodilator system and blood flow. Physiol Rev 40(Suppl 4):69–76, 1960.

Journal Articles

Guyton AC, TG Coleman, AW Cowley Jr., RD Manning Jr, RA Norman Jr and JD Ferguson. A systems analysis approach to understanding long-range arterial blood pressure control and hypertension. Circ. Res. 35:159–176, 1974.

Jacobsen TN, Morgan BJ, Scherrer U, et al: Relative contributions of cardiopulmonary and sinoaortic baroreflexes in causing sympathetic stimulation in the human skeletal muscle circulation during orthostatic stress. Circ Res 73:367–378, 1993.

Mellander S: Comparative studies on the adrenergic neuro-humeral control of resistance and capacitance blood vessels in the cat. Acta Physiol Scand 50(Suppl):176:1–86, 1960.

Morales D, Madigan J, Cullinane S, et al: Reversal by vasopressin of intractable hypotension in the late phase of hemorrhagic shock. Circulation 100:226–229, 1999.

Smith OA Jr, Rushmer RF, Lasher EP: Similarity of cardiovascular responses to exercise and to diencephalic stimulation. Am J Physiol 198:1139–1142, 1960.

Starling EH: On the circulatory changes associated with exercise. J R Army Med Corps 34: 258–275, 1920.

V

The Respiratory System

CHAPTER 25

Organization of the Respiratory System

Walter F. Boron

COMPARATIVE PHYSIOLOGY OF RESPIRATION

External Respiration Is the Exchange of O_2 and CO_2 Between the Atmosphere and the Mitochondria

For millennia, people have regarded life as being synonymous with breathing. Life begins and ends with breathing. The Bible states that God "breathed into [Adam's] nostrils the breath of life," and then later used part of Adam's ventilatory apparatus—a rib—to give life to Eve. In the fourth and fifth centuries BC, writings attributed to Hippocrates suggested that the primary purpose of breathing is to cool the heart.

It was not until the 18th century that the true role of breathing began to emerge as several distinguished investigators studied the chemistry of gases. At the time, chemists recognized similarities between combustion and breathing, but thought that both involved the production of a "fire-essence" principle called "phlogiston." According to their theory, neither combustion nor life could be supported once air became saturated with phlogiston.

In the 1750s, the Scottish scientist Joseph Black found that heating calcium carbonate produces a gas he called "fixed air," now known to be **carbon dioxide** (CO_2). This work revolutionized chemistry. It showed that a chemical reaction can involve a gas, and it further demonstrated that other gases exist besides ordinary "air." Shortly thereafter, Cavendish, working in England, showed that fermentation and putrefaction produce "fixed air." His countryman Priestley discovered several new gases between the late 1760s and mid-1770s, including "dephlogistonated air," co-discovered by the Swedish chemist Scheele. Priestley found that combustion, putrefaction, and breathing all *consume* "dephlogistonated air," and all reduce the volume of room air by approximately 20%. Conversely, he found that green plants *produce* "dephlogistonated air," which he could quantitate by reacting it with nitric oxide (a colorless gas) to produce nitrogen dioxide (a red gas).

In the mid-1770s, Priestley toured the Continent and presented his findings to the Frenchman Lavoisier, who is often regarded as the father of modern chemistry. Lavoisier quickly put Priestley's empirical observations into a theoretical framework that he used to demolish the phlogiston theory, which Priestley held to his death. Lavoisier recognized that dephlogistonated air, which he named **oxygen** (O_2), represents the 20% of room air consumed by combustion in Priestley's experiments, leaving behind "non-vital" air, or **nitrogen**. Furthermore, he proposed that O_2 is consumed because it reacts with one substance to produce another substance. Spallanzani, working in Italy during the late 1790s, confirmed Lavoisier's prediction that O_2 consumption and CO_2 production occur not in the lungs, but in isolated tissues.

Therefore, by the end of the 18th century, chemists/physiologists appreciated that combustion, putrefaction, and respiration all involve chemical reactions that consume O_2 and produce CO_2. Subsequent advances in the chemistry of gases by Boyle, Henry, Avogadro, and others laid the theoretical foundation for dealing with the physiology of O_2 and CO_2. Thus, respiration was a unifying theme in the early histories of physiology, chemistry, and biochemistry.

Later work showed that mitochondrial respiration (i.e., the oxidation of carbon-containing compounds to form CO_2) is responsible for the O_2 consumption and CO_2 production observed by Spallanzani. This aspect of respiration is often called **internal respiration** or oxidative phosphorylation (p. 1220).

In the chapters on respiratory physiology, we focus on **external respiration**, the dual processes of (1) transporting O_2 from the atmosphere to the mitochondria and (2) transporting CO_2 from the mitochondria to the atmosphere. We will also see that CO_2 transport is intimately related to acid-base homeostasis.

Diffusion Is the Major Mechanism of External Respiration for Small Aquatic Organisms

The most important and the most fundamental mechanism of O_2 and CO_2 transport is **diffusion** (p. 56). The random movements of molecules such as O_2 and CO_2, whether in a gaseous phase or dissolved in water, result in a net movement of the substance from regions of high concentration to regions of low concentration (Fig. 25–1A, *inset*). No expenditure of energy is involved. The driving force for diffusion is the concentration gradient.

Imagine a unicellular organism, suspended in a beaker of water at 37°C. We will equilibrate the water with an atmosphere that has the usual composition of O_2 and CO_2 (Table 25–1). The partial pressures of O_2 (Po_2) and of CO_2 (Pco_2) in the dry air are slightly higher than their corresponding values in the wet air immediately above the surface of the water (see the box on Wet Gases). It is

FIGURE 25–1. Diffusion of O_2 and CO_2 for a single-celled organism. In *A* through *D*, the y-axis of grids shows the dissolved concentration (or partial pressure) of O_2 and CO_2. The x-axis represents distance (not to scale). In *D*, the broken red and blue lines and the enclosed violet triangles represent the magnitude of the gradients driving O_2 and CO_2 diffusion. The red (O_2) and blue (CO_2) pathways represent the circuit of blood from the pulmonary capillaries to the systemic capillaries, and back again.

TABLE 25–1

COMPOSITION OF AIR

GAS	DRY AIR Atmosphere		WET AIR Trachea	
	Fraction in Air (%)	Partial Pressure at Sea Level (mm Hg)	Fraction in Air (%)	Partial Pressure at Sea Level (mm Hg)
Nitrogen	78.09	593.48	73.26	556.78
Oxygen	20.95	159.22	19.65	149.37
Carbon dioxide	0.03	0.23	0.03	0.21
Argon	0.93	7.07	0.87	6.63
Water	0	0	6.18	47
Total	100	760	100	760

these partial pressures in wet air that determine the concentrations of dissolved O_2 ($[O_2]_{Dis}$) and dissolved CO_2 ($[CO_2]_{Dis}$) in the water (see the box on Henry's Law). Thus, the P_{O_2} in the wet air—as well as the water beneath it—will be approximately 149 mm Hg (or torr), and the P_{CO_2} will be an almost negligible 0.2 mm Hg. These numbers describe the composition of the water in the **bulk phase**, at some distance from the organism. However, because the mitochondria within the organism continuously consume O_2 and produce CO_2, the P_{O_2} at the surface of the mitochondria will be lower than the

bulk-phase P_{O_2}, whereas the P_{CO_2} at the mitochondrial surface will be higher than the bulk-phase P_{CO_2}. These differences in partial pressure cause O_2 to diffuse from the bulk fluid toward the mitochondria, and the CO_2 to diffuse in the opposite direction.

The diffusion of O_2 follows a gradient of decreasing P_{O_2} (see Fig. 25–1A). The region over which P_{O_2} falls gradually from the bulk fluid toward the organism's outer surface is the **extracellular unstirred layer**, so named because no convective mixing occurs in this zone. A similar gradual decline in P_{O_2} drives O_2 diffusion through the

---

"WET GASES": PARTIAL PRESSURES OF O_2 AND CO_2 IN SOLUTIONS THAT ARE EQUILIBRATED WITH WET AIR

Imagine that a beaker of water is equilibrated with a normal atmosphere, both at a temperature of 37°C. For **dry air** (i.e., air containing no water vapor), O_2 makes up approximately 21% of the total gas by volume (see Table 25–1). Thus, if the barometric pressure (P_B) is 760 mm Hg, the partial pressure of O_2 (P_{O_2}) is 21% of 760 mm Hg, or 159 mm Hg (Fig. 25–2A). However, if the air-water interface is reasonably stationary, then water vapor will saturate the air immediately adjacent to the liquid. What is the P_{O_2} in this **wet air**? At 37°C, the partial pressure of water (P_{H_2O}) is 47 mm Hg. Thus, of the total pressure of the wet air, P_{H_2O} makes up 47 mm Hg, and the components of the dry air make up the remaining 760 − 47, or 713 mm Hg. The partial pressure of O_2 in this wet air is:

$$\underset{\substack{\text{Fraction of dry} \\ \text{air that is } O_2 \\ \downarrow}}{P_{O_2} = F_{O_2}} \times (P_B - P_{H_2O})$$

$$= (21\%) \times (760 \text{ mm Hg} - 47 \text{ mm Hg})$$

$$= 149 \text{ mm Hg}$$

The CO_2 composition of dry air is approximately 0.03% (see Table 25–1). Thus, the partial pressure of CO_2 in wet air is:

$$P_{CO_2} = F_{CO_2} \times (P_B - P_{H_2O})$$

$$= (0.03\%) \times (760 \text{ mm Hg} - 47 \text{ mm Hg})$$

$$= 0.21 \text{ mm Hg}$$

These examples are realistic for respiratory physiology: As we inhale relatively cool and dry air, the nose and other upper respiratory passages rapidly warm and moisturize the passing air so that it assumes the composition of wet air given in Table 25–1.

A PARTIAL PRESSURE OF O_2 IN WET AIR

B HENRY'S LAW

C DIFFUSION OF DISSOLVED GAS

FIGURE 25–2. Partial pressures.

intracellular unstirred layer, from the organism's inner surface to the mitochondria. The final remarkable feature of the PO_2 profile is the abrupt fall in PO_2 at the organism's surface. The profile for PCO_2 is similar, but has the opposite orientation.

The rate at which O_2 or CO_2 moves across the surface of the organism is the **flow** (units: moles/s). According to a simplified version of **Fick's Law** (p. 56), the flow is proportional to the concentration difference across this barrier. Because we know from Henry's Law that the concentration of a dissolved gas is proportional to its partial pressure in the gas phase, the flow is also proportional to the partial-pressure difference (ΔP):

Equation 25–1
$$\text{Flow} \propto \Delta P$$

Simple diffusion is the mechanism by which O_2 and CO_2 move *short* distances in the respiratory system: between the air and the blood in the **alveoli**, and between the mitochondria and the blood of the peripheral circulation.

Convection Enhances Diffusion by Producing Steeper Gradients Across the Diffusion Barrier

A purely diffusive system can establish only a relatively small ΔP across the gas-exchange barrier of the organism

(see Fig. 25–1A). Yet, for small organisms, even this relatively small ΔP is adequate to meet the demands for O_2 uptake and CO_2 removal. However, when the organism's diameter exceeds approximately 1 mm, simple diffusion becomes inadequate for gas exchange. One way of ameliorating this problem is to introduce a mechanism for local **convection** on the outside surface of the organism. For a paramecium, the beating cilia bring bulk-phase water—having a PO_2 of approximately 154 mm Hg at 25°C and a PCO_2 of approximately 0.2 mm Hg—very near to the cell's surface. This mixing reduces the size of the extracellular unstirred layer, thereby increasing the PO_2 and decreasing the PCO_2 on the outer surface of the organism. The net effect is that the partial-pressure gradients for both O_2 and CO_2 increase across the gas-exchange barrier (see Fig. 25–1B), leading to a proportionate increase in the flow of both substances.

A filter feeder, such as an oyster or a clam, pumps bulk-phase water past its organ of gas exchange. Because of the relatively low solubility of O_2 in water, such an organism may need to pump 16,000 ml of water to extract a mere 1 ml of O_2 gas. In fish, which are far more efficient, the ratio is considerably lower, approximately 400:1.

In mammals, the bulk phase is the atmosphere and the external convective system is an air pump consisting of the lungs, the airways, and the respiratory muscles. **Ventilation** is the process of moving air into and out of the

PARTIAL PRESSURES AND HENRY'S LAW

Respiratory physiologists generally express the concentration of a gas, whether mixed with another gas (e.g., O_2 and N_2, as is the case for air) or dissolved in an aqueous solution (e.g., O_2 dissolved in water), in terms of partial pressure. **Dalton's Law** states that the total pressure (P_{Total}) of a mixture of gases is the sum of their individual **partial pressures**. Imagine that we are dealing with an ideal gas (Z) mixed with other gases. Because the ratio of the partial pressure of Z (P_Z) to the total pressure (P_{Total}) is its mole fraction (X_Z),

$$P_Z = X_Z \cdot P_{Total}$$

Thus, if P_Z were twice as high in one sample of gas than in another, X_Z (i.e., concentration of Z) would also be twice as high.

It may not be immediately obvious why partial pressures are also useful for expressing concentrations when dealing with situations in which Z is dissolved in aqueous solutions. According to **Henry's Law**, the concentration of O_2 dissolved in water ($[O_2]_{Dis}$) is proportional to the P_{O_2} in the gas phase:

$$[O_2]_{Dis} = s \times P_{O_2}$$

The proportionality constant s is known as the **solubility**; for O_2, this value is approximately 0.0013 mM/mm Hg at 37°C for a solution mimicking arterial blood plasma. The solubility of CO_2 is approximately 23-fold higher. Consider a beaker of water at 37°C equilibrated with an atmosphere having a P_{O_2} of 100 mm Hg, the partial pressure in mammalian *arterial* blood plasma (see Fig. 25–2B, solution #1). Thus,

$$[O_2]_{Dis} = 0.0013 \text{ mM/mm Hg} \times 100 \text{ mm Hg}$$
$$= 0.13 \text{ mM}$$

Now imagine that we have a second beaker equilibrated with an atmosphere having a P_{O_2} of 40 mm Hg, the partial pressure of O_2 in *mixed-venous* blood (see Fig. 25–2B, solution #2). For this solution,

$$[O_2]_{Dis} = 0.0013 \text{ mM/mm Hg} \times 40 \text{ mm Hg}$$
$$= = 0.05 \text{ mM}$$

If we were to place samples of each of these two solutions on opposite sides of a semipermeable barrier in a closed container (see Fig. 25–2C), the O_2 gradient across this barrier expressed in terms of concentrations ($\Delta[O_2]$) would be 0.13 − 0.05 or 0.08 mM. Expressed in terms of partial pressures (ΔP_{O_2}), this same gradient would be 100 − 40 = 60 mm Hg.

Imagine now that we take a 5-ml sample of each of the solutions in the beakers in Figure 25–2B, drawing the fluid up into syringes, sealing the syringes, putting them on ice, and sending them to a clinical laboratory for analysis—as is routinely done with samples of arterial blood. Even though there is no gas phase in equilibrium with either of the solutions in the syringes, the laboratory will report the O_2 levels in "mm Hg." These are the partial pressures of O_2 with which the solutions *were* or *would have to be* equilibrated to achieve the $[O_2]_{Dis}$ in the samples.

CONVENTIONS FOR MEASURING VOLUMES OF GASES

Gases within the lung are saturated with water vapor at 37°C (310°K). At this temperature, the partial pressure of water is 47 mm Hg. The total pressure of the air in the lungs is equal to barometric pressure, which we will assume to be 760 mm Hg. We can be certain that alveolar pressure equals barometric pressure if the glottis is open and no air is flowing. Thus, the partial pressure of the dry gases in the lungs is (760 − 47) = 713 mm Hg. Whereas the air in the lungs is at "Body Temperature and Pressure, Saturated with Water" (BTPS), this same air, when expelled from the lungs into the spirometer (p. 606), is at "Ambient Temperature and Pressure, Saturated" (ATPS). Thus, we must correct the volume change (ΔV_{ATPS}) registered by the spirometer (at ATPS) to have an accurate measure of the volume (ΔV_{BTPS}) that this same gas had previously occupied in the lungs (at BTPS). According to the ideal gas law:

$$\frac{P_{BTPS} \cdot \Delta V_{BTPS}}{T_{BTPS}} = \frac{P_{ATPS} \cdot \Delta V_{ATPS}}{T_{ATPS}}$$

or

$$\Delta V_{BTPS} = \frac{P_{ATPS}}{P_{BTPS}} \cdot \frac{T_{BTPS}}{T_{ATPS}} \cdot \Delta V_{ATPS}$$

We will assume that the ambient temperature is 25°C (or 298°K). The partial pressure of the dry gases at 25°C is simply the total barometric pressure minus the vapor pressure of water at 25°C, 24 mm Hg. Thus, substituting real numbers into the previous equation:

$$\Delta V_{BTPS} = \frac{(760 - 24)}{(760 - 47)} \cdot \frac{310°K}{298°K} \cdot \Delta V_{ATPS} = 1.074 \cdot \Delta V_{ATPS}$$

Thus, the same dry gas that occupies 1000 ml in the spirometer at ATPS, occupies 1074 ml in the body at BTPS.

lungs. Amphibians move air into their lungs by swallowing it. Reptiles, birds, and mammals expand their lungs by developing a negative pressure inside the thorax. Because of the much higher O_2 content of air (about 210 ml O_2/liter of air at standard temperature and pressure/dry or STPD), as opposed to water (about 35 ml O_2/liter of water), humans need to move far less air than oysters need to move water. For example, a human may ventilate his/her alveoli with 4000 ml of fresh air every minute, and extract from this air 250 ml of O_2 gas, a ratio of 16:1.

Although we are 1000-fold more efficient than oysters, the principle of external convective systems is the same: ensure that the external surface of the gas-exchange barrier is in close contact with a fluid whose composition matches—as closely as is practical—that of the bulk phase. How "closely" is "practical"? The composition of alveolar air approaches that of wet inspired air as alveolar ventilation approaches infinity (p. 692). Because high ventilatory rates have a significant metabolic cost, the body must trade off optimizing alveolar PO_2 and PCO_2 on the one hand, against minimizing the work of ventilation on the other. In the average adult human, the compromise that has evolved is an alveolar ventilation of approximately 4000 ml/min, an alveolar PO_2 of approximately 100 mm Hg (*versus* 149 mm Hg in a wet atmosphere at 37°C) and an alveolar PCO_2 of approximately 40 mm Hg (*versus* 0.2 mm Hg).

A clinical example in which the external convective system fails is barbiturate poisoning. Here, drug intoxication inhibits the respiratory-control centers in the medulla (p. 712), so that ventilation slows or even stops. From a theoretical perspective, the consequence is that the unstirred layer between the bulk-phase atmosphere and the alveolar blood-gas barrier becomes extremely large (i.e., the distance between the nose and the alveoli). As a result, alveolar PO_2 falls to such low levels that the ΔPO_2 across the alveolar wall cannot support an O_2 flow and an arterial $[O_2]$ that is compatible with life. Cessation of ventilation also causes the alveolar PCO_2 to rise to such high levels that the CO_2 flow from blood to alveolar air is unacceptably low and arterial $[CO_2]$ rises to lethal levels.

An *external* convective system maximizes gas exchange by continuously supplying bulk-phase water or air to the external surface of the gas-exchange barrier, thereby maintaining a high external PO_2 and a low external PCO_2. A **circulatory system** is an *internal* convective system that maximizes the flow of O_2 and CO_2 across the gas-exchange barrier by delivering, to the inner surface of this barrier, blood that has as low a PO_2 and as high a PCO_2 as practical. **Perfusion** is the process of delivering blood to the lungs. Figure 25–1C shows a very primitive—and hypothetical—internal convective system, one that essentially stirs the entire internal contents of the organism, so that the PO_2 of the bulk internal fluids is uniform, right up to the surface of the mitochondria. The result is that the ΔPO_2 across the gas-exchange barrier is rather large, but the ΔPO_2 between the bulk internal fluid and the mitochondria is rather small.

Figure 25–1D summarizes the PO_2 and PCO_2 profiles for a sophisticated circulatory system built around a four-chambered heart and separate pulmonary and systemic circulations. The circulatory system carries (by convec-

tion) low-PO_2 blood from a systemic capillary near the mitochondria to the alveolar wall. At the beginning of a pulmonary capillary, a high alveolar-to-blood PO_2 gradient ensures a high O_2 inflow (by diffusion), and blood PO_2 rises to match the alveolar (i.e., external) PO_2 by the time the blood leaves the pulmonary capillary. Finally, the systemic arterial blood carries (by convection) this high-PO_2 blood to the systemic capillaries, where a high blood-to-mitochondria PO_2 gradient maximizes the O_2 flux into the mitochondria (by diffusion). The opposite happens with CO_2. Thus, separate pulmonary and systemic circulations ensure maximal gradients for gas diffusion at the level of both the alveoli and the peripheral mitochondria.

The scenario outlined in Figure 25–1D requires the four-chambered heart characteristic of mammals as well as advanced reptiles and birds. The right ventricle pumps low-PO_2/high-PCO_2 blood received from the peripheral veins to the lungs, whereas the left ventricle pumps high-PO_2/low-PCO_2 blood received from pulmonary veins to the periphery (i.e., mitochondria). Maintaining maximal gradients for O_2 and CO_2 diffusion at both the gas-exchange barrier and at the mitochondria requires that right- and left-ventricular blood not mix. However, this sort of mixing is exactly what occurs in fish and amphibians, whose hearts have a common ventricle. In these animals, the aortic blood has PO_2 and PCO_2 values that are intermediate between the extreme values of venous blood returning from the systemic circulation and the blood returning from the gas-exchange-barrier circulation. The result is less-than-optimal PO_2 and PCO_2 gradients at both the gas-exchange barrier and the mitochondria.

In humans, the internal convective system may fail when diseased heart valves cause a decrease in cardiac output. Another example is the shunting of blood between the pulmonary and the systemic circulations, as may occur in newborns with congenital anomalies (e.g., atrial or ventricular septal defects). The result is the same sort of mixing of systemic venous and gas-exchange-barrier blood that occurs in amphibians and fish. Thus, patients with shunts cannot establish normal PO_2 and PCO_2 gradients in the pulmonary and peripheral capillaries, and thus cannot generate normal fluxes of O_2 and CO_2.

Surface-Area Amplification Enhances Diffusion

The passive flow of O_2 or CO_2 across a barrier is proportional not only to the concentration gradient, but also to the area of the barrier:

Equation 25–2

$$Flow \propto \Delta P \times Area$$

Indeed, higher animals have increased their ability to exchange O_2 and CO_2 with their environment by increasing the **surface area** across which gas exchange takes place. For example, molluscs (e.g., squid) and fish have gills, which they form by evaginating the gas-exchange barrier, thus greatly amplifying its surface area. Higher land animals amplify their gas-exchange barriers by invaginating them, forming lungs. In an amphibian such as the adult frog, the lungs are simple air sacs with a relatively small surface area. Not surprisingly, a large portion of their gas exchange must occur across the skin. The gas-exchange barrier is considerably more sophisticated in reptiles, which line their lungs with alveoli, or even sub-divide them with alveoli-lined barriers. The net effect is that the surface-to-volume ratio of the lungs is greatly increased. Mammals increase the area available for diffusion even more, by developing highly complex lungs with bronchi and a large number of alveoli.

In humans, the lung surface is so large and so thin that O_2 and CO_2 transport across the alveolar wall is approximately three-fold faster than necessary when cardiac output is normal. Nevertheless, this redundancy is extremely important during exercise (when cardiac output can increase markedly), life at high altitude (where the P_{O_2} is low), and in old age (when lung function diminishes). A substantial decrease in surface area, or thickening of the barrier, can be deleterious. Examples are the surgical removal of a lung (which reduces the total surface for gas exchange by about half) and pulmonary edema (which increases the effective thickness of the barrier). Thus, if an individual with a thickened barrier loses a lung, the remaining surface area may not be large enough to sustain normal rates of gas exchange and normal blood levels of O_2 and CO_2.

Respiratory Pigments Such as Hemoglobin Increase the Carrying Capacity of the Blood for Both O_2 and CO_2

In mammals, the external convective system (i.e., ventilatory apparatus), the internal convective system (i.e., circulatory system), and the barrier itself (i.e., alveolar wall) are so efficient that the diffusion of O_2 and CO_2 is not what limits the exchange of gases, at least not in healthy subjects at sea level.

Imagine what would happen if the mixed-venous blood flowing down a pulmonary capillary contained only water and salts. The diffusion of O_2 from the alveolar air space into the "blood" would be so fast—and the solubility of O_2 in saline is so low (see the box on Henry's Law)—that, before the blood could move approximately 1% of the way down the capillary, the P_{O_2} of the blood would match the P_{O_2} of the alveolar air (i.e., all of the O_2 that *could* move *would* have moved). For the remaining approximately 99% of the capillary, the P_{O_2} gradient across the barrier would be nil, and no more O_2 would flow into the blood. As a result, at a normal cardiac output, the "blood" could never carry away enough O_2 from the lungs to the tissues to sustain life. The same is true in reverse for the elimination of CO_2.

Animals solve this problem with respiratory pigments, specialized metalloproteins that greatly increase the carrying capacity of blood for O_2 and CO_2. In some arthropods and molluscs, the pigment is **hemocyanin**, a protein containing copper. Polychaete worms and brachiopods use **hemerythrins**. However, the most common respiratory pigments are the **hemoglobins**, which contain iron. All vertebrates as well as numerous unrelated groups of animals use hemoglobin (Hb), which is the chief component of red blood cells (erythrocytes).

The presence of Hb markedly improves the dynamics of O_2 uptake by blood passing through the lungs. Under normal conditions, Hb reversibly binds approximately 96% of the O_2 that diffuses from the alveolar air spaces to the pulmonary capillary blood, greatly increasing the carrying capacity of blood for O_2. Hemoglobin also plays a key role in the transport or **carriage** of CO_2 by reversibly binding CO_2 and by acting as a powerful pH buffer. In **anemia**, the Hb content of blood is reduced, thus lowering the carrying capacity of blood for O_2 and CO_2. The most common cause of anemia in industrialized societies is a shortage in the diet of the iron necessary to synthesize Hb. An individual with anemia can compensate only if the systemic tissues extract more O_2 from each liter of blood and/or if cardiac output increases. However, there are limits to the amount of O_2 tissues can extract, or to the level to which the heart can increase its output.

Pathophysiology Recapitulates Phylogeny— In Reverse

It should be clear from the pathophysiologic examples discussed that whenever one of the key components of the respiratory system fails in a higher organism, external respiration in that organism becomes more like that of an organism that is lower on the evolutionary ladder. For example, a failure of a mammal's air pump makes this individual behave more like a unicellular aquatic organism without cilia. A reduction in the surface area of the alveoli in a mammal creates the same problems faced by an amphibian with simple sack-like lungs. A major shunt in the circulatory system makes a mammal behave more like a fish. In severe anemia, a mammal faces the same problems as a lower life form that lacks a respiratory pigment in the extracellular fluid.

ORGANIZATION OF THE RESPIRATORY SYSTEM IN HUMANS

Humans Optimize Each of the Processes Involved in External Respiration—Ventilation, Circulation, Area Amplification, Gas Carriage, Local Control, and Central Control

The human respiratory system (Fig. 25–3) has two important characteristics. First, it uses highly efficient convective systems (i.e., ventilatory and circulatory systems) for long-distance transport of O_2 and CO_2. Second, it reserves diffusion exclusively for short-distance movements of O_2 and CO_2. The key components of this respiratory system are:

1. An **air pump**: The external convective system in humans consists of the lungs and other airways, the thoracic cavity and its associated skeletal elements, and the muscles of respiration. These components deliver air to, and remove air from, the alveolar air spaces—**alveolar ventilation**. Inspiration occurs when the muscles of respiration increase the volume of the thoracic cavity, causing the alveoli to expand passively, and lowering alveolar pressure. A quiet expiration occurs when these muscles relax, as discussed in Chapter 26 ("Mechanics of Respiration").

FIGURE 25–3. The respiratory apparatus in humans.

3. A **surface for gas exchange**: The gas-exchange barrier in humans consists of the alveoli, which provide a huge but extremely thin surface area for passive diffusion of gases between the alveolar air spaces and the pulmonary capillaries. The anatomy of the alveoli is discussed later in this chapter, and pulmonary gas exchange is explored in Chapter 29 ("Gas Exchange in the Lungs"). A similar process of gas exchange occurs between the systemic capillaries and mitochondria.

4. A **circulatory system**: The internal convective system in humans consists of a four-chambered heart, and separate systemic and pulmonary circulations. The flow of blood to the lungs—**perfusion**—is discussed in Chapter 30 ("Ventilation and Perfusion of the Lungs").

5. A **mechanism for locally regulating the distribution of ventilation and perfusion**: Neither the delivery of fresh air to the entire population of alveoli nor the delivery of mixed-venous blood to the entire population of pulmonary capillaries is uniform throughout the lungs. Nevertheless, efficient gas exchange requires that, to the extent possible, the ratio of ventilation to perfusion be uniform for all alveoli. The lungs attempt to maximize the uniformity of ventilation/perfusion ratios by using sophisticated feedback-control mechanisms to regulate local air flow and blood flow, as discussed in Chapter 30.

6. A **mechanism for centrally regulating ventilation**: Unlike the rhythmicity of the heart, that of the respiratory system is not intrinsic to the lungs or the chest wall. Instead, respiratory control centers in the **central nervous system** (CNS) rhythmically stimulate the muscles of inspiration. Moreover, these respiratory centers must appropriately modify the pattern of ventilation during exercise or other changes in physical or mental activity. Sensors for arterial P_{O_2}, P_{CO_2}, and pH are part of feedback loops that stabilize these three "blood-gas" parameters. These subjects are the topic of Chapter 31 ("Control of Ventilation").

Respiratory physiologists have agreed on a set of symbols for describing parameters that are important for pulmonary physiology and pulmonary-function tests (Table 25–2).

Conducting Airways Deliver Fresh Air to the Alveolar Spaces

We will discuss lung development on p. 1195. In the embryo, each lung invaginates into a separate pleural sac, which reflects over the surface of the lung.

The **parietal pleura**, the wall of the sac that is farthest from the lung, contains blood vessels that are believed to produce an ultrafiltrate of the plasma called **pleural fluid**. About 10 ml of this fluid normally occupies the virtual space between the parietal and the **visceral pleura**. The latter lies directly on the lung and contains lymphatics that drain the fluid from the pleural space. When the production of pleural fluid exceeds its removal, the volume of pleural fluid increases (**pleural effusion**), limiting the expansion of the lung. Under normal circumstances,

2. **Mechanisms for carrying O$_2$ and CO$_2$ in the blood**: Red blood cells are highly specialized for transporting O$_2$ from the lungs to the peripheral tissues and for transporting CO$_2$ in the opposite direction. They have extremely high levels of hemoglobin and other components (2,3-diphosphoglycerate, carbonic anhydrase; and Cl-HCO$_3$ exchangers) that help to rapidly load and unload huge amounts of O$_2$ and CO$_2$. In the pulmonary capillaries, Hb binds O$_2$, thereby enabling the blood to carry approximately 65-fold more O$_2$ than ordinary saline. At the same time, Hb chemically reacts with approximately 20% of the CO$_2$ produced by the mitochondria and carries this CO$_2$ back to the lungs. Hemoglobin also plays a key role as it buffers the H$^+$ formed as carbonic anhydrase converts CO$_2$ to HCO$_3^-$ and H$^+$. Thus, hemoglobin plays a central role in acid-base chemistry, as discussed in Chapter 27 ("Acid-Base Physiology") as well as for the carriage of O$_2$ and CO$_2$, treated in Chapter 28 ("Transport of Oxygen and Carbon Dioxide in the Blood").

TABLE 25–2

SYMBOL CONVENTIONS IN RESPIRATORY PHYSIOLOGY

	RESPIRATORY MECHANICS		**GAS EXCHANGE**
	Main Symbols		**Main Symbols**
C	Compliance	C	Concentration (or content) in a liquid
f	Respiratory frequency	D	Diffusion capacity
P	Pressure	f	Respiratory frequency
R	Resistance	F	Fraction
V	Volume of gas	P	Pressure
V̇	Flow of gas	Q̇	Flow of blood (perfusion)
		R	Gas-exchange ratio
		S	Saturation of hemoglobin
		V	Volume of gas
		V̇	Ventilation
	Modifiers		**Modifiers**
A	Alveolar	a	Systemic arterial
aw	Airway	A	Alveolar
B	Barometric	B	Barometric
		c	Pulmonary capillary
		E	Expired
		I	Inspired
		v	Systemic venous (in any vascular bed)
		v̄	Mixed systemic venous

Macklem PT: Symbols and abbreviations. In Handbook of Physiology. Section 3: The Respiratory System. Vol 1. Bethesda, MD, American Physiological Society, 1985.

the pleural fluid probably lubricates the pleural space, facilitating physiologic changes in the size and shape of the lung.

The lungs themselves are divided into **lobes**, three in the right lung (i.e., upper, middle, and lower lobes) and two in the left (i.e., upper and lower lobes). The right lung, which is less encumbered than the left by the presence of the heart, makes up approximately 55% of total lung mass and function.

We refer to the progressively bifurcating pulmonary airways by their **generation number** (Fig. 25–4): The zeroth generation is the trachea, the first generation airways are the right and left mainstem bronchi, and so on. Inasmuch as the right mainstem bronchus has a greater diameter than does the left, and is more nearly parallel with the trachea, inhaled foreign bodies more commonly lodge in the right lung than in the left. There is a total of approximately 23 generations of airways. As generation number increases (i.e., as airways become smaller), the amount of cilia, the number of mucus-secreting cells, the presence of submucosal glands, and the amount of cartilage in the airway walls all gradually decrease. The mucus is important for trapping small foreign particles. The cilia sweep the carpet of mucus—kept moist by secretions from the submucosal glands—up toward the pharynx, where swallowing eventually disposes of the mucus. The cartilage is important for preventing airway collapse, which is especially problematic during expiration (p. 630). Airways maintain some cartilage to about the 10th generation, up to which point they are referred to as **bronchi.**

At about the 11th and succeeding generations, the now cartilage-free airways are called **bronchioles.** Because these bronchioles lack cartilage, they can maintain a patent lumen only because the pressure surrounding them may be more negative than the pressure inside, and because of the outward pull (radial traction or tethering) of surrounding tissues. Thus, bronchioles are especially susceptible to collapse during expiration. Up until generation approximately 16, no alveoli are present, and the air cannot exchange with the pulmonary-capillary blood. These alveoli-free airways are the **conducting airways**, which serve only to move air by convection (i.e., like water moving through a pipe) to those regions of the lung that participate in gas exchange. The most distal conducting airways are the **terminal bronchioles** (generation ~16). The total aggregate volume of conducting airways, from the lips/nose to the generation-16 airways, the **anatomic dead space**, amounts to approximately 150 ml in healthy young males and somewhat over 100 ml in females. The anatomic dead space is only a small fraction of the total lung capacity, which averages 5 to 6 liters in adults, depending on the size and health of the individual.

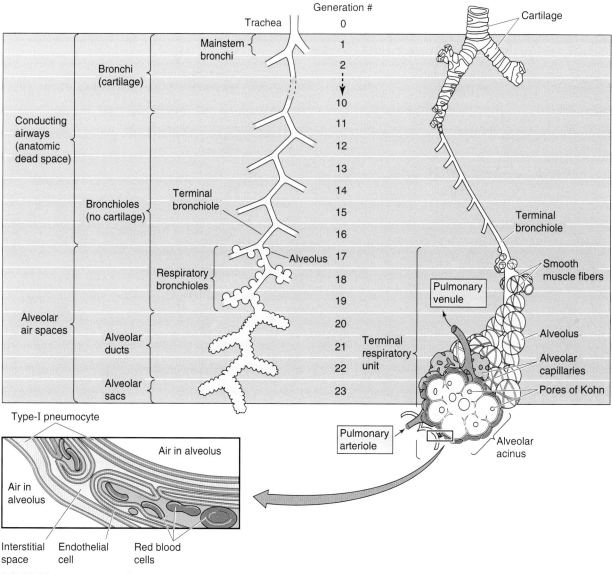

FIGURE 25–4. Generations of airways.

Alveolar Air Spaces Are the Site Of Gas Exchange

Alveoli first appear budding off bronchioles at approximately generation 17. These **respiratory bronchioles** participate in gas exchange over at least part of their surface. Respiratory bronchioles extend from approximately generation 17 to generation 19, the density of alveoli gradually increasing with generation number (see Fig. 25–4). Eventually, alveoli completely line the airways. These **alveolar ducts** (generations 20–22) finally terminate blindly as **alveolar sacs** (generation 23). The aggregation of all airways arising from a single terminal bronchiole (i.e., the respiratory bronchioles, alveolar ducts, and alveolar sacs), along with their associated blood and lymphatic vessels, is a **terminal respiratory unit** or **primary lobule**.

The cross-sectional area of the trachea is approximately 2.5 cm². Unlike the situation in systemic arteries (p. 449), wherein the aggregate cross-sectional area of the branches always exceeds the cross-sectional area of the parent vessel, the aggregate cross-sectional area falls from the trachea through the first four generations of airways (Fig. 25–5). Because all of the air that passes through the trachea also passes through each generation of conducting airways, the product of aggregate cross-sectional area and linear velocity is a constant. Thus, the linear velocity of air in the first four generations is higher than that in the trachea, which may be important during coughing (see p. 732). In succeeding generations, however, the aggregate cross-sectional area rises, at first slowly, and then very steeply. As a result, the linear velocity falls to very low values. For example, at the level of the terminal bronchioles (generation 16), the aggregate cross-sectional area is approximately 180 cm². Thus, the average linear velocity of the air at generation 16 is only (2.5 cm²)/(180 cm²) = 1.4% of the value in the trachea.

As air moves into the respiratory bronchioles and further into the terminal respiratory unit, where the linear velocity is minuscule, convection gradually becomes even less and less important for the movement of gas molecules, and diffusion dominates. Notice that the long-distance movement of gases from lips/nose to the end of the generation-16 airways occurs by *convection*. However, the short-distance movement of gases from generation-17 airways to the farthest reaches of the alveolar ducts occurs by *diffusion*. The movement of gases across the gas-exchange barrier (<0.5 μm) also occurs by *diffusion*. Thus, the distances over which convection occurs are long, whereas the distances over which diffusion takes place are short.

The **alveolus** is the fundamental unit of gas exchange. Alveoli are hemispheric structures with diameters that range from 75 to 300 μm. The approximately 300 million alveoli have a combined surface area of 50 to 100 m² and an aggregate maximal volume of 5 to 6 liters in the two lungs. Both the diameter and the surface area depend on the degree of lung inflation. The lungs have a relatively modest total volume (i.e., approximately 5.5 liters), very little of which is invested in conducting airways (i.e., approximately 0.15 liters). However, the alveolar area is tremendously amplified. For example, a sphere with a volume of 5.5 liters would have a surface area of only 0.16 m², which is far less than 1% of the alveolar surface area.

The alveolar lining consists of two distinct types of epithelial cells, called type-I and type-II alveolar pneumocytes. The cuboidal type-II cells exist in clusters and are responsible for elaborating **pulmonary surfactant**, which substantially eases the expansion of the lungs (p. 618). The type-I cells are much thinner than the type-II cells. Thus, even though the two cell types are present in approximately equal numbers, the type-I cells cover 90% to 95% of the alveolar surface, and represent the shortest route for gas diffusion. After an injury, type-I cells slough and degenerate, whereas type-II cells proliferate and line the alveolar space, re-establishing a continuous epithelial layer. Thus, the type-II cells appear to serve as repair cells.

The pulmonary capillaries are usually sandwiched between two alveolar air spaces. In fact, the flowing blood almost forms an uninterrupted sheet that flows like a twisted ribbon between abutting alveoli. At the type-I cells, the alveolar wall (i.e., pneumocyte plus endothelial cell) is typically 0.15 to 0.30 μm thick. Small holes (**pores of Kohn**) perforate the septum separating two abutting alveoli. The function of these pores, which are surrounded by capillaries, is unknown.

The lung receives two blood supplies: (1) the pulmonary arteries and (2) the bronchial arteries (Fig. 25-6). The **pulmonary arteries**, by far the major blood supply to the lung, carry the relatively deoxygenated mixed-venous blood. After arising from the right ventricle, they bifurcate as they follow the bronchial tree, and their divisions ultimately form a dense, richly anastomosing, hexagonal array of capillary segments that supply the alveoli of the terminal respiratory unit. The pulmonary capillaries have an average internal diameter of approximately 8 μm, and each segment of the capillary network is approximately 10 μm in length. The average erythrocyte spends approximately 0.75 sec in the pulmonary capillaries as it traverses up to three alveoli. After gas exchange in the alveoli, the blood eventually collects in the pulmonary veins.

The **bronchial arteries** are branches of the aorta and thus carry freshly oxygenated blood. They supply the conducting airways. At the level of the respiratory bronchioles, capillaries derived from bronchial arteries anastomose with those derived from pulmonary arteries. Because capillaries of the bronchial circulation drain partially into pulmonary veins, there is some **venous admixture** of the partially deoxygenated blood from the bronchial circulation and the newly oxygenated blood (p. 705). This mixing represents part of a small physiologic **shunt**. A small amount of the bronchial blood drains into the azygos and accessory hemiazygos veins.

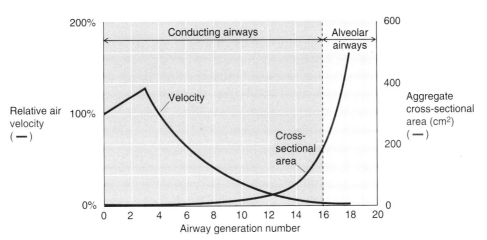

FIGURE 25-5. Dependence of aggregate cross-sectional area and of linear velocity on generation number. At generation 3, the aggregate cross-sectional area has a minimum (not visible), where velocity has its maximum. (Data from Bouhuys A: The Physiology of Breathing. New York, Grune & Stratton, 1977.)

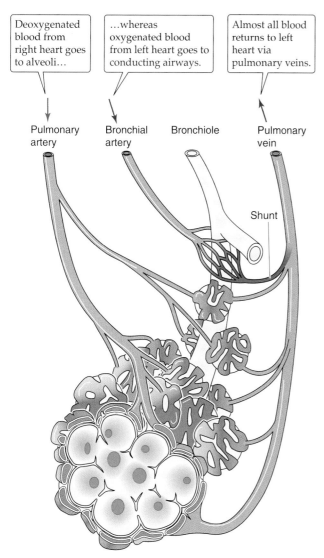

Deoxygenated blood from right heart goes to alveoli…

…whereas oxygenated blood from left heart goes to conducting airways.

Almost all blood returns to left heart via pulmonary veins.

Pulmonary artery

Bronchial artery

Bronchiole

Pulmonary vein

Shunt

FIGURE 25–6. The blood supply to the airways.

The Lungs Play Important Nonrespiratory Roles, Including Filtering the Blood, Serving as a Reservoir for the Left Ventricle, and Performing Several Biochemical Conversions

Although the main function of the lungs is to exchange O_2 and CO_2 between the atmosphere and the blood, the lungs also play important roles that are not directly related to external respiration.

OLFACTION. Ventilation is essential for delivering odorants to the olfactory epithelium (p. 327). Sniffing behavior, especially important for some animals, allows one to sample the chemicals in the air without the risk of bringing potential noxious agents deep into the lungs.

PROCESSING OF INHALED AIR BEFORE IT REACHES THE ALVEOLI. Strictly speaking, the warming, moisturizing, and filtering of inhaled air in the conducting airways is a respiratory function. It is part of the cost of doing the business of ventilation. **Warming** cool, inhaled air is im-

portant so that gas exchange in the alveoli takes place at body temperature. If the alveoli and the associated blood were substantially cooler than body temperature, then the solubility of these alveolar gases in the cool pulmonary capillary blood would be relatively high. As the blood later warmed, the solubility of these gases would decrease, resulting in air bubbles (i.e., emboli) that could lodge in small systemic vessels, and cause infarction. **Moisturizing** is important to prevent the alveoli from becoming desiccated. Finally, **filtering** large particles is important to prevent small airways from being clogged with debris that may also be toxic.

Warming, moisturizing, and filtering are all more efficient with nose breathing, rather than mouth breathing. The nose, including the nasal turbinates, has a huge surface area and a rich blood supply. Nasal hairs tend to filter out large particles (greater than approximately 15 μm in diameter). The turbulence set up by these hairs—as well as the highly irregular surface topography of the nasal passages—increases the likelihood that particles larger than approximately 10 μm in diameter will **impact** and embed themselves in the mucus that coats the nasal mucosa. Moreover, air inspired through the nose must make a right-angle turn as it heads toward the trachea. The inertia of larger particles causes them to strike the posterior wall of the nasopharynx, which coincidentally is endowed with large amounts of lymphatic tissue that can mount an immunologic attack on inspired microbes. Of the larger particles that manage to escape filtration in the upper airways, almost all will impact on the mucus of the trachea and the bronchi.

Smaller particles (2–10 μm in diameter) also may impact a mucus layer. In addition, gravity may cause them to **sediment** from the slowly moving air in small airways and embed themselves in mucus. Particles with diameters below approximately 0.5 μm tend to reach the alveoli suspended in the air as **aerosols**. The airways do not trap most (approximately 80%) of these aerosols, but expel them in the exhaled air.

The lung has a variety of strategies for dealing with particles that remain on the surface of the alveoli or penetrate into the interstitial space. Alveolar macrophages (on the surface) or interstitial macrophages may phagocytize these particles, enzymes may degrade them, or lymphatics may carry them away. In addition, particles suspended in the fluid covering the alveolar surface may flow with this fluid up to terminal bronchioles, where they meet a layer of mucus that the cilia propel up to progressively larger airways. There, they join larger particles—which entered the mucus by impacting or sedimenting—on their journey to the oropharynx. Coughing and sneezing (see Box on p. 732), reflexes triggered by airway irritation, accelerate the movement of particulates up the conducting airways and out of the body.

LEFT-VENTRICULAR RESERVOIR. The highly compliant pulmonary vessels of the typical 70-kg human contain approximately 500 ml of blood (see Table 18–2), which is an important buffer for filling the left ventricle. For example, even if—under experimental conditions—one clamps the pulmonary artery of an experimental animal,

TABLE 25–3

HANDLING OF AGENTS BY THE PULMONARY CIRCULATION

UNAFFECTED	LARGELY REMOVED
PGA_1, PGA_2, PGI_2	PGE_1, PGE_2, $PGF_{2\alpha}$, leukotrienes
Histamine, epinephrine, dopamine	Serotonin
	Bradykinin
Angiotensin II, arginine vasopressin, gastrin, oxytocin	Angiotensin I (converted to angiotensin II)

From Levitzky MG: Pulmonary Physiology, 4th ed. New York, McGraw-Hill, 1999.

so that no blood may enter the lungs, the left heart can suck enough blood from the pulmonary circulation to sustain cardiac output for about two beats.

FILTERING SMALL EMBOLI FROM THE BLOOD. The mixed-venous blood contains microscopic emboli, small particles (e.g., blood clots, fat, air bubbles) capable of occluding a blood vessel. If these emboli were to reach the systemic circulation and lodge in small vessels that feed tissues with no collateral circulation, the consequences—over time—could be catastrophic. Fortunately, the pulmonary vasculature can trap these emboli before they have a chance to reach the left heart. If the emboli are sufficiently few and small, the affected alveoli can recover their function. Keep in mind that alveolar cells do not need the circulation to provide them with O_2 or remove their CO_2. In addition, after a small pulmonary embolism, alveolar cells may obtain nutrients from anas-

tomoses with the bronchial circulation. However, if pulmonary emboli are sufficiently large or frequent, they can cause serious symptoms or even death. A liability of the blood-filtration function is that emboli made up of cancer cells may find the perfect breeding ground for supporting metastatic disease.

BIOCHEMICAL REACTIONS. The entire cardiac output passes through the lungs, exposing the blood to the tremendous surface area of the pulmonary capillary endothelium. It is apparently these cells that are responsible for executing biochemical reactions that selectively remove many agents from the circulation, while leaving others unaffected (Table 25–3). Thus, the lung can be instrumental in determining which signalling molecules in the mixed-venous blood reach the systemic arterial blood. The pulmonary endothelium also plays an important role in converting angiotensin I (a decapeptide) to angiotensin II (an octapeptide), a reaction that is catalyzed by angiotensin converting enzyme (ACE) (p. 866).

REFERENCES

Bouhuys A: The Physiology of Breathing. New York, Grune & Stratton, 1977.

Kellog RH: Laws of physics pertaining to gas exchange. In Handbook of Physiology, Section 3: The Respiratory System, Vol IV. Bethesda, MD, American Physiological Society, 1985, pp. 13–31.

Macklem PT: Symbols and abbreviations. In Handbook of Physiology, Section 3: The Respiratory System, Vol I. Bethesda, MD, American Physiological Society, 1985, p. ix.

Mason RJ, Williams MC: Alveolar type II cells. In Crystal RG, West JB: The Lung. New York, Raven, 1991, pp. 235–246.

Satir P, Sleigh MA: The physiology of cilia and mucociliary interactions. Annu Rev Physiol 52:137–155, 1990.

Schneeberger EE: Alveolar type I cells. In Crystal RG, West JB: The Lung. New York, Raven, 1991, pp. 229–234.

Weibel ER: Lung cell biology. In Handbook of Physiology, Section 3: The Respiratory System, Vol I. Bethesda, MD, American Physiological Society, 1985, pp. 47–91.

CHAPTER 26

Mechanics of Respiration

Walter F. Boron

LUNG VOLUMES AND CAPACITIES

The Spirometer Is a Tool for Measuring All Lung Volumes Except Residual Volume

The maximal volume of all the airways in an adult is typically 5 to 6 liters. This volume includes those of the nasopharynx, the trachea, and all airways down to the alveolar sacs. Respiratory physiologists have defined a series of lung "volumes" and "capacities" that, although not corresponding to a particular anatomic locus, are relatively easy to measure with simple laboratory instruments and that convey useful information for clinical assessment.

A **spirometer** measures the volume of air inspired and expired, and, therefore, the change in lung volume. Spirometers today are complex computers, many so small that they can easily be held in the palm of one hand. The subject blows against a predetermined resistance, and all the calculations and interpretations are done electronically. Nevertheless, the principles of spirometric analysis are very much the same as those for the "old-fashioned" spirometer shown in Figure 26–1A, which is far easier to conceptualize. This simple spirometer has a movable, inverted bell that is partially submerged in water. An air tube extends from the subject's mouth, through the water, and emerges in the bell, just above the water level. Thus, when the subject exhales, air enters the bell and lifts it. The change in bell elevation, which we can record on moving paper, is proportional to the volume of air that the subject exhales. Because air in the lungs is saturated with water vapor at 37°C (body temperature and pressure, saturated with water vapor [BTPS]), and the air in the spirometer is ambient temperature and pressure, saturated with water vapor (ATPS), we must apply a temperature correction to the spirometer reading (see the box, Conventions for Measuring Volumes of Gases, p. 597).

The amount of air entering and leaving the lungs with each breath is the **tidal volume** (V_T). During quiet respirations, the V_T is approximately 500 ml. The initial portion of the spirograph of Figure 26–1B illustrates changes in lung volume during quiet breathing. The product of tidal volume and the frequency of breaths is **total ventilation**, given in liters (BTPS) per minute.

Because, with a typical Western diet, metabolism consumes more O_2 (~250 ml/min) than it produces CO_2 (~200 ml/min; p. 1223), the volume of air entering the lungs with each breath is slightly greater (~1%) than the volume leaving. In reporting changes in lung volume, respiratory physiolo-

A   SIMPLE SPIROMETER

B   SPIROGRAPHIC RECORD

FIGURE 26–1. The workings of a simple spirometer.

Volume and Capacities	Typical ranges (liters)
IRV = Inspiratory reserve volume	1.9–2.5
TV = Tidal volume	0.4–0.5
ERV = Expiratory reserve volume	1.1–1.5
RV = Residual volume	1.5–1.9
TLC = Total lung capacity	4.9–6.4
IC = Inspiratory capacity	2.3–3.0
FRC = Functional residual capacity	2.6–3.4
VC = Vital capacity	3.4–4.5

gists have chosen to measure the volume leaving—the **expired lung volume** (V_E).

At the end of a quiet inspiration, the additional volume of air that the subject *could* inhale with a maximal effort is known as the **inspiratory reserve volume** (IRV). The magnitude of IRV depends on several factors, including:

1. **Current lung volume.** The greater the lung volume after inspiration, the smaller the IRV.
2. **Lung compliance.** A decrease in compliance, a measure of how easy it is to inflate the lungs, will cause IRV to fall as well.
3. **Muscle strength.** If the respiratory muscles are weak, or if their innervation is compromised, IRV will decrease.
4. **Comfort.** Pain associated with injury or disease limits the desire or ability to make a maximal inspiratory effort.
5. **Flexibility of skeleton.** Joint stiffness, caused by diseases such as arthritis and kyphoscoliosis (i.e., curvature of the spine), reduces the maximal volume to which one can inflate the lungs.
6. **Posture.** IRV falls when a subject is in a recumbent position, because it is more difficult for the diaphragm to move the abdominal contents.

After a quiet expiration, the additional volume of air that one can expire with a maximal effort is the **expiratory reserve volume** (ERV). The magnitude of the ERV depends on the same factors listed earlier and on the strength of abdominal and other muscles needed to produce a maximal expiratory effort.

Even after a maximal expiratory effort, a considerable amount of air remains inside the lungs. This amount of air is called the **residual volume** (RV). Because a spirometer can measure only the air entering or leaving the lungs, it obviously is of no use in ascertaining the RV. However, we will see that other methods are available for measuring RV. It might seem inefficient for the lungs to contain air that they cannot exhale. Would it not be better for the lungs to exhale all their air and collapse completely during each expiration? There are two reasons why total collapse would be detrimental. (1) After an airway collapses, it takes an unusually high pressure to inflate it. A modest RV minimizes airway collapse, thereby optimizing the efficiency of ventilation. (2) Blood flow to the lungs and other parts of the body is continuous, even though ventilation is episodic. Thus, even after a maximal expiratory effort, it is beneficial to have a considerable volume of air in the lungs to allow a continuous exchange of gases between mixed-venous blood and alveolar air. If the RV were extremely low, then the composition of blood leaving the lungs would oscillate between a high P_{O_2} at the peak of inspiration, and a low P_{O_2} at the nadir of expiration.

The four primary **volumes** that we have defined—V_T, IRV, ERV, and RV—do not overlap (see Fig. 26–1*B*). Various lung "capacities" are various combinations of these four primary "volumes."

Total lung capacity (TLC) is the sum of all four volumes.

Functional residual capacity (FRC) is the sum of ERV and RV, and is the amount of air remaining inside the respiratory system after a quiet expiration. Because FRC includes RV, we cannot measure it using only a spirometer.

Inspiratory capacity (IC) is the sum of IRV and TV. After a quiet expiration, the IC is the maximal amount of air that one could still inspire.

Vital capacity (VC) is the sum of IRV, TV, and ERV. In other words, VC is the maximal achievable tidal volume and depends on the same factors discussed earlier for IRV and ERV. In patients with pulmonary disease, the physician may periodically monitor VC to follow the progress of the disease.

At the end of the spirographic record in Figure 26–1*B*, the subject made a maximal inspiratory effort and then exhaled as rapidly and completely as possible. The volume of air exhaled in one second under these conditions is the **forced-expiratory volume in one second** (FEV$_1$). In healthy young adults, FEV$_1$ is about 80% of VC. FEV$_1$ depends on all the factors that affect VC, as well as airway resistance. Thus, FEV$_1$ is an extremely important measurement that the physician can use to assess the progression of a variety of pulmonary disorders.

The Volume of Distribution of Helium or Nitrogen in the Lung Is an Estimate of the Residual Volume

As noted earlier, we cannot use a spirometer to measure residual volume, or any "capacity" containing RV (i.e., FRC or TLC). Fortunately, we have at our disposal two general approaches for measuring RV, both based on the **law of conservation of mass**. In the first approach, we compute RV from the volume of distribution of either helium (He) or nitrogen (N_2). However, any other non-toxic gas would do, as long as it does not cross the blood-gas barrier too rapidly. In the second approach, discussed in the next section, we compute RV using Boyle's Law.

The principle underlying the **volume-of-distribution** approach is that the concentration of a substance is the ratio of mass (moles) to volume (liters). If the mass is constant, and if we can measure the mass and concentration, then we can calculate the volume of the physiological compartment in which the mass is distributed. In our case, we ask the subject to breathe a gas that cannot escape from the airways. From the experimentally determined mass and concentration of that gas, we calculate lung volume.

HELIUM-DILUTION TECHNIQUE. We begin with a spirometer containing air with 10% He—this is the *initial* helium concentration, [He]$_{initial}$ = 10% (Fig. 26–2*A*). We use helium because it is poorly soluble in water, and, therefore, diffuses very poorly across the alveolar wall (p. 671). The initial spirometer volume in this example, including all air up to the valve at the subject's mouth, is 2 liters (the initial spirometer volume, $V_{S(initial)}$). The amount of He in the spirometer system at the outset of our experiment is [He]$_{initial} \cdot V_{S(initial)}$, or (10%) $\cdot$ (2 liters) = 0.2 liters.

We now open the valve at the mouth and allow the subject to breathe spirometer air until the He distributes evenly throughout the spirometer and airways. After equilibration, the *final* helium concentration ([He]$_{final}$) is the same in the airways as it is in the spirometer. The volume of the system, which is the spirometer volume (V_S) plus lung volume (V_L), is fixed from the instant that we open the valve between the spirometer and the mouth. When the subject inhales, V_L increases and V_S decreases by equal amounts. When the subject exhales, V_L decreases and V_S increases, but the volume of the system ($V_L + V_S$) remains unchanged. Because the system does not lose He, the total He content after equilibration must be the same as it was at the outset. In our example, let us assume that [He]$_{final}$ is 5%.

If the spirometer volume at the end of the experiment is the same as at the beginning,

$$[He]_{initial} \cdot V_S = [He]_{final} \cdot (V_S + V_L)$$

$$\text{Equation 26–1}$$

Solving for lung volume,

$$V_L = V_S \cdot \left(\frac{[He]_{initial}}{[He]_{final}} - 1 \right)$$

$$\text{Equation 26–2}$$

If we now insert the values from our experiment:

$$V_L = 2 \text{ liters} \cdot \left(\frac{10\%}{5\%} - 1 \right) = 2 \text{ liters}$$

V_L corresponds to the lung volume at the instant we open the mouth valve and allow the He to begin equilibrating. If we wish to measure FRC, we open the valve just after the subject has completed a *quiet* expiration. If the subject has just completed a maximal expiration, then the computed V_L is RV. Because the subject re-breathes the air mixture underneath the spirometer bell until [He] stabilizes, the helium-dilution approach is a **closed-circuit** method.

NITROGEN-WASHOUT METHOD. Imagine that you wanted to rinse a soapy solution out of a glass. Add hot water, swish it around inside the glass, and dump the now soapy water into a graduated cylinder. After repeating this exercise several times, you see that virtually all the soap is now in the graduated cylinder. If you want to know how much soap had been in the glass, simply multiply the volume of soapy water in the graduated cylinder by the concentration of soap in that water. This is the principle behind the nitrogen-washout method.

FIGURE 26–2. Volume-of-distribution and plethysmographic methods for measuring lung volume. In *C*, the spirometer is usually replaced in modern plethysmographs by an electronic pressure gauge. In such instruments, the change in lung volume is computed from the change in pressure inside the plethysmograph (see Fig. 26–11).

Assume that the initial lung volume is V_L, and that the initial concentration of nitrogen gas in the lungs is $[N_2]_{initial}$. Thus, the amount of N_2 in the lungs at the outset is $V_L \cdot [N_2]_{initial}$. We now ask the subject to breathe through a mouthpiece equipped with a special valve (see Fig. 26–2B). During inspiration, the air comes from a reservoir of 100% O_2; the key point is that this inspired air contains no N_2. During expiration, the exhaled air goes to a sack with an initial volume of zero. Each inspiration of 100% O_2 dilutes the N_2 in the lungs. Each expiration sends a fraction of the remaining N_2 into the sack. Thus, the $[N_2]$ in the lungs falls stepwise with each breath until eventually the subject has washed out into the sack virtually all the N_2 that had initially been in the lungs. Also entering the sack are some of the inspired O_2 and all expired CO_2. The standard period for washing out the N_2 with normal breathing is 7 min, after which the sack has a volume of V_{sack} and an N_2 concentration of $[N_2]_{sack}$. Because the amount of N_2 now in the sack is the same as that previously in the lungs:

Equation 26–3
$$[N_2]_{initial} \cdot V_L = [N_2]_{sack} \cdot V_{sack}$$

Thus, the lung volume is:

Equation 26–4
$$V_L = V_{sack} \cdot \frac{[N_2]_{sack}}{[N_2]_{initial}}$$

As an illustration of how to use Equation 26–4, consider an instance in which $[N_2]_{initial}$ is 80%. If the volume of gas washed into the sack is 40 liters, roughly a total ventilation of 6 liters/min for 7 minutes, and $[N_2]_{sack}$ is 4%, then:

Equation 26–5
$$V_L = 40 \text{ liters} \cdot \frac{4\%}{80\%} = 2 \text{ liters}$$

What particular lung volume or capacity does V_L represent? The computed V_L is the lung volume at the instant the subject begins to inhale the 100% O_2. Therefore, if the subject had just finished a quiet expiration before beginning to inhale the O_2, V_L would be FRC, whereas if the subject had just finished a maximal expiratory effort, V_L would represent RV.

The key element in the nitrogen-washout method is the requirement that, during the period of O_2 breathing, all N_2 previously in the lungs—and no more—ends up in the sack. In other words, we assume that there is no substantial diffusion of N_2 from blood into alveolar air during our 7-minute experiment. Because N_2 has a low solubility, and, therefore, the amount dissolved in body fluids is very low at normal barometric pressure, the rate of N_2 diffusion across the alveolar wall is very low (p. 671). Therefore, our assumption about minimal N_2 addition is very nearly correct. In principle, we could preload the lung with any non-toxic, water-insoluble gas (e.g., helium), and then wash it out with any different gas (e.g., room air). Because, in the nitrogen-washout method, the subject inhales from one reservoir and exhales into another, the method is an **open-system** technique.

The Residual Volume Can Also Be Estimated Using a Plethysmograph, Together with Boyle's Law

We also can compute V_L from small *changes* in lung pressure and volume that occur as a subject attempts to inspire through an obstructed airway. This approach is based on **Boyle's Law**, which states that, if the temperature and number of gas molecules are constant, the product of pressure and volume is a constant:

Equation 26–6
$$P \cdot V_L = \text{Constant}$$

To take advantage of this relationship, we have the subject step inside an airtight box called a **plethysmograph** (from the Greek "plethein," to be full), which is similar to a telephone booth. The subject breathes through a tube that is connected to the outside world (see Fig. 26–2C). Connected to this tube is a gauge that registers pressure at the mouth, and an electronically controlled shutter that can, on command, completely obstruct the tube. For the Mead-type plethysmograph in Figure 26–2C, the plethysmograph is attached to a spirometer. As the subject inhales, lung volume and the volume of the subject's body increase by the same amount, displacing an equal volume of air from the plethysmograph into the spirometer, which registers the increase in lung volume (ΔV_L).

As the experiment starts, the shutter is open, and the subject quietly exhales, so that V_L is FRC. Because no air is flowing at the end of the expiration, the alveoli and the mouth are both at barometric pressure, which is registered by the pressure gauge (P). We now close the shutter, and the subject makes a small inspiratory effort, typically only approximately 50 ml, against the closed inlet tube. The subject's inspiratory effort will cause lung volume to increase to a new value, $V_L + \Delta V_L$. However, the number of gas molecules in the airways is unchanged, so this *increase* in volume must be accompanied by a *decrease* in airway pressure (ΔP) to a new value, $P - \Delta P$. Because no air is flowing at the peak of this inspiratory effort, the pressure measured by the gauge at the mouth is once again the same as the alveolar pressure. According to Boyle's Law:

Equation 26–7
$$\underbrace{P \cdot V_L}_{\substack{\text{Initial} \\ \text{PV} \\ \text{product}}} = \underbrace{(P - \Delta P) \cdot (V_L + \Delta V_L)}_{\substack{\text{PV product} \\ \text{at peak of} \\ \text{inspiratory effort}}}$$

Rearranging Equation 26–7 yields the initial lung volume:

Equation 26–8
$$V_L = \Delta V_L \cdot \frac{P - \Delta P}{\Delta P}$$

As an example, assume that ΔV_L at the peak of the inspiratory effort is 50 ml, and that the corresponding

A ELASTIC RECOIL OF LUNGS

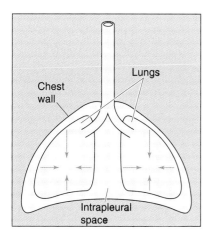

B ELASTIC RECOIL OF CHEST WALL

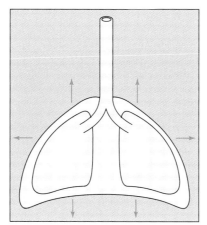

C ELASTIC RECOILS OF LUNGS AND CHEST WALL IN BALANCE

D INTRAPLEURAL PRESSURES

FIGURE 26–3. Opposing elastic recoils of the lungs and chest wall.

pressure decrease in the airways is 12 mm Hg. If the initial pressure (P) was 760 mm Hg,

$$\text{Equation 26–9}$$

$$V_L = 0.050 \text{ liter} \cdot \frac{(760 - 12) \text{ mm Hg}}{12 \text{ mm Hg}} = 3.1 \text{ liters}$$

What particular lung volume or capacity does the 3.1 liters represent? Because, in our example, the inspiratory effort against the closed shutter began after a quiet expiratory effort, the computed V_L is FRC. If it had begun after a maximal expiration, the measured V_L would be RV.

STATIC PROPERTIES OF THE LUNG

The field of **pulmonary mechanics**—the physics of the lungs, airways, and chest wall—deals with how the body moves air in and out of the lungs, producing a *change* in lung volume. When we examine these mechanical properties while no air is flowing, we are studying **static** properties. The situation becomes more complicated under

dynamic conditions, when the lungs are changing volume, and air is flowing either in or out.

The Balance Between the Outward Elastic Recoil of the Chest Wall and the Inward Elastic Recoil of the Lungs Generates a Subatmospheric Intrapleural Pressure

The interaction between the lungs and the thoracic cage determines lung volume. Within the intact thoracic cage, the lungs have a tendency to collapse, which is known as **elastic recoil**. Figure 26–3A depicts lungs at FRC. *Arrows* that pull the lung inward represent elastic recoil. Forces acting in the opposite direction must precisely balance this elastic recoil to prevent lung collapse.

The chest wall has an elastic recoil that is exactly the opposite that of the lungs, tending to pull the thoracic cage outward (see Fig. 26–3B). Thus, the chest cavity can maintain its normal volume only if an equal but opposite force pulls the chest wall inward. The stage is set here for an interaction between the lungs and the chest wall: At equilibrium, the inward elastic recoil of the lungs exactly balances the outward elastic recoil of the chest wall (see

Fig. 26–3C). This interaction between lungs and chest wall does not occur by direct attachment, but via the space between the two, the intrapleural space. Because the lungs and chest wall pull away from each other on opposite sides of the intrapleural space, the pressure inside this space—**intrapleural pressure** (P_{IP})—is less than barometric pressure (P_B); that is, the intrapleural space is a *relative vacuum*. Although we named P_{IP} as if it referred to the intrapleural space, this description is not entirely accurate. Strictly speaking, the **intrapleural space** is the virtual space between the visceral and parietal pleural membranes, a space that usually contains only a thin layer of fluid that may act as a lubricant, allowing the pleural layers to slide past one another as the lungs change volume. However, P_{IP} reflects the pressure in several other regions of the chest cavity:

1. The virtual space between the chest wall or diaphragm and the parietal pleura.
2. The virtual space between the lung and the visceral pleura.
3. The interstitial space surrounding the airways in the lungs.
4. Around the heart and great vessels.
5. Around and inside the esophagus (while it is *not* engaged in peristalsis).

It is helpful to think of P_{IP} as the "intrathoracic pressure"—the pressure everywhere in the thorax except in the lumens of blood vessels, lymphatics, or airways. We could measure P_{IP} by inserting a needle between the parietal and the visceral pleural membranes. However, in practice it is easier and safer to insert a balloon catheter through the mouth and into the esophagus, and use the balloon to measure the intraesophageal pressure.

The vacuum is not uniform throughout the intrapleural space. When the subject is upright, the vacuum is greatest (i.e., P_{IP} is least) near the apex of the lungs, and progressively falls to its lowest value near the bases of the lungs (see Fig. 26–3D). Assuming that P_B is 760 mm Hg and that the subject has finished a quiet expiration, we expect P_{IP} to be approximately 753 mm Hg near the apices of the lungs, and approximately 758 mm Hg near the bases. Thus, P_{IP} is subatmospheric throughout the chest cavity. Because respiratory physiologists historically measured these small pressures with water manometers rather than with less sensitive mercury manometers, it has become customary to express P_{IP} in *cm of H_2O* relative to the barometric pressure. If we define P_B as 0 cm H_2O, then P_{IP} is −10 cm H_2O at the apex and −2.5 cm H_2O at the base of the lungs.

The reasons for the apex-to-base P_{IP} gradient are **gravity** and **posture**. When an individual stands vertically on the surface of the earth, gravity acts on the lungs, pulling them downward and away from the apex of the thoracic cage. This force creates a larger vacuum (i.e., a lower P_{IP}) at the apex. Gravity also tends to push the bases of the lungs into the thoracic cavity, minimizing the vacuum there. For a subject standing on his/her head, these relationships are inverted. Lying on one's side creates a P_{IP} gradient in the transverse direction. In this last instance, the magnitude of the P_{IP} gradient would be much smaller because the transverse dimension of the thorax (and, therefore, the hydrostatic pressure gradient) is smaller than the rostral-caudal dimension. In outer space, there would be no P_{IP} gradient at all. Thus, the local P_{IP} depends on the position within the gravitational field.

For most of the remainder of this chapter, we make the simplifying assumption that P_{IP} is uniform throughout the thorax, with a value of −5 cm H_2O after a quiet expiration.

Contracting the Diaphragm and External Intercostal Muscles Increases the Volume of the Thorax, Producing an Inspiration

We have seen that the opposing elastic recoils of the lungs and chest wall create a negative P_{IP} that keeps the lungs expanded. Any change in the balance between these elastic recoils will cause lung volume to change as well. For example, if the elastic recoil of the lungs increased (as occurs in patients with **pulmonary fibrosis**), P_{IP} would no longer be negative enough to keep the lungs inflated to their normal level, and they would become smaller. As the lungs shrunk, P_{IP} would become more negative, causing chest volume to decrease. In the new equilibrium, the lungs and thorax would be smaller, and P_{IP} would be more negative. Under normal circumstances, the key elastic recoil is the one *we* control: the elastic recoil of the chest wall, which we change moment to moment by modulating the tension of the muscles of respiration.

The **muscles of inspiration** expand the chest, increasing the elastic recoil of the chest wall and making P_{IP} more negative. Responding to this enhanced intrapleural vacuum, the lungs passively expand. The increase in V_L is virtually the same as the increase in the volume of the thoracic cavity. The two muscle groups that produce a quiet inspiration are called the **primary muscles of inspiration**, and include the diaphragm and the many external intercostal muscles.

The most important component of the increase in chest volume is the rise in the chest cavity's rostral-caudal diameter, a result of the action of the **diaphragm**. Stimulated by the phrenic nerves (derived from cervical roots C3–C5), the diaphragm contracts and moves downward toward the abdomen, approximately 1 cm during quiet ventilation.

The **external intercostal muscles** are innervated by segmental spinal nerves and span the space between adjacent ribs. Their contraction has two consequences (Fig. 26–4). First, the rib cage and the tissues between the ribs stiffen and are therefore better able to withstand the increasingly negative P_{IP}. Second, the chest cavity's transverse and anterior-posterior (A-P) diameters increase. The increase in transverse diameter ("bucket-handle effect") occurs as the external intercostal muscles cause ribs 2 through 10 to rotate upward and outward. The increase in A-P diameter ("water-pump–handle effect") occurs as the upper ribs rotate the sternum upward and outward.

During a **forced** inspiration, the **accessory** (or **secondary**) **muscles** of inspiration also come into play:

1. **Scalenes.** These muscles lift the first two ribs.
2. **Sternocleidomastoids.** These muscles lift the sternum outward, contributing to the water-pump–handle effect.

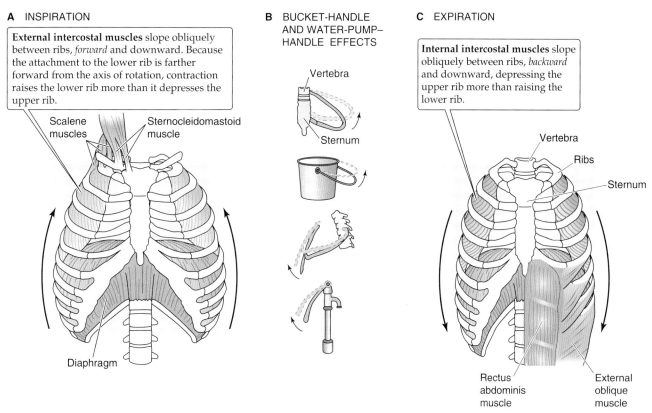

A INSPIRATION

External intercostal muscles slope obliquely between ribs, *forward* and downward. Because the attachment to the lower rib is farther forward from the axis of rotation, contraction raises the lower rib more than it depresses the upper rib.

Scalene muscles

Sternocleidomastoid muscle

Diaphragm

B BUCKET-HANDLE AND WATER-PUMP–HANDLE EFFECTS

Vertebra

Sternum

C EXPIRATION

Internal intercostal muscles slope obliquely between ribs, *backward* and downward, depressing the upper rib more than raising the lower rib.

Vertebra

Ribs

Sternum

Rectus abdominis muscle

External oblique muscle

FIGURE 26–4. Actions of major respiratory muscles.

3. **Neck and back muscles**. These elevate the pectoral girdle (increasing the cross-sectional area of the thorax) and extend the back (increasing the rostral-caudal length).
4. **Upper-respiratory-tract muscles.** The actions of these muscles decrease airway resistance.

Relaxing the Muscles of Inspiration Produces a Quiet Expiration

During a quiet inspiration, normal lungs and airways store enough energy in their elastic recoil to fuel a quiet expiration, just as stretching a rubber band stores enough energy to fuel the return to initial length. Thus, a quiet expiration is normally passive, accomplished simply by relaxing the muscles of inspiration. A corollary to this rule is that *there are no primary muscles of expiration.*

There are two major exceptions to the rule that expiration is entirely passive. The first is a forced expiration in individuals with normal airway resistance. The second is even a quiet expiration of a person with a disease that increases airway resistance (e.g., asthma, chronic bronchitis, emphysema). In either case, the **accessory muscles of expiration** help to make P_{IP} more positive:

1. **Abdominal muscles** (internal and external oblique, rectoabdominal and transverse abdominal muscles). Contracting these muscles increases intra-abdominal pressure and forces the diaphragm upward into the chest cavity, decreasing the rostral-caudal diameter of the thorax and increasing P_{IP}.

2. **Internal intercostals.** The action of these muscles opposes that of the external intercostals, reducing both the A-P and the transverse diameters of the thorax. The internal intercostals are particularly important for coughing.
3. **Neck and back muscles.** Lowering the pectoral girdle reduces the cross-sectional area of the thorax, whereas flexing the trunk reduces the rostral-caudal diameter.

During a forced *inspiration*, the accessory muscles of inspiration use their energy mainly to increase V_L (rather than to overcome resistance to airflow); the lungs store this extra energy in their elastic recoil. During a forced *expiration*, the accessory muscles of expiration use their energy mainly to overcome the resistance to airflow, as discussed later.

Increasing the Static Compliance Makes It Easier to Inflate the Lungs

Imagine that a person suffers a puncture wound to the chest cavity, so that air enters the thorax from the atmosphere, raising P_{IP} to the same level as P_B. This condition is called a **pneumothorax** (from the Greek "pneuma," for "air"). With no vacuum to counter their elastic recoil, alveoli will collapse—a condition known as **atelectasis.** The *upper part* of Figure 26–5A illustrates an extreme, hypothetical case in which pressure is atmospheric throughout the thorax. Even though the lungs are collapsed, lung volume is not zero. The **minimal air volume** is approximately 10% of TLC (~500 ml). The reason air

A PNEUMOTHORAX AND LUNG RE-INFLATION

B STATIC PRESSURE-VOLUME DIAGRAM

FIGURE 26–5. Collapse and re-inflation of the lungs. In *A*, we assume that intrapleural pressure (P_{IP}) rises to barometric pressure (P_B), so that transpulmonary pressure (P_{TP}) falls to zero, collapsing the lungs.

remains inside the lungs even though the P_{IP} is zero is that some larger, proximal airways collapse before smaller ones farther downstream, trapping air.

We now wish to re-expand the collapsed lungs to their original volume (i.e., FRC). What are the forces at work during such a re-expansion? The force responsible for distending an airway is the **transmural pressure** (P_{TM})—the *radial* pressure difference across an airway wall at any point along the tracheobronchial tree:

Equation 26–10

$$P_{TM} = P_{AW} - P_{IP}$$

P_{AW} is the pressure inside the airway (relative to P_B), and P_{IP} is the pressure in the interstitial space surrounding the airway. A special case of P_{TM} is the transmural pressure across the *alveolar* wall, which has a special name—**trans*pulmonary* pressure** (P_{TP}):

Equation 26–11

$$P_{TP} = P_A - P_{IP}$$

P_A is **alveolar pressure**. When the glottis is open and no air is flowing, the lungs are under **static conditions**, and P_A must be 0 cm H_2O:

Equation 26–12

Static conditions: $\quad P_{TP} = 0 - P_{IP} = -P_{IP}$
(glottis open)

In other words, with the glottis open under static conditions, the inflating pressure (P_{TP}) is simply the negative of P_{IP}.

It is important to recognize that we can re-expand the lungs to FRC by any combination of an increase in P_A and a decrease in P_{IP}, as long as P_{TP} ends up at 5 cm H_2O (see Fig. 26–5A, *lower part*). Increasing P_A from 0 to +5 cm H_2O, with P_{IP} fixed at zero, is one way to increase P_{TP}. Decreasing the P_{IP} from 0 to −5 cm H_2O, with P_A fixed at 0, is another.

In an emergency room, a clinician would treat the pneumothorax by inserting a chest tube into the thoracic cavity and gradually pumping out the air as the patient breathes. As P_{IP} becomes more negative, the lung would re-expand. For the sake of illustrating the elastic properties of the lungs, we will do four things that would not be practical for a real patient. First, we will evacuate the air from the chest cavity while the patient is not attempting to breathe. Second, we will use a spirometer to monitor the increase in V_L. Third, we will insert an esophageal balloon to monitor P_{IP}. Fourth, we will evacuate air from the chest cavity in small, discrete steps. Each time the P_{IP} becomes more negative by 1 cm H_2O, we will temporarily stop evacuating the air and record the steady values of V_L and P_{IP}. This stepwise evacuation ensures that we make our measurements under *static conditions*. As a final precaution, we will ensure that the glottis is open, so that the pathway from the atmosphere to the alveoli is uninterrupted. With the glottis open and no airflow, we can be sure that P_A will be 0 during our measurements.

During the stepwise decrease, we can divide the effect on V_L into four stages, starting at the *left end of the lower blue curve* in Figure 26–5B:

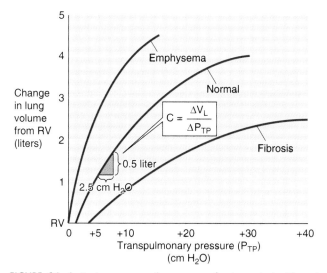

FIGURE 26–6. Static pressure-volume curves for lungs in health and disease.

Stage 1: Stable V$_L$. In the lowest range of P$_{IP}$ values, making P$_{IP}$ more negative has little or no effect on V$_L$. Therefore, if we decrease P$_{IP}$ from 0 to −1 cm H$_2$O (i.e., increase P$_{TP}$ from 0 to +1 cm H$_2$O) and then stop, we record no change in V$_L$. Why? As discussed later, it is very difficult—because of the surface tension created by the air-water interface—to pop open an airway that is almost completely collapsed. Until P$_{TP}$ is large enough to overcome the collapsing effects of surface tension, a decrease in P$_{IP}$ has no effect on V$_L$.

Stage 2: Opening of airways. Stepwise decreases in P$_{IP}$ beyond about −8 cm H$_2$O produce V$_L$ increases that are at first small, and then larger. The first increases in V$_L$ reflect the popping open of the proximal airways with the greatest compliance. Additional increases in V$_L$ reflect the expansion of already-open airways, as well as recruitment of others.

Stage 3: Linear expansion of open airways. When all the airways are already open, making P$_{IP}$ increasingly more negative inflates all airways further, causing V$_L$ to increase in a roughly linear fashion.

Stage 4: Limit of airway inflation. Increases in V$_L$ produced by stepwise decreases in P$_{IP}$ become smaller as V$_L$ approaches TLC. The reasons include decreased airway and chest-wall compliance, and the limits of muscle strength.

What would happen if, having inflated the lungs to TLC, we allowed P$_{IP}$ to increase to 0 cm H$_2$O once again? Obviously, the V$_L$ would decrease. However, the lungs follow a different path during deflation (see Fig. 26–5B, upper blue curve). The difference between the inflation and the deflation paths is known as **hysteresis**, and it exists because a greater pressure difference is required *to open* a previously closed airway than *to keep* an open airway from closing. As an example, the *horizontal line* in Figure 26–5B shows that *inflating* collapsed lungs to FRC requires a P$_{IP}$ of −12 cm H$_2$O, whereas *maintaining* previously inflated lungs at FRC requires a P$_{IP}$ of only −5 cm H$_2$O. During normal respiration, the lungs exhibit much less hysteresis, and the hysteresis loop (see Fig. 26–5B,

green loop) lies close to the deflation limb of the blue loop.

We will now focus on just the upper portion of the "deflation limb" of the blue loop in Figure 26–5B, which is the *middle curve* in Figure 26–6. The average P$_{TP}$ is approximately +5 cm H$_2$O when V$_L$ is at FRC. As the subject makes a normal inspiration with a V$_T$ of 500 ml, P$_{TP}$ increases (i.e., P$_{IP}$ decreases) by 2.5 cm H$_2$O. The ratio of ΔV_L to ΔP_{TP} (i.e., the slope of the P$_{TP}$-V$_L$ curve) is the compliance, and is a measure of the distensibility of the lungs. In our example,

Equation 26–13

$$C = \frac{\Delta V_L}{\Delta P_{TP}} = \frac{0.5 \text{ liter}}{(7.5 - 5.0) \text{ cm H}_2\text{O}} = 0.2 \frac{\text{liter}}{\text{cm H}_2\text{O}}$$

Because we made this measurement under conditions of zero airflow, C is the **static compliance**. The elastance of the lungs, which is a measure of their *elastic recoil*, is the reciprocal of the compliance (E = 1/C). Lungs with a high compliance have a low elastic recoil, and vice versa.

Figure 26–6 also shows representative P$_{TP}$-V$_L$ relationships for lungs of patients with pulmonary fibrosis (*bottom curve*) and emphysema (*top curve*). In **pulmonary fibrosis**, the disease process causes the deposition of fibrous tissue, so that the lung is stiff and difficult to inflate. The same ΔP_{TP} that produces a 500-ml V$_L$ increase in normal lungs produces a substantially *smaller* V$_L$ increase in fibrotic lungs. In other words, static compliance ($\Delta V_L/\Delta P_{TP}$) is much less, or elastic recoil is much greater. As discussed later, static compliance is also low in respiratory distress syndrome (RDS) of the newborn.

In **emphysema**, the situation is reversed. The disease process, a common consequence of cigarette smoking, destroys pulmonary tissue and makes the lungs rather floppy. An important part of the disease process is the destruction of the extracellular matrix, including elastin, by elastase released from macrophages Normal mice that are exposed to cigarette smoke develop emphysema rapidly, whereas the disease does not develop in "smoker" mice lacking the macrophage elastase gene. The same increase in P$_{TP}$ that produces a 500-ml V$_L$ increase in normal lungs produces a substantially *larger* V$_L$ increase in lungs with emphysema. In other words, static compliance is much greater (i.e., much less elastic recoil).

Because it requires work to inflate the lungs against their elastic recoil, one might think that a little emphysema might be a good thing. Although it is true that patients with emphysema exert less effort to inflate their lungs, the cigarette smoker pays a terrible price for this small advantage: The destruction of pulmonary architecture also makes emphysematous airways more prone to collapse during expiration, drastically increasing airway resistance.

Two additional points are worth noting. First, compliance (i.e., slope of P$_{TP}$-V$_L$ curve) decreases as V$_L$ increases from FRC to TLC (Fig. 26–6). Second, the P$_{TP}$-V$_L$ curve is the amalgam of pressure-volume relationships of all alveoli. Different alveoli have different P$_{TP}$-V$_L$ curves and may experience different intrapleural pressures, depending on their position within a gravitational field (see Fig. 26–3D). This inhomogeneity of static parameters contributes

DISEASES AFFECTING VENTILATION

Several diseases can severely reduce total ventilation—that is, the amount of air entering and leaving the lungs per unit of time—by affecting the static properties of the pulmonary system. These fall into four major categories:

INADEQUATE MUSCLE CONTRACTION. The central nervous system may fail to stimulate the respiratory muscles adequately, or the muscles may fail to respond appropriately to stimulation. In **polio**, the virus occasionally attacks respiratory-control centers in the brainstem (p. 714). In **amyotrophic lateral sclerosis** (ALS or "Lou Gehrig's disease"), the disease process leads to the destruction of premotor and motor neurons, including those to the muscles of respiration (p. 712). Indeed, dyspnea on exertion is a common early symptom of ALS. Certain **drug overdoses** (e.g., barbiturate poisoning) may transiently inhibit respiratory-control centers in the brainstem. In the absence of supportive therapy (i.e., mechanical ventilation), the respiratory failure can be fatal. The **pain** that accompanies chest surgery or other injuries to the chest can also severely limit the ability to ventilate.

RIGIDITY OF CHEST WALL. Despite normal neuromuscular performance, chest-wall rigidity makes it difficult to increase thoracic volume. **Ankylosing spondylitis** is an inflammatory disorder of the axial skeleton that may reduce the bucket-handle rotation of the ribs during quiet inspirations, and the flexion and extension of the trunk during forced inspirations and expirations. In **kyphoscoliosis** (angulation and rotation of the spine), deformation of the vertebrae and ribs may reduce ventilation. In both conditions, impairment of coughing predisposes to lung infections.

FLACCIDITY OF CHEST WALL. Local paralysis of the external intercostal muscles allows the enhanced intrathoracic vacuum to suck in intercostal tissues during inspiration. This paradoxical movement reduces the efficiency of inspiration. Paradoxical movement may also occur with broken ribs, a condition also known as **flail chest.**

STIFFNESS OF LUNG PARENCHYMA. "Restrictive" lung diseases (e.g., **pulmonary fibrosis**) decrease lung compliance, and thus require more effort to overcome increased elastic recoil. Patients compensate by making rapid but shallow inspirations.

to regional differences in ventilation, which are discussed on p. 693.

Surface Tension at the Air-Water Interface of the Airways Accounts for Half or More of the Elastic Recoil of the Lungs

What is the basis of the elastic recoil that determines the static compliance of the lungs? The elasticity of pulmonary cells and the extracellular matrix (e.g., elastin and collagen), what we might think of as the "anatomic" component of elastic recoil, generally accounts for less than half. The basis of the other half of the recoil was suggested in 1929 by von Neergaard, who excised lungs from cats and inflated them by applying positive pressure to the trachea under two conditions. When he filled the lungs with air, the P_{TP}-V_L curve looked similar to the one we have seen before (Fig. 26–7A, *blue curve*). However, when von Neergaard degassed the airways and re-inflated them with a saline solution, he found that (1) the P_{TP}-V_L relationship (see Fig. 26–7A, *orange curve*) exhibited far less hysteresis and (2) the static compliance was substantially greater (i.e., much less pressure was required to inflate the lungs). These changes occurred because the saline-filled lungs lacked the air-water interface that generated surface tension in the air-filled lungs. It is this surface tension that is responsible for a large fraction of the lung's elastic recoil.

Surface tension is a measure of the force acting to pull a liquid's surface molecules together at an air-liquid interface. Figure 26–7B shows a cross section through a hypothetical air-water interface. Water molecules in the bulk liquid phase are equally attracted to surrounding water molecules in all directions, so that the net force acting on these "deep" water molecules is zero. However, water molecules at the surface are equally attracted to others in all directions but "up," where no molecules are available to pull surface water molecules toward the air phase. Thus, a net force pulls surface molecules away from the air-water interface toward the bulk water phase.

We can think of the surface water molecules and those diving into the bulk as beads connected by an elastic band. The force that pulls the diving molecule down into the bulk also creates a *tension* between the surface molecules in a direction that is *parallel* to the surface of the water. If we try to overcome this tension and stretch the air-water interface (see Fig. 26–7C), thus increasing its area, we must apply force (F) to bring water molecules from the bulk liquid (a low-energy state) to the surface (a high-energy state). If the body of water on which we tug has a length of ℓ, then the surface tension (T) is:

Equation 26–14

$$T = \frac{F}{\ell}$$

For a simple air-water interface at 37°C, the surface tension is approximately 70 dynes/cm.

Surface tension has important physical and physiological consequences. A drop of water falling through the air tends to form into a sphere because this shape has the smallest surface area, and thus the lowest energy. Put differently, when the drop is spherical, it is impossible for any additional water molecules to leave the surface.

In the reverse scenario, a spherical air bubble surrounded by water (see Fig. 26–7D), unbalanced forces acting on surface water molecules cause them to dive into the bulk, decreasing the surface area and creating tension in the plane of the air-water interface. This surface tension acts like a belt tightening around one's waist. It tends to decrease the volume of compressible gas inside the bubble and increases its pressure. At equilibrium, the tendency of increased pressure to expand the gas bubble balances the tendency of surface tension to collapse it. Laplace's equation describes this equilibrium:

Equation 26–15

$$P = \frac{2T}{r}$$

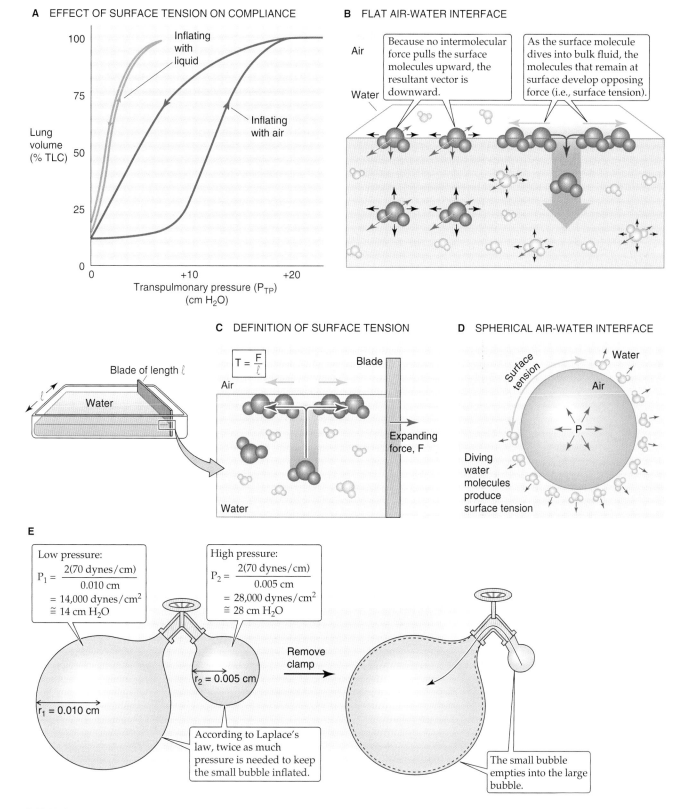

A EFFECT OF SURFACE TENSION ON COMPLIANCE

Inflating with liquid

Lung volume (% TLC)

Inflating with air

Transpulmonary pressure (P_{TP}) (cm H_2O)

B FLAT AIR-WATER INTERFACE

Air

Water

Because no intermolecular force pulls the surface molecules upward, the resultant vector is downward.

As the surface molecule dives into bulk fluid, the molecules that remain at surface develop opposing force (i.e., surface tension).

C DEFINITION OF SURFACE TENSION

Blade of length ℓ

Water

$T = \dfrac{F}{\ell}$

Air

Blade

Expanding force, F

Water

D SPHERICAL AIR-WATER INTERFACE

Surface tension

Water

Air

P

Diving water molecules produce surface tension

E

Low pressure:

$P_1 = \dfrac{2(70 \text{ dynes/cm})}{0.010 \text{ cm}}$

$= 14{,}000 \text{ dynes/cm}^2$

$\cong 14 \text{ cm } H_2O$

High pressure:

$P_2 = \dfrac{2(70 \text{ dynes/cm})}{0.005 \text{ cm}}$

$= 28{,}000 \text{ dynes/cm}^2$

$\cong 28 \text{ cm } H_2O$

$r_2 = 0.005$ cm

$r_1 = 0.010$ cm

Remove clamp

According to Laplace's law, twice as much pressure is needed to keep the small bubble inflated.

The small bubble empties into the large bubble.

FIGURE 26–7. Effect of surface tension on the lung. TLC, total lung capacity.

P is the *dependent* variable; the surface tension *T* is a *constant* for a particular interface, and the bubble radius *r* is the *independent* variable. Therefore, the smaller the bubble's radius, the greater the pressure needed to keep the bubble inflated. See p. 457 for a description of how Laplace's treatment applies to blood vessels.

Our bubble-in-water analysis is important for the lung because a thin layer of water covers the inner surface of the alveoli. Just as surface tension at the air-water interface of our gas bubble causes the bubble to constrict, it also causes alveoli and other airways to constrict, contributing greatly to elastic recoil.

The analogy between air bubbles and alveoli breaks down somewhat because an alveolus only approximates a part of a sphere. A second complicating factor is that not all alveoli are the same size; some may have a diameter that is three to four times larger than others. Third, alveoli are interconnected.

Figure 26–7E shows what would happen if two imaginary air bubbles in water were connected by a tube with a valve that allows us to make or break the connection between the bubbles. Imagine that the valve is initially closed. The first bubble has a radius of 0.010 cm. The second is only half as wide. For both, assume that the surface tension *T* is 70 dynes/cm. At equilibrium, the pressures required to keep the two bubbles inflated are:

Equation 26–16

$$P_1 = \frac{2T}{r} = \frac{2 \times 70 \text{ dynes/cm}}{0.010 \text{ cm}}$$

$$= 14,000 \frac{\text{dynes}}{\text{cm}^2} \cong 14 \text{ cm H}_2\text{O}$$

$$P_2 = \frac{2T}{r} = \frac{2 \times 70 \text{ dynes/cm}}{0.005 \text{ cm}}$$

$$= 28,000 \frac{\text{dynes}}{\text{cm}^2} \cong 28 \text{ cm H}_2\text{O}$$

The pressure inside the smaller bubble is twice that inside the larger bubble. If we now open the valve between the two bubbles, air will flow from the smaller bubble to the larger bubble. To make matters worse for the smaller bubble, the smaller it becomes, the greater is the pressure needed to stabilize its shrinking radius. Because its pressure is less than required, air continues to flow from the smaller to the larger bubble and the smaller bubble implodes completely.

In principle, the lung faces a similar problem. Smaller alveoli tend to collapse into larger alveoli. As we shall see, pulmonary surfactant minimizes this collapsing tendency by lowering surface tension. However, even without surfactant, the collapse of small alveoli could proceed to only so far, because each alveolus is tethered to adjacent alveoli, which help hold it open. This phenomenon is known as the **principle of interdependence**.

Why would it matter if many smaller alveoli collapsed into a few larger alveoli? Such a collapse would reduce the total alveolar surface area available for diffusion of O_2 and CO_2 (p. 671). Thus, from a teleologic point of view,

it is important for the lung to keep the alveoli as uniformly inflated as possible.

Pulmonary Surfactant Is a Mixture of Lipids—Mainly Dipalmitoylphosphatidylcholine—and Apoproteins

As noted earlier, surface tension accounts for more than half the elastic recoil in normal lungs. However, if it were not for the presence of pulmonary surfactant, total elastic recoil would be even higher, and the lungs would be far more difficult to inflate. During quiet breathing, surfactant reduces surface tension to approximately 25 dynes/cm or less, far below the value of 70 dynes/cm that exists at a pure air-water interface.

The term **surfactant** means a surface-active agent. Because surfactant has both a hydro*philic* region (strongly attracted to water) and a hydro*phobic* region (strongly repelled by water), it localizes to the surface of an air-water interface. An example of a synthetic surfactant is dishwashing detergent. As a younger student, you may have done a simple experiment in which you filled a small-diameter cup with water and carefully floated a thin sewing needle—lengthwise—on the surface. The needle, like an insect that walks on water, is held up by surface tension, which pulls in the plane of the air-water interface. When you add a drop of liquid detergent to the surface of the water, the needle instantly sinks. Why? The detergent greatly reduces the surface tension.

Detergent molecules orient themselves so that their hydrophilic heads point toward (and interact with) the most superficial water molecules, whereas the hydrophobic tails point toward the air (Fig. 26–8A). Because the hydrophilic surfactant heads pull strongly upward on the most superficial water molecules, the net force on these surface water molecules is greatly reduced, minimizing their tendency to dive into the bulk water. What prevents surfactant at the air-surfactant interface from diving into the bulk water? The hydrophobic tail exerts a counter force, pulling the surfactant upward toward the air. The situation is not unlike that of a fishing line with a bobber at one end and a sinker at the other: as long as the bobber is sufficiently buoyant, it remains at the water's surface. Thus, unlike surface water molecules, which are subjected to a large net force pulling them into the bulk, surfactant experiences a much smaller net force. The greater the surface density of surfactant molecules at the air-water interface (i.e., the smaller the surface occupied by water molecules), the smaller the surface tension.

Pulmonary surfactant is a complex mixture of lipids and proteins. Type-II alveolar cells (p. 603), cuboidal epithelial cells that co-exist with the much thinner type-I cells, synthesize and secrete pulmonary surfactant. Clara cells in the respiratory bronchioles manufacture at least some components of pulmonary surfactant. Lipid makes up approximately 90% of surfactant and is responsible for the surface-active properties. About half of the lipid is **dipalmitoylphosphatidylcholine** (DPPC) (see Fig. 26–8B), also known as dipalmitoyllecithin, which contains two fully saturated 16-carbon fatty acid chains (i.e., "palmitates"). The second most common lipids in pulmonary

A   EFFECT OF SURFACTANT ON SURFACE TENSION

Surfactant reduces surface tension by decreasing density of water molecules at air-water interface.

Because the hydrophobic tail pulls the surfactant molecule upward, the resultant vector is minimal.

Air

Water

Surfactant

B   DIPALMITOYL PHOSPHATIDYL-CHOLINE (DPPC)

C   THE SURFACTANT APOPROTEIN SP-A

Carbohydrate recognition domains

Collagen-like triple helices

FIGURE 26–8. Effect of a surface-active agent on surface tension.

TABLE 26-1

SURFACTANT APOPROTEINS

APO	SOLUBILITY	ROLE
SP-A	Water	Innate immunity Formation of tubular myelin
SP-B	Lipid	Speeds formation of monolayer Formation of tubular myelin
SP-C	Lipid	Speeds formation of monolayer
SP-D	Water	Innate immunity Metabolism of surfactant?

26–8C) may be important for exerting feedback control that limits surfactant secretion. The two hydrophobic apoproteins, **SP-B** and **SP-C**, are intrinsic membrane proteins that greatly increase the rate at which surfactant enters the air-water interface and then spreads as a surface film. The hereditary absence of SP-B leads to respiratory distress that is fatal unless the newborn receives a lung transplant.

The lipid components of pulmonary surfactant diffuse into type-II cells from the blood stream (Fig. 26–9A). Type-II cells use the secretory pathway (p. 36) to synthesize the four apoproteins, all of which undergo substantial post-translational modification. The final assembly of surfactant occurs in **lamellar bodies**, which are approximately 1 μm in diameter and consist of concentric layers of lipid and protein (see Fig. 26–9B). Some of the material in these lamellar bodies represents newly synthesized components, and some of it represents recycled surfactant components retrieved from the alveolar surface. Each hour, the normal lung secretes into the alveolar space approximately 10% of the material present in the lamellar bodies.

The secretion of pulmonary surfactant occurs by constitutive exocytosis (p. 36). Both synthesis and secretion are quite low until immediately before birth, when a surge in maternal glucocorticoid levels triggers these processes (p. 1195). Infants born prematurely may thus lack sufficient levels of surfactant and may develop **respiratory distress syndrome** (RDS) (see box on p. 1201). In postnatal life, several stimuli enhance the surfactant secretion, including hyperinflation of the lungs (e.g., sighing and yawning), exercise, and pharmacologic agents (e.g., β-adrenergic agonists, Ca^{2+} ionophores).

After its secretion into the thin layer of water that covers the alveolar epithelium, pulmonary surfactant undergoes major structural changes, freed from the physical constraints of confinement to a lamellar body. In this aqueous layer, surfactant takes on the form of a meshwork known as **tubular myelin** (see Fig. 26–9B), which is rich in surfactant apoproteins. It is not clear whether surfactant normally passes through the tubular-myelin state before forming a surface film at the air-water interface. However, tubular myelin is not *required*: SP-A knockout mice lack tubular myelin but have a normal surface film.

Two mechanisms clear components of pulmonary surfactant from the surface of alveoli. Alveolar macrophages

surfactant are phosphatidylcholine molecules with *unsaturated* fatty-acid chains. Compared with cell membranes, phosphatidylglycerol (~11% of lipid) is over-represented in surfactant.

Proteins account for the remaining approximately 10% of pulmonary surfactant. Plasma proteins (mainly albumin) and secretory IgA make up about half of the protein, and four **apoproteins** (SP-A, -B, -C and -D) make up the rest. **SP-A** and **SP-D** are water soluble and have collagen-like domains (Table 26–1). Both contribute to "innate immunity" by acting as opsonins to coat bacteria and viruses, thereby promoting phagocytosis by macrophages resident in the alveoli. In addition, SP-A (see Fig.

A SURFACTANT METABOLISM

B ELECTRON MICOROGRAPH OF LAMELLAR BODIES

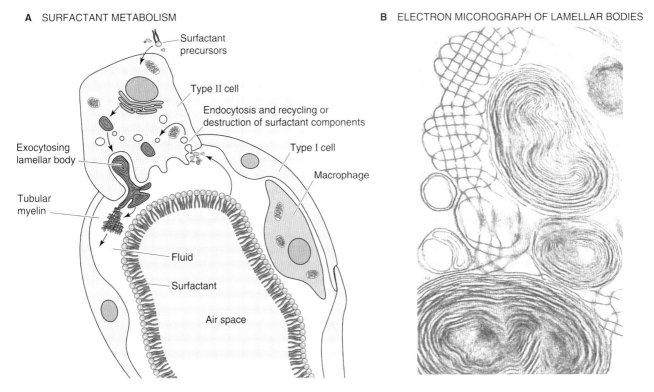

FIGURE 26–9. Generation of pulmonary surfactant. In *B*, the structures with concentric layers are lamellar bodies, which are continuous with tubular myelin (gridlike structures). (*B*, Courtesy of Dr. M.C. Williams, University of California, San Diego.)

degrade some of the surfactant. Type-II cells take up the rest, and either recycle or destroy it.

Pulmonary Surfactant Reduces Surface Tension and Increases Compliance

The pulmonary surfactant present at the alveolar air-water interface has three major effects:

First, because surfactant reduces surface tension, it increases compliance, making it far easier to inflate the lungs. If the surfactant suddenly disappeared from the lungs—mimicking the situation in RDS of the newborn—total elastic recoil would increase (i.e., compliance would *decrease*) twofold or more, causing small airways to collapse partially. The situation would be similar to that described by the "fibrosis" curve in Figure 26–6. Because the compliance of its lungs is far lower than normal, an infant with RDS must produce far larger changes in P_{TP} (or P_{IP}) to achieve the same increase in lung volume, compared with a normal infant. Therefore, infants with low surfactant levels must expend tremendous effort to contract their inspiratory muscles and expand the lungs.

Second, by reducing surface tension, surfactant minimizes fluid accumulation in the alveolus. Normally, Starling forces across the alveolar wall, mainly the negative interstitial hydrostatic pressure (i.e., P_{IP}), favor fluid movement from the alveolar space into the interstitium, keeping the alveoli dry. In the absence of surfactant, the increased surface tension increases the tendency for the "air bubble" inside the alveolus to collapse, thereby drawing fluid into the alveolar space from the interstitium. The

net effect is to increase the distance between air and blood, thereby impairing gas diffusion.

Third, surfactant helps keep alveolar size relatively uniform during the respiratory cycle. Imagine that we start—after a quiet expiration—with two alveoli having the same radius (e.g., 100 μm) and the same surface density of surfactant (to yield a surface tension of 20 dynes/cm), as indicated by the *inner circles* of the two alveoli in Figure 26–10. However, for the lower alveolus, either the anatomic component of compliance is lower (e.g., more fibrous tissue) or the resistance of the airway leading to it is higher. Either way, the lower alveolus will tend to inflate more slowly during inspiration and—at any time—have a smaller volume than the upper one. This size difference has two negative consequences: (1) The total surface area of the two alveoli is less than if they had inflated equally, impairing gas diffusion; (2) Because the final volume increase of the upper alveolus may be greater than that of the lower one, its **ventilation** may be greater. As discussed in Chapter 30, unevenness of ventilation impairs effective gas exchange.

Fortunately, surfactant helps alveoli dynamically adjust their rates of inflation and deflation, thereby tending to equalize ventilation among alveoli. During rapid inflation, alveolar surface area appears to increase more rapidly than additional surfactant can reach the surface from a surfactant pool beneath the surface. As a result, surfactant on the surface is thought to break up like a flow of ice on the sea, with open areas of pure water between clusters of surfactant. The result is an increase in exposed water at the surface, and thus an increase in surface

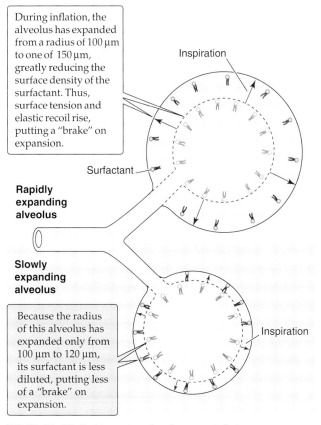

During inflation, the alveolus has expanded from a radius of 100 μm to one of 150 μm, greatly reducing the surface density of the surfactant. Thus, surface tension and elastic recoil rise, putting a "brake" on expansion.

Inspiration

Surfactant

Rapidly expanding alveolus

Slowly expanding alveolus

Because the radius of this alveolus has expanded only from 100 μm to 120 μm, its surfactant is less diluted, putting less of a "brake" on expansion.

Inspiration

FIGURE 26–10. Braking action of surfactant on inflation.

tension. According to estimates, surface tension may double during inspiration, compared with the resting value at FRC. Of course, this effect would be exaggerated in rapidly expanding alveoli, which would rapidly develop a higher surface tension than slowly expanding alveoli. This higher surface tension produces a greater elastic recoil that acts to oppose further expansion. Thus, the dilution of surfactant tends to put more of a "brake" on rapidly expanding airways, slowing their expansion to more nearly match that of alveoli that tend to inflate more slowly.

The opposite appears to happen during expiration, when the surface area of rapidly contracting alveoli falls more rapidly than surfactant can dive back down into the subsurface pool. The compression of surfactant in these more rapidly contracting alveoli causes surface tension to fall precipitously. It has been estimated that surface tension during expiration may fall to half the resting value at FRC. Thus, the more rapidly an alveolus shrinks, the more its surface tension falls, the lower is its elastic recoil, and the greater is its tendency to re-expand. This action puts a "brake" on rapidly contracting alveoli, slowing their rate of shrinkage to more closely match that of slowly contracting alveoli.

DYNAMIC PROPERTIES OF THE LUNG

When air is flowing—that is, under dynamic conditions—one must not only exert the force necessary to maintain the lung and chest wall at a certain volume (i.e.,

"static" component of force), but must also exert an extra force to overcome the inertia and resistance of the tissues and air molecules (i.e., "dynamic" component of force).

Airflow Is Proportional to the Difference Between Alveolar and Atmospheric Pressure, but Inversely Proportional to Airway Resistance

The flow of air through tubes is governed by the same principles governing the flow of blood through blood vessels and the flow of electrical current through wires (see Equation 17–1). Airflow is proportional to driving pressure (ΔP), but inversely proportional to airway resistance (R):

Equation 26–17

$$\dot{V} = \frac{\Delta P}{R} = \frac{P_A - P_B}{R}$$

$\dot{V}$ (measured in liters/sec) is airflow; the dot above the V indicates the time derivative of volume. For the lung, the driving pressure is the difference between the alveolar pressure (P_A) and the barometric pressure (P_B). Thus, for a fixed resistance, more *airflow* requires a greater ΔP (i.e., more effort). Another way of looking at it is that to achieve a desired airflow, more *resistance* requires a greater ΔP.

Equation 26–17 is valid only when airflow is laminar—that is, air molecules move smoothly in the same direction. Under such conditions, Poiseuille's law states that airway resistance is proportional to the viscosity of the gas (η) and the length of the tube (ℓ), but is inversely proportional to the fourth power of radius:

Equation 26–18

$$R = \frac{8}{\pi} \cdot \frac{\eta \ell}{r^4}$$

This equation is the same as Equation 17–11 for laminar blood flow. Generally, changes in viscosity and length are not very important for the lung, although the resistance while breathing helium is greater than that for nitrogen, the major component of air, because helium has a greater viscosity. However, the key aspect of Equation 26–18 is that airflow is extraordinarily sensitive to changes in airway **radius**. The fourth-power dependence of resistance on radius means that a 10% decrease in radius causes a 52% increase in resistance—that is, a 34% *decrease* in airflow. Although Poiseuille's law strictly applies only to laminar-flow conditions, as discussed later, airflow is even more sensitive to changes in radius when airflow is *not* laminar.

In principle, it is possible to compute the total airway resistance of the tracheobronchial tree from anatomic measurements, applying Poiseuille's law when the flow is laminar and analogous expressions for airways in which the flow is not laminar. In 1915, Rohrer used this approach, along with painstaking measurements of the lengths and diameters of the airways of an autopsy specimen, to calculate the aggregate airway resistance of the tracheobronchial tree. Despite Rohrer's efforts, it is not very practical to *compute* airway resistance values, especially if we are interested in studying how R changes, both physiologically and in the course of disease. Therefore, for both physiologists and physicians, it is important to *measure* resistance directly. Rearranging Equation 26–17, we can obtain the resistance during an inspiration or expiration by simply measuring the driving pressure and the airflow that it produces:

Equation 26–19

$$R = \frac{\Delta P}{\dot{V}} = \frac{P_A - P_B}{\dot{V}} \left(\text{units: } \frac{\text{cm } H_2O}{\text{liters/sec}} \right)$$

We can measure airflow directly with a **flowmeter** (pneumotachometer) built into a tube through which the subject breathes. The driving pressure is more problematic because of the difficulty in measuring P_A during breathing. In 1956, DuBois and colleagues met this challenge by cleverly using Boyle's law and a **plethysmograph** to measure the P_A (Fig. 26–11). For example, if the peak $\dot{V}$ during a quiet inspiration is -0.5 liter/sec—by convention, a negative value denotes inflow—and P_A at the same instant is -1 cm H_2O (from the plethysmograph), then

Equation 26–20

$$R = \frac{\Delta P}{\dot{V}} = \frac{(P_A - P_B)}{\dot{V}} = \frac{-1 \text{ cm } H_2O}{-0.5 \text{ liter/sec}} = 2 \frac{\text{cm } H_2O}{(\text{liters/sec})}$$

In normal individuals, *R* is approximately 1.5 cm H_2O/(liters/sec), but can range from 0.6 to 2.3. Resistance values are higher in patients with respiratory disease and can exceed 10 cm H_2O/(liters/sec) in extreme cases.

The resistance that we measure in this way is the **airway resistance,** which represents approximately 80% of total pulmonary resistance. The remaining 20% represents "tissue resistance"—that is, the friction of pulmonary and thoracic tissues as they slide past one another as the lungs expand or contract.

In the Lung, Airflow Is "Transitional" in Most of the Tracheobronchial Tree

We have seen that when airflow is laminar, it is governed by a relationship that is similar to Ohm's law. What happens when the airflow is not laminar? And how can we predict whether the airflow is likely to be laminar? The flow of a fluid down a tube is **laminar** when particles passing any particular point always have the same speed and direction. Because of their viscosity, real fluids move fastest down the midline of the tube, and velocity falls to 0 as we approach the wall of the tube (Fig. 26–12A), as discussed for blood on p. 430. If the average velocity of the fluid flowing down the tube passes a critical value, flow becomes **turbulent**: Local irregular currents, called vortices, develop randomly, and they greatly increase resistance to flow. Under ideal laboratory conditions, airflow generally is laminar when the dimensionless **Reynolds number (Re)** is less than 2000 (p. 430):

Equation 26–21

$$Re = \frac{2 r \bar{v} \rho}{\eta}$$

r is the radius of the tube, $\bar{v}$ is the velocity of the gas averaged over the cross section of the tube, ρ is the density of the gas, and η its viscosity. When *Re* exceeds approximately 3000, flow tends to be turbulent. Between *Re* values of 2000 and 3000, flow is unstable and may switch between laminar and turbulent.

Reynolds developed Equation 26–21 to predict turbulence when fluid flows through tubes that are long, straight, smooth, and unbranched. Pulmonary airways, however, are short, curved, bumpy, and bifurcated. The branches are especially problematic, because they set up small eddies (see Fig. 26–14B). Although these eddies resolve farther along the airways, the air soon encounters yet other bifurcations, which establish new eddies. This sort of airflow is termed **transitional**. Because of the complex geometry of pulmonary airways, the critical *Re* in the lungs is not the ideal value of 2000, but much lower. In fact, *Re* must be less than approximately 1 for lung airflow to be laminar. Such low *Re* values, and thus laminar flow, are present only in the small airways that are distal to terminal bronchioles (p. 601).

Airflow is transitional throughout most of the tracheobronchial tree. Only in the trachea, where the airway radius is large and linear air velocities may be extremely high (e.g., exercise, coughing) is airflow truly turbulent (see Fig. 26–14C).

A major reason why the distinction among laminar, transitional, and turbulent airflow is important is that these patterns influence how much energy one invests in producing airflow. When airflow is *laminar* (see Equation 26–17), the subject invests relatively little energy in airflow. When flow is *transitional*, one must apply more ΔP to produce the same airflow, because it takes extra energy to produce vortices. Thus, the "effective resistance" increases. When flow is *turbulent*, airflow is proportional not to ΔP, but to $\sqrt{\Delta P}$. Thus, we must apply an even greater ΔP to achieve a given flow (i.e., effective resistance is even greater).

The Smallest Airways Contribute Only Slightly to Total Airway Resistance in Healthy Lungs

As discussed earlier, airway resistance for healthy individuals is approximately 1.5 cm H_2O/(liters/sec). Because effective resistance can increase markedly with increases in airflow—owing to transitional and turbulent airflow—it is customary to measure resistances at a fixed, relatively low flow of approximately 0.5 liter/sec. The second column of Table 26–2 shows how airway resistance varies with position down the tracheobronchial tree for a normal subject as air moves from lips to alveoli during a quiet inspiration. A striking feature is that the greatest aggregate resistance is in the pharynx-larynx, and large airways (diameter > 2 mm, or before about generation 8). In this normal subject, of the total airway resistance of 1.5 cm H_2O/(liters/sec), 0.6 is in the upper air passages,

A SUBJECT AT REST

Plethysmograph

Mouth pressure (P_M)

Shutter

P_A

Pneumotachometer (measures air flow, $\dot{V}$)

P_{BOX}

Box pressure (P_{BOX})

1-liter calibrating syringe

FIGURE 26–11. Measuring alveolar pressure during airflow. This plethysmograph is similar to the one in Figure 26–2C, except that the spirometer is replaced by a sensitive device for measuring the pressure inside the plethysmograph (P_{BOX}). The subject breathes plethysmograph air through a tube that has an electronically controlled shutter, as well as meters for measuring airflow and pressure at the mouth. In B, with the subject making an inspiratory effort against a closed shutter, pressure at the mouth equals alveolar pressure (P_A). We obtain the calibration ratio $\Delta P_A/\Delta P_{BOX}$, which allows us to convert future changes in the P_{BOX} to changes in P_A. In C, the subject inspires through an open shutter. During the first moments of inspiration, the thorax expands before much air enters the lungs. Because alveoli expand without much of an increase in the number of gas molecules, P_A must fall. Conversely, because the thorax encroaches on the plethysmograph air, which has hardly lost any gas molecules to the lungs, P_{BOX} must rise. From the calibration ratio $\Delta P_A/\Delta P_{BOX}$, we calculate ΔP_A from ΔP_{BOX} *during* inspiration. P_A at any point during the respiratory cycle is the sum of the known P_B and the measured ΔP_A.

B SUBJECT BREATHING AGAINST A CLOSED SHUTTER

1 As the subject inhales against a closed shutter…

2 …lung volume increases, causing P_A to decrease.

3 Because there is no airflow, mouth pressure (P_M) equals alveolar pressure (P_A). Thus, ΔP_M equals ΔP_A.

P_M

4 As the expanding lung encroaches on the air in the plethysmograph, P_{BOX} increases by ΔP_{BOX}.

$\uparrow P_{BOX}$

$\downarrow P_A$

P_{BOX}

5 During inspiration, the positive ΔP_{BOX} is proportional to the negative ΔP_A. During expiration, the negative ΔP_{BOX} is proportional to the positive ΔP_A. Thus ΔP_{BOX} provides a measure of ΔP_A.

C SUBJECT BREATHING THROUGH AN OPEN SHUTTER

1 As the subject inhales against an open shutter…

2 … air enters the lungs and the pneumotachometer records a negative $\dot{V}$.

3 The positive ΔP_{BOX} allows us to calculate the negative ΔP_A.

Air flow ($\dot{V}$)

$\downarrow P_A$

Box pressure (P_{BOX})

4 We calculate airway resistance (R):
$$R = \frac{\Delta P_A}{\dot{V}}$$
During expiration, both $\dot{V}$ and ΔP_A are positive.

P_{BOX}

0.6 is in the large airways, and only 0.3 is in the small airways.

Because airway resistance increases with the fourth power of airway radius (see Equation 26–18), it might seem counterintuitive that the small airways have the lowest aggregate resistance. However, although each small airway has a high individual resistance, there are so many of them aligned in parallel that their aggregate resistance is very low. We see this same pattern of resistance in the vascular system, where capillaries make a smaller contribution to aggregate resistance than do arterioles (p. 452).

A LAMINAR FLOW

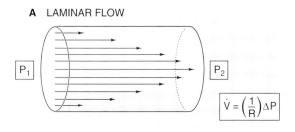

$$\dot{V} = \left(\frac{1}{R}\right)\Delta P$$

B TRANSITIONAL FLOW

C TURBULENT FLOW

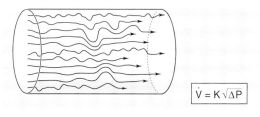

$$\dot{V} = K\sqrt{\Delta P}$$

FIGURE 26–12. Laminar, transitional, and turbulent flow. In *A*, laminar airflow ($\dot{V}$) is proportional to the driving pressure (ΔP). In *C*, where turbulent airflow is proportional to the square root of the driving pressure, a greater ΔP (i.e., effort) is needed to produce the same $\dot{V}$ as in panel *A*.

TABLE 26–2

AGGREGATE AIRWAY RESISTANCE*		
LOCUS	**NORMAL**	**COPD**
Pharynx-Larynx	0.6	0.6
Airways > 2 mm diameter	0.6	0.9
Airways < 2 mm diameter	0.3	3.5
Total airway resistance	1.5	5.0

* Units of resistance, cm H_2O/(liters/sec)
COPD, chronic obstructive pulmonary disease.

gregate resistance, it is within these small airways that disease processes have their greatest and earliest effects. Even a doubling of small-airway resistance from 0.3 to 0.6 cm H_2O/(liter/sec) in the early stages of COPD would produce such a small increment in total airway resistance that it would be impossible to identify the COPD patient in a screening test based on resistance measurements. As discussed on p. 693, approaches that detect the nonuniformity of ventilation are more sensitive for detecting early airway disease. In addition to COPD, the other common cause of increased airway resistance is **asthma** (see the box on Asthma).

Regardless of its cause, increased airway resistance greatly increases the energy required to move air into and out of the lungs. If the increase in resistance is severe enough, it can markedly limit exercise. In extreme cases, even walking may be more exercise than the patient can manage. The reason is obvious from the pulmonary version of Ohm's law (Equation 26–17). For a given ΔP between atmosphere and alveoli, a 3.3-fold increase in *R* (COPD patient in Table 26–2) means a 3.3-fold reduction in $\dot{V}$. Conversely, to maintain a normal $\dot{V}$ in the face of a 3.3-fold increase in resistance, ΔP must increase 3.3-fold. The COPD patient can achieve this ΔP by generating an *alveolar pressure* that is also 3.3-fold higher than normal. Because the patient produces this P_A by contracting the muscles of respiration, compensating for increased airway resistance can require an enormous amount of work.

Vagal Tone, Histamine, and Reduced Lung Volume All Increase Airway Resistance

Even in normal individuals, airway resistance can increase markedly owing to the autonomic nervous system (ANS), humoral factors, and decreases in the volume of the lungs themselves. The vagus nerve, part of the **parasympathetic** division of the ANS, releases acetylcholine, which acts on a muscarinic receptor on bronchial smooth muscle (p. 387). The result is bronchoconstriction and, therefore, an increase in airway resistance. The muscarinic antagonist atropine blocks this action. The bronchoconstriction triggered by such irritants as cigarette smoke (p. 731) is part of a reflex in which the vagus nerve is the efferent limb.

Opposing the action of the vagus nerve is the **sympathetic** division of the ANS, which releases norepinephrine and dilates the bronchi and bronchioles, but reduces

Table 26–2 also shows an example of a patient with moderately severe **chronic obstructive pulmonary disease** (**COPD**), a condition in which emphysema or chronic bronchitis increases airway resistance. COPD is a common and debilitating consequence of cigarette smoking, far more common than the lung cancer that receives so much attention in the lay press. Notice *where* the disease strikes. Even though COPD increases total airway resistance to 5.0 cm H_2O/(liters/sec), or 3.3 times greater than our normal subject, pharynx/larynx resistance does not change at all, and large-airway resistance increases only modestly. Almost all of the incremental increase in total airway resistance is due to a nearly 12-fold increase in the resistance of the smallest airways! According to Equation 26–18, we could produce a 12-fold increase in airway resistance by decreasing radius by about half.

Although small airways normally have a very low ag-

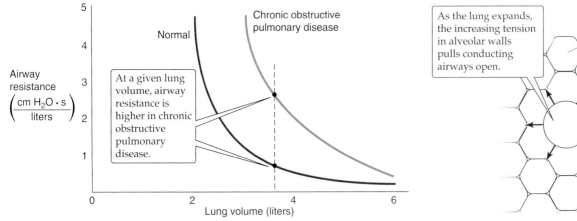

FIGURE 26–13. Airway resistance.

glandular secretions. However, these effects are weak because norepinephrine is a poor agonist of the β_2 adrenergic receptors that mediate this effect via cyclic adenosine monophosphate (cAMP) (p. 388).

Humoral factors include **epinephrine**, released by the adrenal medulla. Circulating epinephrine is a far better β_2 agonist than is norepinephrine and, therefore, a more potent bronchodilator. **Histamine** constricts alveolar ducts and thus increases airway resistance.

One of the most powerful determinants of airway resistance is **lung volume** (V_L). Airway resistance is extremely high at low V_L, but decreases steeply at higher volumes (Fig. 26–13A). One reason for this effect is obvious: all of pulmonary airways expand at high V_L, and resistance falls steeply as radius increases (see Equation 26–18). A second reason is the principle of interdependence (p. 618)—alveoli tend to hold open their neighbors by exerting radial traction or **mechanical tethering** (see Figure 26–13B). This principle is especially important for conducting airways, which account for virtually all of the airway resistance. Because conducting airways have thicker walls than alveoli, their compliance is lower. Thus, at high V_L, alveoli dilate more than the adjacent bronchioles, exerting radial traction and pulling the bronchioles farther open. Patients with obstructive lung disease, by definition, have an increased airway resistance at a given V_L (see Fig. 26–13A). However, because these patients tend to have a higher-than-normal FRC, they breathe at a higher V_L, where airway resistance is—for them—relatively low.

Intrapleural Pressure Has a Static Component ($-P_{TP}$) That Determines Lung Volume and a Dynamic Component (P_A) That Determines Airflow

Earlier, we saw that transpulmonary pressure is, by definition, the difference between alveolar pressure and intrapleural pressure: ($P_{TP} = P_A - P_{IP}$) (see Equation 26–11). What is the physiological significance of these three pressures, and how do we control them?

P_{TP} is a *static* parameter. It does not cause airflow.

Along with compliance, P_{TP} determines *lung volume*, as described by the static pressure-volume relationship in Figure 26–6. Moreover, P_{TP} not only determines V_L under static conditions, when there is no airflow, but also under dynamic conditions (i.e., during inspiration and expiration). However, the body does not directly control P_{TP}.

P_A is a *dynamic* parameter. It does not determine V_L directly. Instead, along with airway resistance, P_A determines *airflow*. When P_A is zero, $\dot{V}$ must be 0, regardless of whether V_L is at RV, FRC, or TLC. But if the P_A is positive and the glottis is open, air flows from alveoli to atmosphere, regardless of V_L. If P_A is negative, air flows in the opposite direction. As is the case with P_{TP}, the body does not directly control P_A.

P_{IP} is the parameter that the brain—through the muscles of respiration—directly controls. If we rearrange the definition of transpulmonary pressure seen in Equation 26–11:

Equation 26–22
$$P_{IP} = (-P_{TP}) + P_A$$

Thus, P_{IP} has two components (Fig. 26–14, *top*). One ($-P_{TP}$) is static and (along with compliance) determines V_L, but it does not directly determine $\dot{V}$. The other (P_A) is dynamic and (along with resistance) determines $\dot{V}$, but it has no direct effect on V_L. As we will see in the next section, P_{TP} and P_A literally flow from P_{IP}.

The *lower left part* of Figure 26–14 is a plot of the lung's *static properties*—like the middle plot of Figure 26–6—and describes how V_L depends on P_{TP}. This P_{TP}-V_L curve describes the pressure required to overcome the elastic (i.e., "static") forces that oppose lung expansion, but makes no statement about $\dot{V}$. The *lower right part* of Figure 26–14 is a plot of the lung's *dynamic properties* and describes how $\dot{V}$ depends on P_A. This P_A-$\dot{V}$ curve describes the P_A required to overcome inertial and resistive (i.e., "dynamic") forces that oppose airflow, but makes no statement about V_L. The slope of this plot is airway **conductance**, the reciprocal of airway resistance. We have assumed that R is constant during a respiratory cycle, so that the P_A-$\dot{V}$ curve is a straight line. However,

ASTHMA

Asthma is a very common condition, occurring in 5% to 10% of the American population. Originally, asthma was thought to be the result of bronchospasm alone, but it is now recognized to be primarily an *inflammatory* disorder, with bronchospasm being secondary to the underlying inflammation. When a susceptible person inhales a trigger (e.g., pollen), inflammatory cells rush into the airways, releasing a multitude of cytokines, leukotrienes, and other humoral substances that induce bronchospasm. Perhaps the most well-known of these substances is histamine.

The patient suffering an acute asthma attack is usually easy to recognize. The classic presentation includes shortness of breath, wheezing, and coughing. Triggers include allergens, heat or cold, a host of occupational irritants, and exercise. The patient can often identify the specific trigger. Spirometry can confirm the diagnosis; the most characteristic feature is a decreased FEV_1. Many asthmatics use peak-flow meters at home because the severity of symptoms does not always correlate with objective measurements of the disease's severity.

The type of treatment depends on the frequency and severity of the attacks. Patients with infrequent attacks that are not particularly severe can often be managed with an inhaled β_2-adrenergic agonist, only when needed. These medications, easily delivered by a metered dose inhaler that can be carried around in one's pocket or purse, act on airway β_2-adrenergic receptors to oppose bronchoconstriction. A patient who requires such an agent more than one or two times a week should receive an inhaled corticosteroid on a regular basis to suppress inflammation. Inhaled corticosteroids generally lack the side-effects of oral corticosteroids, but the latter may be required in a patient with sustained and severe asthma. Many patients rely on regular dosing of long-acting β-agonist inhalers and inhaled corticosteroids to keep their asthma under control. Theophylline (a phosphodiesterase inhibitor that raises $[cAMP]_i$ (p. 91), once a mainstay of asthma therapy, is now used far less commonly. Inhaled anticholinergic agents are more useful with COPD patients than with asthmatics, but can be beneficial in some patients who cannot tolerate the side-effects of β-adrenergic agonists (notably tachycardia). Smooth-muscle relaxants (e.g., cromakalim-related drugs) (p. 198) and other anti-inflammatory agents (e.g., leukotriene inhibitors) also play a role in asthma therapy.

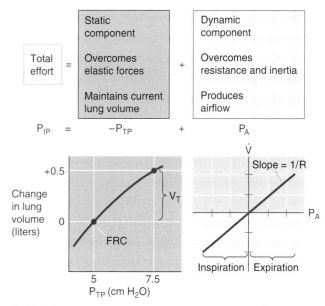

FIGURE 26–14. The static and dynamic components of intrapleural pressure. FRC, functional residual capacity; P_A, alveolar pressure; P_{IP}, intrapleural pressure; P_{TP}, transpulmonary pressure; V_T, tidal volume.

airway resistance changes with lung volume (see Fig. 26–13A) and, as discussed later, airway collapse during expiration causes the airway resistance to be greater during expiration than inspiration.

During Inspiration, a Sustained Negative Shift in P_{IP} Causes P_A to Become Transiently More Negative

During a quiet respiratory cycle—an inspiration of 500 ml, followed by an expiration—the body first generates negative and then positive values of P_A. The four large gray panels of Figure 26–15 show the idealized time courses of five key parameters. The *uppermost panel* is a record of V_L. The *next panel* is a pair of plots, $-P_{TP}$ and P_{IP}. The third shows the record of P_A. The *bottom panel* shows a simultaneous record of $\dot{V}$.

On the *right side* of Figure 26–15 are the static P_{TP}-V_L curve and the dynamic P_A-$\dot{V}$ relationship (both copied from Figure 26–14). On the *left side* is a series of four cartoons that represent snapshots of the key pressures (i.e., P_{IP}, PTP, and P_A) at four points during the respiratory cycle:

a. **Before inspiration begins.** The lungs are under static conditions at a volume of FRC.
b. **Halfway through inspiration.** The lungs are under dynamic conditions, at a volume of FRC + 250 ml.
c. **At the completion of inspiration.** The lungs are once again under static conditions, but at a volume of FRC + 500 ml.
d. **Halfway through expiration.** The lungs are under dynamic conditions, at a volume of FRC + 250 ml.
e. **At the end of expiration/ready for the next inspiration.** The lungs are once again under static conditions, at a volume of FRC.

The V_L record in the *top gray panel* of Figure 26–15 shows that lung volume rises more or less exponentially during inspiration and similarly falls during expiration.

Knowing the time course of V_L, we obtained the P_{TP} values in the *second gray panel* by reading them off the static $P_{TP} - V_L$ diagram to the right, and plotted them as $-P_{TP}$ (for consistency with Equation 26–22). As V_L increases during inspiration, P_{TP} increases (i.e., $-P_{TP}$ becomes more negative). The opposite is true during expiration.

The P_{IP} record in the *second gray panel* shows that P_{IP} is the same as $-P_{TP}$ whenever the lungs are under

FIGURE 26–15. The respiratory cycle. P_B is barometric pressure; P_{IP} is intrapleural pressure; P_{TP} is transpulmonary pressure; and P_A is alveolar pressure (all in cm H_2O). V_L is lung volume and $\dot{V}$ is airflow. The *colored points* (labeled a, b, c, and d) in each of the *central panels* correspond to the illustrations (on *left*) with the same *colored background*. The *two panels* on the *right* are taken from Figure 26–14. FRC, functional residual capacity; V_T, tidal volume.

A   EFFECT OF AIRWAY RESISTANCE ON RATE OF INFLATION

B   EFFECT OF AIRWAY RESISTANCE ON TIDAL VOLUME

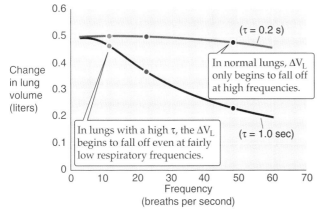

C   EFFECT OF RESPIRATORY FREQUENCY ON TIDAL VOLUME

FIGURE 26–16. Dynamic compliance. In *A* and *B*, the *colored points* represent changes in volume at respiratory frequencies of 12, 24, and 48 breaths per minute.

static conditions (points *a*, *c*, and *a*). During inspiration, P_{IP} rapidly becomes more negative than $-P_{TP}$, but then merges with $-P_{TP}$ by the end of inspiration. The difference between P_{IP} and $-P_{TP}$ is P_A, which must be negative to produce airflow into the lungs. During expiration, P_{IP} is more positive than $-P_{TP}$.

The P_A record in the *third gray panel* shows that alveolar pressure is zero under static conditions (points *a*, *c*, and *a*). During inspiration, P_A rapidly becomes negative, but then relaxes to 0 by the end of inspiration. The opposite is true during expiration. The P_A values in this

plot represent the differences between the P_{IP} and $-P_{TP}$ plots in the *previous panel*.

We computed $\dot{V}$ (*bottom gray panel*) from the relationship $\dot{V} = \Delta P/R$, assuming that R was fixed during the respiratory cycle at 1 cm H_2O/(liters/sec). Thus, the $\dot{V}$ record has the same time course as P_A.

The key message in Figure 26–15 is that during inspiration, the negative shift in P_{IP} has two effects. The body invests some of the energy represented by ΔP_{IP} into transiently making P_A more negative (dynamic component). The result is that air *flows* into the lungs, and V_L increases. But this investment in P_A is only transient. Throughout inspiration, the body invests an increasingly greater fraction of its energy in making P_{TP} more positive (static component). The result is that the body *maintains* the new, higher V_L. By the end of inspiration, the body invests all of the energy represented by ΔP_{IP} into maintaining V_L and none into further expansion. The situation is not unlike that faced by Julius Caesar as he, with finite resources, conquered Gaul. At first, he invested all of his resources in expanding his territory at the expense of the feisty Belgians. But as the conquered territory grew, he was forced to invest an increasingly greater fraction of his resources in maintaining the newly conquered territory. In the end, he necessarily invested all of his resources into maintaining his territory, and was unable to expand further.

The Dynamic Compliance of the Lung Falls as the Respiratory Frequency Increases

In the previous section, we examined pressure, volume, and flow changes during a respiratory cycle of 5 seconds, which corresponds to a respiratory frequency of 12/min. What would happen to ventilation if the frequency were much higher? The top curve in Figure 26–16*A* shows a normal V_L time course during an inspiration. As for any exponential process, the **time constant** (τ) is the interval required for ΔV_L to be approximately 63% complete. For healthy lungs, τ is approximately 0.2 sec. Thus, for inspiration, the increase in V_L is 63% complete after 0.2 sec, 86% complete after 0.4 sec, 95% complete after 0.6 sec, and so on.

A respiratory frequency of 12/min allows 5 sec for each cycle. We will make the simplifying assumption that the time available for inspiration is half this time or 2.5 sec, which represents more than 12 time constants! Thus, if the V_T after infinite time were 500 ml, the ΔV_L measured 2.5 sec after initiating inspiration would also be approximately 500 ml. In Figure 26–16*B*, we plot this value as the green point at a frequency of 12/min on the top curve (i.e., normal lungs).

For a respiratory frequency of 24/min, 1.25 sec is available for inspiration. At the end of this time, the ΔV_L is approximately 499 ml (see Fig. 26–16*B*, *blue point* on the top curve).

If we further increase the respiratory frequency to 48/min, only 0.625 sec is available for inspiration. At the end of this period, only slightly more than three time constants, the ΔV_L is approximately 478 ml (see Fig. 26–16*B*, *red point* on top curve). Thus, over a wide range of frequencies, ΔV_L is largely unchanged. Only when respiratory frequency approaches extremely high values does ΔV_L begin to fall off.

The situation is very different for a subject with substantially increased airway resistance. If R increased fivefold, τ would also increase fivefold to 1 sec. As a result, the trajectory of V_L also would slow by a factor of 5 (see Fig. 26–16A, bottom curve). If we could wait long enough during an inspiration, these unhealthy lungs would eventually achieve a ΔV_L of 500 ml. The problem is that a person cannot wait that long. Therefore, if the frequency is 12/min and inspiration terminates after only 2.5 sec (i.e., only 2.5 time constants), the ΔV_L would be only 459 ml (see Fig. 26–16B, *green point* on bottom curve). Thus, even at a relatively low frequency, the patient with increased airway resistance achieves a ΔV_L that is substantially below normal.

For a respiratory frequency of 24/min, when only 1.25 sec is available for inspiration, the ΔV_L is only 357 ml (see Fig. 26–16B, *blue point* on bottom curve). At a respiratory frequency of 48/min, when only 0.625 sec is available for inspiration, the ΔV_L is only 232 ml (see Fig. 26–16B, *red point* on the bottom curve). Thus, the ΔV_L for the subject with increased airway resistance falls rapidly as frequency increases.

We can represent the *change* in lung volume during cyclic breathing by a parameter called **dynamic compliance**:

Equation 26–23

$$C_{Dynamic} = \frac{\Delta V_L}{-\Delta P_{IP}}$$

Note that $C_{Dynamic}$ is not a constant but is proportional to ΔV_L in Figure 26–16B. Under truly static conditions (i.e., frequency of 0), ΔP_{IP} is the same as $-\Delta P_{TP}$, and *dynamic* compliance is the same as *static* compliance (i.e., Equation 26–23 reduces to Equation 26–13). As frequency increases above 0, $C_{Dynamic}$ falls below static compliance. The degree of divergence increases when resistance increases. For the normal lung in Figure 26–16B, ΔV_L and thus $C_{Dynamic}$ only falls by approximately 5% as frequency rises from zero to 48/min. However, for the lung with a fivefold increased airway resistance, $C_{Dynamic}$ falls by more than 50% as frequency rises from zero to 48/min.

The above pathologic pattern is typical of a patient with asthma, where R is elevated, but static compliance is relatively normal. In a patient with emphysema, both airway resistance and static compliance are elevated. Thus, a plot of $C_{Dynamic}$ versus frequency would show that $C_{Dynamic}$ is initially greater than static compliance at low respiratory frequencies, but it falls below static compliance as frequency increases. What do these frequency-dependent decreases in $C_{Dynamic}$ mean for a patient? The greater the respiratory frequency, the less time is available for inspiration or expiration, and the smaller the V_T (see Fig. 26–16C).

This analysis tremendously oversimplifies what happens in the lungs of real people. Although we have treated the lungs as if there were one value for R and one for C,

each airway has its own R and its own C, and these values vary with parameters such as lung volume, posture, and hormonal status. As a result, some airways have greater time constants than others. Airway pathology may make some of these time constants substantially higher. As the respiratory frequency increases, airways with relatively high time constants will have less and less time to undergo volume changes. As a result, these "slow" airways will make a progressively smaller and smaller contribution to the overall ventilation of the lungs compared with the "faster" airways. At sufficiently high frequencies, very slow airways may drop out of the picture entirely.

Transmural Pressure Differences Cause Airways to Dilate During Inspiration and Compress During Expiration

We discussed two major factors that affect airway caliber: (1) humoral substances (e.g., neurotransmitters) that act on airway smooth muscle, and (2) lung volume *per se* (see Fig. 26–13). A third factor that modulates airway resistance is flow of air through the airway. At a given V_L, airflow creates a pressure difference across the walls of airways, and this **transmural pressure** (P_{TM}) can cause them to dilate or collapse. Figure 26–17A through C depicts the pressures along a single hypothetical airway, extending from the level of the alveolus to the lips, under three conditions: during inspiration (Fig. 26–17A), at rest (Fig. 26–17B), and during expiration (Fig. 26–17C). In all three cases, the lung is at the same volume, FRC; the only difference is whether air is flowing into the lung, not flowing at all, or flowing out of the lung. Because V_L is at FRC, we can assume that the P_{TP}—the P_{TM} for the alveoli—is 5 cm H_2O in all three cases.

First consider what happens under **static conditions** (see Fig. 26–17B). In the absence of airflow, the pressures inside all airways must be 0. Because P_{TP} is 5 cm H_2O and the P_A is 0, we can conclude that the P_{IP} must be -5 cm H_2O. We will ignore the effects of gravity on P_{IP}, and thus assume that P_{IP} is uniform throughout the chest cavity. The P_{IP} of -5 cm H_2O acts not only on the alveoli, but on *all* conducting airways within the thoracic cavity. For each of these, P_{TM} at any point is the difference between the pressure inside the airway (P_{AW}) and P_{IP} (see Equation 26–10):

Equation 26–24

$$P_{TM} = P_{AW} - P_{IP} = 0 - (-5 \text{ cm } H_2O) = +5 \text{ cm } H_2O$$

In other words, a transmural pressure of $+5$ cm H_2O acts on *all* the thoracic airways (but *not* the trachea in the neck, for example), tending to expand them to the extent that their compliance permits.

Now consider what happens during a vigorous **inspiration** (see Fig. 26–17A). We first exhale to a V_L below FRC and then vigorously inhale, so that the P_A will be -15 cm H_2O as V_L passes through FRC. Because the lung is at FRC for our analysis, P_{TP} is $+5$ cm H_2O. The P_{IP} needed to produce a P_A of -15 cm H_2O is therefore

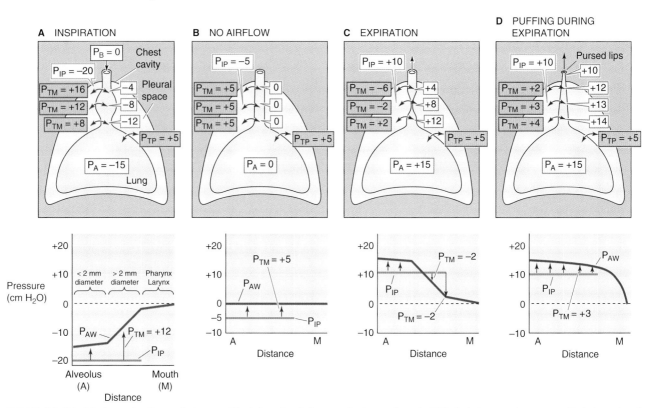

FIGURE 26–17. Dilation and collapse of airways with airflow. In all four panels, lung volume is FRC. P_B is barometric pressure; P_{IP} is intrapleural pressure; P_{TP} is transpulmonary pressure; P_{TM} is the transmural pressure across conducting airways; P_A is alveolar pressure; and P_{AW} (airway pressure) and values in *pale blue balloons* are pressures inside conducting airways (all in cm H_2O). Graphs at *bottom* show P_{AW} profiles along airways (*blue curve*) from alveolus to mouth. P_{IP} is constant throughout the thorax (*green curve*). The *upward arrows* tend to expand the airways, whereas the *downward arrows* tend to squeeze them.

$$P_{IP} = (-P_{TP}) + P_A$$

Equation 26–25

$$= -5 \text{ cm } H_2O + (-15 \text{ cm } H_2O)$$

$$= -20 \text{ cm } H_2O$$

This "inspiring" P_{IP} of -20 cm H_2O is just enough to produce airflow and simultaneously maintain the alveolus at precisely the same volume that it had under static conditions. But how does this exceptionally negative P_{IP} affect airways upstream from the alveolus? The airway pressures must gradually decay from -15 cm H_2O in the alveolus to 0 at the lips. The farther we move from the alveolus, the less negative is P_{AW}, and thus the greater is P_{TM}.

As an illustration, consider a point about halfway up the airway's resistance profile, where P_{AW} is -8 cm H_2O:

Equation 26–26

$$P_{TM} = P_{AW} - P_{IP}$$

$$= -8 \text{ cm } H_2O - (-20 \text{ cm } H_2O)$$

$$= +12 \text{ cm } H_2O$$

Thus, the transmural pressure opposing the elastic recoil at this point has increased from $+5$ cm H_2O at rest (see Fig. 26–17*B*) to $+12$ cm H_2O during this vigorous inspiration (see Fig. 26–17*A*). Because P_{TM} has increased, the airway will tend to dilate. The tendency to dilate becomes greater as we move from the alveolus to the larger airways: As shown in the graph in the *lower part of the panel*, P_{AW} (and thus P_{TM}, as indicated by the *upward arrows*) gradually increases. It is important to recognize that the very positive P_{TM} values that develop in the larger airways only determine the *tendency* to dilate. The extent to which the airway *actually* dilates also depends on its compliance. The amount of cartilage supporting the airways gradually increases from none for 11th-generation airways to a substantial amount for the trachea, and the increased amount of cartilage in the larger airways decreases their compliance and reduces the change in caliber produced by changes in P_{TM}.

As might be expected, the airways tend to collapse during **expiration** (see Fig. 26–17*C*). We first inhale to a V_L above FRC, and then vigorously exhale, so that the P_A is $+15$ cm H_2O as V_L passes through FRC. Because the lung is at FRC for our analysis, the P_{TP} is $+5$ cm H_2O. The P_{IP} needed to produce a P_A of $+15$ cm H_2O is

Equation 26–27

$$P_{IP} = (-P_{TP}) + P_A$$

$$= -5 \text{ cm } H_2O + (+15 \text{ cm } H_2O)$$

$$= +10 \text{ cm } H_2O$$

This P_{IP} of $+10$ cm H_2O is 5 less than the P_A, and thus maintains the alveolus at the same volume that prevailed under static conditions and during inspiration. However, what is the effect of this very positive P_{IP} on the upstream airways? The airway pressures must decrease gradually from +15 cm H_2O in the alveolus to 0 at the lips. The farther we move from the alveolus, the lower the P_{AW}, and thus the lower the P_{TP}. At a point about halfway up the airway's resistance profile, where P_{AW} is +8 cm H_2O:

Equation 26–28

$$P_{TM} = P_{AW} - P_{IP}$$
$$= +8 \text{ cm } H_2O - (+10 \text{ cm } H_2O)$$
$$= -2 \text{ cm } H_2O$$

Thus, at this point during a vigorous expiration, the transmural pressure opposing elastic recoil has fallen sharply from +5 cm H_2O at rest (which tends to mildly inflate, compared with a P_{TM} of 0) to −2 cm H_2O during expiration (which tends to frankly squeeze the airway). As we move from the alveolus to the larger airways, P_{AW} gradually decreases. Thus, P_{TM} gradually shifts from an ever-decreasing inflating force (positive values) to an ever-increasing squeezing force (negative values), as indicated by the change in the orientation of the *arrows* in the *lower panel* of Figure 26–17C. Fortunately, these larger airways, where the collapsing tendency is greatest, have the most cartilage. Thus, in healthy lungs, the cartilage content of the larger airways partially compensates for the natural collapsing tendency that develops during expiration. Nevertheless, total airway resistance is greater during expiration than it is during inspiration.

The problem of airway compression during expiration is exaggerated in patients with **emphysema**, a condition in which the alveolar walls break down. This process results in fewer and larger air spaces with fewer points of attachment and less mutual buttressing of air spaces. Although the affected airways have an increased compliance and thus have a larger diameter at the end of an inspiration, they are flimsy and exert less mechanical tethering on the conducting airways they surround. Thus, during expiration, emphysematous airways are less able to resist the tendency to collapse. As a result, these patients can have great difficulty exhaling. However, these patients make their expirations easier in three ways. We could predict them all from our knowledge of dynamic respiratory mechanics:

1. **They exhale slowly.** A low $\dot{V}$ during expiration translates to a less-positive P_A, which in turn translates to a less-positive P_{IP} and minimizes the tendency to collapse.
2. **They breathe at higher lung volumes.** A high V_L maximizes the mechanical tethering that opposes airway collapse during expiration, and thus minimizes airway resistance (see Fig. 26–13A).
3. **They exhale through pursed lips.** This maneuver, also known as "puffing," creates an artificial, high resistance at the lips. Because the greatest pressure drop occurs at the location of the greatest resistance, puffing causes a greater share of the P_{AW} drop to occur across the lips, rather than along collapsible, cartilage-free airways. As a result, airway pressures are maintained higher, farther along the tracheobronchial tree (Fig.

26–17D). Collapsing tendencies are reduced throughout, and the greatest collapsing tendencies are reserved for the largest airways that have the most cartilage (p. 601).

Because of Airway Collapse, Expiratory Flow Rates Become Independent of Effort at Low Lung Volumes

Cartilage and mechanical tethering from neighboring airways oppose the tendency of conducting airways to collapse during expiration. Because this tethering increases as V_L increases, we would expect the airways to better resist collapse when V_L is high. To see if this is true, we will work through a series of experiments to determine how expiratory airflow varies with "effort" (i.e., alveolar pressure) at different lung volumes.

Imagine that a subject makes a maximal inspiration and then holds his/her breath with glottis open (Figure 26–18A). P_A is 0 because of the static conditions, P_{TP} is +30 cm H_2O to maintain TLC, and P_{IP} is, therefore, −30 cm H_2O. Now, starting from TLC, the subject makes a maximal expiratory effort. Figure 26–18B summarizes the pressures in the airways and thorax at the instant the subject begins exhaling, but before V_L has had time to change. P_{TP} is still +30 cm H_2O, but P_A is now +40 cm H_2O (to produce a maximal expiration) and P_{IP} is therefore +10 cm H_2O. As V_L decreases during the course of the expiration, we will monitor $\dot{V}$ with a flowmeter, monitor the decrease in V_L with a spirometer, monitor P_A using a plethysmograph (see Fig. 26–11).

The *top curve* in Figure 26–18C shows how $\dot{V}$ changes as a function of V_L when, starting from TLC, the subject makes a "maximal" expiratory effort. Notice that $\dot{V}$ rises to its maximal value at a V_L that is somewhat less than TLC, and then gradually falls to 0 as V_L approaches RV. The data in this top curve, obtained with *maximal expiratory effort* (i.e., at very high P_A), will help us determine how expiratory flow varies with effort. To get the rest of the necessary data, we will repeat our experiment by having the subject again inhale to TLC and then exhale to RV. However, with each trial, we ask the subject to exhale with less and less effort (i.e., at smaller and smaller P_A), efforts that we will label as "high," "medium," and "low" in Figure 26–18C.

If we draw a *vertical line* upward from a V_L of 5 liters in Figure 26–18C, we see that, at this very high V_L, $\dot{V}$ gets larger and larger as the effort increases from "low" to "medium" to "high" to "maximal." Because these efforts correspond to increasing P_A values, we can plot these four $\dot{V}$ data points (all obtained at a V_L of 5 liters) versus P_A (see Fig. 26–18D, *top curve*). Because $\dot{V}$ increases continuously with the P_A, flow is **effort dependent** at a V_L of 5 liters. If the airways were made of steel, then this plot of $\dot{V}$ versus P_A in Figure 26–18D would be a straight line. Because the actual plot bends downward at higher values of P_A (i.e., greater "efforts"), airway resistance must have increased with effort (i.e., the airways collapsed somewhat).

Returning to Figure 26–18C, we see that an important characteristic of these data is that the $\dot{V}$ versus V_L *curve*

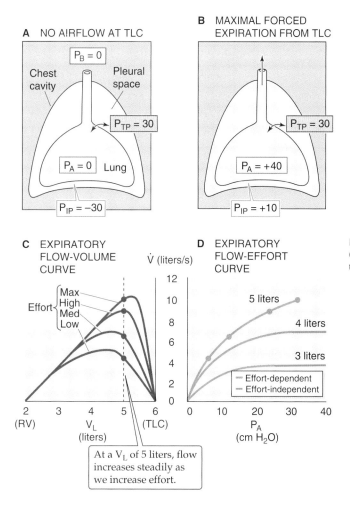

A NO AIRFLOW AT TLC

B MAXIMAL FORCED EXPIRATION FROM TLC

C EXPIRATORY FLOW-VOLUME CURVE

D EXPIRATORY FLOW-EFFORT CURVE

At a V_L of 5 liters, flow increases steadily as we increase effort.

FIGURE 26-18. Maximal expiratory effort from total lung capacity (TLC). P_B is barometric pressure; P_{IP} is intrapleural pressure; P_{TP} is transpulmonary pressure; and P_A is alveolar pressure (all in cm H_2O).

for *maximal* expiratory effort defines an envelope that none of the other *three curves* could penetrate. Thus, at a V_L of 4 liters, $\dot{V}$ is approximately 7 liters/sec, regardless of whether the expiratory effort is "high" or "maximal" (i.e., the two points overlie one another on the graph). At a V_L of 3 liters, the *four curves* have practically merged, so that $\dot{V}$ is approximately 3.5 liters/sec regardless of effort. Thus, at lung volumes that are below 3 liters, it does not matter how much effort the subject makes; the expiratory flow can never exceed a certain value defined by the envelope.

Shifting back to Figure 26-18D, we see that for the *lower two* $\dot{V}$ versus P_A plots, $\dot{V}$ increases with P_A —up to a point. However, further increases in effort are to no avail because the increase in effort (i.e., P_A) is matched by a proportional increase in the airway resistance because of expiration-induced airway collapse. Thus, the more positive values of P_{IP} not only produce more positive values of P_A, but also tend to increase R, so that P_A/R, and thus $\dot{V}$, remains constant.

At low lung volumes, flow becomes **effort independent** because the reduced mechanical tethering cannot oppose the tendency toward airway collapse that always occurs during expiration. Moreover, at progressively lower and lower lung volumes, the flow becomes effort independent earlier. In other words, particularly at low lung volumes, it simply does not pay to try any harder.

REFERENCES

Books and Reviews

Floros J, Kala P: Surfactant proteins: Molecular genetics of neonatal pulmonary diseases. Annu Rev Physiol 60:365–384, 1998.

Gross NJ: Extracellular metabolism of pulmonary surfactant: The role of a new serine protease. Annu Rev Physiol 57:135–150, 1995.

Haagsman HP, van Golde LMG: Synthesis and assembly of lung surfactant. Annu Rev Physiol 53:441–464, 1991.

Macklem PT, Mead J (eds): Handbook of Physiology. Section 3: The Respiratory System, Vol III. Bethesda MD, American Physiological Society, 1986.

Stamenovic D: Micromechanical foundations of pulmonary elasticity. Physiol Rev 70:1117–1134, 1990.

Wright JR: Immunomodulatory functions of surfactant. Physiol Rev 77: 931–962, 1997.

Journal Articles

Avery ME, Mead J: Surface properties in relation to atelectasis and hyaline membrane disease. Am J Dis Child 97:517–523, 1959.

Clements JA: Surface tension of lung extracts. Proc Soc Exp Biol Med 95:170–172, 1957.

DuBois AB, Botelho SY, Comroe J, Jr: A new method for measuring airway resistance in man using a body plethysmograph: Values in normal subjects and in patients with respiratory disease. J Clin Invest 35:327–335, 1956.

Mead J, Whittenberger JL, Radford EP, Jr: Surface tension as a factor in pulmonary volume-pressure hysteresis. J Appl Physiol 10:191–196, 1957.

Perkins WR, Dause RB, Parente RA: Role of lipid polymorphism in pulmonary surfactant. Science 273:330–332, 1996.

CHAPTER 27

Acid-Base Physiology

Walter F. Boron

The study of acid-base physiology is really the study of the proton, or hydrogen ion (H^+). Although protons are present in exceedingly low concentrations in most intracellular and extracellular fluids, they nevertheless have a major impact on biochemical reactions and on a variety of physiological processes that are critical for the homeostasis of the entire body and individual cells. For this reason, the body has evolved sophisticated systems for maintaining plasma and intracellular $[H^+]$ values within narrow and precise ranges.

pH AND BUFFERS

pH Values Vary Enormously Among Different Intracellular and Extracellular Compartments

According to Brønsted's definition, an **acid** is any chemical substance (e.g., CH_3COOH, NH_4^+) that can donate a hydrogen ion. A **base** is any chemical substance (e.g., CH_3COO^-, NH_3) that can accept a hydrogen ion. The term **alkali** can be used interchangeably with the term **base**.

$[H^+]$ varies over a large range in biologic solutions, from more than 100 mM in gastric secretions to less than 10 nM in pancreatic secretions. In 1909, the chemist Sørensen introduced the **pH scale** in an effort to simplify the notation in experiments in which he was examining the influence of $[H^+]$ on enzymatic reactions. The "p" in pH stands for power, and indeed the pH scale is based on powers of 10:

Equation 27–1

$$pH \equiv -\log_{10} [H^+]$$

Thus, when $[H^+]$ is 10^{-7} M, the pH is 7.0. The higher the $[H^+]$, the lower the pH (Table 27–1). It is worth remembering that a 10-fold change in $[H^+]$ corresponds to a pH shift of 1, whereas a 2-fold change in $[H^+]$ corresponds to a pH shift of approximately 0.3.

Even small changes in pH can have significant physiologic consequences, because most biologically important molecules contain chemical groups that can either donate an H^+ (e.g., $R\text{-}COOH \rightarrow R\text{-}COO^- + H^+$) and thereby act as a weak acid, or accept an H^+ (e.g., $R\text{-}NH_2 + H^+ \rightarrow R\text{-}NH_3^+$) and thus behave as a weak base. To the extent that these groups donate or accept protons, a pH shift causes their net electrical charge to change. This change in valence, in turn, can alter a molecule's conformation, and thus its biologic activity.

TABLE 27–1

	RELATIONSHIP BETWEEN [H$^+$] AND pH VALUES		
	[H$^+$] (M)	**pH**	
$\times$ 10	1 $\times$ 10^{-6}	6.0	1 pH unit
	1 $\times$ 10^{-7}	7.0	
	8 $\times$ 10^{-8}	7.1	
	4 $\times$ 10^{-8}	7.4	
$\times$ 2	2 $\times$ 10^{-8}	7.7	0.3 pH unit
	1 $\times$ 10^{-8}	8.0	

pH-sensitive molecules include a variety of enzymes, receptors and their ligands, ion channels, transporters, and structural proteins. For most proteins, pH sensitivity is modest. For example, the activity of the Na-K pump (p. 61) falls by about half when the pH shifts by approximately 1 pH unit from the optimum pH, which is near the cell's normal, resting pH. However, the activity of phosphofructokinase, a key glycolytic enzyme (p. 1220), falls by approximately 90% when pH decreases by only 0.1. The overall impact of pH changes on cellular processes can be impressive. Therefore, cell proliferation in response to mitogenic activation is maximal at the normal, resting intracellular pH, but may fall as much as 85% when intracellular pH falls by only 0.4.

Table 27–2 summarizes the pH values in several body fluids. The pH of neutral water at 37°C is 6.81. Thus, most major body compartments are more alkaline than neutral water.

Because pH can be such an important parameter for many physiologic processes, it is not surprising that sophisticated mechanisms exist to regulate pH in various body compartments. As discussed later, the pH of blood plasma and, by extension, the pH of interstitial fluid is under the dual control of the respiratory system and the kidneys. The control of cerebrospinal fluid pH is dis-

cussed in Chapter 31. We discuss some aspects of intracellular pH regulation at the end of this chapter.

Buffers Minimize the Size of the pH Changes Produced by Adding Acid or Alkali to a Solution

A **buffer** is any substance that reversibly consumes or releases H$^+$. In this way, it helps to stabilize the pH. Buffers do not *prevent* pH changes, they only help to *minimize* them.

Consider a hypothetical buffer B for which the protonated form HB$^{(n+1)}$, with a valence of $n+1$, is in equilibrium with its deprotonated form B$^{(n)}$, which has the valence of n:

Equation 27–2

$$HB^{(n+1)} \rightleftharpoons B^{(n)} + H^+$$

Here, HB$^{(n+1)}$ is a **weak acid**, and B$^{(n)}$ is its **conjugate weak base**. The **total buffer concentration**, [TB], is the sum of the concentrations of the protonated and unprotonated forms:

Equation 27–3

$$[TB] = [HB^{(n+1)}] + [B^{(n)}]$$

The valence of the acidic (i.e., protonated) form can be positive, zero, or negative:

Equation 27–4

Weak Acid (HB$^{(n+1)}$)		Conjugate Weak Base (B^n)	
NH$_4^+$	$\rightleftharpoons$	NH$_3$	+ H$^+$
H$_2$CO$_3$	$\rightleftharpoons$	HCO$_3^-$	+ H$^+$
H$_2$PO$_4^-$	$\rightleftharpoons$	HPO$_4^{2-}$	+ H$^+$

In these examples, NH$_4^+$ (ammonium), H$_2$CO$_3$ (carbonic acid), and H$_2$PO$_4^-$ ("monobasic" inorganic phosphate) are all weak acids, whereas NH$_3$ (ammonia), HCO$_3^-$ (bicarbonate), and HPO$_4^{2-}$ ("dibasic" inorganic phosphate) are the respective conjugate weak bases. Each buffer reaction is governed by a **dissociation constant**, K:

Equation 27–5

$$K = \frac{[B^{(n)}][H^+]}{[HB^{(n+1)}]}$$

TABLE 27–2

APPROXIMATE pH VALUES OF VARIOUS BODY FLUIDS	
COMPARTMENT	**pH**
Gastric secretions (under conditions of maximal acidity)	0.7
Lysosome	5.5
Chromaffin granule	5.5
Neutral H$_2$O at 37°C	6.81
Cytosol of a typical cell	7.2
Cerebral spinal fluid (CSF)	7.3
Arterial blood plasma	7.4
Mitochondrial inner matrix	7.5
Secreted pancreatic fluid	8.1

FIGURE 27-1. Interaction of CO_2 with water.

If we add a small amount of strong acid such as HCl to a physiologic solution, the buffers in the solution consume almost all added H^+:

$$\text{Equation } 27-6$$
$$H^+ + Cl^- + B^{(n)} \longrightarrow HB^{(n+1)} + Cl^-$$

The tiny amount of H^+ that is *not buffered* remains free in solution and is responsible for the decrease in pH. If we instead titrate this same solution with a strong base such as NaOH, H^+ derived from $HB^{(n+1)}$ neutralizes almost all the added OH^-:

$$\text{Equation } 27-7$$
$$Na^+ + OH^- + HB^{(n+1)} \longrightarrow Na^+ + B^{(n)} + H_2O$$

The tiny amount of added OH^- that is not neutralized by the buffer equilibrates with H^+ and H_2O and is responsible for an increase in pH. For each H^+ buffered, one $B^{(n)}$ is *consumed*; for each OH^- buffered, one $B^{(n)}$ is *formed*. Because almost all of the added H^+ or OH^- is buffered, the change in the concentration of the unprotonated form of the buffer (i.e., $\Delta[B^{(n)}]$) is a good index of the amount of strong acid or base added per liter of solution:

$$\text{Equation } 27-8$$
$$\Delta[B^{(n)}] \cong - \underbrace{\Delta[\text{Strong Acid}]}_{\substack{\text{Amount of} \\ \text{Strong Acid} \\ \text{added per liter}}}$$

$$\text{Equation } 27-9$$
$$\Delta[B^{(n)}] \cong \underbrace{\Delta[\text{Strong Base}]}_{\substack{\text{Amount of} \\ \text{Strong Base} \\ \text{added per liter}}}$$

We can quantitate the strength of a buffer by determining its **buffering power** (β), which is the number of moles of strong base (e.g., NaOH) that one must add to a liter of solution to increase pH by one pH unit. This value is equivalent to the amount of strong acid (e.g.,

HCl) that one must add to decrease the pH by one pH unit. Thus, buffering power is:

$$\text{Equation } 27-10$$
$$\beta \equiv \overbrace{\frac{\Delta[\text{Strong Base}]}{\Delta pH}}^{\text{moles/liter}} = - \overbrace{\frac{\Delta[\text{Strong Acid}]}{\Delta pH}}^{\text{moles/liter}}$$

In the absence of CO_2/HCO_3^-, the buffering power of whole blood (which contains erythrocytes, leukocytes, and platelets) is approximately 25 mM/pH unit. This value is known as the **non-HCO_3^- buffering power** ($\beta_{\text{non-}HCO_3^-}$). In other words, we would have to add 25 mmole of NaOH to a liter of whole blood to increase the pH by one unit, assuming that β is constant over this wide pH range. For blood plasma, which lacks the cellular elements of whole blood, the non-HCO_3^- buffering power is only approximately 5 mM/pH unit, which means that only about one fifth as much strong base would be needed to produce the same pH increase.

According to the Henderson-Hasselbalch Equation, pH Depends on the Ratio $[HCO_3^-]/[CO_2]$

The most important physiological buffer pair is CO_2 and HCO_3^-. The strength of this buffer pair is due to the volatility of CO_2, which allows the lungs to maintain stable CO_2 concentrations in the blood plasma, despite ongoing metabolic and buffer reactions that produce or consume CO_2. Imagine that a beaker contains an aqueous solution of 145 mM NaCl (pH = 6.81), but no buffers. We now expose this solution to an atmosphere containing CO_2 (Fig. 27-1). The concentration of dissolved CO_2 ($[CO_2]_{\text{Dis}}$) is governed by **Henry's Law** (see box on p. 597):

$$\text{Equation } 27-11$$
$$[CO_2]_{\text{Dis}} = s \cdot P_{CO_2}$$

At the temperature (37°C) and ionic strength of mammalian blood plasma, the **solubility coefficient**, s, is approximately 0.03 mM/mm Hg. Because the alveolar air with which arterial blood equilibrates has a P_{CO_2} of approximately 40 mm Hg, or torr, $[CO_2]_{\text{Dis}}$ in arterial blood is

$$\text{Equation } 27-12$$
$$[CO_2]_a = (0.03 \text{ mM/mm Hg}) \cdot 40 \text{ mm Hg} = 1.2 \text{ mM}$$

So far, the entry of CO_2 from the atmosphere into the aqueous solution has had *no effect* on pH. The reason is that we have neither generated nor consumed H^+. CO_2 itself is neither an acid nor a base. If we were considering dissolved N_2 or O_2, our analysis would end here because these gases do not further interact with simple aqueous solutions. The aqueous chemistry of CO_2, however, is more complicated, because CO_2 reacts with the solvent (i.e., H_2O) to form carbonic acid:

$$\text{Equation } 27-13$$
$$CO_2 + H_2O \xrightarrow{\text{slow}} H_2CO_3$$

This **CO$_2$ hydration reaction** is very slow. In fact, it is far too slow to meet certain physiologic needs. The enzyme **carbonic anhydrase**, present in erythrocytes and elsewhere, catalyzes a reaction that effectively bypasses this slow hydration reaction (see the box on Carbonic Anhydrases). Carbonic acid is a weak acid that rapidly dissociates into H$^+$ and HCO$_3^-$:

Equation 27-14

$$H_2CO_3 \xrightarrow{\text{fast}} H^+ + HCO_3^-$$

This **dissociation reaction** is the first point at which pH falls. Note that the formation of H$^+$ is accompanied by formation of HCO$_3^-$ (the conjugate weak base of H$_2$CO$_3$) in a stoichiometry of 1:1. The observation that pH decreases, even while the weak base HCO$_3^-$ is produced, is sometimes confusing. A safe way to reason through such an apparent paradox is to focus always on the fate of the proton: If the reaction forms H$^+$, pH falls. Thus, even though the dissociation of H$_2$CO$_3$ leads to generation of a weak base, pH falls because H$^+$ forms along with the weak base.

Unlike the hydration of CO$_2$, the dissociation of H$_2$CO$_3$ is extremely fast. Thus, in the absence of carbonic anhydrase, the slow CO$_2$ hydration reaction limits the speed at which increased [CO$_2$]$_{Dis}$ leads to the production of H$^+$. HCO$_3^-$ can accept a proton to form its conjugate weak acid (i.e., H$_2$CO$_3$) or release a second proton to form its conjugate weak base (i.e., CO$_3^{2-}$). Because this latter reaction generally is of only minor physiologic significance for buffering in mammals, we will not discuss it further.

We may treat the hydration and dissociation reactions that occur when we expose water to CO$_2$ as if only one reaction were involved:

Equation 27-15

$$CO_2 + H_2O \rightleftharpoons H_2CO_3 \rightleftharpoons H^+ + HCO_3^-$$
$$CO_2 + H_2O \rightleftharpoons H^+ + HCO_3^-$$

Moreover, we can define a dissociation constant for this pseudo-equilibrium:

Equation 27-16

$$K = \frac{[H^+][HCO_3^-]}{[CO_2]}$$

In logarithmic form, this equation becomes:

Equation 27-17

$$pH = pK + \log \frac{[HCO_3^-]}{[CO_2]}$$

Finally, we may express [CO$_2$] in terms of P$_{CO_2}$, recalling from Henry's Law that [CO$_2$] = s · P$_{CO_2}$:

Equation 27-18

$$pH = pK + \log \frac{[HCO_3^-]}{s \cdot P_{CO_2}}$$

This is the **Henderson-Hasselbalch** equation, a logarithmic restatement of the CO$_2$/HCO$_3^-$ equilibrium. Its central message is that pH depends not on [HCO$_3^-$] or P$_{CO_2}$ per se, but on their ratio. Human arterial blood has

a P$_{CO_2}$ of approximately 40 mm Hg and a [HCO$_3^-$] of approximately 24 mM. If we assume that the pK governing the CO$_2$/HCO$_3^-$ equilibrium is 6.1 at 37°C, then

Equation 27-19

$$pH = 6.1 + \log \frac{24 \text{ mM}}{(0.03 \text{ mM/mm Hg}) \times 40 \text{ mm Hg}} = 7.40$$

Thus, the Henderson-Hasselbalch equation correctly predicts the normal pH of arterial blood.

CO$_2$/HCO$_3^-$ Has a Far Higher Buffering Power in an Open Than in a Closed System

The buffering power of a weak acid/weak base buffer pair depends on three factors:

1. **Total concentration of the buffer pair, [TB].** Other things being equal, β is proportional to [TB].
2. **The pH of the solution.** The precise dependence on pH will become clear later.
3. **Whether the system is open or closed.** That is, whether one member of the buffer pair can equilibrate between the "system" (the solution in which the buffer is dissolved) and the "environment" (everything else).

If neither member of the buffer pair can enter or leave the system, then HB$^{(n+1)}$ can become B$^{(n)}$, and vice versa, but [TB] is fixed. This is a **closed system**. An example of a closed-system buffer is inorganic phosphate in a beaker of water, or a titratable group on a protein in blood plasma. In a closed system, the buffering power is:

Equation 27-20

$$\beta_{closed} = 2.3[TB] \frac{[H^+] \cdot K}{([H^+ + K])^2}$$

Two aspects of Equation 27-20 are of interest. First, at a given [H$^+$] (i.e., a fixed pH), β_{closed} is proportional to [TB]. The main reason that the buffering power of whole blood is so much higher than that of blood plasma is that whole blood has a high concentration of buffer groups that are part of hemoglobin. Second, at a given [TB], β_{closed} has a bell-shaped dependence on pH (Fig. 27-2A). β_{closed} is maximal when [H$^+$] = K (i.e., when pH = pK). Most non-HCO$_3^-$ buffers in biologic fluids behave as if they are in a closed system. Although many fluids are actually *mixtures* of several non-HCO$_3^-$ buffers, the total buffering power in such a mixture is the sum of their β_{closed} values, each described by Equation 27-20. Figure 27-2B shows how total buffering power varies with pH for a solution containing a mixture of nine buffers, each present at a [TB] of 1 mM, with pK values evenly spaced at intervals of 0.5 pH unit. In this example, total buffering power is remarkably stable over a broad pH range. Whole blood is a complex mixture of many non-HCO$_3^-$ buffers. The most important of these are titratable groups on hemoglobin and, to a far lesser extent, other proteins. Even less important than the "other proteins" are small molecules such as inorganic phosphate. The [TB] values for these many buffers are not identical, and the pK values are not evenly spaced. Nevertheless,

CARBONIC ANHYDRASES

The carbonic anhydrases (CAs) are a family of zinc-containing enzymes with at least 16 members among mammals; Table 27–3 lists some of these isoforms. Physiologically, the CAs catalyze the interconversion of CO_2 and HCO_3^-, although they also can cleave aliphatic and aromatic ester linkages. Carbonic anhydrase I (CA I) is present mainly in the cytoplasm of erythrocytes. CA II is a ubiquitous cytoplasmic enzyme. CA IV is a GPI-linked enzyme (p. 15) found, for example, on the outer surface of the apical membrane of the renal proximal tubule (p. 853). A hallmark of many CAs is their inhibition by sulfonamides (e.g., acetazolamide).

Before considering the action of carbonic anhydrase, it is instructive to examine the interconversion of CO_2 and HCO_3^- in the absence of enzyme. As illustrated by Equation 27–13 and Equation 27–14, when $[CO_2]$ increases,

Equation A

$$CO_2 + H_2O \xrightarrow{slow} H_2CO_3 \xrightarrow{fast} H^+ + HCO_3^-$$

CO_2 can also form HCO_3^- by directly combining with OH^-, a reaction that becomes important at high pH values, when $[OH^-]$ is also high:

Equation B

$$CO_2 + OH^- \longrightarrow HCO_3^-$$
$$H_2O \xrightarrow{\quad} H^+$$

Because the dissociation of H_2O replenishes the consumed OH^-, the two mechanistically distinct pathways for HCO_3^- formation are functionally equivalent. Of course, both reaction sequences are reversible. However, in the absence of CA, the overall speed of the interconversion between CO_2 and HCO_3^- is slow at physiological pH. In fact, it is possible to exploit this slowness experimentally to generate CO_2/HCO_3^- solutions that are temporarily out of equilibrium. Unlike normal (i.e., equilibrated) solutions, such out-of-equilibrium solutions can have virtually any combination of $[CO_2]$, $[HCO_3^-]$, and pH in the physiological range.

Structural biologists have solved the crystal structures of several CAs. At the reaction site, three histidines coordinate a zinc atom that, along with a threonine, plays a critical role in binding CO_2 and HCO_3^-. In CA II, the fastest of the carbonic anhydrases, a fourth histidine acts as a proton acceptor/donor. Extensive site-directed muta-

genesis studies have provided considerable insight into the mechanism of the CA reaction. The carbonic anhydrases have the *effect* of catalyzing the slow CO_2 hydration in Equation A. Actually, these enzymes catalyze the top reaction in Equation B, the direct combination of CO_2 with OH^- to form HCO_3^-. CA II catalyzes *both* reactions in Equation B:

$$(His)Enzyme - Zn - OH^- + CO_2$$
$$\rightleftharpoons (His)Enzyme - Zn - HCO_3^-$$

$$(His)Enzyme - Zn - HCO_3^- + H_2O$$
$$\rightleftharpoons (His)Enzyme - Zn - H_2O + HCO_3^-$$

$$(His)Enzyme - Zn - H_2O$$
$$\rightleftharpoons (H^+ - His)Enzyme - Zn - OH^-$$

$$(H^+ - His)Enzyme - Zn - OH^-$$
$$\rightleftharpoons (His)Enzyme - Zn - OH^- + H^+$$

CA II has one of the highest turnover numbers of any known enzyme: Each second, one CA II molecule can convert more than one million CO_2 molecules to HCO_3^- ions. In the erythrocyte, this rapid reaction is important for the carriage of CO_2 from the peripheral blood vessels to the lungs (p. 663). In the average cell, carbonic anhydrases are important for allowing the rapid buffering of H^+ by the CO_2/HCO_3^- buffer pair. In addition, CA II appears to bind to several HCO_3^- transporters, where it may promote transport.

In humans, the homozygous absence of normal CA II causes **CA II deficiency syndrome**, characterized by osteopetrosis, renal tubular acidosis, and cerebral calcification. At least seven different mutations can cause genetic defects. The mutation that is common in patients of Arabic descent causes mental retardation, but less severe osteopetrosis. Other patients may carry two different mutations. Indeed, the first three patients described with CA II deficiency syndrome, sisters in the same family, were compound heterozygotes, having received one mutation from their mother and a second from their father.

Although **CA I deficiency** exists, the homozygous condition has no obvious consequences because CA I and CA II normally contribute about equally to the CA activity in red blood cells.

---

the buffering power of whole blood is nearly constant near the physiologic pH.

The second physiologically important condition under which a buffer can function is in an **open system**. Here, one buffer species (e.g., CO_2) equilibrates between the system and the environment. A laboratory example of an open-system buffer is a solution containing CO_2 and HCO_3^-, in which dissolved CO_2 equilibrates with gaseous CO_2 in the atmosphere (see Fig. 27–1). A physiological example is blood plasma, in which dissolved CO_2 equilibrates with gaseous CO_2 in the alveoli. In either case, $[CO_2]_{Dis}$ is fixed during buffering reactions. However, the **total CO_2** ($[CO_2] + [HCO_3^-]$, in this case) can vary

widely. Because total CO_2 can rise to very high values, CO_2/HCO_3^- in an open system can be an extremely powerful buffer. Consider, for example, a liter of a solution having a pH of 7.4, a P_{CO_2} of 40 mm Hg (1.2 mM CO_2), and 24 mM HCO_3^-—but *no other buffers* (Fig. 27–3, *stage 1*). What happens when we add 10 mmole of HCl? Available HCO_3^- neutralizes almost all of the added H^+, forming nearly 10 mmole H_2CO_3 and then nearly 10 mmole CO_2 plus nearly 10 mmole H_2O (see Fig. 27–3, *stage 2A*). The CO_2 that forms does not accumulate, but evolves to the atmosphere so that $[CO_2]_{Dis}$ is constant. What is the final pH? If $[CO_2]_{Dis}$ remains at 1.2 mM in our open system, and if $[HCO_3^-]$ decreases by exactly

TABLE 27–3

SOME HUMAN CARBONIC ANHYDRASES*

ISOFORM	MOLECULAR MASS (kDa)	CELLULAR LOCATION	TISSUE DISTRIBUTION	RELATIVE ACTIVITY	SENSITIVITY TO SULFONAMIDES (e.g., ACETAZOLAMIDE)
I	29	Cytosol	RBCs and GI tract	15%	High
II	29	Cytosol	Nearly ubiquitous	100%	High
III	29	Cytosol	8% of soluble protein in slow-twitch (type I) muscle	1%	Low
IV	35	Extracellular surface of membrane (GPI-linked)	Widely distributed, including acid-transporting epithelia	~100%	Moderate
XII	44	Catalytic domain on extracellular surface†	Certain cancers	~30%	(Binds ACZ with unknown affinity)
XIV	54	Catalytic domain on extracellular surface†	Kidney, heart, skeletal muscle, Brain	?	?

* Several additional carbonic anhydrases have been cloned. In some cases they have not been functionally characterized.
†Integral membrane protein with one membrane-spanning segment.
ACZ, acetazolamide; GPI, glycosyl phosphatidylinositol; RBC, red blood cell.

10 mM (i.e., the amount of added H^+), from 24 to 14 mM, the Henderson-Hasselbalch equation predicts a fall in pH from 7.40 to 7.17, corresponding to an increase in free $[H^+]$ of:

Equation 27–21

$$\Delta[H^+] = (10^{-7.17} - 10^{-7.40})$$
$$= 0.000,068 \text{ mM} - 0.000,040 \text{ mM}$$
$$= 0.000,028 \text{ mM}$$

Therefore, even though we have added 10 *millimoles* HCl to 1 liter, $[H^+]$ increased by only 28 *nano*molar (see Fig. 27–3, *stage 3A*). Therefore, the open-system buffer has neutralized 9.999,972 mM of the added 10 mM H^+. The buffering provided by CO_2/HCO_3^- in an *open system* (β_{open}) is so powerful because only depletion of HCO_3^- limits neutralization of H^+. The buildup of CO_2 is not a limiting factor because the atmosphere is an infinite sink for newly produced CO_2.

The opposite acid-base disturbance occurs when we add a strong base such as NaOH. Here, the buffering reactions are just the reverse of those in the previous example. If we add 10 mmole of NaOH to 1 liter of solution, almost all added OH^- combines with H^+ derived from CO_2 that enters from the atmosphere (see Fig. 27–3, *stage 2B*). One HCO_3^- ion forms for each OH^- neutralized. Buffering power in this *open system* is far higher than that in a closed system because CO_2 availability does not limit neutralization of added OH^-. Only the buildup of HCO_3^- limits neutralization of more OH^-. In this example, even though we added 10 *millimolar* NaOH, free $[H^+]$ decreased by only 12 *nano*molar (see Fig. 27–3, *stage 3B*) as pH rose from 7.40 to 7.55.

Whether CO_2/HCO_3^- neutralizes an acid or a base, the open-system buffering power is:

Equation 27–22

$$\beta_{open} = 2.3 \cdot [HCO_3^-]$$

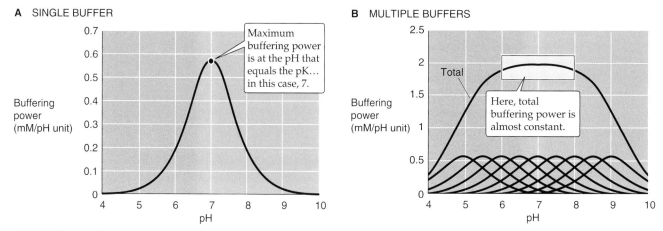

A SINGLE BUFFER

Maximum buffering power is at the pH that equals the pK... in this case, 7.

Buffering power (mM/pH unit)

B MULTIPLE BUFFERS

Total

Here, total buffering power is almost constant.

Buffering power (mM/pH unit)

FIGURE 27–2. Buffering power in a closed system. In *B*, the solution contains nine buffers, each at a concentration of 1 mM and with pK values evenly spaced 0.5 pH unit apart.

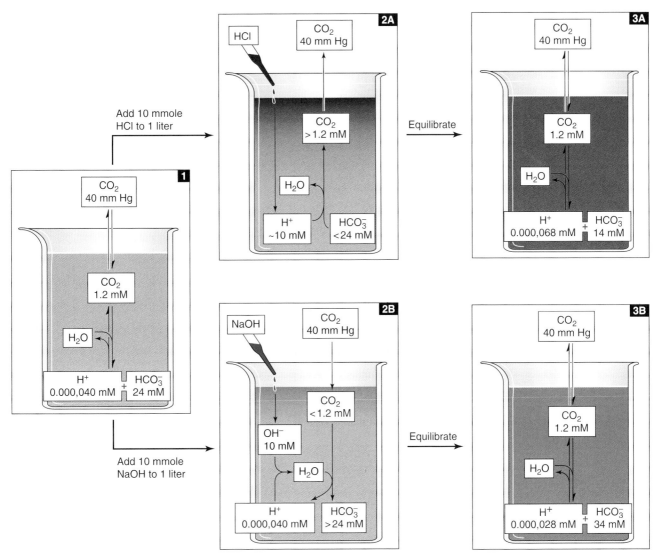

FIGURE 27–3. Buffering of strong acids and bases by CO_2/HCO_3^- in an open system.

FIGURE 27–4. Buffering power of the CO_2/HCO_3^- system. At pH 7.4 on the blue curve, the solution has the same composition as does arterial blood plasma: a Pco_2 of 40 mm Hg and an $[HCO_3^-]$ of 24 mM. If the system is "open" (i.e., CO_2 equilibrates with atmosphere), β_{open} is approximately 55 mM/pH unit at pH 7.40 and rises exponentially with pH (see Equation 27–22). If the system is closed, β_{closed} is only approximately 2.6 mM/pH unit at pH 7.4 and is maximal at the pK of the buffer (see Equation 27–20).

Notice that β_{open} does not have a maximum. Because β_{open} is proportional to $[HCO_3^-]$, β_{open} rises exponentially with pH when Pco_2 is fixed (Fig. 27–4, *blue curve*). In normal arterial blood (i.e., $[HCO_3^-]$ = 24 mM), β_{open} is approximately 55 mM/pH unit. As we have already noted, the buffering power of all non-HCO_3^- buffers ($\beta_{non-HCO_3^-}$) in whole blood is approximately 25 mM/pH unit. Thus, in whole blood, β_{open} represents more than two thirds of the total buffering power. The relative contribution of β_{open} is far more striking in interstitial fluid, which lacks the cellular elements of blood and also has a lower protein concentration.

CO_2/HCO_3^- does not *necessarily* behave as an open-system buffer: In the previous example, we could have added NaOH to a CO_2/HCO_3^- solution in a capped syringe. In such a closed system, not only does accumulation of HCO_3^- limit neutralization of OH^-, but the availability of CO_2 is limiting as well. Indeed, for fluid having the composition of normal arterial blood, the *closed-system* CO_2/HCO_3^- buffering power is only 2.6 mM/pH unit (see Fig. 27–4, *black curve*), less than 5% of the β_{open} value of

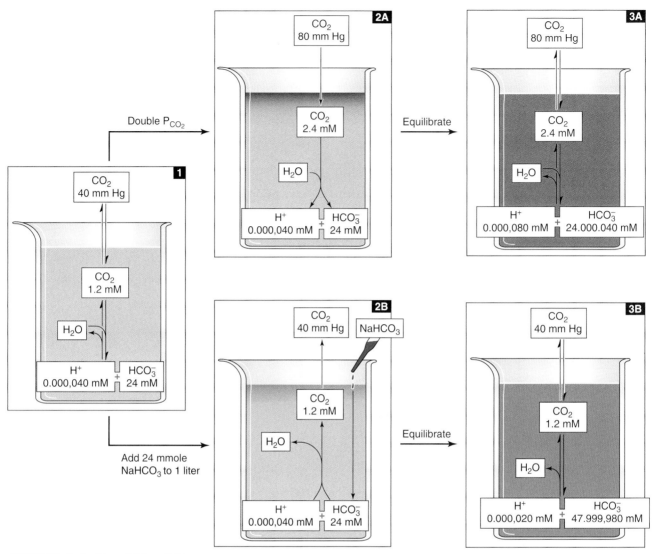

FIGURE 27–5. Doubling of CO_2 or HCO_3^- concentrations.

55 mM/pH unit. You might think that the only reason the closed-system buffering power was so low in this example is that the pH of 7.4 was 1.3 pH units above the pK. However, even if pH were equal to the pK of 6.1, the closed-system CO_2/HCO_3^- buffering power in our example would be only approximately 14 mM/pH unit, about one quarter of the open-system value at pH 7.4. A physiological example in which the CO_2/HCO_3^- system is "poorly open" is **ischemia**, wherein a lack of blood flow minimizes the equilibration of tissue CO_2 with blood CO_2. Thus, ischemic tissues are especially susceptible to large pH shifts.

ACID-BASE CHEMISTRY WHEN CO_2/HCO_3^- IS THE ONLY BUFFER

In this section, we consider buffering by CO_2 and HCO_3^- when these are the *only* buffers present in the solution. We defer to the following section the more complex ex-

ample, in which *both* CO_2/HCO_3^- and non-HCO_3^- buffers are present in the same solution.

In the Absence of Other Buffers, Doubling P_{CO_2} Causes pH to Fall by 0.3, but Causes Almost No Change in $[HCO_3^-]$

Figure 27–5 represents 1 liter of a solution with the same CO_2/HCO_3^- composition as arterial blood plasma, but no buffers other than CO_2/HCO_3^-. What are the consequences of increasing P_{CO_2} in the gas phase? The resulting increase in $[CO_2]_{Dis}$ causes the CO_2/HCO_3^- equilibrium to shift toward formation of H^+ and HCO_3^-. This disturbance is an example of a **CO_2 titration**, because we initiated it by altering P_{CO_2}. More specifically, it is a **respiratory acidosis**—"acidosis" because pH falls, and "respiratory" because pulmonary problems (Table 27–4) are the most common causes of an increase in the P_{CO_2} of arterial blood (p. 691).

In the absence of non-HCO_3^- buffers, how far pH falls

TABLE 27–4

THE FOUR MAJOR ACID-BASE DISORDERS

DISORDER	PROXIMATE CAUSE(S)	CLINICAL CAUSES 🕷	CHANGES IN ARTERIAL ACID-BASE PARAMETERS
Respiratory acidosis	Increased P_{CO_2}	Decreased alveolar ventilation (e.g., drug overdose) ↓ Lung-diffusing capacity (e.g., pulmonary edema) Ventilation-perfusion mismatch	pH: ↓ [HCO_3^-]: ↑ P_{CO_2}: ↑
Respiratory alkalosis	Decreased P_{CO_2}	Increased alveolar ventilation caused by: Hypoxia (e.g., acclimatization to high altitude) Anxiety Aspirin intoxication	pH: ↑ [HCO_3^-]: ↓ P_{CO_2}: ↓
Metabolic acidosis	Addition of acids other than CO_2 or H_2CO_3 Removal of alkali (fixed P_{CO_2})	↓ Urinary secretion of H^+ (e.g., renal failure) Ketoacidosis (e.g., diabetes mellitus) Lactic acidosis (e.g., shock) HCO_3^- loss (e.g., severe diarrhea)	pH: ↓ [HCO_3^-]: ↓ P_{CO_2}: No change
Metabolic alkalosis	Addition of alkali Removal of acids other than CO_2 or H_2CO_3 (fixed P_{CO_2})	HCO_3^- load (e.g., $NaHCO_3$ therapy) Loss of H^+ (e.g., severe vomiting)	pH: ↑ [HCO_3^-]: ↑ P_{CO_2}: No change

during respiratory acidosis depends on the initial pH and P_{CO_2}, as well as on the final P_{CO_2}. For example, doubling P_{CO_2} from 40 mm Hg (see Fig. 27–5, *stage 1*) to 80 mm Hg causes $[CO_2]_{Dis}$ to double to 2.4 mM (see Fig. 27–5, *stage 2A*). At this point, the 1-liter system is far *out* of equilibrium, and can return to equilibrium only if some CO_2 (*x* mM) combines with *x* H_2O to form *x* H^+ and *x* HCO_3^-. Thus, according to Equation 27–16, the following must be true at equilibrium:

Equation 27–23

$$\underbrace{\begin{matrix}10^{-6.1}\text{ M}\\ \text{or}\\ 10^{-3.1}\text{ mM}\end{matrix}}_{K} = \frac{\overbrace{(0.000,040\text{ mM}+x)}^{[H^+]}\overbrace{(24\text{ mM}+x)}^{[HCO_3^-]}}{\underbrace{2.4\text{ mM}}_{[CO_2]}}$$

Solving this equation for *x* yields an extremely small value, nearly 40 nM, or 0.000,040 mM. *x* represents the **flux** of CO_2 that passes through the reaction sequence $CO_2 + H_2O \rightarrow H_2CO_3 \rightarrow H^+ + HCO_3^-$ to re-establish the equilibrium. CO_2 from the atmosphere replenishes the CO_2 consumed in this reaction, so that $[CO_2]_{Dis}$ remains at 2.4 mM after the new equilibrium is achieved (see Fig. 27–5, *stage 3A*). The reason that the flux *x* is so small is that, with no other buffers present, every H^+ formed remains free in solution. Thus, only a minuscule amount of H^+ need be formed before $[H^+]$ nearly doubles from 40 to nearly 80 nM. However, $[HCO_3^-]$ undergoes only a tiny fractional increase, from 24 to 24.000,040 mM. The doubling of the denominator in Equation 27–23 is matched by a doubling of the numerator, nearly all of which is due to the near-doubling of $[H^+]$. The final pH in this example of respiratory acidosis is:

Equation 27–24

$$pH = -\log(80\text{ nM}) = 7.10$$

Another way of arriving at the same answer is to insert the final values for $[HCO_3^-]$ and P_{CO_2} into the Henderson-Hasselbalch equation:

Equation 27–25

$$pH = 6.1 + \log\frac{24.000,040\text{ mM}}{(0.03\text{ mM/mm Hg})\cdot(80\text{ mm Hg})} = 7.10$$

The opposite acid-base disturbance, in which P_{CO_2} falls, is **respiratory alkalosis**. In a solution containing no buffers other than CO_2/HCO_3^-, reducing P_{CO_2} by half, from 40 to 20 mm Hg, would cause all of the aforementioned reactions to shift in the opposite direction, so that pH would rise by 0.3, from 7.4 to 7.7. We could produce respiratory alkalosis in a beaker by lowering the P_{CO_2} in the gas phase. In humans, hyperventilation (see Table 27–4) lowers alveolar and thus arterial P_{CO_2} (p. 691).

Thus, in the absence of non-HCO_3^- buffers, doubling $[CO_2]$ causes pH to fall by 0.3, whereas halving $[CO_2]$ causes pH to rise by 0.3 (see Table 27–1). Remember, the log of 2 is 0.3.

In the Absence of Other Buffers, Doubling [HCO_3^-] Causes pH to Rise by 0.3

What would happen if we double $[HCO_3^-]$, rather than P_{CO_2}? Starting with a solution that has the ionic composition of arterial blood (see Fig. 27–5, *stage 1*), adding 24 mM of HCO_3^- (e.g., $NaHCO_3$) to a liter of this solution drives the CO_2/HCO_3^- equilibrium towards CO_2 (see Fig. 27–5, *stage 2B*). The new equilibrium is achieved when *x* mM of HCO_3^- combine with *x* H^+ to produce *x* CO_2 and *x* H_2O. Because the system is *open to CO_2*, the generation of *x* mM CO_2 causes no change in $[CO_2]_{Dis}$;

the newly formed CO_2 simply evolves into the atmosphere. Thus, according to Equation 27–16, the following must be true at equilibrium:

Equation 27–26

Solving this equation yields an x of nearly 0.000,020 mM. Thus, in the absence of other buffers, an initial doubling of $[HCO_3^-]$ from 24 to 48 mM causes $[H^+]$ to fall by nearly half, from 40 to 20 nM. Although $[HCO_3^-]$ also decreases by 20 nM, its fractional change from 48 to 47.999,980 mM is insignificant. The final pH is:

Equation 27–27
$$pH = -\log(20 \text{ nM}) = 7.70$$

The Henderson-Hasselbalch yields the same result:

Equation 27–28
$$pH = 6.1 + \log \frac{47.999,980 \text{ mM}}{(0.03 \text{ mM/mm Hg}) \cdot (40 \text{ mm Hg})} = 7.70$$

Thus, in the absence of non-HCO_3^- buffers, doubling $[HCO_3^-]$ causes pH to increase by approximately 0.3. Rather than adding HCO_3^-, we could produce an identical effect by adding the same amount of strong base (e.g., NaOH), as we did in Figure 27–3, *stages 2B and 3B*, or by *removing* the same amount of strong acid (e.g., HCl). Removing HCl may seem artificial for a solution in a beaker. However, the loss of gastric HCl due to vomiting (leaving $NaHCO_3$ behind in the blood) is clinically important (see Table 27–4). We also could add a *weak* base (e.g., NH_3) or remove any *weak* acid (e.g., lactic acid) other than CO_2 or H_2CO_3. However, to produce the same alkali load, we would have to add/remove more than for a *strong* base/acid. All of these maneuvers, carried out at a fixed PCO_2, are examples of **metabolic alkalosis**—"alkalosis" because the pH increases, and "metabolic" because derangements in metabolism are common causes.

The opposite acid-base disturbance—in which we remove HCO_3^- or another alkali, or add an acid other than CO_2 or H_2CO_3—is **metabolic acidosis**. Starting with a solution having the ionic composition of arterial blood, halving HCO_3^- or removing 12 mM NaOH or adding 12 mM HCl would cause all of the aforementioned reactions to shift in the opposite direction, so that pH would fall by 0.3, from 7.4 to 7.1. Common causes of metabolic acidosis in humans are renal failure and metabolic problems (see Table 27–4).

We saw in Equation 27–18 that the pH of a CO_2/HCO_3^- solution does not depend on $[HCO_3^-]$ or PCO_2 per se, but on their ratio. Because it is the kidney that controls $[HCO_3^-]$ in the blood plasma (see Chapter 38), and because the lung controls PCO_2 (see Chapter 30), the pH of blood plasma is under the dual control of both

organ systems, a concept embodied by a whimsical variant of the Henderson-Hasselbalch equation:

Equation 27–29
$$pH = \text{Constant} + \frac{\text{Kidney}}{\text{Lungs}}$$

ACID-BASE CHEMISTRY IN THE PRESENCE OF CO_2/HCO_3^- AND NON-HCO_3^- BUFFERS—THE DAVENPORT DIAGRAM

So far, our discussion has focused on a simple system in which CO_2/HCO_3^- is the only pH buffer. Under these circumstances, predicting the effects of altering either PCO_2 or $[HCO_3^-]$ is relatively easy. In real biologic systems, many buffers are present in addition to CO_2/HCO_3^-, and analyzing acid-base disturbances is more complex. For both metabolic and respiratory acid-base disturbances, one is faced with multiple competing equilibria—the CO_2/HCO_3^- reactions that we have already discussed and the reactions of all non-HCO_3^- buffers. Although it is impossible to obtain a precise solution to such clinically relevant problems, one can use a graphical approach to estimate the final pH. The Davenport diagram is the best such tool.

The Davenport Diagram Is a Graphical Tool for Interpreting Acid-Base Disturbances in Blood

We have already seen that doubling PCO_2 in the absence of other buffers causes pH to fall by 0.3. Reaching this conclusion was relatively straightforward because we needed to consider only one equilibrium. However, blood is a complex mixture that includes many non-HCO_3^- buffers. How do we approach a problem in which blood PCO_2 doubles? We simplify matters by lumping together the actions of all non-HCO_3^- buffers, so that $H^+ + B^{(n)} \rightleftharpoons HB^{(n+1)}$ represents the reactions of all non-HCO_3^- buffers. When we raise PCO_2, the newly formed H^+ can react with $B^{(n)}$ to form $HB^{(n+1)}$:

Equation 27–30

In this simplified approach, the final pH depends on two competing buffer reactions—one involving CO_2/HCO_3^-, and the other involving $HB^{(n+1)}$/$B^{(n)}$. Computing the final pH requires solving two simultaneous equations, each describing one of the equilibria.

The first equation that we must solve simultaneously describes the **CO_2/HCO_3^- buffer**, and is a rearrangement of the Henderson-Hasselbalch equation:

TABLE 27–5

RELATIONSHIP BETWEEN [HCO₃⁻] AND pH AT THREE FIXED LEVELS OF P$_{CO_2}$

pH	[HCO₃⁻] (mM)		
	P$_{CO_2}$ = 20 mm Hg	P$_{CO_2}$ = 40 mm Hg	P$_{CO_2}$ = 80 mm Hg
7.1	6 mM	12 mM	24 mM
7.2	8	15	30
7.3	10	19	38
7.4	12	**24**	48
7.5	15	30	60
7.6	19	38	76
7.7	24	48	96

Equation 27–31

$$[HCO_3^-] = s \cdot P_{CO_2} \cdot 10^{(pH - pK_{CO_2})}$$

For a P$_{CO_2}$ of 40 mm Hg, the equation requires that [HCO₃⁻] be 24 mM when pH is 7.40—as in normal arterial blood plasma. If pH decreases by 0.3 at this same P$_{CO_2}$, Equation 27–31 states that [HCO₃⁻] must fall by half to 12 mM. Conversely, if pH increases by 0.3, [HCO₃⁻] must double to 48 mM. The blue column of Table 27–5 lists the [HCO₃⁻] values that Equation 27–31 predicts for various pH values when P$_{CO_2}$ is 40 mm Hg. Plotting these [HCO₃⁻] values against pH yields the blue curve labeled "P$_{CO_2}$ = 40 mm Hg" in Figure 27–6A. This curve, which is known as a CO_2 isobar or **isopleth**, represents all possible combinations of [HCO₃⁻] and pH at a P$_{CO_2}$ of 40 mm Hg. Table 27–5 also summarizes [HCO₃⁻] values prevailing at P$_{CO_2}$ values of 20 and

80 mm Hg. Note that at a P$_{CO_2}$ of 20, representing respiratory alkalosis, [HCO₃⁻] values are half those for a P$_{CO_2}$ of 40 at the same pH. At a P$_{CO_2}$ of 80, representing respiratory acidosis, [HCO₃⁻] values are twice those at a P$_{CO_2}$ of 40. Each of the isopleths in Figure 27–6A rises exponentially with pH. The slope of an isopleth also rises exponentially with pH, and represents β_{open} for CO_2/HCO₃⁻. At a particular pH, the slope of the isopleth is steeper for a higher P$_{CO_2}$ (i.e., a higher [HCO₃⁻]), as Equation 27–22 predicts.

The second of the two equations that we must solve simultaneously describes the lumped reaction of all **non-HCO₃⁻ buffers**. This equation describes a line whose slope is the negative of $\beta_{non-HCO_3^-}$. In Figure 27–6A, this red non-HCO₃⁻ buffer line (representing $\beta_{non-HCO_3^-}$ for whole blood, 25 mM/pH unit) intersects with the CO_2 isopleth for a P$_{CO_2}$ of 40 at the point labeled *Start*, which represents the initial conditions for arterial blood. At this intersection, both CO_2/HCO₃⁻ and non-HCO₃⁻ buffers are simultaneously in equilibrium.

We are now in a position to answer the question raised at the beginning of this section: What will be the final pH when we increase the P$_{CO_2}$ of whole blood from 40 to 80 mm Hg? The final equilibrium conditions for this case of *respiratory acidosis* must be described by a point that lies simultaneously on the non-HCO₃⁻ buffer line and the isopleth for 80 mm Hg. Obtaining the answer using the Davenport diagram requires a three-step process:

Step 1: Identify the point at the intersection of the initial P$_{CO_2}$ isopleth and the initial non-HCO₃ buffer line (Figure 27–6A, *Start*).

Step 2: Identify the isopleth describing the *final* P$_{CO_2}$ (80 mm Hg in this case).

Step 3: Follow the non-HCO₃⁻ buffer line to its intersection with the final P$_{CO_2}$ isopleth. In Figure 27–6A, this intersection occurs at point A, which

FIGURE 27–6. Davenport diagram. In *A*, the *red arrow* represents the transition from a normal acid-base status ("Start") for blood to respiratory acidosis (*point A*) produced by raising P$_{CO_2}$ to 80 mm Hg. *Point B* represents respiratory alkalosis produced by lowering P$_{CO_2}$ to 20 mm Hg. In *B*, the labeled points represent the results of respiratory acidosis when the non-HCO₃⁻ buffering power ($\beta_{non-HCO_3^-}$) is zero (*point A₁*), 25 mM/pH (*point A*) and infinity (*point A₂*).

TABLE 27–6

RELATIONSHIP BETWEEN NON-HCO_3^- BUFFERING POWER, AND THE AMOUNT OF HCO_3^- FORMED IN RESPONSE TO A DOUBLING OF P_{CO_2}					
NON-HCO_3^- BUFFERING POWER	ΔpH	HCO_3^- FORMED (mM)	FRACTIONAL $\Delta[H^+]$	FRACTIONAL $\Delta[HCO_3^-]$	FRACTIONAL $\Delta[HCO_3^-] \times \Delta[H^+]$
0	-0.30	0.000,040	1.999,997	1.000,002	2.00
25	-0.21	5.25	1.71	1.17	2.00
∞	0	24.0	1.00	2.00	2.00

corresponds to a pH of 7.19 and an $[HCO_3^-]$ of 29.25 mM.

As discussed earlier, in the *absence* of non-HCO_3^- buffers, this same doubling of P_{CO_2} causes a larger pH decrease, from 7.4 to 7.1.

By following three similar steps, we can use the Davenport diagram to predict the final pH and $[HCO_3^-]$ under conditions of a *respiratory alkalosis*. For example, what would be the effect of decreasing P_{CO_2} by half, from 40 to 20 mm Hg? Follow the non-HCO_3^- buffer line from *Start* to its intersection with the gold-colored isopleth for a P_{CO_2} of 20 mm Hg (point *B*), which corresponds to a pH of 7.60 and an $[HCO_3^-]$ of 19 mM. If the solution had *not* contained non-HCO_3^- buffers, halving the P_{CO_2} would have caused a larger pH increase, from 7.4 to 7.7.

The Amount of HCO_3^- Formed or Consumed During "Respiratory" Acid-Base Disturbances Increases with the Non-HCO_3^- Buffering Power

Although it is reasonable to focus on CO_2 during respiratory acid-base disturbances, it would be wrong to assume that $[HCO_3^-]$ is constant. For example, in Figure 27–6A, where $\beta_{\text{non-HCO}_3^-}$ is 25 mM/pH unit, increasing P_{CO_2} from 40 to 80 mm Hg causes $[HCO_3^-]$ to increase from 24 to 29.25 mM. Thus, in each liter of solution, 5.25 mmole CO_2 combines with 5.25 mmole H_2O to form 5.25 mmole HCO_3^- (which we see as the $\Delta[HCO_3^-]$ value between *Start* and *A*) and 5.25 mmole H^+. Nearly all of this H^+ disappears as nearly 5.25 mmole of the deprotonated non-HCO_3^- buffers ($B^{(n)}$) consumes H^+ to form nearly 5.25 mmole of their conjugate weak acids ($HB^{(n+1)}$). Thus, the flux through the reaction sequence in Equation 27–30 is nearly 5.25 mmole in each liter of solution.

Equation 27–32

Thus, the non-HCO_3^- buffers drive the conversion of CO_2 to HCO_3^-: These buffers minimize the increase in free $[H^+]$ that a given flux of CO_2 can produce. Thus, with a high $\beta_{\text{non-HCO}_3^-}$, a large amount of CO_2 must "flux" through Equation 27–32 before the free concentrations of HCO_3^- and H^+ rise sufficiently to satisfy the CO_2/HCO_3^- equilibrium (Equation 27–16).

Non-HCO_3^- buffering power varies with the hemoglobin content of blood. Thus, patients with anemia have a low $\beta_{\text{non-HCO}_3^-}$, whereas patients with polycythemia have a high $\beta_{\text{non-HCO}_3^-}$. Figure 27–6B illustrates the importance of $\beta_{\text{non-HCO}_3^-}$.

If $\beta_{\text{non-HCO}_3^-}$ is zero, the non-HCO_3^- buffer line is horizontal, and the Davenport diagram predicts that doubling P_{CO_2} from 40 to 80 mm Hg should not change $[HCO_3^-]$ significantly (Fig. 27–6B, point A_1), verifying our earlier conclusion (see Fig. 27–5, stage 3A). Simultaneously, pH falls by 0.3, which corresponds to a near-doubling of $[H^+]$. Thus, doubling $[CO_2]$ leads to a doubling of the product $[HCO_3^-] \cdot [H^+]$, so that the ratio $[HCO_3^-][H^+]/[CO_2]$—the equilibrium constant, K—is unchanged (Table 27–6, top row). Figure 27–6B also shows what happens if $\beta_{\text{non-HCO}_3^-}$ has the normal value of 25 mM/pH unit. Here, point *A* is the same as *A* in Figure 27–6A, and it shows that $[HCO_3^-]$ increases by 5.25 mM, or 17% (see Table 27–6, middle row). Finally, if $\beta_{\text{non-HCO}_3^-}$ were ∞, the non-HCO_3^- buffer line would be vertical. Thus, doubling P_{CO_2} would not change pH at all (point A_2 in Fig. 27–6B). In this case, $[HCO_3^-]$ would double, so that the doubling of the product $[HCO_3^-] \cdot [H^+]$ would match the doubling of P_{CO_2} (see Table 27–6, bottom row).

Adding or Removing an Acid or Base—at a Constant P_{CO_2}—Produces a "Metabolic" Acid-Base Disturbance

Earlier, we examined the effect of adding HCl in the *absence* of other buffers (see Fig. 27–3). Predicting the pH change for such an acid-base disturbance was straightforward, because the titration of HCO_3^- to CO_2 consumed all buffered H^+. However, the situation is more complex when the solution also contains non-HCO_3^- buffers (Fig. 27–7, stage 1). When we add 10 mmoles of HCl to 1 liter of solution, the open-system CO_2/HCO_3^- buffer pair neutralizes most of the added H^+, non-HCO_3^- buffers handle some, and a minute amount of added H^+ remains free and lowers pH (see Fig. 27–7, stage 2A). Because the

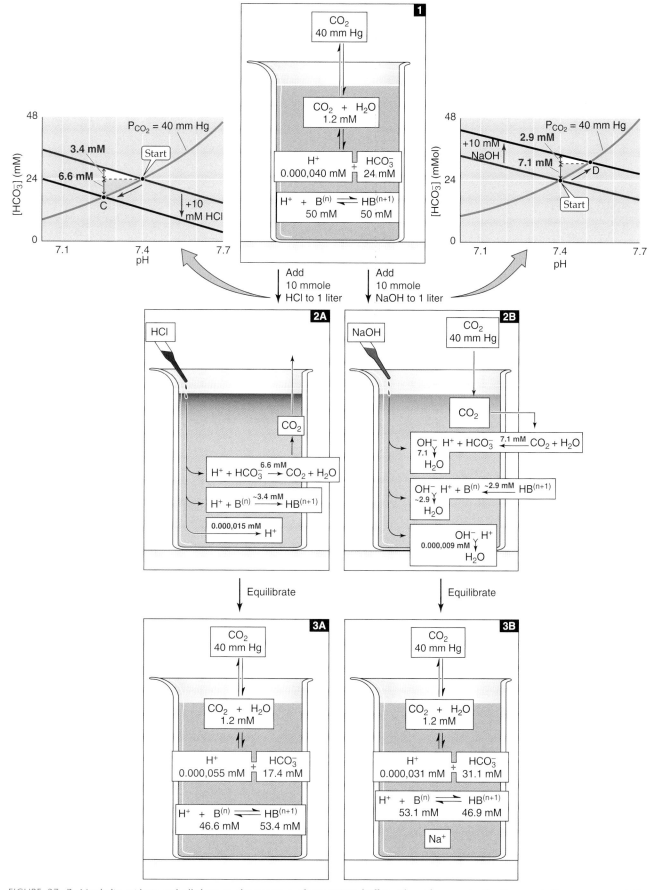

FIGURE 27–7. Metabolic acidosis and alkalosis in the presence of non-HCO_3^- buffers. The red arrows in the Davenport diagrams represent the transition to metabolic acidosis (point *C*) and metabolic alkalosis (point *D*). This example differs from Figure 27–3, in which the solution contained no buffers other than CO_2/HCO_3^-.

TABLE 27–7

BUFFERING PRODUCED BY CO_2/HCO_3^- AND NON-HCO_3^- BUFFERS*						
ADDITION	**ΔpH**	**$\Delta[HCO_3^-]$**	$\beta_{open} = \dfrac{\Delta[HCO_3^-]}{\Delta pH}$	**$\Delta[B^{(n)}]$**	$\beta_{non\text{-}HCO_3^-} = \dfrac{\Delta[B^{(n)}]}{\Delta pH}$	**β_{Total}**
+10 mmole H^+	~−0.14	~6.6 mM	47 mM/pH unit	~3.4 mM	25 mM/pH unit	72 mM/pH
+10 mmole OH^-	~+0.11	~7.1 mM	65 mM/pH unit	~2.9 mM	25 mM/pH unit	89 mM/pH

*The "additions" are made to 1 liter of solution. Initial pH = 7.40, P_{CO_2} = 40 mm Hg, $[HCO_3^-]$ = 24 mM. $\beta_{non\text{-}HCO_3^-}$ assumed to be 25 mM/pH unit.

system is open, the CO_2 formed during buffering of the added H^+ escapes to the atmosphere. If this buffering reaction were occurring in the blood, the newly formed CO_2 would escape first into the alveolar air, and then into the atmosphere.

How much of the added H^+ (Δ[Strong Acid] = 10 mM) follows each of the three pathways in this example of *metabolic acidosis*? Answering this question requires dealing with two competing equilibria, the CO_2/HCO_3^- and the non-HCO_3^- buffering reactions. As for respiratory acid-base disturbances, we cannot precisely solve the equations governing metabolic acid-base disturbances. However, we can use the Davenport diagram on the *left* of Figure 27–7 to obtain a graphical estimate of the final pH and $[HCO_3^-]$ through a three-step process:

Step 1: Identify the point describing the initial conditions (Fig. 27–7, *Start, graph on left*).
Step 2: Generate a new non-HCO_3^- buffer line, parallel to the initial one, but displaced downward (in the direction of decreased $[HCO_3^-]$) by 10 mM—the concentration of added H^+.
Step 3: Follow the original P_{CO_2} isopleth to its intersection with the newly created non-HCO_3^- buffer line. In Figure 27–7, *left*, this intersection occurs at point C, which corresponds to a pH of 7.26 and an $[HCO_3^-]$ of 17.4 mM.

We now can return to the question of how much of the added H^+ follows each of the three pathways in Figure 27–7, *stage 2A*. Because $[HCO_3^-]$ decreased by 24 − 17.4 = 6.6 mM, the amount of H^+ buffered by CO_2/HCO_3^- must have been 6.6 mmole in each liter. Almost all of the remaining H^+ that we added, nearly 3.6 mmole, must have been buffered by non-HCO_3^- buffers. A tiny amount of the added H^+, approximately 0.000,015 mmole, must have remained unbuffered, and was responsible for decreasing pH from 7.40 to 7.26 (see Fig. 27–7, *stage 3A*).

Figure 27–7 also shows what would happen if we added 10 mmole of a strong base such as NaOH to our 1-liter solution. The open-system CO_2/HCO_3^- buffer pair neutralizes most of the added OH^-, non-HCO_3^- buffers handle some, and a minute amount of added OH^- remains unbuffered, thus raising pH (see Fig. 27–7, *stage 2B*). The Davenport diagram on the *right* of Figure 27–7 shows how much of the added OH^- follows each of the three pathways in this example of *metabolic alkalosis*. The approach is similar to the one we used earlier for metabolic acidosis, except that in this case, we generate a new

non-HCO_3^- buffer line that is displaced 10 mM *above* the original one. We follow the P_{CO_2} isopleth to its intersection with the new non-HCO_3^- buffer line at point D, which corresponds to a final pH of 7.51, and an $[HCO_3^-]$ of 31.1 mM. Thus, $[HCO_3^-]$ rose by 31.1 − 24.0 = 7.1 mM. This is the amount of added OH^- that CO_2/HCO_3^- buffered. Non-HCO_3^- buffers must have buffered almost all of the remaining OH^- that we added, approximately 2.9 mmole in each liter. The unbuffered OH^-, which was responsible for the pH increase, must have been in the nanomolar range (see Fig. 27–7, *stage 3B*).

During Metabolic Disturbances, CO_2/HCO_3^- Makes a Greater Contribution to Total Buffering When pH and P_{CO_2} Are High, and When $\beta_{non\text{-}HCO_3^-}$ Is Low

In Figure 27–7, CO_2/HCO_3^- neutralized 7.1 mmole of the 10 mmole of OH^- added to 1 liter ($\Delta pH = +0.11$), but only 6.6 mmole of the added 10 mmole H^+ ($\Delta pH = -0.14$). The reason for this difference is that the buffering power of CO_2/HCO_3^- in an open system increases exponentially with pH (see Fig. 27–4, *blue curve*). In the Davenport diagram, this pH dependence of β_{open} appears as the slope of the CO_2 isopleth, which increases exponentially with pH. *Thus, adding alkali will always cause a smaller pH change than adding an equivalent amount of acid.* In our example of metabolic alkalosis, the mean β_{open} is (7.1 mM)/(0.11 pH unit) = 65 mM/pH unit in the pH range 7.40 to 7.51 (Table 27–7). On the other hand, in the pH range 7.26 to 7.40, the mean β_{open} is (6.6 mM)/(0.14 pH unit) = 47 mM/pH unit, substantially less than in the more alkaline range. Because $\beta_{non\text{-}HCO_3^-}$ is 25 mM/pH unit over the entire pH range, β_{total} is greater in the alkaline pH range.

We have already seen that β_{open} is proportional to $[HCO_3^-]$ (Equation 27–22), and that—at a fixed pH—$[HCO_3^-]$ is proportional to P_{CO_2} (Equation 27–31). Thus, other things being equal, the contribution of β_{open} to total buffering increases with P_{CO_2}. Patients with a high P_{CO_2} due to respiratory failure will, therefore, have a higher buffering power than normal individuals at the same pH.

Because CO_2/HCO_3^- and non-HCO_3^- buffers compete for added OH^- or H^+, the contribution of CO_2/HCO_3^- to total buffering also depends on $\beta_{non\text{-}HCO_3^-}$. Figure 27–8 illustrates the effects of adding 10 mmole NaOH to our standard 1-liter CO_2/HCO_3^- solution at $\beta_{non\text{-}HCO_3^-}$ values of 0, 25 mM/pH unit, and ∞. We discussed the comparable

A NON-HCO$_3^-$ BUFFERING POWER OF ZERO

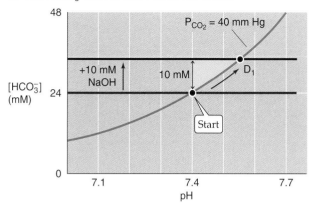

B NON-HCO$_3^-$ BUFFERING POWER OF 25 mM/pH unit

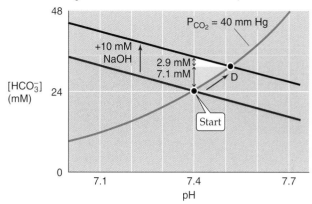

C NON-HCO$_3^-$ BUFFERING POWER OF INFINITY

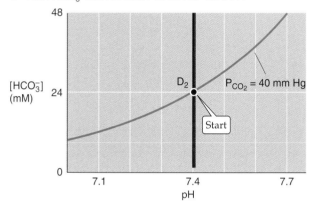

FIGURE 27–8. The effect of non-HCO$_3^-$ buffering power on the pH increase caused by metabolic alkalosis.

examples for *respiratory* acidosis in Figure 27–6B and their implications for patients with altered hemoglobin levels. We also noted in Figure 27–3 (*Stage 3B*) that adding 10 mmole NaOH to a 1-liter solution containing CO_2/HCO$_3^-$ but no other buffers causes [HCO$_3^-$] to increase from 24 to 34 mM, and pH to increase from 7.40 to 7.55. To use a Davenport diagram to solve the same problem (see Fig. 27–8A), we generate a pair of non-HCO$_3^-$ buffering lines with slopes of zero—one through the *Start* point and a "new" one displaced 10 mM higher. Following the blue P_{CO_2} = 40 isopleth from *Start* to the point where the isopleth intersects with the new non-HCO$_3^-$ buffer line at point D_1, we see that—as expected—the final pH is 7.55 and the final [HCO$_3^-$] is 34 mM. Thus, CO_2/HCO$_3^-$ must buffer virtually all 10 mmole of OH$^-$ added to 1 liter. Because the total buffering power is simply β_{open}, the pH increase must be rather large, 0.15.

When $\beta_{non\text{-}HCO_3^-}$ is 25 mM/pH unit, as in the Davenport diagram on the *upper right panel* of Figure 27–7 (replotted in Fig. 27–8B), CO_2/HCO$_3^-$ can buffer only 7.1 mmole because other buffers neutralize 2.9 mmole. With the increased total buffering power, the pH increase is only 0.11.

Finally, when $\beta_{non\text{-}HCO_3^-}$ is ∞, the new, vertical non-HCO$_3^-$ buffer line lies right on top of the original (see Fig. 27–8C). Thus, neither [HCO$_3^-$] nor pH changes at all. However, [B$^{(n)}$] increases by 10 mM because the infinitely powerful non-HCO$_3^-$ buffers do all of the buffering.

A Metabolic Change Can Compensate for a Respiratory Disturbance

Thus far, we have considered what happens during *primary* respiratory and metabolic acid-base disturbances. When challenged by such acid or alkaline loads in the blood plasma, the body **compensates** by altering [HCO$_3^-$] or P_{CO_2}, returning pH toward its initial value and minimizing the magnitude of the overall pH change.

Let us revisit the example in Figure 27–6A (replotted in Fig. 27–9A), wherein we produced a primary respiratory acidosis by increasing P_{CO_2} from 40 to 80 mm Hg. The arrow in Figure 27–9A between *Start* and point A (pH 7.19) represents the respiratory acidosis. The only way we can restore pH toward its initial value of 7.40 is to add an alkali (e.g., HCO$_3^-$ or OH$^-$) or remove an acid (e.g., H$^+$), all of which are equivalent. Adding 10 mmole of OH$^-$ to 1 liter, for example, would superimpose a metabolic *alkalosis* on the primary respiratory *acidosis*, and thereby produce a **metabolic compensation to respiratory acidosis.**

We can use a Davenport diagram to predict the consequences of adding 10 mmole of OH$^-$ to 1 liter. Starting at point A, we generate a new non-HCO$_3^-$ buffer line with the same slope as the original, but displaced upward by 10 mM. Point A_1, at the intersection between this new non-HCO$_3^-$ buffer line and the P_{CO_2} isopleth for 80 mm Hg, represents a final pH of 7.29, still lower than the

FIGURE 27–9. Metabolic compensation to primary respiratory acid-base disturbances.

normal 7.40, but much higher than the 7.19 prevailing before compensation. If we instead add 24 mmole of OH^- to 1 liter, pH returns to exactly its initial value of 7.40 (point A_2 in Fig. 27–9A). In other words, we can compensate for doubling P_{CO_2} from 40 to 80 mm Hg by shifting the non-HCO_3^- buffer line up by 24 mM, which doubles $[HCO_3^-]$ from its value at *Start*. *Perfect* compensation of respiratory acidosis is an example of **isohydric hypercapnia** (i.e., *same* pH at a *higher* P_{CO_2}):

Equation 27–33

$$pH = 6.1 + \log \frac{\overbrace{48 \text{ mM}}^{\text{Doubled } [HCO_3^-]}}{(0.03 \text{ mM/mm Hg}) \times \underbrace{80 \text{ mm Hg}}_{\text{Doubled } P_{CO_2}}} = 7.4$$

Table 27–4 lists some common causes of respiratory acidosis in humans. To produce a metabolic compensation, the kidneys respond to high P_{CO_2} or low blood pH by increasing acid secretion into the urine (p. 856). The net effect is to increase plasma $[HCO_3^-]$ and raise pH. The renal compensation to respiratory acidosis generally is not perfect, so that pH remains below the normal value of 7.40.

The kidneys can also perform a **metabolic compensation to a respiratory alkalosis**. We again revisit Figure 27–6A, but now replotted in Figure 27–9B, for the example of a primary respiratory alkalosis produced by decreasing P_{CO_2} from 40 to 20 mm Hg. In Figure 27–9B, we represent this disturbance by the transition from *Start* to point B (pH 7.60). We can partially compensate for this respiratory alkalosis by adding 10 mmole of HCl to each liter of solution, or by removing 10 mmole $NaHCO_3$ or NaOH, all of which produce the same effect. Starting at point B, we generate a new non-HCO_3^- buffer line parallel to the original one, but displaced downward by 10 mM. Point B_1 (pH 7.44), at the intersection of this

new non-HCO_3^- buffer line with the P_{CO_2} isopleth for 20 mm Hg, represents a partial compensation.

We could achieve a perfect compensation by adding a total of 12 mmole of HCl to each liter, represented by point B_2 (pH 7.40). Why is this amount so much less than the 24 mmole of NaOH that we added to each liter to compensate perfectly for a *doubling* of P_{CO_2}? When we double P_{CO_2}, perfect compensation requires doubling $[HCO_3^-]$ from its normal value of 24 to 48, whereas when we halve P_{CO_2}, we need only to add enough HCl to halve $[HCO_3^-]$ from its normal value of 24 to 12 mM.

Table 27–4 lists some common causes of respiratory alkalosis in humans. In response to a primary respiratory alkalosis, the kidneys secrete less acid into the urine (p. 857). The net effect is a decrease in plasma $[HCO_3^-]$, a compensatory metabolic acidosis.

A Respiratory Change Can Compensate for a Metabolic Disturbance

Just as metabolic changes can compensate for respiratory disturbances, respiratory changes can compensate for metabolic ones. Let us return to the example on the *left* of Figure 27–7 (replotted in Fig. 27–10A), where we added 10 mmole of HCl to 1 liter of normal arterial blood plasma. In Figure 27–10A, we represent this metabolic acidosis by creating a new non-HCO_3^- buffer line 10 mM below the original one, and following the P_{CO_2} isopleth for 40 mm Hg from *Start* until it intersects with the new buffer line at point C (pH 7.26). We can counteract the acid-base disturbance by reducing P_{CO_2}, a **respiratory compensation to a metabolic acidosis**. What happens when we reduce P_{CO_2} from 40 to, say, 35 mm Hg? Starting at C, follow the new non-HCO_3^- buffer line from the P_{CO_2} isopleth for 40 mm Hg to point C_1 on the new isopleth for 35 mm Hg. This respiratory alkalosis brings pH to 7.30, and represents a *partial* compensation.

A RESPIRATORY COMPENSATION TO METABOLIC ACIDOSIS

B RESPIRATORY COMPENSATION TO METABOLIC ALKALOSIS

FIGURE 27–10. Respiratory compensation to primary metabolic acid-base disturbances.

If we instead reduce P_{CO_2} to 23 mm Hg, we produce a perfect compensation, which we represent in Figure 27–10A by moving along the new non-HCO_3^- buffer line from C until we reach pH 7.40 at point C_2, which is on the P_{CO_2} isopleth for 23 mm Hg. Note that with perfect compensation, we reduce P_{CO_2} by the same fraction that we had originally reduced $[HCO_3^-]$.

Table 27–4 lists some causes of primary metabolic acidosis in humans. The low plasma pH or $[HCO_3^-]$ stimulates the peripheral chemoreceptors (p. 723) and, if sufficiently long-standing, also the central chemoreceptors (p. 726). The result is an increase in alveolar ventilation, which lowers P_{CO_2}, and thus provides the respiratory compensation.

The body achieves a **respiratory compensation to a primary metabolic alkalosis** in just the opposite manner. We revisit the right side of Figure 27–7, but now replotted in Figure 27–10B, for the example of a primary metabolic alkalosis caused by adding 10 mmole of NaOH to 1 liter. In Figure 27–10B, we represent this primary acid-base disturbance by point D (pH 7.51). If we now increase P_{CO_2} from 40 to 45 mm Hg, we partially compensate for the metabolic alkalosis by moving from D to D_1 (pH 7.48). If we instead raise P_{CO_2} to 57 mm Hg, the compensation is perfect, and pH returns to 7.40 (D_2).

Table 27–4 lists causes of metabolic alkalosis in humans. The compensatory response is to decrease alveolar ventilation and thereby raise P_{CO_2}. However, compensatory respiratory acidosis in response to a primary metabolic alkalosis is the least complete of the four types of compensation we have discussed. The reason is that one can decrease alveolar ventilation—and oxygenation—only so far before compromising one's very existence.

In a real person, each of the four primary acid-base disturbances—points A, B, C, and D in Figure 27–9 and Figure 27–10—occurs in the extracellular fluid. In each case, the body's first and almost instantaneous response is to use extracellular buffers to neutralize part of the acid or alkaline load. In addition, cells rapidly take up some of the acid or alkaline load, and thus participate in the buffering, as discussed later. Furthermore, renal-tubule cells may respond to a *metabolic* acidosis (e.g., diabetic ketoacidosis) or alkalosis (e.g., vomiting). Thus, points C and D include the effects of actual acid or alkaline load, extracellular and intracellular buffering, and any renal (i.e., "metabolic") response.

Position on a Davenport Diagram Defines the Nature of an Acid-Base Disturbance

The only tools needed for characterizing acid-base status (i.e., pH, $[HCO_3^-]$, and P_{CO_2}) are a Davenport diagram and electrodes for measuring pH and P_{CO_2}. From these last two parameters, we can compute $[HCO_3^-]$ from the Henderson-Hasselbalch equation. The acid-base status of blood plasma—or of any aqueous solution—must fall into one of five major categories:

1. **Normal.** For arterial blood, pH is 7.40, $[P_{CO_2}]$ is 24 mM, and P_{CO_2} is 40 mm Hg. This point was *Start* in the previous figures, and is the central point in Figure 27–11A to D.
2. **One of the four primary (or uncompensated) acid-base disturbances**. If the coordinates for pH and $[HCO_3^-]$ are on the original non-HCO_3^- buffer line, but off the 40–mm Hg isopleth, then the disturbance must be an uncompensated respiratory acidosis (point A, Fig. 27–11A) or alkalosis (point B). On the other hand, if the coordinates fall on the 40–mm Hg isopleth, but off the original non-HCO_3^- buffer line, the disturbance must be an uncompensated metabolic acidosis (point C) or alkalosis (point D).
3. **A partially compensated disturbance.** The coordinates for pH and $[HCO_3^-]$ fall in any of the four colored regions of Figure 27–11B. For example, point A_1 in the blue region represents a partially compensated respiratory acidosis. In a subject for whom a respiratory acidosis has existed for longer than a few

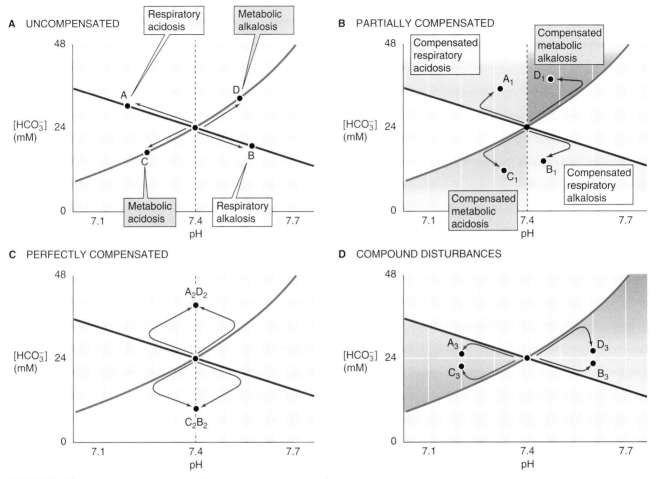

FIGURE 27–11. Acid-base states represented by position on a Davenport diagram.

hours, it is likely that increased renal H^+ excretion has already begun producing a metabolic compensation. Thus, depending on the extent of the original acidosis and the degree to which the compensation has had time to develop, point A_1 could lie anywhere in the blue region. The same is true for the other three disturbances/compensations.

4. **A perfectly compensated disturbance.** The point falls on the vertical line through pH 7.4. As indicated by point A_2D_2 in Figure 27–11C, a perfect compensation following respiratory acidosis is indistinguishable from that following metabolic alkalosis. In either case, the final outcome is isohydric hypercapnia. Similarly, point B_2C_2 represents a perfect compensation from either metabolic acidosis or respiratory alkalosis (isohydric hypocapnia).

5. **A compound respiratory/metabolic disturbance.** The point falls in one of the two colored regions in Figure 27–11D. For example, points A_3 and C_3 represent a respiratory acidosis complicated by metabolic acidosis, or vice versa. The second disturbance causes the pH to move even further away from "normal," as might occur in an individual with both respiratory and renal failure (see Table 27–4). Of course, it is impossible to determine if one of the two compounding disturbances developed before the other.

pH REGULATION OF INTRACELLULAR FLUID

Clinicians focus on the acid-base status of blood plasma, the fluid compartment whose acid-base status is easiest to assess. However, the number of biochemical reactions and other processes that occur *outside* a cell pales in comparison to the number of those that occur *inside*. It stands to reason that the most important biologic fluid for pH regulation is the cytosol. It is possible to monitor intracellular pH (pH_i) continuously in isolated cells and tissues using pH-sensitive dyes or microelectrodes. Moreover, using magnetic resonance techniques, one can monitor pH_i in living humans (e.g., skeletal muscle). The pH of cells both influences, and is influenced by, extracellular pH.

Ion Transporters at the Plasma Membrane Closely Regulate the pH Inside of Cells

Figure 27–12A shows a cell with two acid-base transporters, a Na-H exchanger and a Cl-HCO$_3$ exchanger. We will use the Na-H exchanger (p. 68) as a prototypic example of an **acid extruder**, a transporter that tends to make intracellular pH (pH_i) increase. The Na-H exchanger is a secondary active transporter that uses the energy of the Na^+ gradient to move H^+ out of the cell. We will

A RESPONSE TO
METABOLIC ACIDOSIS

B RECORD OF INTRACELLULAR pH

C pH$_i$ DEPENDENCE OF ACID EXTRUDERS

D RESPONSE TO
METABOLIC ALKALOSIS

E RECORD OF INTRACELLULAR pH

F pH$_i$ DEPENDENCE OF ACID LOADERS

FIGURE 27–12. Recovery of a cell from intracellular acid and alkali loads.

take the Cl-HCO$_3$ exchanger (p. 69) as the prototypic example of an **acid loader**. This exchanger, driven by the steep out-to-in Cl$^-$ gradient, moves HCO$_3^-$ out of the cell. In Chapter 3, we discussed other acid extruders and acid loaders that help regulate pH$_i$. The intracellular acid loading produced by Cl-HCO$_3$ exchange is an example of a **chronic acid load**; it tends to acidify the cell as long as the transporter is active. In the normal steady state, the chronic acid-extruding effect of Na-H exchange balances the chronic acid-loading effect of Cl-HCO$_3$ exchange.

Imagine that we use a micropipette to inject HCl into this cell (Fig. 27–12A). This injection of an **acute acid load**—a one-time-only introduction of a fixed quantity of acid—causes an immediate fall in pH$_i$ (Fig. 27–12B, *black curve*), an example of **intracellular metabolic acidosis**. If we add HCl to a beaker, the pH remains low indefinitely. However, when we acutely acid-load a cell, pH$_i$ spontaneously recovers to the initial value. The pH$_i$

recovery from an acid load cannot be due to passive H$^+$ efflux out of the cell, inasmuch as the electrochemical gradient for H$^+$ (p. 72) usually favors H$^+$ influx. Hence, the pH$_i$ recovery must reflect one or more active transport processes that extrude acid from the cell. This pH$_i$ recovery is thus a *metabolic compensation to a metabolic acid load*.

During the recovery of pH$_i$ from the acid load in Figure 27–12B, the Na-H exchanger not only must extrude the quantity of H$^+$ previously injected into the cell (the *acute* acid load), it also must counteract whatever acid loading the Cl-HCO$_3$ exchanger continues to impose on the cell (the *chronic* acid load).

Acid-extrusion rates are greatest at low pH$_i$ values, and they fall off as pH$_i$ approaches its resting value, as shown for Na-H exchanger by the *black curve* in Figure 27–12C. As discussed later, low pH$_i$ also *inhibits* Cl-HCO$_3$ exchange and thus acid loading. The response to low pH$_i$

A RESPONSE OF CELL   **B** TIME COURSE OF pH CHANGES

FIGURE 27–13. Response of cell to extracellular respiratory acidosis. In *A*, respiratory acidosis sends conflicting messages to the acid-base transporters. The rise in [CO_2] leads to a fall in intracellular pH (pH_i), which stimulates the Na-H exchanger but inhibits the Cl-HCO_3 exchanger—tending to cause pH_i to recover. However, the low extracellular pH (pH_o) directly inhibits the Na-H exchanger but stimulates the Cl-HCO_3 exchanger. In *B*, the low pH_o initially hampers the ability of the cell to recover from the acid load. The delayed recovery of pH_o, through its effects on the transporters, leads to an additional recovery of pH_i as well.

therefore involves two feedback loops controlled in a push-pull fashion, so that low pH_i both stimulates acid extrusion and inhibits acid loading.

In addition to pH_i, hormones, growth factors, oncogenes, cell volume, and extracellular pH (pH_o) all can modulate these transporters. For acid-base physiology, the pH_o effect is especially important. In general, a low pH_o slows the rate of pH_i recovery from acute acid loads and reduces the final steady-state pH_i (see Fig. 27–12*B*, *red curve*), whereas a high pH_o does the opposite (*blue curve*). The underlying cause of these pH_o effects is a shift of the pH_i dependence of acid extrusion (see Fig. 27–12*C*, *red* and *blue curves*) and, as we shall see, changes in acid loading.

Cells also spontaneously recover from acute alkaline loads. If we inject a cell with potassium hydroxide (KOH) (see Fig. 27–12*D*), pH_i rapidly increases but then slowly recovers to its initial value (see Fig. 27–12*E*, *black curve*), reflecting stimulation of acid loading and inhibition of acid extrusion. The injection of OH^- represents a metabolic alkalosis, whereas increased Cl-HCO_3 exchange represents a metabolic compensation. The Cl-HCO_3 exchanger is most active at high pH_i values (see Fig. 27–12*F*). As discussed previously, increases in pH_i generally inhibit acid extruders. Thus, the response to alkaline loads—like the response to acid loads—includes dual feedback loops controlled in a push-pull fashion. Here, alkalinization both stimulates acid loading and inhibits acid extrusion. During the pH_i recovery from an acute

alkaline load, Cl-HCO_3 exchange not only must neutralize the alkali previously injected into the cell (the acute alkali load), but also must counteract the alkalinizing effect of acid extruders such as the Na-H exchanger.

Like the Na-H exchanger, the Cl-HCO_3 exchanger is under the control of hormones and growth factors. It also probably has a pH_o sensitivity that is opposite to that of the acid extruders, with low pH_o enhancing Cl-HCO_3 exchange. We would expect that extracellular metabolic acidosis, with its simultaneous fall in *both* pH_o and [HCO_3^-]$_o$ (see Table 27–4), should stimulate Cl-HCO_3 exchange.

Indirect Interactions Between K^+ and H^+ Make It Appear As If Cells Have a K-H Exchanger

Clinicians have long known that extracellular acidosis leads to a release of K^+ from cells, and thus hyperkalemia. Conversely, hyperkalemia leads to the exit of H^+ from cells, resulting in extracellular acidosis. These observations, which one can duplicate at the level of single cells, led to the suggestion that cells generally have a K-H exchanger. It is true that specialized cells in the stomach (p. 894) and kidney (p. 853) do have an ATP-driven pump that extrudes H^+ in exchange for K^+. Moreover, the K/HCO_3 cotransporter described in certain cells could, in some ways, mimic a K-H exchanger. Nevertheless, the effects that long ago led to the K-H−exchange hypothesis probably reflect indirect interactions of H^+ and K^+.

One example of apparent K-H exchange is that hyperkalemia causes an intracellular alkalosis. Not only is this effect *not* due to a 1:1 exchange of K^+ for H^+, it is not even due to the increase in $[K^+]_o$ per se. Instead, the high $[K^+]_o$ depolarizes the cell, and this positive shift in membrane voltage can promote the net uptake of HCO_3^- via the electrogenic Na/HCO_3 cotransporter (p. 67), and thus a rise in pH_i—a **depolarization-induced alkalinization**. In other cases, the depolarization indirectly stimulates other transporters that alkalinize the cell. We discuss the converse example of acidemia causing hyperkalemia on p. 816: Extracellular acidosis lowers pH_i and inhibits transporters responsible for K^+ uptake, leading to K^+ release from cells. Although we have no evidence that a K-H exchanger exists in humans, imagining that it exists is sometimes a helpful tool for quickly predicting interactions of H^+ and K^+ in a clinical setting.

Changes in Intracellular pH Are Often a Sign of Changes in Extracellular pH, and Vice Versa

Steady-state pH_i depends on the balance between specialized transporters that extrude acid (e.g., Na-H exchange) and others that load the cell with acid (e.g., Cl-HCO_3 exchange). By definition, acid extrusion equals acid loading in the steady state. Anything that disturbs this balance shifts pH_i. For example, an extracellular *metabolic* acidosis inhibits acid extrusion and stimulates acid loading, thus lowering steady-state pH_i. This intracellular acidosis is not instantaneous, but develops over several minutes. Conversely, an extracellular metabolic alkalosis leads to a slow increase in steady-state pH_i. Generally, a change in pH_o will shift pH_i in the same direction, but ΔpH_i is usually only 20% to 60% of ΔpH_o. In other words, an extracellular metabolic acidosis causes a net transfer of acid from the extracellular to the intracellular space, and an extracellular metabolic alkalosis has the opposite effect. An important side effect is that cells participate in buffering extracellular acid and alkali loads.

How would extracellular *respiratory* acidosis affect pH_i? The increase in extracellular $[CO_2]_{Dis}$ creates an inwardly directed gradient for CO_2. Because almost all cell membranes are highly permeable to CO_2, this dissolved gas rapidly enters the cell (see Fig. 27−13A) and produces HCO_3^- and H^+. The result is an **intracellular respiratory acidosis**, which manifests itself as a rapid fall in pH_i (see Fig. 27−13B, *lower panel*). Carbonic anhydrase (see box earlier) greatly accelerates the formation of HCO_3^- and H^+ from CO_2, so that pH_i can complete its decline in just a few seconds. To what extent the cell recovers from this acid load depends on the status of the cell's acid-extruding and acid-loading mechanisms. As shown in Fig. 27−12, the accompanying decrease in pH_o inhibits acid extrusion and stimulates acid loading. As a result, the cell's ability to recover from the acid load is severely impaired, and pH_i may recover only partially if at all.

In response to extracellular respiratory acidosis, the kidney upregulates acid-base transporters and thus stimulates urinary acid secretion (p. 856). The net effect is an extracellular metabolic compensation that causes pH_o to increase gradually. As pH_o rises, it gradually relieves the inhibition of Na-H exchange and other acid extruders, and cancels the stimulation of Cl-HCO_3 exchange and other acid loaders. Thus, *intracellular* pH recovers in parallel with *extracellular* pH, albeit by only 20% to 60% as much as pH_o (see Fig. 27−13B). The pH_i recovery represents an **intracellular metabolic compensation** to the intracellular respiratory acidosis.

Not all cell types have the same resting pH_i. Moreover, different cell types often have very different complements of acid-base transporters, and very different ways of regulating these transporters. Nevertheless, the example in Figure 27−13 illustrates that the fate of pH_i is closely intertwined with that of interstitial fluid, and thus blood plasma. During respiratory acid-base disturbances, the lungs generate the insult, and virtually every other cell in the body must defend itself against it. In the case of metabolic acid-base disturbances, however, some cells may generate the insult, whereas the others must attempt to defend themselves against it. From a teleologic point of view, one can imagine that the primary reason that the body regulates the pH of the blood plasma and extracellular fluids is to allow the cells to properly regulate their pH_i. The primary reason why the clinical assessment of blood acid-base parameters can be useful is that these parameters tend to parallel cellular acid-base status.

REFERENCES

Books and Reviews

Bevensee MO, Alper S, Aronson PS, Boron WF: Control of intracellular pH. In Seldin DW, Giebisch G (eds): The Kidney: Physiology and Pathophysiology, 3rd ed. Philadelphia, JB Lippincott, 2000, pp. 391−442.

Davenport HW: The ABC of Acid Base Chemistry, 6th ed. Chicago, University of Chicago Press, 1974.

Roos A, Boron WF: Intracellular pH. Physiol Rev 61:296−434, 1981.

Sly WS, Hu PY: Human carbonic anhydrases and carbonic anhydrase deficiencies. Annu Rev Biochem 64:375−401, 1995.

Busa WB, Nuccitelli R: Metabolic regulation via intracellular pH. Am J Physiol 246:R409−R438, 1984.

Wakabayashi S, Shigekawa M, Pouysségur J: Molecular physiology of vertebrate Na^+/H^+ exchangers. Physiol Rev 77:51−74, 1997.

Journal Articles

Boron WF, De Weer P: Intracellular pH transients in squid giant axons caused by CO_2, NH_3, and metabolic inhibitors. J Gen Physiol 67:91−112, 1976.

Sørensen SPL: Über die Messung und die Bedeutung der Wasserstoffionenkonzentration bei enzymatischen Prozessen. Biochem Z 21:131−200 and 201−304, 1909.

Thomas RC: The effect of carbon dioxide on the intracellular pH and buffering power of snail neurones. J Physiol 255:715−735, 1976.

Zhao J, Hogan EM, Bevensee MO, Boron WF: Out-of-equilibrium CO_2/HCO_3^- solutions and their use in characterizing a novel K/HCO_3 cotransporter. Nature 374:636−639, 1995.

CHAPTER 28

Transport of Oxygen and Carbon Dioxide in the Blood

Walter F. Boron

CARRIAGE OF O_2

The Amount of O_2 Dissolved in Blood Is Far Too Small to Meet the Metabolic Demands of the Body

Blood carries oxygen in two forms: More than 98% of the O_2 normally binds to hemoglobin within the erythrocytes (also known as red blood cells or RBCs); a tiny fraction physically dissolves in the aqueous phases of both blood plasma and the cytoplasm of blood cells (predominantly RBCs). What is the significance of the O_2 that is bound to hemoglobin?

Imagine that we expose a liter of blood plasma, initially free of O_2, to an atmosphere having the same P_{O_2} as alveolar air—100 mm Hg. Oxygen will move from the atmosphere to the plasma until an equilibrium is established, at which time the concentration of **dissolved O_2** ($[O_2]_{Dis}$) in the blood obeys **Henry's Law** (see box on p. 597):

Equation 28-1

$$[O_2]_{Dis} = kO_2 \cdot P_{O_2}$$

If we express P_{O_2} in mm Hg and $[O_2]_{Dis}$ in ml of O_2 gas (measured at standard temperature and pressure or STP) per 100 ml (or dl) of blood, then the **solubility** kO_2 is approximately 0.003 ml O_2 for each dl of blood and each mm Hg of O_2 partial pressure at 37°C. For arterial blood,

Equation 28-2

$$[O_2]_{Dis} = \frac{0.003 \text{ ml } O_2}{100 \text{ ml blood} \cdot \text{mm Hg}} \cdot 100 \text{ mm Hg}$$

$$= 0.3 \text{ ml } O_2/100 \text{ ml blood}$$

Is such an O_2-carrying capacity adequate for supplying O_2 to the systemic tissues? If these tissues could extract all the O_2 dissolved in arterial blood so that none remained in venous blood, and if cardiac output (p. 428) were 5000 ml/min, then—according to the Fick principle (p. 442)—the delivery of dissolved O_2 to the tissues would be:

Equation 28-3

$$\underbrace{\dot{V}_{O_2}}_{O_2 \text{ delivery}} = \underbrace{\frac{5000 \text{ ml blood}}{\text{min}}}_{\substack{\text{Blood} \\ \text{flow}}} \cdot \underbrace{\frac{0.3 \text{ ml } O_2}{100 \text{ ml}}}_{\substack{O_2 \text{ concentration} \\ \text{in plasma}}}$$

$$= 15 \text{ ml } O_2/\text{min}$$

A HEMOGLOBIN TETRAMER

C CONFORMATIONAL CHANGES WITH O_2 BINDING

F helix of Hb

B HEME

2
As the Fe^{2+} moves downward, it pulls the attached histidine and F helix downward as well, causing the Hb to switch from the tensed (T) to the relaxed (R) state.

His
His

0.6Å

Heme

Heme ring Fe^{2+}

1
When O_2 binds to the Fe^{2+}, the heme changes from a dome-like to a planar conformation, pulling the Fe^{2+} downward.

O_2

Fe^{++}

Figure 28–1. The structure of hemoglobin.

However, the average 70-kg human at rest consumes O_2 at the rate of approximately 250 ml/min. Dissolved O_2 could supply the body's metabolic demands only if cardiac output increased by a factor of 250/15, or nearly 17-fold! Thus, the body cannot rely on dissolved O_2 as a mechanism for O_2 carriage.

Hemoglobin Consists of Two α and Two β Subunits, Each of Which Has an Iron-Containing "Heme" and a Polypeptide "Globin"

Normal adult **hemoglobin** (Hb) is a tetramer having a molecular weight of approximately 68 kDa, each monomer consisting of a heme and a globin (Fig. 28–1A). The heme is a porphyrin compound coordinated to a single iron atom. The globin is a polypeptide, either an α chain (141 amino acids) or a β chain (146 amino acids). The homology between the α and β chains is sufficient that they have similar conformations, a series of seven helices enveloping a single heme. Thus, the complete Hb molecule has the stoichiometry $[\alpha \ (Heme)]_2 \ [\beta \ (Heme)]_2$ and can bind as many as four O_2 molecules, one for each iron atom. The erythrocyte-precursor cells that synthesize Hb closely coordinate the production of α chains, β chains, and heme.

Heme is a general term for a metal ion chelated to a porphyrin ring. In the case of hemoglobin, the metal is iron in the Fe^{2+} or ferrous state (see Fig. 28–1B). The porphyrin consists of four linked pyrrole rings that, through their nitrogen atoms, coordinate a single, centrally located Fe^{2+}. Because the iron-porphyrin complex is rich in conjugated double bonds, it absorbs photons of relatively low energy (i.e., light in the visible range). The interaction among O_2, Fe^{2+}, and porphyrin causes the complex to have a red color when fully saturated with O_2 (e.g., arterial blood) and a purple color when devoid of O_2 (e.g., venous blood).

Hemoglobin can bind O_2 only when the iron is in the Fe^{2+} state. The Fe^{2+} in Hb can become oxidized to ferric iron (Fe^{3+}), either spontaneously or under the influence of compounds such as nitrites or sulfonamides. The result of such an oxidation is **methemoglobin** (metHb), which is incapable of binding O_2. Inside the RBC, the heme-containing enzyme **methemoglobin-reductase** uses the reduced form of nicotinamide-adenine dinucleotide phosphate (NADPH) to reduce metHb back to Hb, so that only about 1.5% of total Hb is in the metHb state. In the rare case in which a genetic defect results in a deficiency of this enzyme, metHb may represent 25% or more of the total Hb. Such a deficiency results in a decreased O_2-carrying capacity, leading to tissue hypoxia.

The environment provided by the **globin** portion of Hb is crucial to the physiology of the O_2-heme interaction. To be useful, this interaction must be fully reversible, allowing repetitive capture and release of O_2. The interaction of O_2 with free Fe^{2+} normally produces Fe^{3+}, the simplest example of which is rust. Even with isolated heme, O_2 *irreversibly* oxidizes Fe^{2+} to Fe^{3+}. However, when heme is part of Hb, interactions with approximately 20 amino acids cradle the heme in the globin, so that O_2 loosely and *reversibly* binds to Fe^{2+}. The crucial residue is a histidine that bonds to the Fe^{2+} and donates negative charge that stabilizes the Fe^{2+}-O_2 complex. This histidine is also crucial for transmitting, to the rest of the Hb tetramer, the information that an O_2 molecule has bound to the Fe^{2+}. When the four hemes of Hb are each devoid of O_2, each Fe^{2+} is approximately 0.06 nm above the *plane of its porphyrin ring* in Figure 28–1C (i.e., toward the histidine). In addition, the porphyrin ring itself is distorted, tenting upward at its center toward the Fe^{2+} and histidine. Thus, the Fe^{2+}-histidine bond is under strain in deoxyhemoglobin, a strain that it transmits to the rest of the α or β subunit, and thence to the rest of the Hb molecule. Indeed, the various components of the Hb tetramer are so tightly interlinked, as if by a snugly fitting system of levers and joints, that no one subunit can leave this **tensed (T) state** unless they all leave it together. Because the shape of the heme in the T state sterically inhibits the approach of O_2, empty Hb has a very low affinity for O_2.

When one O_2 binds to one of the Fe^{2+} atoms, the Fe^{2+} tends to move down into the plane of the porphyrin ring. If the Fe^{2+} actually *could* move, it would flatten the ring and relieve the strain on the Fe^{2+}-histidine bond. When enough O_2 molecules bind, enough energy builds up, such that all four subunits of the Hb simultaneously snap into the **relaxed (R) state**, whether or not they are bound to O_2. In this R state, with its flattened heme, the Hb molecule has an O_2 affinity that is approximately 150-fold greater than that in the T state. Thus, when P_{O_2} is zero, all Hb molecules are in the T state and have a low O_2 affinity. When P_{O_2} is very high, all Hb molecules are in the R state and have a high O_2 affinity. At intermediate P_{O_2} values, an equilibrium exists between Hb molecules in the T and R states.

Myoglobin (Mb) is another heme-containing, O_2-binding protein, which is specific for muscle (p. 251). The globin portion of Mb arose in a gene duplication event from a primordial globin. Additional duplications along the nonmyoglobin branch of the globin family led first to the α and β chains of Hb, and then to other α-like and β-like chains (see the box, Forms of Hemoglobin). Mb functions as a *monomer*, homologous to either an α or a β chain of Hb. Although capable of binding only a single O_2, Mb has a much higher O_2 affinity than Hb. In the capillaries, Hb can thus hand off O_2 to an Mb inside a muscle cell; this Mb then transfers its O_2 to the next Mb, and so on, speeding diffusion of O_2 through the muscle cell. Because of the low solubility of O_2, this action is essential: There is insufficient dissolved O_2, by itself, to establish an intracellular O_2 gradient large enough to deliver adequate O_2 to mitochondria.

The Hemoglobin-O_2 Dissociation Curve Has a Sigmoidal Shape Because of Cooperativity Among the Four Subunits of the Hemoglobin Molecule

Imagine that we perform the experiment introduced at the beginning of this chapter, during which we exposed blood plasma to a gas phase with a P_{O_2} of 100 mm Hg. However, we now introduce two crucial differences. First, we will replace blood plasma with whole blood (Fig. 28–2). Second, we will examine how establishing different P_{O_2} values affects the O_2 content of blood. For example, we could incubate the blood with a P_{O_2} of 40 mm Hg, typical of mixed-venous blood, and centrifuge a sample to separate plasma from erythrocytes, as one would for determining **hematocrit** (p. 51). Next, we individually determine the O_2 content of the plasma (i.e, dissolved O_2) and packed RBCs. If we know how much water is inside the RBCs, we can subtract the amount of O_2 dissolved in this water from the total O_2, arriving at the amount of O_2 bound to Hb.

By repeating the previous exercise over a range of P_{O_2} values, we obtain the red curve in Figure 28–3. The right-hand ordinate gives the O_2 bound to Hb in the units "ml O_2/dl blood." The left-hand ordinate gives the same data in terms of **% saturation** of Hb. The P_{O_2} at which the Hb is half saturated is known as the P_{50}. To compute saturation, we need to know the maximal amount of O_2 that can bind to Hb at extremely high P_{O_2} values. Expressed in terms of grams of Hb protein, this **O_2 capacity** is approximately 1.39 ml O_2/g Hb—assuming that no metHb is present. In real life, the O_2 capacity may be closer to 1.35 ml O_2/g Hb because O_2 cannot bind to Hb that either is in the Fe^{3+} state (e.g., MetHb) or is, as discussed later, bound to carbon monoxide. We can easily translate this O_2 capacity to a value for the maximal amount of O_2 that can bind to Hb in 100 ml of blood. If the Hb content is 15 g Hb/dl blood (i.e., normal for an adult male), then

Equation 28–4

Maximal O_2 bound to Hb

$$= [O_2 \text{ capacity of Hb}] \times [\text{Hb content of blood}]$$

$$= \frac{1.35 \text{ ml } O_2}{\text{g Hb}} \cdot \frac{15 \text{ g Hb}}{\text{dl blood}}$$

$$= {\sim}20.3 \text{ (ml } O_2)/\text{dl blood}$$

The percent saturation of Hb is simply

Equation 28–5

$$\% \text{ Saturation of Hb} = \frac{O_2 \text{ actually bound to Hb}}{O_2 \text{ capacity of Hb}} \cdot 100$$

Notice that the curve in Figure 28–3 is sigmoidal or "S-shaped," owing to the **cooperativity** among the four O_2-binding sites on the Hb molecule. At low P_{O_2} values, increases in P_{O_2} produce relatively small increases in O_2 binding, reflecting the relatively low O_2 affinity of Hb in the T state. At moderate P_{O_2} values, the amount of bound O_2 increases more steeply with increases in P_{O_2}, reflecting the increased O_2 affinity as more Hb molecules shift to

FORMS OF HEMOGLOBIN

The normal **adult form of hemoglobin** ($\alpha_2\beta_2$), known as HbA, is only one of several normal forms that are present in prenatal or postnatal life. Some of these other hemoglobins contain naturally occurring α-like chains (e.g., α and ζ) or β-like chains (e.g., β, γ, δ, and ϵ), whereas others reflect post-translational modifications. Three genes for α-**like chains** (all encoding 141 amino acids) are clustered on chromosome 16: At the 5′ end of the cluster is one gene for a ζ chain, followed by *two* for the α chain. Pseudogenes for ζ and α are also present. Five genes for β-**like chains** (all encoding 146 amino acids) are clustered on chromosome 11: Starting at the 5′ end is one gene for ϵ, followed by two for γ (one encoding for glycine at position 136, the other for alanine), and one each for δ and β. A pseudogene for β is also present. A locus-control region regulates the expression of these β-like chains during development (p. 121).

The four **prenatal hemoglobins** (Table 28–1) consist of various combinations of two α-like chains (e.g., α and ζ) and two β-like chains (e.g., ϵ and γ). Very early in life, when erythropoiesis occurs in the yolk sac, the Hb products are the three **embryonic hemoglobins**. When erythropoiesis shifts to the liver and spleen at approximately 10 weeks' gestation, the Hb product is **fetal hemoglobin,** or HbF ($\alpha_2\gamma_2$). Erythrocytes containing HbF have a higher O_2 affinity than those containing HbA, owing to special properties of γ chains. The newborn's blood contains both HbA and HbF; the latter gradually falls by 1 year of age to the minute levels that are characteristic of the adult (rarely more than 1% to 2% of total Hb). With severe stress to the erythroid system—such as marked hemolysis, bone marrow failure, or recovery from bone marrow transplantation—immature erythroid precursors may be forced to mature before they have differentiated sufficiently to produce HbA. In these conditions, circulating levels of HbF may increase considerably. In some hereditary cases, normal HbF persists in the adult, with no clinically significant consequences.

Even adult blood contains several normal **minor-component hemoglobins** (Table 28–2), which account for 5% to 10% of the total blood Hb. In HbA$_2$ ($\sim$2.5% of total Hb), δ chains replace the β chains of HbA. Although the physiologic significance of HbA$_2$ is unknown, the δ chains reduce the sickling of sickle hemoglobin (see later). Three other minor-component hemoglobins are the result of the nonenzymatic glycosylation of HbA. HbA$_{1a}$, HbA$_{1b}$, and HbA$_{1c}$ form when intracellular glucose-6-phosphate reacts with the terminal amino groups of the β chains of HbA. In poorly controlled diabetes mellitus, a disease characterized by decreased insulin or insulin sensitivity (p. 1084), blood glucose concentrations rise, and with them, the intracellular concentration of glucose-6-phosphate. As a result, glycosylated hemoglobins may represent 10% or more of the total Hb. Because Hb glycosylation is irreversible, and because the RBC has a mean lifetime of 120 days, levels of these glycosylated hemoglobins are clinically useful for assessing the long-term control of blood glucose levels in diabetics.

Numerous abnormal hemoglobins exist, most of which are caused by single-amino-acid substitutions on one of the polypeptide chains. One of the most clinically important is HbS, or **sickle** hemoglobin, in which a valine replaces the glutamate normally present at position 6 of the β chain. Although oxygenated HbS has a normal solubility, deoxygenated HbS is only about half as soluble as deoxygenated HbA. As a result, in low-O_2 environments, HbS can crystallize into long fibers, giving the cells a sickle-like appearance. The sickled erythrocytes may disrupt blood flow in small vessels, causing many of the acute symptoms of "sickle cell crisis," including pain, renal dysfunction, retinal bleeding, and aseptic necrosis of bone. In addition, sickle cells are prone to hemolysis (mean lifetime <20 days), leading to a chronic **hemolytic anemia**.

TABLE 28–1

SUBUNIT STRUCTURES OF PRENATAL AND MINOR-COMPONENT HEMOGLOBINS			
HEMOGLOBIN	**α-LIKE SUBUNIT**	**β-LIKE SUBUNIT**	**TIME OF EXPRESSION**
Gower 1	ζ	ϵ	Embryonic
Gower 2	α	ϵ	Embryonic
Portland	ζ	γ	Embryonic
HbF (fetal)	α	γ	Fetal
HbA$_2$	α	δ	Postnatal
HbA (adult)	α	β	Postnatal

TABLE 28–2

MAKE-UP OF TOTAL HEMOGLOBIN IN ADULT HUMAN BLOOD	
HEMOGLOBIN TYPE	**FRACTION OF TOTAL HEMOGLOBIN**
HbA	$\sim$92%
HbA$_{1a}$	0.75%
HbA$_{1b}$	1.5%
HbA$_{1c}$	3–6%
HbA$_2$	2.5%
Total	100%

Figure 28–2. Determination of O_2 content in blood plasma and erythrocytes. RBC, red blood cells; WBC, white blood cells.

the R state. Finally, the Hb-O_2 versus P_{O_2} curve flattens out at high P_{O_2} values as the Hb saturates. The difference in Hb saturation at low versus high P_{O_2} values is the basis for an important clinical tool, the pulse oximeter (see box on p. 660).

At the P_{O_2} prevailing in normal arterial blood (Pa_{O_2}), which is approximately 100 mm Hg, the Hb saturation (Sa_{O_2}) is approximately 97.5%. In mixed-venous blood, in which P_{O_2} ($P\bar{v}_{O_2}$) is approximately 40 mm Hg, the Hb saturation ($S\bar{v}_{O_2}$) is approximately 75%. From these val-

ues, we can calculate the amount of O_2 that leaves the blood in the systemic capillary beds. This a $-$ $\bar{v}$ difference for O_2 bound to Hb is

Equation 28–6

$$a - \bar{v} \text{ difference for Hb–}O_2$$
$$= (97.5\% - 75\%) \cdot \frac{\sim 20.3 \text{ ml } O_2}{\text{dl blood}}$$
$$\cong 4.5 \text{ ml } O_2/(\text{dl blood})$$

We can obtain the a $-$ $\bar{v}$ difference for dissolved O_2 from Henry's Law:

Equation 28–7

$$a - \bar{v} \text{ difference for dissolved } O_2$$
$$= (100 - 40 \text{ mm Hg}) \cdot \frac{0.003 \text{ ml } O_2}{\text{dl blood} \times \text{mm Hg}}$$
$$\cong 0.2 \text{ ml } O_2/(\text{dl blood})$$

Thus, of the total a $-$ $\bar{v}$ difference of 4.7 ml O_2/dl, Hb provides 4.5 ml O_2/dl or nearly 96% of the O_2 that systemic tissues extract from blood (Table 28–3). Is this a $-$ $\bar{v}$ difference in O_2 content enough to satisfy the metabolic demands of the body (i.e., $\sim$250 ml O_2/min)? Using the Fick principle, as we did in Equation 28–3, we see that the combination of a cardiac output of 5 liters/min and an a $-$ $\bar{v}$ difference of 4.7 ml/dl would be nearly adequate:

Equation 28–8

$$\dot{V}_{O_2} = \frac{5000 \text{ ml blood}}{\text{min}} \cdot \left(\frac{20.0 \text{ ml } O_2}{100 \text{ ml}} - \frac{15.3 \text{ ml } O_2}{100 \text{ ml}} \right)$$

where the braces label $\dot{V}_{O_2}$ as "O_2 consumption by tissues," the blood-flow term as "Blood flow," the first content term as "O_2 content of arterial blood," and the second as "O_2 content of mixed-venous blood."

$$= \sim 235 \text{ ml } O_2/\text{min}$$

By either increasing cardiac output by approximately 6% or decreasing the P_{O_2} of mixed-venous blood, the body could meet a demand of 250 ml O_2/min.

Because the plot of $[O_2]_{Dis}$ versus P_{O_2} is linear (see Fig. 28–3, *yellow curve*), there is no theoretical maximum to the amount of O_2 that can dissolve in blood plasma. Thus, breathing 100% O_2 would raise arterial P_{O_2} by approximately 6-fold, so that approximately 1.8 ml of O_2 would be dissolved in each deciliter of arterial blood. Although dissolved O_2 would make a correspondingly greater contribution to overall O_2 carriage under such unphysiological conditions, Hb would still carry the vast majority of O_2. Hence, a decrease in hemoglobin content of the blood—known as **anemia**—can markedly reduce O_2 carriage. The body can compensate for decreased Hb content in the same two ways that, in the earlier example, we increased the $\dot{V}_{O_2}$ from 235 to 250 ml O_2/min. First, it can increase cardiac output. Second, it can increase O_2 extraction, thereby reducing mixed-venous O_2 content. Anemia leads to pallor of the mucous membranes and

Figure 28–3. A normal Hb-O_2 dissociation curve. The *y axis* on the *right* shows O_2 content. For the *red curve* (O_2 content of hemoglobin), we assume 15 g Hb per dl of blood. The *y axis* on the *left*, which pertains only to the *red curve*, gives the percentage of Hb saturation. Hb, hemoglobin.

skin, reflecting the decrease in the red Hb pigment. Impaired O_2 delivery may cause lethargy and fatigue. The accompanying increase in cardiac output may manifest itself as palpitations and a systolic murmur. Shortness of breath may also be a part of the syndrome.

If decreased Hb levels are detrimental, then increasing Hb content should increase the maximal O_2 content, thus providing a competitive advantage for athletes. Even in normal individuals, [Hb] in RBC cytoplasm is already extremely high. Hypoxia (e.g., adaptation to high altitude) leads to the increased production of erythropoietin (see the box on Erythropoietin, p. 664), a hormone that somewhat increases the amount of Hb per erythrocyte, but especially increases their number. Indeed, a few instances have been highly publicized in the international press in which elite athletes have infused themselves with erythrocytes or injected themselves with recombinant erythropoietin. However, an excessive increase in hematocrit—**polycythemia**—has the adverse effect of increasing blood viscosity, and thus vascular resistance (p. 432). The consequences include increased blood pressure in both the systemic and pulmonary circulations and a mismatch of ventilation to perfusion within the lung. Such a ventilation-perfusion mismatch leads to hypoxia (p. 705), and thus *desaturation* of arterial Hb. Thus, the optimal hematocrit—presumably approximately 45%—is one that achieves a high maximal O_2 content, but at a reasonable blood viscosity.

The purplish color of desaturated Hb produces the physical sign known as **cyanosis**, a purplish coloration of the skin and mucous membranes. Cyanosis results not from the *absence* of saturated or oxygenated Hb, but from the *presence* of desaturated Hb. Thus, an anemic patient with poorly saturated Hb might have too little unsaturated Hb for it to manifest as cyanosis. The physician's ability to detect cyanosis also depends on other factors, such as the subject's skin pigmentation and the lighting conditions for the physical examination.

Increases in Temperature, [CO_2], and [H^+], All of Which Are Characteristic of Metabolically Active Tissues, Cause Hemoglobin to Dump O_2

Metabolically active tissues not only have a high demand for O_2, they also are warm, produce large amounts of CO_2, and are acidic. The hemoglobin molecule is intrinsically sensitive to each of these three parameters: High temperature, high P_{CO_2}, and low pH of metabolically active tissues all decrease the O_2 affinity of Hb by acting at nonheme sites and shifting the equilibrium between the T and R states of Hb more toward the low-affinity T state. The net effect is that metabolically active tissues can signal Hb in the *systemic* capillaries to release more O_2

TABLE 28–3

	P_{O_2} (mm Hg)	Hb SATURATION	O_2 BOUND TO Hb (ml/dl)	O_2 DISSOLVED (ml/dl)	TOTAL O_2 CONTENT (ml/dl)
SUMMARY OF a − v̄ DIFFERENCE IN O_2 COMPOSITION OF BLOOD					
a	100	97.5%	19.7	0.3	20.0
v̄	40	75%	15.2	~0.1	15.3
a − v̄ difference	60	22.5%	4.5	~0.2	4.7

MEASURING THE OXYGEN SATURATION OF HEMOGLOBIN CLINICALLY: THE PULSE OXIMETER

The different colors of venous and arterial blood reflect the difference in light absorbance between oxygenated and deoxygenated hemoglobin. Clinicians now routinely exploit these differences to obtain simple, noninvasive measurements of the O_2 saturation of Hb in patients. The **pulse oximeter** has a probe that one attaches to the ear, finger, or any part of the body at which pulsating blood vessels are accessible externally. On one side of the pulsating vascular bed, the pulse oximeter shines red and infrared light; on the other side, it detects the light transmitted through the bed, and then calculates absorbance. This *total* absorbance has two components, *(1)* a *constant* one that represents the stationary tissues and nonpulsating blood inside the capillaries and veins, and *(2)* a *pulsatile* component that represents blood inside arterioles and arteries. The difference between the total and constant absorbance is thus the pulsatile component, which represents only arterial or oxygenated blood. Because both oxygenated and deoxygenated forms of Hb absorb red and infrared light differently, the pulse oximeter can calculate O_2 saturation from the ratio of pulsatile light absorbed at the two wavelengths. The pulse oximeter accomplishes this magic by using a sophisticated microprocessor and software to produce results that strongly agree with those provided by blood-gas analysis of a sample of arterial blood.

The pulse oximeter measures O_2 saturation in *arterial* blood. Because systemic capillaries and veins do not pulsate, they do not contribute to the measurement. Thus, a patient with peripheral cyanosis (e.g., purple fingertips caused by cold-induced vasoconstriction) may have a perfectly normal "central" (i.e., arterial) O_2 saturation. It is worth noting that the absorbance spectrum of carboxyhemoglobin is similar to that for Hb saturated with O_2. Thus, pulse oximetry cannot detect carbon monoxide poisoning.

Health professionals widely employ pulse oximetry in hospitalized patients, particularly those in intensive care units, where continuous monitoring of O_2 saturation is critical. These patients include those on mechanical ventilators and others, less severely ill, who suffer some degree of respiratory compromise. Pulse oximetry has also become popular as an outpatient tool for assessing the presence of hypoxemia during sleep, and thus screening for the condition called **sleep apnea** (see box on Sleep Apnea on p. 733). The latter is a common disorder associated with severe and excessive snoring, poor and interrupted sleep, daytime somnolence, and behavioral changes, possibly leading ultimately to hypertension and cardiac arrhythmias. Because of the insidious nature of hypoxia, pilots of light aircraft have begun to use pulse oximeters to detect developing hypoxia at high altitudes.

than usual, whereas less active tissues can signal Hb to release less. In the *pulmonary* capillaries—where temperature is lower than in active tissues, PCO_2 is relatively low and pH is high—these same properties promote O_2 uptake by Hb.

TEMPERATURE. Increasing the temperature causes the Hb-O_2 dissociation curve to **shift to the right**, whereas decreasing the temperature has the opposite effect (Fig. 28–4). Comparing the three Hb-O_2 dissociation curves in Figure 28–4 at the PO_2 of mixed-venous blood (40 mm Hg), we see that the amount of O_2 bound to Hb becomes progressively less at higher temperatures. In other words, high temperature decreases the O_2 affinity of Hb, thus releasing O_2. One mechanism of this temperature effect may be small shifts in the pK values of various amino acid side chains, which cause shifts in net charge, and thus a conformational change.

The maximal temperatures achieved in active muscle are approximately 40°C. Of course, very low temperatures can prevail in the skin of extremities exposed to extreme cold.

ACID. In 1904, Christian Bohr, a physiologist and father of atomic physicist Niels Bohr, observed that respiratory acidosis (p. 640) shifts the Hb-O_2 dissociation curve to the right (Fig. 28–5A). This decrease in O_2 affinity has come to be known as the **Bohr effect**. A mild respiratory acidosis occurs physiologically as erythrocytes enter the systemic capillaries. There, the increase in extracellular PCO_2 causes CO_2 to enter erythrocytes, leading to a fall in intracellular pH (p. 653). Other acidic metabolites may also lower extracellular and, therefore, intracellular pH. Thus, this intracellular respiratory acidosis has two components—a decrease in pH and an increase in PCO_2. We now appreciate that *both* contribute to the rightward shift of the Hb-O_2 dissociation curve observed by Bohr.

The effect of acidosis per se on the Hb-O_2 dissociation curve (see Fig. 28–5B), sometimes called the **pH-Bohr effect**, accounts for most of the overall Bohr effect. One can readily demonstrate the pH-Bohr effect in a solution of Hb by imposing a metabolic acidosis (e.g., decreasing pH at a fixed PCO_2). It should not be surprising that Hb is sensitive to changes in pH because Hb is an outstanding H^+ buffer (p. 636):

Equation 28–9

$$Hb + H^+ \rightleftharpoons Hb\text{-}H^+$$

Although Hb has many titratable groups, the only ones important here are those with pK values in the physiologic pH range. As we acidify the solution, raising the ratio [Hb-H^+]/[Hb] for susceptible groups, we change the conformation of the Hb molecule, thus lowering its O_2 affinity:

Equation 28–10

$$Hb(O_2)_4 + 2H^+ \rightleftharpoons Hb(H^+)_2 + 4\,O_2$$

This is an extreme example in which we added enough H^+ to cause Hb to dump *all* of its O_2. Under more physiologic conditions, the binding of approximately 0.7

mole of H⁺ causes Hb to release 1 mole of O_2. This property is important in the systemic tissues, where $[H^+]$ is high. The converse is also true: O_2 binding causes a conformational change in the Hb molecule, which lowers the affinity of Hb for H⁺.

CARBON DIOXIDE. The isolated effect of hypercapnia per se on the Hb-O_2 dissociation curve (see Fig. 28–5C) represents a small portion of the overall Bohr effect. Demonstrating such a **CO₂-Bohr effect** requires that we study the O_2 affinity of Hb at a fixed pH, increasing P_{CO_2} and $[HCO_3^-]$ proportionally—an example of **isohydric hypercapnia** (p. 648). As P_{CO_2} increases, CO_2 combines with unprotonated amino groups on Hb (Hb-NH_2) to form **carbamino groups** (Hb-NH-COO⁻). Although Hb has other amino groups, only the four amino termini of the globin chains are susceptible to appreciable carbamino formation, the β chains more so than the α chains. Because amino groups exist in a protonated form (Hb-NH_3^+) in equilibrium with an unprotonated form, the reaction of CO_2 with Hb-NH_2 tends to shift Hb away from the Hb-NH_3^+ form and toward the Hb-NH-COO⁻ form:

Equation 28–11

$$Hb\text{-}NH_3^+ \xrightarrow{\ H^+\ } Hb\text{-}NH_2 \xrightarrow{\ CO_2\ \ H^+\ } Hb\text{-}NH\text{-}COO^-$$

The overall effect of carbamino formation is therefore a negative shift in the charge on one amino acid side chain, causing a shift in the conformation of Hb, and reducing its O_2 affinity:

Equation 28–12

$$(O_2)_4Hb\text{-}NH_3^+ + CO_2 \rightleftharpoons (O_2)_3Hb\text{-}NH\text{-}COO^- + O_2 + 2H^+$$

Thus, an increased P_{CO_2} causes Hb to unload O_2, which is important in the systemic tissues. Conversely, an increased P_{O_2} causes Hb to unload CO_2, which is important in the lungs.

In conclusion, the Hb-O_2 dissociation curve shifts to the right under conditions prevailing in the capillaries of metabolically active systemic tissues—increased temperature (see Fig. 28–4), decreased pH (see Fig. 28–5B), and increased P_{CO_2} (see Fig. 28–5C). These right shifts are synonymous with decreased O_2 affinity. Thus, high metabolic rates promote the unloading of O_2 from Hb. Clearly, blood cannot unload O_2 unless the blood gets to the tissues. Indeed, in most systemic arterioles, local hypercapnia and acidosis also are powerful stimuli for vasodilation (p. 559), enhancing O_2 *delivery* to metabolically active tissues.

2,3-Diphosphoglycerate Reduces the Affinity of Adult, but Not of Fetal, Hemoglobin

The affinity of hemoglobin for O_2 is very sensitive to the presence of the glycolytic metabolite 2,3-diphosphoglycerate (2,3-DPG) and, to a lesser extent, organic phosphates such as adenosine triphosphate (ATP). The concentration of **2,3-DPG** is about the same as that of Hb. Indeed, 2,3-DPG binds to hemoglobin in a 1:1 stoichiometry, interacting with a central cavity formed by the two β chains. At physiological pH, 2,3-DPG has an average of approximately 3.5 negative charges, which interact with eight positively charged amino acid residues in this central cavity. O_2 binding, however, changes the shape of the central cavity, destabilizing DPG-bound Hb. As a result, the 2,3-DPG affinity of oxygenated Hb is only about 1% as great as that of deoxygenated Hb. Conversely, binding of 2,3-DPG to Hb destabilizes the interaction of Hb with O_2, shifting the following reaction to the right and releasing O_2:

Equation 28–13

$$Hb(O_2)_4 + 2,3\text{-DPG} \rightleftharpoons Hb(2,3\text{-DPG}) + 4\,O_2$$

The result is a right shift in the Hb-O_2 dissociation curve (Fig. 28–6). This effect of 2,3-DPG on the O_2 affinity of Hb is important both in hypoxia and in understanding the physiology of fetal Hb.

Decreasing the P_{O_2} of RBCs stimulates glycolysis, leading to increased levels of 2,3-DPG. Indeed, chronic hypoxia, anemia, and acclimation to high altitude are all associated with an increase in 2,3-DPG levels, thus lower-

Figure 28–4. The effect of temperature changes on the Hb-O_2 dissociation curve.

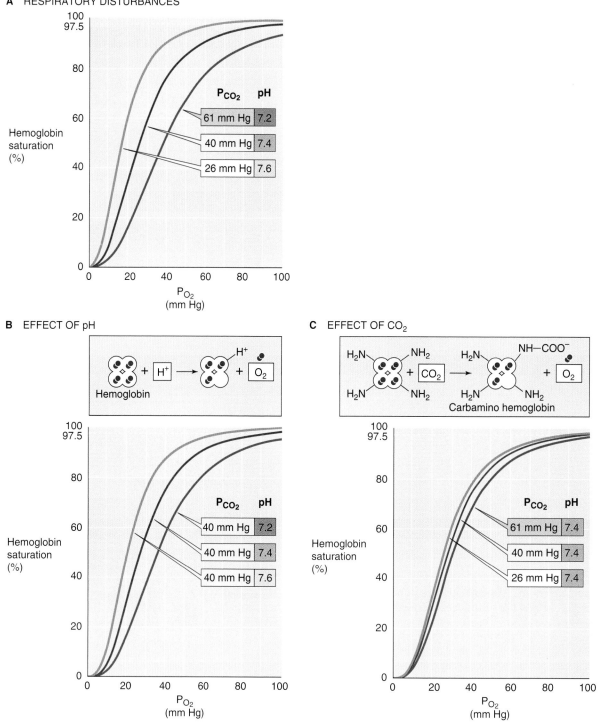

Figure 28–5. The effect of acidosis and hypercapnia on the Hb-O_2 dissociation curve (Bohr effect).

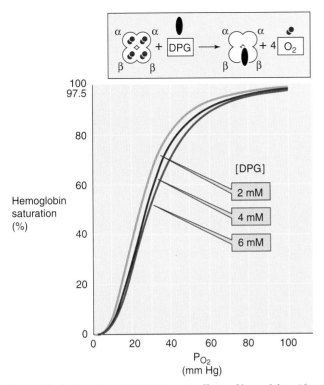

Figure 28–6. The effect of 2,3-DPG on O_2 affinity of hemoglobin. After lowlanders spent about 2 days at an altitude of approximately 4500 m, their cytosolic [2,3-DPG] increased by approximately 50%, shifting the Hb-O_2 dissociation curve to the right. DPG, 2,3-diphosphoglycerate.

ing the O_2 affinity of Hb. Reducing the affinity is a two-edged sword. At the relatively high P_{O_2} in alveoli, where the Hb-O_2 dissociation curve is fairly flat, this decrease in O_2 affinity reduces O_2 uptake only slightly. However, at the low P_{O_2} in systemic tissues, where the Hb-O_2 dissociation curve is steep, this decrease in O_2 affinity markedly increases the release of O_2. Thus, increasing 2,3-DPG may reduce O_2 uptake in the lungs only slightly, while substantially enhancing O_2 unloading in the metabolizing tissues.

Figure 28–7 shows the Hb-O_2 dissociation curve of pure or "stripped" Hb (i.e., in the absence of CO_2, 2,3-DPG, and other organic phosphates). The O_2 affinity of pure Hb is quite high, as evidenced by the left shift of the Hb-O_2 dissociation curve. Adding only CO_2 or only 2,3-DPG to the solution shifts the curve somewhat to the right, but still not to its normal position. However, adding both yields a curve that is indistinguishable from that for intact RBCs under physiologic conditions.

The Hb inside fetal erythrocytes (HbF) (see box on p. 657) has a higher O_2 affinity than the Hb inside adult RBCs (HbA). This difference is crucial for the fetus, whose blood must abstract O_2 from maternal blood in the placenta (p. 1176). The difference in O_2 affinities does not, however, reflect differences in O_2 affinities of *stripped* HbA and HbF, which are nearly identical. The crucial difference is that the γ chains of HbF bind 2,3-DPG less

avidly than do the β chains of HbA. With less 2,3-DPG bound, the dissociation curve of HbF is left-shifted, similar to the *HbA curve* labeled "Hb + CO_2" in Figure 28–7.

O_2 is not the only gas that can bind to the Fe^{2+} of Hb; carbon monoxide (CO), nitric oxide (NO), and H_2S can also bind to Hb and snap it into the R state. In **carbon monoxide poisoning**, CO binds to Hb with an affinity that is approximately 200-fold greater than that of O_2, thus reducing the blood's carrying capacity for O_2. However, the major reason that CO is toxic is that, as it snaps Hb into the R state, it increases the O_2 affinity of Hb and shifts the Hb-O_2 dissociation curve to the left. Thus, when Hb reaches the systemic capillaries in CO poisoning, its tenacity for O_2 is so high that it tends to hold on to the O_2 it is carrying. Thus, although blood is bright red in carbon monoxide poisoning, the Hb cannot release enough O_2 to the tissues.

CARRIAGE OF CO_2

Blood Carries "Total CO_2" Mainly as HCO_3^-

The blood carries carbon dioxide and related compounds in five forms (Table 28–4). Together, they constitute the **total CO_2**:

1. **Dissolved carbon dioxide.** $[CO_2]_{Dis}$ follows Henry's Law (see box on p. 597), and it is in the millimolar range in both blood plasma and blood cells. It makes up only approximately 5% of the total CO_2 of arterial blood.

2. **Carbonic acid.** H_2CO_3 can form either from CO_2 and H_2O, or from H^+ and HCO_3^- (p. 636). Because the equilibrium constant governing the reaction $CO_2 + H_2O \rightleftharpoons H_2CO_3$ is approximately 0.0025, $[H_2CO_3]$ is only 1/400th as large as $[CO_2]$. Thus, H_2CO_3 is not quantitatively important for CO_2 carriage.

3. **Bicarbonate.** HCO_3^- can form in three ways. First, H_2CO_3 can dissociate into HCO_3^- and H^+. Second, CO_2 can combine directly with OH^- to form HCO_3^-, the reaction catalyzed by carbonic anhydrase (see box on p. 637). Third, HCO_3^- forms when carbonate combines with H^+. In arterial blood, $[HCO_3^-]$ is approximately 24 mM, so that HCO_3^- represents approximately 90% of total CO_2.

4. **Carbonate.** CO_3^{2-} forms from the dissociation of bicarbonate: $HCO_3^- \rightarrow CO_3^{2-} + H^+$. Because the pK of this reaction is so high (~10.3), $[CO_3^{2-}]$ is only approximately 1/1000th as high as $[HCO_3^-]$ at pH 7.4. Thus, like H_2CO_3, CO_3^{2-} is not quantitatively important for CO_2 carriage.

5. **Carbamino compounds.** By far the most important carbamino compound is carbamino hemoglobin (Hb-NH-COO$^-$), which forms rapidly and reversibly as CO_2 reacts with free amino groups on Hb. In arterial blood, carbamino compounds account for approximately 5% of total CO_2.

The reason we group together the previously listed five CO_2-related compounds under the term "total CO_2" is

ERYTHROPOIETIN

Erythropoietin (EPO) is an approximately 34-kDa glycoprotein made mainly in the kidney by fibroblast-like type I interstitial cells in the cortex and outer medulla (p. 746). EPO is a growth factor related to other cytokines, and it acts through a tyrosine kinase-associated receptor (p. 111) to stimulate the production of proerythroblasts in the bone marrow, as well as the development of red cells from their progenitor cells. In fetal life, the liver rather than the kidney produces EPO. Even in the adult, Kupffer cells in the liver produce some EPO.

Four lines of evidence indicate that it is a decrease in *local* P_{O_2} that triggers an increase in EPO synthesis. First, synthesis of EPO increases with anemia. Second, EPO production increases with lowered renal blood flow. Third, EPO synthesis increases with central hypoxia (i.e., low arterial P_{O_2}), such as may occur with pulmonary disease or with living at high altitude (p. 1262). In all three of these cases, local P_{O_2} falls as tissues respond to a fall in O_2 delivery by extracting more O_2 from each volume of blood that passes through the kidney. Finally, EPO production increases in cases where Hb has a high O_2 affinity. Here, the renal cells must lower P_{O_2} substantially before O_2 dissociates from Hb. Thus, mutant hemoglobins with high O_2 affinities, stored blood (which has low 2,3-DPG levels), and alkaline blood all lead to increased EPO production.

Besides local hypoxia, several hormones and other agents stimulate EPO production. For example, prostaglandin E_2 (PGE_2) and adenosine appear to stimulate EPO synthesis by increasing intracellular levels of cyclic adenosine monophosphate (cAMP). Norepinephrine and thyroid hormone also stimulate EPO release. Finally, androgens promote—whereas estrogens inhibit—EPO synthesis, explaining at least in part why women in their child-bearing years have lower hematocrit levels than men do.

Because the kidneys are the major source of EPO, renal failure leads to reduced EPO levels and anemia. The development of recombinant EPO has had a major impact in ameliorating the anemia of chronic renal failure.

that the method Van Slyke introduced in the 1920s—which remains the basis for assaying blood HCO_3^- in modern clinical laboratories—measures all five.

CO_2 Transport Depends Critically on Carbonic Anhydrase, the Cl-HCO_3 Exchanger, and Hemoglobin

The total CO_2 concentration of arterial blood is approximately 26 mM, or approximately 48 ml of CO_2 gas per dl (measured at STP; see Table 28–4). As blood courses through the systemic capillary beds, it picks up approximately 4 ml/dl of CO_2, so that the total CO_2 of mixed-venous blood is approximately 52 ml/dl. In what forms does blood carry this *incremental* 4 ml/dl of CO_2 to the

lungs? About 10% of the incremental CO_2 moves as dissolved CO_2, approximately 69% as HCO_3^-, and approximately 21% as carbamino compounds (Fig. 28–8). Therefore, dissolved CO_2 and carbamino CO_2 are far more important for carrying *incremental* CO_2 to the lungs than we might have surmised, given their contribution to *total* CO_2 in arterial blood.

Figure 28–9 summarizes the events that occur as incremental CO_2 enters systemic capillaries. As fast as biologic oxidations in the mitochondria produce CO_2, this gas diffuses out of cells, through the extracellular space, across the capillary endothelium, and into the blood plasma. Some of the incremental CO_2 (~11%) remains in blood plasma throughout its journey to the lungs, but most (~89%), at least initially, enters the RBCs. This breakdown of 11% versus 89% is based on a hematocrit of 40%.

The approximately 11% of the incremental CO_2 in plasma travels in three forms:

1. **Dissolved CO_2.** About 6% of incremental CO_2 remains dissolved in blood plasma.
2. **Carbamino compounds.** An insignificant amount forms carbamino compounds with plasma proteins.
3. **Bicarbonate.** About 5% of incremental CO_2 forms HCO_3^- in the plasma and remains in the plasma: CO_2 + H_2O → H_2CO_3 → H^+ + HCO_3^-. The amount of HCO_3^- that follows this path depends critically on non-HCO_3^- buffering power (p. 644), which is very low in plasma (~5 mM/pH unit).

The approximately 89% of incremental CO_2 that initially enters the red blood cells also has three fates:

1. **Dissolved CO_2.** About 4% of incremental CO_2 remains dissolved inside the RBC.
2. **Carbamino compounds.** About 21% of incremental CO_2 forms carbamino compounds with hemoglobin. Why does so much CO_2 travel as carbamino compounds inside the red cell, whereas so little does in the blood plasma? First, the Hb concentration inside RBCs (~33 g/dl) is far higher than that of albumin and globulins in plasma (~7 g/dl). Second, Hb forms carbamino compounds far more easily than do major plasma proteins. Moreover, Hb forms carbamino compounds even more easily as it loses O_2 in the systemic capillaries (reverse of CO_2-Bohr effect). Finally, Hb is a far better buffer than the plasma proteins for the H^+ produced during carbamino formation. Moreover, Hb becomes an even better buffer as it loses O_2 in the systemic capillaries (reverse of the pH-Bohr effect).
3. **Bicarbonate.** About 64% of the incremental CO_2 forms HCO_3^-. Why does so much more CO_2 form HCO_3^- in the erythrocyte than in plasma? First, erythrocytes contain a high level of carbonic anhydrase (see box on p. 637), greatly accelerating the conversion of CO_2 to HCO_3^-. In the absence of enzyme, hardly any HCO_3^- would form inside erythrocytes during the brief time that the cells spend during their passage through a typical systemic capillary. Second, the Cl-HCO_3 exchanger AE1 (p. 69) transports some of the newly formed HCO_3^- out of the cell, promoting formation of more HCO_3^-. This uptake of Cl^- in exchange for HCO_3^- is known as the chloride or **Hamburger shift**.

TABLE 28–4

COMPONENTS OF "TOTAL CO₂"

COMPONENT		ARTERIAL BLOOD (Pco₂ = 40 mm Hg)			MIXED-VENOUS BLOOD (Pco₂ = 46 mm Hg)		
		Concentration	Contribution to Total CO₂ (ml/dl)	Fraction of Total CO₂ (%)	Concentration	Contribution to Total CO₂ (ml/dl)	Fraction of Total CO₂ (%)
Physically dissolved carbon dioxide	CO_2	1.2 mM	2.4	5	1.4 mM	2.8	5.3
Carbonic acid	H_2CO_3	3 µM	~0	~0	~3.5 µM	~0	~0
Bicarbonate	HCO_3^-	24 mM	43.2	90	25.6 mM	46.0	88.5
Carbonate	CO_3^{2-}	30 µM	~0	~0	30 µM	~0	~0
Carbamino compounds	R-NH-COO⁻	1.2 mM	2.4	5	1.6 mM	3.2	6.2
Total		26.4 mM	48	100	28.6 mM	52	100

Third, intracellular buffers, primarily Hb, buffer the H^+ produced during HCO_3^- formation.

The combined effects of the described intracellular and extracellular events is that approximately 10% of incremental CO_2 formed in systemic tissues moves to the lungs as dissolved CO_2, 6% in plasma and 4% inside erythrocytes. Approximately 21% moves as carbamino compounds, almost exclusively inside erythrocytes as carbamino Hb. Finally, approximately 69% of incremental CO_2 moves as HCO_3^-, 5% that forms in plasma and 64% that forms inside the RBC. Because H_2O enters the cell during HCO_3^- formation, erythrocytes swell as they pass through systemic capillaries.

When mixed-venous blood (with a Pco₂ of ~46 mm Hg) reaches the pulmonary capillaries (surrounded by alveoli with a Pco₂ of only ~40 mm Hg), CO_2 moves from the erythrocytes and blood plasma into the alveolar air space. All of the reactions discussed earlier reverse. In the process, Cl^- and H_2O leave the erythrocytes, and the cells shrink.

The High Po₂ in the Lungs Causes the Blood to Dump CO₂

Total CO_2 carriage in the blood depends on the three blood-gas parameters—Pco₂, plasma pH, and Po₂. Figure 28–10 illustrates some quantitative aspects of these

Figure 28–7. The effect of adding CO_2 or 2,3-DPG to stripped hemoglobin. The *four brown curves* are Hb-O₂ dissociation curves for pure hemoglobin (2 mM) in artificial solutions. "Stripped Hb" is devoid of both CO_2 and 2,3-DPG. When CO_2 or 2,3-DPG was present, Pco₂ was 40 mm Hg and [2,3-DPG] was 2.4 mM. The cytosol of erythrocytes in blood (*red curve*) had the same composition as the artificial solutions. DPG, 2,3-diphosphoglycerate.

Figure 28–8. Constituents of "total CO_2 in blood." The *left bar* (a) represents arterial blood; the *middle bar* (v̄), mixed-venous blood; and the *right bar*, the incremental CO_2 that the blood picks up in the systemic capillaries.

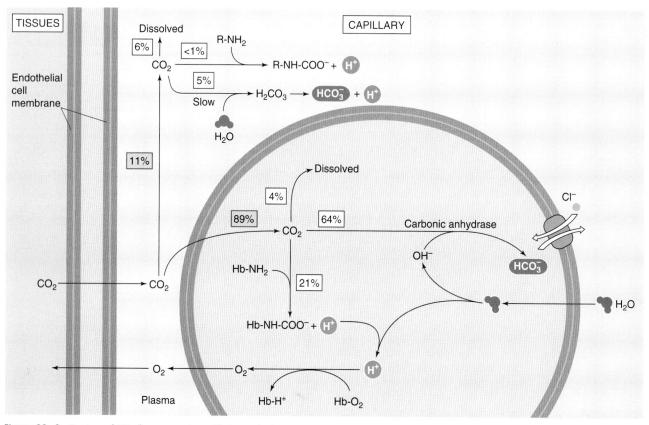

Figure 28–9. Carriage of CO_2 from systemic capillaries to the lungs.

relationships in terms of three **CO_2 dissociation curves**. Each is a curvilinear plot showing how changes in P_{CO_2} affect the total CO_2 content of blood. Although pH per se does not appear in this diagram, pH decreases as P_{CO_2} increases along the x-axis (i.e., respiratory acidosis; p. 640). The *blue plot* is the CO_2 dissociation curve when P_{O_2} is zero (i.e., 0% Hb saturation). The *next two plots* are CO_2 dissociation curves for P_{O_2} values of 40 mm Hg (i.e., ~75% saturation; *purple*) and 100 mm Hg (i.e., ~97.5% saturation; *red*). The *green line* at the bottom of Figure 28–10 shows that the *dissolved* component of total CO_2 rises only slightly with increases in P_{CO_2}.

Three features of the CO_2 dissociation curves in Figure 28–10 are noteworthy:

1. **Quasi-linear relationship between total CO_2 content and P_{CO_2}.** In the physiological range of P_{CO_2} values (i.e., 40–46 mm Hg), the CO_2 dissociation curve is more linear (see Fig. 28–10, *inset*) than is the O_2 dissociation curve in its physiologic range (i.e., 40–100 mm Hg).

2. **Up-shift of curve with decreasing P_{O_2}.** At any P_{CO_2}, total CO_2 content increases as P_{O_2} (or Hb saturation) falls. This inverse relationship between CO_2 content and P_{O_2} is known as the **Haldane effect**. Thus, as blood enters systemic capillaries and releases O_2, the CO_2-carrying capacity rises so that blood picks up extra CO_2. Conversely, as blood enters the pulmonary capillaries and binds O_2, the CO_2-carrying capacity falls so that blood dumps extra CO_2 (Table 28–5). The Haldane effect is the flip side of the coin from the

CO_2-Bohr and pH-Bohr effects. First, just as carbamino formation lowers the O_2 affinity of Hb (Equation 28–12), O_2 binding destabilizes carbamino Hb (Hb-NH-COO⁻), promoting CO_2 release. Second, just as H⁺ binding lowers the O_2 affinity of Hb (Equation 28–10), O_2 binding destabilizes protonated hemoglobin (Hb-H⁺), promoting H⁺ release. By mass action, this H⁺ reduces CO_2−carrying capacity by favoring the formation of CO_2 from both carbamino Hb and HCO₃⁻ (see Fig. 28–9).

3. **Steep relationship between total CO_2 content and P_{CO_2}.** In the physiologic range of partial pressures, the CO_2 dissociation curve (see Fig. 28–10) is much steeper than the O_2 dissociation curve (see Fig. 28–3). Because the O_2 dissociation curve is less steep, P_{O_2} must increase from approximately 40 mm Hg (mixed venous) to approximately 100 mm Hg (arterial) in order to increase the O_2 content of blood by approximately 5 ml/dl, as required to deliver adequate O_2 to the systemic tissues. As discussed later, P_{CO_2} needs to increase from 40 to only 46 mm Hg to increase the CO_2 content by the required approximately 4 ml/dl of CO_2.

The inset to Figure 28–10 shows the physiologically relevant portions of the plots. Point *a* on the *red curve* represents arterial blood, with a P_{CO_2} of 40 mm Hg and a P_{O_2} of 100 mm Hg (i.e., ~97.5% saturation). Point v̄ on the purple curve represents mixed-venous blood, with a P_{CO_2} of 46 mm Hg, but a P_{O_2} of only 40 mm Hg (i.e., ~75% saturation). The difference between the total CO_2

TABLE 28–5

FACTORS AFFECTING THE AMOUNT OF TOTAL CO_2 CARRIED BY BLOOD	
PARAMETER	**EFFECTS OF INCREASING THE "PARAMETER"**
PCO_2	(i) Increased $[CO_2]_{Dis}$ (Henry's Law). (ii) Increased formation of HCO_3^- ($CO_2 + H_2O \rightarrow HCO_3^- + H^+$). (iii) Increased formation of carbamino ($CO_2 + Hb\text{-}NH_3^+ + \rightarrow Hb\text{-}NH\text{-}COO^- + 2H^+$).
[Plasma protein]	Increased plasma buffering power. The increased capacity for consuming H^+ indirectly promotes formation of HCO_3^-.
Plasma pH	(i) Increased formation of HCO_3^- in plasma (Henderson-Hasselbalch equation). (ii) Increased pH inside red cell, promoting formation of HCO_3^- and carbamino hemoglobin.
[Hemoglobin]	(i) Increased formation of carbamino hemoglobin (*direct*). (ii) Increases buffering power inside erythrocyte. The increased capacity for consuming H^+ *indirectly* promotes formation of HCO_3^- and carbamino hemoglobin.
PO_2	(i) Decreased buffering power of hemoglobin (inverse of pH-Bohr effect). The decreased capacity for consuming H^+ indirectly restrains formation of HCO_3^- and carbamino hemoglobin. (ii) Decreased formation of carbamino hemoglobin (inverse of CO_2-Bohr effect).

contents represented by the two points (i.e., 52 versus 48 ml/dl) represents the 4 ml/dl of CO_2 the blood takes up as it passes through systemic capillaries. If it were not for the Haldane effect, the blood would remain on the *red curve*, and the PCO_2 increase would cause the CO_2 content to increase by only approximately 2.7 ml/dl. Thus, at a PCO_2 of 46 mm Hg, the fall in PO_2 that occurs as blood flows through systemic capillaries allows the blood to pick up approximately 50% more CO_2 (i.e., 4 versus 2.7 ml/dl). Viewed differently, if it were not for the Haldane effect, mixed-venous PCO_2 would have to increase to approximately 49 mm Hg for blood to carry 4 ml/dl of CO_2. Table 28–5 summarizes how changes in blood parameters can influence the amount of total CO_2 that the blood is able to carry.

The O_2-CO_2 Diagram Describes the Interaction of PO_2 and PCO_2 in the Blood

We have seen that hemoglobin plays a key role in transporting O_2 from the lungs to peripheral tissues, transporting CO_2 in the opposite direction, and buffering H^+. These functions are all intimately interrelated: PCO_2 and pH influence the O_2-Hb dissociation curve (Bohr effects; see Fig. 28–5), and PO_2 influences the CO_2 dissociation curve (Haldane effect; see Fig. 28–10). A useful way of illustrating this mutual dependence is the **O_2-CO_2 diagram**, which we will revisit on p. 702 to understand regional differences between alveolar PO_2 and PCO_2.

On a coordinate system in which PCO_2 is on the ordinate and PO_2 on the abscissa, each *blue curve* in Figure

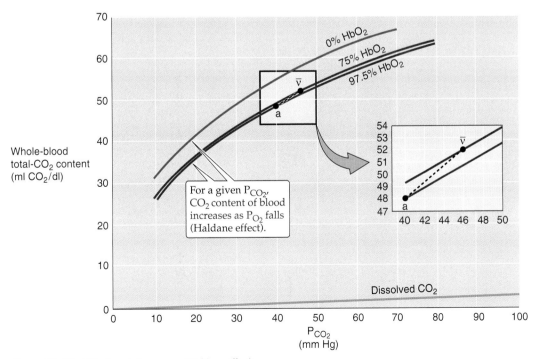

Figure 28–10. CO_2 dissociation curves (Haldane effect).

Figure 28–11. The O_2-CO_2 diagram.

28–11 represents all the points with the same O_2 content in whole blood. These curves are thus **isopleths of identical O_2 content** (from the Greek "isos," equal + "plethein," to be full). For example, arterial blood (point **a**) lies on the isopleth for an O_2 content of 20.0 ml/dl, with coordinates of P_{O_2} = 100 mm Hg and P_{CO_2} = 40 mm Hg. Following the same isopleth from a P_{CO_2} of 40 mm Hg (point **a**) to, say, 46 mm Hg, we see that the blood could carry the same 20.0 ml/dl of O_2 only if we increase P_{O_2} from 100 to nearly 105 mm Hg. *Thus, as P_{CO_2} increases, the O_2-carrying capacity of the blood decreases (Bohr effect).* If it were not for the Bohr effect, all the *blue curves* would be vertical lines. Mixed-venous blood (point $\bar{v}$) is on the O_2-content isopleth for 15.3 ml/dl, at a P_{O_2} of 40 mm Hg and a P_{CO_2} of 46 mm Hg. If blood were equilibrated with inspired air (point **I**), it would have a P_{O_2} of 150 mm Hg and a P_{CO_2} of 0.

The *red curves* are **isopleths of identical CO_2 content**. Arterial blood (point **a**) lies on the CO_2-content isopleth for 48 ml/dl. Similarly, mixed-venous blood (point $\bar{v}$) lies on the CO_2-content isopleth for 52 ml/dl. Following this 52-ml/dl isopleth from a P_{O_2} of 40 mm Hg (point $\bar{v}$) to, say, 100 mm Hg, we see that the blood could carry the same 52 ml/dl of CO_2 only if we increase P_{CO_2} from 46 to nearly 50 mm Hg. *Thus, as the P_{O_2} increases, the CO_2-carrying capacity of the blood decreases (Haldane effect).* If it were not for the Haldane effect, all the *red curves* would be horizontal lines. Blood equilibrated with inspired air (point **I**) would have a CO_2-content of 0.

In Figure 28–11, the *green curve* connecting the points

$\bar{v}$, **a**, and **I** represents all possible combinations of P_{O_2} and P_{CO_2} in normal lungs.

REFERENCES

Books and Reviews

Bauer C: Structural biology of hemoglobin. In Crystal RG, West JB (eds): The Lung. New York, Lippincott-Raven, 1991 pp 1215–1223.

Baumann R, Bartels H, Bauer C: Blood oxygen transport. In Handbook of Physiology, Section 3, The Respiratory System, Vol 1. Bethesda, MD, American Physiological Society, 1985 pp 147–172.

Jelkmann W: Erythropoietin: Structure, control of production, and function. Physiol Rev 72:449–487, 1992.

Kilmartin JV, Rossi-Bernardi L: Interactions of hemoglobin with hydrogen ion, carbon dioxide and organic phosphates. Physiol Rev 53:836–890, 1973.

Klocke RA: Carbon dioxide. In Crystal RG, West JB (eds): The Lung. New York, Lippincott-Raven, 1991 pp 1233–1239.

Winslow RM, Rossi-Bernardi L: Oxygen-hemoglobin dissociation curve. In Crystal RG, West JB (eds): The Lung. New York, Lippincott-Raven, 1991 pp 1225–1231.

Journal Articles

Arnone A: X-ray diffraction study of binding of 2,3-diphosphoglycerate to human deoxyhaemoglobin. Nature 237:146–149, 1972.

Arnone A: X-ray studies of the interaction of CO_2 with human deoxyhaemoglobin. Nature 247:143–145, 1974.

Benesch R, Benesch RE: Intracellular organic phosphates as regulators of oxygen release by haemoglobin. Nature 221:618–622, 1969.

Perutz MF, Lehmann H: Molecular pathology of human haemoglobin. Nature 219:902–909, 1968.

Perutz MF, Kilmartin JV, Nishidura K, et al: Identification of residues contributing to the Bohr effect of human haemoglobin. J Mol Biol 138:649–670, 1980.

CHAPTER 29

Gas Exchange in the Lungs

Walter F. Boron

The complex anatomy of the pulmonary tree, the mechanics of the respiratory system, and the sophisticated carriage mechanisms for O_2 and CO_2 combine to serve two essential purposes: to allow the ready diffusion of O_2 from the alveoli to the pulmonary-capillary blood, and the comparable movement of CO_2 in the opposite direction. In this chapter, we consider the principles that govern these diffusive events and factors that, in certain diseases, can limit gas exchange.

DIFFUSION OF GASES

The Flow of Gas Across a Barrier Is Proportional to Its Diffusing Capacity (D_L) and to Its Concentration Gradient Across the Barrier (Fick's Law)

Although, at one time, physiologists debated whether the lung actively transports O_2, we now know that the movements of both O_2 and CO_2 across the alveolar blood-gas barrier occur by simple **diffusion** (p. 56). Random motion alone causes a net movement of molecules from an area of high concentration to one of low concentration. Although diffusion involves no expenditure of energy, over long distances it can be extremely slow.

Suppose that a barrier that is permeable to O_2 separates two air-filled compartments, each of which contains O_2 (Fig. 29–1A). The partial pressures of O_2 on the two sides are P_1 and P_2. Because the partial pressure of a gas is proportional to its concentration (see box on p. 597), the odds that an O_2 molecule on side 1 will collide with the barrier is proportional to P_1. Once an O_2 molecule has collided with the barrier, it is equally likely to return to side 1 as to traverse the barrier to side 2. Thus, the odds that O_2 moves from side 1 to side 2 are proportional to P_1:

Equation 29–1

$$Flow_{1 \to 2} \propto P_1$$

The **unidirectional movement** of O_2 in the opposite direction, from side 2 to side 1, is proportional to the partial pressure of O_2 on side 2:

Equation 29–2

$$Flow_{2 \to 1} \propto P_2$$

The **net movement** of O_2 from side 1 to side 2 is the difference between the two unidirectional flows:

A DRY, HOMOGENEOUS BARRIER

B ALVEOLAR WALL

C EFFECT OF BARRIER THICKNESS

Figure 29–1 Diffusion of a gas across a barrier.

Equation 29–3

$$\text{Flow}_{\text{Net}} \propto (P_1 - P_2)$$

Note that the net flow is proportional to the absolute difference in partial pressures, not their ratio. Thus, when P_1 is 100 mm Hg (or torr) and P_2 is 95 mm Hg (a 5% PO_2 difference), the net flow is fivefold greater than when P_1 is 2 mm Hg and P_2 is 1 mm Hg (a 100% PO_2 difference).

The term **flow** describes the number of O_2 molecules moving across the entire area of the barrier per unit time (units: moles/sec). If we normalize flow for the area of the barrier, the result is a **flux** (units: moles/{cm² · s}). Respiratory physiologists usually measure the flow of a gas such as O_2 as the volume of gas (measured at standard temperature and pressure/dry, p. 598) moving per unit

time. V refers to the volume and $\dot{V}$ is its time derivative (volume of gas moving per unit time), or flow.

The proportionality constant in Equation 29–3 is the **diffusing capacity** for the lung, D_L (units: ml/[min · mm Hg]). Thus, the flow of gas becomes

Equation 29–4

$$\dot{V}_{\text{net}} = D_L \cdot (P_1 - P_2)$$

This equation is a restatement of a simplified version of **Fick's law** (p. 56), which states that the net flow is proportional to the concentration gradient, in this case expressed as the partial pressure gradient.

Applying Fick's law to the diffusion of gas across the alveolar wall requires that we extend our model somewhat. Rather than a simple barrier separating two compartments filled with dry gas, a wet barrier covered with a film of water on one side will separate a volume filled with moist air from a volume of blood plasma at 37° (see Fig. 29–1B). Now we can examine how the physical characteristics of the gas and the barrier contribute to D_L.

Two *properties of the gas* contribute to D_L—molecular weight (MW) and solubility in water (s). First, the mobility of the gas should decrease as its molecular weight increases. Indeed, **Graham's law** states that diffusion is inversely proportional to the square root of molecular weight. Second, Fick's law states that the flow of the gas across the wet barrier is proportional to the *concentration* gradient of the gas dissolved in water. According to **Henry's law** (see box on p. 597), these concentrations are proportional to the respective partial pressures, and the proportionality constant is the solubility of the gas. Therefore, poorly soluble gases (e.g., nitrogen, helium) diffuse poorly across the alveolar wall.

Two *properties of the barrier* in Figure 29–1A contribute to D_L—area (A) and thickness (a). First, the net flow of O_2 is proportional to the **area** of the barrier, describing the odds that an O_2 molecule will collide with the barrier. Second, the net flow is inversely proportional to the **thickness** of the barrier. The thicker the barrier, the smaller the O_2 partial pressure gradient ($\Delta PO_2/a$) through the barrier (see Fig. 29–1C). An analogy is the slope of the trail that a skier takes from the peak of a mountain to the base. Whether the skier takes a steep "expert" trail or a shallow "beginner's" trail, the endpoints of the journey are the same. However, the trip is much faster along the steeper trail!

Finally, a combined property of both the barrier and the gas also contributes to D_L, a proportionality constant k that describes the interaction of the gas with the barrier.

Replacing D_L in Equation 29–4 with an area, solubility, thickness, molecular weight, and the proportionality constant (k):

Equation 29–5

$$\dot{V}_{net} = \underbrace{\left[k \frac{A \cdot s}{a\sqrt{MW}} \right]}_{D_L} (P_1 - P_2)$$

Equation 29–4 and Equation 29–5 are analogous to **Ohm's law** for electricity:

Equation 29–6

$$I = \left(\frac{1}{R} \right) \cdot \Delta V$$

Electrical current (I) in Ohm's law corresponds to the net flow of gas ($\dot{V}_{net}$), the reciprocal of resistance (i.e., conductance) corresponds to diffusing capacity (D_L), and the voltage difference (ΔV) driving the electrical current corresponds to the pressure difference ($P_1 - P_2$ or ΔP).

The Total Flux of a Gas Between Alveolar Air and Blood Is the Summation of Multiple Diffusion Events Along Each Pulmonary Capillary During the Respiratory Cycle

Equation 29–5 describes O_2 diffusion between two compartments whose properties are uniform both spatially and temporally. Can we use these equations to predict

gas diffusion between alveolar air and pulmonary-capillary blood? If we assume that the alveolar air, blood-gas barrier and pulmonary-capillary blood are uniform spatially and temporally, then the net diffusion of O_2 ($\dot{V}_{O_2}$) from alveolar air to pulmonary-capillary blood is:

Equation 29–7

$$\dot{V}_{O_2} = \underbrace{\left[k \frac{A \cdot s}{a\sqrt{MW}} \right]}_{D_{L_{O_2}}} (P_{A_{O_2}} - P_{C_{O_2}})$$

$D_{L_{O_2}}$ is the diffusing capacity for O_2, $P_{A_{O_2}}$ is the O_2 partial pressure in the alveolar air, and $P_{C_{O_2}}$ is the comparable parameter in pulmonary-capillary blood. Although Equation 29–7 may seem sophisticated, a closer examination reveals that $D_{L_{O_2}}$, $P_{A_{O_2}}$, and $P_{C_{O_2}}$ are all more complicated than they at first appear.

$D_{L_{O_2}}$. Among the five terms that make up $D_{L_{O_2}}$, two vary both temporally (during the respiratory cycle) and spatially (from alveolus to alveolus). As far as *temporal* changes are concerned, during inspiration, lung expansion causes the surface area (A) available for diffusion to increase and the thickness of the barrier (a) to decrease (Fig. 29–2A). Therefore, $\dot{V}_{O_2}$ should be maximal at the end of inspiration. Considering *spatial* differences, alveolar dimensions differ from one alveolus to the next, both at rest and during the respiratory cycle.

$P_{A_{O_2}}$. Like area and thickness, $P_{A_{O_2}}$ varies both temporally and spatially. As far as *temporal* effects are concerned (see Fig. 29–2B), in any given alveolus, $P_{A_{O_2}}$ is greatest during inspiration (when O_2-rich air enters the lungs) and least just before the initiation of the next inspiration (after perfusion has maximally drained O_2 from the alveoli). Considering *spatial* effects, when an individual is standing, $P_{A_{O_2}}$ is greatest near the lung apex and least near the base (p. 702). Therefore, O_2 diffusion would be greatest near the end of inspiration at the apex of the lung.

$P_{C_{O_2}}$. Capillary P_{O_2} varies with distance along the pulmonary capillary (see Fig. 29–2C). As discussed later, as the blood flows down the capillary, $P_{C_{O_2}}$ rises to match $P_{A_{O_2}}$. Therefore, O_2 diffusion will be maximal at the beginning of the pulmonary capillary and gradually fall to zero further along the capillary.

The complications that we have raised for O_2 diffusion apply as well to CO_2 diffusion. Of these complications, by far the most serious is the last: the change in $P_{C_{O_2}}$ with distance along the pulmonary capillary. How, then, can we use Fick's law to understand the diffusion of O_2 and CO_2? Clearly, we cannot insert a single set of fixed values for $D_{L_{O_2}}$, $P_{A_{O_2}}$, and $P_{C_{O_2}}$ into Equation 29–7 and hope to describe the overall flow of O_2 and CO_2 between all alveoli and all pulmonary capillaries throughout the entire respiratory cycle. However, Fick's law does describe gas flow between air and blood at a *single point* in the lung and at a *single time* during the respiratory cycle. For O_2:

Equation 29–8

$$\dot{V}_{O_2} \text{ at one point and one time} = \underbrace{\left[k \frac{A \cdot s}{a\sqrt{MW}} \right]}_{D_{L_{O_2}}} (P_{A_{O_2}} - P_{C_{O_2}})$$

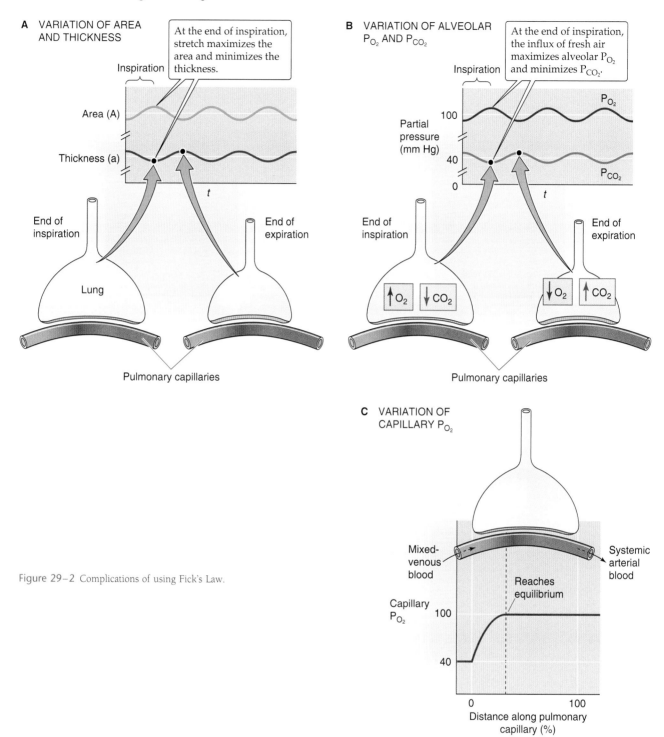

Figure 29–2 Complications of using Fick's Law.

At one point in space and one instant in time, A, a, $P_{A_{O_2}}$, and $P_{C_{O_2}}$ will each have well-defined values. The total amount of O_2 flowing from all alveoli to all pulmonary capillaries throughout the entire respiratory cycle is simply the sum of all individual diffusion events, added up over all pieces of alveolar wall (i.e., for each point along each capillary for all alveoli) and over all times in the respiratory cycle:

Equation 29–9

$$\text{Overall } \dot{V}_{O_2} = \overset{\substack{\text{All pieces} \\ \text{of alveolar} \\ \text{wall}}}{\sum} \overset{\substack{\text{All times} \\ \text{in respi-} \\ \text{ratory cycle}}}{\sum} \left(\underbrace{\left[k \, \frac{A \cdot s}{a\sqrt{MW}} \right]}_{D_{L_{O_2}}} (P_{A_{O_2}} - P_{C_{O_2}}) \right)$$

Here, $D_{L_{O_2}}$ is the "microscopic" diffusing capacity at one point in one alveolus, and at one time. Thus, Fick's law

Figure 29-3 Transport of O_2 from alveolar air to hemoglobin. The 10 diffusion constants (D_1–D_{10}) govern 10 diffusive steps. Hb is hemoglobin and $\theta \cdot V_C$ describes how fast O_2 binds to hemoglobin.

does indeed describe O_2 diffusion from alveolar air to pulmonary-capillary blood, as well as CO_2 diffusion of CO_2 in the opposite direction.

Although we cannot use a simple version of Fick's law of diffusion (Equation 29–7) to predict the uptake of O_2 by the lung, we can easily compute the uptake of O_2 *that has already taken place* using the **Fick principle** (p. 442). The rate of O_2 uptake by the lungs is the difference between the rate O_2 leaves the lungs via the pulmonary veins and the rate O_2 enters the lungs via the pulmonary arteries. For example, the rate of O_2 *departure from* the lungs is the product of blood flow (i.e., cardiac output, $\dot{Q}$) and the O_2 content of the pulmonary-venous blood, which is virtually the same as the O_2 content of systemic arterial blood (Ca_{O_2}). Remember that "content" is the sum of free (i.e., dissolved) O_2 and O_2 bound to hemoglobin (Hb) (p. 656). Similarly, the rate of O_2 *delivery to* the lungs is the product of $\dot{Q}$ and the O_2 content of the pulmonary arterial blood, which is the same as that of the mixed-venous blood ($C\bar{v}_{O_2}$). Thus, the difference between the rates of O_2 departure and O_2 delivery is

Equation 29–10

$$\text{Overall } \dot{V}_{O_2} = \overbrace{\dot{Q} \cdot Ca_{O_2}}^{\substack{\text{Rate of} \\ O_2 \text{ departure} \\ \text{from lung}}} - \overbrace{\dot{Q} \cdot C\bar{v}_{O_2}}^{\substack{\text{Rate of} \\ O_2 \text{ delivery} \\ \text{to lung}}}$$
$$= \dot{Q} \cdot (Ca_{O_2} - C\bar{v}_{O_2})$$

For a cardiac output of 5 liters/min, a Ca_{O_2} of 20 ml O_2/dl blood, and a $C\bar{v}_{O_2}$ of 15 ml O_2/dl blood, the rate of O_2 uptake by the pulmonary-capillary blood is

Equation 29–11

Rate of O_2 uptake

$$= \frac{5000 \text{ ml of blood}}{\text{min}} \times (20 - 15) \frac{\text{ml } O_2}{100 \text{ ml blood}}$$

$$= 250 \text{ ml } O_2/\text{min}$$

Obviously, the amount of O_2 that the lungs take up must be the same regardless of whether we *calculate* it after the fact using the Fick principle (Equation 29–10) or *predict* it by repeatedly applying Fick's law of diffusion (Equation 29–9):

Equation 29–12

$$\text{Overall } \dot{V}_{O_2} = \dot{Q} \cdot (Ca_{O_2} - C\bar{v}_{O_2})$$

$$= \overset{\substack{\text{All pieces} \\ \text{of alveolar} \\ \text{wall}}}{\sum} \overset{\substack{\text{All times} \\ \text{in respi-} \\ \text{ratory cycle}}}{\sum} \left(D_{L_{O_2}} \cdot (P_{A_{O_2}} - P_{C_{O_2}}) \right)$$

The Flow of O_2, CO, and CO_2 Between Alveolar Air and Blood Depends on the Interaction of These Gases with Red Blood Cells

We have been treating O_2 transport as if it involved only the diffusion of the gas across a homogeneous barrier. In fact, O_2 transport from alveolar air into the blood requires that O_2 first diffuses across a complex series of barriers and then, finally, combines with an O_2 buffer—Hb (Fig. 29–3, *upper panel*). One could imagine at least 10 discrete steps involving O_2 diffusion across various barriers. Oxygen must diffuse across or through:

1–3. The two membranes and cytoplasm of the type I alveolar pneumocyte (i.e., epithelial cell),
4. The interstitium (including alveolar and capillary basement membranes),
5–7. The two membranes and cytoplasm of the capillary endothelial cell,
8. The blood plasma,
9–10. The membrane and cytoplasm of the erythrocyte.

The total distance across the type I alveolar pneumocyte and the capillary endothelial cell is normally extremely short (0.15–0.30 μm), although it can increase substantially in disease. A diffusing capacity governs each of the above 10 steps. Together, these 10 diffusing capacities (D_1–D_{10}) contribute to a membrane diffusing capacity, designated $\mathbf{D_M}$ because it primarily describes how O_2 diffuses through various membranes. How do these 10 individual diffusing capacities contribute to D_M? Returning to our electrical model (Equation 29–6), we recognize that D is analogous to the reciprocal of resistance. Therefore, we can represent the 10 diffusive steps by 10 resistors in series. Because the total resistance is the sum of the individual resistances, the reciprocal of D_M is the sum of the reciprocals of the 10 individual diffusing capacities:

Equation 29–13

$$\frac{1}{D_M} = \frac{1}{D_1} + \frac{1}{D_2} + \frac{1}{D_3} + \cdots + \frac{1}{D_8} + \frac{1}{D_9} + \frac{1}{D_{10}}$$

Of course, D_M and its 10 components vary with location in the lung and position in the respiratory cycle.

For most of the O_2 entering the blood, the final step is binding to Hb. The interaction of O_2 with Hb is very complex (p. 655), and takes place at a finite rate:

Equation 29–14

Rate of O_2 uptake by erythrocytes = $(\theta \cdot V_C)$ PO_2

θ is a rate constant that describes how many ml of O_2 gas bind to the Hb in 1 ml of blood each minute, and for each mm Hg of partial pressure. V_C is the volume of blood in the pulmonary *capillaries*. The product $\theta \cdot V_C$ has the same dimensions as does D_M (units: ml/[min · mm Hg]), and both contribute to the overall diffusing capacity:

Equation 29–15

$$\frac{1}{D_L} = \frac{1}{D_M} + \frac{1}{\theta \cdot V_C}$$

Because O_2 binds to Hb so rapidly, its "Hb" term $1/(\theta \cdot V_C)$ is probably only approximately 5% as large as its "membrane" term $1/D_M$. However, for the test gas carbon monoxide (CO), which also binds to Hb (p. 663)—but far more slowly than O_2 binds—the slow equilibration of the gas with Hb is far more serious. The overall uptake of CO, which—as discussed later—pulmonary specialists use to compute D_L, seems to depend approximately equally on the two terms.

As far as the movement of CO_2 is concerned, one might expect the D_L for CO_2 to be substantially higher than that for O_2, inasmuch as the solubility of CO_2 in water is about 23-fold higher than for O_2 (p. 597). However, actual measurements show that $D_{L_{CO_2}}$ is only three- to fivefold greater than $D_{L_{O_2}}$. The reason for the lower-than-expected value for $D_{L_{CO_2}}$ is that the interaction of CO_2 with the red blood cell is even more complicated than that for O_2, involving interactions with Hb, carbonic anhydrase, and the Cl-HCO_3 exchanger (p. 663).

In summary, the movement of O_2, CO, and CO_2 between the alveolus and the pulmonary capillary involves not only diffusion, but also interactions with Hb. Although these interactions have only a minor effect on the

diffusing capacity for O_2, they are extremely important for CO and CO_2. Although we will hereafter refer to "diffusing capacity" as if it represented only the diffusion across a homogeneous barrier, one must keep in mind its more complex nature.

DIFFUSION AND PERFUSION LIMITATIONS ON GAS TRANSPORT

The Diffusing Capacity Normally Limits the Uptake of Carbon Monoxide from Alveolar Air to Blood

Imagine that a subject breathes air containing a very low level of carbon monoxide (CO), say 0.1%, for a brief period of time. Breathing higher levels of CO for longer periods could be fatal, because CO, which binds to Hb with an affinity that is 200 to 300 times higher than that for O_2, prevents Hb from releasing O_2 to the tissues (p. 663). If we assume that barometric pressure (P_B) is 760 mm Hg, and that P_{H_2O} is 47 mm Hg at 37°C, then we can compute the P_{CO} of the wet inspired air entering the alveoli (see the box on partial pressures on p. 595):

Equation 29–16

$$P_{CO} = \overbrace{F_{CO}}^{\substack{\text{Fraction of dry} \\ \text{air that is CO}}} \cdot (P_B - P_{H_2O})$$
$$= 0.1\% \cdot (760 - 47) \text{ mm Hg}$$
$$= \sim 0.7 \text{ mm Hg}$$

If the subject smokes cigarettes or lives in a polluted environment, CO will be present in the mixed-venous blood—and, therefore, the alveolar air—even before our test begins. If not, the initial P_{CO} of the mixed-venous blood entering the pulmonary capillaries will be approximately 0 mm Hg. Thus, a small gradient (~0.7 mm Hg) drives CO diffusion from alveolar air into blood plasma (Fig. 29–4A). As CO enters the blood plasma, it diffuses into the cytoplasm of the erythrocytes, where Hb binds it avidly. The flow of CO from alveolus to erythrocyte is so slow, and the ability of Hb to bind CO is so great, that Hb binds almost all incoming CO. Because only a small fraction of the total CO in the pulmonary-capillary blood remains free in solution, the aqueous phase of the blood remains nearly a perfect sink for CO. That is, P_{CO} in the capillary (Pc_{CO}), which is proportional to *free* [CO] in the capillary, rises only slightly above 0 mm Hg as the blood courses down the capillary (see Fig. 29–4B). Thus, by the time the blood reaches the end of the capillary (~0.75 sec later), Pc_{CO} is still far below alveolar P_{CO} ($P_{A_{CO}}$). In other words, CO fails to reach **diffusion equilibrium** between the alveolus and the blood.

There are three reasons why Pc_{CO} rises so slowly as blood flows down the pulmonary capillary:

1. $\mathbf{D_{L_{CO}}}$ is not even greater than it already is.
2. **A low alveolar P_{CO}.** Because we chose to use an extremely low inspired P_{CO}, the alveolar P_{CO} and thus the ΔP_{CO} driving CO diffusion from alveolar air into blood plasma is likewise small.
3. **The ability of Hb to bind CO.** The high affinity

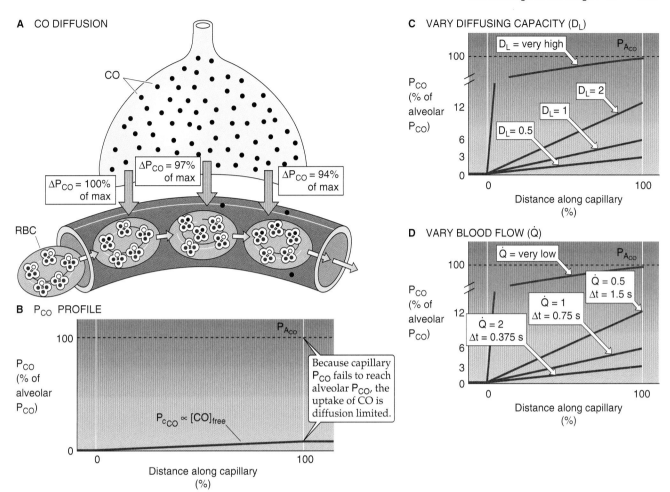

A CO DIFFUSION

CO

$\Delta P_{CO} = 100\%$ of max

$\Delta P_{CO} = 97\%$ of max

$\Delta P_{CO} = 94\%$ of max

RBC

B P_{CO} PROFILE

$P_{A_{CO}}$

P_{CO} (% of alveolar P_{CO})

Because capillary P_{CO} fails to reach alveolar P_{CO}, the uptake of CO is diffusion limited.

$P_{c_{CO}} \propto [CO]_{free}$

Distance along capillary (%)

C VARY DIFFUSING CAPACITY (D_L)

D_L = very high

$P_{A_{CO}}$

P_{CO} (% of alveolar P_{CO})

$D_L = 2$

$D_L = 1$

$D_L = 0.5$

Distance along capillary (%)

D VARY BLOOD FLOW ($\dot{Q}$)

$\dot{Q}$ = very low

$P_{A_{CO}}$

P_{CO} (% of alveolar P_{CO})

$\dot{Q} = 0.5$ $\Delta t = 1.5$ s

$\dot{Q} = 1$ $\Delta t = 0.75$ s

$\dot{Q} = 2$ $\Delta t = 0.375$ s

Distance along capillary (%)

Figure *29-4* Diffusion of CO. In *A*, ΔP_{CO} is CO partial-pressure gradient from alveolar air to pulmonary-capillary blood. As the red blood cell (RBC) enters the capillary, O_2 occupies three of the four sites on hemoglobin. In *B*, $P_{A_{CO}}$ is alveolar P_{CO}. In *C*, the blood flow $\dot{Q}$ has a relative value of 1. In *D*, the diffusing capacity D_L has a relative value of 1. Because P_{CO} is very low in *B–D*, we are on the linear portion of the Hb-CO dissociation curve. Thus, the CO content at the end of the capillary is approximately proportional to the capillary P_{CO}.

and high capacity of Hb for binding CO ensures that nearly all incoming CO disappears from the aqueous phase.

We might now explore factors that influence how much CO the blood takes up as it flows down the capillary. The principles that we develop here will apply equally well to O_2 and CO_2. First, we will use the Fick Principle (Equation 29–10) to quantitate, after the fact, how much CO has entered the blood:

Equation 29–17

$$\text{Overall } \dot{V}_{CO} = \dot{Q} \cdot (Cc'_{CO} - C\bar{v}_{CO})$$

Overall $\dot{V}_{CO}$ is the total flow of CO along the entire length of all capillaries throughout the lungs, $\dot{Q}$ is cardiac output, Cc'_{CO} is the CO content of blood at the end of the pulmonary capillary (dissolved and bound to Hb), and $C\bar{v}_{CO}$ is the CO content of mixed-venous blood at the *beginning* of the capillary. If we assume that $C\bar{v}_{CO}$ is 0, then Equation 29–17 simplifies to:

Equation 29–18

$$\text{Overall } \dot{V}_{CO} = \dot{Q} \cdot Cc'_{CO}$$

Of course, this overall $\dot{V}_{CO}$, computed from the Fick Principle, must be the same as the sum of the individual diffusion events, computed from Fick's law (see Equation 29–12), that took place as CO entered the blood that moved down the pulmonary capillaries:

Equation 29–19

$$\text{Overall } \dot{V}_{CO} = \dot{Q} \cdot Cc'_{CO}$$

$$= \underset{\substack{\text{All pieces} \\ \text{of alveolar} \\ \text{wall}}}{\sum} \underset{\substack{\text{All times} \\ \text{in respir-} \\ \text{atory cycle}}}{\sum} (D_{L_{CO}} \cdot (P_{A_{CO}} - P_{c_{CO}}))$$

How does CO uptake depend on $D_{L_{CO}}$ and $\dot{Q}$? For *basal conditions*, we can assume that when D_L and $\dot{Q}$ each have relative values of 1, the *third curve from top* in Figure 29–4*C* describes the course of $P_{c_{CO}}$. As a result, Cc'_{CO} will also have a relative value of 1. According to the Fick principle, the total amount of CO that moves into the blood along the capillary is:

Equation 29–20

$$\text{Overall } \dot{V}_{CO} = \dot{Q} \cdot Cc'_{CO}$$

$$= 1 \cdot 1$$

$$= 1$$

TABLE 29–1

ALVEOLAR TRANSPORT OF CO						
	DL_{CO}	$\dot{Q}$	×	Cc'_{CO}	=	$\dot{V}_{CO}$
Vary D_L (Q constant)	2	1		2		2
	1	1		1		1
	$\frac{1}{2}$	1		$\frac{1}{2}$		$\frac{1}{2}$
Vary $\dot{Q}$ (D_L constant)	1	$\frac{1}{2}$		2		1
	1	1		1		1
	1	2		$\frac{1}{2}$		1

DL_{CO} is the diffusing capacity of the lungs for CO. $\dot{Q}$ is the cardiac output. Cc'_{CO} is the CO content of the blood at the end of the capillary. $\dot{V}_{CO}$ is the overall rate of CO uptake by the pulmonary capillary blood. The values in the table are all relative to "control" values of unity.

What would happen if we keep $\dot{Q}$ constant, but change D_L? If we doubled D_L, then Fick's law (Equation 29–19) predicts that the flow of CO into the blood for each diffusion event along the capillary would double. Thus, along the entire capillary, Pc_{CO} would rise twice as steeply (see Fig. 29–4C, *second curve from top*) as before. As a result, Cc'_{CO} and thus $\dot{V}_{CO}$ would also double.

Halving D_L would have the opposite effect: Cc'_{CO} and thus $\dot{V}_{CO}$ would also halve (see Fig. 29–4C, *bottom curve*). Therefore, CO uptake is proportional to D_L over a wide range of D_L values (Table 29–1, *upper half*). Of course, if it were possible to make D_L extremely high, then capillary P_{CO} would rise so fast that CO would saturate the Hb before the end of the capillary, and capillary P_{CO} would reach alveolar P_{CO} (see Fig. 29–4C, *top curve*). However, for realistic values of D_L—as well as low alveolar P_{CO} levels and normal Hb concentrations—CO would fail to reach equilibrium by the end of the capillary.

How would altering blood flow affect $\dot{V}_{CO}$? If $\dot{Q}$ were halved and the dimensions of the capillary remained constant, then the contact time of the blood with the alveolus would double. Therefore, at any distance down the capillary, twice as much time would be available for CO diffusion. As a result, the profile of capillary P_{CO} *versus* distance would be twice as steep (see Fig. 29–4D, *second curve from top*) as in the basal state, and Cc'_{CO} would also be twice as great. However, because we achieved this increase in Cc'_{CO} by cutting $\dot{Q}$ in half, the product $\dot{Q} \cdot Cc'_{CO} = \dot{V}_{CO}$ would be the same as that in the basal state (see Table 29–1, *lower half*). Doubling blood flow would cause capillary P_{CO} to rise only half as steeply (see Fig. 29–4D, *bottom curve*) as in the basal state, but still have no effect on $\dot{V}_{CO}$. Thus, for the range of D_L and $\dot{Q}$ values in this example, *CO uptake is unaffected by changes in blood flow*. Of course, if we were to reduce $\dot{Q}$ to extremely low values, then capillary P_{CO} would reach alveolar P_{CO} by the end of the capillary (see Fig. 29–4D, *top curve*).

In our example, we have assumed that the Pc_{CO} profile along the capillary is linear, and the capillary dimensions are unaffected by changes in $\dot{Q}$. In fact, these assumptions are not entirely valid. Nevertheless, the uptake of CO is more or less proportional to the D_L for CO, and rather insensitive to perfusion. Therefore, we say that the uptake of CO is **diffusion limited** because it is the diffusing capacity that predominantly limits CO transport. We can judge whether or not the transport of a gas is predominantly diffusion limited by comparing the partial pressure of the gas at the end of the pulmonary capillary with the alveolar partial pressure. *If the gas does not reach diffusion equilibrium (i.e., if the end-capillary partial pressure fails to reach the alveolar partial pressure), then transport is predominantly diffusion limited.* However, if the gas does reach diffusion equilibrium, then its transport is perfusion limited, as discussed next.

Perfusion Normally Limits the Uptake of Nitrous Oxide from Alveolar Air Space to Blood

Unlike carbon monoxide, nitrous oxide (laughing gas, N_2O) does not bind to Hb. Therefore, when a subject inhales N_2O, the gas enters the blood plasma and the erythrocyte's cytoplasm, but has nowhere else to go (Fig. 29–5A). Consequently, as blood courses down the pulmonary capillary, the concentration of free N_2O—and thus capillary P_{N_2O} (Pc_{N_2O})—rises very rapidly (see Fig. 29–5B). By the time the blood is approximately 10% of the way along the capillary, Pc_{N_2O} has reached the alveolar P_{N_2O} (PA_{N_2O}), and N_2O is thus in diffusion equilibrium between alveolus and blood. The reason N_2O reaches diffusion equilibrium is not that its D_L is high, or that we chose a high inspired P_{N_2O}. The key difference is that Hb does not bind to N_2O.

How does N_2O uptake by the lungs depend on DL_{N_2O} and $\dot{Q}$? If we assume that the N_2O content of the mixed-venous blood entering the pulmonary capillary ($C\bar{v}_{N_2O}$) is 0:

Equation 29–21

$$\text{Overall } \dot{V}_{N_2O} = \dot{Q} \cdot Cc'_{N_2O}$$

Cc'_{N_2O} is the N_2O content of the blood at the end of the pulmonary capillary and represents entirely N_2O physically dissolved in blood, which according to Henry's law (p. 597) is proportional to Pc_{N_2O}. The overall $\dot{V}_{N_2O}$ computed from the Fick Principle in Equation 29–21 is the sum of individual diffusion events along the capillary:

Equation 29–22

$$\text{Overall } \dot{V}_{N_2O} = \dot{Q} \cdot Cc'_{N_2O}$$

$$= \sum_{\substack{\text{All pieces} \\ \text{of alveolar} \\ \text{wall}}} \sum_{\substack{\text{All times} \\ \text{in respi-} \\ \text{ratory cycle}}} (DL_{N_2O} \cdot (PA_{N_2O} - Pc_{N_2O}))$$

Because N_2O reached diffusion equilibrium at approximately 10% of the way down the capillary, the individual diffusion terms from Equation 29–22 equal 0 for 90% of the capillary!

We can approach the uptake of N_2O the same way we did the uptake of CO. We begin, under basal conditions, with relative values of 1 for D_L, $\dot{Q}$, and the end-capillary N_2O content. Thus, the initial $\dot{V}_{N_2O}$ is $\dot{Q} \times Cc'_{N_2O} = 1$.

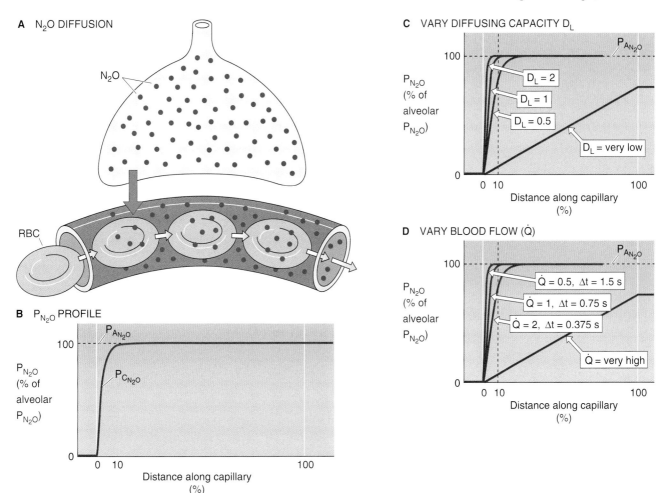

Figure 29–5 Diffusion of N_2O. In *B*, PA_{N_2O} is alveolar P_{N_2O} and PC_{N_2O} is capillary P_{N_2O}. In *C*, the blood flow $\dot{Q}$ has a relative value of 1. In *D*, the diffusing capacity D_L has a relative value of 1. The N_2O content at the end of the capillary is proportional to P_{N_2O}.

Figure 29–5*C* shows that doubling D_L doubles the flow of N_2O into the blood for each diffusion event, causing PC_{N_2O} to rise twice as steeply as before along the capillary. However, even though this doubling of D_L causes N_2O to come into diffusion equilibrium twice as fast as before, it has no effect on either the N_2O content of end-capillary blood or on $\dot{V}_{N_2O}$, both of which remain at 1. Cutting D_L in half also would have no effect on $\dot{V}_{N_2O}$. Thus, N_2O uptake is insensitive to changes in D_L, at least over the range of D_L values that we examined (Table 29–2, *upper half*). In other words, the *uptake of N_2O is not diffusion limited*.

What would be the effect of reducing $\dot{Q}$ by half, while holding D_L constant? If we assume that capillary dimensions remain constant, then halving $\dot{Q}$ would double the contact time of blood with the alveolus and make the PC_{N_2O} profile along the capillary twice as steep as before (see Fig. 29–5*D*). Nevertheless, Cc'_{N_2O} remains unchanged at 1. However, because we reduced $\dot{Q}$ by half, $\dot{V}_{N_2O}$ also falls by half. Conversely, doubling $\dot{Q}$ causes $\dot{V}_{N_2O}$ to double. Thus, N_2O uptake is more or less proportional to blood flow (i.e., perfusion) over a wide range of $\dot{Q}$ values (see Table 29–2, *lower half*). For this reason, we say that N_2O transport is predominantly **perfusion limited**. *The transport of a gas is predominantly perfusion limited if the gas in the capillary comes into equilibrium with the gas in the alveolar air by the end of the capillary.*

In Principle, CO Transport Could Become Perfusion Limited, and N_2O Could Become Diffusion Limited, Under Special Conditions

Although under normal circumstances CO transport is predominantly diffusion limited, and N_2O transport is predominantly perfusion limited, changes in certain parameters could, at least in theory, make CO uptake perfu-

TABLE 29–2

ALVEOLAR TRANSPORT OF N_2O				
	DL_{N_2O}	$\dot{Q}$	× Cc'_{N_2O}	= $\dot{V}_{N_2O}$
Vary D_L ($\dot{Q}$ constant)	2	1	1	1
	1	1	1	1
	$\frac{1}{2}$	1	1	1
Vary $\dot{Q}$ (D_L constant)	1	$\frac{1}{2}$	1	$\frac{1}{2}$
	1	1	1	1
	1	2	1	2

sion limited, or make N_2O uptake diffusion limited. To illustrate this concept, we introduce an analogy (Fig. 29–6): workers at a railroad siding trying to load boxes (the transport of a gas) onto the cars of a passing train. Each worker (the diffusive event) has a limited rate for putting boxes on the train. Each railway car (the blood) has a limited capacity for holding boxes. Finally, because the train is moving (the perfusion rate), a limited time is available to load each railway car.

First consider the situation in which the speed of the train perfectly matches the number of workers (see Fig. 29–6A). Thus, all workers are always fully occupied, and the railway cars depart the siding fully loaded; the last box is put on each car just as the car leaves the siding. Any decrease in worker number, any increase in the carrying capacity of each car, or any increase in train speed will cause the railway cars to leave the siding at least partially empty. Thus, if we fix train speed at "normal," *decreasing the number of workers* below "normal" (see Fig. 29–6B) would cause a proportional decrease in the shipping rate—the number of boxes the train carries away per hour. In other words, when the number of workers is between 0 and normal, the shipping rate is worker (diffusion) limited.

Now return to the original "perfect-match" condition in which both worker number and train speed are normal. Increasing worker number at constant train speed will have no effect on either the number of boxes loaded onto each railway car (which will remain filled to capacity) or on the shipping rate (see Fig. 29–6C). In this higher range of worker numbers, the shipping rate is no longer limited by the workers, but by the speed of the train or by the carrying capacity of the railway cars. Thus, we could say that the shipping rate is speed (perfusion) limited, although it would be equally true to say that it is carrying-capacity (hemoglobin) limited.

Let us return again to the original condition in which worker number perfectly matches train speed. Increasing train speed while fixing worker number at the normal value will cause railway cars to leave the siding partially empty (see Fig. 29–6D). However, shipping rate is unaffected because the normal number of boxes is simply distributed over a greater number of cars. Under these conditions, shipping rate is again worker (diffusion) limited, because increasing the number of workers would proportionally increase shipping rate. In fact, whenever you see cars leaving the siding only partially filled, you can conclude that shipping rate is worker (diffusion) limited, regardless of whether this situation arose because of a decrease in worker number, an increase in train speed, or an increase in car carrying-capacity.

Finally, let us again return to the perfectly matched initial condition and now decrease train speed while holding worker number fixed at the normal value. As velocity decreases below normal, shipping rate decreases proportionally (see Fig. 29–6E), even though the railway cars leave the siding fully loaded. Thus, shipping rate is speed (perfusion) limited. It would be equally true to characterize the system as being limited by carrying capacity (hemoglobin). In fact, whenever you see cars leaving the siding fully filled, you can conclude that shipping rate is speed (perfusion) limited, regardless of whether this situa-

tion arose because of an increase in worker number, a decrease in train speed, or a decrease in car carrying-capacity.

We are now in a position to consider factors that could render CO transport predominantly *perfusion* limited, or N_2O transport *diffusion* limited. At least six changes to the system would cause CO transport to be no longer limited by $D_{L_{CO}}$ (Table 29–3). That is, these changes would cause pulmonary capillary P_{CO} to reach alveolar P_{CO} by the end of the capillary. Similarly, the transport of N_2O, normally perfusion limited, could become diffusion limited by any of at least four changes (Table 29–4) that would cause capillary P_{N_2O} to fail to reach alveolar P_{N_2O} by the end of the pulmonary capillary.

The Uptake of Carbon Monoxide Provides an Estimate of D_L

Because the **pulmonary diffusing capacity** (D_L) plays such an important role in determining the partial pressure profile of a gas along the pulmonary capillary, it would be extremely valuable to estimate D_L in a living person. Moreover, an approach that is easily applicable to patients could be useful both as a diagnostic tool and to follow the progression of diseases affecting D_L.

We have already seen (Equation 29–9) that we can use Fick's law to compute the overall uptake of a gas if we summate many individual diffusion events for all pieces of alveolar wall and all times in the respiratory cycle:

Equation 29–23

$$\text{Overall } \dot{V}_{gas} = \overset{\substack{\text{All pieces} \\ \text{of alveolar} \\ \text{wall}}}{\sum} \; \overset{\substack{\text{All times} \\ \text{in respi-} \\ \text{ratory cycle}}}{\sum} \left(D_{L_{gas}} \cdot [P_{A_{gas}} - P_{C_{gas}}] \right)$$

If it were reasonable to ignore the spatial and temporal nonuniformities, then we could eliminate the two troublesome Σ symbols, and compute an *overall* $D_{L_{gas}}$ from the *overall* $\dot{V}_{gas}$. For example, we could accommodate modest spatial and temporal variations in $P_{A_{gas}}$ by computing an *average* alveolar partial pressure ($\overline{P}_{A_{gas}}$). Furthermore, if the partial pressure of the gas did not vary much along the capillary, it would be reasonable to use an *average* capillary partial pressure ($\overline{P}_{C_{gas}}$) as well. If we could choose a gas for which these assumptions are reasonable, then we could greatly simplify Equation 29–23, and in fact arrive at an expression that is very similar to the version of Fick's law that we started with at the beginning of this chapter (Equation 29–7):

Equation 29–24

$$\text{Overall } \dot{V}_{gas} = D_{L_{gas}} \cdot (\overline{P}_{A_{gas}} - \overline{P}_{C_{gas}})$$

Which gas could we use? If we are interested in estimating the diffusing capacity (D_L), we certainly do *not* want to use N_2O, whose uptake is perfusion limited. After all, $\dot{V}_{N_2O}$ is more or less proportional to changes in $\dot{Q}$, but virtually insensitive to changes in D_L (see Table 29–2). Another way of looking at the problem is that the driving pressure (ΔP_{N_2O}) between alveolus and capillary profile is highly non-uniform (see Fig. 29–5B). Thus, it

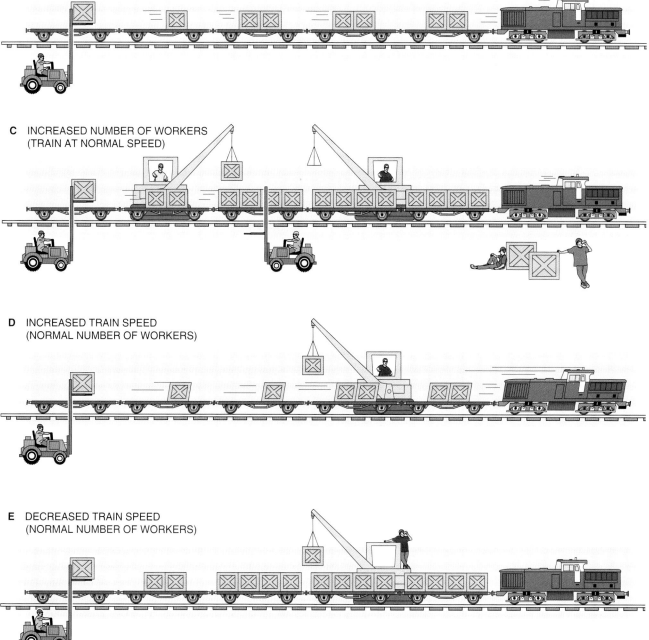

Figure 29–6 Railway car analogy. Workers represent the diffusion of O_2 across the alveolar wall. Railway cars represent capacity of blood to carry O_2. The speed of the train represents blood flow.

TABLE 29–3

CHANGES THAT COULD THEORETICALLY MAKE THE TRANSPORT OF A DIFFUSION-LIMITED GAS (CO) BECOME PERFUSION LIMITED

CHANGE*	WHY CHANGE MAKES TRANSPORT PERFUSION LIMITED
↑ D_L (↑ Number of workers)	If CO could enter rapidly enough, it could load the Hb with CO and cause free [CO] to rise rapidly.
↓ [hemoglobin] (↓ Size of each car)	Because carrying capacity for CO is reduced, a given rate of CO transport causes the concentration of free CO to rise rapidly.
↑ $C\bar{v}_{CO}$ (Partially pre-load cars with dummy boxes)	If the Hb were sufficiently preloaded with CO, not much additional CO would need to enter to fully load the Hb.
↓ $\dot{Q}$ (↓ Train speed)	If the contact time of blood with alveolar air were sufficiently long, enough CO could enter to load the Hb, causing the concentration of free CO to rise rapidly.
↑ Capillary length (Lengthen loading dock)	By increasing the contact time of blood with alveolar air, Hb would eventually become loaded, as described above.
↑ Capillary diameter at fixed $\dot{Q}$ (↓ Train speed)	As above, contact time would increase.

*Expression in parentheses refers to railway car analogy in Figure 29–6.

would be very difficult to pick a reasonable value for the *average* capillary P_{N_2O} to insert into Equation 29–24. However, CO is an excellent choice. In the first place, its uptake is diffusion limited, so that changes in the parameter of interest (i.e., D_L) have nearly a proportionate effect on $\dot{V}_{CO}$. Moreover, the profile of capillary P_{CO} is nearly ideal, varying only slightly as blood courses down the pulmonary capillary (see Fig. 29–4B). Thus, we might solve Equation 29–24 for $D_{L_{CO}}$:

$$\text{Equation 29–25}$$

$$D_{L_{CO}} = \frac{\dot{V}_{CO}}{(\bar{P}_{A_{CO}} - \bar{P}_{c_{CO}})}$$

It is good to remember that $D_{L_{CO}}$ and $\dot{V}_{CO}$ are *average* values that reflect properties of all alveoli throughout both lungs at all times in the respiratory cycle. Regarding $\bar{P}_{A_{CO}}$, although $P_{A_{CO}}$ may not vary much during the respiratory cycle, it probably varies from alveolus to alveolus owing to local differences in ventilation and perfusion (p. 702). Finally, as far as $\bar{P}_{c_{CO}}$ is concerned, P_{CO} is 0 in the blood at the beginning of the pulmonary capillaries for non-

smokers who live in a nonpolluted environment. Thus, we often can ignore $\bar{P}_{c_{CO}}$.

We will discuss two general methods for estimating $D_{L_{CO}}$, the steady-state technique and the single-breath test. These tests, both utilizing CO, are useful for estimating pulmonary diffusing capacity in a clinical setting, even among very ill patients in the intensive care unit.

In the **steady-state technique** (Fig. 29–7A), the subject breathes a low-CO air mixture (e.g., 0.1%–0.2%) for approximately a dozen breaths to allow $P_{A_{CO}}$ to stabilize. Calculating $D_{L_{CO}}$ requires at least two measurements: $\dot{V}_{CO}$ and $\bar{P}_{A_{CO}}$. After the subject's first dozen breaths, one computes the rate of CO uptake from the difference between the amounts of CO in inspired versus expired air over time. The experimenter directly measures $\bar{P}_{A_{CO}}$ in an alveolar air sample (p. 688). D_L is then $\dot{V}_{CO}/P_{A_{CO}}$. If the subject happens to be a smoker or live in a polluted environment, an accurate measurement of D_L requires a venous blood sample to estimate the mixed-venous P_{CO}. In this case, one calculates D_L from the more complete expression in Equation 29–25.

TABLE 29–4

CHANGES THAT COULD THEORETICALLY MAKE THE TRANSPORT OF A PERFUSION-LIMITED GAS (N₂O) BECOME DIFFUSION LIMITED

CHANGE*	WHY CHANGE MAKES TRANSPORT PERFUSION LIMITED
↓ D_L (↓ Worker number)	If N₂O entered slowly enough, $P_{c_{N_2O}}$ would fail to reach $P_{A_{N_2O}}$ by the end of the capillary.
↑ $\dot{Q}$ (↑ Train speed)	If the contact time of blood with alveolar air were sufficiently brief, not enough N₂O would enter the blood to cause $P_{c_{N_2O}}$ to reach $P_{A_{N_2O}}$ by the end of the capillary
↓ Capillary length (Shorten loading dock)	By decreasing contact time of blood with alveolar air, N₂O would fail to reach diffusion equilibrium, as described above.
↓ Capillary diameter at constant $\dot{Q}$ (↑ Train speed)	As above, contact time would decrease.

*Expression in parentheses refers to railway car analogy in Figure 29–6.

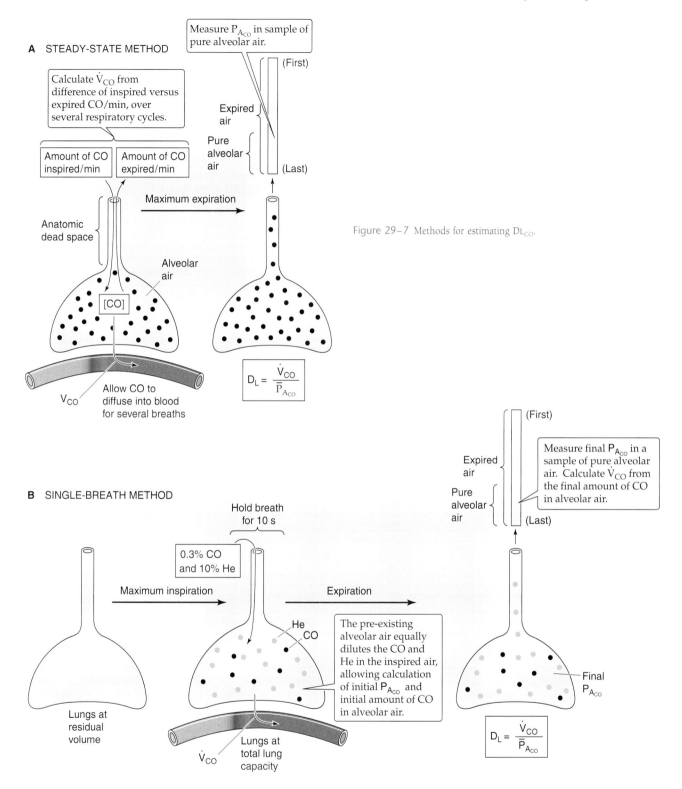

A   STEADY-STATE METHOD

Measure $P_{A_{CO}}$ in sample of pure alveolar air.

Calculate $\dot{V}_{CO}$ from difference of inspired versus expired CO/min, over several respiratory cycles.

(First)

Expired air

Pure alveolar air

(Last)

Amount of CO inspired/min | Amount of CO expired/min

Maximum expiration

Anatomic dead space

Alveolar air

[CO]

$$D_L = \frac{\dot{V}_{CO}}{\overline{P}_{A_{CO}}}$$

V_{CO} Allow CO to diffuse into blood for several breaths

Figure 29–7 Methods for estimating $D_{L_{CO}}$.

B   SINGLE-BREATH METHOD

Hold breath for 10 s

0.3% CO and 10% He

Maximum inspiration

Expiration

He
CO

Lungs at residual volume

$\dot{V}_{CO}$

Lungs at total lung capacity

The pre-existing alveolar air equally dilutes the CO and He in the inspired air, allowing calculation of initial $P_{A_{CO}}$ and initial amount of CO in alveolar air.

(First)

Expired air

Pure alveolar air

(Last)

Measure final $P_{A_{CO}}$ in a sample of pure alveolar air. Calculate $\dot{V}_{CO}$ from the final amount of CO in alveolar air.

Final $P_{A_{CO}}$

$$D_L = \frac{\dot{V}_{CO}}{\overline{P}_{A_{CO}}}$$

In the **single-breath technique** (see Fig. 29–7*B*), the subject makes a maximal expiratory effort, thus decreasing lung volume to residual volume (p. 607), and then makes a maximal inspiration of air containing CO. During a 10-sec period of breath-holding, some of the inhaled CO diffuses into the pulmonary blood. Again, calculating $D_{L_{CO}}$ requires at least two measurements: $\dot{V}_{CO}$ and $\overline{P}_{A_{CO}}$.

The inhaled air is a mixture of dilute CO (e.g., 0.3%) plus a gas such as helium. Because the water solubility of gases such as helium is very low, their transport across the blood-gas barrier is negligible (see Equation 29–5). We can, therefore, use helium to compute the extent to which the inhaled CO/He mixture is diluted as it first enters the alveoli, and also to calculate the alveolar vol-

TABLE 29–5

FACTORS THAT AFFECT THE DIFFUSING CAPACITY FOR CARBON MONOXIDE

FACTOR	EFFECT	EXPLANATION
Body size	↑ Size → ↑ $D_{L_{CO}}$	With ↑ in lung size, diffusion area (A) and volume of pulmonary capillary blood (V_C) both ↑.
Age	↑ Age → ↓ $D_{L_{CO}}$	$D_{L_{CO}}$ decreases by ~2% per year after age 20.
Sex	Male → ↑ $D_{L_{CO}}$	Corrected for age and body size, $D_{L_{CO}}$ is about 10% greater in men than women
Lung volume	↑ Volume → ↑ $D_{L_{CO}}$	In an individual, ↑ in lung volume causes an ↑ in volume of pulmonary capillary blood (V_C), an ↑ in diffusion area (A), and a ↓ in diffusion distance (a).
Exercise	Exercise → ↑ $D_{L_{CO}}$	An ↑ in $\dot{Q}$ causes dilation of pulmonary capillaries, which in turn causes an ↑ in area for diffusion (A) and volume of pulmonary capillary blood (V_C).
Body position	$D_{L_{CO}}$: supine > sitting > standing	Changes in posture presumably ↑ volume of pulmonary capillary blood (V_C).
$P_{A_{O_2}}$	↑ $P_{A_{O_2}}$ → ↓ $D_{L_{CO}}$	O_2 lowers the rate at which CO combines with hemoglobin.
$P_{A_{CO_2}}$	↑ $P_{A_{CO_2}}$ → ↑ $D_{L_{CO}}$	CO_2 causes an ↑ in volume of pulmonary capillary blood (V_C)

$D_{L_{CO}}$, diffusion capacity of carbon monoxide; $P_{A_{O_2}}$, partial pressure of oxygen in arterial blood.

ume into which the CO/He mixture distributes (p. 608). This information allows us to calculate the values of two crucial parameters at the *beginning* of the breath-holding period: (1) the $P_{A_{CO}}$ and (2) the amount of CO in the alveoli. During the 10 seconds of breath-holding, some of the inhaled CO diffuses into the blood. The greater the $D_{L_{CO}}$, the greater the loss of CO, and the more $P_{A_{CO}}$ falls. As the subject exhales, we obtain a sample of alveolar air. This sample allows us to determine the values of two crucial parameters at the *end* of the breath-holding period: (1) the $P_{A_{CO}}$ and (2) the amount of CO in the alveoli. The initial and final $P_{A_{CO}}$ values allow us to compute $\overline{P}_{A_{CO}}$. The initial and final alveolar CO amounts allow us to compute $\dot{V}_{CO}$ over the 10-sec breath-holding period.

Bear in mind that the value of $D_{L_{CO}}$ determined using either of the above methods is an *average* pulmonary diffusing capacity. As discussed in Chapter 30, pulmonary disease can cause ventilation to become nonuniform, making it difficult to obtain alveolar-air samples that are representative of the entire lung. Also, $D_{L_{CO}}$ depends on factors other than D_M (i.e., the "membrane" or truly diffusive component of D_L). A normal value for $D_{L_{CO}}$ is approximately 25 ml CO taken up per minute for each mm Hg of partial pressure driving CO diffusion, and for each ml of blood having a normal Hb content. *For CO transport*, D_M and $\theta \cdot V_C$ in Equation 29–15 are each approximately 50 ml CO/(min · ml blood):

Equation 29–26

$$\frac{1}{D_{L_{CO}}} = \frac{1}{50} + \frac{1}{50} = \frac{1}{25}$$

Thus, $1/(\theta \cdot V_C)$ makes a major contribution to the final $D_{L_{CO}}$. Because the V_C term in $\theta \cdot V_C$ is proportional to the Hb content of the blood, and because Hb content is decreased in **anemia**, a subject can have a reduced $D_{L_{CO}}$

even though the diffusion pathways in the lung (i.e., D_M) are perfectly normal. It is interesting to recall that $1/(\theta \cdot V_C)$ makes an insignificant contribution to the calculation of D_L for O_2. Nevertheless, it is the D_L for CO—and not that for O_2—that one uses for a clinical index of diffusing capacity. Table 29–5 summarizes several factors that can affect the calculated $D_{L_{CO}}$.

For Both O_2 and CO_2, Transport Is Normally Perfusion Limited

Blood enters the pulmonary capillaries (Fig. 29–8A) with the P_{O_2} of mixed-venous blood, typically 40 mm Hg. Capillary P_{O_2} reaches the alveolar P_{O_2} of approximately 100 mm Hg one third of the way along the capillary (see Fig. 29–8B, *black curve*). This partial-pressure profile for O_2 along the pulmonary capillary is intermediate between that of CO (which fails to reach diffusion equilibrium) and N_2O (which reaches diffusion equilibrium at ~10% of the way along the capillary). The transport of O_2 is similar to that of CO in that both molecules bind to Hb. However, in our foregoing CO example in Figure 29–4, the Hb was not preloaded with CO. Thus, the Hb had not only an extremely high affinity for CO, but also a high binding capacity. Moreover, in our example in Figure 29–4, the alveolar P_{CO} was very low, so that the diffusion of CO from alveolus to blood was very slow. Together, these factors ensured that Hb bound virtually all the slowly arriving CO and that P_{CO} increased very slowly along the capillary.

The uptake of O_2 differs from that of CO in three important respects. First, Hb is heavily preloaded with O_2; that is, Hb in mixed-venous blood is approximately 75% saturated with O_2 (p. 658), and, consequently, the available O_2-binding capacity of Hb is relatively low. Sec-

A O₂ DIFFUSION

O₂

RBC

B AT REST

$P_{A_{O_2}}$

Capillary P_{O_2} (mm Hg)

60

$D_L = 2$

$D_L = 1$

$D_L = 0.5$

Initial P_{O_2} gradient

Distance along capillary (%)

C EXERCISE

$P_{A_{O_2}}$

$\dot{Q} = 1$
$D_L = 1$

Capillary P_{O_2} (mm Hg)

$\dot{Q} = 3$
$D_L = 1$

$\dot{Q} = 3$
$D_L = 0.5$

Distance along capillary (%)

D HIGH ALTITUDE

Capillary P_{O_2} (mm Hg)

$P_{A_{O_2}}$

Initial P_{O_2} gradient

30

Exercise

Figure 29–8 Diffusion of O₂. In *A*, as the red blood cell (RBC) enters the capillary, O₂ occupies three of the four sites on hemoglobin. In *B–D*, $P_{A_{O_2}}$ is alveolar P_{O_2}. In *B* and *D*, $\dot{Q}$ is constant.

ond, because the alveolar P_{O_2} is rather high (i.e., ~100 mm Hg), the alveolar-blood P_{O_2} gradient is large (i.e., ~60 mm Hg) and the initial diffusion of O₂ from the alveolus into pulmonary-capillary blood is correspondingly high. Third, D_L for O₂ is higher than that for CO, owing to a greater $\theta \cdot V_C$. As a result, the Hb in pulmonary-capillary blood rapidly approaches its carrying capacity for O₂, so that capillary P_{O_2} reaches alveolar P_{O_2} about one third of the way along the capillary. Because capillary P_{O_2} reaches alveolar P_{O_2}, O₂ transport is primarily **perfusion limited**, as is the case for N₂O. Because O₂ reaches diffusion equilibrium so soon along the capillary, the lung has a tremendous D_L reserve for O₂. Even if we reduce $D_{L_{O_2}}$ by half, O₂ still reaches diffusion equilibrium about two thirds of the way along the capillary (see Fig. 29–8B, *blue curve*). If we could double $D_{L_{O_2}}$, O₂ would reach diffusion equilibrium much earlier than usual (see Fig. 29–8B, *red curve*). However, neither change in $D_{L_{O_2}}$ would affect O₂ uptake, which is *not* diffusion limited. However, even in healthy individuals, severe exercise or high altitude can stress O₂ transport.

The D_L reserve for O₂ is extremely important in the case of **exercise**, where cardiac output can increase by up to a factor of five (p. 425), substantially decreasing the contact time of the blood with the pulmonary capillaries. Even so, the contact time appears not to decrease by more than a factor of approximately 3, probably because the slightly increased pressure recruits and distends the pulmonary vessels (p. 698). As a result, even with vigorous exercise, $P_{C_{O_2}}$ reaches virtual equilibrium with the alveolar air by the end of the capillary (see Fig. 29–8C, *green curve*)—except in some elite athletes. Thus, the increase in $\dot{Q}$ during exercise leads to a corresponding increase in $\dot{V}_O$, which carries obvious survival benefits. In patients with pulmonary disease, however, thickening of the alveolar blood-gas barrier can reduce $D_{L_{O_2}}$ sufficiently that equilibration of P_{O_2} fails to occur by capillary's end during exercise (see Fig. 29–8C, *brown curve*). In this case, O₂ transport becomes diffusion limited.

At **high altitude**, barometric pressure and ambient P_{O_2} decrease proportionally (p. 1262). Therefore, compared with the situation at sea level, P_{O_2} will be low in both the alveoli and the mixed-venous blood entering the pulmonary capillaries, and the alveolar-capillary P_{O_2} gradient will be low as well (see Fig. 29–8D, *red curve*). For a subject at high altitude, O₂ transport tends to become more like CO transport (see Fig. 29–4) for two reasons. First, the magnitude of the P_{O_2} gradient from alveolus to capillary is smaller at altitude than at sea level, reducing the absolute O₂ transport rate. Second, because mixed-venous P_{O_2} is lower, the unused O₂-binding capacity of Hb is not so low as at sea level. Therefore, exercise at high altitude, with its attendant limitation in the contact time of the blood with the alveoli, can cause O₂ transport to become diffusion limited even in healthy individuals (Fig. 29–8D, *green curve*). If the subject also has a pathological condition that lowers $D_{L_{O_2}}$, then transport may become diffusion limited even more readily at altitude. Obviously, any combination of exercise, high altitude, and a reduced $D_{L_{O_2}}$ compounds the problems for O₂ transport.

As far as the transport of **carbon dioxide** is concerned, mixed-venous blood entering the pulmonary capillary has

A CO₂ DIFFUSION

B P_CO₂ PROFILE

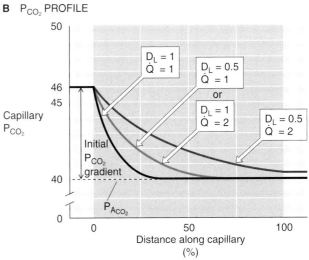

Figure 29–9 Diffusion of CO₂. In B, P_ACO₂ is alveolar P_CO₂.

a P_{CO_2} of approximately 46 mm Hg, whereas the alveolar P_{CO_2} is approximately 40 mm Hg (Fig. 29–9A). What is the P_{CO_2} profile along the pulmonary capillary? One factor tends to speed the equilibration of CO_2. As noted on p. 674, the D_L for CO_2 is threefold to fivefold greater than that for O_2. However, two factors tend to slow the equilibration of CO_2. First, the blood's carrying capacity for CO_2 at physiological P_{CO_2} values is more than twice as large as for O_2 (p. 666). Second, the initial P_{CO_2} gradient across the blood-gas barrier is only approximately 6 mm Hg at the beginning of the capillary, approximately 10% as large as the initial P_{O_2} gradient. Thus, a smaller gradient counteracts the larger D_L and greater CO_2 carrying capacity. Many authors believe that capillary P_{CO_2} reaches alveolar P_{CO_2} about one third of the way along the pulmonary capillary (as is the case for O_2), whereas others have suggested that CO_2 may just reach diffusion equilibrium by the end of the pulmonary capillary. In either case, a decrease in D_L seen in certain lung diseases (see later) or heavy exercise may cause the transport of CO_2 to become diffusion limited.

Pathological Changes That Reduce D_L Do Not Necessarily Produce Hypoxia

The measured pulmonary diffusing capacity for CO is reduced in disease states accompanied by a thickening of the alveolar blood-gas barrier, a reduction in the surface area (i.e., capillaries) available for diffusion, or a decrease in the amount of **Hb** in the pulmonary capillaries. Examples of pathology accompanied by a decrease in D_L include:

Diffuse interstitial pulmonary fibrosis, which is a fibrotic process causing a thickening of the interstitium, thickening of alveolar walls, and destruction of capillaries. Sometimes causing marked decreases in D_L, fibrosis occurs in such disorders as sarcoidosis, scleroderma, and asbestosis.

Chronic obstructive pulmonary disease, which leads to a destruction of pulmonary capillaries, and thus a reduction in both the surface area available for diffusion and total pulmonary-capillary Hb content (p. 624).

Loss of functional lung tissue, as caused by either a tumor or surgery. Surgical removal of lung tissue reduces D_L because of both a decrease in surface area and a decrease in total pulmonary-capillary Hb content.

Anemia, in which there is a reduction in total Hb content, and thus a decrease in the $\theta \cdot V_C$ component of $D_{L_{CO}}$.

Although there is little doubt that pulmonary diseases that cause hypoxemia (i.e., a decrease in arterial P_{O_2}) can also cause a decrease of D_L, it is not necessarily true that the decrease in D_L is the sole or even the major cause of the hypoxemia. The same diseases that lower D_L also upset the distribution of ventilation and perfusion throughout the lung. As discussed in Chapter 30, mismatching ventilation to perfusion among various regions of the lungs can be a powerful influence leading to hypoxemia. Furthermore, because the lung has a sizable D_L reserve for O_2 (and perhaps for CO_2 as well), $D_{L_{O_2}}$ would have to decrease to about one third of its normal value before O_2 became diffusion limited. Thus, in a disease causing both a decrease in D_L and disturbances in the distribution of ventilation and perfusion, it is difficult to determine the extent to which the reduction of D_L is responsible for the resulting hypoxemia.

REFERENCES

Books and Reviews

Cerretelli P, Di Prampero PE: Gas exchange in exercise. In Handbook of Physiology, Section 3: The Respiratory System, Vol. 1. Bethesda, MD, American Physiological Society, 1985, pp 297–339.

Forster RE: Exchange of gases between alveolar air and pulmonary capillary blood: Pulmonary diffusion capacity. Physiol Rev 37:391–452, 1957.

Hlastala MP: Diffusing-capacity heterogeneity. In Handbook of Physiology, Section 3: The Respiratory System, Bethesda, MD, American Physiological Society, 1985, pp 217–232.

Weibel ER: Morphological basis of alveolar-capillary gas exchange. Physiol Rev 53:419–495, 1973.

Journal Articles

Crapo JD, Crapo RO: Comparison of total lung diffusion capacity and the membrane component of diffusion capacity as determined by physiologic and morphometric techniques. Respir Physiol 51:181–194, 1983.

Krogh M: The diffusion of gases through the lungs of man. J Physiol 49:271–300, 1914–1915.

Ogilvie CM, Forster RE, Blakemore WS, Morton JW: A standardized breath-holding technique for the clinical measurement of the diffusing capacity of the lung for carbon monoxide. J Clin Invest 36:1–17, 1957.

Roughton FJW, Forster RE: Relative importance of diffusion and chemical reaction rates in determining rate of exchange of gases in the human lung, with special reference to true diffusing capacity of pulmonary membrane and volume of blood in the lung capillaries. J Appl Physiol 11:290–302, 1957.

Torre-Bueno JR, Wagner PD, Saltzman HA, et al: Diffusion limitation in normal humans during exercise at sea level and simulated altitude. J Appl Physiol 58:989–995, 1985.

Wagner PD, West JB: Effects of diffusion impairment on O_2 and CO_2 time courses in pulmonary capillaries. J Appl Physiol 33:62–71, 1972.

CHAPTER 30

Ventilation and Perfusion of the Lungs

Walter F. Boron

Although diffusion is at the very heart of gas exchange, two other parameters are also extremely important: the convective movement of air (i.e., ventilation) that exchanges gases between the atmosphere and the alveoli, and the convective movement of blood (i.e., perfusion) that carries the gases to and from the lung. In this chapter, we first examine the importance of ventilation as a whole. We next consider that even under physiological conditions, both ventilation and perfusion vary from one group of alveoli to the next. More importantly, we explore the fact that the distribution of the ventilation-perfusion ratio among alveolar units is critically important for gas exchange and thus for the composition of the arterial blood gases: PO_2, PCO_2, and pH.

VENTILATION

About 30% of Total Ventilation in a Respiratory Cycle Is Wasted Ventilating Anatomic Dead Space (i.e., Conducting Airways)

Ventilation is the movement of air into and out of the lungs. More quantitatively, **total ventilation** ($\dot{V}_T$) is the volume of air moved out of the lungs per unit of time:

Equation 30–1

$$\dot{V}_T = \frac{V}{t}$$

Here V is the volume of air exiting the lungs during a *series of breaths*. Note that we are using "$\dot{V}$" differently than in Chapter 26, where "$\dot{V}$" represented flow through an airway at a particular *instant* in time. A practical definition is that $\dot{V}_T$ is the product of tidal volume (TV or V_T) and the respiratory frequency (*f*). Thus, for someone with a tidal volume of 0.5 liter, breathing 12 breaths/min,

Equation 30–2

$$\dot{V}_T = V_T \cdot f$$
$$= (0.5 \text{ liter}) \cdot (12/\text{min})$$
$$= 6 \text{ liters/min}$$

Because total ventilation usually is reported as liters/min, it is sometimes called **minute ventilation**.

686

FIGURE 30–1. Ventilation of dead space and alveolar space during a respiratory cycle.

Of a normal inspiration of approximately 500 ml, only the first approximately 350 ml of "fresh" inspired air reaches the alveoli. The remaining 150 ml of fresh air remains in the conducting airways (i.e., nose, pharynx, larynx, trachea, and other airways without alveoli)— that is, the **anatomic dead space**. These figures are typical for a 70-kg person; V_T and V_D are roughly proportional to body size.

Before an inspiration, the conducting airways are filled with "stale" air having the same composition as alveolar air (Fig. 30–1, *step 1*); we will see why shortly. During inspiration, 500 ml of "fresh" atmospheric air (high P_{O_2}/ low P_{CO_2}) enters the body (*step 2*). However, only the first 350 ml reaches the alveoli; the final 150 ml remains in the conducting airways. Simultaneously, 500 ml of air enters the alveoli. However, the first 150 ml is stale air previously in the conducting airways; only the final 350 ml is "fresh" air. By the end of inspiration, the 500 ml of air that entered the alveoli (150 ml of stale air plus 350 ml of fresh air) has mixed by diffusion with the pre-existing alveolar air (*step 3*). During expiration (*step 4*), the first 150 ml of air emerging from the nose is the fresh air left in the conducting airways from the previous inspiration. As the expiration continues, 350 ml of stale alveolar air sequentially moves into the conducting airways, and then exits the body—for a total of 500 ml of air leaving the body. Simultaneously, 500 ml of air leaves the alveoli. The first 350 ml is the same 350 ml that exited the body. The final 150 ml of stale air to exit the alveoli remains in the conducting airways, as we are ready to begin the next inspiration.

Thus, with each 500-ml inspiration, only the *initial* 350 ml of fresh air entering the nose/mouth reaches the alveoli. With each 500-ml expiration, only the *final* 350 ml of air exiting the nose/mouth comes from the

alveoli. In effect, 150 ml of *fresh air* shuttles back and forth between the atmosphere and conducting airways. Another 150 ml of *stale air* also shuttles back and forth between the conducting airways and alveoli. **Dead space ventilation** ($\dot{V}_D$) is the volume of the "stale" air so shuttled per minute. **Alveolar ventilation** ($\dot{V}_A$) is the volume of "fresh" air per minute that actually reaches the alveoli, or the volume of stale alveolar air that reaches the atmosphere. Thus, total ventilation—a reflection of the work invested in breathing—is the sum of wasted dead space ventilation and alveolar ventilation. In our example,

Equation 30–3

			liters	breaths	liters
			breath	min	min
$\dot{V}_D =$	$V_D \cdot f$	$=$	0.150 ·	12	$= 1.8$
$\dot{V}_A = (V_T - V_D) \cdot f$		$=$	0.350 ·	12	$= 4.2$
$\dot{V}_T =$	$V_T \cdot f$	$=$	0.500 ·	12	$= 6.0$

so that the dead space ventilation is 30% of the total ventilation.

The inset of Figure 30–1 illustrates how inspiration and expiration lead to small fluctuations in the alveolar partial pressures for O_2 and CO_2. Just before an inspiration, alveolar P_{O_2} has fallen to its low point, and alveolar P_{CO_2} has risen to its high point. After the inspiration and mixing of a new bolus of inspired "fresh" air, alveolar P_{O_2} reaches its highest value during the respiratory cycle, and conversely alveolar P_{CO_2} falls to its lowest. During and after the expiration, as the flow of blood through the pulmonary capillaries continuously draws O_2 out of the alveolar air and adds CO_2, alveolar P_{O_2} and P_{CO_2} gradually drift to the values that we saw at the start of the respiratory cycle. Assuming that functional residual capacity (FRC) is approximately 3 liters and that each breath adds only 350 ml of fresh air, one can calculate that alveolar P_{O_2} oscillates with an amplitude of approximately 5 mm Hg, whereas alveolar P_{CO_2} oscillates with an amplitude of approximately 4 mm Hg.

Fowler's Single-Breath N₂ Washout Estimates Anatomic Dead Space

In 1948, Ward Fowler introduced an approach for estimating the anatomic dead space, based on the washout from the lungs of N_2. The key concept is that N_2 is physiologically inert. After the subject has been breathing room air, the alveolar air is approximately 75% N_2. The subject then makes a quiet expiration (Fig. 30–2A, *step 1*). Starting from a lung volume of FRC, he or she takes a single, normal-sized breath (~500 ml) of 100% O_2, although, in principle we could use any gas mixture lacking N_2. The *first portion* of inspired O_2 enters the alveolar spaces (*step 2*), where it rapidly mixes by diffusion and dilutes the N_2 and other gases remaining after the previous breaths of room air (*step 3*). The *last portion* of the inspired O_2 (~150 ml) remains in the conducting airways, which have a P_{N_2} of zero.

The subject now exhales approximately 500 ml of air (*step 4*). If no mixing occurred between the N_2-free air in the most distal conducting airways and the N_2-containing air in the most proximal alveolar spaces, then the first approximately 150 ml of air emerging from the body would have an $[N_2]$ of zero (see Fig. 30–2B). After this would come a sharp transition to a much higher $[N_2]$ for

the final approximately 350 ml of expired air. Thus, the expired volume with an $[N_2]$ of zero would represent air from the conducting airways (anatomic dead space), whereas the remainder would represent air from the alveoli.

In reality, some mixing occurs between the air in the conducting airways and alveoli, so that the transition is S-shaped (see Fig. 30–2C). A vertical line drawn through the S-shaped curve, so that *area a* is the same as *area b*, marks the idealized transition between air from the conducting and alveolar airways—as in Figure 30–2B. The expired lung volume at the point of this vertical line is thus the anatomic dead space. In Figure 30–2C, the part of the S-shaped curve with an expired $[N_2]$ of zero represents pure dead space air, the part where $[N_2]$ gradually rises represents a mixture of dead space and alveolar air, and the part where $[N_2]$ is high and flat represents pure alveolar air. This plateau is important, because it is during this plateau that one obtains an **alveolar gas sample**.

Bohr's Expired-[CO₂] Approach Estimates Physiological Dead Space

In principle, we could compute the dead space using *any* gas whose expiration profile looks like that of N_2. Nitrogen was useful, because we could easily create an artificial situation (i.e., a single breath of 100% O_2) in which no N_2 was present in the dead space, but plenty remained in the alveoli from previous inspirations of room air. However, the concentration profile of CO_2 during expira-

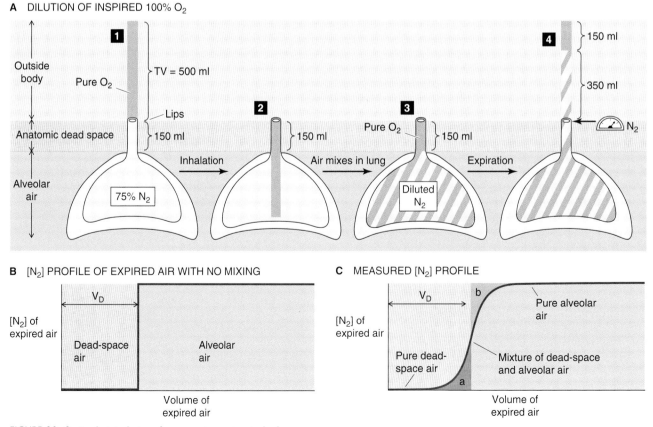

FIGURE 30–2. Fowler's technique for measuring anatomic dead space.

A   DILUTION OF INSPIRED ROOM AIR

B   [CO₂] PROFILE OF EXPIRED AIR

C   EFFECT OF ALVEOLAR DEAD-SPACE VENTILATION ON EXPIRED-CO₂ PROFILE

FIGURE 30–3. Bohr's method for measuring physiological dead space.

tion is similar to that of N_2, and we do not need to use any special tricks to get it to work. Practically no CO_2 is present in the inspired room air, and yet plenty is in the alveoli, where it is deposited by the incoming mixed venous blood. Thus, after a quiet expiration (Fig. 30–3A, step 1), the P_{CO_2} of the alveolar air will be virtually the same as the P_{CO_2} of the arterial blood (p. 684), approximately 40 mm Hg. The subject now inhales a normal tidal volume (~500 ml) of room air, although any CO_2-free gas would do. The first portion enters the alveoli (step 2), where it rapidly dilutes the CO_2 and other gases remaining after the previous breath (step 3). The rest (~150 ml) remains in the conducting airways, which now have a P_{CO_2} of approximately zero. When the subject now expires (step 4), the first air that exits the body is the CO_2-free gas that had filled the conducting airways, followed by the CO_2-containing alveolar air. Thus, the idealized profile of expired [CO_2] (Fig. 30–3B) is similar to the idealized [N_2] record in the Fowler method (see Fig. 30–2B). In particular, the volume of expired air at the vertical line in Figure 30–3B is the estimated *anatomic* dead space.

In principle, then, one could use the record of expired [CO_2] during a single-breath CO_2 washout, rather than

the N_2 that Fowler used to measure anatomic dead space. Indeed, long before the days of rapidly responding N_2 and CO_2 meters, Bohr also used data from a single-breath CO_2 washout to compute dead space. However, Bohr's approach differs from Fowler's in an important way: Bohr analyzed the average P_{CO_2} in the *mixed*-expired air (i.e., averaged over the dead space plus expired alveolar air).

The principle of Bohr's approach is that the amount of CO_2 present in the volume of mixed-expired air (V_E) is the sum of the CO_2 contributed by the volume of air from the dead space (V_D) plus the CO_2 contributed by the volume of air coming from the *alveoli* ($V_E − V_D$). As summarized in Figure 30–3B:

1. The amount of CO_2 coming from the **dead space** is the product of V_D and [CO_2] in this dead space air. Because [CO_2]$_D$ is zero, the area beneath V_D is also zero.
2. The amount of CO_2 coming from **alveolar air** is the product of ($V_E − V_D$) and alveolar [CO_2] and is represented by the rose and violet areas in Figure 30–3B.
3. The total amount of CO_2 in the **mixed-expired air** is the product of V_E and the average [CO_2] in this air and is represented by the blue and violet areas in Figure 30–3B.

Because the rose plus violet areas in Figure 30–3B must equal the blue plus violet areas, and because the alveolar and expired $[CO_2]$ values are proportional to their respective P_{CO_2} values, it is possible to show that

Equation 30–4

$$\frac{V_D}{V_E} = \frac{P_{A_{CO_2}} - P_{E_{CO_2}}}{P_{A_{CO_2}}}$$

This is the **Bohr equation**. Typically, V_D/V_E ranges between 0.20 and 0.35. For a V_D of 150 ml and a V_E of 500 ml, V_D/V_E would be 0.30. To illustrate how we can compute this ratio, if the alveolar P_{CO_2} is 40 mm Hg and the mixed-expired P_{CO_2} is 28 mm Hg, then

Equation 30–5

$$\frac{V_D}{V_E} = \frac{40 - 28}{40} = 30\%$$

Equation 30–4 makes good intuitive sense. In an imaginary case in which we reduced V_D to zero, the expired air would be entirely from the alveoli, so that

Equation 30–6

$$\frac{V_D}{V_E} = \frac{40 - 40}{40} = 0\%$$

On the other hand, if we reduced the tidal volume to a value at or below the dead space volume, then *all* of the expired air would be dead space air. Thus, the $P_{E_{CO_2}}$ would have to be zero, and

Equation 30–7

$$\frac{V_D}{V_E} = \frac{40 - 0}{40} = 100\%$$

Two examples of this principle are of practical importance. During **panting**, the respiratory frequency is very high, but the tidal volume is only slightly greater than the anatomic dead space. Thus, most of the total ventilation is wasted as dead space ventilation. If the tidal volume were reduced below V_D, then there would be no alveolar ventilation at all! During **snorkeling**, a swimmer breathes through a tube that increases V_D. If the snorkeling tube had a volume of 350 ml and the dead space within the body of the swimmer were 150 ml, then a tidal volume of 500 ml would produce no alveolar ventilation. Consequently, the swimmer would suffocate, even though total ventilation was normal! Thus, the fractional dead space (V_D/V_E) depends critically on tidal volume.

It is important to recognize that although Fowler's and Bohr's methods yield about the same estimate for V_D in healthy individuals, the two techniques actually measure somewhat different things. Fowler's approach measures **anatomic dead space**—the volume of the conducting airways from the mouth/nose up to the point where N_2 in the alveolar gas rapidly dilutes inspired 100% O_2. Bohr's approach, on the other hand, measures the **physiological dead space**—the volume of airways *not* receiving CO_2 from the pulmonary circulation, and, therefore, *not* engag-

ing in gas exchange. In a healthy person, the anatomic and **physiological** dead spaces are identical—the volume of the conducting airways. However, if some alveoli are ventilated but not perfused by pulmonary capillary blood, these unperfused alveoli, like conducting airways, do not contain CO_2. The air in such unperfused alveoli, known as **alveolar dead space**, contributes to the physiological dead space:

Equation 30–8

$$\underbrace{\text{Physiological dead space}}_{\text{Bohr's method}} = \underbrace{\text{Anatomic dead space}}_{\text{Fowler's method}} + \text{Alveolar dead space}$$

Fowler's and Bohr's methods could yield very different results in a patient with a **pulmonary embolism**, a condition in which a mass such as a blood clot wedges into and obstructs a part of the pulmonary circulation. Alveoli downstream from the embolus are ventilated but not perfused; that is, they are alveolar dead space (Fig. 30–3C). Thus, Bohr's method—but not Fowler's method—could detect an increase in the **physiological** dead space caused by a pulmonary embolism.

Alveolar Ventilation Is the Rate of CO₂ Production Divided by the Mole Fraction of CO₂ in the Alveolar Air

As discussed, one way of computing alveolar ventilation is to subtract the dead space from the tidal volume, and multiply the difference by the respiratory frequency (see Equation 30–3). Although, this approach is conceptually the most straightforward for computing $\dot{V}_A$, we can also calculate $\dot{V}_A$ from alveolar P_{CO_2}. The body produces CO_2 via oxidative metabolism at a rate of approximately 200 ml/min. In the steady state, this rate of CO_2 production ($\dot{V}_{CO_2}$) must equal the rate at which the alveoli evolve CO_2. All 200 ml/min of evolved CO_2 must be diluted in the alveolar air, which we exhale at a rate of approximately 4200 ml/min. Therefore, collecting all air exiting the alveoli in 1 minute, the 200 ml of CO_2 gas would be diluted in 4200 ml of alveolar air, from which we would conclude that approximately 5% of the alveolar air is CO_2 gas:

Equation 30–9

$$\frac{\begin{matrix}\text{Volume of } CO_2 \\ \text{leaving alveoli} \\ \text{in 1 min}\end{matrix}}{\begin{matrix}\text{Volume of air} \\ \text{leaving alveoli} \\ \text{in 1 min}\end{matrix}} = \left(\begin{matrix}\text{Fraction of} \\ \text{alveolar air} \\ \text{that is } CO_2\end{matrix}\right) = (\text{Fraction } CO_2)_A$$

$$\frac{\dot{V}_{CO_2}}{\dot{V}_A} = \frac{200 \text{ ml}}{4,200 \text{ ml}} = \sim 5\%$$

Rearranging the foregoing equation and solving for $\dot{V}_A$ yields

FIGURE 30–4. Dependence of alveolar CO_2 and O_2 on alveolar ventilation. As alveolar ventilation increases, alveolar PO_2 and PCO_2 approach their values in inspired air. At extremely low or high $\dot{V}_A$, where O_2 consumption and CO_2 production do not remain constant, these idealized curves are no longer valid.

Equation 30–10

$$\dot{V}_A = \frac{\dot{V}CO_2}{(\text{Fraction } CO_2)_A} = k \frac{\dot{V}CO_2}{PA_{CO_2}}$$

The constant k indicates that the alveolar PCO_2 is proportional to the mole fraction of CO_2 in alveolar air. This equation is true only when we *measure all parameters under the same conditions*. This obvious point would hardly be worth noting if respiratory physiologists had not managed, by historical accident, to measure the three terms in Equation 30–10 under three different conditions:

1. Body temperature and pressure, saturated with water vapor (BTPS, p. 597) for $\dot{V}_A$.
2. Standard temperature and pressure, dry (STPD, p. 598) for $\dot{V}CO_2$.
3. 37°C for PA_{CO_2}.

Thus, in *practical* applications, we must replace k in Equation 30–10 by a conversion factor that accounts for the different conditions for measuring $\dot{V}_A$, $\dot{V}CO_2$, and PA_{CO_2}:

Equation 30–11

$$\dot{V}_A = 0.863 \cdot \frac{\dot{V}CO_2}{PA_{CO_2}}$$

(liters/min, BTPS)   (mm Hg · liters/ml)   (mm Hg)   (ml/min, STPD)

This is the **alveolar ventilation equation**, which we can use to compute $\dot{V}_A$ if we know the rate of CO_2

production and the alveolar PCO_2. We determine $\dot{V}CO_2$ by collecting a known volume of expired air over a fixed time period and analyzing its CO_2. For a 70-kg human, $\dot{V}CO_2$ is approximately 200 ml/min. We can determine PA_{CO_2} from a sample of alveolar air, obtaining the **end-tidal PCO_2** (see Fig. 30–2C), which is 40 mm Hg. In practice, clinicians generally measure *arterial* PCO_2 (Pa_{CO_2}), and assume that alveolar and arterial PCO_2 are identical (p. 684). Inserting these values into the alveolar ventilation equation, we have

Equation 30–12

$$\dot{V}_A = 0.863 \cdot \frac{\dot{V}CO_2}{PA_{CO_2}} = 0.863 \cdot \frac{200 \text{ ml/min}}{40 \text{ mm Hg}}$$
$$= 4.315 \text{ liters/min}$$

For the sake of simplicity—and consistency with our example in Equation 30–3—we round this figure to 4.2 liters/min.

Although it is usually safe to regard $\dot{V}CO_2$ as being constant for a person at rest, a clinical example in which $\dot{V}CO_2$ can increase markedly is **malignant hyperthermia** (see box on p. 243), which is associated with increased oxidative metabolism. One hallmark of this clinical catastrophe is that the increase in $\dot{V}CO_2$ leads to an increase in PA_{CO_2} even though $\dot{V}_A$ is normal.

Alveolar and Arterial PCO₂ Are Inversely Proportional to Alveolar Ventilation

Viewing Equation 30–11 from a different perspective illustrates one of the most important concepts in all of respiratory physiology: Other things being equal, alveolar PCO_2 is inversely proportional to alveolar ventilation. This conclusion makes intuitive sense because the greater the $\dot{V}_A$, the more that the fresh, inspired air dilutes the alveolar CO_2. Rearranging Equation 30–11 yields

Equation 30–13

$$PA_{CO_2} = 0.863 \cdot \frac{\dot{V}CO_2}{\dot{V}_A}$$

In other words, if CO_2 production is fixed, then doubling $\dot{V}_A$ causes PA_{CO_2} to fall to half of its initial value. Conversely, halving $\dot{V}_A$ causes PA_{CO_2} to double. Because, at least under ideal circumstances, *arterial* PCO_2 is virtually the same as *alveolar* PCO_2, changes in $\dot{V}_A$ affect not only PA_{CO_2}, but also Pa_{CO_2}.

Figure 30–4 helps illustrate the principle. Imagine that your tissues are producing 200 ml of CO_2 each minute. In a steady state, your lungs must blow off 200 ml of CO_2 each minute. Also, imagine that your lungs are expelling 4200 ml of alveolar air each minute. Because the 200 ml of expired CO_2 must dissolve in the 4200 ml of expired alveolar air, Equation 30–13 tells us that your alveolar PCO_2 (and thus your Pa_{CO_2}) must be approximately 40 mm Hg.

Now, what would happen if the excitement of reading about respiratory physiology caused your alveolar ventilation to double, to 8400 ml/min? This is an example of

hyperventilation. You could double $\dot{V}_A$ either by doubling your respiratory frequency or by increasing your tidal volume, or a combination of the two (see Equation 30–3). Immediately on doubling $\dot{V}_A$, you would blow off twice the previous volume of alveolar air per unit time, and also twice the volume of CO_2 (i.e., 400 ml/min). Because your body would continue to produce only 200 ml CO_2 per minute—assuming that doubling $\dot{V}_A$ does not increase $\dot{V}CO_2$—you would initially blow off CO_2 faster than you made it, causing CO_2 levels throughout your body to fall. However, the falling PCO_2 of mixed venous blood would cause alveolar PCO_2 to fall as well, and thus the rate at which you blow off CO_2 would fall. Eventually, you would reach a new steady state in which the rate at which you blow off CO_2 would exactly match the rate at which you produce CO_2 (i.e., 200 ml/min). At this point, the PCO_2 values in your mixed-venous blood, arterial blood, and alveolar air would be stable. But what would be the $P_{A_{CO_2}}$? Because each minute you now are blowing off 8400 ml of alveolar air (i.e., twice normal) but still only 200 ml of CO_2, your alveolar PCO_2 must be half normal, or approximately 20 mm Hg. Not only does the hyperventilation cause *alveolar* PCO_2 to fall by half, it also causes *arterial* PCO_2 to fall by half. Thus, hyperventilation leads to **respiratory alkalosis** (p. 641). This respiratory alkalosis causes the arterioles in the brain to constrict (p. 561), reducing blood flow to the brain, which causes dizziness.

What would happen if, instead of doubling alveolar ventilation, you halved it from 4200 to 2100 ml/min? This is an example of **hypoventilation**. At the instant you began hypoventilating, the volume of CO_2 expired per unit time would fall by half, to 100 ml/min, even though CO_2 production by the tissues would remain at 200 ml/min. Thus, CO_2 would build up throughout the body, causing $P_{A_{CO_2}}$ to rise. To what value would $P_{A_{CO_2}}$ have to increase before you would reach a new steady state? Because each minute you must exhale 200 ml of CO_2, but this can be diluted in only 2100 ml or half the usual amount of alveolar air, the alveolar $[CO_2]$ must double from approximately 40 to 80 mm Hg. Of course, this doubling of *alveolar* PCO_2 is paralleled by a doubling of *arterial* PCO_2, leading to a **respiratory acidosis** (p. 640).

Therefore, the steady-state alveolar PCO_2 is inversely proportional to alveolar ventilation. The higher the $\dot{V}_A$, the lower the $P_{A_{CO_2}}$. If $\dot{V}_A$ were infinitely high, then $P_{A_{CO_2}}$ would theoretically fall to zero, the PCO_2 of inspired air.

Alveolar and Arterial PO₂ Depend on Alveolar Ventilation, Alveolar PCO₂, and the Respiratory Quotient

Alveolar ventilation also influences O_2 levels. As $\dot{V}_A$ increases, alveolar PO_2 approaches the inspired PO_2. Therefore, $P_{A_{O_2}}$ rises rather than falls with increasing $\dot{V}_A$. At an infinite $\dot{V}_A$, $P_{A_{O_2}}$ would theoretically approach the PO_2 of inspired air, approximately 149 mm Hg.

Although alveolar PO_2 obviously depends critically on $\dot{V}_A$, it is also influenced to a lesser extent by alveolar gases other than O_2—namely H_2O, N_2, and CO_2. The partial pressure of H_2O at 37°C is 47 mm Hg, and P_{H_2O}

will not change unless the subject's temperature changes. The partial pressures of all of the other gases "fit" into what remains of barometric pressure (P_B) after P_{H_2O} has claimed its mandatory 47 mm Hg. We can think of N_2 as a "spectator molecule," because it is not metabolized; P_{N_2} is whatever it has to be to keep the total pressure of the dry alveolar air at $760 - 47 = 713$ mm Hg. That leaves us to deal with CO_2. Because inspired air contains virtually no CO_2, we can think of the alveolar CO_2 as coming exclusively from metabolism. However, $\dot{V}CO_2$ depends not only on how fast the tissues burn O_2 but also on the *kind of fuel* they burn. If the fuel is carbohydrate, then the tissues produce one molecule of CO_2 for each O_2 consumed (p. 1223). This ratio is termed the **respiratory quotient** [RQ]:

$$\text{Equation 30–14}$$

$$RQ = \frac{\dot{V}CO_2}{\dot{V}O_2}$$

In this case the RQ is 1, which is a good place to start when considering how alveolar PCO_2 affects alveolar PO_2. If we consider only the *dry* part of the inspired air that enters the alveoli (see Table 25–1), then the $P_{I_{N_2}}$ is $713 \times 0.78 = 557$, the $P_{I_{O_2}}$ is $713 \times 0.2095 = 149$ mm Hg, the $P_{I_{CO_2}}$ is approximately zero. Eventually, the pulmonary capillary blood takes up all incoming O_2, replacing it with an equal number of CO_2 molecules (RQ = 1). Because the exchange of O_2 for CO_2 is precisely 1 for 1, alveolar PO_2 is what is left of the inspired PO_2 after metabolism replaces some alveolar O_2 with CO_2 ($P_{A_{CO_2}} = 40$ mm Hg):

$$\text{Equation 30–15}$$

$$\begin{aligned} P_{A_{O_2}} &= P_{I_{O_2}} - P_{A_{CO_2}} \\ &= 149 - 40 \\ &= 109 \text{ mm Hg} \end{aligned}$$

On the other hand, a typical fat-containing diet in industrialized nations produces an RQ of approximately 0.8 (p. 1224), so that 8 molecules of CO_2 replace 10 molecules of O_2 in the alveolar air. This 8-for-10 replacement has two consequences. First, the volume of alveolar air falls slightly during gas exchange. Because the non-H_2O pressure remains at 713 mm Hg, this volume contraction concentrates the N_2 and dilutes the O_2. Second, the volume of *expired* alveolar air is slightly less than the volume of *inspired* air. The **alveolar gas equation** describes how alveolar PO_2 depends on RQ:

$$\text{Equation 30–16}$$

$$RQ = 1:$$
$$P_{A_{O_2}} = P_{I_{O_2}} - P_{A_{CO_2}}$$

$$\text{Equation 30–17}$$

Variable RQ:
$$P_{A_{O_2}} = P_{I_{O_2}} - P_{A_{CO_2}} \cdot \left(F_{I_{O_2}} + \frac{1 - F_{I_{O_2}}}{RQ} \right)$$

$F_{I_{O_2}}$ is the fraction of inspired *dry* air that is O_2. A simplified version of this equation, which is nearly as accurate, is

Equation 30–18

Variable RQ: $P_{A_{O_2}} = P_{I_{O_2}} - \dfrac{P_{A_{CO_2}}}{RQ}$

For room air, $F_{I_{O_2}}$ is 0.21 (see Table 25–1). Note that when RQ is 1, the term in parentheses becomes unity, and Equation 30–17 collapses to Equation 30–16. The term in parentheses in Equation 30–17 also becomes unity, regardless of RQ, if $F_{I_{O_2}}$ is 100% (i.e., the subject breathes pure O_2)—in this case, there is no N_2 to dilute the O_2.

The concepts developed in the last two sections have important practical consequences. Together, we can use Equations 30–13 and 30–17 to compute both the alveolar P_{CO_2} and P_{O_2}. The approach is to first use Equation 30–13 to calculate $P_{A_{CO_2}}$ from $\dot{V}_{CO_2}$ and $\dot{V}_A$, and then use Equation 30–17 to calculate $P_{A_{O_2}}$ from $P_{A_{CO_2}}$ and RQ. Imagine that we first found that $P_{A_{CO_2}}$ is 40 mm Hg, and that we know that RQ is 0.8. What is $P_{A_{O_2}}$?

Equation 30–19

Variable RQ:

$$P_{A_{O_2}} = P_{I_{O_2}} - P_{A_{CO_2}} \cdot \left(F_{I_{O_2}} + \frac{1 - F_{I_{O_2}}}{RQ} \right)$$

$$P_{A_{O_2}} = 149 - 40 \cdot \left(\underbrace{0.21 + \frac{1 - 0.21}{0.8}}_{1.2} \right)$$

$$= 149 - 40 \cdot$$

$$= 149 - 48$$

$$= 101 \text{ mm Hg}$$

If $P_{A_{CO_2}}$ is 40 and $P_{A_{O_2}}$ is 101, then, by default, the partial pressure of N_2 and other gases (e.g., argon) is $713 - 40 - 101 = 572$ mm Hg. For simplicity, we round down this $P_{A_{O_2}}$ to 100 mm Hg in our examples.

Because of the Action of Gravity on the Lung of an Upright Subject, Regional Ventilation Normally Is Greater at the Base Than at the Apex

Until now, we have assumed that all alveoli are ventilated to the same extent. We could test this hypothesis by using an imaging technique for assessing the uniformity of ventilation. Imagine that a subject who is standing up is breathing air containing [133]Xe. Because Xe has very low water solubility, it (like He and N_2) has a very low diffusing capacity (p. 671). Thus, inhaled ^{133}Xe remains almost entirely within the alveoli.

Imaging the ^{133}Xe radioactivity immediately after a single breath of ^{133}Xe provides an index of *absolute regional ventilation* (Fig. 30–5A). However, [^{133}Xe] might be low in a particular region either because the tissue is truly hypoventilated or because that region has relatively little tissue. Therefore, we normalize the *absolute* data to the maximal regional alveolar volume by having the subject continue to breathe the ^{133}Xe until [^{133}Xe] values stabilize throughout the lungs. When the subject now makes a maximal inspiratory effort (V_L = Total lung capacity [TLC]), the level of radioactivity detected over any region reflects that region's maximal volume. Dividing the single-breath image by the steady-state image at TLC yields a ratio that describes *regional ventilation per unit volume.*

This sort of analysis shows that alveolar ventilation in a standing person gradually falls from the base to the apex of the lung (see Fig. 30–5B). Why? The answers are **posture** and **gravity**. In Chapter 26 we saw that, because of the lung's weight, intrapleural pressure (P_{IP}) is more negative at the apex than at the base when the subject is upright (see Fig. 30–5C). The practical consequences of this P_{IP} gradient become clear when we examine a static pressure-volume diagram not for the lungs as a whole (as we did in Fig. 26–6), but rather for a small piece of lung (see Fig. 30–5D). We assume that the intrinsic mechanical properties of the airways are the same, regardless of whether the tissue is at the base or at the apex. At the base, where P_{IP} might be only −2.5 cm H_2O at FRC, the alveoli are relatively underinflated compared to tissues at the apex, where P_{IP} might be −10 cm H_2O and the alveoli are relatively overinflated. However, because the base of the lung is underinflated at FRC, it is on a steeper part of the pressure-volume curve (i.e., it has a greater **static compliance**) than the overinflated apex. Thus, during an inspiration, the same ΔP_{IP} (e.g., 2.5 cm H_2O) produces a larger ΔV_L near the base than near the apex. Keep in mind that it is the *change* in volume per unit time, not the initial volume, that defines ventilation.

The relationship between ventilation and basal versus apical location in the lung would be reversed if the subject stood on his or her head. Similarly, if a person were reclining on the right side, then he or she would ventilate the dependent lung tissue on the right side better than the elevated lung tissue on the left side. Of course, the right-to-left P_{IP} gradient in the reclining subject would be smaller than the apex-to-base P_{IP} gradient in the standing subject, reflecting the smaller distance (i.e., smaller hydrostatic pressure difference). For subjects under microgravity conditions (p. 1266), such as astronauts aboard the International Space Station, there are no P_{IP} gradients, and thus no gravity-dependent regional differences in ventilation.

Pathologic Processes Exacerbate the Nonuniformity of Ventilation by Altering Compliance or Increasing Resistance

Even in microgravity, where we would expect ventilation to be *macroscopically* uniform throughout the lungs, ventilation would still be nonuniform at the *microscopic* level, because of minor local differences in static compliance (C) and airway resistance (R). Moreover, pathologic changes in compliance and resistance can substantially increase the nonuniformity of ventilation.

RESTRICTIVE PULMONARY DISEASE. "Restrictive" lung diseases decrease compliance and make it more difficult to inflate alveoli. Examples include pulmonary edema (fluid buildup in the interstitial space and, eventually, the alveoli) and diffuse interstitial pulmonary fibrosis (deposition of fibrous tissue). Figure 30–6A shows a hypothetical example in which R is normal and disease has halved the static compliance of one lung, but left the other unaffected. Thus, for the usual change in P_{IP}, the final volume

A DETECTION OF INSPIRED ^{133}Xe

^{133}Xenon in O$_2$

Radioactivity counters

Apex

Apex

Middle

Base

Base

Lungs

B REGIONAL DISTRIBUTION OF VENTILATION

$$\frac{\dot{V}_A}{\text{Unit volume}}$$
(Arbitrary units)

100
80
60
40
20
0

Base   Middle   Apex
Location in lung

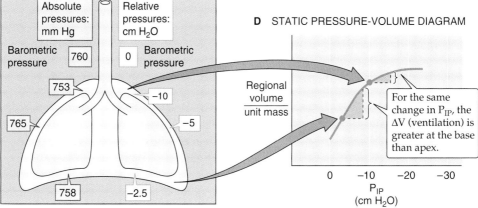

C INTRAPLEURAL PRESSURES

Absolute pressures: mm Hg

Relative pressures: cm H$_2$O

Barometric pressure   760

0   Barometric pressure

753

−10

765

−5

758

−2.5

D STATIC PRESSURE-VOLUME DIAGRAM

$$\frac{\text{Regional volume}}{\text{unit mass}}$$

For the same change in P$_{IP}$, the ΔV (ventilation) is greater at the base than apex.

0   −10   −20   −30
P$_{IP}$
(cm H$_2$O)

FIGURE 30–5. Distribution of ventilation. (Data from West JB: Respiratory Physiology—The Essentials, 4th ed. Baltimore, Williams & Wilkins, 1990.)

change (ΔV) of the diseased lung is only half normal, so that its ventilation is also halved. Because the ventilation of the other unit is normal, decreased compliance has increased the nonuniformity of ventilation.

OBSTRUCTIVE PULMONARY DISEASE. Lung diseases in which airway resistance is abnormally high are referred to as "obstructive." The two most obvious causes of increased resistance are a mass in the lumen of a conducting airway (e.g., aspiration of a foreign body, buildup of mucus), and constriction of the airway lumen (e.g., smooth muscle contraction in asthma, thickening of airway wall in bronchitis). Airway resistance also increases when emphysema destroys the lung parenchyma, thereby reducing the mechanical tethering that opposes the airway collapse during expiration (p. 631). Scar tissue or local masses, such as tumors, can also occlude a conducting airway or compress it from the outside. Regardless of its etiology, an increase in R causes the time constant τ for alveolar filling or emptying to increase (see Fig. 30–6B, *lower curve*). An isolated increase in R has no effect on

the ΔV that would be achieved if sufficient time were available for the inspiration. However, if sufficient time is not available, then alveoli with an elevated τ will not completely fill or empty, and their ventilation will decrease. Of course, the mismatching of ventilation between the two units worsens as respiratory frequency increases, as we saw in our discussion of dynamic compliance (p. 629).

MASSES. Even if a mass has no effect on resistance or compliance, it can prevent alveoli from expanding fully. Within the parenchyma of a lung, an enlarged lymph node, scar tissue, or a tumor can limit the expansion of some airways, thereby decreasing local ventilation. Outside the parenchyma of the lung, a buildup in the intrapleural space of either air (pneumothorax) or fluid (pleural effusion) can restrict the expansion of a much larger amount of pulmonary tissue. Figure 30–6C shows how blocking the full expansion of an airway reduces its ventilation and thereby contributes to the nonuniformity of ventilation.

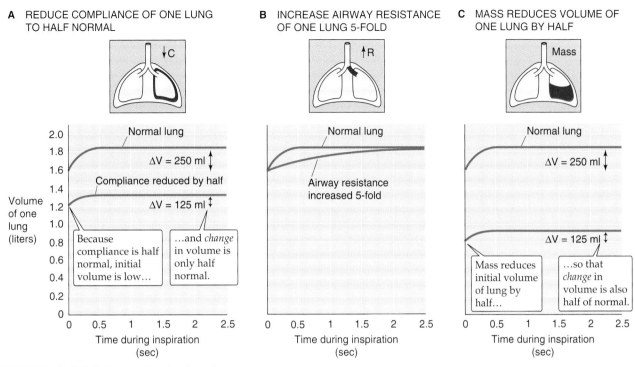

A REDUCE COMPLIANCE OF ONE LUNG TO HALF NORMAL

B INCREASE AIRWAY RESISTANCE OF ONE LUNG 5-FOLD

C MASS REDUCES VOLUME OF ONE LUNG BY HALF

FIGURE 30–6. Pathologic nonuniformity of ventilation.

PERFUSION OF THE LUNG

The Pulmonary Circulation Has Low Pressure and Resistance but High Compliance

The pulmonary circulatory system handles the same cardiac output as the systemic circulation, but in a very different way. The systemic circulation is a *high-pressure* system. This high pressure is necessary to pump blood to the top of the brain while standing, or even to a maximally elevated fingertip. The systemic circulation also needs to be a high-pressure system because it is a high-

resistance system. It uses this high resistance to control the distribution of blood flow. Thus at rest, a substantial fraction of the systemic capillaries are closed, giving the system the flexibility to redistribute large amounts of blood (e.g., to muscle during exercise). The mean pressure of the aorta is approximately 95 mm Hg (Table 30–1). At the opposite end of the circuit is the right atrium, which has a mean pressure of approximately 2 mm Hg. Thus the driving pressure for blood flow through the systemic circulation is approximately 93 mm Hg. Given a cardiac output ($\dot{Q}$) of 5 liters/min or 83 ml/s, we can compute the resistance of the systemic system using an Ohm's law–like equation (see Equation 17–10):

Equation 30–20

$$R_{Systemic} = \frac{\Delta P}{\dot{Q}} = \frac{93 \text{ mm Hg}}{83 \text{ ml blood/s}}$$
$$= 1.1 \text{ PRU}$$

PRU is a peripheral resistance unit (p. 429), which has the dimensions mm Hg/(ml/s). We shall see that, compared to the value for the pulmonary system, $R_{systemic}$ is quite high.

In contrast, the pulmonary circulation is a *low-pressure* system. It can afford to be a low-pressure system because it needs to pump blood only to the top of the lung. Moreover, it *must* be a low-pressure system to avoid the consequences of Starling forces (p. 469), which would otherwise flood the lung with edema fluid. The mean pressure in the pulmonary artery is only approximately 15 mm Hg. Because the mean pressure of the left atrium, at the other end of the circuit, is approximately 8 mm

TABLE 30–1

COMPARISON OF PRESSURES IN THE PULMONARY AND SYSTEMIC CIRCULATORY SYSTEM			
PULMONARY CIRCULATION		**SYSTEMIC CIRCULATION**	
	Mean Pressure (mm Hg)		**Mean Pressure (mm Hg)**
Pulmonary artery	15	Aorta	95
Beginning of capillary	12	Beginning of capillary	35
End of capillary	9	End of capillary	15
Left atrium	8	Right atrium	2
Net driving pressure	15 − 8 = 7	Net driving pressure	95 − 2 = 93

Hg, and because the cardiac output of the right side of the heart is the same as for the left side, we have

Equation 30–21

$$R_{Pulmonary} = \frac{\Delta P}{\dot{Q}} = \frac{7 \text{ mm Hg}}{83 \text{ ml blood/s}}$$
$$= 0.08 \text{ PRU}$$

Thus, the total resistance of the pulmonary circulation is less than one-tenth that of the systemic system, which explains how the pulmonary circulation accomplishes its mission at such low pressures. Unlike in the systemic circulation, where most of the pressure drop occurs in the arterioles (i.e., between the terminal arteries and beginning of the capillaries), in the pulmonary circulation almost the entire pressure drop occurs rather uniformly between the pulmonary artery and the end of the capillaries. In particular, the arterioles make a much smaller contribution to resistance in the pulmonary circulation than in the systemic circulation.

What are the properties of the pulmonary vasculature that give it such a low resistance? First, let us examine the complete circuit. The **pulmonary artery** arises from the right ventricle, bifurcates, and carries relatively deoxygenated blood to each lung. The two main branches of the pulmonary artery follow the two mainstem bronchi into the lungs and bifurcate along with the bronchi and bronchioles. A single pulmonary arteriole supplies all of the capillaries of a terminal respiratory unit (p. 602). Together, the two lungs have about 300 *million* alveoli. However, they may have as many as 280 *billion* highly anastomosing capillary segments (each looking like the edge of a hexagon in a piece of chicken wire), or nearly 1000 such capillary segments per alveolus—creating a surface for gas exchange of approximately 100 m². It is easy to imagine why some have described the pulmonary capillary bed as a nearly continuous flowing sheet of blood surrounding the alveoli. At rest, the erythrocytes spend approximately 0.75 second navigating this capillary bed, which contains approximately 75 ml of blood. During exercise, the capillary blood volume may increase to approximately 200 ml. Pulmonary venules collect the oxygenated blood from the capillary network, converge, course between the lobules, converge some more, and eventually enter the left atrium via the pulmonary veins. The total circulation time through the pulmonary system is 4 to 5 seconds.

Pulmonary blood vessels are generally shorter and wider than their counterparts on the systemic side. Arterioles are also present in much higher numbers in the pulmonary circulation. Although the pulmonary arterioles contain smooth muscle and can constrict, these vessels are far less muscular than their systemic counterparts, and their resting tone is low. These properties combine to produce a system with an unusually **low resistance**.

The walls of pulmonary vessels have another key property: thinness, like the walls of veins elsewhere in the body. The thin walls and paucity of smooth muscle give the pulmonary vessels a **high compliance**. One consequence of this high compliance is that pulmonary vessels can accept relatively large amounts of blood that shift from the legs to the lungs when a person moves from a standing to a recumbent position. In addition, as we discuss later, the high compliance also allows the vessels to dilate in response to modest increases in pulmonary arterial pressure. A third effect of the pulmonary vessels' high compliance is that in the pulmonary system, the pulse pressure is rather low (on an absolute scale). The systolic/diastolic pressures in the pulmonary artery are typically 25/8 mm Hg, yielding a **pulse pressure** of approximately 17 mm Hg. In contrast, the systolic/diastolic pressures in the aorta are approximately 120/80 mm Hg, for a pulse pressure of approximately 40 mm Hg. Nonetheless, relative to the *mean* pulmonary artery pressure of 15 mm Hg, the pulmonary pulse pressure of 17 mm Hg is quite high.

Increasing Lung Volume from Residual Volume to Total Lung Capacity First Decreases, Then Increases, Overall Pulmonary Vascular Resistance

Because pulmonary blood vessels are so compliant, they are especially susceptible to deformation by external forces. These forces are very different for vessels that are surrounded by alveoli (i.e., "alveolar" vessels) compared with those that are not (i.e., "extra-alveolar" vessels). In both types, the key consideration is whether these external forces pull vessels open or crush them.

ALVEOLAR VESSELS. Alveolar vessels include the capillaries, as well as slightly larger vessels that are also surrounded on all sides by alveoli (Fig. 30–7A). The resistance of these alveolar vessels depends on both the transmural pressure gradient and lung volume.

We have already introduced the **transmural pressure gradient** (P_{TM}) in our discussions of systemic blood vessels (p. 428) and conducting airways (p. 629). For alveolar vessels, P_{TM} is the difference between the pressures in the vessel *lumen* and in the surrounding *alveoli* (P_A). For the sake of simplicity, we consider the factors affecting P_{TM} at a fixed lung volume.

The pressure inside these vessels varies with the *cardiac* cycle; indeed, the pulmonary capillary bed is one of the few in which flow is pulsatile (p. 516). The pressure inside the alveolar vessels also depends greatly on their vertical position relative to the left atrium; the higher the vessel, the lower the pressure.

The pressure in the alveoli varies with the *respiratory* cycle. With no airflow and the glottis open, P_A is the same as P_B (i.e., 0 cm H_2O). On the other hand, P_A is negative during inspiration and positive during expiration. A combination of a high intravascular pressure and a negative P_A tends to dilate the compliant alveolar vessels, lowering their resistance. But a combination of a low intravascular pressure and a positive P_A crushes these vessels, raising their resistance.

Changes in lung volume (V_L) have characteristic effects on alveolar vessels. For the sake of simplicity, here we assume that each time we examine a new V_L, airflow has stopped, so that P_A is zero. As V_L increases, the alveolar walls become more stretched out. Consequently, the alveolar vessels become stretched along their longitudinal axis but crushed when viewed in cross-section. Both of these effects tend to raise vessel resistance. Thus, as V_L increases, the resistance of the alveolar vessels also increases (see Fig. 30–7B).

EXTRA-ALVEOLAR VESSELS. Because they course through the lung parenchyma (i.e., they are not surrounded by alveoli), the extra-alveolar vessels are sensitive to intrapleural pressure (Fig. 30–7A). Again for the sake of simplicity, we examine the effect of changing V_L after airflow has already stopped. The increasingly negative values of P_{IP} needed to achieve increasingly higher lung volumes also increase the P_{TM} of the extra-alveolar vessels and tend to dilate them. Thus as V_L increases, the resistance of the extra-alveolar vessels decreases (see Fig. 30–7B).

In summary, increases in V_L tend to crush alveolar vessels and thus increase their resistance, but to expand extra-alveolar vessels and thus decrease their resistance. Thus, the net effect on overall pulmonary vascular resistance of increasing V_L from residual volume (RV) to TLC is biphasic. Starting at RV, an increase in V_L first causes pulmonary vascular resistance to fall, as the dilation of extra-alveolar vessels dominates. Pulmonary vascular resistance reaches its minimum value at about FRC. Further increases in V_L (as during a normal inspiration) increase overall resistance, as the crushing of alveolar vessels dominates.

During Exercise, Slight Increases in Pulmonary Arterial Pressure Greatly Reduce Pulmonary Vascular Resistance, Owing to "Recruitment" and "Distention" of Pulmonary Capillaries

Although the pulmonary circulation is normally a low-resistance system under resting conditions, it has a remarkable ability to lower its resistance even further. During exercise, twofold to threefold increases in cardiac output may elicit only a minor increase in mean pulmonary artery pressure. In other words, a slight increase in pulmonary arterial pressure is somehow able to markedly

decrease resistance (Fig. 30–8A), and thus markedly *increase* flow (Fig. 30–8B). This behavior is a general property of a passive/elastic vascular bed (see Fig. 18–7A, red curve). Two "passive" mechanisms—that is, mechanisms not related to "active" changes in vascular smooth-muscle tone—are at work here: the recruitment and distention of pulmonary capillaries. However, before we can understand either change, we must more completely describe the pulmonary capillaries at "rest."

Under "resting" conditions (i.e., at relatively low values of pulmonary arterial pressure), some pulmonary capillaries are open and conducting blood, others are open but not conducting substantial amounts of blood, and still others are closed (Fig. 30–8C). Why should some capillaries be **open** but have no flow? In a highly anastomosing capillary network, tiny differences in driving pressure might exist. In addition, seemingly random differences in the dimensions of parallel capillaries may lead to differences in resistance. In low-pressure systems, such slight differences in absolute resistance allow pathways with relatively low resistances to steal flow from neighbors with slightly higher resistances, leaving some "open" pathways heavily underutilized. A practical example is a type of garden hose used to drizzle water on a flower bed; this hose is closed at its distal end, but perforated with hundreds of tiny holes. If water pressure is low, only some of the holes conduct water.

Why should some parallel vessels be **closed**? Popping open a previously closed vessel requires that the perfusion pressure overcome the tone of the vascular smooth muscle and reach that vessel's **critical closing pressure** (p. 455), which presumably varies from vessel to vessel. As we discuss later, alveolar vessels also may be closed because the alveolar pressure exceeds intravascular pressure, thereby crushing the vessel.

RECRUITMENT. Imagine that the pressure inside a pulmonary arteriole starts out at a fairly low level. As pressure increases, capillaries that previously had been *open*

A AT END OF INSPIRATION

Expanded alveoli encroach on alveolar vessels.

More negative intrapleural pressure pulls open extra-alveolar vessels.

P_{IP}

$P_A = 0$
Alveolus

Extra-alveolar blood vessel

Alveolar blood vessels

P_{IP}

P_A
Alveolus

Interstitial space

B DEPENDENCE OF VASCULAR RESISTANCE ON LUNG VOLUME

Total resistance is sum of alveolar and extra-alveolar resistances.

Total

Alveolar blood vessels

Pulmonary vascular resistance

Extra-alveolar blood vessels

RV   FRC   TLC
Static lung volume

FIGURE 30–7. Pulmonary vascular resistance. (*B*, Data from Murray JF: *The Normal Lung*, 2nd ed. Philadelphia, WB Saunders, 1986.) FRC, functional residual capacity; RV, respiratory volume; TLC, total lung capacity.

A EFFECT OF PULMONARY ARTERIAL PRESSURE ON VASCULAR RESISTANCE

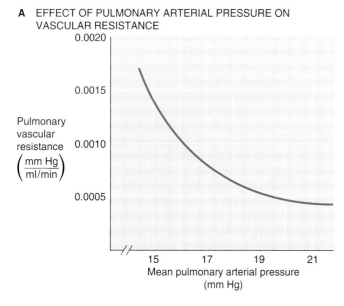

B EFFECT OF PULMONARY ARTERIAL PRESSURE ON BLOOD FLOW

C RECRUITMENT AND DISTENTION OF ALVEOLAR VESSELS

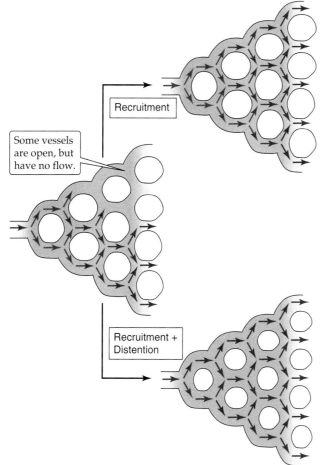

Recruitment

Some vessels are open, but have no flow.

Recruitment + Distention

FIGURE 30–8. Effects of perfusion pressure on pulmonary hemodynamics.

but not conducting now begin to conduct blood (see Fig. 30–8*C, upper right*). Similarly, some vessels that were completely *closed* may now open. The greater the increase in perfusion pressure, the greater the number of vessels that open and conduct. This recruitment of additional parallel capillary pathways reduces overall vascular resistance.

DISTENTION. Once a vessel is open and conducting, further pressure increases will increase P_{TM} and thus cause the vessel to dilate (see Fig. 30–8C, *lower right*). The net effect is a reduction in overall pulmonary resistance. Although a pressure increase can simultaneously recruit and distend various vessels, distention probably tends to occur later; that is, distention is the primary mechanism for lowering resistance under conditions in which the initial pressure was already fairly high.

Hypoxia Is a Strong Vasoconstrictor, Opposite to Its Effect in the Systemic Circulation

In addition to lung volume and perfusion pressure, several other factors can modulate pulmonary vascular resistance.

OXYGEN. The effects of changes in P_{O_2}, P_{CO_2}, and pH on pulmonary vascular resistance are opposite to those observed in the systemic circulation. Thus, hypoxia causes pulmonary vasoconstriction. What appears to be critical is not so much the P_{O_2} in the lumen of the arterioles and venules, but rather the P_{O_2} in the *alveolar air* adjacent to the vessel. Indeed, perfusing the pulmonary vasculature with a hypoxic solution is far less effective than ventilating the airways with a low-P_{O_2} air mixture.

Hypoxic vasoconstriction occurs in isolated lung tissue, and thus does not rely on either the nervous system or systemic hormones. Rather, the low P_{O_2} is generally believed to act directly on the pulmonary vascular smooth muscle cells. How this occurs is unknown, but hypothesized mechanisms include all those proposed for the sensing of hypoxia by the peripheral chemoreceptor, which we discuss on p. 725. Somehow, the hypoxia inhibits one or more K^+ channels, causing the V_m of the vascular smooth muscle cells to move away from E_K, and thus to depolarize. This positive shift in V_m opens voltage-gated Ca^{2+} channels, leading to an influx of Ca^{2+} and smooth-muscle contraction (p. 242).

CARBON DIOXIDE AND LOW pH. High P_{CO_2} and/or low interstitial pH promote vasoconstriction, although with far less potency than hypoxia. Thus, like the effect of hypoxia, the effects of high P_{CO_2} and low pH are opposite those in the systemic circulation. Elevated P_{CO_2} may produce its effect by decreasing the pH of either the extracellular or intracellular fluid. Following a general pattern that is repeated in the control of ventilation (p. 730), hypoxia makes the vascular smooth muscle cells more sensitive to respiratory acidosis.

AUTONOMIC NERVOUS SYSTEM. The sympathetic and parasympathetic innervation of the pulmonary vasculature is far less impressive than that of the systemic circulation. Increased sympathetic tone seems to reduce the compliance of (i.e., stiffen) the pulmonary artery walls without increasing resistance per se. Increased parasympathetic tone causes a mild vasodilation, the relevance of which is unknown.

HORMONES AND OTHER HUMORAL AGENTS. The pulmonary blood vessels are relatively *unresponsive* to hormones and other signaling molecules. Table 30–2 summarizes the actions of some of factors that modify pulmonary vascular resistance.

Because of the Action of Gravity on the Blood of an Upright Subject, Regional Perfusion Normally Is Far Greater Near the Base Than at the Apex of the Lung

Are all alveoli perfused to the same extent? We could answer this question by using a ^{133}Xe imaging technique to assess the uniformity of perfusion. In Figure 30–5A, we used ^{133}Xe inhalation to measure the uniformity of *ventilation*. In Figure 30–9A, we equilibrate a saline solution with ^{133}Xe and then inject the solution intravenously. When the ^{133}Xe reaches the lungs, it rapidly enters the alveolar air, inasmuch as Xe is poorly soluble in water. A lung scan is obtained as the patient holds his or her breath while the ^{133}Xe collects in the alveoli. The distribution of radioactivity now reflects the distribution of *perfusion*. If we normalize the ^{133}Xe to account for differences in regional lung volume—as we did for the ventilation scan—then we can obtain a graph showing how blood flow varies from the bottom to the top of the lung of an upright subject.

The results of such a ^{133}Xe perfusion study show that when the patient is upright, perfusion ($\dot{Q}$) is greatest near the base of the lungs and falls toward low levels near the apex. Note that although regional $\dot{Q}$ is highest near the base of the lung, $\dot{Q}$ falls off somewhat from this peak as we approach the extreme base. With exercise, perfusion increases in all regions of the lung, but more so near the apex, so that the nonuniformity of perfusion is less. Why should $\dot{Q}$ have this peculiar height dependence? The basic answers are the same as those when we raised a similar question about the physiological nonuniformity of *ventilation*: **posture** and **gravity**. Thus, if the subject is upside down, then the flow-height relationship is largely reversed, and we would expect height-related differences in flow to be minimal in microgravity conditions.

TABLE 30–2

AGENTS THAT AFFECT PULMONARY VASCULAR RESISTANCE	
DILATORS	**CONSTRICTORS**
↑ $P_{A_{O_2}}$	↓ $P_{A_{O_2}}$
↓ $P_{A_{CO_2}}$	↑ $P_{A_{CO_2}}$
↑ pH	↓ pH
Histamine, H_2 agonists	Histamine, H_1 agonists
PGI_2 (prostacyclin), PGE_1	Thromboxane A_2, $PGF2_\alpha$, PGE_2
β-adrenergic agonists (e.g., isoproterenol)	α-adrenergic agonists
Bradykinin	Serotonin
Theophylline	Angiotensin II
Acetylcholine	
NO	

Figure 30–9C shows how we can divide the upright lung into as many as four zones based on the relationships among various pressures. We define the first three zones based on how *alveolar* blood vessels are affected by the relative values of three different pressures: alveolar pressure (P_A), the pressure inside pulmonary arterioles (P_{PA}), and the pressure inside pulmonary venules (P_{PV}). In the fourth zone, we instead focus on how extra-alveolar vessels are affected by intrapleural pressure (P_{IP}).

ZONE 1: $P_A > P_{PA} > P_{PV}$. Zone 1 conditions prevail at the apex of the lung under certain conditions. The defining characteristic of a zone-1 alveolar vessel is that P_{PA} and P_{PV} are so low that they have fallen below P_A. The *mean* pulmonary arterial pressure is approximately 15 mm Hg. Because mercury is 13.6-fold more dense than water, this value of P_{PA} corresponds to approximately 20 cm H_2O. Similarly, mean P_{PV} is 8 mm Hg, or approximately 11 cm H_2O. As we move upward from the level of the left atrium (the reference point for these values) closer to the apex of an upright lung, the actual pressures in the lumens of pulmonary arterioles and venules fall by 1 cm H_2O for each 1 cm of vertical ascent. If human lungs extended 20 cm or so above the level of the left atrium, then we would eventually reach a level at which the mean P_{PA} would fall to 0 cm H_2O. At the same level, P_{PV} would be about -9 cm H_2O. The pressure inside the pulmonary capillary (P_c) would fall somewhere in between, perhaps -5 cm H_2O. In principle, blood would still flow through this capillary—the driving pressure would be approximately 9 cm H_2O—if it were not for the pressure inside the alveoli, which is 0 cm H_2O between breaths. Therefore, because P_A is much higher than P_c, the negative P_{TM} would crush the capillary and prevent blood flow.

Fortunately, zone 1 conditions do not exist for normal people at rest. However, they can arise if there is either a sufficient decrease in P_{PA} (e.g., in hemorrhage), or a sufficient increase in P_A (e.g., in **positive-pressure ventilation**).

ZONE 2: $P_{PA} > P_A > P_{PV}$. Zone 2 conditions prevail at the apex to the middle of the lung. The defining characteristic of zone 2 is that mean P_{PA} and P_{PV} have risen enough so that they sandwich P_A. Thus, at the arteriolar end, the positive P_{TM} causes the alveolar vessel to dilate. Further down the capillary, though, luminal pressure gradually falls below P_A, so that the negative P_{TM} squeezes the vessel. This distal squeezing does not completely prevent flow—it merely raises resistance and thus reduces flow. As we move downward in zone 2, the crushing force decreases because the hydrostatic pressures in the arteriole, capillary, and venule all rise in parallel by 1 cm H_2O for each 1 cm of descent. Simultaneously, the resistance decreases and blood flow gradually increases. The conversion of a closed vessel to a conducting one by increased P_{PA} and P_{PV} is an example of **recruitment**.

The arrangement in which a variable P_{TM} controls flow is known as a **Starling resistor**. Keep in mind that the driving force ($P_{PA} - P_{PC}$) is constant in all of the zones.

ZONE 3: $P_{PA} > P_{PV} > P_A$. Zone 3 conditions prevail in the middle to lower lung. The defining characteristic of zone

3 is that mean P_{PA} and P_{PV} are so high that they both exceed P_A. Thus, P_{TM} is positive along the entire length of the alveolar vessel, tending to dilate it. As we move downward in zone 3, the hydrostatic pressures in the arteriole, capillary, and venule all continue to rise by 1 cm H_2O for each 1 cm of descent. Because P_A does not vary with height in the lung, the gradually increasing pressure of the alveolar vessel produces a greater and greater P_{TM}, causing the vessel (i.e., the Starling resistor) to dilate more and more—an example of **distention**. This distention causes a gradual decrease in resistance of the capillaries as we move downward in zone 3. Hence, although the driving force ($P_{PA} - P_{PV}$) remains constant, perfusion increases toward the base of the lung.

ZONE 4: $P_{PA} > P_{PV} > P_A$. Zone 4 conditions prevail at the extreme base of the lungs. In zone 4, the *alveolar vessels* behave the same as in zone 3; they dilate more as we descend toward the base of the lung. However, the *extra-alveolar vessels* behave differently. At the base of the lung, P_{IP} is least negative (see Fig. 30–5C). Thus, as we approach the extreme base of the lung, the distending forces acting on the extra-alveolar blood vessels fade, and the resistance of these extra-alveolar vessels increases. Recall that we saw a similar effect—at the level of the whole lung (see Fig. 30–7A)—where resistance of the extra-alveolar vessels increased at low lung volume. Because these extra-alveolar vessels feed or drain the alveolar vessels, $\dot{Q}$ begins to fall from its peak as we approach the extreme base of the lungs (see Fig. 30–9B).

These lung zones are *physiological*, not anatomic. The boundaries between the zones are neither fixed nor sharp. For example, the boundaries can move downward with positive-pressure ventilation (which increases P_A) and can move upward with exercise (which increases P_{PA}). In our discussion of lung zones, we have tacitly assumed that P_A is always zero and that P_{PA} and P_{PV} both have stable values that are determined by the height in the lung. In real life, of course, things are more complicated. During the respiratory cycle, P_A becomes negative during inspiration (promoting dilation of pulmonary capillaries), but positive during expiration. During the cardiac cycle, the pressure inside the arterioles and pulmonary capillaries is greatest during systole (promoting dilation of the vessel), and lowest during diastole. Thus, we would expect blood flow through an alveolar vessel to be greatest when inspiration coincides with systole.

MATCHING VENTILATION AND PERFUSION

The Greater the Ventilation-Perfusion Ratio, the Higher the P_{O_2} and the Lower the P_{CO_2} in the Alveolar Air

In Figure 30–4 we saw that, all other factors being equal, alveolar ventilation determines alveolar P_{O_2} and P_{CO_2}. The greater the ventilation, the more closely $P_{A_{O_2}}$ and $P_{A_{CO_2}}$ approach their respective values in inspired air. However, in Figure 30–4 we were really focusing on *total* alveolar ventilation and how this influences the *average*,

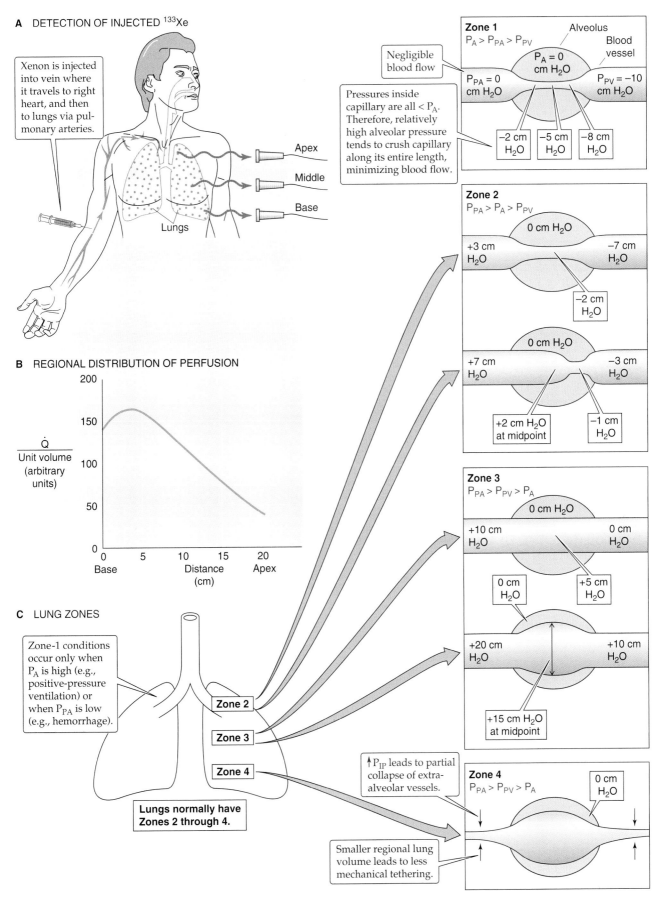

A DETECTION OF INJECTED ^{133}Xe

Xenon is injected into vein where it travels to right heart, and then to lungs via pulmonary arteries.

Apex

Middle

Base

Lungs

Zone 1
$P_A > P_{PA} > P_{PV}$

Alveolus

Blood vessel

Negligible blood flow

$P_A = 0$ cm H_2O

$P_{PA} = 0$ cm H_2O

$P_{PV} = -10$ cm H_2O

Pressures inside capillary are all < P_A. Therefore, relatively high alveolar pressure tends to crush capillary along its entire length, minimizing blood flow.

−2 cm H_2O

−5 cm H_2O

−8 cm H_2O

B REGIONAL DISTRIBUTION OF PERFUSION

$\frac{\dot{Q}}{\text{Unit volume}}$ (arbitrary units)

200

150

100

50

0

0　5　10　15　20
Base　Distance　Apex
(cm)

Zone 2
$P_{PA} > P_A > P_{PV}$

0 cm H_2O

+3 cm H_2O

−7 cm H_2O

−2 cm H_2O

0 cm H_2O

+7 cm H_2O

−3 cm H_2O

+2 cm H_2O at midpoint

−1 cm H_2O

C LUNG ZONES

Zone-1 conditions occur only when P_A is high (e.g., positive-pressure ventilation) or when P_{PA} is low (e.g., hemorrhage).

Zone 2

Zone 3

Zone 4

Lungs normally have Zones 2 through 4.

Zone 3
$P_{PA} > P_{PV} > P_A$

0 cm H_2O

+10 cm H_2O

0 cm H_2O

0 cm H_2O

+5 cm H_2O

+20 cm H_2O

+10 cm H_2O

+15 cm H_2O at midpoint

↑P_{IP} leads to partial collapse of extra-alveolar vessels.

Zone 4
$P_{PA} > P_{PV} > P_A$

0 cm H_2O

Smaller regional lung volume leads to less mechanical tethering.

FIGURE 30–9. Physiological nonuniformity of pulmonary perfusion.

or idealized, alveolar P_{O_2} and P_{CO_2}. In fact, we have already learned that both ventilation and perfusion vary among alveoli. In any group of alveoli, the greater the local ventilation, the more closely the local alveolar air approaches the composition of the inspired air. Similarly, because blood flow removes O_2 from the alveolar air and adds CO_2, the greater the perfusion, the more closely local alveolar air approaches the composition of mixed venous blood. Thus, the local **ventilation-perfusion ratio** ($\dot{V}_A/\dot{Q}$) determines the local $P_{A_{O_2}}$ and $P_{A_{CO_2}}$.

You might view the alveoli as a battlefield where ventilation and perfusion are engaged in a continuous struggle over control of the composition of alveolar air. To the extent that ventilation gains the upper hand, $P_{A_{O_2}}$ rises and $P_{A_{CO_2}}$ falls. To the extent that perfusion holds sway, these parameters change in the opposite direction.

As a physical analog of this struggle over control of alveolar P_{O_2}, consider water flowing (analogous to $\dot{V}_A$) from a faucet into a sink (alveoli); the water exits ($\dot{Q}$) through a drain with an adjustable opening. If the drain opening is in midposition and we allow the water to flow moderately fast, thn the water level ($P_{A_{O_2}}$) will gradually increase and reach a steady state. Increasing the inflow of water ($\dot{V}_A$) wil cause the water level ($P_{A_{O_2}}$) to rise until the product of pressure head and drain conductance is high enough to drive water down the drain as fast as the water flows in. If we increase the drain opening and thus the outflow of water ($\dot{Q}$), then the water level ($P_{A_{O_2}}$) will fall until the decrease in the pressure head matches the increase in drain conductance, so that once again water inflow and outflow are balanced. In a similar way, a high $\dot{V}_A/\dot{Q}$ ratio will increase alveolar P_{O_2}.

Because of the Action of Gravity on an Upright Subject, the Local Ventilation-Perfusion Ratio ($\dot{V}_A/\dot{Q}$) Is Greater at the Apex of the Lung Than at the Base

We have already seen that when a subject is upright in a gravitational field, ventilation falls from the base to the apex of the lung (see Fig. 30–5B), and that perfusion similarly (although more steeply) falls from the base to the apex (see Fig. 30–9B). Thus, it is not surprising that the ratio $\dot{V}_A/\dot{Q}$ itself varies with height in the lung (Fig. 30–10A). $\dot{V}_A/\dot{Q}$ is lowest near the base, where $\dot{Q}$ exceeds $\dot{V}_A$. The ratio gradually increases to 1 at about the level of the third rib, and further increases toward the apex, where $\dot{Q}$ falls more precipitously than $\dot{V}_A$.

Table 30–3 shows how differences in $\dot{V}_A/\dot{Q}$ at the apex and base of the lungs influence the composition of alveolar air. At the apex, where $\dot{V}_A/\dot{Q}$ is highest, alveolar P_{O_2} and P_{CO_2} most closely approach their values in inspired air. Because both O_2 and CO_2 transport across the blood–gas barrier are **perfusion limited** (p. 682), O_2 and CO_2 have completely equilibrated between the alveolar air and the blood by the end of the pulmonary capillaries. Thus blood leaving the apex has the same high P_{O_2} and low P_{CO_2} as the alveolar air. Of course, the relatively low P_{CO_2} produces a *respiratory alkalosis* (p. 641) in the blood leaving the apex.

The situation is just the opposite near the base of the lung. Because $\dot{V}_A/\dot{Q}$ here is lowest, alveolar P_{O_2} and P_{CO_2} tend toward their values in mixed venous blood. What impact do these different regions of the lung, each with its own $\dot{V}_A/\dot{Q}$ ratio, have on the composition of systemic arterial blood? Each region makes a contribution that is proportional to its blood flow (see the rightmost column in Table 30–3). Because the apex is poorly perfused, receiving only 0.07 liter/min (or 1.4% of the total 5 liters/min of cardiac output) in this example, it makes only a small contribution to the overall composition of arterial blood. On the other hand, an equal mass of pulmonary tissue at the base of the lungs, which receives approximately 26% of total cardiac output, makes a major contribution. As a result, the average composition of blood exiting the lung more closely reflects the composition of the blood that had equilibrated with the air in the base of the lung.

The **O_2–CO_2 diagram** introduced as Figure 28–11 is a helpful tool for depicting how different $\dot{V}_A/\dot{Q}$ ratios throughout the lung produce different blood-gas compositions. The curve in Figure 30–10B represents all possible combinations of P_{O_2} and P_{CO_2} in the alveolar air and/or end-pulmonary capillary blood. The H_2O-saturated **inspired air** ($P_{O_2} = 149$, $P_{CO_2} = \sim 0$ mm Hg) represents the rightmost extreme of the diagram. By definition, the $\dot{V}_A/\dot{Q}$ ratio of inspired air is ∞, because it does not come into contact with pulmonary capillary blood. The **mixed venous blood** ($P_{O_2} = 40$, $P_{CO_2} = 46$ mm Hg) represents the other extreme. By definition, the $\dot{V}_A/\dot{Q}$ ratio of mixed venous blood is 0, because it has not yet come into contact with alveolar air. With the endpoints of the diagram established, we can now predict—with the help of the alveolar gas equation (Equation 30–17), the Bohr effect (p. 660), and the Haldane effect (see p. 666)—all possible combinations of P_{O_2} and P_{CO_2} throughout the lung. As shown in Figure 30–10B, the base, midportion, and apex of the lungs correspond to points along the O_2–CO_2 diagram between mixed venous blood at one extreme and inspired air at the other.

When Alveoli Are Ventilated but Not Perfused (Alveolar Dead Space Ventilation), Local $\dot{V}_A/\dot{Q}$ Increases to Infinity, Triggering Compensatory Bronchoconstriction and a Fall in Surfactant Production

The effects of gravity on ventilation and perfusion cause $\dot{V}_A/\dot{Q}$ to vary widely, even in idealized lungs (see Fig. 30–10A). However, physiological and pathologic variations in ventilation and perfusion can cause even greater mismatches of $\dot{V}_A/\dot{Q}$, the extremes of which are alveolar dead space ventilation (this section) and shunt (next section).

ALVEOLAR DEAD SPACE VENTILATION. At one end of the spectrum of $\dot{V}_A/\dot{Q}$ mismatches is the elimination of blood flow to a group of alveoli. For example, if we were to ligate the pulmonary artery feeding one lung, then the affected alveoli would receive no perfusion even though ventilation would initially continue normally (Fig. 30–11A). Earlier, we saw that this alveolar dead space to-

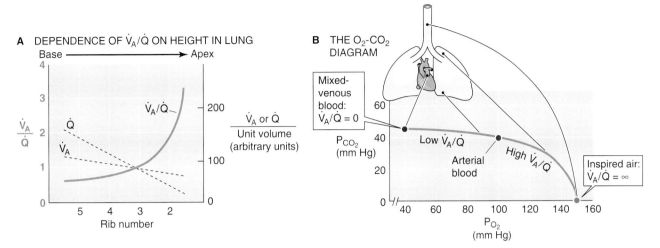

FIGURE 30–10. Regional differences in $\dot{V}_A/\dot{Q}$ ratio and alveolar gas composition. (Data from West JB: Ventilation/Blood Flow and Gas Exchange. Oxford, UK, Blackwell, 1985.)

gether with the anatomic dead space constitute the physiological dead space (see Equation 30–8). The ventilation of the unperfused alveoli is called *alveolar dead space ventilation* because, although they are ventilated, the alveoli do not engage in gas exchange. Thus, these alveoli behave like conducting airways.

A natural cause of alveolar dead space ventilation is a pulmonary embolism, which obstructs blood flow to a group of alveoli. Because one task of the lung is to filter small emboli from the blood (p. 605), the lung must deal with small regions of alveolar dead space ventilation on a recurring basis. At the instant the blood flow ceases, the alveoli supplied by the affected vessel(s) contain normal alveolar air. However, each cycle of inspiration and expiration replaces some stale alveolar air with fresh, inspired air. Because no exchange of O_2 and CO_2 occurs between these unperfused alveoli and pulmonary capillary blood, the alveolar gas gradually achieves the composition of moist inspired air, with alveolar P_{O_2} rising to approximately 149 mm Hg and P_{CO_2} falling to approx-

imately 0 mm Hg (see Fig. 30–11A, *step 2*). By definition, alveolar dead space has a $\dot{V}_A/\dot{Q}$ ratio of infinity and is represented by the "inspired air" point on the x-axis of an O_2–CO_2 diagram.

REDIRECTION OF BLOOD FLOW. Blocking blood flow to one group of alveoli diverts blood to "normal" parts of the lung, which then become somewhat hyperperfused. Thus, the blockage not only increases $\dot{V}_A/\dot{Q}$ in alveoli downstream from the blockage, but also decreases $\dot{V}_A/\dot{Q}$ in other regions. Redirection of blood flow thus accentuates the nonuniformity of ventilation.

REGULATION OF LOCAL VENTILATION. Because alveolar dead space ventilation causes local alveolar P_{CO_2} to fall to approximately 0 mm Hg, it leads to a respiratory alkalosis (p. 641) in the surrounding interstitial fluid. These local changes trigger a compensatory **bronchiolar constriction** in the adjacent tissues (see Fig. 30–11B), so that over a period of seconds to minutes, airflow partially diverts away from the unperfused alveoli and toward normal al-

TABLE 30–3

EFFECT OF $\dot{V}_A/\dot{Q}$ ON THE COMPOSITION OF ALVEOLAR AIR AND PULMONARY CAPILLARY BLOOD LEAVING THE LUNG*

LOCATION	FRACTION OF TOTAL LUNG VOLUME	$\dot{V}_A/\dot{Q}$	P_{O_2} (mm Hg)	P_{CO_2} (mm Hg)	pH	$\dot{Q}$ (liters/min)
Apex	7%	3.3	132	28	7.55	0.07
Base	13%	0.6	89	42	7.38	1.3
Overall	100%	0.84*	100	40	7.40	5.0

*If the overall alveolar ventilation for the two lungs is 4.2 liters/min, and if the cardiac output (i.e., perfusion) is 5 liters/min, then the overall $\dot{V}_A/\dot{Q}$ ratio for the two lungs is (4.2 liters/min)/(5 liters/min) = 0.84.
  Modified from West JB: Ventilation/Blood Flow and Gas Exchange. Oxford, UK, Blackwell, 1989.

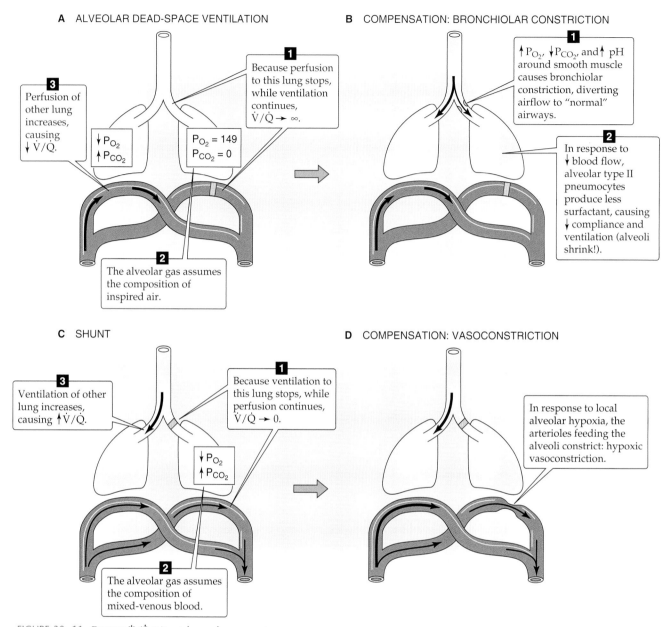

A   ALVEOLAR DEAD-SPACE VENTILATION

1 Because perfusion to this lung stops, while ventilation continues, $\dot{V}/\dot{Q} \rightarrow \infty$.

3 Perfusion of other lung increases, causing ↓ $\dot{V}/\dot{Q}$.

↓ P_{O_2}
↑ P_{CO_2}

$P_{O_2} = 149$
$P_{CO_2} = 0$

2 The alveolar gas assumes the composition of inspired air.

B   COMPENSATION: BRONCHIOLAR CONSTRICTION

1 ↑ P_{O_2}, ↓ P_{CO_2}, and ↑ pH around smooth muscle causes bronchiolar constriction, diverting airflow to "normal" airways.

2 In response to ↓ blood flow, alveolar type II pneumocytes produce less surfactant, causing ↓ compliance and ventilation (alveoli shrink!).

C   SHUNT

1 Because ventilation to this lung stops, while perfusion continues, $\dot{V}/\dot{Q} \rightarrow 0$.

3 Ventilation of other lung increases, causing ↑ $\dot{V}/\dot{Q}$.

↓ P_{O_2}
↑ P_{CO_2}

2 The alveolar gas assumes the composition of mixed-venous blood.

D   COMPENSATION: VASOCONSTRICTION

In response to local alveolar hypoxia, the arterioles feeding the alveoli constrict: hypoxic vasoconstriction.

FIGURE 30–11. Extreme $\dot{V}_A/\dot{Q}$ mismatches and compensatory responses.

veoli, to which blood flow is also being diverted. This compensation makes teleologic sense, because it tends to correct the $\dot{V}_A/\dot{Q}$ shift in both the unperfused and normal alveoli. The precise mechanism of bronchiolar constriction is unknown, although bronchiolar smooth muscle may contract—at least in part—in response to a high extracellular pH.

A second consequence of alveolar dead space ventilation is that, downstream from the blockage, alveolar type II pneumocytes become starved for various nutrients, including the lipids they need to make surfactant. However, these cells never become starved for O_2! As a result of the decreased blood flow, *surfactant production falls* over a period of hours to days. The result is a local decrease in

compliance, further reducing local ventilation. These compensatory responses—bronchiolar constriction and reduced surfactant production—work well only if the alveolar dead space is relatively small, so there is an ample volume of healthy tissue into which the airflow can divert.

When Alveoli Are Perfused but Not Ventilated (Shunt), the Local $\dot{V}_A/\dot{Q}$ Ratio Falls to Zero, Triggering a Compensatory Hypoxic Vasoconstriction

SHUNT. Alveolar dead space ventilation is at one end of the spectrum of $\dot{V}_A/\dot{Q}$ mismatches. At the opposite end is shunt—the elimination of airflow to a group of alveoli. The initial effect is that the alveoli are perfused but not ventilated. For example, if we ligate a mainstem bronchus, then inspired air cannot refresh the air distal to the obstruction (see Fig 30–11C). As a result, mixed venous blood "shunts" from the right side to the left side of the heart, without benefit of ventilation. When the low-O_2 shunted blood mixes with high-O_2 unshunted blood (which is ventilated), it decreases the PO_2, causing hypoxia in the systemic arteries. It is possible to calculate the extent of the shunt from the degree of hypoxia.

Natural causes of airway obstruction include aspiration of a **foreign body** or the presence of a **tumor** in the lumen of a conducting airway. The collapse of alveoli (**atelectasis**) also produces a right-to-left shunt, a pathologic example of which is pneumothorax (p. 613). Atelectasis also occurs naturally in dependent regions of the lungs, where P_{IP} is not so negative (see Fig. 30–5C) and surfactant levels gradually decline. Sighing or yawning stimulates surfactant release (p. 619) and can reverse physiological atelectasis.

Imagine that an infant aspirates a peanut. Initially, the air trapped distal to the obstruction has the composition of normal alveolar air. However, pulmonary capillary blood gradually extracts O_2 from the trapped air and adds CO_2. Eventually, the PO_2 and PCO_2 of the trapped air drift to their values in **mixed venous blood**. If the shunt is small, so that it does not affect the PO_2 or PCO_2 of the systemic arterial blood, then the alveoli will have a PO_2 of 40 mm Hg and a PCO_2 of 46 mm Hg. By definition, shunted alveoli have a $\dot{V}_A/\dot{Q}$ of 0 and are represented by the "mixed venous blood" point on an O_2–CO_2 diagram.

REDIRECTION OF AIRFLOW. Blocking airflow to one group of alveoli simultaneously diverts air to normal parts of the lung, which then become somewhat hyperventilated. Thus, shunt not only decreases $\dot{V}_A/\dot{Q}$ in unventilated alveoli, but also increases $\dot{V}_A/\dot{Q}$ in other regions. The net effect is a widening of the nonuniformity of $\dot{V}_A/\dot{Q}$ ratios.

ASTHMA. Although less dramatic than complete airway obstruction, an incomplete occlusion will also decrease $\dot{V}_A/\dot{Q}$. An example is asthma, in which hyperreactivity of airway smooth muscle increases local airway resistance and decreases ventilation of alveoli distal to the pathology.

NORMAL ANATOMIC SHUNTS. The **thebesian veins** drain some of the venous blood from the heart muscle, particularly the left ventricle, directly into the corresponding cardiac chamber. Thus, delivery of deoxygenated blood from thebesian veins into the left ventricle (<1% of cardiac output) represents a right-to-left shunt. The **bronchial arteries**, branches of the aorta that carry approximately 2% of the cardiac output, supply the *conducting* airways (p. 603). After passing through capillaries, about half of the bronchial blood drains into a systemic vein—the azygos vein—and then to the right heart. The other half (~1% of cardiac output) anastomoses with oxygenated blood in pulmonary venules, and thus represents part of the anatomic right-to-left shunt (p. 426).

PATHOLOGIC SHUNTS. In Chapter 56, we discuss examples of right-to-left shunts. Respiratory distress syndrome of the newborn (see box on p. 1201) can cause airway collapse. Generalized hypoxemia in the newborn can constrict the pulmonary vasculature, as we will see in the next paragraph, leading to pulmonary hypertension and the shunting of blood via the foramen ovale (p. 1202) or a patent ductus arteriosus (p. 1203).

REGULATION OF LOCAL PERFUSION. The alveoli that derive from a single terminal bronchiole surround the pulmonary arteriole that supplies these alveoli. Thus the vascular smooth muscle cells (VSMCs) of this pulmonary arteriole are bathed in an interstitial fluid whose composition reflects that of the local alveolar gas. In the case of shunt, VSMCs sense a decrease in PO_2, an increase in PCO_2, and a fall in pH. The decrease in local alveolar PO_2 triggers a compensatory **hypoxic pulmonary vasoconstriction** (p. 699), which the accompanying respiratory acidosis augments (see Fig. 30–11D). Note that this response is just the opposite of that of *systemic* arterioles, which *dilate* in response to hypoxia (p. 478). Hypoxic pulmonary vasoconstriction makes teleologic sense because it diverts blood flow away from unventilated alveoli toward normal alveoli, to which airflow is also being diverted. This compensation tends to correct the $\dot{V}_A/\dot{Q}$ shift in both the unventilated and normal alveoli.

If the amount of pulmonary tissue involved is sufficiently small (<20%), then hypoxic vasoconstriction has a minimal effect on overall pulmonary vascular resistance. The vasoconstriction causes a slight increase in pulmonary arterial pressure, which recruits and distends pulmonary vessels outside of the shunt zone. In contrast, *global* alveolar hypoxia—caused by, for example, ascending to high altitude—produces a generalized hypoxic vasoconstriction that may cause the resistance of the pulmonary vasculature to more than double. In susceptible individuals, the result can be acute mountain sickness (p. 1264).

Even If Overall $\dot{V}_A$ And $\dot{Q}$ Are Normal, a $\dot{V}_A/\dot{Q}$ Mismatch Leads to Hypoxia and Respiratory Acidosis

The sophisticated compensatory responses to alveolar dead space ventilation and shunt help protect the body from the consequences of $\dot{V}_A/\dot{Q}$ mismatches: respiratory acidosis and hypoxia. To illustrate how $\dot{V}_A/\dot{Q}$ mismatches produce these consequences, here we examine CO_2 and O_2 handling in a normal individual and then in two extreme, idealized examples: alveolar dead space ventilation and shunt.

NORMAL LUNGS. Figure 30–12 shows how an individual with a normal $\dot{V}_A/\dot{Q}$ in each lung handles CO_2 and O_2. We assume that total $\dot{V}_A$ (4.2 liters/min) and $\dot{Q}$ (5 liters/min) are normal and divided equally between the two lungs. Each lung eliminates half of the 200 ml/min of CO_2 produced by metabolism (Fig. 30–12A), and each takes up half of the 250 ml/min of O_2 consumed by metabolism (Fig. 30–12B). As a result, alveolar PCO_2 is approximately 40 mm Hg in each lung, and alveolar PO_2 is approximately 100 mm Hg. Because the fluxes of CO_2

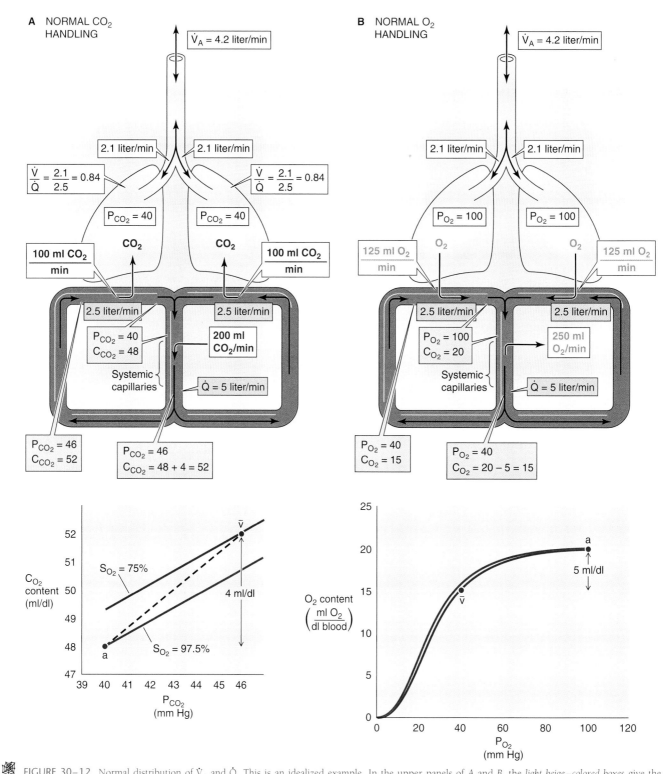

FIGURE 30–12. Normal distribution of $\dot{V}_A$ and $\dot{Q}$. This is an idealized example. In the upper panels of *A* and *B*, the *light beige–colored boxes* give the alveolar ventilation to each lung, as well as the total alveolar ventilation ($\dot{V}_A$). The *pink boxes* give the blood flow to each lung, as well as the total cardiac output ($\dot{Q}$). The *white boxes* give the rates of CO_2 or O_2 transport (ml/min) at either the pulmonary or systemic capillaries. The blue boxes give the CO_2 and O_2 partial pressures (mm Hg) in alveolar air. The *lavendar boxes* give the CO_2 partial pressure (mm Hg) and CO_2 content (ml/dl) in the mixed-venous blood, in the blood leaving each of the lungs, and in the mixed-arterial blood. The *dark beige–colored boxes* give the same information for O_2. The lower panel of *A* shows hypothetical plots of how total CO_2 content varies with P_{CO_2} at the Hb-O_2 saturations typical of arterial blood (*red line*) and mixed-venous blood (*violet line*). The vertical arrow indicates the decrease in total CO_2 content between the mixed-venous and arterial blood (4 ml/dl). The lower panel of *B* shows comparable plots for how total O_2 content varies with P_{O_2} at the pH and P_{CO_2} values typical of mixed-venous blood (*violet curve*) and arterial blood (*red curve*). The vertical arrow indicates the increase in total O_2 content between the mixed-venous and arterial blood (5 ml/dl).

and O_2 across the alveolar blood-gas barrier are each perfusion limited (p. 682), the CO_2 and O_2 partial pressures in the systemic arterial blood are the same as in the alveoli, and arterial pH is normal.

How do $\dot{V}_A/\dot{Q}$ mismatches affect arterial blood gases? The general principle is extremely simple: uncompensated $\dot{V}_A/\dot{Q}$ abnormalities lead to respiratory acidosis and hypoxia. Of course, compensation at the level of the lung (e.g., bronchiolar constriction, decreased surfactant production, hypoxic vasoconstriction) and at the level of the entire respiratory system (i.e., increased ventilation) would help reduce the untoward consequences of the $\dot{V}_A/\dot{Q}$ mismatch. In the following discussion we examine the effects of $\dot{V}_A/\dot{Q}$ mismatches in the absence of any local or system-wide compensation.

ALVEOLAR DEAD SPACE VENTILATION AFFECTING ONE LUNG. To simulate alveolar dead space ventilation (Fig. 30–13) in the laboratory, we can surgically ligate the left pulmonary artery, thereby eliminating all *perfusion to the left lung*. Total $\dot{Q}$ remains at its normal 5 liters/min, but all of it goes to the right lung. $\dot{V}_A$ remains at its normal 4.2 liters/min and is evenly distributed between the two lungs. Thus the $\dot{V}_A/\dot{Q}$ to the left lung is 2.1/0, or infinity, whereas the $\dot{V}_A/\dot{Q}$ to the right lung is 2.1/5, or 0.42. The overall $\dot{V}_A/\dot{Q}$ is normal, 0.84. The key question is whether a combination of a high $\dot{V}_A/\dot{Q}$ in the abnormal lung and a low $\dot{V}_A/\dot{Q}$ in the normal lung can yield normal blood gases.

The normal right lung must now eliminate all of the CO_2—that is, the right lung must eliminate CO_2 at twice the rate that it normally does. However, the right lung has its usual $\dot{V}_A$ of 2.1 liters/min. Because a normal amount of alveolar air must carry away twice as much CO_2 in the new steady state, the right lung's alveolar P_{CO_2} doubles to approximately 80 mm Hg (Fig. 30–13A). Because the entire cardiac output perfuses the normal right lung, arterial P_{CO_2} is also approximately 80 mm Hg. *Thus, even with the severe $\dot{V}_A/\dot{Q}$ abnormality produced by alveolar dead space ventilation, the lung is able to expel the usual 200 ml/min of CO_2, but at a tremendous price: a very high arterial P_{CO_2} and thus respiratory acidosis.*

The normal right lung must also supply all of the body's O_2—delivering O_2 to the blood at twice its normal rate. However, because the right lung still has its normal $\dot{V}_A$ of 2.1 liters/min, its alveolar P_{O_2} falls to approximately 51 mm Hg in the new steady state. The blood leaving the right lung, which is identical to systemic arterial blood, also has a P_{O_2} of approximately 51 mm Hg. *Thus, even with a severe $\dot{V}_A/\dot{Q}$ abnormality, the lung is able to import the usual 250 ml/min of O_2, but at a tremendous price: a very low arterial P_{O_2} (hypoxia).*

We can now answer the question that we posed earlier: The hyperperfused "good" lung cannot make up for the deficit incurred by the hypoperfused "bad lung." In our example, the fundamental problem was that ventilating unperfused alveoli in the left lung reduced the effective alveolar ventilation by half. In real life, the body would respond with bronchiolar constriction and decreased surfactant production in the abnormal left lung (see Fig. 30–11B), thereby diminishing its alveolar dead space ventilation and increasing the true alveolar ventilation to the normal, right lung. In addition, as we discuss in the next

chapter, the respiratory acidosis and hypoxia would stimulate chemoreceptors to increase ventilation. If the body could double $\dot{V}_A$ to the right lung—and if this right lung has a normal diffusing capacity—then all resting blood gas parameters would return to normal. A clinical example is the surgical removal of an entire lung.

A massive pulmonary embolism that obstructs the left pulmonary artery is superficially similar to the example that we have just discussed. However, other associated problems (e.g., right-heart failure secondary to an increase in pulmonary vascular resistance, release of vasoactive agents) make the pulmonary embolism potentially fatal.

SHUNT AFFECTING ONE LUNG. Imagine that an object occludes the left mainstem bronchus, *eliminating all ventilation to the left lung*. Total $\dot{V}_A$ remains at 4.2 liters/min, all of which goes to the right lung. Thus, the $\dot{V}_A/\dot{Q}$ to the left lung is 0/2.5, or 0, whereas the $\dot{V}_A/\dot{Q}$ to the right lung is 4.2/2.5, or 1.68. The overall $\dot{V}_A/\dot{Q}$ is normal, 0.84. Again, the key question is whether a combination of a low $\dot{V}_A/\dot{Q}$ in the abnormal lung and a high $\dot{V}_A/\dot{Q}$ in the normal lung can yield normal blood gases.

The normal right lung must now eliminate CO_2 at twice the rate that it normally does. However, the right lung also has twice its normal $\dot{V}_A$. Because twice the normal amount of alveolar air carries away twice the normal amount of CO_2, the right lung's new steady-state alveolar P_{CO_2} is normal, approximately 40 mm Hg (Fig. 30–14A). The blood leaving the normal lung also has a P_{CO_2} of approximately 40 mm Hg. However, the unventilated lung has the P_{CO_2} of *mixed venous blood*, approximately 51 mm Hg in this example. After the two streams of blood mix—known as **venous admixture**, because venous blood combines with blood from ventilated alveoli—arterial blood in the left ventricle has a CO_2 content that is midway between the CO_2 contents of the two streams of blood, corresponding to an arterial P_{CO_2} of approximately 46 mm Hg. *Thus, even with the severe $\dot{V}_A/\dot{Q}$ abnormality produced by shunt, the lung is once again able to expel the usual 200 ml/min of CO_2, but once again at a price: a high arterial P_{CO_2} (respiratory acidosis).*

The normal right lung must also deliver O_2 to the blood at twice the rate that it normally does. However, because the right lung's $\dot{V}_A$ is also twice its usual value, its new steady-state alveolar P_{O_2} is normal, approximately 100 mm Hg. The blood leaving the right lung also has a P_{O_2} of approximately 100 mm Hg, a hemoglobin (Hb) saturation (S_{O_2}) of approximately 97.5%, and an O_2 content of approximately 20 ml/dl. However, the unventilated lung has a P_{O_2} of mixed venous blood, approximately 29 mm Hg in this example. Thus, the blood leaving the shunted lung has an S_{O_2} of approximately 49% and an O_2 content of approximately 10 ml/dl. After venous admixture, arterial O_2 content is $(20 + 10)/2$ or 15 ml/dl, which corresponds to an arterial S_{O_2} (Sa_{O_2}) of 73 and a P_{O_2} of approximately 40 mm Hg. *Thus, even with the severe $\dot{V}_A/\dot{Q}$ abnormality caused by shunt, the lung is able to import the usual 250 ml/min of O_2, but at the price of an extremely low arterial P_{O_2} (hypoxia).*

Why did the $\dot{V}_A/\dot{Q}$ mismatch caused by shunt lead to only a mild respiratory acidosis but a severe hypoxia? The

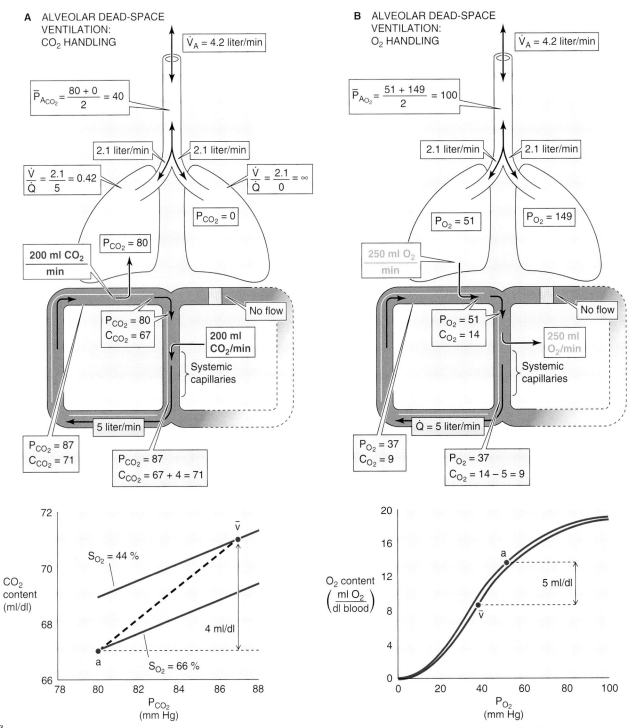

FIGURE 30–13. Alveolar dead space ventilation. The numbers in this idealized example refer to a time after the individual has achieved a new steady state. In the upper panels of A and B, the *light beige–colored boxes* give the alveolar ventilation to each lung, as well as the total alveolar ventilation ($\dot{V}_A$). The *pink boxes* give the blood flow to each lung, as well as the total cardiac output ($\dot{Q}$). The *white boxes* give the rates of CO_2 or O_2 transport (ml/min) at either the pulmonary or systemic capillaries. The *blue boxes* give the CO_2 and O_2 partial pressures (mm Hg) in alveolar air. The *lavender boxes* give the CO_2 partial pressure (mm Hg) and CO_2 content (ml/dl) in the mixed-venous blood, in the blood leaving each of the lungs, and in the mixed-arterial blood. The *dark beige–colored boxes* give the same information for O_2. The lower panel of A shows plots of how total-CO_2 content in this example varies with P_{CO_2} at the Hb-O_2 saturations of arterial blood (*red line*) and mixed-venous blood (*violet line*). Despite the severe respiratory acidosis, the decrease in total CO_2 content between the mixed-venous and arterial blood is normal (4 ml/dl). The lower panel of B shows comparable plots for how total O_2 content varies with P_{O_2} at the pH and P_{CO_2} values of mixed-venous blood (*violet curve*) and arterial blood (*red curve*). Despite the severe hypoxia, the increase in total O_2 content between the mixed-venous and arterial blood is normal (5 ml/dl).

FIGURE 30–14. Shunt. The numbers in this idealized example refer to a time after the individual has achieved a new steady state. In the upper panels of A and B, the *light beige–colored* boxes give the alveolar ventilation to each lung, as well as the total alveolar ventilation ($\dot{V}_A$). The *pink boxes* give the blood flow to each lung, as well as the total cardiac output ($\dot{Q}$). The *white boxes* give the rates of CO_2 or O_2 transport (ml/min) at either the pulmonary or systemic capillaries. The *blue boxes* give the CO_2 and O_2 partial pressures (mm Hg) in alveolar air. The *lavender boxes* give the CO_2 partial pressure (mm Hg) and CO_2 content (ml/dl) in the mixed-venous blood, in the blood leaving each of the lungs, and in the mixed-arterial blood. The *dark beige–colored* boxes give the same information for O_2. The lower panel of A shows plots of how total CO_2 content in this example varies with P_{CO_2} at the Hb-O_2 saturations for unshunted blood at the end of the pulmonary capillary (*red line*), for shunted/mixed-venous blood (*violet line*), and for mixed-arterial blood (*green line*). Because of the 50% shunt, the decrease in total CO_2 content between mixed-venous blood (point $\bar{v}$) and unshunted blood (point c) must be twice normal (8 ml/dl) to produce a normal decrease (4 ml/dl) between mixed-venous blood ($\bar{v}$) and mixed-arterial blood (point a). The lower panel of B shows comparable plots for how total O_2 content varies with P_{O_2} at the pH and P_{CO_2} values of mixed-venous blood (*violet curve*) and arterial blood (*red curve*). Because of the 50% shunt, the increase in total O_2 content between mixed-venous blood (point $\bar{v}$) and unshunted blood (point c) must be twice normal (10 ml/dl) to produce a normal increase (5 ml/dl) between mixed-venous blood (point $\bar{v}$) and mixed-arterial blood (point a).

CLINICAL APPROACHES FOR DIAGNOSING A $\dot{V}_A/\dot{Q}$ MISMATCH

Rather simple diagnostic methods are available for detecting the presence of a $\dot{V}_A/\dot{Q}$ mismatch, assessing its severity, and identifying a shunt.

DIAGNOSIS OF EXCLUSION
The physician can often diagnose a pathologic nonuniformity of $\dot{V}_A/\dot{Q}$ by excluding other possibilities. In a patient with a low arterial P_{O_2} but normal respiratory mechanics, the hypoxia could be due to either a decrease in the diffusing capacity (D_L) or a $\dot{V}_A/\dot{Q}$ mismatch. Because D_L is normally approximately threefold greater than necessary for achieving diffusion equilibrium for O_2 and CO_2 (p. 682), a problem with D_L is unlikely in the absence of a positive history. By default, the most likely cause is a $\dot{V}_A/\dot{Q}$ defect.

ALVEOLAR-ARTERIAL DIFFERENCES FOR O_2 AND CO_2
The difference between the mean alveolar P_{O_2} and the systemic arterial P_{O_2} is known as the **alveolar-arterial (A-a) difference for P_{O_2}**. In our "normal" example in Figure 30–12B, both mean alveolar P_{O_2} and arterial P_{O_2} were 100 mm Hg. In real life, however, physiological and normal anatomic shunts cause arterial P_{O_2} to be 5 to 15 mm Hg below the mean alveolar value.

A defining characteristic of $\dot{V}_A/\dot{Q}$ mismatches is that they widen the A-a P_{O_2} difference. In our example of alveolar dead space in Figure 30–13B, the mean alveolar P_{O_2} was $(51 + 149)/2 = 100$ mm Hg, whereas the systemic arterial P_{O_2} was 51 mm Hg, for an A-a difference of 49 mm Hg. In our example of shunt in Figure 30–14B, the mean alveolar P_{O_2} was 100 mm Hg, whereas the arterial P_{O_2} was only 40 mm Hg—an A-a difference of 60 mm Hg. Thus, the A-a difference for P_{O_2} is an index of the severity of the $\dot{V}_A/\dot{Q}$ mismatch.

BREATHING 100% O_2
Once a $\dot{V}_A/\dot{Q}$ mismatch has been identified, it is important to distinguish between a shunt, which might be corrected surgically, and other causes. Imagine two patients with similar degrees of hypoxia. In one case, the cause is a nonuniformity of ventilation, with one lung relatively hypoventilated (low $\dot{V}_A/\dot{Q}$) and the other relatively hyperventilated (high $\dot{V}_A/\dot{Q}$). However, no alveoli are shunted. In the second case, the cause of hypoxia is a complete shunting of blood through one unventilated lung (a $\dot{V}_A/\dot{Q}$ of 0, as in Fig. 30–14). The normal lung has a high $\dot{V}_A/\dot{Q}$. We can distinguish between the two cases by having both subjects inspire 100% O_2.

When the patient without predominant shunt breathes 100% O_2, the P_{O_2} of the blood leaving both lungs will be far higher than normal (Fig. 30–15A). Blood leaving the hypoventilated lung has a P_{O_2} somewhat lower than that of the blood leaving the hyperventilated lung. However, because the P_{O_2} is on the flat part of the Hb-O_2 dissociation curve in both cases, the S_{O_2} values are virtually identical. The miniscule difference in O_2 contents between the two streams of blood is due to a difference in dissolved O_2. Thus, the mixed systemic arterial blood will have a slightly elevated O_2 content, a SaO_2 of approximately 100%, and a markedly elevated P_{O_2}.

The situation is very different in the patient with a severe shunt (see Fig. 30–15B). Because blood leaving the shunted lung does not equilibrate with the alveoli ventilated with 100% O_2, it has the low P_{O_2}, S_{O_2}, and O_2 content characteristic of mixed venous blood. Although blood leaving the normal lung will have an extremely high P_{O_2}, the S_{O_2} and O_2 content will be only slightly above normal—just as we saw for the hyperventilated lung in Figure 30–15A. Thus, when one stream of blood with a slightly increased O_2 content ("normal" lung) mixes with another stream with a markedly decreased O_2 content ("shunted" lung), the mixed-systemic arterial blood has a lower-than-normal O_2 content. This low O_2 content translates to a low SaO_2, and thus to a low systemic arterial P_{O_2}. Thus, unlike subjects with other kinds of $\dot{V}_A/\dot{Q}$ mismatches that do not include substantial shunt (e.g., alveolar dead space ventilation in Fig. 30–13), those with shunts will have low arterial P_{O_2} values, even while breathing 100% O_2. Because breathing 100% O_2 greatly increases mean alveolar P_{O_2} without substantially increasing arterial P_{O_2}, this maneuver greatly exaggerates the A-a difference for P_{O_2}.

---

fundamental problem is that the Hb-O_2 dissociation curve (see Fig. 28–3) is nearly saturated at the normal arterial P_{O_2}. If O_2 content were proportional to P_{O_2}, then mixing unshunted blood ($P_{O_2} = 100$ mm Hg) with shunted blood ($P_{O_2} = 29$ mm Hg) would have yielded arterial blood with a P_{O_2} of $(100 + 29)/2 = \sim65$ mm Hg, which is far higher than the arterial P_{O_2} of approximately 40 mm Hg in our example.

In response to respiratory acidosis and hypoxia, a patient would increase $\dot{V}_A$, thus lowering P_{CO_2} and raising P_{O_2} in the normal right lung. In fact, even a modest increase in $\dot{V}_A$ would be sufficient to lower arterial P_{CO_2} to 40 mm Hg. However, even if $\dot{V}_A$ approached infinity (raising the right lung's alveolar P_{O_2} to the inspired P_{O_2} of approximately 149 mm Hg), arterial P_{O_2} would be well under 100 mm Hg. In fact, even if the inspired air were 100% O_2, the arterial P_{O_2} would still fail to reach 100 mm Hg; because of the shape of the Hb-O_2 dissociation curve, an increased alveolar P_{O_2} can increase the O_2 content of blood only marginally.

MIXED $\dot{V}_A/\dot{Q}$ MISMATCHES. Alveolar units in a normal person may have $\dot{V}_A/\dot{Q}$ values ranging from approximately 0.6 to 3.3 (see Table 30–3). Pathologic $\dot{V}_A/\dot{Q}$ mismatches cause this range of $\dot{V}_A/\dot{Q}$ ratios to broaden. In realistic examples of mismatches, some alveoli may be true alveolar dead space (i.e., perfusion absent, $\dot{V}_A/\dot{Q} = \infty$), but others are more modestly underperfused. Some alveoli may be truly shunted (i.e., ventilation absent, $\dot{V}_A/\dot{Q} = 0$), but others are more modestly underventilated. Thus, the left ventricle receives a mixture of blood from alveoli with $\dot{V}_A/\dot{Q}$ ratios from ∞ to 0, corresponding to all of the

A V̇A/Q̇ MISMATCH WITHOUT PREDOMINANT SHUNT

	High ↑V̇A/Q̇	Low ↓V̇A/Q̇
Po₂	693	653
% Sat	100	100
Co₂	22.4	22.2

Pulmonary veins	
Systemic arterial	
Co₂	22.3
% Sat	100
Po₂	673

B V̇A/Q̇ MISMATCH CAUSED BY SHUNT

	Un-shunted (High V̇A/Q̇)	Shunted (V̇A/Q̇ = 0)
Po₂	673	34
% Sat	100	60
Co₂	22.3	12.3

Pulmonary veins	
Systemic arterial	
Co₂	17.3
% Sat	85
Po₂	52

FIGURE 30–15. Analyzing V̇A/Q̇ mismatch by administering 100% O₂.

points along the O_2–CO_2 diagram in Figure 30–10B. What is the composition of this mixed blood? The principles that we developed in our simplified examples of alveolar dead space ventilation and shunt still hold. Even if total $\dot{V}_A$ and total $\dot{Q}$ remain normal, pathologically high $\dot{V}_A/\dot{Q}$ ratios in some alveoli cannot make up for pathologically low ratios in others, and vice versa. The result of uncompensated pathologic $\dot{V}_A/\dot{Q}$ mismatching is always respiratory acidosis and hypoxia.

REFERENCES

Books and Reviews

Anthonisen NR, Fleetham JA: Ventilation: Total, alveolar, and dead space. In Farhi LE, Tenney SM (eds): Handbook of Physiology, Section 3: The Respiratory System, vol IV. Bethesda, MD, American Physiological Society, 1985, pp 113–129.

Deffeback ME, Widdicombe J: The bronchial circulation. In Crystal RG, West JB (eds): The Lung. New York, Raven Press, 1991, pp 741–758.

Drazen JM, Gaston B, Shore SA: Chemical regulation of pulmonary airway tone. Annu Rev Physiol 57:151–170, 1995.

Farhi LE: Ventilation-perfusion relationship. In Farhi LE, Tenney SM (eds): Handbook of Physiology, Section 3: The Respiratory System, vol IV. Bethesda, MD, American Physiological Society, 1985, pp 199–215.

Forster RE, BuBois AB, Briscoe WA, Fisher AB: The Lung: Physiological Basis of Pulmonary Function Tests, 3rd ed. Chicago: Year Book, 1986.

Hughes JMB: Distribution of pulmonary blood flow. In Crystal RG, West JB: The Lung. New York, Raven Press, 1991, pp 1135–1145.

Milic-Emili J: Topographical inequality of ventilation. In Crystal RG, West JB: The Lung. New York, Raven Press, 1991, pp 1043–1052.

Journal Articles

Fowler W: Lung function studies II. The respiratory dead space. Am J Physiol 154:405–416, 1948.

Lenfant C: Measurement of ventilation/perfusion distribution with alveolar-arterial differences. J Appl Physiol 18:1090–1094, 1963.

Riley RL, Cournand A: Analysis of factors affecting partial pressures of O_2 and CO_2 in gas and blood of lungs: Theory. J Appl Physiol 4:77–101, 1951.

Riley RL, Cournand A, Donald KW: Analysis of factors affecting partial pressures of O_2 and CO_2 in gas and blood of lungs: Methods. J Appl Physiol 4:102–120, 1951.

West JB, Dollery CT, Naimark A: Distribution of blood flow in isolated lung: Relation to vascular and alveolar pressures. J Appl Physiol 19:713–724, 1964.

CHAPTER 31

Control of Ventilation

George B. Richerson and Walter F. Boron

OVERVIEW OF THE RESPIRATORY CONTROL SYSTEM

Breathing is one of those things in life that you almost never think about until something goes wrong with it. However, those with pulmonary disease become intensely aware of breathing, as do people who overexert themselves, especially at high altitude. The feeling of dyspnea that they experience (see box titled Dyspnea) is one of the most unpleasant sensations in life. Swimmers and SCUBA divers, professional singers, practitioners of the Lamaze technique, and anyone with a bed partner who snores also focus intensely on breathing. It is common for respiratory output to be the last brain function to be lost in comatose patients, in which case its cessation marks the onset of brain death. Thus, despite our common tendency to ignore it, control of ventilation is one of the most important of all brain functions.

The ventilatory control mechanism must be able to accomplish two tasks. First, it must establish the *automatic rhythm* for contraction of the respiratory muscles. Second, it must adjust this rhythm to accommodate changing *metabolic* demands (as reflected by changes in blood P_{O_2}, P_{CO_2}, and pH), varying *mechanical* conditions (e.g., changing posture), and a range of episodic, *nonventilatory* behaviors (e.g., speaking, sniffing, eating).

Automatic Centers in the Brain Stem Drive the Respiratory Muscles Rhythmically and Subconsciously

The rhythmic output of the central nervous system (CNS) to muscles of ventilation normally occurs automatically, without any conscious effort. Neurons within the medulla generate signals that are distributed appropriately to various pools of cranial and spinal motor neurons (p. 250), which directly innervate the respiratory muscles (Fig. 31–1). The specific site containing the neurons that generate the respiratory rhythm—the **central pattern generator** (CPG; p. 365)—under normal conditions is still unknown. A vast array of neurons—located primarily in the medulla, but also in the pons and other regions of the brain stem—fire more action potentials during specific parts of the respiratory cycle. For example, some neurons have peak activity during inspiration, and others, during expiration. These neurons are called **respiratory-related neurons** (RRNs) because their activity patterns correlate with breathing. Some of these RRNs are **interneurons** (i.e., making local connections), others are **premotor neurons** (i.e., innervating motor neurons), and still others are **motor neurons** (i.e., innervating muscles of respiration).

DYSPNEA

Dyspnea is the feeling of being short of breath, or the unpleasant conscious awareness of difficulty in ventilation. Some causes of dyspnea are adaptive responses. For example, when arterial P_{O_2} falls or P_{CO_2} rises from breath-holding, asphyxia, or pulmonary disease, dyspnea leads to efforts to increase ventilation and thus restore blood gases to normal. However, dyspnea can occur even with a normal arterial P_{O_2} and P_{CO_2}. For example, increased airway resistance can cause dyspnea, even if blood gases do not change. Intense exercise also causes dyspnea, even though P_{CO_2} usually falls. Other causes of dyspnea seem maladaptive. For example, claustrophobia and panic attacks can induce the feeling of suffocation—that is, dyspnea—despite normal ventilatory parameters. The central neural mechanisms and pathways responsible for dyspnea are unknown.

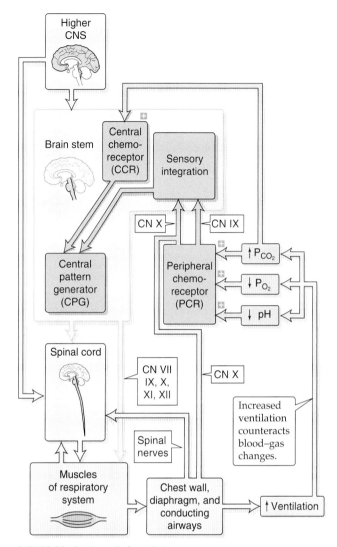

FIGURE 31–1. Control of ventilation.

The most important respiratory motor neurons are those that send axons out from the phrenic nerve to innervate the diaphragm (Table 31–1), one of the *primary muscles of inspiration* (p. 612). When respiratory output increases (e.g., during exercise), activity also appears in motor neurons that innervate a wide variety of *accessory* muscles of inspiration and expiration (p. 612).

Each of these muscles is active at different times within the respiratory cycle, and the brain can alter this timing depending on prevailing conditions. It is the job of the premotor neurons to orchestrate the appropriate patterns of activity among the different pools of motor neurons. The pattern of alternating inspiratory and expiratory activity that occurs under normal conditions during sleep, at rest, and during moderate exercise is called **eupnea**. During eupnea, neural output to respiratory muscles is highly regular, with rhythmic bursts of activity during inspiration only to the diaphragm and external intercostal muscles. Expiration occurs purely as a result of cessation of inspiration and passive elastic recoil of the lungs. During exercise, the amplitude and frequency of phrenic nerve activity increase, and additional activity appears in nerves that supply accessory muscles of inspiration. With this increased effort, the accessory muscles of expiration also become active, thereby producing more rapid exhalation and permitting increased respiratory frequency.

Peripheral and Central Chemoreceptors— Which Sense P_{O_2}, P_{CO_2}, and pH—Drive the Central Pattern Generator

The CPG for breathing is the clock that times the automatic cycling of inspiration and expiration. In some cases, the CPG stops "ticking" in the absence of **tonic drive** inputs, resulting in the absence of ventilation, or **apnea**. Although this tonic drive comes from many sources, the most important are the central and peripheral chemoreceptors, which monitor O_2, CO_2, and pH. Unlike a clock, the respiratory CPG changes with the strength of the drive from the chemoreceptors, resulting in changes in both depth and frequency of ventilation.

The **peripheral chemoreceptors**, located in the carotid and aortic bodies, are primarily sensitive to decreases in arterial P_{O_2}, although high P_{CO_2} and low pH enhance their sensitivity to hypoxia. They convey their sensory information to the medulla via the glossopharyngeal nerve (CN IX) and vagus nerve (CN X). The **central chemoreceptors**, located on the "brain" side of the blood-brain barrier (p. 408), are sensitive only to increases in arterial P_{CO_2} and—much more slowly—decreases in arterial pH, but not arterial P_{O_2}. All three signals trigger an increase in alveolar ventilation that tends to return these arterial blood-gas parameters to normal. Thus, the peripheral and central chemoreceptors, in addition to supplying tonic drive to the CPG, form the critical sensory end of a **negative-feedback system** that uses respiratory output to stabilize arterial P_{O_2}, P_{CO_2}, and pH (see Fig. 31–1).

TABLE 31–1

INNERVATION OF THE PRIMARY AND SOME SECONDARY MUSCLES OF RESPIRATION

MUSCLES	NERVE	LOCATION OF CELL BODY OF MOTOR NEURON
Primary Muscles of Inspiration		
Diaphragm	Phrenic nerve	Phrenic motor nuclei in ventral horn of spinal cord, C3–C5
External intercostal muscles	Intercostal nerves	Ventral horn of thoracic spinal cord
Secondary Muscles of Inspiration		
Larynx and pharynx	Vagus (CN X) and glossopharyngeal (CN IX) nerves	Primarily within the nucleus ambiguus
Tongue	Hypoglossal nerve (CN XII)	Hypoglossal motor nucleus
Sternocleidomastoid and trapezius muscles	Accessory nerve (CN XI)	Spinal accessory nucleus, C1–C5
Nares	Facial nerve	Facial motor nucleus
Secondary Muscles of Expiration		
Internal intercostal muscles	Intercostal nerves	Ventral horn of thoracic spinal cord
Abdominal muscles	Spinal nerves	Ventral horn of lumbar spinal cord

Other Receptors, As Well As Higher Brain Centers, Also Modulate Ventilation

If left alone, the respiratory CPG would tick regularly for an indefinite period. However, many inputs to the CPG reset the clock. For example, respiratory output is often highly irregular during many behaviors that use the respiratory muscles (e.g., eating, talking, yawning). During sleep or quiet wakefulness, and with anesthesia, the CPG is unperturbed and *does* run regularly; it is under these conditions that neuroscientists usually study mechanisms of respiratory control.

A variety of receptors in the lungs and airways provide sensory feedback that the medulla integrates and uses to alter respiratory output. Stretch receptors monitor pulmonary mechanics (e.g., lung volume, muscle length) and may help to optimize breathing parameters during changes in posture or activity. Activation of pulmonary stretch receptors also can terminate inspiratory efforts, thereby preventing overinflation. Other sensors that detect the presence of foreign bodies or chemicals in the airways are important for protecting the lungs by triggering a cough or a sneeze. Still others detect the movement of joints, which may be important for up-regulating ventilation to track exercise. The mechanoreceptors and chemoreceptors from the lungs and lower airways send their sensory information to the respiratory neurons of the medulla via CN X, and those from the upper airways send information via CN IX.

Nonrespiratory brainstem nuclei and higher centers in the CNS also interact with respiratory control centers, allowing the ventilatory system to accommodate such activities as speaking, playing a musical instrument, swallowing, and vomiting. These interconnections also allow respiratory control to be highly integrated with the autonomic nervous system, the sleep-wake cycle, emotions, and other aspects of brain function.

In the remainder of this chapter, we examine: (1) respiratory neurons, (2) how these neurons generate the automatic rhythm of ventilation, (3) the control of ventilation by blood gases (i.e., arterial P_{O_2}, P_{CO_2}, and pH), and

(4) how afferent feedback and higher CNS centers modulate ventilation.

LOCATION OF NEURONS THAT CONTROL RESPIRATORY OUTPUT

The Neurons That Generate the Respiratory Rhythm Are Located in the Medulla

A classic method for determining which parts of the CNS are responsible for controlling respiratory output is to transect the neuraxis at different levels and observe changes in breathing. Using this approach in the 2nd century, Galen performed the first experiments to determine the location of the respiratory controller. As a physician for gladiators in the Greek city of Pergamon, he observed that breathing stopped after a sword blow to the high cervical spine. A similar blow to the lower cervical spine paralyzed the arms and legs, but allowed respiration to continue. He reproduced these lesions in live animals and correctly concluded that the brain sends information via the midcervical spinal cord to the diaphragm. Eighteen centuries later, Lumsden used a similar approach in cats. He found that transecting the CNS between the medulla and spinal cord (Fig. 31–2, *spino-medullary transection*) causes ventilation to cease as a result of loss of the descending input to phrenic and intercostal motor neurons in the spinal cord. However, even after a spino-medullary transection, respiratory activity continues in muscles innervated by motor neurons whose cell bodies reside in the brain stem. During the period that would have been an inspiration, the nostrils continue to flare, and the muscles of the tongue, pharynx, and larynx continue to maximize airway caliber. Spino-medullary transection blocks ventilation by interrupting output to the diaphragm, not by eliminating the respiratory rhythm. Thus, the neural machinery driving ventilation lies above the spinal cord.

If a similar transection is made between the pons and the medulla (see Fig. 31–2, *ponto-medullary transection*), one of two things may happen. Lumsden noticed in the

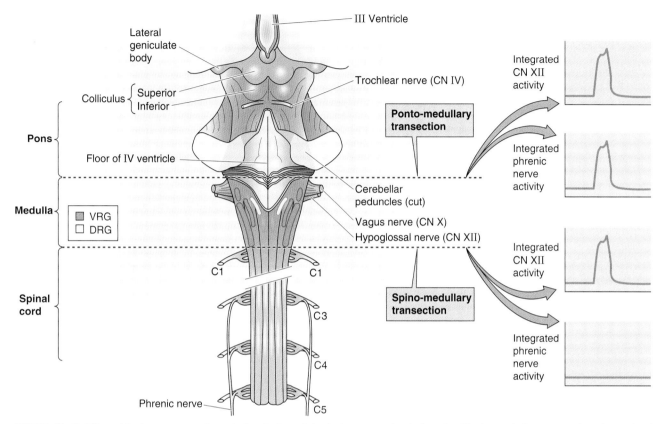

FIGURE 31–2. Effect of brainstem transections. A dorsal view of the brain stem and spinal cord, with the cerebellum removed, and records of integrated nerve activity over one respiratory cycle, following the indicated transection. During inspiration, *integrated nerve activity* (a moving average of the amplitude and frequency of action potentials) increases in the nerves to the tongue (e.g., CN XII) and the diaphragm (e.g., phrenic nerve). CN, cranial nerve; DRG, dorsal respiratory group; VRG, ventral respiratory group.

1940s that breathing continued, but with an abnormal "gasping" pattern. Others have since found that normal breathing continues after a transection at this level, indicating that the medulla contains all the neurons required for eupnea—that is, the respiratory CPG resides in the medulla. The most likely explanation for the gasping seen by Lumsden is that surgery to the rostral medulla can easily damage the respiratory CPG, and techniques were not very refined at the time.

There are actually two identical respiratory CPGs—one on each side of the medulla. All of the elements of the respiratory controller—drive inputs, sensory feedback, RRNs, and motor neurons—are bilateral. Thus, after a midsagittal transection, each side of the medulla generates an independent respiratory rhythm.

The respiratory CPG probably evolved in fish, where blood-gas exchange across the gills requires pumping by *branchial* structures, thus explaining why the CPG is located in the medulla. CPGs generate all repetitive motor activities (p. 366). In invertebrates, these include swimming in sea slugs and movements of the stomach in lobsters. The mechanisms of rhythm generation discovered in these systems have led to establishment of general principles that have been valuable in promoting understanding of CPGs in mammals.

Apneustic and Pneumotaxic Centers in the Pons Modulate—but Are Not Essential for—Normal Respiratory Output

Although the medulla alone can generate the basic eupneic respiratory rhythm, both higher CNS centers and sensory inputs fine-tune this rhythm. For example, the pons contains two regions that affect respiratory output—the apneustic and pneumotaxic centers.

Lumsden found that transecting the brain stem at the midpons has only a modest effect—an increase in tidal volume and a slight decrease in respiratory rate. Interrupting the two vagus nerves, which carry sensory information from pulmonary stretch receptors, has a similar, but modest effect. However, combining a midpons transection *with* cutting of the two vagus nerves causes the animal to make prolonged inspiratory efforts (**inspiratory apneuses**) that are interrupted by only brief expirations. Lumsden found that transecting the brain stem above the pons did not alter the basic respiratory pattern of eupnea. Recall that Lumsden incorrectly concluded that transecting the brain stem between the medulla and pons (see Fig. 31–2, *ponto-medullary transection*) causes gasping. This collection of observations led to the proposal that (1) the medulla is capable only of gasping, (2) the caudal

NORMAL AND ABNORMAL RESPIRATORY PATTERNS

The respiratory pattern can become abnormal for a variety of reasons. Several of these abnormal patterns have recognizable characteristics:

Apnea: Cessation of respiration.

Apneusis (inspiratory): Prolonged inspirations separated by brief expirations.

Ataxic breathing: Highly irregular inspirations, often separated by long periods of apnea. Usually seen with medullary lesions.

Biot breathing: First described in patients with meningitis by Biot (in 1876) as a variant of cluster breathing (see later), with breaths of nearly equal volume separated by periods of apnea. Biot breathing is considered to be a variant of ataxic breathing.

Central neurogenic hyperventilation: Rapid, deep breathing causing a decrease in arterial P_{CO_2}. Although described in some patients with focal brain lesions, this pattern may actually reflect coexisting lung disease or other systemic illness.

Cheyne-Stokes respiration: A benign respiratory pattern. Cycles of a gradual increase in tidal volume, followed by a gradual decrease in tidal volume, and then a period of apnea. Seen with bilateral cortical disease or congestive heart failure, or in healthy people during sleep at high altitude.

Cluster breathing: Groups of breaths, often of differing amplitude, separated by long periods of apnea. Seen with medullary or pontine lesions.

Eupnea: Normal breathing.

Gasping: Maximal, brief inspiratory efforts separated by long periods of expiration. Seen in severe anoxia, as well as a terminal, agonal breathing pattern in patients with brainstem lesions.

Hyperventilation: An increase in ventilation that decreases arterial P_{CO_2}. Seen in pregnancy and cirrhosis (due to increased progesterone), in panic attacks, and in metabolic acidosis.

Kussmaul breathing: Refers to extremely deep, rapid breathing seen with metabolic acidosis, such as in diabetic ketoacidosis (see box on p. 1084).

Sighs: Larger than normal breaths (p. 732) that occur automatically at regular intervals in normal subjects.

Tachypnea: An increase in respiratory rate.

Vagal breathing: Slow, deep inspirations caused by interruption of vagus nerve input to the brain stem.

Yawn: An exaggerated sigh (p. 732).

Most of the abnormalities due to clinical diseases seen in humans also can be experimentally induced in animals (Fig. 31–3). Therefore, observations on experimental animals provide important insight into the neural control of ventilation, as well as into the mechanisms that underlie abnormal breathing patterns in humans.

pons contains an **apneustic center** (i.e., it causes an apneusis), and (3) the rostral pons contains a **pneumotaxic center** (i.e., it promotes coordinated respirations). He believed that all three of these regions are required for coordinated rhythmic breathing.

How do we now interpret these results? The pneumotaxic center is located in the **nucleus parabrachialis medialis** (NPBM) and adjacent **Kölliker-Fuse nucleus** (KF) in the rostral pons. However, one can induce apneuses with lesions in many locations *outside* the rostral pons. Thus, the pneumotaxic center is not unique. Moreover, even apneuses induced by lesions in the pneumotaxic center can be reversed by simply increasing the temperature. The pneumotaxic center plays a general role in a variety of autonomic functions but is not required for generating eupnea. Thus, the terms "apneustic center" and "pneumotaxic center" are used primarily because of their historical significance.

The Dorsal and Ventral Respiratory Groups Contain High Densities of Neurons That Fire in Phase with the Respiratory Cycle

In the 1940s, Robert Pitts and colleagues used electrophysiological techniques to localize respiratory regions. Based on changes in breathing induced by electrical *stimulation* within the medulla, they described "inspiratory and expiratory half-centers." However, the stimuli they used were very large, and these half-centers were probably regions of axons, not neuronal cell bodies.

A more widely used approach has been to use microelectrode *recordings* from individual respiratory neurons. In the 1930s, Gesell and colleagues used extracellular microelectrode recordings to monitor single neurons and found that many neurons within the medulla increase their firing rate during one of the phases of the respiratory cycle. Some of these neurons fire more frequently during inspiration, whereas others fire more often during expiration.

Not all neurons that fire in phase with the respiratory cycle are involved in respiration. For example, because they are located within the chest cavity, aortic baroreceptors (p. 536) produce an output that varies with lung inflation, but they are primarily involved in the control of cardiovascular—not respiratory—function. Conversely, some neurons whose firing does not correlate with the respiratory cycle may be essential for respiratory control. For example, central chemoreceptors may fire tonically (i.e., they do not burst during inspiration), and yet are critical for maintaining respiratory output by providing tonic drive (see earlier). Thus, not all respiratory-related neurons (e.g., those stimulated by the aortic baroreceptor) play a *direct* role in respiration, and respiratory control probably involves more than just RRNs (e.g., chemoreceptor neurons). To avoid confusion, it is preferable to use the term "respiratory-*related* neurons" (see earlier) rather than "respiratory neurons."

Although the functional mapping of RRNs cannot define *all* neurons necessary for producing respiratory output, this mapping has proved very useful in defining neurons that are candidates for *controlling* ventilation. RRNs are present in many regions of the brain stem. However, on each side of the medulla, two large concentrations of RRNs—the dorsal and ventral respiratory groups—are grossly organized into sausage-shaped columns, oriented along the long axis of the medulla (Fig. 31–4). Many neurons of these two regions also tend to

A INTEGRATED PHRENIC NERVE ACTIVITY

B LUNG VOLUME

FIGURE 31–3. Respiratory patterns in experimental animals.

FIGURE 31–4. Motor output of dorsal and ventral respiratory groups. *A,* Inspiratory output. *B,* Expiratory output. These are dorsal views of the brain stem and spinal cord, with the cerebellum removed. The dorsal respiratory group (DRG) includes the nucleus tractus solitarius (NTS). The ventral respiratory group (VRG) includes the Bötzinger complex (Böt.C), nucleus ambiguus (NA), nucleus para-ambigualis (NPA), and nucleus retroambigualis (NRA). The color coding indicates whether the neurons are primarily inspiratory (*red*) or primarily expiratory (*green*).

TABLE 31–2

PROPERTIES OF THE DRG AND VRG

| | | VRG | | |
PROPERTY	**DRG**	**Rostral**	**Intermediate**	**Caudal**
Location	Dorsal medulla	Midway between dorsal and ventral surfaces of medulla		
Major component	Nucleus tractus solitarius (NTS)	Nucleus retrofacialis (NRF) or Bötzinger complex	Nucleus ambiguus (NA) and nucleus para-ambigualis (NPA)	Nucleus retroambigualis (NRA)
Dominant activity	Inspiratory	Expiratory	Inspiratory	Expiratory
Major input	Sensory via CN IX & X	—	—	Rostral VRG
Major output	(a) Pre-motor neurons → spinal cord → primary muscles of inspiration (b) Interneurons → VRG	Interneurons → DRG and caudal VRG	(a) Motor (via CN IX and X) → accessory muscles of inspiration (b) Premotor → spinal cord → primary and accessory muscles of inspiration	Premotor → spinal cord → accessory muscles of expiration

DRG, dorsal respiratory group; VRG, ventral respiratory group.

fire exclusively during either inspiration or expiration, which is not the case for RRNs from some other regions of the brain stem.

There are also two major groups of respiratory-related neurons in the pons—one rostral and the other caudal. Neurons in these regions do not *produce* the normal respiratory rhythm but presumably depend on input from the CPG in the medulla. Nevertheless, these pontine centers can influence respiratory output. Indeed, they may correspond to the pneumotaxic and apneustic centers defined in lesion studies.

The Dorsal Respiratory Group Processes Sensory Input and Contains Primarily Inspiratory Neurons

The **dorsal respiratory group** (DRG) primarily contains inspiratory neurons (Table 31–2). It extends for about ⅓ of the length of the medulla, and is located bilaterally in and around the **nucleus tractus solitarius** (NTS), which receives *sensory* input from all viscera of the thorax and abdomen and is one of the key nuclei of the autonomic nervous system (p. 393). The NTS is viscerotopically organized, with the respiratory portion of the NTS being ventrolateral to the **tractus solitarius**, just beneath the floor of the caudal end of the fourth ventricle (see Fig. 31–4). These NTS neurons, as well as some immediately adjacent neurons in the dorsal medulla, make up the DRG.

As might be surmised from the sensory role of the NTS, one of the major functions of the DRG is the *integration* of sensory information from the respiratory system. Indeed, some of the DRG neurons receive sensory input—via the glossopharyngeal (CN IX) and vagus (CN X) nerves—from peripheral chemoreceptors, as well as from respiratory-related receptors in the lungs and airways (see earlier). Some of the RRNs in the DRG are local *interneurons*. Others are *premotor neurons*, projecting di-

rectly to various pools of motor neurons in the spinal cord and ventral respiratory group (VRG; see Fig. 31–4). For example, an interneuron in the DRG may synapse on a DRG premotor neuron, which, in turn, may descend into the spinal cord and reach one of the paired phrenic motor nuclei in the ventral horn of the spinal cord. There, the premotor neuron synapses on the cell bodies of phrenic motor neurons, whose axons follow the phrenic nerve to the diaphragm.

The Ventral Respiratory Group Is Primarily Motor and Contains Both Inspiratory and Expiratory Neurons

The **ventral respiratory group** (VRG) contains both inspiratory-related and expiratory-related neurons (see Table 31–2). It is ventral to the DRG, about midway between the dorsal and ventral surfaces of the medulla (see Fig. 31–4). The VRG is considerably longer than the DRG, extending almost the entire length of the medulla; it consists of three parts: A small *rostral* region is primarily expiratory; an *intermediate* region is mostly inspiratory, and the *caudal* region of the VRG is almost exclusively expiratory.

As in the DRG, some VRG neurons are local *interneurons*, and others are *premotor* neurons. However, in contrast to the DRG, the VRG also contains *motor* neurons that leave the CNS to innervate muscles of the pharynx and larynx, as well as viscera of the thorax and abdomen. Sensory information related to pulmonary function comes indirectly via the DRG. Thus, the VRG plays more of an efferent role, whereas the DRG primarily plays an afferent role.

Like the DRG, the VRG is defined by the electrophysiology of its neurons, not on the basis of neuroanatomy. In fact, the VRG is not associated with a single anatomic nucleus, but lies within and around a series of four adjacent nuclei (see Table 31–2). Together these nuclei form a column of neurons within the ventral medulla extend-

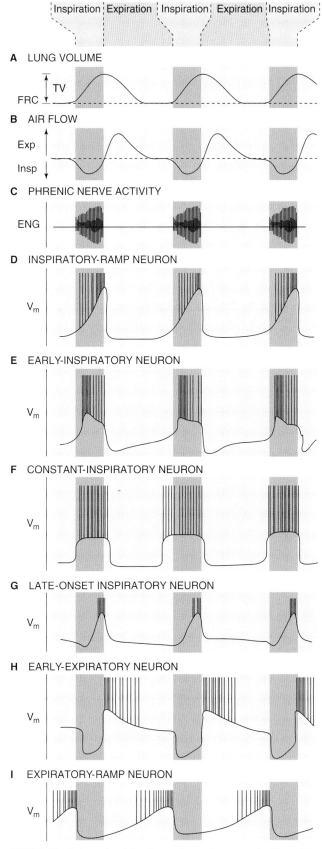

FIGURE 31–5. Neural activity during the respiratory cycle. The activity of respiratory-related neurons in the medulla (examples of which are shown in *D* to *I*) leads to the phasic activity of the phrenic nerve (*C*) and other respiratory nerves, which produces airflow (*B*), causing lung volume to change (*A*). ENG, electroneurogram; Exp, expiration; FRC, functional residual capacity; Insp, inspiration; TV, tidal volume; V_m, membrane potential.

ing from the pons nearly to the spinal cord (see Fig. 31–4).

The three regions of the VRG perform specific functions. The *rostral* region (also known as the Bötzinger complex) drives the expiratory activity of the caudal region. The *intermediate* region contains somatic motor neurons whose axons leave the medulla via CN IX and CN X. These fibers supply the pharynx, larynx, and other structures, thus maximizing the caliber of the upper airways during inspiration. The intermediate VRG also contains premotor neurons that project to inspiratory motor neurons in the spinal cord and medulla. Within the rostral pole of the intermediate VRG, there is a group of inspiratory neurons defined as the pre-Bötzinger complex, which, as we will see later, may be involved in generating the respiratory rhythm. Finally, the *caudal* region of the VRG contains premotor neurons that travel down the spinal cord to synapse on motor neurons that innervate accessory muscles of *expiration*, such as the internal intercostal and abdominal muscles (p. 613).

MECHANISMS OF GENERATION OF RHYTHMIC RESPIRATORY OUTPUT

Different Respiratory-Related Neurons Fire at Different Times During Inspiration and Expiration

Eupneic breathing is highly stereotyped and consists of two phases—inspiration and expiration (Fig. 31–5A–B). During the **inspiratory phase**, phrenic nerve output to the diaphragm gradually increases in activity over 0.5 to 2 seconds, followed by a precipitous decline at the onset of expiration (see Fig. 31–5C). The ramp increase in activity helps to ensure a smooth increase in lung volume. During the **expiratory phase**, the phrenic nerve is inactive, except—in some cases—for a brief burst at the onset. During a quiet expiration, which is normally a passive event, the accessory muscles of expiration are also inactive. However, during a forced expiration, the accessory muscles of expiration become active (p. 613).

Underlying the activity of the phrenic nerve—and the other motor nerves supplying the muscles of inspiration and expiration—is a spectrum of firing patterns of different respiratory-related neurons located within the DRG and VRG (see earlier). RRNs can be broadly classified as inspiratory or expiratory, but each class includes many subtypes, based on their firing patterns, some of which are shown in Figure 31–5D–I. Each subtype presumably plays a unique role in generating and shaping respiratory output—that is, the activity of the nerves to each of the respiratory muscles. RRNs may be further subclassified based on their responses to afferent inputs, such as lung inflation and changes in arterial P_{CO_2}.

Both Intrinsic Membrane Properties and Patterned Synaptic Input Determine the Firing Pattern of RRNs

What are the mechanisms for generating the varied firing patterns of RRNs within the brain stem? Two complementary mechanisms appear to contribute to the patterns of

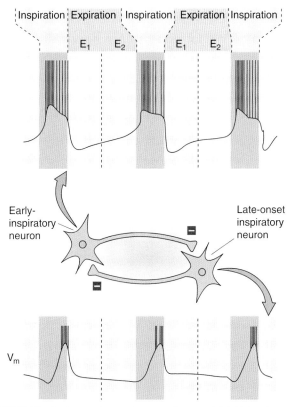

FIGURE 31–6. Patterned synaptic input: Reciprocal inhibition. Because of reciprocal inhibition between the early-burst neuron and the late-onset inspiratory neuron, only one can be maximally active at a time.

activity: (1) intrinsic membrane properties of RRNs and (2) patterned synaptic input. The intrinsic membrane properties include the complement and distribution of ion channels present in a neuron, and how these channels affect firing patterns in response to synaptic input. The patterned synaptic input includes the excitatory postsynaptic potentials (EPSPs) and the inhibitory postsynaptic potentials (IPSPs) that arrive at the appropriate time in the respiratory cycle—and have the appropriate waveform—to generate a specific firing pattern. The combination of intrinsic membrane properties and synaptic input causes the RRN to have a characteristic firing pattern that enables the neuron to do its job. For example, if the RRN is a premotor neuron, its firing pattern must be appropriate for driving a motor neuron, such as one in the phrenic nerve nucleus.

INTRINSIC MEMBRANE PROPERTIES. Many neurons in respiratory nuclei have intrinsic membrane properties that influence the types of firing patterns they are able to produce. For example, many DRG neurons have a large K^+ current called a **transient A-type current** (p. 194). If we first hyperpolarize and then depolarize such a neuron, it responds with a **delayed activation**; that is, it begins firing action potentials, but only after a delay. The hyperpolarization removes the inactivation of the A-type current, and the subsequent depolarization transiently activates the A-type current. Because the A-type current is a K^+ current, it transiently slows depolarization of the membrane and inhibits generation of action potentials

(see Fig. 7–18C). If the A-type current is large, the neuron cannot begin to fire until after the A-type current sufficiently inactivates (see Fig. 7–18D). The delay in firing of a neuron with A-type current mimics the pattern of activity of the late-onset inspiratory activity we have already seen in Figure 31–5G. This neuron receives EPSPs continuously during inspiration. However, it fires action potentials only late in the inspiration phase. The presence of A-type current could provide a mechanism for this delay and would eliminate the need for synaptic input (i.e., the EPSPs) to be rigidly patterned.

A second type of neuron in the DRG has a large amount of **Ca^{2+}-activated K^+ current** (p. 194). After the neuron fires several action potentials, the accumulation of Ca^{2+} inside the cell slowly activates this K_{Ca} channel, hyperpolarizing the cell and limiting the firing rate. Thus, suddenly depolarizing such a neuron triggers a burst of firing that tapers off as K_{Ca} channels activate. The decrease in firing rate, called "spike-frequency adaptation," mimics the early-burst activity of some RRNs (see Fig. 31–5E). Like the A-type current, K_{Ca} channels could cause these neurons to have an appropriate firing pattern, even in the absence of rigidly patterned synaptic input.

PATTERNED SYNAPTIC INPUT. Independent of intrinsic membrane properties, the patterned synaptic input that many RRNs receive from other respiratory neurons can also influence the firing pattern. For example, the early-burst activity of the neuron in Figure 31–5E parallels the strong excitatory synaptic input that the neuron receives during the early part of inspiration, as well as the inhibitory synaptic input that it receives during expiration.

Some firing patterns of RRNs result in part from inhibitory connections between neurons. For example, the early-burst inspiratory neurons in the preceding paragraph appear to inhibit late-onset inspiratory neurons, and vice versa (Fig. 31–6). As a result of this reciprocal inhibition, only one of the two subtypes of inspiratory neurons can be maximally active at any one time.

In addition to patterned synaptic input from RRNs, respiratory neurons also receive input from other neuronal systems, allowing the respiratory system to respond appropriately to challenges and to be integrated with many different brain functions. Some of the neurotransmitters released onto respiratory neurons—both by RRNs and by neurons from other regions of the CNS—are listed in Table 31–3.

In summary, both intrinsic membrane properties and patterned synaptic input can cause RRNs to fire in their characteristic patterns. In theory, either of these properties might be sufficient to ensure that these neurons have the right firing pattern. The presence of both properties illustrates a general concept that appears to be important in critical biologic systems: redundancy. For those body systems critical for life support, use of multiple mechanisms may ensure that normal functioning will occur despite severe perturbations.

Intrinsic Membrane Properties and Synaptic Interactions May Also Contribute to Generation of the Respiratory Rhythm

INTRINSIC MEMBRANE PROPERTIES. The simplest pattern generators are single cells whose membrane properties

TABLE 31–3

NEUROTRANSMITTERS RELEASED ONTO RESPIRATORY NEURONS

Glutamate

GABA (gamma aminobutyric acid)

Serotonin (5-HT, 5-hydroxytryptamine)

Norepinephrine

Dopamine

Acetylcholine

Thyrotropin-releasing hormone (TRH)

Substance P

Corticotropin-releasing hormone (CRH)

Endorphins

Enkephalins

endow them with pacemaker properties (p. 367). For example, isolated cardiac myocytes produce rhythmic activity via "pacemaker currents" (p. 489). Unlike heart cells, which generate a single spike for each cardiac cycle, some pacemaker neurons can spontaneously generate rhythmic bursts of spikes during each cycle of activity (i.e., bursting pacemaker activity).

The first evidence for pacemaker activity in a mammalian respiratory nucleus was obtained in the laboratory of Peter Getting. In brain slices from the guinea pig, putative premotor respiratory neurons in the NTS fire erratically at a low rate, with no apparent respiratory rhythm. However, adding thyrotropin-releasing hormone (TRH; p. 1044) to the bathing medium causes these neurons to generate bursts of action potentials (Fig. 31–7A), similar to inspiratory bursts in RRNs of the DRG during eupnea (see Fig. 31–7B). In the NTS, TRH is present in synaptic terminals of axons that come from the medullary raphe nuclei (p. 301). Thus, when raphe neurons increase their firing rate, the release of TRH would be expected to induce bursting pacemaker activity in NTS neurons. This pacemaker activity might either contribute to generation of the respiratory rhythm or augment respiratory output generated within another site. Pacemaker activity is also present in neurons within another respiratory nucleus—the pre-Bötzinger complex (see later).

SYNAPTIC INPUTS. Neural circuits *without* pacemaker neurons also can generate rhythmic output (p. 367). Indeed, synaptic connections within and between the DRG and VRG establish neural circuits and generate EPSPs and IPSPs with a timing that could explain the neurons' oscillatory behavior during the respiratory cycle (see Fig. 31–6). Computational neurobiologists have proposed a variety of pure **network models** of respiratory rhythm generation. According to these models, the CPG that produces the respiratory rhythm depends solely on synaptic connections between subtypes of RRNs, and not at all on the pacemaker activity of individual neurons. Thus, the rhythm would be an *emergent property* of the network.

FIGURE 31–7. Pacemaker activity in respiratory-related neurons. (*A*, data from Dekin MS, Richerson GB, Getting PA: Thyrotropin-releasing hormone induces rhythmic bursting in neurons of the nucleus tractus solitarius. Science 229:67, 1985; *B*, data from Richerson GB, Getting PA: Maintenance of complex neural function during perfusion of the mammalian brain. Brain Res 409:128, 1987.) DRG, dorsal respiratory group; ENG, electroneurogram; TRH, thyrotropin-releasing hormone.

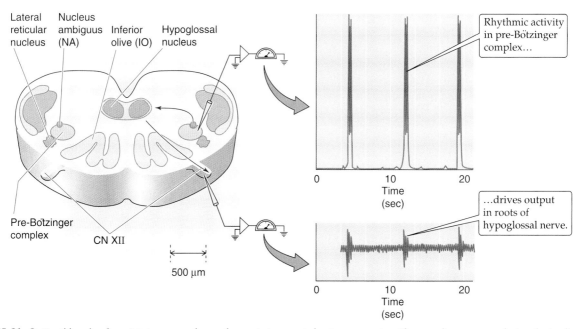

FIGURE 31–8. Possible role of pre-Bötzinger complex as the respiratory central-pattern generator. The recordings were made in a brain slice. (Data from Smith JC, Ellenberger HH, Ballanyi K, et al: Pre-Bötzinger complex: A brainstem region that may generate respiratory rhythm in mammals. Science 254:726, 1991.)

One of the difficulties with network models is that the exact identity of each of the components of the model is not certain. Many of these network models do not take into account the presence of the rich complement of intrinsic membrane properties that exist in the component neurons. As a result, *pure* network models have become increasingly complex in order to explain all aspects of the normal respiratory rhythm. Including intrinsic membrane properties (e.g., pacemaker activity) in network models allows them to be simpler. Moreover, from an evolutionary perspective, it is reasonable to infer that pacemaker cells may have driven primitive respiratory systems (e.g., gills).

The Respiratory Central Pattern Generator for Eupnea Could Be in a Single Restricted Site or Distributed Among Several Sites, or It Could Be an Emergent Property of the Respiratory Network

Where is the respiratory CPG? In 1851, Flourens proposed a *noeud vital* ("vital node") in the medulla, a small region that is the sole site producing respiratory output. In 1909, the neuroanatomist Santiago Ramon y Cajal reported that neurons in the NTS receive afferents from pulmonary stretch receptors, and that NTS neurons project directly to the phrenic motor nucleus. He concluded that the NTS was the site of respiratory rhythm generation. This simple proposal was never proved, and—in spite of considerable progress—the questions of where in the medulla the CPG is located and how the rhythm is generated remain unanswered. Here we discuss three major proposals for the location of the CPG that generates the eupneic respiratory rhythm.

RESTRICTED SITE MODEL. Suzue first introduced the in vitro brainstem/spinal-cord preparation from the neonatal rat, and Jeffrey Smith and Jack Feldman further developed this preparation to study the generation of respiratory output. In this preparation, a small region in the rostral VRG—the **pre-Bötzinger complex**—generates rhythmic motor output in the phrenic nerve and hypoglossal nerve (CN XII, which innervates the tongue, an accessory muscle of inspiration). Destroying the pre-Bötzinger complex in the isolated brain stem causes respiratory output to cease. When the preparation is limited to a brain slice (Fig. 31–8) containing the pre-Bötzinger complex, a piece of the hypoglossal nucleus, and some rootlets of the hypoglossal nerve, the pre-Bötzinger complex generates rhythmic bursts of activity that one can record from the hypoglossal nerve rootlets. The role this region plays in generating eupnea in adult mammals has not yet been proved. However, these and other experiments are consistent with the hypothesis that the pre-Bötzinger complex is the sole site of the respiratory CPG.

DISTRIBUTED OSCILLATOR MODEL. Another possibility is that there is more than one CPG, any one of which could take over the job of generating the respiratory rhythm, depending on the conditions. As was already discussed, TRH can induce bursting pacemaker activity in DRG neurons, suggesting that they could contribute to the generation of rhythmic activity. One interpretation of these results is that various groups of respiratory neurons are *latent* CPGs and that the *dominant* CPG for eupnea is not always in the same place. The location of the dominant

CPG could shift during different behaviors, and a particular respiratory neuron could transiently become a part of the respiratory CPG. A second interpretation is that the presence of rhythmicity in many different respiratory neurons represents a redundancy, ensuring that respiratory output does not fail. This design would be analogous to initiation of the heartbeat, in which many cells within the sinoatrial node can be the first to fire, and cells in other parts of the heart can take over if the sinoatrial node is damaged (p. 489). In this model, some respiratory neurons with intrinsic oscillatory behavior would contribute to rhythm generation only under unusual conditions (e.g., hypoxia, anesthesia, early in development); under these conditions, the neurons might generate abnormal or pathologic respiratory output (e.g., gasping). A third interpretation is that only one CPG exists for eupnea, and that other respiratory neurons with pacemaker activity augment the output of the CPG, making it more robust.

EMERGENT PROPERTY MODEL. The most common early explanation for generation of the respiratory rhythm (e.g., that proposed by Lumsden) is that no individual region of the DRG or VRG is *sufficient* to generate the rhythm, but that many of them are *necessary*. A normal rhythm would require the component neurons in multiple brainstem regions to be "wired up" in a specific way.

None of the previously mentioned theories is universally accepted, and some of their elements are not mutually exclusive. The challenges in proving any of these hypotheses include the complexity of the CNS even at the level of the medulla, the technical difficulty in studying neurons of the mammalian brain stem, and the large number of nonrespiratory neurons in the medulla. Yet, because it is primitive both ontogenetically and phylogenetically, the respiratory CPG will probably prove to be far easier to define than most other mammalian neural networks, such as those responsible for consciousness or memory.

CHEMICAL CONTROL OF VENTILATION

In fulfilling its mission to exchange O_2 and CO_2 between the atmosphere and the capillaries of the systemic circulation, the respiratory system attempts to regulate the blood-gas parameters, that is, the arterial levels of O_2, CO_2, and pH. These are overwhelmingly the most important influences on breathing. The body senses these parameters via two sets of chemoreceptors—the peripheral chemoreceptors and the central chemoreceptors. Hypoxia, hypercapnia, and acidosis all cause an increase in ventilation, which tends to raise PO_2, lower PCO_2, and raise pH, thereby correcting deviations in the three blood-gas parameters. Although small variations in arterial PCO_2 and PO_2 occur with activities such as sleep, exercise, talking, and panting, the control of blood gases is so tight in normal individuals that it is rare for arterial PCO_2 to change from the normal 40 mm Hg by more than a few mm Hg. Thus, the peripheral and central chemoreceptors form the vital sensory arm of a negative-feedback mechanism that stabilizes arterial PO_2, PCO_2, and pH.

PERIPHERAL CHEMORECEPTORS

The Peripheral Chemoreceptors—the Carotid and Aortic Bodies—Respond to Hypoxia, Hypercapnia, and Acidosis

The peripheral chemoreceptors are primarily sensitive to decreases in arterial PO_2. Increases in PCO_2 and decreases in pH also stimulate these receptors to a lesser extent but make them more responsive to hypoxia.

SENSITIVITY TO DECREASED ARTERIAL PO₂. Perfusing the carotid body with blood having a low PO_2—but a normal PCO_2 and pH—causes a prompt and reversible increase in the firing rate of axons in the carotid sinus nerve. Figure 31–9A shows a comparable experiment on an isolated chemoreceptor cell of the carotid body. Under normal acid-base conditions, increasing PO_2 above the normal value of approximately 100 mm Hg has only trivial effects on the firing rate of the nerve. However, at normal values of PCO_2 and pH (see Fig. 31–9B, *blue curve*), decreasing PO_2 to values below 100 mm Hg causes a progressive increase in the firing rate.

SENSITIVITY TO INCREASED ARTERIAL PCO₂. The carotid body can sense hypercapnia in the absence of hypoxia or acidosis. It is possible to maintain a constant extracellular pH (pH_o) while increasing PCO_2 by keeping the ratio $[HCO_3^-]/PCO_2$ constant (p. 648). The *maroon curve* in Figure 31–9C shows the results of experiments in which graded increases in PCO_2—at a fixed blood pH of 7.45 and a fixed PO_2 of 80 mm Hg—produced graded increases in the firing rate of the carotid sinus nerve. Thus, hypercapnia per se stimulates the carotid body to increase ventilation.

SENSITIVITY TO DECREASED ARTERIAL pH. The carotid body also senses acidosis in the absence of hypoxia or hypercapnia. The *green curve* in Figure 31–9C shows the results of experiments that are the same as those represented by the *maroon curve*, except that blood pH was fixed at 7.25 rather than at 7.45. Over the entire range of PCO_2 values, the firing rate of the carotid sinus nerve is greater at a pH of 7.25 than at 7.45. Thus, metabolic acidosis (p. 642) stimulates the carotid body.

In summary, besides being sensitive to hypoxia, the carotid body is sensitive to *both* components of respiratory acidosis (p. 640)—high PCO_2 and low pH. In fact, respiratory acidosis makes the carotid body more sensitive to hypoxia (see Fig. 31–9B, *orange curve*), whereas respiratory alkalosis has the opposite effect (see Fig. 31–9B, *red curve*).

The Glomus Cell Is the Chemosensor in the Carotid and Aortic Bodies

The body has two sets of peripheral chemoreceptors—the **carotid bodies**, one located at the bifurcation of each of the common carotid arteries, and the **aortic bodies**, scattered along the underside of the arch of the aorta (Fig. 31–10A). The carotid *bodies* should not be confused with the carotid *sinus* (p. 536), which is the bulbous initial portion of the internal carotid artery that serves as a

A   EFFECT OF ANOXIA ON SINGLE, ISOLATED GLOMUS CELL

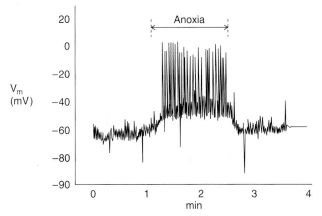

B   EFFECT OF RESPIRATORY ACID-BASE DISTURBANCES
     ON O_2 SENSITIVITY

C   EFFECT OF pH CHANGES ON CO_2 SENSITIVITY

FIGURE 31–9. Chemosensitivity of the carotid body. *A,* Effect of anoxia on a single, isolated glomus cell. Anoxia elicits a depolarization and small action potentials, as measured with a patch pipette. *B,* Effect of respiratory acid-base disturbances on O_2 sensitivity. *C,* Effect of pH changes on CO_2 sensitivity. In *B* and *C,* the y-axis represents the frequency of action potentials in single sensory fibers from the carotid body. (*A,* data from Buckler KJ, Vaughan-Jones RD: Effects of hypoxia on membrane potential and intracellular calcium in rat neonatal carotid body type I cells. J Physiol 476:423–428, 1994; *B,* data from Cunningham DJC, Robbins PA, Wolff CB: Integration of respiratory responses to changes in alveolar partial pressures of CO_2 and O_2 and in arterial pH. In Cherniack NS, Widdicombe J: Handbook of Physiology; Section 3, The Respiratory System. Vol II. American Physiological Society, Bethesda, MD 1986. pp. 475–528; *C,* data from Biscoe TJ, Purves MJ, Sampson SR: The frequency of nerve impulse in single carotid body chemoreceptor afferent fibers recorded in vivo with intact circulation. J Physiol 208:121–131, 1970.)

baroreceptor. Similarly, the aortic *bodies* should not be confused with baroreceptors of the aortic arch.

The major function of the carotid and aortic bodies is to sense hypoxia in the arterial blood, and then to signal cells in the medulla to increase ventilation. This signaling occurs via afferents of the glossopharyngeal nerve (CN IX) for the carotid bodies, and of the vagus nerve (CN X) for the aortic bodies. The carotid bodies have been more extensively studied than the aortic bodies, which are smaller and less accessible. The first description of their function as chemoreceptors was provided by Corneille Heymans, for which he was awarded the 1938 Nobel Prize for Physiology or Medicine.

Aside from their chemosensitivity, three features characterize the carotid bodies. First, they are extremely small: Each weighs only approximately 2 mg. Second, for their size, they receive an extraordinarily high blood flow—the largest of any other tissue in the body. Their blood flow, normalized for weight, is approximately 40-fold higher than that of the brain. Third, they have a very high metabolic rate, two- to threefold greater than that of the brain. Thus, even though the metabolic rate is high, the blood flow is so much higher that the composition of the blood (e.g., P_{O_2}, P_{CO_2}, and pH) in the carotid body capillaries is virtually the same as in the systemic arteries.

The chemosensitive cells of the carotid body are the type I, or **glomus cells**, which are approximately 10 μm in diameter and roughly spherical in shape and occur in clusters (see Fig. 31–10*B*). Adjacent glomus cells may communicate with each other via gap junctions. Embryologically, the glomus cell is neuroectodermal in origin, and shares many characteristics with neurons of the peripheral nervous system, as well as with adrenal chromaffin cells (p. 1061). Indeed, glomus cells have four neuron-like characteristics: First, some are innervated by preganglionic sympathetic neurons. Second, glomus cells have a variety of voltage-gated ion channels. Third, depolarizing the cell triggers action potentials. Fourth, glomus cells have numerous intracellular vesicles containing a variety of neurotransmitters. Stimulating glomus cells causes them to release acetylcholine, dopamine, norepinephrine, substance P, and met-enkephalin. The release of these neurotransmitters controls firing of the nerve endings.

Impinging on glomus cells are *sensory endings* of the carotid sinus nerve (a branch of CN IX). Neurotransmitter release from the glomus cells triggers action potentials in the carotid sinus nerve, which makes its first synapse on neurons of the NTS (part of the DRG), thereby signalling the medulla that the systemic arterial blood has a low P_{O_2}, a high P_{CO_2}, and/or a low pH. Curiously, the sensory endings of the carotid sinus nerve also contain vesicles, so the synapse formed with glomus cells may be bidirectional. The function of this synapse from the carotid sinus nerve onto the glomus cells is unknown.

Surrounding individual clusters of glomus cells are the type II, or **sustentacular cells** (see Fig. 31–10*B*), which are supporting cells similar to glia. Also in close proximity to the glomus cells is a dense network of fenestrated **capillaries**. Therefore, the glomus cells are in an ideal position to monitor arterial blood gases.

Both the sympathetic and parasympathetic divisions of the autonomic nervous system (ANS) innervate the ca-

A LOCATION OF CAROTID AND AORTIC BODIES

B MICROSCOPIC ANATOMY OF CAROTID BODY

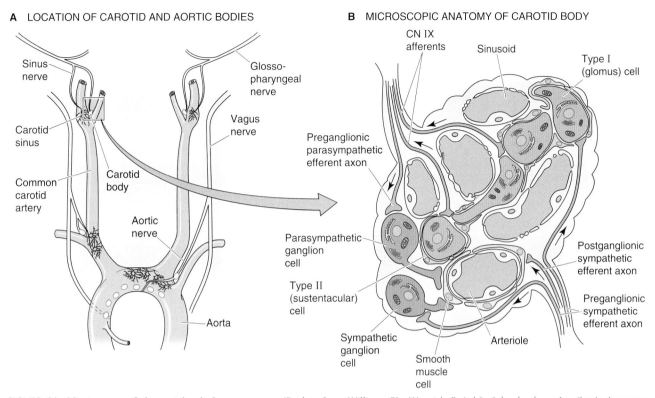

FIGURE 31–10. Anatomy of the peripheral chemoreceptors. (B, data from Williams PL, Warwick R (eds): Splanchnology. In: Gray's Anatomy. Philadelphia, WB Saunders, 1980.)

rotid body. As has already been noted, preganglionic sympathetic neurons synapse on glomus cells, and presumably can alter their function. Autonomic fibers also contact blood vessels; increased sympathetic tone decreases local blood flow. Because the metabolic rate of the carotid body is high, a large decrease in blood flow produces a local fall in PO_2 near the glomus cells, even when systemic arterial PO_2 remains constant. Increased sympathetic tone thus "fools" the carotid body into behaving as if a hypoxic state existed. Hence, by modulating blood flow to the carotid body, the ANS can fine-tune the response of the peripheral chemoreceptors.

The aortic bodies also include scattered glomus cells that presumably have a similar function to those in the carotid bodies. However, there are distinct differences between their responses to stimuli and the effects they have on ventilation. For the purposes of this section, we focus our discussion here on the carotid bodies, about which more is known.

The Common Transduction Pathway for Hypoxia, Hypercapnia, and Acidosis Is Inhibition of K+ Channels, a Rise in Glomus Cell [Ca²⁺]ᵢ, and Release of Neurotransmitters

The sensitivity of the glomus cell to hypoxia, hypercapnia, and acidosis is a special case of chemoreception that we discussed in connection with sensory transduction (p. 326). It is interesting that one cell type—the glomus cell—is able to sense all three blood-gas modalities. The final common pathway for the response to all three stimuli (Fig. 31–11) is an inhibition of K+ channels, depolarization of the glomus cell, possible firing of action potentials, opening of voltage-gated Ca^{2+} channels, an increase in $[Ca^{2+}]_i$, secretion of neurotransmitters, and stimulation of the afferent nerve fiber. What differs among the three pathways is how the stimulus inhibits K+ channels.

HYPOXIA. Investigators have proposed three mechanisms by which low PO_2 might inhibit K+ channels. First, some evidence suggests that the O_2 sensor is a heme-containing protein that, when it loses its O_2, decreases the open probability of closely associated K+ channels. Second, in rabbit glomus cells, hypoxia induces a rise in $[cAMP]_i$, which inhibits a cAMP-sensitive K+ current. Third, other evidence suggests that small decreases in PO_2 inhibit NADPH oxidase in mitochondria of glomus cells, thus increasing the ratio of reduced glutathione (GSH) versus oxidized glutathione (GSSG), which directly inhibits certain K+ channels. There is some controversy—which may reflect species differences—about which K+ channel is the target of hypoxia. Regardless of how hypoxia inhibits K+ channels, the resulting depolarization activates voltage-gated Ca^{2+} channels, as was outlined previously.

HYPERCAPNIA. An increase in PCO_2 causes CO_2 to move into the glomus cell, thereby generating H+ (p. 653) and leading to a virtually instantaneous fall of intracellular pH (pHᵢ). As pHᵢ decreases, the protons appear to inhibit high-conductance K_{Ca} channels by displacing Ca^{2+}

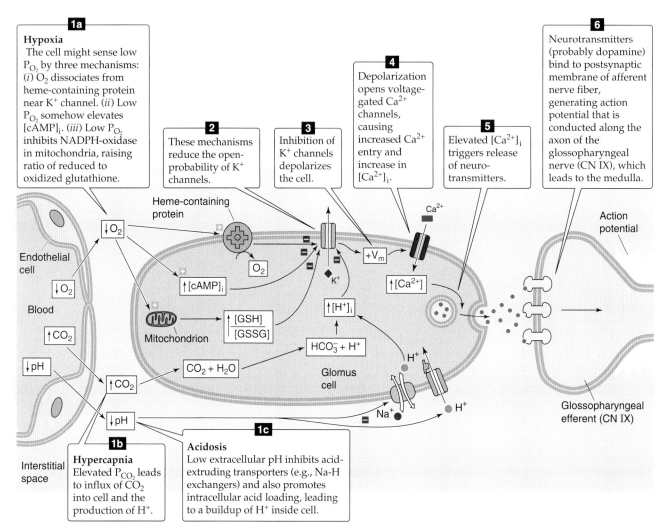

1a
Hypoxia
The cell might sense low P_{O_2} by three mechanisms: (*i*) O_2 dissociates from heme-containing protein near K^+ channel. (*ii*) Low P_{O_2} somehow elevates $[cAMP]_i$. (*iii*) Low P_{O_2} inhibits NADPH-oxidase in mitochondria, raising ratio of reduced to oxidized glutathione.

2
These mechanisms reduce the open-probability of K^+ channels.

3
Inhibition of K^+ channels depolarizes the cell.

4
Depolarization opens voltage-gated Ca^{2+} channels, causing increased Ca^{2+} entry and increase in $[Ca^{2+}]_i$.

5
Elevated $[Ca^{2+}]_i$ triggers release of neuro-transmitters.

6
Neurotransmitters (probably dopamine) bind to postsynaptic membrane of afferent nerve fiber, generating action potential that is conducted along the axon of the glossopharyngeal nerve (CN IX), which leads to the medulla.

1b
Hypercapnia
Elevated P_{CO_2} leads to influx of CO_2 into cell and the production of H^+.

1c
Acidosis
Low extracellular pH inhibits acid-extruding transporters (e.g., Na-H exchangers) and also promotes intracellular acid loading, leading to a buildup of H^+ inside cell.

FIGURE 31–11. Response of glomus cell to hypoxia, hypercapnia, and acidosis. cAMP, cyclic adenosine monophosphate; CN, cranial nerve; GSH, reduced glutathione; GSSG, oxidized glutathione.

from their binding sites. The result is a depolarization, which leads to the release of neurotransmitter.

EXTRACELLULAR ACIDOSIS. A decrease in pH_o inhibits acid-base transporters (e.g., Na-H exchangers) that elevate pH_i, and stimulates acid-base transporters (e.g., Cl-HCO$_3$ exchangers) that lower pH_i, thereby leading to a slow fall in pH_i (p. 653). Thus, extracellular acidosis—at a constant P_{CO_2}—triggers the same cascade of events as was outlined earlier for hypercapnia, albeit more slowly. Thus, metabolic acidosis (i.e., a fall in pH at a fixed P_{CO_2}) and respiratory acidosis (i.e., a fall in pH due to a rise in P_{CO_2}) both stimulate glomus cells via a fall in pH_i.

CENTRAL CHEMORECEPTORS

When the blood-gas parameters are nearly normal, the central chemoreceptors are the primary source of feedback for assessing the effectiveness of ventilation, and also the major source of tonic drive for breathing. Just as the peripheral chemoreceptors are primarily sensitive to arterial hypoxia, the neurons that act as central chemoreceptors are primarily sensitive to arterial *hypercapnia*, which

generally presents itself as respiratory acidosis (i.e., a decrease in pH_o brought about by a rise in P_{CO_2}; p. 640). However, the actual parameter sensed appears to be a low pH in and/or around the chemoreceptor neurons. Although it has long been clear that central chemoreceptors exist, based on experiments on whole animals, it is only recently that physiologists have begun to identify candidate chemoreceptor neurons.

The Blood-Brain Barrier Separates the Central Chemoreceptors in the Medulla from Arterial Blood

In the 1950s, Isidore Leusen—working on dogs with denervated peripheral chemoreceptors—found that perfusing the cerebral ventricles with an acidic solution with a high P_{CO_2} increased ventilation. Because the resultant hyperventilation caused a respiratory *alkalosis* in the blood, the *local acidosis* in the brain must have been responsible for the increased ventilation. From this and later experiments, we now believe that the primary stimu-

A EFFECT OF BREATHING CO₂ ON VENTILATION

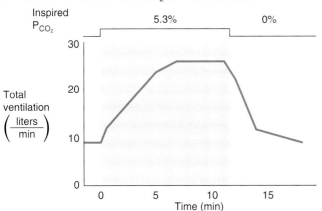

B DEPENDENCE OF CSF pH ON BLOOD pH

C DEPENDENCE OF VENTILATION ON CSF pH

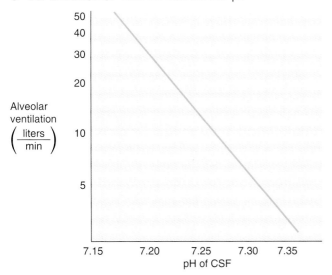

FIGURE 31–12. Effect of arterial hypercapnia on brain pH and ventilation. (*A,* data from Padget P: The respiratory response to carbon dioxide. Am J Physiol 83:384–389, 1928. *B,* data from Fencl V: Acid-base balance in cerebral fluids. In Cherniack NS, Widdicombe J: Handbook of Physiology, Section 3, The Respiratory System. Vol II, Part 1. Bethesda, MD, American Physiological Society, 1986, pp 115–140. *C,* data from Fencl V, Miller TB, Pappenheimer JR: Studies on the respiratory response to disturbances of acid-base balance, with deductions concerning the ionic composition of cerebral interstitial fluid. Am J Physiol 210: 459–472, 1966.)

lus driving respiration during respiratory acidosis is not actually an increase in arterial P_{CO_2}, but probably the ensuing pH decrease within brain tissue. Most evidence indicates that the central chemoreceptors are at a site within the brain parenchyma that responds to changes both in arterial P_{CO_2} and cerebrospinal fluid (CSF) pH.

Starting from normal blood-gas parameters, increasing the arterial P_{CO_2} from 40 to approximately 45 mm Hg (an increase of only ~12.5%) doubles ventilation. By contrast, hypoxia doubles ventilation only if P_{O_2} falls by approximately 50%. If P_{CO_2} increases suddenly, the increase in ventilation begins rapidly, augmenting first the *depth* and later the *frequency* of inspirations. However, the response may take as long as 10 minutes to develop fully (Fig. 31–12*A*). If, instead, the acid-base disturbance in arterial blood is a *metabolic* acidosis (i.e., a decrease in pH_o and $[HCO_3^-]_o$ at a fixed P_{CO_2}; p. 642) of comparable magnitude, ventilation increases much more slowly and the steady-state increase is substantially less.

The reason for these observations is that the central chemoreceptors are located within the brain parenchyma and are bathed in **brain extracellular fluid** (BECF), which is separated from arterial blood by the **blood-brain barrier** (BBB). The BBB has a high permeability to small, neutral molecules such as O_2 and CO_2, but a low permeability to ions such as Na^+, Cl^-, H^+, and HCO_3^- (p. 410). Because CO_2 is freely diffusible across most cell membranes, an increase in arterial P_{CO_2} rapidly leads to a P_{CO_2} increase of similar magnitude in the BECF, in the CSF, and inside brain cells. The result is an acidosis in each of these compartments. In fact, because the protein concentration of CSF or BECF is lower than that of blood plasma (see Table 16–1), the non-HCO_3^- buffering power (p. 635) of CSF and BECF is also substantially less. Thus, at least initially, raising P_{CO_2} produces a larger signal (i.e., pH decrease) in the CSF and BECF than in the blood.

Although raising arterial P_{CO_2} causes the pH of the BECF and CSF to fall rapidly, the choroid plexus (p. 404) and perhaps the BBB partially restore the pH of these compartments by actively transporting HCO_3^- from the blood into the CSF. Thus, after many hours or days of respiratory acidosis in the arterial blood, the low-pH signal in the BECF and CSF gradually becomes attenuated. Even so, respiratory acid-base disturbances lead to substantial changes in the steady-state pH of the BECF and CSF (see Fig. 31–12*B*).

In contrast to its permeability to CO_2, the BBB is much less permeable to ions such as H^+ and HCO_3^-. In addition, because the BBB actively regulates the pH of the BECF and CSF, when blood pH changes during *metabolic* acid-base disturbances, brain pH in the new steady state changes only 10% to 35% as much as during *respiratory* acid-base disturbances (see Fig. 31–12*B*). Therefore, changes in arterial $[H^+]$ and $[HCO_3^-]$ have less effect on the pH of the BECF; as a result, ventilation is much less sensitive to changes in arterial pH and $[HCO_3^-]$ at constant arterial P_{CO_2}. Ventilation correlates uniquely with the pH of the BECF (see Fig. 31–12*C*), regardless of whether respiratory or metabolic acid-base disturbances produce the pH changes in the BECF.

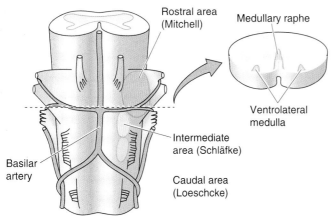

A CHEMOSENSITIVE REGIONS

B NEURONS STIMULATED BY ACIDOSIS

5% CO_2

9% CO_2

C NEURONS INHIBITED BY ACIDOSIS

3% CO_2

9% CO_2

FIGURE 31–13. Chemosensitive neurons in the ventrolateral medulla and raphe. Illustrated in *A* is a ventral view of a cat medulla showing chemosensitive areas named after the three physiologists that first described them. The slice to the right shows the location of serotonergic neurons in the ventrolateral medulla and medullary raphe nuclei. *B* and *C* are patch-pipette recordings of neurons cultured from the medullary raphe of rats. Those that are stimulated by acidosis are serotonergic, and those that are inhibited do not contain serotonin. (*A*, data from Dermietzel R: Central chemosensitivity, morphological studies. In: Loeschke HL, ed. Acid-base Homeostasis of the Brain Extracellular Fluid and the Respiratory Control System. Stuttgart: Thieme Edition/Publishing Sciences Group, pp. 52–66, 1976. *B* and *C*, data from Wang W, Pizzonia JH, Richerson GB: Chemosensitivity of rat medullary raphe neurones in primary tissues culture. J of Physiol 511:433–450, 1998.)

Central Chemoreceptors Are Located in the Ventrolateral Medulla and Other Brainstem Nuclei/Areas

Early work on the central chemoreceptor by Hans Loeschke, Marianne Schläfke, and Robert Mitchell identified candidate regions near the surface of the ventrolateral medulla (VLM; Fig. 31–13A). Applying acidic solutions to the rostral or caudal VLM leads to a prompt increase in ventilation. Moreover, focally cooling these areas to 20° C to reversibly inhibit neurons—or placing lesions to permanently destroy the neurons—blunts the ventilatory response to respiratory acidosis. This and other work led to the conclusion that the central chemoreceptors are located near the surface of the VLM. However, this inference has been controversial because many superficial arteries that penetrate the VLM surface could carry low-pH solutions to deeper nuclei. Moreover, the cooling and the lesions could likewise affect deeper regions of the medulla.

More recent studies on brain slices and cultured cells show that acidosis stimulates neurons in many brainstem nuclei. These include the ventrolateral medulla noted earlier, the medullary raphe (see Fig. 31–13A, inset), the nucleus ambiguus, and the nucleus tractus solitarius—all in the medulla—as well as the locus caeruleus and hypothalamus. Experiments in the laboratory of Eugene Nattie suggest that focal acidosis within many of these areas stimulates breathing in intact animals. At least some of these acidosis-stimulated neurons are probably respiratory chemoreceptors.

It is not clear whether all of these chemosensitive areas play a role in the control of ventilation. If they do, multiple sensors may be another example of redundancy in a critical system. Some may come into play only under special circumstances, such as during severe acid-base disturbances; others may be responsible for arousal from sleep only when airways are obstructed.

Many Neurons of the Medullary Raphe and Ventrolateral Medulla Are Unusually Sensitive to Low pH

Medullary raphe neurons are good candidates for central chemoreceptors because they are unusually pH sensitive. In brain slices and in tissue culture, a small decrease in pH increases the firing rate of one subset of medullary raphe neurons (see Fig. 31–13B) and decreases the firing rate of another (see Fig. 31–13C). In both types of chemosensitive raphe neurons, metabolic and respiratory disturbances have similar effects on firing, indicating that the primary stimulus is a decrease in either extracellular or intracellular pH, rather than an increase in PCO_2. Both types or raphe neurons may be chemoreceptors, acting in opposite ways to control respiratory output. For example, when arterial PCO_2 rises, acidosis-stimulated neurons may stimulate breathing as an accelerator does on a car, whereas acidosis-inhibited neurons may decrease the inhibition of breathing, as when one is letting off on the brake.

The two types of chemosensitive neurons have other distinguishing properties, including different shapes, basal firing patterns, and neurotransmitter content. For example, the neurons stimulated by acidosis contain the neurotransmitter serotonin, whereas those that are inhibited by acidosis do not. Neurons that contain serotonin are also present in the ventrolateral medulla. Serotonergic neurons in both the medullary raphe and ventrolateral medulla project throughout the brain stem and are the major source of serotonin to brainstem respiratory nuclei.

The medullary raphe is located very close to the basilar artery, the major artery to the brain stem, and is highly perfused by penetrating arteries. Many serotonergic neurons lie in close apposition to blood vessels in this region. This perivascular location would provide an obvious advantage for sensing arterial PCO_2. Thus, serotonergic neurons of the raphe and VLM have many properties that would be expected of central respiratory chemoreceptors.

INTEGRATED RESPONSES TO HYPOXIA, HYPERCAPNIA, AND ACIDOSIS

In real life, it is rare for arterial PO_2 to fall without accompanying changes in PCO_2 and pH. In addition, changes in individual blood-gas parameters may independently affect both the peripheral and the central chemoreceptors. How does the respiratory system as a whole respond to changes in multiple blood-gas parameters?

The Acute Response to Respiratory Acidosis Is Accentuated by Hypoxia

RESPIRATORY ACIDOSIS. When the blood-gas parameters are near normal, the effect of respiratory acidosis (increased PCO_2/decreased pH) on ventilation is greater than the effect of hypoxia. If an animal breathes an air mixture containing CO_2, the resultant respiratory acidosis causes ventilation to increase rapidly. Because both peripheral and central chemoreceptors respond to respiratory acidosis, both could contribute to the response. It is possible to isolate the function of the two sets of chemo-

CHRONIC HYPERCAPNIA IN PULMONARY DISEASE

Chronic hypercapnia occurs in many people with lung disease (e.g., emphysema—destruction of alveoli and loss of proper gas exchange) or with muscular weakness (e.g., amyotrophic lateral sclerosis, neuropathies, and myopathies). An increase in PCO_2 leads to an immediate respiratory acidosis in the arterial blood and brain. If CO_2 remains elevated, the pH of the CSF/BECF then slowly recovers (i.e., increases) over the following 8 to 24 hours. The mechanism of this pH_{CSF} increase is probably an increase in HCO_3^- flux into the CSF/BECF across the choroid plexus and BBB, representing a metabolic compensation to the respiratory acidosis (p. 647). The increased CSF pH shifts the CO_2 response curves in Figure 31–14A to the right because, compared with reference conditions, a higher PCO_2 is needed to produce a given degree of CSF acidity (i.e., ventilatory drive). Such a resetting of the central chemoreceptors may be important clinically. Many pulmonary patients, for one reason or another, chronically retain CO_2. Even though PCO_2 may be quite high, adaptation of the CSF/BECF restores pH_{CSF} toward normal. With central chemoreceptor drive for ventilation now decreased, the main drive for ventilation may become hypoxia via peripheral chemoreceptors. Administering supplemental O_2 to such a patient may remove the hypoxic drive as well, such that ventilation decreases and PCO_2 rises to very high levels (e.g., $PCO_2 > 100$ mm Hg). At such high levels, CO_2 acts as a narcotic, depressing respiration. This "CO_2 narcosis" then directly inhibits ventilation and can cause death from hypoventilation—a classic example of "too much of a good thing."

A DEPENDENCE ON P_{CO_2}

B DEPENDENCE ON P_{O_2}

FIGURE 31–14. Integrated ventilatory response to changes in P_{CO_2} (A) and P_{O_2} (B). (A, data from Nielsen M, Smith H: Studies on the regulation of respiration in acute hypoxia. Acta Physiol Scand 24:293–313, 1952. B, data from Loeschcke HH, Gertz KH: Einfluss des O_2-Druckes in der Einatmungsluft auf die Atemtätigkeit der Menschen, geprüft unter Konstanthaltung des alveolaren CO_2-Druckes. Pflugers Arch Ges Physiol 267:460–477, 1958.)

receptors by (1) denervating the peripheral chemoreceptors to study the response of the central chemoreceptors alone, or (2) perfusing the carotid bodies to study the response of the peripheral chemoreceptors alone. Based on approaches such as these, it appears that the central chemoreceptors account for 80% to 90% of the integrated response to respiratory acidosis. However, the response of the peripheral chemoreceptors is considerably more rapid than that of the central chemoreceptors, which require several minutes to develop a full-blown response.

At an alveolar P_{O_2} that is somewhat higher than normal, increasing the alveolar P_{CO_2} causes a linear increase in steady-state ventilation (Fig. 31–14A, *lower right curve*). Lowering the alveolar P_{O_2} has two effects (see Fig. 31–14A, *other two curves*). First, at a given P_{CO_2}, hypoxia increases ventilation, reflecting the response of the peripheral chemoreceptors to hypoxia. Second, hypoxia increases the *sensitivity* of the integrated response to respiratory acidosis. That is, the slopes of the curves increase as P_{O_2} decreases. At least part of the explanation for this increase in slopes is that the peripheral chemoreceptor itself—as judged by the activity of the carotid sinus nerve—becomes more sensitive to respiratory acidosis with coexisting hypoxia.

METABOLIC ACIDOSIS. Severe metabolic acidosis (e.g., diabetic ketoacidosis) leads to profound hyperventilation, known as **Kussmaul breathing**. This hyperventilation can drive arterial P_{CO_2} down to low levels, in an attempt to compensate for the metabolic acidosis. Acutely, the main stimulus for hyperventilation comes from the peripheral chemoreceptors. Because a severe decrease in arterial pH

does produce a small fall in CSF pH, the central chemoreceptors are also involved in this response. If the insult persists for many hours or days, CSF pH falls even farther, such that the central chemoreceptor drive becomes more prominent.

The Acute Response to Hypoxia Is Accentuated by Respiratory Acidosis

If an animal breathes an O_2-free air mixture, the resulting hypoxia causes ventilation to increase rapidly. As was already discussed, the peripheral chemoreceptors respond primarily to hypoxia. To what extent do central mechanisms contribute to the integrated response to acute hypoxia? In an animal with denervated peripheral chemoreceptors, hypoxia actually *depresses* respiratory output. Thus, the integrated response actually underestimates the stimulatory contribution of the peripheral chemoreceptors.

At an arterial P_{CO_2} that is slightly lower than normal, lowering alveolar P_{O_2} has very little effect on ventilation until P_{O_2} falls below 50 mm Hg (see Fig. 31–14B, *bottom curve*). The eventual response at very low P_{O_2} values indicates that the peripheral chemoreceptors play a vital, fail-safe role in responding to extreme hypoxia, as at high altitudes (p. 1263). Increasing the arterial P_{CO_2} (i.e., respiratory acidosis) has two effects (see Fig. 31–14B, *other two curves*). First, at any given P_{O_2}, respiratory acidosis increases ventilation, reflecting the dual contributions of the peripheral and central chemoreceptors to hypercapnia and acidosis. Second, respiratory acidosis increases the *sensitivity* of the integrated response to hypoxia. That

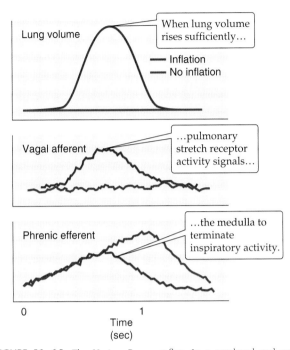

Lung volume

When lung volume rises sufficiently...

— Inflation
— No inflation

Vagal afferent

...pulmonary stretch receptor activity signals...

Phrenic efferent

...the medulla to terminate inspiratory activity.

0   1
Time
(sec)

FIGURE 31–15. The Hering–Breuer reflex. In a paralyzed and artificially ventilated animal, preventing lung inflation during inspiratory activity (*blue curves*) leads to prolonged phrenic nerve output (i.e., if the animal were not paralyzed, then tidal volume would be large). Inflating the lungs during inspiratory activity (*red curves*) produces feedback that shortens the duration of inspiratory activity (i.e., if the animal were not paralyzed, then the tidal volume would be smaller) and also causes the next breath to occur earlier (respiratory frequency would increase). (Data from von Euler C: Brain stem mechanisms for generation and control of breathing pattern. In Cherniack NS, Widdicombe J: Handbook of Physiology, Section 3, The Respiratory System. Vol II, Part 1. Bethesda, MD, American Physiological Society, 1986, pp. 1–67.)

is, the steepness of the curves gradually increase as P_{CO_2} increases. These effects on the integrated response (see Fig. 31–14B) are very similar to—although more exaggerated than—the effects of respiratory acidosis on the response of the peripheral chemoreceptor to hypoxia (see Fig. 31–9B).

MODULATION OF RESPIRATORY OUTPUT

The major parameters that feed back on the respiratory control system are the classical blood gases—P_{O_2}, P_{CO_2}, and pH. In addition to these, the respiratory system receives input from two other major sources: (1) a variety of stretch and chemical/irritant receptors that monitor the size of the airways and the presence of noxious agents, and (2) higher CNS centers that modulate respiratory activity for the sake of nonrespiratory activities.

Stretch and Chemical/Irritant Receptors in the Airways and Lung Parenchyma Provide Feedback About Lung Volume As Well As the Presence of Irritants

Sensors within the lungs and upper airways detect the presence of foreign bodies, chemical irritants, or immunologic challenges, and help to protect the lungs—one of the few

organs that has direct access to the outside world. Sensors also detect changes in lung volume to help control output to the respiratory muscles. Respiratory afferent fibers from the thorax travel with CN X, and those from the upper airways travel with CN IX. Both synapse within the dorsal respiratory group of neurons in the medulla (p. 718).

SLOWLY ADAPTING PULMONARY STRETCH RECEPTORS (PSRs). Within the tracheobronchial tree are mechanoreceptors that detect changes in lung volume by sensing stretch of the airway walls. One type of PSR—the slowly adapting PSR—responds to stretch with an increase in firing that then decays very slowly over time. One of their functions may be to inform the brain about lung volume to optimize respiratory output.

A classic example of a reflex that involves slowly adapting PSRs is the **Hering-Breuer reflex**, one of the first examples in physiology of negative feedback. In 1868, Hering and Breuer found that lung inflation inhibits the output of phrenic motor neurons (Fig. 31–15), thereby protecting the lungs from overinflation. Because the reflex also increases respiratory frequency, it maintains a constant alveolar ventilation. This reflex may be important in controlling tidal volume during eupnea in human infants. In adults, this reflex does not occur until lung volume is greater than during a normal inspiration. However, the sensor may provide feedback that the medulla uses to choose a combination of tidal volume and respiratory frequency to minimize the work of breathing.

RAPIDLY ADAPTING PULMONARY STRETCH (IRRITANT) RECEPTORS. A second type of PSR responds to a sudden, maintained inflation with a rapid increase in firing rate, which then decreases within 1 second to 20% or less of the initial rate. Unlike slowly adapting PSRs, rapidly adapting PSRs are very sensitive to a variety of chemical stimuli, hence the term **irritant receptors**. These agents include serotonin, prostaglandins, bradykinin, ammonia, cigarette smoke, and ether. An important function of these receptors may be to detect pathophysiological processes in the airway, such as chemical irritation, congestion, and inflammation. These receptors also detect histamine, which produces bronchoconstriction in asthma.

C-FIBER RECEPTORS. A rich network of small, unmyelinated axons (C fibers) innervate receptors in the alveoli (**juxtacapillary** or **J receptors**) and conducting airways. Like the slowly adapting PSRs, which are innervated by myelinated fibers, these C-fiber receptors respond to both chemical and mechanical stimuli. Stimulation of C-fiber receptors elicits a triad of rapid, shallow breathing, bronchoconstriction, and increased secretion of mucus into airways, all of which may be defense mechanisms. Bronchoconstriction and rapid, shallow breathing would enhance turbulence (p. 622), favoring the deposition of foreign substances in mucus higher up in the bronchial tree, where mucus-secreting cells are located.

Higher Brain Centers Coordinate Ventilation with Other Behaviors, and Can Override the Brain Stem's Control of Breathing

The role of the CNS in controlling ventilation is far more complex than generating a regular pattern of inspirations

SIGHS, YAWNS, COUGHS, AND SNEEZES

The respiratory apparatus engages in a variety of motor behaviors that help maintain normal lung function and gas exchange by protecting the alveoli from collapse or preventing obstruction of the upper airways.

Sigh, or "augmented breath." A sigh is a slow and deep inspiration, held for just a moment, followed by a longer-than-normal expiratory period (see Fig. 31–3A). A normal person sighs approximately 6 times per hour. Local collapse of alveoli (atelectasis) may initiate a sigh, which is an important mechanism for stimulating release of surfactant (p. 619) and thus reopening these alveoli. Hypoxia and respiratory acidosis increase the number of sighs per hour, consistent with the idea that sighs counteract decreased alveolar ventilation.

Yawn. A yawn is an exaggerated sigh that takes lung volume to total lung capacity for several seconds. The mouth is fully open. In the extreme case, the arms are stretched upward, the neck is extended to elevate the pectoral girdle, and the back is extended—maneuvers that maximize lung volume (p. 612). Yawning is even more effective than sighing in opening up the most resistant atelectatic alveoli. Everyone knows that yawns are contagious. Surprisingly little research has been done on this phenomenon, but there is some evidence that this is actually true. It is possible that yawns serve both to minimize atelectasis as one prepares for a long period of sleep or anticipates sleep (as during a boring cell biology lecture), and to reverse—on arousal—the atelectasis that has accumulated during sleep.

Cough reflex. A cough plays an important role in ridding the tracheobronchial tree of inhaled foreign substances. There is probably no single class of "cough receptors." Mechanosensitive and irritant receptors in the larynx can trigger either coughing or apnea. The tickling sensation that is relieved by a cough is analogous to the cutaneous itch, and is probably mediated by C-fiber receptors. Thus, a cough is a respiratory scratch.

When *lower airway* receptors trigger a cough, it begins with a small inspiration that increases the coughing force

When *laryngeal* receptors trigger the cough, the inspiration is absent, minimizing the chances that the offending foreign body will be forced lower into the lungs. A forced expiratory effort against a closed glottis raises intrathoracic and intra-abdominal pressures to very high levels. The glottis then opens suddenly, and the pressure inside the larynx falls almost instantaneously to near-atmospheric levels. This sudden drop in pressure produces dramatic increases in both the *axial* (alveolus to trachea) pressure gradient that drives air flow (p. 621) and the *radial* (across the tracheal wall) pressure gradient that influences airway diameter (p. 630). This radial gradient translates to a tremendous collapsing pressure on the trachea, which is especially effective on the membranous (i.e., noncartilaginous) part of the trachea, causing the tracheal cross-sectional area to fall to as little as 1/6 of its original value. The net effect is a brief but violent rush of air out of the trachea at velocities near 800 km/hr, or approximately 65% of the speed of sound, which loosens mucus or foreign bodies and moves them upward. Protracted bouts of severe coughing can lead to syncope (lightheadedness) due to a fall in cardiac output because the high intrathoracic pressure decreases venous return (p. 550).

Sneeze. Sensors in the nose detect irritants and can evoke a sneeze. Curiously, these same receptors are probably also responsible for apnea in response to water applied to the face or nose, which is part of the **diving reflex** that evolved in diving mammals such as the seal to prevent aspiration during submersion. A sneeze differs from a cough in that a sneeze is almost always preceded by a deep inspiration. Like a cough, a sneeze involves an initial buildup of intrathoracic pressure behind a closed glottis. Unlike a cough, a sneeze involves pharyngeal constriction during the buildup phase, and an explosive forced expiration via the nose, as well as the mouth. This expiration is accompanied by contraction of facial and nasal muscles, so that the effect is to dislodge foreign bodies from the nasal mucosa.

and expirations, and then modifying this pattern in response to input from mechanical and chemical sensors. The CNS also must balance the need to control PO_2, PCO_2, and pH, with the need to control ventilation for nonrespiratory purposes, such as speaking, sniffing, and regulating temperature (e.g., panting in dogs). In addition, the CNS must coordinate breathing with behaviors that require the *absence* of airflow, such as chewing, swallowing, and vomiting.

Many nonrespiratory regions of the CNS tonically stimulate or inhibit respiration. For example, the **reticular activating system** in the brain stem is one of the sources of tonic drive to the respiratory CPG. An increase in this drive is seen during arousal from sleep, when a *general alerting reaction* increases ventilation and heart rate and activates the electroencephalogram.

COORDINATION OF VOLUNTARY BEHAVIORS THAT USE THE RESPIRATORY MUSCLES. Numerous voluntary actions

initiated in the cerebral cortex involve a change in airflow—voluntarily hyperventilating, breath-holding, speaking, singing, whistling, and playing musical wind instruments. Although voluntary control over muscles of respiration can be exquisitely precise, this control is not absolute. For example, voluntary breath-holding can last only so long before it is overwhelmed by ventilatory drive from chemoreceptors. Control of the respiratory system by the cerebral cortex is achieved by at least two major mechanisms. First, some cortical neurons send axons to the respiratory centers in the medulla. Second, some cortical premotor neurons send axons to motor neurons that control muscles of respiration. One consequence of this dual control mechanism is that lesions in specific areas of the cerebral cortex can cause the inability to voluntarily hold the breath, a condition known as **respiratory apraxia.** Another consequence is that small CNS lesions may specifically knock out one set of connections. For example, patients with intractable pain are sometimes treated with partial transection of the upper cervical ven-

ONDINE'S CURSE, SLEEP, AND SLEEP APNEA

Ondine's curse. Ondine was a water nymph in a German legend immortalized in the fairy tale by Friedrich Heinrich Karl, Baron de la Motte-Fouqué, in 1811. In the play *Ondine* by Jean Giraudoux in 1939, Ondine married a mortal man, Hans, with the understanding that he would never marry a mortal woman. However, when Ondine later returned to the sea, her husband did remarry. Ondine's father punished Hans by requiring him to make a continuous conscious effort to maintain lung ventilation (and all other automatic bodily functions). If he fell asleep, he would stop breathing and die. Hans explained to Ondine how hard it is to live with his curse: "One moment of inattention and I shall forget to hear, to breathe. They will say he died because breathing bored him." Rare patients have been identified who have the same disorder—minus the relationship with a water nymph. These patients can be treated with a ventilator when they sleep, and can maintain normal ventilation on their own while awake.

Sleep. Sleep, or even closing ones eyes, has powerful effects on the breathing pattern and CO_2 responsiveness. During non–rapid eye movement (NREM) sleep, there is an increase in the regularity of eupneic breathing; also, the sensitivity of the respiratory system to CO_2 decreases compared with wakefulness, and the outflow to the muscles of the pharynx decreases. During rapid eye movement (REM) sleep, there is a further decrease in the sensitivity of the respiratory system to CO_2, but now the pattern of breathing becomes markedly irregular, sometimes with no discernible rhythm. The result is that CO_2 levels often increase during NREM sleep, and usually even more so during REM sleep. **Barbiturates** at low doses depress drive to the respiratory system and, if superimposed on normal sleep, can halt ventilation altogether.

Sleep apnea. The collection of disorders in which ventilation ceases during deeper stages of sleep, particularly during REM sleep, is known as sleep apnea. Some cases of sleep apnea are related to Ondine's curse and are due to a lack of central drive (central sleep apnea). However, most cases are due to collapse of the airway with sleep (obstructive sleep apnea), usually in obese people. The airway collapse is due to an exaggeration of the normal decrease in airway tone during sleep, superimposed on the structural problem of reduced airway diameter due to obesity.

ing, sucking, defecating, grunting, and vomiting. During yawning and vomiting, for example, groups of neurons orchestrate an array of simultaneous actions, only some involving the respiratory system. The premotor neurons that project from medullary respiratory centers to respiratory motor neurons are probably distinct from descending pathways involved in these complex nonventilatory behaviors.

THE LIMBIC SYSTEM AND AFFECTIVE STATES. Fear, horror, rage, and passion can be associated with major and highly characteristic changes in the respiratory pattern. For example, if a child runs in front of a car you are driving, the sudden application of the brakes is almost always accompanied by an equally sudden and rapid inspiration, with mouth open widely, increasing lung volume to nearly total lung capacity. The tendency of prevarications to be associated with changes in the breathing pattern is the basis for one part of the polygraph test used as a **lie detector**. Descending pathways from the limbic structures of the forebrain may mediate these emotional effects on breathing.

BALANCING CONFLICTING DEMANDS OF GAS EXCHANGE AND VARIOUS BEHAVIORS. Ventilation, or lack thereof, is involved in a wide variety of behaviors, many of which have nothing to do with alveolar gas exchange per se. How is it that the brain is able to weigh the need for alveolar gas exchange against these competing demands on the respiratory system? Playing a musical wind instrument is an example in which respiratory and nonrespiratory needs are reconciled. Musicians must make rapid and deep inspirations, followed by slow and prolonged expirations that can lead to considerable breath-to-breath variations in alveolar P_{CO_2}. Nevertheless, these variations balance out, so that professionals can follow a musical score for prolonged periods without significant changes in average alveolar ventilation.

In other cases, conflicting demands are not so easily resolved. In infants, suckling relegates alveolar ventilation to a lower priority, and P_{CO_2} rises. Subjects reading aloud tend to increase their alveolar ventilation by approximately 25%, and P_{CO_2} falls. Thus, during speech, chemical drive is overwhelmed by voluntary behavior. On the other hand, when strenuous exercise increases the need for alveolar ventilation, the CNS permits only brief gasps for speech—the ability of voluntary behavior to subvert body homeostasis can only go so far.

trolateral spinal cord to cut axons carrying pain sensation to the thalamus (spinothalamic tract). When this procedure inadvertently involves respiratory projections within the reticulospinal tract, patients breathe properly while awake but experience respiratory failure while asleep (**Ondine's curse;** see box). The lesion may cut automatic premotor neurons descending to the spinal cord from respiratory centers in the medulla, but not voluntary ones from the cortex.

COORDINATION OF COMPLEX NONVENTILATORY BEHAVIORS. One of the jobs of the brain is to coordinate complex behaviors such as yawning, chewing, swallow-

REFERENCES

Books and Reviews

Cherniack NS, Longobardo GS: Abnormalities in respiratory rhythm. In Cherniack NS, Widdicombe J: Handbook of Physiology; Section 3, The Respiratory System. Vol II. American Physiological Society, Bethesda, MD, 1986, pp 729–749.

Coleridge HM, Coleridge JCG: Pulmonary reflexes: Neural mechanisms of pulmonary defense. Annu Rev Physiol 56:69–91, 1994.

Feldman JL: Neurophysiology of breathing in mammals. In Bloom FE: Handbook of Physiology; Section 1: The Nervous System Vol IV. American Physiological Society. 1986, pp 463–525.

Peers C, Buckler KJ: Transduction of chemostimuli by the Type I carotid body cell. J Membrane Biol 144:1–9, 1995.

Loeschcke HH: Central chemosensitivity and the reaction theory. J Physiol 332:1–24, 1982.

Richerson GB: Serotonergic neurons as carbon dioxide sensors that maintain pH homeostasis. *Nature Rev Neurosci* 5:449–461, 2004.

Journal Articles

Fencl V, Miller TB, Pappenheimer JR: Studies on the respiratory response to disturbances of acid-base balance, with deductions concerning the ionic composition of cerebral interstitial fluid. Am J Physiol 210:459–472, 1966.

Gray PA, Janczewski WA, Mellen N, et al: Normal breathing requires pre-Bötzinger complex neurokinin-1 receptor-expressing neurons. Nature Neurosci 4(9):1–4, 2001.

Pappenheimer, JR, Fencl V, Heisey SR, Held D: Role of cerebral fluids in control of respiration as studied in unanesthetized goats. Am J Physiol 208:436–450, 1965.

Schläfke ME, See WR, Loeschcke HH: Ventilatory response to alterations of H⁺ ion concentration in small areas of the ventral medullary surface. Resp Physiol 10:198–212, 1970.

Wang W, Zaykin AV, Tiwari JK et al: Acidosis-stimulated neurons of the medullary raphe are serotonergic. J Neurophysiol 85:2224–2235, 2001.

VI

The Urinary System

CHAPTER 32

Organization of the Urinary System

Gerhard Giebisch and Erich Windhager

The kidneys serve three essential functions. First, they function as filters, removing metabolic products and toxins from the blood and excreting them through the urine. Second, they play a key homeostatic role by regulating the body's fluid status, electrolyte balance, and acid–base balance. Third, the kidneys produce hormones that are involved in erythrogenesis, calcium metabolism, and the regulation of blood pressure and blood flow.

FUNCTIONAL ANATOMY OF THE KIDNEY

We begin this discussion with a macroscopic view and progress to the microscopic level as we describe the **nephron**, the functional unit of the kidney that is repeated approximately 1 million times within each kidney.

The Kidneys Are Paired, Retroperitoneal Organs That Comprise a Complex Mixture of Vascular and Epithelial Elements

The human kidneys are paired, bean-shaped structures that lie behind the peritoneum on each side of the vertebral column (Fig. 32–1A). They extend from the twelfth thoracic vertebra to the third lumbar vertebra. The two kidneys together comprise somewhat less than 0.5% of the total body weight; in adult males, each kidney weighs 125 to 170 g, whereas in adult females, each kidney weighs 115 to 155 g.

A fibrous, almost nondistensible capsule covers each kidney (Fig. 32–1B). In the middle of the concave surface is a slit in the capsule that is called the hilus. The **hilus** serves as the port of entry for the renal artery and nerves and as the site of exit for the renal vein, the lymphatics, and the ureter. The hilus opens into a shallow space called the **renal sinus**, which is completely surrounded by renal parenchyma except where it connects with the upper end of the ureter. The renal sinus includes the urine-filled spaces: the **renal pelvis** proper and its extensions, the **major** and the **minor calyces**. Blood vessels and nerves also pass through the sinus. The renal capsule reflects into the sinus at the hilus so that its inner layers line the sinus, and the outer layers anchor to the blood vessels and renal pelvis.

A cut section of the kidney (see Fig. 32–1B) reveals two basic layers, the cortex (granular outer region) and the medulla (darker inner region). The

A URINARY SYSTEM

B KIDNEY

C MAJOR BLOOD VESSELS IN KIDNEY

FIGURE 32–1. Structure of the urinary system.

granularity of the **cortex** is due to the presence of glomeruli, microscopic tufts of capillaries, and a large number of highly convoluted epithelial structures in the form of tubules. The **medulla** lacks glomeruli and consists of a parallel arrangement of tubules and small blood vessels.

The medulla is subdivided into 8 to 18 conically shaped **renal pyramids**, whose bases face the cortical-medullary border; the tip of each pyramid terminates in the renal pelvis. At the tip of each pyramid are perforations, almost invisible to the naked eye, through which urine escapes into the minor calyces of the renal sinus.

The Kidneys Are Unique in Having a Very High Blood Flow and Glomerular Capillaries That Are Bounded by Upstream and Downstream Arterioles

Although the kidneys comprise less than 0.5% of total body weight, they receive approximately 20% of the car-

diac output. This high blood flow provides the blood plasma necessary for forming an ultrafiltrate in the glomeruli. The renal circulation has a unique sequence of vascular elements: a high-resistance arteriole (the afferent arteriole), followed by a high-pressure glomerular capillary network for filtration, followed by a second high-resistance arteriole (the efferent arteriole), which is followed by a low-pressure capillary network that surrounds the renal tubules (peritubular capillaries) and takes up the fluid absorbed by these tubules.

The main features of the renal vascular system are illustrated in Figures 32–1*B* and 32–1*C*. A single **renal artery** enters the hilus and quickly divides into anterior and posterior branches, which give rise to interlobar arteries and then arcuate arteries. The latter skirt the corticomedullary junction, where they branch into ascending interlobular arteries that enter the cortex and give rise to numerous **afferent arterioles**. These give rise to glomerular capillaries that rejoin to form **efferent arterioles**. For nephrons in the *superficial* portion of the cortex, the efferent arterioles are the origin of a dense peritubular capillary network that supplies oxygen and nutrients to the tubules in the cortex. These afferent and efferent arterioles determine the hydrostatic pressure in the interposed glomerular capillaries. The tone of both arterioles is under the control of a rich sympathetic innervation, as well as a wide variety of chemical mediators.

Very small branches of the arcuate artery, or the proximal portion of the interlobular artery, supply a subpopulation of "juxtamedullary" nephrons whose glomeruli are located at the junction of cortex and medulla. The efferent arterioles of these nephrons descend into the renal papillae to form hairpin-shaped vessels called the **vasa recta**, which provide capillary networks for tubules located in the medulla. Some 90% of the blood entering the kidney perfuses superficial glomeruli and cortex; only approximately 10% perfuses juxtamedullary glomeruli and medulla.

Lymph vessels, which drain the interstitial fluid of the cortex and may contain high concentrations of renal hormones such as renin, leave the kidney by following ar-

teries towards the hilus. Lymphatics are absent from the renal medulla, where they would otherwise tend to drain the medulla of its high-osmolality interstitial fluid, which is necessary for producing a concentrated urine.

The Functional Unit of the Kidney Is the Nephron

Each kidney consists of 800,000 to 1,2000,000 nephrons. Each is an independent entity until the point at which its collecting duct merges with the collecting duct(s) from one or more other nephrons.

A nephron consists of a glomerulus and a tubule. The **glomerulus** is a cluster of blood vessels from which the filtrate forms. The **tubule** is an epithelial structure consisting of many subdivisions, designed to convert the blood filtrate into urine. These two entities—vascular and epithelial—meet at a structure called **Bowman's capsule**, which surrounds the glomerulus and contains Bowman's space, which is contiguous with the lumen of the tubule. It is here that filtrate passes from the vascular system into the tubule system.

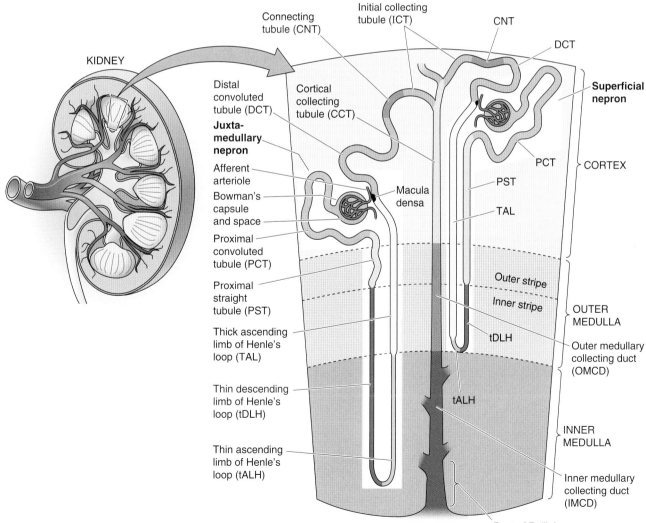

FIGURE 32–2. Structure of the nephron.

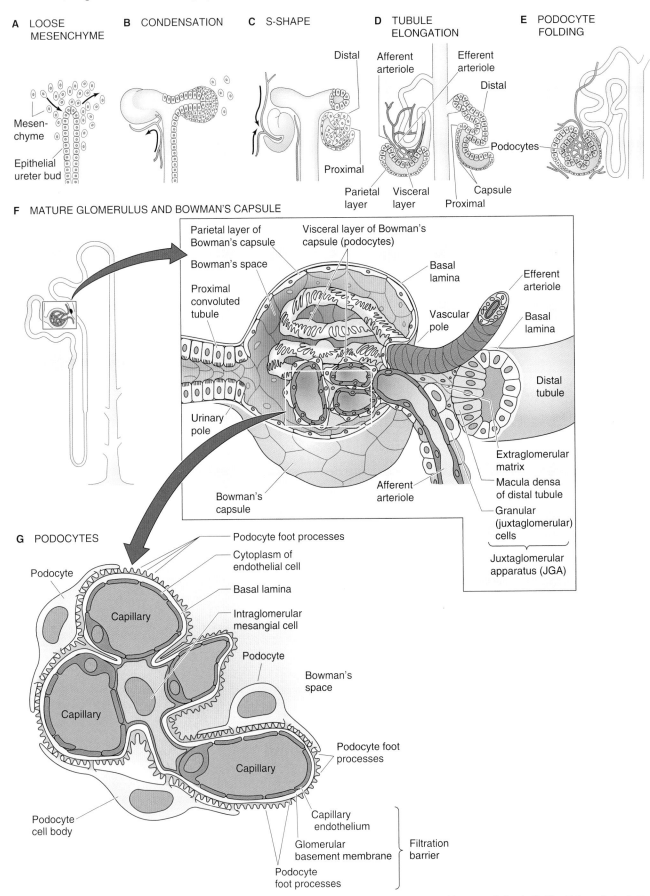

A LOOSE MESENCHYME

Mesenchyme

Epithelial ureter bud

B CONDENSATION

C S-SHAPE

Distal

Proximal

D TUBULE ELONGATION

Afferent arteriole

Efferent arteriole

Distal

Podocytes

Capsule

Proximal

Parietal layer

Visceral layer

E PODOCYTE FOLDING

F MATURE GLOMERULUS AND BOWMAN'S CAPSULE

Parietal layer of Bowman's capsule

Bowman's space

Proximal convoluted tubule

Visceral layer of Bowman's capsule (podocytes)

Basal lamina

Vascular pole

Efferent arteriole

Basal lamina

Distal tubule

Urinary pole

Bowman's capsule

Afferent arteriole

Extraglomerular matrix

Macula densa of distal tubule

Granular (juxtaglomerular) cells

Juxtaglomerular apparatus (JGA)

G PODOCYTES

Podocyte

Capillary

Capillary

Podocyte cell body

Podocyte foot processes

Cytoplasm of endothelial cell

Basal lamina

Intraglomerular mesangial cell

Podocyte

Bowman's space

Podocyte foot processes

Capillary

Capillary endothelium

Glomerular basement membrane

Podocyte foot processes

Filtration barrier

FIGURE 32–3. Development of glomerulus and Bowman's capsule. (*A–E*, Data from Ekblom P: In Seldin DW, Giebisch G: The Kidney, 2nd ed. New York, Raven Press, 1992, pp 475–501.)

FIGURE 32–4. Glomerular capillaries covered by the foot processes of podocytes. This scanning electron micrograph shows a view of glomerular capillaries from the vantage point of Bowman's space. The outer surfaces of the capillary endothelial cells are covered by a layer of interdigitating foot processes of the podocytes. The podocyte cell body links to the foot processes by leg-like connections. (From Kriz W, Kaissling B: In Seldin DW, Giebisch G (eds): The Kidney: Physiology and Pathophysiology, 3rd ed. New York, Raven Press, 2000, pp 587–854.)

The remainder of the nephron consists of the various subdivisions of the tubule (Fig. 32–2). The epithelial elements of the nephron include the Bowman capsule, the proximal tubule, thin descending and thin ascending limbs of the loop of Henle, thick ascending limb of the loop of Henle, the distal convoluted tubule, and the connecting tubule. The connecting tubule leads further into the initial collecting tubule, the cortical collecting tubule, and medullary collecting ducts.

Within the renal cortex, as noted earlier, one can distinguish two populations of nephrons (see Fig. 32–2). **Superficial nephrons** have short loops extending to the boundary between outer and inner medulla. The **juxtamedullary nephrons**, which play a special role in the production of a concentrated urine, have long loops that extend as far as the tip of the medulla.

The Renal Corpuscle Has Three Components: Vascular Elements, the Mesangium, and the Bowman Capsule and Space

The **renal corpuscle,** the site of formation of the glomerular filtrate, comprises a capillary tuft (the source of the filtrate), the Bowman space (where the filtrate goes), and

the Bowman capsule (the modified initial portion of the proximal tubule).

During the development of the kidney, the interaction between the ureteric bud—which gives rise to the urinary system from the collecting duct to the ureters—and the surrounding loose mesenchyme (Fig. 32–3A) leads to the branching of the ureteric bud and condensation of the mesenchyme (Fig. 32–3B). These condensed cells differentiate into an epithelium, which forms a hollow, S-shaped tubular structure (Fig. 32–3C) that gives rise to the nephron's tubular elements between the Bowman capsule and the connecting segment. The distal portion of the S-shaped tubular structure elongates and connects with branches of the developing ureteric bud (Fig. 32–3D). At the same time, the blind proximal end of this S-shaped tubule closely attaches to the arterial vascular bundle that develops into the glomerular capillary tuft. Thinning of the epithelium on one circumference of the blind end of the S-shaped tubule leads to the emergence of the future parietal layer of Bowman's capsule. In contrast, the opposite visceral layer thickens and attaches to the glomerular capillaries (Fig. 32–3D). These visceral epithelial cells later fold and develop into podocytes (Fig. 32–3E).

In the mature kidney (Fig. 32–3F), foot processes of the podocytes cover the glomerular capillaries. These podocytes, modified epithelial cells, thus represent the *visceral* layer of the Bowman capsule. Beginning at the vascular pole, the podocytes are continuous with the *parietal* layer of the Bowman capsule. Glomerular filtrate drains into the space between these two layers (the Bowman space) and flows into the proximal tubule at the urinary pole of the renal corpuscle.

The glomerular filtration barrier between the glomerular tuft of capillaries and the Bowman capsule comprises three elements with different functional properties (Fig. 32–3G): (1) endothelial cells, (2) the glomerular basement membrane, and (3) the layer of epithelial podocytes.

FIGURE 32–5. Inner aspect of glomerular capillaries, showing fenestrations of endothelial cells. This scanning electron micrograph shows a view of the glomerular capillary wall from the vantage point of the capillary lumen. Multiple fenestrations, each approximately 70 nm in diameter, perforate the endothelial cells. (From Kriz W, Kaissling B: In Seldin DW, Giebisch G (eds): The Kidney: Physiology and Pathophysiology, 3rd ed. New York, Raven Press, 2000, pp 587–854.)

A GLOMERULUS AND BOWMAN'S CAPSULE

Efferent arteriole

Distal tubule

Afferent arteriole

Basal lamina

Podocytes

Proximal convoluted tubule

Bowman's capsule

B COMPONENTS OF FILTRATION BARRIER

CL

CB

FIGURE 32–6. Filtration barrier of the glomerulus. *B*, This transmission electron micrograph shows a cross section through the filtration barrier. From *left to right*, note the capillary lumen (CL); the capillary endothelium with large fenestrations; the lamina rara interna; the lamina densa; the lamina rara externa; multiple foot processes of the podocyte, separated by slit diaphragms (*arrows*); Bowman's space; and finally a portion of the overarching podocyte cell body (CB). (*B* from Kriz W, Kaissling B: In Seldin DW, Giebisch G (eds): The Kidney: Physiology and Pathophysiology, 3rd ed. New York, Raven Press, 2000, pp 587–854.)

The **endothelial cells** of the glomerular capillaries are almost completely surrounded by the glomerular basement membrane and a layer of podocyte foot processes (Fig. 32–4). The exception is a small region toward the center of the glomerulus, where the endothelial cells have neither basement membrane nor podocytes and come into direct contact with smooth-muscle-like mesangial cells. Filtration occurs away from the mesangial cells, at the peripheral portion of the capillary wall, which is covered with basement membrane and podocytes. The endothelial cells contain large **fenestrations**, 70-nm holes that provide no restriction to the movement of water and small solutes—including proteins or other large molecules—out of the lumen of the capillary (Fig. 32–5). Thus, the endothelial cells probably serve only to limit the filtration of cellular elements (e.g., erythrocytes).

The **basement membrane**, located between endothelial cells and podocyte foot processes, separates the endothelial layer from the epithelial layer in all parts of the glomerular tuft (Fig. 32–6A). The basement membrane itself consists of three layers: (1) an inner thin layer (*lamina rara interna*); (2) a thick layer (*lamina densa*), and (3) an outer thin layer (*lamina rara externa*), as shown in Figure 32–6B. The basement membrane makes an important contribution to the permeability characteristics of the filtration barrier by restricting intermediate- to large-sized solutes (molecular weight > 1 kDa). The basement membrane is also the site of strongly anionic charges, a result of the sialic and dicarboxylic amino acid residues that are present in basement membrane proteoglycans.

The **podocytes** have foot processes that interdigitate

and cover the basement membrane (see Fig. 32–4). These foot processes are separated from each other by **filtration slits** (see Fig. 32–6B), which are connected by a thin diaphragmatic structure (the "slit diaphragm") with pores ranging in size from 4 to 14 nm. Glycoproteins with negative charges cover the podocytes, filtration slits, and slit diaphragms. The negative charges at both the basement-membrane and podocyte layers favor the filtration of positively charged solutes.

Supporting the glomerular capillary loops is a network

TABLE 32–1

TUBULE SEGMENTS OF THE NEPHRON	
TUBULE SEGMENT	**ABBREVIATION**
Proximal convoluted tubule	PCT
Proximal straight tubule	PST
Thin descending limb of loop of Henle	tDLH
Thin ascending limb of loop of Henle	tALH
Thick ascending limb of loop of Henle	TAL
Distal convoluted tubule	DCT
Connecting tubule	CNT
Initial collecting tubule	ICT
Cortical collecting tubule	CCT
Outer medullary collecting duct	OMCD
Inner medullary collecting duct	IMCD

of contractile **mesangial cells**, which secrete the extracellular matrix. This network is continuous with the smooth-muscle cells of the afferent and efferent arterioles. The matrix extends into a region of the "extraglomerular matrix." The **juxtaglomerular apparatus** (JGA) includes this extraglomerular matrix, the macula densa, and the granular cells. The **macula densa** is a region of specialized epithelial cells of the thick ascending limb where it contacts its glomerulus (see Fig. 32–3F). Macula densa cells differ from the other cells of the thick ascending limb. They have strikingly large cell nuclei and are closely packed, thus causing the appearance of a plaque, which has led to the term "macula densa." The **granular cells**—also called juxtaglomerular cells—in the wall of afferent arterioles are specialized smooth-muscle cells that are the site of production, storage, and regulated release of **renin**, an important renal hormone. The JGA is part of a complex feedback mechanism that regulates not only renal blood flow and filtration rate (p. 769), but also indirectly modulates Na$^+$ balance (p. 866) and systemic blood pressure (p. 555).

The Tubule Components of the Nephron Include the Proximal Tubule, the Loop of Henle, the Distal Tubule, and the Collecting Duct

Figure 32–7 illustrates the ultrastructure of the cells of the different tubule segments. Table 32–1 lists these segments and their abbreviations.

Based on its appearance at relatively low magnification, the **proximal tubule** can be divided into a convoluted part, the proximal convoluted tubule (PCT) (Fig. 32–7A, B), and a straight part, the proximal straight tubule (PST) (Fig. 32–7B). However, based on ultrastructure, the proximal tubule can alternatively be subdivided into three segments: S1, S2, and S3. The S1 segment starts at the glomerulus and includes the first portion of the PCT. The S2 segment starts within the second half of the PCT and continues into the first half of the PST. Finally, the S3 segment includes the distal half of the PST that extends into the medulla.

Both the apical (luminal) and basolateral (peritubular) membranes of proximal-tubule cells are extensively amplified (see Fig. 32–7A, B). Therefore, the apical membrane shows infoldings in the form of a well-developed *brush border* system. This enlargement of the apical surface area correlates with the main function of this nephron segment, namely, the reabsorption of the bulk of the filtered fluid back into the circulation. From the S1 to the S3 segments, cell complexity progressively declines, correlating with a gradual decrease of reabsorptive rates along the tubule. Thus, the cells exhibit a progressively less developed brush border system, diminished complexity of lateral cell interdigitations, a lower basolateral cell membrane area, and a decrease in the number of mitochondria.

The *basolateral membranes* of adjacent proximal-tubule cells form numerous interdigitations, bringing abundant mitochondria in close contact with the plasma membrane. The interdigitations of the lateral membranes also form an extensive extracellular compartment bounded by the tight junctions at one end, and by the basement membrane of the epithelium at the other end. Proximal-tubule cells contain lysosomes, endocytic vacuoles, and a well-developed system of endoplasmic reticulum. Proximal-tubule cells are also characterized by a prominent Golgi apparatus (p. 23), which is important for synthesizing many membrane components, sorting them, and targeting them to specific surface sites.

In comparison with the S3 segment of the proximal tubule, the cells lining the **descending** and **ascending thin limbs** of the loop of Henle are far less complex (see Fig. 32–7C, D), with few mitochondria and little cell-membrane amplification. The *thin ascending* limbs are poorly developed in short loops of superficial nephrons. However, they form a major part of the long loops of the juxtamedullary nephrons.

Epithelial cells lining the **thick ascending limb** of the loop of Henle, which terminates at the macula densa, are characterized by tall interdigitations and numerous mitochondria within extensively invaginated basolateral membranes (see Fig. 32–7E). This complex cell machinery correlates with the key role these cells play in generating a hyperosmotic medium in the renal medullary interstitium.

Until the latter part of the 20th century, morphologists defined the "**classic distal tubule**"—on the basis of light microscopic studies—as the segment of the nephron stretching from the macula densa to the first confluence of two nephrons in the collecting duct system. Today, we subdivide the classic distal tubule into three segments, based on ultrastructural studies: the distal convoluted tubule (starting at the macula densa), the connecting tubule, and the initial collecting duct. What was classically termed the "early" distal tubule is mainly the DCT, whereas the classically termed "late" distal tubule is mainly the initial collecting duct.

The **distal convoluted tubule** begins at the macula densa and ends at the transition to the connecting tubule (Fig. 32–7F). The cells lining the DCT are similar in structure to those of the thick ascending limb. However, significant cell heterogeneity characterizes the tubule segments that follow.

The **connecting tubule**, which ends at the transition to the initial collecting tubule, consists of two cell types—connecting-tubule cells and intercalated cells. Connecting-tubule cells (see Fig. 32–7G) are unique in that they produce and release renal **kallikrein**, a local hormone whose precise function is still uncertain. We will discuss intercalated cells below.

The two segments following the connecting tubule, the **initial collecting tubule** (up to the first confluence) and **cortical collecting tubule** (after the confluence), are identical. They are composed of intercalated and principal cells, which exhibit striking morphologic and functional differences. **Intercalated cells**, similar in structure to the intercalated cells of the connecting tubule, make up about one third of the lining of these collecting-tubule segments (see Fig. 32–7H, I). Distinct subpopulations of these cells secrete H$^+$ (A- or α-intercalated cells) or HCO$_3^-$ (B- or β-intercalated cells) and reabsorb K$^+$. **Principal cells** make up about two thirds of the cells of the initial and cortical

FIGURE 32–7. Structure of tubule cells along the nephron. Because of the variability among tubule segments, the cross sections of the tubule are not to scale.

collecting tubules (see Fig. 32–7H, I). Their invaginations of the basolateral cell membrane are only modestly developed, and their number of mitochondria is less than that of intercalated cells. Principal cells, easily recognized by a central *cilium* on the apical cell membrane, reabsorb Na$^+$ and Cl$^-$ and secrete K$^+$.

The **medullary collecting duct** is lined mostly by one cell type that increases in cell height towards the papilla (see Fig. 32–7J, K). The number of intercalated cells diminishes, beginning at the medullary collecting duct. Cells in this segment continue the transport of electrolytes and participate in the hormonally regulated transport of water and of urea. At the extreme end of the medullary collecting duct (i.e., "papillary" collecting duct or duct of Bellini), the cells are extremely tall.

The Tightness of Tubule Epithelia Increases from the Proximal to the Medullary Collecting Tubule

Epithelia may be either "tight" or "leaky," depending on the permeability of their tight junctions (p. 83). In general, the tightness of the tubule epithelium increases from the proximal tubule to the collecting duct. The proximal tubule, a leaky epithelium, has shallow junctional complexes (p. 46). In freeze-fracture studies, these junctions show only a few strands of fused membrane. On the other hand, the collecting tubule, a relatively tight epithelium, has long, tight junctions that extend deeper into the intercellular space and consist of multiple strands of fused membranes. Tubule segments with tight junctions consisting of only one strand have a low electrical resistance and are highly permeable, whereas the presence of several strands of apposing membranes correlates with a high electrical resistance and lower ion permeability.

Gap junctions (p. 164) provide intercellular contact between some, but not all, neighboring tubule cells. These gap junctions are located at various sites between the basement membrane and the tight junctions, and probably represent the morphologic basis of low-resistance pathways between cells. Electrical coupling exists among proximal-tubule cells, but not among heterogenous cell types, such as those found in the connecting and collecting tubules.

MAIN ELEMENTS OF RENAL FUNCTION

The Nephron Forms an Ultrafiltrate of the Blood Plasma and Then Selectively Reabsorbs the Tubule Fluid or Secretes Solutes Into It

As they do for capillaries elsewhere in the body, Starling forces (p. 469) govern the flow of fluid across the capillary walls in the **glomerulus** and result in a net filtration. However, in the case of the glomerular capillaries, the filtrate flows not into the interstitium, but into the Bowman space, which is contiguous with the lumen of the proximal tubule.

The main function of the tubule elements of the kidney is to recover most of the fluid and solutes filtered from the glomerulus. If the fluid were not recovered, the kidney would excrete the volume of the entire blood plasma in less than half an hour. The retrieval of the largest fraction of glomerular filtrate occurs in the **proximal tubule**, which reabsorbs NaCl and NaHCO$_3$, as well as an osmotically obligated volume of water. In addition, the proximal tubule reabsorbs filtered nutrients such as glucose and amino acids. Furthermore, this nephron segment reabsorbs divalent ions, such as Ca^{2+}, HPO$_4^{2-}$, and SO$_4^{2-}$. The proximal tubule also plays a role in the regulation of acid-base balance by reabsorbing the bulk of filtered HCO$_3^-$ and by secreting NH$_4^+$. Finally, several organic anion and cation transporters secrete a variety of endogenous and exogenous solutes into the proximal-tubule lumen.

The main function of the **loop of Henle** (i.e., tDLH, tALH, TAL) is to participate in forming a concentrated or dilute urine. The loop does this by pumping NaCl into the interstitium of the medulla, thus making it hypertonic. This hypertonicity is exploited downstream as fluid flowing down the medullary collecting duct is either allowed—or not allowed—to lose water to the hypertonic interstitium by osmosis. In humans, only approximately 15% of the nephrons have long loops that descend to the tip of the papilla. Nevertheless, this *subpopulation* of juxtamedullary nephrons (see Fig. 32–2) is extremely important for creating the osmotic gradients within the papilla that allow water movement out of the lumen of the *entire population* of medullary collecting ducts. As a result of this water movement, urine osmolality in the collecting ducts can far exceed that in the plasma.

The TAL cells secrete the Tamm-Horsfall mucoprotein. Normal subjects excrete 30 to 50 mg/day into the urine, accounting—along with albumin (<20 mg/day)—for most of the protein in the urine. The function of the Tamm-Horsfall protein is unknown, but it constitutes the matrix of all urinary "casts"; a cast is cylindrically shaped debris in the urine that has taken the shape of the tubule lumen in which it was formed.

The classic **distal tubule** and the **collecting duct system** are sites for the fine control of salt and water excretion. Although only small fractions of the glomerular filtrate reach these most distally located nephron sites, the role of these tubule segments is important. Several hormones (e.g., aldosterone, arginine vasopressin) exert their main effects on electrolyte and water excretion at these sites.

The Juxtaglomerular Apparatus Is a Region Where Each Thick Ascending Limb Contacts Its Glomerulus

Elements of the JGA provide the basis for two important regulatory mechanisms. First, if the amount of fluid and NaCl delivered to the **macula densa** of a nephron increases (see Fig. 32–3F), the glomerular filtration rate of *that nephron* falls markedly. This phenomenon of **tubuloglomerular feedback** occurs as increased NaCl delivery to the macula densa triggers constriction of the afferent arteriole, reducing the glomerular filtration rate.

The second regulatory mechanism comes into play during a decrease in the pressure of the renal artery feeding the various afferent arterioles. The afferent arteriole, which acts as a baroreceptor, senses decreased stretch in its wall, and directs neighboring granular cells to increase their release of renin into the general circulation—an endocrine effect. Because renin converts angiotensinogen into angiotensin I (p. 866), the subsequent production of angiotensin II, a powerful vasoconstrictor, provides an effective feedback mechanism for increasing **systemic arterial blood pressure**. This sequence of events is the primary mechanism for controlling plasma renin levels.

Sympathetic Nerve Fibers to the Kidney Regulate Renal Blood Flow, Glomerular Filtration, and Tubule Reabsorption

The autonomic innervation to the kidneys is entirely from the **sympathetic division** of the autonomic nervous system; the kidneys lack a supply of parasympathetic nerve fibers. The sympathetic supply to the kidneys originates from the celiac plexus (see Fig. 15–3), and generally follows the arterial vessels into the kidney. The varicosities of the sympathetic fibers release norepinephrine and dopamine into the loose connective tissue near the smooth-muscle cells of the vasculature (i.e., renal artery as well as afferent and efferent arterioles) and near the proximal tubules. Sympathetic stimulation to the kidneys has three major effects. First, the catecholamines cause vasoconstriction. Second, the catecholamines strongly enhance Na^+ reabsorption proximal-tubule cells. Third, as a result of the dense accumulation of sympathetic fibers near the granular cells of the JGA, increased sympathetic nerve activity dramatically stimulates renin secretion.

Renal nerves also include afferent (i.e., sensory) fibers. A few myelinated nerve fibers conduct baroreceptor and chemoreceptor impulses that originate in the kidney. Increased perfusion pressure stimulates renal **baroreceptors** in the interlobar arteries and afferent arterioles. Renal ischemia and abnormal ion composition of the interstitial fluid stimulate **chemoreceptors** located in the renal pelvis. These pelvic chemoreceptors probably respond to high levels of K^+ and H^+, and may elicit changes in capillary blood flow.

The Kidneys Are Also Endocrine Organs: They Produce Renin, the Biologically Active Form of Vitamin D, Erythropoietin, Prostaglandins, and Bradykinin

Besides the production of renin by the JGA granular cells, the kidney plays several other endocrine roles. Proximal-tubule cells convert circulating 25-hydroxyvitamin D to the active metabolite, **1,25-dihydroxyvitamin D**. This hormone controls calcium and phosphorus metabolism by acting on the intestines, the kidneys, and bone (p. 1095), and it is important for developing and maintaining bone structure.

Fibroblast-like cells in the interstitium of the cortex and outer medulla secrete **erythropoietin** (EPO) in re-

sponse to a fall in the local tissue P_{O_2} (see box on p. 664). EPO stimulates the development of red blood cells by action on hematopoietic stem cells in bone marrow, and it is an important therapeutic agent in the treatment of severe anemias that develop in chronic renal failure and particularly in dialysis patients.

The kidney releases **prostaglandins** and several **kinins**, which act as local hormones for the control of circulation within the kidney. In general, they are vasodilators and may play a protective role when renal blood flow is compromised. In addition, tubule cells secrete angiotensin, bradykinin, cyclic adenosine monophosphate, and adenosine triphosphate into the lumen, but the precise function of such local secretion is poorly understood.

MEASURING RENAL CLEARANCE AND TRANSPORT

Numerous tests are available for assessing renal function. Some of these are applicable only in animal experiments. Other tests are useful in clinical settings, and fall into two general categories:

1. Modern imaging techniques provide outstanding macroscopic views of renal blood flow, filtration, and excretory function.
2. Measurements of the so-called "renal clearance" of various substances evaluate the ability of the kidneys to handle solutes and water.

This subchapter focuses on clearance measurements. The clearance approach compares the rate at which the glomeruli filter a substance (water or a solute) with the rate at which the kidneys excrete it into the urine. By measuring—for a particular substance—the difference between the amounts filtered and excreted, we can estimate the net amount reabsorbed or secreted by the renal tubules, and thus gain insight into the three basic functions of the kidney—glomerular **filtration**, tubule **reabsorption**, and tubule **secretion**. Although they are widely used, clearance methods have the inherent limitation that they measure *overall* nephron function. This function is "overall" in two different senses. First, clearance sums many individual transport operations occurring sequentially at different sites along a single nephron. Second, clearance sums the output of all 2 million nephrons in parallel. Hence, clearance cannot provide information on precise sites and mechanisms of transport. Such information can, however, come from studies of individual nephrons, tubule cells, or cell membranes.

One can also apply the clearance concept to other problems, such as the clearance of bile by the liver (p. 995) or clearance of hormones from the blood.

The "Clearance" of a Solute Is the Virtual Volume of Blood That Would Be Totally Cleared of a Solute in a Given Time

All solutes excreted into the urine ultimately come from the blood perfusing the kidney. Thus, the rate at which the kidney excretes a solute into the urine equals the rate at which the solute disappears from the blood plasma. Imagine that, during 1 minute, 700 ml of blood plasma flow through the kidney. This blood contains 0.7 liter × 142 mM or approximately 100 millimoles of Na^+. The kidney removes only a tiny amount of Na^+—approximately 0.14 millimoles—from this blood and excretes it into the urine. These 0.14 millimoles of Na^+ could hypothetically have come from only 1 ml of plasma, had all Na^+ ions been removed (i.e., "cleared") from this volume. The **clearance** of a solute is defined as the virtual volume of blood plasma (per unit time) needed to supply that amount of the solute to the urine. Thus, in our example, Na^+ clearance was 1 ml/min, even though 700 ml of plasma flowed through the kidney.

Renal clearance methods are based on the principle of mass balance and the special anatomy of the kidney (Fig. 32–8). For any solute (X) that the kidney neither metabolizes nor produces, the only route of entry to the kidney is the renal artery, and the only two routes of exit are the renal vein and the ureter. Because the input of X equals the output of X,

Equation 32–1

$$\underbrace{P_{X,a} \cdot RPF_a}_{\frac{mmole}{ml} \quad \frac{ml}{min}} = \underbrace{(P_{X,v} \cdot RPF_v)}_{\frac{mmole}{ml} \quad \frac{ml}{min}} + \underbrace{(U_X \cdot \dot{V})}_{\frac{mmole}{ml} \quad \frac{ml}{min}}$$

$$\text{Arterial input of X} \qquad \text{Venous output of X} \qquad \text{Urine output of X}$$

In the above equation, $P_{X,a}$ and $P_{X,v}$ are the plasma concentrations of X in the renal artery and renal vein, respectively. RPF_a and RPF_v are the rates of renal plasma flow in the renal artery and vein, respectively. U_X is the concentration of X in the urine. $\dot{V}$ is the urine flow (the "dot" represents the time derivative of volume). The product $U_X \cdot \dot{V}$ is the **urinary excretion rate**—the amount of X excreted in the urine per unit time.

In developing the concept of renal clearance, we can transform Equation 32–1 in two ways. First, because we assume that the kidney clears all of X from an incoming volume of arterial blood, we can replace RPF_a with the "virtual input volume" (i.e., the "clearance" of X, C_X) that is sufficient to provide just that amount of X that appears in the urine. Second, again because we assume that the kidney removes all of X from the incoming volume of blood, we assign the "virtual venous output" a value of zero. Thus, Equation 32–1 becomes:

Equation 32–2

$$\begin{array}{ccc} \text{Virtual} & = \text{Virtual} & + \text{Actual} \\ \text{arterial input} & \text{venous output} & \text{urine output} \end{array}$$

$$P_{X,a} \cdot C_X \quad = \quad 0 \quad + \quad (U_X \cdot \dot{V})$$

Solving for clearance,

Equation 32–3

$$C_X = \frac{U_X \cdot \dot{V}}{P_X}$$

This is the classic clearance equation that describes the virtual volume of plasma that would be *totally cleared* of a solute in a given time (Table 32–2A). We need to know only three parameters to compute the clearance of a solute X: (1) the concentration of X in the urine (U_X), (2) the volume of urine formed in a given time ($\dot{V}$), and (3) the concentration of X in systemic blood plasma (P_X). This last parameter is the same as $P_{X,a}$ that we used in Equation 32–1.

Together, the three basic functions of the kidney—glomerular filtration, tubule reabsorption, and tubule secretion—determine the renal clearance of a solute. In the special case in which the kidneys completely clear X from plasma during a *single passage* through the kidneys ($P_{X,v} = 0$ in Equation 32–1), the renal clearance of X equals arterial renal plasma flow (RPF_a in Equation 32–1); **p-aminohippurate (PAH)** is just such a special solute. Thus, the clearance of PAH is a good estimate of **renal plasma flow** (Table 32–2B), which we discuss on p. 767. Note that RPF is the same as RPF_a in Equation 32–1. For all solutes that *do not* behave like PAH, the renal venous plasma still contains some X. Thus, the virtual volume cleared of X in a given time is less than the total renal plasma flow. For most solutes, then, clearance describes a virtual volume of blood that would be *totally cleared* of a solute, whereas in reality a much larger volume of blood is *partially cleared* of the solute.

We can use a clearance approach to estimate another important renal parameter: **glomerular filtration rate** (GFR), which is the volume of fluid filtered into the Bowman capsule per unit time. Imagine a solute X that fulfills two criteria. First, X is freely filtered (i.e., concentration of X in Bowman's space is the same as that in

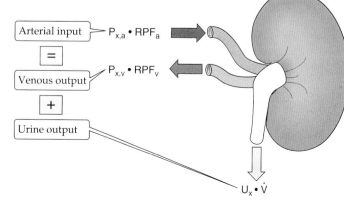

FIGURE 32–8. Solute mass balance in the kidney.

TABLE 32–2

RENAL CLEARANCE

A. Clearance of Any Substance X

$$C_X = \frac{U_X \cdot \dot{V}}{P_X} = \frac{(mg \text{ or } moles/ml) \cdot (ml/min)}{mg \text{ or } moles/ml} = \frac{ml}{min}$$

C_X may vary between zero, for a substance that does not appear in the urine (e.g., glucose), and approximately 700 ml/min (i.e., total RPF) for a substance (e.g., PAH) that is totally removed from the blood in a single pass through the kidney.

B. Clearance of PAH Approximates RPF (at Low Plasma PAH Concentration)

$$C_{PAH} = RPF = \frac{U_{PAH} \cdot \dot{V}}{P_{PAH}}$$

C. Clearance of Inulin (In) Approximates GFR

$$C_{In} = GFR = \frac{U_{In} \cdot \dot{V}}{P_{In}}$$

GFR, glomerular filtration rate; PAH, para-aminohippurate; RPF, renal plasma flow.

blood plasma). Second, the tubules do not absorb, secrete, or metabolize X. Thus, the amount of X that appears in the urine per unit time ($U_X \cdot \dot{V}$) is the same as the amount of X that the glomerulus filters per unit time ($P_X \cdot GFR$):

Equation 32–4

$$\overbrace{P_X \cdot GFR}^{\substack{\text{Input to} \\ \text{Bowman} \\ \text{space}}} = \overbrace{U_X \cdot \dot{V}}^{\substack{\text{Output into} \\ \text{urine}}}$$

The input to the Bowman space is also known as the **filtered solute load** and is generally given in millimoles (or mg) per minute. Rearranging Equation 32–4,

Equation 32–5

$$GFR = \frac{U_X \cdot \dot{V}}{P_X}$$

Equation 32–5 is in exactly the same form as the classic clearance equation (Equation 32–3). In other words, GFR is C_X if X has the required properties. As discussed on p. 758, **inulin** is just such a solute (Table 32–2C).

A Solute's Urinary Excretion Is the Algebraic Sum of Its Filtered Load, Reabsorption by Tubules, and Secretion by Tubules

The homeostasis of body fluids critically depends on the ability of the kidneys to decide how much of what substances to excrete in the urine. Renal excretion in general is determined by three factors (Fig. 32–9):

1. The rate of filtration of X (i.e., filtered load), which is the product of GFR and plasma concentration of X,
2. The rate of reabsorption of X by the tubules,
3. The rate of secretion of X by the tubules.

This interrelationship is expressed quantitatively by

Equation 32–6

$$\begin{array}{c} \text{Amount} \\ \text{excreted} \\ \text{per unit} \\ \text{time} \end{array} = \begin{array}{c} \text{Amount} \\ \text{filtered} \\ \text{per unit} \\ \text{time} \end{array} - \begin{array}{c} \text{Amount} \\ \text{reabsorbed} \\ \text{per unit} \\ \text{time} \end{array} + \begin{array}{c} \text{Amount} \\ \text{secreted} \\ \text{per unit} \\ \text{time} \end{array}$$

As noted earlier, for some substances (e.g., inulin), there is no reabsorption or secretion. For most substances, *either* reabsorption *or* secretion determines the amount present in the final urine. However, for some substances, *both* reabsorption *and* secretion determine excretion.

If a solute is only reabsorbed, *but not secreted*, the rate of **reabsorption** can be obtained by rearranging Equation 32–6:

Equation 32–7

$$\begin{array}{c} \text{Reabsorption} \\ \text{rate} \\ \text{(mg/min)} \end{array} = \begin{array}{c} \text{Filtered} \\ \text{load} \\ \text{(mg/min)} \end{array} - \begin{array}{c} \text{Rate of} \\ \text{excretion} \\ \text{(mg/min)} \end{array}$$

$$= GFR \cdot P_X - U_X \cdot \dot{V}$$

Conversely, if a solute is only secreted, *but not reabsorbed*, the rate of **secretion** is:

Equation 32–8

$$\begin{array}{c} \text{Secretion} \\ \text{rate} \\ \text{(mg/min)} \end{array} = \begin{array}{c} \text{Rate of} \\ \text{excretion} \\ \text{(mg/min)} \end{array} - \begin{array}{c} \text{Filtered} \\ \text{load} \\ \text{(mg/min)} \end{array}$$

$$= U_X \cdot \dot{V} - GFR \cdot P_X$$

In applying Equation 32–7 and Equation 32–8, we must keep in mind two important limitations. First, to estimate the rate at which a substance appears in the filtrate—the filtered load—from the product $GFR \cdot P_X$, we must assume that P_X represents the *freely filterable* concentration of X. Indeed, many substances—particularly univalent electrolytes, urea, glucose, and amino acids—are freely filterable. However, if the solute binds to protein, for example, then it will not be freely filterable. For these solutes—including calcium, phosphate, magnesium, and PAH—it is necessary to measure plasma binding and correct for the nonfilterable fraction of the solute. Second, for us to apply the mass balance equation (Equation 32–6), the kidney must neither synthesize nor degrade the solute. An example of a solute that is synthesized by the kidney is ammonium. Examples of solutes degraded by the kidney include glutamate and glutamine (which are converted to ammonium) as well as several other amino acids and monocarboxylic and dicarboxylic acids.

If the kidney both *reabsorbs* and *secretes* a substance, clearance data are inadequate to describe the renal han-

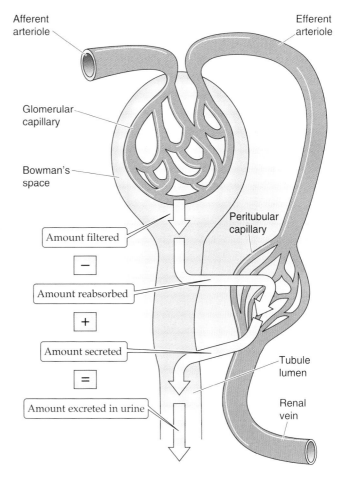

FIGURE 32–9. Factors contributing to the net urinary excretion of a substance.

dling. For example, if a solute were completely reabsorbed in the proximal tubule, and some secreted later in the nephron, clearance data alone would imply that only filtration and reabsorption occurred. We would have no reason to suspect that secretion was involved at all. Conversely, if a solute were secreted and a lesser amount reabsorbed, clearance data would suggest that only filtration and secretion had occurred. Complex combinations of reabsorption and secretion occur with potassium, uric acid, and urea.

Another useful parameter for gauging how the kidney handles a freely filtered solute is the **fractional excretion** (FE). The fractional excretion is the ratio of the amount excreted in the urine ($U_X \cdot \dot{V}$) to the filtered load ($P_X \cdot$ GFR):

Equation 32–9

$$FE_X = \frac{U_X \cdot \dot{V}}{P_X \cdot GFR}$$

According to Equation 32–3, however, the term ($U_X \cdot \dot{V} / P_X$) is simply the clearance of X (C_X):

Equation 32–10

$$FE_X = \frac{C_X}{GFR}$$

As discussed on p. 758, one estimates GFR by measuring the clearance of inulin (C_{In}). Thus, fractional excretion of a freely filterable solute is the same as the **clearance ratio**:

Equation 32–11

$$FE_X = \frac{C_X}{C_{In}}$$

Microscopic Techniques Make It Possible to Measure Single-Nephron Rates of Filtration, Absorption, and Secretion

Because clearance methods treat the kidney as a "black box," it is very difficult to determine which nephron segments are responsible for which transport processes. It is also impossible to determine which nephrons are responsible for overall urinary excretion. To learn how single nephrons function, and also to understand how individual segments of the nephron contribute to overall nephron function, renal physiologists have developed a series of invasive techniques for studying the function of renal cells in the research laboratory (Fig. 32–10).

The rationale for investigating renal function at the single-nephron level is that total kidney function, studied by the macroscopic methods discussed in the previous sections, reflects the activity of many single nephrons and nephron segments. To apply the concept of clearance to a single nephron site, one uses the free-flow micropuncture approach (Fig. 32–10A) and measures the concentration of the solute in the tubule fluid at that site (TF_X), volume flow at that site (i.e., the collection rate), and plasma concentration (P_X). By analogy with the *macroscopic* clearance equation, we can write a clearance equation for a single nephron:

$$\text{Equation 32-12}$$

$$C_X = \frac{TF_X \times \text{Volume collection rate}}{P_X}$$

Compared with Equation 32-3, here TF_X replaces U_X and "Volume collection rate" replaces $\dot{V}$. We can use this basic equation to compute the amount of fluid that a single nephron filters, as well as the amounts of fluid and solutes that a single tubule segment handles.

SINGLE-NEPHRON GLOMERULAR FILTRATION RATE (SNGFR). If X in Equation 32-12 is a marker for GFR (e.g., inulin or "In"), one can calculate SNGFR using an equation that is similar to that in Table 32-2C to calculate total GFR:

$$\text{Equation 32-13}$$

$$SNGFR = \frac{TF_{In} \times \text{Volume collection rate}}{P_{In}}$$

Using the numeric values for rat kidney shown in Figure 32-11, we can use Equation 32-13 to compute the SNGFR:

$$\text{Equation 32-14}$$

$$SNGFR = \frac{(3 \text{ mg/ml}) \times (10 \text{ nl/min})}{(1 \text{ mg/ml})} = 30 \text{ nl/min}$$

HANDLING OF H_2O BY TUBULE SEGMENTS IN A SINGLE NEPHRON. We also can use the same information that we used to compute SNGFR to calculate the rate of water reabsorption between the glomerulus and the micropuncture site. The **fraction of filtered water remaining** at the micropuncture site is

$$\text{Equation 32-15}$$

$$\begin{array}{c} \text{Fraction of} \\ \text{filtered water} \\ \text{remaining} \end{array} = \frac{\text{Volume collection rate}}{SNGFR}$$

Substituting the expression for SNGFR (Equation 32-13) into Equation 32-15, we have

A FREE-FLOW MICROPUNCTURE

A pipette is inserted into a superficially located tubule in the kidney; in this case, the proximal tubule.

Connecting tubule   Pipette

Capsule

B STOPPED-FLOW MICROPERFUSION

A droplet of oil is pipetted into the tubule through one barrel of a double-barrelled pipette, and split...

...by an aqueous solution introduced through the second barrel.

Oil — Saline

Oil block

Oil

Collected saline

Oil block

Later, a second pipette with a single barrel samples the fluid that the tubule has modified.

C CONTINUOUS MICROPERFUSION

The tubule undergoes continuous perfusion through a pipette, as does the adjacent capillary.

A downstream pipette continuously collects the fluid.

Oil block

Capillary   Tubule

Voltage measurements are taken from either the tubule lumen...

Record   Record   ...or cell interior.

D ISOLATED PERFUSED TUBULE

One isolates a tubule from any segment of any nephron.

The lumen of the tubule, as well as its basolateral surface, are continuously perfused.

This pipette collects the fluid.

FIGURE 32-10. Methods for studying renal function in the research laboratory.

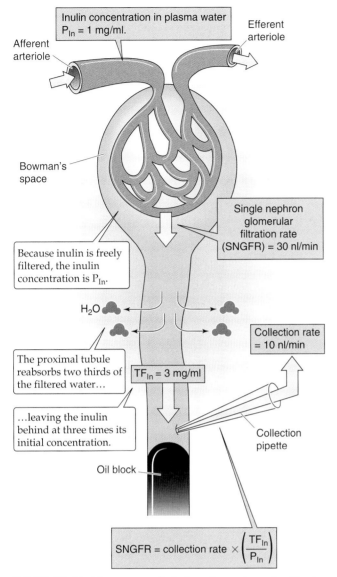

Inulin concentration in plasma water
P_{In} = 1 mg/ml.

Efferent
arteriole

Afferent
arteriole

Bowman's
space

Single nephron
glomerular
filtration rate
(SNGFR) = 30 nl/min

Because inulin is freely
filtered, the inulin
concentration is P_{In}.

H_2O

Collection rate
= 10 nl/min

The proximal tubule
reabsorbs two thirds of
the filtered water...

TF_{In} = 3 mg/ml

...leaving the inulin
behind at three times its
initial concentration.

Collection
pipette

Oil block

$$SNGFR = collection\ rate \times \left(\frac{TF_{In}}{P_{In}}\right)$$

FIGURE 32–11. Measurement of single-nephron glomerular filtration rate. Data are for the rat.

Equation 32–16

$$\begin{aligned} \text{Fraction of} \\ \text{filtered water} \\ \text{remaining} \end{aligned} = \frac{\text{Volume collection rate}}{(TF_{In} \times \text{Volume collection rate})/P_{In}}$$

$$= \frac{P_{In}}{TF_{In}}$$

Thus, to know the *fraction* of filtered water remaining at the collection site, we do not need to know the collection rate, only the concentrations of inulin in blood plasma and at the collection site. In the example of Figure 32–11, in which the tubule reabsorbed two thirds of the fluid, the fraction of filtered water remaining at the sampling site is (1 mg/ml)/(3 mg/ml) or approximately 0.33.

The **fraction of filtered water reabsorbed** is 1 minus the fraction of filtered water remaining:

Equation 32–17

$$\text{Fraction of filtered water reabsorbed} = 1 - \frac{P_{In}}{TF_{In}}$$

In our example, the fraction of filtered water reabsorbed is 1– 0.33 or approximately 0.67.

HANDLING OF SOLUTES BY TUBULE SEGMENTS IN A SINGLE NEPHRON. We can use the same concepts of single-nephron clearance to quantitate the reabsorption or secretion of any *solute* along the tubule. The first step is to estimate the fraction of the filtered solute remaining at the puncture site. This parameter—the **fractional solute excretion**—is the ratio of the amount of solute appearing at the micropuncture site to the amount of solute filtered at the glomerulus (i.e., **single-nephron filtered load**):

Equation 32–18

$$\begin{aligned} \text{Fractional} \\ \text{solute} \\ \text{excretion} \end{aligned} = \frac{\begin{aligned} \text{Rate of solute} \\ \text{delivery to} \\ \text{micropuncture site} \end{aligned}}{\text{Single-nephron filtered load}}$$

The numerator is the product of volume collection rate and tubule solute concentration (TF_X), and the denominator is the product of SNGFR and the plasma solute concentration (P_X):

Equation 32–19

$$\begin{aligned} \text{Fractional} \\ \text{solute} \\ \text{excretion} \end{aligned} = \frac{\text{Volume Collection Rate} \times TF_X}{\text{SNGFR} \times P_X}$$

In Equation 32–15 and Equation 32–16, we saw that the ratio (Volume Collection Rate/SNGFR) is (P_{In}/TF_{In}). Making this substitution in Equation 32–19, we obtain an alternative expression for fractional solute excretion:

Equation 32–20

$$\text{Fractional solute excretion} = \frac{TF_X/P_X}{TF_{In}/P_{In}}$$

The advantage of Equation 32–20 over Equation 32–19 is that no precise measurements of collection rates are required.

Equation 32–20 is important for understanding the transport of a solute along the nephron. If (TF_X/P_X)/(TF_{In}/P_{In}) is greater than 1, **secretion** has occurred. The mere observation that the *concentration* of a solute in tubule fluid increases progressively along the length of the nephron does not necessarily mean that the tubule secreted the solute; the concentration would also increase if water were reabsorbed. Secretion occurs only if the concentration of the solute in tubule fluid, relative to its concentration in filtrate, exceeds the concentration ratio of inulin. However, if (TF_X/P_X)/(TF_{In}/P_{In}) is less than 1, **reabsorption** has occurred.

Rather than referring to the fraction of the solute excreted (i.e., remaining) up to the point of the micropuncture site, we can also refer to the **fractional solute reabsorption** at the puncture site. By analogy to Equation

32–17 for water, this parameter for a solute is merely 1 minus the fractional solute excretion:

Equation 32–21

$$\text{Fractional solute reabsorption} = 1 - \frac{\text{TF}_X/\text{P}_X}{\text{TF}_{In}/\text{P}_{In}}$$

Thus, applying the principles of clearance and mass balance to a single nephron, we can calculate SNGFR as well as the fractional reabsorption of water and solutes at a particular point along the nephron (i.e., the micropuncture site).

THE URETERS AND BLADDER

As discussed in Chapters 43 and 44, the epithelium of the gastrointestinal (GI) system continues to modify the contents of the GI tract up until the point where the contents finally exit the body. The situation is very different in the mammalian urinary system. By the time the tubule fluid leaves the most distal portion of the collecting duct, the fluid has the composition of final urine. Thus, the epithelia downstream to the tip of the papilla—the pelvis, ureters, bladder, and urethra—do not substantially modify the urine.

The Ureters Propel Urine from the Renal Pelvis to the Bladder by Peristaltic Waves Conducted Along a Syncytium of Smooth Muscle Cells

The **ureters** serve as conduits for the passage of urine from the renal pelvis into the urinary bladder (see Fig. 32–1A). Located in the retroperitoneum, each ureter loops over the top of the common iliac artery and vein on the same side of the body and courses through the

pelvis. The ureters enter the lower, posterior portion of the bladder (**ureterovesical junction**), pass obliquely through its muscular wall, and empty into the bladder lumen 1 to 2 cm above, and lateral to, the orifice of the urethra (Fig. 32–12A). The two ureteral orifices, connected by a ridge of tissue, and the urethral orifice form the corners of a triangle (**bladder trigone**). A flaplike mucous-membrane valve covers each ureteral orifice. This anatomic valve, in conjunction with the physiological valvelike effect created by the ureter's oblique pathway through the bladder wall, prevents reflux of urine back into the ureters during contraction of the bladder.

The lumen of each ureter is lined by **transitional epithelium**, which is above a submucosal layer of connective tissue, as well as an inner longitudinal and an outer circular layer of smooth muscle. Because ureteral **smooth muscle** functions as a syncytium, it is an example of unitary smooth muscle (p. 232). Gap junctions (p. 164) conduct electrical activity from cell to cell at a velocity of 2 to 6 cm/sec. Mechanical stimuli (stretch), chemical stimuli, or conduction of a suprathreshold membrane depolarization may trigger an **action potential** (see Fig. 32–12B) of the "plateau" type (p. 232).

Contraction of ureteral smooth muscle occurs by mechanisms that are characteristic of other smooth muscle (p. 242), where a Ca^{2+}-calmodulin complex activates myosin light chain kinase (MLCK). cAMP-dependent protein kinase (PKA) can phosphorylate MLCK, lowering the affinity of the MLCK for Ca^{2+}-calmodulin, thus impairing the phosphorylation of myosin light chains. This mechanism may, at least in part, account for the relaxing effect of cAMP on smooth muscle.

Ureteral **peristaltic waves** originate from electrical **pacemakers** in the proximal portion of the pelvis of the kidney. These waves propel urine along the ureters and into the bladder in a series of spurts, at frequencies of 2 to 6 per minute. The intra-ureteral hydrostatic pressure is 0 to 5 cm H_2O at baseline, but increases to 20 to 80 cm H_2O during peristaltic waves. Blocking ureteral outflow to

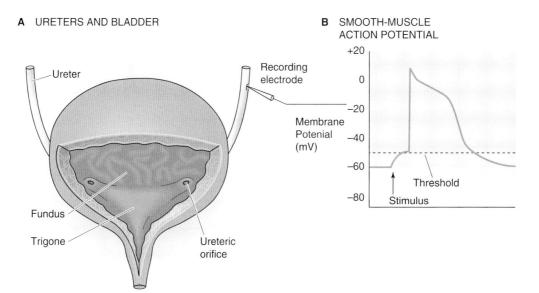

A   URETERS AND BLADDER

Ureter

Fundus

Trigone

Ureteric orifice

B   SMOOTH-MUSCLE ACTION POTENTIAL

Recording electrode

Membrane Potential (mV)

+20

0

−20

−40

−60

−80

Threshold

Stimulus

FIGURE 32–12. Anatomy of the ureters and bladder. In *B*, ureteral smooth-muscle cells generally have a resting membrane potential of about −60 mV, mainly determined by a high K^+ permeability. Na^+ channels speed the upstroke of the action potential, although Ca^{2+} channels are mainly responsible for the action potential.

the bladder, as by a kidney stone, causes the ureters to dilate and increases the baseline hydrostatic pressure to 70 to 80 cm H$_2$O over a period of 1 to 3 hours. This pressure is transmitted in retrograde fashion back to the nephrons, creating a "stopped-flow" condition in which glomerular filtration nearly comes to a halt. **Hydronephrosis**, dilation of the pelvis and calyces of the kidney, can evolve over hours to days. Patients will complain of severe pain (renal colic) due to distention of involved structures. If the obstruction is not cleared, consequences can include marked renal dysfunction and even acute renal failure. Interestingly, with persistent obstruction, the pressure inside the ureter declines to a level that is only

slightly higher than the normal baseline level. Even though the patient produces no urine ("anuria"), glomerular filtration continues, albeit at a markedly reduced rate, indicating that fluid reabsorption by the tubules matches this filtration.

Ureteral peristalsis can occur without innervation. Nevertheless, the autonomic nervous system can modulate peristalsis. As in other syncytial smooth muscle, autonomic control of the ureters occurs by diffuse transmitter release from multiple varicosities formed as the postganglionic axon courses over the smooth-muscle cell. *Sympathetic* input (via the aortic, hypogastric, and ovarian or spermatic plexuses) modulates ureteral contractility as

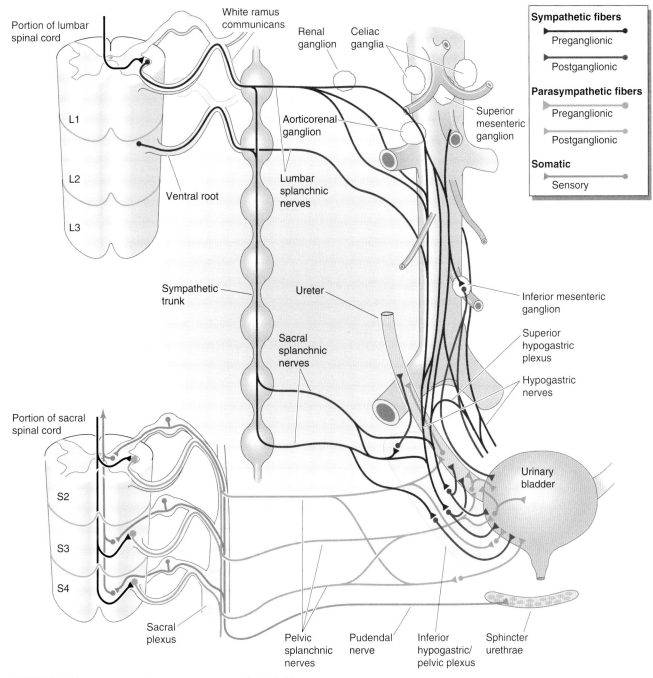

FIGURE 32–13. Autonomic and somatic innervation of the bladder.

norepinephrine acts via excitatory α-adrenergic receptors and inhibitory β-adrenergic receptors. *Parasympathetic* input enhances ureteral contractility via acetylcholine (ACh), either by direct stimulation of muscarinic cholinergic receptors (i.e., ACh receptors coupled to G proteins) or by causing postganglionic sympathetic fibers to release norepinephrine, which then can stimulate α-adrenoceptors. Some of the autonomic nerve fibers innervating the ureters are afferent **pain fibers**. In fact, the pain of renal colic associated with violent peristaltic contractions proximal to an obstruction is one of the most severe pains encountered in clinical practice.

The Urinary Bladder and Its Sphincters Are Innervated by Sympathetic, Parasympathetic, and Somatic Nerve Fibers

The urinary bladder is a hollow viscus, consisting of a main portion (body) that collects the urine, and a funnel-shaped extension (neck) that connects with the urethra (see Fig. 32–12A). A transitional epithelium lines the bladder lumen. Three poorly defined layers of smooth muscle make up the bulk of the bladder wall, the so-called **detrusor muscle**. At the lower tip of the trigone is the opening of the bladder lumen into the posterior urethra (i.e., distal part of bladder neck), which extends over 2 to 3 cm. The wall of the posterior urethra contains *smooth* muscle fibers of the detrusor muscle interspersed with elastic tissue, together forming the **internal sphincter** (Table 32–3). Immediately adjacent is the **external sphincter**, made up of voluntary, mainly slow-twitch *striated* muscle fibers.

In humans, bladder smooth muscle appears to lack gap junctions, suggesting the absence of electrotonic coupling between cells. Thus, the bladder smooth muscle is probably "multiunit" (p. 231), with a 1:1 ratio between nerve endings and smooth-muscle cells. Contraction of smooth muscle occurs by the same mechanisms found in other types of smooth-muscle cells, such as the ureteral smooth muscle described earlier.

The bladder and sphincters receive sympathetic and parasympathetic (autonomic) as well as somatic (voluntary) innervation (Fig. 32–13).

The **sympathetic innervation** to the bladder and internal sphincter arises from neurons in the intermediolateral cell column of the tenth thoracic to the second lumbar spinal cord segment (p. 379). The preganglionic fibers then pass via lumbar splanchnic nerves to the superior hypogastric plexus, where they give rise to left and right hypogastric nerves. These nerves lead to the inferior hypogastric/pelvic plexus, where preganglionic sympathetic fibers synapse with postganglionic fibers. After the synapses, these postganglionic fibers continue to the bladder wall via the distal portion of the hypogastric nerve. This distal portion also contains the preganglionic *parasympathetic* axons discussed in the next paragraph.

The **parasympathetic innervation** of the bladder originates from the intermediolateral cell column in segments S2 through S4 of the sacral spinal cord. The *parasympathetic* fibers approaching the bladder via the pelvic splanchnic nerve are still preganglionic. They synapse with postganglionic neurons in the body and neck of the urinary bladder.

TABLE 32–3

THE URETHRAL SPHINCTERS		
	INTERNAL SPHINCTER	**EXTERNAL SPHINCTER**
Type of muscle	Smooth	Skeletal
Nerve reaching the structure	Hypogastric	Pudendal
Nature of innervation	Autonomic	Somatic

The **somatic innervation** originates from motor neurons arising from segments S2 to S4. Via the pudendal nerve, these motor neurons innervate and control the voluntary skeletal muscle of the external sphincter (not shown in Fig. 32–13).

Filling the Bladder Triggers Stretch Receptors That Initiate the Micturition Reflex, a Spinal Reflex Arc That Is Also Under the Control of Higher Central Nervous System Centers

Bladder **tone** is defined by the relationship between bladder volume and internal ("intravesical") pressure. One can measure the volume-pressure relationship by first inserting a catheter through the urethra and emptying the bladder, and then recording the pressure while filling the bladder with 50-ml increments of water. The record of the relationship between volumes and pressure values is called a **cystometrogram** (Fig. 32–14, *blue curve*). Increasing bladder volume from 0 to approximately 50 ml produces a moderately steep increase in pressure. Additional increases in volume, up to approximately 300 ml, produce almost no pressure increase; this high compliance reflects relaxation of bladder smooth muscle. Above 400 ml, additional increases in volume produce steep increases in the "passive" pressure. Bladder tone—up to the point of triggering the micturition reflex—is independent of extrinsic bladder innervation.

Cortical and suprapontine centers in the brain normally

FIGURE 32–14. A cystometrogram.

PATHOPHYSIOLOGY OF MICTURITION

Lesions in the nervous system can lead to bladder dysfunction, the characteristics of which will depend on the site of the neural lesion. Three major classes of lesions can be distinguished.

1. **Combined afferent and efferent lesions.** Severing both afferent and efferent nerves initially causes the bladder to become distended and flaccid. In the chronic state of the so-called "decentralized bladder," many small contractions of the progressively hypertrophied bladder muscles replace the coordinated micturition events. Although small amounts of urine can be expelled, a residual volume of urine remains in the bladder after urination.

2. **Afferent lesions.** When only the sacral dorsal roots (sensory fibers) are interrupted, reflex contractions of the bladder, in response to stimulation of the stretch receptors, are totally abolished. The bladder frequently becomes distended, the wall thins, and bladder tone decreases. However, some residual contractions remain because of the intrinsic contractile response of smooth muscle to stretch. As a rule, a residual urine volume is present after urination.

3. **Spinal-cord lesions.** The effects of spinal-cord transection (e.g., in paraplegic patients) include the initial state of **spinal shock** in which the bladder becomes overfilled and exhibits sporadic voiding ("overflow incontinence"). With time, the voiding reflex is re-established, but with no voluntary control. Bladder capacity is often reduced and reflex hyperactivity may lead to a state called "spastic neurogenic bladder." Again, the bladder cannot empty completely, resulting in the presence of significant residual urine. Urinary-tract infections are frequent because the residual urine volume in the bladder serves as an incubator for bacteria. In addition, during the period of "overflow incontinence," before the voiding reflex is re-established, these patients have to be catheterized frequently, further predisposing to urinary tract infections.

exert an inhibitory influence on the micturition reflex, which the pontine micturition center (PMC) coordinates. The PMC controls both the bladder detrusor muscle and the urinary sphincters. During the **storage phase**, stretch receptors in the bladder send afferent information to the brain via the pelvic splanchnic nerves. One first senses the urge for voluntary bladder emptying at a volume of approximately 150 ml, and senses fullness at 400 to 500 ml. Nevertheless, until a socially acceptable opportunity to void presents itself, efferent impulses from the brain—in a learned reflex—inhibit presynaptic parasympathetic neurons in the sacral spinal cord that would otherwise stimulate the detrusor muscle in the bladder. In addition, voluntary contraction of the external urinary sphincter probably also contributes to storage.

The **voiding phase** begins with a voluntary relaxation of the external urinary sphincter, followed by the internal sphincter. When a small amount of urine reaches the proximal (posterior) urethra, afferents signal the cortex

that voiding is imminent. The micturition reflex now continues as suprapontine and pontine centers no longer inhibit the parasympathetic preganglionic neurons that innervate the detrusor muscle. As a result, the detrusor muscle of the bladder wall contracts, expelling urine. Once this micturition reflex has started, the initial contractions of the bladder lead to further trains of sensory impulses from stretch receptors, thus initiating a self-regenerating process (Fig. 32–14, *red spikes moving to the left*). At the same time, the cortical centers inhibit the external sphincter muscles. Voluntary urination also involves the voluntary contraction of abdominal muscles, which further raises bladder pressure and thus contributes to voiding and complete bladder emptying.

The basic bladder reflex that we have just discussed, although inherently an autonomic spinal cord reflex, may be either facilitated or inhibited by higher centers in the central nervous system that set the level at which the threshold for voiding occurs.

Because of the continuous flow of urine from the kidneys to the bladder, the function of the various sphincters, and the near-complete emptying of the bladder during the micturition, the entire urinary system is normally sterile.

REFERENCES

Books and Reviews

Seldin DW, Giebisch G (eds): The Kidney: Physiology and Pathophysiology, 3rd ed. Philadelphia, Lippincott Williams & Wilkins, 2000.

Ekblom P: Renal Development. In Seldin DW, Giebisch G (eds): The Kidney: Physiology and Pathophysiology, 2nd ed. New York, Raven Press, 1992.

Kriz W, Bankir L: A standard nomenclature for structures of the kidney. Kidney Int 33:1–7, 1988.

Moss NG, Colindres RE, Gottschalk CW: Neural control of renal function. In Windhager EE (ed): Handbook of Physiology, Section 8: Renal Physiology, Vol I. New York, Oxford University Press, 1992, pp 1061–1128.

Schuster V, Seldin DW: Renal Clearance. In Seldin DW, Giebisch G (eds): The Kidney: Physiology and Pathophysiology, 2nd ed. New York, Raven Press, 1992, pp 943–978.

Smith H: The Kidney: Structure and Function in Health and Disease. New York, Oxford University Press, 1951.

Tisher CC, Madsen KM: Anatomy of the kidney. In Brenner BM, Rector FC, Jr, (eds): The Kidney, 4th ed. Philadelphia, WB Saunders, 1992, pp 3–75.

Weiss RW: Physiology and pharmacology of the renal pelvis and ureter. In Walsh PC, Rettig AB, Vaughan E, Wein AJ (eds): Campbell's Urology, 7th ed. Philadelphia, WB Saunders, 1998, pp 839–870.

Journal Articles

Maxwell PH, Osmond MK, Pugh CW, et al: Identification of the renal erythropoietin-producing cells using transgenic mice. Kidney Internat 44:1149–1162, 1993.

Shannon JA: The excretion of inulin by the dog. Am J Physiol 112:405–413, 1935.

Smith HW, Finklestein N, Aliminosa L, et al: The renal clearances of substituted hippuric acid derivatives and other aromatic acids in dog and man. J Clin Invest 24:388–404, 1945.

Tamm I and FL Horsfall, Jr. A mucoprotein derived from human urine which reacts with influenza, mumps, and Newcastle disease viruses. J. Exp. Med. 95:71–97, 1952.

Walker AM, Bott PA, Oliver J, MacDowell MC: The collection and analysis of fluid from single nephrons of the mammalian kidney. Am J Physiol 134:580–595, 1941.

CHAPTER 33

Glomerular Filtration and Renal Blood Flow

Gerhard Giebisch and Erich Windhager

GLOMERULAR FILTRATION

A High Glomerular Filtration Rate Is Essential for Maintaining Stable and Optimal Extracellular Levels of Solutes and Water

Qualitatively, the filtration of blood plasma by the renal glomeruli is the same as the filtration of blood plasma across capillaries in other vascular beds (p. 470). Glomerular ultrafiltration results in the formation of a fluid with solute concentrations that are similar to those in plasma water; the exceptions are proteins and other high–molecular-weight compounds, which are present at reduced concentration. The glomerular filtrate, like filtrates formed across other body capillaries, is free of formed blood elements, such as red and white blood cells.

Quantitatively, the filtration that occurs in the glomeruli greatly exceeds that in all the other capillaries of the circulation combined. Compared with other organs, the kidneys receive an extraordinarily large amount of blood flow—normalized to the mass of the organ—and filter an unusually high fraction of this blood flow. Under normal conditions, the **glomerular filtration rate** (GFR; p. 747) of the two kidneys is 125 ml/min or 180 liters/day. Such a large rate of filtrate formation is required to expose the entire extracellular fluid frequently (more than 10 times a day) to the scrutiny of the renal-tubule epithelium. If it were not for such a high turnover of the extracellular fluid, only small volumes of blood would be "cleared" per unit time (p. 746) of certain solutes and water. Such a low clearance would have two harmful consequences for the renal excretion of solutes that renal tubules *cannot adequately secrete*.

First, in the face of a sudden increase in the plasma level of a toxic material—originating either from metabolism or food/fluid intake—the excretion of the material would be delayed. A high blood flow and high GFR allow the kidneys to eliminate harmful materials rapidly by filtration.

A second consequence of low clearance would be that steady-state plasma levels would be very high for waste materials that depend on filtration for excretion. The following example by Robert Pitts, a major contributor to renal physiology, illustrates the importance of this concept. Consider two individuals on a diet that contains 70 g/day of protein, one with normal renal function (e.g., GFR of 180 liters/day), the other a renal patient with sharply reduced glomerular filtration (e.g., GFR of 18 liters/day). Each individual produces 12 g/day of nitrogen in the form of urea

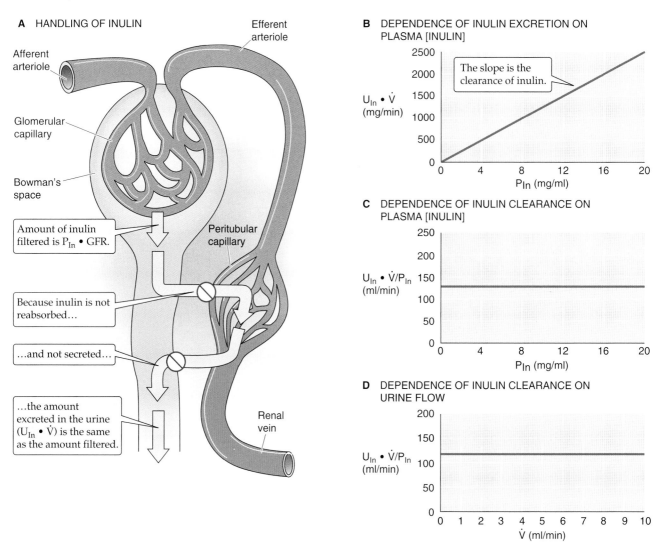

FIGURE 33–1. Clearance of inulin. GFR, glomerular filtration rate; P_{In}, plasma inulin concentration; U_{In}, urine inulin concentration; $\dot{V}$, urine flow.

("urea nitrogen") derived from dietary protein and must excrete this into the urine. However, these two individuals achieve urea balance at very different blood urea levels. We will make the simplifying assumption that the tubules neither absorb nor secrete urea, so that *only* filtered urea can be excreted, and *all* filtered urea is excreted. The normal individual can excrete 12 g/day of urea nitrogen from 180 liters of blood plasma having a [blood urea nitrogen] of 12 g/180 liters, or 6.7 mg/dl. In the patient whose GFR is reduced to 10% of normal, excreting 12 g/day of urea nitrogen requires that each of the 18 liters of filtered blood plasma has a [blood urea nitrogen] that is 10 times higher, or 67 mg/dl. Thus, excreting the same amount of urea nitrogen—to maintain a steady state—requires a much higher plasma [blood urea nitrogen] in the patient than in the normal individual.

The Clearance of Inulin Is a Measure of Glomerular Filtration Rate

Any substance X that has the same concentration in the glomerular filtrate as in plasma, and is neither reabsorbed

nor secreted along the nephron, could serve as a **glomerular marker** for measuring GFR (Fig. 33–1A). In Equation 32–4, we saw that:

$$\text{Equation 33–1}$$

$$\underbrace{P_X \cdot GFR}_{\substack{\text{Input into} \\ \text{Bowman's space}}} = \underbrace{U_X \cdot \dot{V}}_{\substack{\text{Output into} \\ \text{urine}}}$$

Units: (mg/ml) (ml/min) (mg/ml) (ml/min)

P_X is the concentration of the solute in plasma, *GFR* is the sum of volume flow from the plasma into all Bowman's spaces, U_X is the urine concentration of the solute, and $\dot{V}$ is the urine flow. Rearranging this equation,

$$\text{Equation 33–2}$$

$$GFR = \frac{U_X \cdot V}{P_X}$$

Units: $\dfrac{\text{ml}}{\text{min}} = \dfrac{(\text{mg/ml}) \cdot (\text{ml/min})}{(\text{mg/ml})}$

Note that Equation 33–2 has the same form as the

TABLE 33–1

CRITERIA FOR USE OF A SUBSTANCE TO MEASURE GFR

1. Substance must be freely filterable in the glomeruli.

2. Substance must be neither reabsorbed nor secreted by the renal tubules.

3. Substance must be neither metabolized nor produced by the kidney.

4. Substance must be physiologically inert (not toxic and without effect on renal function).

GFR, glomerular filtration rate.

clearance equation (Equation 32–3) and is identical to Equation 32–5. Thus, the plasma clearance of a glomerular marker is the *glomerular filtration rate*.

Inulin is an exogenous starch-like fructose polymer that is extracted from the Jerusalem artichoke and has a molecular weight of 5000. Inulin is freely filtered at the glomerulus, but neither reabsorbed nor secreted by the renal tubules. Additional requirements for a glomerular marker, which inulin also fulfills, are that the substance is not metabolized or synthesized by the kidney, is nontoxic, and has no effects on GFR (Table 33–1).

Assuming that GFR does not change, three tests prove that inulin clearance is an accurate marker of GFR. First, as shown in Figure 33–1B, the rate of inulin excretion $(U_{In} \cdot \dot{V})$ is directly proportional to the plasma inulin concentration (P_{In}), as implied by Equation 33–2. The slope in Figure 33–1B is the inulin clearance. Second, inulin clearance is independent of the plasma inulin concentration (see Fig. 33–1C). This conclusion was already implicit in Figure 33–1B, where the slope (i.e., inulin clearance) does not vary with P_{In}. Third, inulin clearance is independent of urine flow (see Fig. 33–1D). Given a particular P_{In}, after the renal corpuscles filter the inulin, the total amount of inulin in the urine does not change. Thus, diluting this glomerular marker in a large amount of urine or concentrating it in a small volume, does not affect the total amount of inulin excreted $(U_{In} \cdot \dot{V})$. If the urine flow is high, the urine inulin concentration will be proportionally low, and vice versa. Because $(U_{In} \cdot \dot{V})$ is fixed, $(U_{In} \cdot \dot{V})/P_{In}$ is also fixed.

Two lines of evidence provide direct proof that inulin clearance represents GFR. First, by collecting filtrate from single glomeruli, Richards and coworkers showed in 1941 that the concentration of inulin in Bowman's space of the mammalian kidney is the same as in plasma. Thus, inulin is freely filtered. Second, by perfusing single tubules with known amounts of labeled inulin, Marsh and Frasier showed that the renal tubules neither secrete nor reabsorb inulin.

Although the inulin clearance is the most reliable method for measuring GFR, it is not practical for clinical use. One must administer inulin intravenously to achieve reasonably constant plasma inulin levels. Another deterrent is that the chemical analysis for determining inulin levels in plasma and urine is sufficiently demanding to

render inulin unsuitable for routine use in a clinical laboratory.

The normal value for GFR in a 70-kg adult male is approximately 125 ml/min. Population studies show that GFR is proportional to body surface area. Because the surface area of an average 70-kg male is 1.73 m², the normal GFR in males is often reported as 125 ml/min per 1.73 m² of body surface area. In females, this figure is 110 ml/min per 1.73 m². Age is a second variable. GFR is very low in the newborn, owing to incomplete development of functioning glomerular units. Beginning at about age 2 years, GFR normalizes for body surface area and gradually falls off with age as a consequence of progressive loss of functioning nephrons.

The Clearance of Creatinine Is a Useful Clinical Index of GFR

Because inulin is not a convenient marker for routine clinical testing, nephrologists use other compounds that can be labeled with radioisotopes and that have clearances that are similar to those of inulin. The most commonly used compounds in human studies are ^{125}I-iothalamate, radioactive vitamin B_{12} ([57]Co- or [58]Co-cyanocobalamin) and ^{51}Cr-ethylenediaminetetraacetic acid (EDTA). However, these compounds are of limited reliability in GFR measurements because of variable binding to proteins and the loss of labeled iodine from the iothalamate.

The problems of intravenous infusion of a GFR marker can be completely avoided by using an *endogenous* substance with inulin-like properties. **Creatinine** is such a substance, and its clearance is a reasonable estimate of GFR in humans, but not all species. Tubules, to variable degree, secrete creatinine, which, by itself, would lead to an approximately 20% overestimate of GFR in humans. However, because commonly used colorimetric methods overestimate plasma creatinine concentrations, the calculated creatinine clearance turns out to be close to the inulin clearance. Thus, the effects of these two errors (i.e., tubule secretion and overestimated plasma levels) tend to cancel each other out. In clinical practice, determining the creatinine clearance is an easy and reliable means of assessing the GFR, and such determination avoids the need to inject anything into the patient. One merely obtains samples of venous blood and urine, analyzes them for creatinine concentration, and makes a simple calculation.

The source of plasma creatinine is the normal metabolism of **creatine phosphate** in muscle. In men, this metabolism generates creatinine at the rate of 20 to 25 mg/kg body weight per day (i.e., ~1.5 g/day in a 70-kg male). In women, the value is 15 to 20 mg/kg body weight per day (i.e., ~1.2 g/day in a 70-kg female), owing to a lower muscle mass. In the steady state, the rate of urinary creatinine excretion equals this rate of metabolic production. Therefore, to avoid errors in estimating the GFR from the creatinine clearance, one must take care to exclude non–steady state pathologic conditions of creatinine release, such as hyperthermia or other conditions of muscle wasting or damage. Ingestion of meat, which has a high creatinine content, also pro-

FIGURE 33–2. Dependence of plasma creatinine and blood urea nitrogen on the glomerular filtration rate (GFR). In the steady state, the amount of creatinine appearing in the urine per day ($U_{Cr} \cdot \dot{V}$) equals the production rate. Because all filtered creatinine ($P_{Cr} \cdot C_{Cr}$) appears in the urine, ($P_{Cr} \cdot C_{Cr}$) equals ($U_{Cr} \cdot \dot{V}$), which is constant. Thus, P_{Cr} must increase as C_{Cr} (i.e., GFR) decreases, and vice versa. If we assume that the kidney handles urea in the same way that it handles inulin, then a plot of blood urea nitrogen versus GFR will have the same shape as that of creatinine concentration versus GFR.

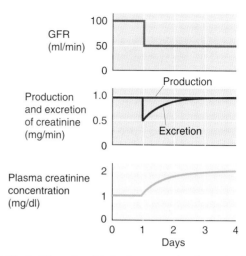

FIGURE 33–3. Effect of suddenly decreasing the glomerular filtration rate on plasma creatinine concentration.

duces non–steady state conditions. To minimize the effects of such an ingestion, the patient collects urine over an entire 24-hour period, and the plasma sample is obtained by venipuncture in the morning prior to breakfast.

Frequently, clinicians use the **endogenous plasma concentration of creatinine**, normally 1 mg/dl, as an instant index of GFR. This use rests on the inverse relationship between the plasma creatinine concentration (P_{Cr}) and the creatinine clearance (C_{Cr}):

Equation 33–3

$$C_{Cr} = \frac{U_{Cr} \cdot \dot{V}}{P_{Cr}}$$

In the steady state, when metabolic production in muscle equals the urinary excretion rate ($U_{Cr} \cdot \dot{V}$) of creatinine, and both remain fairly constant, this equation predicts that a plot of P_{Cr} versus C_{Cr} (i.e., P_{Cr} versus GFR) is a rectangular hyperbola (Fig. 33–2). For example, in a healthy person whose GFR is 100 ml/min, plasma creatinine is approximately 1 mg/dl. The product of GFR (100 ml/min) and P_{Cr} (1 mg/dl) is thus 1 mg/min, which is the rate of both creatinine production and of creatinine excretion. If GFR suddenly drops to 50 ml/min (Fig. 33–3, *top*), the kidneys will initially filter and excrete less creatinine (Fig. 33–3, *middle*), although the production rate is unchanged. As a result, the plasma creatinine level will rise to a new steady state, which is reached at a P_{Cr} of 2 mg/dl (see Fig. 33–3, *bottom*). At this point, the product of the reduced GFR (50 ml/min) and the elevated P_{Cr} (2 mg/dl) will again equal 1 mg/min, the rate of endogenous production of creatinine. Similarly, if GFR were to fall to one quarter of normal, P_{Cr} would rise to 4 mg/dl. This concept is reflected in the right-rectangular hyperbola of Figure 33–2.

Molecular Size, Electrical Charge, and Shape Determine the Filterability of Solutes across the Glomerular Filtration Barrier

The glomerular filtration barrier consists of three elements (p. 741): (1) endothelial cells, (2) the glomerular base-

ment membrane, and (3) epithelial podocytes. The latter two layers are covered with negative charges. Table 33–2 summarizes the permselectivity of the glomerular barrier for different solutes, as estimated by the ratio of solute concentration in the ultrafiltrate versus the plasma (UF_X/P_X). The ratio UF_X/P_X, also known as the **sieving coefficient** for the solute X, depends on molecular weight and effective molecular radius. Investigators have used two approaches to estimate UF_X/P_X. The first, which is valid for all solutes, is the **micropuncture** technique (see Fig. 32–10A). Sampling fluid from Bowman's space yields a direct measurement of UF_X, from which we can compute UF_X/P_X. The second approach, which is only valid for solutes that the kidney neither absorbs nor secretes, is to compute the **clearance ratio** (p. 749), the ratio of the clearances of X (C_X) and inulin (C_{In}).

Inspection of Table 33–2 shows that substances of low **molecular weight** (<5500 Da) and small **effective molecular radius**—such as water, urea, glucose, and inulin—appear in the filtrate in the same concentration as in plasma ($UF_X/P_X = 1$). In these instances, there is no sieving of the contents of the fluid moving through the glomerular "pores," so that the water moving through the filtration slits by convection carries the solutes with it. As a result, the concentration of the solute in the filtrate is the same as in bulk plasma. The situation is different for substances with a molecular weight that is above approximately 14 kDa, such as lysozyme. Larger and larger macromolecules are increasingly restricted from passage, so that only traces of plasma albumin (69 kDa) are normally present in the glomerular filtrate.

In addition to molecular weight and radius, **electrical charge** also makes a major contribution to the permselectivity of the glomerular barrier. Figure 33–4A is a plot of the clearance ratio for uncharged, positively charged, and negatively charged dextran molecules of varying molecular size. Two conclusions can be drawn from these data. First, *neutral* dextrans below an effective molecular radius of 2 nm pass readily across the glomerular barrier. For dextrans with a larger radius, the clearance ratio decreases with an increase in molecular size, so that passage ceases

TABLE 33–2

PERMSELECTIVITY OF THE GLOMERULAR BARRIER

SUBSTANCE	MOLECULAR WEIGHT (Da)	EFFECTIVE MOLECULAR RADIUS* (nm)	RELATIVE CONCENTRATION IN FILTRATE (UF$_X$/P$_X$)
Na$^+$	23	0.10	1.0
K$^+$	39	0.14	1.0
Cl$^-$	35.5	0.18	1.0
H$_2$O	18	0.15	1.0
Urea	60	0.16	1.0
Glucose	180	0.33	1.0
Sucrose	342	0.44	1.0
Polyethylene glycol	1,000	0.70	1.0
Inulin	5,200	1.48	0.98
Lysozyme	14,600	1.90	0.8
Myoglobin	16,900	1.88	0.75
Lactoglobulin	36,000	2.16	0.4
Egg albumin	43,500	2.80	0.22
Bence Jones protein	44,000	2.77	1.0
Hemoglobin	68,000	3.25	0.03
Serum albumin	69,000	3.55	<0.01

*The effective molecular radius is the Einstein-Stokes radius, which is the radius of a sphere that diffuses at the same rate as the substance under study.

Modified from Pitts RF: Physiology of the Kidney and Body Fluids, 3rd ed. Chicago, Year Book Medical Publishers, 1974.

when the radius exceeds 4.2 nm. Second, *anionic* dextrans (i.e., dextran sulfates) are restricted from filtration, whereas *cationic* dextrans (i.e., diethylaminoethyl dextrans) pass more readily into the filtrate. For negatively charged dextrans, the relationship between charge and filterability is characterized by a left shift of the curve relating molecular size to clearance ratio, whereas the opposite is true for positively charged dextrans.

The previously discussed results suggest that the glomerular filtration barrier carries a net negative charge that restricts the movement of anions but enhances the movement of cations. In experimental glomerulonephritis, in which the glomerular barrier loses its negative charge, the permeability of the barrier to negatively charged macromolecules is enhanced. Figure 33–4*B* compares clearance ratios of dextran sulfate in normal rats and in rats with nephrotoxic serum nephritis. Clearance ratios of dextran sulfate are uniformly greater in the animals with nephritis. Thus, the disease process destroys negative charges in the filtration barrier and accelerates the passage of negatively charged dextrans. Because albumin is also negatively charged at physiological pH, loss of negative charge in the glomerular barrier probably contributes in an important way to the development of albuminuria in the early stages of renal diseases such as glomerulonephritis.

Finally, the **shape** of macromolecules also affects the permselectivity of the glomerular barrier. Rigid or globular molecules have lower clearance ratios (i.e., sieving coeffi-

cients) than molecules of a similar size, such as dextrans, which are highly deformable.

The Hydrostatic Pressure in the Glomerular Capillary Favors Glomerular Ultrafiltration, Whereas the Oncotic Pressures in the Capillary and the Hydrostatic Pressure in Bowman' Space Oppose It

As is the case for filtration in other capillary beds (p. 470), glomerular ultrafiltration depends on the product of the ultrafiltration coefficient (K$_f$) and net Starling forces.

Equation 33–4

$$GFR = K_f \cdot [\underbrace{(P_{GC} - P_{BS}) - (\pi_{GC} - \pi_{BS})}_{P_{UF}}]$$

Figure 33–5*A* provides a schematic overview of the driving forces affecting ultrafiltration. P_{GC} is the hydrostatic pressure in the glomerular capillary, which favors ultrafiltration. P_{BS} is the hydrostatic pressure in Bowman's space, which opposes ultrafiltration. π_{GC} is the oncotic pressure in the glomerular capillary, which opposes ultrafiltration. Finally, π_{BS} is the oncotic pressure of the filtrate in Bowman's space, which favors ultrafiltration. Thus, two

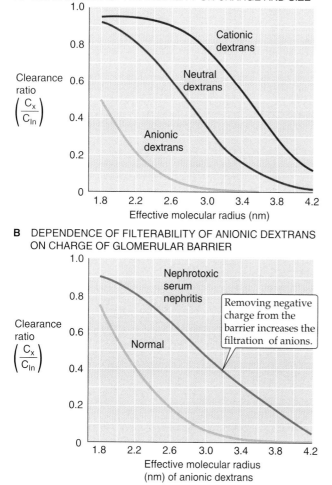

A DEPENDENCE OF FILTERABILITY ON CHARGE AND SIZE

B DEPENDENCE OF FILTERABILITY OF ANIONIC DEXTRANS
ON CHARGE OF GLOMERULAR BARRIER

FIGURE 33–4. Clearance ratio of dextrans. C_{In}, inulin clearance; C_X, clearance. (Data from Brenner BM, Hostetter TH, Humes HD: Molecular basis of proteinuria of glomerular origin. New England J Med 298:826–833, 1978.)

forces favor filtration (P_{GC} and π_{BS}), and two oppose it (P_{BS} and π_{GC}).

The **net driving force favoring ultrafiltration** (P_{UF}) at any point along the glomerular capillaries is the difference between the hydrostatic pressure difference and the oncotic pressure difference between the capillary and Bowman's space. Thus, the glomerular filtration rate is proportional to the net **hydrostatic force** ($P_{GC}-P_{BS}$) minus the net **oncotic force** ($\pi_{GC}-\pi_{BS}$). The first term of the hydrostatic pressure difference is the **pressure in the capillary lumen** (P_{GC}). As we will see later, the unique arrangement in which afferent and efferent arterioles flank the glomerular capillary keep P_{GC} at approximately 50 mm Hg (see Fig. 33–5B), a value that is twice as high as in most other capillaries. Moreover, direct measurements of pressure in rodents show that P_{GC} decays very little between the afferent and efferent ends of glomerular capillaries. The second term of the hydrostatic pressure difference is **the hydrostatic pressure in Bowman's space** (P_{BS}). This pressure is approximately 10 mm Hg, and does not vary along the capillary.

As far as the oncotic driving forces are concerned, the

first term is **the oncotic pressure in Bowman's space** (π_{BS}), which is very small (see Fig. 33–5B). The **oncotic pressure in the glomerular capillary** (π_{GC}) starts off at 25 mm Hg at the beginning of the capillary. As a consequence of the continuous production of a protein-free glomerular filtrate, the oncotic pressure of the fluid left behind in the glomerular capillary progressively rises along the capillary.

Figure 33–5C compares the two forces *favoring* ultrafiltration ($P_{GC} + \pi_{BS}$) with the two forces *opposing* ultrafiltration ($P_{BS} + \pi_{GC}$) and shows how they vary along the glomerular capillary. The rapid increase in the oncotic pressure of capillary blood (π_{GC}) is the major reason why the forces favoring and opposing filtration may balance each other at a point some distance before the end of the glomerular capillary. Beyond this point, P_{UF} is zero and the system is said to be in **filtration equilibrium** (i.e., no further filtration).

Note that K_f in Equation 33–4 is the product of the hydraulic conductivity of the capillary (L_p) and the effective surface area available for filtration (S_f), as defined earlier (p. 475). We use K_f because it is experimentally difficult to assign values to either L_p or S_f. Whereas P_{UF} is of similar order of magnitude in glomerular and systemic capillaries, the value of K_f of the glomerular filtration barrier exceeds—by more than an order of magnitude—the K_f of all other systemic capillary beds combined. This difference in K_f values underlies the tremendous difference in filtration, approximately 180 liters/day in the kidneys (which receive ~20% of the cardiac output) compared with approximately 20 liters/day in the combined *arteriolar* ends of capillary beds in the rest of the body (which receive the other ~80%). Of course, approximately 17 liters/day is reabsorbed at the *venular* end of these systemic capillaries owing to Starling forces, so that the net formation of lymph is approximately 3 liters/day (p. 475).

Alterations in the glomerular capillary surface area—owing to changes in mesangial-cell contractility (p. 743)—can produce substantial changes in the S_f component of K_f. These cells respond to extrarenal hormones such as systemically circulating angiotensin II, arginine vasopressin, and parathyroid hormone. Mesangial cells also produce several vasoactive agents, such as prostaglandins and angiotensin II.

RENAL BLOOD FLOW

Renal blood flow (RBF) is approximately 1 liter/min out of the total cardiac output of 5 liters/min. Normalized for weight, this blood flow amounts to approximately 350 ml/min for each 100 g of tissue, which is sevenfold higher than the normalized blood flow to the brain (p. 560). Renal *plasma* flow (RPF) is

Equation 33–5
$$RPF = (1 - Hct) \cdot RBF$$

Given a hematocrit (Hct) of 0.40 (p. 51), the "normal" RPF is approximately 600 ml/min.

A FORCES AFFECTING ULTRAFILTRATION

Afferent arteriole

Efferent arteriole

Bowman's space

P_{GC} π_{GC}

Two forces filter fluid out.

Two forces oppose ultrafiltration.

π_{BS} P_{BS}

P_{GC} = Glomerular capillary hydrostatic pressure
π_{BS} = Bowman's space oncotic pressure
P_{BS} = Bowman's space hydrostatic pressure
π_{GC} = Glomerular capillary oncotic pressure

B STARLING FORCES ALONG THE GLOMERULAR CAPILLARIES

Pressure (mm Hg)

P_{GC}
π_{GC}
P_{BS}
π_{BS}

C P_{UF} ALONG THE GLOMERULAR CAPILLARIES

Pressure (mm Hg)

P_{UF}

Favors filtration
$P_{GC} + \pi_{BS}$

When the forces balance, there is no filtration.

Opposes filtration
$P_{BS} + \pi_{GC}$

Afferent arteriole — Distance along glomerular capillary network → Efferent arteriole

FIGURE 33–5. Glomerular ultrafiltration. In *B*, the oncotic pressure of the glomerular capillary (π_{GC}), which starts off at the value of normal arterial blood, rises as ultrafiltration removes fluid from the capillary. In *C*, P_{UF} is the net driving force favoring ultrafiltration.

Increased Glomerular Plasma Flow Leads to an Increase in GFR

At low glomerular plasma flow (Fig. 33-6A), **filtration equilibrium** occurs halfway down the capillary. At higher plasma flow (i.e., normal for humans), the profile of net ultrafiltration forces (P_{UF}) along the glomerular capillary stretches out considerably to the right (see Fig. 33–6B) so that the point of equilibrium would be reached at a site actually beyond the end of the capillary. Failure to reach equilibrium (**filtration *disequilibrium***) occurs because the increased delivery of plasma to the capillary outstrips the ability of the filtration apparatus to remove fluid and simultaneously increase capillary oncotic pressure. As a result, π_{GC} rises more slowly along the length of the capillary.

The shift of filtration equilibrium toward the efferent arteriole has two important consequences. First, as one progresses along the capillary, P_{UF} (and hence filtration) remains greater. Second, filtration occurs along a greater stretch of the glomerular capillary, thereby increasing the useful surface area for filtration. Thus, the end of the capillary that is "wasted" at low plasma flow rates really is "in reserve" to contribute at higher rates.

A further increase in plasma flow stretches out the π_{GC} profile even more, so that P_{UF} is even higher at each point along the capillary (see Fig. 33–6C). Single-nephron glomerular filtration rate (SNGFR) is the sum of indi-

vidual filtration events along the capillary. Thus, SNGFR is proportional to the *yellow area* that represents the product of P_{UF} and effective (i.e., nonwasted) length along the capillary. Because the *yellow areas* progressively increase from Figure 33–6A to Figure 33–6C, SNGFR increases with glomerular plasma flow. However, this increase is not linear. Compared with the normal situation, the GFR summed for both kidneys increases only moderately with *increasing* RPF, but decreases greatly with *decreasing* RPF (see Fig. 33–6D).

The relationship between GFR and RPF also defines a parameter known as the **filtration fraction** (FF), which is the volume of filtrate that forms from a given volume of plasma entering the glomeruli:

Equation 33–6

$$FF = \frac{GFR}{RPF}$$

Because the "normal" GFR is approximately 125 ml/min and the normal RPF is approximately 600 ml/min, the normal FF is approximately 0.2. Because GFR saturates at high values of RPF, FF is greater at low plasma flows than it is at high plasma flows.

The dependence of GFR on plasma flow through the glomerular capillaries is similar to the dependence of alveolar O_2 and CO_2 transport on pulmonary blood flow (p. 682).

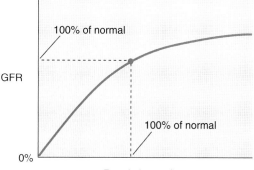

FIGURE 33–6. Dependence of the glomerular filtration rate (GFR) on plasma flow.

Afferent and Efferent Arteriolar Resistances Control Both Glomerular Plasma Flow and GFR

The renal microvasculature has two unique features. First, this vascular bed has two major sites of resistance control, the afferent and the efferent arterioles. Second, it has two capillary beds in series, the glomerular and the peritubular capillaries. As a consequence of this unique architecture, significant pressure drops occur in both arterioles (Fig. 33–7), glomerular-capillary pressure is relatively high throughout, and peritubular-capillary pressure is relatively low. Selective constriction or relaxation of the afferent and efferent arterioles allows for highly sensitive control of the hydrostatic pressure in the intervening glomerular capillary, and thus of glomerular filtration.

Figure 33–8A illustrates an idealized example in which we reciprocally change afferent and efferent arteriolar re-

sistance, while keeping total arteriolar resistance—and thus glomerular plasma flow—constant. Compared with an initial condition in which the afferent and efferent arteriolar resistances are the same (see Fig. 33–8A, *top panel*), constricting the *afferent* arteriole—while relaxing the efferent arteriole—lowers P_{GC} (see Fig. 33–8A, *middle panel*). Conversely, constricting the *efferent* arteriole—while relaxing the afferent arteriole—raises P_{GC} (see Fig. 33–8A, *lower panel*). From these idealized P_{GC} responses, one might predict that an increase in afferent arteriolar resistance would decrease the GFR and that an increase in efferent arteriolar resistance should have the opposite effect. However, physiological changes in the afferent and efferent arteriolar resistance usually do not keep overall arteriolar resistance constant. Thus, changes in arteriolar resistance generally lead to changes in glomerular plasma flow, which, as discussed earlier, can influence GFR independent of glomerular-capillary pressure.

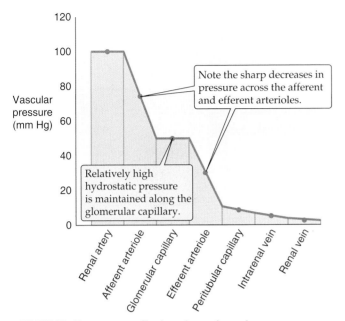

FIGURE 33–7. Pressure profile along the renal vasculature.

often leads to a significant fall in GFR. If we imagine that the peak of the GFR curve in Figure 33–8C represents the patient before treatment, then reducing the resistance of the efferent arteriole would indeed cause GFR to decrease.

The Peritubular Capillaries Provide Nutrients for Tubules and Retrieve the Fluid the Tubules Reabsorb

Peritubular capillaries originate from the efferent arterioles of the superficial and juxtamedullary glomeruli (see Fig. 32–1C). The capillaries from the superficial glomeruli form a dense network in the cortex, and those from the juxtamedullary glomeruli follow the tubules down into the medulla, where the capillaries are known as the vasa recta (p. 739). The peritubular capillaries have two main functions. First, these vessels deliver oxygen and nutrients to the epithelial cells. Second, they are responsible for taking up from the interstitial space the fluid that the renal tubules reabsorb.

The Starling forces that govern filtration in other capillary beds apply here as well (Fig. 33–9A). However, in peritubular capillaries, the pattern is unique. In "standard" systemic capillaries, Starling forces favor filtration at the arteriolar end and absorption at the venular end (p. 470). Glomerular capillaries resemble the early part of these "standard" capillaries: the Starling forces always favor filtration (see Fig. 33–9B, *yellow area*). The peritubular capillaries are like the late part of "standard" capillaries: the Starling forces always favor absorption (see Fig. 33–9C, *brown area*).

What makes peritubular capillaries unique is that glomerular capillaries and the efferent arteriole precede them. Glomerular filtration elevates the oncotic pressure of blood entering the peritubular capillary network (π_{PC}) to approximately 35 mm Hg. In addition, the resistance of the efferent arteriole decreases the intravascular hydrostatic pressure (P_{PC}) to approximately 20 mm Hg (see Fig. 33–9A). Interstitial oncotic pressure (π_o) is 4 to 8 mm Hg, and interstitial hydrostatic pressure (P_o) is probably 6 to 10 mm Hg. The net effect is a large net absorptive pressure at the beginning of the peritubular capillary. Along the peritubular capillary, π_{PC} falls modestly because of the reabsorption of protein-poor fluid from the interstitium into the capillary, and hydrostatic pressure probably falls modestly as well. Even so, the Starling forces remain solidly in favor of absorption along the entire length of the peritubular capillary, falling from approximately 17 mm Hg at the arteriolar end to approximately 12 mm Hg at the venular end (see Fig. 33–9C).

The net absorptive force at the beginning of the peritubular capillaries is subject to the vagaries of glomerular fluid dynamics. For instance, expansion of the extracellular fluid volume (Fig. 33–10) inhibits the renin-angiotensin system (p. 866), leading to a relatively larger decrease in efferent than in afferent arteriolar resistance and therefore a rise in P_{PC}. The fall in total arteriolar resistance causes a rise in RPF that is larger than the rise in GFR, resulting in a fall in filtration fraction. Thus, more fluid remains inside the glomerular capillary, and

Figures 33–8B and 33–8C show somewhat more realistic effects on RPF and GFR as we change the resistance of a *single* arteriole. With a selective increase of *afferent* arteriolar resistance (see Fig. 33–8B), both capillary pressure and RPF decrease, leading to a monotonic decline in the GFR. In contrast, a selective increase of *efferent* arteriolar resistance (see Fig. 33–8C) causes a steep increase in glomerular capillary pressure but also a decrease in RPF. As a result, over the lower range of resistances, GFR increases with efferent resistance as an increasing P_{GC} dominates. On the other hand, at higher resistances, GFR begins to fall as the effect of a declining RPF dominates. These opposing effects on glomerular capillary pressure and RPF account for the biphasic dependence of GFR on efferent resistance.

The examples in Figures 33–8B and 33–8C, in which only afferent or efferent resistance increased, are still somewhat artificial. During sympathetic stimulation, or in response to angiotensin II, both afferent *and* efferent resistances increase. Thus, RPF decreases. The generally opposing effects on GFR of increasing both afferent resistance (see Fig. 33–8B) and efferent resistance (see Fig. 33–8C) explain why the combination of both keeps GFR fairly constant despite a decline in RPF.

There are realistic examples in which changes in either the afferent or the efferent arteriolar resistance dominates. A striking case in which a decrease in *afferent arteriolar* resistance dominates is the large increase in RPF that occurs with the loss of renal tissue, as after a nephrectomy in a kidney donor. GFR in the **remnant kidney** nearly doubles, owing primarily to a dramatic *decrease* in the resistance of the afferent arteriole (see Fig. 33–8B).

An example of a predominantly *efferent arteriolar* effect is seen after administration of angiotensin II inhibitors (e.g., captopril) to patients with hypertension that is due to increased endogenous angiotensin levels. Administering such agents not only decreases blood pressure, but also

A RECIPROCAL CHANGES IN AFFERENT AND
EFFERENT ARTERIOLAR RESISTANCE

B CONSTRICTION OF ONLY *AFFERENT* ARTERIOLE   **C** CONSTRICTION OF ONLY *EFFERENT* ARTERIOLE

FIGURE 33–8. Role of afferent and efferent arteriolar resistance on pressure and flows. In *A*, the sum of afferent and efferent arteriolar resistance is always 2, whereas in *B* and *C*, the total resistance changes. GFR, glomerular filtration rate; RPF, renal plasma flow.

the blood entering the peritubular capillaries has an oncotic pressure that is below normal. The fall in efferent arteriolar resistance also raises the hydrostatic pressure in the peritubular capillaries. As a consequence of the low π_{PC} and high P_{PC}, the peritubular capillaries take up less interstitial fluid. An additional consequence, discussed in Chapter 34, is that the altered interstitial forces reduce fluid absorption—from the tubule lumen to the interstitium—by the proximal tubule. Thus, a change in glomerular dynamics leads to a decrease in uptake of interstitial fluid. The reverse sequence of events takes place during volume contraction and in chronic heart failure. We discuss the effect of such hemodynamic changes on Na$^+$ and fluid transport on page 784.

Lymphatic capillaries are mainly found in the cortex.

They provide an important route for removing protein from the interstitial fluid. Proteins leak continuously from the peritubular capillaries into the interstitial fluid. Total renal lymph flow is small and amounts to less than 1% of RPF.

Blood Flow in the Renal Cortex Exceeds That in the Renal Medulla

Measurements of regional blood flow in the kidney show that approximately 90% of the blood leaving the glomeruli in efferent arterioles perfuses cortical tissue. The remaining 10% perfuses the renal medulla, with only 1% to 2% reaching the papilla. The relatively low blood flow

A GLOMERULAR AND PERITUBULAR CAPILLARIES

B P_{UF} ALONG GLOMERULAR CAPILLARIES

C NET ABSORPTIVE PRESSURE ALONG PERITUBULAR CAPILLARIES

FIGURE 33–9. Starling forces along the *peritubular* capillaries. BS, Bowman's space; GC, glomerular capillary; O, interstitial fluid; P, hydrostatic pressure; PC, peritubular capillary; π, colloid osmotic pressure; P_{UF}, ultrafiltration pressure.

FIGURE 33–10. Effect of volume expansion on fluid uptake by peritubular capillaries.

through the medulla, a consequence of the high resistance of the long vasa recta, is important for minimizing wash-out of the hypertonic medullary interstitium, and thus for producing a concentrated urine (p. 837).

The Clearance of Para-Aminohippurate Is a Measure of Renal Plasma Flow

As discussed in Chapter 32, for any solute (X) that the kidney neither metabolizes nor produces, the only route of entry to the kidney is the renal artery, and the only two routes of exit are the renal vein and the ureter (p. 747):

Equation 33–7

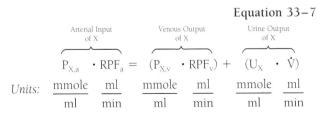

$$\underbrace{P_{X,a} \cdot RPF_a}_{\substack{\text{Arterial Input}\\\text{of X}}} = \underbrace{(P_{X,v} \cdot RPF_v)}_{\substack{\text{Venous Output}\\\text{of X}}} + \underbrace{(U_X \cdot \dot{V})}_{\substack{\text{Urine Output}\\\text{of X}}}$$

Units: $\dfrac{mmole}{ml} \quad \dfrac{ml}{min} \qquad \dfrac{mmole}{ml} \quad \dfrac{ml}{min} \qquad \dfrac{mmole}{ml} \quad \dfrac{ml}{min}$

The above equation (a restatement of Equation 32–1)

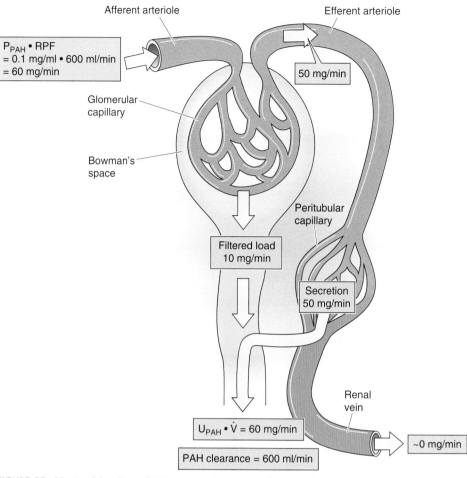

FIGURE 33–11. Renal handling of PAH. P_{PAH} and U_{PAH} are plasma and urine concentrations of PAH. RPF, renal plasma flow; $\dot{V}$, urine flow.

is an application of the Fick principle used for measurements of regional blood flow (p. 442). To estimate renal arterial plasma flow (RPF_a)—or, more simply, RPF—we could in principle use the clearance of *any substance* that the kidney measurably excretes into the urine, as long it is practical to obtain samples of systemic arterial plasma, renal venous plasma, and urine. The problem, of course, is sampling blood from the renal vein.

However, we can avoid the need for sampling the renal vein if we choose a substance that the kidneys clear so efficiently that they leave almost *none* in the renal vein. **Para-aminohippuric acid** (PAH) is just such a substance (p. 747). Because PAH is an organic acid that is not normally present in the body, PAH must be administered by continuous intravenous infusion. Some PAH binds to plasma proteins, but a significant amount remains freely dissolved in the plasma, and therefore filters into Bowman's space. However, the kidney filters only approximately 20% of the renal plasma flow (i.e., FF = ~0.2), and a major portion of the PAH remains in the plasma that flows out of the efferent arterioles. PAH diffuses out of the peritubular capillary network and reaches the basolateral surface of the proximal-tubule cells. These cells have a high capacity to secrete PAH from blood into the tubule lumen against large concentration gradients.

This PAH-secretory system (p. 799) is so efficient that—as long as we do not overwhelm it by infusing too much PAH—almost no PAH (~10%) remains in the renal venous blood. We assume that all of the PAH presented to the kidney appears in the urine:

Equation 33–8
$$\begin{matrix} \text{PAH excreted} & = & \text{PAH filtered} & + & \text{PAH secreted} \\ \text{in urine} & & \text{in glomerulus} & & \text{by tubules} \end{matrix}$$

In the example of Figure 33–11, the concentration of filterable PAH in the arterial blood plasma (P_{PAH}) is 10 mg/dl or 0.1 mg/ml. If RPF is 600 ml/min, then the arterial load of PAH to the kidney is 60 mg/min. Of this amount, 10 mg/min appears in the glomerular filtrate. If the tubules secrete the remaining 50 mg/min, then the entire 60 mg/min of PAH presented to the kidney appears in the urine. That is, the kidneys clear the entire quantity of PAH that is presented to them during a single passage of blood. In practice, the kidneys excrete approximately 90% of the arterial load of PAH when P_{PAH} does not exceed 12 mg/dl.

As long as we do not infuse too much PAH—that is, as long as virtually no PAH remains in the renal venous

FIGURE 33–12. Autoregulation of renal blood flow and glomerular filtration rate (GFR). (Data from Arendshorst WJ, Finn WF, Gottschalk CW: Autoregulation of renal blood flow in the rat kidney. *Am J Physiol* 228:127–133, 1975.)

blood—Equation 33–7 reduces to the equation for the clearance of PAH, as introduced in Table 32–2B:

$$\text{Equation 33–9}$$

$$C_{PAH} = RPF = \frac{U_{PAH} \cdot \dot{V}}{P_{PAH}}$$

If we apply this equation to the example in Figure 33–11:

$$\text{Equation 33–10}$$

$$C_{PAH} = RPF = \frac{60 \text{ mg/min}}{10 \text{ mg/dl}}$$

$$= \frac{60 \text{ mg/min}}{0.1 \text{ mg/ml}} = 600 \text{ ml/min}$$

To compute RPF, we need to collect a urine sample to obtain ($U_{PAH} \cdot \dot{V}$) and a blood sample to obtain P_{PAH}. However, the blood sample need not be arterial. For example, one can obtain venous blood from the arm, inasmuch as skeletal muscle extracts negligible amounts of PAH.

CONTROL OF RENAL BLOOD FLOW AND GLOMERULAR FILTRATION

Autoregulation, Which Involves Both a Renal Myogenic and a Tubuloglomerular Feedback Mechanism, Keeps Renal Blood Flow and GFR Relatively Constant

An important feature of the renal circulation is its remarkable ability to maintain RBF and GFR within narrow limits, even though mean arterial pressure may vary between approximately 80 and 170 mm Hg (Fig. 33–12, *middle and bottom panels*). Stability of blood flow—known as **autoregulation** (p. 480)—is also a property of the vascular beds serving two other vital organs, the brain and the heart. Perfusion to all three of these organs must be preserved in emergency situations, such as hypotensive

shock. Autoregulation of the renal blood supply is independent of the influence of renal nerves and circulating hormones, and persists even when one perfuses isolated kidneys with erythrocyte-free solutions. Autoregulation of RBF—and, consequently, autoregulation of GFR, which depends on RBF (see Fig. 33–6D)—stabilizes the filtered load of solutes that reach the tubules over a wide range of arterial pressures. Autoregulation of RBF also protects the fragile glomerular capillaries against increases in perfusion pressure that might lead to structural damage.

The kidney autoregulates RBF by responding to a rise in renal arterial pressure with a proportional increase in the resistance of the afferent arterioles. Autoregulation comes into play during alterations in arterial pressure that occur, for example, during changes in posture, light to moderate exercise, and sleep. It is the *afferent arteriole* where the autoregulatory response occurs, and where the resistance to flow rises with increasing perfusion pressure (see Fig. 33–12, *top panel*). In contrast, *efferent* arteriolar resistance, capillary resistance and venous resistance all change very little over a wide range of renal arterial pressures.

Two basic mechanisms— equally important—underlie renal autoregulation: a myogenic response of the smooth muscle of the afferent arterioles and a tubuloglomerular feedback mechanism.

MYOGENIC RESPONSE. The afferent arterioles have the inherent ability to respond to changes in vessel-wall tension by contracting or relaxing, a myogenic response (p. 478). It appears that an increase in vessel diameter opens stretch-activated, nonselective cation channels in vascular smooth muscle, depolarizing the cell and leading to an influx of Ca^{2+} that stimulates contraction.

TUBULOGLOMERULAR FEEDBACK. The juxtaglomerular apparatus (JGA; p. 743) mediates the tubuloglomerular feedback (TGF) mechanism. The **macula densa** cells in the thick ascending limb sense an increase in GFR and, in classical feedback fashion, translate this to an increase in the tone of the afferent arteriole, and hence a decrease in GFR.

Experimental evidence for the existence of a TGF mechanism rests on measurements of SNGFR. One introduces a wax block into the lumen of the proximal tubule to block luminal flow (Fig. 33–13A). Upstream from the wax block, a pipette collects the fluid needed to compute SNGFR (see Equation 32–13). Downstream to this oil block, another pipette perfuses the loop of Henle with known solutions and at selected flows. The key observation is that an inverse relationship exists between the late-proximal perfusion rate (i.e., fluid delivery to macula densa) and SNGFR (see Fig. 33–13B).

The mechanism of this TGF is thought to be the following. An increase in arterial pressure leads to increases in glomerular-capillary pressure, RPF and GFR. The increase in GFR leads to an increased delivery of Na^+ and Cl^- and fluid into the proximal tubule and, ultimately, to the macula densa cells of the JGA. The macula densa does not sense flow per se, but the higher luminal $[Na^+]$ or $[Cl^-]$ resulting from high flow. Because of high Na/K/Cl cotransporter activity at the apical membrane of the macula-densa cell, increases in luminal $[Na^+]$ and $[Cl^-]$ trans-

A EXPERIMENTAL PREPARATION

B DEPENDENCE OF SNGFR ON DISTAL-TUBULE FLOW

FIGURE 33–13. Tubuloglomerular feedback. SNGFR, single nephron glomerular filtration rate. (Data from *B* is modified from Navar LG: Regulation of renal hemodynamics *Adv Physiol Educ* 20:S221–S235, 1998.)

TABLE 33–3

MODULATION OF TUBULOGLOMERULAR FEEDBACK

Factors That *Increase* Sensitivity of TGF
Volume Contraction

Adenosine

PGE₂

Thromboxane

HETE

Angiotensin II

Factors That *Decrease* Sensitivity of TGF
Volume Expansion

ANP

NO

cAMP

PGI₂

High-protein diet

ANP, atrial natriuretic peptide; cAMP, cyclic adenosine mono-phosphate; HETE, hydroxyeicosatetraenoic [acid]; NO, nitric oxide; PGE₂, prostaglandin E₂; PGI₂, prostaglandin I₂.

late to parallel increases in intracellular concentrations of these two ions. Indeed, blocking the Na/K/Cl cotransporter with furosemide (p. 67) not only blocks the uptake of Na^+ and Cl^- into the macula densa cells, but also interrupts tubuloglomerular feedback. The rise in $[Cl^-]_i$, in conjunction with a Cl^- channel at the basolateral membrane, apparently leads to a depolarization, which activates a nonselective cation channel, which in turn allows Ca^{2+} to enter the macula densa cell. The result is an increase in $[Ca^{2+}]_i$ that causes the macula densa cell to release paracrine agents (perhaps adenosine triphosphate, adenosine, thromboxane, or other substances) that may trigger contraction of nearby vascular smooth-muscle cells. A1 adenosine receptors on the smooth muscle cells may be particularly important in this response. The net effect is an increase in afferent arteriolar resistance and a decrease in GFR, thereby counteracting the initial increase in GFR.

Several factors increase or decrease the sensitivity of the TGF mechanism (see Fig. 33–13B). Indeed, investigators have suggested that several of these factors may be physiological signals from the macula densa cells or that they modulate these signals (Table 33–3).

Volume Expansion and a High-Protein Diet Increase GFR by Reducing Tubuloglomerular Feedback

The **sensitivity** of TGF is defined as the change in SNGFR for a given change in the perfusion rate of the

TABLE 33–4

HEMODYNAMIC ACTIONS OF ANGIOTENSIN II ON THE KIDNEY

SITE	ACTION	PROPERTIES
Renal artery and afferent arteriole	Constriction	▷ Ca^{2+} influx through voltage-gated channels ▷ Inhibited by prostaglandins
Efferent arteriole	Constriction	▷ May depend on Ca^{2+} mobilization from internal stores ▷ Insensitive to Ca^{2+}-channel blockers ▷ Prostaglandins may counteract the constriction during volume contraction or low effective circulating volume
Mesangial cells	Contraction with reduction in K_f	▷ Ca^{2+} influx ▷ Ca^{2+} mobilization from internal stores
Tubuloglomerular feedback mechanism	Increased sensitivity	▷ Increased responsiveness of afferent arteriole to signal from macula densa
Medullary blood flow	Reduction	▷ May be independent of changes in cortical blood flow

Modified from Arendshorst WJ, Navar LG. In Schrier RW, Gottschalk CW: Diseases of The Kidney, Vol 1, 5th ed. Boston, Little, Brown, 1993, pp. 65–117.

loop of Henle. Thus, sensitivity is the absolute value of the slope of the curves in Figure 33–13B. The **set point** of the feedback system is defined as the loop-perfusion rate at which SNGFR falls by 50%.

Both the intrinsic sensitivity of the macula densa mechanism and the initial set point for changes in flow are sensitive to changes in the extracellular fluid volume. Expansion of the extracellular fluid decreases the sensitivity (i.e., steepness) of the overall feedback loop. Conversely, volume contraction increases the sensitivity of TGF, helping preserve fluid by reducing GFR.

Of clinical importance may be the observation that a **high-protein diet** increases the GFR and RPF by indirectly lowering the sensitivity of the TGF mechanism. A high-protein diet somehow enhances NaCl reabsorption along the thick ascending limb, so that luminal [NaCl] at the macula densa falls. As a consequence, the flow in the loop of Henle (and thus GFR) must be higher to raise [NaCl] to a particular level at the macula densa. A high-protein diet may decrease tubuloglomerular feedback, and thus increase glomerular capillary pressure. This sequence of events may lead, particularly in the presence of intrinsic renal disease, to permanent glomerular damage.

Four Factors That Modulate RBF and GFR Play Key Roles in Regulating Effective Circulating Volume

Changes in effective circulating volume (p. 556) trigger responses in four parallel effector pathways that ultimately modulate either renal hemodynamics or renal Na^+ reabsorption. The four effector pathways are: (1) the renin-angiotensin-aldosterone axis, (2) the sympathetic nervous system, (3) arginine vasopressin, and (4) atrial natriuretic peptide. In Chapter 39, we discuss the integrated control of effective circulating volume. Here, we focus on the direct actions of the four effector pathways on renal hemodynamics.

RENIN-ANGIOTENSIN-ALDOSTERONE AXIS. In terms of renal hemodynamic effects, the most important part of this axis is its middle member, the peptide hormone angiotensin II (p. 866). ANG II has multiple actions on renal hemodynamics (Table 33–4), the overall effect of which is to reduce blood flow and GFR.

SYMPATHETIC DIVISION OF THE AUTONOMIC NERVOUS SYSTEM. Sympathetic tone to the kidney may increase either as part of a general response—as occurs with pain, stress, trauma, hemorrhage or exercise—or as part of a more selective renal response to a decrease in effective circulating volume (p. 867). In either case, sympathetic nerve terminals release **norepinephrine** into the interstitial space. At relatively high levels of nerve stimulation, both afferent and efferent arteriolar resistances rise, generally decreasing RBF and GFR. The observation that the RBF may fall more than the GFR is consistent with a preferential *efferent* arteriolar constriction. With maximal nerve stimulation, however, afferent vasoconstriction predominates and leads to drastic reductions in both RBF and GFR.

In addition, sympathetic stimulation triggers granular cells to increase their release of renin, raising levels of ANG II (p. 867), which acts as described earlier. Finally, sympathetic tone signals tubule cells to increase their reabsorption of Na^+ (p. 787).

ARGININE VASOPRESSIN. In response to increases in the osmotic pressure of the extracellular fluid, the posterior pituitary releases arginine vasopressin (AVP)—also known as antidiuretic hormone (p. 840). Although the principal effect of this small polypeptide is to increase water absorption in the collecting duct, AVP also increases vascular resistance. Despite physiological fluctuations of circulating AVP levels, total RBF and GFR remain nearly constant. Nevertheless, AVP may decrease blood flow to the renal *medulla*, thereby minimizing the washout of the hypertonic medulla; this hypertonicity is essential for forming a concentrated urine.

In amphibians, reptiles, and birds, the generalized vascular effects of AVP are more pronounced than they are in mammals. In humans, severe decreases in effective circulating volume (e.g., shock) cause a massive release of AVP via nonosmotic stimuli (p. 586). Only under these conditions does AVP produce a systemic vasoconstriction and thus contribute to maintaining systemic blood pressure (p. 555).

ATRIAL NATRIURETIC PEPTIDE. Atrial myocytes release atrial natriuretic peptide (ANP) in response to increased atrial pressure, and thus effective circulating volume (p. 867). The major effect of ANP is hemodynamic: it markedly vasodilates afferent and efferent arterioles, thereby increasing cortical and medullary blood flow, and lowers the sensitivity of the TGF mechanism (see Table 33–3). The net effect is an increase in RPF and GFR. ANP also affects renal hemodynamics indirectly, by inhibiting secretion of renin (thus lowering ANG II levels) and AVP. At higher levels, ANP decreases systemic arterial pressure and increases capillary permeability. ANP plays a role in the diuretic response to the redistribution of extracellular fluid and plasma volume into the thorax that occurs during space flight and water immersion (p. 1266).

Other Vasoactive Agents Modulate RBF and GFR

Many vasoactive agents—in addition to the ones discussed in the previous section—modulate RBF and GFR when infused systemically or applied locally to the renal vasculature. Despite considerable research on such hemodynamic actions, the precise role of individual vasoactive agents in the response to physiological and pathophysiological stimuli remains uncertain. At least three kinds of observations have complicated our understanding: (1) several agents with opposing actions are often released simultaneously; (2) blocking a specific vasoactive messenger may have relatively little effect on renal hemodynamics; (3) a single vasoactive agent may have different, or even opposing, actions at low and high concentrations. Nevertheless, renal and extrarenal agents may cooperate to provide a full and physiologically adequate response to a wide spectrum of challenges.

EPINEPHRINE. Released by the chromaffin cells of the adrenal medulla (p. 1061), epinephrine exerts dose-dependent effects on the kidney that are similar to those of norepinephrine (see earlier).

DOPAMINE. Dopaminergic nerve fibers terminate in the kidney, and dopamine receptors are present in renal blood vessels. The renal effect of dopamine is to vasodilate, which is opposite to the effects of epinephrine and norepinephrine.

ENDOTHELINS. The endothelins are peptides with a strong vasoconstrictor action (p. 480), but a very short half-life. The hemodynamic actions of endothelins are limited to local effects, because little of this hormone escapes into the general circulation. In the kidney, several agents—ANG II, epinephrine, higher does of AVP, thrombins, and shear stress—trigger release of endothelins from the endothelium of renal cortical vessels and mesangial cells. The endothelins act locally to constrict smooth muscles of renal vessels and thus most likely are a link in the complex network of local messengers between endothelium and smooth muscle. When administered systemically, endothelins constrict the afferent and efferent arterioles and reduce the ultrafiltration coefficient (K_f). The result is a sharp reduction in both RBF and GFR.

PROSTAGLANDINS. In the kidney, vascular smooth-muscle cells, endothelial cells, mesangial cells, and tubule and interstitial cells of the renal medulla are particularly important for synthesizing the locally acting prostaglandins from arachidonic acid, via the cyclooxygenase pathway (p. 104). The effects of prostaglandins are complex and depend on the baseline vasoconstriction exerted by ANG II. Indeed, prostaglandins appear mainly to be protective and are important under conditions when the integrity of the renal circulation is threatened. In particular, local intrarenal effects of prostaglandins provide a buffer against excessive vasoconstriction, especially during increased sympathetic outflow to the kidney or activation of the renin-angiotensin system. Accelerated prostaglandin synthesis and release are responsible for maintaining fairly constant blood flow and GFR in conditions of high ANG II levels—for example, during surgery, following blood loss, or in the course of salt depletion.

LEUKOTRIENES. Probably in response to inflammation, the renal vascular smooth-muscle cells and glomeruli—as well as leukocytes and blood platelets—synthesize several leukotrienes from arachidonic acid, via the lipoxygenase pathway (p. 106). These locally acting vasoactive agents are strong vasoconstrictors; their infusion reduces RBF and GFR.

NITRIC OXIDE. The endothelial cells of the kidney use nitrous oxide synthase (NOS) to generate NO from L-arginine (p. 110). NO has a strong smooth-muscle–relaxing effect and—under physiological, unstressed conditions—produces significant renal vasodilation. NO probably defends against excess vasoconstrictor effects of agents such as ANG II and epinephrine. Injecting NOS inhibitors into the systemic circulation constricts afferent and efferent arterioles, increasing renal vascular resistance and producing a sustained fall of RBF and GFR. Moreover, NOS inhibitors blunt the vasodilatation that is triggered by low rates of fluid delivery to the macula-densa part of the TGF mechanism.

REFERENCES

Books and Review

Maddox DA, Brenner BM: Glomerular ultrafiltration. In Brenner BM (ed): The Kidney, 6th ed. Philadelphia, WB Saunders, 2000, pp 319–374.

Navar LG, Inscho WE, Majid DSA, et al: Paracrine regulation of the renal microcirculation. Physiol Rev 76: 425–537, 1996.

Schnermann J, Traynor T, Yang T, et al: Tubuloglomerular feedback: New concepts and developments. Kidney Int 54:S40–S45, 1998.

Seldin DW, Giebisch G (eds): The Kidney: Physiology and Pathophysiology, 3rd ed. Philadelphia, Lippincott Williams & Wilkins, 2000.

Stockand JD, Sansom SC: Glomerular mesangial cells: Electrophysiology and regulation of contraction. Physiol Rev 78:723–744, 1998.

Journal Articles

Arendshorst WJ, Finn WF, Gottschalk CW: Autoregulation of renal blood flow in the rat kidney. Am J Physiol 228:127–133, 1975.

Brenner BM, Troy JL, Daugharty TM, et al: Dynamics of glomerular ultrafiltration in the rat. II. Plasma flow dependence of GFR. Am J Physiol 223:1184–1190, 1972.

Lapointe J-Y, Laamarti A, Bell PD: Ionic transport in macula densa cells. Kidney Int 54:S58–S64, 1998.

Robertson CR, Deen WM, Troy JL, Brenner BM: Dynamics of glomerular ultrafiltration in the rat. III. Hemodynamics and autoregulation. Am J Physiol 223:1191–1200, 1972.

Wilcox CS, Welch WJ, Murad F, et al: Nitric oxide synthase in macula densa regulates glomerular capillary pressure. Proc Natl Acad Sci USA 89:11993–11997, 1992.

CHAPTER 34

Transport of Sodium and Chloride

Gerhard Giebisch and Erich Windhager

The kidneys help to maintain the body's extracellular fluid (ECF) volume by regulating the amount of Na^+ in the urine. Sodium is the most important contributor to the overall osmolality of the ECF; hence, where Na^+ goes, water follows. This chapter focuses on how the kidneys maintain the ECF volume by regulating Na^+ and its most prevalent anion, Cl^-.

The normal daily urinary excretion of Na^+ is only a tiny fraction of the total Na^+ filtered by the kidneys (Fig. 34–1). The filtered load of Na^+ is the product of the glomerular filtration rate (GFR, ~180 liters/day) and the plasma Na^+ concentration (~142 mM; see Table 3–2), or approximately 25,500 mmole/day. This amount is equivalent to the Na^+ in approximately 1.5 kg of table salt, more than nine times the total quantity of Na^+ present in the body fluids! With a typical Western diet containing approximately 120 mmole of Na^+, the kidneys reabsorb approximately 99.6% of the filtered Na^+ by the time the tubule fluid reaches the renal pelvis. Therefore, even minute variations in the fractional reabsorptive rate could lead to changes in total-body Na^+ that markedly alter ECF volume and, hence, body weight. Thus, it is not surprising that each nephron segment makes its own unique contribution to Na^+ homeostasis.

Na^+ AND Cl^- TRANSPORT BY THE NEPHRON

Na^+ and Cl^- Reabsorption Is Largest in the Proximal Tubule, followed by Henle's Loop, the Classic Distal Tubule, and the Collecting Tubules and Ducts

Figure 34–2 summarizes the segmental distribution of Na^+ reabsorption along the nephron. The **proximal tubule** reabsorbs the largest fraction of filtered Na^+ (~67%). Because [Na^+] in *tubule fluid* (or TF_{Na}) remains the same as that in *plasma* (i.e., TF_{Na}/P_{Na} = 1.0; p. 751) throughout the length of the proximal tubule, it follows that the [Na^+] in the *reabsorbate* is the same as that in plasma. Because Na^+ salts are the dominant osmotically active solutes in the filtrate, reabsorption must be a near isosmotic process.

The **loop of Henle** reabsorbs a smaller but significant fraction of filtered Na^+ (~25%). Because of the low water permeability of the thick ascending limb (TAL), this nephron segment reabsorbs Na^+ faster than it reabsorbs water, so that [Na^+] in the tubule fluid entering the distal convoluted tubule has decreased substantially ($TF_{Na}/P_{Na} \cong 0.45$).

The **classic distal tubule** (p. 743) and **collecting ducts** reabsorb smaller

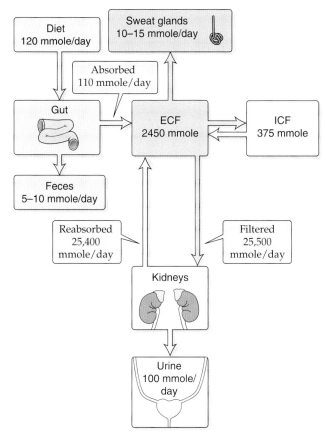

FIGURE 34–1. Distribution and balance of Na$^+$ throughout the body. ECF, extracellular fluid; ICF, intracellular fluid.

fractions of filtered Na$^+$ and water than do more proximal segments. The segments between the distal convoluted tubule (DCT) and the cortical collecting tubule (CCT), inclusive, reabsorb approximately 5% of the filtered Na$^+$ load. Finally, the medullary collecting duct reabsorbs approximately 3% of the filtered Na$^+$ load. Although the distal nephron reabsorbs only small amounts of Na$^+$, it can establish a steep transepithelial concentration gradient and respond to several hormones, including mineralocorticoids and arginine vasopressin (AVP).

The Tubule Reabsorbs Na$^+$ Via Both the Transcellular and the Paracellular Pathways

The tubule can reabsorb Na$^+$ and Cl$^-$ via both transcellular and paracellular pathways (Fig. 34–3A). In the **transcellular pathway**, Na$^+$ and Cl$^-$ sequentially traverse the apical and basolateral membranes before entering the blood. In the **paracellular pathway**, these ions move entirely by an extracellular route, through the tight junctions between cells. In the transcellular pathway, transport rates depend on the electrochemical gradients, ion channels, and transporters at the apical and basolateral membranes. However, in the paracellular pathway, transepithelial electrochemical driving forces and permeability properties of the tight junctions govern ion movements.

TRANSCELLULAR Na$^+$ REABSORPTION. The basic mechanism of transcellular Na$^+$ reabsorption is similar in all nephron segments and is a variation on the classic two-membrane model of epithelial transport (p. 84). The *first step* is the passive entry of Na$^+$ into the cell across the **apical** membrane. Because the intracellular Na$^+$ concentration ($[Na^+]_i$) is low and the cell voltage is negative with respect to the lumen, the electrochemical gradient is favorable for passive Na$^+$ entry across the apical membrane (see Fig. 34–3B). However, different tubule segments use different mechanisms of passive Na$^+$ entry across the apical membrane. The proximal tubule, the TAL, and the DCT all use a combination of Na$^+$-coupled cotransporters and exchangers to move Na$^+$ across the apical membrane; however, in the cortical and medullary collecting ducts, Na$^+$ enters the cell through epithelial Na$^+$ channels (ENaC).

The *second step* of transcellular Na$^+$ reabsorption is the active extrusion of Na$^+$ out of the cell across the basolateral membrane (see Fig. 34–3B). This Na$^+$ extrusion is mediated by the Na-K pump (p. 61), which keeps $[Na^+]_i$ low (~15 mM) and $[K^+]_i$ high (~120 mM). Because the basolateral membrane is primarily permeable to K$^+$, it develops a voltage of approximately 70 mV, with the cell interior negative with respect to the interstitial space. Across the apical membrane, the cell is negative with respect to the lumen. The magnitude of the apical membrane voltage may be either lower or higher than that of the basolateral membrane, depending on the nephron segment and its transport activity.

PARACELLULAR Na$^+$ REABSORPTION. The basic mechanism of paracellular Na$^+$ transport is similar among nephron segments: the transepithelial electrochemical gradient for Na$^+$ drives transport. However, both the transepithelial voltage and luminal $[Na^+]$ vary along the nephron (Table 34–1). As a result, the net driving force for Na$^+$ is positive—favoring passive Na$^+$ reabsorption—only in the S2 and S3 segment of the proximal tubule, and the TAL. In the other segments, the net driving force is negative—favoring passive Na$^+$ diffusion from blood to lumen ("backleak"). In addition to the purely passive, paracellular reabsorption of Na$^+$ in the S2 and S3 segments and TAL, Na$^+$ can also move uphill from lumen to blood via **solvent drag** across the tight junctions. In this case, the movement of H$_2$O—energized by the active transport of Na$^+$ into the lateral intercellular space—from the lumen to the lateral intercellular space also sweeps Na$^+$ and Cl$^-$ in the same direction.

Nephron segments also vary in their **leakiness** to Na$^+$ ions. This leakiness is largely a function of the varying ionic conductance of the paracellular pathway between cells across the tight junction. In general, the leakiness of the paracellular pathway decreases along the nephron from the proximal tubule (the most leaky) to the papillary collecting ducts. However, even the tightest renal epithelia have only what might be regarded as a moderate degree of tightness compared with truly "tight" epithelia, such as the skin, the gastric mucosa, and the urinary bladder (p. 82).

The leakiness of an epithelium has serious repercus-

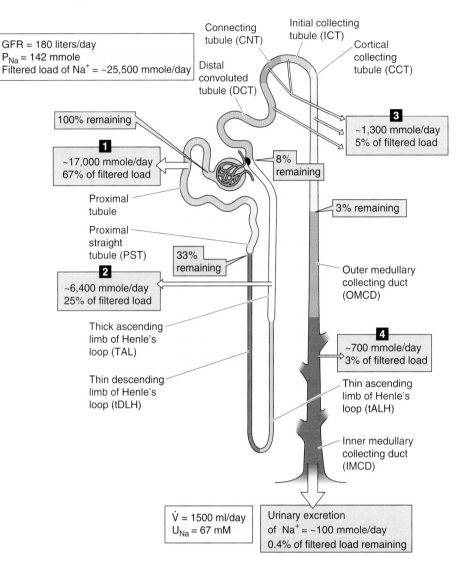

FIGURE 34-2. Renal handling of Na$^+$ along the nephron. The *numbered yellow boxes* indicate the absolute amount of Na$^+$—as well as the fraction of the filtered load—that various nephron segments reabsorb. The *green boxes* indicate the fraction of the filtered load that remains in the lumen at these sites. P$_{Na}$, plasma sodium concentration; U$_{Na}$, urine sodium concentration.

sions for the steepness of the ion gradients that the epithelium can develop and maintain. For both Na$^+$ and Cl$^-$, the ability of specific nephron segments to establish large concentration gradients correlates with the degree of tightness, which limits the backflux of ions between cells. Thus, the luminal fluid in the distal nephron attains much lower concentrations of Na$^+$ and Cl$^-$ than it does in the proximal tubule.

An important consequence of a highly leaky paracellular pathway is that it provides a mechanism by which the basolateral membrane voltage can generate a current that flows through the tight junctions and charges up the apical membrane, and vice versa (see Fig. 34–3B). For example, hyperpolarization of the basolateral membrane leads to a hyperpolarization of the apical membrane. A consequence of this **electrical "crosstalk"** is that the apical membrane of a leaky epithelium, such as the proximal tubule, has a membrane voltage that is negative (-67 mV in Fig. 34–3B) and close to that of the basolateral membrane (-70 mV in Fig. 34–3B), whereas one would expect that, based on the complement of channels and ion gradients at the apical membrane, the apical membrane

would have a far less negative voltage. A practical benefit of this crosstalk is that it helps couple the activity of the basolateral electrogenic Na-K pump to the passive entry of Na$^+$ across the apical membrane. If the Na-K pump rate increases, not only does [Na$^+$]$_i$ decrease, enhancing the *chemical* Na$^+$ gradient across the apical membrane, but also the basolateral membrane hyperpolarizes (i.e., the cell becomes more negative with respect to the blood). Electrical crosstalk translates this basolateral hyperpolarization to a concomitant apical hyperpolarization, thus also enhancing the electrical gradient favoring apical Na$^+$ entry.

Different Nephron Segments Use Different Apical Transporters or Channels for Transcellular Na$^+$ Reabsorption

PROXIMAL TUBULE. Along the first half of the tubule (Fig. 34–4A), a variety of cotransporters in the *apical membrane* couples the downhill uptake of Na$^+$ to the uphill uptake of solutes such as glucose, amino acids,

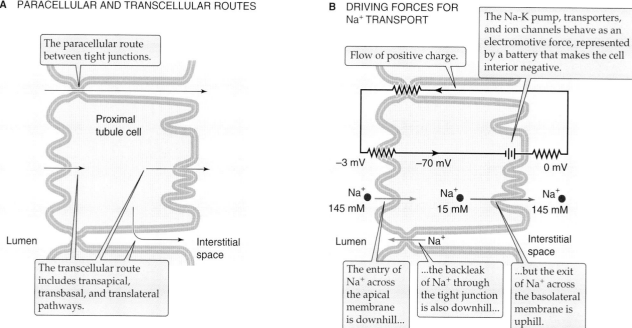

A PARACELLULAR AND TRANSCELLULAR ROUTES

The paracellular route between tight junctions.

Proximal tubule cell

Lumen

Interstitial space

The transcellular route includes transapical, transbasal, and translateral pathways.

B DRIVING FORCES FOR Na⁺ TRANSPORT

The Na-K pump, transporters, and ion channels behave as an electromotive force, represented by a battery that makes the cell interior negative.

Flow of positive charge.

−3 mV   −70 mV   0 mV

Na⁺   Na⁺   Na⁺
145 mM   15 mM   145 mM

Lumen   Na⁺   Interstitial space

The entry of Na⁺ across the apical membrane is downhill...

...the backleak of Na⁺ through the tight junction is also downhill...

...but the exit of Na⁺ across the basolateral membrane is uphill.

FIGURE 34–3. Transcellular and paracellular mechanisms of Na⁺ and Cl⁻ reabsorption. The example in *B* illustrates the electrochemical driving forces for Na⁺ in the early proximal tubule. The equivalent circuit demonstrates that the flow of positive charge across the apical membrane makes the apical membrane voltage more negative.

phosphate, sulfate, lactate, and other monocarboxylic and dicarboxylic acids. Many of these Na⁺-driven cotransporters are electrogenic, carrying net positive charge into the cell. Thus, both the low [Na⁺]ᵢ and the negative apical membrane voltage fuel the secondary active uptake of these other solutes, which we discuss in Chapter 35. In addition to the cotransporters, Na⁺ entry is also coupled to the extrusion of H⁺ through the electroneutral **Na-H exchanger** (NHE-3). The role of NHE-3 in renal acid secretion is discussed on p. 852.

Both cotransporters and exchangers exploit the downhill Na⁺ gradient across the apical cell membrane that is

established by the **Na-K pump** in the *basolateral membrane*. The Na-K pump—and, to a lesser extent, the electrogenic Na/HCO₃ cotransporter (NBC)—is also responsible for the second step in Na⁺ reabsorption, moving Na⁺ from cell to blood. The presence of K⁺ channels in the basolateral membrane is important for two reasons. First, these channels establish the negative voltage across the basolateral membrane and establish a similar negative voltage across the apical membrane via electrical crosstalk. Second, these channels permit the recycling of K⁺ that had been transported into the cell by the Na-K pump.

Because of a lumen-negative voltage in the early proxi-

TABLE 34–1

TRANSEPITHELIAL DRIVING FORCES FOR Na⁺

	LUMINAL [Na⁺]	TRANSEPITHELIAL CHEMICAL DRIVING FORCE*‡	TRANSEPITHELIAL VOLTAGE (i.e., ELECTRICAL DRIVING FORCE)†‡	TRANSEPITHELIAL ELECTROCHEMICAL DRIVING FORCE‡
Proximal tubule, S1	142 mM	0 mV	−3 mV	−3 mV
Proximal tubule, S3	142 mM	0 mV	+3 mV	+3 mV
TAL	100 mM	−9 mV	+15 mV	+6 mV
DCT	70 mM	−19	−5 to +5 mV	−24 to −14 mV
CCT	40 mM	−34 mV	−40 mV	−74 mV

CCT, cortical collecting tubule; DCT, distal convoluted tubule; TAL; thick ascending limb.
*The chemical driving force is calculated assuming a plasma [Na⁺] of 142 mM, and is given in mV.
†A negative value indicates that the lumen is negative with respect to the blood.
‡A negative value promotes passive Na⁺ movement from blood to lumen (i.e., backleak or secretion), whereas a positive value promotes passive Na⁺ movement from lumen to blood (i.e., reabsorption).

FIGURE 34–4. Cell models of Na$^+$ reabsorption. ATP, adenosine triphosphate; PCT, proximal convoluted tube.

mal tubule, as well as a paracellular pathway that is permeable to Na$^+$, approximately one third of the Na$^+$ that is transported from lumen to blood by the transcellular pathway diffuses back to the lumen by the *paracellular pathway* ("backleak").

THIN LIMBS OF HENLE'S LOOP. Na$^+$ transport by the thin descending and thin ascending limbs of Henle's loop is almost entirely passive and paracellular (p. 833).

THICK ASCENDING LIMB. Two major pathways contribute to Na$^+$ reabsorption in the TAL: transcellular and paracellular (see Fig. 34–4B). The *transcellular pathway* includes two major mechanisms for taking up Na$^+$ across the apical membrane. The **Na/K/Cl cotransporter** (NKCC2) couples the inward movement 1 Na$^+$, 1 K$^+$, and 2 Cl$^-$ ions in an electroneutral process driven by the downhill concentration gradients of Na$^+$ and Cl$^-$ (p. 67). The second entry pathway for Na$^+$ is an **Na-H exchanger**. As in the proximal tubule, the basolateral Na-K pump keeps [Na$^+$]$_i$ low and moves Na$^+$ to the blood.

Two features of the apical step of Na$^+$ reabsorption in the TAL are noteworthy. First, the **"loop diuretics"** (e.g., furosemide and bumetanide) inhibit Na/K/Cl cotransport.

Second, a large fraction of the K$^+$ that the Na/K/Cl cotransporter brings into the cell recycles to the lumen via apical K$^+$ channels. These channels are essential for adequate turnover of the Na/K/Cl cotransporter.

A key aspect of the *paracellular pathway* for Na$^+$ reabsorption in the TAL is a lumen-positive voltage (see Fig. 34–4B). Nearly all other epithelia have a lumen-negative voltage because the apical membrane voltage is less negative than the basolateral membrane voltage (see Fig. 3–18D). The TAL is just the opposite. Because of a high density of K$^+$ channels in the apical membrane, the voltage of the TAL apical membrane is more negative than the basolateral membrane voltage, resulting in a lumen-positive voltage. The lumen-positive voltage provides the driving force for the diffusion of Na$^+$ across the tight junctions, accounting for about half of the Na$^+$ reabsorption by the TAL. The lumen-positive voltage also drives the passive reabsorption of K$^+$ (p. 821), Ca^{2+} (p. 807), and Mg^{2+} (p. 811) via the paracellular pathway. Because the TAL has a low water permeability, removing luminal NaCl leaves the remaining tubule fluid *hypoosmotic.* Hence, the TAL is sometimes referred to as the "diluting segment."

DISTAL CONVOLUTED TUBULE. Na$^+$ reabsorption in the DCT occurs almost exclusively by the transcellular route (see Fig. 34–4C). The *apical step* of Na$^+$ uptake is mediated by an electroneutral Na/Cl cotransporter (NCC; see p. 67) that is in the same family as that of the Na/K/Cl cotransporter in the TAL. However, the Na/Cl cotransporter differs from the Na/K/Cl cotransporter in being independent of K$^+$ and highly sensitive to thiazide diuretics. Although the thiazides produce less diuresis than the loop diuretics do, the thiazides are nevertheless effective in removing excess Na$^+$ from the body. The *basolateral step* of Na$^+$ reabsorption, as in other cells, is mediated by the Na-K pump.

INITIAL AND CORTICAL COLLECTING TUBULES. Na$^+$ reabsorption in these nephron segments is transcellular, and mediated by the majority cell type, the **principal cell** (see Fig. 34–4D). The neighboring β-intercalated cells are important for reabsorbing Cl$^-$, as discussed later. Na$^+$ crosses the *apical membrane* of the principal cell via the **ENaCs**, which are distinct from the voltage-gated Na$^+$ channels seen in excitable tissues (p. 186). ENaC is a heteromer comprising homologous α, β, and γ subunits, each of which has two membrane-spanning segments. These ENaCs are unique in that low levels of the diuretic drug **amiloride** block them in a specific way. This compound is a relatively mild diuretic because Na$^+$ reabsorption along the collecting duct is modest. The *basolateral step* of Na$^+$ reabsorption is mediated by the Na-K pump, which also provides the electrochemical driving force for the apical entry of Na$^+$.

The unique transport properties of the apical and basolateral membranes of the principal cells are also the basis for the lumen-negative transepithelial potential difference of approximately −40 mV in the CCT (see Table 34–1). In addition to ENaC Na$^+$ channels, the CCT has both apical and basolateral K$^+$ channels, which play a key role in K$^+$ transport (p. 822). The apical entry of Na$^+$ (which tends to make the lumen negative) and the basolateral exit of K$^+$ (which tends to make the cell negative) are, in effect, two batteries of identical sign in series. In principle, these two batteries could add up to a transepithelial voltage of approximately 100 mV (lumen negative). However, under most conditions, K$^+$ *exit* from cell to lumen partially opposes the lumen-negative potential generated by Na$^+$ *entry*. The net effect of these three batteries is a transepithelial voltage of about −40 mV (lumen negative).

The transepithelial voltage of the CCT can fluctuate considerably, particularly because of changes in the apical Na$^+$ battery owing to, for example, changes in luminal [Na$^+$]. In addition, changing levels of aldosterone or AVP may modulate the *number* of ENaCs that are open in the apical membrane and thus affect the relative contribution of this Na$^+$ battery to apical membrane voltage.

MEDULLARY COLLECTING DUCT. The inner and outer medullary collecting ducts reabsorb only a minute amount of Na$^+$, approximately 3% of the filtered load (see Fig. 34–2). It is likely that ENaCs mediate the apical entry of Na$^+$ in these segments and that the Na-K pump extrudes Na$^+$ from the cell across the basolateral membrane (see Fig. 34–4D).

Cl$^-$ Reabsorption Involves Paracellular Diffusion as Well as Transcellular Movements Via Transporters and Channels

Most of the filtered Na$^+$ is reabsorbed with Cl$^-$. However, the segmental handling of Cl$^-$ differs somewhat from that of Na$^+$. Both transcellular and paracellular pathways participate in Cl$^-$ reabsorption.

PROXIMAL TUBULE. The proximal tubule reabsorbs Cl$^-$ by both the transcellular and the paracellular routes, with the *paracellular* believed to be the dominant one in the early proximal tubule (Fig. 34–5A). The *transcellular pathway* is dominant in the late proximal tubule (see Fig. 34–5B), where the energetically uphill movement of Cl$^-$ across the apical membrane probably occurs via an exchange of luminal Cl$^-$ for cellular anions (e.g., formate, oxalate, HCO$_3^-$ and OH$^-$). When this anion is a base, Cl-anion exchange is an example of *tertiary* active transport: the apical Na-H exchanger, itself a *secondary* active transporter (p. 61), provides the H$^+$ that neutralizes base in the lumen, thereby sustaining the gradient for Cl-anion exchange. The basolateral exit step for transcellular Cl$^-$ movement may occur in part via a **Cl$^-$ channel** that is analogous in function to cystic fibrosis transmembrane conductance regulator (CFTR; p. 916). In addition, the basolateral membrane of the proximal tubule may also have a **K/Cl cotransporter** (KCC), which is in the same family as the Na/K/Cl and Na/Cl cotransporters.

Passive Cl$^-$ reabsorption via the *paracellular pathway* is driven by different electrochemical Cl$^-$ gradients in the early versus the late proximal tubule. The S1 segment initially has no Cl$^-$ concentration gradient between lumen and blood. However, the lumen-negative voltage (see Table 34–1)—generated by electrogenic Na/glucose and Na/amino-acid cotransport—establishes a favorable *electrical* gradient for passive Cl$^-$ reabsorption. Solvent drag also makes a contribution in the S1 segment. In the S2 and S3 segments, the lumen-positive voltage opposes paracellular Cl$^-$ absorption (see Table 34–1). However, preferential HCO$_3^-$ reabsorption in the earlier portions of the proximal tubule leaves Cl$^-$ behind (p. 850), so that [Cl$^-$] in the lumen becomes higher than that in the blood. This favorable lumen-to-blood *chemical* gradient for Cl$^-$ overcomes the electrical gradient so that paracellular movement of Cl$^-$ in the late proximal tubule proceeds in the reabsorptive direction.

The *upper part* of Figure 34–6 shows the profile of the ratio of concentrations in tubule fluid versus plasma (TF/P) (p. 751) for the major solutes in tubule fluid along the proximal tubule. Only minor changes occur in the total osmolality of the tubule fluid or inulin (In) TF$_{Na}$. Because the tubule does not reabsorb In, the substantial increase in TF$_{In}$ indicates net fluid reabsorption. The fall in TF$_{HCO_3}$ mirrors an increase in TF$_{Cl}$ because the tubule reabsorbs HCO$_3^-$ more rapidly than it does Cl$^-$. The early proximal

FIGURE 34–5. Cell models of Cl⁻ transport. In *B*, base may include formate, oxalate, HCO₃⁻ and OH⁻. HBase represents the conjugate weak acid (e.g., formic acid). ATP, adenosine triphosphate.

tubule avidly reabsorbs glucose and amino acids, leading to sharp decreases in the concentrations of these substances in the tubule fluid.

An important characteristic of the proximal tubule is that the transepithelial voltage reverses polarity between the S1 and the S2 segments (see Fig. 34–6, *lower panel*). The early proximal tubule is lumen negative because it reabsorbs Na⁺ electrogenically, both via electrogenic apical Na⁺ transporters (e.g., Na/glucose cotransporter) and the basolateral Na-K pump. The late proximal tubule

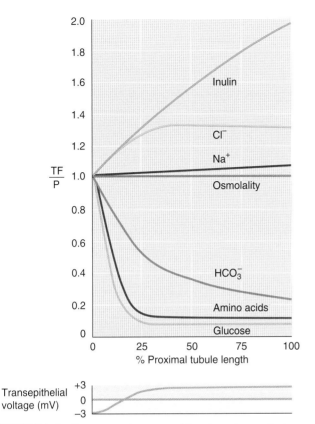

FIGURE 34–6. Changes in solute composition along the proximal tubule. In the *upper panel*, TF/P is the ratio of concentration or osmolality in tubule fluid (TF) versus blood plasma (P). Because we assume that the proximal tubule reabsorbs half of the filtered water, TF_{In}/P_{In} rises from 1 to 2. The *lower panel* shows the transition of transepithelial voltage from a negative to a positive value.

reabsorbs Na^+ at a lower rate. Moreover, because TF_{Cl} is greater than P_{Cl}, the paracellular diffusion of Cl^- from lumen to bath generates a lumen-positive potential that facilitates passive Na^+ reabsorption via the same paracellular route.

THICK ASCENDING LIMB. Cl^- reabsorption in the TAL takes place largely by Na/K/Cl cotransport across the apical membrane (see Fig. 34–5C), as we already noted in our discussion of Na^+ reabsorption (see Fig. 34–4B). The exit of Cl^- across the basolateral cell membrane via Cl^- channels of the ClC family (see Table 6–2, #15) overwhelms any entry of Cl^- via the Cl-HCO$_3$ exchanger. You may recall that only *half* of the Na^+ reabsorption by the TAL is transcellular, whereas *all* of Cl^- reabsorption is transcellular. Overall, Na^+ and Cl^- reabsorption are identical because the apical Na/K/Cl cotransporter moves two Cl^- for each Na^+.

DISTAL CONVOLUTED TUBULE. Cl^- reabsorption by the DCT (see Fig. 34–5D) occurs by a mechanism that is somewhat similar to that in the TAL, except that the apical step occurs via the Na/Cl cotransporter, as discussed earlier in connection with Na^+ reabsorption by the DCT (see Fig. 34–4C). Cl^- channels that are probably

similar to those in the TAL mediate the basolateral Cl^- exit step.

COLLECTING DUCTS. The initial cortical and cortical collecting tubules reabsorb Cl^- by two mechanisms. First, the principal cell generates a transepithelial voltage ($\sim$40 mV, lumen negative) that is favorable for *paracellular* diffusion of Cl^- (see Fig. 34–5E). Second, the β-type intercalated cells reabsorb Cl^- using a *transcellular* process that involves Cl-HCO$_3$ exchange across the apical membranes and Cl^- channels in the basolateral membrane (see Fig. 34–5F). Neither the α-type intercalated cells nor the principal cells are involved in transcellular Cl^- reabsorption.

Water Reabsorption Is Always Passive and Secondary to Solute Transport

PROXIMAL TUBULE. If water reabsorption by the proximal tubule were to follow solute reabsorption *passively*, then one might expect the osmolality inside the peritubular capillaries to be greater than that in the luminal fluid. Indeed, investigators have found that the lumen is slightly hypoosmolar.

If, on the other hand, proximal-tubule water reabsorption were active, one might expect it to be independent of Na^+ reabsorption. Actually, the opposite was found by Windhager and colleagues in 1959. Using the stationary microperfusion technique, they introduced solutions having various [Na^+] values into the proximal-tubule lumen, keeping luminal osmolality constant by adding mannitol (which is poorly reabsorbed). Because these experiments were performed on amphibian proximal tubules, the maximal [Na^+] was only 100 mM, the same as that in blood plasma. After a known time interval, they measured the volume of fluid remaining in the tubule lumen and calculated the rate of fluid reabsorption (J_V). They also measured [Na^+] of the luminal fluid and calculated the rate of Na^+ reabsorption (J_{Na}). These experiments showed that both J_V and J_{Na} are directly proportional to the initial luminal [Na^+] (Fig. 34–7). Moreover, over the entire range of [Na^+] values, they found that the *final* luminal [Na^+] was about the same as the *initial* one. Thus, the concentration of Na^+ and water in the reabsorbed fluid is about the same as that originally present in the lumen. In other words, Na^+ reabsorption is approximately **isosmotic** to the composition in the lumen.

Windhager and colleagues also found that at a luminal [Na^+] of 100 mM, the J_{Na} and J_V were large and in the reabsorptive direction. When luminal [Na^+] was only 65 mM, both J_{Na} and J_V were zero. At lower luminal [Na^+] values, both J_{Na} and J_V reversed; that is, the tubule secreted both Na^+ and water. At these low luminal [Na^+] values, active transcellular movement of Na^+ from lumen to blood cannot overcome the increasing paracellular backleak of Na^+, resulting in net "secretion" of an isosmotic NaCl solution. This experiment shows that Na^+ can move uphill from lumen to blood, as long as the opposing Na^+ gradient is not too steep, and also suggests that the movement of water is not active, but passively follows the reabsorption of Na^+.

OSMOTIC DIURESIS

Normally, luminal [Na⁺] does not change along the proximal tubule. The only exception is **osmotic diuresis**, a state in which poorly permeable substances are present in the plasma and, therefore, in the glomerular filtrate. Examples are the infusion of sucrose and mannitol. Another is untreated diabetes mellitus (see box on p. 1084), when the blood sugar level may become too high for the capacity of renal tubules to reabsorb the highly elevated glucose load. Glucose then acts as a poorly reabsorbed substance and as an osmotic diuretic. Because the proximal tubule must reabsorb isosmotic Na⁺ salts from a luminal mixture of Na⁺ salts and poorly reabsorbable solutes (e.g., mannitol), luminal [Na⁺] progressively falls, luminal [mannitol] rises, but luminal osmolality does not change (Fig. 34–8).

Because, as we have seen, the rate of Na⁺ and fluid reabsorption falls as the luminal [Na⁺] falls (Fig. 34–7), the proximal tubule reabsorbs progressively less Na⁺ and fluid as the fluid travels along the tubule. This decrease in Na⁺ and water reabsorption leaves a larger volume of tubule fluid behind, producing the osmotic diuresis. Clinicians use osmotic diuretics in several settings. For example, mannitol osmotically draws water out of brain tissue into the vascular system, for ultimate excretion by the kidneys. For this reason, osmotic diuresis has proven useful in treating patients with acutely increased intracranial pressure from an expanding tumor or abscess, hematoma or hemorrhage, or edema. Mannitol also reduces the risk of radiocontrast-induced acute renal failure in susceptible patients (e.g., those with underlying renal disease, volume depletion, diabetes mellitus, or congestive heart failure) who must undergo radiologic procedures that require a substantial dye load.

It is common to distinguish between two types of diuresis, solute and water diuresis. The above example of **solute or osmotic diuresis** is characterized by excretion of a larger-than-normal volume of urine that is rich in solutes. In contrast, **water diuresis** leads to excretion of larger than normal volumes of urine that is dilute (i.e., poor in solutes).

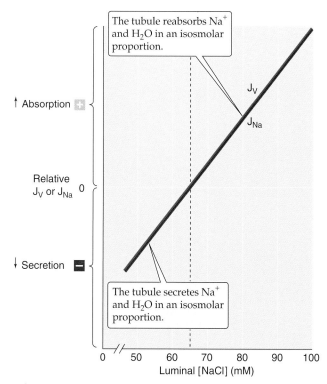

FIGURE 34–7. Isosmotic water reabsorption in the proximal tubule. J_V and J_{Na} are the rates of fluid (or *volume*) and Na⁺ reabsorption, respectively, in stationary microperfusion experiments.

ence of a high density of AQP1 **water channels** in both the apical and basolateral membranes.

LOOP OF HENLE AND DISTAL NEPHRON. Two features distinguish water and Na⁺ transport in the distal nephron. First, the TAL and all downstream segments have a relatively low water permeability in the absence of AVP (or antidiuretic hormone). The upregulation of this water permeability by AVP is discussed in Chapter 37. Second, the combination of NaCl reabsorption and low water permeability allows these nephron segments to generate a low luminal [Na⁺] and osmolality with respect to the surrounding interstitial fluid. Given this large osmotic gradient across the epithelium, the distal nephron is poised to reabsorb water passively from a hypoosmotic luminal fluid into the isosmotic blood when AVP increases the water permeability.

The Kidney's High Oxygen Consumption Reflects a High Level of Active Na⁺ Transport

Because virtually all Na⁺ transport ultimately depends on the activity of the ATP-driven Na-K pump, and, therefore, on the generation of ATP by oxidative metabolism, it is not surprising that renal O_2 consumption is large and parallels Na⁺ reabsorption. Despite their low weight (less than 0.5% of body weight), the kidneys are responsible for 7% to 10% of total O_2 consumption. Although it might seem that the high O_2 consumption would necessitate a large arteriovenous difference in P_{O_2}, actually the renal blood flow is so large that the artery–vein P_{O_2}

If water movement is passive, why is the difference in osmolality so small between the proximal-tubule lumen and blood? The answer is that, because the water permeability of the proximal-tubule epithelium to water is so high, the osmolality gradient needed to generate the observed passive reabsorption of water is only 2 to 3 mOsm. A somewhat greater osmolality gradient probably exists between the lumen and an inaccessible basolateral compartment comprising the lateral intercellular space and the microscopic unstirred layer that surrounds the highly folded basolateral membrane of the proximal-tubule cell.

The pathway for water movement across the proximal-tubule epithelium is a combination of transcellular and paracellular transit, with the transcellular route dominating. The reason for the high rate of water movement through the proximal-tubule cell appears to be the pres-

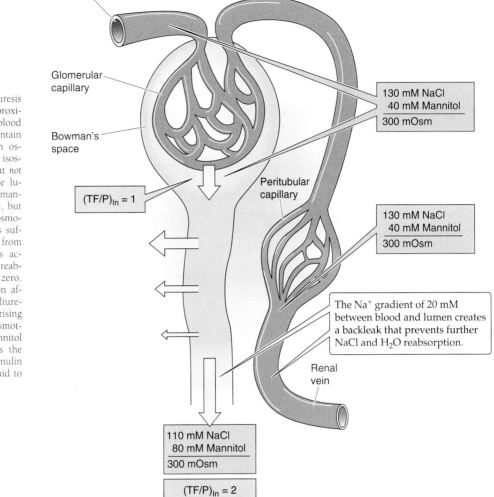

FIGURE 34–8. Osmotic diuresis and luminal [Na⁺] along the proximal tubule. In this example, blood and glomerular filtrate both contain 40 mM mannitol and have an osmolality of 300 mOsm. The isosmotic reabsorption of NaCl (but *not* mannitol) from proximal-tubule lumen to blood causes luminal [mannitol] to rise and [NaCl] to fall, but causes no change in luminal osmolality. Once luminal [Na⁺] falls sufficiently, the Na⁺ backleak from peritubular capillaries balances active Na⁺ reabsorption, and net reabsorption of NaCl and water is zero. The absence of fluid absorption after this point causes osmotic diuresis. Viewed another way, the rising luminal [mannitol], with the osmotically obligated water the mannitol holds in the lumen, produces the diuresis. (TF/P)$_{In}$, the ratio of inulin concentrations in the tubule fluid to plasma.

Labels within the figure:
Renal artery
Glomerular capillary
Bowman's space
130 mM NaCl / 40 mM Mannitol / 300 mOsm
Peritubular capillary
(TF/P)$_{In}$ = 1
130 mM NaCl / 40 mM Mannitol / 300 mOsm
The Na⁺ gradient of 20 mM between blood and lumen creates a backleak that prevents further NaCl and H₂O reabsorption.
Renal vein
110 mM NaCl / 80 mM Mannitol / 300 mOsm
(TF/P)$_{In}$ = 2

difference is actually much smaller than that in cardiac muscle or brain.

If one varies Na⁺ reabsorption experimentally and measures renal O_2 consumption, the result is a straight-line relationship (Fig. 34–9). Note, however, that the kidneys continue to consume a modest but significant amount of O_2 even in the complete absence of net Na⁺ reabsorption. This transport-independent component reflects the basic metabolic needs for the maintenance of cell viability.

REGULATION OF Na⁺ AND Cl⁻ TRANSPORT

The body regulates Na⁺ transport using three major mechanisms.

1. Changes in renal hemodynamics alter the Na⁺ load presented to the kidney and modulate the rate of NaCl reabsorption in the proximal tubule by a process known as glomerulotubular (GT) balance. We will discuss these hemodynamic effects in the next three sections.
2. Three factors that increase "effective circulating vol-

ume" (p. 556) do so in part by increasing Na⁺ reabsorption, as we will see in the fourth section of this subchapter.
3. Five natriuretic humoral factors can decrease Na⁺ reabsorption, as we will see in the final section.

Glomerulotubular Balance Stabilizes the Fractional Na⁺ Reabsorption by the Proximal Tubule in the Face of Changes in the Filtered Na⁺ Load

When the Na⁺ load presented to the nephron varies because of hemodynamic changes that alter GFR (e.g., those caused by changes in the intake of Na⁺, protein, or by severe exercise, pain or anesthesia), the *proximal* tubules respond by reabsorbing a *constant fraction* of the Na⁺ load that is presented to them. This constancy of fractional Na⁺ reabsorption along the proximal tubule—defined as **glomerulotubular balance**—is independent of external neural and hormonal control, and thus safeguards Na⁺ balance.

Figure 34–10A shows how the *absolute reabsorption* of Na⁺ increases proportionally with increases in the filtered

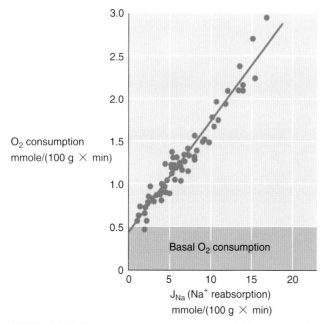

FIGURE 34–9. Dependence of O_2 consumption on Na^+ transport. Na^+ reabsorption (J_{Na}) was varied by changing GFR, administering diuretics, or imposing hypoxia. O_2 consumption was computed from the arteriovenous P_{O_2} difference.

Na^+ load, achieved by varying GFR at a constant plasma $[Na^+]$. The amount of Na^+ remaining in the lumen at the end of the proximal tubule also increases linearly with filtered Na^+ load. The impact of such altered Na^+ delivery to more distally located nephron segments is discussed later.

If excessive Na^+ loss (e.g., sweating) contracts the ECF volume, the reduced renal perfusion pressure causes GFR to fall. In response, the proximal tubule excretes a constant fraction of Na^+ and water, which corresponds to a smaller absolute amount. Thus, GT balance helps prevent additional Na^+ and water loss. However, if Na^+ retention expands ECF (causing GFR to rise), the proximal tubule excretes a constant fraction of filtered Na^+, which corresponds to an increased absolute amount. This response tends to correct the volume expansion.

At the level of the whole kidney, GT balance is not perfect, mainly because distal-nephron Na^+ absorption is under neural and hormonal control.

The Proximal Tubule Achieves GT Balance by both Peritubular and Luminal Mechanisms

How do the proximal-tubule cells know that the GFR has changed? Both peritubular and luminal control mechanisms contribute, although there is no agreement concerning their relative roles.

PERITUBULAR FACTORS IN THE PROXIMAL TUBULE. As discussed in the previous chapter, Starling forces across the peritubular capillaries determine the uptake of interstitial fluid, and thus net reabsorption of NaCl and fluid from tubule lumen into the peritubular capillaries (p.

765). These peritubular *physical factors* also play a role in GT balance. We can distinguish a sequence of three transport steps as reabsorbed fluid moves from the tubule lumen into the blood (see Fig. 34–10*B*):

Step 1: Via the transcellular pathway, solutes and water first enter a tubule cell across the apical membrane, and then exit across the basolateral membrane.

Step 2: The solute and water (i.e., "reabsorbate") enters an intercellular compartment (i.e., **lateral interspace**) that is bounded by the apical tight junction, the basolateral tubule-cell membranes, and a basement membrane that does not discriminate between solutes and solvent.

Step 3: The reabsorbate can either "backleak" into the lumen or move sequentially into the interstitial space and then into the blood.

At normal GFR (see Fig. 34–10*B*), reabsorptive forces—the low hydrostatic and high oncotic pressure in the capillaries—lead to an extensive uptake of reabsorbate into the capillaries.

In GT balance, alterations in GFR lead to changes in the peritubular pressures (both hydrostatic and oncotic) that, in turn, modulate the forces that govern Step 3. This mechanism of GT balance comes into play only when the changes in GFR are associated with alterations in **filtration fraction** (FF = GFR/RPF; p. 763). For example, consider a situation in which we increase GFR at constant glomerular plasma flow, leading to an increase in FF (see Fig. 34–10*C*). We can produce this effect by increasing efferent arteriolar resistance while concomitantly decreasing afferent arteriolar resistance (see Fig. 33–8*A, lower panel*). The result is an increase in glomerular capillary pressure (i.e., net filtration pressure) without a change in overall arteriolar resistance. These changes have two important consequences for the peritubular capillaries. First, the increase in GFR translates to less fluid remaining in the efferent arteriole, so that peritubular *oncotic pressure* (π_{PC}) rises proportionally. Second, because of the increased glomerular filtration, blood flow into the efferent arteriole falls, decreasing *hydrostatic pressure* in the peritubular capillaries (P_{PC}). As a consequence, the net driving force increases for the transport of fluid from the lateral interspace into the capillaries, leading to a more effective absorption of fluid and NaCl.

LUMINAL FACTORS IN THE PROXIMAL TUBULE. Luminal factors also contribute to GT balance, as evidenced by the observation that increased flow along the proximal tubule—without any peritubular effects—leads to an increase in fluid and NaCl reabsorption. The luminal concentrations of solutes such as glucose, amino acids and HCO_3^- fall along the length of the proximal tubule, as the tubule reabsorbs these solutes (see Fig. 34–6). Increasing luminal flow would, for instance, cause $TF_{Glucose}$ to fall less steeply along the tubule length, and more glucose would be available for reabsorption at distal sites. The net effect is that, integrated over the entire proximal tubule, the reabsorption of Na^+, glucose, and other Na^+-coupled solutes increases at higher luminal flows.

A second luminal mechanism—a hypothetical humoral

A   DEPENDENCE OF Na⁺ REABSORPTION ON LOAD

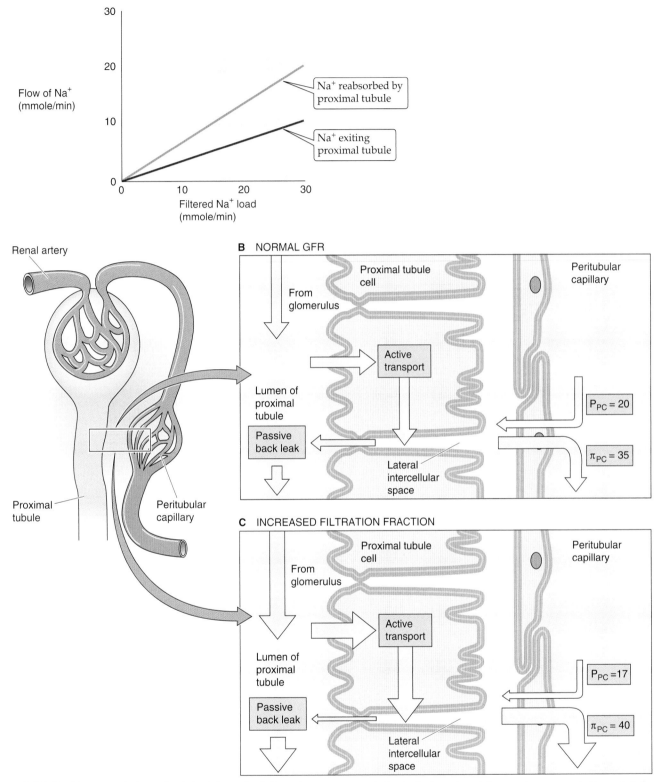

FIGURE 34–10. Proximal glomerulotubular balance. In B, P_{PC} and π_{PC} are, respectively, the hydrostatic and the oncotic pressures in the peritubular capillaries. At the level of the tubule, the net Na⁺ reabsorption is the difference between active transport and passive backleak. At the level of the peritubular capillary, net fluid absorption is the difference between fluid absorption (driven by π_{PC}) and fluid filtration (driven by P_{PC}). In C, increasing the filtered fraction has effects on both the tubule and the peritubular capillaries. At the level of the tubule, the increased concentrations of Na⁺–coupled solutes (e.g., glucose) increase active transport. At the level of the capillaries, the lower P_{PC} and higher protein concentration (π_{PC}) pull more H₂O from the interstitium. The net effect is reduced passive backleak. GFR, glomerular filtration rate.

FIGURE 34–11. Flow dependence of Na$^+$ transport in the distal nephron. *A* and *B* are idealized representations of the effect of increased flow (V) on luminal [Na$^+$] and Na$^+$ reabsorption rate (J$_{Na}$) along the TAL. Limiting [Na] is the theoretical minimal value that the tubule could achieve at zero flow. *C* summarizes the effect of flow on cumulative Na$^+$ reabsorption between the late proximal tubule and the late portion of the classical distal tubule.

factor—may also contribute to GT balance. If one harvests tubule fluid and injects it into a single proximal tubule, Na$^+$ reabsorption increases. Angiotensin II (ANG II)—a peptide hormone that is small enough to be filtered in the glomeruli, and that is also secreted by proximal-tubule cells—increases Na$^+$ reabsorption in the proximal tubule at physiological concentrations. Moreover, luminal breakdown and re-uptake would cause luminal ANG II levels to fall. If increased luminal flow stretched out the ANG II concentration profile, then increased flow would lead to enhanced reabsorption.

The Distal Nephron Also Increases Na$^+$ Reabsorption in Response to an Increased Na$^+$ Load

The tubules of the distal nephron, like their proximal counterparts, also increase their absolute magnitude of Na$^+$ reabsorption in response to increased flow. The principle is the same as that for glucose transport in the proximal tubule, except here it is luminal [Na$^+$] that falls less steeply when flow increases (Fig. 34–11A). Because the transport mechanisms responsible for Na$^+$ reabsorption by the distal nephron work faster at higher luminal [Na$^+$] values, the reabsorption at any site is higher at higher flows (Fig. 34–11B). Thus, in contrast to GT balance in the proximal tubule, increasing flow by a factor of four in the distal nephron may cause cumulative Na$^+$ reabsorption to rise by only a factor of two (Fig. 34–11C).

The opposite changes in Na$^+$ and fluid transport occur when GFR—and thus distal flow—acutely *falls*, as in **circulatory shock**. Because of GT balance, the proximal nephron reabsorbs a constant fraction of Na$^+$, delivering a lower absolute amount of Na$^+$ to the distal convoluted tubule. Distal reabsorption lowers luminal [Na$^+$] even further—under the influence of neural and humoral factors discussed below—so that the final urine may contain only traces of Na$^+$.

Aldosterone, the Sympathetic Division of the Autonomic Nervous System, and Arginine Vasopressin All Increase Na$^+$ Reabsorption

GT balance is only one element in a larger, complex system for controlling Na$^+$ balance. As we will see in Chapter 39, the control of effective circulating volume (i.e., Na$^+$ content) is under the powerful control of four parallel effectors (p. 864): the renin-angiotensin-aldosterone axis, the sympathetic nervous system, AVP, and atrial natriuretic peptide. In the previous chapter, we saw how these factors modulate renal blood flow and GFR (p. 771). In this section, we will discuss the first three of these effectors, all of which stimulate Na$^+$ reabsorption.

RENIN-ANGIOTENSIN-ALDOSTERONE AXIS. Aldosterone—the final element in the renin-angiotensin-aldosterone axis (p. 866)—stimulates Na$^+$ reabsorption by initial and cortical-collecting tubules, and by medullary collecting ducts. Normally, only 2% to 3% of the filtered Na$^+$ load is under humoral control by aldosterone. Nevertheless, the sustained loss of even such a small fraction exceeds significantly the daily Na$^+$ intake. Accordingly, the lack of aldosterone that occurs in adrenal insufficiency (Addison's disease) can lead to severe Na$^+$ depletion, contraction of the extracellular fluid volume, and circulatory insufficiency.

Figure 34–12 shows the renal effects of intravenously administered aldosterone. The acute effects include significant decreases in Na$^+$ and Cl$^-$ excretion, as well as increases in K$^+$ and NH$_4^+$ excretion. The reverse changes occur in adrenalectomy, and the administration of **mineralocorticoids** (e.g., aldosterone) promptly reverses these deficiencies.

Aldosterone acts on the **principal cells** of the collecting ducts (Fig. 34–13A). The cellular mechanisms of aldosterone action include activation of apical ENaC Na$^+$ channels, apical K$^+$ channels, the basolateral Na-K pump, and mitochondrial metabolism. Physiological increases in

Aldosterone

Na$^+$ urinary excretion (mmole/day)

Cl$^-$ urinary excretion (mmole/day)

K$^+$ urinary excretion (mmole/day)

NH$_4^+$ urinary excretion (mmole/day)

Day number

FIGURE 34–12. Acute effects of intravenously administered aldosterone on electrolyte excretion in humans. Data from Liddle, G.W. Aldosterone antagonists. Arch. Intern. Med. 102:998–1005, 1958.

aldosterone concentration raise the product of number of channels and open probability (NP$_o$). The simultaneous activation of apical Na$^+$ entry and basolateral Na$^+$ extrusion ensures that, even with very high levels of Na$^+$ reabsorption, [Na$^+$]$_i$ and cell volume are stable. All of these changes require a few hours to manifest themselves because they depend on the increased production of aldosterone-induced proteins. Aldosterone binds to cytoplasmic mineralocorticoid receptors (MR) that translocate to the nucleus and upregulate transcription (p. 112 and p. 131). Chronic exposure to aldosterone leads to the targeting of newly synthesized Na-K pumps to the basolateral membrane, and to amplification of the basolateral membrane area.

Because mineralocorticoid receptors distinguish poorly between glucocorticoids and mineralocorticoids, and because plasma concentrations of glucocorticoids greatly exceed that of aldosterone, one might expect that glucocorticoids would exert a mineralocorticoid effect and cause Na$^+$ retention. Under normal conditions, this does not happen because of the enzyme **11β-hydroxysteroid dehydrogenase** (11β-HSD), which co-localizes with intracellular adrenal steroid receptors (see Fig. 34–13B). This enzyme converts cortisol into cortisone, an inactive metabolite with low affinity for mineralocorticoid receptors.

In sharp contrast, the enzyme does not metabolize aldosterone. Thus, 11β-HSD enhances the apparent specificity of the mineralocorticoid receptor by protecting the receptors from illicit occupancy by cortisol. As may be expected, an 11β-HSD deficiency may mimic a mineralocorticoid excess. Carbenoxolone, a specific inhibitor of 11β-HSD, prevents the metabolism of cortisol in the target cell, permitting abnormal activation of mineralocorticoid receptors by this glucocorticoid (see Fig. 34–13C). Another inhibitor of 11β-HSD is glycyrrhetinic acid, the active component of **licorice**. Thus, licorice can cause abnormal Na$^+$ retention and hypertension, a condition referred to as **mineralocorticoid excess syndrome** (MES).

SYMPATHETIC DIVISION OF THE AUTONOMIC NERVOUS SYSTEM. Sympathetic nerve terminals in the kidney release norepinephrine, which has three major effects on Na$^+$ reabsorption. First, high levels of sympathetic stimulation markedly reduce renal blood flow and, therefore, GFR (p. 771). As a result of proximal GT balance (see Fig. 34–10), as well as the flow response of the distal nephron (see Fig. 34–11), Na$^+$ excretion decreases. Second, norepinephrine stimulates granular cells to release renin, activating the renin-angiotensin-aldosterone axis (see earlier). Third, even low levels of sympathetic stimulation activate α-adrenergic receptors on renal-tubule cells to increase Na$^+$ reabsorption, independent of any hemodynamic effects. This increase results from the activation of both the apical Na-H exchanger (NHE3) and the basolateral Na-K pump in the proximal tubule (see Fig. 34–4A).

ARGININE VASOPRESSIN OR ANTIDIURETIC HORMONE. Released by the posterior pituitary, AVP binds to a G$_s$-linked receptor at the basolateral membrane of target cells, leading to an increase in [cAMP]$_i$ (p. 97). The overall renal effect of AVP in humans is to produce urine with a high osmolality and thereby retain water. AVP achieves this action mainly by increasing the water permeability of the collecting tubules and ducts, allowing water to exit the tubule lumen and enter the hypertonic medullary interstitium (p. 840). However, AVP also stimulates Na$^+$ reabsorption. In the TAL, AVP stimulates the apical Na/K/Cl cotransporter and K$^+$ channels, thus enhancing the generation of the hypertonic interstitium. In principal cells of the initial and cortical collecting tubules, AVP stimulates Na$^+$ transport by increasing the number of open Na$^+$ channels (NP$_o$) in the apical membrane. This effect may reflect fusion of Na$^+$-channel-containing vesicles with the apical cell membrane or activation of preexisting Na$^+$ channels in the membrane by cAMP-dependent protein kinase.

Natriuretic Factors—such as Atrial Natriuretic Peptide (ANP), Endogenous ATPase Inhibitor, Prostaglandins, Bradykinin, and Dopamine—All Decrease Na$^+$ Reabsorption

Five humoral agents have significant natriuretic action, in part due to inhibition of Na$^+$ reabsorption at the level of the tubule cell.

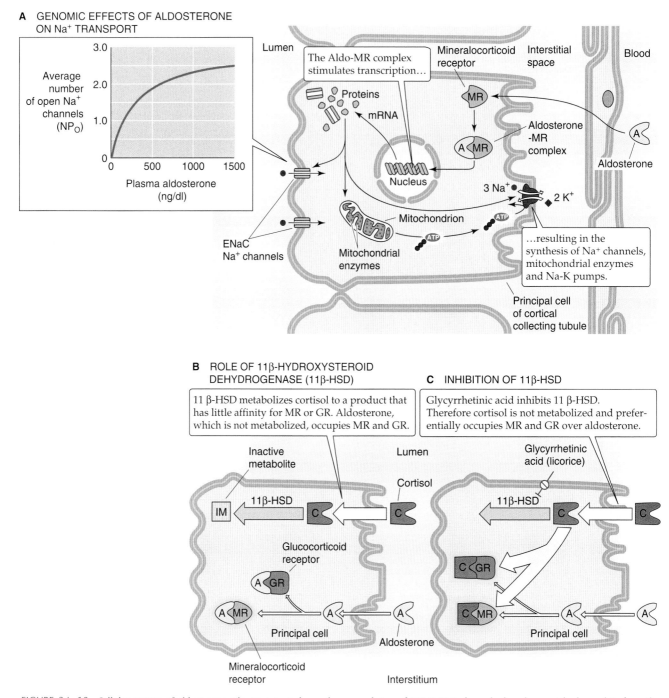

A   GENOMIC EFFECTS OF ALDOSTERONE ON Na+ TRANSPORT

B   ROLE OF 11β-HYDROXYSTEROID DEHYDROGENASE (11β-HSD)

11 β-HSD metabolizes cortisol to a product that has little affinity for MR or GR. Aldosterone, which is not metabolized, occupies MR and GR.

C   INHIBITION OF 11β-HSD

Glycyrrhetinic acid inhibits 11 β-HSD. Therefore cortisol is not metabolized and preferentially occupies MR and GR over aldosterone.

FIGURE 34–13. Cellular actions of aldosterone. The *inset* in *A* shows the upregulation of ENaC Na+ channels, based on patch-clamp data from the rat cortical collecting tubule. N is the number of channels in the patch and P_O is the open probability. In *B*, 11β-HSD prevents cortisol (a glucocorticoid), which is present at high plasma concentrations, from having mineralocorticoid effects in the target cell. In *C*, with the enzyme blocked, cortisol acts as a mineralocorticoid. ATP, adenosine triphosphate; GR, glucocorticoid receptor; MR, mineralocorticoid; mRNA, messenger RNA.

ATRIAL NATRIURETIC PEPTIDE. Atrial natriuretic peptide (ANP) is the fourth of the four parallel effectors (p. 867) that control effective circulating volume, and the only one that promotes Na+ excretion. A polypeptide released by atrial cardiac myocytes (p. 549), ANP stimulates a receptor guanylyl cyclase to generate cyclic guanosine monophosphate (cGMP; p. 108). The hemodynamic actions of ANP—increased GFR, increased cortical and medullary blood flow, and decreased release of renin and AVP—promote natriuresis. In addition, ANP also directly inhib-

its Na+ transport in the inner medullary collecting duct. Patch-clamp studies show that cGMP directly decreases the activity of nonselective cation channels in the apical membrane of the medullary collecting duct.

ENDOGENOUS ADENOSINE TRIPHOSPHATASE INHIBI-TOR. Recent evidence indicates that human plasma contains an endogenous, ouabain-like steroid that inhibits Na-K pumps in a wide variety of cells. This natural Na-K pump inhibitor increases with salt loading and is present in high levels in patients with hypertension. The general hypothesis is that, in response to Na$^+$ loading, the body increases levels of this inhibitor, which presumably would bind preferentially to Na-K pumps of collecting-duct cells, thereby enhancing Na$^+$ excretion.

PROSTAGLANDINS AND BRADYKININ. Produced locally in the kidney, these agents act through protein kinase C (p. 102) to inhibit Na$^+$ reabsorption, probably by phosphorylating K$^+$ or Na$^+$ channels. In the TAL, PGE$_2$ inhibits the apical *K$^+$ channel*, depolarizing the apical and basolateral membranes, and diminishing passive Cl$^-$ efflux across the basolateral membrane. [Cl$^-$]$_i$ therefore rises, impeding the turnover of the apical Na/K/Cl cotransporter (see Fig. 34–4*B*). Also, the transepithelial voltage becomes less lumen positive, thus decreasing the driving force for passive paracellular reabsorption of Na$^+$ and other cations. In the cortical collecting tubule, both PGE$_2$ and bradykinin inhibit ENaC *Na$^+$ channels* (see Fig. 34–4*D*).

DOPAMINE. The kidney forms dopamine locally from circulating L-dopa. Na$^+$ loading increases the synthesis and urinary excretion rate of dopamine, whereas a low Na$^+$ diet has the opposite effect. As noted earlier, dopamine causes renal vasodilation (p. 772), which increases Na$^+$ excretion. In addition, dopamine directly inhibits Na$^+$ reabsorption at the level of tubule cells. Indeed, D$_1$ and D$_2$ dopamine receptors are present in the renal cortex, where they both apparently lead to an increase in [cAMP]$_i$. The result is an inhibition of both the apical Na-H exchanger and the basolateral Na-K pump in proximal-tubule and TAL cells. Indeed, administering low doses of dopamine to humans leads to natriuresis, at least in part by inhibiting Na-H exchangers and Na-K pumps.

REFERENCES

Books and Reviews

Aronson PS, Giebisch G: Mechanisms of chloride transport in the proximal tubule. Am J Physiol 273:F179–F192, 1997.

Benos DL, Fuller DM, Shlyonsky VG, et al: Amiloride-sensitive Na$^+$ channels: Insights and outlooks. News Physiol Sci 12:55–61, 1997.

Garcia NH, Ramsey CR, Knox FG: Understanding the role of paracellular transport in the proximal tubule. News Physiol Sci 13:38–243, 1998.

Reilly RF, Ellison DH: The mammalian distal tubule: Physiology, pathophysiology, and molecular anatomy. Physiol Rev 80:277–313, 2000.

Seldin DW, Giebisch G (eds): The Kidney: Physiology and Pathophysiology, 3rd ed. Philadelphia, Lippincott Williams & Wilkins, 2000.

Wilcox CS, Baylis C, Wingo C: Glomerulo-Tubular Balance and Proximal Regulation. In Seldin DW, Giebisch G (eds): The Kidney: Physiology, 2nd ed, Vol 2. New York, Raven Press, 1992, pp 1805–1841.

Wright FS: Flow-dependent transport processes: Filtration, absorption, secretion. Am J Physiol 243:F1–F11, 1982.

Journal Articles

Alpern RJ, Howlin KJ, Preisig P: Active and passive components of chloride transport in the rat proximal convoluted tubule. J Clin Invest 76:1360–1366, 1985.

Green R, Giebisch G: Osmotic forces driving water reabsorption in the proximal tubule of the rat kidney. Am J Physiol 257:F669–F675, 1989.

Lewy J, Windhager EE: Peritubular control of proximal tubular fluid reabsorption in the rat kidney. Am J Physiol 214:943–954, 1968.

CHAPTER 35

Transport of Urea, Glucose, Phosphate, Calcium, Magnesium, and Organic Solutes

Gerhard Giebisch and Erich Windhager

The kidney plays a central role in controlling the plasma levels of a wide range of solutes that are present at low concentrations in the body. The renal excretion of a solute depends on three processes—filtration, reabsorption, and secretion (p. 746). The kidney filters and then totally reabsorbs some of the substances we discuss in this chapter (e.g., glucose). Others, it filters and also secretes (e.g., the organic anion p-aminohippurate [PAH]). Still others, the kidney filters, reabsorbs, and secretes (e.g., urea).

UREA

The Kidney Filters, Reabsorbs, and Secretes Urea

The liver generates urea from NH_4^+, the primary nitrogenous end product of amino acid catabolism (p. 997). The primary route for urea excretion is the urine, although some urea exits through the stool and sweat. The normal plasma concentration of urea is 2.5 to 6 mM. Clinical laboratories report plasma urea levels as **blood urea nitrogen** (BUN) in the units "mg of elemental nitrogen per dl plasma"; normal values are 7 to 18 mg/dl. For a 70-kg human on a typical Western diet, and producing 1.5 to 2 liters/day of urine, the urinary excretion of urea is approximately 450 mmole/day.

The kidney freely filters urea at the glomerulus, and then it both reabsorbs and secretes it. Because the tubules reabsorb more urea than they secrete, the amount of urea excreted in the urine is less than the quantity filtered. In the example shown in Figure 35–1A (i.e., average urine flow), the kidneys excrete approximately 40% of the filtered urea. The primary sites for urea reabsorption are the proximal tubule and the medullary collecting duct, whereas the primary sites for secretion are the thin limbs of the loop of Henle.

In the very early **proximal tubule** (Fig. 35–1B), [urea] in the lumen is the same as in blood plasma. However, paracellular fluid reabsorption along the proximal tubule sweeps some urea along with it via **solvent drag** (p. 469). In addition, water leaves the lumen through the tubule cells, leaving behind urea, and generating a favorable transepithelial gradient for urea that drives its reabsorption by **diffusion** via the transcellular or paracellular pathway. The greater the fluid reabsorption along the proximal tubule, the greater is the reabsorption of urea via both solvent drag and diffusion.

In *juxtamedullary* nephrons, as the tubule fluid in the **thin descending limb** (tDLH) approaches the tip of the loop of Henle, [urea] is higher in

A HANDLING OF UREA ALONG NEPHRON

B PROXIMAL TUBULE

C THIN DESCENDING LIMB (tDLH)

D THIN ASCENDING LIMB (tALH)

E INNER MEDULLARY COLLECTING DUCT (IMCD)

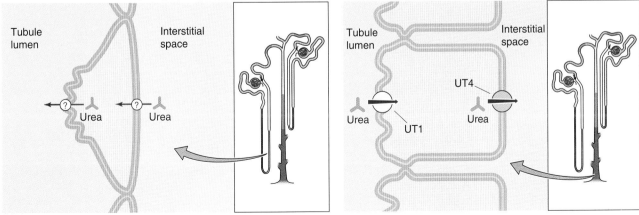

FIGURE 35–1. Urea handling by the kidney. In *A*, we assume a normal urine flow, and thus a urea excretion of 40% of the filtered load. The *numbered yellow boxes* indicate the fraction of the filtered load that various nephron segments *reabsorb*. The thin ascending limb (tALH) and the tip of the thin descending limb (tDLH) in juxtamedullary nephrons secrete urea. In superficial nephrons, the entire tDLH may secrete urea. The *red box* indicates the fraction of the filtered load jointly *secreted* by both nephron types. The *green boxes* indicate the fraction of the filtered load that remains in the lumen after these segments are secreted. UT, urea transporter.

FIGURE 35–2. Urea excretion versus urine flow. GFR, glomerular filtration rate. (Data from Austin JH, Stillman E & Van Slyke DD: Factors governing the excretion rate of urea. *J Biol Chem* 46:91–112, 1921.)

the medullary interstitium than in the lumen (p. 835). Thus, the deepest portion of the tDLH, which has a urea transporter known as **UT2**, *secretes* urea via facilitated diffusion (Fig. 28–1C). As the fluid turns the corner to flow up the **thin ascending limb** (tALH), the tubule cells continue to secrete urea into the lumen, probably also by facilitated diffusion (Fig. 28–1D).

The tDLH of *superficial* nephrons is located in the inner stripe of the outer medulla. Here, the interstitial [urea] is higher than the luminal [urea] because the vasa recta carry urea from the inner medulla. Because the tDLH cells of these superficial nephrons appear to have UT2 along their entire length, these cells *secrete* urea. Thus, both superficial and juxtamedullary nephrons contribute to urea secretion, raising urea delivery to approximately 110% of the filtered load at the level of the cortical collecting ducts.

Finally, the **inner medullary collecting duct** (IMCD) *reabsorbs* urea via a transcellular route that is unusual in that both the apical and basolateral steps occur via facilitated diffusion (Fig. 35–1E). The **UT1** urea transporter moves urea across the apical membrane of the IMCD cell, whereas **UT4** probably mediates urea movement across the basolateral membrane. Arginine vasopressin (AVP)—also known as antidiuretic hormone (ADH)—stimulates UT1 but not UT4. In Chapter 37, we discuss the role of urea transport in the urinary concentrating mechanism (p. 836).

UT2, the prototypical member of the UT family, is a 43-kDa integral membrane protein with 10 putative membrane-spanning segments. UT2 is unusual among membrane proteins in that it is extremely hydrophobic; except for a large extracellular loop, almost the entire central portion of the protein may be embedded within the membrane. UT1, a splice variant of the same gene, is a 102-kDa protein with 20 membrane-spanning segments. UT1 is nearly a tandem repeat of UT2, with the two UT2-like domains linked by an intracellular loop. This loop has several putative phosphorylation sites for protein kinase A (PKA), which explains why AVP—which acts through cyclic adenosine monophosphate (cAMP) (p. 97)—stimulates only UT1. As is discussed in Chapter 37, **UT3**, which is closely related to UT2, is present in the descending limb of the vasa recta (p. 838).

Urea Excretion Rises with Increasing Urinary Flow

Because urea transport depends primarily on urea concentration differences across the tubule epithelium, changes in urine flow unavoidably affect renal urea handling (Fig. 35–2). At low urine flow, when the tubule reabsorbs considerable water and, therefore, much urea, the kidneys excrete only approximately 15% of filtered urea (see Fig. 37–5). However, the kidneys may excrete as much as 70% of filtered urea at high urine flow, when the tubules reabsorb relatively less water and urea. During the progression of renal disease, the decline of the glomerular filtration rate (GFR) leads to a low urine flow and urea retention, and thus an increase in BUN.

In clinical conditions such as *volume depletion*, in which the urine flow declines sharply (p. 864), urea excretion decreases out of proportion to the fall in GFR. The resulting high BUN can thus serve as laboratory confirmation of dehydration. The flow dependence of urea clearance contrasts with the behavior of creatinine clearance, which, like inulin clearance (p. 759), is largely independent of urine flow. Consequently, in patients with reduced effective circulating volume (p. 556), and thus a low urine flow, the plasma [BUN]/[creatinine] ratio increases from its normal value of approximately 10 (both concentrations in mg/dl).

GLUCOSE

The Proximal Tubule Reabsorbs Glucose via an Apical, Electrogenic Na/Glucose Cotransporter (SGLT) and a Basolateral Facilitated Diffusion Mechanism (GLUT)

Glucose is normally present in plasma at concentrations of 4 to 5 mM (70–100 mg/dl), a range that insulin and other hormones carefully regulate. The kidneys freely filter glucose at the glomerulus and then reabsorb it, so that only trace amounts normally appear in the urine (Fig. 35–3A). The *proximal tubule* reabsorbs nearly all the filtered load of glucose, mostly along the first third of this

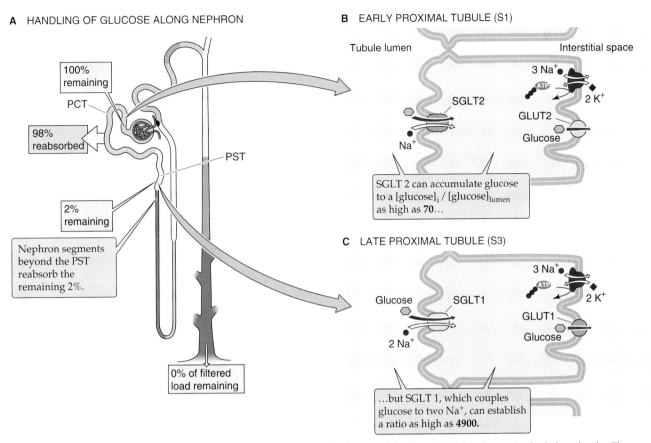

A HANDLING OF GLUCOSE ALONG NEPHRON

100% remaining

PCT

98% reabsorbed

PST

2% remaining

Nephron segments beyond the PST reabsorb the remaining 2%.

0% of filtered load remaining

B EARLY PROXIMAL TUBULE (S1)

Tubule lumen   Interstitial space

3 Na$^+$

ATP

2 K$^+$

SGLT2

GLUT2

Glucose

Na$^+$

SGLT 2 can accumulate glucose to a [glucose]$_i$ / [glucose]$_{lumen}$ as high as **70**...

C LATE PROXIMAL TUBULE (S3)

3 Na$^+$

ATP

2 K$^+$

Glucose   SGLT1

GLUT1

Glucose

2 Na$^+$

...but SGLT 1, which couples glucose to two Na$^+$, can establish a ratio as high as **4900.**

FIGURE 35–3. Glucose handling by the kidney. The *yellow box* indicates the fraction of the filtered load that the proximal tubule reabsorbs. The *green boxes* indicate the fraction of the filtered load that remains in the lumen at various sites. GLUT, glucose transporter (which mediates facilitated diffusion); PCT, proximal convoluted tubule; PST, proximal straight tubule; SGLT, Na/glucose cotransporter.

segment. More distal segments reabsorb almost all of the remainder. In the proximal tubule, luminal [glucose] is initially equal to plasma [glucose]. As the early proximal tubule reabsorbs glucose, luminal [glucose] drops sharply, falling to levels far below those in the interstitium. Accordingly, glucose reabsorption occurs against a concentration gradient and must, therefore, be active.

Glucose reabsorption is transcellular; glucose moves from the lumen to the proximal tubule cell via Na/glucose cotransport, and from cytoplasm to blood via facilitated diffusion (Fig. 35–3B, C). At the apical membrane, a member of the **Na/glucose cotransporter** family (p. 66) couples the movements of the electrically neutral D-glucose (but not L-glucose) and Na$^+$. Phloridzin, extracted from the root bark of certain fruit trees (e.g., cherry, apple), inhibits the SGLTs. The basolateral Na-K pump maintains intracellular [Na$^+$] ([Na$^+$]$_i$) below the [Na$^+$] of the tubule fluid. Moreover, the electrically negative cell interior establishes a steep electrical gradient that favors the passage of Na$^+$ from lumen to cell. Thus, the electrochemical gradient of Na$^+$ drives the uphill transport of glucose into the cell (i.e., secondary active transport), concentrating glucose in the cytoplasm (Fig. 35–4).

In the early part of the proximal tubule (S1 segment), a high-capacity/low-affinity transporter called SGLT2 mediates apical glucose uptake (see Fig. 35–3B). This cotransporter has an Na$^+$:glucose stoichiometry of 1:1. In the later part of the proximal tubule (S3 segment), a high-affinity/low-capacity cotransporter called SGLT1 is responsible for apical glucose uptake (Fig. 35–3C). Because this cotransporter has an Na$^+$/glucose stoichiometry of 2:1 (i.e., far more energy per glucose), it can generate a far larger glucose gradient across the apical membrane (p. 66). Paracellular glucose permeability progressively diminishes along the proximal tubule, further contributing to the tubule's ability to maintain high transepithelial glucose gradients and to generate near-zero glucose concentrations in the fluid emerging from the proximal tubule.

Once inside the cell, glucose exits across the basolateral membrane via a member of the **GLUT** family of glucose transporters (p. 60). These transporters are Na$^+$-*independent* and move glucose by facilitated diffusion. Thus, the GLUTs are quite distinct from the SGLTs. Like the apical SGLTs, the basolateral GLUTs differ between early and late proximal tubule segments, with GLUT2 in the early proximal tubule (see Fig. 35–3B) and GLUT1 in the late proximal tubule (see Fig. 35–3C). In contrast to the apical SGLTs, the basolateral GLUTs have a much lower sensitivity to phloridzin.

Glucose Excretion in the Urine Occurs Only When the Plasma Concentration Exceeds a Threshold

The relationship between plasma [glucose] and the rate of glucose reabsorption is the **glucose titration curve**. Figure 35–5A shows how rates of glucose filtration (*orange curve*), excretion (*green*), and reabsorption (*red*) vary when

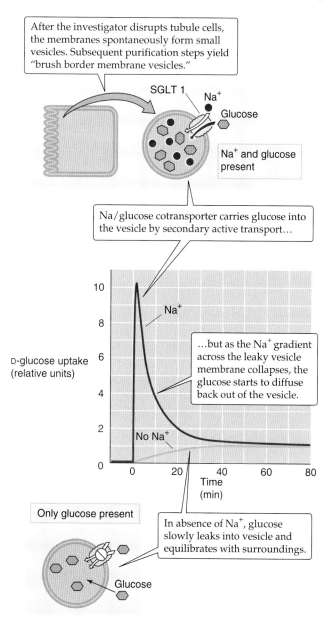

After the investigator disrupts tubule cells, the membranes spontaneously form small vesicles. Subsequent purification steps yield "brush border membrane vesicles."

SGLT 1

Na⁺ and glucose present

Na/glucose cotransporter carries glucose into the vesicle by secondary active transport...

...but as the Na⁺ gradient across the leaky vesicle membrane collapses, the glucose starts to diffuse back out of the vesicle.

Only glucose present

In absence of Na⁺, glucose slowly leaks into vesicle and equilibrates with surroundings.

FIGURE 35–4. Glucose uptake into brush-border membrane vesicles. SGLT, Na/glucose cotransporter.

one increases plasma [glucose] by infusing intravenous glucose. As plasma [glucose] rises from control levels to approximately 250 mg/dl, glucose excretion remains zero. It is only above a **threshold** of approximately 250 mg/dl (~14 mM) that glucose appears in the urine. Glucose excretion rises linearly as plasma [glucose] increases further. Because the threshold is considerably higher than the normal plasma [glucose] of approximately 100 mg/dl (~5.5 mM), and because the body effectively regulates plasma [glucose] (p. 1069), healthy people do not excrete any glucose in the urine, even after a meal. Likewise, patients with *diabetes mellitus*, who have chronically elevated plasma glucose concentrations, do not experience glucosuria until the blood sugar level exceeds this threshold value.

The glucose titration curve shows a second property — **saturation**. The rate of glucose reabsorption reaches a

plateau (T_m) at approximately 400 mg/min. The reason for the T_m value is that the low-capacity Na/glucose cotransporter (i.e, SGLT1) in the late proximal tubule—and perhaps even the high-capacity cotransporter (i.e., SGLT2) in the early proximal tubule—now become fully saturated. Therefore, these transporters cannot respond to further increases in filtered glucose.

Figure 35–5A also shows that the rate of glucose reab-

FIGURE 35–5. The effect of increasing plasma glucose concentrations on glucose excretion and clearance. In *A*, T_m is the transport maximum for reabsorption.

sorption reaches the T_m gradually, not abruptly. This **splay** in the titration curve probably reflects both anatomic and kinetic differences among nephrons. Therefore, a particular nephron's filtered load of glucose may be mismatched to its capacity to reabsorb glucose. For example, a nephron with a larger glomerulus has a larger load of glucose to reabsorb. Different nephrons may have different distributions and densities of SGLT2 and SGLT1 along the proximal tubule. Accordingly, saturation in different nephrons may occur at different plasma levels.

At low filtered glucose loads, when no glucose appears in the urine (see Fig. 35–5A), the *clearance* (p. 746) of glucose is zero. As the filtered load increases beyond the threshold, and glucose excretion increases linearly with plasma [glucose], the clearance of glucose progressively increases. At extremely high glucose loads, when the amount of glucose reabsorbed becomes small compared with the filtered load, glucose behaves more like inulin (i.e., it remains in the tubule lumen). Thus, if we replot the glucose-excretion data in Figure 35–5A as *clearance* (i.e., excretion divided by plasma [glucose]), we see that, as the filtered glucose load rises, glucose clearance (see Fig. 35–5B, *red curve*) approaches inulin clearance (*orange*).

The four key characteristics of glucose transport—(1) threshold, (2) saturation (T_m), (3) splay, and (4) clearance approaching GFR at infinite plasma concentrations—ap-

ply to several other solutes as well, including amino acids, Krebs cycle intermediates (e.g., acetate, citrate, and α-ketoglutarate), PAH, and phosphate.

OTHER ORGANIC SOLUTES

The Proximal Tubule Reabsorbs Amino Acids Using Apical and Basolateral Transporters Mediating Secondary Active Transport or Facilitated Diffusion

The total concentration of amino acids in the blood is approximately 2.4 mM. These L-amino acids are largely those absorbed by the GI tract (p. 956), although they may be the products of protein catabolism or of the de novo synthesis of nonessential amino acids.

The glomeruli freely filter amino acids (Fig. 35–6A). Because amino acids are important nutrients, it is advantageous to retrieve them from the filtrate. The proximal tubule reabsorbs more than 98% of these amino acids via a transcellular route, using a wide variety of amino acid transporters (see Table 44–3). At the *apical* membrane, Na⁺-dependent cotransporters mediate the active uptake of many amino acids, although Na⁺-independent, facilitated diffusion mediates the uptake of others (Fig. 35–

A HANDLING OF AMINO ACIDS ALONG NEPHRON

B GENERIC MODEL OF AMINO-ACID REABSORPTION BY PROXIMAL TUBULE

C REABSORPTION OF Glu⁻, Lys⁺, AND Pro BY PROXIMAL TUBULE

FIGURE 35–6. Amino-acid handling by the kidney. In *A*, the *yellow box* indicates the fraction of the filtered load that the proximal tubule reabsorbs. The *green boxes* indicate the fraction of the filtered load that remains in the lumen at various sites. PCT, proximal convoluted tubule; PST, proximal straight tubule. In *C*, Glu⁻ is glutamate, Lys⁺ is lysine, and Pro is proline.

HYPERAMINOACIDURIAS

In general, an increase in the renal excretion of an amino acid (**hyperaminoaciduria**) may occur when the plasma concentration increases owing to any of several metabolic derangements, or when the carrier-mediated reabsorption of the amino acid decreases abnormally.

Prerenal (i.e., the defect is *before* the kidney) **hyperaminoacidurias. Hyperargininemia** (Table 35–1*A*), an inherited condition in which a metabolic defect leads to an increase in plasma arginine (Arg) levels, which in turn increases the filtered load of Arg. Although the reabsorption of Arg increases, the filtered load exceeds the T_m, and the renal excretion increases.

Competition. Because the same transporter (y^+ or CAT in Table 44–3) that carries Arg across the apical membrane also transports lysine (Lys) and ornithine, competition from Arg decreases the reabsorption of the other two (Table 35–1*B*). As a result, the urinary excretion of Lys and ornithine also increases. Because the metabolic production of Lys and ornithine does not change, plasma concentrations of these two amino acids, in contrast to that of Arg, usually fall.

Renal aminoacidurias. This category of diseases results from an autosomal recessive defect in an amino acid transporter (Table 35–1*C*), and thus also affects absorption in the GI tract (see box on p. 958). In **Hartnup disease**, the defective apical membrane transporter normally handles neutral and ring-structured amino acids (e.g., Ala, Ser, Phe, Trp). In **cystinuria,** the affected transporter normally is present in the apical-membrane, and it carries cystine (Cys-S-S-Cys), Arg, Lys, and ornithine. An increased filtered load of one of these amino acids leads to increased excretion of all of them. Nephrolithiasis (i.e., kidney stones) may be a consequence of the increased excretion of the poorly soluble cystine.

Generalized proximal tubule dysfunction. The Fanconi syndrome (Table 35–1*D*), which can be inherited or acquired, is characterized by a generalized loss of proximal tubule function. The kidney fails to appropriately reabsorb not only amino acids, but also Na$^+$, Cl$^-$, HCO$_3^-$, glucose, and water.

6B). At the *basolateral* membrane, most amino acids exit the cell via facilitated diffusion. Particularly in the late proximal tubule and "postproximal" nephron segments, where the availability of luminal amino acids is low, Na$^+$-dependent amino acid uptake across the basolateral membrane is important for metabolism or nutrition of the cells. For example, a basolateral Na$^+$-dependent transporter takes up glutamine—the precursor for NH$_4^+$ synthesis and gluconeogenesis in proximal tubule cells.

Although the proximal tubule reabsorbs most amino acids by one of the generic pathways illustrated in Figure 35–6*B*, it reabsorbs others using alternate mechanisms. For example, the apical glutamate transporter moves not only Na$^+$ but also H$^+$ into the cell, and moves K$^+$ out (Fig. 35–6*C*). Glutamate probably exits across the basolateral membrane via facilitated diffusion. The positively

charged lysine crosses the apical membrane by facilitated diffusion driven by the cell-negative voltage. However, lysine exits across the basolateral membrane in *exchange* for Na$^+$, rather than jointly with Na$^+$. Proline transport also does not fit the generic model because it enters together with H$^+$, rather than with Na$^+$. Proline exits across the basolateral membrane via facilitated diffusion.

Because the same carrier can reabsorb structurally similar amino acids, *competitive inhibition* may occur in the presence of two related amino acids. This effect may explain why the tubules do not fully reabsorb some amino acids (e.g., glycine, histidine, and some nonproteogenic amino acids, such as 1-methylhistidine and taurine), even though the transporter itself is normal. Competition can also occur in patients with hyperargininemia (see the box, Hyperaminoacidurias).

Apparent competition between transported solutes occurs when they compete for the same energy source. Because the apical uptake of a large number of organic solutes and some inorganic solutes (e.g., phosphate, sulfate) depends on the electrochemical Na$^+$ gradient, increasing the activity of one such transporter can slow others. Thus, glucose loading may compromise the reabsorption of amino acids and other solutes. This competitive behavior occurs for two reasons. First, solute-coupled Na$^+$ entry through one transporter raises [Na$^+$]$_i$ and thus diminishes the chemical Na$^+$ gradient for other Na$^+$-driven transporters. Second, some Na$^+$-driven transporters carry net positive charge into the cell, causing the membrane voltage across the apical membrane to become more positive, thus decreasing the electrical energy available for unrelated electrogenic transporters that carry "competing" solutes.

With a few exceptions, the kinetics of amino acid reabsorption resembles that of glucose: The titration curves show saturation and transport maxima (T_m). In contrast to the case of glucose, where the T_m is relatively high, the T_m values for amino acids are generally low. As a consequence, when plasma levels of amino acids increase, the kidneys excrete the amino acids in the urine, thus limiting the maximal plasma levels.

An H$^+$-Driven Cotransporter Takes Up Oligopeptides Across the Apical Membrane, Whereas Endocytosis Takes Up Proteins and Other Large Organic Molecules

OLIGOPEPTIDES. The proximal tubules effectively reabsorb approximately 99% of filtered oligopeptides (Fig. 35–7*A*). Segments beyond the proximal tubule contribute little to peptide transport.

Several peptidases are present at the outer surface of the brush border membrane of proximal tubule cells (Fig. 35–7*B*), just as they are in the small intestine (p. 955). These brush border enzymes (e.g., γ-glutamyltransferase, aminopeptidases, endopeptidases, and dipeptidases) hydrolyze many peptides, including angiotensin II (p. 866), releasing into the tubule lumen the free constituent amino acids and oligopeptides. Tubule cells reabsorb the resulting free amino acids as described in the previous section. The cell also absorbs the resulting oligopeptides—as well

TABLE 35–1

PATTERNS OF HYPERAMINOACIDURIAS

	DISEASE	AMINO ACIDS	MECHANISM
A. Prerenal hyperaminoaciduria ("overflow")	Hyperargininemia	Arg	Elevated plasma concentration and thus elevated filtered load overwhelms T_m.
B. Competition	Side effect of hyper-argininemia	Lys Ornithine	High filtered load of one amino acid (e.g., Arg) inhibits the reabsorption of another, in this case carried by same transporter.
C. Renal aminoaciduria	Anionic aminoaciduria	Glu Asp	Amino acid transporter (EAAT3) is defective, impairing reabsorption. Rare autosomal-recessive disease.
	Hartnup disease (neutral aminoaciduria)	Neutral and ring-structure amino acids (e.g., phenylalanine)	Amino acid transporter (ATB⁰) is defective, impairing reabsorption. Autosomal-recessive disease.
	Cystinuria (cationic aminoaciduria)	Cystine (Cys-S-S-Cys)	The amino acid transporter (D2 or rBAT) is defective. Autosomal-recessive disease.
D. Generalized proximal tubule dysfunction	Fanconi syndrome	All amino acids	Metabolic, immune or toxic conditions (inherited or acquired) that impair function of the proximal tubule cell.

as other peptides (e.g., carnosine and aminopeptides) that are resistant to brush border enzymes—using an apical H/oligopeptide cotransporter (PepT1; p. 67). Driven by the lumen-to-cell H^+ gradient, this transporter takes up small peptides, two to four amino acids in length.

Once inside the cell, the oligopeptides undergo hydrolysis by cytosolic peptidases; this pathway is involved in the degradation of neurotensin and bradykinin. The distinction between which oligopeptides the cells fully digest in the lumen, and which they take up via PepT1 is not clear-cut. Those oligopeptides that are more resistant to hydrolysis by peptidases are probably more likely to enter via PepT1.

PROTEINS. Although the glomerular filtration barrier (p. 741) generally prevents the filtration of large amounts of protein, this restriction is incomplete (p. 760). For example, the albumin concentration in the filtrate is very low (4 to 20 mg/liter), which is only 0.01% to 0.05% of the plasma albumin concentration. Nevertheless, given a GFR of 180 liters/day, the filtered albumin amounts to 0.7 to 3.6 g per day. In contrast, albumin excretion in the urine normally is only approximately 30 mg per day. Thus, the tubules reabsorb some 96% to 99% of filtered albumin (Fig. 35–7C). In addition to albumin, the tubules extensively reabsorb other proteins (e.g., lysozyme, light chains of immunoglobulins, and β_2-microglobulin), SH-containing peptides (e.g., insulin), and other polypeptide hormones (e.g., parathyroid hormone [PTH], atrial natriuretic peptide [ANP], and glucagon). It is not surprising that tubule injury can give rise to proteinuria even in the absence of glomerular injury.

Proximal tubule cells use **receptor-mediated endocytosis** (p. 42) to reabsorb proteins and polypeptides (Fig. 35–7D). The first step is binding to components of the apical membrane, followed by internalization into

clathrin-coated endocytotic vesicles. Factors that interfere with vesicle formation or internalization, such as metabolic inhibitors and cytochalasin B, inhibit this selective absorption. The vesicles fuse with endosomes; this fusion recycles the vesicle membrane to the apical surface and targets their content for delivery to lysosomes. At the lysosomes, acid-dependent proteases largely digest the contents over a period that is on the order of minutes for peptide hormones, and many hours or even days for other proteins. The cells ultimately release the low-molecular-weight end products of digestion, largely amino acids, across the basolateral membrane into the peritubular circulation. Although the proximal tubule hardly reabsorbs any protein in an intact state, a small subset of proteins avoids the lysosomes and move by transcytosis for release at the basolateral membrane.

In addition to the apical absorption and degradation pathway, the kidney has two other pathways for protein degradation. The first may be important for several bioactive proteins, particularly those for which receptors are present on the basolateral membrane (e.g., insulin, ANP, AVP, and PTH). After transcytosis, the proximal tubule cell partially hydrolyzes peptide hormones at the basolateral cell membrane. The resulting peptide fragments reenter the circulation, where they are available for glomerular filtration and ultimate handling by the apical absorption/degradation pathway. The second alternative pathway for protein degradation involves receptor-mediated endocytosis by endothelial cells of the renal vascular and glomerular structures. This pathway participates in the catabolism of small peptides, such as ANP.

In conclusion, the kidney plays a major role in the metabolism of small proteins and peptide hormones. Renal extraction rates may be large, and they account for as much as 80% of the total metabolic clearance. Thus, it is not surprising that end-stage renal disease can lead to

A HANDLING OF OLIGOPEPTIDES
     ALONG NEPHRON

PCT

99% reabsorbed

100% remaining

PST

1% remaining

0% of filtered load remaining

B PROXIMAL TUBULE: OLIGOPEPTIDES

Oligopeptides hydrolyzed by brush border enzymes

$(AA)_n$
Angiotensin
Glutathione

Brush border enzymes

Amino acids (AA)

Na^+

AA

AA

Tubule lumen

Metabolism

Interstitial space

$3\ Na^+$

ATP

$2\ K^+$

PepT 1

H^+

Oligopeptide

AA

AA

$(AA)_n$
Carnosine

Short peptides (n=2 to 4) reabsorbed by oligopeptide cotransporter

Intracellular peptidase

C HANDLING OF PROTEIN
     ALONG NEPHRON

99% reabsorbed

100% remaining

~1% of filtered load remaining

D PROXIMAL TUBULE: PROTEIN

Tubule lumen

Proteins (e.g., albumin)
Peptide hormones (e.g., insulin)

Coated vesicle

Lysosome

Multivesicular body

Interstitial space

Free amino acids

Clathrin-coated pit

Endosome

Multivesicular endosome

Proximal tubule cell

?

FIGURE 35–7. Oligopeptide and protein handling by the kidney. In *A* and *C*, the *yellow box* indicates the fraction of the filtered load that the proximal tubule reabsorbs. The *green boxes* indicate the fraction of the filtered load that remains in the lumen at various sites. PCT, proximal convoluted tubule; PST, proximal straight tubule.

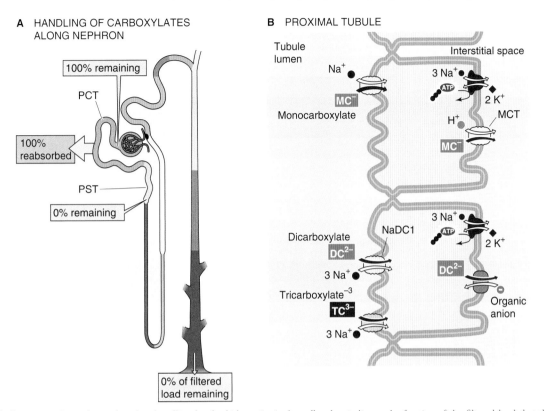

A HANDLING OF CARBOXYLATES ALONG NEPHRON

B PROXIMAL TUBULE

FIGURE 35–8. Mono-, di-, and tricarboxylate handling by the kidney. In *A*, the *yellow box* indicates the fraction of the filtered load that the proximal tubule reabsorbs. The *green boxes* indicate the fraction of the filtered load that remains in the lumen at various sites. MCT, H+/monocarboxylate cotransporter.

elevated levels of glucagon, parathyroid hormone, gastrin, and ANP. Under physiologic conditions, glomerular filtration represents the rate-limiting step for the removal of low-molecular-weight proteins from the circulation—apical absorption by the tubules, intracellular hydrolysis, and peritubular hydrolysis do not saturate over a wide range of filtered loads.

Two Separate Apical Na+-Driven Cotransporters Reabsorb Monocarboxylates and Di/Tricarboxylates

The combined concentration of carboxylates in the blood plasma is a few millimolars, of which lactate represents the largest fraction. The monocarboxylates pyruvate and lactate are products of anaerobic glucose metabolism (p. 1220). The dicarboxylates and tricarboxylates include intermediates of the **citric acid cycle**. Because these carboxylates are important for energy metabolism, their loss in the urine would be wasteful. Normally, the proximal tubule reabsorbs virtually all of these substances (Fig. 35–8*A*).

At least two distinct Na+-dependent cotransporters carry carboxylates across the apical membranes (Fig. 35–8*B*). One system is specific for monocarboxylates, including lactate, pyruvate, acetoacetate, and β-hydroxybutyrate. A second cotransporter (NaDC1) carries dicarboxylates and tricarboxylates, such as α-ketoglutarate, malate, succinate, and citrate. Once inside the cell, the monocarboxylates exit across the basolateral membrane via an

H+/monocarboxylate cotransporter (MCT). Because monocarboxylates enter across the apical membrane coupled to Na+, and then exit across the basolateral membrane coupled to H+, monocarboxylate reabsorption leads to an accumulation of Na+ by the cell and a rise in intracellular pH.

Dicarboxylates exit the cell across the basolateral membrane via multiple organic anion–carboxylate exchangers (e.g., the renal organic anion transporter ROAT1; p. 69) that may overlap in substrate specificity, or even carry anions of different valence. Because the molecular identities and stoichiometries of some of these transporters are unknown, we present organic anion exchangers in a generic sense in this and the next three sections.

Although the proximal tubule normally reabsorbs carboxylates fully, they may appear in the urine when their plasma levels are elevated. Urinary excretion may occur when the filtered load of acetoacetate and β-hydroxybutyrate—ketone bodies (p. 1083) produced during starvation or during low-insulin states (diabetes mellitus)—exceeds the T_m in the proximal tubule.

The Handling of Para-Aminohippurate Is an Example of a T_m-Limited Secretory Mechanism

The kidneys handle para-aminohippurate (PAH, a monovalent anion), as well as many organic anions (e.g., many metabolites of endogenous compounds and administered drugs), by both filtration and secretion (Fig. 35–9A). The synthetic anion PAH is somewhat unusual in that approximately 20% of it binds to plasma proteins, largely albumin. Thus, only about 80% of PAH is available for filtration. Assuming a filtration fraction (p. 763) of 20%, only 80% × 20%, or 16%, of the arterial load of PAH appears in Bowman's space. Nevertheless, the kidneys excrete into the urine nearly all (~90%) of the PAH entering the renal arteries, so that very little PAH remains in the renal veins. Because the kidneys almost completely clear it from the blood in a single passage, PAH is useful for measuring renal plasma flow (p. 767).

The nephron secretes PAH mainly in the late proximal tubule (S3 segment), and does so via the transcellular route, against a sizable electrochemical gradient. PAH uptake across the *basolateral* membrane is energetically uphill, and an example of tertiary active transport. The transporter responsible for PAH uptake is ROAT1, an organic anion exchanger driven by the outward gradient of dicarboxylates, such as α-ketoglutarate (see Fig. 35–9B). Creating this outward dicarboxylate gradient is the task of a basolateral Na/dicarboxylate cotransporter (i.e., *secondary active transport*)—similar to the *apical* Na/dicarboxylate cotransporter (NaDC1) in the lower cell of Figure 35–8B—that carries dicarboxylates from blood to cell. Finally, the basolateral Na-K pump (i.e., *primary active transport*) establishes the Na^+ gradient used to drive the accumulation of dicarboxylates.

The apical step of PAH secretion occurs via carrier-mediated exchange for luminal anions such as urate. Several anionic drugs (e.g., probenecid) that compete at the basolateral PAH-anion exchanger or the apical PAH-anion exchanger inhibit PAH secretion from blood to lumen.

Just as glucose reabsorption saturates at its T_m as one increases plasma [glucose], PAH secretion (Fig. 35–10A, *red curve*) saturates at a sufficiently high plasma [PAH]. Starting from an initially low value, increasing plasma [PAH] causes excretion (*green*) to rise much faster than filtration (*orange*). Subtracting the amount filtered from the amount excreted, we see that the rate of PAH secretion at first rises rapidly with plasma [PAH]. However, as plasma [PAH] approaches approximately 20 mg/dl, the amount of secreted PAH reaches a plateau (T_m), typically 60 to 80 mg/min, indicating saturation of secretory mechanisms.

After plasma [PAH] has increased enough to reach the T_m, further increases in plasma [PAH] increase urinary excretion, but only as a consequence of the increase in the filtered load—not because of increased tubule secretion. At these high plasma PAH levels, the kidneys can no longer fully remove PAH from the blood in a single pass through the kidney, and therefore it would no longer be appropriate to use PAH secretion to estimate renal plasma flow. At low plasma [PAH] values (<12 mg/dl), PAH extraction from plasma flowing through the kidney is nearly complete (~90%), forming the basis for using PAH clearance as a measure of renal plasma flow.

Recall that as plasma [glucose] increases, glucose clearance *rises* to approach inulin clearance (see Fig. 35–5B). In contrast, PAH clearance (Fig. 35–10B, *red curve*) *decreases* with increasing plasma [PAH], and falls to approach the inulin clearance (*orange*). The reason is that, as plasma [PAH] increases, secreted PAH forms a progressively smaller fraction of the PAH appearing in the urine.

A HANDLING OF PAH ALONG NEPHRON

PCT

100% remaining

PST

500% secreted

600% remaining

600% of filtered load remaining

B LATE PROXIMAL TUBULE (S3)

Tubule lumen

Interstitial space

● 3 Na⁺

DC^{2-}

DC^{2-}

Dicarboxylate

Anion ⊖

PAH^-

PAH^-

FIGURE 35–9. PAH handling by the kidney. In *A*, the *red box* indicates the fraction of the filtered load secreted by the proximal tubule. The *green boxes* indicate the fraction of the filtered load that remains in the lumen at various sites when plasma [PAH] is low (<12 mg/dl). PAH, para-aminohippurate; PCT, proximal convoluted tubule.

FIGURE 35–10. The effect of increasing plasma PAH concentrations on PAH excretion and clearance. In A, T_m is the transport maximum for reabsorption. PAH, para-aminohippurate.

Transporters Similar to Those That Secrete PAH Also Secrete a Variety of Organic Anions

In addition to PAH, the late proximal tubule secretes a wide variety of organic anions. These anions include (Table 35–2): (1) Endogenous anions, such as oxalate and bile salts; (2) exogenous anions such as the drugs penicillin and furosemide; and (3) uncharged molecules *conjugated* to anionic groups such as sulfate or glucuronate (p. 987). The proximal tubule secretes these anions into the lumen using basolateral and apical anion exchangers that are similar to those involved in PAH secretion (see Fig. 35–9B). At the apical membrane, the secreted anion appears to exchange for luminal Cl^-, urate, or OH^-.

Although the Proximal Tubule Both Reabsorbs and Secretes Urate, Reabsorption Usually Dominates

Urate, a monovalent anion, is the end product of purine catabolism. Plasma [urate] is typically 3 to 7 mg/dl (0.2–0.4 mM), and is elevated in gout. The kidneys filter urate, and then the proximal tubule successively reabsorbs, secretes, and again reabsorbs urate (Fig. 35–11A). Reabsorption is the more important transport pathway, so that the kidneys excrete only approximately 10% of filtered urate.

Reabsorption of urate occurs by both a paracellular route involving passive diffusion and a transcellular route involving active transport (Fig. 35–11B). The transcellular mechanism predominates in the early proximal tubule. The active apical step does not involve Na^+ cotransport,

but rather the exchange of luminal urate for any of a host of intracellular anions. In pathway #1 in Figure 35–11B, luminal urate exchanges for OH^- or HCO_3^- (*tertiary active transport*) in parallel with the apical Na-H exchanger (*secondary active transport*). In pathway #2, luminal urate exchanges for monocarboxylates (e.g., lactate, β-hydroxybutyrate) or dicarboxylates (*tertiary active transport*), in parallel with Na^+-driven carboxylate cotransport (*secondary active transport*). In pathway #3, luminal urate exchanges for anions like PAH (*tertiary active transport*), in series with the basolateral uptake of the PAH-like anion (*secondary active transport*). Once inside the cell, urate exits across the basolateral membrane, probably in exchange for an anion; in an experimental setting, PAH supports this exchange.

The drugs DIDS (which inhibits many HCO_3^- transporters, probenecid, and salicylate all inhibit the *apical* urate exchanger, and thus cause urate excretion to increase. Indeed, probenecid is useful in the treatment of gout. Probenecid and similar drugs are termed **uricosuric** agents.

Under certain conditions, renal urate excretion exceeds the quantity filtered, indicating net secretion. The active step of urate *secretion* is probably basolateral urate uptake, mediated by an anion exchanger similar to (but different from) the one that mediates basolateral PAH uptake (see Fig. 35–9B). Urate probably exits the cell across the apical membrane by reversal of one of the transport processes shown in Figure 35–11B.

States of extracellular volume depletion and enhanced proximal tubule fluid reabsorption are often associated with decreased urate excretion and thus high plasma levels of urate.

TABLE 35–2

ORGANIC ANIONS AND CATIONS SECRETED BY THE LATE PROXIMAL TUBULE		
	ANIONS	**CATIONS**
Endogenous	cAMP & cGMP	Epinephrine
	Bile salts	Acetylcholine
	Hippurate	Choline
	Oxalate	Dopamine
	α-ketogluta-rate	Histamine
	Short-chain fatty acids	Serotonin
	Prostaglandins (e.g., PGE_2)	Thiamine
	Urate	Guanidine
	Creatinine (zwitterion)	Creatinine (zwitterion)
	Uremic organic anions*	
Exogenous	Acetazolamide	Atropine
		Quinine
	Chlorothiazide	Amiloride
	Furosemide	Cimetidine
	PAH	NMN
	Penicillin G	Morphine
	Probenecid	Paraquat
	Saccharin	Procainamide
	Salicylate	Tetraethylammonium
	Indomethacin	Chlorpromazine
Conjugated (endogenous and exogenous)	Glucuronate conjugates†	
	Glutathione conjugates†	
	Sulfate conjugates†	

* Hippurate-like aryl organic anions that interfere with PAH transport.
† See p. 987.
cAMP, cyclic adenosine monophosphate; cGMP, cyclic guanosine monophosphate; NMN, *N*-methylnicotinamide; PAH, p-aminohippurate; PGE_2, prostaglandin E_2.

The Late Proximal Tubule Secretes Several Organic Cations

The late proximal tubule (Fig. 35–12A) is also responsible for secreting a wide range of both endogenous and exogenous organic *cations* (see Table 35–2). Some of the most important endogenous organic cations are the monoamine neurotransmitters such as dopamine, epinephrine, norepinephrine, and histamine (p. 304). Exogenous secreted organic cations include the morphine, quinine, and the diuretic amiloride (p. 779).

Several polyspecific organic cation transporters (OCT1–3; p. 61) are responsible for the *basolateral* uptake of these organic cations (Fig. 35–12B). OCT1 mediates facilitated diffusion and is electrogenic.

At the *apical* membrane, an organic cation-H^+ exchanger moves these cations from the cell to the lumen.

The energy for the extrusion of the organic cation is the H^+ electrochemical gradient across the apical membrane, from lumen to cell. Because the apical Na-H exchanger (*a secondary active transporter*) is largely responsible for establishing this H^+ gradient, the cation-H exchange is an example of tertiary active transport.

An organic cation–secreting mechanism is also responsible for secreting creatinine, the breakdown product of phosphocreatine. Despite this modest secretion, creatinine is a useful index of GFR (p. 759).

The Nonionic Diffusion of Neutral Weak Acids and Bases Promotes Their Transport Across Tubules and Explains Why Their Excretion Is pH Dependent

Many cations or anions are, in fact, weak acids or bases in equilibrium with a neutral species (p. 634), which generally diffuses across a membrane much faster than the corresponding cation or anion. This rapid diffusion usually occurs because the neutral species is far more soluble in the lipid bilayer of cell membranes than is the charged species.

Changing the luminal pH can substantially affect the overall transport of a buffer pair. For example, acidifying the tubule lumen promotes the reabsorption of a neutral weak acid and the secretion of a neutral weak base. In the case of a neutral weak acid such as salicylic acid (Fig. 35–13A), the glomerular filtrate contains both the neutral weak acid (HA) and its conjugate weak base, which is an anion (A^-). The secretion of H^+ into the lumen (p. 852) titrates the A^- to HA, raising luminal [HA] above intracellular [HA], so that HA rapidly diffuses across the apical membrane—by the process of **nonionic diffusion**—into the tubule cell and across the basolateral membrane into the blood. The more acidic the luminal fluid, the greater the titration of A^- to HA, and the greater the nonionic diffusion of HA from lumen to blood.

In the case of a weak base such as ammonia (Fig. 35–13B), the glomerular filtrate contains both the neutral weak base (B) and the cationic species (BH^+). The secretion of H^+ into the lumen titrates B to BH^+, lowering luminal [B] below intracellular [B], so that B rapidly diffuses from cell to lumen. The resulting fall in intracellular [B] sets up a gradient for B to diffuse from blood to cell. The more acidic the luminal fluid, the greater the titration of B to BH^+, and the greater the nonionic diffusion of B from blood to lumen.

A striking example of how luminal pH affects the clearance of a weak acid is the renal handling of salicylic acid and its anion species, salicylate. At a urinary pH of approximately 7.5, the amount of "total salicylate" (salicylic acid + salicylate anion) excreted is the same as the filtered load (Fig. 35–13C); that is, the clearance of total salicylate ($C_{Salicylate}$) equals GFR. Lower urinary pH values favor the titration of luminal salicylate anion to salicylic acid, which the tubule readily reabsorbs. Hence, lowering pH causes the fractional excretion of total salicylate ($FE_{Salicylate} = C_{Salicylate}/GFR$; p. 749) to fall below unity. At very low urinary pH values, the kidney reabsorbs virtually

A HANDLING OF URATE ALONG NEPHRON

B PROXIMAL TUBULE: URATE REABSORPTION

FIGURE 35–11. Urate handling by the kidney. In *A*, the *yellow arrows* indicate reabsorption, whereas the *red arrow* indicates secretion. The *green boxes* indicate the fraction of the filtered load remaining at various sites. The molecular identities of the apical and basolateral urate transporters are unknown. PAH, para-aminohippurate; PCT, proximal convoluted tubule.

FIGURE 35–12. Organic cation handling by the kidney. In *A*, the *red arrow* indicates secretion. The *green boxes* indicate the fraction of the filtered load remaining at various sites. OCT, organic cation transporter.

A HANDLING OF ORGANIC CATIONS ALONG NEPHRON

B LATE PROXIMAL TUBULE (S3)

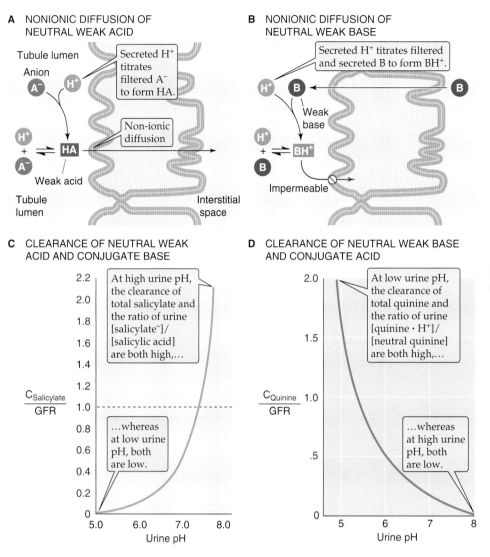

A NONIONIC DIFFUSION OF NEUTRAL WEAK ACID

B NONIONIC DIFFUSION OF NEUTRAL WEAK BASE

C CLEARANCE OF NEUTRAL WEAK ACID AND CONJUGATE BASE

D CLEARANCE OF NEUTRAL WEAK BASE AND CONJUGATE ACID

FIGURE 35–13. Nonionic diffusion. GFR, glomerular filtration rate.

all salicylate, and $FE_{Salicylate}$ approaches zero. However, at urinary pH values above approximately 7.5, $FE_{Salicylate}$ increases markedly because the alkalinity keeps luminal levels of the salicylate anion high and levels of salicylic acid low, so that the neutral weak acid now diffuses from blood to lumen.

It is possible to treat overdoses of salicylate or acetylsalicylate (i.e., aspirin) by alkalinizing the urine with HCO_3^- or by increasing urine flow with diuretics. The reason is that both high pH and high urine flow keep luminal levels of salicylic acid low, maintaining a sink for salicylic acid in the lumen. Both treatments enhance the urinary excretion of the drug and lower plasma concentrations.

The converse example of urinary pH dependence is seen in the excretion of a neutral weak base, such as ammonia or quinine (Fig. 35–13D).

PHOSPHATE

As discussed in Chapter 51, the metabolism of inorganic phosphate depends on bone, the gastrointestinal tract, and kidneys (p. 1088). About half of total plasma phosphate (Table 35–3) is in an ionized form, and the rest is either complexed to small solutes (~40%) or bound to protein (10%–15%). The plasma concentration of total inorganic phosphate varies rather widely, between 0.8 and 1.5 mM (2.5–4.5 mg/dl of elemental phosphorus). Thus, the filterable phosphate (i.e., both the ionized and complexed) varies between about 0.7 and 1.3 mM. At a nor-

TABLE 35–3

COMPONENTS OF TOTAL PLASMA PHOSPHATE			
	mg/dl	**mM**	**% OF TOTAL**
Ionized $H_2PO_4^-$ and HPO_4^{2-}	2.1	0.7	50
Diffusible phosphate complexes	1.5	0.5	40
Nondiffusible (protein-bound) phosphate	0.6	0.2	10
Total phosphate	4.2	1.4	100

mal blood pH of 7.4, 80% of the ionized plasma phosphate is HPO_4^{2-}, and the rest is $H_2PO_4^-$. Assuming that the total plasma phosphate concentration is 4.2 mg/dl, that only the free and complexed phosphate is filterable, and that the GFR is 180 liters/day, each day the kidneys filter approximately 7000 mg of phosphate. Because this amount is more than an order of magnitude greater than the total extracellular pool of phosphate (p. 1088), it is clear that the kidney must reabsorb most of the phosphate filtered in the glomerulus.

The Proximal Tubule Reabsorbs Phosphate via an Apical Na/Phosphate Cotransporter (NaPi)

The proximal tubule reabsorbs approximately 80% of the filtered phosphate (Fig. 35–14A). The loop of Henle and the collecting ducts reabsorb only negligible amounts of phosphate, but the "classical distal tubule" (p. 743) reabsorbs approximately 10% of the filtered load. The kidneys excrete the remaining approximately 10% in the urine.

The proximal tubule reabsorbs most of the filtered phosphate by the transcellular route (Fig. 35–14B). Phosphate ions enter the cell across the *apical* membrane by secondary active transport, energized by the apical electrochemical Na^+ gradient. The apical NaP_i cotransporter (NaP_i, type II) translocates three Na^+ ions and one phosphate ion (either HPO_4^{2-} or $H_2PO_4^-$). Thus, in either case,

the process is electrogenic (net positive charge into the cell). As pH along the proximal tubule falls, the relative concentration of $H_2PO_4^-$ increases, and overall phosphate uptake becomes even more electrogenic.

Apical phosphate uptake is under the control of intracellular pH as well as luminal pH and $[Na^+]$. Intracellular H^+ appears to stimulate NaP_i allosterically. However, *luminal* H^+ is a competitive inhibitor of Na^+ binding to the extracellular face of NaP_i, so that when luminal pH falls, it is more difficult for Na^+ to bind. In addition, even when luminal $[Na^+]$ is saturating, an acidic luminal pH inhibits phosphate uptake, possibly by shifting the phosphate equilibrium toward $H_2PO_4^-$, which NaP_i may not transport as well as HPO_4^{2-}.

The passive exit of phosphate across the *basolateral* membrane occurs by a mechanism that is not well understood. The basolateral membrane also has a *type III* NaP_i cotransporter that carries three Na^+ with each phosphate. It thus mediates electrogenic *uptake* of phosphate — presumably for nutrition of the tubule cells — rather than exit across the basolateral membrane.

Although it is clear that the proximal tubule reabsorbs almost all filtered phosphate at low filtered loads, the role of the distal nephron in phosphate handling is controversial. When experimental animals are maintained on a low-phosphate diet, the classical distal tubule absorbs a significant fraction of the filtered load of phosphate, thus minimizing phosphate loss in the urine.

A   HANDLING OF PHOSPHATE ALONG NEPHRON

B   PROXIMAL TUBULE

FIGURE 35–14. Phosphate handling by the kidney. In *A*, the *numbered yellow boxes* indicate the fraction of the filtered load that various nephron segments reabsorb. The *green boxes* indicate the fraction of the filtered load that remains in the lumen after these segments. In *B*, the *top cell* illustrates reabsorption of divalent phosphate (HPO_4^{2-}), and the *bottom cell* illustrates the reabsorption of monovalent phosphate ($H_2PO_4^-$). PCT, proximal convoluted tubule; PST, proximal straight tubule.

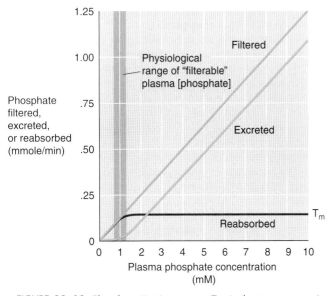

FIGURE 35–15. Phosphate titration curves. Tm is the transport maximum for reabsorption. The plasma phosphate concentration is the filterable phosphate (i.e., ionized plus complexed to small solutes).

TABLE 35–4

FACTORS THAT MODULATE PHOSPHATE EXCRETION

↓ REABSORPTION ↑ EXCRETION	↑ REABSORPTION ↓ EXCRETION
PTH	1,25-dihydroxyvitamin D
Extracellular volume expansion	High Ca^{2+} intake
High dietary phosphate intake	Phosphate deprivation
High plasma (phosphate)	
Glucocorticoids	Insulin
Acidosis	Alkalosis
Calcitonin	Thyroid hormone
ANP	Growth hormone
Dopamine	
Diuretics	
PTHrP	
Fasting	
Acute renal denervation	
Autosomal and X-linked hypophosphatemia	

ANP, atrial natriuretic peptide; PTH, parathyroid hormone; PTHrP, parathyroid hormone–related protein.

Phosphate Excretion in the Urine Already Occurs at Physiologic Plasma Concentrations

Phosphate handling by the kidney shares some of the properties of renal glucose handling, including threshold, saturation with T_m kinetics, and splay (Fig. 35–15). However, there are important differences. First, some phosphate excretion (*green curve*) occurs even at normal levels of plasma [phosphate]. Thus, a small increment in the plasma [phosphate] results in significant acceleration of phosphate excretion (i.e., to higher values along the *green curve*), whereas plasma [glucose] must double before glucose excretion even commences. Accordingly, the kidney plays an important role in the regulation of plasma [phosphate], but does not normally modulate plasma [glucose]. Second, the kidney reaches the T_m for phosphate (*red curve*) at the high end of normal plasma [phosphate] values, whereas the kidney reaches the T_m for glucose at levels that are far above physiologic plasma [glucose] levels. Third, the renal phosphate T_m is sensitive to a variety of stimuli, including hormones and acid-base balance, whereas the glucose T_m is insensitive to regulators of glucose metabolism, such as insulin.

Parathyroid Hormone, the Key Regulator of Phosphate Excretion, Inhibits Apical Na/Phosphate Uptake

Table 35–4 summarizes the major hormones and other factors that regulate phosphate transport by the proximal tubule. Although these factors affect phosphate transport via many different signalling pathways, they fall into two major categories. Some act rapidly and independently of protein synthesis. Others act more slowly, through mechanisms requiring protein synthesis.

The most important hormonal regulator is **parathyroid hormone** (PTH), which inhibits phosphate reabsorption (p. 1093) and thus promotes phosphate excretion. PTH is a classic example of a rapid regulator that does *not* require protein synthesis. PTH binds to PTH 1R receptors, which appear to couple to *two* heterotrimeric G proteins (p. 1093). The first ($G\alpha_s$) activates adenylyl cyclase and, via cAMP, stimulates protein kinase A (PKA; p. 97). The second ($G\alpha_q$), particularly at low PTH levels, activates phospholipase C (PLC), and then protein kinase C (PKC; p. 102). Once activated, PKA and PKC promote endocytotic removal of NaPi from the apical membrane, thus reducing phosphate reabsorption. Conversely, when PTH levels decrease, a net insertion of membrane vesicles containing NaPi occurs, leading to an increase in phosphate reabsorption.

Another inhibitor of phosphate reabsorption, ANP (p. 867), may also activate protein kinase, but does so via cyclic guanosine monophosphate (cGMP) rather than cAMP. An additional example of a rapid effect on phosphate reabsorption is extracellular fluid expansion, which accelerates proximal phosphate excretion along with Na^+ excretion (p. 784).

Several modulators of phosphate transport are slow, acting by controlling protein synthesis and thus NaPi-cotransporter mRNA levels. High dietary phosphate intake decreases phosphate reabsorption, even without changes in PTH levels. Changes in plasma [phosphate], such as those that occur in phosphate depletion or loading, also modulate the balance between retrieval and insertion of NaP$_i$ cotransporters. Both phosphate depletion and 1,25 (OH)$_2$ vitamin D (p. 1098) upregulate the cotransporter. Glucocorticoid excess and metabolic acidosis downregulate the cotransporter; the latter effect is synergistic with the direct effects of H$^+$ on the NaPi protein (see earlier). Because phosphate is a pH buffer, the factors that increase urinary [phosphate] (e.g., acidosis) increase the titratable acidity component of renal acid excretion (p. 849).

CALCIUM

Binding of Plasma Proteins and Formation of Calcium-Anion Complexes Influence the Filtration and Reabsorption of Calcium

Whole-body calcium balance—as well as the hormonal control of free, ionized plasma calcium (Ca^{2+}) levels—is the subject of Chapter 51. The *total* concentration of calcium in plasma is normally 2.2 to 2.7 mM (8.8–10.6 mg/dl). Table 35–5 summarizes the forms of total calcium in the plasma. Some 40% binds to plasma proteins, mainly albumin, and constitutes the nonfilterable fraction. The **filterable** portion, approximately 60% of total plasma calcium, consists of two moieties. The first, approximately 15% of the total, complexes with small anions such as carbonate, citrate, phosphate, and sulfate. The second, approximately 45% of total calcium, is the ionized Ca^{2+} that one may measure with Ca^{2+}-sensitive electrodes or dyes. It is the concentration of this free, ionized calcium that the body tightly regulates; plasma [Ca^{2+}] normally is 1.0 to 1.3 mM (4.0–5.2 mg/dl).

The distribution among the various forms of total calcium is not fixed. Because H$^+$ competes with Ca^{2+} for binding to anionic sites on proteins or small molecules, acidosis generally increases plasma [Ca^{2+}]. Thus, the decrease in luminal pH that occurs along the nephron (p. 850) makes additional Ca^{2+} available for recovery. In addition, Ca^{2+} binding to proteins in the plasma depends on the concentration of proteins, particularly albumin. A change in the level of the anions with which Ca^{2+} can form complexes also affects the distribution of differ-

ent calcium entities. Tubule cells probably reabsorb Ca-anion complexes poorly. However, because the concentration of these anions declines along the nephron owing to anion reabsorption, free Ca^{2+} becomes available for transport.

The Proximal Tubule Reabsorbs a Large Fraction of Filtered Ca^{2+}, with the Thick Ascending Limb and Distal Convoluted Tubule Reabsorbing Smaller Amounts

The kidney reabsorbs approximately 99.5% of the filtered load of calcium, principally at the proximal tubule, the thick ascending limb, and the distal convoluted tubule (Fig. 35–16A).

PROXIMAL TUBULE. The proximal tubule reabsorbs approximately 65% of the filtered Ca^{2+}, a process that is *not* subject to hormonal control. A small part of the Ca^{2+} reabsorbed by the proximal tubule (~20% of the 65%) moves via the *transcellular* route that we will discuss in the next section. However, most proximal tubule Ca^{2+} reabsorption (~80% of the ~65%) occurs via the paracellular route (Fig. 35–16B). The evidence for a large component of *paracellular Ca^{2+} transport* is the high Ca^{2+} permeability of the tubule, as well as the sensitivity of net Ca^{2+} transport to changes in the transepithelial electrochemical gradient for Ca^{2+}. For example, imposing a lumen-negative transepithelial voltage induces Ca^{2+} secretion, whereas a lumen-positive voltage induces reabsorption. Because the S2 and S3 segments of the proximal tubule normally have a small lumen-positive voltage, it is not surprising that they are responsible for reabsorbing a large fraction of filtered Ca^{2+} by the paracellular route. In addition to Ca^{2+} *diffusion* through tight junctions, proximal Ca^{2+} reabsorption parallels that of Na$^+$ and water, implying participation of *solvent drag* (p. 469).

THICK ASCENDING LIMB. The thick ascending limb (TAL) reabsorbs approximately 25% of the filtered Ca^{2+} (Fig. 35–16C). Under normal conditions, about half of the Ca^{2+} reabsorption in the TAL occurs passively via a paracellular route, driven by the lumen-positive voltage. Thus, it is not surprising that hormones such as AVP, which make the transepithelial voltage more positive, indirectly increase Ca^{2+} reabsorption. The other half of Ca^{2+} reabsorption by the TAL occurs via the transcellular pathway (see next section), which PTH stimulates.

DISTAL CONVOLUTED TUBULE. This segment reabsorbs approximately 8% of the filtered Ca^{2+} load (Fig. 35–16D). Despite the relatively small amount of Ca^{2+} delivered, the distal convoluted tubule (DCT) is a major regulatory site for Ca^{2+} excretion. In contrast to the proximal tubule and TAL, the DCT reabsorbs Ca^{2+} predominantly via an active, transcellular route (see next section). Evidence against a substantial component of paracellular Ca^{2+} reabsorption is that—under a variety of experimental maneuvers (p. 810)—it is easy to dissociate Ca^{2+} transport in the DCT from Na$^+$ and water reabsorption.

The quantitative contribution of the collecting ducts

TABLE 35–5

COMPONENTS OF TOTAL PLASMA CALCIUM			
	mg/dl	**mM**	**% OF TOTAL**
Ionized Ca^{2+}	4.7	1.2	~45%
Diffusible calcium complexes	1.4	0.3	~15%
Nondiffusible (protein-bound) calcium	3.9	1.0	~40%
Total calcium	10.0	2.5	100

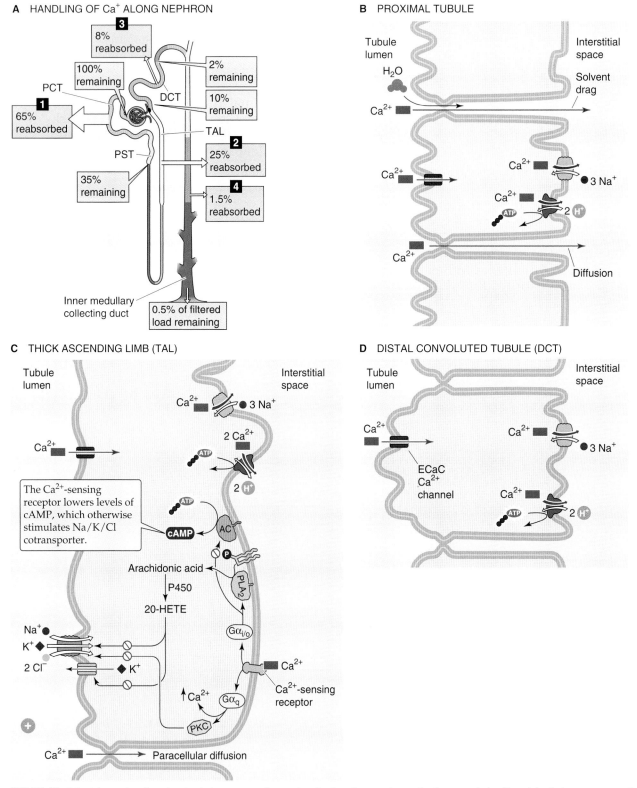

A HANDLING OF Ca⁺ ALONG NEPHRON

B PROXIMAL TUBULE

C THICK ASCENDING LIMB (TAL)

D DISTAL CONVOLUTED TUBULE (DCT)

FIGURE 35–16. Calcium handling by the kidney. In *A*, the *numbered yellow boxes* indicate the fraction of the filtered load that various nephron segments *reabsorb*. The *green boxes* indicate the fraction of the filtered load that remains in the lumen after these segments. AC, adenylyl cyclase; ATP, adenosine triphosphate; cAMP, cyclic adenosine monophosphate; HETE, hydroxyeicosatetraenoic acid; PKC, protein kinase C.

TABLE 35–6

FACTORS AFFECTING Ca²⁺ REABSORPTION ALONG THE NEPHRON

SITE	INCREASE REABSORPTION	DECREASE REABSORPTION
Proximal tubule	Volume contraction	Volume expansion
Thick ascending limb	PTH Calcitonin	Furosemide and related diuretics
Distal convoluted tubule	PTH Vitamin D AVP Alkalosis Thiazide diuretics	Phosphate depletion
Collecting duct	Amiloride	—

AVP, arginine vasopressin; PTH, parathyroid hormone.

and tubules to Ca^{2+} reabsorption is quite small (~1.5% of the filtered load), and their role in regulating renal Ca^{2+} excretion is not well defined.

Transcellular Ca²⁺ Movement Is a Two-Step Process, Involving Passive Ca²⁺ Entry Through Apical Channels and Basolateral Extrusion by Electrogenic Na/Ca Exchange and an ATP-Driven Ca²⁺ Pump

We have seen that the contribution of the transcellular route to Ca^{2+} reabsorption increases steadily from the proximal tubule to the TAL and to the DCT. Regardless of the nephron segment, tubule cells apparently use the same general mechanism to move Ca^{2+} through the cell from lumen to blood (Fig. 35–16B–D).

Because $[Ca^{2+}]_i$ is only approximately 100 nM (~10,000-fold less than in extracellular fluid), and because the membrane voltage across the apical membrane is about −70 mV, a steep electrochemical gradient favors Ca^{2+} entry across *the apical membrane*. Work on the DCT shows that apical Ca^{2+} entry is passive and is mediated not by a voltage-gated Ca^{2+} channel, but by an epithelial Ca^{2+} channel (ECaC). This Ca^{2+} channel, has consensus phosphorylation sites for PKA, PKC, and cGMP-stimulated protein kinase (PKG), as well as interaction sites for ankyrin (p. 21), a component of the cytoskeleton. Mg^{2+} competes with Ca^{2+} for entry into the cytoplasm, and extracellular H^+ blocks channel activity. Whether similar Ca^{2+} channels play a role in transcellular Ca^{2+} reabsorption in the proximal tubule and TAL is unknown.

As Ca^{2+} enters the tubule cell across the apical membrane, Ca^{2+}-binding proteins buffer the Ca^{2+}, helping to keep $[Ca^{2+}]_i$ low, and maintaining a favorable gradient for Ca^{2+} influx. In addition, Ca^{2+} may temporarily enter certain organelles, particularly the endoplasmic reticulum and mitochondria. In the steady state, however, the cell must extrude across the basolateral membrane all the Ca^{2+} that enters across the apical membrane. Both primary and secondary active transporters participate in this Ca^{2+} extrusion against a steep electrochemical gradient. The primary active transporter is an ATP-driven plasma-

membrane Ca^{2+} ATPase or pump (PMCA; p. 64). PMCA is present in several nephron segments, with its highest density in the basolateral membrane of the DCT. Increases in $[Ca^{2+}]_i$—such as those triggered by PTH via PLC and inositol triphosphate (IP_3), (p. 100)—activate calmodulin (p. 102) and thus stimulate PMCA.

In addition to the Ca^{2+} pump, an Na-Ca exchanger (NCX; p. 68) also extrudes Ca^{2+} across the basolateral membrane of tubule cells. At physiologically low $[Ca^{2+}]_i$ levels, when the Na-Ca exchanger is not very active, the major pathway for Ca^{2+} extrusion is the Ca^{2+} pump. Only when $[Ca^{2+}]_i$ increases does the Na-Ca exchanger begin to make a significant contribution. On the other hand, if the $[Ca^{2+}]_i$ is normal and the inward Na^+ electrochemical gradient falls (e.g., $[Na^+]_i$ rises), the Na-Ca exchanger can reverse direction and load the cell with Ca^{2+}.

Parathyroid Hormone and Vitamin D Stimulate—Whereas High Plasma Ca²⁺ Inhibits—Ca²⁺ Reabsorption

Table 35–6 summarizes factors that modulate Ca^{2+} handling by various segments of the nephron.

PARATHYROID HORMONE. The most important regulator of renal Ca^{2+} reabsorption is **PTH**, which stimulates Ca^{2+} reabsorption in the thick ascending limb, the distal convoluted tubule, and the connecting tubule. PTH appears to increase the open probability of apical Ca^{2+} channels (see Fig. 35–16C, D). Such an increase in Ca^{2+} permeability would increase $[Ca^{2+}]_i$, which in turn would stimulate basolateral Ca^{2+} extrusion mechanisms, increase Ca^{2+} reabsorption, and raise plasma $[Ca^{2+}]$.

As we saw in our discussion of phosphate handling, PTH acts by binding to the PTH 1R receptor, which apparently couples to *two* heterotrimeric G proteins and activates two kinases (p. 1093). Activation of $G\alpha_s$ raises $[cAMP]_i$ and stimulates PKA (p. 97). Activation of $G\alpha_q$ ultimately stimulates a PKC (p. 102) that is unusual in being *in*sensitive to phorbol esters. Both pathways are essential for the action of PTH on apical Ca^{2+} entry. Like PTH, **calcitonin** at low concentrations also increases Ca^{2+} reabsorption via cAMP in both the TAL and the DCT.

VITAMIN D. Acting on gene transcription, vitamin D (p. 1095) increases Ca^{2+} reabsorption in the distal nephron, complementing the major Ca^{2+}-retaining action of vitamin D, which is on Ca^{2+} absorption in the gastrointestinal tract (p. 971). In renal tubule cells, vitamin D upregulates the Ca^{2+}-binding protein, which contributes to enhanced Ca^{2+} reabsorption by keeping $[Ca^{2+}]_i$ low during increased Ca^{2+} traffic through the cell.

PLASMA Ca²⁺ LEVELS. The kidney, similar to the parathyroid gland (p. 1092), responds directly to changes in extracellular $[Ca^{2+}]$. In the cortical TAL, an increase in basolateral $[Ca^{2+}]$ inhibits both the Na/K/Cl cotransporter and K^+ channels on the apical membrane (Fig. 35–16C), resulting in a decrease in the lumen-positive transepithelial potential, and thus a reduction in paracellular Ca^{2+} reabsorption. The mechanism appears to be the following: Extracellular Ca^{2+} binds to a basolateral Ca^{2+}-sensing receptor (CaSR), which couples to at least two G proteins. First, activation of $G\alpha_i$ decreases $[cAMP]_i$, reducing stimulation of Na/K/Cl cotransport by cAMP (p. 787). Second, activation of a member of the G_i/G_o family stimulates PLA_2 (p. 103), increasing levels of arachidonic acid and one of its P450 metabolites, probably 20-hydroxyeicosatetraenoic acid (HETE). The latter inhibits apical Na/K/Cl cotransporters and K^+ channels. Third, CaSR activates $G\alpha_q$, elevating $[Ca^{2+}]_i$ and stimulating PKC (p. 102), which also inhibits Na/K/Cl cotransport. Thus, an increase in plasma $[Ca^{2+}]$ directly inhibits Na^+ and K^+ reabsorption, and indirectly—by reducing the lumen-positive voltage generated by apical K^+ recycling—inhibits the paracellular reabsorption of Ca^{2+} and Mg^{2+} (see later). The Ca^{2+}-sensing receptor is also present in the proximal tubule, the medullary thick ascending limb, the distal convoluted tubule, and the collecting ducts.

An interesting consequence of reduced Na^+ reabsorption induced by high plasma $[Ca^{2+}]$ is an inhibition of the kidney's ability to generate a concentrated urine (p. 833). Indeed, chronic hypercalcemia results in a dilute urine, a form of nephrogenic diabetes insipidus (see box on p. 843). By keeping urine $[Ca^{2+}]$ relatively low, this effect may help avoid Ca^{2+} stones under conditions of high Ca^{2+} excretion.

EFFECTIVE CIRCULATING VOLUME. A reduction in effective circulating volume triggers four parallel effector pathways (p. 864) that act to restore volume. One of these pathways—the sympathetic division of the ANS—increases Na^+ reabsorption by the proximal tubule (p. 787). Because proximal tubule Ca^{2+} reabsorption depends largely on transepithelial voltage and solvent drag (p. 807), which in turn depend on Na^+ reabsorption, it is not surprising that volume contraction, which increases Na^+ reabsorption, also increases Ca^{2+} reabsorption. Volume expansion has the opposite effects on both Na^+ and Ca^{2+} reabsorption.

ACID-BASE BALANCE. Metabolic alkalosis increases renal Ca^{2+} reabsorption (i.e., decreases excretion) at the level of the distal convoluted tubule, probably by relieving the inhibition of apical ECaC Ca^{2+} channels by H^+. This effect is independent of the PTH status, as well as of Na^+ transport. The latter observation suggests that factors such as solvent drag and diffusion are not involved.

PHOSPHATE DEPLETION. Chronic phosphate depletion impairs Ca^{2+} reabsorption at both proximal and distal sites. The effects are independent of the decrease in PTH secretion that follows phosphate depletion; the basis for the effect is otherwise unknown.

DIURETICS. Among diuretics, those acting on the thick ascending limb, such as furosemide, decrease Ca^{2+} reabsorption, whereas those acting on the distal nephron, such as thiazides and amiloride, increase Ca^{2+} reabsorption. Thus, of these drugs, only the powerful loop diuretic furosemide is appropriate for treating hypercalcemic states. In the TAL, **furosemide** (p. 778) reduces the lumen-positive voltage, and thus the driving force for passive, paracellular Ca^{2+} reabsorption. Accordingly, urinary Ca^{2+} excretion increases in parallel with Na^+ excretion.

In contrast, the effects of thiazides and amiloride are exceptions to the general rule that Ca^{2+} and Na^+ excretion parallel each other. **Thiazide diuretics** (p. 779) inhibit Na/Cl cotransport and stimulate Ca^{2+} reabsorption in the distal convoluted tubule. Inhibiting apical Na/Cl cotransport lowers $[Cl^-]_i$ in the DCT cell, thus hyperpolarizing the cell. The steeper electrical gradient increases apical Ca^{2+} entry, secondarily stimulating basolateral Ca^{2+} extrusion. **Amiloride** (p. 779) inhibits apical Na^+ channels in the initial and cortical collecting tubules and hyperpolarizes the apical membrane. Thus, like the thiazides, amiloride augments Ca^{2+} reabsorption by enhancing the gradient for apical Ca^{2+} entry. The stimulatory effects of thiazides and of amiloride on apical Ca^{2+} uptake require physiologic PTH levels to keep the apical Ca^{2+} channels open.

MAGNESIUM

Most Mg²⁺ Reabsorption Takes Place Along the Thick Ascending Limb

About 99% of the total body stores of magnesium reside either within bone (~54%) or within the intracellular compartment (~45%), mostly muscle. Renal magnesium excretion plays an important role in maintaining physiological plasma magnesium levels. The body maintains the total magnesium concentration in blood plasma within narrow limits, 0.8 to 1.0 mM (1.8–2.2 mg/dl). Of this total, approximately 30% is protein-bound (Table 35–7). The remaining approximately 70% of total magnesium, which is filterable, is made up of two components. Less than 10% is complexed to anions such as phosphate, citrate, and oxalate, leaving approximately 60% of the total as free, ionized magnesium (Mg^{2+}).

Disturbances of Mg^{2+} metabolism usually involve ab-

TABLE 35–7

COMPONENTS OF TOTAL PLASMA MAGNESIUM

	mg/dl	mM	% OF TOTAL
Ionized Mg^{2+}	1.3	0.56	62
Diffusible magnesium complexes	0.1	0.06	7
Nondiffusible (protein-bound) magnesium	0.6	0.28	31
Total magnesium	2.0	0.90	100

normal *losses*, and these occur most frequently during gastrointestinal malabsorption (p. 972) and diarrhea, in the course of renal disease, and following the administration of diuretics. Clinical manifestations of Mg^{2+} depletion include neurologic disturbances such as tetany (especially when associated with hypocalcemia), cardiac arrhythmias, and increased peripheral vascular resistance. On the other hand, increased Mg^{2+} intake may lower blood pressure and lower the incidence of hypertension. Severe hypermagnesemia, which may occur following excessive intake or renal failure, results in a toxic syndrome involving nausea, hyporeflexia, respiratory insufficiency, and cardiac arrest.

Normally, 5% or less of the filtered magnesium load appears in the urine (Fig. 35–17A). In contrast to the predominantly "proximal" reabsorption pattern of the major components of the glomerular filtrate, Mg^{2+} reabsorption occurs mainly along the TAL. In all segments, Mg^{2+} reabsorption is mainly paracellular.

Normally, the **proximal tubule** reabsorbs only approximately 15% of the filtered magnesium load (Fig. 35–17B). Water reabsorption along the proximal tubule causes luminal $[Mg^{2+}]$ to double compared with the value in Bowman's space, establishing a favorable Mg^{2+} electrochemical gradient for passive, paracellular Mg^{2+} reabsorption. Solvent drag may also contribute to the paracellular reabsorption of Mg^{2+}.

The **thick ascending limb** absorbs approximately 70% of the filtered magnesium load, and is also the main site of *control* of Mg^{2+} transport (Fig. 35–17C). The driving force for paracellular Mg^{2+} reabsorption is the lumen-positive voltage of the TAL. Reabsorption of Mg^{2+} in both the proximal tubule and the TAL closely follows the reabsorption of NaCl and water, as expected for Mg^{2+} reabsorption by the paracellular route. In states of Mg^{2+} depletion (see later), the TAL may reabsorb some Mg^{2+} by a *transcellular* route.

In the TAL, a specific tight junction protein called **claudin 16** (paracellin-1) is necessary for paracellular Mg^{2+} reabsorption. A mutation of the paracellin-1 gene leads to an autosomal-recessive disorder characterized by severe renal Mg^{2+} wasting. Thus, it appears that paracellin-1 controls the paracellular Mg^{2+} permeability.

Magnesium reabsorption along the **distal convoluted tubule** and the **collecting tubules** and **ducts** accounts for only approximately 10% of the filtered load.

Magnesium Reabsorption Increases with Depletion of Magnesium or Calcium, Extracellular Fluid Contraction, and Parathyroid Hormone

Table 35–8 shows the site of action of factors modulating renal Mg^{2+} excretion.

MAGNESIUM DEPLETION. In response to low plasma $[Mg^{2+}]$, the TAL increases its reabsorption of Mg^{2+}, independent of Na^+ and Ca^{2+} transport. This observation has been taken to suggest that a fraction of Mg^{2+} reabsorption may be *transcellular* and involve an active transport step. Because $[Mg^{2+}]_i$ in TAL cells is relatively low (0.5–0.6 mM) and the apical membrane voltage is negative, the apical electrochemical gradient favors passive Mg^{2+} uptake. It is likely that cation-selective channels, perhaps ECaC, mediate apical Mg^{2+} uptake. The basolateral step for transcellular Mg^{2+} reabsorption is also uncertain, but may include a unique ATP-dependent Mg^{2+} pump or an Na-Mg exchanger.

HYPERMAGNESEMIA AND HYPERCALCEMIA. The kidney seems to discriminate poorly between increases in plasma $[Mg^{2+}]$ and $[Ca^{2+}]$. Thus, *each* of these disturbances inhibits the reabsorption of both Mg^{2+} and Ca^{2+} in the TAL, leading to increased urinary excretion of both Mg^{2+} and Ca^{2+}. It is likely that high plasma $[Mg^{2+}]$ and $[Ca^{2+}]$ each diminish Mg^{2+} reabsorption because each can bind to the Ca^{2+}-sensing receptor.

EFFECTIVE CIRCULATING VOLUME. As is true for Ca^{2+}, a decrease in effective circulating volume leads to an increase in Na^+ reabsorption, and an increase in the forces that drive Mg^{2+} reabsorption via paracellular pathways. Thus, volume contraction increases Mg^{2+} reabsorption, whereas volume expansion has the opposite effect.

HORMONES. PTH is the most important hormone for Mg^{2+} regulation and increases both proximal and distal Mg^{2+} reabsorption. When tested separately in hormone-depleted animals, AVP, glucagons, and calcitonin all stimulate Mg^{2+} reabsorption in the TAL, acting via cAMP and PKA. Many of these hormones probably act by modulating passive Mg^{2+} movement through the paracellular pathway, either by changing NaCl transport and transepithelial voltage or by increasing paracellular permeability.

ACID-BASE BALANCE. As is the case for Ca^{2+}, alkalosis increases Mg^{2+} reabsorption. However, for Mg^{2+}, the effect is at the level of the TAL.

DIURETICS. In general, diuretics decrease Mg^{2+} reabsorption and thus enhance Mg^{2+} excretion. This statement is particularly true for diuretics targeting the TAL. Similar to their effects on Ca^{2+}, loop diuretics act by depressing the lumen-positive voltage, and thus the gradient for the passive, paracellular Mg^{2+} reabsorption. Osmotic diuretics, such as mannitol, also reduce Mg^{2+} reabsorption along the loop of Henle.

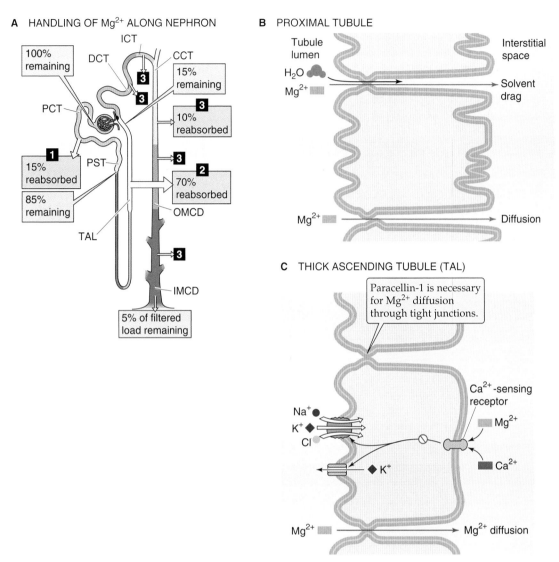

FIGURE 35–17. Magnesium handling by the kidney. In *A*, the *numbered yellow boxes* indicate the fraction of the filtered load that various nephron segments reabsorb. The DCT, ICT, CCT, OMCD and IMCD together reabsorb 10% of the filtered load. The *green boxes* indicate the fraction of the filtered load that remains in the lumen after these segments. CCT, cortical collecting tubule; DCT, distal convoluted tubule; ICT, initial collecting tubule; IMCD, inner medullary collecting duct; Mg^{2+}, magnesium; OMCD, outer medullary collecting duct.

TABLE 35–8

FACTORS AFFECTING Mg^{2+} REABSORPTION ALONG THE NEPHRON

SITE	INCREASE REABSORPTION	DECREASE REABSORPTION
Proximal tubule	Volume contraction	Volume expansion
Thick ascending limb	PTH, calcitonin, glucagon, AVP Low plasma $[Mg^{2+}]$ Metabolic alkalosis	Furosemide and related loop diuretics Mannitol High plasma $[Mg^{2+}]$ or $[Ca^{2+}]$
Distal convoluted tubule and collecting tubules/ducts	PTH, calcitonin, glucagon, AVP, aldosterone, PGE_2 Low plasma $[Mg^{2+}]$ Amiloride	High plasma $[Mg^{2+}]$ or $[Ca^{2+}]$ Metabolic acidosis K^+ or phosphate depletion

AVP, arginine vasopressin; PTH, parathyroid hormone.

REFERENCES

Books and Reviews

Daniel H, Herget M: Cellular and molecular mechanisms of renal peptide transport. Am J Physiol 42:F1–F8, 1997.

DeRouffignac C, Quamme G: Renal magnesium handling and its hormonal control. Physiol Rev 74:305–322, 1994.

Hediger MA, Rhoads DB: Molecular physiology of sodium-glucose cotransporters. Physiol Rev 74:993–1026, 1994.

Hoenderop JGJ, Willems PHGM, Bindels RJM: Toward a comprehensive molecular model of active calcium reabsorption. Am J Physiol 278:F352–F360, 2000.

Koepsell H, Busch A, Gorboulev V, Arndt P: Structure and function of renal organic cation transporters. News Physiol Sci 13: 11–16, 1998.

Murer H, Hernando N, Forster I, Biber J: Proximal tubular phosphate reabsorption: Molecular mechanisms. Physiol Rev 80:1373–1409, 2000.

Palacin M, Estevez R, Bertran J, Zorzano A: Molecular biology of mammalian plasma membrane amino acid transporters. Physiol Rev 78: 969–1054, 1998.

Seldin DW, Giebisch G, eds: The Kidney: Physiology and Pathophysiology, 3rd ed. Philadelphia, Lippincott Williams & Wilkins, 2000.

Journal Articles

Forster IC, Wagner CA, Busch AE, et al: Electrophysiological characterization of the flounder type II Na/Pi cotransporter (NaPi-5) expressed in *Xenopus laevis* oocytes. J Membr Biol 160:9–25, 1997.

Fei YJ, Kanai Y, Nussberger S, et al: Expression cloning of a mammalian proton-coupled oligopeptide transporter. Nature 368:563–566, 1994.

Hediger MA, Coady MJ, Ikeda IS, Wright EM: Expression cloning and cDNA sequencing of the Na^+/glucose transporter. Nature 330:379–381, 1987.

Simon DB, Lu Y, Choate KA, et al: Paracellin-1, a renal tight junction protein required for paracellular Mg^{2+} resorption. Science 285:103–106, 1999.

You G, Smith CP, Kanai Y, et al: Expression cloning and characterization of the vasopressin-regulated urea transporter. Nature 365:844–847, 1993.

CHAPTER 36

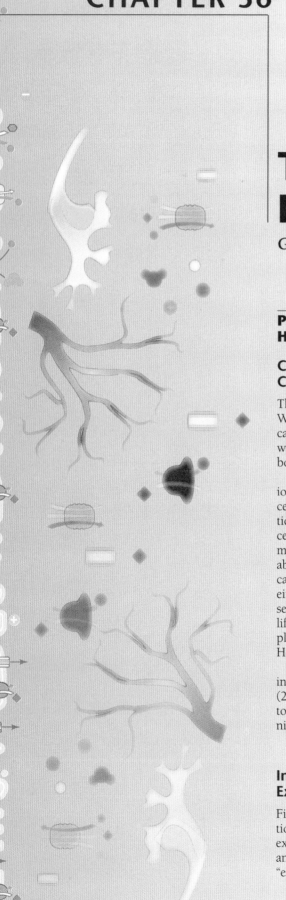

Transport of Potassium

Gerhard Giebisch and Erich Windhager

POTASSIUM BALANCE AND THE OVERALL RENAL HANDLING OF POTASSIUM

Changes in K⁺ Concentrations Can Have Major Effects on Cell and Organ Function

The distribution of K^+ in the body differs strikingly from that of Na^+. Whereas Na^+ is largely extracellular, K^+ is the most abundant intracellular cation. Some 98% of the total-body K^+ content (50–55 mmole/kg body-weight) is inside cells; only 2% is in the extracellular fluid (ECF). The body tightly maintains the plasma $[K^+]$ at 3.5 to 5.0 mM.

Table 36–1 summarizes the most important physiologic functions of K^+ ions. A *high* $[K^+]$ inside cells and mitochondria is essential for maintaining cell volume, regulating intracellular pH and controlling cell-enzyme function, DNA and protein synthesis, and cell growth. The relatively *low* extracellular $[K^+]$ is necessary for maintaining the steep K^+ gradient across cell membranes that is largely responsible for the membrane potential of excitable and nonexcitable cells. Therefore, changes in extracellular $[K^+]$ can cause severe disturbances in excitation and contraction. As a general rule, either doubling the normal plasma $[K^+]$ or reducing it by half results in severe disturbances in skeletal and cardiac muscle function. The potentially life-threatening disturbances of cardiac rhythmicity that result from a rise of plasma $[K^+]$ are particularly important (see the box Hyperkalemia and the Heart).

Chronic K^+ depletion leads to several metabolic disturbances. These include (1) inability of the kidney to form a concentrated urine (p. 843); (2) a tendency to develop metabolic alkalosis (p. 853); and, closely related to this acid-base disturbance, (3) a striking enhancement of renal ammonium excretion (p. 859).

Ingested K⁺ Moves Transiently into Cells for Storage Before Excretion by the Kidney

Figure 36–1 illustrates processes that govern K^+ balance and the distribution of K^+ in the body: (1) gastrointestinal intake, (2) renal and extrarenal excretion, and (3) the internal distribution of K^+ between the intracellular and extracellular fluid compartments. The first two processes accomplish "external" K^+ balance (i.e., between body and environment), whereas the

TABLE 36-1

PHYSIOLOGICAL ROLE OF POTASSIUM IONS

A. Roles of Intracellular K+

Cell-volume Maintenance	Net loss of $K^+ \rightarrow$ Cell shrinkage
	Net gain of $K^+ \rightarrow$ Cell swelling
Intracellular pH Regulation	Net loss of $K^+ \rightarrow$ Cell acidosis
	Net gain of $K^+ \rightarrow$ Cell alkalosis
Cell Enzyme Functions	K^+ dependence of enzymes: e.g., some ATPases, succinic dehydrogenase
DNA/Protein Synthesis, Growth	Lack of $K^+ \rightarrow$ reduction of protein synthesis, stunted growth

B. Roles of Transmembrane [K+] Ratio

Resting Cell Membrane Potential	Reduced $[K^+]_i/[K^+]_o \rightarrow$ membrane depolarization
	Increased $[K^+]_i/[K^+]_o \rightarrow$ membrane hyperpolarization
Neuromuscular Activity	Low plasma K^+: muscle weakness, muscle paralysis, intestinal distention, peripheral vasodilation, respiratory failure
	High plasma K^+: increased muscle excitability; later, muscle weakness (paralysis)
Cardiac Activity	Low plasma K^+: slowed conduction of pacemaker activity, arrhythmias
	High plasma K^+: conduction disturbances, ventricular arrhythmias and ventricular fibrillation
Vascular Resistance	Low plasma K^+: vasoconstriction
	High plasma K^+: vasodilation

ATP, adenosine triphosphate.

last achieves "internal" K^+ balance (i.e., between intracellular and extracellular fluids).

EXTERNAL K+ BALANCE. The relationship between dietary K^+ intake and K^+ excretion determines external K^+ balance. The *dietary intake* of K^+ is approximately equal to that of Na^+, 80 to 120 mmole/day. This K^+ intake is more than the entire K^+ content of the ECF, which is only about 70 mmole. For the plasma K^+ content to remain constant, the body must excrete K^+ via renal and extrarenal mechanisms at the same rate as K^+ ingestion. Moreover, because dietary K^+ intake can vary over a wide range, it is important that these K^+ excretory mechanisms be able to adjust appropriately to variable K^+ intake. The kidney is largely responsible for K^+ excretion, although the gastrointestinal tract plays a minor role. The kidneys excrete 90% to 95% of the daily K^+ intake; the colon excretes 5% to 10%. Although the colon can adjust its K^+ excretion in response to some stimuli (e.g., adrenal hormones, changes in dietary K^+, decreased capacity of the kidneys to excrete K^+), the colon—by itself—is incapable of increasing K^+ secretion sufficiently to maintain external K^+ balance.

INTERNAL K+ BALANCE. Maintaining normal intracellular and extracellular $[K^+]$ requires not only the external K^+ balance just described, but also the appropriate distribution of K^+ within the body. Most of the K^+ is inside cells, particularly muscle cells, with smaller quantities in liver, bone, and red blood cells. The markedly unequal distribution between the intracellular and extracellular K^+ content has important quantitative implications. Of the total intracellular K^+ content of approximately 3.5 mole, shut-

tling as little as 1% to or from the ECF would cause a 50% change in extracellular $[K^+]$, with severe consequences for neuromuscular function (see Table 36–1).

What happens when the body is presented with a K^+ load? By far, the most common source of a K^+ load is dietary K^+. When one ingests K^+ salts, both the small intestine (p. 940) and the colon (p. 943) absorb the K^+. In addition to external sources of K^+, substantial amounts of K^+ may enter the ECF from damaged tissues (see the box on p. 826). Such K^+ release from intracellular to extracellular fluid can lead to a severe, even lethal, increase in plasma $[K^+]$ (i.e., **hyperkalemia**). However, even a large meal presents the body with a K^+ load that could produce hyperkalemia if it were not for mechanisms that buffer and ultimately excrete this K^+.

Absorbed K^+ is not immediately excreted. Instead, some four fifths of the ingested K^+ temporarily moves into cells, so that plasma $[K^+]$ rises only modestly. Were it not for this translocation, plasma $[K^+]$ could reach dangerous levels.

The most important factors modulating extrarenal K^+ distribution are hormones: insulin, β-adrenergic agonists (e.g., epinephrine), and aldosterone all promote the transfer of K^+ from extracellular to intracellular fluid via the ubiquitous Na-K pump. Figure 36–3A shows how these hormones increase K^+ transfer into cells in response to high plasma $[K^+]$. The lack of **insulin** (in diabetes) or a deficient renin-angiotensin-**aldosterone** system (in diabetes and some forms of hypertension) can significantly compromise tolerance to K^+ loading, and predispose to hyperkalemia. Similarly, administering β-adrenergic blockers (in treatment of hypertension) or α-adrenergic agonists impairs the extrarenal sequestra-

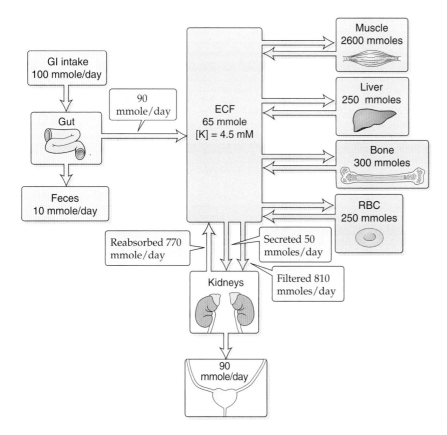

FIGURE 36–1. Distribution and balance of K⁺ throughout the body. ECF, extracellular fluid; GI, gastrointestinal; RBC, red blood cell.

tion of an acute K⁺ load. For example, during exercise, overactivation of α receptors may contribute to hyperkalemia.

Acid-base disturbances also affect internal K⁺ distribution. As a rule, acidemia leads to hyperkalemia as tissues release K⁺. One can think of this K⁺ release as an "exchange" of intracellular K⁺ for extracellular H⁺, although a single transport protein generally does not mediate this "exchange" (p. 652). Extracellular acidosis probably leads to loss of cellular K⁺ because the resulting decrease in intracellular pH lessens the binding of K⁺ to non-diffusible intracellular anions (see Fig. 36–3B). Moreover, intracellular acidosis compromises both the Na-K pump and the Na/K/Cl cotransporter, both of which move K⁺ into cells. Interestingly, for the same degree of acidemia, mineral acids produce a greater degree of hyperkalemia than do organic acids.

Alkalemia causes cells to take up K⁺, leading to **hypokalemia**. Although the mechanism is not known, high HCO_3^- levels—even in the absence of extracellular pH changes—induce hypokalemia by stimulating K⁺ transfer into cells. Another example of this apparent exchange of K⁺ for H⁺ is the effect of K⁺ on acid-base homeostasis. As discussed on p. 859, K⁺ depletion causes intracellular acidosis and extracellular alkalosis.

In some clinical conditions, an increase of the **extracellular osmolality** induces the transfer, not only of water, but also of K⁺ into the extracellular space. The rise in plasma K⁺ following infusion of hypertonic mannitol solutions is an example of this phenomenon.

Following a K⁺ load, the time course of K⁺ transfer into cells by the mechanisms discussed is much faster than the renal excretory response (Fig. 36–4). Whereas

the hormonally mediated redistribution between intracellular and extracellular fluid is rapid and almost complete after an hour, the renal response takes hours to excrete the surfeit of K⁺.

HYPERKALEMIA AND THE HEART

An electrocardiogram (ECG)—a measure of the electrical activity of the myocardial cells (p. 493)—can be clinically useful for detecting a rising plasma [K⁺].

As plasma [K⁺] begins to rise (Fig. 36–2, *6 mM*), the T wave becomes tall and peaked, assuming a symmetric, "tented" shape. The P-R interval becomes prolonged, and the P wave gradually flattens. Eventually, the P wave disappears (Fig. 36–2, *8 mM*). Moreover, the QRS complex, which represents depolarization of the ventricles, widens and merges with the T wave, forming a sine-wave pattern. At higher concentrations, ventricular fibrillation, a lethal arrhythmia, may develop (Fig. 36–2, *10 mM*). These electrocardiographic changes do not always occur in this precise order, and some patients with hyperkalemia may progress very rapidly to ventricular fibrillation. Any change in the ECG resulting from hyperkalemia requires immediate clinical attention.

Decreases in plasma [K⁺] also affect the ECG. For example, moderate decreases in [K⁺] to ~3 mM cause the QT interval to lengthen and the T wave to flatten. Lower values of [K⁺] lead to the appearance of a U wave (Fig. 36–2, *1.5 mM*), which represents the delayed repolarization of the ventricles.

FIGURE 36–2. Effect of changes in plasma [K^+] on the ECG. These five traces show electrocardiographic (ECG) recordings from the precordial V_4 lead.

achieve K^+ balance, the kidneys normally need to excrete 10% to 15% of the filtered K^+. Under conditions of low dietary K^+ intake, the kidneys excrete 1% to 3% of filtered K^+, so that—with a normal- or low-K^+ diet—the kidneys could achieve K^+ balance by *filtration* and *reabsorption* alone. Considering only the filtered K^+ load and external K^+ balance, we would have no reason to suspect that the kidneys might be capable of K^+ secretion. However, with a chronically high dietary K^+, when the kidneys must rid the body of excess K^+, urinary K^+ excretion may exceed 150% of the total amount of filtered K^+. Therefore, even if the tubules reabsorbed none of the filtered K^+, they must be capable of secreting an amount equivalent to at least 50% of the filtered K^+ load.

As discussed later, even in the absence of a large dietary K^+ load, K^+ *secretion* by the tubules is an important component of urinary K^+ excretion. Therefore, K^+ handling is a complex combination of K^+ filtration at the glomerulus as well as both K^+ reabsorption and secretion by the renal tubules.

POTASSIUM HANDLING BY DIFFERENT SEGMENTS OF THE NEPHRON

The Proximal Tubule Consistently Reabsorbs the Bulk of the Filtered K^+, Whereas the Distal Nephron May Reabsorb or Secrete K^+, Depending on Dietary K^+

Figure 36–5 summarizes the pattern of K^+ transport along the nephron under conditions of low or normal/high K^+ intake. In either case, the kidney filters K^+ in the glomerulus and then extensively reabsorbs it along the proximal tubule (~80%) and the loop of Henle (~10%), so that only approximately 10% of the filtered K^+ enters the distal convoluted tubule (DCT). Also, in either case, the medullary collecting duct reabsorbs K^+. The K^+ handling depends critically on dietary K^+ in five nephron segments: the DCT, the connecting tubule (CNT), the initial collecting tubule (ICT), the cortical collecting tubule (CCT), and the medullary collecting duct (MCD).

LOW DIETARY K^+. When the body is trying to conserve K^+, the "classic distal tubule" (i.e., DCT, CNT, and ICT) and CCT all reabsorb K^+, so that only a small fraction of the filtered load (1%–3%) appears in the urine (see Fig. 36–5A). In states of K^+ depletion, this additional K^+ reabsorption can be life saving, retrieving from the tubule lumen precious K^+ that escaped reabsorption along the proximal tubule and loop of Henle. Despite the degree to which the kidneys can enhance K^+ reabsorption, they cannot restrict K^+ loss in the urine as effectively as they can restrict Na^+ loss; therefore, hypokalemia may eventually develop in individuals in whom K^+ intake has been abnormally low for prolonged periods of time.

NORMAL OR HIGH DIETARY K^+. When external K^+ balance demands that the kidneys excrete K^+, the ICT, CCT and the more proximal portion of the MCD *secrete* K^+ into the tubule lumen (see Fig. 36–5B). Together, these segments, known as the **distal K^+-secretory system**, account for most of the urinary excretion of K^+. It is also this distal K^+-secretory system that responds to many

The Kidney Excretes K^+ by a Combination of Filtration, Reabsorption, and Secretion

At a normal glomerular filtration rate and at physiological levels of plasma [K^+], the kidney filters approximately 800 mmole of K^+ per day, far more than the usual dietary intake of 80 to 120 mmole/day. Therefore, to

A RESPONSE TO HIGH PLASMA [K⁺]

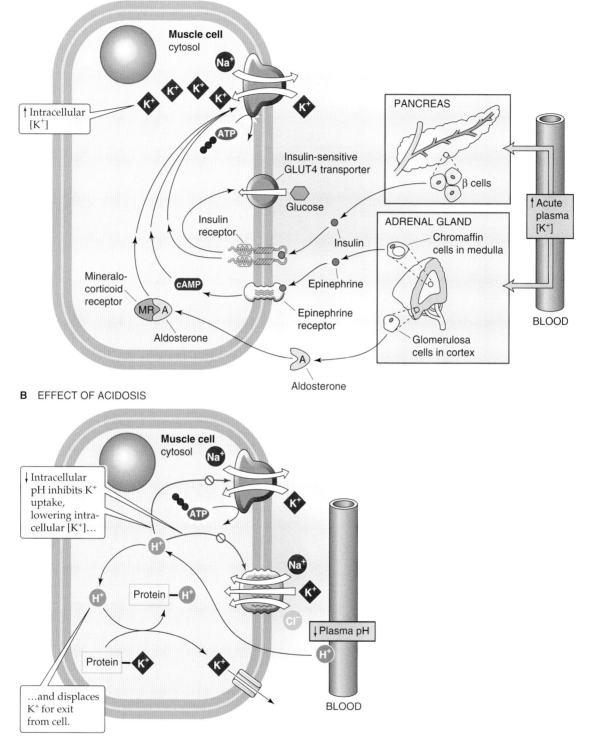

B EFFECT OF ACIDOSIS

FIGURE 36–3. Control of K⁺ uptake into cells. ATP, adenosine triphosphate; cAMP, cyclic adenosine monophosphate.

stimuli that modulate K⁺ excretion. Note that even at normal rates of K⁺ excretion (10%–15% of the filtered load), the proximal tubules and loop of Henle first absorb very large amounts of K⁺ (~90% of the filtered load), so that the K⁺ appearing in the urine may largely represent K⁺ secreted by more distal segments of the nephron.

Medullary Trapping of K⁺ Helps to Maximize K⁺ Excretion when K⁺ Intake Is High

Regardless of whether the distal K⁺-secretory system reabsorbs K⁺ (see Fig. 36–5A) or secretes K⁺ (see Fig. 36–5B), the *medullary* collecting ducts reabsorb some K⁺. The

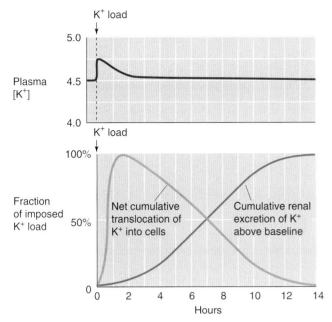

FIGURE 36–4. K⁺ handling following an acute K⁺ load. (Data from Cogan, M.G. Fluid & Electrolytes: Physiology & Pathophysiology. Appleton & Lange, Norwalk, CT, 1991.)

net effect of this K⁺ loss from the lumen of the medullary collecting ducts is that [K⁺] rises in the medullary interstitium.

The pattern of K⁺ transport in **juxtamedullary nephrons** differs somewhat from that in superficial nephrons, whose loops of Henle do not dip into the inner medulla (p. 741). In addition to the distal K⁺-secretory system present in superficial nephrons, juxtamedullary nephrons also secrete K⁺ in the thin descending limb of the loop of Henle (tDLH). Analysis of fluid collected from the hairpin bend of the loop of Henle of juxtamedullary nephrons shows that the amount of K⁺ delivered to the collection site at the hairpin bend can exceed not only the amount of K⁺ present at the end of the proximal tubule, but also the amount of K⁺ filtered.

This K⁺ secretion by the tDLH is the first step of a process known as **medullary K⁺ recycling** (Fig. 36–6). The second step is K⁺ reabsorption by the thin and thick ascending limbs, which deposits K⁺ in the medullary interstitium. This K⁺ deposited in the interstitium by the ascending limbs represents part of the K⁺ that entered the lumen of the tDLH. The rest of the K⁺ that entered the

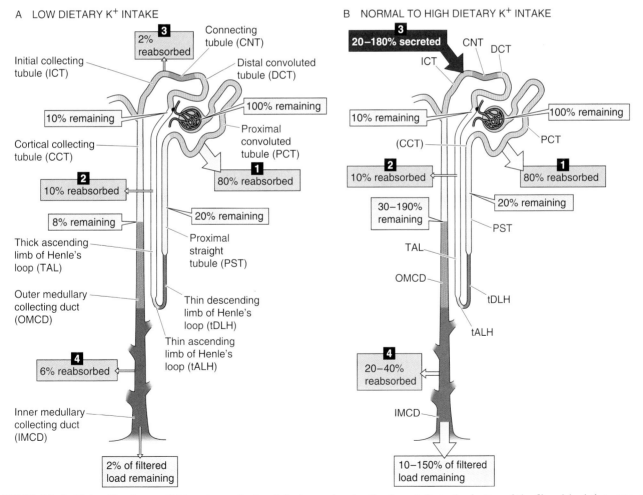

FIGURE 36–5. K⁺ handling in superficial nephrons. In *A* and *B*, the numbered *yellow boxes* indicate the fraction of the filtered load that various nephron segments reabsorb, whereas the *red box* in *B* indicates the fraction of the filtered load secreted by the ICT and CCT. The green boxes indicate the fraction of the filtered load that remains in the lumen after these segments.

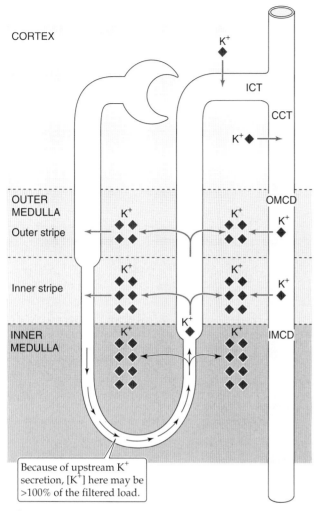

CORTEX

K$^+$

ICT

CCT

K$^+$

OUTER
MEDULLA

OMCD

Outer stripe

K$^+$ K$^+$ K$^+$

Inner stripe

K$^+$ K$^+$ K$^+$

K$^+$

INNER
MEDULLA

K$^+$ K$^+$ IMCD

Because of upstream K$^+$
secretion, [K$^+$] here may be
>100% of the filtered load.

FIGURE 36–6. Medullary recycling of K$^+$ by juxtamedullary nephrons.

tDLH is the K$^+$ deposited in the medullary interstitium by the medullary collecting ducts, as described earlier (the *third step* in medullary recycling). Together, the thin and thick *ascending* limbs of a juxtamedullary loop reabsorb more K$^+$ than the *descending* limb secretes, so that net K$^+$ reabsorption occurs along the loop. The net effect of these three steps is the *trapping of K$^+$ in the medullary interstitium*, with the interstitial [K$^+$] being highest at the tip of the papilla and falling towards the cortex.

One might think that—with respect to K$^+$ excretion—medullary K$^+$ recycling is inefficient, because K$^+$ exits the medullary collecting duct only to re-enter the nephron upstream, in the tDLH. However, medullary recycling and concomitant K$^+$ trapping may be important in maximizing the excretion of K$^+$ when K$^+$ intake is high. Under these conditions, K$^+$ secretion by the distal K$^+$-secretory system is intense, so that luminal [K$^+$] in the medullary collecting duct may rise to 200 mM or higher. Thus, the high [K$^+$] in the medullary interstitium minimizes the [K$^+$] difference between the collecting-duct lumen and its peritubular environment, thus reducing the passive loss of K$^+$ from the medullary collecting duct.

POTASSIUM TRANSPORT AT THE CELLULAR AND MOLECULAR LEVEL

K$^+$ Reabsorption Along the Proximal Tubule Is Largely Passive and Follows the Movement of Na$^+$ and Fluid

The proximal tubule reabsorbs most of the filtered K$^+$ via two paracellular mechanisms: solvent drag and simple diffusion (Figure 36–7). **Solvent drag** (p. 469) occurs along the entire length of the proximal tubule. Active Na$^+$ transport (p. 776) drives net fluid reabsorption across the proximal-tubule epithelium via the paracellular shunt pathway, entraining K$^+$ along with the fluid. Indeed, one of the distinguishing features of proximal-tubule K$^+$ reabsorption is its strong dependence on net fluid reabsorption. Thus, interventions that depress fluid reabsorption almost always inhibit K$^+$ reabsorption.

As fluid flows down the proximal tubule, the luminal voltage shifts from negative to positive (p. 780). By the late proximal tubule, the transepithelial voltage is sufficiently positive to provide a favorable gradient for K$^+$ **diffusion** through the low-resistance paracellular pathway, from lumen to blood.

Although the proximal tubule reabsorbs K$^+$ by paracellular mechanisms, the proximal tubule has several cellular pathways for K$^+$ movement that do not directly participate in K$^+$ reabsorption (see Fig. 36–7A): (1) a basolateral Na-K pump, a feature common to all tubule cells, (2) apical and basolateral K$^+$ channels, and (3) a basolateral K/Cl cotransporter.

The K$^+$ conductance of the basolateral membrane greatly exceeds that of the apical membrane, and it appears that different channels are responsible for the K$^+$ conductances in these two membranes. The open probability of the *basolateral* K$^+$ channel increases sharply with the turnover rate of the Na-K pump. Accordingly, most of the K$^+$ taken up via the Na-K pump recycles across the basolateral membrane via K$^+$ channels and a K/Cl cotransporter, and does not appear in the lumen. This basolateral K$^+$ channel belongs to the class of inwardly rectifying K$^+$ channels characterized by adenosine triphosphate (ATP) sensitivity: a decrease in [ATP]$_i$ enhances channel activity (p. 198). This regulation by [ATP]$_i$ is most likely involved in the coupling between basolateral Na-K pumps and K$^+$ channels. An increase in pump rate—which might occur when increased apical Na$^+$ entry increases [Na$^+$]$_i$—would lower [ATP]$_i$, relieving inhibition of the K$^+$ channels. Were it not for this interaction between basolateral Na-K pump and K$^+$ channels, the K$^+$ content of proximal-tubule cells would fluctuate dramatically during alterations in net Na$^+$ transport.

In contrast to the high state of activity of the basolateral K$^+$ channels, *apical* K$^+$ channels are largely quiescent under normal conditions. They appear to become active, however, when tubule cells swell, possibly when entry of Na$^+$ from the lumen increases rapidly. These channels, which may be activated by membrane stretch, then allow K$^+$ to leave the cell, a process that causes cells to shrink toward their original volume (a volume-regulatory decrease; p. 77).

A PROXIMAL TUBULE

B THICK ASCENDING LIMB (TAL)

C CORTICAL COLLECTING TUBULE (CCT):
α INTERCALATED CELL

D CORTICAL COLLECTING TUBULE (CCT):
PRINCIPAL CELL

FIGURE 36–7. Cellular models of K^+ transport along the nephron. ATP, adenosine triphosphate; ENaC, epithelial Na^+ channel.

Even if the apical K^+ channels were open more often, uptake of K^+ across the apical membrane would not occur, because the electrochemical K^+ gradient favors K^+ movement from cell to lumen. Because K^+ cannot enter across the apical membrane, there can be no transcellular reabsorption of K^+. Thus, proximal-tubule K^+ reabsorption must occur exclusively via the paracellular pathway.

K^+ Reabsorption Along the Thick Ascending Limb Occurs via Both a Passive Paracellular Route and a Transcellular Route That Exploits Secondary Active Na/K/Cl Cotransport

As discussed earlier, the **thin descending limbs** of the loop of Henle, particularly those originating from juxtamedullary nephrons, *secrete* K^+ (see Fig. 36–6). This secretion of K^+ from the medullary interstitium into the tDLH lumen is passive, driven by the high $[K^+]$ of the medullary interstitium and made possible by a substantial K^+ permeability. Both the tDLH lumen and the interstitium become increasingly K^+-rich toward the tip of the papilla.

In the **thin ascending limb** (tALH), K^+ moves from lumen to interstitium passively, via the paracellular pathway. The major driving force for this passive reabsorption of K^+ is the lumen-to-interstitium K^+ gradient, which

becomes progressively larger as the fluid moves towards the cortex because interstitial $[K^+]$ becomes progressively lower towards the cortex.

The **thick ascending limb** of the loop of Henle (TAL) reabsorbs K^+ by both paracellular and transcellular mechanisms (see Fig. 36–7B). The lumen-positive voltage, together with the relatively high paracellular K^+ permeability, allows passive K^+ reabsorption to occur via the *paracellular* pathway. The lumen-positive voltage develops because of a substantial difference in the ion permeabilities of the apical and basolateral membranes. The *apical* membrane is K^+-selective, so that the apical membrane potential depends mainly on the cell-to-lumen $[K^+]$ gradient. In contrast, the TAL *basolateral* membrane is permeable to both K^+ and Cl^-. Hence, the basolateral membrane potential lies between the equilibrium potentials of Cl^- (approximately −50 mV) and K^+ (about −90 mV), so that it is less negative than if the basolateral membrane were permeable only to K^+. Because the apical membrane potential is more negative than the basolateral membrane potential, the transepithelial voltage is lumen-positive. This potential provides a substantial driving force for the passive, paracellular reabsorption of cations such as K^+ and Na^+. Half of the K^+ reabsorbed by the TAL exits via this paracellular pathway, with the lumen-positive potential being the main driving force.

The other half of K$^+$ reabsorption by the TAL occurs via a *transcellular* pathway, using the apical Na/K/Cl cotransporter NKCC2 (p. 67). The major evidence for such a mechanism is the mutual interdependence of Na$^+$, Cl$^-$, and K$^+$ transport. Removing any of the three cotransported ions from the lumen abolishes transcellular K$^+$ reabsorption. However, because inhibiting the Na/K/Cl cotransporter also abolishes the lumen-positive potential (p. 778), this inhibition also blocks passive, paracellular K$^+$ reabsorption.

The apical NKCC2 is a typical example of a "secondary" active transporter (p. 61). Expressed in electrical terms, the apical membrane potential is some 10 to 12 mV more positive than the K$^+$ equilibrium potential, so that K$^+$ would tend to passively diffuse from cell to lumen. Because the combined inward gradients of Na$^+$ and Cl$^-$ across the apical membrane greatly exceed that of K$^+$, the energy is adequate for the coupled uptake of all three ion species. Ultimately, a primary active transporter (i.e., Na-K pump) at the basolateral membrane drives the secondary active transport of K$^+$ in the apical membrane. Inhibiting the basolateral Na-K pump leads to an increase in [Na$^+$]$_i$ and [Cl$^-$]$_i$, so that apical Na/K/Cl transport ceases. A characteristic feature of the Na/K/Cl cotransporter is its sensitivity to a class of diuretics that have their main site of action in the TAL. Therefore, administering so-called **loop diuretics** such as furosemide or bumetanide blocks net reabsorption of Na$^+$, Cl$^-$, and K$^+$.

The apical K$^+$ conductance mentioned earlier—which mainly represents a K$^+$ channel called ROMK2—is also important for the function of the Na/K/Cl cotransporter (see Fig. 36–7B). The major function of the apical K$^+$ channel is to provide a mechanism for recycling much of the K$^+$ from cell to lumen, so that luminal [K$^+$] does not fall too low to sustain Na/K/Cl cotransport (p. 778). Nevertheless, some of the K$^+$ entering the cell via the Na/K/Cl cotransporter exits across the basolateral membrane, accounting for transcellular K$^+$ reabsorption. The presence of apical K$^+$ channels also explains why inhibiting Na/K/Cl cotransport—either with loop diuretics (e.g., furosemide) or by deleting from the lumen of any of the cotransported ions—causes the TAL to engage in net K$^+$ *secretion*. Active K$^+$ uptake no longer opposes the K$^+$ leak from the cell to lumen.

K$^+$ Reabsorption by Intercalated Cells Occurs via Apical K$^+$ Uptake Mediated by an H-K Pump, Followed by Passive Efflux of K$^+$ across the Basolateral Membrane

Ultrastructurally, the initial and cortical collecting tubules are nearly identical (p. 743), being made up of approximately 70% principal cells (which secrete K$^+$) and approximately 30% intercalated cells (some of which reabsorb K$^+$).

As discussed earlier, the ICT, CCT, and MCD reabsorb K$^+$ in response to K$^+$ depletion (see Fig. 36–5A). This K$^+$ reabsorption is a transcellular process (see Fig. 36–7C), mediated by α **intercalated cells**, a subpopulation of intercalated cells that are interspersed among the principal cells. These cells are also responsible for H$^+$ secretion (p. 852).

Net K$^+$ reabsorption by intercalated cells requires two elements: (1) an active K$^+$ pump to move K$^+$ into the cell

across the apical membrane and (2) a K$^+$ channel to allow the K$^+$ to leak out across the basolateral membrane. The K$^+$ pump is thought to be an ATP-driven H-K pump (p. 63) similar to that present at the apical membrane of the parietal cells in the gastric gland (p. 894). The coupling of K$^+$ reabsorption to H$^+$ secretion helps to explain why K$^+$ depletion, a condition in which the abundance of H-K pumps increases dramatically, is often associated with accelerated secretion of H$^+$ and the development of hypokalemic alkalosis.

K$^+$ Secretion by Principal Cells of the ICT and CCT Occurs by Active K$^+$ Uptake Across the Basolateral Membrane, Followed by Passive Diffusion Through Apical K$^+$ Channels

The *early* portion of the classical distal tubule (i.e., DCT) secretes K$^+$ but at a relatively low rate. However, K$^+$ secretion into the tubule fluid is one of the distinguishing features of *late* portions of the classic distal tubule (i.e., ICT) and of the CCT. Of the two cell types in the ICT and CCT, it is the **principal cell** that secretes K$^+$, doing so by a transcellular process (see Fig. 36–7D). The three key elements of the principal cell are: (1) an Na-K pump for active K$^+$ uptake at the basolateral membrane, (2) a relatively high (and variable) apical K$^+$ permeability, and (3) a favorable electrochemical driving force for K$^+$ exit across the apical membrane. In addition, K$^+$ may move from cell to lumen via the apical K/Cl cotransporter (KCC) (p. 67). The net effect is the active movement of K$^+$ from blood to cell, and the passive movement of K$^+$ from cell to lumen. Changes in any of the three elements can affect the secretion of K$^+$.

K$^+$ Reabsorption along the Medullary Collecting Duct Is Passive

The capacity for K$^+$ *secretion* diminishes from the cortical to the medullary collecting duct. Indeed, the **medullary collecting duct** is responsible for K$^+$ *reabsorption*, which contributes to medullary K$^+$ recycling (see Fig. 36–6). This K$^+$ loss from the nephron lumen can occur by passive reabsorption along a favorable concentration gradient across the MCD epithelium. In addition, especially during low K$^+$ intake, apical K-H pumps may mediate K$^+$ absorption. The luminal [K$^+$] of the medullary collecting duct is high for two reasons. First, the segments just upstream (i.e., distal K$^+$-secretory system) may have secreted K$^+$. Second, the continuing reabsorption of fluid in the medullary collecting tubules, particularly in the absence of diuresis, further increases luminal [K$^+$]. This high luminal [K$^+$] constitutes the driving force for the passive reabsorption of K$^+$ by the medullary collecting duct. Moreover, the medullary collecting duct has a significant transepithelial K$^+$ permeability.

REGULATION OF RENAL POTASSIUM EXCRETION

Table 36–2 summarizes factors that modulate K$^+$ secretion. These may be grouped into luminal and peritubular (i.e., bathing basolateral membrane) factors.

TABLE 36–2

LUMINAL AND PERITUBULAR FACTORS THAT MODULATE K⁺ SECRETION BY THE DISTAL K⁺-SECRETORY SYSTEM*

LUMINAL FACTORS

Stimulators	Inhibitors
↑ Flow rate	↑ $[K^+]$
↑ $[Na^+]$	↑ $[Cl^-]$
↓ $[Cl^-]$	↑ $[Ca^{2+}]$
↑ $[HCO_3^-]$	Ba^{2+}
Negative luminal voltage	Amiloride
Diuretics acting upstream of ICT/CCT	

PERITUBULAR FACTORS

Stimulators:	Inhibitors
↑ K^+ intake	↓ pH
↑ $[K^+]$	Epinephrine
↑ pH	
Aldosterone	
Arginine vasopressin (AVP)	

*Initial and cortical collecting tubules, and proximal portion of medullary collecting duct.
CCT, cortical collecting tubule; ICT, initial collecting tubule.

Increased Luminal Flow Increases K⁺ Secretion

One of the most potent stimuli of K⁺ secretion is the rate of fluid flow along the distal K⁺-secretory system (i.e., ICT and CCT). Under almost all circumstances, an increase in luminal flow increases K⁺ secretion (Fig. 36–8) and a similar relationship holds between final urine flow and K⁺ excretion. Accordingly, the increased urine flow that occurs with extracellular volume expansion, osmotic diuresis, or administration of several diuretic agents (e.g., furosemide, thiazides, acetazolamide) leads to enhanced K⁺ excretion (**kaliuresis**). Almost uniformly, increased urinary flow is associated with increased Na⁺ excretion (natriuresis) as well, so that both solutes appear in increased amounts in the urine.

The strong flow-dependence of distal K⁺ secretion is a consequence of the high apical K⁺ permeability of principal cells (see Fig. 36–7D). When luminal flow is low, then as K⁺ moves from the principal cell to the lumen, luminal $[K^+]$ rises rapidly to a steady-state level, inhibiting further K⁺ diffusion from the cell. Thus, total K⁺ secretion is relatively low. When luminal flow is high, it sweeps newly secreted K⁺ downstream. The resulting fall in luminal $[K^+]$ steepens the K⁺ gradient across the apical membrane, and thus increases passive K⁺ flux from cell to lumen.

Increased luminal flow also increases the Na⁺ delivery to tubule cells, thus raising luminal $[Na^+]$ and enhancing Na⁺ uptake. This incremental supply of Na⁺ to the principal cell stimulates its Na-K pump, increasing basolateral K⁺ uptake and further increasing K⁺ secretion. The Na⁺ sensitivity of K⁺ secretion is most pronounced when luminal $[Na^+]$ is below 35 mM, as is often the case in the CCT.

An Increased Lumen-Negative Transepithelial Potential Increases K⁺ Secretion

The apical step of K⁺ secretion in the ICT and CCT occurs by diffusion of K⁺ from the principal cell to the lumen, which depends on the apical electrochemical K⁺ gradient (see Fig. 36–7D). Increases in luminal $[Na^+]$—enhancing apical Na⁺ entry through ENaC channels (p. 779)—depolarize the apical membrane, favoring the exit of K⁺ from cell to lumen (i.e., K⁺ secretion). Conversely, a fall in luminal $[Na^+]$ hyperpolarizes the apical membrane, inhibiting K⁺ secretion.

The diuretic **amiloride** (p. 779) has the same effect on K⁺ secretion as decreasing luminal $[Na^+]$. By blocking apical ENaC Na⁺ channels, amiloride hyperpolarizes the apical membrane, reducing the electrochemical gradient for K⁺ secretion. Thus, amiloride is a K⁺-sparing diuretic.

Low Luminal [Cl⁻] Enhances K⁺ Secretion

Lowering luminal Cl⁻—replacing it with an anion (e.g., SO_4^{2-} or HCO_3^-) that the tubule reabsorbs poorly—promotes K⁺ loss into the urine, independent of changes in the lumen-negative voltage. Underlying this effect may be the K/Cl cotransporter in the apical membrane of the principal cell (see Fig. 36–7D). Lowering luminal $[Cl^-]$ increases the cell-to-lumen Cl⁻ gradient, which presumably stimulates K/Cl cotransport, and thus K⁺ secretion.

When luminal $[Cl^-]$ in the DCT is low, thiazide diuretics may indirectly *inhibit* K⁺ secretion. These drugs inhibit Cl⁻ uptake by a luminal Na/Cl cotransporter in the DCT (p. 779), thus presenting a *higher* luminal $[Cl^-]$ to the downstream K⁺-secretory sites in the ICT and CCT. This elevation in luminal $[Cl^-]$ secondarily inhibits K⁺ efflux from the principal cell via the K/Cl cotransporter (see Fig. 36–7D), and thus reduces K⁺ secretion.

Aldosterone Increases K⁺ Secretion

Both mineralocorticoids (p. 1057) and glucocorticoids (p. 1049) cause kaliuresis. Primary hyperaldosteronism leads

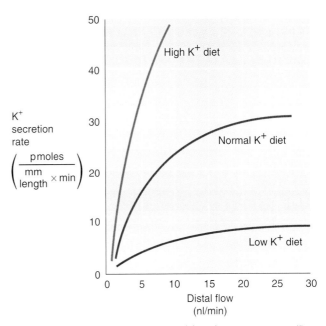

FIGURE 36–8. Effect of flow (i.e., Na⁺ delivery) on K⁺ excretion. (Data from Stanton BA, Giebisch, G: Renal potassium transport. *In* Handbook of Physiology: Renal Physiology, E. Windhager, ed., Oxford University Press, 813–874, 1992.)

to K⁺ wasting and hypokalemia, whereas adrenocortical insufficiency (i.e., deficiency of both mineralocorticoids and glucocorticoids) leads to K⁺ retention and hyperkalemia.

MINERALOCORTICOIDS. Aldosterone, the main native mineralocorticoid, induces K⁺ secretion in the ICT and CCT, particularly when its effects are prolonged (see Fig. 34–12). Either aldosterone or desoxycorticosterone acetate (DOCA), a powerful synthetic mineralocorticoid, increases the transcription of genes that enhance Na⁺ reabsorption and, secondarily, K⁺ secretion in the *principal cells* of the ICT and CCT (p. 786). Three factors act in concert to promote K⁺ secretion. First, over a period of a few hours, aldosterone increases the basolateral K⁺ uptake by stimulating the Na-K pump. Over a few days, elevated aldosterone also leads to a marked amplification of the area of the basolateral membrane of principal cells, as well as to a corresponding increase in the number of Na-K pump molecules. Conversely, adrenalectomy causes a significant reduction in basolateral surface area and Na-K pumps in principal cells. Second, mineralocorticoids stimulate apical ENaC channels, depolarizing the apical membrane and increasing the driving force for K⁺ diffusion from cell to lumen. Third, aldosterone increases the K⁺ conductance of the apical membrane.

Considering its mechanisms of action, we might expect aldosterone to stimulate both K⁺ secretion and Na⁺ reabsorption. Therefore, one might think that the renal excretion of K⁺ and Na⁺ should always be inversely related. However, the extent to which aldosterone increases K⁺ excretion depends strongly on Na⁺ excretion. For example, if Na⁺ intake and excretion are low, the Na⁺ retention induced by aldosterone reduces luminal flow and Na⁺ delivery to such low levels that K⁺ excretion fails to increase. In contrast, under high-flow conditions (e.g., with a high Na⁺ load or following administration of diuretics that act on the TAL or the DCT), aldosterone increases K⁺ excretion.

Chronically administering mineralocorticoids leads to a sequence of events known as **aldosterone escape**. Aldosterone leads to Na⁺ retention, and thus volume expansion. Eventually, the volume expansion causes proximal Na⁺ reabsorption to fall (see Fig. 33–11), increasing Na⁺ delivery to the ICT and CCT, and ultimately raising Na⁺ excretion toward pre-aldosterone levels. Thus, the kidney can "escape" the Na⁺-retaining effect of aldosterone, albeit at the price of expanding the extracellular volume. The situation is different with respect to K⁺, because the increased Na⁺ delivery to the distal K⁺-secretory system continues to stimulate K⁺ secretion. Once the body has become depleted of K⁺, the aldosterone-stimulated K⁺ secretion eventually wanes, and the distal nephron may return to net K⁺ reabsorption.

GLUCOCORTICOIDS. Under physiologic conditions, glucocorticoids enhance K⁺ excretion. Corticosterone and dexamethasone, a synthetic glucocorticoid, produce this effect largely by increasing flow along the distal K⁺-secretory system (i.e., ICT and CCT). Because glucocorticoids increase the glomerular filtration rate (GFR) and probably lower the water permeability of the distal K⁺-secretory system, they increase the amounts of fluid and Na⁺ remaining in these segments. These two flow effects, by themselves, increase K⁺ secretion. Indeed, when one perfuses the distal K⁺-secretory system at a *constant rate*, glucocorticoids have no effect on K⁺ transport.

In addition, administering unphysiologically high doses of glucocorticoids may stimulate K⁺ transport directly as glucocorticoids bind to *mineralocorticoid* receptors, despite the presence of 11β-HSD in aldosterone target cells (p. 787).

High K⁺ Intake Promotes Renal K⁺ Secretion

DIETARY K⁺ LOADING. An increase in dietary K⁺ intake causes, after some delay, an increase in urinary K⁺ excretion (see Fig. 36–5B). If the period of high-K⁺ intake is prolonged, a condition of tolerance ("K⁺ adaptation") develops in which the kidneys can now efficiently excrete large doses of K⁺—even previously lethal doses—with only a small rise in plasma [K⁺].

The kaliuresis following an acute or chronic K⁺ load is the result of increased K⁺ secretion in the ICT and CCT (compare the *three curves* in Fig. 36–8 at a single flow), which occurs by three mechanisms. First, a transient rise in plasma [K⁺], even if maintained for only short periods, is an effective stimulus for K⁺ excretion. The mechanism is an increased K⁺ uptake across the basolateral membrane of principal cells by the Na-K pump, a response shared by most of the cells of the body. As is the case with mineralocorticoid stimulation, the ultrastructure of the ICT and CCT correlates with changes in the rate of K⁺ transport induced by high dietary K⁺. Therefore, a high-K⁺ diet—independent of the effects of aldosterone—causes surface amplification of the basolateral membrane of principal cells. Second, the increased plasma [K⁺] stimulates glomerulosa cells in the adrenal cortex to synthesize and release aldosterone (p. 1060). This mineralocorticoid is a potent stimulus for K⁺ secretion both in the kidney by principal cells (see earlier) and in the colon (p. 942). Third, acute K⁺ loading inhibits proximal Na⁺ and fluid reabsorption and increases the flow and Na⁺ delivery to the distal K⁺-secretory system, which stimulates K⁺ secretion.

DIETARY K⁺ DEPRIVATION. In response to K⁺ restriction, the kidneys retain K⁺ (see Fig. 36–5A). The rate of urinary K⁺ excretion may fall to 1% to 3% of the filtered load, reflecting the action of two mechanisms at the level of the ICT and CCT. First, the low plasma [K⁺] suppresses K⁺ secretion by the principal cells (Fig. 36–8, *lower curve*) by both reducing basolateral K⁺ uptake by principal cells and by reducing aldosterone secretion. Second, the low plasma [K⁺] stimulates K⁺ reabsorption by intercalated cells via H-K pumps (see Fig. 36–7C), causing the [K⁺] of the final urine to fall sharply, sometimes to levels below that of the plasma. In addition, the medullary collecting duct responds to K⁺ depletion by increasing its reabsorption of K⁺, by enhancing both the activity of its apical K-H pump and its paracellular K⁺ permeability. As a result, the [K⁺] of the final urine falls sharply, sometimes to levels below that of the plasma.

Whereas states of high-K⁺ secretion (i.e., aldosterone or high-K⁺ diet) amplify the basolateral membrane of principal cells, K⁺ deprivation amplifies the *apical* membrane of

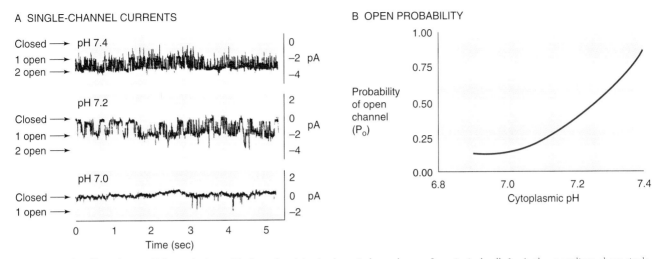

FIGURE 36–9. Effect of intracellular acidosis on K⁺-channel activity in the apical membrane of a principal cell. In *A*, the recordings show single-channel K⁺ currents from inside-out patches, with different pH values on the "cytoplasmic" side. As shown in *B*, channels are almost never open at pH values at 7.0 or below. (Data from Wang W, Geibel J, Giebisch G: Regulation of small conductance K channel in the apical membrane of rat cortical collecting tubule. *Am J Physiol* 259:F494–F502, 1990.)

α intercalated cells. Moreover, K⁺ depletion causes an increased incorporation of rod-shaped particles in the apical membrane of *α* intercalated cells, and the density of these particles correlates well with enhanced K⁺ reabsorption. These morphologic changes probably underlie the increased active K⁺ reabsorption and H⁺ secretion mediated by H-K pumps.

Acidosis Decreases K⁺ Secretion

Acid-base disturbances have marked effects on renal K⁺ transport. In general, either metabolic alkalosis (p. 642) or respiratory alkalosis (p. 641) leads to increased K⁺ excretion. Conversely, acidosis reduces K⁺ excretion, although this response is more variable than that to alkalosis. Changes in systemic acid-base parameters affect K⁺ transport mainly by acting on the distal K⁺-secretory system.

As discussed, alkalosis leads to hypokalemia (p. 816),

owing to K⁺ uptake by cells throughout the body. Despite this fall in plasma [K⁺], alkalosis *stimulates* K⁺ secretion in the distal K⁺-secretory system, worsening the hypokalemia. Conversely, K⁺ secretion falls in acidosis despite the shift of K⁺ from cells to ECF and the concomitant rise in plasma [K⁺].

The cellular events underlying the renal response to acid-base disturbances most likely involve effects of intracellular pH (pH$_i$) on both the basolateral Na-K pump and the apical K⁺ channels of the principal cells in the ICT and CCT. Tubule-perfusion studies with ⁴²K indicate that decreasing the extracellular pH—which also decreases pH$_i$—inhibits the Na-K pump and thus K⁺ secretion. Even more important is that the decrease in pH$_i$ also reduces the permeability of the apical K⁺ channels, which are exquisitely sensitive to acidification (Figs. 36–9*A* and 36–9*B*). The reverse changes occur in alkalosis.

Changes in tubule flow (i.e., fluid delivery to the distal K⁺-secretory system) that occur in acid-base disturbances

FIGURE 36–10. Interaction of opposing factors on K⁺ secretion. ADH, antidiuretic hormone; ECF, extracellular fluid; GFR, glomerular filtration rate.

CLINICAL IMPLICATIONS: EVALUATING HYPOKALEMIA AND HYPERKALEMIA IN THE PATIENT

We can directly apply the physiological principles discussed in this chapter to understanding the common causes and treatment of hypokalemia and hyperkalemia.

HYPOKALEMIA

The body can lose K^+ from three sites: the kidneys, the GI tract, and the skin. Renal losses occur most commonly in patients taking diuretics (e.g., furosemide and thiazides) that act at sites upstream to the distal K^+-secretory system (i.e., ICT, CCT, and proximal portion of MCD). K^+ losses can also occur in individuals with renal-tubule disorders or alterations in the renin-angiotensin-aldosterone system (e.g., hyperaldosteronism). Because gastric and intestinal secretions have a high $[K^+]$, vomiting and severe diarrhea are common causes of hypokalemia. Significant K^+ depletion through the skin can occur in two situations: (1) strenuous exercise on a hot, humid day can cause dehydration and hypokalemia from the loss of many liters of perspiration, and (2) severe and extensive burns can result in the transudation of vast amounts of K^+-containing fluid through the skin.

A low plasma $[K^+]$ can also develop as the result of altered K^+ distribution within the body, without any net loss of whole-body K^+. Common causes include alkalosis, a catecholamine surge (as, for instance, during any acute stress to the body, such as an acute myocardial infarction), and excessive insulin administration during the treatment of diabetic ketoacidosis.

Patients may develop hypokalemia because of inadequate dietary K^+ intake. Patients receiving large amounts of intravenous saline (which lacks K^+) may also waste K^+. Some persons in rural areas ingest clay (a behavior called pica), which binds K^+ in the GI tract and prevents K^+ absorption.

HYPERKALEMIA

Probably the most common cause of a high laboratory value for plasma $[K^+]$ is **pseudohyperkalemia**, a falsely elevated value that results from traumatic hemolysis of red blood cells during a blood drawing. Red blood cells release their intracellular stores of K^+ in the blood sample, and the laboratory reports a falsely elevated plasma $[K^+]$. Patients with myeloproliferative disorders associated with greatly increased numbers of platelets or white blood cells can also show a falsely elevated $[K^+]$ because of K^+ released during clot formation within the blood-sample tube.

Excessive intake of K^+ rarely causes hyperkalemia in persons with healthy kidneys. However, even in these individuals, a large K^+ bolus can cause a transient hyperkalemia (see Fig. 36–4, *top*), often from an ill-advised intravenous line. Altered distribution of K^+ can lead to elevated plasma levels in patients with acidosis and, rarely, as a result of β-adrenergic blockade. Digitalis, a cardiac glycoside that inhibits the Na-K pump (p. 63), is another rare cause of hyperkalemia caused by K^+ redistribution. Massive breakdown of cells can release large amounts of K^+ into the extracellular space. This release can occur with intravascular hemolysis (e.g., from a mismatched blood transfusion), burns, crush injuries, rhabdomyolysis (massive muscle destruction such as can be seen with trauma or sepsis), gastrointestinal bleeding with subsequent intestinal absorption of K^+-rich fluid, or destruction of tumor tissue or leukemic blood cells by chemotherapy.

Impaired renal excretion of K^+ is the primary cause of a sustained increase in plasma $[K^+]$. Hypoaldosteronism, high doses of amiloride, and distal renal tubular acidosis can be responsible, but advanced renal failure itself from any of a myriad number of disorders is the most common cause.

The treatment of hyperkalemia depends on the severity of the problem. For severe hyperkalemia (i.e., a $[K^+]$ greater than 8 mM) with accompanying ECG changes, the physician immediately infuses calcium gluconate intravenously to counter the electrophysiological effects of the hyperkalemia. (Ca^{2+} raises the threshold for action potentials and lessens membrane excitability). One may also simultaneously administer $NaHCO_3$, glucose, and often insulin to move some of the K^+ from the extracellular to the intracellular space. These are all temporizing measures. To actually remove the excess K^+ from the body, the physician introduces a nonabsorbable Na-K cation exchange resin (e.g., sodium polystyrene sulfonamide) either orally or as an enema. The resin binds the K^+ and carries it out of the body via the GI tract. However, the resin takes several hours to work. Thus, for patients with hyperkalemia and ECG changes, the temporizing measures buy time for the resin to act. For patients with end-stage renal failure, dialysis is often necessary to return the plasma $[K^+]$ to normal.

CCT, cortical collecting tubule; ECG, electrocardiogram; ICT, initial collecting tubule; GI, gastrointestinal; MCD, medullary collecting duct.

---

may modulate the effects of pH changes per se. For example, metabolic alkalosis increases the flow by delivering a HCO_3^--rich solution to the ICT and CCT. By itself, this increased flow will enhance K^+ secretion, and thus *potentiate* the effect of alkalosis *per se*. In contrast, acidosis also increases distal flow, in this case by inhibiting proximal fluid reabsorption, with the consequence that the tendency of increased flow to increase K^+ secretion *opposes* the effect of acidosis per se to decrease it. Therefore, the net effect of acidosis on K^+ excretion is variable.

Epinephrine Reduces K^+ Excretion

By both extrarenal and renal mechanisms, **epinephrine** lowers K^+ excretion. First, epinephrine enhances K^+ uptake by extrarenal tissues (p. 815), lowering plasma $[K^+]$ and reducing the filtered K^+ load. Second, catecholamines directly inhibit K^+ secretion in nephron segments downstream of the ICT.

Although it is not a major regulator of K^+ excretion, **arginine vasopressin** ([AVP], also known as antidiuretic hormone [ADH]) can stimulate the distal K⁺-secretory system by two mechanisms (see Fig. 36–7D): (1) AVP increases the apical Na⁺ conductance, depolarizing the apical membrane and providing a larger driving force for K⁺ efflux from cell to lumen. (2) AVP increases apical K⁺ permeability. However, AVP also reduces urine flow, which inhibits K⁺ secretion. Therefore, the two opposing effects—a direct stimulation of K⁺ secretion and a flow-related reduction of K⁺ secretion—may cancel each other.

Effects on Distal Flow May Either Augment or Diminish the Direct Effects of "Regulatory Factors" on K⁺ Secretion

It should be apparent from the above discussion that the net effect of a specific disturbance on K⁺ excretion in the final urine often represents a result of two or more interacting factors. Changes in flow often indirectly amplify or attenuate the direct response of the distal K⁺-secretory system to a given stimulus. Figure 36–10 shows four examples of **attenuating effects**. The first three (acidosis, volume expansion, and high water intake) are characterized by the competition between a direct depressing effect on K⁺ secretion and an indirect stimulating effect of increased flow (Fig. 36–10A through C).

Extracellular-volume contraction (see Fig. 36–10D) has three effects. First, it decreases distal flow, which inhibits the distal K⁺-secretory system. Second, volume contraction increases angiotensin II (ANG II) levels, which in turn *increases* aldosterone release and, thus, K⁺ secretion. Third, volume contraction also produces a small rise in plasma [K⁺], the magnitude of which might normally not evoke much of an increase in aldosterone release. However, in the presence of elevated ANG II, even such a small increase in plasma [K⁺] is a potent stimulus for aldosterone release (p. 1060). Thus, the potentiation between K⁺ and angiotensin II ensures continued K⁺ excretion, even when low fluid delivery to the distal K⁺-secretory system would have the opposite effect.

In some instances, the direct actions of an agent and flow-related effects may have **additive effects**. Three examples follow.

First, metabolic alkalosis—as discussed—directly stimulates the distal K⁺-secretory system. In addition, the delivery of the poorly reabsorbable HCO₃⁻ in metabolic alkalosis increases distal flow, potentiating K⁺ excretion.

Second, hyperkalemia directly stimulates the distal K⁺-secretory system. In addition, because increased plasma [K⁺] inhibits Na⁺ and fluid reabsorption in the proximal tubule, distal flow increases, again potentiating K⁺ excretion.

Third, administering diuretics that act on a site upstream of the initial and cortical collecting tubules increase Na⁺ delivery to the distal K⁺-secretory system, stimulating K⁺ secretion. In addition, the volume contraction induced by the diuretic raises aldosterone levels, again potentiating K⁺ excretion. Hypokalemia is thus a possible harmful side effect of diuretic treatment.

REFERENCES

Books and Reviews

Giebisch G: Renal potassium transport: Mechanisms and regulation. Am J Physiol 274:F817–F833, 1998.

Jamison RL: Potassium recycling. Kidney Int 31:695–703, 1987.

Seldin DW, Giebisch G (eds): The Kidney: Physiology and Pathophysiology, 3rd ed. Philadelphia, JB Lippincott, 2000.

Wingo CS, Cain BD: The renal H-K-ATPase: Physiological significance and role in potassium homeostasis. Annu Rev Physiol 55:323–347, 1993.

Wang W, Hebert SC, Giebisch G: Renal K⁺ channels: Structure and function. Annu Rev Physiol 59:413–436, 1997.

Journal Articles

Greger R, Schlatter E: Presence of luminal K⁺, a prerequisite for active NaCl transport in the cortical thick ascending limb of Henle's loop of rabbit kidney. Pflugers Arch 392:92–94, 1981.

Ho K, Nichols CG, Lederer WJ, et al: Cloning and expression of an inwardly rectifying ATP-regulated potassium channel. Nature 362:31–38, 1993.

Malnic G, Klose R, Giebisch G: Micropuncture study of renal potassium excretion in the rat. Am J Physiol 206:674–686, 1964.

Stokes J: Consequences of potassium recycling in the renal medulla: Effects on ion transport by the medullary thick ascending limb of Henle's loop. J Clin Invest 70:219–229, 1982.

Wade JB, O'Neil RG, Pryor JL, Boulpaep EL: Modulation of cell membrane area in renal cortical collecting tubules by corticosteroid hormones. J Cell Biol 81:439–445, 1979.

CHAPTER 37

Urine Concentration and Dilution

Gerhard Giebisch and Erich Windhager

The Kidney Can Generate a Urine as Dilute as 30 mOsm (1/10 of Plasma Osmolality) or as Concentrated as 1200 mOsm (4× Plasma Osmolality)

In the steady state, water intake and output must be equal (Table 37–1). The body's three major sources of water are (1) water consumed as a liquid, (2) water contained within foods that we eat, and (3) water produced by aerobic metabolism as mitochondria convert foodstuffs and O_2 to CO_2 and H_2O (p. 1220).

The major route of water loss is usually through the kidneys, the organs that play the central role in regulating water balance. The feces are usually a minor route of water output (p. 934). Although the production of sweat can increase markedly during exercise or at high temperatures, sweat production is geared to help regulate body core temperature (p. 1237), not body water balance. Water also evaporates from the skin and is lost in the humidified air exhaled from the lungs and air passages. The figures summarized in Table 37–1 will obviously vary, depending on diet, physical activity, and the environment (e.g., temperature and humidity).

The kidney adjusts its water output to compensate for either abnormally high or abnormally low water intake, or for abnormally high water losses via other routes. The kidney excretes a variable amount of solute, depending especially on salt intake. But, for a normal diet, the excreted solute is approximately 600 milliosmoles per day. For average conditions of water and solute intake and output, these 600 mosmole are dissolved in a daily urine output of 1500 ml. However, a key principle is that, regardless of the volume of water they excrete, the kidneys must excrete approximately 600 mosmole/day. Stated somewhat differently, the product of urine osmolality and urine output is approximately constant:

Equation 37–1

$$\text{Osmoles excreted/day} = \underbrace{U_{osm}}_{\text{Urine osmolality}} \cdot \underbrace{\dot{V}}_{\text{Urine output}}$$

Therefore, to excrete a wide range of water volumes, the human kidney must produce urine having a wide range of osmolalities. For example, when the kidney excretes the 600 mosmole dissolved in 1500 ml of urine each day, urine osmolality must be 400 mOsm:

TABLE 37–1

INPUT AND OUTPUT OF WATER

INPUT Source	Amount (ml)
Ingested fluids	1200
Ingested food	1000
Metabolism	300
Total	2500

OUTPUT Route	Amount (ml)
Urine	1500
Feces	100
Skin/Sweat	550
Exhaled air	350
Total	2500

Modified from Valtin H: Renal Dysfunction: Mechanisms Involved in Fluid and Solute Imbalance. Boston, Little, Brown, 1979; p 21.

$$\text{Equation } 37-2$$
$$U_{osm} = \frac{\text{Osmole excreted/day}}{\dot{V}} = \frac{600 \text{ mosmole/day}}{1.5 \text{ liters/day}}$$
$$= 400 \text{ mOsm}$$

When the intake of water is especially high, the human kidney can generate urine having an osmolality as low as approximately 30 mOsm. Because the kidneys might still need to excrete 600 mosmole of solutes, the urine volume in an extreme **water diuresis** would be as high as 20 liters!

$$\text{Equation } 37-3$$
$$\dot{V} = \frac{\text{Osmole excreted/day}}{U_{osm}} = \frac{600 \text{ mosmole/day}}{30 \text{ mOsm}}$$
$$= 20 \text{ liters/day}$$

However, when it is necessary to conserve water (e.g., with restricted water intake; excessive loss by sweat or stool), the kidney is capable of generating urine with an osmolality as high as approximately 1200 mOsm. Therefore, with an average solute load, the minimal urine volume can be as low as approximately 0.5 liter:

$$\text{Equation } 37-4$$
$$\dot{V} = \frac{\text{Osmole excreted/day}}{U_{osm}} = \frac{600 \text{ mosmole/day}}{1200 \text{ mOsm}}$$
$$= 0.5 \text{ liter/day}$$

Therefore, the kidney is capable of diluting the urine approximately 10-fold with respect to blood plasma, but is capable of concentrating the urine only fourfold.

The Free-Water Clearance (C_{H_2O}) Is Positive if the Kidney Produces Urine That Is Less Concentrated Than Plasma, and Negative if the Kidney Produces Urine That Is More Concentrated Than Plasma

A urine sample can be thought of as consisting of two moieties: (1) The volume that would be necessary to dissolve all the excreted solutes at a concentration that is isosmotic with blood plasma. (2) The volume of pure or solute-free water—or, simply, **free water**—that one must add (or subtract) to the previous volume to account for the entire urine volume. As discussed later, the kidney generates free water in the tubule lumen by reabsorbing solutes, mainly NaCl, in excess of water along nephron segments with low water permeability. When the kidney generates free water, the urine becomes dilute (hypoosmotic). Conversely, when the kidney removes water from an isosmotic fluid, the urine becomes concentrated (hyperosmotic). When the kidney neither adds nor subtracts free water from the isosmotic moiety, the urine is isosmotic with blood plasma.

The urine output is the sum of the rate at which kidney excretes the isosmotic moiety of urine (**osmolal clearance**, C_{osm}) and the rate at which it excretes "free water" (**free-water clearance**, C_{H_2O}):

$$\text{Equation } 37-5$$
$$\dot{V} = C_{osm} + C_{H_2O}$$

Of course, C_{H_2O} is "negative" (i.e., excretion of "negative free water") if the kidney removes free water and produces a concentrated urine. We compute C_{osm} in the same way we would compute the clearance of any substance from the blood (p. 746):

$$\text{Equation } 37-6$$
$$C_{osm} = \frac{U_{osm} \cdot \dot{V}}{P_{osm}}$$

P_{osm} is the osmolality of blood plasma. The osmolal clearance is the hypothetical volume of blood (in ml) that the kidneys fully clear of solutes (or osmoles) per unit time. For example, if the daily solute excretion ($U_{osm} \cdot \dot{V}$) is fixed at 600 mosmole/day, and P_{osm} is 300 mosmole/liter, then Equation 37–6 tells us that C_{osm} has a fixed value of 2 liters/day.

We can only obtain the free water clearance by subtraction:

$$\text{Equation } 37-7$$
$$C_{H_2O} = \dot{V} - C_{osm}$$

Indeed, "free-water clearance" does not conform to the usual definition of "clearance" because C_{H_2O} is not ($U_{H_2O} \cdot \dot{V}/P_{H_2O}$). Nevertheless, this apparent misnomer has been accepted by renal physiologists and nephrologists.

The range of C_{H_2O} values for the human kidney is related to the extremes in urine osmolality, as shown for these three examples:

ISOSMOTIC URINE. If the osmolalities of the urine and plasma are the *same* ($U_{osm} = P_{osm}$), then osmolal clearance is the same as urine flow:

Equation 37–8

$$C_{osm} = \frac{U_{osm} \cdot \dot{V}}{P_{osm}} = \frac{300 \text{ mosmole/liter} \times 2 \text{ liters/day}}{300 \text{ mosmole/liter}}$$

$$= 2 \text{ liters/day} = \dot{V}$$

Therefore, Equation 37–7 tells us that the free-water clearance must be zero.

DILUTE URINE. If the urine is more dilute than plasma ($\dot{V} > C_{osm}$), the difference between $\dot{V}$ and C_{osm} is the **"positive" free-water clearance**. When the kidney *maximally dilutes* the urine to 30 mOsm, the total urine flow ($\dot{V}$) must be 20 liters/day (see Equation 37–3):

Equation 37–9

$$C_{H_2O} = \qquad \dot{V} \qquad - \qquad C_{osm}$$

Maximal dilution: $C_{H_2O} = 20 \text{ liters/day} - 2 \text{ liters/day}$

$$= 18 \text{ liters/day}$$

CONCENTRATED URINE. If the urine is more concentrated than plasma ($\dot{V} < C_{osm}$), the difference between $\dot{V}$ and C_{osm} is a negative number, the **"negative" free-water clearance**. When the kidney *maximally concentrates* the urine to 1200 mOsm, the total urine flow must be 0.5 liter/day (see Equation 37–4):

Equation 37–10

$$C_{H_2O} = \qquad \dot{V} \qquad - \qquad C_{osm}$$

Maximal
concentration: $C_{H_2O} = \quad 0.5 \text{ liter/day} \quad - 2 \text{ liters/day}$

$$= -1.5 \text{ liters/day}$$

Thus, the kidneys can generate a free-water clearance of as much as +18 liters/day under maximally diluting conditions, or as little as −1.5 liters/day under maximally concentrating conditions. This wide range of free-water clearances represents the kidneys' attempt to stabilize the osmolality of extracellular fluid in the face of changing loads of solutes or water. From the extreme free-water clearances that the kidneys can achieve, we can conclude that the organism is better able to withstand a challenge of an excessive water load than a deficit of water (dehydration).

SITES OF WATER MOVEMENT

The Kidney Generates a Concentrated Urine by Using Osmosis to Drive Water from the Tubule Lumen, Across a Water-Permeable Epithelium, into a Hypertonic Interstitium

The kidney generates a *dilute* urine by pumping salts out of the lumen of tubule segments that are impermeable to water. What is left behind is a tubule fluid that is hypoosmotic (dilute) with respect to the blood.

How does the kidney generate a *concentrated* urine? One approach might be to actively pump water out of the tubule lumen. However, water pumps do not exist (p. 72). Instead, the kidney uses osmosis as the driving force to concentrate the contents of the tubule lumen.

The kidney generates the osmotic gradient by creating a hypertonic interstitial fluid in a confined compartment, the renal medulla. The final step for making a hyperosmotic urine is to thread a water-permeable tube—the medullary collecting duct—through this hyperosmolar compartment. The result is that the fluid in the tubule lumen can equilibrate with the hypertonic interstitium, thus generating a concentrated urine.

Although net absorption of H_2O occurs all along the nephron, not all segments alter the osmolality of the tubule fluid. The proximal tubule, *regardless of the final osmolality of the urine*, reabsorbs two thirds of the filtered fluid isosmotically (i.e., the fluid reabsorbed has the same osmolality as plasma). The loop of Henle reabsorbs salt in excess of water, so that the fluid entering the distal convoluted tubule (DCT) is hypoosmotic. *Whether the final urine is dilute or concentrated* depends on whether water reabsorption occurs in more distal segments: the initial and cortical collecting tubules (ICT and CCT) and the outer and inner medullary collecting ducts (OMCD and IMCD). **Arginine vasopressin** (AVP)—also called antidiuretic hormone (ADH)—regulates the variable fraction of water reabsorption in these four nephron segments.

Tubule Fluid Is Isosmotic in the Proximal Tubule, Becomes Dilute in the Loop of Henle, and Then Either Remains Dilute or Becomes Concentrated by the End of the Collecting Duct

Figure 37–1 shows two examples of how tubule-fluid osmolality (expressed as the ratio TF_{Osm}/P_{Osm}) changes along the nephron. The first is a case of water restriction, in which the kidneys maximally concentrate the urine and excrete a minimal volume of water (**antidiuresis**). The second is a case of ingestion of excess water, in which the kidneys produce a large volume of dilute urine (**water diuresis**). In both cases, the tubule fluid does not change in osmolality along the proximal tubule, and becomes hypotonic to plasma by the end of the thick ascending limb of the loop of Henle (TAL), also known as the "diluting segment" (p. 778). Therefore, the fluid entering the DCT is hypoosmotic with respect to plasma, regardless of the final urine osmolality.

Under conditions of restricted water intake or **hydropenia**, elevated levels of AVP increase the water permeability of the nephron from the ICT to the end of the IMCD. As a result, the osmolality of the tubule fluid increases along the ICT (see Fig. 37–1, *red curve*), achieving the osmolality of the cortical interstitium—which is the same as the osmolality of plasma (~290 mOsm)—by the end of this nephron segment. No additional increase in osmolality occurs along the CCT, because the tubule fluid is already in osmotic equilibrium with the surrounding cortical interstitium. However, in the medullary collecting ducts, the luminal osmolality rises sharply as the tubule fluid equilibrates with the surrounding medullary interstitium, which becomes increasingly more hyperosmotic from the corticomedullary junction to the papillary tip. Eventually the tubule fluid reaches osmolalities that are as much as four times higher than the plasma. Thus,

FIGURE 37–1. Relative osmolality of the tubule fluid along the nephron. Plotted on the y-axis is the ratio of the osmolality of the tubule fluid (TF) to the osmolality of the plasma (P); plotted on the x-axis is a representation of distance along the nephron. The *red* record is the profile of relative osmolality (i.e., TF/P$_{osmolality}$) for water restriction, whereas the *blue* record is the profile for high water intake. (Data from Gottschalk CW: Micropuncture studies of tubular function in the mammalian kidney. Physiologist 4:33–55, 1961.)

the medullary collecting ducts are responsible for concentrating the final urine.

In summary, the two key elements in producing a concentrated urine are the hyperosmotic medullary interstitium that provides the osmotic gradient and the AVP that raises the water permeability of the distal nephron. How the kidney generates this interstitial hyperosmolality is discussed in the next subchapter, and the role of AVP is discussed in the last subchapter.

Under conditions of **water loading**, depressed AVP levels cause the water permeability of the distal nephron to remain low. However, the continued reabsorption of NaCl along the distal nephron effectively separates salt from water, leaving a relatively hypotonic fluid behind in the tubule lumen. Thus, the tubule fluid becomes increasingly hypotonic from the distal convoluted tubule throughout the remainder of the nephron (see Fig. 37–1, *blue curve*).

GENERATING A HYPEROSMOTIC MEDULLA AND URINE

Understanding the mechanisms involved in forming a hypertonic or hypotonic urine requires knowing (1) the solute and water permeability characteristics of each tubule segment, (2) the osmotic gradient between the tubule lumen and its surrounding interstitium, (3) the transport mechanisms that generate the hyperosmotic

medullary interstitium, and (4) the "exchange" mechanisms that act among the tubules, the interstitium, and the blood vessels that sustain the hyperosmotic medullary compartment.

The Renal Medulla Is Hyperosmotic to Blood Plasma During Both Antidiuresis (Low Urine Flow) and Water Diuresis

The loop of Henle plays a key role in both the osmotic dilution and the concentration of the urine. The main function of the loop is to remove NaCl—more so than water—from the lumen and deposit this NaCl in the interstitium of the renal medulla. By separating tubule NaCl from tubule water, the loop of Henle participates *directly* in forming an osmotically dilute urine. Conversely, because the TAL deposits this NaCl into the medullary interstitium, making it hyperosmotic, the loop of Henle is *indirectly* responsible for elaborating an osmotically concentrated urine. As discussed later, urea also contributes to the hypertonicity of the medulla.

Figure 37–2A shows approximate values of osmolality in the tubule fluid and interstitium during an *antidiuresis* produced, for example, by water restriction. Figure 37–2B, however, illustrates the comparable information during a *water diuresis* produced, for example, by high water intake. In *both* conditions, interstitial osmolality progressively rises from the cortex to the tip of the medulla

A WATER RESTRICTION (ANTIDIURESIS)

B HIGH WATER INTAKE (WATER DIURESIS)

FIGURE 37–2. Nephron and interstitial osmolalities. *A*, Water restriction (antidiuresis). *B*, High water intake (water diuresis). The numbers in boxes are osmolalities (mOsm) along the lumen of the nephron and along the corticomedullary axis of the interstitium. The outflow of blood from the vasa recta is greater than the inflow, reflecting the uptake of water reabsorbed from the collecting ducts.

("corticomedullary osmolality gradient"). The difference between the two conditions is that the maximal interstitial osmolality during antidiuresis, approximately 1200 mOsm (see Fig. 37–2*A*), is more than twice that achieved during water diuresis, approximately 500 mOsm (see Fig. 37–2*B*).

Because of the NaCl pumped out of the rather water-impermeable TAL, the tubule fluid at the end of this segment is hypoosmotic to the cortical interstitium during both antidiuresis and water diuresis. However, beyond the TAL, luminal osmolalities differ considerably between antidiuresis and diuresis. In *antidiuresis*, the fluid becomes progressively more concentrated from the ICT to the end of the nephron (see Fig. 37–2*A*). In contrast, during *water diuresis*, the hypotonicity of the tubule fluid is further accentuated as the fluid passes along segments from the distal convoluted tubule to the end of the nephron segments that are relatively water impermeable and continue to pump NaCl out of the lumen (see Fig. 37–2*B*). During *antidiuresis*, the tubule fluid in the ICT, CCT, OMCD, and IMCD more or less equilibrates with the interstitium, but fails to do so during *water diuresis*. This marked difference in osmotic equilibration reflects the action of AVP, which increases water permeability in each of the previously mentioned four segments.

Although NaCl Transport Generates a Gradient of Only Approximately 200 mOsm Across Any Portion of the Ascending Limb, the "Countercurrent" System Can "Multiply" This "Single Effect" to Produce a 900-mOsm Gradient Between the Cortex and the Papilla

Developing and maintaining the hyperosmolality of the medullary interstitium depends on the net transport of NaCl across the rather water-impermeable wall of the ascending limb of the loop of Henle, from lumen to interstitium. This salt reabsorption increases the osmolality of the interstitium and decreases the osmolality of the fluid within the lumen. The limiting NaCl concentration gradient that the tubule can develop at any point along its length is only approximately 200 mOsm, and this concentration alone could not explain the ability of the kidney to raise the osmolality of the papilla to 1200 mOsm. The kidney can achieve such high solute levels only because the hairpin loops of Henle create a countercurrent flow mechanism that multiplies the "single" *transverse* gradient of 200 mOsm. The result is an osmotic gradient of 900 mOsm along both the axis of the lumen of the ascending limb and the corticomedullary axis of the interstitium. In addition to the hairpin shape of the loop of Henle, osmotic multiplication also depends on a distinct pattern of salt and water permeabilities along the loop of Henle.

Figure 37–3 illustrates a simplified, schematized model of a **countercurrent-multiplier** system. The kidney in this example establishes a longitudinal osmotic gradient of 300 mOsm from cortex (300 mOsm) to papilla (600 mOsm) by iterating (i.e., "multiplying") a "single effect" that is capable of generating a transepithelial osmotic gradient of only 200 mOsm. Of course, if we had used more

cycles, we could have generated a corticomedullary gradient that was even greater. For example, after 39 cycles in our example, the interstitial osmolality at the tip of the loop of Henle would be approximately 1200. Therefore, the countercurrent arrangement of the loop of Henle magnifies the osmotic work that a single ascending-limb cell can perform. Among mammals, the length of the loop of Henle—compared with the thickness of the renal cortex—determines the maximal osmolality of the medulla.

In the *last panel* of Figure 37–3, we include the collecting duct in the model to show the final event of urine concentration: allowing the fluid in the collecting duct to osmotically equilibrate with the hyperosmotic interstitium produces a concentrated urine.

The "Single Effect" Is the Result of Passive NaCl Reabsorption in the Thin and Active NaCl Reabsorption in the Thick Ascending Limb

So far, we have treated the "ascending limb" as a functionally uniform epithelium that is capable of generating a 200-mOsm gradient between lumen and interstitium, across a relatively water-impermeable barrier. However, the bottom of the ascending limb is "thin" (tALH), whereas the top is "thick" (TAL). Both the tALH and the TAL separate salt from water, but transport the NaCl by very different mechanisms. The **thick ascending limb** moves NaCl from lumen out to interstitium using a combination of transcellular and paracellular pathways (see Fig. 34–4*B*). For the transcellular pathway, the TAL cell takes up Na^+ and Cl^- via an apical Na/K/Cl cotransporter and exports these ions to the blood using basolateral Na-K pumps and Cl^- channels. For the paracellular pathway, the lumen-positive transepithelial voltage drives Na^+ from lumen to blood via the tight junctions. Using these two pathways, the TAL can generate a "single effect" as large as 200 mOsm.

In contrast, the movement of Na^+ and Cl^- from the lumen to the interstitium of the **thin ascending limb of the loop of Henle** appears to be an entirely passive process. During the debate on the mechanism of NaCl reabsorption in the tALH, several investigators pointed out that it was difficult to imagine how the extraordinarily thin cells of the tALH, with their paucity of mitochondria, could perform intensive active solute transport. The prevailing view is that tALH cells produce a "single effect" because the concentration of NaCl is greater in the lumen than it is in the interstitium of the inner medulla, leading to passive NaCl reabsorption. The key question for this model is: How did the luminal [NaCl] in the tALH get so high in the first place?

The work of concentrating the NaCl in the lumen was performed earlier, when the fluid was in the thin *descending* limb (tDLH) of juxtamedullary nephrons. This tDLH has three features that allow it to concentrate luminal NaCl: (1) the tDLH has a high water permeability; (2) the tDLH has a low permeability to NaCl and—over most of its length—to urea; and (3) the interstitium of the inner medulla has a very high [NaCl] and [urea]. It is these high interstitial concentrations of NaCl and urea that pro-

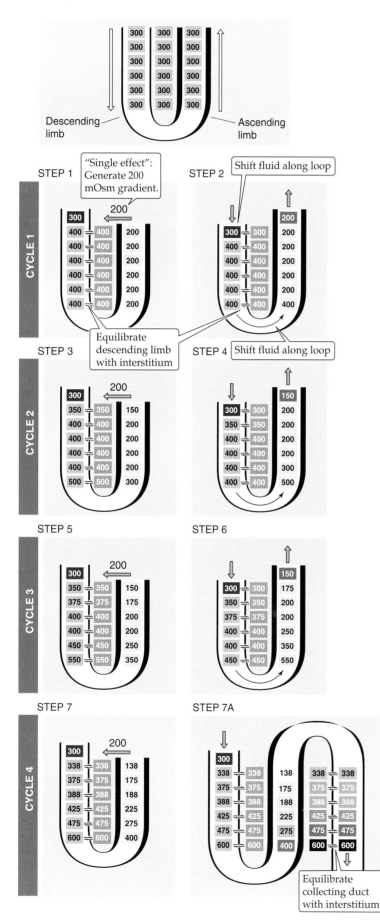

FIGURE 37–3. Stepwise generation of a high interstitial osmolality by a countercurrent multiplier. This example illustrates in a stepwise fashion how a countercurrent-multiplier system in the loop of Henle increases the osmolality of the medullary interstitium. Heavy boundaries of ascending limb and early distal convoluted tubule indicate that these nephron segments are rather impermeable to water, even in the presence of arginine vasopressin (AVP). The numbers refer to the osmolality (mOsm) of tubule fluid and interstitium. The top panel shows the starting condition (step 0), with isosmotic fluid (~300 mOsm) throughout the ascending and descending limbs and in the interstitium. Each cycle comprises two steps. Step 1 is the "single effect": NaCl transport from the lumen of the ascending limb to the interstitium, which instantaneously equilibrates with the lumen of the descending limb (steps 1, 3, 5, and 7). Step 2 is an "axial shift" of tubule fluid along loop of Henle (steps 2, 4, and 6), with an instantaneous equilibration between the lumen of the descending limb and the interstitium. Beginning with the conditions in step 0, the first single effect is NaCl absorption across the rather water-impermeable *ascending* limb. At each level, we assume that this single effect creates a 200-mOsm *difference* between the ascending limb (which is water *impermeable*) and a second compartment: the combination of the interstitium and descending limb (which is water *permeable*). Thus, the osmolality of ascending limb falls to 200 mOsm, whereas the osmolality of the interstitium and descending limb rise to 400 mOsm (step 1). The shift of new isosmotic fluid (~300 mOsm) from the proximal tubule in the cortex into the descending limb pushes the column of tubule fluid along the loop of Henle, *decreasing* osmolality at the top of the descending limb and *increasing* osmolality at the bottom of the ascending limb. Through instantaneous equilibration, the interstitium—with an assumed negligible volume—acquires the osmolality of the descending limb, thereby diluting the top of the interstitium (step 2). A second cycle starts with net NaCl transport out of the ascending limb (step 3), again generating an osmotic gradient of 200 mOsm—at each transverse level—between the ascending limb on the one hand and the interstitium and descending limb on the other. After the axial shift of tubule fluid and instantaneous equilibration of the descending limb with the interstitium (step 4), osmolality at the bottom of the ascending limb exceeds that of preceding cycle. With successive cycles, interstitial osmolality at tip of the loop of Henle rises progressively from 300 (step 0) to 400 (step 1) to 500 (step 3) to 550 (step 5) and then to 600 (step 7). Thus, in this example, the kidney establishes a longitudinal osmotic gradient of 300 mOsm from the cortex (300 mOsm) to the papilla (600 mOsm) by iterating (i.e., "multiplying") a "single effect" that is capable of generating a transepithelial osmotic gradient of only 200 mOsm. Step 7A adds the collecting duct and shows the final event of urine concentration: allowing the fluid in the collecting duct to osmotically equilibrate with the hyperosmotic interstitium, producing a concentrated urine. (Based on a model by Pitts RF: Physiology of the Kidney and Body Fluids. Chicago, Year Book, 1974.)

A   CONCENTRATION PROFILES

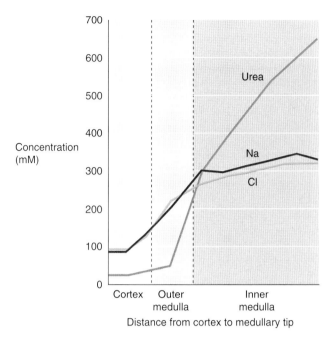

B   PASSIVE MODEL FOR "SINGLE EFFECT" IN tALH

FIGURE 37–4. Role of urea in the urine concentrating mechanism. In A, the data are from hydropenic dogs. In B, which refers to antidiuresis, the numbers in *violet boxes* refer to osmolality (in mOsm) due to NaCl in the lumen. The numbers in the *green boxes* refer to osmolality due to NaCl or urea in the interstitium. The "forbidden" icon (*red circle with slash*) indicates a lack of permeability. This simplified model assumes that the thin ascending limb is impermeable to urea. (A, data from Ullrich KJ, Kramer K, Boylan JW: Present knowledge of the counter-current system in the mammalian kidney. Progr Cardiovasc Dis 3:395–431, 1961.)

vide the osmotic energy for passively reabsorbing water, which secondarily concentrates NaCl in the lumen of the tDLH.

In the interstitium, [Na⁺], [Cl⁻], and [urea] all rise along the axis from the cortex to the papillary tip of the renal medulla (Fig. 37–4A). In the *outer* medulla, it is the rise in interstitial [Na⁺] and [Cl⁻]—owing to the pumping of NaCl out of the TAL (p. 778)—that is largely responsible for producing the hypertonicity. Although urea makes only a minor contribution in the outermost portion of the outer medulla, [urea] rises steeply from the middle of the outer medulla to the papilla. Therefore, at the tip of the papilla, interstitial [urea] is about twice the interstitial [NaCl], and urea contributes—at least in dogs—about half of the interstitial osmolality. As discussed in the next section, this characteristic [urea] profile is the result of the unique water and urea permeabilities of the collecting tubules and ducts.

Knowing that NaCl and urea contribute to the high

osmolality of the inner medullary interstitium, we can understand how the tDLH "passively" elevates [NaCl] in the lumen above that in the interstitium. We illustrate this effect with a simplified model (see Fig. 37–4B) in which urea is absent from the outer medulla. As luminal fluid in the tDLH crosses the border between outer and inner medulla, luminal [Na⁺] + [Cl⁻] produces an osmolality of 600 mOsm, the same as the osmolality of the interstitial [Na⁺] + [Cl⁻]. As the luminal fluid descends more deeply into the medulla, interstitial osmolality becomes progressively higher, and the luminal fluid still osmotically equilibrates with the interstitium. However, here two solutes—NaCl and urea—contribute to the interstitial osmolality. For example, when the interstitial osmolality is 900 mOsm, 600 represents [Na⁺] + [Cl⁻], and 300 represents [urea]. At this level, the exit of water from the lumen of the tDLH will continue until luminal osmolality rises to 900 mOsm—almost all contributed by the Na⁺ and Cl⁻ that was previously in the proximal tubule. The result is osmotic equilibrium, but a decided *disequilibrium* with respect to the concentrations of Na^+, Cl^-, and urea. Thus, luminal $[Na^+] + [Cl^-]$ increases along the tDLH, just as [urea] increases in the interstitium. At the tip of the loop in our example, interstitial osmolality is 1200 mOsm, 600 from $[Na^+] + [Cl^-]$ and 600 from [urea]. Again, osmotic equilibration between interstitium and lumen raises luminal osmolality to 1200 mOsm—almost all of which represents $[Na^+] + [Cl^-]$. Therefore, by the time we reach the hairpin of the loop of Henle, 600 mM of urea in the interstitium balances 600 mM of the 1200 mM of $[Na^+] + [Cl^-]$ in the lumen.

As the luminal fluid turns the corner and moves up the tALH, it encounters a very different epithelium, one that is now impermeable to water but permeable to NaCl. Therefore, at the level where the interstitial osmolality is 1200 mOsm and the interstitial $[Na^+] + [Cl^-]$ is 600 mM, the luminal $[Na^+] + [Cl^-]$ of 1200 mM provides a substantial gradient driving the passive reabsorption of Na^+ and Cl^-. Similarly, at the level where interstitial osmolality is 900 mOsm and interstitial $[Na^+] + [Cl^-]$ is 600 mM, the luminal $[Na^+] + [Cl^-]$ of 900 mM still drives passive NaCl reabsorption. Thus, the energy for "passive" NaCl reabsorption across the wall of the tALH ultimately comes from the presence in the interstitium of a high concentration of a solute other than NaCl, namely, urea. We discuss the generation of this urea gradient in the next section. Even though the mechanism of the "single effect" is different in the tALH and the TAL, the result is the same: At any level, osmolality in the lumen of the ascending limb is lower than it is in the interstitium.

Although the "passive model" described earlier explains almost all of the experimental data, the issue of how the kidney produces a "single effect" in the inner medulla is not entirely settled. Some investigators suggest that other structures in the inner medulla (i.e., tDLH, IMCD) produce a single effect, that solutes other than urea are involved, that solute transport by the tALH is more complex than has been envisaged, or that mechanisms may differ among species.

The Inner Medullary Collecting Duct Reabsorbs Urea, Producing High Levels of Urea in the Interstitium of the Inner Medulla

As just discussed, urea appears to play a pivotal role in the "single effect" of NaCl transport by the *thin* ascending limb. Because urea comes from protein breakdown, urea delivery to the kidney, and, therefore, the contribution of urea to the medullary hyperosmolality, is larger with protein-rich diets. Indeed, investigators have long known that the higher the dietary protein content, the greater the concentrating ability.

UREA HANDLING. The renal handling of urea is complex (p. 790). The kidney filters urea in the glomerulus and reabsorbs about half in the proximal tubule. In juxtamedullary nephrons, the tALH as well as the deepest portion of the tDLH secretes urea into the tubule lumen. Finally, the inner medullary collecting duct reabsorbs urea. The net effect is that the kidney excretes less urea into the urine than it filters. Depending on urine flow (see Fig.

35–2), the fractional excretion may be as low as 15% (minimal urine flow) or as high as 60% or more (maximal urine flow). Because we are interested in understanding the role of urea in establishing a hypertonic medullary interstitium, in Figure 37–5 we will consider an example in which maximal AVP produces minimal urine flow (i.e., antidiuresis).

As the tubule fluid enters the TAL, the [urea] is several-fold higher than it is in the plasma because about 100% of the filtered load of urea remains, even though earlier nephron segments have reabsorbed water. All nephron segments from TAL to the OMCD, inclusive, have low permeabilities to urea. In the presence of AVP, however, all segments from the ICT to the end of the nephron have high water permeabilities and continuously reabsorb fluid. As a result, luminal [urea] gradually rises, beginning at the ICT and reaching a concentration as much as eightfold to 10-fold higher than that in blood plasma by the time the tubule fluid reaches the end of the OMCD.

The **inner medullary collecting duct** differs in an important way from the three upstream segments: Although AVP increases *only water permeability* in the ICT, CCT, and OMCD, AVP increases water *and urea permeability* in the IMCD. In the IMCD, the high luminal [urea] and the high urea permeabilities of the apical membrane (via the urea transporter UT1) and basolateral membrane (via UT4) promote the outward facilitated diffusion of urea from the IMCD lumen, through the IMCD cells, and into the medullary interstitium. As a result, urea accumulates in the interstitium and contributes about half of the total osmolality in the deepest portion of the inner medulla.

Because of the accumulation of urea in the inner medullary interstitium, [urea] is higher in the interstitium than it is in the lumen of the **thin ascending limb** of juxtamedullary (i.e., long-loop) nephrons. This concentration gradient drives urea into the tALH, probably via an as-yet unidentified transporter. In addition, urea also moves into the deepest portion of the tDLH, probably mediated by UT2. In contrast to the thin *ascending* limb of juxtamedullary nephrons, the main portion of the thin *descending* limb is poorly permeable to urea, as it must be for [NaCl] to rise along the tDLH in the inner medulla as it approaches the hairpin turn of the loop of Henle (see Fig. 37–4*B*). The secretion of urea into the tALH accounts for two important observations: First, more urea (i.e., a greater fraction of the filtered load) emerges from the tALH than entered the tDLH. Second, as noted earlier, [urea] in the TAL is considerably higher than that in blood plasma.

UREA RECYCLING. The processes that we have just described—(1) absorption of urea from IMCD into the interstitium, (2) secretion of urea from interstitium into the tALH, and (3) carriage of urea up into the cortex and back down via nephron segments from the tALH to the IMCD—are the three elements of a closed loop. According to the "passive model," this **urea recycling** is responsible for the buildup of a high [urea] in the inner medulla. A small fraction of the urea that the IMCD deposits in the interstitium moves into the vasa recta, which removes it from the medulla and returns it either to superficial nephrons or to the general circulation.

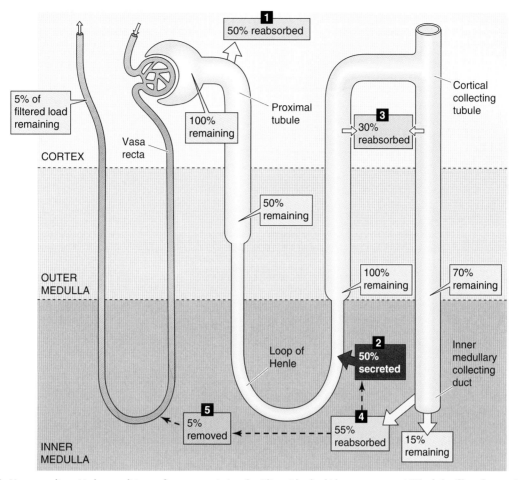

FIGURE 37–5. Urea recycling. Under conditions of water restriction (antidiuresis), the kidneys excrete ~15% of the filtered urea. The numbered *yellow boxes* indicate the fraction of the filtered load that various nephron segments *reabsorb*. The single *red box* indicates the fraction of the filtered load *secreted* by the thin ascending limb and the single *brown box* indicates the fraction of the filtered load *carried away* by the vasa recta. The *green boxes* indicate the fraction of the filtered load that remains in the lumen after these segments.

ENERGY SOURCE FOR UREA ACCUMULATION. Because urea moves from the IMCD to the interstitium by facilitated diffusion, one might ask where the energy comes from that concentrates the urea in the medullary interstitium. Working our way backwards, we see that the driving force for urea to enter the interstitium was the high [urea] in the IMCD lumen, which was the consequence of preferentially removing water—in the presence of AVP—from tubule segments between the ICT and the OMCD. In turn, this water removal depended on active NaCl reabsorption from the ICT to the OMCD. Thus, the work of actively reabsorbing NaCl in the cortex and outer medulla translates to a different sort of work (i.e., osmotic work of concentrating urea) in a different part of the kidney (i.e., interstitium of inner medulla).

The preceding discussion focused on the situation in *antidiuresis*, in which AVP levels are high and the kidney concentrates urea in the inner medulla. The converse situation pertains in *water diuresis*, when circulating levels of AVP are low. The kidney reabsorbs *less* water along the ICT, CCT, OMCD, and IMCD. Furthermore, with low AVP levels, the IMCD has a *lower* permeability to both urea and water. Therefore, during water diuresis, the interstitial [urea] is lower, and more urea appears in the urine.

The Vasa Recta's Countercurrent-Exchange Mechanism and Relatively Low Blood Flow Minimize the Washout of the Medullary Hypertonicity

The simplified scheme for the countercurrent multiplier presented in Figure 37–3 did not include blood vessels. If we were simply to introduce a straight, permeable blood vessel running from papilla to cortex, or vice versa, the blood flow would soon wash away the papillary hypertonicity that is critical for concentrating urine. Figure 37–6A shows a hypothetical, poorly designed kidney with only *descending* vasa recta. Here, blood would flow from cortex to papilla and then exit the kidney. Because the blood vessel wall is permeable to small solutes and water, the osmolality of the blood would gradually increase from 300 to 1200 mOsm during transit from cortex to papilla, reflecting a loss of water or a gain of solutes. Because these movements occur at the expense of the medullary interstitium, the interstitium's hyperosmolality would be washed out into the blood. The greater the blood flow through this straight/unlooped blood vessel, the greater the medullary washout.

The kidney solves the medullary-washout problem in two ways. First, compared with the blood flow in the

A HYPOTHETICAL STRAIGHT-TUBE EXCHANGER **B** HYPOTHETICAL COUNTERCURRENT EXCHANGER

FIGURE 37–6. Countercurrent exchange. *A*, If blood simply flows from the cortex to the medulla through a straight tube, then the blood exiting the medulla will have a high osmolality (750 mOsm), washing out the osmolality gradient of the medullary interstitium. The numbers in the *yellow boxes* indicate the osmolality (in mOsm) inside the vasa recta, and the numbers in *green boxes* indicate the osmolality of the interstitial fluid. *B*, If blood flows into and out of the medulla through a hairpin loop, then the water will leave the vessel and solute will enter along the entire descending vessel and part of the ascending vessel. Along the rest of the ascending vessel, the fluxes of water and solute are reversed. The net effect is that the blood exiting the medulla is less hypertonic than that in *A* (450 vs. 750 mOsm), so that the kidney better preserves the osmotic gradient in the medulla. (Data from a model by Pitts RF: Physiology of the Kidney and Body Fluids. Chicago, Year Book, 1974.)

renal cortex, which is one of the highest (per gram of tissue) of any tissue in the body, the blood flow through the medulla is relatively low, corresponding to no more than 5% to 10% of total renal plasma flow. This low flow represents a compromise between the need to deliver nutrients to the medulla and the need to avoid washout of medullary hypertonicity.

Second, and far more significant, the kidney uses a hairpin configuration, with the descending and ascending vasa recta both entering and leaving through the same region, thus creating an efficient **countercurrent-exchange mechanism** (see Fig. 37–6*B*) in the blood vessels. The vasa recta have a hairpin configuration, but no capacity for active transport. We start with the osmotic stratification in the medullary interstitium that the countercurrent multiplier generated in the presence of high AVP levels. This osmotic stratification is due in part to a gradient of [Na$^+$] + [Cl$^-$], but also to a similarly directed cortex-to-papilla gradient of [urea] (see Fig. 37–4*A*). As isosmotic blood enters the hyperosmotic milieu of the medulla, which has high concentrations of NaCl and urea, NaCl and urea diffuse into the lumen of the descending vasa recta, whereas water moves in the opposite direction. This entry of urea into the descending vasa recta occurs via facilitated diffusion, mediated by the UT3 urea transporter (p. 792). The result is that the osmolality of the blood increases as the blood approaches the tip of the hairpin loop. As the blood rounds the curve and heads up toward the cortex inside the ascending vasa

recta, that blood will eventually have a higher solute concentration than the surrounding interstitium. As a consequence, NaCl and urea now diffuse from the lumen of the vasa recta into the interstitium, while water moves into the ascending vasa recta.

Viewed as a whole, these passive exchange processes cause the descending vasa recta to gain solute and lose water, but cause the ascending vessels to lose solute and gain water. Thus, at any level, the descending and ascending vessels exchange solutes and water via—and at the expense of—the medullary interstitium. Solute recirculates from the ascending vessel, through the interstitium, to the descending vessel. Conversely, the countercurrent-exchange mechanism also "short-circuits" the water, but in the opposite direction, from the descending vessel, through the interstitium, to the ascending vessel. The net effect is that the countercurrent exchanger tends to trap solutes in the medulla and minimize the dissipation of the corticomedullary osmolality gradient.

The total mass of solute and water leaving the medulla each minute via the *ascending* vasa recta must exceed the total inflow of solute and water into the medulla via the *descending* vasa recta. With regard to *solute balance*, the renal tubules continuously deposit NaCl and urea in the medullary interstitium. Thus, in the steady state, the vasa recta must remove these solutes lest they form crystals of NaCl and urea in the medullary interstitium. Almost all the urea in the interstitium of the inner medulla comes from the IMCD, and in the steady state most of this leaves the interstitium by way of the tALH (see Fig. 37–5, *red box*). The blood of the vasa recta carries away the balance or "excess" urea (see Fig. 37–5, *brown box*). The blood must also carry off the excess NaCl that enters the interstitium from the ascending limb of the loop of Henle and, to some extent, from the medullary collecting ducts.

With regard to *water balance* within the medulla, the descending limb of the loop of Henle and—in the presence of AVP—the medullary collecting duct continuously give up water to the medullary interstitium as the tubule fluid becomes more concentrated. Therefore, in the steady state, the ascending vasa recta must also remove excess water from the medulla.

The net effect of managing both solute and water balance in the medulla is that the ascending vasa recta carry out more salt and more water than the descending vasa recta carry in. Although there have been no precise measurements, it is likely that the osmolality of blood leaving the ascending vasa recta exceeds that of the blood entering the descending vessels by a fairly small amount, perhaps 10 to 30 mOsm.

The Medullary Collecting Duct Produces a Concentrated Urine by Osmosis, Driven by the [NaCl] Gradient Between the Medullary Interstitium and the Lumen

In contrast to the loop of Henle, which acts as a *counter-current multiplier*, and the loop-shaped vasa recta, which act as a *counter*current exchanger, the medullary collecting duct is an unlooped or straight-tube exchanger. The wall of the medullary collecting duct has three important permeability properties: (1) in the absence of AVP, it is relatively impermeable to water, urea, and NaCl along its entire length; (2) AVP increases its water permeability along its entire length; and (3) AVP increases its urea permeability along just the terminal portion of the tube (IMCD). The collecting duct traverses a medullary interstitium that has a stratified, ever-increasing osmolality from the cortex to the tip of the papilla. Thus, along the entire length of the tubule, an osmotic gradient across the collecting-duct epithelium favors the reabsorption of water from lumen to interstitium.

A complicating factor is that two solutes—NaCl and water—contribute to the osmotic gradient across the tubule wall. As fluid in the collecting-duct lumen moves from the cortico-medullary junction to the papillary tip, the [NaCl] gradient across the tubule wall always favors the osmotic reabsorption of water (Fig. 37–7). For urea, the situation is just the opposite. However, because the ICT, CCT, and OMCD are all relatively impermeable to urea, water reabsorption predominates in the presence of AVP and gradually causes luminal [urea] to increase in these segments. Because the interstitial [urea] is low in the cortex, a rising luminal [urea] in the ICT and CCT *opposes* water reabsorption in these segments. Even when the tubule crosses the cortico-medullary junction, courses toward the papilla, and is surrounded by interstitial fluid with an ever-increasing [urea], the transepithelial urea gradient still favors water movement into the lumen.

Thus, the presence of urea per se in the lumen of the collecting tubules and ducts is actually a handicap for the osmotic concentration of the urine, because the luminal urea tends to pull water back into the tubule lumen. Fortunately, the IMCD partially compensates for this problem by having a relatively low reflection coefficient for urea (σ_{urea}), thus converting any transepithelial difference in urea concentration into a smaller difference in effective osmotic pressure (p. 470). The σ for urea is 0.74, whereas that for NaCl is 1.0. Thus, water reabsorption continues in the inner medullary collecting duct even though [urea] in tubule fluid exceeds that in the interstitium. The combination of a high interstitial [NaCl] and high σ_{NaCl} promotes NaCl-driven water *absorption*. A low σ_{urea} minimizes urea-driven water *secretion*.

The kidney also compensates for having a high [urea] in the lumen of the medullary collecting ducts by having a high interstitial [urea], which—to some extent—osmotically balances the urea in the lumen of the papillary collecting ducts. Were it not for urea accumulation in the medullary interstitium, interstitial [NaCl] would have to be much higher, which in turn would require increased NaCl transport in the TAL.

If luminal urea opposes the formation of a concentrated urine, why did the mammalian kidney evolve to have high levels of urea in the lumen of the collecting tubules and ducts? There are at least two reasons. First, because urea is the body's major excretable nitrogenous waste, the kidney's ability to achieve a high urinary [urea] reduces the necessity to excrete large volumes of water for excreting nitrogenous waste. Second, as we have already seen, the kidney actually takes advantage of urea to generate a maximally concentrated urine. Thus, in the presence of AVP, the permeability of the IMCD to urea is high, so that large amounts of urea can enter the medullary interstitium. The high interstitial [urea] energizes the increase in luminal [NaCl] in the tDLH, which in turn fuels the "single effect" in the tALH, thus creating the high inner-medullary [NaCl] that is *directly* responsible for concentrating the urine.

As discussed, the composition of the inner medullary interstitium determines the composition of the final urine. However, to some extent, the composition of the final urine, as well as the rate of urine flow, also influences the composition of the interstitium. Figure 37–2 shows that the medullary interstitial osmolality is much lower, and the stratification of osmolality from cortex to papillary tip is much less, during water diuresis than during antidiuresis. Two factors contribute to the lesser degree of osmotic stratification under conditions of water diuresis, when levels of AVP are low. First, less urea moves from the IMCD lumen to the interstitium, both because of the low urea permeability of the IMCD and because of the low water permeability of the upstream segments that would otherwise concentrate urea. Second, the medullary collecting ducts reabsorb some water despite the low AVP levels, and this water dilutes the medullary interstitium. The reasons for this apparent paradox are: (1) even when AVP is low, the water permeability is not zero; (2) the ICT and CCT present a much larger fluid volume to the medullary collecting duct, because they reabsorb less water when AVP levels are low; and (3) the tubule fluid is

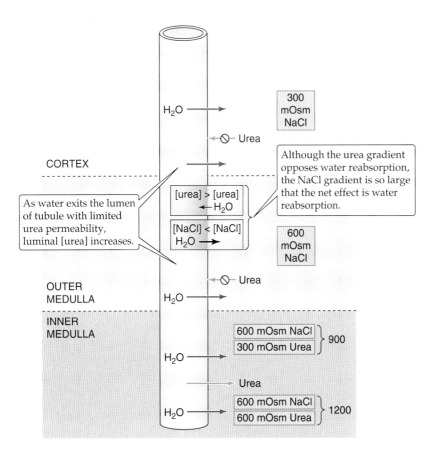

As water exits the lumen of tubule with limited urea permeability, luminal [urea] increases.

Although the urea gradient opposes water reabsorption, the NaCl gradient is so large that the net effect is water reabsorption.

FIGURE 37–7. Opposing effects of NaCl and urea gradients on urine concentrating ability during antidiuresis. The numbers in the *green boxes* indicate the osmolalities (in mOsm) of the interstitial fluid.

more hypotonic, so that there is a larger osmotic gradient for transepithelial water movement. With low AVP levels, this larger osmotic gradient overrides the effect of the lower water permeability.

Table 37–2 summarizes factors that modulate urinary concentration ability.

REGULATION BY ARGININE VASOPRESSIN

Large-bodied neurons in the paraventricular and supraoptic nuclei of the hypothalamus synthesize arginine vasopressin, a nonapeptide also known as antidiuretic hormone. These neurons package the AVP and transport it along their axons to the posterior pituitary, where they release AVP through a breech in the blood-brain barrier into the systemic circulation (p. 871). In Chapter 39, we discuss how increased plasma osmolality and decreased effective circulating volume increase AVP release. AVP has synergistic effects on two target organs. First, at rather high circulating levels, such as those seen in hypovolemic shock, AVP acts on vascular smooth muscle to cause *vasoconstriction* (p. 555) and thus increase blood pressure. Second, and more importantly, AVP acts on the kidney, where it is the major regulator of water excretion. AVP increases water reabsorption by enhancing the water permeabilities of the collecting tubules and ducts, and also by stimulating urea transport across the cells of the inner medullary collecting duct.

Arginine Vasopressin Increases Water Permeability in All Nephron Segments Beyond the Distal Convoluted Tubule

Of the water remaining in the distal convoluted tubule, the kidney reabsorbs a variable fraction in the segments from the initial collecting tubule to the end of the nephron. Absorption of this final fraction of water is under the control of circulating AVP. In the kidney, AVP (1) increases water permeability in all the segments beyond the DCT, (2) increases urea permeability in the IMCD, and (3) increases active NaCl reabsorption in the thick ascending limb.

Figure 37–8 summarizes the water permeability of various nephron segments. The water permeability is highest in the proximal tubule and thin descending limb of the loop of Henle. The high water permeability in these segments reflects the abundant presence of **aquaporin 1** (AQP1) water channels (p. 58) in the apical and basolateral cell membranes.

In marked contrast to the proximal tubule and tDLH, the following few segments—from the thin ascending limb to the connecting tubule—have very low water permeabilities. In the absence of AVP, the next tubule segments, the ICT and CCT, have rather low water permeabilities, whereas the medullary collecting ducts are virtually impermeable to water. However, AVP dramatically increases the water permeabilities of the collecting tubules (ICT and CCT) and ducts (OMCD and IMCD) by causing AQP2 water channels to insert into the apical

TABLE 37–2

FACTORS THAT MODULATE URINARY CONCENTRATION AND DILUTION

1) **Osmotic gradient of medullary interstitium from cortico-medullary junction to papilla:**
   a) **Length of loops of Henle:** Species with long loops (e.g., desert rodents) concentrate more than those with short loops (e.g., beaver).
   b) **Rate of active NaCl reabsorption in the TAL:** Increased luminal Na^+ delivery to TAL (high GFR or filtration fraction, and low proximal-tubule Na^+ reabsorption) enhances NaCl reabsorption, whereas low Na^+ delivery (low GFR, increased proximal Na^+ and fluid reabsorption) reduces concentrating ability. High Na-K pump turnover enhances NaCl reabsorption, whereas inhibiting transport (e.g., loop diuretics) reduces concentrating ability.

2) **Protein content of diet:** High protein diet, up to a point, promotes urea accumulation in the inner medullary interstitium, and increased concentrating ability.

3) **Medullary blood flow:** Low blood flow promotes high interstitial osmolality. High blood flow washes out medullary solutes.

4) **Osmotic permeability of the collecting tubules and ducts to water:** AVP enhances water permeability and thus water reabsorption.

5) **Luminal flow in the loop of Henle and the collecting duct:** High flow (osmotic diuresis) diminishes the efficiency of the countercurrent multiplier, and thus reduces the osmolality of the medullary interstitium. In the medullary collecting duct, high flow reduces the time available for equilibration of water and urea.

6) **Pathophysiology:** Central or nephrogenic diabetes insipidus either reduces plasma AVP levels or renal responsiveness to AVP (see box titled "Diabetes Insipidus").

membrane (see later). A third type of water channel, AQP3, is present in the basolateral cell membranes of medullary collecting ducts. Like AQP1, AQP3 is *insensitive* to AVP.

Given the favorable osmotic gradients discussed in the preceding subchapter, high levels of AVP cause substantial water reabsorption to occur in AVP-sensitive nephron segments. In contrast, when circulating levels of AVP are low, for instance after ingestion of large amounts of water, the water permeability of these nephron segments remains low. Therefore, the fluid leaving the DCT remains hypotonic as it flows down more distal nephron segments. In fact, in the absence of AVP, continued NaCl

absorption makes the tubule fluid even more hypotonic, resulting in a large volume of dilute urine (see Fig. 37–1).

Arginine Vasopressin, Acting Through Cyclic Adenosine Monophosphate, Causes Vesicles Containing Aquaporin 2 Water Channels to Fuse with the Apical Membrane of Principal Cells of the Collecting Tubules and Ducts

AVP binds to V_2 receptors in the basolateral membrane of the principal cells from the ICT to the end of the nephron (Fig. 37–9). Receptor binding activates the G_s hetero-

FIGURE 37–8. Water permeability in different nephron segments. Note that the x-axis scale is logarithmic. AVP, arginine vasopressin. (From Knepper MA, Rector FC: Urine concentration and dilution. In Brenner BM [ed]: The Kidney. Philadelphia, WB Saunders, 1996, pp 532–570.)

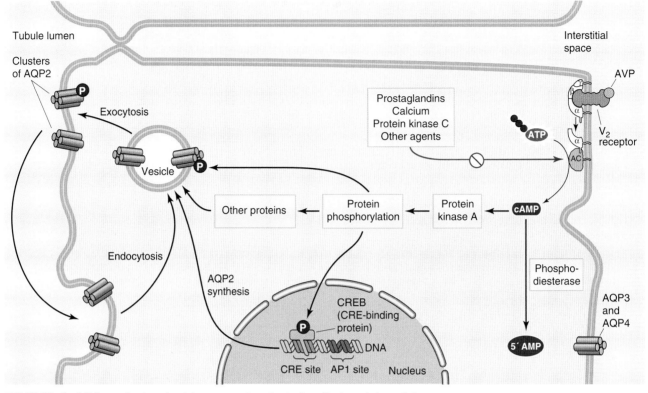

FIGURE 37–9. Cellular mechanism of arginine vasopressin action in the collecting tubules and ducts.

trimeric G protein, stimulating adenylyl cyclase to generate cyclic adenosine monophosphate (cAMP) (p. 97). The latter activates protein kinase A, which phosphorylates unknown proteins that play a role in the trafficking of intracellular vesicles containing AQP2 and the fusion of these vesicles with the apical membrane. These water channels are "AVP-sensitive," not in the sense that AVP modulates their single-channel water conductance, but rather their *density* in the apical membrane. In conditions of low AVP, AQP2 water channels are mainly in the membrane of intracellular vesicles just beneath the apical membrane. In the membrane of these vesicles, the AQP2 water channels are present as **aggregophores**—aggregates of AQP2 proteins. Under the influence of AVP, the vesicles containing AQP2 move to the apical membrane of principal cells of the collecting tubules and ducts. By exocytosis (p. 36), these vesicles fuse with the apical membrane, thus increasing the density of AQP2. When AVP levels in the blood decline, endocytosis retrieves the water channel–containing aggregates from the apical membrane and shuttles them back to the cytoplasmic vesicle pool.

The apical water permeability of principal cells depends not only on AVP levels, but on a number of other factors. For example, high $[Ca^{2+}]_i$ and high $[Li^+]$ both inhibit adenylyl cyclase, thus decreasing $[cAMP]_i$, reducing water permeability, and producing a diuresis. A similar inhibition of AQP2 insertion, and thus a decrease in water permeability, occurs when agents such as colchicine disrupt the integrity of the cytoskeleton. Conversely, inhibitors of phosphodiesterase (e.g., theophylline), which in-

crease $[cAMP]_i$, tend to increase the osmotic water permeability.

Arginine Vasopressin Enhances the Urinary-Concentrating Mechanism by Stimulating the Urea Transporter UT1 in the Inner Medullary Collecting Ducts, Thus Increasing Urea Reabsorption

AVP promotes water reabsorption not only by increasing the water permeability of the collecting tubules and ducts, but also by enhancing the osmotic gradients across the walls of the inner and perhaps the outer medullary collecting duct.

In the *outer* medulla, AVP acts through the cAMP pathway to increase NaCl reabsorption by the TAL. AVP acts by stimulating apical Na/K/Cl cotransport and K^+ recycling across the apical membrane (p. 787). The net effect is to increase the osmolality of the outer medullary interstitium, and thus enhance the osmotic gradient favoring water reabsorption by the OMCD. In addition, AVP stimulates the growth of TAL cells in animals that are genetically devoid of AVP. This hormone also stimulates Na^+ reabsorption in the CCT, largely by activating apical Na^+ channels (ENaC). These observations on the TAL and CCT were all made on rodents. In humans these TAL and CCT mechanisms may have only minor significance.

In the *inner* medulla, AVP enhances the urea permeability of the terminal two thirds of the inner medullary collect duct (p. 836). The AVP-dependent increase in

DIABETES INSIPIDUS

Diabetes insipidus (DI) is a fairly rare disorder that occurs in two varieties: (1) Neurogenic or *central* **diabetes insipidus** is caused by failure of AVP secretion. The lesion can be either at the level of the hypothalamus (where neurons synthesize AVP) or the pituitary gland (where neurons release AVP). Central DI can be idiopathic, familial, or caused by any disorder of the hypothalamus or pituitary, such as injury, a tumor, infection, or autoimmune processes. (2) In *nephrogenic* **diabetes insipidus**, the kidneys respond inadequately to normal or even elevated levels of circulating AVP. Nephrogenic DI can also be idiopathic or familial and may be associated with electrolyte abnormalities (e.g., states of K^+ depletion or high plasma $[Ca^{2+}]$), the renal disease associated with sickle cell anemia, and various drugs (notably Li^+ and colchicine).

In both central and nephrogenic DI, patients present with polyuria and polydipsia. If allowed to progress unchecked, the disorder can result in marked hypernatremia, hypotension, and shock. Often the physician first suspects the diagnosis when the patient is deprived of access to water or other fluids. The patient may then quickly become dehydrated and a random determination of plasma $[Na^+]$ may yield a very high value.

The physician can confirm the diagnosis of DI most easily by a fluid-deprivation test. The patient will continue to produce a large output of dilute urine, despite the need to conserve fluids. If the patient has *central* DI, administering a subcutaneous dose of AVP will rapidly increase urine osmolality by more than 50%. In patients with *nephrogenic* DI, on the other hand, the increase in

urine osmolality will be less. Simultaneous measurements of plasma AVP levels may confirm the diagnosis.

The treatment for central DI is desmopressin acetate (DDAVP) (see Fig. 55–8), a synthetic AVP analog that patients can take intranasally. Nephrogenic DI, in which the kidneys are resistant to the effects of the hormone, will not respond to DDAVP. In these patients, it is best to treat the underlying disease and also to reduce the elevated plasma $[Na^+]$ by administering a diuretic (to produce a natriuresis) and by restricting dietary Na^+.

The high urine flow in DI is associated with low rates of solute excretion. Therefore, the physician must distinguish DI from states of **polyuria** accompanied by high rates of solute excretion in the urine (**osmotic diuresis**). The most frequent cause is **chronic renal failure**, when a decreasing population of nephrons is charged with excreting the daily load of solutes or other renal diseases associated with compromised proximal fluid and solute transport. Polyuria with excretion of a solute-rich urine also occurs in untreated **diabetes mellitus**. In that case, the polyuria occurs because the high plasma [glucose] leads to the filtration of an amount of glucose that exceeds the capacity of the proximal tubule to retrieve it from the lumen (p. 793). A third cause of osmotic diuresis is the administration of poorly reabsorbable solutes, such as mannitol or HCO_3^-.

In an entirely distinct class of polyurias is **primary polydipsia**, a psychoneurotic disorder in which patients drink large amounts of fluid. Whereas simple water deprivation will benefit a patient with primary polydipsia, it will aggravate the condition of a patient with DI.

ROLE OF AQUAPORINS IN RENAL WATER TRANSPORT

Whereas aquaporin 1 (AQP1) is the water channel responsible for a large amount of transcellular fluid movement in the proximal tubule and the tDLH, three related isoforms of the water-channel protein—AQP2, AQP3 and AQP4—are present in the principal cells of the collecting ducts. These channels regulate water transport in collecting tubules and ducts. Apical AQP2 is the basis for AVP-regulated water permeability. AQP3 and AQP4 are present in the basolateral membrane of principal cells, where they provide an exit pathway for water movement into the peritubular fluid.

Both short-term and long-term regulation of water permeability depend on an intact AQP2 system. In short-term regulation, AVP—via cAMP—causes water channel-containing vesicles from a subapical pool to fuse with the apical membrane (see Fig. 37–9). As a result, the number of channels and the water permeability sharply increase. In long-term regulation, AVP—by enhancing transcription of the AQP2 gene—increases the abundance of AQP2 protein in principal cells.

Mutations of several aquaporin genes lead to loss of function and marked abnormalities of water balance. Examples include sharply decreased fluid absorption along the proximal tubule in AQP1 knock-out animals and nephrogenic diabetes insipidus (see other box on this page) in patients with mutations of the gene for AQP2. An interesting situation may develop during the third trimester of pregnancy, when elevated plasma levels of vasopressinase—a placental aminopeptidase that degrades AVP—may lead to a clinical picture of central DI.

An acquired increase of AQP2 expression often accompanies states of abnormal fluid retention, such as congestive heart failure, hepatic cirrhosis, the nephrotic syndrome, and pregnancy. Conversely, some conditions—including acute and chronic renal failure, primary polydipsia, a low protein diet, and SIADH (see the box, Syndrome of Inappropriate Antidiuretic Hormone Secretion)—are associated with increased AQP2 levels in the apical membrane.

SYNDROME OF INAPPROPRIATE ANTIDIURETIC HORMONE SECRETION

The syndrome of inappropriate antidiuretic hormone secretion (SIADH) is the opposite of diabetes insipidus. Patients with SIADH secrete levels of antidiuretic hormone (i.e., arginine vasopressin [AVP]) or AVP-like substances that are inappropriately *high*, given the plasma osmolality. Thus, the urine osmolality is inappropriately high as the kidneys salvage inappropriately large volumes of water from the urine. As a result, total body water increases, the blood becomes hypoosmolar, and plasma [Na⁺] drops (**hyponatremia**). If plasma [Na⁺] falls substantially, the patient can develop headaches, nausea, vomiting, and behavioral changes. Eventually, stupor, coma, and seizures may ensue.

Before making the diagnosis of SIADH, the physician must rule out other causes of hyponatremia in which AVP levels may be appropriate. In Chapter 39, we discuss how plasma osmolality (p. 870) and effective circulating volume (p. 867) *appropriately* regulate AVP secretion. SIADH has four major causes:

1. Certain **malignant tumors** (e.g., bronchogenic carcinoma, sarcomas, lymphomas and leukemias) release AVP or AVP-like substances.
2. **Cranial disorders** (e.g., head trauma, meningitis, and brain abscesses) can increase AVP release.
3. **Non-malignant pulmonary disorders** (e.g., tuberculosis, pneumonia, and abscesses) and positive-pressure ventilation also can cause SIADH.
4. Several **drugs** can either stimulate AVP release (e.g., clofibrate, phenothiazines), increase the sensitivity of renal tubules to AVP (e.g., chlorpropamide), or both (e.g., carbamazepine).

Treatment is best directed at the underlying disorder, combined, if necessary and clinically appropriate, with fluid restriction. Patients with a plasma [Na⁺] that is below 110 mM must receive urgent attention. Infusing hypertonic Na⁺ is usually effective, but the correction must be gradual or severe neurologic damage can result owing to rapid changes in the volume of neurons, especially in the pontine area of the brainstem.

[cAMP]$_i$ that triggers the apical insertion of AQP2-containing vesicles also leads to a phosphorylation of UT1 (p. 792), increasing its activity. In addition, cAMP also stimulates the insertion of vesicles containing UT1. The result is a substantial increase in urea reabsorption, and thus the high interstitial [urea] that is indirectly responsible for generating the osmotic gradient that drives water reabsorption in the inner medulla.

Segments of the nephron other than the IMCD have varying degrees of urea permeability. However, AVP increases urea permeability only in the apical membrane of the IMCD. In particular, AVP has no effect on other urea transporters: UT2 (in tDLH), UT3 (in vasa recta), or UT4 (basolateral membrane of the IMCD).

REFERENCES

Books and Reviews

Agre P, Preston GM, Smyth BL, et al: Aquaporin CHIP: The archetypal molecular water channel. Am J Physiol 265:F463–F476, 1993.

Greger R: Transport mechanisms in thick ascending limb of Henle's loop of mammalian nephron. Physiol Rev 65:760–797, 1985.

Knepper MA, Valtin H, Sands JM: Renal action of vasopressin. In Fray JCS, Goodman HM (eds): Handbook of Physiology, Section 7, The Endocrine System. American Physiological Society, Washington 2000, pp 496–529.

Sasaki W, Ishibashi K, Marumo F: Aquaporin-2 and -3: Representatives of two subgroups of the aquaporin family colocalized in the kidney collecting duct. Annu Rev Physiol 60:199–220, 1998.

Seldin DW, Giebisch G (eds): The Kidney: Physiology and Pathophysiology, 3rd ed. Philadelphia, Lippincott Williams and Wilkins, 2000.

Tsukaguchi H, Shayakul C, Berger UV, Hediger MA: Urea transporters in kidney: Molecular analysis and contribution to the urinary concentrating process. Am J Physiol 275:F319–F324, 1998.

Journal Articles

Gottschalk CW, Mylle M: Micropuncture study of composition of loop of Henle fluid in desert rodents. Am J Physiol 204:532–535, 1959.

Grantham JJ, Burg MB: Effect of vasopressin and cyclic AMP on permeability of isolated collecting tubules. J Clin Invest 49:1815–1826, 1970.

Deen PMT, Verdijk MAJ, Knoers NVAM, et al: Requirement of human renal water channel AQP-2 for vasopressin-dependent concentration of urine. Science 264:92–95, 1994.

Lassiter WE, Gottschalk CW, Mylle M: Micropuncture study of net transtubular movement of water and urea in nondiuretic kidney. Am J Physiol 200:1139–1146, 1964.

Sanjana VM, Robertson CR, Jamison RL: Water extraction from the inner medullary collecting tubule system: A role for urea. Kidney Int 10: 139–146, 1976.

CHAPTER 38

Transport of Acids and Bases

Gerhard Giebisch and Erich Windhager

The lungs and the kidneys are largely responsible for regulating the acid-base balance of the blood (p. 642). They do so by independently controlling the two major components of the body's major buffering system: CO_2 and HCO_3^- (Fig. 38–1). Chapter 30 focuses on how the lungs control plasma $[CO_2]$. In this chapter we will see how the kidneys control plasma $[HCO_3^-]$.

ACID-BASE BALANCE AND THE OVERALL RENAL HANDLING OF H$^+$

Although the Lungs Excrete a Large Amount of CO$_2$, a Potential Acid Formed by Metabolism, the Kidneys Are Crucial For Excreting Nonvolatile Acids

The kidneys play a critical role in helping the body rid itself of excess acid that accompanies the intake of food or that forms in certain metabolic reactions. By far, the largest potential source of acid is **CO_2 production** (Table 38–1A), which arises during oxidation of carbohydrates, fats, and most amino acids (p. 1220). An adult ingesting a typical Western diet produces approximately 15,000 mmole/day of CO_2. This CO_2 would act as an acid if it went on to form H^+ and HCO_3^- (p. 636). Fortunately, the lungs excrete this prodigious amount of CO_2 by diffusion across the respiratory epithelia (p. 682), preventing the CO_2 from forming H^+.

However, metabolism also generates **nonvolatile acids**—such as sulfuric acid, phosphoric acid, and various organic acids—that the lungs cannot handle (see Table 38–1B). Metabolism also generates **nonvolatile bases**, which end up as HCO_3^- (see Table 38–1C). Subtracting the metabolically generated base from the metabolically generated acid leaves a net endogenous H^+ production of approximately 40 mmole/day for a person weighing 70 kg. The strong acids contained in a typical Western acid-ash diet (20 mmole/day of H^+ gained) as well as the obligatory loss of bases in stool (10 mmole/day of OH^- lost) represent an additional acid load to the body of 30 mmole/day. Thus, the body is faced with a total load of nonvolatile acids (i.e., not CO_2) of approximately 70 mmole/day—or about 1 mmole/kg body weight—derived from metabolism, diet, and intestinal losses. The kidneys handle this acid load by "dividing" 70 mmole/day of carbonic acid (H_2CO_3): excreting approximately 70 mmole/day of H^+ into the urine and simultaneously transporting 70 mmole/day of new HCO_3^- into the blood.

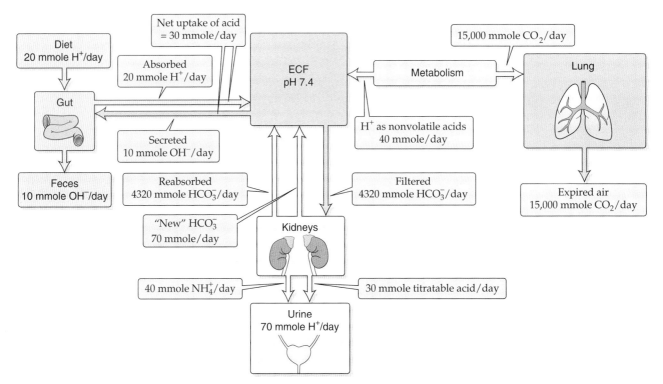

FIGURE 38–1. Acid-base balance. All values are for a 70-kg human on a typical "Western" acid-ash diet.

Once in the blood, this new HCO_3^- neutralizes the daily load of 70 mmole of nonvolatile acid.

Were it not for the tightly controlled excretion of H^+ by the kidney, the daily load of approximately 70 mmole of nonvolatile acids would progressively lower plasma pH

and, in the process, exhaust the body's stores of bases, especially HCO_3^-. The result would be death by relentless acidification. Indeed, one of the characteristic symptoms of renal failure is severe acidosis caused by acid retention. The kidneys continuously monitor the acid-base parameters of the extracellular fluid and adjust their rate of acid secretion to maintain the pH of extracellular fluid within narrow limits.

In summary, although the lungs excrete an extremely large amount of a *potential* acid in the form of CO_2, the kidneys play an equally essential role in the defense of the normal acid-base equilibrium, because they are the sole effective route for neutralizing *nonvolatile* acids.

To Maintain Acid-Base Balance, the Kidney Must Not Only Reabsorb Virtually All Filtered HCO_3^-, But Must Also Secrete Into the Urine the Daily Production of Nonvolatile Acids

As discussed, the major job of the kidney, in terms of acid-base balance, is to secrete acid into the urine and thus neutralize the nonvolatile acids that metabolism produces. However, before the kidney can begin to accomplish this task, it has to deal with a related and even more serious problem: retrieving from the tubule fluid virtually all HCO_3^- filtered by the glomeruli.

Each day, the glomeruli filter 180 liters of blood plasma, each liter containing 24 mmole of HCO_3^-, so that the daily filtered load of HCO_3^- is 180 liters × 24 mM = 4320 mmole. If this filtered HCO_3^- were all left behind in the urine, the result would be equivalent to an acid load in the blood of 4320 mmole, a catastrophic metabolic acidosis (p. 642). The kidneys deal with this problem by

TABLE 38–1

METABOLIC SOURCES OF NONVOLATILE ACIDS AND BASES

A. REACTIONS PRODUCING CO_2 (MERELY A POTENTIAL ACID)
1. Complete oxidation of neutral carbohydrate and fat → CO_2 + H_2O
2. Oxidation of *most* neutral amino acids → Urea + CO_2 + H_2O

B. REACTIONS PRODUCING NONVOLATILE ACIDS
1. Oxidation of sulfur-containing amino acids → Urea + CO_2 + H_2O + H_2SO_4 → 2 H^+ + SO_4^{2-} (Examples: methionine, cysteine)
2. Metabolism of phosphorus-containing compounds → H_3PO_4 → H^+ + $H_2PO_4^-$
3. Oxidation of *cationic* amino acids → Urea + CO_2 + H_2O + H^+ (Examples: lysine$^+$, arginine$^+$)
4. Production of non-metabolizable organic acids → HA → H^+ + A^- (Examples: uric acid, oxalic acid)
5. Incomplete oxidation of carbohydrate and fat → HA → H^+ + A^- (Examples: lactic acid, keto-acids)

C. REACTIONS PRODUCING NONVOLATILE BASES
1. Oxidation of *anionic* amino acids → Urea + CO_2 + H_2O + HCO_3^- (e.g., glutamate$^-$, aspartate$^-$)
2. Oxidation of organic anions → CO_2 + H_2O + HCO_3^- (e.g., lactate$^-$, acetate$^-$)

TABLE 38–2

	1	**2**	**3**
Net urinary acid excretion =	Excreted H^+ bound to phosphate (as $H_2PO_4^-$), creatinine and uric acid	+ Excreted H^+ bound to NH_3 (as NH_4^+)	− Excretion of filtered HCO_3^-

reclaiming virtually all of the filtered HCO_3^-. As discussed in the next section, the kidney accomplishes this task by secreting H^+ into the tubule lumen and titrating the 4320 mmole/day of filtered HCO_3^- to CO_2 and H_2O.

After the kidney reclaims virtually all the filtered HCO_3^- (i.e., 4320 mmole/day), how does it deal with the acid load of 70 mmole/day produced by metabolism, diet, and intestinal losses? If we simply poured 70 mmole of nonvolatile acid into the approximately 1.5 liters of "unbuffered" urine produced each day, urinary $[H^+]$ would be 0.070 mole/1.5 liters = 0.047 M, which would correspond to a pH of approximately 1.3. The lowest urine pH that the kidney can achieve is approximately 4.4, which corresponds to an $[H^+]$ that is three orders of magnitude lower than required to excrete the 70 mmole/day of nonvolatile acids. The kidneys solve this problem by binding the H^+ to buffers that the kidney can excrete within the physiologic range of urinary pH values. Some of these buffers the kidney *filters*—for example, phosphate, creatinine and urate. Because of its favorable pK of 6.8 and its relatively high rate of excretion, phosphate is the most important nonvolatile filtered buffer. The other major urinary buffer is NH_3/NH_4^+, which the kidney *synthesizes*. After diffusing into the tubule lumen, the NH_3 reacts with secreted H^+ to form NH_4^+. Through adaptive increases in the synthesis of NH_3 and excretion of NH_4^+, the kidneys can respond to the body's need to excrete increased loads of H^+.

Does the kidney eliminate the 70 mmole/day of nonvolatile acids by simply filtering and then excreting them in the urine? After the 70-mmole/day **acid challenge** presents itself to the extracellular fluid, the body deals with this challenge in three steps:

Step 1: Extracellular HCO_3^- neutralizes *most* of the H^+ load:

$$\text{Equation 38–1}$$
$$HCO_3^- + \underbrace{H^+}_{\text{Acid Load}} \longrightarrow CO_2 + H_2O$$

Thus, HCO_3^- decreases by an amount that is equal to the H^+ it consumes, producing an equal amount of CO_2 in the process. Non-HCO_3^- buffers ($B^- + H^+ \rightleftharpoons BH$; p. 643) in the blood neutralize most of the remaining H^+ load:

$$\text{Equation 38–2}$$
$$B^- + \underbrace{H^+}_{\text{Acid Load}} \longrightarrow BH$$

Thus, B^-, too, decreases by an amount that is equal to the H^+ it consumes. A very tiny fraction of the H^+ load—less than 0.001% (p. 638)—escapes buffering by either HCO_3^- or B^-. This remnant H^+ is responsible for a small drop in the extracellular pH.

Step 2: The lungs excrete the CO_2 formed in Equation 38–1. The body does not excrete the HB generated in Equation 38–2, but rather converts it back into B^-, as discussed later.

Step 3: The kidneys regenerate the HCO_3^- and B^- in the extracellular fluid by creating new HCO_3^- at a rate that is equal to the rate of H^+ production (i.e., ~70 mmole/day). Thus, over the course of a day, 70 mmole more HCO_3^- exits the kidneys via the renal veins than entered via the renal arteries. Most of this new HCO_3^- replenishes the HCO_3^- consumed by the neutralization of nonvolatile acids, maintaining extracellular $[HCO_3^-]$ at approximately 24 mM. The remainder of this new HCO_3^- regenerates B^-:

$$\text{Equation 38–3}$$
$$HCO_3^- + BH \longrightarrow \underbrace{B^-}_{\substack{\text{Regenerated} \\ \text{Base}}} + CO_2 + H_2O$$

Again, the lungs excrete the CO_2 formed in Equation 38–3, just as they excrete the CO_2 formed in Equation 38–1. Thus, by generating new HCO_3^-, the kidneys maintain constant levels of both HCO_3^- and the deprotonated forms of non-HCO_3^- buffers (B^-) in the extracellular fluid.

Table 38–2 summarizes the three components of net urinary acid excretion. Historically, *component #1* is referred to as **titratable acid**, the amount of base one must add to a sample of urine to bring its pH back up to the pH of blood plasma. The titratable acid does *not* include the H^+ the kidneys excrete as NH_4^+, which is *component #2*. Because the pK of the NH_3/NH_4^+ equilibrium is greater than 9, almost all of the ammonium buffer in the urine is in the form of NH_4^+, and titrating urine from an acid pH to a pH of 7.4 will not appreciably convert NH_4^+ to NH_3. If no filtered HCO_3^- were lost in *component #3*, the generation of new HCO_3^- by the kidneys would be the sum of *#1 + #2*. To the extent that filtered HCO_3^- is lost in the urine, the new HCO_3^- must exceed the sum of *#1 + #2*.

The kidneys also can control HCO_3^- and B^- following an **alkaline challenge**, produced, for example, by ingesting alkali or by vomiting (which leads to a loss of HCl). The kidney responds by decreasing net acid excretion—that is, by sharply reducing the excretion rates of titratable acid and NH_4^+. The result is a decrease in the production of new HCO_3^-. With an extreme alkali challenge, the excretion of urinary HCO_3^- also increases and may exceed

A HCO_3^- REABSORPTION

Tubule lumen

Interstitial space

Carbonic anhydrases

CAIV

CAII

CO_2

CO_2

OH^-

H^+

H^+

OH^-

H_2O

HCO_3^-

Retrieved HCO_3^-

B FORMATION OF TITRATABLE ACID

Tubule lumen

Interstitial space

CO_2 CAII

OH^-

HCO_3^-

New HCO_3^-

H^+

H^+

HPO_4^{2-}

$H_2PO_4^-$

C AMMONIUM EXCRETION

Tubule lumen

Interstitial space

CO_2 CAII

HCO_3^-

New HCO_3^-

H^+

H^+

NH_3

NH_3

NH_4^+

OH^-

Metabolism

NH_4^+

FIGURE 38–2. Titration of luminal buffers by secreted H^+. *A* and *B*, Generic models of H^+ secretion at various sites along the nephron. The *red arrows* represent diverse transport mechanisms. *C*, Ammonium handling by the proximal tubule.

the combined rates of titratable acid and NH_4^+ excretion. In other words, *component #3* in Table 38–2 exceeds the sum of *#1* and *#2*, so that "net acid excretion" becomes negative, and the kidney becomes a net excretor of alkali. In this case, the kidneys return less HCO_3^- to the extracellular fluid via the renal veins than entered the kidneys via the renal arteries.

Secreted H^+ Titrates HCO_3^- to CO_2 (HCO_3^- Reabsorption) and Also Titrates Filtered Non-HCO_3^- Buffers and Endogenously Produced NH_3 (Nonvolatile Acid Excretion)

As we have seen, the kidney can reabsorb nearly all of the filtered HCO_3^- and excrete additional acid into the urine as both titratable acid and NH_4^+. The common theme of these three processes is **H^+ secretion** from the blood into the lumen. Thus, the secreted H^+ can have three fates. It can titrate (1) filtered HCO_3^-; (2) filtered phosphate (or other filtered buffers that contribute to the "titratable acid"); and (3) NH_3, both secreted and, to a lesser extent, filtered.

TITRATION OF FILTERED HCO_3^- ("HCO_3^- REABSORPTION"). Extensive reabsorption reclaims almost all of the filtered HCO_3^- (more than 99.9%). As discussed in the next subchapter, the kidney reabsorbs HCO_3^- at specialized sites along the nephron. However, regardless of the site, the basic mechanism of HCO_3^- reabsorption is the same (Fig. 38–2*A*): H^+ transported into the lumen by the tubule cell titrates filtered HCO_3^- to CO_2 plus H_2O. One way that this titration can occur is by H^+ interacting with HCO_3^- to form H_2CO_3, which in turn dissociates to yield H_2O and CO_2. However, the reaction $H_2CO_3 \rightarrow H_2O + CO_2$ is far too slow to convert the entire filtered load of HCO_3^- to CO_2 plus H_2O. The enzyme carbonic anhydrase (see box on p. 637) which is present in many tubule segments, bypasses this slow reaction by splitting HCO_3^- into CO_2 and OH^- (see Table 38–1). The secreted H^+ neutralizes this OH^- so that the net effect is to accelerate the production of H_2O and CO_2.

The apical membranes of these H^+-secreting tubules are highly permeable to CO_2, so that CO_2 produced in the lumen, as well as the H_2O, diffuses into the tubule cell. Inside the tubule cell, the CO_2 and H_2O regenerate intracellular H^+ and HCO_3^- with the aid of carbonic anhydrase. Finally, the cell exports these two products, moving the H^+ out across the apical membrane into the tubule lumen and the HCO_3^- out across the basolateral membrane into the blood. Thus, for each H^+ secreted into the lumen, one HCO_3^- disappears from the lumen, and one HCO_3^- appears in the blood. However, the HCO_3^- disappearing from the lumen and the HCO_3^- appearing in the blood are *not* the same molecule! To secrete H^+ and yet keep intracellular pH within narrow physiological limits (p. 650), the cell closely coordinates the apical secretion of H^+ and the basolateral exit of HCO_3^-.

Two points are worth re-emphasizing. First, HCO_3^- reabsorption does not represent net H^+ excretion into the urine. It merely prevents the loss of the filtered alkali. Second, even though HCO_3^- reabsorption is merely a reclamation effort, this process consumes by far the largest

TABLE 38–3

TITRATION OF BUFFERS

pH	% PROTONATED BUFFER		
	Phosphate (pK = 6.8)	Urate (pK = 5.8)	Creatinine (pK = 5.0)
7.4	20.1	2.5	0.4
6.2	79.9	28.5	5.9
4.4	99.6	96.2	79.9

fraction of the H^+ secreted into the tubule lumen. For example, reclaiming the 4320 mmole of HCO_3^- filtered each day requires 4320 mmole of H^+ secretion, far more than the additional 70 mmole/day of H^+ secretion necessary for neutralizing nonvolatile acids.

TITRATION OF FILTERED NON-HCO_3^- BUFFERS ("TITRATABLE-ACID" FORMATION). The H^+ secreted into the tubules can interact with buffers other than HCO_3^- and NH_3. The titration of the non-NH_3, non-HCO_3^- buffers (B^-)— mainly HPO_4^-, creatinine, and urate—to their conjugate weak acids (BH) constitutes the "titratable acid" discussed earlier.

$$H^+ + B^- \longrightarrow BH$$

Equation 38–4

The major proton acceptor in this category of buffers excreted in the urine is HPO_4^{2-}, although creatinine also makes an important contribution; urate and other buffers contribute to a lesser extent. Figure 38–2B shows the fate of H^+ as it protonates phosphate from its divalent form (HPO_4^{2-}) to its monovalent form ($H_2PO_4^-$). Because low luminal pH inhibits the apical Na/phosphate cotransporter (NaPi) in the proximal tubule, and NaPi carries $H_2PO_4^-$ less well than HPO_4^{2-} does (p. 805), the kidneys tend to excrete H^+-bound phosphate in the urine. For each H^+ it transfers to the lumen to titrate HPO_4^{2-}, the tubule cell generates one new HCO_3^- and transfers it to the blood (see Fig. 38–2B).

How much does the "titratable acid" contribute to net acid excretion? Three factors determine the rate at which these buffers act as vehicles for excreting acid:

1. **The amount of the buffer in the glomerular filtrate and final urine**. The filtered load of HPO_4^{2-}, for example, is the product of plasma [HPO_4^{2-}] and the glomerular filtration rate (GFR) (p. 748). Plasma phosphate levels may range from 0.8 to 1.5 mM (p. 1088). Therefore, increasing plasma [HPO_4^{2-}] allows the kidneys to excrete more H^+ in the urine as $H_2PO_4^-$. Conversely, decreasing the GFR (as in chronic renal failure) reduces the amount of HPO_4^{2-} available for buffering, lowers the excretion of titratable acid, and thus contributes to metabolic acidosis. Ultimately, the key parameter is the amount of buffer excreted in the urine. In the case of phosphate, the fraction of the filtered load that the kidney excretes increases markedly as plasma [phosphate] exceeds the T_m (p. 806). For a plasma [phosphate] of 1.3 mM, the kidneys

reabsorb approximately 90%, and approximately 30 mmole/day appear in the urine.

2. **The pK of the buffer**. To be most effective at accepting H^+, the buffer (e.g., phosphate, creatinine, urate) should have a pK value that is between the pH of the glomerular filtrate and the pH of the final urine. For example, if blood plasma has a pH of 7.4, then only approximately 20% of its phosphate (pK = 6.8) will be in the form of $H_2PO_4^-$ (Table 38–3). Even if the final urine were only mildly acidic, having a pH of 6.2, approximately 80% of the phosphate in the urine would be in the form of $H_2PO_4^-$. In other words, the kidney would have titrated approximately 60% of the filtered phosphate from HPO_4^{2-} to $H_2PO_4^-$. Because creatinine has a pK of 5.0, lowering the pH of the tubule fluid from 7.4 to 6.2 increases the fractional protonation of creatinine from approximately 0.4% to only approximately 6%. However, urate has a pK of 5.8, so lowering pH from 7.4 to 6.2 would increase its fractional protonation from 2.5% to 28.5%.

3. **pH of the urine**. Regardless of the pK of the buffer, the lower the urinary pH, the more protonated is the buffer, and the greater is the amount of acid excreted with this buffer. As discussed, lowering the pH of the tubule fluid from 7.4 to 6.2 increases the protonation of creatinine from 0.4% to only approximately 6%. However, if the final-urine pH is 4.4, the fractional protonation of creatinine increases to approximately 80% (see Table 38–3). Thus, creatinine becomes a much more effective buffer during acidosis, when the kidney maximally acidifies the urine.

TITRATION OF FILTERED AND SECRETED NH_3 ("AMMONIUM EXCRETION"). The third class of buffer titrated by luminal H^+ is NH_3. However, unlike either HCO_3^- or the bases that give rise to "titratable acid" (e.g., HPO_4^{2-}), most of the luminal NH_3 is not filtered in the glomerulus. Instead, most NH_3 diffuses into the lumen from the tubule cell (see Fig. 38–2C), and some NH_4^+ may enter the lumen directly via the apical Na-H exchanger NHE3. In the case of the proximal tubule, the conversion of glutamine to α-ketoglutarate generates two NH_4^+ ions, which form two NH_3 and two H^+ ions. In addition, the metabolism of α-ketoglutarate generates two OH^- ions, which carbonic anhydrase converts to HCO_3^- ions. This new HCO_3^- then enters the blood.

In summary, when renal-tubule cells secrete H^+ into the lumen, this H^+ simultaneously titrates three kinds of buffers: (1) HCO_3^-, (2) HPO_4^{2-} and other buffers that become the "titratable acid," and (3) NH_3. Each of these three buffers competes with the other two for available H^+. In our example, each day the kidney must secrete 4390 mmole of H^+ into the tubule lumen. The kidney uses most of this secreted acid—4320 mmole/day or about 98% of the total—to reclaim filtered HCO_3^-. The balance of the total H^+ secreted, 70 mmole/day, the kidney uses to generate new HCO_3^-.

ACID-BASE HANDLING BY DIFFERENT SEGMENTS OF THE NEPHRON

Most nephron segments secrete H^+ to varying degrees.

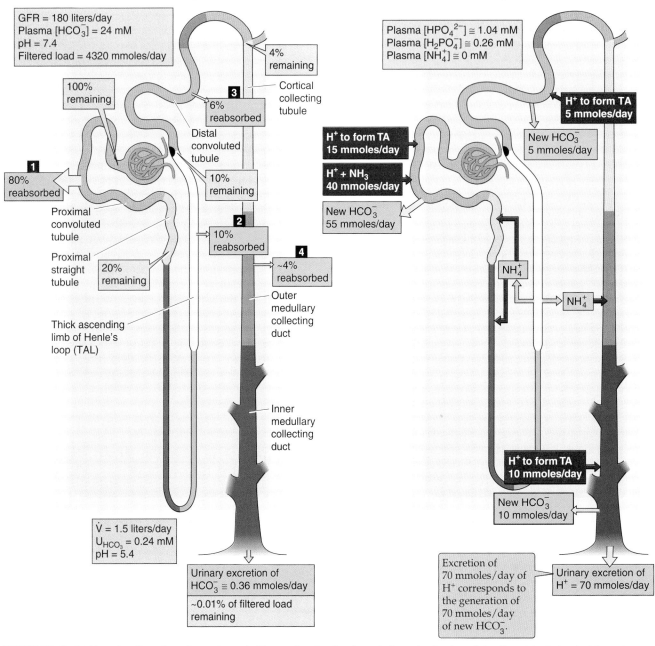

A RECLAMATION OF FILTERED HCO$_3^-$ ALONG THE NEPHRON

GFR = 180 liters/day
Plasma [HCO$_3^-$] = 24 mM
pH = 7.4
Filtered load = 4320 mmoles/day

100% remaining

80% reabsorbed **1**

Proximal convoluted tubule

Proximal straight tubule

20% remaining

Thick ascending limb of Henle's loop (TAL)

Distal convoluted tubule

6% reabsorbed **3**

4% remaining

Cortical collecting tubule

10% remaining

10% reabsorbed **2**

~4% reabsorbed **4**

Outer medullary collecting duct

Inner medullary collecting duct

$\dot{V}$ = 1.5 liters/day
U$_{HCO_3}$ = 0.24 mM
pH = 5.4

Urinary excretion of HCO$_3^-$ ≅ 0.36 mmoles/day

~0.01% of filtered load remaining

B GENERATION OF NEW HCO$_3^-$

Plasma [HPO$_4^{2-}$] ≅ 1.04 mM
Plasma [H$_2$PO$_4^-$] ≅ 0.26 mM
Plasma [NH$_4^+$] ≅ 0 mM

H$^+$ to form TA 5 mmoles/day

New HCO$_3^-$ 5 mmoles/day

H$^+$ to form TA 15 mmoles/day

H$^+$ + NH$_3$ 40 mmoles/day

New HCO$_3^-$ 55 mmoles/day

NH$_4^+$

NH$_4^+$

H$^+$ to form TA 10 mmoles/day

New HCO$_3^-$ 10 mmoles/day

Excretion of 70 mmoles/day of H$^+$ corresponds to the generation of 70 mmoles/day of new HCO$_3^-$.

Urinary excretion of H$^+$ = 70 mmoles/day

FIGURE 38–3. Acid-base handling along the nephron. *A*, The numbered *yellow boxes* indicate the fraction of the filtered load absorbed by various nephron segments. The *green boxes* indicate the fraction of the filtered load that remains in the lumen after these segments. *B*, The *red boxes* indicate the moieties of acid secretion associated with either the formation of titratable acid or the secretion of NH$_4^+$. The *yellow boxes* indicate the formation of new HCO$_3^-$ or NH$_4^+$ reabsorption by the thick ascending limb.

The Nephron Reclaims Virtually All of the Filtered HCO$_3^-$ in the Proximal Tubule (~80%), Thick Ascending Limb (~10%), and Distal Nephron (~10%)

The kidney reabsorbs the largest fraction of filtered HCO$_3^-$ (~80%) along the proximal tubule (Fig. 38–3A). By the end of the proximal tubule, luminal pH falls to approximately 6.8, which represents only a modest transepithelial H$^+$ gradient, compared with the plasma pH of 7.4. Thus, the proximal tubule is a high-capacity, low-gradient system for H$^+$ secretion. The thick ascending limb of the

loop of Henle (TAL) reabsorbs an additional 10% of filtered HCO$_3^-$, so that by the time the tubule fluid reaches the distal convoluted tubule (DCT), the kidney has reclaimed approximately 90% of the filtered HCO$_3^-$. The rest of the distal nephron—from the DCT to the inner medullary collecting duct—reabsorbs almost all of the remaining approximately 10% of the filtered HCO$_3^-$. Although the latter portion of the nephron reabsorbs only a small fraction of the filtered HCO$_3^-$, it can lower luminal pH to approximately 4.4. Thus, the collecting tubules and ducts are a low-capacity, high-gradient system for H$^+$ transport.

TABLE 38-4

TITRATABLE ACIDITY OF CREATININE AND PHOSPHATE ALONG THE NEPHRON*

| | pH | PHOSPHATE | | CREATININE | | Sum of Titratable Acid Due to Phosphate and Creatinine (mmole/day) |
		Filtered Load Remaining (%)	Titratable Acid Due to P_i (mmole/day)	Filtered Load Remaining (%)	Titratable Acid Due to Creatinine (mmole/day)	
Bowman space	7.4	100	0	100	0	0
End of PT	6.8	20	14.0	120†	0.2	14.2
End of ICT	6.0	10	15.5	120	1.7	17.2
Final urine	5.4	10	17.8	120	5.5	23.3

*Note that other buffers in the urine contribute to the *total* titratable acid, which increases with the excreted amount of each buffer and with decreases in urine pH. In this example, we assume a plasma [phosphate] of 1.3 mM, a plasma [creatinine] of 0.09 mM, and a GFR of 180 liters/day.

†We assume that the proximal tubule secretes an amount of creatinine that is equivalent to 20% of the filtered load.

GFR, glomerular filtration rate; ICT, initial collecting tubule; P_i, inorganic phosphate; PT, proximal tubule.

The amount of HCO_3^- lost in the urine depends on urine pH. If the $[CO_2]$ in the urine were the same as that in the blood, and if urine pH were 5.4, the $[HCO_3^-]$ in the urine would be 0.24 mM, which is 1% of the 24 mM in blood (p. 636). For a urine production of 1.5 liters/day, the kidneys would excrete 0.36 mmole/day of HCO_3^-. For a filtered HCO_3^- load of 4320 mmole/day, this loss represents a fractional excretion of approximately 0.01%. In other words, the kidneys reclaim approximately 99.99% of the filtered HCO_3^-. Similarly, at a nearly maximally acidic urine pH of 4.4, urine $[HCO_3^-]$ would be only 0.024 mM. Therefore, the kidneys would excrete only 36 μmoles/day of filtered HCO_3^-, and reabsorb approximately 99.999%.

The Nephron Generates New HCO_3^-, Mostly in the Proximal Tubule

The kidney generates new HCO_3^- in two ways (see Fig. 38-3B). It titrates filtered buffers such as HPO_4^{2-} to produce "titratable acid," and it titrates secreted NH_3 to NH_4^+. In healthy people, NH_4^+ excretion is the more important of the two, contributing approximately 60% of *net* acid excretion or new HCO_3^-.

FORMATION OF TITRATABLE ACID. The extent to which a particular buffer contributes to titratable acid (see Fig. 38-2B) depends on the amount of buffer in the lumen and luminal pH. The titratable acid due to *phosphate* is already substantial at the end of the proximal tubule (Table 38-4), even though the proximal tubule reabsorbs approximately 80% of the filtered phosphate. The reason is that the luminal pH equals the pK of the buffer at the end of the proximal tubule. The titratable acid due to phosphate rises only slightly along the "classical distal tubule" (i.e., distal convoluted tubule [DCT], connecting tubule [CNT], initial collecting tubule [ICT]), because the effect of that of acid secretion slightly exceeds phosphate reabsorption. The titratable acid due to phosphate rises further as luminal pH falls to 4.4 along the collecting ducts in the absence of significant phosphate reabsorption.

Although the late proximal tubule secretes creatinine, the titratable acid due to *creatinine* (see Table 38-4) is minuscule at the end of the proximal tubule, because luminal pH is so much higher than creatinine's pK. However, the titratable acidity due to creatinine increases substantially along the collecting ducts as luminal pH plummets. The urine contains other small organic acids (e.g., uric, lactic, pyruvic, and citric acids) that also contribute to titratable acid.

NH_4^+ EXCRETION. Of the new HCO_3^- that the nephron generates, approximately 60% (~40 mmole/day) is the product of NH_4^+ excretion (see Fig. 38-3B). The proximal tubule secretes slightly larger quantities of H^+ and NH_3 than the 40 mmole/day of NH_4^+ that ultimately appears in the urine. However, the TAL reabsorbs some NH_4^+ and deposits it in the interstitium. Some of this interstitial NH_4^+ represents NH_4^+ secreted by the proximal tubule. Some of the vasa recta washes out, and some enters the lumen of the collecting duct. Thus, the total new HCO_3^- that is attributable to NH_4^+ excretion is the NH_4^+ secreted by the proximal tubule, less the NH_4^+ that is reabsorbed by the TAL, plus the NH_4^+ secreted by the collecting ducts.

ACID-BASE TRANSPORT AT THE CELLULAR AND MOLECULAR LEVEL

The secretion of acid from the blood to the lumen—whether for reabsorption of filtered HCO_3^-, formation of titratable acid, or NH_4^+ excretion—requires at least three components:

1. Transport of H^+ from tubule cell to lumen, resulting in the production of intracellular OH^-.
2. Conversion of intracellular OH^- to HCO_3^-, catalyzed by carbonic anhydrase.
3. Transport of newly formed HCO_3^- from tubule cell to blood.

FIGURE 38–4. Cell models of H⁺ secretion. ATP, adenosine triphosphate.

In addition, because the buffering power of filtered non-HCO₃⁻ buffers is not high enough for these buffers to accept sufficient luminal H⁺, the formation of new HCO₃⁻ requires that the kidney generate buffer *de novo*. This buffer is NH₃.

H⁺ Moves Across the Apical Membrane From Tubule Cell to Lumen by Three Mechanisms: Na-H Exchange, Electrogenic H⁺ Pumping, and K-H Pumping

Although the kidney could, in principle, acidify the tubule fluid either by secreting H⁺ or by reabsorbing OH⁻ or HCO₃⁻, the secretion of H⁺ appears to be solely responsible for acidifying tubule fluid. At least three mechanisms can extrude H⁺ across the apical membrane; not all of these are present in any one cell.

THE Na-H EXCHANGER (NHE). The Na-H exchanger (p. 68) is responsible for the largest fraction of net H⁺ secretion. This exchanger is present not only throughout the proximal tubule (Fig. 38–4*A*, *B*) but also in the TAL (Fig. 38–4*C*) and DCT.

Of the known isoforms of the Na-H exchanger, NHE3 is particularly relevant for the kidney because it moves more H⁺ from tubule cell to lumen than any other transporter. The apical **NHE3** secretes H⁺ in exchange for

luminal Na⁺. Because a steep lumen-to-cell Na⁺ gradient drives this exchange process (p. 61), apical H⁺ secretion ultimately depends on the activity of the basolateral Na-K pump.

The carboxy termini of the NHEs have phosphorylation sites for various protein kinases. Protein kinase C (PKC) phosphorylates all isoforms, whereas protein kinase A (PKA) phosphorylates only the apical NHE3. In the proximal tubule, PKC activates the apical Na-H exchanger, but PKA inhibits it. For example, parathyroid hormone inhibits NHE3 via PKA.

THE ELECTROGENIC H⁺ PUMP. A second mechanism for apical H⁺ secretion by tubule cells is the electrogenic H⁺ pump, which appears to be a vacuolar-type adenosine triphosphatase (ATPase) (p. 64). Mutations in the gene encoding one of the subunits of this H⁺ pump cause a metabolic acidosis (p. 642) in the blood. The ATP-driven H⁺ pump can establish steep transepithelial H⁺ concentration gradients, lowering the urine pH to about 4.0 to 5.0. In contrast, the Na-H exchanger, which depends on the 10-fold Na⁺ gradient across the apical membrane, cannot generate an H⁺ gradient in excess of approximately 1 pH unit.

The apical electrogenic H⁺ pumps are located mainly in a subpopulation of intercalated cells (*α* cells) of the cortical collecting tubule (CCT) and in cells of the inner and outer medullary collecting ducts (IMCD and OMCD; see

Fig. 38–4D). However, H$^+$ pumps are also present in the apical membrane of the proximal tubule (see Figs. 38–4A, B), the TAL (see Fig. 38–4C), and DCT. In addition, an electrogenic H$^+$ pump is also present in the basolateral membrane of β intercalated cells.

The regulation of the apical H$^+$ pump probably involves several mechanisms. First, the transepithelial electrical potential appears to modulate the H$^+$ pump rate. For instance, aldosterone induces increased apical Na$^+$ uptake by the principal cells in the CCT (p. 786), causing an increase in the lumen-negative potential, which in turn stimulates the H$^+$ pump. Second, aldosterone stimulates the H$^+$ pump independently of changes in voltage. Third, acidosis increases the recruitment and targeting of pump molecules to the apical membranes of α intercalated cells in the ICT and CCT, whereas alkalosis has the opposite effect.

THE H-K EXCHANGE PUMP. A third type of H$^+$-secretory mechanism is present in the ICT, the CCT, and the OMCD (see Fig. 38–4D): an electroneutral H-K pump (p. 63) that is related to the Na-K pump. Several isoforms of the H-K pump are present in the kidney, and exhibit differential sensitivities to inhibition by drugs such as omeprazole, SCH-28080, and ouabain. The H-K pump retrieves luminal K$^+$ in animals on a low-K$^+$ diet (p. 824) and, as a side effect, produces enhanced H$^+$ secretion that contributes to the generation of hypokalemic metabolic alkalosis.

Carbonic Anhydrases in the Lumen and Cytosol Stimulate H$^+$ Secretion by Accelerating the Interconversion of CO$_2$ and HCO$_3^-$

The carbonic anhydrases (see Table 27–3) play an important role in renal acidification by catalyzing the interconversion of CO$_2$ to HCO$_3^-$. Inhibition of carbonic anhydrase (CA) by sulfonamides, such as acetazolamide, profoundly slows acid secretion. CA may act at three distinct sites of acid-secreting tubule cells (see Fig. 38–4): the extracellular face of the apical membrane; the cytoplasm; and the extracellular face of the basolateral membrane. Two CA isoforms are especially important for tubule cells. The soluble CA-II is present in the cytoplasm, whereas a GPI linkage (p. 15) anchors CA-IV to the outside of the apical membrane, predominantly in proximal cells.

APICAL ACTION OF CARBONIC ANHYDRASE (CA-IV). In the absence of apical CA, the H$^+$ secreted accumulates in the lumen, thus inhibiting Na-H exchange and H$^+$ secretion. By promoting the conversion of luminal HCO$_3^-$ to CO$_2$ plus OH$^-$, apical carbonic anhydrase prevents the lumen from becoming overly acidic and thus substantially relieves this inhibition. Thus, CA promotes high rates of HCO$_3^-$ reabsorption along the early proximal tubule (see Fig. 38–4A).

In the distal nephron (see Fig. 38–4D), H$^+$ secretion is less dependent on luminal CA than it is in the early proximal tubule for two reasons. First, the H$^+$ secretion rate is lower than that in the proximal tubule. Thus, the

uncatalyzed conversion of luminal H$^+$ and HCO$_3^-$ to CO$_2$ and H$_2$O can more easily keep up with the lower H$^+$ secretion rate. Second, in the collecting tubules and ducts the electrogenic H$^+$ pump can extrude H$^+$ against a very high gradient. Therefore, even in the absence of CA, the collecting ducts can raise luminal [H$^+$] substantially, thus accelerating the uncatalyzed reaction by mass action.

CYTOPLASMIC ACTION OF CARBONIC ANHYDRASE (CA-II). Cytoplasmic CA accelerates the conversion of intracellular CO$_2$ and OH$^-$ to HCO$_3^-$ (see Fig. 38–4). As a result, CA-II increases the supply of H$^+$ for apical H$^+$ extrusion and the supply of HCO$_3^-$ for the basolateral HCO$_3^-$ exit step. In the ICT and CCT, the intercalated cells (which engage in acid-base transport) contain CA-II, whereas the principal cells do not.

BASOLATERAL ACTION OF CARBONIC ANHYDRASE. The role played by basolateral CA is not yet settled.

INHIBITION OF CARBONIC ANHYDRASE. The administration of drugs that block carbonic anhydrase, such as acetazolamide, strongly inhibits HCO$_3^-$ reabsorption along the nephron, leading to the excretion of an alkaline urine. Because acetazolamide reduces the reabsorption of Na$^+$, HCO$_3^-$, and water, this drug is also a **diuretic** (i.e., it promotes the excretion of urine). However, a small amount of H$^+$ secretion and HCO$_3^-$ reabsorption remains despite the complete inhibition of CA. This remaining transport is due in part to the slow uncatalyzed hydration-dehydration reactions, and in part to a buildup of luminal H$_2$CO$_3$, which might diffuse into the cell across the apical membrane (i.e., mimicking the uptake of CO$_2$ and H$_2$O).

Bicarbonate Efflux Across the Basolateral Membrane Takes Place by Electrogenic Na/HCO$_3$ Cotransport and Cl-HCO$_3$ Exchange

The regulation of the intracellular pH of acid-secreting tubule cells requires that H$^+$ secretion across the apical membrane be tightly linked to, and matched by, the extrusion of HCO$_3^-$ across the basolateral membrane. Two mechanisms are responsible for HCO$_3^-$ transport from the cell into the peritubular fluid: electrogenic Na/HCO$_3$ cotransport and Cl-HCO$_3$ exchange.

ELECTROGENIC Na/HCO$_3$ COTRANSPORT (NBC). In proximal-tubule cells, the electrogenic Na/HCO$_3$ cotransporter NBC (p. 67) is responsible for much of the HCO$_3^-$ transport across the basolateral membrane. The electrogenic Na/HCO$_3$ cotransporter is expressed at highest levels in the S1 portion of the proximal tubule (see Fig. 38–4A) and gradually becomes less abundant in the more distal proximal-tubule segments (see Fig. 38–4B). NBC, which is a member of the superfamily of HCO$_3^-$ transporters, is a 1035 amino-acid protein with a molecular weight of ~130 kDa. 4,4′-diisothiocyanostilbene-2,2′-disulfonate (DIDS), an inhibitor of most HCO$_3^-$ transporters, also inhibits NBC. Because, in proximal-tubule cells, this transporter usually transports three HCO$_3^-$ ions for each Na$^+$, the electrochemical driving forces cause it to carry these ions from cell to blood. Note that renal NBC carries two *net* negative charges and is, thus, electrogenic. Accordingly, cell depolarization inhibits Na/HCO₃ efflux or can even reverse the direction of transport and cause Na/HCO₃ uptake.

Chronic metabolic and respiratory acidosis, hypokalemia, and hyperfiltration all increase NBC activity. As might be expected, several factors cause parallel changes in the activities of the apical Na-H exchanger and basolateral Na/HCO₃ cotransporter, minimizing changes in cell pH and [Na⁺]. Thus, angiotensin II (ANG II) and PKC stimulate both transporters, whereas parathyroid hormone and PKA markedly inhibit both.

Cl-HCO₃ EXCHANGE (AE). In the S3 segment of the proximal tubule, as well as in the TAL and collecting tubules and ducts, Cl-HCO₃ exchangers participate in transepithelial acid-base transport. The AEs (p. 69) are in the same superfamily of HCO₃⁻ transporters as are the NBCs and are inhibited by DIDS. The AE1 isoform is found in the basolateral membranes of α intercalated cells of the CNT, the ICT, and the CCT (see Fig. 38–4D). Basolateral AE2 is present in the TAL (see Fig. 38–4C) and DCT.

Ammonium Is Synthesized From Glutamine by Proximal Tubules, Partly Reabsorbed in the Loop of Henle, and Secreted Passively Into Papillary Collecting Ducts

The **proximal tubule** is the main site of renal ammonia synthesis, although almost all other tubule segments have the capacity to form ammonia. Ammonia (NH_3) is a weak base that can combine with H^+ to form ammonium (NH_4^+). Because the pK of the NH_3/NH_4^+ equilibrium is approximately 9.2, the NH_3/NH_4^+ ratio is 1:100 at a pH of 7.2. Whereas the cationic NH_4^+ is only poorly soluble in lipid membranes and, therefore, cannot readily diffuse across cell membranes, NH_3 is relatively lipid soluble and readily crosses most, but not all, cell membranes. When NH_3 diffuses from a relatively alkaline proximal-tubule or collecting-duct cell into the more acidic lumen, the NH_3 becomes "trapped" in the lumen after combining with H^+ to form the relatively impermeant NH_4^+ (Fig. 38–5A).

The proximal tubule forms NH_4^+ largely from glutamine (Fig. 38–5A), which enters tubule cells both from luminal and peritubular fluid via Na^+-coupled cotransporters. Inside the mitochondria, glutaminase splits glutamine into NH_4^+ and glutamate, and then glutamate dehydrogenase splits the glutamate into α-ketoglutarate and a second NH_4^+. The two NH_4^+ dissociate intracellularly into H^+ and NH_3. The NH_3 diffuses into the lumen (Fig. 38–5A). In addition, the apical Na-H exchanger may directly secrete some NH_4^+ into the proximal tubule lumen (with NH_4^+ taking the place of H^+). The α-ketoglutarate and two H^+ ions go on to form "half" a glucose (i.e., two α-ketoglutarates and four H^+ form one glucose). The consumption of two H^+ ions with each α-ketoglutarate is equivalent to forming two HCO_3^- ions. Accordingly, for each NH_4^+ secreted into the tubule lumen, the cell secretes one new HCO_3^- into the peritubular fluid.

In juxtamedullary nephrons, which have long loops of Henle, the **thin descending limb** may both secrete and

reabsorb NH_3. Tubule fluid may become alkaline along the tDLH, titrating NH_4^+ to NH_3 and promoting NH_3 efflux from the tubule lumen (i.e., reabsorption). On the other hand, reabsorption of NH_4^+ by the TAL (see following paragraph) creates a gradient favoring NH_3 diffusion into the lumen of the tDLH. Modeling of these processes predicts net secretion of NH_3 into the tDLH in the outer medulla (see Fig. 38–5D) and net absorption in the inner medulla (not shown). In the **thin ascending limb**, NH_4^+ reabsorption may occur by direct diffusion of NH_4^+ into the interstitium.

In contrast to the earlier segments, the **thick ascending limb** *reabsorbs* NH_4^+ (see Fig. 38–5C). Thus, much of the NH_4^+ secreted by the proximal tubule and tDLH does not reach the DCT. Because the apical membrane of the TAL is unusual in having a very low NH_3 permeability, the TAL takes up NH_4^+ across the apical membrane using two transport mechanisms, the Na/K/Cl cotransporter and the K^+ channels. Indeed, inhibiting the Na/K/Cl cotransporter blocks a significant fraction of NH_4^+ reabsorption, suggesting that NH_4^+ can replace K^+ on the cotransporter. Ammonium leaves the cell across the basolateral membrane as NH_3, leading to accumulation of NH_4^+ in the renal medulla.

The NH_4^+ that has accumulated in the interstitium of the medulla has three possible fates (see Fig. 38–5D). First, some dissociates into H^+ and NH_3. The late proximal tubule and the early tDLH take up this NH_3 by nonionic diffusion and trap it as NH_4^+ (see Fig. 38–5B). Thus, NH_4^+ **recycles** between the proximal tubule/tDLH and the TAL.

Second, some of the interstitial NH_4^+ that dissociates into NH_3 enters the lumen of the cortical and medullary collecting ducts by nonionic diffusion. There, H^+ secreted into the lumen titrates the NH_3 to NH_4^+ (see Fig. 38–5E). In addition, the Na-K pump may carry NH_4^+ into cells of the medullary collecting ducts, substituting NH_4^+ for K^+. To the extent that NH_4^+ moves directly from the TAL to the medullary collecting duct, it represents a **bypass** of the cortical portions of the distal nephron. This bypass prevents cortical portions of the distal nephron from losing NH_3 by diffusion from the lumen into the cortical interstitium, and thus preventing the toxic NH_3 from entering the circulation. Therefore, the kidney excretes NH_4^+ into the urine by a combination of synthesis and secretion by the proximal tubule, accumulation in the renal medulla, and transport by nonionic diffusion into the most terminal nephron segments.

The third fate of medullary NH_4^+ is **washout**, the return of a small fraction of the NH_4^+ to the systemic circulation for eventual detoxification by the liver. In the steady state, the buildup of NH_4^+ in the medulla leads to a sharp increase of [NH_4^+] along the corticomedullary axis.

Because it is the liver that synthesizes glutamine (p. 997), the main starting material for NH_4^+ production in the kidney, hepatorenal interactions are important in the overall process of NH_4^+ excretion (Fig. 38–6). The liver disposes of approximately 1000 mmole/day of amino groups during the catabolism of amino acids. Some of these amino groups become NH_4^+ via deamination reactions, and some end up as amino groups on either glutamate or aspartate via transamination reactions.

A EARLY PROXIMAL TUBULE

Tubule lumen

Glutamine

Na^+

$2\ NH_3$ ← $2\ NH_3$

ATP

H^+ ← → H^+

H^+ H^+

Na^+

$2\ NH_4^+$

Mitochondrion

Glutamine

Na^+ Glutamine

Glutaminase

NH_4^+ → $2\ NH_4^+$

$2\ OH^-$ → $2\ HCO_3^-$ → $3\ HCO_3^-$ CAII

$2\ CO_2$

H_2O → $2\ H^+$

Glutamate$^-$

NH_4^+

Glutamate dehydrogenase

NH_4^+

α-ketoglutarate

NBC

Na^+

GLUT

½ Glucose

$3\ Na^+$

ATP $2\ K^+$

Interstitial space

B DESCENDING LIMB OF HENLE (tDLH)

Tubule lumen | Interstitial space

NH_3

H^+ NH_3

NH_4^+

C THICK ASCENDING LIMB (TAL)

NH_4^+ → NH_4^+

$3\ Na^+$

ATP $2\ K^+$

$2\ Cl^-$ H^+

Na^+ NH_3 → NH_3

NH_4^+ H^+

NH_4^+

To the liver
$2\ NH_4^+ + 2HCO_3^- \rightarrow$ Urea + CO_2

D FATES OF MEDULLARY NH_4^+

NH_3

1 **2**

3 To liver

NH_3

40 mmoles/day $NH_3 \rightleftarrows NH_4^+$

E MEDULLARY COLLECTING DUCT

Tubule lumen | Interstitial space

NH_3 ← NH_3

NH_3

H^+ ← H^+ $3\ Na^+$

ATP NH_4^+ $2\ NH_4^+$

NH_4^+ ATP

FIGURE 38–5. Ammonium handling. *B,* In juxtamedullary nephrons, the secretion of NH_4^+ into the tubule lumen of the tDLH occurs mainly in the outer portion of the medulla. In *D,* the three numbered boxes indicate the three fates of the NH_4^+ reabsorbed by TAL. ATP, adenosine triphosphate.

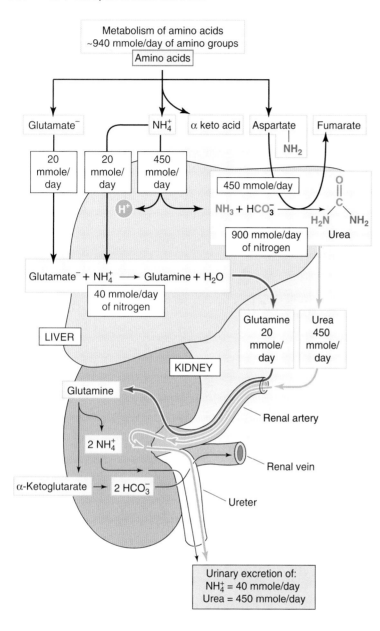

FIGURE 38–6. Cooperation between the liver and kidney in excreting nitrogen derived from amino acid breakdown. In this example, we assume a release of 940 mmoles/day of amino groups, resulting in the urinary excretion of 450 mmoles/day of urea (900 mmoles/day of amino nitrogen) and 40 mmoles/day of NH_4^+.

Of the approximately 1000 mmole/day of catabolized amino groups, the liver detoxifies approximately 95% by producing urea (p. 997), which the kidneys excrete (p. 790). Half of the -NH_2 in urea comes from NH_4^+ that dissociates to form NH_3 and H^+, whereas the other half comes from aspartate, resulting in the consumption of one HCO_3^-. Thus, urea formation generates two acid equivalents.

The liver detoxifies the remaining approximately 5% of catabolized amino groups by converting NH_4^+ and glutamate to glutamine. This reaction does not generate acid-base equivalents. The proximal-tubule cells take up this hepatic glutamine and use it as the source of the NH_4^+ that they secrete into the tubule lumen as they generate one new HCO_3^- (see Fig. 38–5A).

Thus, the two hepatorenal mechanisms for disposing of catabolized amino groups have opposite effects on HCO_3^-. For each catabolized amino group excreted as urea, the liver *consumes* the equivalent of one HCO_3^-. For each catabolized amino group excreted as NH_4^+ via the glutamine pathway, the proximal tubule *produces* one new

HCO_3^- (see Fig. 38–6). To the extent that the kidney excretes NH_4^+, the liver consumes less HCO_3^- as it synthesizes urea.

REGULATION OF RENAL ACID SECRETION

A variety of physiological and pathophysiological stimuli can modulate renal H^+ secretion as well as NH_3 synthesis. Most of these factors produce coordinated changes in apical and basolateral acid-base transport, as well as in NH_3 production.

Respiratory Acidosis Stimulates Renal H^+ Secretion

The four fundamental pH disturbances are respiratory acidosis and alkalosis, and metabolic acidosis and alkalosis (see Fig. 27–11). In each case, the initial and almost

TABLE 38-5

THE EFFECTS OF CHRONIC ACIDOSIS ON PROXIMAL-TUBULE FUNCTION

*Enhanced Na citrate reabsorption is a defense against acidosis by conversion of citrate to HCO_3^-. The price paid is enhanced stone formation because luminal citrate reduces stones. Indeed, acidotic patients tend to get calcium-containing kidney stones.
NBC, electrogenic Na/HCO_3 cotransporter; NHE3, Na-H exchanger 3.

instantaneous line of defense is the action of buffers—both in the extracellular and intracellular compartments—to *minimize* the magnitude of the pH changes (p. 634). However, *restoring* the pH to a value as close to "normal" as possible requires slower, compensatory responses from the lungs or kidneys.

In respiratory acidosis, where the primary disturbance is an increase in arterial P_{CO_2}, the compensatory response is an increase in renal H^+ secretion, which translates to increased production of new HCO_3^- via NH_4^+ excretion. The opposite occurs in respiratory alkalosis. These changes in H^+ secretion tend to correct the distorted $[HCO_3^-]/[CO_2]$ ratios that occur in primary respiratory acid-base derangements.

Respiratory acidosis stimulates H^+ secretion in at least two ways. First, an *acute* elevated P_{CO_2} directly stimulates proximal-tubule cells to secrete H^+, as shown by applying solutions in which it is possible to change P_{CO_2} without altering basolateral pH or $[HCO_3^-]$. However, isolated changes in basolateral pH (i.e., without an accompanying change in $[HCO_3^-]$ or P_{CO_2}), which also produce large changes in intracellular pH (pH_i), have a negligible effect in the short term. Thus, proximal-tubule cells seem to have a mechanism for sensing CO_2. Second, *chronic* respiratory acidosis leads to adaptive responses that upregulate acid-base transporters. For example, activities of the apical Na-H exchanger and basolateral Na/HCO_3 cotransporter are elevated in membrane vesicles that have been isolated from animals who were previously exposed to high P_{CO_2} levels. These adaptive changes persist for some time, even after P_{CO_2} levels have returned to normal. Such a sustained increase in transporter activity may help explain why, once H^+ secretion has adapted, reversing the original respiratory acidosis may produce a rebound metabolic alkalosis.

Metabolic Acidosis Stimulates Both Proximal H^+ Secretion and NH_3 Production

The first response to metabolic acidosis is increased alveolar ventilation, which blows off CO_2 (p. 723) and thus corrects the distorted $[HCO_3^-]/[CO_2]$ ratio in a primary metabolic acidosis. The kidneys can also participate in the compensatory response, assuming, of course, that the aci-

dosis is not the consequence of renal pathology. An *acute* fall in basolateral $[HCO_3^-]$ stimulates proximal H^+ secretion, probably by enhancing HCO_3^- efflux from the proximal-tubule cell via the Na/HCO_3 cotransporter and also by reducing HCO_3^- backleak via tight junctions from interstitial fluid to tubule lumen.

In *chronic* metabolic acidosis, the adaptive responses of the proximal tubule are probably similar to those outlined above for chronic respiratory acidosis. These include upregulation of apical Na-H exchange and electrogenic H^+ pumping, as well as basolateral Na/HCO_3 cotransport (Table 38–5). For example, when one isolates brush border membranes from the renal cortex of animals who have been made chronically acidotic, NHE3 activity is significantly increased. Therefore, the proximal-tubule cell adapts to chronic acidosis, possibly by increasing the number of transporters. The up-regulation appears to involve activation of PKC, a serine/threonine kinase (p. 102). In proximal-tubule cells, chronic intracellular acidosis also stimulates a member of the Src family of receptor-associated tyrosine kinases (p. 111). Indeed, herbimycin, a tyrosine-kinase inhibitor, blocks upregulation of NHE3 in chronic acidosis. Endothelin appears to be essential for the upregulation of NHE3 in chronic metabolic acidosis.

The parallel activation of apical and basolateral transporters minimizes changes in pH_i, while increasing transepithelial HCO_3^- reabsorption. An important and still unresolved question concerns how tubule cells continue to respond to a chronic acidosis even after the coordinated stimulation of apical and basolateral acid-base transporters has returned pH_i to normal.

In addition to the increased H^+ secretion, the other ingredient needed to produce new HCO_3^- is enhanced NH_3 production. Together, the two increase NH_4^+ excretion. Indeed, the excretion of NH_4^+ into the urine increases markedly as a result of the adaptive response to chronic metabolic acidosis (Fig. 38–7A). Thus, the ability to increase NH_3 synthesis is an important element in the kidney's defense against acidotic challenges. Indeed, as a chronic metabolic acidosis develops, the kidneys progressively excrete a larger fraction of urinary H^+ as NH_4^+. As a consequence, the excretion of titratable acid becomes a progressively smaller fraction of total acid excretion.

The adaptive stimulation of NH_3 synthesis, which oc-

A EFFECT OF CHRONIC METABOLIC ACIDOSIS ON TOTAL NH_4^+ EXCRETION INTO FINAL URINE

B EFFECT OF BASOLATERAL ALKALOSIS ON H^+ SECRETION BY PROXIMAL TUBULES

FIGURE 38-7. (*A*, Data from RF Pitts: Renal excretion of acid. Fed Proc 7:418–426, 1948. *B*, Data from Alpern RJ, Cogan MG, Rector FC: Effects of extracellular fluid volume and plasma bicarbonate concentration on proximal acidification in the rat. J Clin Invest 71:736–746, 1983.)

curs in response to a fall in pH_i, involves a stimulation of both glutaminase and phosphoenolpyruvate carboxykinase (PEPCK). The stimulation of mitochondrial glutaminase increases the conversion of glutamine to NH_4^+ and glutamate (see Fig. 38–5A). The stimulation of PEPCK enhances gluconeogenesis and thus the conversion of α-ketoglutarate (the product of glutamate deamination) to glucose.

Metabolic Alkalosis Reduces Proximal H^+ Secretion and, in the Cortical Collecting Tubule, May Even Provoke HCO_3^- Secretion

We can illustrate the response of the proximal tubule to metabolic alkalosis by considering an artificial experimental maneuver. The *upper curve* in Figure 38–7B summarizes the results of experiments in which investigators perfused single proximal tubules with solutions having progressively higher HCO_3^- concentrations, while maintaining $[HCO_3^-]$ in the peritubular capillaries at a *physiologic level*. The rate of H^+ secretion increases steeply up to a luminal $[HCO_3^-]$ of approximately 45 mM, but levels off thereafter. The reason H^+ secretion increases with increased luminal $[HCO_3^-]$ is that the incremental HCO_3^- represents an additional buffer that helps keep luminal pH relatively alkaline in the vicinity of the apical H^+ transporters.

The *lower curve* in Figure 38–7B shows the results from experiments that were similar, except that the peritubular blood had a higher-than-physiological $[HCO_3^-]$; that is, there was a metabolic alkalosis on the basolateral side of the cells. HCO_3^- reabsorption is uniformly lower during alkalosis: for a given luminal $[HCO_3^-]$, the tubules secrete less H^+. The likely explanation is that the increase in blood $[HCO_3^-]$ (1) depresses the rate at which the Na/

HCO_3 cotransporter moves HCO_3^- from cell to blood and (2) increases paracellular HCO_3^- backleak from interstitium to lumen.

So far, we have discussed the effect of metabolic alkalosis on H^+ secretion by the proximal tubule. In the initial and cortical collecting tubule, metabolic alkalosis can cause the tubule to switch from secreting H^+ to secreting HCO_3^- into the lumen. The α **intercalated cells** in the ICT and CCT secrete H^+, using an apical H^+ pump and a basolateral Cl-HCO_3 exchanger (see Fig. 38–4D). Metabolic alkalosis, over a period of days, shifts the intercalated-cell population, increasing the proportion of β **intercalated cells** at the expense of α cells. Because β cells have the opposite apical-versus-basolateral distribution of H^+ and HCO_3^- transporters, they *secrete* HCO_3^- into the lumen. Thus, the CCT now switches from net HCO_3^- reabsorption to net HCO_3^- secretion. Increased activity of β intercalated cells may correct metabolic alkalosis by accelerating Cl-HCO_3 exchange. HCO_3^- secretion can also be stimulated by increased luminal delivery of Cl^- to the exchanger.

By Increasing HCO_3^- Delivery to the Tubules, an Increased Glomerular Filtration Rate Enhances HCO_3^- Reabsorption (Glomerulotubular Balance for HCO_3^-)

Increasing either luminal flow or luminal $[HCO_3^-]$ significantly enhances HCO_3^- reabsorption, probably by raising effective $[HCO_3^-]$ (and thus pH) in the microenvironment of H^+ transporters in the brush-border microvilli. Because a high luminal pH stimulates the Na-H exchangers and H^+ pumps located in the microvilli of the proximal tubule, increased flow translates to enhanced H^+ secretion.

This flow-dependence, an example of glomerulotubular (G-T) balance (p. 783), is important because it minimizes HCO_3^- loss, and thus the development of a metabolic acidosis, when GFR increases. Conversely, this G-T balance of HCO_3^- reabsorption also prevents metabolic *alkalosis* when GFR decreases. The flow dependence of HCO_3^- reabsorption also accounts for the stimulation of H^+ transport that occurs after uninephrectomy (i.e., surgical removal of one kidney), when GFR in the remnant kidney rises in response to the loss of renal tissue.

Volume Contraction Stimulates Renal H⁺ Secretion by Increasing Levels of Angiotensin II, Aldosterone, and Sympathetic Activity

As discussed in Chapter 39, a decrease in *effective circulating volume* stimulates Na^+ reabsorption by four parallel pathways (p. 864), including activation of the renin-angiotensin-aldosterone axis (and thus an increase in ANG II levels) and stimulation of renal sympathetic nerves (and thus the release of norepinephrine). Both ANG II and norepinephrine stimulate Na-H exchange in the proximal tubule. Because the proximal tubule couples Na^+ and H^+ transport, volume contraction not only increases Na^+ reabsorption but H^+ secretion as well. Volume expansion has the opposite effect. On a longer time scale, volume depletion also increases aldosterone levels, enhancing H^+ secretion in cortical and medullary collecting ducts (see later). Thus, the regulation of effective circulating volume takes precedence over the regulation of plasma pH.

Decreased *dietary* Na^+ *intake* increases apical Na-H exchange activity, even if one assesses the activity in brush-border membrane vesicles removed from the animal. A high-Na^+ diet has the opposite effect.

Hypokalemia Increases Renal H⁺ Secretion

As discussed on page 816, acid-base disturbances can cause changes in K^+ homeostasis. The opposite is also true. Because a side effect of K^+ depletion is increased renal H^+ secretion, K^+ depletion is frequently associated with metabolic alkalosis. Several lines of evidence indicate that, in the proximal tubule, hypokalemia leads to a marked increase in apical Na-H exchange and basolateral Na/HCO_3 cotransport. As in other cells, the pH of tubule cells falls during K^+ depletion (p. 652). The resulting chronic cell acidification may lead to adaptive responses that activate Na-H exchange and electrogenic Na/HCO_3 cotransport, presumably by the same mechanisms that stimulate H^+ secretion in chronic acidosis (Table 38–5). In the proximal tubule, K^+ depletion also markedly increases NH_3 synthesis and NH_4^+ excretion, thus increasing urinary H^+ excretion as NH_4^+. Finally, K^+ depletion stimulates apical K-H exchange in α intercalated cells of the ICT and CCT (p. 824), enhancing H^+ secretion as a side effect of K^+ retention.

Just as hypokalemia can cause metabolic alkalosis, hyperkalemia is often associated with metabolic *acidosis*. An important contributory factor may be reduced NH_4^+ excretion, perhaps because of lower synthesis in proximal-tubule cells and reduced NH_4^+ accumulation in the medullary interstitium. High luminal $[K^+]$ in the TAL may compromise NH_4^+ reabsorption because the K^+ competes with NH_4^+ for uptake by apical Na/K/Cl cotransporters and K^+ channels. Reduced NH_4^+ levels in the medullary interstitium provide less NH_3 for diffusion into the medullary collecting duct, leading to less NH_4^+ excretion and thus to acidosis.

Both Glucocorticoids and Mineralocorticoids Stimulate Acid Secretion

Prolonged adrenal insufficiency (p. 786) leads to acid retention and, potentially, to life-threatening metabolic acidosis. Both glucocorticoids and mineralocorticoids stimulate H^+ secretion, but at different sites along the nephron.

Glucocorticoids (e.g., cortisol) enhance the activity of Na-H exchange in the proximal tubule and thus stimulate H^+ secretion. In addition, they inhibit phosphate reabsorption, raising the luminal availability of buffer anions for titration by secreted H^+.

Mineralocorticoids (e.g., aldosterone) stimulate H^+ secretion by three coordinated mechanisms—one direct and two indirect. First, mineralocorticoids *directly* stimulate H^+ secretion in the collecting tubules and ducts by increasing the activity of the apical electrogenic H^+ pump and basolateral $Cl-HCO_3$ exchanger (see Fig. 38–4D). Second, mineralocorticoids *indirectly* stimulate H^+ secretion by enhancing Na^+ reabsorption in the collecting ducts (p. 786), thus increasing the lumen-negative voltage. This increased negativity may stimulate the apical electrogenic H^+ pump in α intercalated cells to secrete acid. Third, mineralocorticoids—particularly when administered for longer periods of time and accompanied by high Na^+ intake—cause K^+ depletion, *indirectly* increasing H^+ secretion (see previous section).

Diuretics Can Increase or Decrease H⁺ Secretion, Depending on How They Affect Transepithelial Voltage, Extracellular Fluid Volume, and Plasma [K⁺]

The effects of diuretics on renal H^+ secretion vary substantially from one diuretic to another, depending both on the site and mechanism of action. From the point of view of acid-base balance, diuretics fall broadly into two groups, those that promote the excretion of a relatively alkaline urine and those that have the opposite effect.

To the first group belong carbonic-anhydrase inhibitors and K^+-sparing diuretics. The **CA inhibitors** lead to excretion of an alkaline urine by inhibiting H^+ secretion. Their greatest effect is in the proximal tubule, but they also inhibit H^+ secretion by the TAL and DCT. **K⁺-sparing diuretics**—including amiloride, triamterene, and the spironolactones—also alkalinize the urine. Both amiloride and triamterene inhibit the apical epithelial Na^+ channels (ENaC) (p. 779) in the collecting tubules and ducts, thus hyperpolarizing the apical membrane and making it more difficult for the electrogenic H^+ pump to secrete H^+ ions into the lumen. Spironolactones decrease H^+ secretion by interfering with the action of aldosterone.

The second group of diuretics—which tend to *increase* urinary acid excretion and often induce alkalosis—includes **loop diuretics** such as furosemide (which inhibits the apical Na/K/Cl cotransporter in the TAL) and **thiazide diuretics** such as chlorthiazide (which inhibits the apical Na/Cl cotransporter in the DCT). These diuretics act by three mechanisms. First, all cause some degree of volume contraction, and thus lead to increased levels of ANG II and aldosterone (p. 866), both of which enhance H^+ secretion. Second, these diuretics enhance Na^+ delivery to the collecting tubules and ducts, thus increasing the electrogenic uptake of Na^+, thus increasing the lumen-negative voltage, and thus enhancing H^+ secretion. Third, this group of diuretics causes K^+ *wasting*; as discussed earlier, K^+ depletion enhances H^+ secretion.

REFERENCES

Books and Reviews

Alpern RJ: Endocrine Control of Acid-Base Balance. In Fray JCS, Goodman HM (eds): Handbook of Physiology: Endocrine. Vol. 3, Section 7: Endocrine Regulation of Water and Electrolyte Balance. New York, Oxford University Press, pp 570–606, 2000.

Good DW: Ammonium Transport by the Thick Ascending Limb of Henle's Loop. Annu Rev Physiol 56:623–647, 1994.

Rose BD, Post TW: Clinical Physiology of Acid-Base and Electrolyte Disorders, 5th ed. New York, McGraw-Hill, 2001.

Seldin DW, Giebisch G (eds): The Kidney: Physiology and Pathophysiology, 3rd ed. Philadelphia, Lippincott Williams & Wilkins, 2000.

Stone DK, Xie XS: Proton Translocating ATPases: Issues in Structure and Function. Kidney Int 33:767–774, 1988.

Wakabayashi S, Shigekawa M, Pouysségur J: Molecular physiology of vertebrate Na^+/H^+ exchangers. Physiol Rev 77:51–74, 1997.

Journal Articles

Aronson PS, Nee J, Suhm MA: Modifier role of internal H in activating the Na-H exchanger in renal microvillus membrane vesicles. Nature 299:161–163, 1982.

Boron WF, Boulpaep EL: Intracellular pH regulation in the renal proximal tubule of the salamander: basolateral HCO_3^- transport. J Gen Physiol 81:53–94, 1983.

Geibel J, Giebisch G, Boron WF: Angiotensin II stimulates both Na-H exchange and Na/HCO_3 cotransport in the rabbit proximal tubule. Proc Natl Acad Sci USA 87:7917–7920, 1990.

Karet FE, Finberg KE, Nelson RD, et al: Mutations in the gene encoding B1 subunit of H^+-ATPase cause renal tubular acidosis with sensorineural deafness. Nat Genet 21:84–90, 1999.

McKinney TD, Burg MB: Bicarbonate transport by rabbit cortical collecting tubules: Effect of acid and alkali loads *in vivo* on transport *in vitro*. J Clin Invest 60:766–768, 1977.

Romero MF, Hediger MA, Boulpaep EL, Boron WF: Expression cloning of the renal electrogenic Na/HCO_3 cotransporter. Nature 387:409–413, 1997.

Wang T, Malnic G, Giebisch G, Chan YL: Renal bicarbonate reabsorption in the rat. IV. Bicarbonate transport mechanisms in the early and late distal tubule. J Clin Invest 91:2776–2784, 1993.

CHAPTER 39

Integration of Salt and Water Balance

Gerhard Giebisch and Erich Windhager

Two separate but closely interrelated control systems regulate the volume and osmolality of the extracellular fluid (ECF). It is important to regulate the **extracellular fluid volume** to maintain blood pressure, which is essential for adequate tissue perfusion and function. The body regulates ECF volume by monitoring and adjusting the total-body content of NaCl. It is important to regulate the **extracellular osmolality** because hypotonic or hypertonic osmolalities cause changes in cell volume (p. 76) that seriously compromise cell function, especially in the central nervous system (CNS). The body regulates extracellular osmolality by monitoring and adjusting total-body water content. These two homeostatic mechanisms—for ECF volume and osmolality—use different sensors, different hormonal transducers, and different effectors (Table 39–1). However, they have one thing in common: some of their effectors, although different, are located in the kidney. In the case of the ECF volume, the control system modulates the urinary excretion of Na^+. In the case of osmolality, the control system modulates the urinary excretion of water.

Na^+ BALANCE. The maintenance of the ECF volume, or Na^+ balance, depends on signals that reflect the adequacy of the circulation—the so-called effective circulating volume, discussed later. Low- and high-pressure baroreceptors in the circulation send afferent signals to the brain (p. 536), which translates this "volume signal" into several responses that can affect ECF over either the short or the long term. The short-term effects (over a period of seconds to minutes) occur as the autonomic nervous system and humoral mechanisms modulate the heart and blood vessels to control blood pressure. The long-term effects (over a period of hours to days) occur as nervous, humoral, and hemodynamic mechanisms modulate the kidney to control Na^+ excretion. Chapter 34 treats Na^+ excretion. In the first part of this chapter, we discuss the entire feedback loop, of which Na^+ excretion is merely the end point.

Why is the Na^+ content of the body the main determinant of the ECF volume? Na^+, with its associated anions, Cl^- and HCO_3^-, is the main osmotic constituent of the ECF volume; when Na^+ moves, water must move with it. Because the body generally maintains ECF osmolality within narrow limits (e.g., ~290 mosmole/kg or mOsm), it follows that whole-body Na^+ content—which the kidneys control—must be the major determinant of the ECF volume. A simple example illustrates the point. If the kidney were to enhance the excretion of Na^+ and its accompanying anions by 145 milliequivalents (meq) each—the amount of solute normally present in one liter of ECF—the kidneys would have to excrete an additional liter of urine to prevent a serious fall in osmolality. Alternatively,

TABLE 39–1

COMPARISON OF THE SYSTEMS CONTROLLING EXTRACELLULAR FLUID VOLUME AND OSMOLALITY

	REGULATION OF ECF VOLUME	REGULATION OF OSMOLALITY	
What Is Sensed?	*Effective Circulating Volume*	*Plasma Osmolality*	
Sensors	Carotid sinus, aortic arch, renal afferent arteriole, atria	Hypothalamic osmoreceptors	
Efferent Pathways	Renin-angiotensin-aldosterone axis, sympathetic nervous system, AVP, ANP	AVP	Thirst
Effector	*Short term:* Heart, blood vessels *Long term:* Kidney	Kidney	Brain: drinking behavior
What Is Affected?	*Short term:* Blood pressure *Long term:* Na$^+$ excretion	Renal water excretion	Water intake

ANP, atrial natriuretic peptide; AVP, arginine vasopressin; ECF, extracellular fluid.

adding 145 mmole of "dry" NaCl to the ECF obligates adding one liter of water to the ECF; this addition can be accomplished by drinking water or reducing renal excretion of solute-free water. Relatively small changes in Na$^+$ excretion lead to marked alterations in the ECF volume. Thus, precise and sensitive control mechanisms are needed to safeguard and regulate the body's content of Na$^+$.

WATER BALANCE. The maintenance of osmolality, or water balance, depends on receptors in the hypothalamus that detect changes in the plasma osmolality. These receptors send signals to areas of the brain that (1) control thirst, thus regulating water intake, and (2) control the production of arginine vasopressin (AVP)—also known as antidiuretic hormone (ADH)—thus regulating water excretion by the kidneys. We discussed renal water excre-

tion in Chapter 37. In the second part of this chapter, we discuss the entire feedback loop, of which water excretion is merely the end point.

Why is the water content of the body the main determinant of osmolality? Total-body osmolality is defined as the ratio of total-body osmoles to total-body water (p. 50). Although the ECF-volume control system can regulate the amount of *extracellular* osmoles, it has little effect on *total-body* osmoles. Total-body osmoles are largely a function of the *intracellular* milieu because the intracellular compartment is large and its solute composition is highly regulated. Total-body osmoles do not change substantially except during growth or during certain disease states, such as diabetes mellitus (in which excess glucose increases total-body osmolality). Only by controlling water independent of Na$^+$ control can the body control osmolality.

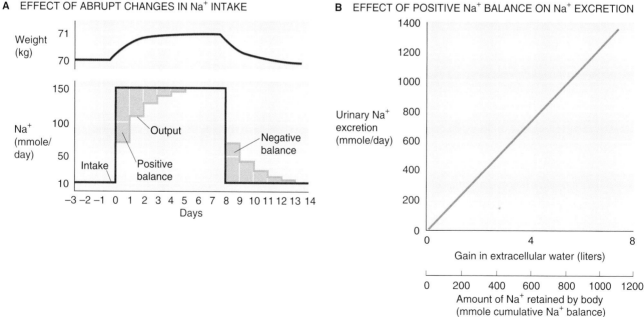

A   EFFECT OF ABRUPT CHANGES IN Na$^+$ INTAKE

B   EFFECT OF POSITIVE Na$^+$ BALANCE ON Na$^+$ EXCRETION

FIGURE 39–1. Na$^+$ balance. In *A*, the *red curve* shows the time course of dietary Na$^+$ intake, and the *green curve* shows Na$^+$ excretion. The *golden area* between the *two curves at the beginning* of the experiment corresponds to the accumulated total-body Na$^+$ of 140 mmole. This additional Na$^+$, dissolved in approximately 1 liter of extracellular fluid, accounts for the 1-kg gain in body weight (*blue curve*). (*B*, Data from Walser M: Phenomenological analysis of renal regulation of sodium and potassium balance. Kidney Int 27:837–841, 1985.)

CONTROL OF EXTRACELLULAR FLUID VOLUME

In the Steady State, Na⁺ Intake via the Gastrointestinal Tract Equals Na⁺ Output from Renal and Extrarenal Pathways

The two principal solutes in the ECF are Na^+ and Cl^-. **Sodium** is the most abundant ion in the body, totaling some 58 meq/kg body weight. About 65% of the total Na^+ is located in the ECF, and an additional 5 to 10% in the intracellular fluid. Extracellular and intracellular Na^+, comprising 70% to 75% of the total-body pool, is readily "exchangeable," as defined by its ability to equilibrate rapidly with injected radioactive Na^+. The remaining 25% to 30% of the body's Na^+ pool is bound as Na^+-apatites in bone. The concentration of Na^+ in the plasma and interstitial fluid typically ranges between 135 and 145 mM.

Chloride totals approximately 33 meq/kg body weight. Approximately 85% is extracellular, and the remaining 15% is intracellular. Thus, all of Cl^- is readily exchangeable. The $[Cl^-]$ of plasma and interstitial fluid normally varies between 100 and 108 mM. Changes in total-body Cl^- are usually influenced by the same factors, and in the same direction, as changes in total-body Na^+. Exceptions arise during acid-base disturbances, when Cl^- metabolism may change independently of Na^+.

By definition, in the steady state, the total-body content of water and electrolytes is constant. Focusing on Na^+,

Equation 39–1

Oral Na^+ intake = Renal Na^+ output
$$+ \text{ Extrarenal } Na^+ \text{ output}$$

Under normal circumstances, extrarenal Na^+ output is negligible. However, large fluid losses from the GI tract (e.g., vomiting, diarrhea) or skin (e.g., excessive sweating, extensive burns) can represent substantial extrarenal Na^+ losses. The kidney responds to such deficits by reducing renal Na^+ excretion. On the other hand, in conditions of excessive Na^+ intake, the kidneys excrete the surfeit of Na^+.

The Kidneys Increase Na⁺ Excretion in Response to an Increase in Extracellular Fluid Volume, not an Increase in Extracellular Na⁺ Concentration

In contrast to many other renal mechanisms of electrolyte excretion, the renal excretion of Na^+ depends on the *amount* of Na^+ in the body and not on the Na^+ *concentration* in ECF. Because the amount of Na^+ is the product of ECF volume and the extracellular Na^+ concentration, and because the osmoregulatory system keeps plasma osmolality constant within very narrow limits, it is actually the *volume* of ECF that acts as the signal for Na^+ homeostasis.

Figure 39–1A demonstrates the renal response to an abrupt "step" increase and a "step" decrease in Na^+ intake. A subject weighing 70 kg starts with an unusually low Na^+ intake of 10 mmole/day, matched by an equally low urinary output. When the individual abruptly increases dietary Na^+ intake from 10 to 150 mmole/day—and maintains it at this level for several days—urinary Na^+ output also increases, but at first lags behind intake.

This initial period during which Na^+ intake exceeds Na^+ output is a state of **positive Na⁺ balance**. After approximately 5 days, urinary Na^+ output rises to match dietary intake, after which total-body Na^+ does not increase further. In this example, we assume that the cumulative retention of Na^+ amounts to 140 mmole.

The abrupt increase in dietary Na^+ initially elevates plasma osmolality, stimulating thirst and release of AVP. Because the subject has free access to water, and because the kidneys salvage water in response to AVP (p. 840), the volume of solute-free water rises. This increase in "free water" not only prevents a rise in $[Na^+]$ and osmolality, but also produces a weight gain that—in this example—is 1 kg (see Fig. 39–1A). This weight gain corresponds, in our example, to the accumulation of 140 mmole of Na^+ and the accompanying free water, which makes 1 liter of isotonic saline. Note that, in the new steady state, only *extracellular* compartment has increased in volume. *Intracellular* volume does not change because, in the end, there is no driving force for water to cross cell membranes (i.e., extracellular osmolality is normal). It is the slight expansion of the extracellular volume that signals the kidney to increase its rate of Na^+ excretion. The extracellular Na^+ *concentration* is unchanged during this period, and thus cannot be the signal to increase Na^+ excretion.

When the subject in our example later reduces Na^+ intake to the initial level of 10 mmole/day (see Fig. 39–1A), Na^+ excretion diminishes until the initial balanced state (input = output) is re-established once again. Immediately after the reduction in Na^+ intake, Na^+ is temporarily out of balance. This time, it is a period of **negative Na⁺ balance**, where output exceeds input. During this period, the ECF volume falls by 1 liter, and body weight returns to normal. Note again that the extracellular Na^+ *concentration* is unchanged during this transient period.

Ingesting increasingly larger amounts of Na^+ results in *retaining* progressively larger amounts in the steady state, and thus accumulating progressively more ECF volume. Urinary Na^+ excretion increases linearly with this rise in ECF volume or body weight; the *slope* in Figure 39–1B is idealized for the subject in Figure 39–1A. The control system that so tightly links urinary Na^+ excretion to ECF volume is extremely sensitive. In our example (see Fig. 39–1A)—a 70-kg individual with an initial ECF volume of 17 liters—expanding ECF volume by 1 liter, or approximately 6%, triggers a 15-fold increase in steady-state urinary Na^+ excretion (i.e., from 10 mmole/day to 150 mmole/day in Fig. 39–1A). Normal individuals can be in Na^+ balance on a nearly Na^+-free diet (1–2 mmole/day) without overt signs of ECF volume depletion. Conversely, even on a high Na^+ diet (200 mmole/day versus the "normal" approximately 100 mmole/day for a Western diet), clinical signs of ECF volume excess, such as edema, are absent.

It Is Not the Extracellular Fluid Volume As a Whole, but "Effective Circulating Volume," That Regulates Na⁺ Excretion

Although we have referred to the overall expansion of the ECF volume as the signal for increased urinary Na^+ excretion, this is an oversimplification. Only certain regions

VOLUME EXPANSION
AND CONTRACTION

When Na$^+$ intake persists in the face of impaired renal Na$^+$ excretion (e.g., during renal failure), the body retains isosmotic fluid. The result is an expansion of plasma volume and the interstitial fluid compartment. In the extreme, the interstitial-volume increase can become so severe that the subepidermal tissues swell (e.g., around the ankles). When the physician presses with a finger against the skin, and then removes the finger, the finger imprint remains in the tissue ("**pitting edema**"). Not all cases of lower-extremity edema reflect Na$^+$ and fluid retention. Particularly in the elderly, peripheral vascular insufficiency is a common cause and does not reflect total body fluid overload, but rather a local malfunction, usually of the veins. These patients should elevate their feet whenever possible, and use compression stockings.

Fluid can also accumulate in certain "transcellular" spaces (p. 52), such as the pleural cavity (pleural effusion) or the peritoneal cavity (ascites), reflecting derangements of local Starling forces (see box on p. 473) that determine the fluid distribution between the plasma and the extracellular fluid (ECF). In cases of abnormal Na$^+$ retention, putting the subject on a low-Na$^+$ diet can partially correct the edema. Diuretics can also reduce volume overload, as long as the kidney retains sufficient function to respond to them.

An excessive loss of Na$^+$ into the urine can be caused by disturbances of Na$^+$ reabsorption along the nephron, leading to a dramatic shrinkage of the ECF volume. Because the plasma volume is part of the ECF volume, significant reductions can severely affect the circulation, culminating in **hypovolemic shock** (p. 586). Renal causes of reduced ECF volume include the prolonged use of powerful "loop" diuretics (p. 778) and osmotic diuretics (p. 782) and various renal-tubule malfunctions, including proximal renal tubular acidosis and the recovery phase following acute renal failure.

of the extracellular compartment are important for this signalling. For an expansion in ECF volume to stimulate Na$^+$ excretion, the expansion must make itself evident in the part of the ECF compartment where the "ECF-volume sensors" are located.

The thoracic blood vessels appear to be the site of greatest importance. For example, in congestive heart failure, particularly when edema is extensive, the total extracellular volume is greatly increased. However, the low cardiac output fails to expand the thoracic blood vessels. As a result, Na$^+$ reabsorption by the renal tubules remains high (i.e., urinary Na$^+$ excretion is inappropriately low compared with Na$^+$ intake), exacerbating the systemic congestion.

Another example of the importance of the thoracic vessels for regulating renal Na$^+$ excretion is the effect of gravity in modulating venous return. Urinary Na$^+$ excretion is lowest when one is standing (when thoracic perfusion is lowest), higher when one is lying down (recumbency), and highest when immersing one's self up to the chin for several hours in warm water. During immersion, the hydrostatic pressure of the water compresses the tissues—and thus the vessels, particularly the veins—in the extremities and abdomen, enhancing venous return to the thorax. The thoracic vessels are immune to this compression because their extravascular pressure (i.e., intrapleural pressure) (p. 612) is unaffected by the water. Thus, it is the enhanced venous return alone that stimulates vascular sensors to increase Na$^+$ excretion.

In the above three examples of the effects of gravity, Na$^+$ excretion varies widely even though the total ECF volume is the same. Thus, *extracellular fluid volume* per se is not the critical factor in regulating renal Na$^+$ excretion. Recumbency—and, to a greater extent, water immersion—shifts blood into the thoracic vessels, increasing the so-called "central blood volume" (p. 450). In contrast, the upright position depletes the intrathoracic blood volume. This example clearly demonstrates that only special portions within the ECF compartment play critical roles in the sensing of ECF volume.

The critical parameter that the body recognizes as an index of changes in Na$^+$ content is the **effective circulating volume**. The effective circulating volume is not something that can be identified anatomically. Rather, it is a *functional* blood volume that reflects the extent of tissue perfusion in specific regions, as evidenced by the fullness or pressure within their blood vessels. Normally, changes in the effective circulatory volume parallel those in total ECF volume. However, this relationship may be distorted in certain diseases. For example, in patients with congestive heart failure (see earlier), nephrotic syndrome, or liver cirrhosis, *total* ECF volume is grossly expanded (e.g., edema or ascites). In contrast, the *effective* circulatory volume is low, resulting in Na$^+$ retention.

Low- and High-Pressure Baroreceptors Sense Decreases in Effective Circulating Volume and Use Four Parallel Effector Pathways to Decrease Renal Na$^+$ Excretion

Figure 39–2 summarizes the elements of the feedback loop that controls the effective circulating volume. As summarized in Table 39–2, sensors that monitor changes in effective circulating volume are **baroreceptors** located in both high-pressure (p. 535) and low-pressure (p. 548) areas of the circulation. Although most are located within the vascular tree of the thorax, additional baroreceptors are present in the kidney—particularly in the afferent arterioles (p. 746)—central nervous system, and liver. These sensors generate four distinct hormonal or neural signals (see Figure 39–2, *pathways 1–4*).

In the first pathway, a reduced effective circulating volume directly stimulates a hormonal effector pathway, the **renin-angiotensin-aldosterone system**.

The second and third effector pathways are neural. Baroreceptors detect decreases in effective circulating volume and communicate these via afferent neurons to the medulla of the brain stem. From the medulla, two types of efferent signals emerge that ultimately act on the kidney. In one, increased activity of the **sympathetic division** of the autonomic nervous system reduces renal

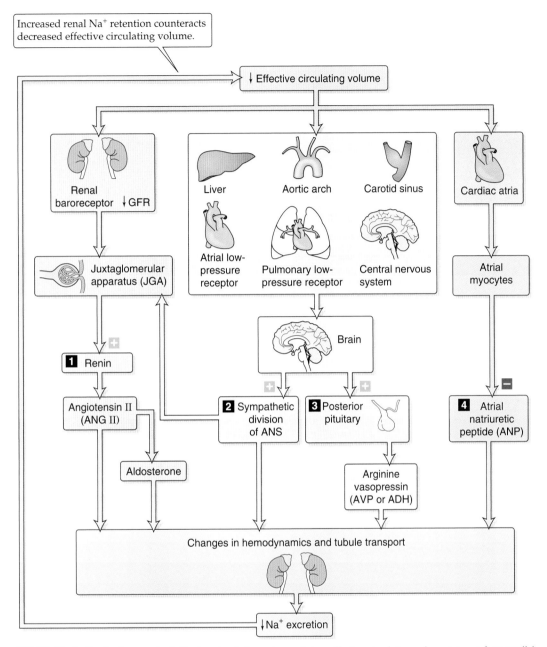

FIGURE 39–2. Feedback control of effective circulating volume. A low effective circulating volume triggers four parallel effector pathways (numbered *1–4*) that act on the kidney, either by changing the hemodynamics or by changing Na$^+$ transport by the renal tubule cells. ANS, autonomic nervous system; GFR, glomerular filtration rate.

blood flow, and thus reduces Na$^+$ excretion. In the other effector pathway, the **posterior pituitary** increases its secretion of AVP, and thus conserves water. The latter mechanism becomes active only after large declines in effective circulating volume.

The final pathway is hormonal. Reduced effective circulating volume decreases the release of **atrial natriuretic peptide** (ANP), thus reducing Na$^+$ excretion.

All four parallel effector pathways modulate renal Na$^+$ excretion, correcting the primary change in effective circulating blood volume. Thus, an increase in effective circulatory volume promotes Na$^+$ excretion (thus reducing ECF volume), whereas a decrease in effective circulatory volume inhibits Na$^+$ excretion (thus raising ECF volume).

An important feature of renal Na$^+$ excretion is the two-way redundancy of control mechanisms. First, several efferent pathways may act in concert on a single effector within the kidney. For instance, both sympathetic input and hemodynamic/physical factors often act on proximal tubules. Second, one efferent pathway may act at different effector sites—for example, regulating Na$^+$ reabsorption *directly* by modulating Na$^+$ transport by tubule cells and *indirectly* by modulating renal hemodynamic parameters. In particular, angiotensin II (ANG II) enhances Na$^+$ retention not only by stimulating Na-H exchange in tubule cells, but also by lowering renal plasma flow (p. 765).

The next two sections are focused on the four parallel effector pathways. In the third, we discuss how purely

TABLE 39–2

ECF VOLUME RECEPTORS

"Central" vascular sensors
Low-pressure (very important)
Cardiac atria
Pulmonary vasculature
High-pressure (less important)
Carotid sinus
Aortic arch
Juxtaglomerular apparatus (renal afferent arteriole)

Sensors in the CNS (less important)

Sensors in the liver (less important)

CNS, central nervous system; ECF, extracellular fluid.

hemodynamic/physical factors modulate effective circulating volume.

Increased Activity of the Renin-Angiotensin-Aldosterone Axis Is the First of Four Parallel Pathways That Correct a Low Effective Circulating Volume

The **renin-angiotensin-aldosterone** axis (Fig. 39–3) promotes Na$^+$ retention via the actions of both ANG II and aldosterone. In Chapter 49, we discuss this axis in the context of the physiology of the adrenal cortex (p. 1059).

Angiotensinogen, also known as "renin substrate," is an α_2-globulin that is synthesized by the liver and released into the systemic circulation. The liver contains only small stores of angiotensinogen. Another protein, **renin**, is produced and stored in distinctive granules by the **granular cells** of the juxtaglomerular apparatus (JGA) of the kidney (p. 743). As discussed later, decreases in effective circulating volume stimulate these cells to release

renin, which is a protease that catalyzes the conversion of angiotensinogen to the decapeptide, **angiotensin I** (ANG I). **Angiotensin-converting enzyme** (ACE) rapidly converts the physiologically inactive ANG I to the physiologically active octapeptide **ANG II**. ACE is present on the luminal surface of vascular endothelia throughout the body and is abundantly present in the endothelium-rich lungs. ACE in the kidney—particularly in the endothelial cells of the afferent and efferent arterioles—can produce enough ANG II to exert *local* vascular effects. Thus, the kidney receives ANG II from two sources: (1) Systemic ANG II comes from the general circulation and originates largely from the pulmonary region. (2) Local ANG II forms from the renal conversion of systemic angiotensin I. In addition, the proximal tubule secretes ANG II into its lumen, achieving intraluminal concentrations in excess of those in the general circulation. ANG II in the circulation has a short half-life (~2 min) because aminopeptidases further cleave it to the heptapeptide ANG III, which is still biologically active.

The principal factor controlling ANG II levels is renin release from the granular cells of the JGA. A decrease in effective circulating volume manifests itself to the JGA—and thus stimulates renin release—in three ways (see Fig. 39–2):

1. **Decreased systemic blood pressure (sympathetic effect on JGA).** A low effective circulating volume, sensed by baroreceptors located in the central arterial circulation (p. 536), signals medullary control centers to increase sympathetic outflow to the JGA, thus increasing renin release. Renal denervation or β-adrenergic blocking drugs (e.g., propranolol) inhibit renin release.
2. **Decreased NaCl concentration at macula densa ("NaCl sensor").** Independent of renal-nerve activity, changes in luminal [NaCl] at the macula densa directly modulate renin release.

FIGURE 39–3. The renin-angiotensin-aldosterone axis. ACE, angiotensin-converting enzyme; JGA, juxtaglomerular apparatus.

3. **Decreased renal perfusion pressure ("renal" barore-ceptor).** Stretch receptors in the granular cells (p. 743) of the *afferent* arterioles sense the decreased distention associated with low effective circulating volume. Decreased stretch of these receptors lowers $[Ca^{2+}]_i$, leading to an increase in renin release and initiating the cascade that tends to increase blood pressure. Conversely, increased distention (high extracellular volume) inhibits renin release.

The above stimulation of renin release by a *decrease* in $[Ca^{2+}]_i$ is unusual. In contrast to most Ca^{2+}-activated secretory processes, in which an increase in $[Ca^{2+}]_i$ stimulates secretion (p. 222), an increase in $[Ca^{2+}]_i$ in granular cells inhibits renin secretion. Another example is the chief cell of the parathyroid gland, in which an increase in $[Ca^{2+}]_i$ inhibits secretion of parathyroid hormone (p. 1092).

In addition to Ca^{2+}, intracellular cyclic adenosine monophosphate (cAMP) also appears to be a second messenger for renin release. Thus, agents that activate adenylyl cyclase (e.g., forskolin, β-adrenergic agonists, A_2 adenosine receptor agonists, dopamine, and glucagon), exogenous cAMP, and phosphodiesterase inhibitors all enhance renin secretion, presumably through protein kinase A. The question whether the effects of $[cAMP]_i$ and $[Ca^{2+}]_i$ are independent or sequential remains open.

Additional factors also modulate renin release. Prostaglandins E_2 and I_2 and endothelin all activate renin release. Agents that blunt renin release include ANG II (which represents a short feedback loop), AVP, thromboxane A_2, high plasma levels of K^+, and NO.

Angiotensin II has several important actions:

1. **Stimulation of aldosterone release from glomerulosa cells in the adrenal cortex** (p. 1059). In turn, aldosterone promotes Na^+ reabsorption in the collecting tubules and ducts (p. 786).
2. **Vasoconstriction of renal and other systemic vessels.** ANG II increases Na^+ reabsorption by altering renal hemodynamics, probably in two ways (Fig. 39–4). First, at high concentrations, ANG II constricts the efferent more than the afferent arterioles, thus increasing filtration fraction and reducing the *hydrostatic pressure* in the downstream peritubular capillaries. The increased filtration fraction also increases the protein concentration in the downstream blood, and hence increases the *colloid osmotic pressure* of the peritubular capillaries. The combination of these two Starling forces favors uptake of the reabsorbate from the peritubular interstitium into the peritubular capillaries (p. 784), and hence enhances the reabsorption of Na^+ and fluid by the proximal tubule. Second, ANG II decreases medullary blood flow through vasa recta. Low blood flow decreases the medullary washout of NaCl and urea (p. 837), thus raising the urea concentration in the medullary interstitium and enhancing Na^+ reabsorption along the thin ascending limb of the loop of Henle (p. 833).
3. **Enhanced tubuloglomerular feedback.** ANG II raises the sensitivity and lowers the set point of the tubuloglomerular feedback mechanism (p. 769), so that an increase in Na^+ and fluid delivery to the macula densa elicits a more pronounced fall in the glomerular filtration rate (GFR).

4. **Enhanced Na-H exchange.** ANG II stimulates the Na-H exchangers in the proximal tubule and thick ascending limb, as well as in the Na^+ channels in the initial collecting tubule. The effect is to promote Na^+ reabsorption.
5. **Renal hypertrophy.** ANG II induces hypertrophy of renal-tubule cells.
6. **Stimulated thirst and AVP release.** ANG II acts on the hypothalamus, where it increases the sensation of thirst and stimulates the secretion of AVP from the posterior pituitary, both of which increase total-body free water. Thus, this ANG II effect represents an intersection between the systems for regulating effective circulating volume and osmolality.

Increased Sympathetic Nerve Activity and Arginine Vasopressin, As Well As Decreased Atrial Natriuretic Peptide, Are the Other Three Parallel Pathways That Correct a Low Effective Circulating Volume

RENAL SYMPATHETIC NERVE ACTIVITY. The second of the four parallel effector pathways for the control of effective circulating volume is the sympathetic nervous system. Enhanced activity of the renal sympathetic nerves has three major effects (p. 787): (1) increased renal vascular resistance, (2) enhanced renin release from granular cells (see previous section), and (3) increased tubule reabsorption of Na^+. Taken together, the multiple actions of sympathetic traffic to the kidney retain Na^+, and thus increase effective circulating volume, by reducing the GFR and by enhancing Na^+ reabsorption.

In everyday life (i.e., the unstressed state), the role of sympathetic nerve activity in kidney function appears to be modest at best. However, sympathetic innervation may play a role during challenges to volume homeostasis. For example, low Na^+ intake triggers reduced renal Na^+ excretion; renal denervation blunts this response. Another example is hemorrhage, where renal sympathetic nerves emerge as important participants in preserving ECF volume. However, expansion of the intravascular volume increases renal Na^+ excretion; renal denervation sharply reduces this response as well.

ARGININE VASOPRESSIN (ANTIDIURETIC HORMONE). The posterior pituitary releases AVP primarily in response to increases in extracellular *osmolality*. Indeed, AVP mainly increases distal-nephron water permeability, thus promoting water retention (p. 840). However, the posterior pituitary also releases AVP in response to large reductions in effective circulating volume (e.g., hemorrhage), and a secondary action of AVP, promoting Na^+ retention (p. 787), is appropriate for this stimulus.

ATRIAL NATRIURETIC PEPTIDE. As discussed, renal sympathetic nerve activity, AVP, and the renin-angiotensin-aldosterone axis all contribute to Na^+ retention (see Fig. 39–2). In contrast, ANP, as its name implies, promotes **natriuresis** (i.e., Na^+ excretion). Atrial myocytes synthesize and store ANP and release ANP in response to stretch (a low-pressure volume sensor) (p. 549). Thus, reduced effective circulating volume inhibits the release of ANP, and reduces Na^+ excretion. ANP plays a role in the

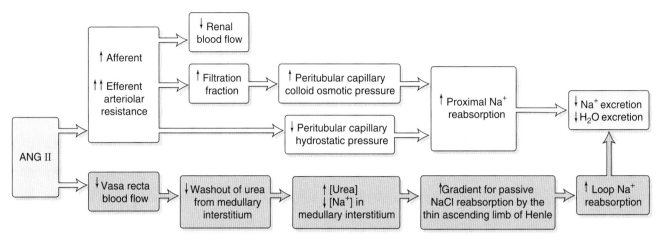

FIGURE 39–4. Hemodynamic actions of ANG II on Na⁺ reabsorption. ANG, angiotensin.

RENAL HYPERTENSION

In the 1930s, Goldblatt produced hypertension experimentally in unilaterally nephrectomized animals by placing a surgical clip around the renal artery of the remaining kidney (**one-kidney Goldblatt hypertension**). The constriction can be adjusted so that it does not result in renal ischemia, but only in a reduction of the perfusion pressure distal to the clip. This maneuver stimulates the renal baroreceptors, leading to a rapid increase in synthesis and secretion of renin from the clipped kidney. The renin release reaches a peak after 1 hour. As renin cleaves angiotensin I from angiotensinogen, systemic angiotensin I levels rise quickly. Angiotensin converting enzyme (ACE), present mainly in the lungs but also in the kidneys, then rapidly converts angiotensin I (ANG I) into angiotensin II (ANG II). Thus, within minutes of clamping the renal artery, one observes a sustained rise in systemic arterial pressure. The newly established stable elevation in systemic pressure will then normalize the pressure in the renal artery downstream from the constriction. From this time on, circulating renin and ANG II levels will decline toward normal over 5 to 7 days, while the systemic arterial pressure remains abnormally high. The early rise in blood pressure is the result of the renin-angiotensin vasoconstrictor mechanism, which is activated by the experimentally induced reduction in pressure and flow in the renal artery distal to the constriction. The later phase of systemic hypertension is the result of aldosterone release and the retention of salt and water.

Unilateral partial clamping of a renal artery in an otherwise healthy animal also produces hypertension (**two-kidney Goldblatt hypertension**). As in the one-kidney model, the clipped kidney increases its synthesis and secretion of renin. Renin then causes ANG II levels to increase systemically and will, in addition to the effect on the clamped kidney, cause the nonclamped, contralateral kidney to retain salt and water. As in the one-kidney model, the resulting hypertension has an early vasoconstrictive phase and a delayed volume-dependent phase.

In both types of Goldblatt hypertension, administration of ACE inhibitors can lower arterial blood pressure. However, inhibiting the converting enzyme is therapeutically effective even after circulating renin and ANG II levels have normalized. Maintaining the hypertension must involve an increased *intrarenal* conversion of ANG I to ANG II (via renal ACE), with the ANG II enhancing proximal Na⁺ reabsorption. Indeed, direct measurements show that, even after *circulating* renin and ANG II levels have returned to normal, the *intrarenal* levels of ACE and ANG II are elevated.

These experimental models serve as paradigms for some forms of human hypertension, including renin-secreting tumors of the juxtaglomerular apparatus and all cases of pathologic impairment of renal arterial blood supply. Thus, coarctation of the aorta, in which the aorta is constricted above the renal arteries but below the arteries to the head and upper extremities, invariably leads to hypertension. Renal hypertension also results from stenosis of a renal artery, caused, for example, by arteriosclerotic thickening of the vessel wall. However, the most common form of renal hypertension occurs, in parts of the kidney, when inflammatory or fibrotic lesions stenose preglomerular arteries or arterioles. Such local intrarenal vasoconstriction may lead to local ischemia, while some parts of the kidney remain entirely normal. This pattern, therefore, closely resembles the two-kidney Goldblatt hypertension model. In fact, high levels of ANG II may be encountered in such patients. The administration of ACE inhibitors is generally beneficial because they lower ANG II levels, systemically and within the kidney itself.

FIGURE 39–5. Sites of action of atrial natriuretic peptide. ANG, angiotensin; GFR, glomerular filtration rate; U_{Na}, urine sodium concentration. (Data from Atlas SA, Maack T: Atrial natriuretic factor. In Handbook of Physiology: Renal Physiology, E, Windhager, Ed., Oxford University Press, N.Y. 1992, pp 1577–1674.)

diuretic response to the redistribution of ECF and plasma volume into the thorax that occurs during water immersion and space flight (p. 1266).

ANP binds to a receptor guanylyl cyclase, elevating intracellular levels of cyclic guanosine monophosphate (cGMP) (p. 108). ANP has many synergistic effects that promote renal Na^+ and water excretion. Figure 39–5 provides an overview of the hemodynamic and transport effects of ANP along the nephron. ANP may have direct effects on Na^+ transport in the medullary collecting duct (p. 788). However, the major effect of ANP is **hemodynamic**. ANP causes renal vasodilation, massively increasing blood flow to both the cortex and the medulla. Increased blood flow to the *cortex* raises GFR and increases the Na^+ load to the proximal tubule and to the thick ascending limb of the loop of Henle (p. 772). Increased blood flow to the *medulla* washes out the medullary interstitium (p. 837), decreasing its osmolality, and ultimately reducing passive Na^+ reabsorption in the thin ascending limb (p. 833). The combined effect of increasing cortical and medullary blood flow is to increase the Na^+ load to the distal nephron, and thus increase urinary Na^+ excretion.

Increases of Arterial Pressure Lead to an Increase of Na⁺ Excretion by Purely Hemodynamic/Physical Mechanisms, Independent of Changes in Effective Circulating Volume

We have seen that expanding the effective circulating volume stimulates sensors that increase Na^+ excretion via four parallel effector pathways (see Fig. 39–2). However, the kidney can also increase Na^+ excretion in response to purely hemodynamic changes. We consider two examples in which changes in arterial blood pressure modulate Na^+ excretion.

LARGE, ACUTE DECREASE IN ARTERIAL BLOOD PRESSURE. Acutely lowering the GFR by partial clamping of the aorta causes a steep decrease in urinary Na^+ excretion (Fig. 39–6, *red curve*). If GFR falls sufficiently, the kidneys excrete only traces of Na^+ in a small volume of urine. If glomerulotubular balance (p. 783) were perfect, Na^+ excretion would fall linearly with GFR (see Fig. 39–6, *blue line*). However, Na^+ excretion, in fact, falls much more steeply. This response primarily reflects the trans-

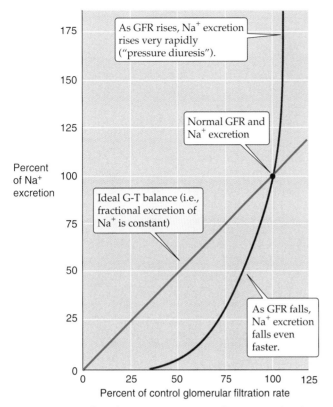

FIGURE 39-6. Effect of changes in glomerular filtration rate (GFR) on urinary Na⁺ excretion. The *blue line* represents ideal glomerulotubular (G–T) balance. The *red curve* summarizes data from dogs. The investigators reduced GFR by inflating a balloon in the aorta, above the level of the renal arteries. They increased GFR by compressing the carotid arteries, and thus increased blood pressure. (Data from Thompson DD, Pitts RF: Effects of alterations of renal arterial pressure on sodium and water excretion. Am J Physiol 168:490–499, 1952.)

port of the distal tubule (p. 786), which continues to reabsorb Na⁺ at a high rate despite the decreased Na⁺ delivery.

LARGE, CHRONIC INCREASE IN ARTERIAL PRESSURE. In some cases, an increased effective circulating volume is accompanied by an increase in the arterial pressure. An example is the hypertension of Liddle's disease, a state of abnormally high distal Na⁺ reabsorption. By a phenomenon known as **pressure diuresis**, the kidney responds to the hypertension by increasing Na⁺ excretion. The hypertension increases GFR, increasing the filtered load of Na⁺, which even alone would increase urinary Na⁺ excretion (see Fig. 39–6, *blue line*). In addition, at least four mechanisms reduce Na⁺ reabsorption along the nephron, further enhancing Na⁺ excretion (see Fig. 39–6, *red curve*). First, the increased effective circulating volume inhibits the renin-angiotensin-aldosterone axis, and thus reduces Na⁺ reabsorption (p. 786). Second, the high blood pressure augments blood flow in the vasa recta, washing out medullary solutes and reducing interstitial hypertonicity in the medulla (p. 837), ultimately reducing passive Na⁺ reabsorption in the thin ascending limb (p. 833). Third, an acute increase in arterial pressure leads, by an unknown mechanism, to a prompt reduction in the number of apical Na-H exchangers in the proximal tubule. Normalizing the blood pressure rapidly reverses this effect.

Finally, the renal vasculature partly transmits high blood pressure to the peritubular capillaries, reducing proximal-tubule reabsorption according to the physical factor theory (p. 784).

CONTROL OF WATER CONTENT (EXTRACELLULAR OSMOLALITY)

Water accounts for half or more of body weight—approximately 60% in men and 50% in women—and is distributed between the intracellular and extracellular fluid compartments (p. 50). Changes in whole-body water content lead to changes in osmolality, to which the CNS is extremely sensitive. Osmolality deviations of ± 15% lead to severe disturbances of CNS function. Thus, osmoregulation is critical.

Two elements control water content, and thus whole-body osmolality: (1) the kidneys, which control water excretion (p. 840), and (2) thirst mechanisms, which control the oral intake of water. These two effector mechanisms are part of negative feedback loops that begin within the hypothalamus. An increase in osmolality stimulates separate osmoreceptors to secrete AVP (which reduces renal excretion of free water) and to trigger thirst (which, if fulfilled, increases intake of free water). As a result, the two complementary feedback loops stabilize osmolality and thus [Na⁺].

Increased Plasma Osmolality Stimulates Osmoreceptors in the Hypothalamus That Trigger the Release of Arginine Vasopressin, Which Inhibits Water Excretion

An increase in the osmolality of the ECF is the primary signal for the secretion of AVP from the posterior pituitary gland. An elegant series of animal studies by Verney in the 1940s established that infusing a hyperosmotic NaCl solution into the *carotid artery* abruptly terminates an established water diuresis (Fig. 39–7A). Infusing hyperosmotic NaCl into the *peripheral circulation* has no effect because the hyperosmolar solution becomes diluted by the time it reaches the cerebral vessels. Therefore, the osmosensitive site is intracranial. Surgically removing the posterior pituitary abolishes the effect of infusing hyperosmotic NaCl into the carotid artery (see Fig. 39–7B). However, injecting posterior-pituitary extracts into the animal inhibits the diuresis, regardless of whether the posterior pituitary is intact. Later work showed that Verney's posterior-pituitary extract contained an "antidiuretic hormone"—now known to be AVP—that the posterior pituitary secretes in response to increased plasma osmolality. When the plasma osmolality falls owing to the intake of large volumes of water, AVP levels fall.

In healthy individuals, plasma osmolality is approximately 290 mOsm. The **threshold** for AVP release is somewhat lower, approximately 280 mOsm (Fig. 39–8, *red curve*). Increasing the osmolality by only 1% above this level is sufficient to produce a detectable increase in plasma [AVP], which rises steeply with further increases in osmolality. Thus, hyperosmolality leads to increased

A BEFORE REMOVAL OF POSTERIOR PITUITARY

B AFTER REMOVAL OF POSTERIOR PITUITARY

FIGURE 39–7. Sensing of blood osmolality in the dog brain. i.a., intra-arterial injection; i.v., intravenous injection; p.o., oral intake. (Data from Verney EG: The antidiuretic hormone and the factors which determine its release. Proc Royal Soc, Lond B 135:25–106, 1947.)

levels of AVP, which completes the feedback loop by instructing the kidneys to retain water (p. 840).

Although it is a change in plasma [NaCl] that is usually responsible for a change in plasma osmolality, other solutes can do the same. For example, hypertonic mannitol resembles NaCl in stimulating AVP release. However, an equivalent increase in extracellular osmolality by urea has little effect on plasma AVP levels. The reason is that urea

FIGURE 39–8. Dependence of arginine vasopressin (AVP) release on plasma osmolality. (Data from Robertson GL, Aycinena P, Zerbe RL: Neurogenic disorders of osmoregulation. Am J Med 72:339–353, 1982.)

has a low effective osmolality or tonicity (p. 77) and is thus ineffective in shrinking cells.

Special Neurons in the Hypothalamus Synthesize Arginine Vasopressin and Transport it Along their Axons to the Posterior Pituitary, Where They Store It in Nerve Terminals Prior to Release

The osmoreceptors of the CNS appear to be located in two areas that breech the blood-brain barrier: the organum vasculosum of the lamina terminalis (OVLT) and the subfornical organ (SFO), two of the "circumventricular organs" (p. 409). Neurons in these regions (Fig. 39–9) are thus able to sense changes in *plasma* osmolality. They apparently behave as osmometers, responding to elevated osmolality by increasing the activity of mechanosensitive cation channels located in their cell membranes, resulting in significant membrane depolarization that increases the frequency of action potentials. Hypoosmolality results in a striking depression of electrical activity. The osmosensitive neurons project to large-diameter neurons in the supraoptic and paraventricular nuclei of the anterior hypothalamus (see Fig. 39–9). These neurons synthesize AVP, package it into granules, and transport the granules along their axons to nerve terminals in the posterior lobe of the pituitary, which is part of the brain (p. 1012). When stimulated by the osmosensitive neurons, these magnocellular neurons release the stored AVP into the posterior pituitary—an area that also lacks a blood-brain barrier—and AVP enters the general circulation.

In humans and most mammals, the antidiuretic hormone is AVP, which is encoded by the messenger RNA for **preproneurophysin** II. After cleavage of the signal peptide, the resulting prohormone contains AVP, neurophysin II (NpII), and a glycopeptide. Cleavage of the prohormone within the secretory granule yields these three components. AVP has nine amino acids, with a disulfide bridge connecting two cysteine residues. Mutations of NpII impair AVP secretion, suggesting that NpII assists in the processing or secretion of AVP.

Levels of circulating AVP depend on both the rate of AVP release from the posterior pituitary and the rate of AVP degradation. The major factor controlling *AVP release* is plasma osmolality. However, as discussed later, other factors also can modulate AVP secretion.

Two organs, the liver and the kidney, contribute to the *breakdown of AVP* and the rapid decline of AVP levels when secretion has ceased. The half-life of AVP in the circulation is 18 minutes. Diseases of the liver and kidney may impair AVP degradation and thus contribute to fluid retention. For example, the congestion of the liver and impairment of renal function that accompany heart failure can compromise AVP breakdown and lead to inappropriately high circulating levels of AVP.

Increased Osmolality Stimulates a Second Group of Osmoreceptors That Trigger Thirst, Which Promotes Water Intake

The second efferent pathway of the osmoregulatory system is **thirst**, which regulates the oral intake of water.

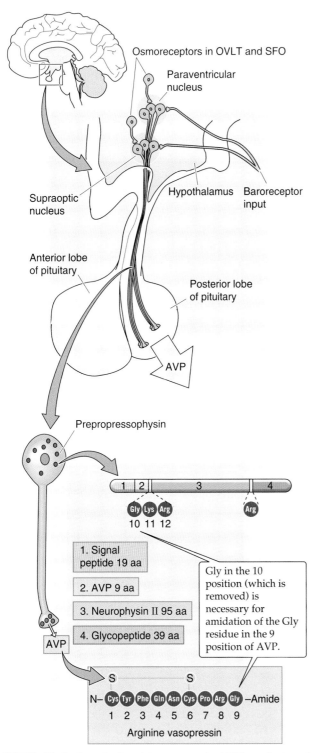

FIGURE 39–9. Control of arginine vasopressin (AVP) synthesis and release by osmoreceptors. Osmoreceptors are located in the organum vasculosum laminae terminalis (OVLT) and subfornical organ (SFO), two areas that breech the blood-brain barrier.

Like the osmoreceptors that trigger AVP release, the osmoreceptors that trigger thirst are located in two circumventricular organs, the OVLT and the SFO. Also like the osmoreceptors that trigger AVP release, those that trigger thirst respond to the cell shrinkage that is caused by

hyperosmolar solutions. However, these "thirst osmoreceptor" neurons are distinct from the adjacent "AVP osmoreceptor" neurons in the OVLT and SFO.

Hyperosmolality triggers two parallel feedback-control mechanisms that have a common end point (Fig. 39–10): an increase in whole-body free water. In response to hyperosmolality, the AVP osmoreceptors in the hypothalamus trigger other neurons to release AVP. The result is the insertion of aquaporin 2 (AQP2) water channels in the collecting duct of the kidney, an increase in the reabsorption of water, and, therefore, a reduced *excretion* of free water. In response to hyperosmolality, the thirst osmoreceptors stimulate an appetite for water, which leads to the increased *intake* of free water. The net effect is an increase in whole-body free water and, therefore, a reduction in osmolality.

Several Nonosmotic Stimuli Also Enhance Arginine Vasopressin Secretion

Although an increase in plasma osmolality is the primary trigger for AVP release, several other stimuli increase AVP release, including a decrease in effective circulating volume or **arterial pressure** and pregnancy. Conversely, volume expansion diminishes AVP release.

REDUCED EFFECTIVE CIRCULATING VOLUME. As noted earlier, a mere 1% rise in plasma *osmolality* stimulates AVP release by a detectable amount. However, fairly large reductions in effective circulating volume (5%–10%) are required to stimulate AVP release of similar amounts. However, once the rather high threshold for nonosmotic release of AVP is exceeded, AVP release rises steeply with further volume depletion. The interaction between osmotic and volume stimuli on AVP release is illustrated in Figure 39–8, which shows that the effective circulating volume modifies the **slope** of the relationship between plasma AVP levels and osmolality, as well as the osmotic **threshold** for AVP release. At a fixed osmolality, volume contraction (Fig. 39–8, *green curve*) increases the rate of AVP release. Therefore, during volume depletion, a low plasma osmolality that would normally inhibit the release of AVP allows AVP secretion to continue. This leftward shift of the osmolality threshold for AVP release is accompanied by an increased slope, reflecting an increased sensitivity of the osmoreceptors to changes in osmolality.

The *left side* of Figure 39–10 summarizes the pathways by which decreased effective circulating volume and low arterial pressure enhance AVP release. A reduction in left atrial pressure—produced by volume depletion—via low-pressure receptors in the left atrium decreases the firing rate of vagal afferents (p. 548). These afferents signal brainstem neurons, causing neurons in the hypothalamus to release AVP. Indeed, at constant osmolality, AVP secretion varies inversely with left-atrial pressure. In addition, low effective circulating volume triggers granular cells in the JGA to release renin, which leads to the formation of ANG II, which acts on receptors in the OVLT and the SFO to stimulate AVP release. Even more important, a fall in the arterial pressure causes high-pressure carotid-sinus baroreceptors to similarly stimulate AVP release (p. 535).

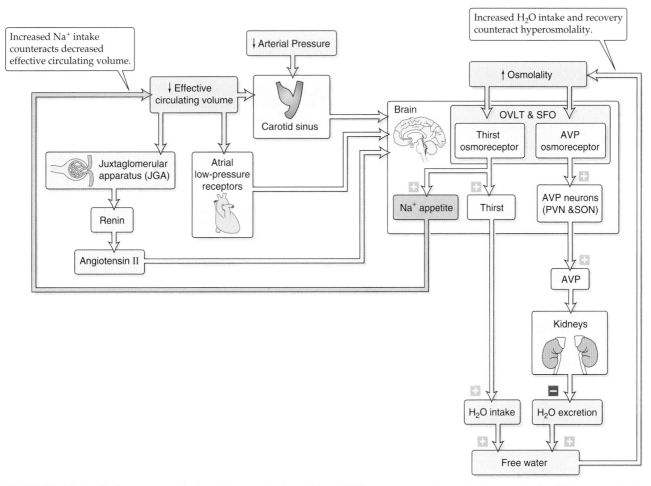

FIGURE 39–10. Feedback systems involved in the control of osmolality. OVLT, organum vasculosum laminae terminalis; PVN, paraventricular nucleus; SFO, subfornical organ; SON, supraoptic nucleus of the hypothalamus.

Two clinical examples in which reduced effective circulating volume leads to increases in AVP are severe **hemorrhagic shock** and **hypovolemic shock** (e.g., shock due to excessive loss of ECF, as in cholera). In both cases, the water retention caused by AVP release accounts for the accompanying hyponatremia. In the first part of this chapter, we said that the appropriate renal response to decreased effective circulating volume is to retain Na$^+$ (i.e., isotonic saline). Why is it that, in response to shock, the body also retains free water? Compared with isotonic saline, free water is less effective as an expander of the ECF volume (p. 79). Nevertheless, in times of profound need, the body uses free water retention to help expand extracellular (and plasma) volume. Clearly, the body is willing to tolerate some hypoosmolality of the body fluids as the price for maintaining an adequate blood volume.

A clinical example in which reduced effective circulating volume can lead to an *inappropriate* increase in AVP levels is **congestive heart failure** (p. 864). In this situation, the water retention may be so severe that the patient develops **hyponatremia** (i.e., hypoosmolality).

VOLUME EXPANSION. In contrast to volume contraction, chronic volume *expansion* reduces AVP secretion, as a consequence of the rightward shift of the threshold to higher osmolalities and of a decline in the slope (Fig. 39–8, *blue curve*). In other words, volume expansion decreases the sensitivity of the central osmoreceptors to changes in plasma osmolality. A clinical example is **hyperaldosteronism**. With normal thirst and water excretion, the chronic Na$^+$ retention resulting from the hyperaldosteronism would expand the ECF volume isotonically, leaving plasma [Na$^+$] unchanged. However, because chronic volume expansion downregulates AVP release, the kidneys do not retain adequate water, resulting in **hypernatremia** (i.e., elevated plasma [Na$^+$]) and hyperosmolality.

PREGNANCY. A leftward shift in the threshold for AVP release and thirst often occurs during pregnancy. These changes probably reflect the action of chorionic gonadotrophin on the sensitivity of the osmoreceptors. Pregnancy is, therefore, often associated with a decrease of 8 to 10 mOsm in plasma osmolality. A similar but smaller change may also occur in the late phase of the menstrual cycle.

OTHER FACTORS. Pain, nausea, and several drugs (e.g., morphine, nicotine, and high doses of barbiturates) *stimulate* AVP secretion. In contrast, alcohol and drugs that block the effect of morphine (opiate-antagonists) inhibit AVP secretion, promoting diuresis. Of great clinical importance is the hypersecretion of AVP that may occur

DIURETICS

Diuretics reversibly inhibit Na^+ reabsorption at specific sites along the nephron, increasing the excretion of Na^+ and water, creating a state of negative Na^+ balance and thereby reducing the volume of extracellular fluid (ECF). Clinicians use diuretics to treat edema (see box on p. 473) in patients with heart failure, cirrhosis of the liver, or nephrotic syndrome. Common to these edematous diseases is an abnormal shift of ECF away from the *effective* circulating volume, thereby activating the feedback pathways. The result is Na^+ retention and expansion of *total* extracellular volume. However, this expansion, which results in edema formation, falls short of correcting the underlying decrease in the *effective* circulating volume. Why most of this "added" extracellular volume remains "ineffective"—and does not restore the effective circulating volume—is not intuitive but reflects the underlying pathology that initiated the edema in the first place. Thus, treating these diseases requires generating a negative Na^+ balance, which can often be achieved by rigid dietary Na^+ restriction and/or the use of diuretics. Diuretics are also useful in treating hypertension. Even though the primary cause of the hypertension may not always be an increase in the effective circulating volume, enhanced Na^+ excretion is frequently effective in lowering blood pressure.

CLASSIFICATION OF DIURETICS
The site and mechanism of a diuretic's action determines the magnitude and nature of the response (Table 39–3). Both chemically and functionally, diuretics are very heterogeneous. For example, acetazolamide produces diuresis by inhibiting carbonic anhydrase and thus the component of proximal-tubule Na^+ reabsorption that is coupled to HCO_3^- reabsorption. The diuretic effect of hydrochlorothiazide is largely due to its ability to inhibit Na/Cl cotransport in the distal convoluted tubule. Spironolactone (which resembles aldosterone) competitively inhibits mineralocorticoid receptors in principal cells of the initial and cortical collecting tubule. Mannitol (reduced fructose) is a powerful osmotic diuretic that reduces net Na^+ transport along water-permeable nephron segments by retaining water in the lumen.

An "ideal" diuretic should promote the excretion of urine whose composition resembles that of the ECF. Such diuretics do not exist. In reality, diuretics not only inhibit the reabsorption of Na^+ and its osmotically obligated water, but also interfere with the renal handling of Cl^-, H^+, K^+, and Ca^{++}, as well as with urinary concentrating ability. Thus, many diuretics disturb the normal plasma electrolyte pattern. Table 39–4 summarizes the most frequent side effects of diuretic use on the electrolyte composition of the ECF. These electrolyte derangements are the predictable consequences of the mechanism of action of individual diuretics at specific tubule sites.

DELIVERY OF DIURETICS
Diuretics generally inhibit transporters or channels at the apical membrane of tubule cells. How do the diuretics get there? Plasma proteins bind many diuretics so that the free concentration of the diuretic in plasma water may be fairly low. Thus, glomerular filtration may deliver only a modest amount to the tubule fluid. However, organic-anion or organic-cation transporters in the S3 segment of the proximal tubule can secrete diuretics and thereby produce high luminal concentrations. For example, the basolateral organic-*anion* transporter system that carries PAH (p. 799) also secretes the diuretics furosemide, ethacrynic acid, and spironolactone. The organic *cation* transporter (p. 802) secretes amiloride. The subsequent reabsorption of fluid in the loop of Henle and downstream nephron segments further concentrates diuretics in the tubule lumen. Not surprisingly, renal disease may compromise the delivery of diuretics.

RESPONSE OF NEPHRON SEGMENTS DOWNSTREAM FROM A DIURETIC'S SITE OF ACTION
The proximal tubule reabsorbs the largest fraction of filtered Na^+, with the loop of Henle, the distal convoluted tubule, and the collecting ducts retrieving smaller fractions. Thus, intuition might suggest that the proximal tubule would be the best target for diuretics. However, secondary effects in "downstream" nephron segments can substantially mitigate the primary effect of a diuretic. Inhibiting Na^+ transport by the proximal tubule raises Na^+ delivery to downstream segments and almost always stimulates Na^+ reabsorption there (p. 786). As a result of this downstream Na^+ reclamation, the overall diuretic action of proximally acting diuretics (e.g., acetazolamide) is relatively weak.

A diuretic is most potent if it acts downstream of the proximal tubule, a condition met by "loop" diuretics, which inhibit Na^+ transport along the thick ascending limb of Henle's loop (TAL). Although the TAL normally reabsorbs only 15% to 25% of the filtered load of Na^+, the reabsorptive capacity of the more distal nephron segments is limited. Thus, the loop diuretics are presently the most powerful diuretic agents. Because nephron segments distal to the TAL have only modest rates of Na^+ reabsorption, diuretics that target these segments are not as potent as the loop diuretics. Nevertheless, distally acting diuretics are important because their effects are long lasting and because they are "K^+-sparing" (i.e., they tend to conserve body K^+).

It is sometimes advantageous to use two diuretics that act at different sites along the nephron, generating a synergistic effect. Thus, if a loop diuretic alone is providing an inadequate diuresis, one could complement its action with acetazolamide, which can deliver a larger Na^+ load to the inhibited loop.

BLUNTING OF DIURETIC ACTION WITH CHRONIC USE
The prolonged administration of a diuretic may lead to a sustained loss of body weight, but only a transient natriuresis. Most of the decline in Na^+ excretion occurs because the drug-induced fall in effective circulating volume triggers Na^+ retention mediated by increased sympathetic outflow to the kidneys (which lowers GFR), increased secretion of aldosterone and AVP, and decreased secretion of ANP. Hypertrophy and/or increased activity of tubule segments downstream of the main site of action of the diuretic can also contribute to the diminished efficacy of the drug during chronic administration.

TABLE 39–3

ACTION OF DIURETICS

SITE	TARGET	DRUG	PHYSIOLOGICAL REGULATION OF "TARGET"		TEXT REFERENCE TO TARGET
			Stimulator	Inhibitor	
PCT	Carbonic anhydrase	Acetazolamide			p. 853
PCT	Na-H exchanger	Dopamine	ANG II, Sympathetic nerve activity, α-adrenergic agonists	Dopamine	p. 852
TAL	Na/K/Cl cotransporter	"Loop Diuretics": Furosemide Bumetanide Ethacrynic acid	Aldosterone	PGE_2	p. 778
DCT	Na/Cl cotransporter	Thiazides Metolazone	Aldosterone		p. 779
CCT	Na^+ channel	Amiloride Triamterene Spironolactone	Aldosterone		p. 779
IMCD	cGMP-gated cation channel	Amiloride	Aldosterone	ANP	p. 788
Water-permeable segments	Water channels	Osmotic diuretics (mannitol)	Physical factors, AVP		Box on p. 782

ANG II, angiotensin II; ANP, atrial natriuretic peptide; AVP, arginine vasopressin; cGMP, cyclic guanosine monophosphate; CCT, cortical collecting tubule; DCT, distal convoluted tubule; IMCD, inner meduallary collecting duct; PCT, proximal convoluted tubule; PGE_2, prostaglandin E_2; TAL, thick ascending limb of the loop of Henle.

TABLE 39–4

COMPLICATIONS OF DIURETIC THERAPY

COMPLICATION	CAUSATIVE DIURETIC	SYMPTOMS	CAUSATIVE FACTORS
Extracellular volume depletion	Loop diuretics and thiazides	Lassitude, thirst, muscle cramps, hypotension	Rapid reduction of plasma volume
K^+ depletion	Acetazolamide, loop diuretics, thiazides	Muscle weakness, paralysis, cardiac arrhythmias	Flow and Na^+-related stimulation of distal K^+ secretion
K^+ retention	Amiloride, triamterene, spironolactone	Cardiac arrhythmias, muscle cramps, and paralysis	Blocking ENaC in the collecting duct
Hyponatremia	Thiazides, furosemide	CNS symptoms, coma	Block of Na^+ transport in water-impermeable nephron segment
Metabolic alkalosis	Loop diuretics, thiazides	Cardiac arrhythmias, CNS symptoms	Excessive Cl^- excretion, secondary volume contraction
Metabolic acidosis	Acetazolamide, amiloride, triamterene	Hyperventilation, muscular and neurologic disturbances	Interference with H^+ secretion
Hypercalcemia	Thiazides	Abnormal tissue calcification, disturbances of nerve and muscle function	Increased Ca^{2+} reabsorption in distal convoluted tubule
Hyperuricemia	Thiazides, loop diuretics	Gout	Consequence of decreased ECV that activates proximal fluid and uric acid reabsorption

CNS, central nervous system; ECV, extracellular volume; ENaC, epithelial Na^+ channel.

after surgery. Also, ectopic metastases of some malignant tumors secrete large amounts of AVP. Such secretion of inappropriate amounts of "antidiuretic hormone" leads to pathologic retention of water with dilution of the plasma electrolytes, particularly Na^+. If progressive and uncorrected, this condition may lead to life-threatening deterioration of cerebral function (see the box on p. 844).

Decreased Effective Circulating Volume and Low Arterial Pressure Also Trigger Thirst

Large decreases in effective circulating volume and blood pressure not only stimulate the release of AVP, they also profoundly stimulate the sensation of thirst. In fact, hemorrhage is one of the most powerful stimuli of hypovolemic thirst: "Thirst among the wounded on the battlefield is legendary" (Fitzsimons). Therefore, three distinct stimuli—hyperosmolality, profound volume contraction, and large decreases in blood pressure—lead to the sensation of thirst. Low effective circulating volume and low blood pressure stimulate thirst centers in the hypothalamus via the same pathways by which they stimulate AVP release (see Fig. 39–10).

In addition to thirst, some of these hypothalamic areas are also involved in stimulating the desire to ingest salt (i.e., Na^+ appetite). In Chapter 57, we discuss the role of the hypothalamus in the control of appetite (p. 1227).

Defense of the Effective Circulating Volume Has Priority over the Osmolality

Under physiologic conditions, the body regulates plasma *volume* and plasma *osmolality* independently. However, as discussed, this clear separation of defense mechanisms against volume and osmotic challenges breaks down when more dramatic derangements of fluid or salt metabolism occur. In general, the body defends volume at the expense of osmolality. Examples include severe reductions in absolute blood volume (e.g., hemorrhage) and decreases in effective circulating volume even when absolute ECF volume may be expanded (e.g., congestive heart failure, nephrotic syndrome, and liver cirrhosis). All are conditions that strongly stimulate both Na^+ *and* water retaining mechanisms. However, hyponatremia can be the consequence.

An exception to the rule of defending volume over osmolality occurs during severe water loss (i.e., dehydration). In this case, the hyperosmolality that accompanies the dehydration maximally stimulates AVP secretion and thirst (see Fig. 39–10). Of course, severe dehydration also reduces total-body volume. However, this loss of "free water" occurs at the expense of both intracellular water (60%) and extracellular water (40%). Thus, dehydration does not put the effective circulating volume at as great a risk as the acute loss of an equivalent volume of blood. Because dehydration reduces effective circulating volume, you might think that the renin-angiotensin-aldosterone axis would lead to Na^+ retention during dehydration. However, the opposite effect may occur, possibly because hyperosmolality makes the glomerulosa cells of the adrenal medulla less sensitive to ANG II, thus reducing the release of aldosterone. Thus, the kidneys fail to retain Na^+ appropriately. Accordingly, in severe dehydration, the net effect is an attempt to correct hyperosmolality by both water intake and retention, as well as by the loss of Na^+ (i.e., natriuresis) that occurs because aldosterone levels are inappropriately low for the effective circulating volume. Therefore, in severe dehydration, the body violates the principle of defending volume over osmolality.

REFERENCES

Books and Reviews

Bourque CW, Oliet SHR: Osmoreceptors in the central nervous system. Annu Rev Physiol 59:601–619, 1997.

DiBona GF, Kopp UC: Neural control of renal function. Physiol Rev 77: 75–197, 1997.

Fitzsimons JT: Angiotensin, thirst and sodium appetite. Physiol Rev 78: 583–686, 1998.

Gutkowska J, Antunes-Rodrigues J, McCann SM: Atrial natriuretic peptide in brain and pituitary gland. Physiol Rev 77:465–515, 1997.

Nader PC, Thompson JR, Alpern RJ: Complications of diuretic use. Semin Nephrol 8:365–387, 1988.

Navar LG, Zou L, Von Thun A, et al: Unraveling the mystery of Goldblatt hypertension. News Physiol Sci 13:170–176, 1998.

Rolls BJ, Rolls ET: Thirst. Cambridge, England, Cambridge University Press, 1982.

Journal Articles

Chou CL, Marsh DJ: Role of proximal convoluted tubule in pressure diuresis in the rat. Am J Physiol 251:F283–F289, 1986.

Mason WT: Supraoptic neurones of rat hypothalamus are osmosensitive. Nature 287:154–157, 1980.

Oliet SHR, Bourque CW: Mechanosensitive channels transduce osmosensitivity in supraoptic neurons. Nature 364:341–343, 1993.

Rabkin R, Share L, Payne PA, et al: The handling of immunoreactive vasopressin by the isolated perfused rat kidney. J Clin Invest 63:6–13, 1979.

Verney EG: The antidiuretic hormone and the factors which determine its release. Proc R Soc London B Biol Sci 135:25–106, 1947.

VII

The Gastrointestinal System

CHAPTER 40

Organization of the Gastrointestinal System

Henry J. Binder

OVERVIEW OF DIGESTIVE PROCESSES

The Gastrointestinal Tract Is a Tube That Is Specialized Along Its Length for the Sequential Processing of Food

The gastrointestinal (GI) tract consists of both the series of hollow organs stretching from the mouth to the anus and the several accessory glands and organs that add secretions to these hollow organs (Fig. 40–1). Each of these hollow organs, separated from each other at key locations by sphincters, has evolved to serve a specialized function. The mouth and oropharynx are responsible for chopping food into small pieces, lubricating it, initiating carbohydrate and fat digestion, and propelling the food into the esophagus. The esophagus acts as a conduit to the stomach. The stomach (see Chapter 41) temporarily stores food and also initiates digestion by churning and by secreting proteases and acid. The small intestine (see Chapters 43 and 44) continues the work of digestion and is the primary site for the absorption of nutrients. The large intestine (see Chapters 43 and 44) reabsorbs fluids and electrolytes and also stores the fecal matter before expulsion from the body. The accessory glands and organs include the salivary glands, pancreas, and liver. The pancreas (Chapter 42) secretes digestive enzymes into the duodenum, in addition to secreting HCO_3^- to neutralize gastric acid. The liver secretes bile (see Chapter 45), which the gallbladder stores for future delivery to the duodenum during a meal. Bile contains bile acids, which play a key role in the digestion of fats.

Although the anatomy of the wall of the GI tract varies along its length, certain organizational themes are common to all segments. Figure 40–2, a cross section through a generic piece of stomach or intestine, shows the characteristic layered structure of mucosa, submucosa, muscle, and serosa.

The **mucosa** consists of the epithelial layer, as well as an underlying layer of loose connective tissue known as the **lamina propria**, which contains capillaries, enteric neurons, and immune cells (e.g., mast cells), as well as a thin layer of smooth muscle known as the *lamina muscularis mucosae* (literally, the muscle layer of the mucosa). The surface area of the epithelial layer is amplified by several mechanisms. Most cells have microvilli on their apical surfaces. In addition, the layer of epithelial cells can be evaginated to form villi or invaginated to form glands (or crypts). Finally, on a grosser scale, the mucosa is organized into large folds.

The **submucosa** consists of loose connective tissue and larger blood vessels. The submucosa may also contain glands that secrete material into the GI lumen.

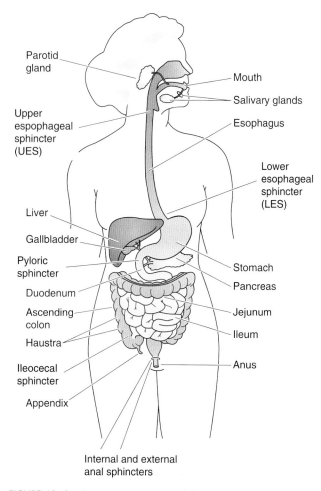

FIGURE 40–1. The major components of the human digestive system.

The **muscle layer**, the *muscularis externa*, includes two layers of smooth muscle. The inner layer is circular, whereas the outer layer is longitudinal. These muscles are responsible for peristalsis, which is a progressive wave of relaxation, followed by contraction. Enteric neurons are present between these two muscle layers.

The **serosa** is an enveloping layer of connective tissue that is covered with squamous epithelial cells.

Assimilation of Dietary Food Substances Requires Digestion As Well As Absorption

The sedentary human body requires approximately 30 kcal/kg body weight each day (p. 1211). This nutrient requirement is normally acquired by the oral intake of multiple food substances that the GI tract then assimilates. Although antigenic amounts of protein enter the body via the skin and across the pulmonary epithelium, caloric uptake via routes other than the GI tract is not thought to occur. Both the small and large intestine absorb water and electrolytes, but only the small intestine absorbs lipids, carbohydrates, and amino acids. It should be noted, however, that even without effective GI function, parenteral (i.e., intravenous) alimentation can provide sufficient calories to sustain adults and to support growth in premature infants. Total parenteral nutrition

has been used successfully on a long-term basis in many clinical settings where oral intake is impossible or undesirable.

Food substances are not necessarily consumed in a chemical form that the small intestine can directly absorb. To facilitate absorption, the GI tract digests the food by both mechanical and chemical processes.

Mechanical disruption of ingested food begins in the mouth with chewing (mastication). Individuals without teeth usually require their solid food to be cut into smaller pieces before eating. The mechanical processes that alter food composition to facilitate absorption continue in the stomach (p. 893), both to initiate protein and lipid enzymatic digestion and to allow passage of gastric contents through the pylorus into the duodenum. This change in the size and consistency of gastric contents is necessary because solids that are greater than 2 mm in diameter do not pass through the pylorus.

The chemical form in which different nutrients are ingested and absorbed varies according to the specific nutrient in question. For example, although most lipids are consumed in the form of triglycerides, it is fatty acids and monoglycerides, *not* triglycerides, that are absorbed by the small intestine. Thus, a complex series of chemical reactions (i.e., lipid digestion) are required to convert dietary triglycerides to these smaller lipid forms (p. 960). Similarly, amino acids are present in food as proteins and large peptides, but only amino acids and small peptides—primarily dipeptides and tripeptides—are absorbed by the small intestine. Carbohydrates are present in the diet as starch, disaccharides, and monosaccharides (e.g., glucose). However, because the small intestine absorbs all carbohydrates as monosaccharides, many dietary carbohydrates require chemical digestion before their absorption.

Digestion Requires Enzymes Secreted in the Mouth, Stomach, Pancreas, and Small Intestine

Digestion involves the conversion of dietary food nutrients to a form that the small intestine can absorb. For carbohydrates and lipids, these digestive processes are initiated in the mouth by salivary and lingual enzymes: amylase for carbohydrates and lipase for lipids. Protein digestion is initiated in the stomach by gastric proteases (i.e., pepsins), whereas additional lipid digestion in the stomach occurs primarily as a result of the lingual lipase that is swallowed, although some gastric lipase is also secreted. Carbohydrate digestion does not involve any secreted gastric enzymes.

Digestion is completed in the small intestine by the action of both pancreatic enzymes and enzymes at the brush border of the small intestine. Pancreatic enzymes, which include lipase, chymotrypsin, and amylase, are critical for the digestion of lipids, protein, and carbohydrates, respectively. The enzymes on the luminal surface of the small intestine (e.g., brush-border disaccharidases and dipeptidases) complete the digestion of carbohydrates and proteins. Digestion by these brush-border enzymes is referred to as "membrane digestion."

A MACROSCOPIC VIEW OF THE WALL OF THE DUODENUM

B MICROSCOPIC VIEW OF THE WALL OF THE COLON

FIGURE 40–2. The wall of the gastrointestinal tract. *A,* The wall of a generic segment of the gastrointestinal tract consists of the following structures, from inside to outside: an epithelial layer with crypts, lamina propria, muscularis mucosae, submucosa, the circular and then the longitudinal layer of the muscularis externa, and serosa. *B,* The colon has the same basic structure as the small intestine. Some of the epithelial cells are on the surface, and others are in the crypts that penetrate into the wall of the colon.

The material presented to the small intestine includes both dietary intake and secretory products. The food material entering the small intestine differs considerably from that of the ingested material because of the mechanical and chemical changes just discussed. The load to the small intestine is also significantly greater than that of the ingested material. Dietary fluid intake is 1.5 to 2.5 liters/day, whereas the fluid load presented to the small intestine is 8 to 9 liters/day. The increased volume is due to substantial quantities of salivary, gastric, biliary, pancreatic, and small intestinal secretions. These secretions contain large amounts of protein, primarily in the form of the digestive enzymes discussed earlier.

Ingestion of Food Initiates Multiple Endocrine, Neural and Paracrine Responses

Digestion of food involves multiple secretory, enzymatic, and motor processes that are closely coordinated with one another. The necessary control is achieved by neural and hormonal processes that are initiated by dietary food substances; the result is a coordinated series of motor and secretory responses. For example, chemoreceptors, osmoreceptors, and mechanical receptors in the mucosa in large part generate the afferent stimuli that induce gastric and pancreatic secretions. These receptors sense the luminal contents and initiate a neurohumoral response.

Endocrine, neural, and paracrine mechanisms all contribute to digestion. All three include sensor and transmitter processes. An **endocrine** mechanism (p. 88) involves the release of a transmitter (e.g., peptide) into the blood. For example, protein in the stomach stimulates the release of gastrin from antral G cells. Gastrin then enters the blood and stimulates H^+ release from parietal cells in the body of the stomach. A **neural** mechanism involves the activation of nerves and neurotransmitters that influence either secretory or motor activity. Neural transmission of these responses may involve the enteric nervous system (ENS; see later) or the central nervous system (CNS). An example of neural control is activation of the vagus nerve in response to the smell of food. The resultant release of the neurotransmitter acetylcholine also releases H^+ from parietal cells in the stomach.

The third mechanism of neurohumoral control is **paracrine** (p. 88). In this mechanism, a transmitter is released from a sensor cell, and it affects adjacent cells without either entering the blood or activating neurons. For example, paracrine mechanisms help regulate gastric-acid secretion by parietal cells: the histamine released from so-called enterochromaffin-like (ECL) cells in the body of the stomach stimulates H^+ release from neighboring parietal cells.

In addition to the primary response that leads to the release of one or more digestive enzymes, other signals terminate these secretory responses. Enteric neurons are important throughout the initiation and termination of the responses.

Although the endocrine, neural, and paracrine responses are most often studied separately, with considerable effort made to isolate individual events, it is important to remember that these responses never occur as isolated events. Rather, they are each part of an integrated response that results in food digestion and absorption. This entire series of events that results from the ingestion of food can best be described as an integrated response to a meal that includes both afferent and efferent limbs.

In Addition to Its Function in Nutrition, the Gastrointestinal Tract Plays Important Roles in Excretion, Fluid and Electrolyte Balance, and Immunity

Although its primary role is digesting and absorbing dietary calories and nutrients, the GI tract also excretes **waste material**. Fecal material includes nondigested/nonabsorbed dietary food products, colonic bacteria and their metabolic products, and several excretory products. These excretory products include: (1) heavy metals such as iron and copper, whose major route of excretion is in bile; and (2) several organic anions and cations, including drugs, that are excreted in bile but are either poorly or not at all reabsorbed by either the small or large intestine.

As noted earlier, the small intestine is presented with 8 to 9 liters/day of fluid, an amount that includes approximately 1 liter/day that the small intestine itself secretes. Almost all this water is reabsorbed in the small and large intestine; therefore, stool has relatively small amounts of water (~0.1 liter/day). Diarrhea (an increase in stool liquidity and weight, >200 g/day) results from either increased fluid secretion by the small or large intestine, or decreased fluid reabsorption by the intestines. An important clinical example of diarrhea is cholera—especially in developing countries. Cholera can be fatal because of the water and electrolyte imbalance that it creates. Thus, the GI tract plays a crucial role in maintaining overall **fluid and electrolyte balance** (see Chapter 43).

The GI tract also contributes to **immune function**. The mucosal immune system, or gut-associated lymphoid tissue (**GALT**), consists of both organized aggregates of lymphoid tissue (e.g., Peyer patches; see Fig. 40–2B) and diffuse populations of immune cells. The latter include lymphocytes that reside between the epithelial cells lining the gut, as well as lymphocytes and mast cells in the lamina propria. GALT has two primary functions: (1) protect against potential microbial pathogens, including bacteria, protozoans, and viruses, and (2) permit immunologic *tolerance* to both the potentially immunogenic dietary substances and bacteria that normally reside primarily in the lumen of the large intestine.

The mucosal immune system is important because the GI tract has the largest area of the body in potential direct contact with infectious, toxic, and immunogenic material. Approximately 80% of the immunoglobulin-producing cells are found in the small intestine. Although GALT has some interaction with the systemic immune system, operationally, GALT is distinct. Finally, there is evidence of communication between the GALT and mucosal immune systems at other mucosal surfaces, such as the pulmonary epithelia.

Certain **nonimmunologic defense** processes are also important in protecting against potential luminal pathogens and in limiting the uptake of macromolecules from the GI tract. The nonimmunologic mechanisms that are critical in maintaining the ecology of intestinal flora include gastric-acid secretion, intestinal mucin, peristalsis, and the epithelial-cell permeability barrier. Thus, whereas relatively low levels of aerobic bacteria are present in the lumen of the small intestine of normal subjects, individuals with impaired small-intestinal peristalsis often have substantially higher levels of both aerobic and anaerobic bacteria in their small intestine. A consequence may be diarrhea or steatorrhea (i.e., increased fecal fat excretion). The clinical manifestation of impaired intestinal peristalsis is referred to as either "blind loop syndrome" or "stagnant bowel syndrome."

REGULATION OF GASTROINTESTINAL FUNCTION

The Enteric Nervous System Is a "Minibrain" with Sensory Neurons, Interneurons, and Motor Neurons

The ENS is the primary neural mechanism that controls GI function and, as described in Chapter 15, is one of the three divisions of the autonomic nervous system (ANS), along with the sympathetic and parasympathetic divisions. One indication of the importance of the ENS is the number of neurons consigned to it. The ENS consists of ap-

proximately 100 million neurons, roughly the number in the spinal cord or in the rest of the entire ANS. The ENS is located solely within GI tissue, but it can be modified by input from the brain. Neurons of the ENS are primarily, but not exclusively, clustered in one of two collections of neurons (Fig. 40–3A): the submucosal plexus and the myenteric plexus. The **submucosal (or Meissner's) plexus** is found in the submucosa only in the small and large intestine. The **myenteric (or Auerbach's) plexus** is located between the circular and longitudinal muscle layers throughout the GI tract from the proximal end of the esophagus to the rectum.

The ENS is a complete reflex circuit and can operate totally within the GI tract, without the participation of either the spinal cord or the cephalic brain. As is the case for other neurons, the activity of the ENS is the result of the generation of action potentials by single neurons and the release of chemical neurotransmitters that affect either other neurons or effector cells (i.e., epithelial or muscle cells). The ENS consists of sensory circuits, interneuronal connections, and secretomotor neurons (see Fig. 40–3B). Sensory (or **afferent**) neurons monitor changes in luminal activity, including distention (i.e., smooth-muscle tension), chemistry (e.g., pH, osmolality, specific nutrients), and mechanical stimulation. These sensory neurons in turn activate **interneurons**, which relay signals that activate **efferent** secretomotor neurons. The latter stimulate or inhibit a wide range of effector cells: smooth muscle

A LOCATION OF THE ENS

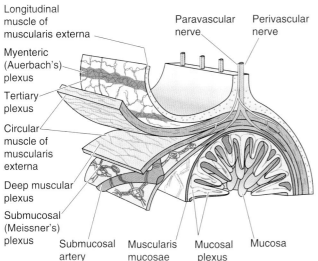

B CONNECTIONS OF ENS NEURONS

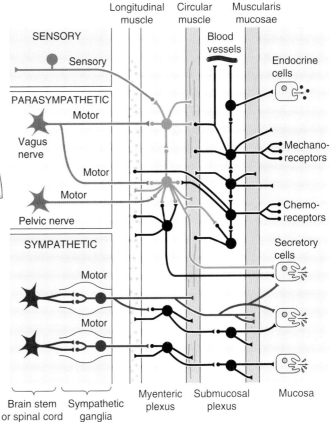

FIGURE 40–3. Schematic representation of enteric nervous system. *A*, The submucosal (or Meissner's) plexus is located between the muscularis mucosae and the circular muscle of the muscularis externa. The myenteric (or Auerbach's) plexus is located between the circular and longitudinal layers of the muscularis externa. In addition to these two plexuses that have ganglia, three others—mucosal, deep muscular, and tertiary plexus—are also present. *B*, The ENS consists of sensory neurons, interneurons, and motor neurons. Some sensory signals travel centrally from the ENS. Both the parasympathetic and the sympathetic divisions of the autonomic nervous system modulate the ENS. This figure illustrates some of the typical circuitry of ENS neurons. ENS, enteric nervous system.

cells, epithelial cells that secrete or absorb fluid and electrolytes, submucosal blood vessels, and enteric endocrine cells.

The largely independent function of the ENS has given rise to the concept of a GI "minibrain." Because the efferent response to several different stimuli is often quite similar, a generalized concept has developed that the ENS possesses multiple preprogrammed responses. For example, both mechanical distention of the jejunum and the presence of a bacterial enterotoxin in the jejunum can elicit identical responses: stimulation of profuse fluid and electrolyte secretion, together with propagated, propulsive, coordinated smooth-muscle contractions. Such preprogrammed efferent responses are probably initiated by sensory input to the enteric interneuronal connections. However, efferent responses controlled by the ENS may also be modified by input from autonomic ganglia, which are in turn under the influence of the spinal cord and brain (p. 395). In addition, the ENS receives input directly from the brain via parasympathetic nerves (i.e., the vagus nerve).

Acetylcholine, Peptides, and Bioactive Amines Are the ENS Neurotransmitters That Regulate Epithelial and Motor Function

Acetylcholine (ACh) is the primary preganglionic and postganglionic neurotransmitter regulating both secretory function and smooth-muscle activity in the GI tract. In addition, many other neurotransmitters are present in enteric neurons. Among the peptides, vasoactive intestinal peptide (VIP) has an important role in both inhibition of intestinal smooth muscle and stimulation of intestinal fluid and electrolyte secretion. Although VIP was first identified in the GI tract, it is now appreciated that it is also an important neurotransmitter in the brain (Table 12–1). Other substances probably also play an important role in GI regulation. These substances include other peptides, such as the enkephalins, somatostatin, and substance P; amines such as serotonin (5-hydroxytryptamine [5-HT]); and nitric oxide (NO).

The field of ENS neurotransmitters is rapidly evolving, with the list of agonists growing ever longer. In addition, substantial species differences exist. Frequently, chemical neurotransmitters are identified in neurons without a clear-cut demonstration of their physiologic role in the regulation of organ function. More than one neurotransmitter has been identified within single neurons, thus suggesting that regulation of some cell functions may require more than one neurotransmitter.

The Brain-Gut Axis Is a Bidirectional System That Controls Gastrointestinal Function via the Autonomic Nervous System, Gastrointestinal Hormones, and the Immune System

Well recognized, but poorly understood, is the modification of several different aspects of GI function by the brain. In other words, neural control of the GI tract is a function of not only intrinsic nerves (i.e., the ENS), but also nerves that are extrinsic to the GI tract. These extrinsic pathways are composed of both the parasympathetic—and, to a lesser extent, the sympathetic—nervous system and are under the control of autonomic centers in the brain stem (p. 393).

Parasympathetic innervation of the GI tract from the pharynx to the distal colon is through the vagus nerve; the distal third of the colon receives its parasympathetic innervation from the pelvic nerves (see Fig. 15–4). The preganglionic fibers of the parasympathetic nerves use acetylcholine as their neurotransmitter and synapse on some neurons of the ENS (see Fig. 40–3B). These ENS neurons are thus postganglionic parasympathetic fibers, and their cell bodies are, in a sense, the parasympathetic ganglion. These postganglionic parasympathetic fibers use mainly ACh as their neurotransmitter; however, as noted in the previous section, many other neurotransmitters are also present. The result of parasympathetic stimulation is—after one or more synapses in a very complex ENS network—increased secretion and motility. The parasympathetic nerves also contain afferent fibers (p. 381) that carry information to autonomic centers in the medulla from chemoreceptors, osmoreceptors, and mechanical receptors in the mucosa. The loop that is initiated by these afferents, integrated by central autonomic centers, and completed by the aforementioned parasympathetic efferents, is known as a vagovagal reflex.

The preganglionic sympathetic fibers to the GI tract synapse on postganglionic neurons in the prevertebral ganglia (see Fig. 15–4); the neurotransmitter at this synapse is ACh (p. 385). The postganglionic sympathetic fibers either synapse in the ENS or directly innervate effector cells (see Fig. 40–3B).

In addition to the control that is entirely within the ENS, as well as control via autonomic centers in the medulla, the GI tract is also under the control of higher CNS centers. Examples of cerebral function that affects GI behavior include the flight-or-fight response, which reduces blood flow to the GI tract, and the sight and smell of food, which increases gastric-acid secretion.

Communication between the GI tract and higher CNS centers is bidirectional. For example, cholecystokinin from the GI tract mediates, in part, the development of food satiety in the brain. In addition, gastrin-releasing peptide, a neurotransmitter made in ENS cells (p. 900), inhibits gastric-acid secretion when experimentally injected into the ventricles of the brain. Table 40–1 summarizes peptide hormones made by the GI tract, as well as their major actions.

In addition to the "hard-wired" communications involved in sensory input and motor output, communication via the gut-brain axis also requires significant participation of the immune system. Neuroimmune regulation of both epithelial and motor function in the small and large intestine primarily involves mast cells in the lamina propria of the intestine. Because the mast cells are sensitive to neurotransmitters, they can process information from the brain to the ENS and can also respond to signals from interneurons of the ENS. Mast cells also monitor sensory input from the intestinal lumen by participating in the immune response to foreign antigens. In turn, chemical mediators released by mast cells (e.g., his-

TABLE 40–1

GASTROINTESTINAL PEPTIDE HORMONES

HORMONE	SOURCE	TARGET	ACTION
Cholecystokinin	I cells in duodenum and jejunum and neurons in ileum and colon	Pancreas	↑ Enzyme secretion
		Gallbladder	↑ Contraction
Gastric-inhibitory peptide	K cells in duodenum and jejunum	Pancreas	Exocrine: ↓ fluid absorption Endocrine: ↑ insulin release
Gastrin	G cells, antrum of stomach	Parietal cells in body of stomach	↑ H^+ secretion
Gastrin-releasing peptide	Vagal nerve endings	G cells in antrum of stomach	↑ Gastrin release
Glucagon	α Cells of pancreatic islets of Langerhans	Liver	↑ Glycogenolysis ↑ Gluconeogenesis
Guanylin	Ileum and colon	Small and large intestine	↑ Fluid absorption
Motilin	Endocrine cells in upper GI tract	Esophageal sphincter Stomach Duodenum	↑ Smooth-muscle contraction
Neurotensin	Endocrine cells, widespread in GI tract	Intestinal smooth muscle	Vasoactive stimulation of histamine release
Peptide YY	Endocrine cells in ileum and colon	Stomach	↓ Vagally mediated acid secretion
		Pancreas	↓ Enzyme and fluid secretion
Secretin	S cells in small intestine	Pancreas	↑ HCO_3 and fluid secretion by pancreatic ducts
		Stomach	↓ Gastric-acid secretion
Somatostatin	D cells of stomach and duodenum, δ cells of pancreatic islets	Stomach	↓ Gastrin release
		Intestine	↑ Fluid absorption/ ↓ secretion ↑ Smooth-muscle contraction
		Pancreas	↓ Endocrine/exocrine secretions
		Liver	↓ Bile flow
Substance P	Enteric neurons	Enteric neurons	Neurotransmitter
Vasoactive intestinal peptide	ENS neurons	Small intestine	↓ Smooth-muscle relaxation ↑ Secretion by small intestine
		Pancreas	↑ Secretion by pancreas

ENS, enteric nervous system; GI, gastrointestinal.

tamine) directly affect both intestinal smooth-muscle cells and epithelial cells. Our understanding of how the immune system modulates the neural control of GI function is rapidly evolving.

In conclusion, three parallel components of the gut-brain axis—the ENS, GI hormones, and the immune system—control GI function, an arrangement that provides substantial redundancy. Such redundancy permits fine-tuning of the regulation of digestive processes and provides "backup" or "fail-safe" mechanisms that ensure the integrity of GI function, especially at times of impaired function (i.e., during disease).

GASTROINTESTINAL MOTILITY

Tonic and Rhythmic Contractions of Smooth Muscle Are Responsible for Gastrointestinal Motility

The motor activity of the GI tract performs three primary functions. First, it produces segmental contractions that are associated with nonpropulsive movement of the luminal contents. The result is the increased mixing (or churning) that enhances the digestion and absorption of dietary nutrients. Second, GI motor activity produces peristaltic contractions that cause propulsion, or the propagated movement of food and its digestive products in a caudal direction. The result is elimination of nondigested, nonabsorbed material. Third, motor activity allows some hollow organs—particularly the stomach and large intestine—to act as **reservoirs** for holding the luminal content. This reservoir function is made possible by **sphincters** that separate the organs of the GI tract. All these functions are primarily accomplished by the coordinated activity of **smooth muscle** (see Chapter 9).

The electrical and mechanical properties of intestinal smooth muscle needed for these functions include both tonic (i.e., sustained) contractions and rhythmic contractions (i.e., alternating contraction and relaxation) of individual muscle cells. The intrinsic rhythmic contractility is a function of the membrane voltage (V_m) of the smooth-muscle cell. V_m can either oscillate in a subthreshold range at a low frequency (several per minute), referred to as **slow-wave activity**, or reach a threshold for initiating a true **action potential** (see Fig. 9–3). The integrated effect of the slow waves and action potentials determines the smooth muscle activity of the GI tract. Slow-wave activity apparently occurs as voltage-gated Ca^{2+} channels depolarize the cell and increase $[Ca^{2+}]_i$, followed by the opening of Ca^{2+}-activated K^+ channels, which repolarize the cell (p. 234).

These activities are regulated, in large part, by both neural and hormonal stimuli. Modulation of intestinal smooth-muscle contraction is largely a function of $[Ca^{2+}]_i$ (p. 250). Several agonists regulate $[Ca^{2+}]_i$ either by: (1) activating G-protein–linked receptors, which results in the formation of inositol 1,4,5-triphosphate (IP_3) and the release of Ca^{2+} from intracellular stores; or by (2) opening and closing plasma-membrane Ca^{2+} channels. Both excitatory and inhibitory neurotransmitters can modulate smooth-muscle $[Ca^{2+}]_i$ and thus contractility. In general, ACh is the predominant neurotransmitter of *excitatory* motor neurons, whereas VIP and NO are the neurotransmitters of *inhibitory* motor neurons. Different neural or hormonal inputs probably increase (or decrease) the frequency with which V_m exceeds threshold and produces an action potential and thus increases (or decreases) muscle contractility.

An additional unique factor in the aforementioned regulatory control is that luminal food and digestive products activate mucosal chemical and mechanical receptors, as discussed earlier, thus inducing hormone release or stimulating the ENS and controlling smooth-muscle function. For example, gastric contents with elevated osmolality or a high lipid content entering the duodenum activates mucosal osmoreceptors and chemoreceptors that increase the release of cholecystokinin and thus delay gastric emptying (p. 907).

Segments of the Gastrointestinal Tract Have Both Longitudinal and Circular Arrays of Muscles and Are Separated by Sphincters That Consist of Specialized Circular Muscles

The muscle layers of the GI tract consist almost entirely of smooth muscle. Exceptions are the striated muscle of the upper esophageal sphincter (which separates the hypopharynx from the esophagus), the upper third of the esophagus, and the external anal sphincter. As shown earlier in Figure 40–2, the two smooth-muscle layers are arranged as an inner circular layer and an outer longitudinal layer. The myenteric ganglia of the ENS are located between the two muscle layers.

The segments of the GI tract through which food products pass are hollow, low-pressure organs that are separated by specialized circular muscles or **sphincters**. These sphincters function as barriers to flow by maintaining a positive **resting pressure** that serves to separate the two adjacent organs, in which lower pressures prevail. Sphincters thus regulate both antegrade (forward) and retrograde (reverse) movement. For example, the resting pressure of the pyloric sphincter controls, in part, the emptying of gastric contents into the duodenum. On the other hand, the resting pressure of the lower esophageal sphincter (LES) serves to prevent gastric contents from refluxing back into the esophagus and causing gastroesophageal reflux disease (GERD). As a general rule, stimuli proximal to a sphincter cause sphincteric relaxation, whereas stimuli distal to a sphincter induce sphincteric contraction. Changes in sphincter pressure are coordinated with the smooth-muscle contractions in the organs on either side. This coordination depends on both the intrinsic properties of sphincteric smooth muscle and neurohumoral stimuli.

Sphincters effectively serve as one-way valves. Thus, the act of deglutition (or swallowing) induces relaxation of the upper esophageal sphincter, whereas the LES remains contracted. Only when the UES returns to its initial pressure does the LES begin to relax, approximately 3 sec after the start of deglutition. Disturbances in sphincter activity are often associated with alterations in one or more of these regulatory processes.

Location of a Sphincter Determines Its Function

Six sphincters are present in the GI tract (see Fig. 40–1), each with different resting pressures and different responses to various stimuli. An additional sphincter, the sphincter of Oddi, regulates movement of the contents of the common bile duct into the duodenum.

UPPER ESOPHAGEAL SPHINCTER. Separating the pharynx and the upper part of the esophagus is the UES, which consists of striated muscle and has the highest resting pressure of all the GI sphincters. Control of the swallow-

ACHALASIA

Achalasia is a relatively uncommon condition associated with difficulty swallowing (dysphagia) and a dilated esophagus proximal to a narrowed, tapered area at the gastroesophageal junction. The term *achalasia* is derived from Greek words meaning "absence of relaxation." The distal narrowed area of the esophagus suggests the presence of a stricture. However, it is easy to introduce an esophagoscope into the stomach through the narrowed area. Subsequent studies of esophageal motility in which investigators measured intraesophageal pressure demonstrated the presence of two defects in patients with achalasia: (1) failure of the lower esophageal sphincter (LES) to relax, and (2) impaired peristalsis in the distal two thirds of the body of the esophagus—that is, the portion that consists of *smooth* muscle. Peristalsis is intact in the proximal third of the esophagus, which consists of *striated* muscle. In essence, the smooth-muscle portions of the esophagus behave as a denervated structure. The fundamental defect in achalasia is unknown but is probably due to selective loss of inhibitory neurons that regulate the LES, the neurotransmitters of which are vasoactive intestinal peptide (VIP) and nitric oxide (NO). Treatment is either physical distention (or stretching) of the LES with a pneumatic-bag dilator or surgical cutting of the LES (i.e., an esophageal myotomy or Heller procedure).

LES is mediated both by the vagus nerve and by intrinsic properties of the smooth muscle, including important inhibitory effects by VIP and by NO.

Abnormalities of both resting LES pressure and its relaxation in response to deglutition are often associated with significant symptoms. Thus, a reduced resting LES pressure often results in gastroesophageal reflux, which may cause esophagitis (i.e., inflammation of the esophageal mucosa). A defect in LES relaxation is a major component of a condition called **achalasia** (see the box titled Achalasia), which often results in dilatation of the esophagus (megaesophagus) and is associated with difficulty in swallowing (dysphagia).

Swallowing and the function of the upper and lower esophageal sphincters are closely integrated into the function of the esophagus. Under normal circumstances, esophageal muscle contractions are almost exclusively peristaltic and are initiated by swallowing. Deglutition initiates relaxation of the UES and propagated contractions, first of the UES and then of the muscles along the esophagus (see Fig. 40–4). In the meantime, the LES has already relaxed. The result of the advancing peristaltic wave is the caudad propulsion of a bolus toward the stomach.

Distention of the esophagus (in the absence of swallowing) also initiates propulsive esophageal contractions that

ing mechanism, including the oropharynx and the UES, is largely under the control of the **swallowing center** in the medulla via cranial nerves V (trigeminal), IX (glossopharyngeal), X (vagus), and XII (hypoglossal). Respiration and deglutition are closely integrated (p. 733). The UES is closed during inspiration, thereby diverting atmospheric air to the glottis and away from the esophagus. During swallowing, the situation reverses, with closure of the glottis and inhibition of respiration, but with relaxation of the UES (Fig. 40–4). These changes permit the entry of food contents into the esophagus and not into the airways of the respiratory tract.

LOWER ESOPHAGEAL SPHINCTER. The esophagus is separated from the stomach by the LES, which is composed of specialized smooth muscle that is both anatomically and pharmacologically distinct from adjacent smooth muscle in the distal end of the esophagus and proximal portion of the stomach. The primary functions of the LES are: (1) to permit coordinated movement of ingested food into the stomach from the esophagus after swallowing or deglutition, and (2) to prevent reflux of gastric contents into the esophagus. Either deglutition or distention of the esophagus results in a reduction in LES pressure (see Fig. 40–4) to that of intragastric pressure, thereby permitting entry of food into the stomach. Relaxation of the LES occurs after the UES has already returned to its resting pressure. The LES maintains a resting tone that is the result of both intrinsic myogenic properties of the sphincteric muscle and cholinergic regulation. Relaxation of the

FIGURE 40–4. Esophageal pressures during swallowing. The swallowing center in the medulla that initiates deglutition includes the nucleus ambiguus (CN IX and X), the dorsal motor nucleus of the vagus (CN X), and others. Shown are recordings of intraluminal pressures at different sites along the esophagus, from the upper esophageal sphincter (*record 1*) to the lower esophageal sphincter (*record 6*). The *left side* of the graph shows the pressures at rest. As shown on the *right side*, after a dry swallow, the pressure wave of a "primary peristalsis" moves sequentially down the esophagus. CN, cranial nerve; LES, lower esophageal sphincter; UES, upper esophageal sphincter. (Data from Conklin JL, Christensen J: Motor functions of the pharynx and esophagus. In Johnson LR [ed]: Physiology of the Gastrointestinal Tract, 3rd ed. New York, Lippincott-Raven, 1994, pp 903–928.)

A RECTUM

If passive distention of the rectum is sufficiently large...

Rectal distention

Passive

Active

...it triggers an active contraction of the rectal smooth muscles.

Change in pressure (mm Hg)

40
30
20
10
0

Time

B INTERNAL ANAL SPHINCTER

Passive rectal distention also triggers relaxation of the smooth muscle of the internal anal sphincter (rectosphincteric reflex).

Change in pressure (mm Hg)

0
−10
−20

Time

C EXTERNAL ANAL SPHINCTER

If defecation is not desired, the skeletal muscle of the external anal sphincter contracts by an involuntary reflex.

Change in pressure (mm Hg)

30
15
10
5
0

Time

FIGURE 40–5. Pressure changes initiated by rectal distention. (Data from Schuster MM: Simultaneous manometric recording of internal and external anal sphincteric reflexes. Johns Hopkins Med J 116:70–88, 1965.)

are distal to the site of distention, as well as relaxation of the LES. Reflux of gastric contents into the lower part of the esophagus also produces such a local distention, without a swallow, and elicit the same response: peristaltic contractions that clear the esophagus of refluxed gastric material. Peristalsis that is initiated by swallowing is called **primary peristalsis**, whereas that elicited by distention of the esophagus is referred to as **secondary peristalsis**. Esophageal contractions after a swallow are regulated by the medullary swallowing center, intramural esophageal plexuses, the vagus nerve, and intrinsic myogenic processes.

PYLORIC SPHINCTER. The pylorus is the sphincter that separates the stomach from the duodenum. The pressure of the pyloric sphincter regulates, in part, gastric emptying and prevents duodenal-gastric reflux. However, although a specific pyloric sphincter is present, it is quite

short and is a relatively poor barrier (i.e., it can resist only a small pressure gradient). The stomach, duodenum, biliary tract, and pancreas—which are closely related embryologically—function as a unit. Indeed, coordinated contraction and relaxation of the antrum, pylorus, and duodenum (which is sometimes referred to as the "antroduodenal cluster unit") are probably more important than simply the pressure produced by the pyloric smooth muscle per se. Regulation of gastric emptying is discussed further on p. 907.

ILEOCECAL SPHINCTER. The valve-like structure that separates the ileum and cecum is called the ileocecal sphincter. Similar to other GI sphincters, the ileocecal sphincter maintains a positive resting pressure and is under the control of the vagus nerve, sympathetic nerves, and the ENS. Distention of the ileum results in relaxation of the sphincter, whereas distention of the proximal (ascending) colon causes contraction of the ileocecal sphincter. As a consequence, ileal flow into the colon is regulated by luminal contents and pressure, both proximal and distal to the ileocecal sphincter.

INTERNAL AND EXTERNAL ANAL SPHINCTERS. The "anal sphincter" actually consists of both an internal and an external sphincter. The **internal sphincter** has both circular and longitudinal smooth muscle and is under involuntary control. The **external sphincter**, which encircles the rectum, contains only striated muscle but is controlled by both voluntary and involuntary mechanisms. The high resting pressure of the overall anal sphincter predominantly reflects the resting tone of the *internal* anal sphincter. Distention of the rectum (Fig. 40–5A), either by colonic contents (i.e., stool) or experimentally by balloon inflation, initiates the **rectosphincteric reflex** by relaxing the internal sphincter (see Fig. 40–5B). If defecation is not desired, continence is maintained by an involuntary reflex—orchestrated by the sacral spinal cord—that contracts the external anal sphincter (see Fig. 40–5C). If defecation is desired, a series of both voluntary and involuntary events occur that include relaxation of the external anal sphincter, contraction of abdominal wall muscles, and relaxation of pelvic wall muscles. Flexure of the hips and descent of the pelvic floor then facilitate defecation by minimizing the angle between the rectum and anus. In contrast, if a delay in defecation is needed or desired, voluntary contraction of the external anal sphincter is usually sufficient to override the series of reflexes initiated by rectal distention.

Motility of the Small Intestine Achieves Both Propulsive Movement and Churning, and Its Temporal Pattern Differs in the Fed and Fasted States

Digestion and absorption of dietary nutrients are the primary functions of the small intestine, and the motor activity of the small intestine is closely integrated with its digestive and absorptive roles. One class of small-intestine motor activity is characterized by mixing or churning, which is accomplished by segmental, nonpropulsive contractions. Another class of motor activity is propulsion of

HIRSCHSPRUNG DISEASE

The anal sphincter controls defecation and consists of a smooth-muscle internal sphincter and a striated-muscle external sphincter. Distention of the rectum by inflation of a balloon—which simulates the effect of the presence of solid feces in the rectum—results in relaxation of the internal sphincter and contraction of the external sphincter (see Fig. 40–5). Voluntary control of the external sphincter regulates the timing of defecation.

Hirschsprung disease is a congenital disorder associated with constipation, megacolon, and a narrowed segment of colon in the rectum. Histologic examination of this narrowed segment reveals an absence of ganglion cells from both the submucosal (or Meissner's) and myenteric (or Auerbach's) plexuses (see Fig. 40–3A). The fundamental defect is due to arrest of the caudad migration of neural crest cells, which are the precursors of ganglion cells. Manometric assessment of the internal and external anal sphincters reveals that the smooth-muscle internal sphincter does not relax after rectal distention (Fig. 40–5), but that the external anal sphincter functions normally. The patient's constipation and resulting megacolon are secondary to failure of this "aganglionic" segment to relax in response to proximal distention. Treatment of this condition is usually surgical, with removal of the narrowed segment that is missing the ganglia that normally regulate relaxation of the smooth muscle of the internal anal sphincter.

the bolus of luminal contents and is associated with propagated, peristaltic contractions. **Churning** mixes the luminal contents with pancreatic, biliary, and small intestinal secretions, thus enhancing the digestion of dietary nutrients in the lumen. These segmental contractions also decrease the unstirred water layer that is adjacent to the apical membranes of the small-intestine cells, thus promoting absorption. However, churning does not advance the luminal contents along the small intestine. In contrast, **propulsion** results in caudad movement of the intestinal luminal contents, either for absorption at more distal sites of the small or large intestine or for elimination in stool. It is believed that the circular smooth muscle in the small intestine participates in both churning and propulsion. The exact role of longitudinal smooth muscle in the motor function of small-intestinal movement remains controversial.

As noted earlier and in Chapter 9, the V_m changes of intestinal smooth muscle cells consist of both slow-wave activity and action potentials. The patterns of electrical and mechanical activity differ in the fasting and fed states. In the **fasting state**, the small intestine is relatively quiescent but exhibits synchronized, rhythmic changes in both electrical and motor activity (Fig. 40-6). The interdigestive myoelectric or **migrating motor complex (MMC)** is the term used to describe these rhythmic contractions of the small intestine that are observed in the fasting state. MMCs in humans occur at intervals of 90 to 120 minutes and consist of four distinct phases: (1) a prolonged quiescent period, (2) a period of increasing action-potential frequency and contractility, (3) a period of peak electrical and mechanical activity that lasts a few minutes, and (4)

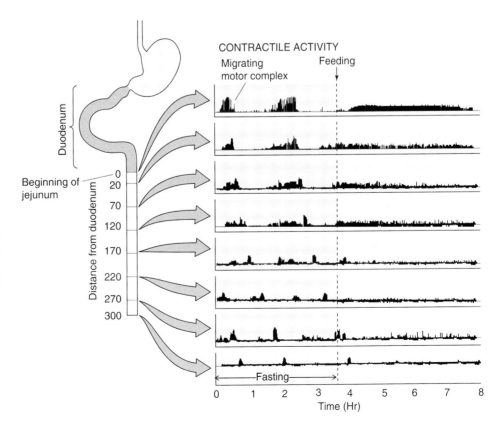

FIGURE 40–6. Mechanical activity in the fasting and fed states. Shown are records of intraluminal pressure along the small intestine of a conscious dog. Before feeding (*left side*), the pattern is one of migrating motor complexes (MMCs). Feeding triggers a switch to a different pattern, characterized by both segmental contractions that churn the contents and peristaltic contractions that propel the contents along the small intestine. (Data from Itoh Z, Sekiguchi T: Interdigestive motor activity in health and disease. Scand J Gastroenteral Suppl 82:121–134, 1983.)

a period of declining activity that merges into the next quiescent period. During the interdigestive period, particles greater than 2 mm in diameter can pass from the stomach into the duodenum, thus permitting emptying of ingested material from the stomach (e.g., bones, coins) that could not be reduced in size below 2 mm. The slow propulsive contractions that characterize phases 2 to 4 of the MMCs clear the small intestine of its residual content, including undigested food, bacteria, desquamated cells, and intestinal and pancreatic biliary secretions. MMCs usually originate in the stomach and often travel to the distal end of the ileum, but approximately 25% are initiated in the duodenum and proximal part of the jejunum.

Feeding terminates MMCs and initiates the appearance of the "fed motor pattern" (see Fig. 40–6). The latter is less well characterized than MMCs but, as noted earlier, consists of both segmental contractions ("churning"), which enhance digestion and absorption, and peristaltic contractions ("propulsion").

Determination of the primary factors that regulate both MMCs and transition to the fed pattern has been hampered by both species differences and complex interactions among the multiple probable mediators. Nonetheless, clear evidence has been presented for a role of the ENS, one or more humoral factors, and extrinsic innervation. A major determinant of the MMC pattern is the hormone **motilin**, a 22–amino-acid peptide that is synthesized in the duodenal mucosa and released just before the initiation of phase 3 of the MMC cycle. Motilin does not appear to have a role in the motor pattern that is observed in the fed state. Factors important in induction of the fed pattern include the vagus nerve (because sham feeding also both terminates MMCs and initiates a fed pattern) and the caloric content, as well as the type of food (e.g., fat more than protein) in the meal.

Motility of the Large Intestine Achieves Both Propulsive Movement and a Reservoir Function

The human large intestine has four primary functions. First, the colon absorbs large quantities of fluid and electrolytes and converts the liquid content of ileocecal material to solid or semisolid stool. Second, the colon avidly absorbs the short-chain fatty acids formed by the catabolism (or fermentation) of dietary carbohydrates that are not absorbed in the small intestine. The abundant colonic microflora accomplish this fermentation. Third, the storage of colonic content represents a reservoir function of the large intestine. Fourth, the colon eliminates its contents in a regulated and controlled fashion, largely under voluntary control. To accomplish these important activities, the large intestine functionally acts as two distinct organs. The proximal (or ascending and transverse) part of the colon is the site where most of the fluid and electrolyte absorption occurs and where bacterial fermentation takes place. The distal (or descending and rectosigmoid) portion of the colon provides final desiccation, as well as reservoir function, and serves as a storage organ for colonic material before defecation.

In contrast to the motor pattern in the small intestine,

no distinct fasting and fed patterns of contractions are seen in the colon. Similar to small-intestinal motor activity, colonic contractions are regulated by myogenic, neurogenic, and hormonal factors. Parasympathetic control of the proximal two thirds of the colon is mediated by the vagus nerve, whereas parasympathetic control of the descending and rectosigmoid colon is mediated by pelvic nerves originating from the sacral spinal cord.

The **proximal colon** has two types of motor activity, nonpropulsive segmentation and mass peristalsis. **Nonpropulsive "segmentation"** is generated by slow-wave activity that produces circular-muscle contractions that churn the colonic contents and move them in an orad direction (i.e., toward the cecum). The segmental contractions that produce the churning give the colon its typical appearance of segments or haustra (see Fig. 40–1). During this mixing phase, material is retained in the proximal portion of the large intestine for relatively long periods, and fluid and electrolyte absorption continues. One to three times a day, a so-called **mass peristalsis** occurs in which a portion of the colonic contents is propelled distally 20 cm or more. Such mass peristaltic contractions are the primary form of propulsive motility in the colon and may be initiated by eating. During mass peristalsis, the haustra disappear; they reappear after the completion of mass peristalsis.

In the **distal colon**, the primary motor activity is nonpropulsive segmentation that is produced by annular or segmental contractions. It is in the distal part of the colon that the final desiccation of colonic contents occurs. It is also here that these contents are stored before an occasional mass peristalsis that propels them into the rectum. The **rectum** itself is kept nearly empty by nonpropulsive segmentation until it is filled by mass peristalsis of the distal end of the colon. As described in Figure 40–5, filling of the rectum triggers a series of reflexes in the internal and external anal sphincters that lead to defecation.

REFERENCES

Books and Reviews

Andrews JM, Dent J: Small intestinal motor physiology. In Feldman M, Friedman LS, Sleisenger MH (eds): Gastrointestinal and Liver Disease, Vol 2, 7th ed. Philadelphia, Saunders, 2002, pp 1665–1678.

Biancani P, Hartnett KM, Behar J: Esophageal motor function. In Yamada T (ed): Textbook of Gastroenterology, Vol 1, 4th ed. Philadelphia, Lippincott, Williams and Wilkins, 2003, pp 166–194.

Cook IJ, Brookes SJ: Motility of the large intestine. In Feldman M, Friedman LS, Sleisenger MH (eds): Gastrointestinal and Liver Disease, Vol 2, 7th ed. Philadelphia, Saunders, 2002, pp 1679–1691.

Johnson LR (ed): Physiology of the Gastrointestinal Tract, 3rd ed. New York, Raven, 1994.

Maklouf GM: Smooth muscle of the gut. In Yamada T (ed): Textbook of Gastroenterology, Vol 1, 4th ed. Philadelphia, Lippincott, Williams and Wilkins, 2003, pp 92–116.

Rehfeld JF: The new biology of gastrointestinal hormones. Physiol Rev 78:1087–1108, 1998.

Surprenant A: Control of the gastrointestinal tract by enteric neurons. Annu Rev Physiol 56:117–140, 1994.

Journal Articles

Itoh Z, Sekiguchi T: Interdigestive motor activity in health and disease. Scand J Gastroenterol Suppl 82:121–134, 1983.

CHAPTER 41

Gastric Function

Henry J. Binder

The stomach plays several important roles in human nutrition and has secretory, motor, and humoral functions. These activities are not separate and distinct, but rather represent integrated functions that are required to initiate the normal digestive process.

The stomach has several specific **secretory** products. In addition to the stomach's best-known product—acid—these products include pepsinogen, mucus, bicarbonate, intrinsic factor, and water. These substances continue the food digestion that was initiated by mastication and the action of salivary enzymes in the mouth. In addition, they help protect the stomach from injury. The stomach also has several important **motor** functions that regulate the intake of food, its mixing with gastric secretions and reduction in particle size, and the exit of partially digested material into the duodenum. Moreover, the stomach produces two important **humoral agents**—gastrin and somatostatin—that have both endocrine and paracrine actions. These peptides are primarily important in the regulation of gastric secretion.

Although these functions are important in the maintenance of good health, the stomach is nevertheless not required for survival. Individuals who have had their entire stomach removed (i.e., total gastrectomy) for non-neoplastic reasons can maintain adequate nutrition and achieve excellent longevity.

FUNCTIONAL ANATOMY OF THE STOMACH

The Mucosa Is Composed of Surface Epithelial Cells and Glands

The basic structure of the stomach wall is similar to that of other regions of the gastrointestinal (GI) tract (see Fig. 40–2); therefore, the wall of the stomach consists of both mucosal and muscle layers. The stomach can be divided, based on its gross anatomy, into three major **segments** (Fig. 41–1): (1) A specialized portion of the stomach called the **cardia** is located just distal to the gastroesophageal junction and is devoid of the acid-secreting parietal cells. (2) The body or **corpus** is the largest portion of the stomach; its most proximal region is called the **fundus**. (3) The distal portion of the stomach is called the **antrum**. The surface area of the gastric mucosa is substantially increased by the presence of **gastric glands**, which consist of a pit, a neck, and a base. These glands contain several cell types, including mucous, parietal, chief, and endocrine cells; endocrine cells are

FIGURE 41–1. Anatomy of the stomach. Shown are the macroscopic divisions of the stomach, as well as two progressively magnified views of a section through the wall of the body of the stomach.

found only in the antrum. The surface epithelial cells, which have their own distinct structure and function, secrete HCO_3^- and mucus.

Marked cellular heterogeneity exists not only *within* segments (e.g., glands versus surface epithelial cells) but also between segments of the stomach. For instance, as discussed later, the structure and function of the mucosal epithelial cells in the antrum and body are quite distinct. Similarly, although the smooth muscle in the proximal and distal portions of the stomach appear structurally similar, their functions and pharmacologic properties differ substantially.

With Increasing Rates of Secretion of Gastric Juice, the H+ Concentration Rises and the Na+ Concentration Falls

The glands of the stomach typically secrete approximately 2 liters/day of a fluid that is approximately isotonic with

blood plasma. As a consequence of the heterogeneity of gastric mucosal function, early investigators recognized that gastric secretion consists of two distinct components: parietal- and nonparietal-cell secretion. According to this hypothesis, gastric secretion consists of (1) an Na+-rich basal secretion that originates from nonparietal cells, and (2) a stimulated component that represents a pure parietal-cell secretion that is rich in H+. This model helps explain the inverse relationship between the luminal concentrations of H+ and Na+ as a function of the rate of gastric secretion (Fig. 41–2). Thus, at high rates of gastric secretion—for example, when gastrin or histamine stimulates parietal cells—intraluminal [H+] is high whereas intraluminal [Na+] is relatively low. At low rates of secretion or in clinical situations in which maximal acid secretion is reduced (e.g., pernicious anemia, see box on p. 971), intraluminal [H+] is low but intraluminal [Na+] is high.

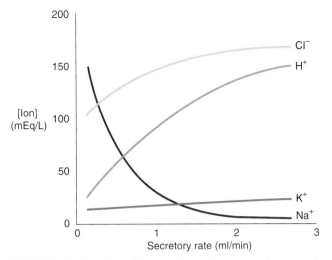

FIGURE 41–2. The effect of the gastric secretion rate on the composition of the gastric juice.

The Proximal Portion of the Stomach Secretes Acid, Pepsinogens, Intrinsic Factor, Bicarbonate, and Mucus, Whereas the Distal Part Releases Gastrin and Somatostatin

CORPUS. The primary secretory products of the proximal part of the stomach—acid (protons), pepsinogens, and intrinsic factor—are made by distinct cells from glands in the corpus of the stomach. The two primary cell types in the gastric glands of the body of the stomach are parietal cells and chief cells.

Parietal cells (or oxyntic cells) secrete both acid and intrinsic factor, a glycoprotein that is required for cobalamin (vitamin B_{12}) absorption in the ileum (p. 970). The parietal cell has a very distinctive morphology (see Fig. 41–1). It is a large triangular cell with a centrally located nucleus, an abundance of mitochondria, intracellular tubulovesicular membranes, and canalicular structures. We discuss H^+ secretion in the next subchapter and intrinsic factor in Chapter 44.

Chief cells (or peptic cells) secrete pepsinogens, but not acid. These epithelial cells are substantially smaller than parietal cells. A close relationship exists among pH, pepsin secretion, and function. Pepsins are endopeptidases (i.e., they hydrolyze "interior" peptide bonds) and initiate protein digestion by hydrolyzing specific peptide linkages. The basal luminal pH of the stomach is 4 to 6; with stimulation, the pH of gastric secretions is usually reduced to less than 2. At pH values that are less than 3, pepsinogens are rapidly activated to pepsins. A low gastric pH also helps prevent bacterial colonization of the small intestine.

In addition to parietal and chief cells, glands from the corpus of the stomach also contain **mucus-secreting cells**, which are confined to the neck of the gland (see Fig. 41–1), and five or six **endocrine cells**. Among the latter are enterochromaffin-like (ECL) cells, which release histamine.

ANTRUM. The glands in the antrum of the stomach do not contain parietal cells. Therefore, the antrum does not secrete either acid or intrinsic factor. Glands in the antral mucosa contain **chief cells** and **endocrine cells**; the endocrine cells include the so-called G cells and D cells, which secrete gastrin and somatostatin, respectively (see Table 40–1). These two peptide hormones function as both endocrine and paracrine regulators of acid secretion. As discussed in more detail later, **gastrin** stimulates gastric-acid secretion by two mechanisms and is also a major trophic or growth factor for GI epithelial-cell proliferation. As discussed more fully later, **somatostatin** also has several important regulatory functions, but its primary role in gastric physiology is to inhibit both gastrin release and parietal-cell acid secretion.

In addition to the cells of the gastric glands, the stomach also contains superficial epithelial cells that cover the gastric pits, as well as the surface in between the pits. These cells secrete HCO_3^-.

The Stomach Accommodates Food, Mixes It with Gastric Secretions, Grinds It, and Empties the Chyme into the Duodenum

In addition to its secretory properties, the stomach also has multiple motor functions. These functions are the result of gastric smooth-muscle activity, which is integrated by both neural and hormonal signals. Gastric motor functions include both propulsive and retrograde movement of food and liquid, as well as a nonpropulsive movement that increases intragastric pressure.

Similar to the heterogeneity of gastric epithelial cells, considerable diversity is seen in both the regulation and contractility of gastric smooth muscle. The stomach has at least two distinct areas of motor activity; the proximal and distal portions of the stomach behave as separate, but coordinated, entities. At least four events can be identified in the overall process of gastric filling and emptying: (1) receiving and providing temporary storage of dietary food

GASTRIC pH AND PNEUMONIA

Many patients hospitalized in the intensive care unit (ICU) receive prophylactic antiulcer treatment (e.g., histamine-2 receptor antagonists, such as cimetidine) that either neutralize existing acid or block its secretion and thereby raise gastric pH. Patients in the ICU who are mechanically ventilated or have coagulopathies are highly susceptible to hemorrhage from gastric stress ulcers, a complication that can contribute significantly to overall morbidity and mortality. These different antiulcer regimens do effectively lessen the risk of developing stress ulcers. However, by raising gastric pH, these agents also lower the barrier to gram-negative bacterial colonization of the stomach. Esophageal reflux and subsequent aspiration of these organisms are common in these very sick patients, many of whom are already immunocompromised or even mechanically compromised by the presence of a ventilator tube. If these bacteria are aspirated into the airway, pneumonia can result. The higher the gastric pH, the greater the risk of pneumonia.

and liquids; (2) mixing of food and water with gastric secretory products, including pepsin and acid; (3) grinding of food so that particle size is reduced to enhance digestion and permit passage through the pylorus; and (4) regulating the exit of retained material from the stomach into the duodenum (i.e., gastric emptying of "chyme") in response to various stimuli.

The mechanisms by which the stomach receives and empties liquids and solids are significantly different. Emptying of *liquids* is primarily a function of the smooth muscle of the *proximal* part of the stomach, whereas emptying of *solids* is regulated by *antral* smooth muscle.

ACID SECRETION

The Parietal Cell Has a Specialized Tubulovesicular Structure That Increases Apical Membrane Area When the Cell Is Stimulated to Secrete Acid

In the basal state, the rate of acid secretion is low. Tubulovesicular membranes are present in the apical portion of the resting, nonstimulated parietal cell and contain the H-K pump (or H,K-adenosinetriphosphatase [ATPase]) that is responsible for acid secretion. Upon stimulation, cytoskeletal rearrangement causes the tubulovesicular membranes that contain the H-K pump to fuse into the canalicular membrane (Fig. 41–3). The result is a substantial increase (50- to 100-fold) in the surface area of the apical membrane of the parietal cell, as well as the appearance of microvilli. This fusion is accompanied by insertion of the H-K pumps, as well as K$^+$ and Cl$^-$ channels, into the canalicular membrane. The large number of mitochondria in the parietal cell is consistent with the high rate of glucose oxidation and O$_2$ consumption that is needed to support acid secretion.

An H-K Pump Is Responsible for Gastric Acid Secretion by Parietal Cells

The parietal cell H-K pump is a member of the gene family of P-type ATPases (p. 63) that includes the ubiquitous Na-K pump (Na,K-ATPase), which is present at the

FIGURE 41–4. Acid secretion by parietal cells. When the parietal cell is stimulated, H-K pumps (fueled by ATP hydrolysis) extrude H$^+$ into the lumen of the gastric gland in exchange for K$^+$. The K$^+$ recycles back into the lumen via K$^+$ channels. Cl$^-$ exits through channels in the luminal membrane, completing the net process of HCl secretion. The H$^+$ needed by the H-K pump is provided by the entry of CO$_2$ and H$_2$O, which are converted to H$^+$ and HCO$_3^-$ by carbonic anhydrase. The HCO$_3^-$ exits across the basolateral membrane via the Cl-HCO$_3$ exchanger. ATP, adenosine triphosphate.

basolateral membrane of virtually all mammalian epithelial cells and at the plasma membrane of nonpolarized cells. Similar to other members of this ATPase family, the parietal cell H-K pump requires both an α subunit and a β subunit for full activity. The catalytic function of the H-K pump resides in the α subunit; however, the β subunit is required for targeting to the apical membrane. The two subunits form a heterodimer with close interaction at the extracellular domain.

The activity of these P-type ATPases, including the gastric H-K pump, is affected by inhibitors that are clinically important in the control of gastric acid secretion. The two types of gastric H-K pump inhibitors are (1) substituted benzimidazoles (e.g., omeprazole), which act by binding covalently to cysteines on the extracytoplasmic surface, and (2) substances that act as competitive inhibitors of the K$^+$ binding site (e.g., the experimental drug Schering 28080). **Omeprazole** (see the box titled Gastrinoma or Zollinger-Ellison Syndrome) is a potent inhibitor of parietal-cell H-K pump activity and is an extremely effective drug in the control of gastric-acid secretion in both normal subjects and patients with hypersecretory states. In addition, H-K pump inhibitors have been useful in furthering understanding of the function of these pumps. Thus, ouabain, a potent inhibitor of the Na-K pump, does not inhibit the gastric H-K pump, whereas omeprazole does not inhibit the Na-K pump. The *colonic* H-K pump, whose α subunit has an amino-acid sequence that is similar to that of both the Na-K pump and the parietal-cell H-K pump, is partially inhibited by ouabain but not by omeprazole.

According to the model presented in Figure 41–4, the

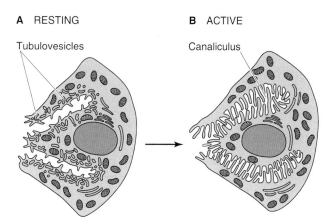

A RESTING

Tubulovesicles

B ACTIVE

Canaliculus

FIGURE 41–3. Parietal cell: resting and stimulated.

key step in gastric-acid secretion is extrusion of H^+ into the lumen of the gastric gland in exchange for K^+. The K^+ taken up into the parietal cells is recycled to the lumen through K^+ channels. The final component of the process is passive movement of Cl^- into the gland lumen. The apical membrane H-K pump energizes the entire process, the net result of which is the active secretion of HCl. Secretion of acid across the apical membrane by the H-K pump results in a rise in parietal cell pH. The adaptive response to this rise in pH includes passive uptake of CO_2 and H_2O, which the enzyme **carbonic anhydrase** (see box on p. 637) converts to HCO_3^- and H^+. The H^+ is the substrate of the H-K pump. The HCO_3^- exits across the basolateral membrane via the $Cl-HCO_3$ exchanger. This latter process also provides the Cl^- required for net HCl movement across the apical/canalicular membrane. The basolateral Na-H exchanger may participate in intracellular pH regulation, especially in the basal state.

Three Secretagogues (Acetylcholine, Gastrin, and Histamine) Directly and Indirectly Induce Acid Secretion by Parietal Cells

The action of secretagogues on gastric-acid secretion occurs via at least two parallel and perhaps redundant mechanisms (Fig. 41–5). In the first, acetylcholine (ACh), gastrin, and histamine bind **directly** to their respective membrane receptors on the parietal cell and synergistically stimulate and potentiate acid secretion. ACh (see Fig. 15–8) is released from endings of the vagus nerve (cranial nerve X), and as we shall see in the next section, gastrin is released from D cells. Histamine is synthesized from histidine (see Fig. 12–9). The documented presence of ACh, gastrin, and histamine receptors, at least on the canine parietal cell, provides the primary support for this view. In the second mechanism, ACh and gastrin **indirectly** induce acid secretion as a result of their stimulation of histamine release from enterochromaffin-like

(ECL) cells and possibly from mast cells (histaminocytes) in the lamina propria. The central role of histamine and ECL cells is consistent with the observation that histamine-2 receptor antagonists (i.e., H_2 blockers), such as cimetidine and ranitidine, not only block the direct action of histamine on parietal cells but also substantially inhibit the acid secretion stimulated by ACh and gastrin. The effectiveness of H_2 blockers in controlling acid secretion after stimulation by most agonists is well established in studies of both humans and experimental animals. These drugs are widely prescribed to treat active peptic ulcer disease.

The Three Acid Secretagogues Act Through Either Ca^{2+}/Diacylglycerol or Cyclic Adenosine Monophosphate

Stimulation of acid secretion by ACh, gastrin, and histamine, is mediated by a series of intracellular signal-transduction processes similar to those responsible for the action of other agonists in other cell systems. All three secretagogues bind to specific G-protein–coupled receptors on the parietal-cell membrane (Fig. 41–6).

Acetylcholine binds to an M_3 muscarinic receptor (p. 387) on the parietal cell basolateral membrane. This ACh receptor couples to a guanosine triphosphate (GTP)-binding protein ($G\alpha_q$) and activates phospholipase C (PLC), which converts phosphatidylinositol 4,5-biphosphate (PIP_2) to inositol 1,4,5-triphosphate (IP_3) and diacylglycerol (DAG, p. 100). IP_3 causes internal stores to release Ca^{2+}, which then probably acts via calmodulin-dependent protein kinase (p. 102). DAG activates protein kinase C (PKC). The M_3 receptor also activates a Ca^{2+} channel.

Gastrin binds to a specific parietal-cell receptor that has been identified as the gastrin-cholecystokinin B (CCK_B) receptor. Two related CCK receptors have been identified, CCK_A and CCK_B. Their amino-acid sequences are approximately 50% identical, and both are G-protein

FIGURE 41–5. The direct and indirect actions of the three acid secretagogues: acetylcholine, gastrin, and histamine. ACh, acetylcholine; CCK_B, cholecystokinin B; ECL, enterochromaffin-like; ENS, enteric nervous system.

FIGURE 41–6. Receptors and signal-transduction pathways in the parietal cell. The parietal cell has separate receptors for three acid secretagogues. Acetylcholine (ACh) and gastrin each bind to specific receptors (M₃ and CCK_B, respectively) that are coupled to the G protein Gα_q. The result is activation of phospholipase C (PLC), which ultimately leads to the activation of protein kinase C (PKC) and the release of Ca²⁺. The histamine binds to an H₂ receptor, coupled through Gα_s to adenylyl cyclase (AC). The result is production of cAMP and activation of PKA. Two inhibitors of acid secretion also act directly on the parietal cell. Somatostatin and prostaglandins bind to separate receptors that are linked to Gα_i. These agents thus oppose the actions of histamine. cAMP, cyclic adenosine monophosphate; CCK_B, cholecystokinin B; DAG, diacylglycerol; ER, endoplasmic reticulum; PIP₂, phosphatidyl inositol 4,5-biphosphate.

coupled. The CCK_B receptor has equal affinity for both gastrin and CCK. In contrast, the CCK_A receptor's affinity for CCK is three orders of magnitude higher than its affinity for gastrin. These observations and the availability of receptor antagonists are beginning to clarify the parallel, but at times opposite, effects of gastrin and CCK on various aspects of GI function. The CCK_B receptor couples to Gα_q and activates the same PLC pathway as ACh does, which leads to both an increase in [Ca²⁺]_i and activation of PKC.

The **histamine** receptor on the parietal cell is an H₂ receptor that is coupled to the Gα_s GTP-binding protein. Histamine activation of the receptor complex stimulates the enzyme adenylyl cyclase, which in turn generates cyclic adenosine monophosphate (cAMP). The resulting activation of protein kinase A leads to the phosphorylation of a number of parietal-cell–specific proteins, including the H-K pump.

Gastrin Is Released by Both Antral and Duodenal G Cells, and Histamine Is Released by Enterochromaffin-Like Cells in the Corpus

The presence of a gastric hormone that stimulates acid secretion was initially proposed in 1905. Direct evidence of such a factor was obtained in 1938, and in 1964 Gregory and Tracey isolated and purified gastrin and determined its amino-acid sequence. Gastrin has three major effects on GI cells: (1) stimulation of acid secretion by parietal cells (see Fig. 41–5), (2) release of histamine by ECL cells, and (3) regulation of mucosal growth in the corpus of the stomach, as well as in the small and large intestine.

Gastrin exists in several different forms, but the two major forms are G-17, or "little gastrin," a 17–amino acid linear peptide (Fig. 41–7A), and G-34, or "big gastrin," a 34–amino acid peptide (see Fig. 41–7B). A single gene encodes a peptide of 101 amino acids. Several cleavage steps and C-terminal amidation (i.e., addition of a -NH₂

FIGURE 41–7. Amino acid sequences of the gastrins and CCK. *A,* A single gene encodes a 101-amino-acid peptide that is processed to both G-17 and G-34. The N-terminal glutamine is modified to create a pyroglutamyl residue. The C-terminal phenylalanine is amidated. These modifications make the hormone resistant to carboxy- and aminopeptidases. *B,* The final 16 amino acids of G-34 are identical to the final 16 amino acids in G-17. Both G-17 and G-34 may be either *not sulfated* (Gastrin I) or *sulfated* (Gastrin II). *C,* The five final amino acids of CCK are identical to those of G-17 and G-34. CCK, cholecystokinin.

to the C terminus) occur during gastrin's post-translational modification, a process that occurs in the endoplasmic reticulum, trans-Golgi apparatus, and both immature and mature secretory granules. The final product of this post-translational modification is either G-17 or G-34. The tyrosine residue may be either sulfated (so-called gastrin II) or nonsulfated (gastrin I); the two forms are equally active and are present in equal amounts. Gastrin and **cholecystokinin**, a related hormone, have identical C-terminal tetrapeptide sequences (see Fig. 41–7C) that possess all the biologic activities of both gastrin and CCK. Both G-17 and G-34 are present in blood plasma, and their plasma levels primarily reflect their degradation rates. Thus, although G-17 is more active than G-34, the

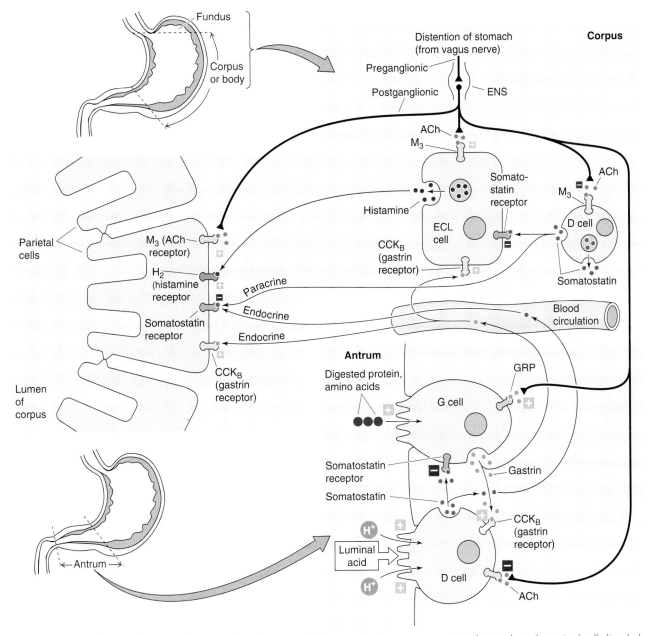

FIGURE 41–8. Regulation of gastric-acid secretion. In the **corpus** of the stomach, the vagus nerve not only stimulates the parietal cell directly by releasing ACh, it also stimulates both ECL and D cells. Vagal stimulation of the ECL cells enhances gastric-acid secretion via increased histamine release. Vagal stimulation of the D cells also promotes gastric-acid secretion by inhibiting the release of somatostatin, which would otherwise inhibit—by paracrine mechanisms—the release of histamine from ECL cells and the secretion of acid by parietal cells.

In the **antrum** of the stomach, the vagus stimulates both G cells and D cells. The vagus stimulates the G cells via GRP (gastrin-releasing peptide), promoting gastrin release. This gastrin promotes gastric-acid secretion by two endocrine mechanisms: directly via the parietal cell and indirectly via the ECL cell, which releases histamine. The vagal stimulation of D cells via ACh inhibits the release of somatostatin, which would otherwise inhibit—by paracrine mechanisms—the release of gastrin from G cells and—by an endocrine mechanism—acid secretion by parietal cells. Luminal H⁺ directly stimulates the D cells to release somatostatin, which inhibits gastrin release from the G cells, thereby reducing gastric-acid secretion (negative feedback). In addition, products of protein digestion (i.e., peptides and amino acids) directly stimulate the G cells to release gastrin, which stimulates gastric-acid secretion (positive feedback). ACh, acetylcholine; CCK_B, cholecystokinin B; ECL, enterochromaffin-like; ENS, enteric nervous system.

latter is degraded at a substantially lower rate than G-17. As a consequence, the infusion of equal amounts of G-17 or G-34 produces comparable increases in gastric-acid secretion.

Specialized endocrine cells (**G cells**) in both the antrum and duodenum make each of the two gastrins. Antral G cells are the primary source of G-17, whereas duodenal G cells are the primary source of G-34. Antral G cells are unusual in that they respond to both luminal and basolateral stimuli (Fig. 41–8). Antral G cells have microvilli on their apical membrane surface and are referred to as an "open-type" endocrine cell. These G cells release gastrin in response to luminal peptides and amino acids, as well as in response to **gastrin-releasing peptide** (GRP), a 27–amino acid peptide that is released by vagal nerve endings. As discussed later, gastrin release is inhibited by somatostatin, which is released from adjacent D cells.

Somatostatin, Released by Gastric D Cells, Is the Central Mechanism of Inhibition of Acid Secretion

Gastric-acid secretion is under close control of not only the stimulatory pathways discussed earlier but also the inhibitory pathways. The major inhibitory pathway involves the release of **somatostatin**, a polypeptide hormone made by D cells in the antrum and corpus of the stomach. Somatostatin is also made by the δ cells of the pancreatic islets (p. 1084) and by neurons in the hypothalamus (p. 1026). Somatostatin exists in two forms, SS-28 and SS-14, which have identical C termini. SS-28 is the predominant form in the GI tract.

Somatostatin inhibits gastric-acid secretion by both direct and indirect mechanisms (see Fig. 41–8). In the **direct pathway**, somatostatin coming from two different sources binds to a $G\alpha_i$-coupled receptor (SST) on the basolateral membrane of the parietal cell and inhibits adenylyl cyclase. The net effect is to antagonize the stimulatory effect of histamine and thus inhibit gastric-acid secretion by parietal cells. The source of this somatostatin can either be *paracrine* (i.e., D cells present in the corpus of the stomach, near the parietal cells) or *endocrine* (i.e., D cells in the antrum). However, there is a major difference in what triggers the D cells in the corpus and antrum. Neural and hormonal mechanisms stimulate D cells in the *corpus* (which cannot sense intraluminal pH), whereas low intraluminal pH stimulates D cells in the *antrum*.

Somatostatin also acts via two **indirect pathways**, both of which are paracrine in nature. In the corpus of the stomach, D cells release somatostatin that inhibits the release of *histamine* from ECL cells (see Fig. 41–8). Because histamine is an acid secretagogue, somatostatin thus reduces gastric-acid secretion. In the antrum of the stomach, D cells release somatostatin that inhibits the release of *gastrin* from G cells. Because gastrin is another acid secretagogue, somatostatin also reduces gastric-acid secretion by this route. Note that the gastrin released by the G cell feeds back on itself by stimulating D cells to release the inhibitory somatostatin.

The presence of multiple mechanisms by which soma-

tostatin inhibits acid secretion is another example of the *redundant regulatory pathways* that control acid secretion. An understanding of the regulation of somatostatin release from D cells is slowly evolving, but it appears that gastrin stimulates somatostatin release whereas cholinergic agonists inhibit somatostatin release.

Several Enteric Hormones ("Enterogastrone") and Prostaglandins Inhibit Gastric-Acid Secretion

Multiple processes in the duodenum and jejunum participate in the negative-feedback mechanisms that inhibit gastric-acid secretion. Fat, acid, and hyperosmolar solutions in the duodenum are potent inhibitors of gastric-acid secretion. Of these inhibitors, lipids are the most potent, but acid is also quite important. Several candidate hormones have been suggested as the prime mediator of this acid inhibition (Table 41–1). These include CCK (p. 920), secretin (p. 921), vasoactive intestinal peptide (VIP), gastric inhibitory peptide (GIP p. 899), neurotensin, and peptide YY (p. 924). Although each inhibits acid secretion after systemic administration, none has been *unequivocally* established as the sole physiologic "enterogastrone."

Evidence suggests that **secretin**, which is released by duodenal S cells, may have a prime role in inhibiting gastric acid secretion after the entry of fat and acid into the duodenum. Secretin appears to reduce acid secretion by at least three mechanisms: (1) inhibition of antral gastrin release, (2) stimulation of somatostatin release, and (3) direct downregulation of the parietal-cell H^+ secretory process.

The presence of luminal fatty acids causes enteroendocrine cells in the duodenum and the proximal part of the

TABLE 41–1

ENTERIC HORMONES THAT INHIBIT GASTRIC H^+ SECRETION	
HORMONE	**SOURCE**
CCK (cholecystokinin)	I cells of duodenum and jejunum and neurons in ileum and colon
Secretin	S cells in small intestine
VIP (vasoactive intestinal peptide)	ENS neurons
GIP (gastric inhibitory peptide, or glucose-dependent insulinotropic polypeptide)	K cells in duodenum and jejunum
Neurotensin	Endocrine cells in ileum
Peptide YY	Endocrine cells in ileum and colon
Somatostatin	D cells of stomach and duodenum, δ cells of pancreatic islets

ENS, enteric nervous system.

small intestine to release both GIP and CCK. **GIP** reduces acid secretion directly by inhibiting parietal-cell acid secretion and indirectly by inhibiting the antral release of gastrin. GIP also has the important function of stimulating insulin release from pancreatic islet cells in response to duodenal glucose and fatty acids and is therefore often referred to as glucose-dependent insulinotropic polypeptide (p. 1073). CCK participates in feedback inhibition of acid secretion by directly reducing parietal-cell acid secretion. Finally, some evidence indicates that a neural reflex elicited in the duodenum in response to acid also inhibits gastric-acid secretion.

Prostaglandin E$_2$ (PGE$_2$) inhibits parietal-cell acid secretion, probably by inhibiting histamine's activation of parietal-cell function at a site that is distal to the histamine receptor. PGE$_2$ appears to bind to an EP3 receptor on the basolateral membrane of the parietal cell (see Fig. 41–6) and stimulates Gα_i, which in turn inhibits adenylyl cyclase. In addition, prostaglandins also indirectly inhibit gastric-acid secretion by reducing histamine release from ECL cells and gastrin release from antral G cells.

Acid Secretion Occurs in Four Phases: A Basal (or Interdigestive) Phase and Three Phases Associated with Eating

BASAL STATE. Gastric-acid secretion occurs throughout the day and night. Substantial increases in acid secretion occur after meals, whereas the rate of acid secretion between meals is low (i.e., the interdigestive phase). This interdigestive period follows a circadian rhythm; acid secretion is lowest in the morning before awakening and highest in the evening. Acid secretion is a direct function of the number of parietal cells, which is also influenced, at least in part, by body weight. Thus, men have higher rates of basal acid secretion than women do. Considerable

variability in basal acid secretion is also seen among normal individuals, and the resting intragastric pH can range from 3 to 7.

In contrast to the low rate of acid secretion during the basal or interdigestive period, acid secretion is enhanced several-fold by eating (Fig. 41–9). It is important to note that regulation of gastric-acid secretion is most often studied in the fasting state, a state in which intragastric pH is relatively low because of the basal H$^+$ secretory rate and the absence of food that would otherwise buffer the secreted gastric acid. Experimental administration of a secretagogue in the fasted state thus stimulates parietal cells and further lowers intragastric pH. However, the time course of intragastric pH after a meal can vary considerably despite stimulation of acid secretion. The reason is that intragastric pH depends not only on gastric-acid secretion but also on the buffering power (p. 635) of food and the rate of gastric emptying of both acid and partially digested material into the duodenum.

Regulation of acid secretion during a meal can be best characterized by three separate, but interrelated phases: the cephalic, the gastric, and the intestinal phases. The cephalic and gastric phases are of primary importance. Regulation of acid secretion includes both the stimulatory and inhibitory mechanisms that we discussed earlier (see Fig. 41–8). ACh, gastrin, and histamine all promote acid secretion whereas somatostatin inhibits gastric-acid secretion.

Note that although dividing acid secretion during a meal into three phases has been used for decades, it is somewhat artificial because of considerable overlap in the regulation of acid secretion. For example, the vagus nerve is the central player in the cephalic phase, but it is also important for the vagovagal reflex that is part of the gastric phase. Similarly, gastrin release is a major component of the gastric phase, but vagal stimulation during the

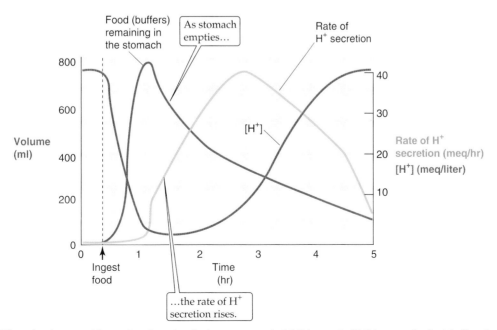

FIGURE 41–9. Effect of eating on acid secretion. Ingesting food causes a marked fall in gastric [H$^+$] because the food buffers the pre-existing H$^+$. However, as the food leaves the stomach and as the rate of H$^+$ secretion increases, [H$^+$] slowly rises to its "interdigestive" level.

cephalic phase also induces the release of antral gastrin. Finally, the development of a consensus model has long been hampered by considerable differences in regulation of the gastric phase of acid secretion in humans, dogs, and rodents.

CEPHALIC PHASE. The smell, sight, taste, thought, and swallowing of food initiate the cephalic phase, which is primarily mediated by the vagus nerve (see Fig. 41–8). Although the cephalic phase has long been studied in experimental animals, especially dogs, recent studies of sham feeding have confirmed and extended the understanding of the mechanism of the cephalic phase of acid secretion in humans. The aforementioned sensory stimuli activate the **dorsal motor nucleus of the vagus nerve** in the medulla (p. 381), thus activating parasympathetic preganglionic efferent nerves. Insulin-induced hypoglycemia also stimulates the vagus nerve and in so doing promotes acid secretion.

Stimulation of the vagus nerve results in four distinct physiological events—which we have already introduced in Figure 41–8—that together result in enhanced gastric-acid secretion. First, in the body of the stomach, vagal postganglionic muscarinic nerves release acetylcholine, which stimulates parietal-cell H^+ secretion directly. Second, in the lamina propria of the body of the stomach, the ACh released from vagal endings triggers histamine release from ECL cells, which stimulates acid secretion. Third, in the antrum, *peptidergic* postganglionic parasympathetic vagal neurons, as well as other enteric nervous system (ENS) neurons, release GRP, which induces gastrin release from antral G cells. This gastrin stimulates

FIGURE 41–11. Intestinal phase of gastric-acid secretion. Digested protein fragments (peptones) in the proximal small intestine stimulate gastric-acid secretion by three major mechanisms.

gastric-acid secretion both directly by acting on the parietal cell and indirectly by promoting histamine release from ECL cells. Fourth, in both the antrum and the corpus, the vagus nerve inhibits D cells, thus reducing their release of somatostatin and reducing the background inhibition of gastrin release. Thus, the cephalic phase stimulates acid secretion directly and indirectly by acting on the parietal cell. The cephalic phase accounts for *approximately 30% of total acid secretion* and occurs before the entry of any food into the stomach.

One of the surgical approaches for the treatment of peptic ulcer disease is cutting the vagus nerves (vagotomy) to inhibit gastric-acid secretion. Rarely performed, largely because of the many effective pharmacologic agents available to treat peptic ulcer disease, the technique has nevertheless proved to be effective in selected cases. Because vagus-nerve stimulation affects several GI functions besides parietal-cell acid secretion, the side effects of vagotomy include a delay in gastric emptying and diarrhea. To minimize these untoward events, there have been successful attempts to perform more "selective" vagotomies, severing *only those* vagal fibers going to the parietal cell.

GASTRIC PHASE. Entry of food into the stomach initiates the two primary stimuli for the gastric phase of acid secretion (Fig. 41–10). First, the food distends the gastric mucosa, which activates a vagovagal reflex as well as local ENS reflexes. Second, partially digested proteins stimulate antral G cells.

Distention of the gastric wall—both in the corpus and antrum—secondary to entry of food into the stomach elicits two distinct neurally mediated pathways. The first is activation of a **vagovagal reflex** (p. 884), in which gastric-wall distention activates a vagal *afferent* pathway, which in turn stimulates a vagal *efferent* response in the

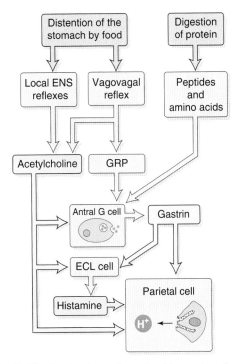

FIGURE 41–10. Gastric phase of gastric-acid secretion. Food in the stomach stimulates gastric-acid secretion by two major mechanisms: mechanical stretch and the presence of digested protein fragments ("peptones"). ECL, enterochromaffin-like; ENS, enteric nervous system; GRP, gastrin-releasing peptide.

dorsal nucleus of the vagus nerve. Stimulation of acid secretion in response to this vagal efferent stimulus occurs via the same four parallel pathways that are operative when the vagus nerve is activated during the cephalic phase (see Fig. 41–8). Second, gastric-wall distention also activates a **local ENS pathway** that releases ACh, which in turn stimulates parietal-cell acid secretion.

The presence of **partially digested proteins** (peptones) or amino acids in the antrum directly stimulates G cells to release gastrin (see Fig. 41–8). Intact proteins have no effect. Acid secretion and activation of pepsinogen are linked in a positive-feedback relationship. As discussed later, low pH enhances the conversion of pepsinogen to pepsin. Pepsin digests proteins to peptones, which promote gastrin release. Finally, gastrin promotes acid secretion, which closes the positive-feedback loop. There is little evidence that either carbohydrate or lipid participate in the regulation of gastric-acid secretion. Components of wine, beer, and coffee stimulate acid secretion by this G-cell mechanism.

In addition to the two stimulatory pathways acting during the gastric phase, a third pathway *inhibits* gastric-acid secretion by a classic negative feedback mechanism, already noted earlier in our discussion of Figure 41–8.

GASTRINOMA OR ZOLLINGER-ELLISON SYNDROME

On rare occasion, patients with one or more ulcers have very high rates of gastric-acid secretion. The increased acid secretion in these patients is most often a result of elevated levels of serum gastrin, released from a pancreatic islet cell adenoma or "gastrinoma" (Table 41–2). This clinical picture is also known as the **Zollinger-Ellison (ZE) syndrome.** Because gastrin released from these islet cell adenomas is not under physiological control, but rather is continuously released, acid secretion is substantially increased under basal conditions. However, the intravenous administration of pentagastrin—a synthetic gastrin consisting of the last four amino acids of gastrin plus β-alanine—produces only a modest increase in gastric-acid secretion. Omeprazole, a potent inhibitor of the parietal-cell H-K pump, is now an effective therapeutic agent to control the marked enhancement of gastric-acid secretion in gastrinoma patients, and thus helps heal their duodenal and gastric ulcers.

In contrast to patients with gastrinoma or ZE syndrome, other **duodenal ulcer** patients have serum gastrin levels that are near normal. Their basal gastric-acid–secretion rates are modestly elevated, but increase markedly in response to pentagastrin. Patients with **pernicious anemia** (see Box on pernicious anemia on p. 971) lack parietal cells and thus cannot secrete H^+. In the absence of a low luminal pH, the antral D cell is not stimulated by acid (see Fig. 41–10*B*). Consequently, the release of somatostatin from the D cell is low, and there is minimal tonic inhibition of gastrin release from G cells. It is not surprising, then, that these patients have very high levels of serum gastrin, but virtually no H^+ secretion (see Table 41–2).

TABLE 41–2

SERUM GASTRIN LEVELS AND GASTRIC ACID SECRETION RATES

	SERUM GASTRIN (pg/ml)	H^+ SECRETION (meq/hr)	
		Basal	After Pentagastrin
Normal	35	0.5–2.0	20–35
Duodenal ulcer	50	1.5–7.0	25–60
Gastrinoma	500	15–25	30–75
Pernicious anemia	350	0	0

Low intragastric pH stimulates antral D cells to release somatostatin. Because somatostatin inhibits the release of gastrin by G cells, the net effect is a reduction in gastric-acid secretion. The effectiveness of low pH in inhibiting gastrin release is emphasized by the following observation: Although peptones are normally a potent stimulus for gastrin release, they fail to stimulate gastrin release either when the intraluminal pH of the antrum is maintained at 1.0 or when somatostatin is infused.

The gastric phase of acid secretion, which occurs primarily as a result of gastrin release, accounts for *50% to 60% of total gastric acid secretion.*

THE INTESTINAL PHASE. The presence of amino acids and partially digested peptides in the proximal portion of the small intestine stimulates acid secretion by three mechanisms (Fig. 41–11). First, these peptones stimulate duodenal G cells to secrete gastrin, just as peptones stimulate antral G cells in the gastric phase. Second, peptones stimulate an unknown endocrine cell to release an additional humoral signal that has been referred to as "enterooxyntin." The chemical nature of this agent has not yet been identified. Third, amino acids absorbed by the proximal part of the small intestine stimulate acid secretion by mechanisms that require further definition.

Of interest, gastric-acid secretion mediated by the intestinal phase is enhanced after a portacaval shunt. Such a shunt—which is used in the treatment of portal hypertension caused by chronic liver disease—diverts the portal blood that drains the small intestine around the liver on its return to the heart. Thus, the signal released from the small intestine during the "intestinal phase" is probably—in normal individuals—removed in part by the liver before reaching its target, the corpus of the stomach.

Approximately 5% to 10% of total gastric acid secretion is a result of the intestinal phase.

PEPSINOGEN SECRETION

Chief Cells, Triggered by Both cAMP and Ca^{2+} Pathways, Secrete Multiple Pepsinogens That Initiate Protein Digestion

The chief cells in gastric glands, as well as mucous cells, secrete **pepsinogens**, a group of proteolytic proenzymes (i.e., zymogens or inactive enzyme precursors) that belong to the general class of aspartic proteinases. They are activated to pepsins by cleavage of an N-terminal peptide. **Pepsins** are endopeptidases that initiate the hydrolysis of ingested protein in the stomach. Although eight pepsinogen isoforms were initially identified on electrophoresis, recent classifications are based on immunologic identity, so pepsinogens are most often classified as group I pepsinogens, group II pepsinogens, and cathepsin E. Group I pepsinogens predominate. They are secreted from chief cells located at the base of glands in the corpus of the stomach. Group II pepsinogens are also secreted from chief cells but, in addition, are secreted from mucous neck cells in the cardiac, corpus, and antral regions.

Pepsinogen secretion in the basal state is approximately 20% of its maximal secretion after stimulation. Although pepsinogen secretion generally parallels the secretion of acid, the ratio of maximal to basal pepsinogen secretion is considerably less than that for acid secretion. Moreover, the cellular mechanism of pepsinogen release is quite distinct from that of H^+ secretion by parietal cells. Release of pepsinogen across the apical membrane is the result of a novel process called **compound exocytosis**, in which secretory granules fuse with both the plasma membrane and other secretory granules. This process permits rapid and sustained secretion of pepsinogen. After stimulation, the initial peak in pepsinogen secretion is followed by a persistent lower rate of secretion. This pattern of secretion has been interpreted as reflecting an initial secretion of *preformed* pepsinogen, followed by the secretion of *newly synthesized* pepsinogen. However, recent in vitro studies suggest that a feedback mechanism may account for the subsequent reduced rate of pepsinogen secretion.

Two groups of agonists stimulate chief cells to secrete pepsinogen. One group acts through adenylyl cyclase and cAMP, and the other acts through increases in $[Ca^{2+}]_i$.

AGONISTS ACTING VIA cAMP. Chief cells have receptors for **secretin/VIP**, β_2**-adrenergic** receptors, and EP2 receptors for **PGE$_2$**. All these receptors activate adenylyl cyclase. At lower concentrations than those required to *stimulate* pepsinogen secretion, PGE$_2$ can also *inhibit* pepsinogen secretion, probably by binding to another receptor subtype.

AGONISTS ACTING VIA Ca^{2+}. Chief cells also have M$_3$ muscarinic receptors for **acetylcholine,** as well as receptors for the **gastrin/CCK** family of peptides. Unlike gastric-acid secretion, which is stimulated via the CCK$_B$ receptor, pepsinogen secretion is stimulated via the CCK$_A$ receptor, which has a much higher affinity for CCK than for gastrin. Activation of both the M$_3$ and CCK$_A$ receptors causes Ca^{2+} release from intracellular stores via IP$_3$ and thereby raises $[Ca^{2+}]_i$. However, uncertainty exists about whether increased Ca^{2+} influx is also required and about whether PKC also has a role.

Of the agonists just listed, the most important for pepsinogen secretion is ACh released in response to vagal stimulation. Not only does ACh stimulate chief cells to release pepsinogen, it also stimulates parietal cells to secrete acid. This gastric acid produces additional pepsinogen secretion via two different mechanisms. First, in the

stomach, a fall in pH elicits a local cholinergic reflex that results in further stimulation of chief cells to release pepsinogen. Thus, the ACh that stimulates chief cells can come both from the vagus and from the local reflex. Second, in the duodenum, acid triggers the release of secretin from S cells. By an endocrine effect, this secretin stimulates the chief cells to release more pepsinogen. The exact role or roles of histamine and gastrin in pepsinogen secretion are unclear.

Low pH Is Required for Both Pepsinogen Activation and Pepsin Activity

Pepsinogen is inactive and requires activation to a protease, pepsin, to initiate protein digestion. This activation occurs by spontaneous cleavage of a small N-terminal peptide fragment (the activation peptide), but only at a pH that is less than 5.0 (Fig. 41–12). Between pH 5.0 and 3.0, spontaneous activation of pepsinogen is slow, but it is extremely rapid at a pH that is less than 3.0. In addition, pepsinogen is also autoactivated; that is, newly formed pepsin itself cleaves pepsinogen to pepsin.

Once pepsin is formed, its *activity* is also pH dependent. It has optimal activity at a pH between 1.8 and 3.5; the precise optimal pH depends on the specific pepsin, type and concentration of substrate, and osmolality of the solution. pH values above 3.5 *reversibly* inactivate pepsin, and pH values above 7.2 *irreversibly* inactivate the enzyme. These considerations are sometimes useful for establishing optimal antacid treatment regimens in peptic ulcer disease.

Pepsin is an endopeptidase that initiates the process of protein digestion in the stomach. Pepsin action results in the release of small peptides and amino acids (peptones) that, as noted earlier, stimulate the release of gastrin from antral G cells; these peptones also stimulate CCK release from duodenal I cells. As previously mentioned, the peptones generated by pepsin stimulate the very acid secretion required for pepsin activation and action. Thus, the peptides that pepsin releases are important in initiating a coordinated response to a meal. However, most protein entering the duodenum remains as large peptides, and nitrogen balance is not impaired after total gastrectomy.

Digestive products of both carbohydrates and lipid are also found in the stomach, although secretion of their respective digestive enzymes either does not occur or is not a major function of gastric epithelial cells. Carbohy-

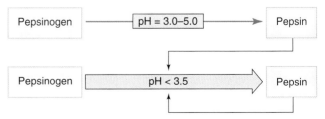

FIGURE 41–12. Activation of the pepsinogens to pepsins. At pH values from 5 to 3, pepsinogens spontaneously activate to pepsins by the removal of an N-terminal "activation peptide." This spontaneous activation is even faster at pH values that are below 3. The newly formed pepsins themselves—which are active only at pH values below 3.5— also can catalyze the activation of pepsinogens.

drate digestion is initiated in the mouth by **salivary amylase**. However, after this enzyme is swallowed, the stomach becomes a more important site for starch hydrolysis than the mouth. There is no evidence of gastric secretion of enzymes that hydrolyze starch or other saccharides. Similarly, although lipid digestion is also initiated in the mouth by lingual lipase, significant lipid digestion occurs in the stomach as a result of both the **lingual lipase** that is swallowed and **gastric lipase**, both of which have an acid pH optimum (p. 962).

PROTECTION OF THE GASTRIC SURFACE EPITHELIUM AND NEUTRALIZATION OF ACID IN THE DUODENUM

At maximal rates of H^+ secretion, the parietal cell can drive the intraluminal pH of the stomach to 1 or less (i.e., $[H^+] > 100$ mM) for long periods. The gastric epithelium must maintain an H^+ concentration gradient of over a million-fold because the intracellular pH of gastric epithelial cells is approximately 7.2 (i.e., $[H^+] \cong 60$ nM) and plasma pH is about 7.4 (i.e., $[H^+] \cong 40$ nM). Simultaneously, there is a substantial plasma-to-lumen Na^+-concentration gradient of approximately 30 because plasma $[Na^+]$ is 140 mM whereas intragastric $[Na^+]$ can reach values as low as 5 mM, but only at high secretory rates (see Fig. 41–2). How is the stomach able to maintain these gradients? How is it that the epithelial cells are not destroyed by this acidity? Moreover, why do pepsins in the gastric lumen not digest the epithelial cells? The answer to all three questions is the so-called **gastric diffusion barrier**.

Although the nature of the gastric diffusion barrier had been controversial, it is now recognized that the diffusion barrier is both physiologic and anatomic. Moreover, it is apparent that the diffusion barrier represents at least three components: (1) relative impermeability to acid of the apical membrane and epithelial cell tight junctions in the gastric glands; (2) a mucous-gel layer varying in thickness between 50 and 200 μm overlying the surface epithelial cells; and (3) an HCO_3^--containing microclimate adjacent to the surface epithelial cells that maintains a relatively high local pH.

Vagal Stimulation and Irritation Stimulate Gastric Mucous Cells to Secrete Mucin, a Glycoprotein That Is Part of the Mucosal Barrier

The mucus layer is largely composed of mucin, phospholipids, electrolytes, and water. **Mucin** is the high-molecular-weight glycoprotein (p. 40) that contributes to the formation of a protective layer over the gastric mucosa. Gastric mucin is a tetramer consisting of four identical peptides joined by disulfide bonds. Each of the four peptide chains is linked to long polysaccharides, which are often sulfated and thus mutually repulsive. The ensuing high carbohydrate content is responsible for the viscosity of mucus, which explains, in large part, its protective role in gastric mucosal physiology.

Mucus is secreted by three different mucous cells: surface mucous cells (i.e., on the surface of the stomach), mucous neck cells (i.e., at the point where a gastric pit joins a gastric gland), and glandular mucous cells (i.e., in the gastric glands in the antrum). The type of mucus secreted by these cells differs; mucus that is synthesized and secreted in the glandular cells is a neutral glycoprotein, whereas the mucous cells on the surface and in the gastric pits secrete both neutral and acidic glycoproteins. Mucin forms a **mucous-gel layer** in combination with phospholipids, electrolytes, and water. This mucous-gel layer provides protection against injury from noxious luminal substances, including acid, pepsins, bile acids, and ethanol. Mucin also lubricates the gastric mucosa to minimize the abrasive effects of intraluminal food.

The mucus barrier is not static. Abrasions can remove pieces of mucus. When mucus comes in contact with a solution with a very low pH, the mucus precipitates and sloughs off. Thus, the mucous cells must constantly secrete mucus. Regulation of mucus secretion by gastric mucosal cells is less well understood than is regulation of the secretion of acid, pepsinogens, and other substances by gastric cells. The two primary stimuli for inducing mucus secretion are vagal stimulation and physical and chemical irritation of the gastric mucosa by ingested food. The current model of mucus secretion suggests that vagal stimulation induces the release of ACh, which leads to increases in $[Ca^{2+}]_i$ and thus stimulates mucus secretion. In contrast to acid and pepsinogen secretion, cAMP does not appear to be a second messenger for mucus secretion.

Gastric Surface Cells Secrete HCO_3^-, Stimulated by Acetylcholine, Acids, and Prostaglandins

Surface epithelial cells both in the corpus and in the antrum of the stomach secrete HCO_3^-. Despite the relatively low rate of HCO_3^- secretion—in comparison to acid secretion—HCO_3^- is extremely important as part of the gastric mucosal protective mechanism. The mucus-gel layer provides an unstirred layer under which the secreted HCO_3^- remains trapped and maintains a local pH of approximately of 7.0 versus an intraluminal pH in the bulk phase of 1 to 3. As illustrated in Figure 41–13A, an electrogenic Na/HCO_3 cotransporter (NBC) appears to mediate the uptake of HCO_3^- across the basolateral membrane of surface epithelial cells. The mechanism of HCO_3^- exit from the cell into the apical mucus layer is unknown but may be mediated by a channel.

Similar to the situation for mucus secretion, relatively limited information is available about the regulation of HCO_3^- secretion. The present model suggests that *vagal stimulation* mediated by ACh leads to an increase in $[Ca^{2+}]_i$, which in turn stimulates HCO_3^- secretion. Sham feeding is a potent stimulus for HCO_3^- secretion via this pathway. A second powerful stimulus of gastric HCO_3^- secretion is *intraluminal acid*. The mechanism of stimulation by acid appears to be secondary to both activation of neural reflexes and local production of PGE_2. Finally, evidence suggests that a humoral factor may also be involved in the induction of HCO_3^- secretion by acid.

A NORMAL SURFACE EPITHELIUM

B DAMAGED MUCOSAL BARRIER

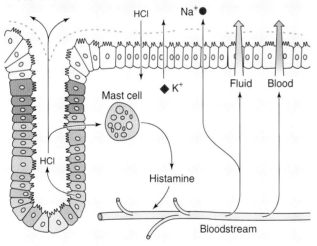

FIGURE 41–13. Diffusion barrier in the surface of the gastric mucosa. *A*, The mucus secreted by the surface cells serves two functions. First, it acts as a diffusion barrier for H$^+$ and also pepsins. Second, the mucus layer traps a relatively alkaline solution of HCO$_3^-$. This HCO$_3^-$ titrates any H$^+$ that diffuses into the gel layer from the stomach lumen. The alkaline layer also inactivates any pepsin that penetrates into the mucus. *B*, If H$^+$ penetrates into the gastric epithelium, it damages mast cells, which release histamine and other agents, setting up an inflammatory response. If the insult is mild, the ensuing increase in blood flow can promote the production of both mucus and HCO$_3^-$ by the mucus cells. If the insult is more severe, the inflammatory response leads to a decrease in blood flow and thus to cell injury.

Mucus Protects the Gastric Surface Epithelium by Trapping an HCO$_3^-$-Rich Fluid Near the Apical Border of These Cells

Mucous cells on the surface of the stomach, as well as in the gastric pits and neck portions of the gastric glands, secrete both HCO$_3^-$ and mucus. Why is this barrier so effective? First, the secreted mucus forms a mucous-gel layer that is relatively impermeable to the *diffusion* of H$^+$ from the gastric lumen to the surface cells. Second, beneath this layer of mucus is a microclimate that contains fluid with a high pH and high [HCO$_3^-$], the result of HCO$_3^-$ secretion by gastric surface epithelial cells (see Fig. 41–13*A*). Thus, this HCO$_3^-$ neutralizes most acid that diffuses through the mucus layer. Mucosal integrity, including that of the mucosal diffusion barrier, is also

maintained by PGE$_2$, which—as we saw in the previous section—stimulates mucosal HCO$_3^-$ secretion.

Deep inside the gastric gland, where no obvious mucus layer protects the parietal, chief, and ECL cells, the impermeability of the cells' apical barrier appears to exclude H$^+$ even at pH values as low as 1. The paradox of how HCl secreted by the parietal cells emerges from the gland and into the gastric lumen may be explained by a process known as **viscous fingering**. Because the liquid emerging from the gastric gland is both extremely acidic and presumably under pressure, it can tunnel through the mucous layer covering the opening of the gastric gland onto the surface of the stomach. However, this stream of acid apparently does not spread laterally, but rather rises to the surface as a "finger" and thus does not neutralize the

HCO_3^- in the microenvironment between the surface epithelial cells and the mucus.

The mucous-gel layer and the trapped alkaline HCO_3 solution protect the surface cells not only from H^+ but also from pepsin. The mucus per se acts as a pepsin-diffusion barrier. The relative alkalinity of the trapped HCO_3^- inactivates any pepsin that penetrates into the mucus. Recall that pepsin is reversibly inactivated at pH values that are above approximately 3.5 and irreversibly inactivated by pH values approximately above 7.2. Thus, the mucus/HCO_3^- layer plays an important role in preventing "autodigestion" of the gastric mucosa.

Entry of Acid into the Duodenum Induces the Release of Secretin From S Cells, Thus Triggering the Secretion of HCO_3^- by the Pancreas and Duodenum, Which in Turn Neutralizes Gastric Acid

The overall process of regulating gastric-acid secretion involves not only stimulation and inhibition of acid secretion—which we discussed earlier—but also neutralization of the gastric acid that passes from the stomach into

---

BREAKDOWN OF THE GASTRIC BARRIER

Integrity of the gastric-epithelial barrier can be conveniently judged by maintenance of a high lumen-negative transepithelial potential difference (PD) of about -60 mV. Several agents that cause mucosal injury, including mucosal ulceration, can alter the mucosal diffusion barrier. Salicylates, bile acids, and ethanol all impair the mucosal diffusion barrier and result in H^+ (acid) backdiffusion, an increase in intraluminal $[Na^+]$, a fall in PD, and mucosal damage (see Fig. 41–13B). Three decades ago, Davenport proposed an attractive model to explain how H^+, after having breached the mucosal diffusion barrier, produces injury to the gastric mucosa. Although several details of this original model have been modified during the ensuing years, it is still believed that entry of acid into the mucosa damages mast cells, which release histamine and other mediators of **inflammation.** The histamine and other agents cause a local vasodilatation that increases blood flow. If the damage is not too severe, this response allows the surface cells to maintain their production of mucus and HCO_3^-. However, if the injury is more severe, inflammatory cells release a host of agents—including platelet-activating factor (PAF), leukotrienes, endothelins, thromboxanes, and oxidants—that reduce blood flow (ischemia) and result in tissue injury, including capillary damage.

Prostaglandins play a central role in maintaining mucosal integrity. For example, prostaglandins prevent or reverse mucosal injury secondary to salicylates, bile, and ethanol. This protective effect of prostaglandins is the result of several actions, including their ability to inhibit acid secretion, stimulate both HCO_3^- and mucus secretion, increase mucosal blood flow, and modify the local inflammatory response induced by acid.

HELICOBACTER PYLORI

During the past decade, our understanding of the etiology of duodenal and gastric ulcers has radically changed. Abundant evidence now indicates that the majority of peptic ulcers are an infectious disease in that most (but not all) ulcers are caused by *H. pylori*, a gram-negative bacillus that colonizes the antral mucosa. Nonsteroidal anti-inflammatory drugs (NSAIDs) are responsible for approximately 20% of ulcers. Although almost all ulcers that are not associated with NSAID use are secondary to *H. pylori* infestation, many, if not most, individuals with evidence of *H. pylori* infestation do not have peptic ulcer disease. The factor or factors responsible for *H. pylori*–induced inflammation or ulceration are not known. However, the increase in gastric-acid secretion that is present in most patients with duodenal ulcers may occur because *H. pylori*–induced antral inflammation inhibits the release of somatostatin by antral D cells. Because somatostatin normally inhibits gastrin release by antral G cells, the result would be increased gastrin release and thus increased gastric-acid secretion. Indeed, as noted in Table 41–2, serum gastrin levels are modestly elevated in patients with duodenal ulcers.

Inhibition of acid secretion heals, but does not cure *H. pylori*–induced peptic ulcers. However, antibiotic therapy that eradicates *H. pylori* cures peptic ulcer disease.

---

the duodenum. The amount of secreted gastric acid is reflected by a fall in intragastric pH. We have already seen that this fall in pH serves as the signal to antral D cells to release somatostatin and thus inhibit further acid secretion, a classic negative-feedback process. Likewise, low pH in the duodenum serves as a signal for the secretion of alkali to neutralize gastric acid in the duodenum.

The key player in this neutralization process is **secretin**, the same secretin that inhibits gastric-acid secretion and promotes pepsinogen secretion by chief cells. A low duodenal pH, with a threshold of 4.5, triggers the release of secretin from **S cells** in the duodenum. However, the S cells are probably not pH sensitive themselves but, instead, may respond to a signal from other cells that are pH sensitive. As discussed in Chapter 42, secretin stimulates the secretion of fluid and HCO_3^- by the pancreas, thus leading to intraduodenal neutralization of the acid load from the stomach. Maximal HCO_3^- secretion is a function of the amount of acid entering the duodenum, as well as the length of duodenum exposed to acid. Thus, high rates of gastric-acid secretion trigger the release of large amounts of secretin, which greatly stimulates pancreatic HCO_3^- secretion; the increased HCO_3^- in turn neutralizes the increased duodenal acid load.

In addition to *pancreatic* HCO_3^- secretion, the duodenal acid load resulting from gastric-acid secretion is partially neutralized by *duodenal* HCO_3^- secretion. This duodenal HCO_3^- secretion occurs in the proximal—but not the distal—part of the duodenum under the influence of prostaglandins. Attention has been focused on duodenal epithelial cells (villus and/or crypt cells) as the cellular source of HCO_3^- secretion, but the possibility that duodenal HCO_3^- originates, at least in part, from duodenal submucosal Brunner glands has not been excluded. Patients with duodenal ulcer disease tend to have both increased gastric-acid secretion and reduced duodenal HCO_3^- secretion. Thus, the increased acid load in the duodenum is only partially neutralized, so the duodenal mucosa has increased exposure to a low-pH solution.

FILLING AND EMPTYING OF THE STOMACH

Gastric Motor Activity Plays a Role in Filling, Churning, and Emptying

Gastric motor activity has three functions: (1) The receipt of ingested material represents the **reservoir function** of the stomach and occurs as smooth muscle relaxes. This response occurs primarily in the proximal portion of the stomach. (2) Ingested material is **churned** and thus altered to a form that rapidly empties from the stomach through the pylorus and facilitates normal jejunal digestion and absorption. Thus, in conjunction with gastric acid and enzymes, the motor function of the stomach helps initiate digestion. (3) The pyloric antrum, pylorus, and proximal part of the duodenum function as a single unit for **emptying** into the duodenum the modified gastric contents ("chyme"), consisting of both partially digested food material and gastric secretions. Gastric filling and emptying are accomplished by the coordinated activity of smooth muscle in the esophagus, lower esophageal sphincter, and proximal and distal portions of the stomach, as well as the pylorus and duodenum.

The pattern of gastric smooth-muscle activity is distinct during fasting and after eating. The pattern during fasting is referred to as the **migrating myoelectric (or motor) complex** (MMC), which we already discussed in connection with the small intestine (p. 889). This pattern is terminated by eating, at which point it is replaced by the so-called **fed pattern**. Just as the proximal and distal regions of the stomach differ in secretory function, they also differ in the motor function responsible for storing, processing, and emptying liquids and solids. The proximal part of the stomach is the primary location for storage of both liquids and solids. The distal portion of the stomach is primarily responsible for churning the solids and generating smaller liquid-like material, which then exits the stomach in a manner that is similar to that of ingested liquids. Thus, the gastric emptying of liquids and solids is closely integrated.

Filling of the Stomach Is Facilitated by Both Receptive Relaxation and Gastric Accommodation

Even a dry swallow relaxes both the lower esophageal sphincter and the proximal part of the stomach. Of course, the same happens when we swallow food. These relaxations facilitate the entry of food into the stomach. Relaxation in the fundus is primarily regulated by a vagovagal reflex and has been called **receptive relaxation**. In

a **vagovagal reflex**, afferent fibers running with the vagus nerve carry information to the central nervous system (CNS), and efferent vagal fibers carry the signal from the CNS to the stomach and cause relaxation via a mechanism that is neither cholinergic nor adrenergic. The result is that intragastric volume increases *without* an increase in intragastric pressure. If vagal innervation to the stomach is interrupted, gastric pressure rises much more rapidly.

Quite apart from the receptive relaxation of the stomach that anticipates the arrival of food after swallowing and esophageal distention, the stomach can also relax in response to gastric filling per se. Thus, increasing intragastric volume, as a result of either food entering the stomach or gastric secretion, does not produce a proportionate increase in intragastric pressure. Instead, small increases in volume do not cause increases in intragastric pressure until a threshold is reached, after which intragastric pressure rises steeply (Fig. 41–14A). This phenomenon is due to *active* dilatation of the fundus and has been called **gastric accommodation**. Vagotomy abolishes a major portion of gastric accommodation, so increases in intragastric volume produce greater increases in intragastric pressure. However, the role of the vagus nerve in gastric

FIGURE 41–14. Gastric filling and emptying. (*Panel B*, data from Dooley CP, Reznick JB, Valenzuela JE: Variations in gastric and duodenal motility during gastric emptying of liquid meals in humans. Gastroenterology 87:1114–1119, 1984.)

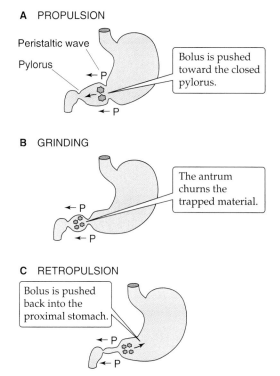

A PROPULSION

Peristaltic wave

Pylorus

Bolus is pushed toward the closed pylorus.

B GRINDING

The antrum churns the trapped material.

C RETROPULSION

Bolus is pushed back into the proximal stomach.

FIGURE 41–15. Mechanical actions of the stomach on its contents.

accommodation is one of modulation. It is generally believed that the **enteric nervous system** (p. 883) is the primary regulator permitting the storage of substantial amounts of solids and liquids in the proximal part of the stomach without major increases in intragastric pressure.

The Stomach Churns Its Contents Until the Particles Are Small Enough to Be Gradually Emptied into the Duodenum

The substance most rapidly emptied by the stomach is isotonic saline or water. Emptying of these liquids occurs without delay and is faster the greater the volume of fluid. Acidic and caloric fluids leave the stomach more slowly, and fatty materials exit even more slowly (see Fig. 41–14B). Solids do not leave the stomach as such, but must first be reduced in size (i.e., trituration). Particles greater than 2 mm in size do not leave the stomach during the immediate postprandial digestive period. The delay in gastric emptying of solids occurs because solids must be reduced in size to less than 2 mm; at that point, they are emptied by mechanisms that are similar to those of liquids.

Movement of solid particles toward the antrum is accomplished by the interaction of propulsive gastric contractions and occlusion of the pylorus, a process termed **propulsion** (Fig. 41–15A). Gastric contractions are initiated by the gastric pacemaker, which is located on the greater curvature, approximately at the junction of the proximal and middle portions of the stomach. These contractions propel the luminal contents toward the pylorus, which is partially closed by contraction of the pyloric

musculature before delivery of the bolus. This increase in pyloric resistance represents the coordinated response of antral, pyloric, and duodenal motor activity. Once a bolus of material is trapped near the antrum, it is churned to help reduce the size of the particles, a process termed **grinding** (see Fig. 41–15B). Only a small portion of gastric material—that containing particles smaller than 2 mm—is propelled through the pylorus to the duodenum. Thus, most of the gastric contents are returned to the body of the stomach for pulverization and shearing of solid particles, a process known as **retropulsion** (see Fig. 41–15C). These processes of propulsion, grinding, and retropulsion repeat multiple times until the gastric contents are emptied. Particles larger than 2 mm are initially retained in the stomach but are eventually emptied into the duodenum by MMCs during the interdigestive period that begins approximately 2 hours or more after eating.

Modification of gastric contents is associated with the activation of multiple feedback mechanisms. This feedback usually arises from the duodenum (and beyond) and almost always results in a delay in gastric emptying. Thus, as small squirts of gastric fluid leave the stomach, chemoreceptors and mechanoreceptors—primarily in the proximal but also in the distal portion of the small intestine—sense low pH, a high content of calories, lipid, or some amino acids (i.e., tryptophan), or changes in osmolarity. These signals all decrease the rate of gastric emptying by a combination of neural and hormonal signals, including the vagus nerve, secretin, CCK, and GIP released from duodenal mucosa. Delayed gastric emptying represents: the coordinated function of fundic relaxation; inhibition of antral motor activity; stimulation of isolated, phasic contractions of the pyloric sphincter; and altered intestinal motor activity.

REFERENCES

Books and Reviews

DelValle J, Todisco A: Gastric secretion. In Yamada T (ed): Textbook of Gastroenterology, Vol 1, 4th ed. Philadelphia, Lippincott, Williams and Wilkins, 2003, pp 266–307.

Dockray GJ, Varro A, Dimaline R: Gastric endocrine cells: Gene expression, processing and targeting of active products. Physiol Rev 76:767–798, 1996.

Hasler WL: The physiology of gastric motility and gastric emptying. In Yamada T (ed): Textbook of Gastroenterology, Vol 1, 4th ed. Philadelphia, Lippincott, Williams and Wilkins, 2003, pp 195–219.

Hersey SJ, Sachs G: Gastric acid secretion. Physiol Rev 75:155–189, 1995.

Lichtenberger LM: The hydrophobic barrier properties of gastrointestinal mucus. Annu Rev Physiol 57:565–583, 1995.

Sachs G, Prinz C: Gastric enterochromaffin-like cells and the regulation of acid secretion. News Physiol Sci 11:57–62, 1996.

Sachs G, Zeng N, Prinz C: Physiology of isolated gastric endocrine cells. Annu Rev Physiol 59:243–256, 1997.

Sawada M, Dickinson CJ: The G cell. Annu Rev Physiol 59:273–298, 1997.

Journal Articles

Dooley CP, Reznick JB, Valenzuela JE: Variations in gastric and duodenal motility during gastric emptying of liquid meals in humans. Gastroenterology 87:1114-1119, 1984.

Waisbren SJ, Geibel JP, Modlin IM, Boron WF: Unusual permeability properties of gastric gland cells. Nature 368:332–335, 1994.

CHAPTER 42

Pancreatic and Salivary Glands

Christopher R. Marino and Fred S. Gorelick

OVERVIEW OF EXOCRINE GLAND PHYSIOLOGY

The Pancreas and Major Salivary Glands Are Compound Exocrine Glands

The exocrine pancreas and major salivary glands are compound exocrine glands—specialized secretory organs that contain a branching ductular system through which they release their secretory products. The principal function of these exocrine glands is to aid in the digestion of food. The saliva produced by the salivary glands lubricates ingested food and initiates the digestion of starch. Pancreatic juice, rich in HCO_3^- and digestive enzymes, neutralizes the acidic gastric contents that enter the small intestine and also completes the intraluminal digestion of ingested carbohydrate, protein, and fat. Each of these exocrine glands is under the control of neural and humoral signals that generate a sequential and coordinated secretory response to an ingested meal. We discuss the *endocrine* pancreas in Chapter 50.

Morphologically, the pancreas and salivary glands are divided into small but visible **lobules**, each of which represents a subdivision of the parenchyma and is drained by a single **intralobular duct** (Fig. 42–1A). Groups of lobules separated by connective tissue septa are drained by larger **interlobular ducts**. These interlobular ducts empty into a **main duct** that connects the entire gland to the lumen of the gastrointestinal tract.

Within the lobules reside the microscopic structural and functional secretory units of the gland. Each **secretory unit** is composed of an acinus and a small intercalated duct. The **acinus** represents a cluster of 15 to 100 acinar cells that synthesize and secrete proteins into the lumen of the epithelial structure. In the pancreas, acinar cells secrete approximately 20 different zymogens (inactive enzyme precursors) and digestive enzymes. In the salivary glands, the principal acinar cell protein products are α-amylase, mucins, and proline-rich proteins. Acinar cells from both the pancreas and salivary glands also secrete an isotonic, plasma-like fluid that accompanies the secretory proteins. In all, the final acinar secretion is a protein-rich product known as the primary secretion.

Each acinar lumen is connected to the proximal end of an **intercalated duct**. Distally, the intercalated ducts fuse with other small ducts to form progressively larger ducts that ultimately coalesce to form the intralobular

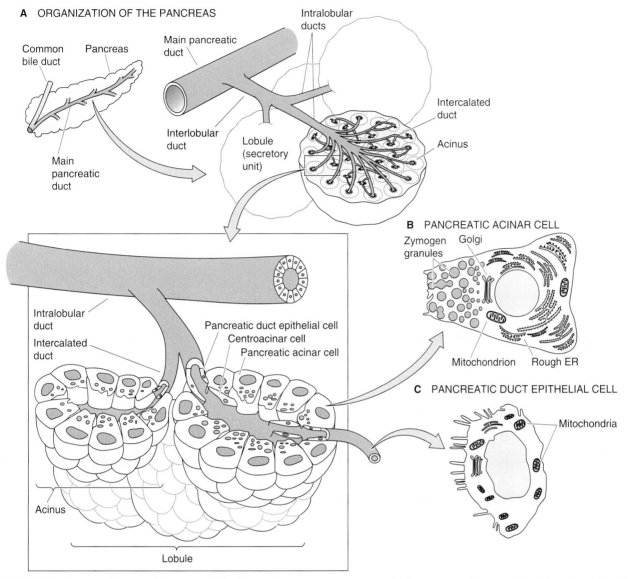

A ORGANIZATION OF THE PANCREAS

Common bile duct

Pancreas

Main pancreatic duct

Intralobular ducts

Interlobular duct

Lobule (secretory unit)

Intercalated duct

Acinus

Main pancreatic duct

Intralobular duct

Intercalated duct

Pancreatic duct epithelial cell
Centroacinar cell
Pancreatic acinar cell

Acinus

Lobule

B PANCREATIC ACINAR CELL

Zymogen granules   Golgi

Mitochondrion   Rough ER

C PANCREATIC DUCT EPITHELIAL CELL

Mitochondria

FIGURE 42–1. Acinus-duct morphology. *A*, The fundamental secretory unit is composed of an acinus and an intercalated duct. Intercalated ducts merge to form intralobular ducts, which in turn merge to form interlobular ducts, and then the main pancreatic duct. *B*, The acinar cell is specialized for protein secretion. Large condensing vacuoles are gradually reduced in size and form mature zymogen granules that store digestive enzymes in the apical region of the acinar cell. *C*, The duct cell is a cuboidal cell with abundant mitochondria. Small microvilli project from its apical membrane.

duct that drains the lobule. Although the ducts provide a conduit for the transport of secretory proteins, it is clear that the epithelial cells lining the ducts also play an important role in modifying the fluid and electrolyte composition of the primary secretion. Thus, the final exocrine gland secretion represents the combined product of two distinct epithelial cell populations, the acinar cell and the duct cell.

In addition to acini and ducts, exocrine glands contain a rich supply of nerves and blood vessels. Postganglionic **parasympathetic** and **sympathetic** fibers contribute to the autonomic regulation of secretion through the release of cholinergic and adrenergic neurotransmitters that bind to receptors on the acinar and duct cells. Both central and reflex pathways contribute to the neural regulation of

exocrine secretion. The autonomic nerves also carry afferent pain fibers that are activated by glandular inflammation and trauma. The vasculature not only provides oxygen and nutrients for the gland but also carries the hormones that help regulate secretion.

Acinar Cells Are Specialized Protein-Synthesizing Cells

Acinar cells are polarized epithelial cells that are specialized for the production and export of large quantities of protein. Thus, the acinar cell is equipped with a well-developed rough endoplasmic reticulum (see Fig. 42–1*B*). However, the most characteristic feature of the acinar cell is the abundance of electron-dense secretory granules at the apical pole of the cell. These granules are storage pools of secretory proteins, and they are poised for releasing their contents after stimulation of the cell by neurohumoral agents. The secretory granules of *pancreatic* acinar cells contain the mixture of enzymes required for digestion. The secretory granules of *salivary* acinar cells contain either α-amylase (in the parotid gland) or mucins (in the submandibular glands). Secretory granules in the pancreas appear uniform, whereas those in the salivary glands often exhibit focal nodules of condensation within the granules known as "spherules."

The pancreatic acinar cell has served as an important model for elucidating protein synthesis and export via the **secretory pathway**. Synthesis of secretory proteins (p. 36) begins with the cellular uptake of amino acids and their incorporation into nascent proteins in the *rough* **endoplasmic reticulum** (Fig. 42–2). Vesicular transport mechanisms then shuttle the newly synthesized proteins to the Golgi complex.

Within the **Golgi complex**, secretory proteins are segregated away from lysosomal enzymes. Most lysosomal enzymes require the mannose 6-phosphate receptor for sorting to the lysosome (p. 41). However, the signals required to direct digestive enzymes into the secretory pathway remain unclear.

Secretory proteins exit the Golgi complex in **condensing vacuoles.** These large membrane-bound structures are acidic and maintain the lowest pH within the secretory pathway.

Maturation of the condensing vacuole to a secretory or zymogen granule is marked by condensation of the proteins within the vacuole and pinching off of the membrane. The diameter of a **zymogen granule** is about two thirds that of a condensing vacuole, and its content is more electron dense. Secretory proteins are stored in zymogen granules that are located in the apical region of the acinar cell. The bottom portion of Figure 42–2 shows the results of a pulse-chase experiment that follows the cellular itinerary of radiolabeled amino acids as they move sequentially through the four major compartments of the secretory pathway.

Exocytosis, the process by which secretory granules release their contents, is a complex series of events that involves the movement of the granules to the apical membrane, fusion of these granules with the membrane, and release of their contents into the acinar lumen. Secretion is triggered by either hormones or neural activity. At the onset of secretion, the area of the apical plasma membrane increases as much as 30-fold. Thereafter, activation of an apical endocytic pathway leads to retrieval of the secretory granule membrane for recycling and a decrease in the area of the apical plasma membrane back to its resting value. Thus, during the steady state of secretion, the secretory granule membrane is simultaneously delivered to and retrieved from the apical membrane.

The cytoskeleton of the acinar cell plays an important role in the regulation of exocytosis. A component of the actin network appears to be required for delivery of the secretory granules to the apical region of the cell. A second actin network, located immediately below the apical membrane, acts as a barrier that blocks fusion of the granules with the apical plasma membrane. Upon stimu-

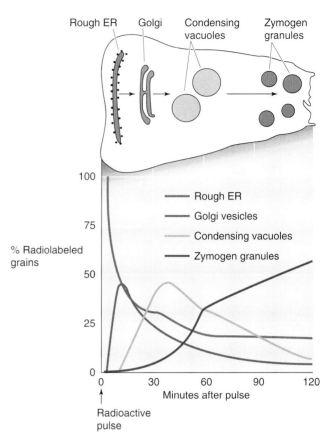

FIGURE 42–2. Movement of newly synthesized proteins through the secretory pathway. The cell model at the *top* illustrates the vectoral movement of nascent proteins through the compartments of the secretory pathway. The four *records* in the graph show the time course of secretory proteins moving through these compartments. To radioactively label newly synthesized proteins, the investigators briefly pulsed the pancreatic acinar cells with ³H-labeled amino acids. At specific times after the pulse, tissues were fixed, and the distribution of the radioactive amino acid was determined using autoradiography. Each of the four *records* shows the number of radiographic grains—as a fraction of all of the grains—found in each compartment at various times after the pulse. ER, endoplasmic reticulum. (Data from Jamieson J, Palade G: Intracellular transport of secretory proteins in the pancreatic acinar cell. J Cell Biol 34:597–615, 1967; and Jamieson J, Palade G: Synthesis, intracellular transport, and discharge of secretory proteins in stimulated pancreatic exocrine cells. J Cell Biol 50:135–158, 1971.)

lation, this second network reorganizes and then releases the blockade to permit the secretory granules to approach the apical plasma membrane. Fusion of the granules with the plasma membrane probably requires the interaction of proteins on both the secretory granules and the apical plasma membrane, as well as various cytosolic factors (p. 39). After fusion, the granule contents are released into the acinar lumen and carried down the ducts into the gastrointestinal tract.

Duct Cells Are Epithelial Cells Specialized for Fluid and Electrolyte Transport

Pancreatic and salivary duct cells are polarized epithelial cells specialized for the transport of electrolytes across distinct apical and basolateral membrane domains. Duct epithelial cells contain specific membrane transporters and an abundance of mitochondria to provide energy for active transport, and they exhibit varying degrees of basolateral membrane infolding that increases membrane surface area (see Fig. 42–1C). Although some duct cells contain prominent cytoplasmic vesicles, or storage granules—an indication of an additional *protein* secretory function—the synthetic machinery (i.e., endoplasmic reticulum and Golgi complex) of the duct cell is, in general, much less developed than that of the acinar cell.

Duct cells exhibit a considerable degree of morphologic heterogeneity along the length of the ductal tree. At the junction between pancreatic acinar and duct cells are small cuboidal epithelial cells known as centroacinar cells. These cells express very high levels of carbonic anhydrase (see box on p. 637) and presumably play a role in HCO_3^- secretion. The epithelial cells of the most proximal (intercalated) duct are squamous or low cuboidal in shape, have an abundance of mitochondria, and tend to lack cytoplasmic vesicles. These features suggest that the primary function of these cells is fluid and electrolyte transport. Progressing distally, the cells become more cuboidal-columnar in shape and contain more cytoplasmic vesicles and granules. These features suggest that these cells are capable of both transport of fluid and electrolytes and secretion of proteins. Functional studies indicate that the types of solute transport proteins within duct cells differ depending on the cell's location in the ductal tree.

Ion transport in duct cells is regulated by neurohumoral stimuli that act through specific receptors that are located on the basolateral membrane. As is the case for cells elsewhere in the body, duct cells can increase transcellular electrolyte movement either by activating individual transport proteins or by increasing the number of transport proteins in the plasma membrane.

Goblet Cells Contribute to Mucin Production in Exocrine Glands

In addition to acinar and duct cells, exocrine glands contain varying numbers of goblet cells. These cells secrete high-molecular-weight glycoproteins known as **mucins**. When hydrated, mucins form **mucus** (p. 40). Mucus has several important functions, including lubrication, hydration, and mechanical protection of surface epithelial cells. Mucins also play an important immunologic role by binding to pathogens and interacting with immune-competent cells. These properties may help prevent pancreatic infections. In the pancreas, mucin-secreting goblet cells are primarily found among the epithelial cells that line the large, distal ducts. They can account for as many as 25% of the epithelial cells in the distal main pancreatic duct of some species. In the salivary gland, goblet cells are also seen in the large distal ducts, although in less abundance than in the pancreas. However, in many salivary glands, mucin is also secreted by acinar cells.

PANCREATIC ACINAR CELL

The Acinar Cell Secretes Digestive Proteins in Response to Stimulation

To study secretion at the cellular level, investigators use enzymes to digest pancreatic connective tissue and obtain *single acini* (small groups of 15 to 100 acinar cells), or they mechanically dissect *single lobules* (groups of 250 to 1000 cells). The measure of secretion is the release of digestive proteins into the incubation medium. The amount released over a fixed time interval is expressed as a percentage of the total content at the outset of the experiment. Because amylase is released in a fully active form, it is common to use the appearance of amylase activity as a marker for secretion by acinar cells.

When the acinar cells are in an unstimulated state, they secrete low levels of digestive proteins via a **constitutive secretory pathway**. Acinar cells stimulated by neurohumoral agents secrete proteins via a **regulated pathway**. Regulated secretion by acini and lobules in vitro is detected within 5 minutes of stimulation and is energy dependent. During a 30- to 60-minute stimulation period, acinar cells typically secrete 5 to 10 times more amylase than with constitutive release. However, during this period of regulated secretion, the cells typically secrete only 10% to 20% of the digestive proteins stored in their granules. Moreover, acinar cells are able to increase their rate of protein synthesis to replenish their stores.

The acinar cell may exhibit two distinct patterns of regulated secretion: monophasic and biphasic (Fig. 42–3A). An agonist that generates a **monophasic** dose-response relationship (e.g., gastrin-releasing peptide [GRP]) causes secretion to reach a maximal level that does not fall with higher concentrations of the agent. In contrast, a secretagogue that elicits a **biphasic** dose-response relationship (e.g., cholecystokinin [CCK] and carbachol) causes secretion to reach a maximal level that subsequently diminishes with higher concentrations of the agent. As discussed later, this biphasic response may reflect the presence of functionally separate high- and low-affinity receptors.

Regulated Secretion of Proteins by Pancreatic Acinar Cells Is Mediated Through Cholecystokinin and Muscarinic Receptors

Although at least a dozen different receptors have been found on the plasma membrane of the pancreatic acinar cell, the most important in regulating protein secretion are the CCK receptors and the muscarinic acetylcholine (ACh) receptors. These receptors have many similarities: both are linked to the $G\alpha_q$ heterotrimeric G protein, use the phospholipase C (PLC)/Ca^{2+} signal-transduction pathway (p. 100), and lead to increased enzyme secretion from the acinar cell.

Two closely related CCK receptors are distinguished by their structure, affinity for ligands, and tissue distribution (p. 895). Although both CCK receptors may be activated by CCK or gastrin, the CCK_A receptor has a much higher affinity for CCK than for gastrin, whereas the CCK_B receptor has approximately equal affinities for CCK and gastrin. It appears that human acinar cells lack the CCK_A receptor.

An important feature of both CCK receptors is their ability to exist in both a high- and a low-affinity state. Low (picomolar) concentrations of CCK activate the high-affinity forms of the CCK receptors and *stimulate* secretion. On the other hand, supraphysiological (10- to 100-

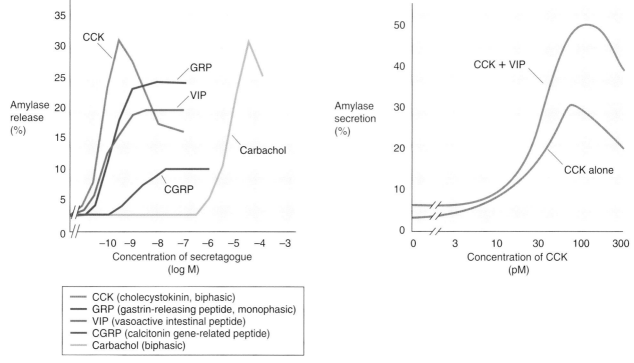

A PANCREATIC SECRETAGOGUES

B POTENTIATED SECRETAGOGUE RESPONSE

--- CCK (cholecystokinin, biphasic)
--- GRP (gastrin-releasing peptide, monophasic)
--- VIP (vasoactive intestinal peptide)
--- CGRP (calcitonin gene-related peptide)
--- Carbachol (biphasic)

FIGURE 42–3. Neurohumoral agents elicit different secretory responses from the pancreatic acinar cell. (*A,* Data from Jensen RT: Receptors on pancreatic acinar cells. In Johnson LR [ed]: Physiology of the Gastrointestinal Tract. New York, Raven Press, 1994, pp 1377–1446. *B,* Data from Burnham DB, McChesney DJ, Thurston KC, Williams JA: Interaction of cholecystokinin and vasoactive polypeptide on function of mouse pancreatic acini in vitro. J Physiol 349:475–482, 1984.)

fold higher) concentrations of CCK activate the low-affinity forms of the receptors and *inhibit* secretion. As we explain in the next section, these two affinity states (i.e., activated by different concentrations of CCK) of each of the two CCK receptors generate distinct second-messenger signalling patterns. It is likely that under physiological conditions, only the high-affinity states of the CCK or muscarinic receptor are activated. Stimulation of the lower-affinity states by supraphysiological concentrations of either CCK or ACh not only inhibits enzyme secretion but may also injure the acinar cell (see the box titled Acute Pancreatitis).

The muscarinic receptor on the acinar cell is probably of the M_3 subtype (p. 387) found in many glandular tissues. Like the CCK receptor, the M_3 receptor is localized to the basolateral membrane of the cell. A number of other receptors, including those for GRP (p. 898), calcitonin-gene–related peptide (CGRP; p. 1099), insulin (p. 1073), secretin (p. 915), somatostatin (p. 898), and vasoactive intestinal polypeptide (VIP; p. 898), are also found on the pancreatic acinar cell. Although these other receptors may also play a role in regulating secretion, protein synthesis, growth, and transformation, their precise physiological function remains to be clearly defined.

Activation of receptors that stimulate *different* signal-transduction pathways may lead to an enhanced secretory response. For example, as shown in Figure 42–3B, simultaneous stimulation of the high-affinity CCK receptor (which acts via $[Ca^{2+}]_i$) and the VIP receptor (which acts via cyclic adenosine monophosphate [cAMP]) generates an additive effect on secretion. Alternatively, acinar cells

that have previously been stimulated may become temporarily refractory to subsequent stimulation. This phenomenon is known as **desensitization**.

Ca²⁺ Is the Major Second Messenger for the Secretion of Proteins by Pancreatic Acinar Cells

Ca²⁺. Much of the pioneering work on the role of intracellular Ca^{2+} in cell signalling has been performed in the pancreatic acinar cell (Fig. 42–4A). Generation of a cytosolic Ca^{2+} signal is a complex summation of cellular events (p. 102) that regulates cytosolic free Ca^{2+} levels ($[Ca^{2+}]_i$). Even when the acinar cell is in the resting state, $[Ca^{2+}]_i$ oscillates slowly. In the presence of maximal stimulatory (i.e., physiological) concentrations of CCK or ACh, the frequency of the oscillations increases (Fig. 42–4B), but little change in their amplitude is noted. This increase in the frequency of $[Ca^{2+}]_i$ oscillations is required for protein secretion by acinar cells. In contrast, supramaximal (i.e., hyperstimulatory) concentrations of CCK or ACh generate a sudden, large spike in $[Ca^{2+}]_i$ and eliminate additional $[Ca^{2+}]_i$ oscillations. This $[Ca^{2+}]_i$ spike plus subsequent absence of oscillations is associated with an *inhibition* of secretion that appears to be mediated by disruption of the cytoskeletal components that are required for secretion.

cGMP. Physiological stimulation of the acinar cell by either CCK or ACh also generates a rapid and prominent increase in intracellular cyclic guanosine monophosphate (cGMP) levels. The increase in $[cGMP]_i$ has been linked

A SIGNAL-TRANSDUCTION PATHWAYS

B CHANGES IN INTRACELLULAR [Ca²⁺]

FIGURE 42–4. Stimulation of protein secretion from the pancreatic acinar cell. *A*, The pancreatic acinar cell has at least two pathways for stimulating the insertion of zymogen granules, and thus releasing digestive enzymes. Acetylcholine (ACh) and cholecystokinin (CCK) both activate $G\alpha_q$, which stimulates phospholipase C (PLC), which ultimately leads to the activation of protein kinase C (PKC) and the release of Ca^{2+}. Elevated $[Ca^{2+}]_i$ also activates calmodulin (CaM), which can activate protein kinases (PK) and phosphatases (PP). Finally, vasoactive intestinal peptide (VIP) and secretin both activate $G\alpha_s$, which stimulates adenylyl cyclase (AC), leading to the production of cAMP and the activation of PKA. *B*, Applying a physiological dose of CCK (i.e., 10 pM) triggers a series of $[Ca^{2+}]_i$ oscillations, as measured by a fluorescent dye. However, applying a supraphysiologic concentration of CCK (1 nM) elicits a single large $[Ca^{2+}]_i$ spike and halts the oscillations. Recall that high levels of CCK also are less effective in causing amylase secretion. (*B*, Data from Tsunoda Y, Stuenkel EL, Williams JA: Characterization of sustained $[Ca^{2+}]_i$ increase in pancreatic acinar cells and its relation to amylase secretion. Am J Physiol 259:G792–G801, 1990.)

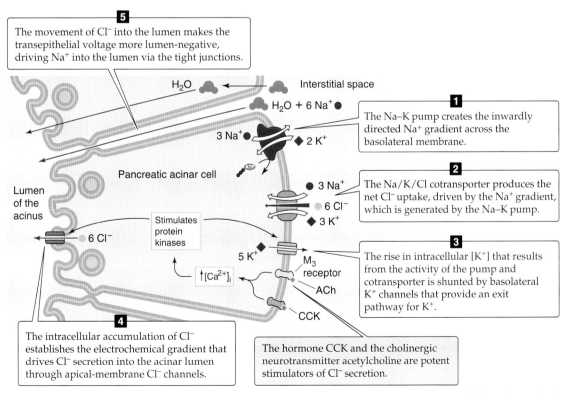

FIGURE 42–5. Stimulation of isotonic NaCl secretion by the pancreatic acinar cell. Both acetylcholine (ACh) and cholecystokinin (CCK) stimulate NaCl secretion, probably by leading to phosphorylation of the basolateral and apical channels.

to nitric oxide metabolism; inhibition of nitric oxide synthase (p. 110) blocks the increase in $[cGMP]_i$ after secretagogue stimulation. Some evidence suggests that cGMP may be involved in regulating Ca^{2+} entry and storage in the acinar cell.

cAMP. Secretin, VIP, and CCK increase cAMP production and thus activate protein kinase A (PKA) activity in pancreatic acinar cells. Low concentrations of CCK cause a transient stimulation of PKA, whereas supraphysiological concentrations of CCK cause a much more prominent and prolonged increase in $[cAMP]_i$ and PKA activity. ACh, however, has little, if any, effect on the cAMP signalling pathway.

EFFECTORS. As summarized in Figure 42–4A, the most important *effectors* of intracellular second messengers are the protein kinases. Stimulation of CCK and muscarinic receptors on the acinar cell leads to the generation of similar Ca^{2+} signals and activation of calmodulin-dependent protein kinases (p. 102) and members of the protein kinase C (PKC) family (p. 102). Activation of secretin or VIP receptors increases $[cAMP]_i$ and thus activates PKA. These second messengers probably also activate protein phosphatases, as well as a number of other protein kinases not depicted in Figure 42–4A. The protein targets of activated kinases and phosphatases in pancreatic acinar cell are largely unknown. However, some are involved in regulating secretion whereas others mediate protein synthesis, growth, transformation, and cell death.

In Addition to Proteins, the Pancreatic Acinar Cell also Secretes a Plasma-Like Fluid

In addition to protein, acinar cells in the pancreas secrete an isotonic, plasma-like fluid (Fig. 42–5). This NaCl-rich fluid hydrates the dense, protein-rich material that the acinar cells secrete. The fundamental transport event is the secretion of Cl^- across the apical membrane.

For transcellular (plasma to lumen) movement of Cl^- to occur, Cl^- must move into the cell across the basolateral membrane. As in many other Cl^--secreting epithelial cells (p. 84), basolateral Cl^- uptake by the acinar cell occurs via an Na/K/Cl cotransporter. The Na-K pump generates the Na^+ gradient that energizes the Na/K/Cl cotransporter. The K^+ entering through the Na-K pump and the Na/K/Cl cotransporter exits through K^+ channels that are also located on the basolateral membrane. Thus, a pump, a cotransporter, and a channel are necessary to sustain the basolateral uptake of Cl^- into the acinar cell.

The rise in $[Cl^-]_i$ produced by basolateral Cl^- uptake drives the secretion of Cl^- down its electrochemical gradient through channels in the apical membrane. As the transepithelial voltage becomes more lumen-negative, Na^+ moves through the cation-selective paracellular pathway (i.e., tight junctions) to join the Cl^- secreted into the lumen. Water also moves through this paracellular pathway, as well as via water channels on the apical and basolateral membranes. Therefore, the net effect of these acinar cell transport processes is the production of an isotonic, NaCl-rich fluid.

Like the secretion of protein by acinar cells, secretion of fluid and electrolytes is stimulated by secretagogues that raise $[Ca^{2+}]_i$. In the pancreas, activation of muscarinic receptors by cholinergic neural pathways and activation of CCK receptors by humoral pathways increase the membrane conductance of the acinar cell. A similar effect is seen with GRP. Apical membrane Cl^- channels and basolateral membrane K^+ channels appear to be the effector targets of the activated Ca^{2+} signalling pathway. Phosphorylation of these channels by Ca^{2+}-dependent kinases is one likely mechanism that underlies the increase in open-channel probability that accompanies stimulation.

PANCREATIC DUCT CELL

The Pancreatic Duct Cell Secretes Isotonic $NaHCO_3$

The principal physiological function of the pancreatic duct cell is to secrete an HCO_3^--rich fluid that alkalinizes and hydrates the protein-rich primary secretions of the acinar cell. The apical step of transepithelial HCO_3^- secretion (Fig. 42–6) is mediated in part by a **Cl-HCO_3 exchanger,** a member of the SAT family (p. 69) that secretes intracellular HCO_3^- into the duct lumen. Luminal Cl^- must be available for this exchange process to occur. Although some luminal Cl^- is present in the primary secretions of the acinar cell, additional Cl^- is provided to the lumen by anion channels on the apical membrane of the duct cell. The most important of these anion channels is the **cystic fibrosis transmembrane conductance regulator (CFTR),** a cAMP-activated Cl^- channel that is present on the apical membrane of pancreatic duct cells, as well as many other epithelial cells. When open, the CFTR allows Cl^- to diffuse from the cytoplasm into the lumen, after which the Cl^- cycles back into the cell via the Cl-HCO_3 exchanger. This process is called "Cl^- recycling." In some species, such as the rat and mouse, pancreatic duct cells also contain a Ca^{2+}-activated Cl^- channel on the apical membrane; this channel also provides Cl^- to the lumen for recycling. Apical Cl^- channels may also directly serve as conduits for HCO_3^- movement from the duct cell to the lumen.

The HCO_3^- that appears inside the duct cell arises from two transport pathways at the basolateral membrane. The first is direct basolateral uptake of HCO_3^- via an electrogenic Na/HCO_3 cotransporter (NBC), which presumably operates with an Na^+/HCO_3^- stoichiometry of $1:2$. The second mechanism is the generation of intracellular HCO_3^- from CO_2 and OH^-, catalyzed by carbonic anhydrase (see box on p. 637). The OH^- in this reaction is derived, along with H^+, from H_2O. Thus, the H^+ that accumulates in the cell must be extruded across the basolateral membrane. One mechanism of H^+ extrusion is Na-H exchange. The second mechanism for H^+ extrusion across the basolateral membrane, at least in some species, is an adenosine triphosphate (ATP)-dependent H^+ pump. Pancreatic duct cells contain acidic intracellular vesicles (presumably containing vacuolar-type H^+ pumps) that are mobilized to the basolateral membrane of the cell after stimulation by secretin, a powerful HCO_3^- secretagogue (see later). Indeed,

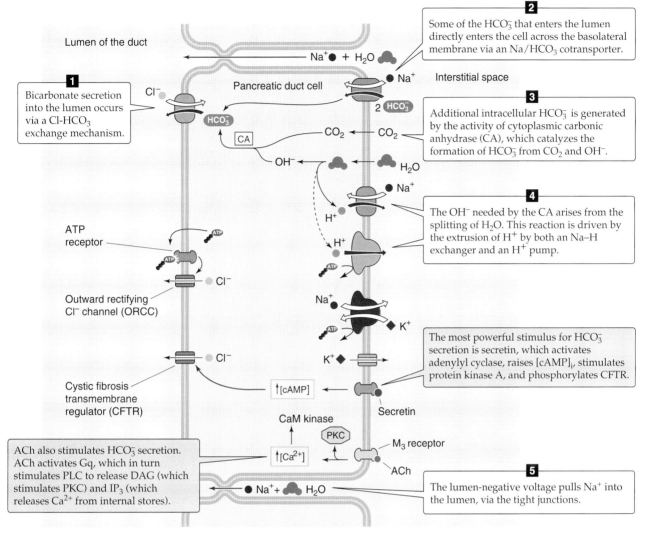

1 Bicarbonate secretion into the lumen occurs via a Cl-HCO$_3$ exchange mechanism.

2 Some of the HCO$_3^-$ that enters the lumen directly enters the cell across the basolateral membrane via an Na/HCO$_3$ cotransporter.

3 Additional intracellular HCO$_3^-$ is generated by the activity of cytoplasmic carbonic anhydrase (CA), which catalyzes the formation of HCO$_3^-$ from CO$_2$ and OH$^-$.

4 The OH$^-$ needed by the CA arises from the splitting of H$_2$O. This reaction is driven by the extrusion of H$^+$ by both an Na–H exchanger and an H$^+$ pump.

The most powerful stimulus for HCO$_3^-$ secretion is secretin, which activates adenylyl cyclase, raises [cAMP]$_i$, stimulates protein kinase A, and phosphorylates CFTR.

ACh also stimulates HCO$_3^-$ secretion. ACh activates Gq, which in turn stimulates PLC to release DAG (which stimulates PKC) and IP$_3$ (which releases Ca^{2+} from internal stores).

5 The lumen-negative voltage pulls Na$^+$ into the lumen, via the tight junctions.

FIGURE 42–6. HCO$_3^-$ secretion by the cells of the pancreatic duct. Secretin is the most important HCO$_3^-$ secretagogue. Secretin somehow stimulates the Na/HCO$_3$ cotransporter and opens the CFTR Cl$^-$ channels via phosphorylation. ACh, acetycholine; ATP, adenosine triphosphate; CaM, calmodulin; cAMP, cyclic adenosine monophosphate; PKC, protein kinase C; PLC, phospholipase C.

H$^+$ pumps are most active under conditions of neurohumoral stimulation.

Thus, three basolateral transporters directly or indirectly provide the intracellular HCO$_3^-$ that pancreatic duct cells need for secretion: (1) the electrogenic Na/HCO$_3$ cotransporter, (2) the Na-H exchanger, and (3) the H$^+$ pump. The physiological importance of these three acid-base transporters in humans has yet to be fully established.

Secretin (via cAMP) and Acetylcholine (via Ca^{2+}) Both Stimulate HCO$_3^-$ Secretion by the Pancreatic Duct

When stimulated, the epithelial cells of the pancreatic duct secrete an isotonic NaHCO$_3$ solution. The duct cells have receptors for secretin, ACh, GRP—all of which stimulate HCO$_3^-$ secretion—and substance P—which inhibits it. Although some evidence indicates that CCK

modulates ductular secretory processes, CCK receptors have not been identified on these cells.

Secretin is the most important humoral regulator of ductal HCO$_3^-$ secretion. Activation of the secretin receptor on the duct cell stimulates adenylyl cyclase, which raises [cAMP]$_i$. Because forskolin and cAMP analogues stimulate ductal HCO$_3^-$ secretion, the secretin response has been attributed to its effect on [cAMP]$_i$ and activation of PKA. However, even low concentrations of secretin that do not measurably increase [cAMP]$_i$ can stimulate HCO$_3^-$ secretion. This observation suggests that the secretin response may be mediated by (1) unmeasurably small increases in total cellular cAMP, (2) cAMP increases that are localized to small intracellular compartments, or (3) activation of alternative second-messenger pathways. Secretin acts by stimulating the apical CFTR Cl$^-$ channel and the basolateral Na/HCO$_3$ cotransporter, without affecting the Na-H exchanger.

HCO$_3^-$ secretion is also regulated by the parasympathetic division of autonomic nervous system (p. 380). The postganglionic parasympathetic neurotransmitter **acetylcholine** increases $[Ca^{2+}]_i$ and activates Ca^{2+}-dependent protein kinases (PKC and the calmodulin-dependent protein kinases) in pancreatic duct cells. The ACh effect is inhibited by atropine, which indicates that this neurotransmitter is acting through **muscarinic receptors** on the duct cell. Although ductular secretion in the rat is also stimulated by **GRP**, the second messenger mediating this effect is not known. Unlike the effect on the acinar cell, GRP does not increase $[Ca^{2+}]_i$ in the duct cell. GRP also does not raise $[cAMP]_i$.

In the rat, both basal and stimulated ductular HCO_3^- secretion is inhibited by **substance P**. The second messenger mediating this effect is also unknown. Because substance P inhibits HCO_3^- secretion regardless of whether the secretagogue is secretin, ACh, or GRP—which apparently act via three different signal-transduction mechanisms—substance P probably acts at a site that is distal to the generation of second messengers.

Apical Membrane Chloride Channels Are Important Sites of Neurohumoral Regulation

In the regulation of pancreatic duct cells by the neurohumoral mechanisms just discussed, the only effector proteins that have been identified as targets of the protein kinases and phosphatases are the apical Cl^- channels, basolateral K^+ channels, and Na/HCO_3 cotransporter.

CFTR, the product of the cystic fibrosis gene, is an approximately 170-kDa intrinsic membrane glycoprotein

A CFTR

FIGURE 42–7. CFTR regulation by ATP. *A*, The CFTR Cl^- channel is a glycoprotein with two membrane-spanning domains (MSD1 and MSD2), each composed of six membrane-spanning segments. A large cytoplasmic regulatory (R) domain separates the two halves of the molecule, each of which has ATP-binding domain (NBD1 and NBD2). The most common mutation in cystic fibrosis is the deletion of the phenylalanine at position 508 (ΔF508) in the NBD1 domain. *B*, The figure shows a widely accepted model of how ATP regulates CFTR both by phosphorylation and ATP hydrolysis. The channel is closed in the three channel states in the *top row* (nothing bound to the nucleotide-binding domains). The channel is in a "flickery" open state as it makes the transition from the *top row* to the *middle row* (NBD1 occupied). Finally, the channel is in a stable or "long" open state in the *third row* (NBD1 and NBD2 occupied). ADP, adenosine monophosphate; ATP, adenosine triphosphate; CFTR, cystic fibrosis transmembrane conductance regulator; MSD, membrane-spanning domain; NBD, nucleotide-binding domain. (*A*, Model adapted from Riordan JR, Rommens JM, Kerem B, et al: Identification of the cystic fibrosis gene: cloning and complementary DNA. Science 245:1066–1073, 1989. *B*, Data from Gadsby DC, Dousmanis AG, Nairn AC: ATP hydrolysis cycles the gating of CFTR Cl^- channels. Acta Physiol Scand Suppl 643:247–256, 1998.)

Illustration continued on following page

B REGULATION OF THE CFTR CHANNEL BY ATP

1 In the resting state, the R domain is dephosphorylated and the channel pore is closed.

2 Secretagogues stimulate PKA, which—in the presence of ATP—phosphorylates the R domain. This phosphorylation leads to a conformational change that makes NBD1 accessible to ATP.

3 Further phosphorylation of the R domain by PKA leads to a further conformational change that also makes NBD2 accessible to ATP.

4 Binding of ATP to NBD1, followed by hydrolysis to ADP + P_i, causes the channel to open.

5 The ADP and P_i soon fall off, causing the channel to close. The brief periods when the ADP and P_i are bound account for the "flickery openings."

6 The binding of a second ATP to NBD2 now locks the channel in an open state.

7 The hydrolysis of the ATP at NBD2 returns the channel to the "flickery opening" state. This hydrolysis is necessary for the ultimate closure of the channel.

FIGURE 42–7. *Continued*

that functions as a low-conductance, apical Cl⁻ channel (Fig. 42–7A). CFTR has two membrane-spanning domains (MSD1 and MSD2), each composed of six membrane-spanning segments. In addition, it has two nucleotide-binding domains (NBD1 and NBD2). Separating the two halves of the molecule is a large cytoplasmic regulatory (R) domain. Because of the presence of the nucleotide-binding domains, CFTR is a member of the superfamily of ABC (or ATP-binding cassette) proteins (p. 65). CFTR is an important target of neurohumoral agents that control fluid and electrolyte secretion by the pancreatic ducts and elsewhere in the body.

The CFTR Cl⁻ channel is regulated by ATP through two types of mechanisms: protein phosphorylation and ATP hydrolysis (see Fig. 42–7B). CFTR is phosphorylated by PKA at several sites within its R domain. Modest phosphorylation causes a conformational change in the R domain that makes NBD1 accessible to ATP. Additional phosphorylation also makes NBD2 accessible to ATP. When ATP binds to NBD1 and is subsequently hydrolyzed, the channel opens, but then rapidly closes once the adenosine diphosphate and phosphate dissociate ("flickery opening"). However, if a second ATP binds to NBD2, the channel is stabilized in its open state ("long opening"). ATP hydrolysis at NBD2 terminates the long opening and is thus necessary for CFTR to return to its *closed state*. Dephosphorylation of the R domain by protein phosphatases returns CFTR to its *resting state*. The control of CFTR by ATP hydrolysis is reminiscent of the control of G-protein activity by GTP hydrolysis (p. 93).

The R domain of CFTR can also be phosphorylated by PKC. PKC enhances the stimulatory effect of PKA on CFTR Cl⁻ transport, but alone it appears to have little direct effect on CFTR function.

In addition to CFTR, pancreatic duct cells in some species have an outwardly rectifying Cl⁻ channel (ORCC) on the apical membrane. This channel, which has been identified in a variety of epithelial cells, can be activated by increases in $[cAMP]_i$ or $[Ca^{2+}]_i$. Recent studies suggest that a part of the effect of cAMP on ORCCs may be indirect and occur through CFTR. The working hypothesis is that stimulation of CFTR somehow promotes ATP efflux from the cell to the lumen and that the ATP binds to an apical purinergic receptor to activate ORCCs in an autocrine/paracrine fashion (see Fig. 42–6).

In rat pancreatic duct cells, Ca^{2+}-sensitive basolateral K⁺ channels seem to be targets of neurohumoral stimulation. Activators of the cAMP pathway stimulate phosphorylation by PKA, thus enhancing the responsiveness of these channels to $[Ca^{2+}]_i$ and increasing their probability of being open.

Pancreatic Duct Cells May also Secrete Glycoproteins

Although the pancreatic duct cells' primary function is to secrete HCO_3^-, they may also synthesize and secrete various high-molecular-weight proteoglycans. Some of these proteins are structurally distinct from the mucin that is produced by the specialized goblet cells in the duct. Un-

like the proteins that are secreted by acinar cells, the glycoproteins synthesized in duct cells are not accumulated in large secretion granules. Rather, they appear to be continuously synthesized and secreted from small cytoplasmic vesicles. Secretin increases the secretion of glycoproteins from these cells, but this action appears to result from stimulation of glycoprotein synthesis rather than stimulation of vesicular transport or exocytosis itself. The role of these proteins may be to protect against protease-mediated injury to mucosal cells.

COMPOSITION, FUNCTION, AND CONTROL OF PANCREATIC SECRETION

Pancreatic Juice Is a Protein-Rich, Alkaline Secretion

Humans produce approximately 1.5 liters of pancreatic fluid each day. The pancreas has the highest rates of protein synthesis and secretion of any organ in the body. Each day the pancreas delivers between 5 and 15 g of protein into the small intestine. The level of pancreatic secretion is determined by a balance between factors that stimulate secretion and those that inhibit it.

The human pancreas secretes over 20 proteins, some of which are listed in Table 42–1. Most of these proteins are either inactive digestive enzyme precursors (i.e., **zymogens**) or active digestive enzymes. The secretory proteins responsible for digestion can be classified according to their substrates: **proteases** hydrolyze proteins, **amylases** digest carbohydrates, **lipases** and phospholipases break down lipids, and **nucleases** digest nucleic acids. The functions of other secretory proteins—such as glycoprotein 2 (GP2), lithostathine, and pancreatitis-associated protein—are less well defined.

GP2 is an unusual protein with an N-terminal glycosyl phosphatidylinositol moiety that links it to the inner leaflet of the zymogen granule membrane. GP2 has been implicated in the regulation of endocytosis. After exocytosis, luminal cleavage of the GP2 linkage to the zymogen granule membrane seems to be necessary for proper trafficking of the zymogen granule membrane back into the cell from the plasma membrane. Under certain circumstances, the released GP2—and also **lithostathine**—may form protein aggregates in the pancreatic juice. This finding is not surprising inasmuch as GP2 is structurally related to the Tamm-Horsfall protein, which is secreted by the renal thick ascending limb (p. 745). The tendency of GP2 and lithostathine to form aggregates may have detrimental clinical consequences in that both proteins have been implicated in the pathologic formation of protein plugs that can obstruct the lumen of acini in patients with cystic fibrosis and chronic pancreatitis.

Pancreatitis-associated protein is a secretory protein that is present in low concentrations in the normal state. However, levels of this protein may increase up to several hundred-fold during the early phases of pancreatic injury. Pancreatitis-associated protein is a bacteriostatic agent that may help prevent pancreatic infection during bouts of pancreatitis.

Pancreatic juice is also rich in Ca^{2+} and HCO_3^-. **Calcium** concentrations are in the millimolar range inside the organelles of the secretory pathway of the acinar cells. These high levels of Ca^{2+} may be required to induce the aggregation of secretory proteins and direct them into the secretory pathway. **Bicarbonate** secreted by duct cells neutralizes the acidic gastric secretions that enter the duodenum and allows digestive enzymes to function properly; HCO_3^- also facilitates the micellar solubilization of lipids and mucosal cell function. The $[HCO_3^-]$ in pancreatic juice increases with increases in the secretory flow rate (Fig. 42–8). In the unstimulated state, the flow is low and the electrolyte composition of pancreatic juice closely resembles that of blood plasma. As the gland is stimulated and flow increases, exchange of Cl^- in the pancreatic juice for HCO_3^- across the apical membrane of the duct cells produces a secretory product that is more alkaline (pH of ~8.1) and has a lower $[Cl^-]$. Concentrations of Na^+ or K^+, however, are not significantly altered by changes in flow.

FIGURE 42–8. Flow dependence of the electrolyte composition of pancreatic fluid. In this experiment on a cat, increasing the level of secretin not only increases the rate at which fluids flow out of the pancreas, but also changes the composition of the fluid. (Data from Case RM, Harper AA, Scratcherd T: The secretion of electrolytes and enzyme by the pancreas of the anaesthetized cat. J Physiol 201:563–596, 1969.)

TABLE 42–1

PANCREATIC ACINAR CELL SECRETORY PRODUCTS

DIGESTIVE PROTEINS	
Zymogens	**Function(s)**
Trypsinogens	digestion
Chymotrypsinogen	digestion
Proelastase	digestion
Proprotease E	digestion
Procarboxypeptidase A	digestion
Procarboxypeptidase B	digestion
Active Enzymes	
α-Amylase	digestion
Carboxyl ester lipase	digestion
Lipase	digestion
RNAase	digestion
DNAase	digestion
Colipase	digestion
Others	
Trypsin inhibitor	Block trypsin activity
Lithostathine	May prevent stone formation; constituent of protein plugs
Glycoprotein 2 (GP-2)	Endocytosis?; formation of protein plugs
Pancreatitis-associated protein	Bacteriostatic?
Na^+, Cl^-, H_2O	Hydrate secretions
Ca^{2+}	?

In the Fasting State, Levels of Secreted Pancreatic Enzymes Oscillate at Low Levels

Pancreatic secretion is regulated in both the fasted and fed states. Under basal conditions, the pancreas releases low levels of pancreatic enzymes (Fig. 42–9). However, during the digestive period (eating a meal), pancreatic secretion increases in sequential phases to levels that are 5- to 20-fold over basal levels. The systems that regulate secretion appear to be redundant; if one system fails, a second takes its place. These mechanisms ensure that the release of pancreatic enzymes corresponds to the amount of food in the small intestine.

Like other organs in the upper gastrointestinal tract, the pancreas has a basal rate of secretion even when food is not being eaten or digested. During this **interdigestive (fasting) period,** pancreatic secretions vary cyclically and correspond to sequential changes in the motility of the small intestine (p. 888). Pancreatic secretion is minimal when intestinal motility is in its quiescent phase (phase I); biliary and gastric secretions are also minimal at this time. As duodenal motility increases (phase II), so does pancreatic secretion. During the interdigestive period, *enzyme secretion* is maximal when intestinal motility—the migrating motor complexes (MMCs; see Fig. 40–6)—is also maximal (phase III). However, even this maximal interdigestive secretory rate is only 10% to 20% of that stimulated by a meal. The peak phase of interdigestive intestinal motor activity and pancreatic secretory activity are followed by a declining period (phase IV). *Fluid and electrolyte secretion* rates during the interdigestive phase are usually less than 5% of maximum levels.

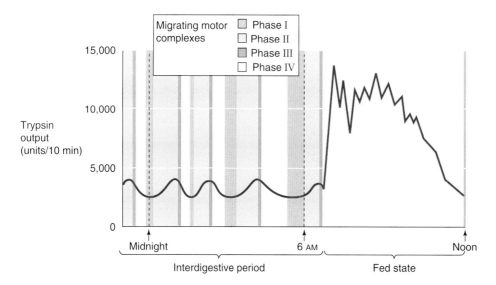

FIGURE 42–9. Time course of pancreatic secretion during fasting and feeding. The interdigestive output of secretory products (e.g., trypsin) by the pancreas varies cyclically and in rough synchrony with the four phases of motor activity (migrating motor complexes) of the small intestine, shown by *colored vertical bands*. During the fed state, there is a massive and sustained increase in trypsin release by the pancreas, as well as a switch of small-intestine motility to the "fed state." (Data from DiMagno EP, Layer P. In Go VLW, DiMagno EP, Gardner JD, et al [eds]: The Pancreas: Biology, Pathobiology and Disease, 2nd ed. New York, Raven Press, pp 275–300, 1993.)

The cyclic pattern of interdigestive pancreatic secretion is mediated by intrinsic and extrinsic mechanisms. The predominant mechanism of pancreatic regulation is through **parasympathetic pathways**. Telenzepine, an antagonist of the M_1 muscarinic ACh receptor, reduces interdigestive enzyme secretion by over 85% during phases II and III. Although cholinergic pathways are the major regulators of interdigestive pancreatic secretion, CCK and adrenergic pathways also play a role. **CCK** appears to stimulate pancreatic enzyme secretion during phases I and II. In contrast, basal α-adrenergic tone appears to suppress interdigestive pancreatic secretion. Although human and canine pancreas denervated during transplantation exhibits cyclic secretion, this secretion is no longer synchronous with duodenal motor activity. These observations support a role for the autonomic nervous system in regulating basal (resting) pancreatic secretion.

Cholecystokinin from Duodenal I Cells Stimulates Enzyme Secretion from the Acini, and Secretin from S Cells Stimulates HCO$_3^-$ and Fluid Secretion by the Ducts

Cholecystokinin plays a central role in regulating pancreatic secretion. CCK is released from neuroendocrine cells (**I cells;** see Table 40–1) present in the duodenal mucosa and acts on pancreatic acinar cells to increase protein secretion (see Fig. 42–4). In response to a meal, plasma CCK levels increase 5- to 10-fold within 10 to 30 minutes. Three lines of evidence show that CCK is a physiologic mediator of pancreatic protein secretion: (1) CCK levels increase in the serum in response to a meal. (2) Administration of exogenous CCK at the same levels produced by a meal stimulates pancreatic protein secretion to higher levels than those generated by a meal (the meal may also stimulate the release of inhibitory factors in addition to CCK). (3) A specific CCK inhibitor reduces pancreatic protein secretion by over 50%.

The most potent stimulator of CCK release from I cells is **lipid.** Protein digestive products (i.e., peptones, amino acids) also increase CCK release, but carbohydrate and acid have little effect. CCK secretion may also be stimulated by **CCK-releasing factors,** which are peptides released by mucosal cells of the duodenum or secreted by the pancreas. The level of these releasing factors may reflect a balance between the relative amounts of nutrients and digestive enzymes that are present in the gut lumen at any one time, so the level of the factors reflects the digestive milieu of the duodenum. In the fasting state, luminal CCK releasing factors are degraded by digestive enzymes that accompany basal pancreatic secretion, so little releasing factor remains to stimulate the I cells. However, during a meal, the digestive enzymes are diverted to the digestion of ingested nutrients entering the gut lumen, and the CCK-releasing factors are spared degradation. Hence, the relative level of proteins to proteases in the small intestine determines the amount of CCK-releasing factor available to drive CCK release and thus pancreatic secretion.

CCK acts on the acinar cell through both direct and indirect pathways: it directly stimulates enzyme secretion through a CCK$_A$ receptor on the acinar cell (see Fig. 42–4), and it may indirectly stimulate enzyme secretion by activating the parasympathetic (cholinergic) nervous system. As we shall see later, the parasympathetic pathway plays a major role in mediating the intestinal phase of pancreatic secretion. Vagal stimulation can drive pancreatic secretion to nearly maximum levels. Atropine, an antagonist of muscarinic ACh receptors (p. 387), reduces the secretion of enzymes and HCO$_3^-$ during the intestinal phase of a meal. Atropine also inhibits secretion in response to stimulation by physiological levels of exogenous CCK. Together, these findings suggest that CCK somehow stimulates the parasympathetic pathway, which in turn stimulates muscarinic receptors on the acinar cell.

Like CCK, **gastrin-releasing peptide**—which is structurally related to bombesin—may also be a physiological regulator of pancreatic enzyme secretion. Stimulation of acinar cells with GRP leads to enzyme secretion. In contrast to the hormone CCK, the major source of GRP appears to be the vagal nerve terminals.

Secretin is the most potent humoral stimulator of fluid and HCO$_3^-$ secretion by the pancreas (see Fig. 42–6).

Secretin is released from neuroendocrine cells (**S cells**) in the mucosa of the small intestine in response to duodenal acidification and, to a lesser extent, bile acids and lipids. Like CCK, secretin levels increase after the ingestion of a meal. However, when these levels are reached experimentally by administration of exogenous secretin, pancreatic HCO_3^- secretion is less than that generated by a meal. These findings suggest that secretin is acting in concert with CCK, ACh, and other agents to stimulate HCO_3^- secretion.

In addition to hormones of intestinal origin, **insulin** secreted by the islets of Langerhans within the pancreas may also influence pancreatic exocrine secretion. Blood flow from the pancreatic islets moves to the exocrine pancreas through a *portal system*. This organization allows high concentrations of islet hormones to interact with pancreatic acinar cells. One result of this arrangement may be that insulin modifies the composition of digestive enzymes within the acinar cell and increases the relative levels of amylase.

Regulation of exocrine pancreatic secretion is complex, and understanding of this process has been made difficult by the following: (1) The tissue levels of an exogenously infused hormone may not match those generated physiologically. (2) Because several neurohumoral factors are released in response to a meal, the infusion of a single agent may not accurately reflect its physiological role. (3) Specific neurohumoral inhibitors are often unavailable. (4) Pancreatic responses may differ depending on the species.

A Meal Triggers Cephalic, Gastric, and Intestinal Phases of Pancreatic Secretion That Are Mediated by a Complex Network of Neurohumoral Interactions

The digestive period has been divided into three phases (Table 42–2) based on the site at which food acts to stimulate pancreatic secretion, just as is the case for gastric secretion (p. 899). These three phases (cephalic, gastric, and intestinal) are sequential and follow the progression of a meal from its initial smell and taste to its

TABLE 42–2

THE THREE PHASES OF PANCREATIC SECRETION			
PHASE	**STIMULANT**	**REGULATORY PATHWAY**	**% OF MAXIMUM ENZYME SECRETION**
Cephalic	Sight Smell Taste Mastication	Vagal pathways	25
Gastric	Distention Gastrin?	Vagal-cholinergic	10–20
Intestinal	Amino acids Fatty acids H^+	Cholecystokinin Secretin Enteropancreatic reflexes	50–80

movement through the gastrointestinal tract (Fig. 42–10). These phases act in a coordinated fashion to maximize efficiency of the digestive process. For example, stimulation of secretion before the entry of food into the small intestine during the cephalic and gastric phases ensures that active enzymes are present when food arrives. On the other hand, suppression of secretion during the late digestive phase suppresses the release of pancreatic enzymes when nutrients are no longer present in the proximal end of the small intestine.

THE CEPHALIC PHASE. During the cephalic phase, the sight, taste, and smell of food usually generates only a modest increase in fluid and electrolyte secretion (see Fig. 42–10A). However, it has a prominent effect on enzyme secretion. In most animal species, enzyme secretion increases to 25% to 50% of the maximum rate evoked by exogenous CCK. In humans, the cephalic phase is short lived and dissipates rapidly when food is removed. The cephalic phase is mediated by neural pathways. In the dog, stimulation of several regions of the hypothalamus (dorsomedial and ventromedial nuclei and the mammillary body) enhances pancreatic secretion. The efferent signal travels along vagal pathways to stimulate pancreatic secretion via ACh, an effect blocked by atropine. The cephalic phase does not depend on gastrin or CCK release, but it is probably mediated by the stimulation of muscarinic receptors on the *acinar cell*.

THE GASTRIC PHASE. During the gastric phase (see Fig. 42–10A), the presence of food in the stomach modulates pancreatic secretion by (1) affecting the release of hormones, (2) stimulating neural pathways, and (3) modifying the pH and availability of nutrients in the proximal part of the small intestine. The presence of specific peptides or amino acids (peptones) stimulates gastrin release from G cells in the antrum of the stomach and, to a much lesser extent, G cells in the proximal part of the duodenum. The gastrin/CCK_B receptor and the CCK_A receptor are closely related (p. 895). Although in some species the gastrin-CCK_B receptor is not present on the pancreatic acinar cell, gastrin can still act—though less well—through the CCK_A receptor. Although physiological concentrations of gastrin can stimulate pancreatic secretion in some species, its importance in regulating secretion in the human pancreas remains unclear. As far as local neural pathways are concerned, gastric distention stimulates low levels of pancreatic secretion, probably through a vagovagal gastropancreatic reflex. Although the presence of food in the stomach affects pancreatic secretion, the most important role for chyme in controlling pancreatic secretion occurs after the gastric contents enter the small intestine.

THE INTESTINAL PHASE. During the intestinal phase, chyme entering the proximal region of the small intestine stimulates a major pancreatic secretory response by three major mechanisms (see Fig. 42–10B). First, gastric acid entering the duodenum—and to a lesser extent, bile acids and lipids—stimulates duodenal **S cells** to release secretin, which stimulates duct cells to secrete HCO_3^- and fluid. The acid stimulates fluid and electrolyte secretion to a greater extent than it stimulates protein secretion. Sec-

A CEPHALIC AND GASTRIC PHASES

B INTESTINAL PHASE

ond, lipids and, to a lesser degree, peptones stimulate duodenal I cells to release CCK, which stimulates acinar cells to release digestive enzymes. Finally, the same stimuli that trigger I cells also activate a vagovagal enteropancreatic reflex that predominantly stimulates acinar cells.

The pattern of enzyme secretion—mediated by the CCK and vagovagal pathways—depends on the contents of the meal. For example, a *liquid* meal elicits a response that is only about 60% of maximal. On the other hand, a *solid* meal, which contains larger particles and is slowly released from the stomach, elicits a prolonged response. Meals rich in *calories* cause the greatest response.

The *chemistry* of the ingested nutrients also affects pancreatic secretion via the CCK and vagovagal pathways. For example, perfusion of the duodenum with carbohydrates has little effect on secretion, whereas lipids are potent stimulators of pancreatic enzyme secretion. As far as **lipids** are concerned, triglycerides do not stimulate pancreatic secretion, but their hydrolytic products—monoglycerides and free fatty acids—do. The longer the chain length of the fatty acid, the greater the secretory response; C-18 fatty acids generate protein secretion that is near the maximum produced by exogenous CCK. Some fatty acids also stimulate pancreatic HCO_3^- secretion. Because fatty acids also reduce gastric acid secretion and delay gastric emptying, they may play an important role in modulating pH conditions in the proximal part of the small intestine. **Protein** breakdown products are intermediate in their stimulatory effect. Nonessential amino acids have little effect on protein secretion, whereas some essential amino acids (p. 1215) stimulate secretion. The most potent amino acid stimulators are phenylalanine, valine, and methionine. Short peptides containing phenylalanine stimulate secretion to the same extent as the amino acid itself. Because gastric digestion generates more peptides than amino acids, it is likely that peptides provide the initial pancreatic stimulation during the intestinal phase.

The relative potency of the different nutrients in stimulating secretion is inversely related to the pancreatic reserves of digestive enzymes. Thus, the pancreas needs to release only a small portion of its amylase to digest the carbohydrate in a meal, and to release only slightly greater portions of proteolytic enzymes to digest the proteins. However, a greater fraction of pancreatic lipase has to be released to efficiently digest the fat in most meals. The exocrine pancreas has the ability to respond to long-term changes in dietary composition by modulating the reserves of pancreatic enzymes. For example, a diet that is relatively high in carbohydrates may lead to a relative increase in pancreatic amylase content.

The Pancreas Has Large Reserves of Digestive Enzymes for Carbohydrates and Proteins, but Not for Lipids

The exocrine pancreas stores more enzymes than are required for digesting a meal. The greatest pancreatic reserves are those required for carbohydrate and protein digestion. The reserves of enzymes required for lipid digestion—particularly for triglyceride hydrolysis—are more limited. Even so, nutrient absorption studies after partial pancreatic resection show that maldigestion of dietary fat does not occur until 80% to 90% of the pancreas has been removed. Similar reserves exist for pancreatic *endocrine* function. These observations have important clinical implications because they indicate that individuals can tolerate large pancreatic resections for tumors without fear of maldigestion or diabetes developing postoperatively. When fat maldigestion or diabetes does develop because of pancreatic disease, the gland must have undergone extensive destruction.

Fat in the Distal Part of the Small Intestine Inhibits Pancreatic Secretion

Once maximally stimulated, pancreatic secretion begins to decrease after several hours. Nevertheless, all the while the levels of secretion remain adequate for digestion. Regulatory systems only gradually return secretion to its basal (interdigestive) state. The regulatory mechanisms that are

TABLE 42–3

MECHANISMS THAT PROTECT THE ACINAR CELL FROM AUTODIGESTION

PROTECTIVE FACTOR	MECHANISM
Packaging of many digestive proteins as zymogens	Precursor proteins lack enzymatic activity
Selective sorting of secretory proteins and storage in zymogen granules	Restricts the interaction of secretory proteins with other cellular compartments
Protease inhibitors in the zymogen granule	Block the action of prematurely activated enzymes
Condensation of secretory proteins at low pH	Limits the activity of active enzymes
Nondigestive proteases	Degrade active enzymes

FIGURE 42–10. Three phases of pancreatic secretion. *A,* During the cephalic phase, the sight, taste, or smell of food stimulates pancreatic acinar cells, via the vagus nerve and muscarinic cholinergic receptors, to release digestive enzymes and, to a lesser extent, stimulates duct cells to secrete HCO_3^- and fluid. The release of gastrin from G cells is not important during this phase. During the gastric phase, the presence of food in the stomach stimulates pancreatic secretions—primarily from the acinar cells—via two routes. First, distention of the stomach activates a vagovagal reflex. Second, protein digestion products (peptones) stimulate G cells in the antrum of the stomach to release gastrin, which is a poor agonist of the CCK_A receptors on acinar cells. *B,* The arrival of gastric acid in the duodenum stimulates S cells to release secretin, which stimulates duct cells to secrete HCO_3^- and fluid. Protein and lipid breakdown products have two effects. First, they stimulate I cells to release CCK, which stimulates acinar cells to release digestive enzymes. Second, they stimulate afferents pathways that initiate a vagovagal reflex that primarily stimulate the acinar cells via M_3 cholinergic receptors. ACh, acetylcholine; CCK, cholecystokinin; GRP, gastrin-releasing peptide.

ACUTE PANCREATITIS

Acute pancreatitis is an inflammatory condition that may cause extensive local damage to the pancreas, as well as compromise the function of other organs such as the lungs. The most common factors that initiate acute pancreatitis in humans are alcohol and gallstones. However, other insults may also precipitate acute pancreatitis. Hypertriglyceridemia, an inherited disorder of lipid metabolism, is one such culprit. Less commonly, toxins that increase acetylcholine levels, such as cholinesterase inhibitors (some insecticides) or the sting of scorpions found in the Caribbean and South and Central America, may lead to pancreatitis. Acetylcholine probably causes pancreatitis by overstimulating the pancreatic acinar cell.

Experimental models of pancreatitis suggest a primary defect in protein processing and acinar cell secretory function. Over 100 years ago it was found that treating animals with doses of acetylcholine that are 10 to 100 times greater than those that elicit maximal enzyme secretion causes "hyperstimulation" pancreatitis. The same type of injury can be generated by cholecystokinin. The

injury in this model appears to be linked to two events within the acinar cell: (1) zymogens are pathologically processed within the acinar cell into active forms. In this model, the protective mechanisms outlined in Table 42–3 are overwhelmed and active enzymes are generated within the acinar cell. (2) Acinar cell secretion is inhibited and the active enzymes are retained within the cell. Although premature activation of zymogens is probably an important step in initiating pancreatitis, other events are important for perpetuating injury, including inflammation, vascular injury, and occlusion that results in decreased blood flow and reduced tissue oxygenation (ischemia).

Knowledge of the mechanisms of acute pancreatitis may lead to effective therapies. In experimental models, serine protease inhibitors that block the activation of pancreatic zymogens improve the course of the acute pancreatitis. In some clinical forms of pancreatitis, prophylactic administration of the protease inhibitor gabexate appears to reduce the severity of the disease.

responsible for this feedback inhibition are less well characterized than those responsible for stimulating pancreatic secretion. The presence of fat in the distal end of the small intestine reduces pancreatic secretion in most animals, including humans. This inhibition may be mediated by **peptide YY (PYY)**, which is present in neuroendocrine cells in the ileum and colon. PYY may suppress pancreatic secretion by acting on inhibitory neural pathways, as well as by decreasing pancreatic blood flow. **Somatostatin** (particularly SS-28; p. 1026), released from intestinal D cells, and **glucagon**, released from pancreatic islet α cells, may also play a role in returning pancreatic secretion to the interdigestive state after a meal.

Several Mechanisms Protect the Pancreas from Autodigestion

Premature activation of pancreatic enzymes within acinar cells may lead to autodigestion and could play a role in initiating pancreatitis. To prevent such injury, the acinar cell has a number of mechanisms for preventing enzymatic activity (Table 42–3). First, many digestive proteins are stored in secretory granules as inactive precursors or zymogens. Under normal conditions, zymogens become activated only after entering the small intestine. There, the intestinal enzyme **enterokinase** converts trypsinogen to trypsin, which initiates the conversion of all other zymogens to their active forms (see Chapter 44). Second, the secretory granule membrane is impermeable to proteins. Thus, the zymogens and active digestive enzymes are sequestered from proteins in the cytoplasm and other intracellular compartments. Third, enzyme inhibitors such as **pancreatic trypsin inhibitor** are copackaged in the secretory granule. Sufficient pancreatic trypsin inhibitor is present in the secretory granules to block 10% to 20% of the potential trypsin activity. Fourth, the condensation of zymogens, the low pH, and the ionic conditions within

the secretory pathway may further limit enzyme activity. Fifth, enzymes that become prematurely active within the acinar cell may themselves be degraded by other enzymes or be secreted before they can cause injury.

Degradation of prematurely active enzymes may be mediated by other enzymes that are present within the secretory granule or by mixing of secretory granule contents with lysosomal enzymes that can degrade active enzymes. Three mechanisms lead to the mixing of digestive proteases and lysosomal enzymes: (1) lysosomal enzymes may be copackaged in the secretory granule; (2) secretory granules may selectively fuse with lysosomes (a process called crinophagy); and (3) secretory granules, as well as other organelles, may be engulfed by lysosomes (a process called autophagy). Failure of these protective mechanisms may result in the premature activation of digestive enzymes within the pancreatic acinar cell.

SALIVARY ACINAR CELL

Different Salivary Acinar Cells Secrete Different Proteins

Unlike the pancreas, the salivary glands contain two acinar cell populations that synthesize and secrete different protein products. The acinar cells of the parotid glands in most species secrete a serous (i.e., watery) product that contains an abundance of α-amylase. The acinar cells of the sublingual glands secrete a mucus product that is composed primarily of **mucin glycoproteins**. The morphologic appearance of these two acinar cell populations differs as well. The submandibular gland of many species contains both mucus-type and serous-type acinar cells. In some species, these two distinct cell types are dispersed throughout the submandibular gland, whereas in other species such as humans, distinct mucus and serous acinar

CYSTIC FIBROSIS

Cystic fibrosis (CF), the most common lethal genetic disease in whites, affects about 1 in 2000. Approximately 1 in 20 whites carry the genetic defect. Clinically, CF is characterized by progressive pancreatic and pulmonary insufficiency resulting from the complications of organ obstruction by thickened secretions. The disease results from mutations in the CF gene (located on chromosome 7) that alter the function of its product, the cystic fibrosis transmembrane conductance regulator (CFTR; see Fig. 42–7). **CFTR** is a cyclic adenosine monophosphate–activated Cl^- channel that is present on the apical plasma membrane of many epithelial cells. In the pancreas, CFTR has been localized to the apical membrane of duct cells, where it functions to provide the luminal Cl^- for $Cl\text{-}HCO_3$ exchange (see Fig. 42–6).

Most CF-gene mutations result in the production of a CFTR molecule that is abnormally folded after its synthesis in the endoplasmic reticulum (ER). The ER quality control system recognizes these molecules as defective, and most mutant CFTR molecules are prematurely degraded before they reach the plasma membrane. Subsequent loss of CFTR expression at the plasma membrane disrupts the apical transport processes of the duct cell and results in decreased secretion of HCO_3^- and water by the ducts. As a result, protein-rich primary (acinar) secretions thicken within the duct lumen and lead to ductal obstruction and eventual tissue destruction. Pathologically, the ducts appear dilated and obstructed, and fibrotic tissue and fat gradually replace the pancreatic parenchyma—hence the original designation "cystic fibrosis." The subsequent deficiency of pancreatic enzymes that occurs leads to the maldigestion of nutrients and thus the excretion of fat in the stool (steatorrhea) by CF patients. Before the development of oral enzyme replacement therapy, many CF patients died of complications from malnutrition.

Now, the major cause of CF morbidity and mortality is progressive pulmonary disease. The pathophysiology of lung disease in CF is more complex than that of pancreatic disease. A major finding is that the airway mucus is thick and viscous as a result of insufficient fluid secretion into the airway lumen. The pulmonary epithelium probably both secretes fluid—in a mechanism that requires CFTR—and absorbs fluid—in a mechanism that requires apical ENaC Na^+ channels. In CF, the reduced activity of CFTR shifts the balance more toward absorption, and a thick mucous layer is generated that inhibits the ciliary clearance of foreign bodies (p. 601). The result is an increased rate and severity of infections and thus inflammatory processes that contribute to the destructive process in the lung.

It is the pulmonary symptoms that bring the patient to the physician's attention in early childhood. Cough and recurrent respiratory infections that are hard to eradicate are usually the first indications of the illness. The child's sputum is particularly thick and viscous. Pulmonary function progressively declines over the ensuing years, and patients may also experience frequent and severe infections, atelectasis (collapse of lung parenchyma), bronchiectasis (chronic dilatation of the bronchi), and recurrent pneumothoraces (air in the intrapleural space). In addition to the pancreatic and pulmonary manifestations, CF also causes a characteristic increase in the [NaCl] of sweat, which is intermediate in heterozygotes.

Pharmacologic approaches that bypass the Cl^--transport defect in a lung with CF are currently being evaluated, and considerable effort is being directed toward the development of *in vivo* gene transfer techniques to correct the underlying genetic defect.

---

units are the rule. In addition to α-amylase and mucin glycoproteins, salivary acinar cells also secrete many proline-rich proteins. Like mucin proteins, proline-rich proteins are highly glycosylated, and like other secreted salivary proteins, they are present in the acinar secretory granules and are released by exocytosis.

Cholinergic and Adrenergic Neural Pathways Are the Most Important Physiological Activators of Regulated Secretion by Salivary Acinar Cells

Unlike the pancreas, where humoral stimulation plays an important role in stimulating secretion, the salivary glands are mostly under autonomic neural control (see Chapter 15). The major agonists of salivary acinar secretion are ACh and norepinephrine, which are released from postganglionic parasympathetic and sympathetic nerve terminals, respectively (see Fig. 15–8). The cholinergic receptor on the salivary acinar cell is the muscarinic M_3 glandular subtype. The adrenergic receptors identified on these cells include both the α and β subtypes. Other receptors identified in salivary tissue include those for substance P

(NK1 receptors), VIP, purinergic agonists (P_{2z} receptors), neurotensin, prostaglandin, and epidermal growth factor (EGF). However, some of these other receptors are found only on specific salivary glands and may be present on duct rather than acinar cells. Significant species variation with regard to surface receptor expression is also seen. Thus, for the salivary glands, it is difficult to discuss the regulation of acinar cell secretion in general terms. It is fair to say, however, that both cholinergic and adrenergic neurotransmitters can stimulate exocytosis by salivary acinar cells.

The Major Second Messenger for Salivary Acinar Secretion Is Ca^{2+}

Protein secretion by the salivary acinar cell has been associated with increases in both $[cAMP]_i$ and $[Ca^{2+}]_i$, as in the pancreatic acinar cell. Activation of the β-adrenergic receptor results in an increase in $[cAMP]_i$ and stimulation of amylase secretion. On the other hand, α-adrenergic stimulation acts by increasing $[Ca^{2+}]_i$. In the parotid acinar cell, treatment with the neurotransmitters ACh, norepinephrine (acting via α adrenoceptors), and substance P causes G-protein–dependent activation of PLC and thus leads to the formation of inositol 1,4,5-trisphosphate (IP$_3$) and diacylglycerol (DAG). IP$_3$ releases Ca^{2+} from intracellular stores and stimulates Ca^{2+}-dependent protein kinases such as PKC (p. 102) and calmodulin kinase (p. 102), whereas DAG directly activates PKC. The repetitive spikes in [Ca^{2+}]$_i$ in salivary acinar cells, as in pancreatic acinar cells, depends on Ca^{2+}-induced Ca^{2+} release from intracellular stores (p. 242) and on the influx of extracellular Ca^{2+}. ATP coreleased with norepinephrine (p. 390) activates a P$_{2z}$ receptor, which is a receptor-gated cation-selective channel that allows Ca^{2+} to enter across the plasma membrane and thus increase [Ca^{2+}]$_i$.

Muscarinic and α-adrenergic agents secondarily increase [cGMP]$_i$, perhaps because increased [Ca^{2+}]$_i$ can stimulate soluble guanylyl cyclase (p. 110).

The mechanisms of fluid and electrolyte secretion by salivary acinar cells are similar to those in pancreatic acinar cells (see Fig. 42–5). In the salivary gland, activation of muscarinic ACh receptors by parasympathetic stimulation and activation of α-adrenergic receptors by sympathetic stimulation induce similar membrane conductance changes. Substance P, acting through its own receptor, also initiates conductance changes in the salivary acinar cell. All these effects seem to be mediated by rises in [Ca^{2+}]$_i$. Apical Cl$^-$ channels and basolateral K$^+$ channels appear to be the effector targets of the activated Ca^{2+}-signalling pathway. Phosphorylation of these channels by Ca^{2+}-dependent kinases may affect the probability of these channels being open and thus increase conductance.

SALIVARY DUCT CELL

Salivary Duct Cells Produce a Hypotonic Fluid That Is Poor in NaCl and Rich in KHCO$_3$

In the salivary glands, as in the pancreas, the duct modifies the composition of the isotonic, plasma-like primary secretion of the acinar cells (Fig. 42–11). In general, salivary duct cells absorb Na$^+$ and Cl$^-$ and, to a lesser extent, secrete K$^+$ and HCO$_3^-$. Because the epithelium is not very water permeable, more water remains within the lumen, which becomes hypotonic. However, significant differences are seen in the various types of salivary glands.

Reabsorption of Na$^+$ by salivary duct cells is a two-step process, as in other epithelia. First, Na$^+$ enters the cell from the lumen through ENaC Na$^+$ channels (p. 84) that are present on the apical membrane. Second, the basolateral Na-K pump extrudes this Na$^+$ across the basolateral membrane, thus providing a transcellular pathway for the movement of Na$^+$ from lumen to plasma.

Reabsorption of Cl$^-$ is also a two-step process. Entry of Cl$^-$ across the apical membrane occurs by means of a Cl-HCO$_3$ exchanger. To a certain extent, apical Cl$^-$ channels, including CFTR, recycle the Cl$^-$ that is absorbed by the Cl-HCO$_3$ exchanger. Duct cells also have basolateral Cl$^-$ channels that provide an exit pathway for Cl$^-$, thus completing the movement from duct lumen to blood.

The apical step in *HCO$_3^-$ secretion* occurs via the same Cl-HCO$_3$ exchanger mentioned before. How HCO$_3^-$ accumulates inside the salivary duct cell is unknown; it may

FIGURE 42–11. Salivary-duct transporters. Na$^+$ absorption occurs as Na$^+$ enters the cell across the apical membrane via the ENaC Na$^+$ channel and probably also the Na-H exchanger. Na$^+$ exits across the basolateral membrane via the Na-K pump. Cl$^-$ absorption occurs as Cl$^-$ enters the cell via the apical Cl-HCO$_3$ exchanger. More Cl$^-$ exits via basolateral than apical Cl$^-$ channels. HCO$_3^-$ secretion occurs as the apical Cl-HCO$_3$ exchanger secretes HCO$_3^-$ into the lumen. The basolateral step of HCO$_3^-$ secretion is not well understood. K$^+$ secretion begins with the basolateral uptake of K$^+$ via the Na-K pump, followed by the exit of K$^+$, possibly via an apical K-H exchanger. ENaC, epithelial Na$^+$ channel.

follow the same routes as in the pancreatic duct cell (see Fig. 42–6).

The basolateral step in *K⁺ secretion* is the uptake of K^+ via the Na-K pump. The apical step has been postulated to result from K-H exchange at the apical membrane, but this mechanism remains controversial.

Parasympathetic Stimulation Decreases Na⁺ Absorption, Whereas Aldosterone Increases Na⁺ Absorption by Duct Cell

Regulation of duct-cell transport processes is less well understood in the salivary glands than in the pancreas. In the intact salivary gland (i.e., acini and ducts), secretion is stimulated primarily by *parasympathetic* input via ACh. In the duct cell, cholinergic agonists, acting through muscarinic receptors, increase $[Ca^{2+}]_i$ and presumably activate Ca^{2+}-dependent regulatory pathways. The effector targets of this Ca^{2+}-signalling pathway are not known. The role played by duct cells in the increased saliva production that occurs in response to cholinergic stimulation seems to be decreased NaCl absorption and decreased K⁺ secretion, with more fluid left behind in the duct lumen.

Salivary glands also receive *sympathetic* input and have both α- and β-adrenergic receptors. The specific effects that adrenergic stimulation has on duct-cell transport activity are unclear. Nevertheless, activation of the β-adrenergic receptor increases $[cAMP]_i$ and activates the CFTR Cl^- channel.

Salivary duct cell function is also regulated by other neurohumoral signals. The mineralocorticoid hormone **aldosterone** stimulates the absorption of NaCl and secretion of K⁺ by salivary duct cells in several species. Although its role has not been well examined in salivary duct cells per se, aldosterone in other Na^+-absorbing epithelia (e.g., kidney and colon) stimulates Na^+ transport by increasing both ENaC and Na-K pump activity (p. 786). Salivary duct cells may also have receptors for certain neuropeptides such as VIP, although their physiological significance remains unknown.

Salivary Duct Cells also Secrete and Take Up Proteins

Duct cells handle proteins in three ways. Some proteins that are synthesized by duct cells are secreted into the lumen, others are secreted into blood, and still others are reabsorbed from the lumen to the cell.

Intralobular duct epithelial cells in rodent submandibular glands synthesize a variety of proteins that are stored in intracellular granules and secreted in response to neurohumoral stimuli. EGF, nerve growth factor, and kallikrein are among the most abundant proteins that are packaged for secretion by these cells. Salivary duct cells may also synthesize, store, and secrete some digestive enzymes (α-amylase and ribonucleases). Degranulation of intralobular duct cells occurs primarily in response to α-adrenergic stimulation, thus suggesting that protein secretion by duct cells is regulated primarily by the sympathetic division.

Although regulatory peptides (i.e., glucagon and soma-tostatin) have also been detected in salivary duct cells, no evidence indicates that they are stored in granules or secreted into the lumen (i.e., they may be basolaterally secreted as peptide hormones). In addition, duct cells synthesize polymeric IgA receptors that are responsible for the basolateral endocytosis of IgA, and they also synthesize a secretory component that facilitates the apical release of IgA.

Salivary duct cells can also remove organic substances from the duct lumen. Endocytosis of acinar proteins and other materials (e.g., ferritin) at the apical pole of the duct cell has been demonstrated immunocytochemically. In addition, salivary duct cells express the transferrin receptor (p. 44) on the apical membrane, thus indicating that some regulated endocytosis also occurs in these cells. The latter process may function to take up specific luminal substances or to traffic ion transporters to and from the apical plasma membrane.

COMPOSITION, FUNCTION, AND CONTROL OF SALIVARY SECRETION

Depending on Protein Composition, Salivary Secretions Can Be Serous, Seromucous, or Mucous

Most saliva (~90%) is produced by the major salivary glands: the parotid, the sublingual, and the submandibular glands. The remaining 10% of saliva comes from numerous minor salivary glands that are scattered throughout the submucosa of the oral cavity. Each salivary gland produces either a serous, a seromucous, or a mucous secretion; the definition of these three types of saliva is based on the glycoprotein content of the gland's final secretory product. In humans and most other mammals, the parotids produce a serous (i.e., low glycoprotein content) secretion, the sublingual and submandibular glands produce a seromucous secretion, and the minor salivary glands produce a mucous secretion.

Serous secretions are enriched in α-amylase, and mucous secretions are enriched in mucin. However, it is important to note that the most abundant proteins in parotid and submandibular saliva are members of the group of **proline-rich proteins**. These proteins have a very high proline content (approximately one third of the total amino acids) and exist in acidic, basic, and glycosylated forms. They have antimicrobial properties and may play an important role in neutralizing dietary tannins, which can damage epithelial cells. In addition to these protective functions, proline-rich salivary proteins contribute to the lubrication of ingested foods and may enhance tooth integrity through their interactions with Ca^{2+} and hydroxyapatite. Saliva also contains smaller amounts of lipase, nucleases, lysozyme, peroxidases, lactoferrin, secretory IgA, growth factors, regulatory peptides, and vasoactive proteases such as kallikrein and renin (Table 42–4).

Saliva functions primarily to prevent dehydration of the oral mucosa and provide lubrication for the mastication and swallowing of ingested food. The sense of taste and, to a lesser extent, smell depend on an adequate supply of

TABLE 42–4

MAJOR ORGANIC COMPONENTS OF MAMMALIAN SALIVA

COMPONENT	CELL TYPE	GLAND(S)	POSSIBLE FUNCTION
Proline-rich proteins	Acinar	P, SM	Enamel formation Ca^{2+} binding Antimicrobial Lubrication
Mucin glycoproteins	Acinar	SL, SM	Lubrication Antimicrobial Protease protective
Enzymes			
α-Amylase	Acinar	P, SM	Starch digestion
Lipase	Acinar	SL	Fat digestion
Ribonuclease	Duct	SM	RNA digestion
Kallikrein	Duct	P, SM, SL	Unknown
Miscellaneous			
Lactoperoxidase	Acinar	SM	Antimicrobial
Lactoferrin	Acinar	Unknown	Antimicrobial
Lysozyme	Duct	SM	Antimicrobial
IgA receptor	Duct	Unknown	Antimicrobial
IgA secretory piece	Duct	Unknown	Antimicrobial
Growth factors	Duct	SM	Unknown

P, parotid; SL, sublingual; SM, submandibular.

saliva. Saliva plays a very important role in maintaining proper oral hygiene. It accomplishes this task by washing away food particles, killing bacteria (lysozyme and IgA activity), and contributing to overall dental integrity. Although α-amylase is a major constituent of saliva and digests a significant amount of the ingested starch, salivary amylase does not appear to be essential for effective carbohydrate digestion in the presence of a normally functioning pancreas. The same can be said for lingual lipase. However, in cases of pancreatic insufficiency, these salivary enzymes can partially compensate for the maldigestion that results from pancreatic dysfunction.

At Low Flow Rates, the Saliva Is Hypotonic and Rich in K⁺, Whereas at Higher Flow Rates, Its Composition Approaches That of Plasma

The composition of saliva varies from gland to gland and from species to species. The primary secretion of the salivary acinar cell at rest is plasma-like in composition. Its osmolality, which is due mostly to Na^+ and Cl^-, is approximately 300 mosmole/kg. The only significant difference from plasma is that the $[K^+]$ of the salivary primary secretion is always slightly higher than that of plasma. In some species, acinar cells may help generate a Cl^--poor, HCO-rich primary secretion after salivary gland stimulation. In most species, however, salivary gland stimulation does not significantly alter acinar cell transport

function or the composition of the primary secretion. The leakiness of the tight junctions between acinar cells contributes to the formation of a plasma-like primary secretory product (p. 83).

The composition of the primary salivary secretion is subsequently modified by the transport processes of the duct cell. At *low (basal) flow rates*, Na^+ and Cl^- are absorbed and K^+ is secreted by the duct cells of most salivary glands (Table 42–5). These transport processes generate a K^+-rich, hypotonic salivary secretion at rest (see Fig. 42–11). The tightness of the ductal epithelium

TABLE 42–5

ELECTROLYTE COMPONENTS OF HUMAN PAROTID SALIVA

COMPONENT	UNSTIMULATED OR BASAL STATE (mM)	STIMULATED (CHOLINERGIC AGONISTS) (mM)
Na^+	15	90
K^+	30	15
Cl^-	15	50
Total CO_2	15	60

From Thaysen JH, Thorn NA, Schwartz IL: Excretion of sodium, potassium, chloride and carbon dioxide in human parotid saliva. Am J Physiol 178:155–159, 1954.

inhibits paracellular water movement and therefore contributes to the formation of a hypotonic secretory product.

At *higher flow rates*, the composition of the final secretory product begins to approach that of the plasma-like primary secretion (Table 42–5). This observation suggests that, as in the case of the renal tubules, the ductular transport processes have limited capacity to handle the increased load that is presented to them as the flow rate accelerates. However, the extent to which the transporters are flow dependent varies from gland to gland and from species to species. Human saliva is always hypotonic, and salivary $[K^+]$ is always greater than plasma $[K^+]$. In humans, increased salivary flow rates cause alkalinization of the saliva and a relative increase in its $[HCO_3^-]$, thus indicating that human salivary glands can be net secretors of HCO_3^-. HCO_3^- secretion and salivary alkalinization in humans neutralize the gastric acid that normally refluxes into the esophagus.

Parasympathetic Stimulation Increases Salivary Secretion

Humans produce about 1.5 liters of saliva each day. Under basal conditions, the salivary glands produce saliva at a rate of approximately 0.5 ml/min, with a much slower flow rate during sleep. After stimulation, flow increases 10-fold over the basal rate. Although the salivary glands respond to both cholinergic and adrenergic agonists in vitro, the parasympathetic nervous system is the most important physiological regulator of salivary secretion in vivo.

PARASYMPATHETIC CONTROL. Parasympathetic innervation to the salivary glands originates in the salivatory nuclei of the brain stem (see Fig. 15–5). Both local and central input to the salivatory nuclei can regulate the parasympathetic signals transmitted to the glands. Taste and tactile stimuli from the tongue are transmitted to the brain stem, where their signals can excite the salivatory nuclei and stimulate salivary gland secretion. Central impulses triggered by the sight and smell of food also excite the salivatory nuclei and can induce salivation before food is ingested. These central effects were best illustrated by the classic experiments of Pavlov, who conditioned dogs to salivate at the sound of a bell.

Preganglionic parasympathetic fibers travel in cranial nerve (CN) VII to the submandibular ganglia, from which postganglionic fibers reach the sublingual and submandibular glands (see Fig. 15–4). Preganglionic parasympathetic fibers also travel in CN IX to the otic ganglia, from which postganglionic fibers reach the parotid glands. In addition, some parasympathetic fibers reach their final destination via the buccal branch of CN V to the parotid glands or via the lingual branches of CN V to the sublingual and submandibular glands. Postganglionic parasympathetic fibers from these ganglia directly stimulate the salivary glands through their release of ACh. The prominent role of the parasympathetic nervous system in salivary function can be readily appreciated by examining the consequences of cholinergic blockage. Disruption of the

parasympathetic fibers to the salivary glands can lead to glandular atrophy. This observation suggests that parasympathetic innervation is necessary for maintaining the normal mass of salivary glands. Clinically, some medications (particularly psychiatric drugs) have "anticholinergic" properties that are most commonly manifested as "dry mouth." For some medications, this effect is so uncomfortable for the patient that use of the medication must be discontinued. Conversely, excessive salivation is induced by some anticholinesterase agents that can be found in certain insecticides and "nerve gases."

SYMPATHETIC CONTROL. The salivary glands are also innervated by postganglionic sympathetic fibers from the superior cervical ganglia that travel along blood vessels to the salivary glands (see Fig. 15–4). Although sympathetic (adrenergic) stimulation increases saliva flow, interruption of sympathetic nerves to the salivary glands has no major effect on salivary gland function in vivo. However, the sympathetic nervous system is the primary stimulator of

---

SJÖGREN SYNDROME

Sjögren syndrome is a chronic and progressive autoimmune disease that affects salivary secretion. Patients with Sjögren syndrome generate antibodies that react primarily with the salivary and lacrimal glands. Lymphocytes infiltrate the glands, with subsequent immunologic injury to the acini leading to a decrease in net secretory function. Expression of the Cl-HCO₃ exchanger is lost in the striated duct cells of the salivary gland. Sjögren syndrome can occur as a primary disease (salivary and lacrimal gland dysfunction only) or as a secondary manifestation of a systemic autoimmune disease, such as rheumatoid arthritis. The disease primarily affects women; systemic disease usually does not develop.

Individuals with Sjögren syndrome have *xerostomia* (dry mouth) and *keratoconjunctivitis sicca* (dry eyes). Loss of salivary function causes these patients to have difficulty tasting, as well as chewing and swallowing dry food. They also have difficulty with continuous speech and complain of a chronic burning sensation in the mouth. On physical examination, patients with Sjögren syndrome have dry, erythematous oral mucosa with superficial ulceration and poor dentition (dental caries, dental fractures, and loss of dentition). Parotid gland enlargement is commonly present.

The proteins that are the targets of the immunologic attack in Sjögren syndrome are not known. Therefore, no specific therapy for the disorder is available. Until the underlying cause of Sjögren syndrome is discovered, patients will have to rely on eyedrops and frequent oral fluid ingestion to compensate for their deficiencies in lacrimal and salivary secretion. Various stimulants of salivary secretion (sialogogues), such as methylcellulose and sour candy, can also be helpful. Patients with severe involvement and functional disability are sometimes treated with corticosteroids and immunosuppressants.

the **myoepithelial cells** that are closely associated with cells of the acini and proximal (intercalated) ducts. These stellate-shaped cells have structural features of both epithelial and smooth-muscle cells. They support the acinar structures and decrease the flow resistance of the intercalated ducts during stimulated secretion. Thus, the net effect of myoepithelial cell activation is to facilitate secretory flow in the proximal regions of the gland, thus minimizing the extravasation of secretory proteins that might otherwise occur during an acute increase in secretory flow.

The sympathetic division can also indirectly affect salivary gland function by modulating blood flow to the gland. However, the relative contribution of this vascular effect to the overall secretory function of the salivary glands is difficult to determine.

In addition to cholinergic and adrenergic regulation of salivary secretion, some autonomic fibers that innervate the salivary glands contain VIP and substance P. Although acinar cells in vitro respond to stimulation by substance P, the physiological significance of these neurotransmitters in vivo has not been established. Salivary secretion is also regulated, in part, by mineralocorticoids. The adrenal hormone aldosterone produces saliva that contains relatively less Na^+ and more K^+. The opposite effect on saliva is seen in patients with adrenal insufficiency caused by **Addison disease**. The mineralocorticoid effect represents the only well-established example of a humoral (i.e., nonneural) agent regulating salivary secretion.

REFERENCES

Books and Reviews

Beger HG, Warshaw AL, Carr-Locke D, et al: The Pancreas. Cambridge, MA, Blackwell, 1998.

Frizzell RA (guest editor of special issue): Physiology of cystic fibrosis. Physiol Rev 79, 1999.

Gadsby DC, Dousmanis AG, Nairn AC: ATP hydrolysis cycles the gating of CFTR Cl^- channels. Acta Physiol Scand Suppl 643:247–256, 1998.

Go VLW, DiMagno EP, Gardner JD, et al: The Exocrine Pancreas, 2nd ed. New York, Raven, 1993.

Johnson LR (ed): Physiology of the Gastrointestinal Tract, 3rd ed. New York, Raven, 1994.

Liddle RA: Cholecystokinin cells. Annu Rev Physiol 59:221–242, 1997.

Turner RJ: Mechanisms of fluid secretion by salivary glands. Ann N Y Acad Sci 694:24–35, 1993.

Williams JA: Intracellular signaling mechanisms activated by cholecystokinin regulating synthesis and secretion of digestive enzymes in pancreatic acinar cells. Annu Rev Physiol 63:77–97, 2001.

Journal Articles

Ashton N, Argent BE, Green R: Characteristics of fluid secretion from isolated rat pancreatic ducts stimulated with secretin and bombesin. J Physiol 435:533–546, 1991.

Ishiguro H, Naruse S, Steward MC, et al: Fluid secretion in interlobular ducts isolated from guinea-pig pancreas. J Physiol 511:407–422, 1998.

Marino CR, Jeanes V, Boron WF, Schmitt BM: Expression and distribution of the Na^+-HCO_3^- cotransporter in human pancreas. Am J Physiol 277:G487–494, 1999.

Marino CR, Matovcik LM, Gorelick FS, Cohn JA: Localization of the cystic fibrosis transmembrane conductance regulator in pancreas. J Clin Invest 88:712–716, 1991.

Zhao H, Xu X, Diaz J, Muallem S: Na^+, K^+, and H^+/HCO_3^- transport in submandibular salivary ducts. J Biol Chem 270:19599–19605, 1995.

CHAPTER 43

Intestinal Fluid and Electrolyte Movement

Henry J. Binder

FUNCTIONAL ANATOMY

The small intestine and large intestine have many similarities in structure and function. In some cases, different regions of the intestinal tract carry out certain functions in much the same manner. In other cases, however, substantial heterogeneity exists between different intestinal segments (e.g., ileum versus jejunum) or between different mucosal areas (i.e., villus versus crypt) in one intestinal segment.

As discussed in Chapter 40, the basic structure of the intestine is a hollow cylinder with columnar epithelial cells lining the lumen, circular and longitudinal layers of smooth muscle in the wall, and with endocrine and neural elements (see Fig. 40–2). Enteric neurons, as well as endocrine and paracrine agonists, regulate both epithelial transport and motor activity during both the interdigestive and the postprandial periods. As a result, the intestines propagate their contents in a caudad direction while either removing fluid and electrolytes from the intestinal lumen (i.e., absorption) or adding these substances to the lumen (i.e., secretion).

Both the Small Intestine and Large Intestine Absorb and Secrete Fluid and Electrolytes, Whereas Only the Small Intestine Absorbs Nutrients

Among mammals, **absorption** of dietary nutrients is an exclusive function of the small intestine. Only during the neonatal period does significant nutrient absorption take place in the large intestine. The small intestine absorbs nonelectrolytes after extensive digestion of dietary nutrients by both luminal and brush border enzymes, as discussed in Chapter 44. In contrast, *both* the small intestine and the large intestine absorb fluid and electrolytes by several different cellular transport processes, which may differ between the small and large intestine and are the subject of this chapter.

Another vitally important function of the intestinal epithelium is the **secretion** of intestinal fluid and electrolytes. On a teleologic basis, fluid secretion may be considered an adaptive mechanism that the intestinal tract uses to protect itself from noxious agents, such as bacteria and bacterial toxins. In general, the cellular mechanisms of intestinal electrolyte secretion

A SMALL INTESTINE

Circular folds (of Kerckring)

Villi

Lamina propria

Crypt of Lieberkühn

Muscularis mucosae

Submucosa

Circular muscle of muscularis externa

Lacteal

Lymphoid nodule

Longitudinal muscle of muscularis externa

Villus

Crypt

Absorptive cell

Goblet cell

Enteric endocrine cell

Stem/progenitor cell

Paneth cell

B LARGE INTESTINE

Haustra

Semilunar folds

Surface epithelium

Crypt of Lieberkühn

Lamina propria

Muscularis mucosae

Submucosa

Circular muscle of muscularis externa

Longitudinal muscle of muscularis externa

Lymphoid nodule (Peyer patch)

Crypt

Absorptive cell

Goblet cell

Microvacuolated columnar cell

Enteric endocrine cell

Stem/progenitor cell

FIGURE 43–1. Microscopic view of the anatomy of small and large intestine. *A,* The surface area of the small intestine is amplified at three levels: (1) macroscopic folds of Kerckring; (2) microscopic villi and crypts of Lieberkühn; and (3) submicroscopic microvilli. *B,* The surface area of the colon is amplified at the same three levels as the small intestine: (1) macroscopic semilunar folds; (2) crypts (but not villi); and (3) microvilli.

in the small intestine and colon are similar, if not identical. Frequently, the adaptive signal that induces the secretory response also stimulates a motor response from the intestinal muscle that results in a propagated propulsive response in an attempt to eliminate the offending toxin.

The Small Intestine Has a Villus-Crypt Organization, Whereas the Colon Has Surface Epithelial Cells with Interspersed Crypts

Both the small intestine and large intestine have a specialized epithelial structure that correlates well with epithelial transport function.

The small intestine (Fig. 43–1*A*) consists of finger-like projections—**villi**— surrounded by the openings of glandular structures called **crypts of Lieberkühn,** or simply crypts. Both villi and crypts are covered by columnar epithelial cells. The cells lining the villi are considered to be the primary cells responsible for both nutrient and electrolyte *absorption*, whereas the crypt cells primarily participate in *secretion*.

The colon (see Fig. 43–1*B*) does not have villi. Instead, the cells lining the large intestine are surface epithelial cells, and interspersed over the colonic surface are numerous apertures of colonic crypts (or glands) that are similar in function and structure to the small-intestinal crypts. Not surprisingly, the surface epithelial cells of the colon are the primary cells responsible for colonic electrolyte *absorption*, whereas colonic gland cells are generally believed to mediate ion *secretion*.

The intestinal mucosa is a dynamic organ with continuous cell proliferation and migration. The zone of cell proliferation is at the base of the crypt in both the small and large intestine. The **progenitor cell** is a stem cell that, in the small intestine, differentiates into vacuolated, goblet, and Paneth cells. The vacuolated cell migrates along the crypt-villus axis and becomes a villous absorptive cell after undergoing substantial changes in its morphologic and functional characteristics. These villous cells migrate until they reach the tips of the villi and then slough into the lumen of the intestine. The overall period from the initiation of cell proliferation to sloughing is approximately 48 to 96 hours. The overall rate of cell migration may increase or decrease: decreased cell turnover occurs during starvation, whereas increased cell turnover occurs during feeding and lactation, as well as after intestinal resection. The compensatory response that follows intestinal resection involves both luminal and hormonal factors.

The Surface Area of the Small Intestine Is Amplified by Folds, Villi, and Microvilli; Amplification Is Less Marked in the Colon

An additional hallmark of both the small and large intestine is the presence of structures that amplify function by increasing the luminal surface area. These structures exist at three levels. In the small intestine, the first level consists of the macroscopic **folds of Kerckring**. The second level consists of the microscopic **villi** and **crypts** that we have already discussed. The third level is the submicro-

TABLE 43–1

STRUCTURAL AND FUNCTIONAL DIFFERENCES BETWEEN THE SMALL AND THE LARGE INTESTINE		
	SMALL INTESTINE	**LARGE INTESTINE**
Length (m)	6	2.4
Area of apical plasma membrane (m²)	~200	~25
Folds	Yes	Yes
Villi	Yes	No
Crypts or glands	Yes	Yes
Microvilli	Yes	Yes
Nutrient absorption	Yes	No
Active Na⁺ absorption	Yes	Yes
Active K⁺ secretion	No	Yes

scopic **microvilli** on the apical surfaces of the epithelial cells. Thus, if the small intestine is thought of as a hollow cylinder, the net increase in total surface area of the small intestine (versus that of a smooth cylinder) is 600-fold. The total surface area of the human small intestine is approximately 200 m², or the surface area of a doubles tennis court (Table 43–1). The colonic surface area is also amplified, but to a more limited extent. Because the colon lacks villi, amplification is a result of only the presence of colonic folds, crypts, and microvilli. Amplification is an effective means of increasing the surface area that is available for intestinal absorption, the primary function of the small and large intestine.

OVERVIEW OF FLUID AND ELECTROLYTE MOVEMENT IN THE INTESTINES

The Small Intestine Absorbs Approximately 6.5 Liters/Day of an Approximately 8.5-Liter Fluid Load That Is Presented to It, and the Colon Absorbs Approximately 1.9 Liters/Day

The fluid content of the average diet is typically 1.5 to 2.5 liters/day. However, the fluid load to the small intestine is considerably greater—8 to 9 liters/day. The difference between these two sets of figures is accounted for by salivary, gastric, pancreatic, and biliary secretions, as well as the secretions of the small intestine itself (Fig. 43–2). Similarly, the total quantity of electrolytes (Na^+, K^+, Cl^-, and HCO_3^-) that enter the lumen of the small intestine also consists of dietary sources plus endogenous secretions from the salivary glands, stomach, pancreas, liver, and small intestine.

We can calculate the absorption of water and electrolytes from the small intestine by comparing the total load that is presented to the lumen of the small intestine (i.e., 7.5 liters/day entering from other organs + 1.0 liter/day secreted by the small intestine = 8.5 liters/day) with that

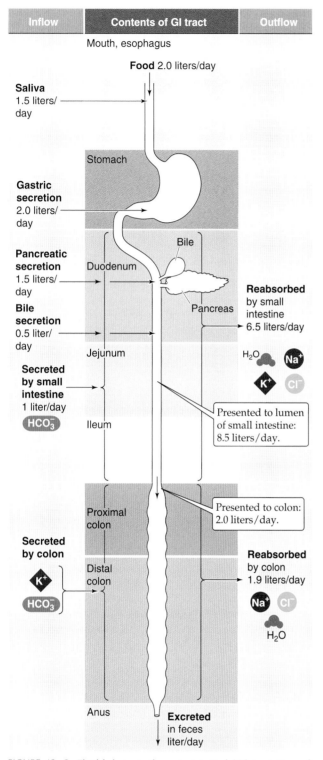

FIGURE 43–2. Fluid balance in the gastrointestinal (GI) tract. For each segment of the GI tract, the figure shows substances flowing into the lumen on the left and substances flowing out of the lumen on the right. Of the approximately 8.5 liters/day that are presented to the small intestine, the small intestine removes approximately 6.5 liters/day, delivering approximately 2 liters/day to the colon. The large intestine removes approximately 1.9 liters/day, leaving approximately 0.1 liter/day in the feces.

leaving the small intestine (i.e., ileocecal flow). The latter is about 2.0 liters/day in normal subjects. Thus, overall small-intestinal water absorption is 8.5 − 2.0, or approximately 6.5 liters/day. Na^+ absorption is approximately 600 meq/day. Maximal small-intestinal fluid absorption has not been directly determined but has been estimated to be as great as 15 to 20 liters/day.

Colonic fluid absorption is the difference between ileocecal flow (∼2.0 liters/day) and stool water, which is usually less than 0.2 liter/day (∼0.1 liter/day). Thus, colonic water absorption is approximately 2.0 − 0.1, or 1.9 liters/day. In contrast, the maximal colonic water **absorptive capacity** is between 4 and 5 liters/day. As a result, a significant increase in ileocecal flow—for example, up to perhaps 5 liters/day, as occurs with a decrease in small-intestinal fluid absorption—will not exceed the absorptive capacity of the large intestine. Thus, a compensatory increase in colonic fluid absorption can prevent an increase in stool water (i.e., diarrhea) despite substantial decreases in fluid absorption by the small intestine.

The Small Intestine Absorbs Net Amounts of Water, Na$^+$, Cl$^-$, and K$^+$ and Secretes HCO$_3^-$, Whereas the Colon Absorbs Net Amounts of Water, Na$^+$, and Cl$^-$ and Secretes Both K$^+$ and HCO$_3^-$

Net ion movement represents the summation of several events. At the level of the entire small or large intestine, there is substantial movement of ions from the intestinal lumen into the blood and from the blood into the lumen. The *net* ion movement across the entire epithelium is the difference between these two unidirectional fluxes.

Fluid and electrolyte transport in the intestine varies considerably in two different axes, both along the length of the intestines ("segmental" heterogeneity) and from the bottom of a crypt to the top of a villus or to the surface cells ("crypt-villus/surface" heterogeneity). A comparison of two different segments of intestine (e.g., duodenum versus ileum) shows that they differ substantially in function. These differences in function reflect **segmental heterogeneity** of ion transport processes along the longitudinal axis of the intestine in different macroscopic regions of both the small and the large intestine; these differences are both qualitative and quantitative. For example, HCO$_3^-$ stimulation of Na$^+$ absorption occurs only in the proximal part of the small intestine. On the other hand the so-called electrogenic Na$^+$ absorption is restricted to the rectosigmoid segment of the colon.

Within an intestinal segment (e.g., a piece of ileum), **crypt-villus/surface heterogeneity** leads to differences in transport function along the radial axis of the intestine wall. For example, it is generally believed that absorptive function is located in villous cells in the small intestine (and surface epithelial cells in the large intestine) whereas secretory processes reside in the crypt cells. Finally, at a certain level within a single villus or crypt—or within a very small area of the colonic surface epithelium—individual cells may demonstrate further heterogeneity (**cellular heterogeneity**), with specific transport mechanisms restricted to different cells.

Overall ion movement in any segment of the intestine

represents the summation of various absorptive and secretory events. These events may be paracellular or transcellular, may occur in the villus or crypt, and may be mediated by a goblet cell or an absorptive cell.

Despite the segmental heterogeneity of small-intestinal electrolyte transport, overall water and ion movement in the proximal and distal portions of the small intestine is similar: in health, the small intestine is a net absorber of water, Na^+, Cl^-, and K^+, but is a net secretor of HCO_3^- (see Fig. 43–2). In general, absorptive processes in the small intestine are enhanced in the postprandial state. The human colon carries out net absorption of water, Na^+, and Cl^- with few exceptions, but carries out net secretion of K^+ and HCO_3^-.

The Intestines Absorb and Secrete Solutes by Both Active and Passive Mechanisms

As discussed in Chapter 3, intestinal epithelial cells are polar; that is, they have two very different membranes— an apical membrane and a basolateral membrane—that are separated from one another by tight junctions. It is important to emphasize that the transport processes present in the small and large intestine are quite similar to those present in other epithelia, such as the renal tubules, with only some organ-specific specialization to distinguish them. The "transepithelial" movement of a solute across the entire epithelium can be either absorptive or secretory. In each case, the movement can be either transcellular or paracellular. In transcellular movement, the solute must cross the two cell membranes in series. In general, movement of the solute across at least one of these membranes must be active (i.e., against an electrochemical gradient). In paracellular movement, the solute moves passively between adjacent epithelial cells via the tight junctions.

All transcellular Na^+ absorption is mediated by the Na-K pump (i.e., Na,K-adenosinetriphosphatase [Na,K-ATPase]) located at the basolateral membrane. This enzyme is responsible for Na^+ extrusion across the basolateral membrane and results in a relatively low $[Na^+]_i$ and an intracellular-negative membrane potential. This Na^+ gradient serves as the driving force, in large part, for Na^+ entry into the epithelial cell across the luminal (apical) membrane, a process mediated either by Na^+ channels or by Na^+-coupled transporters (e.g., Na/glucose cotransport, Na-H exchange). The epithelial cell may also use this Na^+ gradient to energize other transport processes at the apical or basolateral membrane.

Intestinal Fluid Movement Is Always Coupled to Solute Movement, Whereas Solute Movement May Be Coupled to Fluid Movement by "Solvent Drag"

Fluid movement is always coupled to active solute movement. The model of the osmotic coupling of fluid movement to solute movement in the intestine is similar to that in all or most epithelial cells (p. 84). It is uncertain, however, whether the water movement occurs predominantly via a transcellular route or via a paracellular route.

Solute movement is the driving force for fluid movement. However, the converse may also be true: solute movement may be coupled to fluid movement by **solvent drag**, a phenomenon in which the dissolved solute is swept along by bulk movement of the solvent (i.e., water). Solvent drag accounts for a significant fraction of the Na^+ and urea absorbed in the human jejunum (but not in the more distal segments of the small intestine or the large intestine). For all intents and purposes, solvent drag occurs via the paracellular route, and it depends on the permeability properties of the tight junctions ("reflection coefficient"; p. 470) and the magnitude of the convective water flow. Thus, solvent drag contributes primarily to the absorption of relatively small, water-soluble molecules, such as urea and Na^+, and does so mainly in epithelia with relatively high permeability. The transepithelial permeability of the jejunum is considerably greater than that of the ileum or colon, as evidenced by its lower spontaneous transepithelial voltage difference (V_{TE}), higher passive movement of NaCl, and larger apparent pore size.

The Resistance of the Tight Junctions Primarily Determines the Transepithelial Resistance of Intestinal Epithelia

Epithelial permeability is an inverse function of transepithelial resistance. In epithelial structures such as the small and large intestine, transepithelial resistance is determined by cellular resistance and paracellular resistance, which are arranged in parallel (p. 82). Paracellular resistance is considerably lower than transcellular resistance; therefore, overall mucosal resistance depends mainly on paracellular resistance, which in turn depends primarily on the properties of the tight junctions. Therefore, intestinal permeability is essentially a function of tight-junction structure. Just as transport function varies greatly throughout the intestine, major differences in transepithelial permeability and the properties of tight junctions are also present throughout the intestinal tract. In general, resistance increases in the aboral direction (i.e., moving away from the mouth). Thus, the resistance of the jejunum is considerably lower than that of the distal end of the colon. Evidence also indicates that the permeability of the tight junctions in the crypt is greater than that in the villus.

CELLULAR MECHANISMS OF Na$^+$ ABSORPTION

Both the small intestine and the large intestine absorb large amounts of Na^+ and Cl^- daily, but different mechanisms are responsible for this extremely important physiologic process in different segments of the intestine. The villous epithelial cells in the small intestine and the surface epithelial cells in the colon are responsible for absorbing most of the Na^+. Absorption of Na^+ is the result of a complex interplay of both apical and basolateral membrane transport processes. Figure 43–3 summarizes the four fundamental mechanisms by which Na^+ may enter the cell across the apical membrane. In each case, the Na-K pump is responsible, at least in part, for the movement of Na^+ from cell to blood. Also in each case, the driving force for apical Na^+ entry is provided by the

FIGURE 43–3. Modes of active Na^+ absorption by the intestine. *A,* "Nutrient-coupled" Na^+ absorption occurs in the villous cells of the jejunum and ileum and is the primary mechanism for postprandial Na^+ absorption. The thickness of the arrows in the *inset* indicates the relative magnitude of the Na^+-absorptive flux through this pathway. *B,* Electroneutral Na-H exchange at the apical membrane, in the absence of Cl-HCO₃ exchange, is stimulated by the high pH of the HCO_3^--rich luminal contents. *C,* Na-H and Cl-HCO₃ exchange is coupled by a change in intracellular pH that results in "electroneutral NaCl absorption," which is the primary mechanism for interdigestive Na^+ absorption. *D,* In "electrogenic" Na^+ absorption, the apical step of Na^+ movement occurs via the ENaC Na^+ channel. ATP, adenosine triphosphate; CA, carbonic anhydrase.

large, inwardly directed electrochemical gradient for Na^+, which in turn is provided by the Na-K pump.

The following four sections describe these four apical membrane transport processes.

Na/Glucose and Na/Amino Acid Cotransport in the Small Intestine Is a Major Mechanism for Postprandial Na⁺ Absorption

"Nutrient-coupled" Na^+ absorption (see Fig. 43–3A) occurs throughout the small intestine. Although glucose- and amino acid–coupled Na^+ absorption also takes place

in the colon of the newborn, it disappears during the neonatal period. Glucose- and amino acid–coupled Na^+ absorption occurs only in villous epithelial cells and not in crypt epithelial cells (see Fig. 43–1A). This process is the primary mechanism for Na^+ absorption after a meal, but it makes little contribution during the interdigestive period—when only limited amounts of glucose and amino acids are present in the intestinal lumen.

Glucose- and amino acid–coupled Na^+ absorption is mediated by specific apical membrane transport proteins. The Na/glucose cotransporter SGLT1 (p. 66) is responsible for glucose uptake across the apical membrane, as discussed in Chapter 44. Several distinct Na/amino acid cotransporters, each specific for a different class of amino acids (see Table 44–3), are responsible for the Na^+-coupled uptake of amino acids across the apical membrane. Because these transporters couple the energetically downhill movement of Na^+ to the uphill movement of glucose or an amino acid, the transporter processes are examples of **secondary active transport** (p. 61). The glucose and amino acid–coupled uptake of Na^+ entry across the apical membrane increases $[Na^+]_i$, which in turn increases Na^+ extrusion across the basolateral membrane via the Na-K pump. Because the apical Na/glucose and Na/amino acid cotransporters are electrogenic, as is the Na-K pump, the overall transport of Na^+ carries net charge and makes V_{TE} more lumen-negative. Thus, glucose- and amino acid–stimulated Na^+ absorption is an **electrogenic** process. As discussed later, the increase in the lumen-negative V_{TE} provides the driving force for the parallel absorption of Cl^-.

Nutrient-coupled Na^+ transporters, unlike other small-intestinal Na^+-absorptive mechanisms, are not inhibited by either cyclic adenosine monophosphate (cAMP) or $[Ca^{2+}]_i$. Thus, agonists that increase $[cAMP]_i$ (i.e., *Escherichia coli* or cholera enterotoxin) or $[Ca^{2+}]_i$ (i.e., serotonin) do not inhibit glucose- or amino acid–stimulated Na^+ absorption.

Electroneutral Na-H Exchange in the Duodenum and Jejunum Is Responsible for Na^+ Absorption That Is Stimulated by Luminal Alkalinity

Luminal HCO_3^-—the result of pancreatic, biliary, and duodenal secretion—increases Na^+ absorption in the proximal portion of the small intestine by stimulating apical-membrane Na-H exchange (see Fig. 43–3*B*). The Na-H exchanger couples Na^+ uptake across the apical membrane to proton extrusion into the intestinal lumen, a process that is enhanced by both decreases in intracellular pH (pH_i) and increases in luminal pH. The energy for Na-H exchange comes from the Na^+ gradient, a consequence of the ability of the Na-K pump to extrude Na^+, thereby lowering $[Na^+]_i$. This process is characteristically inhibited by *millimolar* concentrations of the diuretic amiloride.

Several isoforms of the Na-H exchanger exist (p. 68), and different isoforms are present on the apical and basolateral membranes. Intestinal epithelial cells also have Na-H exchangers on their basolateral membranes. However, this NHE1 isoform, like its counterpart in nonepithelial cells, regulates pH_i (a "housekeeping" function) and does not contribute to the transepithelial movement of Na^+. In contrast, both the NHE2 and NHE3 exchanger isoforms present on the apical membrane are responsible for both transepithelial Na^+ movement *and* pH_i regulation. Although Na-H exchangers are present on the apical membrane of villous epithelial cells throughout the entire intestine, only in the duodenum and jejunum (i.e., the proximal part of the small intestine) is Na-H exchange present without the parallel presence of Cl-HCO_3 exchangers (see next section). Thus, in the proximal portion

---

ORAL REHYDRATION SOLUTION

The therapeutic use of oral rehydration solution (**ORS**) provides an excellent demonstration of applied physiology. Many diarrheal illnesses (see the later Box titled Secretory Diarrhea, on p. 945) are caused by bacterial exotoxins that induce fluid and electrolyte secretion by the intestine. Hence such a toxin is referred to as an **enterotoxin.** Despite the massive toxin-induced fluid secretion, both intestinal morphology and nutrient-coupled Na^+ absorption are normal. Because nutrient-coupled (e.g., glucose or amino acid) fluid absorption is intact, therapeutically increasing the concentration of glucose or amino acids in the intestinal lumen can enhance absorption. ORS contains varying concentrations of glucose, Na^+, Cl^-, and HCO_3^- and is extremely effective in enhancing fluid and electrolyte absorption in secretory diarrhea when the intestine secretes massive amounts of fluid. Administration of ORS can reverse the dehydration and metabolic acidosis that may occur in severe diarrhea and that are often the primary cause for morbidity and mortality, especially in children younger than 5 years. ORS is the major advance of the past half century in the treatment of diarrheal disease, especially in developing countries. The development of ORS was a direct consequence of research on the physiology of glucose- and amino acid–stimulated Na^+ absorption.

of the small intestine, the Na-H exchanger solely mediates the Na^+ absorption that is stimulated by the alkalinity of the HCO_3^--rich intraluminal contents.

Parallel Na-H and Cl-HCO₃ Exchange in the Ileum and Proximal Part of the Colon Is the Primary Mechanism of Na^+ Absorption During the Interdigestive Period

"Electroneutral" NaCl absorption occurs in portions of both the small and large intestine (see Fig. 43–3*C*). Electroneutral NaCl absorption is not due to an Na/Cl cotransporter, but rather to parallel apical membrane Na-H and Cl-HCO_3 exchangers that are closely linked by small changes in pH_i. In the human colon, DRA (downregulated-in-adenoma; p. 69) mediates this Cl-HCO_3 exchange. This mechanism of NaCl absorption is the primary method of Na^+ absorption between meals (i.e., the interdigestive period), but it does not contribute greatly to postprandial Na^+ absorption, which is mediated primarily by the nutrient-coupled transporters described previously. Electroneutral NaCl absorption occurs in the ileum and throughout the large intestine, with the exception of the most distal segment. It is not affected by either luminal glucose or luminal HCO_3^-. However, aldosterone inhibits electroneutral NaCl absorption.

The overall electroneutral NaCl absorptive process is regulated by both cAMP and cyclic guanosine monophosphate (cGMP), as well as intracellular Ca^{2+}. Increases in each of these three intracellular messengers *reduce* NaCl absorption. Conversely, decreases in $[Ca^{2+}]_i$ *increase* NaCl absorption. Decreased NaCl absorption is important in the pathogenesis of most diarrheal disorders. For example, one of the common causes of "traveler's diarrhea" (see the box titled Secretory Diarrhea) is the heat-labile enterotoxin that is produced by the bacterium *E. coli*. This toxin activates adenylyl cyclase and increases [cAMP]$_i$, which in turn decreases NaCl absorption and stimulates active Cl$^-$ secretion, as discussed later.

Epithelial Na$^+$ Channels Are the Primary Mechanism of "Electrogenic" Na$^+$ Absorption in the Distal Part of the Colon

In "electrogenic" Na$^+$ absorption (see Fig. 43–3D), Na$^+$ entry across the apical membrane occurs via ENaC channels that are highly specific for Na$^+$ (p. 84). Like the Na-H exchanger, these ENaC channels are blocked by the diuretic amiloride, but at *micro*molar rather than *milli*molar concentrations. Na$^+$ absorption in the distal part of the colon is highly efficient. Because this segment of the colon is capable of absorbing Na$^+$ against large concentration gradients, it plays an important role in Na$^+$ conservation. Na$^+$ movement via electrogenic Na$^+$ absorption is not affected by luminal glucose or by HCO$_3^-$, nor is it regulated by cyclic nucleotides. However, it is markedly enhanced by mineralocorticoids (e.g., aldosterone).

Mineralocorticoids increase Na$^+$ absorption in the colon—as in other aldosterone-responsive epithelia, notably the renal collecting duct (p. 786)—via multiple mechanisms. Aldosterone increases electrogenic Na$^+$ absorption by increasing Na$^+$ entry through the apical Na$^+$ channel and by stimulating activity of the Na-K pump. The increase in apical Na$^+$ uptake can occur (1) rapidly (i.e., within seconds) as a consequence of an increase in the opening of apical Na$^+$ channels, (2) more gradually (within minutes) because of the insertion of preformed Na$^+$ channels from subapical epithelial vesicle pools into the apical membrane, or (3) very slowly (within hours) as a result of an increase in the synthesis of both new apical Na$^+$ channels and Na-K pumps.

CELLULAR MECHANISMS OF Cl$^-$ ABSORPTION AND SECRETION

Cl$^-$ absorption occurs throughout the small and large intestine and is often closely linked to Na$^+$ absorption. Cl$^-$ and Na$^+$ absorption may be coupled via either an electrical potential difference or by pH$_i$. However, sometimes *no* coupling takes place, and the route of Cl$^-$ movement may be either paracellular or transcellular.

"Voltage-Dependent" Cl$^-$ Absorption Represents Coupling of Cl$^-$ Absorption to Electrogenic Na$^+$ Absorption in Both the Small and the Large Intestine

Cl$^-$ absorption can be a purely passive process (Fig. 43–4A), driven by the electrochemical gradient for Cl$^-$ either across the tight junctions (paracellular route) or across the individual membranes of the epithelial cell (transcellu-

lar route). In either case, the driving force for Cl$^-$ absorption derives from either of the two electrogenic mechanisms of Na$^+$ absorption described previously—namely, nutrient-coupled transport in the small intestine and epithelial Na$^+$ channels in the distal end of the colon. This process is referred to as "voltage-dependent Cl$^-$ absorption"; it is not an active transport process.

Within the *small intestine*, induction of a lumen-nega-

FIGURE 43–4. Modes of Cl$^-$ absorption by the intestine. *A*, In "voltage-dependent" Cl$^-$ absorption, Cl$^-$ may passively diffuse from lumen to blood across the tight junctions, driven by the lumen-negative transepithelial voltage (paracellular route). Alternatively, Cl$^-$ may diffuse through apical and basolateral Cl$^-$ channels. The thickness of the arrows in the inset indicates the relative magnitude of the Cl$^-$-absorptive flux through this pathway. *B*, In the absence of a parallel Na-H exchanger, "electroneutral Cl-HCO$_3$ exchange" at the apical membrane results in Cl$^-$ absorption and HCO$_3^-$ secretion. *C*, "Electroneutral NaCl" absorption (see Fig. 43–3C) can mediate Cl$^-$ absorption in the interdigestive period. Note that intracellular pH couples the two exchangers. CA, carbonic anhydrase.

tive potential difference by glucose- and amino acid–induced Na^+ absorption (see Fig. 43–3A) provides the driving force for Cl^- absorption. As noted earlier, nutrient-coupled Na^+ absorption primarily represents a villous cell process that occurs in the postprandial period and is insensitive to cyclic nucleotides and changes in $[Ca^{2+}]_i$. Voltage-dependent Cl^- absorption shares these properties. It is uncertain whether the route of voltage-dependent Cl^- absorption is transcellular or paracellular.

In the *large intestine*, especially in the distal segment, electrogenic Na^+ absorption via the ENaC Na^+ channel (see Fig. 43–3D) also induces a lumen-negative potential difference that provides the driving force for colonic voltage-dependent Cl^- absorption. Factors that increase or decrease the voltage difference will similarly affect Cl^- absorption.

Electroneutral Cl-HCO₃ Exchange Results in Cl⁻ Absorption and HCO₃⁻ Secretion in the Ileum and Colon

Electroneutral Cl-HCO_3 exchange, in the absence of parallel Na-H exchange, occurs in villous cells in the ileum and in surface epithelial cells in the large intestine (see Fig. 43–4B). It is not known whether this process occurs in the cells lining the crypts. A Cl-HCO_3 exchanger in the apical membrane is responsible for the 1 : 1 exchange of apical Cl^- for intracellular HCO_3^-. In humans, this Cl-HCO_3 exchanger is DRA (p. 69). The details of Cl^- movement across the *basolateral* membrane are not well understood, but may involve the ClC-2 Cl^- channel (p. 169).

CONGENITAL CHLORIDORRHEA

The congenital absence of an apical Cl-HCO_3 exchanger (which mediates the Cl-HCO_3 involved in electroneutral NaCl absorption) is an autosomal recessive disorder known as **congenital chloridorrhea** or **congenital chloride diarrhea (CLD).** Affected children have diarrhea with an extremely high stool $[Cl^-]$, a direct consequence of absence of the apical membrane Cl-HCO_3 exchanger. In addition, because HCO_3^- secretion is reduced, patients are alkalotic (i.e., have an increased plasma $[HCO_3^-]$). The gene for congenital chloridorrhea is located on chromosome 7q31. The gene product is the same as that of the downregulated-in-adenoma (DRA) gene. DRA (also known as SLC26A3) is a member of the SAT (sulfate anion transporter) family of sulfate transporters (p. 69) and mediates Cl-HCO_3 exchange. In addition, DRA transports sulfate and other anions. However, DRA is distinct from the AE (anion exchanger) gene family that encodes the Cl-HCO_3 exchangers in erythrocytes and several other tissues. Indeed, Cl-HCO_3 exchange in the renal tubule, erythrocytes, and other cells is unaffected in individuals with CLD, as are other intestinal transport processes.

Parallel Na-H and Cl-HCO₃ Exchange in the Ileum and the Proximal Part of the Colon Mediates Cl⁻ Absorption During the Interdigestive Period

"Electroneutral NaCl absorption," discussed in connection with Na^+ absorption (see Fig. 43–3C), also mediates Cl^- absorption in the ileum and proximal part of the colon (see Fig. 43–4C). The apical step of Cl^- absorption by this mechanism is mediated by parallel Na-H and Cl-HCO_3 exchanges, which are coupled via pH_i.

Electrogenic Cl⁻ *Secretion* Occurs in Crypts of Both the Small and the Large Intestine

In the previous three sections, we saw that intestinal Cl^- *absorption* occurs via three mechanisms. The small intestine and the large intestine are also capable of active Cl^- secretion, although Cl^- secretion is believed to occur mainly in the crypts rather than in either the villi or surface cells.

A small amount of Cl^- secretion probably occurs in the "basal" state but is masked by the higher rate of the three Cl^- absorptive processes that are discussed earlier in this subchapter. However, Cl^- secretion is markedly stimulated by secretagogues such as acetylcholine and other neurotransmitters. Moreover, Cl^- secretion is the major component of the ion transport events that occur during most clinical and experimental diarrheal disorders.

The cellular model of active Cl^- secretion is outlined in Figure 43–5 and includes three transport pathways on the basolateral membrane: (1) an Na-K pump, (2) an Na/K/Cl cotransporter, and (3) two types of K^+ channels. In addition, a Cl^- channel is present on the apical membrane. This complex Cl^- secretory system is energized by the Na-K pump, which generates a low $[Na^+]_i$ and provides the driving force for Cl^- entry across the basolateral membrane via Na/K/Cl cotransport. As a result, $[Cl^-]_i$ is raised sufficiently that the Cl^- electrochemical gradient favors the passive efflux of Cl^- across the apical membrane. One consequence of these many transport processes is that the transepithelial voltage becomes more lumen-negative, thereby promoting voltage-dependent Na^+ secretion. This Na^+ secretion that accompanies active Cl^- secretion presumably occurs through the tight junctions (paracellular pathway). Thus, the net result is stimulation of NaCl and fluid secretion.

Normally—that is, in the unstimulated state—the crypts secrete little Cl^- because the apical membrane Cl^- channels are either closed or not present. Cl^- secretion requires activation by cyclic nucleotides or $[Ca^{2+}]_i$, which are increased by any of several **secretagogues**, including (1) bacterial exotoxins (i.e., "enterotoxins"), (2) hormones and neurotransmitters, (3) products of cells of the immune system (e.g., histamine), and (4) laxatives (see Table 43–3).

Some secretagogues initially bind to membrane receptors and stimulate the activation of adenylyl cyclase (vasoactive intestinal peptide [VIP]), guanylyl cyclase (the heat-

FIGURE 43–5. Cellular mechanism of electrogenic Cl⁻ secretion by crypt cells. The basolateral Na/K/Cl cotransporter brings Cl⁻ into the crypt cell; the Cl⁻ exits across the apical Cl⁻ channel. Secretagogues may open pre-existing Cl⁻ channels or cause subapical vesicles to fuse with the apical membrane, thus delivering new Cl⁻ channels. The paracellular pathway allows Na⁺ movement from blood to lumen, driven by the lumen-negative transepithelial voltage. The thickness of the arrows in the *inset* indicates that the magnitude of the Cl⁻-secretory flux through this pathway is the same throughout the intestine. ATP, adenosine triphosphate; cAMP, cyclic adenosine monophosphate.

stable toxin of *E. coli*), or phospholipase C (acetylcholine). Others increase $[Ca^{2+}]_i$ by opening Ca^{2+} channels at the basolateral membrane. The resulting activation of one or more protein kinases—by any of the aforementioned pathways—increases the Cl⁻ conductance of the apical membrane either by activating pre-existing Cl⁻ channels or by inserting into the apical membrane Cl⁻ channels that—in the unstimulated state—are stored in subapical membrane vesicles. In either case, Cl⁻ is now able to exit the cell through apical Cl⁻ channels. The resulting decrease in $[Cl^-]_i$ leads to increased uptake of Na⁺, Cl⁻, and K⁺ across the basolateral membrane via the Na/K/Cl cotransporter. The Na⁺ is recycled out of the cell via the Na-K pump. The K⁺ is recycled via basolateral K⁺ channels that are opened by the same protein kinases that increase Cl⁻ conductance. The net result of all these changes is the initiation of active Cl⁻ secretion across the epithelial cell.

The induction of apical membrane Cl⁻ channels is extremely important in the pathophysiology of many diarrheal disorders. The box Secretory Diarrhea at the end of this chapter discusses the changes in ion transport that occur in secretory diarrheas such as cholera. A central role in **cystic fibrosis** has been posited for the cystic fibrosis transmembrane regulator (CFTR) Cl⁻ channel in the apical membrane (p. 916). However, more than one (and possibly several) Cl⁻ channels are present in the intestine, and CFTR may not be the only Cl⁻ channel associated with active Cl⁻ secretion.

CELLULAR MECHANISMS OF K⁺ ABSORPTION AND SECRETION

Overall Net Transepithelial K⁺ Movement Is Absorptive in the Small Intestine and Secretory in the Colon

The gastrointestinal tract participates in overall K⁺ balance, although when compared with the role of the kidneys, the small intestine and large intestine play a relatively modest role, especially in healthy individuals.

The pattern of intestinal K⁺ movement parallels that of the kidney: (1) the intestines have the capacity for both K⁺ absorption and secretion, and (2) the intestines absorb K⁺ in the proximal segments but secrete it in the distal segments.

Dietary K⁺ furnishes 80 to 120 millimoles/day, whereas stool K⁺ output is only approximately 10 millimoles/day. The kidney is responsible for disposal of the remainder of the daily K⁺ intake (p. 815). Substantial quantities of K⁺ are secreted in gastric, pancreatic, and biliary fluid. Therefore, the total K⁺ load presented to the small intestine is considerably greater than that represented by the diet. The concentration of K⁺ in stool is frequently more than 100 mM. This high stool $[K^+]$ is the result of several factors, including both colonic K⁺ secretion and water absorption, especially in the distal part of the colon.

K⁺ Absorption in the Small Intestine Probably Occurs Via Solvent Drag

Studies in which a plasma-like solution is perfused through segments of the intestine have established that K⁺ is absorbed in the jejunum and ileum of the small intestine and secreted in the large intestine. Although the small intestine absorbs substantial amounts of K⁺, no evidence has been presented to suggest that K⁺ absorption in the jejunum and ileum is an active-transport process or even carrier mediated. Thus, K⁺ absorption in the small intestine is probably passive, most likely a result of **solvent drag** (i.e., pulled along by bulk water movement), as illustrated in Figure 43–6A. Although changes in dietary Na⁺ and K⁺ and alterations in hydration influence K⁺ movement in the *colon*, similar physiological events do not appear to affect K⁺ absorption in the *small intestine*.

Passive K⁺ Secretion Is the Primary Mechanism for Net Colonic Secretion

In contrast to the small intestine, the human colon is a net *secretor* of K⁺. This secretion occurs by two mechanisms: a passive transport process that is discussed in this section and an active process that is discussed in the next. Together, these two K⁺-secretory pathways are greater than a modest component of active K⁺ absorption in the distal part of the colon and thus account for the overall secretion of K⁺ by the colon.

Passive K⁺ secretion, which is the pathway that is primarily responsible for overall net colonic K⁺ secretion,

A PASSIVE K⁺ ABSORPTION

B PASSIVE K⁺ SECRETION

The lumen potential is 25mV.

C ACTIVE K⁺ SECRETION

D ACTIVE K⁺ ABSORPTION

Jejunum

Ileum

Proximal colon

Distal colon

Proximal colon

Distal colon

Distal colon

High transport

Moderate transport

Low transport

Very low transport

is driven by the lumen-negative V_{TE} of 15 to 25 mV. The route of passive K⁺ secretion is predominantly paracellular, not transcellular (see Fig. 43–6B). Because V_{TE} is the primary determinant of passive K⁺ secretion, it is not surprising that passive K⁺ secretion is greatest in the distal end of the colon, where V_{TE} difference is most negative. Similarly, increases in the lumen-negative V_{TE} that occur as an adaptive response to dehydration—secondary to an elevation in aldosterone secretion (see the next section)—result in an enhanced rate of passive K⁺ secretion. Information is not available regarding the distribution of passive K⁺ secretion between surface epithelial and crypt cells.

Active K⁺ Secretion Is Also Present Throughout the Large Intestine and Is Induced Both by Aldosterone and by cAMP

In addition to *passive* K⁺ secretion, *active* K⁺-transport processes—both secretory and absorptive—are also present in the colon. However, active transport of K⁺ is subject to considerable segmental variation in the colon. Whereas active K⁺ *secretion* occurs throughout the colon, active K⁺ *absorption* is present only in the distal segments of the large intestine. Thus, in the rectosigmoid colon, active K⁺ absorption and active K⁺ secretion are both operative and appear to contribute to total-body homeostasis.

The model of active K⁺ secretion in the colon is quite similar to that of active Cl⁻ secretion (see Fig. 43–5) and is also parallel to that of active K⁺ secretion in the renal distal nephron (p. 822). The general paradigm of active K⁺ transport in the colon is a "pump-leak" model (Fig. 43–6C). Uptake of K⁺ across the basolateral membrane is a result of both the Na-K pump and the Na/K/Cl cotransporter, which is energized by the low $[Na^+]_i$ that is created by the Na-K pump. Once K⁺ enters the cell across the basolateral membrane, it may exit either across the apical membrane (K⁺ secretion) or across the basolateral membrane (K⁺ recycling). The cell controls the extent to which secretion occurs, in part by K⁺ channels present in both the apical and the basolateral membranes. When apical K⁺-channel activity is less than basolateral channel activity, K⁺ recycling dominates. Indeed, in the basal

FIGURE 43–6. Cellular mechanisms of K⁺ secretion and absorption. *A*, This mechanism pertains only to the small intestine, which is a net absorber of K⁺ via solvent drag across tight junctions. The thickness of the arrows in the *inset* indicates the relative magnitude of the K⁺ flux through this pathway. *B*, The colon is a net secretor of K⁺. The primary mechanism is passive K⁺ secretion through tight junctions, which occurs throughout the colon. The driving force is a lumen-negative transepithelial voltage. *C*, Another mechanism of K⁺ secretion throughout the colon is a transcellular process that involves the basolateral uptake of K⁺ via the Na-K pump and the Na/K/Cl cotransporter, followed by the efflux of K⁺ through apical K⁺ channels. *D*, Confined to the distal colon is a transcellular mechanism of K⁺ absorption that is mediated by an apical H-K pump.

state, the rate of active K^+ secretion is low because the apical K^+-channel activity is minimal in comparison with the K^+-channel activity in the basolateral membrane.

The rate-limiting step in active K^+ secretion is the apical K^+ channel. Both aldosterone and cAMP increase K^+ channel activity in the apical membrane and thus stimulate active K^+ secretion in the large intestine. However, both aldosterone and cAMP do more than just influence the apical membrane K^+ channels.

ALDOSTERONE. This mineralocorticoid enhances overall net K^+ secretion by two mechanisms. First, it increases **passive** K^+ secretion by increasing Na-K pump activity and thus increasing electrogenic Na^+ absorption (see Fig. 43–3D). The net effect is to increase the lumen-negative V_{TE} and enhance passive K^+ secretion (see Fig. 43–6B). Second, aldosterone stimulates **active** K^+ secretion by increasing the activity of both apical K^+ channels and basolateral Na-K pumps (see Fig. 43–6C).

cAMP AND Ca^{2+}. VIP and cholera enterotoxin both increase $[cAMP]_i$ and thus stimulate K^+ secretion. Increases in $[Ca^{2+}]_i$—induced, for example, by serotonin (or 5-hydroxytryptamine [5-HT])—also stimulate active K^+ secretion. In contrast to aldosterone, neither of these second messengers has an effect on the Na-K pump; rather, they increase the activity of both the apical and the basolateral K^+ channels. Because the stimulation of K^+ channels is greater at the apical than at the basolateral membrane, the result is an increase in K^+ exit from the epithelial cell across the apical membrane (i.e., secretion). Stimulation of K^+ secretion by cAMP and Ca^{2+}, both of which also induce active Cl^- secretion (see Fig. 43–5), contributes to the significant fecal K^+ losses that occur in many diarrheal diseases.

Active K^+ Absorption Is Located Only in the Distal Portion of the Colon and Is Energized by an Apical H-K Pump

As noted earlier, not only does the distal end of the colon actively secrete K^+, it also actively absorbs K^+. The balance between the two processes plays a role in overall K^+ homeostasis. Increases in dietary K^+ enhance both passive and active K^+ *secretion* (see Fig. 43–6B, C). However, dietary K^+ depletion enhances active K^+ *absorption* (see Fig. 43–6D). The mechanism of active K^+ absorption appears to be an exchange of luminal K^+ for intracellular H^+ across the apical membrane, mediated by an H-K pump (p. 63). The colonic H-K pump is approximately 60% identical at the amino acid level with both the Na-K pump and the gastric parietal cell H-K pump. Thus, colonic K^+ movement via the active K^+-absorption process occurs via a transcellular route, in contrast to the paracellular route that characterizes K^+ absorption in the small intestine (see Fig. 43–6A). The mechanism of K^+ exit across the basolateral membrane may involve K/Cl cotransport. Not known is whether active K^+ secretion (see Fig. 43–6C) and active K^+ absorption (see Fig. 43–6D) occur in the same cell or in different cells.

REGULATION OF INTESTINAL ION TRANSPORT

Chemical Mediators from the Enteric Nervous System, Endocrine Cells, and Immune Cells in the Lamina Propria May Be Either Secretagogues or Absorptagogues

Numerous chemical mediators from several different sources regulate intestinal electrolyte transport. Some of these agonists are important both in health and in diarrheal disorders, and at times only quantitative differences separate normal regulatory control from the pathophysiology of diarrhea. These mediators may function in one or more modes: neural, endocrine, paracrine, and perhaps autocrine (p. 88). Most of these agonists (i.e., secretagogues) promote secretion, whereas some others (i.e., absorptagogues) enhance absorption.

The **enteric nervous system** (ENS), discussed in Chapters 15 and 40, is important in the normal regulation of intestinal epithelial electrolyte transport. Activation of enteric secretomotor neurons results in the release of acetylcholine from mucosal neurons and in the induction of active Cl^- secretion (see Fig. 43–5). Additional neurotransmitters, including VIP, 5-HT, and histamine, mediate ENS regulation of epithelial ion transport.

An example of regulation mediated by the **endocrine system** is the release of aldosterone from the adrenal cortex and the subsequent formation of angiotensin II; both dehydration and volume contraction stimulate this renin-angiotensin-aldosterone axis (p. 866). Both angiotensin and aldosterone regulate total-body Na^+ homeostasis by stimulating Na^+ absorption, angiotensin in the small intestine and aldosterone in the colon. Their effects on cellular Na^+ absorption differ. In the small intestine, angiotensin enhances electroneutral NaCl absorption (see Fig. 43–3C), probably by upregulating apical membrane Na-H exchange. In the colon, aldosterone stimulates electrogenic Na^+ absorption (see Fig. 43–3D).

The response of the intestine to angiotensin and aldosterone represents a classic endocrine feedback loop: dehydration results in increased levels of angiotensin and aldosterone, the primary effects of which are to stimulate fluid and Na^+ absorption by both the renal tubules (p. 786) and the intestines, thus restoring total body fluid and Na^+ content.

Regulation of intestinal transport also occurs by **paracrine effects**. Endocrine cells constitute a small fraction of the total population of mucosal cells in the intestines. These endocrine cells contain several peptides and bioactive amines that are released in response to various stimuli. Relatively little is known about the biology of these cells, but gut distention can induce the release of one or more of these agonists (e.g., 5-HT). The effect of these agonists on adjacent surface epithelial cells represents a paracrine action.

Another example of paracrine regulation of intestinal fluid and electrolyte transport is the influence of **immune cells** in the *lamina propria* (see Fig. 43–1). Table 43–2 presents these immune cells and a partial list of the agonists that they release. The same agonist may be released

TABLE 43–2

PRODUCTS OF LAMINA PROPRIA CELLS THAT AFFECT INTESTINAL ION TRANSPORT

CELL	PRODUCT
Macrophages	Prostaglandins
	O_2 radicals
Mast cells	Histamine
Neutrophils	Eicosanoids
	PAF
Fibroblasts	Eicosanoids
	Bradykinin

PAF, platelet-activating factor.

from more than one cell, and individual cells produce multiple agonists. These agonists may activate epithelial cells directly or activate other immune cells or enteric neurons. For example, reactive oxygen radicals released by mast cells affect epithelial cell function by acting on enteric neurons and fibroblasts, and they also have direct action on surface and crypt epithelial cells.

A single agonist usually has multiple sites of action. For example, the histamine released from mast cells can induce fluid secretion as a result of its interaction with receptors on surface epithelial cells (Fig. 43–7). However, histamine can also activate ENS motor neurons, which can in turn alter epithelial cell ion transport, as well as intestinal smooth-muscle tone and blood flow. As a consequence, the effects of histamine on intestinal ion transport are multiple and amplified.

Secretagogues Can Be Classified by Their Type and by the Intracellular Second-Messenger System That They Stimulate

Several agonists induce the accumulation of fluid and electrolytes in the intestinal lumen (i.e., net secretion).

These secretagogues are a diverse, heterogeneous group of compounds, but they can be effectively classified in two different ways: by the type of secretagogue and by the intracellular second messenger that these agonists activate.

Grouped according to "type," the secretagogues fall into four categories: (1) bacterial exotoxins (i.e., enterotoxins), (2) hormones and neurotransmitters, (3) products of cells of the immune system, and (4) laxatives. Table 43–3 provides a partial list of these secretagogues. A **bacterial exotoxin** is a peptide that is produced and excreted by bacteria that can produce effects independently of the bacteria. An **enterotoxin** is an exotoxin that induces changes in intestinal fluid and electrolyte movement. For example, *E. coli* produces two distinct enterotoxins (the so-called heat-labile and heat-stable toxins) that induce fluid and electrolyte secretion via two distinct receptors and second-messenger systems.

We can also classify secretagogues according to the signal-transduction system that they activate after binding to a specific membrane receptor. As summarized in Table 43–3, the second messengers of these signal-transduction systems include cAMP, cGMP, and Ca^{2+}. For example, the **heat-labile** toxin of *E. coli* binds to apical membrane receptors, becomes internalized, and then activates basolateral adenylyl cyclase. The resulting increase in $[cAMP]_i$ activates protein kinase A. VIP also acts by this route (Fig. 43–8). The **heat-stable** toxin of *E. coli* binds to and activates an apical receptor guanylyl cyclase, similar to the atrial natriuretic peptide (ANP) receptor (p. 108). The newly produced cGMP activates protein kinase G and may also activate protein kinase A. The natural agonist for this pathway is guanylin, a 15–amino acid peptide secreted by mucosal cells of the small and large intestine. Still other secretory agonists (e.g., 5-HT) produce their effects by increasing $[Ca^{2+}]_i$ and thus activating protein kinase C or Ca^{2+}-calmodulin–dependent protein kinases. One way that secretagogues can increase $[Ca^{2+}]_i$ is by stimulating phospholipase C, which leads to the production of inositol 1,4,5-triphosphate (IP_3) and the release

FIGURE 43–7. Mast cell activation. Activation of mast cells in the lamina propria triggers the release of histamine, which directly affects epithelial cells, or which stimulates an enteric neuron and thus has an indirect effect. The neuron modulates the epithelium (secretion), intestinal smooth muscle (motility), or vascular smooth muscle (blood flow). ACh, acetylcholine.

TABLE 43–3

MODE OF ACTION OF SECRETAGOGUES

CATEGORY	SECRETAGOGUE	SECOND MESSENGER
Bacterial Enterotoxins	Cholera toxin	cAMP
	Escherichia coli toxins: heat labile	cAMP
	E. coli toxins: heat stable	cGMP
	Yersinia toxin	cGMP
	Clostridium difficile toxin	Ca^{2+}
Hormones and Neurotransmitters	VIP	cAMP
	Guanylin	cGMP
	Acetylcholine	Ca^{2+}
	Bradykinin	Ca^{2+}
	Serotonin (5-HT)	Ca^{2+}
Immune Cell Products	Histamine	cAMP
	Prostaglandins	cAMP
Laxatives	Bile acids	Ca^{2+}
	Ricinoleic acid	?

cAMP, cyclic adenosine monophosphate; cGMP, cyclic guanosine monophosphate; 5-HT, 5-hydroxytryptamine; VIP, vasoactive intestinal peptide.

FIGURE 43–8. Action of secretagogues. Secretagogues (agents that stimulate the net secretion of fluid and electrolytes into the intestinal lumen) act by any of three mechanisms. Some (e.g., VIP, heat-labile toxin) activate adenylyl cyclase, which in turn generates cAMP and thus stimulates protein kinase A (PKA). Others (e.g., heat-stable toxin—also known as ST_a) bind to the guanylin receptor, which is a receptor guanylyl cyclase that generates cGMP and results in the stimulation of protein kinase G (PKG). Others (e.g., serotonin) stimulate the phospholipase C (PLC) pathway, which leads to the generation of IP_3 and DAG. The DAG activates protein kinase C (PKC). The increased $[Ca^{2+}]_i$ stimulates PKC and Ca^{2+}-calmodulin-dependent protein kinase (CaM kinase). These activated kinases stimulate net secretion by phosphorylating apical-membrane transporters or other proteins. AC, adenylyl cyclase; cAMP, cyclic adenosine monophosphate; cGMP, cyclic guanosine monophosphate; DAG, diacylglycerol; ER, endoplasmic reticulum; G_q and G_s, α-subunit types of G proteins; PIP_2, phosphatidylinositol 4,5-biphosphate.

TABLE 43–4

END EFFECTS OF SECOND MESSENGERS ON INTESTINAL TRANSPORT		
SECOND MESSENGER	**INCREASED ANION SECRETION**	**INHIBITED NaCl ABSORPTION**
cAMP	+++	+++
cGMP	+	+++
Ca²⁺	+++	+++

cAMP, cyclic adenosine monophosphate; cGMP, cyclic guanosine monophosphate.

of Ca^{2+} from intracellular stores (p. 100). Secretagogues can also increase [Ca^{2+}]$_i$ by activating protein kinases, which may stimulate basolateral Ca^{2+} channels.

Although the secretagogues listed in Table 43–3 stimulate fluid and electrolyte secretion via one of three distinct second messengers (i.e., cAMP, cGMP, and Ca^{2+}), the *end effects* are quite similar. As summarized in Table 43–4, all three second-messenger systems stimulate active Cl$^-$ secretion (see Fig. 43–5) and inhibit electroneutral NaCl absorption (see Fig. 43–3C). The abilities of cAMP and Ca^{2+} to stimulate Cl$^-$ secretion and inhibit electroneutral NaCl absorption are almost identical. In contrast, cGMP's ability to stimulate Cl$^-$ secretion is somewhat less, although its effects on electroneutral NaCl absorption are quantitatively similar to those of cAMP and Ca^{2+}. Both stimulation of Cl$^-$ secretion and inhibition of electroneutral NaCl absorption have the same overall effect: *net secretion of fluid and electrolytes.* It is uncertain whether the observed decrease in electroneutral NaCl absorption is the result of inhibiting Na-H exchange, Cl-HCO₃ exchange, or both inasmuch as electroneutral NaCl absorption represents the coupling of separate Na-H and Cl-HCO₃ exchange processes via pH$_i$ (see Fig. 43–3C).

Mineralocorticoids, Glucocorticoids, and Somatostatin Are Absorptagogues

Although multiple secretagogues exist, relatively few agonists can be found that *enhance* fluid and electrolyte *absorption.* The cellular effects of these absorptagogues are less well understood than those of the secretagogues. Those few absorptagogues that have been identified increase intestinal fluid and electrolyte absorption by either a paracrine or an endocrine mechanism.

Corticosteroids are the primary hormones that enhance intestinal fluid and electrolyte absorption. **Mineralocorticoids** (e.g., aldosterone) stimulate Na$^+$ absorption and K$^+$ secretion in the distal end of the colon; they do not affect ion transport in the small intestine. Their cellular actions are outlined in Chapter 49. Aldosterone induces both apical membrane Na$^+$ channels (a process that is inhibited by the diuretic amiloride) and basolateral Na-K pumps; this action results in substantial enhancement of colonic "electrogenic" Na$^+$ absorption. Although the effects of glucocorticoids on ion transport have most often been considered a result of crossover binding to the mineralocorticoid receptor (p. 787), it is now evident that

glucocorticoids also have potent actions on ion transport via their own receptor and that these changes in ion transport are distinct from those of the mineralocorticoids: **glucocorticoids** stimulate electroneutral NaCl absorption (Fig. 43–3C) throughout the large and small intestine without any effect on either K$^+$ secretion or electrogenic Na$^+$ absorption. Both corticosteroids act, at least in part, by genomic mechanisms (p. 131).

Other agonists appear to stimulate fluid and electrolyte absorption by stimulating electroneutral NaCl absorption and inhibiting electrogenic HCO₃$^-$ secretion; both these changes *enhance fluid absorption.* Among these absorptagogues are **somatostatin**, which is released from endocrine cells in the intestinal mucosa (p. 898), and the enkephalins and norepinephrine, which are neurotrans-

---

SECRETORY DIARRHEA

Diarrhea is a common medical problem and can be defined as a "symptom" (i.e., an increase in the number of bowel movements or a decrease in stool consistency) or as a "sign" (i.e., an increase in stool volume of more than 0.2 liters per 24 hours). Diarrhea has many causes and can be classified in various ways. One classification divides diarrheas by the causative factor. The causative factor can be a dietary nutrient that is not absorbed, in which case the result is an **"osmotic diarrhea."** An example of osmotic diarrhea is primary lactase deficiency. Alternatively, the causative factor may *not* be a dietary nutrient, but rather endogenous secretions of fluid and electrolytes from the intestine, in which case the result is a **"secretory diarrhea."**

The leading causes of secretory diarrhea include infections with *Escherichia coli* (the major cause of traveler's diarrhea) and cholera (a substantial cause of morbidity and mortality in developing countries). In these infectious diarrheas, an enterotoxin produced by one of many bacterial organisms raises intracellular concentrations of cyclic adenosine monophosphate ([cAMP]$_i$), cyclic guanosine monophosphate ([cGMP]$_i$), or calcium ([Ca^{2+}]$_i$) (see Table 43–3).

A second group of secretory diarrheas include those produced by different, although relatively uncommon, hormone-producing tumors. Examples include tumors that produce vasoactive intestinal peptide (the Verner-Morrison syndrome), glucagon (glucagonomas), and serotonin (the carcinoid syndrome). These secretagogues act by raising either [cAMP]$_i$ or [Ca^{2+}]$_i$ (see Table 43–3). When a tumor produces these secretagogues in abundance, the resulting diarrhea can be copious and explosive.

As we have seen, the secretory diarrheas have in common their ability to increase [cAMP]$_i$, [cGMP]$_i$, or [Ca^{2+}]$_i$. Table 43–4 summarizes the mechanisms by which these second messengers produce the secretory diarrhea. Because the second messengers do not alter the function of nutrient-coupled Na$^+$ absorption, administration of an oral rehydration solution containing glucose and Na$^+$ is effective in the treatment of enterotoxin-mediated diarrhea (see the earlier box titled Oral Rehydration Solution, on p. 937).

mitters of enteric neurons. The limited information available suggests that these agonists affect ion transport by *decreasing* $[Ca^{2+}]_i$, probably by blocking Ca^{2+} channels. Thus, it appears that fluctuations in $[Ca^{2+}]_i$ regulate Na^+ and Cl^- transport in both the absorptive (low $[Ca^{2+}]_i$) and secretory (high $[Ca^{2+}]_i$) directions. Therefore, Ca^{2+} is clearly a critical modulator of intestinal ion transport.

REFERENCES

Books and Reviews

Binder HJ, Sandle GI: Electrolyte transport in the mammalian colon. In Johnson LR (ed): Physiology of the Gastrointestinal Tract, 3rd ed. New York, Raven, 1994, pp 2133–2172.

Field M, Semrad CE: Toxigenic diarrheas, congenital diarrheas, and cystic fibrosis: Disorders of intestinal ion transport. Annu Rev Physiol 55:631–655, 1993.

Greger R, Bleich M, Leipziger J, et al: Regulation of ion transport in colonic crypts. News Physiol Sci 12:62–66, 1997.

Montrose MH, Keely SJ, Barrett KE: Electrolyte secretion and absorption. Small intestine and colon. In Yamada T (ed): Textbook of Gastroenterology, Vol 1, 4th ed. Philadelphia, Lippincott, Williams and Wilkins, 2003, pp 308–340.

Palacin M, Estevez R, Bertran J, Zorzano A: Molecular biology of mammalian plasma membrane amino acid transporters. Physiol Rev 78: 969–1054, 1998.

Rao MC: Oral rehydration therapy: New explanations for an old remedy. Annu Rev Physiol 66:385–417, 2004.

Journal Articles

Canessa CM, Horisberger J-D, Rossier BC: Epithelial sodium channel related to proteins involved in neurodegeneration. Nature 361:467–470, 1993.

Knickelbein RG, Aronson PS, Schron CM, et al: Sodium and chloride transport across rabbit ileal brush border. II. Evidence for Cl-HCO$_3$ exchange and mechanism of coupling. Am J Physiol 249:G236–G245, 1985.

Moseley RH, Hoglund P, Wu GD, et al: Downregulated in adenoma gene encodes a chloride transporter defective in congenital chloride diarrhea. Am J Physiol 276:G185–G192, 1999.

Schulz S, Green CK, Yuen PST, Garbers DL: Guanylyl cyclase is a heat-stable enterotoxin receptor. Cell 63:941–948, 1990.

Singh SK, Binder HJ, Boron WF, Geibel JP: Fluid absorption in isolated perfused colonic crypts. J Clin Invest 96:2373–2379, 1995.

CHAPTER 44

Nutrient Digestion and Absorption

Henry J. Binder and Adrian Reuben

In general, the digestive-absorptive processes for most of the constituents of our diet are highly efficient. For example, normal adult intestine absorbs approximately 95% of dietary lipid. However, we ingest most of the constituents of dietary food in a form that the intestine cannot readily absorb. Multiple digestive processes convert dietary food to a form that can be absorbed—primarily in the small intestine, but also, to a much smaller extent, in the colon.

The **digestive process**—the enzymatic conversion of complex dietary substances to a form that can be absorbed—is initiated by the sight, smell, and taste of food. Although some digestion (that of carbohydrates) begins in the mouth and additional digestion may occur within the lumen of the stomach, the vast majority of digestive processes occur in the small intestine. Digestion within the small intestine occurs either in the *lumen,* mediated by pancreatic enzymes, or at the small intestine *brush-border membrane* ("membrane digestion"), mediated by brush-border enzymes. Several different patterns of luminal, brush-border, and cytosolic digestion exist (Fig. 44–1). Some of the dietary carbohydrate and protein that escape digestion and absorption in the small intestine are altered in the large intestine by bacterial enzymes to short-chain fatty acids that are absorbed by the colon.

The digestive processes for carbohydrates, proteins, and lipids result in the conversion of dietary nutrients to a chemical form for which there are intestinal **absorptive processes.** As a consequence, the digestive-absorptive processes for the several dietary constituents are closely integrated and regulated biologic events that ensure survival. Multiple diseases can alter these digestive-absorptive processes and thereby impair nutrient **assimilation** (i.e., the overall process of digestion and absorption). Because of the substantial segmental distribution of nutrient absorption along the gastrointestinal tract (Fig. 44–2), the clinical manifestations of disease (Table 44–1) often reflect these segmental differences.

CARBOHYDRATE DIGESTION

Carbohydrates, Which Provide Approximately 45% of the Total Energy Needs of Western Diets, Require Hydrolysis to Monosaccharides Before Absorption

We classify dietary carbohydrates into two major groups: the **monosaccharides** (monomers) on the one hand and the **oligosaccharides** (short polymers) and **polysaccharides** (long polymers) on the other. The small intes-

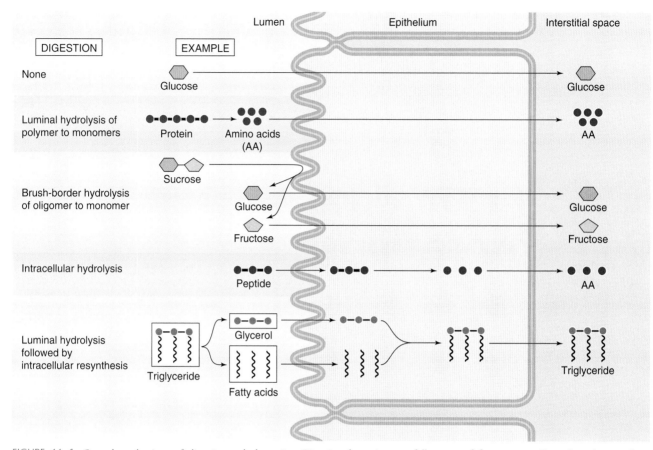

FIGURE 44–1. General mechanisms of digestion and absorption. Digestion-absorption can follow any of five patterns. First, the substance (e.g., glucose) may not require digestion; the intestinal cells may absorb the nutrient as ingested. Second, a polymer (e.g., protein) may be digested in the lumen to its constituent monomers (e.g., amino acids) by pancreatic enzymes prior to absorption. Third, an oligomer (e.g., sucrose) is digested into its constituent monomers (e.g., monosaccharidess) by brush-border enzymes prior to absorption. Fourth, an oligomer (e.g., oligopeptide) may be directly absorbed by the cell and then broken down into monomers (e.g., amino acids) inside the cell. Finally, a substance (e.g., triglyceride) may be broken down into its constituent components prior to absorption; the cell may then resynthesize the original molecule.

TABLE 44–1

MAJOR GASTROINTESTINAL DISEASES AND NUTRITIONAL DEFICIENCIES

DISEASE	ORGAN SITE OF PREDOMINANT PATHOLOGY	DEFECTS IN NUTRIENT DIGESTION/ ABSORPTION
Celiac sprue	Duodenum and jejunum	Fat absorption, lactose hydrolysis
Chronic pancreatitis	Exocrine pancreas	Fat digestion
Surgical resection of ileum; Crohn's disease of ileum	Ileum	Cobalamin and bile-acid absorption
Primary lactase deficiency	Small intestine	Lactose hydrolysis

tine can directly absorb the monomers but not the polymers. Some polymers are **digestible,** that is, the body can digest them to form the monomers that the small intestine can absorb. Other polymers are **nondigestible,** or "fiber." The composition of dietary carbohydrate is quite varied and is a function of culture. The diet of so-called developed countries contains considerable amounts of "refined" sugar and, compared to most developing countries, less fiber. Such differences in the fiber content of the Western diet may account for several diseases that are more prevalent in these societies (e.g., colon carcinoma and atherosclerosis). As a consequence, the consumption of fiber by the health-conscious public in the United States has increased during the past two decades. In general, increased amounts of fiber in the diet are associated with increased stool weight and frequency.

Approximately 45% to 60% of dietary carbohydrate is in the form of **starch,** which is a polysaccharide. Starch is a storage form for carbohydrates that is primarily found in plants, and consists of both amylose and amylopectin. In contrast, the storage form of carbohydrates in animal tissues is glycogen, which is consumed in much smaller amounts. **Amylose** is a straight-chain glucose polymer that typically contains multiple glucose residues, connected by α-1,4 linkages. On the other hand, **amylopec-**

A CARBOHYDRATES, PROTEINS AND LIPIDS

Carbo-hydrates, proteins, lipids

Duodenum
Jejunum
Ileum

B CALCIUM, IRON AND FOLATE

Calcium
Iron
Folate

Duodenum
Calcium
Calcium

High absorption
Moderate absorption
Low absorption
Very low absorption

C BILE ACIDS

Bile acids

Duodenum
Jejunum
Ileum

D COBALAMIN

Cobalamin

Ileum

FIGURE 44–2. Sites of nutrient absorption. *A*, The entire small intestine absorbs carbohydrates, proteins, and lipids. However, the absorption is greatest in the duodenum, somewhat less in the jejunum, and much less in the ileum. The thickness of the arrows in the *inset* indicates the relative magnitude of total absorption at the indicated site in vivo. The maximal absorptive capacity of a specific segment under *optimized* experimental conditions (e.g., substrate concentrations) may be greater. *B*, Some substances are actively absorbed only in the duodenum. *C*, Bile acids are absorbed along the entire small intestine, but active absorption occurs only in the ileum. *D*, The vitamin cobalamin is absorbed only in the ileum.

tin is a massive branched glucose polymer that may contain one million glucose residues. In addition to the α-1,4 linkages, amylopectin has frequent α-1,6 linkages at the branch points. Amylopectins are usually present in much greater quantities (perhaps 4-fold) than amylose. Glycogen—the "animal starch"—also has α-1,4 and α-1,6 linkages like amylopectin. However, glycogen is more highly branched (i.e., α-1,6 linkages).

The majority of dietary oligosaccharides are the disaccharides sucrose and lactose, which represent 30% to 40% of dietary carbohydrates. **Sucrose** is table sugar, derived from sugar cane and sugar beets, whereas **lactose** is the sugar found in milk. The remaining digestible carbohydrates are the monosaccharides **fructose** and **glucose,** which make up 5% to 10% of total carbohydrate intake. There is no evidence of any intestinal absorption of either starches or disaccharides. Because the small intestine can absorb only *monosaccharides,* all dietary carbohydrate must be digested to monosaccharides before absorption. The colon cannot absorb monosaccharides.

Dietary fiber consists of both soluble and insoluble forms and includes lignins, pectins, and cellulose. These fibers are primarily present in fruits, vegetables, and cereals. Cellulose is a glucose polymer connected by β-1,4 linkages, which cannot be digested by mammalian enzymes. However, enzymes from colonic bacteria may de-

grade fiber. This process is carried out with varying efficiency; pectins, gum, and mucilages are metabolized to a much greater degree than either cellulose or hemicellulose. In contrast, lignins, which are aromatic polymers and not carbohydrates, are not altered by microbial enzymes in the colonic lumen and are excreted unaltered in stool.

As we discuss later, the digestive process for dietary carbohydrates is a two-step process: **intraluminal hydrolysis** of starch to oligosaccharides by salivary and pancreatic amylases (Fig. 44–3), and so-called "**membrane digestion**" of oligosaccharides to monosaccharides by brush-border disaccharidases. The resulting carbohydrates are absorbed by transport processes that are specific for certain monosaccharides. These transport pathways are located in the apical membrane of the small-intestine villous epithelial cells.

Luminal Digestion Begins with the Action of Salivary Amylase and Finishes with Pancreatic Amylase

Both salivary and pancreatic acinar cells (p. 909) synthesize and secrete α amylases. These two amylases, unlike most of the pancreatic proteases that we discuss later, are

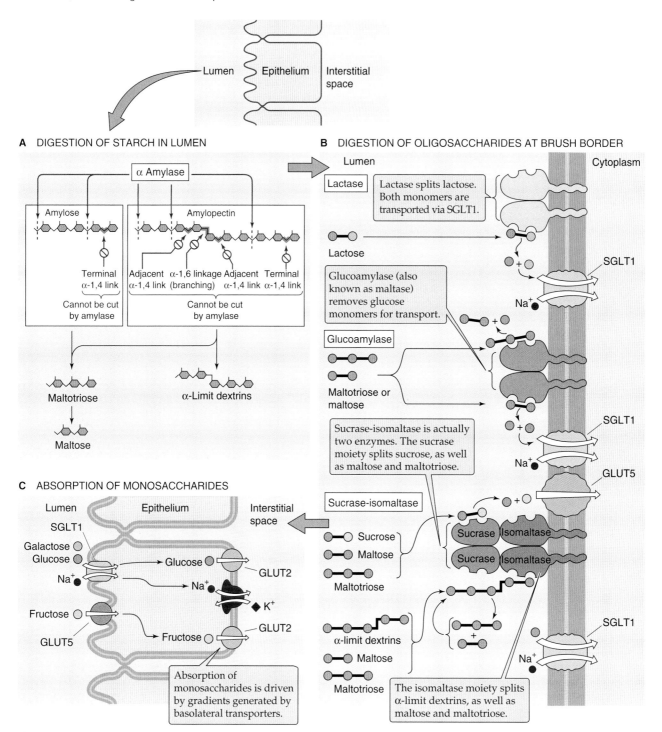

FIGURE 44–3. Digestion of carbohydrates to monosaccharides. *A*, Salivary and pancreatic α amylase are endoenzymes. They can digest the linear "internal" α-1,4 linkages between glucose residues, but cannot break "terminal" α-1,4 linkages (i.e., between the last two sugars in the chain). They also cannot split the α-1,6 linkages at the branch points of amylopectin or the adjacent α-1,6 linkages. As a result, the products of α amylase action are linear glucose oligomers, maltotriose (a linear glucose trimer), maltose (a linear glucose dimer), and α-limit dextrins (which contain an α-1,6 branching linkage). *B*, The brush-border oligosaccharidases are intrinsic membrane proteins with their catalytic domains facing the lumen. The sucrase-isomaltase is actually two enzymes, and, therefore, there are a total of four oligosaccharidases that split the oligosaccharides produced by α amylase into monosaccharides. *C*, SGLT1 is the Na$^+$-coupled transporter that mediates the uptake of glucose or galactose from lumen of the small intestine into the enterocyte. GLUT5 mediates the facilitated diffusion of fructose into the enterocyte. Once the monosaccharides are inside the enterocyte, GLUT2 mediates their efflux across the basolateral membrane into the interstitial space. GLUT, glucose transporter; SGLT, Na/glucose cotransporter.

secreted not in an inactive proenzyme form, but rather in an active form. Salivary and pancreatic α amylases have similar enzymatic function, and their amino acid sequences are 94% identical. **Salivary amylase** in the mouth initiates starch digestion; in healthy adults, this step is of relatively limited importance. Salivary amylase is inactivated by gastric acid, but can be partially protected by complexing with oligosaccharides.

Pancreatic α amylase completes starch digestion in the lumen of the small intestine. Although amylase binds to the apical membrane of enterocytes, this localization does not provide any kinetic advantage for starch hydrolysis. Cholecystokinin (CCK) triggers the secretion of pancreatic α amylase by pancreatic acinar cells (p. 909).

α Amylase is an **endoenzyme** that hydrolyzes *internal* α-1,4 linkages (see Fig. 44–3A). α Amylase does not cleave terminal α-1,4 linkages, α-1,6 linkages (i.e., branch points), or α-1,4 linkages that are immediately adjacent to α-1,6 linkages. As a result, starch hydrolysis products are maltose, maltotriose, and α-limit dextrins. Because α amylase has no activity against terminal α-1,4 linkages, glucose is *not* a product of starch digestion. The intestine cannot absorb these products of amylase digestion of starch, and thus further digestion is required to produce substrates (i.e., monosaccharides) that the small intestine can absorb by specific transport mechanisms.

"Membrane Digestion" Involves Hydrolysis of Oligosaccharides to Monosaccharides by Brush-Border Disaccharidases

The human small intestine has three brush-border "oligosaccharidases": lactase, glucoamylase (most often called maltase), and sucrase-isomaltase. These enzymes are all integral membrane proteins whose catalytic domains face the intestinal lumen (see Fig. 44–3B). Sucrase-isomaltase is actually two enzymes—sucrase and isomaltase (also known as α-dextrinase or debranching enzyme)—bound together. Thus, there are a total of four oligosaccharidases at the brush border. **Lactase** has only one substrate; it breaks lactose into glucose and galactose. The other three enzymes have more complicated substrate spectra. All will cleave the terminal α-1,4 linkages of maltose, maltotriose, and α-limit dextrins. In addition, each of these three enzymes has at least one other activity. **Maltase** can also degrade the α-1,4 linkages in straight-chain oligosaccharides up to nine monomers in length. However, maltase cannot split either sucrose or lactose. The **sucrase** moiety of sucrase-isomaltase is required for the splitting of sucrose into glucose and fructose. The **isomaltase** moiety of sucrase-isomaltase is critical; it is the only enzyme that can split the branching α-1,6 linkages of α-limit dextrins.

The action of the four oligosaccharidases generates several monosaccharides. Maltose is hydrolyzed to two glucose residues, whereas sucrose's hydrolysis products are glucose and fructose. The hydrolysis of lactose by lactase yields glucose and galactose. The activities of the hydrolysis reactions of sucrase-isomaltase and maltase are considerably greater than the rates at which the various transporters can dispose of the resulting monosaccharides. Thus the uptake, not hydrolysis, is the rate-limiting step.

In contrast, lactase activity is considerably less than that of the other oligosaccharidases and is rate-limiting for overall lactose digestion-absorption.

The oligosaccharidases have a varying spatial distribution throughout the small intestine. In general, peak oligosaccharidase distribution and activity occur in the proximal jejunum (i.e., at the ligament of Treitz). Considerably less activity is noted in the duodenum and distal ileum and none in the large intestine. The distribution of oligosaccharidase activity parallels that of active glucose transport.

These oligosaccharidases are affected by developmental and dietary factors in different ways. In many nonwhite ethnic groups, as well as in almost all other mammals, lactase activity markedly decreases after weaning in the postnatal period. The regulation of this decreased lactase activity is genetically determined. The other oligosaccharidases do not decrease in the postnatal period. In addition, chronic feeding of sucrose upregulates sucrase activity. In

LACTASE DEFICIENCY

Primary lactase deficiency is extremely common in nonwhite adults, and also occurs in some whites. Lactase activity decreases after weaning; the time course of its reduction is determined by hereditary factors. Ingestion of lactose in the form of milk and milk products by individuals with decreased amounts of small intestinal lactase activity may be associated with a range of gastrointestinal symptoms, including diarrhea, cramps, and flatus, or with no discernible symptoms. Several factors determine whether individuals with lactase deficiency experience symptoms after ingestion of lactose, including rate of gastric emptying, transit time through the small intestine, and, most importantly, the ability of colonic bacteria to metabolize lactose to short-chain fatty acids, CO_2, and H_2. Figure 44–4A shows the rise of plasma [glucose] following the ingestion of either lactose or glucose in adults *with* normal lactase levels. This figure also shows that the [H_2] in the breath rises only slightly following the ingestion of either lactose or glucose in these individuals with normal lactase levels. Figure 44–4B shows that in individuals with primary lactase deficiency, the ingestion of lactose leads to a much smaller rise in plasma [glucose], although the ingestion of glucose itself leads to a normal rise in plasma [glucose]. Thus, there is no defect in glucose absorption per se, but simply a markedly reduced capacity to hydrolyze lactose to glucose and galactose. In lactase-deficient individuals, breath H_2 is increased after lactose ingestion, because nonabsorbed lactose is metabolized by colonic bacteria to H_2, which is absorbed into the blood and subsequently excreted by the lungs. In contrast, the rise in breath H_2 is normal after the ingestion of glucose in these individuals.

Treatment for symptomatic individuals with primary lactase deficiency is reducing or eliminating milk and milk products, or using milk products treated with a commercial lactase preparation. No other defects in intestinal function or structure are associated with primary lactase deficiency.

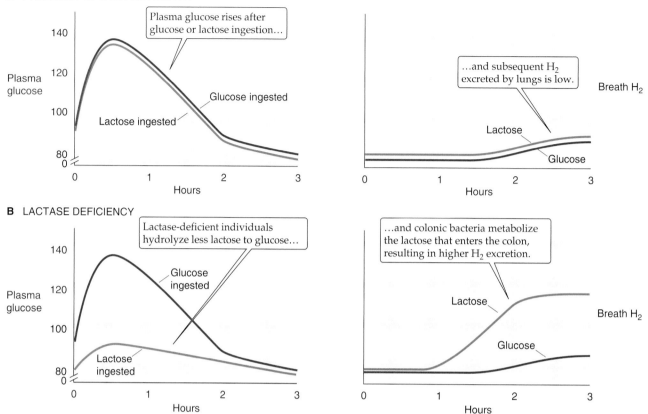

FIGURE 44-4. Effects of lactase deficiency on levels of glucose in the plasma and H_2 in the breath. *A,* In an individual with normal lactase activity, blood glucose levels rise after the ingestion of either glucose or lactose. Thus, the small intestine can split the lactose into glucose and galactose, and absorb the two monosaccharides. At the same time, H_2 in the breath is low. *B,* In an adult with low lactase activity, the rise in blood levels is less pronounced after ingesting lactose. Because the rise is normal after ingesting glucose, we can conclude that the difference is due to lactase activity. Conversely, the individual with lactase deficiency excretes large amounts of H_2 into the breath. This H_2 is the product of lactose catabolism by colonic bacteria.

contrast, sucrase activity is more greatly reduced by fasting than lactase activity. In general, lactase activity is both more susceptible to enterocyte injury and slower to recover from damage than other oligosaccharidase activity. Reduced lactase activity (as a consequence of both genetic regulation and environmental effects) has substantial clinical significance in that lactose ingestion may result in a range of symptoms in affected individuals.

CARBOHYDRATE ABSORPTION

The three monosaccharide products of carbohydrate digestion—**glucose, galactose,** and **fructose**—are absorbed by the small intestine in a two-step process involving their uptake across the apical membrane into the epithelial cell and their coordinated exit across the basolateral membrane (see Fig. 44-3C). The Na/glucose transporter (SGLT1) is the membrane protein responsible for glucose and galactose uptake at the *apical membrane.* The exit of all three monosaccharides across the *basolateral membrane* uses a facilitated sugar transporter (GLUT2). Because SGLT1 cannot carry fructose, the apical step of fructose absorption occurs by the facilitated diffusion of

fructose via GLUT5. Thus, although there are two different apical-membrane transport mechanisms for glucose and fructose uptake, a single transporter (GLUT2) is responsible for the movement of both monosaccharides across the basolateral membrane.

SGLT1 Is Responsible for the Na⁺-Coupled Uptake of Glucose and Galactose Across the Apical Membrane

The uptake of glucose across the apical membrane via SGLT1 (Fig. 44-5A) represents active transport, because the glucose influx occurs against the glucose concentration gradient (p. 66). Glucose uptake across the apical membrane is energized by the electrochemical Na⁺ gradient, which in turn is maintained by the extrusion of Na⁺ across the basolateral membrane by the Na-K pump. This type of Na⁺-driven glucose transport is an example of *secondary active transport* (p. 61). Inhibition of the Na-K pump reduces active glucose absorption by decreasing the apical membrane Na⁺ gradient and thus decreasing the driving force for glucose entry.

The affinity of SGLT1 for glucose is markedly reduced in the absence of Na⁺. The varied affinity of SGLT1 for

GLUCOSE-GALACTOSE MALABSORPTION

Molecular studies have been performed with jejunal mucosa from patients with so-called glucose-galactose malabsorption (or monosaccharide malabsorption). These individuals have diarrhea when they ingest dietary sugars that are normally absorbed by SGLT1. This diarrhea results from both reduced small intestine Na^+ and fluid absorption (as a consequence of the defect in Na^+-coupled monosaccharide absorption) and fluid secretion secondary to the osmotic effects of nonabsorbed monosaccharide. Eliminating the monosaccharides glucose and galactose, as well as the disaccharide lactose (i.e., glucose + galactose), from the diet eliminates the diarrhea. The monosaccharide fructose, which crosses the apical membrane via GLUT5, does not induce diarrhea. Early studies identified the abnormality in this hereditary disorder as a defect at the apical membrane that is presumably related to defective or absent SGLT1. Molecular studies of SGLT1 have revealed multiple mutations that result in single amino acid substitutions in SGLT1, each of which prevents the transport of glucose by SGLT1 in affected individuals. Patients with glucose-galactose malabsorption do not have glycosuria (i.e., glucose in the urine), because glucose reabsorption by the proximal tubule normally occurs via both SGLT1 and SGLT2 (p. 793).

different monosaccharides reflects its preference for specific molecular configurations. SGLT1 has two structural requirements for monosaccharides: (1) a hexose in a D-configuration and (2) a hexose that can form a six-membered pyranose ring (see Fig. 44–5B). SGLT1 will not absorb L-glucose, which has the wrong stereochemistry, and will not absorb D-fructose, which forms a five-membered ring.

The GLUT Transporters Mediate the Facilitated Diffusion of Fructose at the Apical Membrane and of All Three Monosaccharides at the Basolateral Membrane

Early work showed that fructose absorption is independent of Na^+ but has characteristics of both a carrier-mediated and a passive process. These observations show that the small intestine has separate transport systems for glucose and fructose. Subsequent studies established that *facilitated diffusion* is responsible for fructose absorption. Fructose uptake across the *apical membrane* is mediated by **GLUT5** (p. 60), a member of the GLUT family of transport proteins. GLUT5 is present mainly in the jejunum.

The efflux of glucose, fructose, and galactose across the *basolateral membrane* also occurs by facilitated diffusion. The characteristics of the basolateral sugar transporter, identified as **GLUT2**, are similar to those of other sugar transport systems in erythrocytes, fibroblasts, and adipocytes. GLUT2 has no homology to SGLT1 but is 41% identical to GLUT5, which is responsible for the uptake of fructose from the lumen.

A STRUCTURE OF SGLT1

B STRUCTURAL REQUIREMENTS OF SUGAR

Pyranose ring in D configuration.

FIGURE 44–5. The Na^+-coupled glucose transporter, SGLT1. *A*, The SGLT family of proteins is believed to have 12 membrane-spanning segments. The deduced amino acid sequence has an open reading frame of 662 amino acids, predicting a molecular mass of 73 kDa. SGLT1 has a Na^+:sugar stoichiometry of 2:1. *B*, SGLT1 will only transport hexoses in a D-configuration and with a pyranose ring. This figure shows D-glucose; D-galactose is identical, except that the H and OH on C-4 are inverted.

PROTEIN DIGESTION

Proteins Require Hydrolysis to Oligopeptides or Amino Acids Before Absorption in the Small Intestine

With the exception of antigenic amounts of dietary protein that are absorbed intact, proteins must first be digested into their constituent oligopeptides and amino acids before being taken up by the enterocytes. Digestion-absorption occurs through four major pathways. First, several *luminal* enzymes (i.e., proteases) from the stomach and pancreas may hydrolyze proteins to peptides and then to amino acids, which are then absorbed (Fig. 44–6). Second, *luminal* enzymes may digest proteins to peptides, but enzymes present at the *brush border* digest the peptides to amino acids, which are then absorbed. Third, *luminal* enzymes may digest proteins to peptides, which are themselves taken up as oligopeptides by the enterocytes. Further digestion of the oligopeptides by cytosolic enzymes yields intracellular amino acids, which are moved by transporters across the basolateral membrane into the blood. Fourth, luminal enzymes digest dietary proteins to oligopeptides, which are taken up and by enterocytes and moved directly into the blood. Overall

protein digestion-absorption is very efficient; less than 4% of ingested nitrogen is excreted in the stool.

The protein that is digested and absorbed in the small intestine comes from both dietary and endogenous sources. Dietary protein in developed countries amounts to 70 to 100 g/day. This amount is far in excess of minimum daily requirements and represents 10% to 15% of energy intake. In contrast, dietary protein content in developing countries in Africa is often 50 g/day. Deficiency states are rare unless intake is markedly reduced.

Proteins are encoded by mRNA and consist of 20 amino acids. Nine of these amino acids are essential (p. 1215); that is, they are not synthesized in adequate amounts by the body and thus must be derived from either animal or plant protein sources. In addition, cells synthesize additional amino acids by post-translational modifications: γ-carboxyglutamic acid, hydroxylysine, 4-hydroxyproline, and 3-hydroxyproline. Protein digestion is influenced by the amino acid composition of the protein, by the source of protein, and by food processing. Thus, proteins rich in proline and hydroxyproline are digested relatively less completely. Cooking, storage, and dehydration also reduce the completeness of digestion. In general, protein derived from animal sources is digested more completely than plant protein.

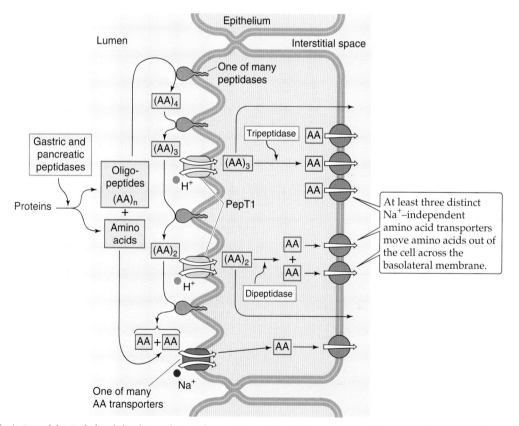

FIGURE 44–6. Action of luminal, brush-border, and cytosolic peptidases. Pepsin from the stomach and the five pancreatic proteases hydrolyze proteins—both dietary and endogenous—to single amino acids, AA, or to oligopeptides, $(AA)_n$. These reactions occur in the lumen of the stomach or small intestine. A variety of peptidases at the brush borders of enterocytes then progressively hydrolyze oligopeptides to amino acids. The amino acids are directly taken up by any of several transporters. The enterocyte directly absorbs some of the small oligopeptides via the action of the H+/oligopeptide cotransporter (PepT1). These small peptides are digested to amino acids by peptidases in the cytoplasm of the enterocyte. Several Na+-independent amino acid transporters move amino acids out of the cell across the basolateral membrane.

TABLE 44–2

PANCREATIC PEPTIDASES				
PROENZYME	**ACTIVATING AGENT**	**ACTIVE ENZYME**	**ACTION**	**PRODUCTS**
Trypsinogen	Enteropeptidase (i.e., enterokinase from jejunum) and trypsin	Trypsin	Endopeptidase	Oligopeptides (2–6 amino acids)
Chymotrypsinogen	Trypsin	Chymotrypsin	Endopeptidase	Oligopeptides (2–6 amino acids)
Proelastase	Trypsin	Elastase	Endopeptidase	Oligopeptides (2–6 amino acids)
Procarboxypeptidase A	Trypsin	Carboxypeptidase A	Exopeptidase	Single amino acids
Procarboxypeptidase B	Trypsin	Carboxypeptidase B	Exopeptidase	Single amino acids

In addition to dietary sources of protein, significant amounts of endogenous protein are secreted into the gastrointestinal tract, then conserved by protein digestion and absorption. Such endogenous sources represent approximately 50% of the total protein entering the small intestine and include enzymes, hormones, and immunoglobulins present in salivary, gastric, pancreatic, biliary, and jejunal secretions. A second large source of endogenous protein is desquamated intestinal epithelial cells; plasma proteins also enter the small intestine.

Neonates can absorb substantial amounts of *intact protein* from colostrum (p. 1204) through the process of endocytosis. This mechanism is developmentally regulated and in humans remains active only until about 6 months of age. In adults, proteins are almost exclusively digested to their constituent amino acids and di- and tri- or tetra-peptides before absorption. However, even adults absorb small amounts of intact proteins. These absorbed proteins can be important in inducing immune responses to dietary proteins.

Luminal Digestion of Protein Involves Both Gastric and Pancreatic Proteases, Yielding Amino Acids and Oligopeptides

Both gastric and pancreatic proteases, unlike the digestive enzymes for carbohydrates and lipids, are secreted as **proenzymes** that require conversion to their active form for protein hydrolysis to occur. As discussed on p. 893, the gastric chief cells secrete **pepsinogen.** Both the activation of pepsinogen to pepsin and the enzymatic activity of pepsin require a low intragastric pH (p. 902). The conversion of pepsinogen to pepsin occurs through the removal of an oligopeptide; this process occurs slowly at pH 3 to 5 and rapidly at pH < 3. Once activated, pepsin can catalyze the additional breakdown of pepsinogen to pepsin. The hydrolytic activity of **pepsin** is maximal at pH 1.8 to 3.5, and pepsin is irreversibly inactivated at pH > 7. Pepsin is an endopeptidase with primary specificity for peptide linkages of aromatic and larger neutral amino acids. Although pepsin in the stomach partially digests 10% to 15% of dietary protein, pepsin hydrolysis is not absolutely necessary; patients with either total gastrectomies or pernicious anemia (who do not secrete acid and

thus whose intragastric pH is always >7) do not have increased fecal nitrogen excretion.

Five pancreatic enzymes (Table 44–2) participate in protein digestion and are secreted as inactive proenzymes. Trypsinogen is initially activated by a jejunal brush-border enzyme, enterokinase (enteropeptidase), by the cleavage of a hexapeptide, yielding trypsin. Trypsinogen is also autoactivated by trypsin. Trypsin also activates the other pancreatic proteolytic proenzymes. The secretion of proteolytic enzymes as proenzymes, with subsequent luminal activation, prevents pancreatic **autodigestion.**

Pancreatic proteolytic enzymes are either exopeptidases or endopeptidases and function in an integrated manner. Trypsin, chymotrypsin, and elastase are **endopeptidases** with affinity for peptide bonds adjacent to specific amino acids, resulting in the production of oligopeptides with two to six amino acids. In contrast, the **exopeptidases**—carboxypeptidase A and carboxypeptidase B—hydrolyze peptide bonds adjacent to the carboxy terminus, resulting in the release of individual amino acids. The coordinated action of these pancreatic proteases converts approximately 70% of luminal amino nitrogen to oligopeptides and approximately 30% to free amino acids.

Brush-Border Peptidases Fully Digest Some Oligopeptides to Amino Acids, Whereas Cytosolic Peptidases Digest Oligopeptides That Directly Enter the Enterocyte

Small peptides present in the small intestinal lumen after digestion by gastric and pancreatic proteases undergo further hydrolysis by peptidases at the brush border (see Fig. 44–6). Multiple peptidases are present on both the brush border and in the cytoplasm of villous epithelial cells. This distribution of cell-associated peptidases stands in contrast to that of the oligosaccharidases, which are found only at the brush border. Because each peptidase recognizes only a limited repertoire of peptide bonds, and because the oligopeptides to be digested contain 24 different amino acids, a great number of peptidases are required to ensure the hydrolysis of peptides.

As we discuss later, a transporter on the apical membrane of enterocytes can take up small oligopeptides, primarily di- and tripeptides. Once inside the cell, these oligopeptides may be further digested by *cytoplasmic* peptidases. The brush-border and cytoplasmic peptidases have substantially different characteristics. For example, the brush-border peptidases have affinity for relatively larger oligopeptides (three to eight amino acids), whereas the cytoplasmic peptidases primarily hydrolyze di- and tripeptides. Because the brush-border and cytoplasmic enzymes often have different biochemical properties (e.g., heat lability and electrophoretic mobility), it is evident that the peptidases in the brush border and cytoplasm are distinct, independently regulated molecules.

Like the pancreatic proteases, each of the several brush-border peptidases is either an endopeptidase, an exopeptidase, or a dipeptidase and has affinity for specific peptide bonds. The exopeptidases are either carboxypeptidases, which release carboxy-terminal amino acids, or aminopeptidases, which hydrolyze the amino acids at the amino-terminal end. There are relatively fewer **cytoplasmic peptidases.**

PROTEIN, PEPTIDE, AND AMINO ACID ABSORPTION

Absorption of Whole Protein by Apical Pinocytosis Occurs Primarily During the Neonatal Period

During the postnatal period, intestinal epithelial cells absorb protein by endocytosis, providing a mechanism for transfer of passive immunity from mother to child. The uptake of intact protein by the epithelial cell ceases by the sixth month; the cessation of this protein uptake, called "closure," is hormonally mediated. For example, administration of corticosteroids during the postnatal period will induce closure and reduce the time that the intestine can absorb significant amounts of whole protein.

The adult intestine can absorb finite amounts of intact protein and polypeptides. Uncertainty exists regarding the cellular route(s) by which they are absorbed, as well as the relationship of the mechanism of protein uptake in adults to that in neonates. Enterocytes can take up by endocytosis a small amount of intact protein, the vast majority of which is degraded in lysosomes (Fig. 44–7). A small amount of intact protein appears in the interstitial space. The uptake of intact proteins also occurs through a second, more specialized route. In the small intestine, immediately overlying the **Peyer's patches** (follicles of lymphoid tissue in the lamina propria), **M cells** replace the usual enterocytes on the surface of the gut. M cells have few microvilli and are specialized for protein uptake. They have limited ability for lysosomal protein degradation; rather, they package ingested proteins (i.e., antigens) in clathrin-coated vesicles, which they secrete at their basolateral membranes into the lamina propria. There, immunocompetent cells process the target antigens and transfer them to lymphocytes to initiate an immune response. Although protein uptake in adults may not have nutritional value, such uptake is clearly important in mucosal immunity and probably is involved in one or more disease processes.

The Apical Absorption of Di-, Tri-, and Tetrapeptides Occurs via an H⁺-Driven Cotransporter

Virtually all absorbed protein products exit the villous epithelial cell and enter the blood as individual amino acids. A substantial portion of these amino acids are released in the lumen of the small intestine by luminal proteases and brush-border peptidases and, as we discuss later, move across the apical membranes of enterocytes via several amino acid transport systems (see Fig. 44–6). However, substantial amounts of protein are absorbed from the intestinal lumen as di-, tri-, or tetrapeptides and then hydrolyzed to amino acids by intracellular peptidases.

The transporter responsible for the uptake of luminal oligopeptides (Fig. 44–8A) is distinct from the various amino acid transporters. Furthermore, administering an amino acid as a peptide (e.g., the dipeptide glycylglycine) results in a higher blood level of the amino acid than administering an equivalent amount of the same amino acid as a monomer (e.g., glycine; see Fig. 44–8B). One possible explanation for this effect is that the oligopeptide cotransporter, which carries multiple amino acids rather than a single amino acid into the cell, may simply be more effective than amino acid transporters in transferring amino acid monomers into the cell. This accelerated peptide absorption has been referred to as a "kinetic advantage" and raises the question of the usefulness of the enteral administration of crystalline amino acids to patients with impaired intestinal function and/or catabolic deficiencies. The evidence for a specific transport process for di-, tri-, and tetrapeptides comes from direct measurements of oligopeptide transport, molecular identification of the transporter, and studies of the hereditary disorders of amino acid transport, cystinuria, and Hartnup disease.

Oligopeptide uptake is an active process driven not by a Na⁺ gradient, but by a proton gradient. Oligopeptide uptake occurs via a **H⁺/oligopeptide cotransporter** known as PepT1 (p. 67), which is also present in the renal proximal tubule. PepT1 also appears to be responsible for the intestinal uptake of certain dipeptide-like antibiotics (e.g., oral amino-substituted cephalosporins). As noted earlier, after their uptake, di-, tri-, and tetrapeptides are usually hydrolyzed by cytoplasmic peptidases to their constituent amino acids, the forms in which they are transported out of the cell across the basolateral membrane. Because peptides are almost completely hydrolyzed to amino acids intracellularly, few peptides appear in the portal vein. Proline-containing dipeptides, which are relatively resistant to hydrolysis, are the primary peptides present in the circulation.

Amino Acids Enter Enterocytes via One or More Group-Specific Apical Membrane Transporters

Multiple amino acid transport systems have been identified and characterized in various nonepithelial cells. The absorption of amino acids across the small intestine requires sequential movement across both the apical and basolateral membranes of the villous epithelial cell. Al-

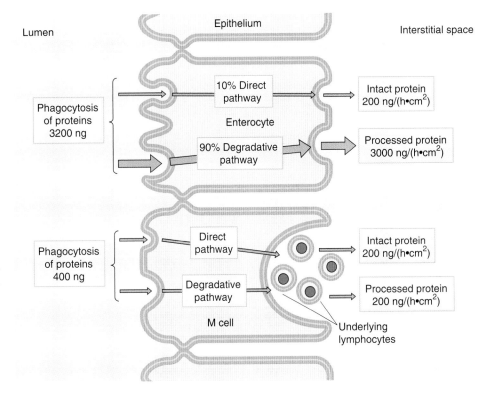

FIGURE 44–7. Absorption of whole proteins. Both enterocytes and specialized M cells can take up intact proteins. The more abundant enterocytes can endocytose far more total protein than can the M cells. However, the lysosomal proteases in the enterocytes degrade about 90% of this endocytosed protein. The less abundant M cells take up relatively little intact protein, but about half of this emerges intact at the basolateral membrane. There, immunocompetent cells process the target antigens and then transfer them to lymphocytes, initiating an immune response.

though the amino acid transport systems have overlapping affinities for various amino acids, there is general agreement that at least seven distinct transport systems are present at the apical membrane (Table 44–3); we discuss the basolateral amino acid transporters in the next section. Whereas many apical amino acid transporters are probably unique to epithelial cells, some of those at the basolateral membrane are probably the same as in nonepithelial cells.

The predominant apical amino acid transport system is **system B** (see Table 44–3) and results in Na^+-dependent uptake of neutral amino acids. As is the case for glucose uptake (p. 952), uphill movement of neutral amino acids is driven by an inwardly directed Na^+ gradient that is main-

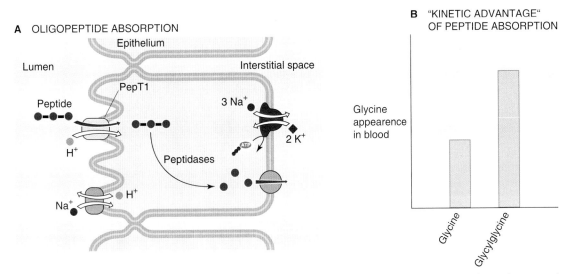

FIGURE 44–8. Absorption of oligopeptides. A, The H^+/oligopeptide cotransporter PepT1 moves dipeptides, tripeptides, and tetrapeptides into the enterocyte, across the apical membrane. Peptidases in the cytoplasm hydrolyze the oligopeptides into their constituent amino acids, which then exit across the basolateral membrane via one of three Na^+-independent amino acid transporters. B, If glycine is present in the lumen only as a free amino acid, then the enterocyte absorbs it only via apical amino acid transporters. However, if the same amount of glycine is present in the lumen in the form of the dipeptide glycylglycine, the rate of appearance of glycine in the blood is about twice as high. Thus, PepT1, which moves several amino acid monomers for each turnover of the transporter, is an effective mechanism for absorbing "amino acids." ATP, adenosine triphosphate.

FIGURE 44–9. Genetic disorders of apical amino acid transport. *A*, In Hartnup disease, an autosomal-recessive disorder, the "system B" apical-membrane amino acid transporter is defective. As a result, the absorption of neutral amino acids such as L-phenylalanine, is reduced. (However, the absorption of L-cystine (i.e., Cys-S-S-Cys) and cationic (i.e., basic) amino acids (e.g., L-arginine) remains intact.) The enterocyte can absorb L-phenylalanine normally if the amino acid is present in the form of the dipeptide L-phenylalanyl-L-leucine, inasmuch as the oligopeptide cotransporter PepT1 is normal. *B*, In cystinuria, an autosomal-recessive disorder, the "system B⁰⁺" or "system b⁰⁺" apical-membrane amino acid transporter is defective. As a result, the absorption of L-cystine (i.e., Cys-S-S-Cys) and cationic (i.e., basic) amino acids (e.g., L-arginine) is reduced. However, the absorption of amino acids that use "System B" (e.g., L-Ala) is normal. The enterocyte can absorb L-arginine, normally if the amino acid is present in the form of the dipeptide L-arginyl-L-leucine.

DEFECTS IN APICAL AMINO ACID TRANSPORT: HARTNUP DISEASE AND CYSTINURIA

Hartnup disease and cystinuria are hereditary disorders of amino acid transport across the apical membrane. These autosomal recessive disorders are associated with both small intestine and renal tubule abnormalities (see box on p. 796) in the absorption of neutral amino acids in the case of Hartnup disease, and cationic (i.e., basic) amino acids and cysteine in the case of cystinuria.

The clinical signs of **Hartnup disease** are most evident in children and include the skin changes of pellagra, cerebellar ataxia, and psychiatric abnormalities. The principal manifestation of **cystinuria** is the formation of kidney stones. In Hartnup disease, the absorption of neutral amino acids by system B in the small intestine is markedly reduced, whereas that of cationic amino acids is intact (Fig. 44–9). In contrast, in cystinuria the absorption of cationic amino acids by system B⁰⁺ or b⁰⁺ is abnormal, but absorption of neutral amino acids is normal. Because neither of these diseases involves the oligopeptide cotransporter, the absorption of oligopeptides containing either neutral or cationic amino acids is nor-

mal in both diseases. Affected individuals do not appear to have any evidence of protein deficiency commonly associated with defects in protein or amino acid absorption. The lack of evidence of protein deficiency is a consequence of the presence of more than one transport system for different amino acids, as well as a separate transporter for oligopeptides. Thus, oligopeptides containing neutral amino acids are absorbed normally in Hartnup disease, and oligopeptides with cationic amino acids are absorbed normally in cystinuria.

These two genetic diseases also emphasize the existence of amino acid transport mechanisms on the basolateral membrane that are distinct and separate from the apical amino acid transporters. Thus, in both Hartnup disease and cystinuria, oligopeptides are transported normally across the apical membrane and are hydrolyzed to amino acids in the cytosol, and the resulting neutral and cationic amino acids are readily transported out of the cell across the basolateral membrane.

TABLE 44–3

AMINO ACID TRANSPORTERS

TRANSPORT SYSTEM*	ISOLATED cDNA	SUBSTRATES	COTRANSPORTED ION
Apical			
B	ATB⁰	Neutral amino acids	Na⁺ (Electrogenic)
B⁰⁺	—	Neutral and cationic (i.e., basic) amino acids + cystine (i.e., Cys-S-S-Cys)	Na⁺ (Electrogenic)
b⁰⁺	rBAT/b⁰⁺ AT (heterodimer)	Neutral and cationic amino acids + cystine	None
y⁺	CAT-1 to -4	Cationic amino acids (i.e., basic) amino acids (e.g., Arg, Lys, His, ornithine)	None, but will cotransport small, neutral amino acids with Na⁺
Imino	—	Imino acids	Na⁺ and Cl⁻
X_{AG}^-	EAAT1 - 5	Anionic (or acidic) amino acids (Glu and Asp)	2 Na⁺, 1 H⁺ inward 1 K⁺ outward (Electrogenic: net + charge)
β		β amino acids:	Na⁺ and Cl⁻
	BGT-1	Betaine (also GABA)	
	pNCT	Taurine	
Basolateral			
A	?	Neutral and imino acids	Na⁺
ASC	ASCT1, 2	Neutral amino acids with 3–4 carbons	Na⁺
asc	—	Neutral amino acids with 3–4 carbons	None
L	—	Neutral, hydrophobic and large amino acids	None
y⁺	CAT-1 to -4	Cationic (i.e., basic) amino acids (e.g., Arg, Lys, His, ornithine)	None, but will cotransport small, neutral amino acids with Na⁺
Not Necessarily Present in GI Tract			
GABA (γ amino acid)	GAT1-4	GABA (also betaine, β-alanine, taurine)	Na⁺ and Cl⁻
Gly	GLYT1, -2	Glycine (also N-methylglycine, i.e., sarcosine)	Na⁺ and Cl⁻

* This historical classification is based on functional characteristics in intact epithelia, intact cells, or membrane vesicles.

tained by the basolateral Na-K pump. The uptake of amino acids by system B is an electrogenic process and represents another example of *secondary active transport*. It transports amino acids with an L-stereo configuration and an amino group in the α position. System B⁰⁺ is similar to system B but has broader substrate specificity. System b⁰⁺ differs from B⁰⁺ mainly in being independent of Na⁺.

Other carrier-mediated transport mechanisms exist for anionic (i.e., acidic), cationic (i.e., basic), β amino acids, and imino acids (see Table 44–3). Because the apical amino acid transporters have overlapping affinities for amino acids, and because there are species differences as well as segmental and developmental differences among the transporters, it has been difficult to establish a comprehensive model of apical membrane amino acid transport in the mammalian small intestine.

At the Basolateral Membrane, Amino Acids Exit Enterocytes via Na⁺-Independent Transporters and Enter via Na⁺-Dependent Transporters

Amino acids appear in the cytosol of intestinal **villous cells** either as the result of their uptake across the apical membrane or the hydrolysis of oligopeptides that had entered the apical membrane (see Fig. 44–6). The enterocyte subsequently uses approximately 10% of the absorbed amino acids for intracellular protein synthesis.

Movement of amino acids across the basolateral membrane is bidirectional; the movement of any one amino acid can occur via one or more amino acid transporters. At least five amino acid transporters are present in the basolateral membrane (see Table 44–3). Three amino

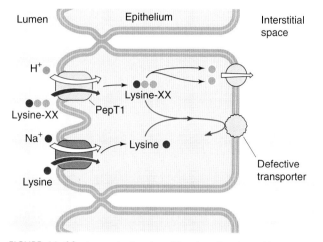

FIGURE 44-10. A genetic disorder of basolateral amino acid transport, lysinuric protein intolerance is an autosomal recessive defect in which the Na$^+$-independent y$^+$ amino acid transporter on the apical and basolateral membranes is defective. However, the absence of y$^+$ at the apical membrane does not present a problem because Na$^+$-dependent amino acid transporters can take up lysine, and PepT1 can take up lysine-containing oligopeptides (Lysine-XX). However, there is no mechanism for moving lysine out of the enterocyte across the basolateral membrane.

acid transport processes on the basolateral membrane mediate amino acid *exit* from the cell into the blood and thus complete the process of protein assimilation. Two other amino acid transporters mediate *uptake* from the blood for the purposes of cell nutrition. It appears that the three Na$^+$-independent amino acid transport systems mediate amino acid movement *out* of the epithelial cell into blood. One of these, y$^+$, is also present on the apical membrane. The two Na$^+$-dependent processes facilitate their movement *into* the epithelial cell. Indeed, these two Na$^+$-dependent transporters resemble those that are also present in nonpolar cells.

In general, the amino acids incorporated into protein within villous cells are derived more from those that enter across the apical membrane than across the basolateral membrane. In contrast, **epithelial cells in the intestinal crypt** derive almost all of their amino acids for protein synthesis from the circulation; crypt cells do not take up amino acids across their apical membrane.

LIPID DIGESTION

Natural Lipids Are Organic Compounds of Biological Origin That Are Sparingly Soluble in Water

Lipids in the diet are derived from animals and/or plants and are composed of carbon, hydrogen, and a smaller amount of oxygen. Some lipids also contain small but functionally important amounts of nitrogen and phosphorus (Fig. 44–11). Lipids are typified by their preferential solubility in organic solvents, compared to water. A widely used indicator of the lipidic nature of a compound is its octanol-water partition coefficient, which for most lipids is between 10^4 and 10^7. The biological fate of lipids depends critically on their chemical structure as well as on their interactions with water and other lipids in aque-

ous body fluids (e.g., intestinal contents and bile). Thus, lipids have been classified according to their physico-chemical interactions with water. Lipids may be either **nonpolar** and completely insoluble in water (e.g., cholesteryl esters and carotene) or **polar** and amphophilic, that is, having both polar (hydrophilic) and nonpolar (hydrophobic) groups. Added in small amounts, polar lipids form stable or unstable monolayers on the surface of water (see Fig. 2–1C), whereas in bulk their physicochemical behavior varies from insolubility (as is the case with triglycerides and cholesterol) to the formation of various macroaggregates, such as liquid crystals and micelles. Less-soluble lipids are incorporated into the macroaggregates of the more-polar lipids and are thus stabley maintained in aqueous solutions. The term "**fat**" is generally used to refer to triglyceride, but it is also loosely used to refer to lipids in general.

Dietary Lipids Are Predominantly Triglycerides, but Food Also Contains Membrane Lipids, Vitamins, and Chemicals from the Environment

Typical adult western diets contain approximately 140 g of fat (providing ~55% of the energy), which is more than the ideal intake of less than 70 g of fat (<30% of energy). Of this fat, more than 90% is **triglycerides**, which are commonly long-chain fatty acyl esters of glycerol, a trihydroxyl alcohol (see Fig. 44–11, A–C). At body temperature, fats are usually liquid droplets. Newborn infants consume three to five times more lipid than adults, relative to body weight. Dietary fat is the body's only source of essential fatty acids, and it acts as a vehicle for the absorption of fat-soluble vitamins (the handling of

---

BASOLATERAL AMINO ACID TRANSPORT DEFECTS: LYSINURIC PROTEIN INTOLERANCE

Lysinuric protein intolerance is a rare autosomal recessive disorder of amino acid transport across the basolateral membrane. There is evidence of impaired cationic amino acid transport and symptoms of malnutrition. It appears that the defect is in the y$^+$ transporter, which is also present on the apical membrane. Nevertheless, lysine can still enter the enterocyte across the apical membrane via other amino acid transporters (Fig. 44–10). Unlike the situation in Hartnup disease or cystinuria, where the enterocytes can absorb the amino acid normally if it is presented as an oligopeptide, in lysinuric protein intolerance the enterocytes cannot absorb the amino acid regardless of whether the amino acid is "free" or part of an oligopeptide. These observations are best explained by hypothesizing that the patients hydrolyze intracellular oligopeptides properly but have a defect in the transport of cationic amino acids across the basolateral membrane. It is of interest that this defect is present not only in the small intestine, but also in hepatocytes and kidney cells, and perhaps in nonepithelial cells as well.

FIGURE 44–11. Chemical formulas of some common lipids. The example in *A* is stearic acid, a fully saturated fatty acid with 18 carbon atoms. In *C*, the left and center fatty acids are palmitic acid, a fully saturated fatty acid with 16 carbon atoms. The rightmost fatty acid is palmitoleic acid, which is also a 16-carbon structure, but with a double bond between carbons 9 and 10. In *F*, the left fatty acid is palmitic acid (16 carbons, fully saturated), and the right fatty acid is palmitoleic acid (16 carbons, double bond between carbons 9 and 10). In *I*, the example is the result of esterifying cholesterol and palmitic acid (16 carbons, fully saturated).

which is discussed on p. 1001). Fat is also the major nutrient responsible for postprandial satiety. The ratio of **saturated** to **unsaturated** fatty acids in triglycerides is high in animal fats and low in plant fats. There is evidence that in so-called developed countries, average fat intake is falling, as is the proportion of fat contributed by saturated fatty acids. Conversely, the proportion of polyunsaturated fats has risen. Certain milk products

contain short-chain fatty acids. Fish contain unusual but metabolically important fatty acids, as well as wax esters.

Approximately 5% (4 to 6 g/day) of dietary lipids come from cell membranes and are **phospholipids.** Most phospholipids are *glycerophospholipids.* They consist of a glycerol backbone that is esterified at the first two positions to fatty acids and at the third position to a phosphate that in turn is esterified to a head group (see Fig. 2–2). One of the *glycerophospholipids,* phosphatidylcholine (lecithin), is the predominant phospholipid (see Fig. 44–11*F*). The other major class of membrane phospholipid is the *sphingolipid,* which has a serine rather than a glycerol backbone.

The diet contains approximately 0.5 g of unesterified **cholesterol** (also derived from animal cell membranes; see Fig. 44–11*H*), whereas esterified cholesterol (see Fig. 44–11*I*) is usually found only in liver or food made from blood products. Traces of lipovitamins and provitamins (e.g., carotene) are present in dietary fat, which may also contain lipid-soluble toxins and carcinogens from the environment. These undesirable lipid-soluble chemicals— which include nitrosamines, aflatoxins and polycyclic hydrocarbons such as benzo(a)pyrene—are all found in margarine, vegetable oils, and other dietary fats. The diet also may contain skin lipids, which are chemically diverse and complex and difficult to digest.

Endogenous Lipids Are Predominantly Lecithin and Cholesterol from Bile and Membrane Lipids from Desquamated Intestinal Epithelial Cells

The bile secreted into the intestine (p. 989) plays a key role in the assimilation of dietary lipids, as we explain later. This bile contains phospholipid (10 to 15 g/day)— also predominantly lecithin—and unesterified cholesterol (1 to 2 g/day). Quantitatively, these biliary lipids exceed those present in the diet by 2- to 4-fold. Membrane lipids from desquamated intestinal cells account for a further 2 to 6 g of lipid for digestion. It has been estimated that approximately 10 g of lipids derive each day from dead bacteria. The majority of bacterial lipids are added in the colon.

Dietary Lipids Are Disrupted Mechanically in the Mouth and Stomach, and the Resulting Lipid Particles Are Stabilized as an Emulsion

The central process in the digestion of lipids is their hydrolysis in the aqueous milieu of the intestinal lumen. Lipid hydrolysis is catalyzed by **lipases** secreted by the glands and cells of the upper gastrointestinal tract. The products of lipolysis diffuse through the aqueous content of the intestinal lumen, traverse the so-called "unstirred water layer" and mucus barrier that line the intestinal epithelial surface, and enter the enterocyte for further processing. Because dietary lipids are insoluble in water, digestive lipases have evolved to act more efficiently at oil-water interfaces than on water-soluble substrates.

A key step preliminary to lipid digestion is the transformation of ingested solid fat and oil masses into an emulsion of fine oil droplets in water. The **emulsification** of dietary fats begins with food preparation (grinding, marinating, blending, and cooking), followed by chewing and gastric churning (p. 906) caused by antral peristalsis against a closed pylorus. Emulsification of ingested lipids is enhanced when muscular movements of the stomach intermittently squirt the gastric contents into the duode-

num and, conversely, when peristalsis of the duodenum propels the duodenal contents retrograde into the stomach through the narrow orifice of a contracted pylorus. The grinding action of the antrum also mixes food with the various digestive enzymes derived from the mouth and stomach. Intestinal peristalsis mixes luminal contents with pancreatic and biliary secretions. Together, these mechanical processes that reduce the size of the lipid droplets also dramatically increase their ratio of surface area to volume, thereby increasing the area of the oil-water interface.

The emulsion, produced by the mechanical processes just outlined, is stabilized by preventing the dispersed lipid particles from coalescing. This is achieved by coating the emulsion droplets with membrane lipids, denatured protein, dietary polysaccharides, certain products of digestion (e.g., fatty acids and monoglycerides), and biliary phospholipids and cholesterol. Phospholipids and cholesterol are well suited as emulsion stabilizers because they dissolve neither in oil nor in water, but have excellent interfacial solubilities at oil-water interfaces. Thus they form a surface monomolecular layer on emulsion particles. The polar groups of the phospholipids project into the water; the charges of the polar groups and their high degree of hydration prevent coalescence of the emulsion particles. The core of the emulsion particle is composed of triglyceride, which also contains cholesteryl esters and other nonpolar or weakly polar lipids. A very small fraction of the triglyceride in the lipid particle localizes to the particle surface. The fat in breast milk is already emulsified by proteins and phospholipids incorporated into the surface of fat droplets during lactation. Foods such as sauces, ice cream, and puddings are stably emulsified during their preparation.

Lingual and Gastric (Acid) Lipase Initiate Lipid Digestion

A small amount of lipid digestion begins in the mouth, mediated by lingual lipase. In the stomach, both **lingual lipase** that is swallowed and a gastric lipase secreted by gastric chief cells digest substantial amounts of lipid. Human **gastric lipase** is a 42-kDa glycoprotein whose secretion is stimulated by gastrin. Gastric lipase secretion is already well established in the neonatal period (unlike pancreatic lipase secretion), and thus gastric lipolysis is important for fat digestion in newborn infants. Gastric and lingual—as well as pharyngeal—lipases belong to a family of serine hydrolases that have acidic pH optima (pH 4), are stable in the acidic environment of the stomach, are resistant to digestion by pepsin, and are not inhibited by the surface layer of membrane lipids (emulsifiers) that envelopes triglyceride droplets. However, acid lipases are readily inactivated by pancreatic proteases (especially in the presence of bile salts) once they reach the small intestine.

In vivo, gastric lipase releases a single **fatty acid** from **triglycerides,** leaving behind intact **diglycerides** (see Fig. 44–11*D*). The carboxyl groups of long-chain fatty acids, released from triglycerides in the stomach, are protonated and insoluble at the acidic pH prevailing in the stomach.

These fatty acids are not absorbed in the stomach, but rather remain in the core of the triglyceride droplets, in whose emulsification they participate in the small intestine. Medium- and short-chain fatty acids are also mainly protonated at the acidic gastric pH. However, because these protonated species are relatively water soluble, they are passively absorbed across the gastric mucosa into portal blood.

In healthy adult humans, approximately 15% of fat digestion occurs in the stomach. In patients with pancreatic insufficiency, however, the lack of pancreatic proteases and HCO_3^- in the duodenal lumen may permit the continued action of gastric lipase after the gastric contents leave the stomach and enter the duodenum. Extended gastric lipase activity partly alleviates fat malabsorption due to pancreatic disease and pancreatic lipase deficiency.

Pancreatic (Alkaline) Lipase, Colipase, Milk Lipase, and Other Esterases—Aided by Bile Salts—Complete Lipid Hydrolysis in the Duodenum and Jejunum

The process of fat digestion that begins in the stomach is completed in the proximal small intestine, predominantly by enzymes synthesized and secreted by pancreatic acinar cells (p. 909), and carried into the duodenum in the pancreatic juice. In humans, a lipase found in human milk—the so-called **bile-salt–stimulated milk lipase**—also digests fat. A similar lipase is found in the milk of relatively few other animal species. Milk lipase is stable during passage through the acid environment of the stomach, yet is active at the alkaline pH of the duodenum and jejunum, where it hydrolyzes diglycerides, monoglycerides, cholesteryl esters, and fat-soluble vitamin esters, as well as triglycerides. Bile salts not only stimulate milk lipase activity but also protect the enzyme from proteolysis in the small intestine. Like gastric lipase, milk lipase is important for fat digestion in breast-fed infants.

Once the fatty acids generated in the stomach reach the duodenum, they trigger the release of **cholecystokinin** and gastric inhibitory polypeptide (GIP) from the duodenal mucosa. CCK stimulates the *flow of bile* into the duodenum by causing the gallbladder to contract and the sphincter of Oddi to relax (p. 993). CCK also stimulates the *secretion of pancreatic enzymes,* including lipases and esterases (p. 911). As we discuss later, long-chain fatty acids also facilitate the lipolytic action of pancreatic lipase.

The major lipolytic enzyme of pancreatic juice is a 48-kDa carboxylic esterase known as **pancreatic (triglyceride) lipase,** sometimes referred to as colipase-dependent pancreatic lipase. In adults but not in infants, this enzyme, which is secreted into the duodenum in its active form in 1000-fold excess, is thought to effectively digest all dietary triglycerides not hydrolyzed in the stomach. Full lipolytic activity of pancreatic lipase requires the presence of a small (10-kDa) protein cofactor called **colipase,** as well as an alkaline pH, bile salts, and fatty acids. The pancreas secretes colipase in the pro- form (i.e., procolipase), which has no intrinsic lipolytic activity. Trypsin cleaves procolipase into colipase and an N-terminal pentapeptide, enterostatin. This cleavage is important because the newly formed colipase is a cofactor of pancreatic lipase, as we discuss later. In addition, the N-terminal pentapeptide may control satiety.

Pancreatic lipase is active only at the oil-water interface of a triglyceride droplet. However, surface emulsifier components (e.g., phospholipids, protein) present at that interface inhibit lipase action. Bile salt micelles also inhibit lipolysis by displacing the lipase from the oil-droplet surface. Binding of colipase reverses this inhibition either by attaching first to the interface and serving as an anchor for the binding of the lipase, or by first forming a colipase–pancreatic-lipase complex that then binds to the lipid interface. Colipase also can penetrate the phospholipid coating of the triglyceride emulsion. Bile salt micelles bring the colipase closer to the interface. Because bile salts are nearby, they can participate in the solubilization and removal of the products of lipolysis released from the emulsion droplet. Fatty acids augment lipolysis, probably by enhancing the binding of the colipase-lipase complex to the lipid interface.

Studies of the crystal structure of pancreatic lipase have shown that when the enzyme is free in solution, the catalytic site of the lipase—located in a cleft in the molecule—is partly covered by a "lid" formed of loop(s) of its peptide chain. The interaction of the colipase and lipase with the interface causes a conformational change in the lipase molecule that moves the lid, thereby allowing lipid substrate to diffuse to the now-exposed catalytic site of the enzyme.

Pancreatic lipase mainly hydrolyzes the ester bonds of triglycerides at the first and third positions of the glycerol backbone. The end products of such reactions are two fatty acids and a single 2-monoglyceride (2-MG) (see Fig. 44–11E).

The pancreas secretes other enzymes that hydrolyze lipid esters. **Carboxyl ester hydrolase** is a pancreatic enzyme whose protein structure is closely related to that of bile salt–stimulated milk lipase. Like milk lipase, carboxyl ester hydrolase lacks substrate specificity and is active against a wide range of esters. Carboxyl ester hydrolase is probably the same enzyme as "pancreatic esterase," "cholesterol esterase," "lysophospholipase," and others. Among the many products of reactions catalyzed by this enzyme are free cholesterol and free glycerol.

The pancreas also secretes **phospholipase A_2** (PLA_2), which is active against glycerophospholipids (but not sphingolipids), from which it releases a single fatty acid to yield lysophospholipids (see Fig. 44–11G). Pancreatic PLA_2, secreted as a proenzyme, is effective at alkaline pH and requires bile salts for activity. PLA_2 in the small intestine may also be derived from Paneth cells, whereas phospholipase found in the colon probably comes from anaerobic flora there. In contrast to the human intestinal lipases, bacterial lipases are nonspecific with respect to substrates, have neutral or slightly acidic pH optima, are not inhibited by bile acids, and do not require cofactors. In the human colon, both triglycerides and phospholipids are totally hydrolyzed by bacteria. Fecal fat is thus generally present as **fatty acid soaps** and sterols. Even in severe fat malabsorption, intact glycerides are rarely found in the stools. The chemical test for stool fat, Sudan-III staining, depends on the property of Sudan III dye to partition into "oils" that contain protonated fatty acids.

LIPID ABSORPTION

Products of Lipolysis Enter the Bulk Water Phase of the Intestinal Lumen as Vesicles, Mixed Micelles, and Monomers

After their secretion in pancreatic juice and bile, respectively, the various activated pancreatic lipases and biliary bile salts, lecithin, and cholesterol adsorb to the surface of the **emulsion droplets** arriving from the stomach (Fig. 44–12A). The lipolytic products—monoglycerides, fatty acids (including long-chain species from gastric lipolysis that are now ionized at alkaline, duodenal pH), lysolecithin, and cholesterol—act as additional emulsifiers. As surface triglycerides are hydrolyzed, they are replaced by triglycerides from the core of the emulsion particle. The emulsion droplets become progressively smaller. Initially, a crystalline calcium–fatty-acid soap phase forms near the surface of the triglyceride droplet, until the local free Ca^{2+} is depleted. At the same time, a multilamellar liquid crystalline layer of fatty acids, monoglycerides, lysolecithins,

cholesterol, and bile salts builds up on the surface of the emulsion particle. This liquid crystalline layer "buds off" as a **multilamellar liquid crystal vesicle** (see Fig. 44–12B), which consist of several lipid bilayers. Bile salt micelles transform these multilamellar vesicles into **unilamellar vesicles** (see Fig. 44–12C), which are single-lipid bilayers, and then into **mixed micelles** (see Fig. 44–12D) composed of bile salts and mixed lipids (i.e., fatty acids, monoglycerides, lysophospholipids, and cholesterol).

Continued digestion by PLA_2 and other esterases can still occur on the mixture of aggregates now present. If intestinal contents taken from humans during fat digestion are centrifuged, three phases separate. An oily layer floats on top and contains fat droplets and lipolytic products that have not been solubilized by bile salts. A middle layer contains lipid vesicles, mixed lipid–bile salt micelles, simple bile salt micelles, and lipid monomers. Finally, a pellet contains debris and precipitated calcium soaps of fatty acids. Whereas most fat absorption in health is from the micellar phase of digested lipid, in

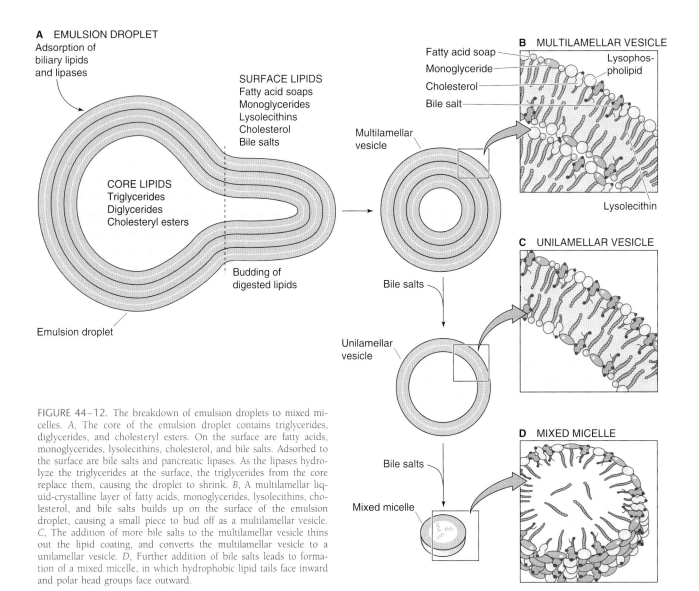

A EMULSION DROPLET

Adsorption of biliary lipids and lipases

SURFACE LIPIDS
Fatty acid soaps
Monoglycerides
Lysolecithins
Cholesterol
Bile salts

CORE LIPIDS
Triglycerides
Diglycerides
Cholesteryl esters

Budding of digested lipids

Emulsion droplet

Multilamellar vesicle

B MULTILAMELLAR VESICLE
Fatty acid soap
Monoglyceride
Cholesterol
Bile salt
Lysophospholipid
Lysolecithin

C UNILAMELLAR VESICLE
Bile salts
Unilamellar vesicle

D MIXED MICELLE
Bile salts
Mixed micelle

FIGURE 44–12. The breakdown of emulsion droplets to mixed micelles. *A*, The core of the emulsion droplet contains triglycerides, diglycerides, and cholesteryl esters. On the surface are fatty acids, monoglycerides, lysolecithins, cholesterol, and bile salts. Adsorbed to the surface are bile salts and pancreatic lipases. As the lipases hydrolyze the triglycerides at the surface, the triglycerides from the core replace them, causing the droplet to shrink. *B*, A multilamellar liquid-crystalline layer of fatty acids, monoglycerides, lysolecithins, cholesterol, and bile salts builds up on the surface of the emulsion droplet, causing a small piece to bud off as a multilamellar vesicle. *C*, The addition of more bile salts to the multilamellar vesicle thins out the lipid coating, and converts the multilamellar vesicle to a unilamellar vesicle. *D*, Further addition of bile salts leads to formation of a mixed micelle, in which hydrophobic lipid tails face inward and polar head groups face outward.

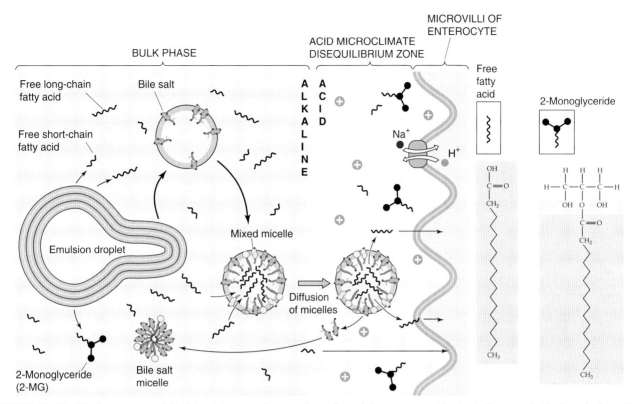

FIGURE 44–13. Micellar transport of lipid breakdown products to the surface of the enterocyte. Mixed micelles carry lipids through the acidic unstirred layer to the surface of the enterocyte. 2-Monoglyceride (2-MG), fatty acids, lysophospholipids, and cholesterol leave the mixed micelle and enter an acidic microenvironment created by an apical Na-H exchanger. The acidity favors the protonation of the free fatty acids. The lipids enter the enterocyte by diffusion, incorporation into the enterocyte membrane ("collision"), or, perhaps, carrier-mediated transport.

situations in which intraluminal bile salt concentrations are low (e.g., in newborns and patients with obstructive jaundice), lipid absorption can occur from vesicles.

Lipids, as Mixed Micelles and Monomers, Diffuse Across the Unstirred Water Layer on the Surface of the Jejunal Mucosa and Cross the Enterocyte Brush Border

To reach the interior of the enterocyte, lipolytic products must cross several barriers. These include (1) the mucous gel layer that lines the intestinal epithelial surface, (2) the unstirred water layer ("disequilibrium zone") contiguous with the enterocyte's apical membrane, and (3) the apical membrane itself. Although the mucous gel that lines the intestine is 95% water, its interstices provide a barrier to the free diffusion—from the "bulk phase" to the unstirred water layer—of lipid macroaggregates, particularly the various vesicles that exist in equilibrium with the mixed micelles and monomers. Because of this diffusion barrier, the unstirred water lying adjacent to the enterocyte's apical membrane is not in equilibrium with the bulk phase of water in the lumen. According to calculations based on the diffusion of various probes under different experimental conditions and luminal fluid flow rates, it was originally estimated that the unstirred water layer was several hundred microns thick and posed a significant barrier to the diffusion of lipid nutrients to the enterocyte brush border. It is now thought that the un-

stirred water layer is likely only approximately 40 μm thick and does not constitute a major absorptive barrier. For short- and medium-chain fatty acids, which are readily soluble in water, diffusion of these monomers through the unstirred water layer to the enterocyte is efficient. As fatty-acid chain length increases, the monomer's solubility in water decreases, whereas its partitioning into micelles increases. It is true that the diffusion of a single monomer through the aqueous barriers is speedier than that of a single micelle or vesicle. However, mixed-lipid micelles give the aqueous solution such a high *effective concentration* of lipid products that the diffusion of these micelles is the most efficient mechanism for bringing lipolytic products to the enterocytes. Calculations suggest that, compared with monomers dissolved in water, vesicular solubilization increases the "concentration" of long-chain fatty acids near the enterocyte's brush border membrane by a factor of 100,000 and micellar solubilization by a factor of 1,000,000.

When the fatty acid/bile salt mixed micelles reach the enterocyte surface, they encounter a low-pH microclimate generated by Na-H exchange at the brush-border membrane. It is postulated that fatty acids now become protonated and leave the mixed micelle to enter the enterocyte, either by "nonionic" diffusion (p. 802) of the uncharged fatty acid or by "collision" and incorporation of the fatty acid into the cell membrane (Fig. 44–13). Similarly, unesterified cholesterol and lysophospholipids must leave the micelle carrier to enter the enterocyte as monomers. It has been suggested that cholesterol derived from bile is better absorbed than dietary cholesterol. After the entry of lipids into enterocytes, the remaining bile salts return to the lumen and are then absorbed passively throughout the small intestine and via active transport in the distal ileum (p. 993). Fatty acids, 2-MG, lysophospholipids, and cholesterol traditionally were assumed to enter the enterocyte by simple diffusion across the apical plasma membrane of the brush border villi. Recently, however, membrane proteins have been identified in both enterocytes and hepatocytes that may be responsible for the transfer of fatty acids, phospholipids, and cholesterol across their respective cell membranes. Such carriers may yet provide a mechanism for facilitated or active absorption of the various products of lipid digestion.

The Enterocyte Re-Esterifies Lipid Components and Assembles Them into Chylomicrons

The assimilation of fats, thus far, has been a process of disassembly of energy-dense, water-insoluble lipid macromolecular aggregates into monomers for intestinal absorption. The enterocyte elegantly reverses this process (Fig. 44–14). After absorbing long-chain fatty acids, monoglycerides, lysophospholipids, and cholesterol, the enterocyte re-esterifies them and assembles the products with specific apoproteins into emulsion-like particles called chylomicrons. The enterocyte then exports the chylomicrons to the lymph (chyle) for ultimate deliver to other organs via the bloodstream.

Chylomicrons are the largest of the five lipoprotein particles in the blood stream. (The other lipoprotein particles—VLDLs, IDLs, LDLs, and HDLs—are discussed on p. 998; see Table 45–5.) Ranging in diameter from 75 to 1200 nm, chylomicrons consist primarily of triglycerides, with smaller amounts of phospholipids, cholesteryl esters, cholesterol, and various apoproteins.

The first step in the enterocyte's reformation of triglycerides is for long-chain fatty acids to bind to a 12-kDa cytosolic protein called **fatty acid–binding protein.** The concentration of fatty acid–binding protein in the intestine is highest in regions where fats are absorbed, namely the villi of the proximal jejunal enterocytes. Fatty acid–binding protein preferentially binds long-chain (rather than medium- or short-chain) fatty acids, minimizing both reflux back into the intestinal lumen and toxic damage to the enterocyte. Fatty acid–binding protein also ensures transfer of fatty acids up to the smooth endoplasmic reticulum (SER) of the enterocyte. The re-esterification to form triglycerides occurs within the SER, using either absorbed 2-MG as a substrate ("monoglyceride pathway") or glycerol-3-phosphate derived from glucose

FIGURE 44–14. Re-esterification of digested lipids by the enterocyte, and the formation and secretion of chylomicrons. The enterocyte takes up short- and medium-chain fatty acids and glycerol and passes them unchanged into the blood capillaries. The enterocyte also takes up long-chain fatty acids and 2-monoglyceride and re-synthesizes them into triglycerides in the smooth endoplasmic reticulum (SER). The enterocyte also processes cholesterol into cholesteryl esters and lysolecithin into lecithin. The fate of these substances, and the formation of chylomicrons, is illustrated by steps 1 to 7. RER, rough endoplasmic reticulum; VLDL, very-low-density lipoprotein.

metabolism ("phosphatidic acid pathway"). As summarized in Figure 57–4, each of these pathways depends on the activation of the fatty acid to acetyl coenzyme A (acetyl CoA), catalyzed by acetyl CoA synthetase. Long-chain fatty acids are the preferred substrate for this enzyme. Fatty acids are esterified mainly by the monoglyceride pathway during fat absorption, and by the phosphatidic acid pathway during fasting, when the enterocyte may take up fatty acids and chylomicron remnants from the bloodstream. The net effect of this series of reactions is the formation of triglycerides in the SER. Triglycerides and fat droplets may be seen in the cisternae of the SER on electron microscopy. The enterocyte also esterifies both **cholesterol** and **lysolecithin.**

Besides the lipids, the other components of the chylomicron are the various apoproteins, which the enterocyte synthesizes in the rough endoplasmic reticulum (RER) (see Table 45–5). These apoproteins move to the lumen of the SER, where they associate with newly synthesized triglycerides (see Fig. 44–14). Besides incorporating apoproteins, the packaging of nascent chylomicrons involves adding esterified cholesterol and a surface coating of lecithin and other phospholipids. It is thought that vesicles derived from the SER carry nascent chylomicrons to the *cis* face of the Golgi apparatus, where they fuse and deliver their contents internally. Enzymes in the Golgi apparatus glycosylate the apoproteins. Vesicles carrying processed chylomicrons bud off from the *trans* face of the Golgi and move toward the basolateral plasma membrane of the enterocyte. There they fuse with the basolateral membrane and leave the enterocyte.

The foregoing discussion focused on the digestion and absorption of *long-chain* triglycerides. The handling of triglycerides with **medium-length fatty acid chains** is very different. In the first place, the uptake into the enterocyte of fatty acids and monoglycerides derived from medium-chain triglycerides does not depend on the presence of either mixed micelles or bile salts. Moreover, the enterocyte does not re-esterify the medium-chain fatty acids but instead transfers them directly into the portal blood. As a result, medium-chain triglycerides are suitable fat substitutes for feeding patients with fat malabsorption.

The Enterocyte Secretes Chylomicrons into the Lymphatic Circulation During Feeding and Secretes Very-Low-Density Lipoproteins During Fasting

As we have described, vesicles carrying mature chylomicrons discharge their contents outside the enterocyte through exocytosis at the basolateral membrane. Chylomicrons are too large to pass through the fenestrae of blood capillaries, and thus they enter **lymph** through the larger interendothelial channels of the lymphatic capillaries. During fasting, the intestine secretes **very-low-density lipoproteins** (VLDLs), which are smaller (30 to 80 nm) than chylomicrons. These lipoprotein particles are of similar protein and lipid composition to chylomicrons (see Table 45–5) but are synthesized independently and carry mainly endogenous lipids. The lymph lacteals originate in the tips of the villi and discharge their contents into the

cisternae chyli. Lymph flows from the cisternae chyli to the thoracic duct, to enter the blood circulation via the left subclavian vein. The protein and lipid composition of both chylomicrons and VLDLs are modified during their passage through lymph and on entry into the blood.

The process of lipid digestion and absorption has great reserve capacity and many redundancies. For example, the mechanical disruption of food is accomplished in several ways by the mouth, stomach, and proximal intestine. Many of the digestive lipases have overlapping functions, and pancreatic lipase in particular is secreted in great excess. Much of the small intestine is not used for fat absorption in healthy individuals. Nonetheless, fat malabsorption does occur in many disease states. A logical classification for these disorders can be devised based on knowledge of the normal physiology. Thus, fat malabsorption may occur because of impairments in intraluminal digestion, intraluminal dispersion, mucosal penetration, and/or transport from enterocyte to the blood circulation. Within each major category are subdivisions. Frequently, the pathophysiology of these disorders is mixed (i.e., more than one step in the digestive or absorptive process is deranged), but nonetheless the defective components can be identified and appropriate therapy given.

DIGESTION AND ABSORPTION OF WATER-SOLUBLE VITAMINS AND MINERALS

Dietary Folate (PteGlu7) Must Be Deconjugated by a Brush-Border Enzyme Before Absorption by an Anion Exchanger at the Apical Membrane

Folate is also referred to as folic acid, or pteroylmonoglutamate (PteGlu1). As we discuss later, the reduced form of folate—tetrahydrofolate (THF)—is a cofactor in biochemical reactions involving the transfer of 1-carbon fragments. The recommended daily allowance (RDA) for folate is 200 μg for males and 180 μg for females (see Table 57–6), but is more than doubled in pregnant women (p. 1182). THF is essential for the synthesis of thymine and purines, which are critical components of DNA. Thus folate deficiency compromises DNA synthesis and cell division, an effect that is most clinically noticeable in the bone marrow, where the turnover of cells is rapid. Because RNA and protein synthesis are not impaired, large red blood cells called megaloblasts are produced. The resultant *megaloblastic anemia* can become quite severe if untreated. Megaloblastic cells also may be seen in other organs with rapid cell turnover, such as the small intestine. Folic acid supplementation during pregnancy also reduces the risk of neural-tube defects.

The medicinal form of folate is PteGlu1, a **monoglutamate.** Figure 44–15A shows the structure of PteGlu1, and also illustrates how folate can act as a methyl acceptor or donor in the interconversion of serine to glycine. Dietary folate exists in several forms, much of it in the form of **folate polyglutamate**, or PteGlu7 (see Fig. 44–15B), which is widely available in the diet, particularly in spinach, beans, and liver. The intestinal absorption of

A MEDICINAL FOLATE (PteGlu1)

Pteridine

p-Aminobenzoate   **Glutamate**

"R"

B FOOD FOLATE (PteGlu7)

Pteroylpolyglutamate

C FOLATE ABSORPTION

Pte(Glu)$_n$

PteGlu1

PteGlu1

Brush border peptidase

Basolateral carrier

PteGlu1

N^5-methyl-THF

OH$^-$

Brush border PteGlu carrier

Interstitial space

Lumen of jejunum   Epithelium

D METHYLATION OF REDUCED FOLATE

Reactive

Ser   Gly

H$^+$ + NADH   NAD$^+$

Reactive

5,10-methylene-THF

dUMP

dTMP → DNA

DHF

Tetrahydrofolate (THF)

N^5-methyl-tetrahydrofolate

FIGURE 44–15. Folate deconjugation and absorption. *A*, Tetrahydrofolate has three parts: the biologically active pteridine moiety, a *p*-aminobenzoate, and a glutamate. PteGlu1 is the oxidized form of folate and is biologically inactive. *B*, Dietary folate is similar to medicinal folate but has several glutamate residues. PteGlu7 is also oxidized and inactive. *C*, In the proximal small intestine, a brush-border peptidase sequentially removes all but the last of the glutamate residues from dietary folate. The enterocyte then absorbs the resulting PteGlu1 using a folate-OH exchanger. Once inside the enterocyte, the PteGlu1 exits across the basolateral membrane via an unknown transporter. The enterocyte may reduce some of the PteGlu1 to dihydrofolate (DHF) and then to tetrahydrofolate (THF), the biologically active form of folate. The enterocyte may then methylate some of the THF to form N^5-methyl-THF, as summarized in *D*. *D*, After the cell has reduced PteGlu1 to THF by adding the four highlighted hydrogens, it first converts THF to 5,10-methylene-THF, breaking down serine to glycine in the process. This 5,10-methylene-THF is the methyl donor in the conversion of the nucleotide dUMP to dTMP in the synthesis of DNA. A second reaction converts this 5,10-methylene-THF to N^5-methyl-THF, which can then act as a methyl donor in the synthesis of methionine (see Fig. 44–16*B*). dTMP, deoxthymidine monophosphate; dUMP, deoxyuridine monophosphate; Gly, glycine; NAD, nicotinamide adenine dinucleotide; NADH, nicotinamide adenine dinucleotide (reduced form); Ser, serine.

FIGURE 44–16. Cobalamin and the role of intrinsic factor in the absorption of cobalamin. *A*, Cyanocobalamin. *B*, Methylation cycle. Cobalamin is the coenzyme for the enzyme homocysteine : methionine methyltransferase, which transfers a methyl group from N^5-methyltetrafolate to homocysteine, thereby forming methionine and tetrahydrofolate. *C*, Steps 1 to 8 show the fate of dietary cobalamin (CBL). Steps 4 to 8 show the role of intrinsic factor (IF). In addition, bile carries cobalamin into the duodenum. *D*, The intrinsic-factor/cobalamin complex is thought to be endocytosed. The cobalamin is liberated within the enterocyte by mechanisms that have not been established. Within the enterocyte, cobalamin binds to transcobalamin II (TCII), which is required for cobalamin's exit from the enterocyte.

A CYANOCOBALAMIN

B METHYLATION CYCLE

C COBALAMIN HANDLING BY THE STOMACH AND PROXIMAL SMALL INTESTINE

D COBALAMIN ABSORPTION BY ILEAL ENTEROCYTE

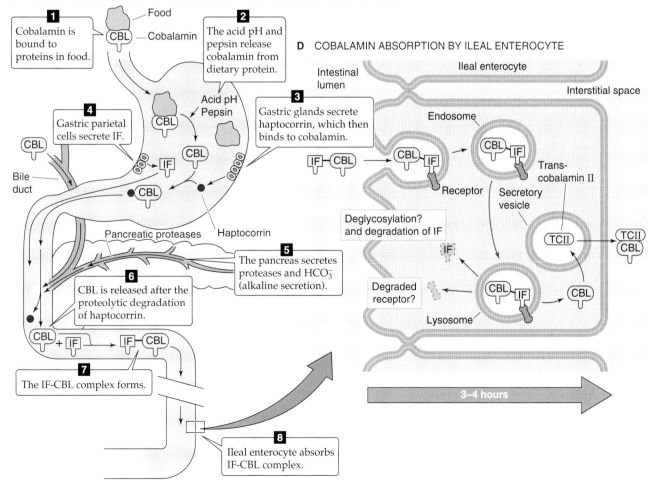

PteGlu7 requires deconjugation by a brush-border peptidase to PteGlu1, which then enters the enterocyte via a transporter (see Fig. 44–15C). This deconjugation is catalyzed by folate conjugase, a zinc-activated exopeptidase present in the brush border. This enzyme removes glutamate residues from PteGlu7 in a stepwise fashion before absorption of PteGlu1. This stepwise hydrolysis of the polyglutamate chain of PteGlu7 is the rate-limiting step in folate digestion-absorption. Both folate deconjugation and absorption occur only in the proximal small intestine and are maximally active at a pH of 5.

PteGlu1 absorption is saturable, shows substrate specificity, and is markedly enhanced at an acid pH. Folate absorption represents an apical-membrane anion exchange process, in which folate uptake is linked to the efflux of OH^- across the apical membrane (i.e., folate-OH exchange). The mechanism of folate movement out of the epithelial cell across the basolateral membrane is not understood.

The PteGlu1 taken up by the enterocyte is not biologically active. The enzyme difolate reductase acts on PteGlu1 to first form dihydrofolate (DHF) and then the biologically active derivative THF. The cell then converts THF to 5,10-methylene-THF (see Fig. 44–15D), the form of folate needed for DNA synthesis. The cell also can transform this 5,10-methylene-THF to the N^5-methyl-THF, which—as we discuss in the next section—can act as a methyl donor in the synthesis of methionine. The circulating, storage, and active forms of folate constitute various reduced (DHF and THF) and methylated derivatives of THF. The liver is the primary site at which dietary pteroylglutamates are reduced and methylated, although the intestinal epithelium may make a small contribution to these reactions.

Vitamin B₁₂ (Cobalamin) Binds to Haptocorrin in the Stomach, and Then to Intrinsic Factor in the Small Intestine, Before Endocytosis by Enterocytes in the Ileum

Cobalamin, or vitamin B_{12} (Fig. 44–16A), is synthesized only by microorganisms, not by mammalian cells. The primary source of cobalamin in humans is the ingestion of animal products—meat, fish, shellfish, eggs, and (to a limited extent) milk. Cobalamin is not present in vegetables or fruit. Therefore, strict vegetarians are at risk of developing dietary cobalamin deficiency.

Cobalamin's primary function is to serve as a coenzyme for homocysteine:methionine methyltransferase (see Fig. 44–16B), which transfers a methyl group from methyltetrafolate to homocysteine, thereby converting homocysteine to methionine. Methionine is an essential amino acid and in an altered form serves as an important donor of methyl groups in a number of important enzymatic reactions. If cobalamin is deficient and methionine levels fall, then the body converts its stores of intracellular "folate" (e.g., PteGlu1, THF, 5,10-methylene-THF) into N^5-methyl-THF (see Fig. 44–15D) in an effort to produce more methionine. As a result, 5,10-methylene-THF (the form of folate needed for DNA synthesis) falls, which explains why folate and cobalamin deficiencies cause

identical hematologic abnormalities (i.e., megaloblastic anemia). In addition, cobalamin deficiency causes various neurologic and psychological abnormalities that are not part of the syndrome of folate deficiency. Some of these abnormalities may be linked to deficient activity of methylmalonyl CoA mutase, another cobalamin-dependent coenzyme.

Cobalamin reaches the stomach bound to proteins in ingested food. In the stomach, pepsin and the low gastric pH release the cobalamin from the ingested proteins (see Fig. 44–16C). The now-free cobalamin binds to **haptocorrin** (formerly known as "R" type binder), a glycoprotein secreted by the salivary and gastric glands. The parietal cells of the stomach secrete a second protein, **intrinsic factor** (IF), crucial for the absorption of cobalamin. But cobalamin and IF do not interact in the acidic milieu of the stomach. Rather, gastric acidity enhances the binding of cobalamin to haptocorrin. When this cobalamin-haptocorrin complex reaches the duodenum, the haptocorrin is degraded by pancreatic proteases (Fig. 44–16C).

After the release of cobalamin from the cobalamin-haptocorrin complex in the proximal small intestine-made alkaline by the secretion of HCO_3^- from the pancreas and duodenum—both dietary cobalamin and cobalamin derived from bile bind to IF. The cobalamin-IF complex is highly resistant to enzyme degradation. As noted earlier, the gastric parietal cells secrete IF, a 45-kDa glycoprotein. Histamine, acetylcholine, and gastrin stimulate gastric-acid secretion (p. 895) and also stimulate IF secretion. Although IF secretion parallels proton secretion, there are three important differences. First, similar to pepsinogen secretion, histamine triggers an IF release that peaks within minutes and then continues at a reduced rate. This secretory pattern is related to the secretion of preformed IF; histamine has no effect on IF synthesis. Second, although cyclic adenosine monophosphate (cAMP) is important in IF secretion, a role for intracellular Ca^{2+} has not as yet been established. Third, H_2 histamine-receptor antagonists block IF secretion, but omeprazole, an inhibitor of the parietal cell H-K pump, does not affect IF secretion.

The next step in the absorption of cobalamin is the binding of the cobalamin-IF complex to specific receptors on the apical membranes of enterocytes in the ileum. Cobalamin without IF neither binds to ileal receptors nor is absorbed. The binding of the cobalamin-IF complex is selective and rapid and requires Ca^{2+}, but it is not energy dependent. The enterocyte next internalizes the cobalamin-IF complex in a process that is energy dependent but has not been well characterized. Inside the cell, cobalamin and IF dissociate; lysosomal degradation may play a role here. Within the enterocyte, cobalamin binds to another transport protein—transcobalamin II—which is required for cobalamin's exit from the enterocyte. The cobalamin exits the ileal enterocyte across the basolateral membrane bound to transcobalamin II, possibly by an exocytotic mechanism. The transcobalamin II-cobalamin complex enters the portal circulation, where it is delivered to the liver for storage and for secretion into the bile.

Total body cobalamin stores are large (~5 mg), particularly when compared to the daily rate of cobalamin absorption and loss. (The daily cobalamin requirement for

FIGURE 44–17. Active Ca^{2+} uptake in the duodenum. The small intestine absorbs Ca^{2+} by two mechanisms. The passive, paracellular absorption of Ca^{2+} occurs throughout the small intestine. This pathway is the predominant one, but is *not* under the control of vitamin D. The second mechanism—the active, transcellular absorption of Ca^{2+}—occurs only in the duodenum. Ca^{2+} enters the cell across the apical membrane via a channel. Inside the cell, the Ca^{2+} is buffered by binding proteins such as calbindin and is also taken up into intracellular organelles, such as the endoplasmic reticulum. The enterocyte then extrudes Ca^{2+} across the basolateral membrane via a Ca^{2+} pump and an Na-Ca exchanger. Thus, the net effect is Ca^{2+} absorption. The active form of vitamin D (1,25 dihydroxy vitamin D) stimulates all three steps of transcellular Ca^{2+} absorption. ATP, adenosine triphosphate; mRNA, messenger RNA.

PERNICIOUS ANEMIA

The close relationship between acid and gastrin release is clearly manifested in individuals with impaired acid secretion. In **pernicious anemia,** atrophy of the gastric mucosa in the corpus and an absence of parietal cells results in the lack in the secretion of both gastric acid and intrinsic factor (IF). Many patients with pernicious anemia exhibit antibody-mediated immunity against their parietal cells, and many of these patients also produce anti-IF autoantibodies.

Because IF is required for cobalamin absorption in the ileum, the result is impaired cobalamin absorption. In contrast, the antrum is normal and gastrin release is unimpaired. However, plasma gastrin levels are markedly elevated as a result of the absence of intraluminal acid, which normally triggers gastric D cells to release somatostatin (see p. 898), which in turn inhibits antral gastrin release (see box on p. 901). Because parietal cells are absent, the elevated plasma gastrin levels are not associated with enhanced gastric acid secretion.

The clinical complications of cobalamin deficiency evolve over a period of years. Patients develop a **megaloblastic anemia** in which the circulating red blood cells are enlarged, a distinctive glossitis, and a neuropathy. The earliest neurologic findings are those of peripheral neuropathy, as manifested by paresthesias and slow reflexes, as well as impaired senses of touch, vibration, and temperature. If untreated, the disease will ultimately involve the spinal cord, particularly the dorsal columns, producing weakness and ataxia. Memory impairment, depression, and dementia can also result. Parenteral administration of cobalamin reverses and prevents the manifestations of pernicious anemia, but does not influence parietal cells or restore gastric secretion of either IF or intraluminal acid.

---

normal adults is only 2 *micro*grams.) The load of cobalamin presented to the small intestine is derived about equally from two sources: the diet and biliary secretions. The latter is the result of the enterohepatic circulation (p. 983) of cobalamin; after its absorption, cobalamin is delivered throughout the body, and the excess is secreted by the liver into the bile, where it once again can be reabsorbed by the small intestine and recirculated.

Cobalamin deficiency has many possible causes. As already mentioned, a strict vegetarian diet is deficient in cobalamin. In **pernicious anemia,** a disorder seen primarily in the elderly, the absence of gastric parietal cells results in the absence of gastric acid and IF secretion. Consequently, cobalamin absorption is markedly reduced, and cobalamin deficiency develops. Other causes of cobalamin deficiency include related problems in the intestine. Bacterial overgrowth in the small intestine as a result of stasis (e.g., multiple jejunal diverticulosis) can be associated with cobalamin deficiency as a consequence of bacterial use of cobalamin. Crohn's disease affecting the ileum and ileal resection are other possible causes of cobalamin malabsorption and deficiency as a result of an absence of ileal receptors for the cobalamin-IF complex.

Calcium Absorption, Regulated Primarily by Vitamin D, Occurs by Active Transport in the Duodenum and by Diffusion Throughout the Small Intestine

The physiological importance and complex regulation of Ca^{2+} and vitamin D are discussed in Chapter 51. The Ca^{2+} load presented to the small intestine comprises dietary sources and digestive secretions. Most of the dietary Ca^{2+} (~1000 mg/day) comes from milk and milk products (see Fig. 51–1), but not all of it is bioavailable. For

HEMOCHROMATOSIS

Hereditary hemochromatosis (HH) is a relatively common inherited disorder (3 to 5 persons per 1000 of northwestern European ancestry are homozygous) in which the body absorbs excessive iron from the diet. This autosomal recessive disease becomes clinically significant only in homozygotes. If left untreated, HH can be fatal. The excess iron is stored in the liver, where it reaches toxic concentrations, eventually causing cirrhosis and greatly increasing the risk of hepatoma. Iron eventually accumulates in other organ systems as well, causing pancreatic damage (diabetes mellitus), a bronze pigmentation of the skin, pituitary and gonadal failure, arthritis, and cardiomyopathy. The disease almost never becomes apparent before the individual enters the third decade of life. Women are relatively protected as long they are premenopausal, because their monthly menstrual flow keeps total body iron stores relatively normal.

The diagnosis can be made by detection of elevated iron and transferrin-saturation levels and an elevated ferritin on blood testing. A liver biopsy is confirmatory.

The treatment, reminiscent of the general medieval approach to disease, is to remove (phlebotomize) one or even several units of blood (1 unit = 500 ml) from the patient on a regular basis until the iron overload is corrected as evidenced by normal plasma-ferritin levels. Afterward, most patients require phlebotomy only once every few months to maintain their low iron stores.

The HFE gene that is associated with HH is related to the major histocompatibility complex (MHC) class I family. More than 80% of patients with HH are homozygous for a *missense* mutation (C282Y) in HFE. However, the role that this mutated gene plays in hemochromatosis is not yet clear because the penetrance of hemochromatosis in individuals with the C282Y allele is very low (<5%). Recent attention has also focused on hepcidin, a newly identified hepatic protein that appears to play a critical role in iron homeostasis.

The *active* transport of Ca^{2+} across the villous epithelial cells of the duodenum is transcellular and under the control of vitamin D—primarily via genomic effects (p. 131). Transcellular Ca^{2+} absorption involves three steps. The uptake of Ca^{2+} across the apical membrane occurs via **Ca^{2+} channels**, driven by the electrochemical gradient between the lumen and the cell. Cytosolic Ca^{2+} then binds to a protein called **calbindin**, which buffers intracellular Ca^{2+}. This step is important because it allows unbound (i.e., free) intracellular Ca^{2+} to remain rather low despite large transcellular fluxes of Ca^{2+}. **A Ca^{2+} pump** and a **Na-Ca exchanger** on the basolateral membrane then extrude the Ca^{2+} from the cell into the interstitial fluid. The active form of vitamin D—1,25-dihydroxy-vitamin D—stimulates all three steps of the transcellular pathway, but its most important effect is to enhance the second step by increasing the synthesis of calbindin.

The passive absorption of Ca^{2+} throughout the small intestine occurs via the paracellular pathway, which is *not* under the control of vitamin D. Calcium absorption is also enhanced by low plasma $[Ca^{2+}]$ and during pregnancy and lactation. Absorption tends to diminish with aging.

Vitamin D itself is a fat-soluble vitamin that is absorbed mainly in the jejunum. Of course, the skin synthesizes vitamin D_3 from cholesterol in a process that requires ultraviolet light (p. 1095). Thus, dietary vitamin D (both vitamin D_2 and D_3) is most important in regions of the world that do not get much sunlight and during long, dark winters.

Magnesium Absorption Occurs by an Active Process in the Ileum

Magnesium is an important intracellular ion that is required as an enzyme cofactor—many enzymes using adenosine triphosphate (ATP) actually require that the ATP be complexed with Mg^{2+}—and is critical for neurotransmission and muscular contractions. Magnesium deficiency can affect neuromuscular, cardiovascular, and gastrointestinal function. Magnesium is also important for the proper secretion of, and end-organ response to, parathyroid hormone. Thus, Mg^{2+} depletion is typically associated with hypocalcemia.

Magnesium is widely available in different foods but is present in particularly large amounts in green vegetables, cereals, and meats. The RDA for Mg^{2+} (see Table 57–6) in young adults is approximately 350 mg/day for males and approximately 280 mg/day for females. The Mg^{2+} load to the small intestine is derived from both dietary sources and digestive secretions.

Mg^{2+} absorption by the gastrointestinal tract is not yet well understood, but it appears to differ substantially from the absorption of the other key divalent cation, Ca^{2+}, in three important respects. First, an active transport process for Mg^{2+} absorption appears to exist in the ileum, rather than in the duodenum, as is the case for Ca^{2+}. Second, 1,25-dihydroxy vitamin D does not consistently increase Mg^{2+} absorption. Third, patients with increased intestinal Ca^{2+} absorption (e.g., absorptive hyper-

---

example, only very little of the Ca^{2+} present in leafy vegetables is absorbed because of the concomitant presence of oxalate, a salt that binds Ca^{2+} and reduces its availability for absorption. The small intestine absorbs about 500 mg/day of Ca^{2+}, and also secretes approximately 325 mg/day of Ca^{2+}. Thus the net uptake is 175 mg/day.

Active, transcellular uptake of Ca^{2+} occurs only in the epithelial cells of the duodenum, but Ca^{2+} is absorbed by passive, paracellular diffusion throughout the small intestine. More Ca^{2+} is absorbed in the jejunum and ileum by diffusion than in the duodenum by active transport; this difference arises largely because the duodenum has a smaller total surface area and because the flow of Ca^{2+}-containing fluid through the duodenum is more rapid (Fig. 44–17).

FIGURE 44–18. Absorption of nonheme and heme iron in the duodenum. Dietary iron is present in two major forms, as part of a heme group or not. The absorption of nonheme iron occurs almost exclusively as Fe^{2+}. This Fe^{2+} enters via DCT1 (or DMT1). An apical ferrireductase (duodenal cytochrome b or Dcytb) reduces any free dietary Fe^{3+} to Fe^{2+} for import via DCT1. Heme enters the enterocyte by an unknown mechanism. Inside the cell, heme oxygenase releases Fe^{3+}, which is then reduced to Fe^{2+}. Regardless of which path the Fe^{2+} takes, cytoplasmic Fe^{2+} then binds to mobilferrin for transit across the cell to the basolateral membrane. Fe^{2+} exits the enterocyte across the basolateral membrane via the IREG1 (or ferroportin) transporter, after which hephaestin oxidizes the Fe^{2+} to Fe^{3+}. Once in the blood plasma, the Fe^{3+} binds to plasma transferrin, which carries the iron to various tissues.

calciuria) have normal Mg^{2+} absorption. Along with active Mg^{2+} absorption in the ileum, the rest of the small intestine absorbs Mg^{2+} passively.

Heme and Nonheme Iron Are Absorbed in the Duodenum by Distinct Cellular Mechanisms

Iron plays several critical roles in human physiology, both in the heme groups of the cytochromes and as a key component of the oxygen-carrying heme moieties of hemoglobin and myoglobin. The most important complication of iron depletion is anemia. Iron overload produces **hemochromatosis,** a not-uncommon genetic disease (see box titled Hemochromatosis).

Dietary iron takes two major forms: iron that is part of a heme moiety and iron that is not. These two types of dietary iron are absorbed by distinctly different mechanisms (Fig. 44–18). Overall iron absorption is low; 10% to 20% of ingested iron is absorbed. Heme iron is absorbed more efficiently than nonheme iron. Body stores of iron are almost exclusively determined by iron absorption, because (except in menstruating women, who require approximately 50% more iron in their diets), very little iron is lost from the body. Dietary iron comes primarily from meat—especially liver and fish—as well as vegetables.

The RDA for iron (see Table 57–6) in young adults is approximately 10 mg/day for males and approximately 15 mg/day for females.

Nonheme iron may be either ferric (Fe^{3+}) or ferrous (Fe^{2+}). Ferric iron tends to form salt complexes with anions quite easily and thus is not readily absorbed; it is not soluble at pH values above 3. Ferrous iron does not complex easily and is soluble at pH values as high as 8. Ascorbic acid (vitamin C) forms soluble complexes with iron and reduces iron from the ferric to the ferrous state, thereby enhancing iron absorption. Tannins, present in tea, form insoluble complexes with iron and lower its absorption.

The absorption of nonheme iron is restricted to the duodenum. The enterocyte takes up nonheme iron across the apical membrane via the **divalent cation transporter DCT1** (or DMT1), which cotransports Fe^{2+} and H^+ into the cell (p. 68). DCT1, as well as the oligopeptide cotransporter that we discussed earlier, is unusual in being energized by the inwardly directed H^+ gradient. DCT1 also efficiently absorbs a host of other divalent metals, including several that are highly toxic (e.g., Cd^{2+}, Pb^{2+}). In the case of dietary ferric iron, a ferrireductase at the extracellular surface of the apical membrane—**Dcytb,** which is related to cytochrome b—can reduce Fe^{3+} to Fe^{2+} for import via DCT1.

After Fe^{2+} moves into the cytoplasm of the enterocyte, it binds to **mobilferrin**, an intracellular protein that ferries the Fe^{2+} to the basolateral membrane. The enterocyte then translocates the Fe^{2+} across the basolateral membrane, possibly via the IREG1 transporter (or ferroportin). The mRNA encoding IREG1 has an iron-responsive element (p. 143) in its 5′ untranslated region; thus, an increase in intracellular iron levels would be expected to decrease IREG1 synthesis. Following the exit of Fe^{2+} from the enterocyte via IREG1, the ferroxidase **hephaestin**—a homolog of the plasma protein ceruloplasmin, which carries copper (p. 1001)—apparently oxidizes the Fe^{2+} to Fe^{3+}, which then binds to plasma **transferrin** (p. 44) for carriage in the blood.

Once in the circulation, nonheme iron is carried to other organs bound to transferrin. Nonheme iron is ultimately deposited in all the tissues of the body, but has a particular predilection for the liver and reticuloendothelial system. Inside these cells, it binds to the protein apoferritin to form **ferritin,** the major storage form of iron. Smaller amounts of storage iron exists in an insoluble form called hemosiderin.

Heme iron, derived from myoglobin and hemoglobin, is also absorbed by duodenal epithelial cells. Heme iron enters the cells either by binding to a brush-border protein or through an endocytotic mechanism. Inside the cell, heme iron is split enzymatically by heme oxygenase, releasing free Fe^{3+}, carbon monoxide, and biliverdin. Biliverdin is metabolized into bile salts (see box on p. 986). The enterocyte reduces the Fe^{3+} to Fe^{2+}, which it then handles in the same manner as nonheme iron.

Iron absorption is tightly regulated by the size of existing body iron stores. In normal subjects, iron absorption is limited but is markedly *increased* in states of iron deficiency, caused most often by gastrointestinal bleeding or excessive menstrual flow. For example, the expression of

DCT1 and IREG1 increase in iron deficiency. Conversely, an increase in iron stores modestly reduces iron absorption.

REFERENCES

Books and Reviews

Carey MC, Hernell O: Digestion and absorption of fat. Semin Gastroenterol 3:189–204, 1992.

Civitelli R, Avioli LV: Calcium, phosphate and magnesium absorption. In Johnson LR (ed): Physiology of the Gastrointestinal Tract, 3rd ed. New York, Raven Press, 1994, pp 2173–2182.

Debnam ES, Srai SKS: Intestinal iron absorption: Cellular mechanism and regulation. News Physiol Sci 12:184–189, 1997.

Farrell JJ: Digestion and absorption of nutrients and vitamins. In Feldman M, Friedman LS, Sleisenger MH (eds): Gastrointestinal and Liver Disease, Vol 2, 7th ed. Philadelphia, Saunders, 2002, pp 1715–1750.

Johnson LR (ed): Physiology of the Gastrointestinal Tract, 3rd ed. New York, Raven Press, 1994.

Hentze MW, Muckenthaler MU, Andrews NC: Balancing acts: Molecular control of mammalian iron metabolism. Cell 117:285–297, 2004.

Palacin M, Estevez R, Bertran J, Zorzano A: Molecular biology of mammalian plasma membrane amino acid transporters. Physiol Rev 78:969–1054, 1998.

Wright EM: The intestinal Na^+/glucose cotransporter. Annu Rev Physiol 55:575–589, 1993.

Journal Articles

Feder JN, Gnirke A, Thomas W, et al: A novel MHC class I-like gene is mutated in patients with hereditary haemochromatosis. Nat Genet 13:399–408, 1996.

Fei YJ, Kanai Y, Nussberger S, et al: Expression cloning of a mammalian proton-coupled oligopeptide transporter. Nature 368:563–566, 1994.

Gunshin H, Mackenzie B, Berger UV, et al: Cloning and characterization of a proton-coupled mammalian metal ion transporter. Nature 388:482–488, 1997.

Shiau YF: Mechanisms of intestinal fatty acid uptake in the rat: The role of an acidic microclimate. J Physiol 421:463–474, 1990.

CHAPTER 45

Hepatobiliary Function

Winita Hardikar and Frederick J. Suchy

OVERVIEW OF LIVER PHYSIOLOGY

The liver weighs between 1200 and 1500 g. Except for the skin, it is the largest organ in the human body, approximately 4% to 5% of body weight in the newborn and 2% to 5% in the adult. The liver is strategically situated in the circulatory system, receiving the portal blood that drains the stomach, small intestine, large intestine, pancreas, and spleen (see Fig. 23–7). In this position, the liver plays a key role in handling foodstuffs assimilated by the small intestine. However, the liver's role is far more diverse; it serves as a chemical factory, an excretory systm, an exocrine gland, and an endocrine gland.

The Liver Biotransforms and Degrades Substances Taken Up from Blood and Either Returns Them to the Circulation or Excretes Them into Bile

A major function of the liver is to metabolize, detoxify, and inactivate both endogenous compounds (e.g., steroids and other hormones) and exogenous substances (e.g., drugs and toxins). In addition, by virtue of its large vascular capacity and abundance of phagocytes (Kupffer cells), the liver provides an important filtering mechanism for the circulation by removing foreign particulate matter, including bacteria, endotoxins, parasites, and aging red blood cells. The Kupffer cells constitute 80% to 90% of the fixed macrophages of the reticuloendothelial system.

The liver has the capacity to convert important hormones and vitamins into a more active form. Examples include the initial hydroxylation of vitamin D and the deiodination of the thyroid hormone thyroxine (T_4) to triiodothyronine (T_3). Moreover, a variety of enzymes in the liver process lipophilic chemicals into more polar, water-soluble metabolites, which are more readily excreted into bile.

Bile is a complex secretory product produced by the liver. Biliary secretion has two principal functions: (1) eliminate many endogenous and exogenous waste products from the body, such as bilirubin and cholesterol, and (2) promote the digestion and absorption of lipids from the intestine. The composition of bile is modified significantly as a result of the absorptive and secretory properties of epithelial cells that line the intrahepatic and extrahepatic bile ducts. Moreover, bile solutes are further concentrated as bile is stored in the gallbladder.

The Liver Stores Carbohydrates, Lipids, Vitamins, and Minerals; It Synthesizes Carbohydrates, Protein, and Intermediary Metabolites

The products of digested food, including carbohydrates, peptides, vitamins, and some lipids, are avidly extracted from portal blood by the liver. Depending on the metabolic requirements of the body, these substrates may be stored by the hepatocytes or released into the bloodstream either unbound (e.g., glucose) or associated with a carrier molecule (e.g., a triglyceride molecule complexed to a lipoprotein).

The liver also synthesizes—in a highly regulated fashion—many substances that are essential to the metabolic demands of the body. These substances include albumin and other plasma proteins, glucose, cholesterol, fatty acids for triglyceride biosynthesis, and phospholipids. The liver must provide a supply of substrates as fuels for other organs, particularly in the fasted state. For example, the liver produces ketone bodies, which can be used by the central nervous system during periods of fasting, thereby sparing about 50% of the amount of glucose that would otherwise be used by this tissue. Thus, the liver has a critical and unique role in the energy metabolism of all nonhepatic organs.

FUNCTIONAL ANATOMY OF THE LIVER AND BILIARY TREE

Hepatocytes Are Secretory Epithelial Cells That Separate the Lumen of the Bile Canaliculi from the Fenestrated Endothelium of the Vascular Sinusoids

One way of looking at the organization of the liver is to imagine that a "classic lobule" is a hexagon in cross section (Fig. 45–1A) with a branch of the hepatic vein at its center and, at each of the six corners, triads composed of branches of the hepatic artery, portal vein, and bile duct. Hepatocytes account for approximately 80% of the parenchymal volume in human liver. Hepatocytes form an epithelium, one cell thick, that constitutes a functional barrier between two fluid compartments with differing ionic compositions: the tiny **canalicular lumen** containing bile and the much larger **sinusoid** containing blood (Fig. 45–1B). Moreover, hepatocytes significantly alter the composition of these fluids by vectorial transport of solutes across the hepatocyte. This vectorial transport depends critically on the polarized distribution of specific transport mechanisms and receptors that are localized to the **apical membrane** that faces the canalicular lumen and the **basolateral membrane** that faces the pericellular space between hepatocytes and the blood-filled sinusoid (Fig. 45–1B, C). As in other epithelia, the apical and basolateral membrane domains of hepatocytes are structurally, biochemically, and physiologically distinct.

The **space of Disse**, or perisinusoidal space, is the extracellular gap between the endothelial cells lining the sinusoids and the basolateral membranes of the hepatocytes. These basolateral membranes have microvilli that project into the space of Disse to facilitate contact with the solutes in sinusoidal blood. The microvilli greatly amplify the basolateral membrane, which accounts for approximately 85% of the total surface area of the hepatocyte.

The bile canaliculi, into which bile is initially secreted, are formed by the apical membranes of adjoining hepatocytes. The apical membrane of the hepatocyte runs as a narrow belt that encircles and grooves into the polygonal hepatocyte (Fig. 45–1B, C). Two adjacent hepatocytes form a canaliculus that is approximately 1 μm in diameter by juxtaposing their groove-like apical membranes along their common face (i.e., one side of the polygon). Because a hepatocyte has many sides and a different neighbor on each side, the canaliculi form a chicken wire–like pattern along the contiguous surfaces of hepatocytes and communicate to form a three-dimensional tubular network. Although the apical membrane belt is very narrow (i.e., ~1 μm), its extensive microvillous structure amplifies its surface area so that the canalicular membrane constitutes as much as 15% of the total membrane surface area. Because of this high surface-to-volume ratio, the total apical surface area available for the movement of water and solutes in the human liver is in excess of 10.5 m².

The seal that joins the apical membranes of two juxtaposed hepatocytes and that separates the canalicular lumen from the pericellular space—which is contiguous with the space of Disse—comprises several elements, including **tight junctions** (Fig. 45–1D) and desmosomes (p. 48). By virtue of their permeability and morphology, hepatic junctions can be classified as having an intermediate tightness, somewhat between tight epithelia (e.g., toad bladder) and leaky epithelia (e.g., proximal tubule). Specialized structures called gap junctions (p. 164) allow functional communication between adjacent hepatocytes.

Hepatocytes do not have a true basement membrane, but rest on a complex scaffolding provided by the **extracellular matrix** in the space of Disse, which includes several types of collagens (I, III, IV, V and VI), fibronectin, undulin, laminin, and proteoglycans. Cells are linked to the matrix through specific adhesion proteins on the cell surface. The extracellular matrix not only provides structural support for liver cells but also seems to influence and maintain the phenotypic expression of hepatocytes and sinusoidal lining cells.

The Liver Contains Endothelial Cells, Macrophages (Kupffer Cells), and Stellate Cells (Ito Cells) Within the Sinusoidal Spaces

Just over 6% of the volume of the liver parenchyma is made up of cells other than hepatocytes, including endothelial cells (2.8%), Kupffer cells (2.1%), and stellate cells (fat-storing or Ito cells, 1.4%). The **endothelial cells** that line the vascular channels or sinusoids form a fenestrated structure with their bodies and cytoplasmic extensions. Plasma solutes, but not blood cells, can move freely into

A CLASSIC HEPATIC LOBULE

Portal triad

Central vein

C HEPATOCYTES AND BILE CANALICULI

Bile canaliculi

Apical membrane facing lumen of canaliculus

Baso-lateral membrane

D TIGHT JUNCTION

Pericellular space

Groove

Ridge

Extracellular space

Strands of trans-membrane proteins

Lumen of bile canaliculus

Cytosol of the hepatocyte

B SECTION OF LOBULE

Sinusoid lumen

Lumen of the bile canaliculus

Basolateral membrane (facing the sinusoid)

Apical membrane (facing the lumen of canaliculus)

Hepatic artery   Portal vein   Bile ducts

Portal triad

Periportal bile ducts

Space of Disse

Sinusoidal capillary

FIGURE 45–1. Hepatocytes, sinusoids, and the intrahepatic bile system.

the space of Disse through pores, or fenestra, in the endothelial cells. Some evidence indicates that the fenestra may regulate access into the perisinusoidal space of Disse by means of their capacity to contract.

The **Kupffer cells** are within the sinusoidal vascular space. This population of fixed macrophages removes particulate matter from the circulation. The **stellate cells** are in the space of Disse and are characterized morphologically by the presence of large fat droplets in their cytoplasm. These cells play a central role in the storage of vitamin A, and evidence suggests that they can be trans-

formed into proliferative, fibrogenic and contractile myofibroblasts. Upon liver injury, these "activated" cells participate in fibrogenesis through remodeling of the extracellular matrix and deposition of type-1 collagen, which can lead to cirrhosis.

The Liver Has a Dual Blood Supply, but a Single Venous Drainage System

The blood supply to the liver has two sources. The **portal vein** contributes approximately 75% of the total circula-

FIGURE 45–2. Blood supply to the liver.

tion to the liver; the **hepatic artery** contributes the other 25% (Fig. 45–2A). Blood from portal venules and hepatic arterioles combines in a complex network of hepatic sinusoids (see Fig. 45–2B). Blood from these sinusoids converge on terminal hepatic venules (or "**central veins**"), which in turn converge to form the **hepatic vein** (see Fig. 45–2C). Branches of the portal vein, hepatic artery, and a bile duct (i.e., the "triad"), as well as lymphatics and nerves, travel together as a **portal tract**.

The arterial supply for the bile ducts arises mainly from the right hepatic artery (Fig. 45–2C). These arterioles give rise to an extraordinarily rich plexus of capillaries that surround the bile ducts as they pass through the portal tracts. Blood flowing through this peribiliary plexus empties into the sinusoids by way of branches of the portal vein so that this blood may pick up solutes from the bile ducts and cycle them back to the hepatocytes. Thus, the peribiliary plexus may provide the means for modifying biliary secretions through the bidirectional exchange of compounds such as proteins, inorganic ions, and bile acids between the bile and blood within the portal tract.

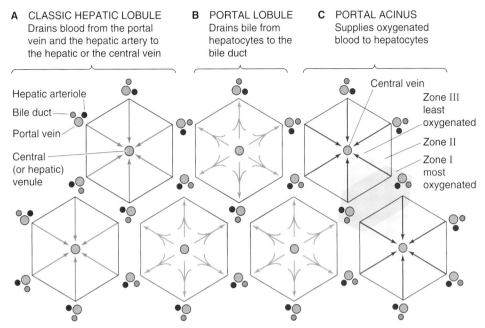

A CLASSIC HEPATIC LOBULE
Drains blood from the portal
vein and the hepatic artery to
the hepatic or the central vein

B PORTAL LOBULE
Drains bile from
hepatocytes to the
bile duct

C PORTAL ACINUS
Supplies oxygenated
blood to hepatocytes

Hepatic arteriole
Bile duct
Portal vein
Central
(or hepatic)
venule

Central vein
Zone III
least
oxygenated
Zone II
Zone I
most
oxygenated

FIGURE 45–3. Zones in the acinus. *A,* The classic lobule includes all hepatocytes drained by a single central vein. At each corner of the hexagon are triads composed of branches of the hepatic artery, portal vein and bile duct. *B,* The portal lobule includes all hepatocytes drained by a bile ductule. *C,* This organization emphasizes the arterial blood supply to the hepatocytes and thus the oxygenation gradient between a branch of the hepatic artery and branches of the hepatic vein (i.e., central vein). The periportal hepatocytes of zone I immediately surround the portal tract and thus have the highest P_{O_2} and the most nutrients. They specialize in oxidative metabolism and certain other functions. The pericentral hepatocytes of zone III surround the central vein and have the lowest P_{O_2}. The zone-III hepatocytes specialize in biotransformations and drug detoxification. Zone II is an intermediate zone between zones I and III.

Hepatocytes Can Be Thought of As Being Arranged As Classic Hepatic Lobules, Portal Lobules, or Acinar Units

The complex structure of the liver makes it difficult to define a single unit—something analogous to the nephron in the kidney—that is capable of performing the functions of the entire liver. One way of viewing the organization of the liver is depicted in Figures 45–1 and 45–2, where we regarded the central vein as the core of the **classic hepatic lobule**. Thus, the classic hepatic lobule (Fig. 45–3A) includes all hepatocytes drained by a single central vein, and it is bounded by two or more portal triads. Alternatively, we can view the liver as though the triad is the core of a **portal lobule** (see Fig. 45–3B). Thus, the portal lobule includes all hepatocytes drained by a single bile ductule and is bounded by two or more central veins. A third way of viewing the liver is to group the hepatocytes according to their supply of arterial blood (Fig. 45–3C). Thus, the **portal acinus** is a small three-dimensional mass of hepatocytes that are irregular in size and shape, with one axis formed by a line between two triads (i.e., high P_{O_2}) and another axis formed by a line between two central veins (i.e., low P_{O_2}).

Periportal Hepatocytes Specialize In Oxidative Metabolism, Whereas Pericentral Hepatocytes Detoxify Drugs

Rappaport first proposed that a zonal relationship exists between cells that constitute the portal acini and their

blood supply (Fig. 45–3C). Hepatocytes close to the vascular core formed by the terminal portal venule and terminal hepatic arteriole are perfused first and thus receive the highest concentrations of oxygen and solutes. These **periportal** hepatocytes are said to reside in **zone I**, and as a consequence of their location, they are the most resistant to the effects of circulatory compromise or nutritional deficiency. They are also more resistant to other forms of cell injury and are the first to regenerate. Hepatocytes in the intermediate **zone II** and the most distal population of **pericentral** hepatocytes located near the terminal hepatic venule ("central vein") in **zone III** are sequentially perfused with blood that is already modified by the preceding hepatocytes; thus, they are exposed to progressively lower concentrations of nutrients and oxygen. The exact boundaries of these zones are difficult to define.

The concept of zonal heterogeneity of liver function has evolved as a result of these differences in access to substrate. Because of the specialized microenvironments of cells in different zones, some enzymes are preferentially expressed in one zone or another (Table 45–1). For example, in zone I, oxidative energy metabolism with β oxidation, amino acid metabolism, ureagenesis, gluconeogenesis, cholesterol synthesis, and bile formation is particularly important. Localized in zone III are glycogen synthesis from glucose, glycolysis, liponeogenesis, ketogenesis, xenobiotic metabolism, and glutamine formation. Molecular techniques have allowed an even more precise definition of which hepatocytes express particular mRNA and proteins. For example, the enzyme glutamine synthe-

TABLE 45–1

ZONAL HETEROGENEITY OF PREFERENTIAL HEPATOCYTE FUNCTION

ZONE I	ZONE III
Amino acid catabolism	Glycolysis
Gluconeogenesis	Glycogen synthesis from glucose
Glycogen degradation	Liponeogenesis
HMG-CoA reductase (cholesterol synthesis)	Cholesterol 7α-hydroxylase (bile acid biosynthesis)
Ureagenesis (all hepatocytes with exception of the last one or two rows encircling the hepatic venules)	Ketogenesis
Bile acid–dependent canalicular bile flow	Glutamine synthesis
Oxidative energy metabolism and probably β oxidation of fatty acids	Bile acid–independent canalicular bile flow
	Biotransformation of drugs

HMG-CoA, hydroxymethylglutaryl-coenzyme A.

tase is expressed exclusively in only one or two hepatocytes immediately adjacent to the hepatic venules. Hepatocytes of zone III also seem to be important for general detoxification mechanisms and the biotransformation of drugs. The zonal distribution of drug-induced toxicity manifested as cell necrosis may be attributed to zone III localization of the enzymatic pathways involved in the biotransformation of substrates by oxidation, reduction, or hydrolysis. Although it appears that each hepatocyte is potentially capable of multiple metabolic functions, the predominant enzymatic activity appears to result from adaptation to the microenvironment provided by the hepatic microcirculation. In some cases, it has been possible to reverse the zone I–to–zone III gradient of hepatocyte function by experimentally reversing the direction of blood supply (i.e., nutrient flow).

Bile Drains From Its Site of Secretion In the Canaliculi into Small Terminal Ductules, Then into Progressively Larger Ducts of the Biliary Tree, and Eventually into the Duodenum via a Single Large Common Duct

As noted earlier, the **canaliculi** into which bile is secreted form a three-dimensional polygonal meshwork of tubes between hepatocytes, with many anastomotic interconnections (see Fig. 45–1). From the canaliculi, the bile enters the small terminal bile ductules, the so-called **canals of Hering**, which have a basement membrane and in cross section are surrounded by three to six ductal epithelial cells or hepatocytes (Fig. 45–4A). The canals of Hering then empty into a system of **perilobular ducts**, which in

turn drain into interlobular bile ducts. The **interlobular bile ducts** form a richly anastomosing network that closely surrounds the branches of the portal vein. These bile ducts are lined by a layer of cuboidal or columnar epithelium that has a microvillous architecture on its luminal surface. The cells have a prominent Golgi apparatus and numerous vesicles, which probably participate in the exchange of substances among the cytoplasm, bile, and blood plasma through exocytosis and endocytosis.

The interlobular bile ducts unite to form larger and larger ducts, first the septal ducts and then the lobar ducts, two hepatic ducts, and finally a common hepatic duct (see Fig. 45–4B). Along the biliary tree, the biliary epithelial cells, or **cholangiocytes**, are similar in their fine structure except for size and height. However, emerging evidence suggests that they differ in their complement of transporters and receptors. Increasing emphasis has been placed on the absorptive and secretory properties of the biliary epithelial cells, properties that contribute significantly to the process of bile formation. As with other epithelial cells, cholangiocytes are highly cohesive, with the lateral plasma membranes of contiguous cells forming tortuous interdigitations. Tight junctions seal contacts between cells that are close to the luminal region and thus limit the exchange of water and solutes between plasma and bile.

The **common hepatic duct** emerges from the porta hepatis after the union of the right and left hepatic ducts. It merges with the cystic duct emanating from the gallbladder to form the common bile duct. In adults, the **common bile duct** is quite large, approximately 7 cm in length and around 0.5 to 1.5 cm in diameter. In most individuals, the common bile duct and the pancreatic duct merge before forming a common antrum known as the **ampulla of Vater**. At the point of transit through the duodenal wall, this common channel is surrounded by a thickening of both the longitudinal and the circular layers of smooth muscle, the so-called **sphincter of Oddi**. This sphincter constricts the lumen of the bile duct and thus regulates the flow of bile.

The Gallbladder Is a Concentrative and Storage Reservoir That Can Deliver Bile Acid in High Concentration and in a Controlled Manner to the Duodenum for the Solubilization of Dietary Lipid

The gallbladder lies in a fossa beneath the right lobe of the liver. This distensible pear-shaped structure has a capacity of 30 to 50 ml in adults. The absorptive surface of the gallbladder is enhanced by numerous prominent folds that are important for concentrative transport activity, as discussed later. The gallbladder is connected at its neck to the **cystic duct**, which empties into the common bile duct (see Fig. 45–4B). The cystic duct maintains continuity with the surface columnar epithelium, lamina propria, muscularis, and serosa of the gallbladder. Instead of a sphincter, the gallbladder has, at its neck, a spiral valve (valve of Heister) formed by the mucous membrane. This valve regulates flow into and out of the gallbladder.

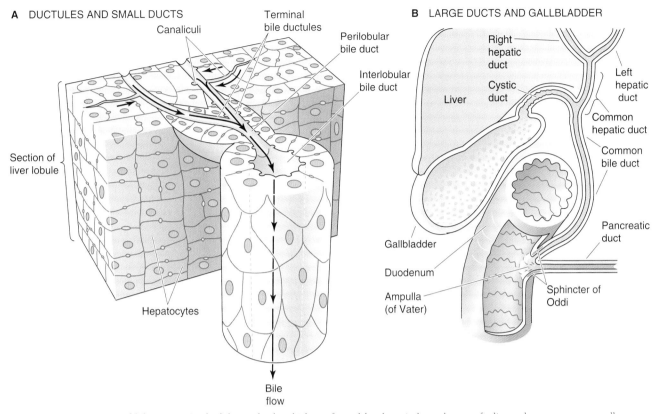

A DUCTULES AND SMALL DUCTS

Canaliculi

Terminal bile ductules

Perilobular bile duct

Interlobular bile duct

Section of liver lobule

Hepatocytes

Bile flow

B LARGE DUCTS AND GALLBLADDER

Right hepatic duct

Left hepatic duct

Liver

Cystic duct

Common hepatic duct

Common bile duct

Pancreatic duct

Gallbladder

Duodenum

Ampulla (of Vater)

Sphincter of Oddi

FIGURE 45–4. Structure of biliary tree. *A*, The bile canaliculi, which are formed by the apical membranes of adjacent hepatocytes, eventually merge with terminal bile ductules (canals of Hering). The ductules eventually merge into perilobular ducts, and then interlobular ducts. *B*, The interlobular ducts merge into septal ducts, lobar ducts, and eventually the right and left hepatic ducts, which combine as the common hepatic duct. The confluence of the common hepatic and the cystic ducts gives rise to the common bile duct. The common bile duct may merge with the pancreatic duct and form the ampulla of Vater before entering the duodenum, as shown in the figure, or have a completely independent lumen. In either case, there is a common sphincter—the sphincter of Oddi—that simultaneously regulates flow out of the common bile duct and the pancreatic duct.

UPTAKE, PROCESSING, AND SECRETION OF COMPOUNDS BY HEPATOCYTES

The liver metabolizes an enormous variety of compounds that are brought to it by the portal and systemic circulations. These compounds include endogenous molecules (e.g., bile salts and bilirubin, which are key ingredients of bile) and exogenous molecules, such as drugs and toxins. The hepatocyte handles these molecules in four major steps (Fig. 45–5*A*): (1) the hepatocyte imports the compound from the blood across its basolateral (i.e., sinusoidal) membrane, (2) the hepatocyte transports the material within the cell, (3) the hepatocyte may chemically modify or degraded the compound intracellularly, and (4) the hepatocyte excretes the molecule or its product or products into the bile across the apical (i.e., canalicular) membrane. Thus, compounds are secreted in a vectorial manner through the hepatocyte.

An Na-K Pump at the Basolateral Membrane of Hepatocytes Provides the Energy for Transporting a Wide Variety of Solutes via Channels and Transporters

Like other epithelial cells, the hepatocyte is endowed with a host of transporters that are necessary for basic housekeeping functions. To the extent that these transporters are restricted to either the apical or basolateral membrane, they have the potential of participating in net transepithelial transport. For example, the Na-K pump (p. 61) at the basolateral membrane of hepatocytes maintains a low $[Na^+]_i$ and high $[K^+]_i$ (see Fig. 45–5*B*). A basolateral, adenosine triphosphate (ATP)-dependent Ca^{2+} pump maintains $[Ca^{2+}]_i$ at an extremely low level, approximately 100 nM, as in other cells. The hepatocyte uses the inwardly directed Na^+ gradient to fuel a variety of active transporters, such as the Na-H exchanger, Na/HCO_3 cotransporter, and Na^+-driven amino acid transporters. As discussed later, the Na^+ gradient also drives one of the bile acid transporters. The hepatocyte takes up glucose via the GLUT2 facilitated-diffusion mechanism (p. 60), which is insensitive to regulation by insulin.

The resting basolateral membrane has a voltage (V_m) of −30 to −40 mV and is endowed with both K^+ and Cl^- channels. Basolateral K^+ conductance helps maintain a negative V_m; the resting V_m is considerably more positive than the equilibrium potential for K^+ (E_K) because of the presence of numerous "leak" pathways, such as the aforementioned electrogenic Na^+-driven transporters, as well as channels for ions other than K^+. For example, Cl^- is passively distributed (i.e., $E_{Cl} = V_m$).

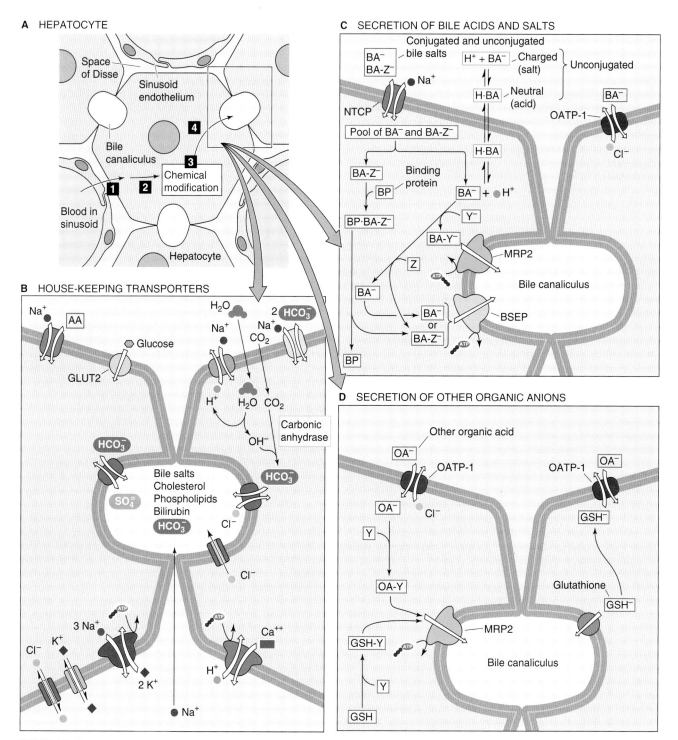

FIGURE 45–5. Transporters in hepatocyte. *A,* The hepatocyte can process compounds in four steps: (1) uptake from blood across the basolateral (i.e., sinusoidal) membrane; (2) transport within the cell; (3) control chemical modification or degradation; and (4) export into the bile across the apical (i.e., canalicular) membrane. *B,* The hepatocyte has a full complement of transporters for maintaining a low $[Na^+]_i$, a high $[K^+]_i$, and a low $[Ca^{2+}]_i$. Various channels establish the membrane voltage. Various acid-base transporters regulate intracellular pH. *C,* Bile acids can enter the hepatocyte in any of several forms: the unconjugated salt (BA^-); the neutral, protonated bile acid ($H \cdot BA$); the bile salt conjugated to taurine or glycine ($BA-Z^-$, where Z represents taurine or glycine). The three pathways for bile acid entry across the basolateral membrane are the Na^+-driven transporter NTCP, which prefers $BA-Z^-$, but also carries BA^-; nonionic diffusion of $H \cdot BA$; and the anion exchanger OATP-1. Binding proteins (BP) may ferry conjugated bile acids across the cytoplasm. Some bile acids are conjugated to sulfate or glucuronate (Y); these exit the cell across the canalicular membrane via the MRP2 transporter. Most bile acids are conjugated to glycine or taurine (Z) prior to their extrusion into the bile via BSEP, an ATP-driven member of the ABC class of proteins. *D,* Organic anions (including bile acids and bilirubin) may enter across the basolateral membrane via OATP-1. After conjugation with sulfate or glucuronate (Y), these compounds may be extruded into the bile by MRP2, an ATP-driven member of the ABC class of proteins. Glutathione (GSH) synthesized in the hepatocyte, after conjugation to Y, can enter the canaliculus via MRP2. Unconjugated GSH can enter the canaliculus via an unidentified transporter. About 90% of the GSH found in the blood exits the hepatocytes across the basolateral membrane via OATP-1. ATP, adenosine triphosphate; BSEP, bile salt export pump; MRP2, multidrug resistance–associated protein 2; OATP, organic anion transport protein.

Hepatocytes Use Several Carrier Mechanisms to Take Up Bile Acids, Other Organic Anions, and Organic Cations Across Their Basolateral (Sinusoidal) Membranes

BILE ACIDS AND SALTS. The primary bile acids are cholic acid and chenodeoxycholic acid, both of which are synthesized by hepatocytes, as described later (Fig. 45–9). Other "secondary" bile acids form in the intestinal tract as bacteria dehydroxylate the primary bile acids. Because the pK values of the primary bile acids are near neutrality, a high fraction of the bile acid molecules are neutral; that is, they are *bile acids* (H · BA), and thus not very water soluble. Of course, some of these molecules are deprotonated, and thus are *bile salts* (BA⁻). The liver may conjugate the primary bile acids and salts to glycine or taurine ("Z" in Fig. 45–5C), as well as to sulfate or glucuronate ("Y" in Fig. 45–5C). Most of the bile acids that the liver secretes into the bile are conjugated, such as taurocholate (the result of conjugating cholic acid to taurine). These conjugated derivatives have a negative charge, and thus they, too, are *bile salts* (BA-Z⁻ and BA-Y⁻). Bile salts are far more water soluble than the corresponding bile acids.

Because the small intestine absorbs some bile acids and salts, they appear in the blood plasma, mainly bound to albumin, and are presented to the hepatocytes for re-uptake. This recycling of bile acids, an example of **enterohepatic circulation**, is discussed later (Fig. 45–13). Dissociation from albumin occurs before uptake. Surprisingly, the presence of albumin actually stimulates Na⁺-dependent taurocholate uptake, perhaps by increasing the affinity of the transporter for taurocholate.

Uptake of bile acids has been studied extensively and is mediated predominantly by an Na⁺-coupled transporter known as Na-taurocholate cotransporting polypeptide (NTCP) (Fig. 45–5C). This transporter is a 50-kDa glycosylated protein, and it appears to have seven membrane-spanning segments. NTCP handles unconjugated bile acids, but it has a particularly high affinity for conjugated bile acids. In addition, NTCP can also transport other compounds, including neutral steroids (e.g., progesterone, 17β-estradiol sulfate), cyclic oligopeptides (e.g., amanitidine and phalloidin), and a wide variety of drugs (e.g., verapamil, furosemide).

As is the case for other transporters, NTCP activity is low in the fetus and neonate and increases with development.

Although NTCP also carries unconjugated bile acids, as much as 50% of these *unconjugated* bile acids may enter the hepatocyte by passive nonionic diffusion (Fig. 45–5B). Because unconjugated bile acids are weak acids of the form

Equation 45–1

$$H \cdot BA \rightleftharpoons H^+ + BA^-$$

the neutral H · BA form can diffuse into the cell. Conjugation of bile acids enhances their hydrophilicity (taurine more so than glycine) and promotes dissociation of the proton from the side chain (i.e., lowering the pK_a), thus raising the concentration of BA⁻. Both properties decrease the ability of bile acid to traverse membranes via passive nonionic diffusion.

ORGANIC ANIONS. The organic anion transport protein **OATP-1** (Fig. 45–5D) is a 75-kDa glycosylated protein that mediates the uptake of bile acids and other organic anions (e.g. bromosulphthalein). It probably contributes little to bilirubin uptake. The ion dependencies of this transporter are quite different from those of NTCP. OATP-1 exchanges Cl⁻ for the anionic form of the bile acid, but the exchange is independent of Na⁺. A second transporter, **OATP-2** (also known as PGT; p. 69), transports various prostanoids (e.g., prostaglandin E₂ [PGE₂], PGF₂α, and thromboxane B₂ [TxB₂]), but not arachidonic acid. Unlike OATP-1, OATP-2 is widely distributed. It is uncertain whether other Na⁺-independent transporters, such as anion exchangers, take up bile acids.

Thus, basolateral uptake of **bile acids** into the hepatocyte is a complex process that involves both an Na⁺-dependent transporter (NTCP) and an Na⁺-*in*dependent transporter (OATP-1), as well as nonionic diffusion of unconjugated bile acids.

BILIRUBIN. Senescent erythrocytes are taken up by macrophages in the reticuloendothelial system, where the degradation of hemoglobin leads to the release of bilirubin into the blood (Fig. 45–6A) (see the box titled Jaundice). Bilirubin arrives at the liver bound to albumin, and uptake of bilirubin across the basolateral membrane of the hepatocyte may be accomplished by as many as three mechanisms (Fig. 45–6B). The first (and minor) component may be Cl⁻-dependent uptake of bilirubin by OATP-1, as mentioned earlier. The second is some electroneutral mechanism. The third is thought to be electrogenic uptake of anionic bilirubin by bilitranslocase, a 37-kDa basolateral membrane protein. Bilitranslocase is also involved in the uptake of nicotinic acid and the antibiotic rifamycin, but not bile acids.

ORGANIC CATIONS. The major organic cations transported by the liver are aromatic and aliphatic amines, including such important drugs as cholinergics, local anesthetics, and antibiotics, as well as endogenous solutes such as choline, thiamine, and nicotinamide (Fig. 45–7). The basolateral membrane of the hepatocyte contains two functionally characterized transport systems, namely, a system for small (i.e., type I) and a system for bulky (i.e., type II) organic cations. OCT1, also present in the kidney (p. 61), mediates the electrogenic uptake of small organic cations (type I). A multispecific transporter that is a product of the *Oatp1* gene to some extent mediates the basolateral uptake of bulky organic cations (type II). Physiological studies have identified proton–organic cation exchangers at both the basolateral and the canalicular membranes; however, the molecular identities of these transporters are currently unknown.

NEUTRAL ORGANIC COMPOUNDS. This group of molecules is also taken up by an Na⁺-independent, energy-dependent process, but the nature of the driving force is not known. The best characterized substrate is ouabain, uptake of which is inhibited by other neutral steroids, such as cortisol, aldosterone, estradiol, and testosterone.

A HEME METABOLISM

B BILIRUBIN SECRETION

FIGURE 45–6. Excretion of bilirubin. *A*, Macrophages phagocytose senescent red blood cells and break the heme down to bilirubin, which travels in the blood, linked to albumin, to the liver. The conversion to the colorless urobilinogen occurs in the terminal ileum and colon, whereas the oxidation to the yellowish urobilin occurs in the urine. *B*, The hepatocyte takes up bilirubin across its basolateral membrane by three mechanisms and then conjugates the bilirubin with one or two glucuronic acid residues. The cell then exports this conjugated form of bilirubin into the bile. After being secreted in the bile, some of the bilirubin glucuronide is converted back to bilirubin by bacteria in the terminal ileum and colon. This bilirubin is further converted to the colorless urobilinogen. If it remains in the colon, the compound is further converted to stercobilin, which is the main pigment of feces. If the urobilinogen enters the plasma and is filtered by the kidney, it is converted to urobilin and gives urine its characteristic yellow color.

FIGURE 45–7. Excretion of organic cations. Small organic cations (type I) enter the hepatocyte across the basolateral (i.e., sinusoidal) membrane via OCT1. Bulky organic cations (type II) enter via a product of the *Oatpl* gene. Organic cations may also enter via a proton-organic–cation exchanger. The organic cations exit the hepatocyte across the apical (i.e., canalicular) membrane via members of the MDR (multidrug resistance) family. It is not clear how important the proton-organic–cation exchanger is for exporting organic cations across the canalicular membrane. ER, endoplasmic reticulum; MRP2, multidrug resistance–associated protein 2; OCT, organic cation transporter; UGT, uridine glucuronosyl transferase.

We will return to Figures 45–5, 45–6, and 45–7 later, when we discuss the movement of solutes into the bile canaliculus.

Inside the Hepatocyte, the Basolateral-to-Apical Movement of Many Compounds Occurs by Vesicular or Protein-Bound Routes

BILE SALTS. Some compounds traverse the cell while bound to intracellular **"binding" proteins** (see Fig. 45–5C). The binding may serve to trap the molecule within the cell or may be involved in intracellular transport. For bile salts, three such proteins have been identified. In humans, the main bile-acid–binding protein appears to be the hepatic **dihydrodiol dehydrogenase**, one of a large family of dehydrogenases, the catalytic and binding properties of which are organ and species specific. The two others are **glutathione-S-transferase B** and **fatty-acid–binding protein**. Intracellular sequestration of bile salts by these proteins may serve an important role in bile acid transport or regulation of bile acid synthesis. Transcellular diffusion of bile salts bound to proteins can be detected within seconds after bile salts are applied to hepatocytes; this mechanism may be the primary mode of cytoplasmic transport under basal conditions.

Intracellular transport of bile salts may also follow the microtubule-dependent **vesicular pathway**, which is

slower and recruited at higher bile-salt loads. Furthermore, the type of bile salt may influence its primary transcellular pathway. For example, a vesicular pathway may be involved in the transcellular traffic of *mono*anionic bile salts, whereas *di*anionic bile salts may traverse the cell via binding proteins.

BILIRUBIN. After uptake at the basolateral membrane, unconjugated bilirubin is transported to the endoplasmic reticulum (ER), where it is conjugated to glucuronic acid (see Fig. 45–6). Because the resulting bilirubin glucuronide is markedly hydrophobic, it was thought that intracellular transport was mediated by binding proteins such as glutathione transferase B. Recently, however, spontaneous transfer of bilirubin between phospholipid vesicles has been observed to occur by rapid movement through the aqueous phase, in the absence of soluble proteins. It has, therefore, been suggested that direct membrane-to-membrane transfer is the principal mode of bilirubin transport within the hepatocyte. In addition, the membrane-to-membrane flux of bilirubin is biased toward the membrane with the higher cholesterol/phospholipid ratio. Hence, the inherent gradient for cholesterol from the basolateral membrane to the ER membrane may direct the flux of bilirubin to the ER.

In Phase I of the Biotransformation of Organic Anions and Other Compounds, Hepatocytes Use Mainly Cytochrome P-450 Enzymes

The liver is responsible for the metabolism and detoxification of many endogenous and exogenous compounds. Some compounds (e.g., proteins and other ligands) taken up by hepatocytes are completely digested within lysosomes. Specific carriers exist for the lysosomal uptake of sialic acid, cysteine, and vitamin B_{12}. Clinical syndromes resulting from an absence of these carriers have also been identified. The lysosomal acid hydrolases cleave sulfates, fatty acids, and sugar moieties from larger molecules.

Hepatocytes handle other compounds by biotransformation reactions that usually occur in two phases. Phase I reactions represent oxidation or reduction reactions in large part catalyzed by the P-450 cytochromes. The diverse array of phase I reactions include hydroxylation, dealkylation, dehalogenation, and others. The common feature of all of these reactions is that one atom of oxygen is inserted into the substrate. Hence these monooxygenases make the substrate a more polar compound, poised for further modification by a phase II reaction. For example, when the phase I reaction creates a hydroxyl group, the phase II reaction may increase the water solubility of ROH by conjugating it to a highly hydrophilic compound such as glucuronate, sulfate, or gluthathione:

Equation 45–2

$$RH \xrightarrow{\text{Phase I}} ROH \xrightarrow{\text{Phase II}} RO\text{-Conjugate}$$

Finally, the conjugated compound is secreted into the blood or bile.

JAUNDICE

Jaundice denotes a yellowish discoloration of body tissues, most notable in the skin and sclera of the eyes. The condition is caused by an accumulation of bilirubin in extracellular fluid, either in free form or after conjugation. Bilirubin is a yellow-green pigment that is the principal degradation product of heme (Fig. 45–6A), the iron-binding portion of hemoglobin. Approximately 65% to 80% of total bilirubin production is derived from the hemoglobin of senescent red cells. Because of avid extraction and conjugation by the liver, the normal plasma concentration of bilirubin, which is mostly of the unconjugated variety, is approximately 0.5 mg/dl or lower. The skin or eyes may begin to appear jaundiced when the bilirubin level rises to 1.5 to 3 mg/dl.

Hemoglobin released into the circulation is phagocytized by macrophages throughout the body and split into globin and heme. Cleavage of the heme ring releases both free iron, which is transported in the blood by transferrin, and a straight chain of 4-pyrrole nuclei (Fig. 45–6A), which is the precursor from which bilirubin is eventually formed. The first product is the compound **biliverdin,** which is rapidly reduced to free bilirubin. This form of bilirubin is often referred to as free or **unconjugated bilirubin** to distinguish it from bilirubin conjugated to glucuronic acid. After release into the circulation, the pigment becomes reversibly bound to albumin and is avidly removed from plasma by the liver (Fig. 45–6B). In the course of its vectorial transport into bile by the hepatocyte, bilirubin is esterified with glucuronic acid to form monoconjugated and diconjugated derivatives. The unconjugated form of bilirubin is extremely insoluble, and the process of conjugation facilitates its excretion into bile. **Conjugated bilirubin** is more soluble and thus suitable for excretion by the liver, but it cannot be absorbed by the biliary or intestinal epithelia.

Jaundice occurs under several circumstances. Increased destruction of red blood cells or hemolysis may occur with rapid release of free, unconjugated bilirubin into the circulation. **Unconjugated hyperbilirubinemia** occurs commonly in neonates not only because of increased production of heme but also because of the immaturity of the pathways for glucuronidation in the liver. Obstruction of the bile ducts or damage to the liver may also result in jaundice. In this setting, **conjugated bilirubin** produced by the liver cannot be excreted in bile and consequently refluxes back into the systemic circulation. Therefore, most of the bilirubin in plasma is the highly soluble conjugated bilirubin, a small amount of which can be filtered by the kidneys, rather than the poorly soluble free form of bilirubin, which is mostly bound to albumin and not excreted by the kidneys. Thus, in obstructive jaundice, conjugated bilirubin imparts a dark yellow color to the urine. Measurement of free and conjugated bilirubin in serum serves as a sensitive test for detecting liver disease.

Under normal conditions, about half of the bilirubin reaching the intestinal lumen is metabolized by bacteria into the colorless **urobilinogen** (see Fig. 45–6A). About 20% of this soluble compound may be reabsorbed through the intestinal mucosa into the portal circulation, extracted by the liver, and then re-excreted by the liver into the gastrointestinal tract. A small fraction (~20% of daily urobilinogen production) may be excreted by the kidneys into the urine. Urobilinogen may be detected in urine by using a clinical dipstick test. On exposure to air, urobilinogen becomes oxidized to yield **urobilin;** in the feces, urobilinogen is metabolized to yield the pigment **stercobilin.** In obstructive jaundice, no bilirubin reaches the intestine to be converted into urobilinogen, and therefore no urobilinogen is reabsorbed into the blood to be available for excretion by the kidney. As a result, tests for urobilinogen in urine are negative in obstructive jaundice. Because of the lack of stercobilin and other bile pigments in obstructive jaundice, the stool becomes clay colored.

The major enzymes involved in phase I reactions are the **P-450 cytochromes**. Cytochromes are colored proteins that contain heme for use in the transfer of electrons. Some cytochromes—not the P-450 system—are essential for the electron transport events that culminate in oxidative phosphorylation in the mitochondria. The P-450 cytochromes, so named because they absorb light at 450 nm when bound to CO, are a diverse, but related group of enzymes that reside mainly in the ER and typically catalyze **hydroxylation** reactions. Over 150 P-450 isoforms have been characterized.

In this text, we encounter P-450 oxidases in two sets of organs. In cells that synthesize steroid hormones—the adrenal cortex (p. 1052), testes (p. 1128), ovary (p. 1153), and placenta (p. 1179)—P-450 oxidases are localized either in the mitochondria or the ER, where they catalyze various steps in steroidogenesis. In the liver, these enzymes are located in the ER, where they catalyze a vast array of hydroxylation reactions involving the me-

tabolism of drugs and chemical carcinogens, bile acid synthesis, and the activation and inactivation of vitamins. The same reactions occur in other tissues, such as the intestines and the lungs.

Hepatic microsomal P-450 enzymes have similar molecular weights (48 to 56 kDa). The functional protein is a holoenzyme that consists of an apoprotein and a heme prosthetic group. The apoprotein region confers substrate specificity, which differs among the many P-450 enzymes. These substrates include RH moieties that are as wide ranging as the terminal methyl group of fatty acids, carbons in the rings of steroid molecules, complex heterocyclic compounds, and phenobarbital. In general, phase I processes add or expose a functional group, a hydroxyl group in the case of the P-450 oxidases, which renders the molecule reactive with phase II enzymes. The metabolic products of phase I may be directly excreted, but more commonly, because of only a modest increment in solubility, further metabolism by phase II reactions is required.

In Phase II of Biotransformation, Hepatocytes Conjugate the Products of Phase I to Make Them More Water Soluble for Secretion into Blood or Bile

In phase II, the hepatocyte conjugates the metabolites generated in phase I to produce more hydrophilic compounds, such as glucuronides, sulfates, and mercapturic acids. These phase II products are readily secreted into the blood or bile. Conjugation reactions are generally considered to be the critical step in detoxification. Either a defect in a particular enzyme, which may result from a genetic defect, or saturation of the enzyme with excess substrate may result in a decrease in the overall elimination of a compound. One example is the "gray syndrome," a potentially fatal condition that occurs after the administration of chloramphenicol to newborns who have low glucuronidation capacity. Infants have an ashen gray appearance and become weak and apathetic, and complete circulatory collapse may ensue.

Hepatocytes use three major conjugation reactions:

CONJUGATION TO GLUCURONATE. The **uridine diphosphate glucuronosyl transferases** (UGTs), which reside in the SER of the liver, are divided into two families based on their substrate specificity. Family 1 consists of at least four members and is encoded by genes that are located on chromosome 2. These UGTs catalyze the conjugation of glucuronic acid with phenols or bilirubin (Fig. 45–6B). Family 2 contains at least five UGTs that are encoded by genes on chromosome 4. These UGTs catalyze the glucuronidation of steroids or bile acids. Because family 1 UGTs are essential for the dual conjugation of bilirubin (Fig. 45–6B) and because only *conjugated* bilirubin can be excreted in bile, congenital absence of bilirubin-UGT activity results in jaundice from birth

and bilirubin encephalopathy, as can be seen in patients with Crigler-Najjar type I syndrome.

CONJUGATION TO SULFATE. The **sulfotransferases**—which are located in the cytosol rather than in the SER—catalyze the sulfation of steroids, catechols, and foreign compounds such as alcohol and metabolites of carcinogenic hydrocarbons. Their substrate specificity is greater than that of the UGTs. The different cellular localization of these two groups of enzymes suggests that they act in a cooperative rather than competitive fashion. In general, sulfates are not toxic and are readily eliminated, with the exception of sulfate esters of certain carcinogens.

CONJUGATION TO GLUTATHIONE. Hepatocytes also conjugate a range of compounds to reduced glutathione (GSH) for excretion and later processing in either the bile ducts or kidney (Fig. 45–8). **Glutathione** is a tripeptide composed of glutamate γ-linked to cysteine, which in turn is α-linked to glycine. The liver has the highest concentration of glutathione (~5 mM), with approximately 90% found in the cytoplasm and 10% in the mitochondria. **Glutathione-S-transferases**, which are mainly cytosolic, catalyze the conjugation of a number of substrates to the cysteine moiety of GSH. Substrates include the electrophilic metabolites of lipophilic compounds (e.g., epoxides of polycyclic aromatic hydrocarbons), products of lipid peroxidation, and alkyl and aryl halides. In some cases, the conjugates are then secreted into bile and further modified by removing the glutamyl residue from the glutathione by γ-glutamyl transpeptidase on the bile duct epithelial cell. The fate of glutathione-*S*-conjugates in bile is largely unknown. Some (e.g., the leukotrienes) undergo enterohepatic circulation. In other cases, the glutathione conjugates are secreted into plasma and filtered by the kidney, where a γ-glutamyl transpepti-

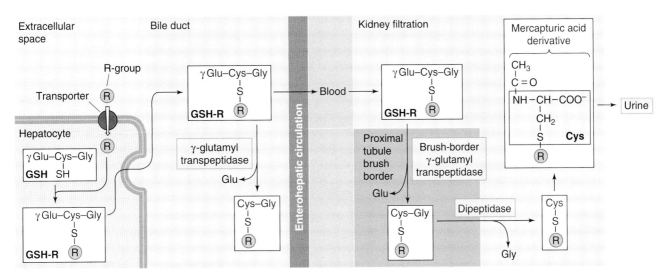

FIGURE 45–8. Conjugation to glutathione (GSH) and formation of mercapturic acids. The hepatocyte detoxifies compounds by chemically linking ("conjugating") them to small molecules, such as GSH, which is a tripeptide. The first step is for glutathione-S-transferase to couple the target compound (R) to the S on the cysteine residue of GSH. After MRP2 transports this GSH conjugate into the canalicular lumen (see Fig. 45–5D), a γ-glutamyl transpeptidase may remove the terminal glutamate residue. Alternatively, the conjugate may reach the blood and be filtered by the kidney where a γ-glutamyl transpeptidase at the brush border and a dipeptidase generate a cysteine derivative of R. Acetylation yields the mercapturic acid derivative, which appears in the urine. MRP2, multidrug resistance–associated protein 2.

dase on the proximal tubule brush border again removes the glutamyl residue. Next, a dipeptidase removes the glycine residue to produce a cysteine-S-conjugate. The cysteine-S-conjugate is either excreted in the urine or acetylated in the kidney or liver to form a mercapturic acid derivative, which is also excreted in the urine.

Although glutathione conjugation is generally considered to be a detoxification reaction, several such conjugates undergo activation into highly reactive intermediates.

OTHER CONJUGATIONS. Other forms of conjugation include methylation (e.g., catechols, amines, and thiols), acetylation (e.g., amines and hydrazines), and conjugation (e.g., bile acids) with amino acids such as taurine, glycine, or glutamine.

The involvement of multiple enzyme systems in these detoxification reactions facilitates the rapid removal of toxic species and provides alternative pathways in the event of failure of the preferred detoxification mechanism.

Hepatocytes Secrete Bile Acids, Organic Anions, and Organic Cations Across Their Apical (Canalicular) Membrane by Channels and Transporters

At the apical membrane, the transport of compounds is generally unidirectional, from cell to canalicular lumen. An exception is certain precious solutes, such as amino acids and adenosine, which are reabsorbed from bile by Na^+-dependent secondary active-transport systems.

BILE SALTS. Bile-salt transport from hepatocyte to canalicular lumen (Fig. 45–5C) occurs via an ATP-dependent transporter called BSEP (bile-salt export pump), also known as SPGP (sister of P-glycoprotein). Like the multidrug resistance protein (MDR)—also known as P-glycoprotein—BSEP is a member of the ABC (ATP-binding cassette) protein family (p. 65). BSEP has a very high affinity for taurocholate. The electrical charge of the side chain is an important determinant of canalicular transport inasmuch as only negatively charged bile salts are effectively excreted. Secretion of bile salts occurs against a significant cell-to-canaliculus concentration gradient, which may range from 1:100 to 1:1000.

ORGANIC ANIONS. Organic anions that are *not bile salts* move from the cytoplasm of the hepatocyte to the canalicular lumen via MRP2 (multidrug resistance–associated protein 2), also known as canalicular multispecific organic anion transporter (cMOAT) (Fig. 45–5D). MRP2 is electrogenic and ATP dependent, but distinct from BSEP. MRP2 has a broad substrate specificity (Table 45–2). Its substrates include bilirubin diglucuronide, sulfated bile acids, and glucuronidated bile acids. In general, transported substrates must have a hydrophobic core and at least two negative charges separated by a specific distance. MRP2 is critical for the transport of GSH conjugates across the canalicular membrane into bile. Although MRP2 has a low affinity for GSH, other mechanisms for GSH transport probably exist as suggested by functional studies. Several animal models have defective MRP2; all these strains have hyperbilirubinemia, which corresponds

TABLE 45–2

SUBSTRATES FOR MRP2

Bilirubin glucuronides

Dianionic bile salts

Glucuronosyl estradiol

Cysteinyl leukotrienes

Glutathione disulfide

Many glucuronate, glutathione, and sulfate conjugates

MRP2, multidrug resistance–associated protein 2.

phenotypically to the Dubin-Johnson syndrome in humans. Other anions, such as HCO_3^- and SO_4^{2-}, are excreted by anion exchangers.

ORGANIC CATIONS. Biliary excretion of organic cations is poorly understood, with the exception of transport that is mediated by the MDR proteins like BSEP that we discussed earlier, the hepatic MDR proteins belong to a larger ABC family of transporters that are energized by ATP hydrolysis (p. 65).

At least two MDR proteins, MDR1 and MDR3, are present in the canalicular membrane, where they mediate the excretion of some organic cations into the bile canaliculus (Fig. 45–7). The nomenclature of the MDRs is especially confusing because different and conflicting numbering systems have been used for different species; we will use the human numbering system. **MDR1** secretes bulky organic cations, including xenobiotics, cytotoxins, anticancer drugs, and other drugs (e.g., colchicine, quinidine, verapamil, cyclosporine). **MDR3** is a "flippase" that promotes the active translocation of phosphatidylcholine from the inner to the outer leaflet of the canalicular membrane. The bile salts then extract this phosphatidylcholine from the outer leaflet so that it becomes a component of bile, where it participates in micelle formation. Indeed, in humans with an inherited deficiency of MDR3, a progressive liver disease develops, characterized by extremely low concentrations of phospholipids in the bile.

Other organic cations appear to be secreted into the canaliculus by a transport process driven by a pH gradient (Fig. 45–7). The presence of an electroneutral H/organic cation exchanger has been demonstrated at the canalicular membrane. However, the importance of this process is uncertain because major H^+ gradients probably do not exist in the bile canaliculus. In some cases, it appears that organic cations passively move across the apical membrane into the canaliculus, where they are sequestered by biliary micelles.

Hepatocytes Take Up Proteins Across Their Basolateral Membrane Both by Specific Receptor-Mediated Endocytosis and by Nonspecific Fluid-Phase Endocytosis

The hepatocyte takes up macromolecules, such as plasma proteins, from the blood plasma via endocytosis, transports these molecules across the cytoplasm, and then secretes them into the bile via exocytosis. Three forms of endocytosis have been identified in the basolateral (sinusoidal) membrane: fluid-phase endocytosis, adsorptive endocytosis, and receptor-mediated endocytosis.

Fluid-phase endocytosis involves the uptake of a small amount of extracellular fluid, with its solutes, and is a result of the constitutive process of membrane invagination and internalization (p. 42). The process is nondiscriminatory and inefficient.

Adsorptive endocytosis involves nonspecific binding of the protein to the plasma membrane before endocytosis, resulting in more efficient protein uptake.

Receptor-mediated endocytosis is quantitatively the most important mechanism for the uptake of macromolecules (p. 42). After endocytosis, the receptor recycles to the plasma membrane, and the ligand may be excreted directly into bile by exocytosis or delivered to lysosomes for degradation. Receptor-mediated endocytosis is involved in the hepatic removal from the blood of proteins such as insulin, polymeric IgA, asialoglycoproteins, and epidermal growth factor.

BILE FORMATION

The Secretion of Canalicular Bile Is Active and Isotonic

The formation of bile occurs in three discrete steps. First, the hepatocytes actively secrete bile into the bile canaliculi. Second, intrahepatic and extrahepatic bile ducts not only transport this bile but also secrete into it a watery, HCO_3^--rich fluid. These first two steps may produce approximately 900 ml/day of so-called hepatic bile (Table 45–3). This production of hepatic bile is termed **choleresis**. Third, between meals, about half the hepatic bile— perhaps 450 ml/day—is diverted to the gallbladder, which stores the bile and isosmotically removes salts and water. The result is that the gallbladder concentrates the key remaining solutes in bile fluid—bile salts, bilirubin, cholesterol, and lecithin—by 10- to 20-fold. The 500 ml/day of bile that reaches the duodenum through the ampulla of Vater is thus a mixture of relatively "dilute" hepatic bile and "concentrated" gallbladder bile.

The first step in bile formation cannot be ultrafiltration because the hydrostatic pressure in the canaliculi is significantly higher than the sinusoidal perfusion pressure. This situation is in marked contrast to glomerular filtration by the kidney (see Chapter 33), which relies predominantly on passive hydrostatic forces for producing the fluid in Bowman's space. Instead, bile formation is an *active process*. It is sensitive to changes in temperature and to metabolic inhibitors. Bile formation by hepatocytes requires the active, energy-dependent secretion of inorganic and organic solutes into the canalicular lumen, followed by the passive movement of water. This movement of water through the tight junctions between hepatocytes carries with it other solutes by the process of solvent drag (p. 469). Canalicular bile is an isosmotic fluid, thus indicating that the intercellular junctions allow the passage of water and small ions. Further down the biliary tree (i.e., ducts and gallbladder), where the pore size of paracellular junctions is significantly smaller, solvent drag is not as important. Organic solutes do not readily enter bile distal to the canaliculi.

Major Organic Molecules in Bile Include Bile Acids, Cholesterol and Phospholipids

Bile has two important functions: (1) bile provides the sole excretory route for many solutes that are not excreted by the kidney, and (2) secreted bile salts and acids are required for normal lipid digestion (p. 963) and absorption (p. 965).

Both hepatic bile and gallbladder bile are complex secretions that are isosmotic with plasma (~300 mosmole/kg) and consist of water, inorganic electrolytes, and a variety of organic solutes, including bilirubin, cholesterol, fatty acids, and phospholipid (see Table 45–3). The predominant cation in bile is Na^+, and the major inorganic anions are Cl^- and HCO_3^-. Solutes whose presence in bile is functionally important include micelle-forming bile acids, phospholipids, and immunoglobulin A.

Bile acids promote dietary lipid absorption through their micelle-forming properties (p. 965). As shown in Figure 45–9, hepatocytes synthesize the so-called **primary bile acids**—cholic acid and chenodeoxycholic acid—from cholesterol. Indeed, biliary excretion of cholesterol and conversion of **cholesterol** to bile acids are the principal routes of cholesterol excretion and catabolism, thus making bile formation pivotal for total-body cholesterol balance. The first step in this conversion is catalyzed by cholesterol 7α-hydroxylase, a specific cyto-

TABLE 45–3

COMPOSITION OF BILE

PARAMETER	HEPATIC BILE	GALLBLADDER BILE
pH	7.5	6.0
Na^+ (mM)	141–165	220
K^+ (mM)	2.7–6.7	14
Ca^{2+} (mM)	1.2–3.2	15
Cl^- (mM)	77–117	31
HCO_3^- (mM)	12–55	19
Total phosphorus (g/liter)	0.15	1.4
Bile acids (g/liter)	3–45	32
Total fatty acids (g/liter)	2.7	24
Bilirubin (g/liter)	1–2	3
Phospholipids (g/liter)	1.4–8.1	34
Cholesterol (g/liter)	1–3.2	6.3
Proteins (g/liter)	2–20	4.5

Data from Boyer JL: Mechanisms of bile secretion and hepatic transport. In Andreoli TE, Hoffman JF, Fanestil DD, Schultz SG (eds): Physiology of Membrane Disorders. New York, Plenum, 1986.

FIGURE 45–9. Synthesis of bile acids. The liver converts cholesterol to the "primary bile acids"—cholic acid and chenodeoxycholic acid—in a series of 14 reactions occurring in four different cellular organelles. The first reaction is the 7α hydroxylation of cholesterol. In addition, the action of bacteria in the terminal ileum and colon may *de*hydroxylate bile acids, yielding the "secondary bile acids" deoxycholic acid and lithocholic acid. The hepatocytes conjugate most of the primary bile acids to small molecules such as glycine and taurine (not shown) before secreting them into the bile. In addition, those secondary bile acids that return to the liver via the enterohepatic circulation may also be conjugated to glycine or taurine, as shown in the figure. The liver may also conjugate some primary and secondary bile acids to sulfate or glucuronate (not shown).

chrome P-450 enzyme that is located in the SER. As we shall see later, **secondary bile acids** are the products of bacterial dehydroxylation in the terminal ileum and colon. After being absorbed and returning to the liver ("entero-hepatic circulation," discussed later), these secondary bile acids may also undergo conjugation. Figure 45–9 shows typical examples of conjugation reactions.

Phospholipids in bile help to solubilize cholesterol as well as diminish the cytotoxic effects of other bile acids on hepatocytes and bile duct cells. **Immunoglobulin A** inhibits bacterial growth in bile.

Excretory or **waste products** found in bile include cholesterol, bile pigments, trace minerals, plant sterols, lipophilic drugs and metabolites, antigen-antibody complexes, and oxidized glutathione.

Bile is also the excretory route for compounds that do not readily enter the renal glomerular filtrate, either because they are associated with proteins such as albumin or because they are associated with formed elements in blood. Although these compounds are generally lipo-philic, they also include the heavy metals. Some bile acids (e.g., the trihydroxy bile acid cholic acid) are only partly bound to serum albumin and may therefore enter the glomerular filtrate. However, they are actively reabsorbed by the renal tubule. In health, bile acids are virtually absent from the urine.

Canalicular Bile Flow Has a Constant Component Driven by the Secretion of Small Organic Molecules and a Component Driven by the Secretion of Bile Acids

Total bile flow is the sum of the bile flow from hepato-cytes into the canaliculi ("canalicular flow") and the addi-tional flow from cholangiocytes into the bile ducts ("duc-tular flow"). In most species, the rate of **canalicular bile secretion** (i.e., milliliters per minute) increases more or less linearly with the rate of bile acid secretion (i.e., moles per minute). Canalicular bile flow is the sum of two components (Fig. 45–10): (1) a "constant" component that is independent of bile acid secretion (bile acid–*independent* flow) and (2) a rising component that in-creases linearly with bile acid secretion (bile acid–*depen-dent* flow). In humans, most of the canalicular bile flow is bile acid dependent. If we now add the **ductular secre-tion**, which is also "constant," we have the **total bile flow** in Figure 45–10. We will discuss the canalicular secre-tion in the remainder of this section, and ductular secre-tion in the following section.

FIGURE 45–10. Components of bile flow.

BILE ACID–INDEPENDENT FLOW IN THE CANALICULI. The secretion of *organic* compounds probably provides the major driving force for bile acid–independent flow. For example, glutathione, present in bile in high concentrations, may generate a potent osmotic driving force for canalicular bile formation.

BILE ACID–DEPENDENT FLOW IN THE CANALICULI. The negatively charged bile salts in bile are in a micellar form and are—in a sense—large polyanions. Thus, they are effectively out of solution and have a low **osmotic activity coefficient**. However, the positively charged counterions accompanying these micellar bile acids are still in aqueous solution and may thus represent the predominant osmotic driving force for water movement in bile acid–dependent flow. If one infuses an animal with a nonphysiological bile acid that does not form micelles or one that forms micelles only at a rather high concentration, the osmotic activity will be higher and thus the exogenous bile acid will be more effective in producing bile acid–dependent flow. In other words, the slope of the *blue* "bile acid–dependent" line in Figure 45–10 would be steeper than for physiological bile acids.

Bile flow does not always correlate with the osmotic activity of the bile acid. In some cases, bile acids increase electrolyte and water flux by other mechanisms, such as by stimulating Na^+-coupled cotransport mechanisms or by modulating the activity of other solute transporters. For example, the bile acid ursodeoxycholic acid produces a substantial increase in bile flow by markedly stimulating biliary HCO_3^- excretion.

Bile acids in the lumen may also stimulate the secretion of other solutes by trapping them in the lumen. These solutes include bilirubin and other organic anions, as well as lipids such as cholesterol and phospholipids. The mixed micelles formed by the bile acids apparently sequester these other solutes, thus lowering their effective luminal concentration and favoring their entry. Thus, excretion of cholesterol and phospholipid is negligible when bile acid output is low, but it increases and approaches maximum values as bile acid output increases.

Secretin Stimulates the Cholangiocytes of Ductules and Ducts to Secrete a Watery, HCO_3^--Rich Fluid

As we saw in the previous section, biliary epithelial cells, or **cholangiocytes**, are the second major source of the fluid in hepatic bile. Experimentally, one can isolate cholangiocytes from normal liver or from the liver of experimental animals in which ductular hyperplasia has been induced by ligating the bile duct. These cholangiocytes have a number of transporters (Fig. 45–11), including an apical Cl-HCO_3 exchanger, and several apical Cl^- channels, including CFTR (p. 916). In a mechanism that may be similar to that in pancreatic duct cells (p. 914), the Cl-HCO_3 exchanger, in parallel with the Cl^- channels for Cl^- recycling, can secrete an HCO_3^--rich fluid.

A complex network of hormones, mainly acting via cAMP, regulate cholangiocyte secretory function. Secretin receptors (p. 902) are present on the basolateral mem-

FIGURE 45–11. Secretion of an HCO_3^--rich fluid by cholangiocytes. The apical step of HCO_3^- secretion by the duct cell is mediated by a Cl-HCO_3 exchanger. The Cl^- recycles back to the lumen via Cl^- channels, such as cystic fibrosis trans-membrane regulator (CFTR). The basolateral step of HCO_3^- secretion probably is mediated in part by the uptake of HCO_3^- via an electrogenic Na/HCO_3 cotransporter. The uptake of CO_2, combined with the extrusion of H^+ via an Na-H exchanger and an H^+ pump generates the rest of the HCO_3^- via carbonic anhydrase (CA). Secretin, glucagon, vasoactive intestinal peptide (VIP), and gastrin-releasing peptide (GRP) all are choleretics. Somatostatin either enhances fluid absorption or inhibits secretion.

branes of cholangiocytes, which explains why **secretin** produces a water-rich choleresis—that is, a bile rich in HCO_3^- (i.e., alkaline) but diluted in bile acids. Similarly, the hormones **glucagon** (p. 1081) and **VIP** (vasoactive intestinal peptide; p. 898) also produce an HCO_3^--rich choleresis at the level of the ducts. These hormones raise $[cAMP]_i$ and thus stimulate apical Cl^- channels and the Cl-HCO_3 exchanger. A Ca^{2+}-activated Cl^- channel is also present in the apical membrane.

Cholangiocytes are also capable of reabsorbing fluid and electrolytes, as suggested by the adaptation that occurs after removal of the gallbladder (i.e., cholecystectomy). Bile found within the common bile duct of cholecystectomized, fasting animals is similar in composition to the concentrated bile typically found in the gallbladder. Thus, the ducts have partially taken over the function of the gallbladder (see later).

The hormone **somatostatin** inhibits bile flow by lowering $[cAMP]_i$, an effect opposite that of secretin. This inhibition may be caused by enhancing fluid reabsorption by bile ducts or by inhibiting ductular secretion of the HCO_3^--rich fluid discussed earlier.

Solutes reabsorbed from bile by cholangiocytes can be returned to the hepatocyte for resecretion. As shown earlier in Figure 45–2, the intralobular bile ducts are endowed with a rich peribiliary vascular plexus that is supplied by the hepatic artery. The blood draining this plexus finds its way into the hepatic sinusoids. This plexus is analogous to the capillaries of the gut, which via the portal vein, also find their way into the hepatic sinusoids. Thus, some solutes, such as the hydrophilic bile acid ursodeoxycholic acid, may be absorbed by the cholangiocytes from bile and returned to the hepatocytes for resecretion, thus inducing significant choleresis.

The Gallbladder Stores and Concentrates Bile and Delivers It to the Duodenum During a Meal

The gallbladder is not an essential structure of bile secretion, but it does serve to concentrate bile acids up to 10- or even 20-fold during interdigestive periods. Tonic contraction of the sphincter of Oddi facilitates gallbladder filling by maintaining a positive pressure within the common bile duct. As we noted earlier, up to 50% of hepatic bile—or approximately 450 ml/day—is diverted to the gallbladder during fasting. The remaining approximately 450 ml/day passes directly into the duodenum. Periods of gallbladder filling between meals are interrupted by brief periods of partial emptying of concentrated bile and probably aspiration of dilute hepatic bile in a process analogous to the function of a bellows.

Bile salts and certain other components of bile are concentrated up to 20-fold within the gallbladder lumen because they are left behind during the isotonic reabsorption of NaCl and NaHCO₃ by the leaky gallbladder epithelium (Figure 45–12). The apical step of NaCl uptake and transport is electroneutral and mediated by parallel Na-H and Cl-HCO₃ exchangers. At the basolateral membrane, Na^+ exits via the Na-K pump, whereas Cl^- most

FIGURE 45–12. Isotonic fluid reabsorption by the gallbladder epithelium. The gallbladder epithelium performs the isotonic absorption of NaCl. The apical step is parallel Na-H exchange and Cl-HCO₃ exchange. Because Na-H exchange is somewhat faster, there is a net secretion of acid into the lumen. The basolateral step of NaCl absorption is mediated by the Na-K pump and Cl⁻ channels. K⁺ channels provide a route for basolateral K⁺ recycling. Water follows passively through the tight junctions and through the basolateral membrane.

likely exits by Cl^- channels. Both water and HCO_3^- move passively from lumen to blood via the tight junctions, which are rather leaky. Water can also move through the cell. The net transport is isotonic, which leaves behind gallbladder bile that is also isotonic but has a higher concentration of bile salts, K^+, and Ca^{2+}. Net fluid and electrolyte transport across the gallbladder epithelium is under hormonal regulation. Both VIP (released from neurons innervating the gallbladder) and serotonin inhibit net fluid and electrolyte absorption. Conversely, α-adrenergic blockade of neuronal VIP release increases fluid absorption.

Although the gallbladder reabsorbs NaCl by parallel Na-H and Cl-HCO₃ exchange at the apical membrane, Na-H exchange outstrips Cl-HCO₃ exchange, with the end result being net secretion of **H⁺ ions**. This action neutralizes the HCO_3^- and acidifies the bile. The H⁺ secreted by the gallbladder protonates the intraluminal contents. This action greatly increases the solubility of calcium salts in bile and reduces the likelihood of calcium salt precipitation and **gallstone formation**. Common "pigment gallstones" contain one or more of several calcium salts, including carbonate, bilirubinate, phosphate, and free fatty acids. The solubility of each of these compounds is significantly increased by the acidification of bile.

Mucus secretion by gallbladder epithelial cells results in the formation of a polymeric gel that protects the apical surface of the gallbladder epithelium from the potentially toxic effects of bile salts. However, excessive mucin synthesis can be deleterious. For example, in animal models of cholesterol cholelithiasis (i.e., formation of gallstones made of cholesterol), a marked increase in mucin release precedes crystal and stone formation.

The Relative Tone of the Gallbladder and Sphincter of Oddi Determines Whether Bile Secreted by the Liver Flows from the Common Hepatic Duct into the Gallbladder or into the Duodenum

Bile exiting the liver and flowing down the common hepatic duct reaches a bifurcation that permits flow either into the cystic duct and then into the gallbladder or into the common bile duct, through the sphincter of Oddi, and into the duodenum (see Fig. 45–4). The extent to which bile takes either path depends on the relative resistance of the two pathways.

The sphincter of Oddi—which also controls the flow of pancreatic secretions into the duodenum—corresponds functionally to a short (4 to 6 mm) zone within the wall of the duodenum. The basal pressure within the lumen of the duct at the level of the sphincter is 5 to 10 mm Hg. The pressure in the lumen of the resting common bile duct is also 5 to 10 mm Hg, compared with a pressure of approximately 0 mm Hg inside the duodenum.

The basal contraction of the sphincter prevents reflux of the duodenal contents into the common bile duct. In its basal state, the sphincter exhibits high-pressure, phasic contractions several times per minute. These contractions are primarily peristaltic and antegrade to provide a motive force toward the duodenum. Thus, the sphincter of Oddi acts principally as an adjustable occluding mechanism and regulator of bile flow.

Both hormonal and cholinergic mechanisms appear to be involved in gallbladder emptying. Dietary lipid stimulates the release of cholecystokinin (CCK) from duodenal I cells (p. 920). This CCK not only stimulates pancreatic secretion but also causes smooth-muscle contraction and evacuation of the gallbladder. The coordinated response to CCK also includes relaxation of the sphincter of Oddi, thus enhancing bile flow into the duodenum.

ENTEROHEPATIC CIRCULATION OF BILE ACIDS

The Enterohepatic Circulation of Bile Acids Is a Loop Consisting of Secretion by the Liver, Reabsorption by the Intestine, and Return To the Liver in Portal Blood for Resecretion into Bile

Bile acids are important for promoting the absorption of dietary lipids in the intestine. The quantity of bile acid that the liver normally *secretes* in a day varies with the number of meals and the fat content of these meals, but it typically ranges between 12 and 36 g. The liver's basal rate of *synthesis* of bile acids from cholesterol (see Fig. 45–9) is only approximately 600 mg/day in healthy humans, sufficient to replace the equivalent losses of bile acid in the feces. Obviously, the gastrointestinal tract must have an extremely efficient mechanism for recycling the bile acids secreted by the liver (Fig. 45–13). This recycling, known as the **enterohepatic circulation**, occurs as the terminal ileum and colon reabsorb bile acids and returns them to the liver in the portal blood. The total pool of bile acids in the gastrointestinal tract is around 3 g. This pool must recirculate about 4 to 12 times per day, or as many as 5 or more times for a single fat-rich meal. If reabsorption of bile acids is defective, which can happen with resection of the ileum, de novo synthesis of bile acids by the liver can be as high as 4 to 6 g/day.

The Intestinal Conservation of Bile Acids Is Extremely Efficient and Mediated Both by Active Apical Absorption in the Terminal Ileum and by Passive Absorption Throughout the Intestinal Tract

Most of the bile secreted into the duodenum is in the conjugated form. Very little of these bile salts are reabsorbed into the intestinal tract until they reach the terminal ileum, an arrangement that allows the bile salts to remain at high levels throughout most of the small intestine, where they can participate in lipid digestion and absorption (see Chapter 44). However, the enterohepatic circulation must eventually reclaim 95% or more of these secreted bile salts. Some of the absorption of bile acids by the intestines is passive and occurs along the entire small intestine and colon. Nevertheless, the major component

---

CHOLESTASIS

Ther term *cholestasis* refers to the suppression of bile secretion. Biliary constituents may therefore be retained within the hepatocyte and regurgitated into the systemic circulation. Cholestasis causes three major groups of negative effects: first, regurgitation of bile components (bile acids, bilirubin) into the systemic circulation gives rise to the symptoms of jaundice and pruritus (itching). Second, cholestasis damages hepatocytes, as evidenced by the release of "liver enzymes" (e.g., alkaline phosphatase) into the plasma. Third, because the bile acids do not arrive in the duodenum, lipid digestion and absorption may be impaired.

Many acute and chronic liver diseases produce cholestasis by mechanically obstructing the **extrahepatic** bile ducts or impairing bile flow at the level of the hepatocytes or **intrahepatic** bile ducts. The mechanisms underlying the obstructive and functional forms of cholestasis are complex and have not been completely defined. Experimental models of cholestasis have produced multiple abnormalities: (1) altered plasma membrane composition and fluidity; (2) inhibition of membrane proteins, including the Na-K pump; (3) reduced expression of genes encoding transporters for bile acids and other organic anions; (4) increased permeability of the paracellular pathway, with backdiffusion of biliary solutes into the plasma; (5) altered function of microfilaments, with decreased contractions of bile canaliculi; and (6) loss of the polarized distribution of some plasma membrane proteins.

FIGURE 45–13. Enterohepatic circulation of bile acids. The bile acids that the liver delivers to the duodenum in the bile are primarily conjugated to taurine or glycine (BA-Z⁻). The vast majority of bile acids are reabsorbed as conjugated bile salts (BA-Z⁻) in the terminal ileum via an Na⁺-coupled cotransporter (ASBT). Also in the terminal ileum and colon, bacteria deconjugate a small amount of these bile salts to form unconjugated bile acids (H · BA ⇌ H⁺ + BA⁻), allowing H · BA to be passively absorbed by nonionic diffusion. Bacteria in the terminal ileum and colon also dehydroxylate primary bile acids to form secondary bile acids (see Fig. 45–9). Some of these are passively absorbed, and the rest are excreted in the feces. The absorbed bile acids return to the liver via the portal blood and are then taken up into the hepatocyte for resecretion.

of bile acid absorption is active and occurs only in the terminal ileum (see Fig. 45–13).

Passive absorption of bile acids occurs along the entire small intestine and colon (see Fig. 45–13), but it is less intensive than the active absorption. The mechanism of bile acid uptake across the apical membrane may consist of either **ionic** or **nonionic diffusion**. Nonionic diffusion—or passive diffusion of the protonated or neutral form of the bile acid—is 10-fold greater than ionic diffusion. The extent of nonionic diffusion for a given bile acid depends on the concentration of its neutral, protonated form, which is maximized when the luminal pH is low and the pK of the bile acid is high. At the normal intestinal pH of 5.5 to 6.5, few of the taurine-conjugated

bile salts are protonated, a small amount of the glycine-conjugated bile salts are protonated, and about 50% of unconjugated bile acids are protonated. Thus, the unconjugated bile acids are in the best position to be reabsorbed by nonionic diffusion, followed by the glycine-conjugated bile acids and then finally by the taurine-conjugated bile acids. Among these unconjugated bile acids, more lipophilic bile acids, such as chenodeoxycholate and deoxycholate, diffuse more readily through the apical membrane than do hydrophilic bile acids such as cholic acid. Nonionic diffusion also depends on the total concentration of the bile acid (i.e., neutral plus charged form), which in turn depends on the maximum solubilizing capacity of bile salt micelles for that bile acid.

Active absorption of bile acids in the intestine is restricted to the *terminal ileum*. This active process preferentially absorbs the negatively charged *conjugated* bile salts—the form *not* well absorbed by the passive mechanisms. Active uptake of bile salts involves saturation kinetics, competitive inhibition, and a requirement for Na^+ (see Fig. 45–13). The Na^+-dependent transporter responsible for the apical step of active absorption is known as the apical Na^+/bile salt transporter (ASBT). ASBT is a 50-kDa protein with seven membrane-spanning segments that displays significant homology to the Na^+-dependent uptake mechanism present at the basolateral membrane of hepatocytes, NTCP (see Fig. 45–5C). Once bile salts have been transported into ileal enterocytes across the apical membrane, they are thought to leave via an Na^+-independent anion exchanger localized to the *basolateral* membrane (see Fig. 45–13).

Because the most polar bile salts are poorly absorbed by nonionic diffusion, it is not surprising that the ASBT in the apical membrane of the enterocytes of the terminal ileum has the highest affinity and maximal transport rates for these salts. For example, ASBT is primarily responsible for absorbing the ionized, taurine-conjugated bile salts in the ileum. Conversely, ASBT in the ileum is relatively poor at absorbing the more lipophilic bile acids, which tend to be absorbed passively in the upper intestine.

Upon their entry into portal blood, the bile acids are predominantly bound to albumin and, to a lesser extent, lipoproteins. The liver removes or "clears" these bile acids from portal blood by the transport mechanisms outlined earlier in Figure 45–5C. Hepatic "clearance" of bile acids is often expressed as the percentage of bile acids removed during a single pass through the liver. The hepatic extraction of bile acids is related to bile acid structure and the degree of albumin binding. It is greatest for hydrophilic bile acids and least for protein-bound, hydrophobic bile acids.

The small fraction of bile acids that escapes active or passive absorption in the small intestine is subject to *bacterial modification* in the *colon*. This bacteria modification takes two forms. First, the bacteria deconjugate the bile. Second, the bacteria perform a 7α-dehydroxylation reaction with the formation of *secondary bile acids*. These secondary bile acids include **deoxycholate** and **lithocholate** (see Fig. 45–9). The deconjugated secondary bile acids may then be either absorbed passively in the colon or excreted in the feces, their fate depending on their physicochemical properties and their binding to luminal contents. Up to one third of the deoxycholate formed in the colon may be reabsorbed by nonionic diffusion. Lithocholate, which is relatively insoluble, is absorbed to a much lesser extent. The secondary bile acids formed by colonic bacteria and recycled back to the liver may undergo biotransformation through conjugation to glycine and taurine.

Thus, the enterohepatic circulation of bile acids is driven by two *mechanical* pumps: (1) the motor activity of the gallbladder, and (2) peristalsis of the intestines to propel the bile acids to the terminal ileum and colon. It is also driven by two *chemical* pumps: (1) energy-dependent transporters located in the terminal ileum, and (2) energy-dependent transporters in the hepatocyte.

GALLSTONES

The majority of gallstones ($\sim$80%) consist mainly of cholesterol. Thus, **cholelithiasis** may be regarded as a disturbance of bile secretion and cholesterol elimination. When cholesterol and phospholipids are secreted together into the bile, they form unilamellar bilayered vesicles. These vesicles become incorporated into mixed micelles that form because of the amphiphilic properties of bile acids. Micellation allows cholesterol to remain in solution in its passage through the biliary tree. However, if the concentration of bile acids is insufficient to maintain all the cholesterol in the form of mixed micelles, the excess cholesterol is left behind as vesicles in the aqueous phase. These cholesterol-enriched vesicles are relatively unstable and prone to aggregate and form large multilamellar vesicles, from which cholesterol crystals nucleate. Growth of crystals may result in the formation of gallstones. An excess of biliary cholesterol in relation to the amount of phospholipids and bile acids can result from hypersecretion of cholesterol, inadequate secretion of bile acids, or both. Cholelithiasis may be further promoted by other factors, such as gallbladder mucin and other nonmucus glycoproteins, as well as by stasis of bile in the gallbladder.

THE LIVER AS A METABOLIC ORGAN

The liver is a metabolically active and highly aerobic organ. It receives approximately 28% of the total blood flow and extracts about 20% of the oxygen used by the body. The liver is responsible for the synthesis and degradation of carbohydrates, proteins, and lipids. The small molecules that are products of digestion are efficiently sorted in the liver for metabolism, storage, or distribution to extrahepatic tissues for energy. The liver provides energy to other tissues mainly by exporting two substrates that are critical for oxidization in the peripheral tissues, glucose and ketone bodies (e.g., acetoacetate).

The Liver Can Serve as Either a Source or a Sink for Glucose

Between meals, when levels of insulin are relatively low and levels of glucagon are high (see Chapter 50), the liver serves as a source of plasma glucose, both by synthesizing glucose and by generating it from the breakdown of glycogen. The de novo synthesis of glucose, or **gluconeogenesis** (see Fig. 50–12), is one of the liver's most important functions; it is essential for maintaining a normal plasma concentration of glucose, which is the primary energy source for most tissues (see Chapter 57). Glucose is synthesized in the lumen of the ER, principally from amino acids and lactate. Dietary fructose and galactose are also largely converted to glucose. Glucose exits the ER by facilitated diffusion (mediated by GLUT7) and then passes into the blood via another facilitated-diffusion mechanism

(GLUT2), which is located in the basolateral membrane of the hepatocyte.

The second way in which the liver delivers glucose to blood plasma is by **glycogenolysis**. Stored glycogen may account for as much as 7% to 10% of the total weight of the liver. Glycogenolysis in the *liver* yields glucose as its major product, whereas glycogen breakdown in *muscle* produces lactic acid (see Chapter 59).

After a meal, when levels of insulin are relatively high, the liver does just the opposite: it acts as a sink for glucose by taking it up from the portal blood and either breaking it down to pyruvate or using it to synthesize glycogen (see Fig. 50–8). Glucose oxidation has two phases. In the anaerobic phase, glucose is broken down to pyruvic acid (**glycolysis**). In the aerobic phase, pyruvic acid is completely oxidized to H_2O and CO_2 via the citric acid cycle.

The liver also consumes glucose by using it for **glycogen synthesis**. Carbohydrate that is not stored as glycogen or oxidized is metabolized to **fat**.

All the aforementioned processes are regulated by hormones such as insulin and glucagon (see Chapter 50), which enable rapid responses to changes in the metabolic requirements of the body.

The Liver Synthesizes a Variety of Important Plasma Proteins (e.g., Albumin, Coagulation Factors, and Carriage Proteins) and Metabolizes Dietary Amino Acids

PROTEIN SYNTHESIS. One of the major functions of the liver is to produce a wide array of proteins for export to the blood plasma (Table 45–4). These products include major **plasma proteins** that are important for maintaining the colloid osmotic pressure of plasma (see Chapter 19). Other products include factors involved in **hemostasis** (blood clotting) and **fibrinolysis** (breakdown of blood clots), **carriage proteins** that bind and transport hormones and other substances in the blood, **prohormones**, and **lipoproteins** (Table 45–5). The liver synthesizes plasma proteins at a maximum rate of 15 to 50 g/day.

AMINO ACID UPTAKE. A major role of the liver is to take up and metabolize dietary amino acids that are absorbed by the gastrointestinal tract (p. 956) and transported to the liver in portal blood. These amino acids are taken up by both Na⁺-*dependent* and Na⁺-*independent* mechanisms. Although the cDNA for all these transporters has not been isolated, transport studies suggest the presence of at least 12 amino acid transporters on the hepatocyte membrane. These transporters are likely to be similar to the amino acid transporters in the small intestine (see Table 44–3). Apart from a few exceptions, liver amino acid transporters appear to be located on both the basolateral and apical membranes. For example, Na⁺-dependent glutamate uptake by the excitatory amino acid transporters EAAT2 (also known as GLT-1) and EAAT3 (also known as EAAC1) occurs primarily at the apical membrane but can be induced at the basolateral membrane by dexamethasone (corticosteroid) treatment.

AMINO ACID METABOLISM. Unlike glucose, which can be stored, amino acids must either be used immediately

---

TABLE 45–4

PROTEINS MADE BY THE LIVER FOR EXPORT

Major Plasma Proteins

Albumin

α_1-Fetoprotein

Plasma fibronectin (an α_2 glycoprotein)

C-reactive protein

α_2-Microglobulin

Various other globulins

Factors Involved in Hemostasis/Fibrinolysis

Coagulation: fibrinogen and all others except for factor VIII

Inhibitors of coagulation: α_1-antitrypsin and antithrombin III, α_2-macroglobulin, protein S, protein C

Fibrinolysis: plasminogen

Inhibitors of fibrinolysis: α_2-antiplasmin

Complement C3

Carriage Proteins ("Binding Proteins")

Ceruloplasmin (p. 1001)

Corticosteroid-binding globulin (CBG, aka transcortin; p. 1053)

GH-binding protein (low affinity form)

Haptoglobin

Hemopexin

IGF-binding proteins (p. 1029)

Retinol-binding protein (p. 1001)

Sex hormone–binding globulin (SHBG; p. 1156)

Thyroid-binding globulin (TBG; p. 1038)

Transferrin

Transthyretin (p. 1038)

Vitamin D–binding protein (p. 1096)

Prohormones

Angiotensinogen (p. 1059)

Apolipoproteins

Apo A-I

Apo A-II

Apo A-IV

Apo B-100

Apo C-II

Apo D

Apo E

GH, growth hormone; IGF, insulin-like growth factor; TBG, thyroxine-binding globulin.

TABLE 45–5

MAJOR CLASSES OF LIPOPROTEINS

	CHYLOMICRONS	VLDL	IDL	LDL	HDL
Density (g/cm³)	<0.95	<1.006	1.006–1.019	1.019–1.063	1.063–1.210
Diameter (nm)	75–1200	30–80	25–35	18–25	50–120
Mass (kDa)	400,000	10,000–80,000	5,000–10,000	2300	175–360
% Protein (surface)	1.5–2.5	5–10	15–20	20–25	40–55
% Phospholipid (surface)	7–9	15–20	22	15–20	20–35
% Free cholesterol (surface)	1–3	5–10	8	7–10	3–4
% Triglycerides (core)	84–89	50–65	22	7–10	3–5
% Cholesteryl esters (core)	3–5	10–15	30	35–40	12
Major apolipoproteins	A-I, A-II, B-48, C-I, C-II, C-III, E	B-100, C-I, C-II, C-III, E	B-100, C-III, E	B-100	A-I, A-II, C-I, C-II, C-III, D, E

HDL, high-density lipoprotein; IDL, intermediate-density lipoprotein; LDL, low-density lipoprotein; VLDL, very-low-density lipoprotein.
Adapted from Voet D, Voet JG: Biochemistry, 2nd ed. New York, John Wiley & Sons, 1995, p 317.

(e.g., for the synthesis of proteins) or broken down. The breakdown of α-amino acids occurs by **deamination** to α-keto acids and NH_4^+ (Fig. 45–14). The α-keto acids ("carbon skeleton"), depending on the structure of the parent amino acid, are metabolized to pyruvate, various intermediates of the citric acid cycle (see Fig. 57–9), acetyl coenzyme A (acetyl CoA), or acetoacetyl CoA. The liver detoxifies approximately 95% of the NH_4^+ through a series of reactions known as the **urea cycle** (see Fig. 45–14); the liver can also use NH_4^+—together with glutamate—to generate glutamine. Individual deficiencies in each of the enzymes involved in the urea cycle have been described and result in life-threatening hyperammonemia.

The urea generated by the urea cycle exits the hepatocyte via a urea channel, which is, in fact, aquaporin 9. The urea then enters the blood and is ultimately excreted by the kidneys (see Chapter 35). The glutamine synthesized by the liver also enters the blood. Some of this glutamine is metabolized by the kidney to yield glutamate and NH_4^+, which is exported in the urine (p. 854).

The liver is also the main site for the synthesis and secretion of **glutathione**. GSH is critical for detoxification (in conjugation reactions in the liver) and for protection against oxidative stress in multiple organs. Thus, erythrocytes that have low levels of GSH are more prone to hemolysis. Because over 90% of the GSH in the circula-

FIGURE 45–14. Amino acid metabolism and urea formation in hepatocytes. When a hepatocyte takes up an α-amino acid, it either must use it immediately in protein synthesis or deaminate it. The deamination reaction transfers the amino group of the α-amino acid to α-ketoglutarate, yielding glutamate and the corresponding α-keto acid. Depending on the backbone of the α-keto acid, it may be metabolized into acetoacetyl CoA, acetyl CoA, pyruvate, or a variety of citric acid cycle intermediates. The NH_4^+ that results from the regeneration of the α-ketoglutarate is consumed in the urea cycle. The other amino group of the urea is derived from the amino group of aspartate. The C = O moiety of urea is derived from CO_2. The liver then exports the urea, which exits the hepatocyte via "aquaporin" 9. CoA, coenzyme A.

tion is synthesized in the liver, GSH efflux across the basolateral membrane from the hepatocyte to the sinusoid is important. OATP-1, which can exchange GSH for organic solutes, provides a pathway for GSH release into blood (see Fig. 45–5D), but it cannot fully account for the total flux of GSH into blood. In addition, some GSH moves across the canalicular membrane into bile, as stated earlier, mediated by MRP2 and an unidentified transporter.

The Liver Obtains Dietary Triglycerides and Cholesterol by Taking Up Remnant Chylomicrons via Receptor-Mediated Endocytosis

As discussed in Chapter 44, enterocytes in the small intestine process fatty acids consumed as dietary triglycerides and secrete them into the lymph primarily in the form of extremely large proteolipid aggregates called chylomicrons (Fig. 45–15). These **chylomicrons**—made up of triglycerides (80% to 90%), phospholipids, cholesterol, and several apoproteins (see Table 45–5)—pass from the lymph to the blood via the thoracic duct. As discussed on page 1215, lipoprotein lipase (LPL) on the walls of the capillary endothelium in adipose tissue and muscle then partially digests the triglycerides in these chylomicrons. The result of this digestion is glycerol, free fatty acids, and smaller or "remnant" chylomicrons, which are triglyceride depleted, and thus enriched in cholesterol. The glycerol and free fatty acids generated by LPL enter adipocytes and muscle cells. The cholesterol-rich **remnant chylomicrons**, on the other hand, remain in the blood and make their way to the liver, where they enter hepatocytes by a process that is saturable, specific, and of high affinity. Although low-density lipoprotein (LDL) receptors can recognize chylomicron remnants, another member of the LDL receptor gene family, the LDL-related receptor, is of greater importance. The chylomicron remnant binds to this receptor on the basolateral membrane, enters the hepatocyte via receptor-mediated endocytosis (p. 42), and is degraded in lysosomes. Thus, chylomicrons transport dietary triglycerides to adipose tissue and muscle, whereas their "remnants" transport dietary triglycerides and cholesterol to hepatocytes.

The hepatocyte can also take up across its basolateral membrane the **long-chain fatty acids** liberated by LPL but not used by other tissues. Fatty-acid uptake occurs by at least two different mechanisms: facilitated uptake and a nonspecific "flip-flop" across the lipid bilayer.

To extract energy from the neutral fats derived from the remnant chylomicrons, hepatocytes must first split the triglycerides into glycerol and fatty acids. The fatty acids thus derived from remnant chylomicrons, as well as those that enter the hepatocyte directly, are metabolized by β oxidation into two-carbon acetyl intermediates that then form acetyl CoA. Acetyl CoA can enter the citric acid cycle, where it is oxidized to produce large amounts of energy. The acetyl CoA that is not used by the liver is converted by the condensation of two molecules of acetyl CoA to yield acetoacetic acid. The liver is the only organ that produces **acetoacetate** for metabolism by muscle,

brain, and kidney, but it does not use this substrate for its own energy needs. In fasting or in poorly controlled diabetes, where the supply of acetyl CoA is in excess, the acetyl CoA is diverted to produce acetoacetate, which in turn can yield β hydroxybutyrate and acetone. Together, acetoacetate, β hydroxybutyrate, and acetone are referred to as **ketone bodies**. Another fate of free fatty acids in the liver is that they can be re-esterified to glycerol, with the formation of triglycerides that can either be stored or exported as **very-low-density lipoproteins** (**VLDLs**) and released into the circulation for use by peripheral tissues.

Cholesterol, Synthesized Primarily in the Liver, Is an Important Component of Cell Membranes and Serves As a Precursor for Bile Acids and Steroid Hormones

The body's major pools of cholesterol include the cholesterol and cholesterol derivatives in bile, cholesterol in membranes, cholesterol carried as lipoproteins in blood (see Table 45–5), and cholesterol-rich tissues. Cholesterol is present in membranes and bile mainly as free cholesterol. In plasma and in some tissues, cholesterol is esterified with long-chain fatty acids. The major *sources* of cholesterol are dietary uptake of cholesterol and de novo synthesis of cholesterol by various cells (Table 45–6). The major *fates* of cholesterol are secretion into bile, excretion in the feces when intestinal cells are sloughed, sloughing of skin, and synthesis of steroid hormones. However, in mammals, the most important route for the elimination of cholesterol is the hepatic conversion of cholesterol into bile acids. In the steady-state, the liver must excrete an amount of sterol (as cholesterol and bile acids) that equals the amount of cholesterol that is synthesized in the various organs and absorbed from the diet.

The liver is the major organ for controlling cholesterol metabolism (see Fig. 45–15). The liver obtains cholesterol from three major sources: (1) The intestine packages dietary cholesterol as chylomicrons, which travel via the lymph to blood vessels in adipocytes and muscle, where LPL hydrolyzes triglycerides to free fatty acids and glycerol. The resultant cholesterol-enriched remnant chylomicrons are then delivered as cholesterol to the liver. (2) The liver synthesizes cholesterol de novo. (3) The liver takes up cholesterol in the guise of **low-density lipoproteins**. However, the liver exports cholesterol in two major ways: (1) The liver uses cholesterol to synthesize bile acids and also includes cholesterol and cholesteryl esters in the bile. (2) The liver also exports cholesterol to the blood in the form of VLDLs.

SYNTHESIS OF CHOLESTEROL. The de novo synthesis of cholesterol occurs in many extrahepatic tissues, as well as in the intestine and liver. The synthesis of cholesterol proceeds from acetyl CoA in a multistep process that takes place in the SER and cytosol (Fig. 45–16). The hepatic synthesis of cholesterol is inhibited by dietary cholesterol and by fasting and is increased with bile drainage (fistula) and bile duct obstruction. The rate-limiting step in cholesterol synthesis is the conversion of 3-hydroxy-3-methylglutaryl-CoA (HMG-CoA) to mevalonate

FIGURE 45–15. Cholesterol metabolism. CETP, cholesteryl ester transfer protein; Chol-E, cholesteryl ester; FFA, free fatty acid; HDL, high-density lipoprotein; IDL, intermediate-density lipoprotein; LCAT, lecithin-cholesterol acyltransferase; LDL, low-density lipoprotein; VLDL, very-low-density lipoprotein.

by **HMG-CoA reductase**, the level of which is decreased—in typical negative feedback fashion—by cholesterol levels in the cell (see the box titled Control of Cholesterol Synthesis). The most potent cholesterol-lowering agents that are clinically available today—the "statins"—are inhibitors of HMG-CoA reductase.

The Liver Is the Organ That Is Principally Responsible for Cholesterol Homeostasis in the Body, As Well As the Synthesis and Degradation of Low-Density Lipoprotein

The liver is the hub of cholesterol metabolism. It is the hub of an "exogenous loop" in which the liver takes up dietary cholesterol as remnant chylomicrons and exports cholesterol and cholesterol metabolites into bile. The liver is also the hub an of "endogenous loop" in which the liver exports cholesterol and other lipids as VLDLs and takes them up from the blood as LDLs. Table 45–5 summarizes the properties of these lipoproteins, as well as two others: the intermediate-density lipoproteins (IDLs) and the **high-density lipoproteins** (HDLs). Notice that as

TABLE 45–6

SOURCES AND FATES OF CHOLESTEROL IN HUMANS

PROCESS	FLOW (g/day for a 70-kg human)
Intestinal absorption	0.1–0.5
Synthesis	1.05
Biliary secretion	0.9
Cholesterol consumed in synthesis of bile acids	0.5
Cholesterol secreted in VLDLs by the liver	0.25–1.75

VLDLs, very-low-density lipoproteins.
Modified from Cooper AD, Ellsworth JL: Lipoprotein metabolism. In Zakim D, Boyer TD (eds): Hepatology. Philadelphia, WB Saunders, 1996.

we move from left to right in Table 45–5, the size of the particles decreases, the density increases (because the fractional mass of protein increases), the fractional amount of triglycerides decreases, and the fractional amount of phospholipids increases.

Regardless of the source of the cholesterol, the liver can package it along with other lipids and apoproteins as **VLDLs**. The VLDLs are large—and therefore less dense—when the availability of triglycerides is high (e.g., obesity, diabetes), but they are small when triglyceride availability is low. VLDLs enter the bloodstream (see Fig. 45–15) and eventually make their way to the blood vessels of adipose tissue and muscle, where the same LPL that degrades chylomicrons degrades the VLDLs on the luminal surface of blood vessel endothelial cells. In the process, free fatty acids are released to the tissues. Thus, VLDLs act as lipid shuttles that transport "endogenous" triglycerides to adipose tissue for storage as fat or to muscle for immediate use. As a result of the LPL activity, the large, buoyant VLDLs rapidly shrink to become the smaller **IDLs** and the even smaller LDLs. The half-life of VLDL is less than an hour. In plasma, only minute amounts of IDLs are present.

Both the liver and extrahepatic tissue can take up LDLs—and to a lesser extent, IDLs—by the process of receptor-mediated endocytosis (p. 44). **LDLs** are the ma-

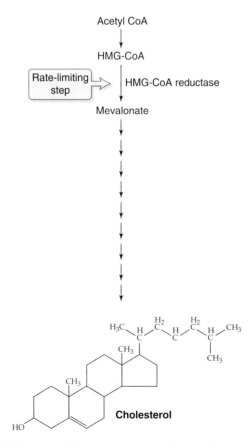

FIGURE 45–16. Cholesterol synthesis. The liver synthesizes cholesterol de novo from acetyl CoA in a multi-step process that occurs in the SER and cytosol. The rate-limiting step is the conversion of 3-hydroxy-3-methylglutaryl (HMG-CoA) to mevalonate by HMG-CoA reductase. CoA, coenzyme A; SER, smooth endoplasmic reticulum.

CONTROL OF CHOLESTEROL SYNTHESIS

3-Hydroxy-3-methylglutaryl-coenzyme A (HMG-CoA) reductase, the rate-limiting enzyme in cholesterol biosynthesis, is a 97-kDa enzyme intrinsic to the endoplasmic reticulum (ER). The protein is anchored in the ER by a 339–amino acid domain that spans the membrane eight times and is required for activity of the protein. In the short term, decreased intracellular levels of adenosine triphosphate lead to phosphorylation of HMG-CoA reductase, which reduces the activity of the enzyme, presumably preserving energy stores in the cell.

Far more important than the short-term regulation of HMA-CoA reductase is the long-term control of the amount of the enzyme, which can increase as much as 200-fold. The amount of HMG-CoA reductase protein increases after cells are depleted of mevalonate or when the demand for mevalonate-derived metabolites is increased. HMG-CoA reductase activity is upregulated by a combination of enhanced gene transcription, increased mRNA translation, and increased stability of the enzyme. These changes are reversed by the addition of cholesterol or mevalonate to the cells. The transmembrane domain of HMG-CoA reductase may serve as a receptor for the regulatory effects of sterols.

Sterol repression of HMG-CoA reductase gene expression—as well as the expression of low-density lipoprotein and HMG-CoA synthase genes—is mediated by specific transcription factors and specific sequence elements within the 5′ upstream region to which *trans*-acting proteins bind. Several related sterol regulatory elements whose activities mediate sterol repression of gene expression, such as SRE-1, provide a specific sequence required for the recognition of DNA binding proteins. These SRE binding proteins (SREBPs) are membrane-bound basic-helix-loop-helix transcriptional activators (p. 125) that control genes involved in the synthesis and receptor-mediated uptake of cholesterol and fatty acids.

jor carriers of cholesterol in plasma. The half-life of LDL is 2 to 3 days. Of course, uptake of LDL by the liver is a major pathway of cholesterol input to the liver. The liver degrades about 40% to 60% of LDL, with no other tissue taking up more than approximately 10%. LDL uptake by other tissues provides a mechanism for the delivery of cholesterol that can be used for the synthesis of cell membranes and steroid hormones or for storage as cholesteryl ester droplets.

The other major player in cholesterol metabolism is **HDL**. The two major apoproteins of HDLs, A-I and A-II, are made by the intestines as part of chylomicrons, as well as by the liver (see Table 45–5). As LPL digests VLDLs on endothelial cells, some excess surface material (i.e., cholesterol and phospholipids) of these rapidly shrinking particles is transferred to the HDLs. The HDLs also play a major role in scavenging cholesterol from extrahepatic tissue. HDLs extract unesterified cholesterol from the plasma membranes of these cells. The enzyme **lecithin cholesterol acyltransferase** (LCAT), which is synthesized in the liver and associated with HDL, then takes an acyl group from lecithin and esterifies it to cholesterol to produce a cholesteryl ester. The HDLs then transfer these cholesteryl esters to the VLDLs, IDLs, and LDLs with assistance by apoprotein D, also known as **cholesteryl ester transfer protein**. Thus, the HDLs— sometimes known as the "good cholesterol"—play a central role in transporting excess cellular cholesterol back to the liver.

The Liver Is the Prime Site For Metabolism and Storage of the Fat-Soluble Vitamins A, D, E, and K

VITAMIN A. Vitamin A (retinol and its derivatives)— like dietary vitamin D, as well as vitamins E and K—is absorbed from the intestine and then transported in newly synthesized chylomicrons or VLDLs. After some peripheral hydrolysis of its triglyceride, the remnant chylomicrons are taken up by the liver. In the hepatocyte, retinyl esters may be hydrolyzed to release free retinol, which can then be transported into the sinusoids bound to **retinol-binding protein** (RBP) and prealbumin. Alternatively, retinyl esters may be stored in the hepatocyte or transported as RBP-bound retinol to stellate (Ito) cells, the storage site of over 80% of hepatic vitamin A under normal conditions. Retinol may also undergo oxidation to **retinal** and conversion to **retinoic acid**, which plays a key role in phototransduction (p. 339). Retinoic acid is conjugated to glucuronide and secreted into bile, where it undergoes enterohepatic circulation and excretion. Liver disease resulting in cholestasis may lead to a secondary vitamin A deficiency by interfering with absorption in the intestine (lack of the bile needed for digestion/absorption of vitamin A) or by impairing delivery to target tissues because of reduced hepatic synthesis of RBP.

VITAMIN D. Skin cells—under the influence of ultraviolet light—synthesize vitamin D_3 (p. 1095). Dietary vitamin D can come from either animal sources (D_3) or plant sources (D_2). In either case, the first step in activation of vitamin D is the 25-hydroxylation of vitamin D, catalyzed by a hepatic cytochrome P-450 enzyme. This hydroxylation is followed by 1-hydroxylation in the kidney to yield a product (1,25-dihydroxyvitamin D) with full biologic activity. Termination of the activity of 1,25-dihydroxyvitamin D also occurs in the liver by hydroxylation at carbon 24, mediated by another cytochrome P-450 enzyme.

VITAMIN E. This fat-soluble vitamin is absorbed from the intestine primarily in the form of α- and γ-tocopherol. It is incorporated into chylomicrons and VLDL with other products of dietary lipid digestion. As noted earlier, these particles reach the systemic circulation via the lymphatics and undergo some triglyceride hydrolysis. In the process, some vitamin E is transferred to other tissues. The α- and γ-tocopherol remaining in the remnant chylomicrons is transported into the liver, which is the major site of discrimination between the two forms. The α-

tocopherol is resecreted as a component of hepatically derived VLDL and perhaps HDL. The γ-tocopherol appears to be metabolized or excreted by the liver. A hepatic tocopherol binding protein may play a role in this discriminatory process.

VITAMIN K. Vitamin K is a fat-soluble vitamin produced by intestinal bacteria. This vitamin is essential for the γ carboxylation of certain glutamate residues in coagulation factors II, VII, IX, and X. Intestinal absorption and handling of vitamin K—which is present in two forms, K_1 and K_2—are similar to that of the other fat-soluble vitamins: A, D, and E. Common causes of vitamin K deficiency, which can lead to a serious bleeding disorder, include extrahepatic or intrahepatic cholestasis, fat malabsorption, biliary fistulas, and dietary deficiency, particularly in association with antibiotic therapy.

The Liver Stores Copper and Iron

COPPER. About half the copper in the diet (the recommended dietary allowance is 1.5 to 3 mg/day) is absorbed in the jejunum and reaches the liver in the portal blood, mostly bound to albumin. A small fraction of plasma copper is also bound to amino acids, especially histidine. Albumin-bound copper is taken up by a specific facilitated transport system at the basolateral membrane. Histidine appears to facilitate the uptake of copper by hepatocytes in the presence of albumin. In this way, 60% to 90% of the copper absorbed in the intestine is taken up into the hepatocyte. Once inside the hepatocyte, copper is initially bound to one of a series of low-molecular-weight proteins called copper chaperones. These transport copper to sites of copper incorporation such as secreted cuproenzymes, mitochondria (for incorporation into cytochrome c oxidase), or superoxide dismutase. Excess copper is transported to the canalicular membrane for excretion into bile. If intake of copper exceeds efflux capacity, free copper induces the production of **metallothioneins,** small cysteine-rich proteins that sequester heavy metals. **Ceruloplasmin**, an α_2-globulin, is the primary carrier by which copper is secreted into the systemic circulation. The precise role of ceruloplasmin is unclear; it may serve as a transporter of copper to extrahepatic tissues, as an oxidase, or as an antioxidant.

More than 80% of the copper absorbed each day is excreted in bile, for a total of 1.2 to 2.4 mg/day. Copper complexed to large proteins, such as metallothioneins, enters bile canaliculi by exocytosis and is the major source of biliary copper. The Cu-protein complex cannot be reabsorbed by the small intestine and hence represents a pathway for copper excretion. Additional pathways for copper excretion into bile may be available because the protein complexes do not account for all biliary copper. Enterohepatic circulation of copper is minimal, and urine, sweat, and menstrual blood represent minor pathways for excretion. Therefore, processes that impair the biliary excretion of copper result in the accumulation of copper, initially in the lysosomal fraction of hepatocytes, with subsequent elevation of plasma copper levels.

Wilson disease (WD) is an autosomally inherited condition in which the buildup of copper causes toxic effects in the liver, brain, kidney, cornea, and other tissues as a result of impaired biliary excretion of copper. The disorder is associated with low serum levels of ceruloplasmin. The gene responsible for WD encodes a P-type copper-transporting ATPase. The WD gene product has been localized to the Golgi apparatus, where it participates in intracellular copper transport through mechanisms that are not fully defined. It is also possible that the WD gene is involved in the regulation of ceruloplasmin production or is required for incorporation of copper into ceruloplasmin, in part by maintaining the metal ion in the correct redox state.

IRON. Dietary iron is absorbed by the duodenal mucosa and then transported through the blood bound to **transferrin** (p. 973), a protein synthesized in the liver. The liver also takes up, secretes, and stores iron. Entry of iron into hepatocytes is mediated through specific cell-surface transferrin receptors (p. 44). Within the cell, a small pool of soluble iron is maintained for intracellular enzymatic reactions, primarily for those involved in electron transport. However, iron is also toxic to the cell. Hence, most intracellular iron is complexed to **ferritin**. The toxicity of iron is clearly evident when normal storage mechanisms become overwhelmed, as occurs in hemochromatosis (see the box on hereditary hemochromatosis on p. 972), an autosomal recessive disease in which regulation of iron absorption is uncoupled from total-body storage levels.

WILSON DISEASE

Wilson disease is inherited as an autosomal recessive illness. It is rare, but must be considered in the differential diagnosis of anyone younger than 30 years with evidence of significant liver disease. Patients most often have neuropsychiatric complications, including ataxia, tremors, increased salivation, and behavioral changes. Slit-lamp examination of the cornea reveals the diagnostic Kayser-Fleischer rings at the limbus of the cornea. The best way to confirm the diagnosis is the detection of a low serum ceruloplasmin level and elevated urinary copper excretion. A few affected patients will have normal ceruloplasmin levels, and the diagnosis must then be sought with a liver biopsy. The disease can be treated by chelating the excess copper with penicillamine.

REFERENCES

Books and Reviews

Boyer JL: Bile duct epithelium: Frontiers in transport physiology. Am J Physiol 270:G1–G5, 1996.

Boyer JL, Graf J, Meier PJ: Hepatic transport systems regulating pH$_i$, cell volume and bile secretion. Annu Rev Physiol 54:415–438, 1992.

Gatmaitan ZC, Arias IN: ATP-dependent transport systems in the canalicular membrane of the hepatocyte. Physiol Rev 75:261–275, 1995.

Hillgartner FB, Salati LM, Goodridge AG: Physiological and molecular mechanisms involved in nutritional regulation of fatty acid synthesis. Physiol Rev 75:47–76, 1995.

Koepsell H: Organic cation transporters in intestine, kidney, liver and brain. Annu Rev Physiol 60:243–266, 1998.

Shulman GI, Landau BR: Pathways of glycogen repletion. Physiol Rev 72:1019–1035, 1992.

Trauner M, Meier PJ, Boyer JL: Molecular pathogenesis of cholestasis. N Engl J Med 39:1217–1227, 1998.

Journal Articles

Bull LN, van Eijk MJT, Pawlikowska L: A gene encoding a P-type ATPase mutated in two forms of hereditary cholestasis. Nat Genet 18:219–224, 1998.

Hagenbuch B, Meier PJ: Molecular cloning, chromosomal localization and functional characterization of a human liver Na$^+$/bile acid cotransporter. J Clin Invest 93:1326–1331, 1994.

Kullak-Ublick GA, Hagenbuch B, Stieger B: Molecular and functional characterization of an organic anion transporting polypeptide cloned from human liver. Gastroenterology 109:1274–1282, 1995.

Oude Elferink RPJ, Meijer DKF, Kuipers F, et al: Hepatobiliary secretion of organic compounds: Molecular mechanisms of membrane transport. Biochim Biophys Acta 1241:215–268, 1995.

VIII

The Endocrine System

CHAPTER 46

Organization of Endocrine Control

Eugene J. Barrett

With the development of multicellular organisms that have specialized tissues and organs, two major systems evolved to communicate and coordinate body functions:

1. The **nervous system** integrates tissue functions by a network of cells and cell processes that constitute the nervous system and all of its subdivisions, as discussed in Chapters 10 through 15.
2. The **endocrine system** integrates organ function via chemicals that are secreted from endocrine tissues or "glands" into the extracellular fluid. These chemicals, called **hormones**, are then carried through the blood to distant target tissues where they are recognized by specific, high-affinity receptors. As discussed in Chapter 4, these receptors may be located either on the surface of the target tissue, within the cytosol, or in the target cell's nucleus. These receptor molecules allow the target cell to recognize a unique hormonal signal from among the numerous chemicals that are carried through the blood and bathe the body's tissues. The accuracy and sensitivity of this recognition are remarkable in view of the very low concentration (10^{-9} to 10^{-12} M) at which many hormones circulate.

Once a hormone is recognized by its target tissue or tissues, it can exert its biologic action by a process known as **signal transduction** (see Chapter 4). In this chapter, we discuss how the signal-transduction cascades couple the hormone to its appropriate end responses (see Chapter 4). Some hormones elicit responses within seconds (e.g., the increased heart rate provoked by epinephrine or the stimulation of hepatic glycogen breakdown caused by glucagon), whereas others may require many hours or days (e.g., the changes in salt retention elicited by aldosterone or the increases in protein synthesis caused by growth hormone [GH]). We also examine the principles underlying the feedback mechanisms that control endocrine function.

In the remainder of the endocrine part of this book, we will see how the principles introduced in this chapter apply to specific endocrine systems.

PRINCIPLES OF ENDOCRINE FUNCTION

Chemical Signalling Can Occur Through Endocrine, Paracrine or Autocrine Pathways

As we saw in Figure 4–1A, in classic **endocrine** signalling, a hormone carries a signal from a secretory gland across a large distance to a target tissue. Hormones secreted into the extracellular space can also regulate nearby cells without ever passing through the systemic circulation. This regulation is referred to as **paracrine** action of a hormone (see Fig 4–1*B*). Finally, chemicals can also bind to receptors on or in the cell that is actually secreting the hormone and thus affect the function of the hormone-secreting cell itself. This action is referred to as **autocrine** regulation (see Fig 4–1*C*). All three mechanisms are illustrated for individual endocrine systems in subsequent chapters. At the outset, it can be appreciated that summation of the endocrine, paracrine, and autocrine actions of a hormone can provide the framework for a complex regulatory system.

ENDOCRINE GLANDS. The major hormones of the human body are produced by one of seven classic endocrine glands: the pituitary, the thyroid, the parathyroids, the testes, the ovary, the adrenal (cortex and medulla), and the endocrine pancreas. In addition, other tissues that are not classically recognized as part of the endocrine system produce hormones and play a vital role in endocrine regulation. These tissues include the central nervous system (CNS), particularly the hypothalamus, and the gastrointestinal tract, liver, heart, kidney, and others.

In some circumstances, particularly with certain neoplasms, nonendocrine tissues can produce hormones that are usually thought to be made only by endocrine glands (see the box titled Neoplastic Hormone Production).

PARACRINE FACTORS. A number of specialized tissues that are not part of the classic endocrine system release "factors" into the extracellular fluid that can signal neighboring cells to effect a biologic response. The interleukins, or lymphokines, are an example of such paracrine factors, as are several of the growth factors, such as platelet-derived growth factor (PDGF), fibroblast growth factor, and others. These factors are not hormones in the usual sense. They are not secreted by glandular tissue, and their sites of action are usually (but not always) within the local environment. However, these signalling molecules share many properties of the classic peptide and amine hormones in that they bind to surface receptors and regulate one or more of the specific intracellular signalling mechanisms described in Chapter 4.

The distinction between the hormones of the classic endocrine systems and other biologically active secreted peptides blurs even further in the case of neuropeptides. As an example, the hormone somatostatin is a 28–amino acid peptide secreted by the δ cells of the pancreatic islet, where it can exert a paracrine action in the regulation of insulin and glucagon secretion (p. 1084). However, somatostatin is also made by hypothalamic neurons. Nerve terminals in the hypothalamus release somatostatin into the pituitary portal bloodstream (p. 1026). This specialized segment of the circulatory system then carries the somatostatin from the hypothalamus to the **anterior pituitary**, where it inhibits the secretion of GH. Somatostatin in the hypothalamus is one of a number of neuropeptides that bridge the body's two major communication systems.

NEOPLASTIC HORMONE PRODUCTION

The ability of nonendocrine tissue to produce hormones first became apparent with the description of clinical syndromes in which some patients with lung cancer were found to make excessive amounts of vasopressin, a hormone usually made by the hypothalamus. Shortly afterward, people with other lung or gastrointestinal tumors were found to make adrenocorticotropic hormone (ACTH), which is normally made only in the pituitary. Subsequently, many neoplastic tissues were described that secrete a variety of hormones. As the ability to measure hormones in tissues has improved and, in particular, as the capability of measuring mRNA that codes for specific peptide hormones has developed, it has become clear that hormone production by neoplastic tissue is quite common, although most tumors produce only small amounts that may have no clinical consequence.

The production of hormones by nonendocrine neoplastic cells has been most clearly defined for cancers of the lung. There are several different types of lung cancer, each deriving from a different cell line, and yet each is capable of producing one or several hormones. The clinical syndromes that result from secretion of these hormones are often called **paraneoplastic syndromes.** Thus lung cancers arising from squamous cells are sometimes associated with hypercalcemia, which results from the secretion of a protein—parathyroid hormone–related peptide—that can mimic the activity of parathyroid hormone (p. 1101). Small-cell lung cancers are notorious for their ability to secrete a variety of hormones, including arginine vasopressin or antidiuretic hormone (with resultant hyponatremia; see box on p. 844), ACTH (with resultant Cushing syndrome; p. 1056), and many others. Still other types of lung cancer produce other paraneoplastic syndromes.

Nearly all these ectopic, neoplastic sources of hormone produce *peptide* hormones. Other sources of hormone production, in addition to lung cancer, include gastrointestinal tumors, renal and bladder cancer, neural tumors, unique tumors called **carcinoid tumors** that can arise almost anywhere in the body, and even lymphomas and melanomas. In some patients, the symptoms and signs resulting from ectopic hormone production may appear before any other reason to suspect an underlying neoplasm, and they may be the key tip-off to the correct diagnosis.

Hormones May Be Peptides, Metabolites of Single Amino Acids, or Metabolites of Cholesterol

Although the chemical nature of hormones is diverse, most commonly recognized mammalian hormones can be grouped into one of several classes. Table 46–1 is a list of many of the recognized classic mammalian hormones, which are divided into three groups based on their chemical structure and how they are made in the body.

TABLE 46–1

CHEMICAL CLASSIFICATION OF SELECTED HORMONES

Peptide Hormones

Adrenocorticotropin (ACTH)

Atrial natriuretic peptide (ANP)

Arginine vasopressin (AVP)
  (also known as antidiuretic hormone [ADH])

Calcitonin

Cholecystokinin (CCK)

Corticotropin-releasing hormone (CRH)

Follicle-stimulating hormone (FSH)

Glucagon

Gonadotropin-releasing hormone (GnRH)

Growth hormone (GH)

Growth hormone–releasing hormone (GHRH)

Inhibin

Insulin

Insulin-like growth factors I and II (IGFs)

Luteinizing hormone (LH)

Oxytocin (OT)

Parathyroid hormone (PTH)

Prolactin (PRL)

Secretin

Somatostatin

Thyrotropin (TSH)

Thyrotropin-releasing hormone (TRH)

Vasoactive intestinal peptide (VIP)

Amino Acid Hormones

Dopamine (DA)

Epinephrine (Epi), aka adrenaline

Norepinephrine (NE), aka noradrenaline

Serotonin, aka 5-hydroxytryptamine (5-HT)

Thyroxine (T_4)

Triiodothyronine (T_3)

Steroid Hormones

Aldosterone

Cortisol

Estradiol (E2)

Progesterone

Testosterone

Peptide hormones include a large group of hormones made by a variety of endocrine tissues. Insulin, glucagon, and somatostatin are made in the pancreas. The pituitary gland makes GH; the two gonadotropin hormones, luteinizing hormone (LH) and follicle-stimulating hormone (FSH); adrenocorticotropic hormone (ACTH); thyrotropin (also called thyroid-stimulating hormone or TSH); and prolactin (PRL). Parathyroid hormone is made in the parathyroid, and calcitonin is made in the thyroid glands.

In addition, other peptide hormones, such as somatostatin and several releasing hormones (e.g., growth hormone–releasing hormone [GHRH]) are made by the hypothalamus. Secretin, cholecystokinin, and other hormones are made by the gastrointestinal tract. Yet these tissues are not considered classic endocrine glands.

A more restricted number of tissues make **catecholamines** and **steroid hormones**. Synthesis of these hormones (from tyrosine and cholesterol, respectively) necessitates a number of enzymatic steps. Only very specialized tissues are capable of the series of enzymatic conversions that are necessary to make active hormone from the starting materials. Synthesis of thyroid hormone is even more complex and is essentially entirely restricted to the thyroid gland.

A number of glands make two or more hormones. Examples are the pituitary, the pancreatic islets, and the adrenal medulla. However, for the most part, individual cells within these glands are specialized to secrete a single hormone. One exception is the gonadotropin-producing cells of the pituitary, which secrete both FSH and LH.

Hormones Can Circulate Either Free or Bound to Carrier Proteins

Once secreted, many hormones circulate freely in the blood until they reach their target tissue. Others form complexes with circulating **binding proteins**; this use of binding proteins is particularly true for thyroid hormones (thyroxine [T_4] and triiodothyronine [T_3]), steroid hormones, insulin-like growth factors I and II (IGF-I and IGF-II), and GH.

Forming a complex with a circulating binding protein serves several functions. First, it provides the blood with a reservoir or pool of the hormone, thus minimizing minute-to-minute fluctuations in hormone concentration. Second, it extends the half-life of the hormone in the circulation. For example, more than 99.99% of T_4 circulates bound to one of three binding proteins (p. 1038); the half-life of circulating T_4 is 7 to 8 days, whereas the half-life of free T_4 is only several minutes. The hormones bound to plasma-binding proteins appear to be those whose actions are *chronic*—in particular, those involving induction of the synthesis of new protein in target tissues. Hormones that play a major *acute* role in the regulation of body metabolism (e.g., catecholamines, many peptide hormones) circulate freely without associated binding proteins.

The presence of plasma binding proteins can affect the total circulating concentration of a hormone without necessarily affecting the concentration of unbound or **free**

hormone in the blood. For example, during pregnancy the liver's synthesis of thyroxine-binding globulin increases. Because this protein avidly binds T_4, the free T_4 concentration would fall. However, the pituitary senses the small decline in free T_4 levels and secretes more TSH. As a result, the thyroid makes more T_4, so plasma levels of total T_4 rise. However, the free T_4 level is unchanged.

Immunoassays Allow Measurement of Circulating Hormones

In the late 1950s, Solomon Berson and Rosalyn Yalow demonstrated that in patients who receive insulin, the body forms antibodies that are directed against the insulin molecule. This observation was important in two respects:

First, it advanced the principle that the body's immune system can react to endogenous compounds; therefore, autoimmunity or reaction to self-antigens does occur. This notion is a fundamental tenet of our current understanding of many autoimmune diseases, among which are endocrine diseases such as type 1 diabetes mellitus, autoimmune hypothyroidism, and Graves' disease, a common form of autoimmune hyperthyroidism. Before the description of insulin autoantibodies, it was thought that the immune system simply did not react to self-antigens.

Second, because antibodies with a high affinity for insulin were induced in patients who were treated with insulin, Berson and Yalow reasoned that these antibodies could be used to measure the amount of insulin in serum. Figure 46–1 illustrates the principle of a **radioimmunoassay** and how it is used to measure the concentration of a hormone (or many other chemicals). If we incubate increasing amounts of a radiolabelled hormone with an antibody to that hormone, the quantity of labelled hormone that is bound to the antibody yields a saturation plot (see Fig. 46–1A). If we now add *unlabelled* hormone to the incubation mixture, less radioactively labelled hormone remains complexed to the antibody as unlabelled hormone takes its place. The more unlabelled hormone we add, the less labelled hormone is bound to the antibody (see Fig. 46–1B). A **displacement curve** is created by plotting the amount of radioactively labelled hormone that is complexed to the antibody as a function of the concentration of unlabelled hormone that is added (see Fig. 46–1C). This displacement curve can then be used as a standard curve to estimate the amount of hormone that is present in unknown samples. This estimate is accurate only if two assumptions hold true: first, that nothing else in the unknown mixture binds with the antibody other than the hormone under study, and second, that nothing in the unknown sample interferes with normal binding of the hormone to the antibody.

Antibodies that are highly specific for the chemical structure of interest can frequently be obtained. Moreover, these antibodies are of sufficiently high affinity to bind even the often minute amounts of hormone that is circulating in blood. Thus, radioimmunoassays—and recent adaptations that substitute chemiluminescent or enzymatic detection for radioactivity—have emerged as a potent and popular tool. Radioimmunoassays are now used for the measurement of virtually all hormones, as well as many

drugs, viruses, and toxins. Much of our understanding of the physiology of hormone secretion and action has been gained by the use of immunoassay methodology. Yalow shared the 1977 Nobel Prize in Medicine or Physiology for the discovery of the radioimmunoassay (Berson died before the honor was bestowed).

Hormones Can Have Complementary and Antagonistic Actions

Regulation of a number of complex physiological functions necessitates the **complementary action** of several hormones. This principle is true both for minute-to-minute homeostasis and for more long-term processes. For example, epinephrine (adrenaline), cortisol, and glucagon each contribute to the body's response to an acute bout of exercise (such as swimming the 50-m butterfly or running the 100-m dash). If one or more of these hormones are missing, exercise performance is adversely affected, and even more seriously, severe hypoglycemia and hyperkalemia (elevated plasma $[K^+]$) may develop. On a longer time scale, GH, insulin, IGF-I, thyroid hormone, and sex steroids are all needed for normal growth. Deficiency of GH, IGF-I, or thyroid hormone results in dwarfism. Deficiency of sex steroids, cortisol, or insulin produces less severe disturbances of growth.

Integration of hormone action can also involve hormones that exert **antagonistic actions**. In this case, the overall effect on an end organ depends on the balance between opposing influences. One example is the counterpoised effects of insulin and glucagon on blood glucose levels. Insulin lowers glucose levels by *inhibiting* glycogenolysis and gluconeogenesis in the liver and by stimulating glucose uptake into muscle and adipose tissue. Glucagon, in contrast, *stimulates* hepatic glycogenolysis and gluconeogenesis. Whereas glucagon does not appear to directly antagonize glucose uptake, epinephrine (which like glucagon is released in response to hypoglycemia) does. Balancing tissue function by opposing humoral effector mechanisms appears to be an important regulatory strategy for fine-tuning the control of many cellular functions.

Endocrine Regulation Occurs Through Feedback Control

The key to any regulatory system is its ability to sense when it should increase or decrease its activity. For the endocrine system, this function is accomplished by feedback control of hormone secretion (Fig. 46–2A). The hormone-secreting cell functions as a "sensor" that continually monitors the circulating concentration of some regulated variable. This variable may be a metabolic variable (e.g., glucose concentration) or the activity of another hormone. When the endocrine gland senses that too much (or too little) of the regulated variable is circulating in blood, it responds by decreasing (or increasing) the rate of hormone secretion. This response in turn affects the metabolic or secretory behavior of the target tissue, which may either directly "feed back" to the sensing cell or stimulate some other cell that eventually signals the

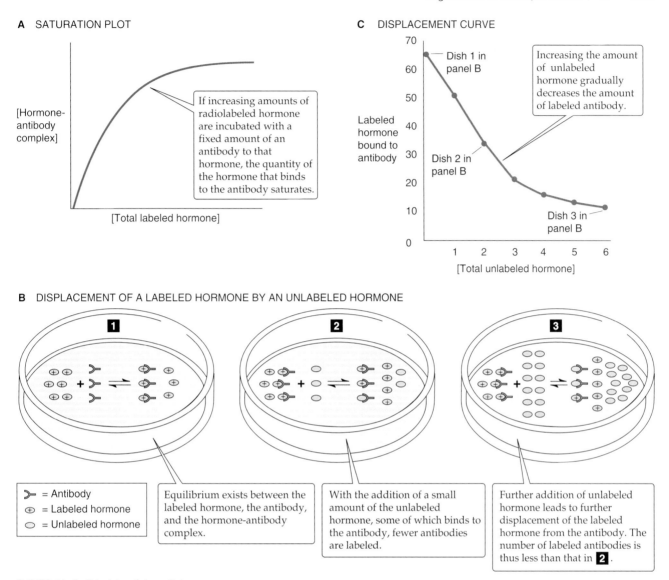

FIGURE 46–1. Principles of the radioimmunoassay.

"sensor" regarding whether the altered function of the endocrine gland has been effective.

A simple example is insulin secretion by the β cells of the pancreas. Increases in plasma [glucose] are "sensed" by the β cell, which secretes insulin in response. The rise in plasma [insulin] acts on the liver to decrease the synthesis of glucose and on the muscle to promote the storage of glucose. As a result, plasma [glucose] falls, and this decrease is sensed by the β cell, which reduces the rate of insulin secretion. This arrangement represents a very simple feedback system. Other systems can be quite complex; however, even this simple system involves the recognition of two circulating signals. The liver and muscle recognize the increase in plasma [insulin] as one signal, and the pancreatic β cell (the cell responsible for insulin secretion) recognizes the signal of a rise or decline in blood [glucose] as the other signal. In each case, the sensing system within a particular tissue is linked to an effector system that transduces the signal to the appropriate biologic response.

Endocrine Regulation Can Involve Hierarchic Levels of Control

Faced with a stress (e.g., a severe infection or extensive blood loss), the cerebral cortex stimulates the hypothalamus to release a neuropeptide called corticotropin-releasing hormone (CRH) (see Fig. 46–2B). Carried by the pituitary portal system (blood vessels that connect the hypothalamus to the anterior pituitary), CRH stimulates the anterior pituitary to release another hormone, ACTH, which in turn stimulates the adrenal cortical cells to synthesize cortisol. Cortisol regulates vascular tone as well as metabolic and growth functions in a variety of tissues.

This "stress response" therefore involves two glands, the pituitary and the adrenal cortex, as well as specialized "neuroendocrine" tissue in the hypothalamus and the CNS. This hierarchic control is regulated by feedback, just as in the simple feedback between plasma [glucose] and insulin. Within this CRH-ACTH-cortisol axis, feedback can occur at several levels. Cortisol inhibits the

A SIMPLE FEEDBACK
LOOP

B HIERARCHICAL
CONTROL

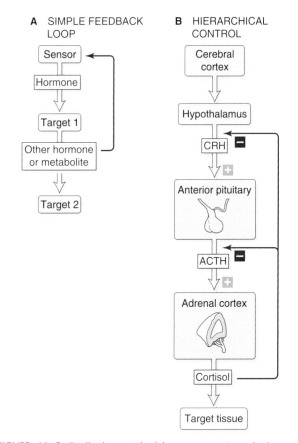

FIGURE 46–2. Feedback control of hormone secretion. *A,* A sensor (e.g., a β cell in a pancreatic islet) detects some regulated variable (e.g., plasma [glucose]) and responds by modulating its secretion of a hormone (e.g., insulin). This hormone, in turn, acts on a target (e.g., liver or muscle) to modulate its production of another hormone or a metabolite (e.g., glucose), which may affect a second target (e.g., making glucose available to the brain). In addition, the other hormone or metabolite feeds back on the original sensor cell. *B,* Under the influence of the cerebral cortex, the hypothalamic releases CRH, which stimulates the anterior pituitary to release ACTH, which in turn stimulates the adrenal cortex to release cortisol. The cortisol acts on a number of effector organs. In addition, the cortisol feeds back on both the anterior pituitary and the hypothalamus. ACTH, adrenocorticotropic hormone; CRH, corticotropin-releasing hormone.

production of CRH by the hypothalamus, as well as the sensitivity of the pituitary to a standard dose of CRH, which directly reduces ACTH release.

Feedback in hierarchic endocrine control systems can be quite complex and frequently involves interaction between the CNS and the endocrine system. Other examples are regulation of the female menstrual cycle (p. 1145) and regulation of GH secretion (p. 1026).

Together, the Hypothalamus and Pituitary Gland Provide Central Control of Multiple Endocrine Organs

Among the classic endocrine tissues, the **pituitary** (also known as the hypophysis) plays a special role (Fig. 46–3). Located at the base of the brain, just below the hypothalamus, the pituitary resides within a saddle-shaped cavity called the "sella turcica" (Latin for "Turkish sad-

dle"), which has bony anterior, posterior, and inferior borders and fibrous tissue that separate it from venous sinuses on either side. The pituitary in humans is composed of both an anterior and a posterior lobe. Through vascular and neural connections, the pituitary bridges and integrates the neural and endocrine mechanisms of homeostasis. The pituitary is a highly vascular tissue. The posterior pituitary receives arterial blood, whereas the anterior pituitary receives only portal venous inflow from the median eminence. The **pituitary portal system** is particularly important in its function of carrying neuropeptides from the hypothalamus and pituitary stalk to the anterior pituitary.

ANTERIOR PITUITARY. Glandular tissue in the anterior lobe of the pituitary synthesizes and secretes six peptide hormones: GH, TSH, ACTH, LH, FSH, and PRL. In each case, secretion of these hormones is under the control of hypothalamic **releasing hormones** (Table 46–2). The sources of these releasing hormones are small-diameter neurons located mainly in the "periventricular" portion of the hypothalamus that surrounds the third ventricle (p. 409). These small-diameter neurons synthesize the releasing hormones and discharge them into the median eminence and neural stalk, where they enter leaky capillaries—which are not part of the blood-brain barrier (p. 409). The releasing hormones then travel via the pituitary portal veins to the anterior pituitary. Once in the anterior pituitary, a releasing factor stimulates specialized cells to release a particular peptide hormone into the systemic bloodstream. The integrative function of the anterior pituitary can be appreciated by realizing that the main target for four of the anterior pituitary hormones (i.e., TSH, ACTH, and LH/FSH) is other endocrine tissue. Thus, these four anterior pituitary hormones are themselves "releasing hormones" that trigger the secretion of specific

FIGURE 46–3. The hypothalamo-pituitary axis. The pituitary (or hypophysis) is actually two glands—an anterior pituitary and a posterior pituitary (or neurohypophysis). Although in both cases the hypothalamus controls the secretion of hormones by the pituitary, the mechanisms are very different. **Anterior pituitary.** Small-bodied neurons in the hypothalamus secrete *releasing* and *inhibitory factors* into a rich funnel-shaped plexus of capillaries that penetrates the median eminence and surrounds the infundibular recess. The cell bodies of these neurons are in several nuclei that surround the third ventricle. These include: the arcuate, the paraventricular and ventromedial nuclei, and the medial preoptic and periventricular regions. The capillaries (primary plexus), which are outside of the blood-brain barrier, coalesce into *long* portal veins that carry the releasing and inhibitory factors down the pituitary stalk to the anterior pituitary. Other neurons secrete their releasing factors into a capillary plexus that is much further down the pituitary stalk; *short* portal veins carry these releasing factors to the anterior pituitary. There, the portal veins break up into the secondary capillary plexus of the anterior pituitary and deliver the releasing and inhibitory factors to the "troph" cells that actually secrete the anterior pituitary hormones (GH, TSH, ACTH, LH, FSH and PRL) that enter the systemic bloodstream and distribute throughout the body. **Posterior pituitary.** Large neurons in the paraventricular and supraoptic nuclei of the hypothalamus actually synthesize the hormones AVP and OT. These hormones travel down the axons of the hypothalamic neurons to the posterior pituitary where the nerve terminals release the hormones, like neurotransmitters, into a rich plexus of vessels. ACTH, adrenocorticotropin hormone; AVP, arginine vasopressin; FSH, follicle-stimulating hormone; GH, growth hormone; LH, luteinizing hormone; OT, oxytocin; PRL, prolactin; TSH, thyroid-stimulating hormone.

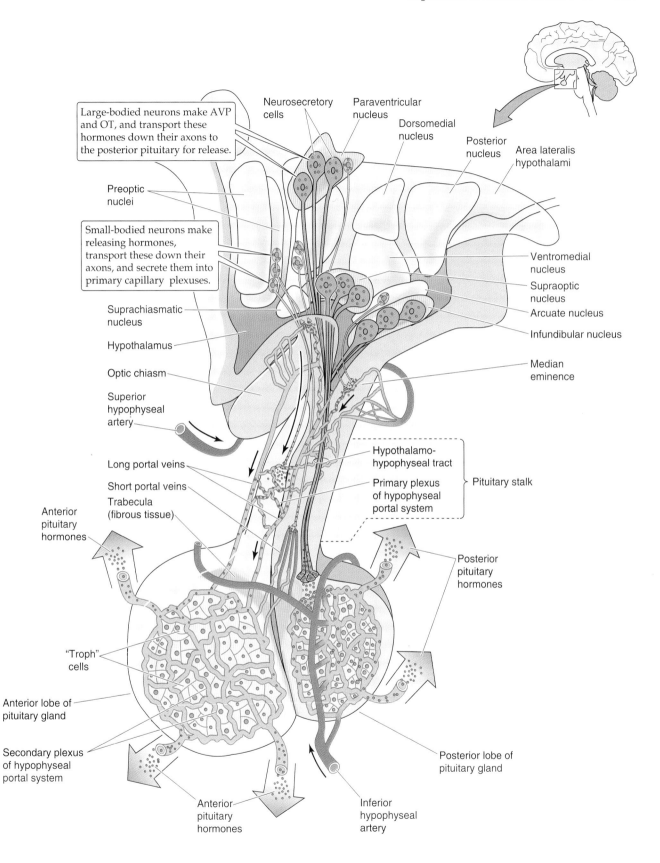

Large-bodied neurons make AVP and OT, and transport these hormones down their axons to the posterior pituitary for release.

Neurosecretory cells

Paraventricular nucleus

Dorsomedial nucleus

Posterior nucleus

Area lateralis hypothalami

Preoptic nuclei

Small-bodied neurons make releasing hormones, transport these down their axons, and secrete them into primary capillary plexuses.

Ventromedial nucleus

Supraoptic nucleus

Arcuate nucleus

Suprachiasmatic nucleus

Infundibular nucleus

Hypothalamus

Optic chiasm

Median eminence

Superior hypophyseal artery

Long portal veins

Hypothalamo-hypophyseal tract

Short portal veins

Primary plexus of hypophyseal portal system

Pituitary stalk

Trabecula (fibrous tissue)

Anterior pituitary hormones

Posterior pituitary hormones

"Troph" cells

Anterior lobe of pituitary gland

Secondary plexus of hypophyseal portal system

Posterior lobe of pituitary gland

Anterior pituitary hormones

Inferior hypophyseal artery

TABLE 46–2

HYPOTHALAMIC AND PITUITARY HORMONES

ANTERIOR PITUITARY

Releasing (Inhibitory) Factor Made by Hypothalamus	Target Cell in Anterior Pituitary	Hormone Released by Anterior Pituitary	Target of Anterior Pituitary Hormone
GHRH (inhibited by somatostatin)	Somatotroph	GH	Multiple somatic tissues
TRH	Thyrotroph	TSH	Thyroid follicular cells, stimulated to make thyroid hormone
CRH	Corticotroph	ACTH	Fasciculata and reticularis cells of the adrenal cortex, to make corticosteroids
GnRH	Gonadotroph	FSH	Ovarian follicular cells, to make estrogens and progestins Sertoli cells, to initiate spermato-genesis
GnRH	Gonadotroph	LH	Ovarian follicular cells, to make estrogens and progestins Leydig cells, to make testosterone
(inhibited by dopamine)	Lactotroph	PRL	Mammary glands, initiates and maintains milk production

POSTERIOR PITUITARY

Hormone Synthesized in Hypothalamus	Hormone Released into Posterior Pituitary	Target of Posterior Pituitary
AVP	AVP	Collecting duct, to increase water permeability
OT	OT	Uterus and breast

ACTH, adrenocorticotropic hormone; AVP, arginine vasopressin; CRH, corticotropin-releasing hormone; FSH, follicle-stimulating hormone; GH, growth hormone; GHRH, GH-releasing hormone; GnRH, gonadotropin-releasing hormone; LH, luteinizing hormone; OT, oxytocin; PRL, prolactin; TRH, thyrotropin-releasing hormone; TSH, thyroid-stimulating hormone.

hormones. For example, TSH causes the follicular cells in the thyroid gland to synthesize and release thyroid hormones. The mechanism by which the pituitary regulates these endocrine glands is discussed in detail in later chapters in the endocrine part of this text.

GH also acts like a "releasing factor" in that it regulates the production of another hormone, IGF-I. IGF-I is made in principally *non*endocrine tissues (e.g., liver, kidney, muscle, and cartilage). Nevertheless, IGF-I in the circulation feeds back on the hypothalamus and on the pituitary to inhibit GH secretion. In this respect, the GH–IGF-I axis is similar to axes involving classic pituitary pathways, such as the thyrotropin-releasing hormone (TRH)-TSH axis.

Regulation of PRL secretion differs from that of other anterior pituitary hormones in that no endocrine "feedback" mechanism has yet been identified. The pituitary secretes **prolactin** at relatively low levels throughout life in both males and females. However, its major biologic action, promotion of lactation, is important only in females and only at specific times in a woman's life. Although PRL is not part of an identified feedback system, its release is controlled. Left to its own devices, the anterior pituitary would secrete high levels of PRL. However, secretion of PRL is normally inhibited by the release of dopamine from the hypothalamus (p. 1187). During breast

stimulation, neural afferents inhibit hypothalamic dopamine release, thus inhibiting release of the inhibitor and permitting lactation to proceed. PRL receptors are present on multiple tissues other than the breast. However, other physiologic actions beyond lactation have not been well characterized.

POSTERIOR PITUITARY. Unlike the anterior pituitary, the posterior lobe of the pituitary is actually part of the brain. The posterior pituitary (or neurohypophysis) contains the nerve endings of *large*-diameter neurons whose cell bodies are in the supraoptic and paraventricular nuclei of the hypothalamus (see Fig. 46–3). Recall that the hypothalamic neurons that produce releasing factors, which act on "troph" cells in the anterior pituitary, are *small*-diameter neurons. The large-diameter hypothalamic neurons synthesize arginine vasopressin and oxytocin and then transport these hormones along their axons to the site of release in the posterior pituitary. Thus, like the anterior pituitary, the posterior pituitary releases peptide hormones. Also like the anterior pituitary, release of these hormones is under ultimate control of the hypothalamus. However, the hypothalamic axons traveling to the posterior pituitary replace both the transport of releasing factors by the portal system of the anterior pituitary, and the synthesis of hormones by the anterior pituitary "troph" cells. Although the posterior pituitary is part of the brain, it is one of the so-called circumventricular organs (p. 409) whose vessels breech the blood-brain barrier and allow the secreted vasopressin and oxytocin to reach the systemic circulation.

Arginine vasopressin (AVP), or antidiuretic hormone (ADH), is a neuropeptide hormone that acts on the collecting duct of the kidney to increase water reabsorption (p. 840). **Oxytocin** is the other neuropeptide secreted by the posterior pituitary. However, its principal biologic action relates to stimulation of smooth muscle contraction by the uterus during parturition (p. 1184) and by the mammary gland during suckling (p. 1189).

PEPTIDE HORMONES

Specialized Endocrine Cells Synthesize, Store, and Secrete Peptide Hormones

Organisms as primitive as fungi secrete proteins or peptides in an effort to respond to and affect their environment. In more complex organisms, peptide hormones play important developmental and other regulatory roles. Transcription of peptide hormones is regulated by both *cis*- and *trans*-acting elements (see Chapter 5). When transcription is active, the mRNA is processed in the nucleus and the capped message moves to the cytosol, where it associates with ribosomes on the rough endoplasmic reticulum. These peptides are destined for secretion because an amino acid signal sequence—the "signal sequence"—present near the N terminus targets the protein to the endoplasmic reticulum while the protein is still associated with the ribosome (Fig. 2–16).

With minor modification, the **secretory pathway** that is illustrated in Figure 2–19 describes the synthesis, processing, storage, and secretion of peptides by a wide variety of endocrine tissues. Once the protein is in the lumen of the endoplasmic reticulum, processing (e.g., glycosylation or further proteolytic cleavage) yields the mature, biologically active hormone. This processing occurs in a very dynamic setting. The protein is first transferred to the *cis*-Golgi domain, then through to the *trans*-Golgi, and finally to the mature, membrane-bound secretory vesicle or granule in which the mature hormone is stored before secretion. This pathway is referred to as the **regulated pathway** of hormone synthesis because external stimuli can trigger the cell to release hormone that is stored in the secretory granule, as well as promote the synthesis of additional hormone. For example, binding of GHRH to somatotrophs causes them to release GH.

A second pathway of hormone synthesis is the "**constitutive pathway.**" Here, secretion occurs more directly from the endoplasmic reticulum or vesicles formed in the *cis*-Golgi. Secretion of hormone, both mature and partially processed, by the constitutive pathway is less responsive to secretory stimuli than is secretion by the regulated pathway.

In both the regulated and constitutive pathways, fusion of the vesicular membrane with the plasma membrane—exocytosis of the vesicular contents—is the final common pathway for hormone secretion. In general, the regulated pathway is capable of secreting much larger amounts of hormone—on demand—than the constitutive pathway is. However, even when stimulated to secrete its peptide hormone, the cell typically secretes only a very small amount of the total hormone present in the secretory granules. To maintain this secretory reserve, many endocrine cells increase the synthesis of peptide hormones in response to the same stimuli that trigger secretion.

Peptide Hormones Bind to Cell-Surface Receptors and Activate a Variety of Signal-Transduction Systems

Once secreted, most peptide hormones exist free in the circulation. As noted earlier, this lack of binding proteins contrasts with the situation for steroid and thyroid hormones, which circulate bound to plasma proteins. IGF-I and IGF-II are an exception to this rule: at least six plasma proteins bind these peptide growth factors.

While traversing the circulation, peptide hormones encounter receptors on the surface of target cells. These receptors are intrinsic membrane proteins that bind the hormone with very high affinity (typically, K_d ranges from 10^{-8} to 10^{-12} M). Examples of several types of peptide hormone receptors are shown in Figure 46–4. Each of these receptors has already been introduced in Chapter 4. The primary sequence of most peptide hormone receptors is known from molecular cloning, mutant receptors have been synthesized, and the properties of native and mutant receptors have been compared to assess primary structural requirements for receptor function. Despite this elegant work, too little information is available on the three-dimensional structure of these membrane proteins for us to know just how the message that a hormone has bound to the receptor is transmitted to the internal surface of the cell membrane. However, regardless of the details, occupancy of the receptor can activate a variety of intracellular signal-transduction systems (Fig. 46–4 and Table 46–3) that transfer the signal of cell activation from the internal surface of the membrane to intracellular targets. The receptor provides the link between a specific extracellular hormone and the activation of a specific signal-transduction system. We have discussed each of these signal-transduction systems in Chapter 4. Here, we briefly review the various signal-transduction systems through which peptide hormones act.

HETEROTRIMERIC G PROTEINS COUPLED TO ADENYLYL CYCLASE. Cyclic adenosine monophosphate (cAMP), the prototypic second messenger, was discovered during investigation of glucagon's action on glycogenolysis in the liver. In addition to playing a role in hormone action, cAMP is involved in such diverse processes as lymphocyte activation, mast-cell degranulation, and even slime mold aggregation!

As summarized in Figure 46–4A, binding of the appropriate hormone (e.g., parathyroid hormone) to its receptor initiates a cascade of events (p. 97): (1) activation of a heterotrimeric G protein (α_s or α_i); (2) activation (by α_s) or inhibition (by α_i) of a membrane-bound adenylyl cyclase; (3) formation of intracellular cAMP from adenosine triphosphate, catalyzed by adenylyl cyclase; (4) bind-

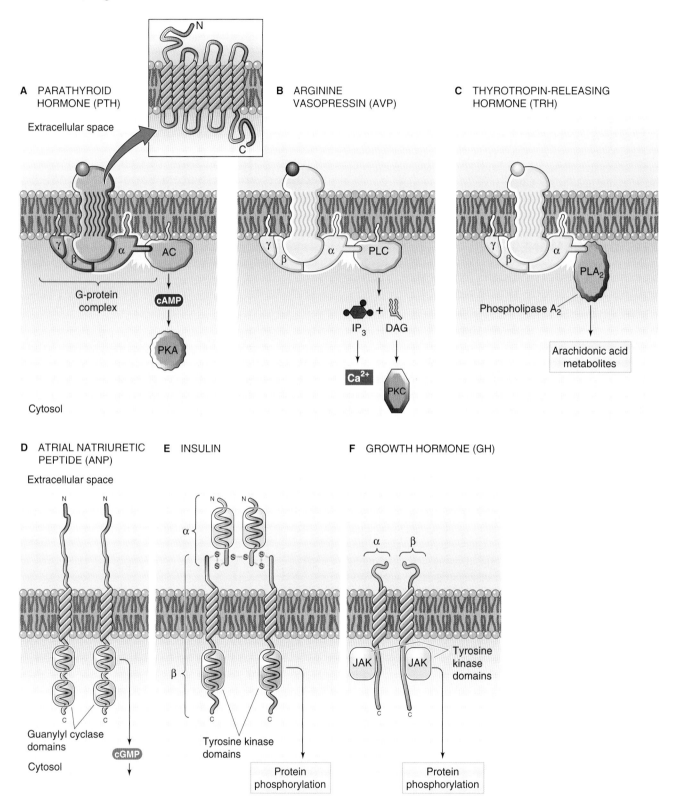

FIGURE 46–4. Receptors and downstream effectors for peptide hormones. AC, adenylyl cyclase; cAMP, cyclic adenosine monophosphate; cGMP, cyclic guanosine monophosphate; DAG, diacylglycerol; IP$_3$, inositol 1,4,5-triphosphate; JAK, Janus kinase or just another kinase; PK, protein kinase; PL, phospholipid.

TABLE 46–3

PEPTIDE HORMONES AND THEIR SIGNAL-TRANSDUCTION PATHWAYS

AGONISTS	RECEPTOR	LINKED ENZYME	SECOND MESSENGER
PTH	Coupled to $G\alpha_s$	Adenylyl cyclase	cAMP
ANG II	Coupled to $G\alpha_i$	Adenylyl cyclase (inhibited)	cAMP
AVP, ANG II, TRH	Coupled to $G\alpha_q$	Phospholipase C	IP_3 and DAG
ANG II	Coupled to G_i/G_o	PLA_2	Arachidonic acid metabolites
ANP	Guanylyl cyclase	Guanylyl cyclase	cGMP
Insulin, IGF-I, IGF-II, EGF, PDGF	Tyrosine kinase	Tyrosine kinase	Phosphoproteins
Growth hormone, erythropoietin, LIF	Associated with tyrosine kinase	JAK/STAT family of tyrosine kinases	Phosphoproteins

ANG II, angiotensin II; ANP, atrial natriuretic peptide; AVP, arginine vasopressin; cAMP, cyclic adenosine monophosphate; cGMP, cyclic guanosine monophosphate; DAG, diacylglycerol; EGF, epidermal growth factor; IGF, insulin-like growth factor; IP_3, inositol 1,4,5-triphosphate; JAK/STAT, Janus kinase/signal transducer and activator of transcription; LIF, leukemia inhibitory factor; PLA_2, phospholipase A_2; PDGF, platelet-derived growth factor; PTH, parathyroid hormone; TRH, thyrotropin-releasing hormone.

ing of cAMP to the enzyme protein kinase A (PKA); (5) separation of the two catalytic subunits of PKA from the two regulatory subunits; (6) phosphorylation of *serine* and *threonine* residues on a variety of cellular enzymes and other proteins by the free catalytic subunits of PKA that are no longer restrained; and (7) modification of cellular function by these phosphorylations. The activation is terminated in two ways. First, phosphodiesterases in the cell degrade cAMP. Second, *serine/threonine*-specific protein phosphatases can dephosphorylate enzymes and proteins that had previously been phosphorylated by PKA.

HETEROTRIMERIC G PROTEINS COUPLED TO PHOSPHOLIPASE C. As summarized in Figure 46–4B, binding of the appropriate peptide hormone (e.g., AVP) to its receptor initiates the following cascade of events (p. 100): (1) activation of $G\alpha_q$; (2) activation of a membrane-bound phospholipase C (PLC); and (3) cleavage of phosphatidylinositol 4,5-biphosphate (PIP_2) by this PLC, with the generation of *two* signalling molecules, inositol 1,4,5-triphosphate (IP_3) and diacylglycerol (DAG). The first step in the IP_3 fork of the pathway is (4) binding of IP_3 to a receptor on the cytosolic surface of the endoplasmic reticulum; (5) release of Ca^{2+} from internal stores, which causes $[Ca^{2+}]_i$ to rise by several-fold; (6) activation of Ca^{2+}-dependent kinases (e.g., Ca^{2+}-calmodulin–dependent protein kinases, protein kinase C [PKC]) by the increases in $[Ca^{2+}]_i$; and (7) alteration of cell function.

The first step in the DAG fork of the pathway is (4) allosteric activation of PKC by DAG (the activity of this enzyme is also stimulated by the increased $[Ca^{2+}]_i$) and (5) phosphorylation of a variety of proteins by PKC, which is activated in the plane of the cell membrane. An example of a hormone whose actions are in part mediated by DAG is TSH.

HETEROTRIMERIC G PROTEINS COUPLED TO PHOSPHOLIPASE A₂. As summarized in Fig. 46–4C, some peptide hormones (e.g., TRH) activate phospholipase A_2 (PLA_2)

through the following cascade (p. 103): (1) activation of $G\alpha_q$ or $G\alpha_{11}$, (2) stimulation of membrane-bound PLA_2 by the activated $G\alpha$, (3) cleavage of membrane phospholipids by PLA_2 to produce lysophospholipid and arachidonic acid, and (4) conversion—by a number of enzymes—of arachidonic acid into a variety of biologically active eicosanoids (e.g., prostaglandins, prostacyclins, thromboxanes, and leukotrienes).

GUANYLYL CYCLASE. Other peptide hormones (e.g., atrial natriuretic peptide) bind to a receptor (see Fig. 46–4D) that is itself a guanylyl cyclase that converts cytoplasmic guanosine triphosphate to cyclic guanosine monophosphate (cGMP) (p. 108). In turn, cGMP can activate cGMP-dependent kinases, phosphatases, or ion channels.

PSEUDOHYPOPARATHYROIDISM

Inasmuch as G proteins are part of the signalling system involved in a large number of hormone responses, molecular alterations in G proteins might be expected to affect a number of signalling systems. In the disorder **pseudohypoparathyroidism,** the key defect is an abnormality in a stimulatory α subunit (α_s) of a heterotrimeric G protein. The result is an impairment in the ability of parathyroid hormone (PTH) to regulate body calcium and phosphorus homeostasis (see Chapter 51). Patients with this disorder have a low serum $[Ca^{2+}]$ and high serum phosphate level, just like patients whose parathyroid glands have been surgically removed. However, patients with pseudohypoparathyroidism have **increased** circulating concentrations of PTH; the hormone simply cannot act normally on its target tissue, hence the term "pseudohypoparathyroidism." These individuals also have an increased risk for hypothyroidism and gonadal dysfunction (the latter in women). These additional endocrine deficiencies arise from the same defect in signalling.

FIGURE 46–5. Catecholamine receptors. The β_1, β_2, and DA-1 receptors all interact with $G\alpha_s$, which activates adenylyl cyclase (AC) and raises levels of cyclic AMP (cAMP). The α_2 and DA-2 receptors interact with $G\alpha_i$, which inhibits AC. Additionally, the α_1 receptor interacts with $G\alpha_q$, which activates phospholipase C (PLC), which in turn converts phophoinositides in the cell membrane to inositol-1,4,5-trisphosphate (IP_3) and diacylglycerol (DAG). ATP, adenosine triphosphate; DA, dopamine.

RECEPTOR TYROSINE KINASES. For some peptide hormones, notably insulin and IGF-I and IGF-II, the hormone receptor (see Fig. 46–4E) itself possesses tyrosine kinase activity (p. 110). This property is also true for other growth factors, including PDGF and epidermal growth factor. Occupancy of the receptor by the appropriate hormone increases kinase activity. For the insulin and IGF-I receptor, as well as for others, this kinase autophosphorylates tyrosines within the hormone receptor, as well as substrates within the cytosol, initiating a cascade of phosphorylation reactions.

TYROSINE KINASE–ASSOCIATED RECEPTORS. Some peptide hormones (e.g., GH) bind to a receptor that, when occupied, activates a cytoplasmic tyrosine kinase (see Fig. 46–4F), such as a member of the JAK (Janus kinase) family of kinases (p. 111). As for the receptor tyrosine kinases, activation of these receptor-associated kinases initiates a cascade of phosphorylation reactions.

AMINE HORMONES

Amine Hormones Are Made from Tyrosine and Tryptophan

Four major amine hormones are recognized. The adrenal medulla makes the catecholamine hormones **epinephrine** and **norepinephrine** from the amino acid tyrosine (see Fig. 12–9C). These hormones are the principal active amine hormones made by the endocrine system. In addition to its role as a hormone, norepinephrine also serves as a neurotransmitter by the CNS (p. 300) and by postganglionic sympathetic neurons (p. 387). **Dopamine**, which is also synthesized from tyrosine, acts as a neurotransmitter (p. 302); it is synthesized in a number of other tissues, but its functional role outside the nervous system is not well clarified. Finally, the hormone **serotonin** is made from tryptophan (see Fig. 12–9B) by endocrine cells that are located within the gut mucosa. Serotonin appears to act locally to regulate both motor and secretory function of the gut.

The **adrenal medulla** in humans secretes principally epinephrine (p. 1062). The final products are stored in vesicles that are called **chromaffin granules**. Secretion of catecholamines by the adrenal medulla appears to be mediated entirely by stimulation of the sympathetic division of the autonomic nervous system (p. 388). Unlike the situation for many peptide hormones, where the circulating concentration of the hormone (e.g., TSH) negatively feeds back on secretion of the releasing hormone (e.g., TRH), the amine hormones do not have such a hierarchic "feedback" system. Rather, the feedback of amine hormones is indirect. The higher control center does not sense circulating levels of the amine hormones (e.g., epinephrine), but rather a physiologic "end effect" of that amine hormone (e.g., blood pressure; see Chapter 22). The "sensor" of the end effect may be a peripheral receptor (e.g., stretch receptor) that communicates to the higher center (e.g., the CNS), and the efferent limb is the sympathetic outflow that determines release of the amine.

Amine Hormones Act via Surface Receptors

Once secreted, circulating epinephrine is free to associate with specific adrenergic receptors or **adrenoceptors** located on the surface membranes of target cells. A variety of types of adrenoceptors exist and are generically grouped as α and β, each of which has several subtypes (see Table 15–2). All adrenoceptors, isolated from a variety of tissues and species, are classic G-protein–coupled receptors. As indicated in Figure 46–5, the intracellular action of a specific catecholamine is determined by the complement of receptors present on the surface of a specific cell. For example, when epinephrine binds to the β_1 receptor, it activates a $G\alpha_s$ protein, which stimulates adenylyl cyclase, promotes increases in $[cAMP]_i$, and thus enhances the activity of PKA (Table 46–4). On the other

TABLE 46–4

CATECHOLAMINE RECEPTORS AND THEIR TRANSDUCTION PATHWAYS

RECEPTOR TYPE	AGONISTS*	G PROTEIN	LINKED ENZYME	SECOND MESSENGER
α_1	NE $\geq$ Epi (phenylephrine)	$G\alpha_q$	PLC	$\uparrow$ IP$_3$ and Ca^{2+} DAG
α_2	NE $\geq$ Epi (clonidine)	$G\alpha_i$	Adenylyl cyclase (inhibited)	$\downarrow$ [cAMP]$_i$
β_1	Epi = NE (dobutamine, isoproterenol)	$G\alpha_s$	Adenylyl cyclase	$\uparrow$ [cAMP]$_i$
β_2	Epi > NE (terbutaline, isoproterenol)	$G\alpha_s$	Adenylyl cyclase	$\uparrow$ [cAMP]$_i$
β_3	NE > Epi (SR 59230A, isoproterenol)	$G\alpha_s$	Adenylyl cyclase	$\uparrow$ [cAMP]$_i$
DA-1	Dopamine	$G\alpha_s$	Adenylyl cyclase	$\uparrow$ [cAMP]$_i$
DA-2	Dopamine	$G\alpha_i$	Adenylyl cyclase	$\downarrow$ [cAMP]$_i$

*Epi is epinephrine and NE is norepinephrine. Selective agonists are in parentheses.
cAMP, cyclic adenosine monophosphate; DAG, diacylglycerol; IP$_3$, inositol 1,4,5-triphosphate; PLC, phospholipase C; SR 59230A, [3-(2-ethyl-phenoxy)-[(1S)-1,2,3,4-tetrahydronaphth-1-ylaminol]-(2S)2-propanol oxalate.

hand, when the same hormone binds to a cell displaying principally α_2 receptors, it activates a $G\alpha_i$ protein, which inhibits adenylyl cyclase, diminishes [cAMP]$_i$, and therefore reduces PKA activity. Thus, the response of a specific tissue to adrenergic stimulation (whether via circulating epinephrine or via norepinephrine released locally by sympathetic neurons) is determined by the receptor repertoire displayed by the cell. The same is true for dopamine; the DA-1 receptor is coupled to $G\alpha_s$ and the DA-2 receptor is linked to $G\alpha_i$.

Epinephrine has a greater affinity for β receptors than for α receptors, whereas norepinephrine acts predominantly via α receptors. The various signal-transduction systems linked to these receptors are discussed in Chapter 4. β-Adrenergic stimulation occurs via the adenylyl cyclase system. The α_2 receptor also usually acts through adenylyl cyclase. However, α_1-adrenergic stimulation is linked to $G\alpha_q$, which activates a membrane-associated PLC that liberates IP$_3$ and DAG. IP$_3$ can release Ca^{2+} from intracellular stores, and DAG directly enhances the activity of PKC. Combined, these actions enhance the cellular activity of Ca^{2+}-dependent kinases, which produce a metabolic response that is characteristic of the specific cell. The response to adrenergic agonists may be, for example, glycogenolysis in the liver or muscle (predominantly a β effect), contraction (an α_1 effect) or relaxation (a β_2 effect) of vascular smooth muscle, a change in the inotropic or chronotropic state of the heart (a β_1 effect), or a variety of other effects.

STEROID AND THYROID HORMONES

Cholesterol Is the Precursor for the Steroid Hormones: Cortisol, Aldosterone, Estradiol, Progesterone, and Testosterone

The family of hormones called "steroids" shares a common biochemical parentage: all are synthesized from cholesterol. Only two tissues in the body possess the enzy-

matic apparatus to convert cholesterol to active hormones. The **adrenal cortex** makes cortisol (the main glucocorticoid hormone), aldosterone (the principal mineralocorticoid in humans), and androgens. The **gonads** make either estrogen and progesterone (ovary) or testosterone (testes). In each case, production of steroid hormones is regulated by trophic hormones released from the pituitary. For aldosterone, the renin-angiotensin system also plays an important regulatory role.

The pathways involved in steroid synthesis are summarized in Figure 46–6. Cells that produce steroid hormones can use, as a starting material for hormone synthesis, the cholesterol that is circulating in the blood in association with low-density lipoprotein (LDL) (p. 1000). Alternatively, these cells can synthesize cholesterol de novo from acetate (Fig. 45–16). In humans, LDL cholesterol appears to furnish approximately 80% of the cholesterol used for steroid synthesis (Fig. 46–6). An LDL particle contains both free cholesterol and cholesteryl esters, in addition to phospholipids and protein. The cell takes up this LDL particle via the LDL receptor and receptor-mediated endocytosis (p. 44) into clathrin-coated vesicles. Lysosomal hydrolases then act on the cholesteryl esters to release free cholesterol. The cholesterol nucleus, whether taken up or synthesized de novo, subsequently undergoes a series of reactions that culminate in the formation of **pregnenolone**, the common precursor of all steroid hormones. Via divergent pathways, pregnenolone is then further metabolized to the major steroid hormones: the mineralocorticoid aldosterone (see Fig. 49–2), the glucocorticoid cortisol (see Fig. 49–2), the estrogen estradiol (see Fig. 54–9), and the androgen testosterone (see Fig. 53–5).

Unlike the peptide and amine hormones that we have considered up to now, steroid hormones are not stored in secretory vesicles before their secretion (Table 46–5). For these hormones, synthesis and secretion are very closely linked temporally. Steroid-secreting cells are capable of increasing the secretion of steroid hormones many-fold within several hours. The lack of a preformed storage pool of steroid hormone does not appear to limit their

FIGURE 46–6. Uptake of cholesterol and synthesis of steroid hormones from cholesterol. The cholesterol needed as the starting material in the synthesis of steroid hormones comes from two sources. Approximately 80% is taken up as LDL particles via receptor-mediated endocytosis. The cell synthesizes the remaining cholesterol de novo from acetyl coenzyme A (Acetyl CoA). LDL, low-density lipoprotein; VLDL, very-low-density lipoprotein.

effectiveness as an endocrine regulatory system. Furthermore, steroid hormones, unlike peptide and amine hormones, mediate nearly all their actions on target tissues by regulating gene transcription. As a result, the response of target tissues to steroids typically occurs over hours to days.

Like cholesterol itself, steroid hormones are poorly soluble in water. On their release into the circulation, steroid hormones associate with specific binding proteins (e.g., sex hormone–binding globulin) that transport the steroid hormones through the circulatory system to their target tissues. The presence of these binding proteins, whose concentration in the circulation can change in response to a variety of physiologic conditions, can complicate efforts to measure the amount of active steroid hormone in the circulation.

Steroid Hormones Bind to Intracellular Receptors That Regulate Gene Transcription

Steroid hormones appear to enter their target cell by simple diffusion across the plasma membrane (Fig. 46–7). Once within the cell, steroid hormones are bound with high affinity (K_d in the range of 1 nM) to receptor proteins located in the cytosol and/or the nucleus. As detailed in Chapter 5, binding of steroid hormone to its receptor results in a change in the receptor conformation so that the "active" receptor-hormone complex now binds with high affinity to specific DNA sequences called **hormone response elements** or **steroid response elements** (SREs) (p. 131). These sequences are within the 5′ region of target genes whose transcription is regulated by the specific steroid hormone–receptor complex. *Termination*

of gene regulation by the steroid hormone–receptor complex is not as well understood as *initiation* of the signal. The receptor protein may be modified in a manner that permits dissociation of the hormone and DNA. The receptor itself could then be recycled and the steroid molecule metabolized or otherwise cleared from the cell.

Steroid receptors are monomeric phosphoproteins with a molecular weight that is between 80 and 100 kDa. A remarkable similarity is seen among receptors for the glucocorticoids, sex steroids, retinoic acid, the steroid-like vitamin 1,25-dihydroxyvitamin D, and thyroid hormone. The receptors for these diverse hormones are considered part of a gene super family (p. 112). Each of these receptors has a similar modular construction with six domains (A through F). The homology among receptors is especially striking for the C domain, particularly the C1 subdomain, which is the part of the receptor molecule that is responsible for binding to DNA.

Steroid hormone receptors dimerize on binding to their target sites on DNA. Dimerization appears essential for the regulation of gene transcription. Within the C1 DNA-binding domain of the steroid receptor monomer are two "zinc fingers" that are involved in binding of the receptor to DNA (p. 131). Note that even receptors with very different biologic actions have a striking sequence similarity in this domain of the receptor. Because the specificity with which genes are regulated by a specific steroid receptor arises from the specificity of the DNA-binding domain, mutations in this region can greatly alter hormone function. For example, substitution of two amino acids in the *glucocorticoid* receptor causes the mutated glucocorticoid receptor to bind to DNA to which the *estrogen* receptor normally binds. In such a system, a glucocorticoid might have an estrogen-like effect.

TABLE 46–5

DIFFERENCES BETWEEN STEROID AND PEPTIDE/AMINE HORMONES		
PROPERTY	**STEROID HORMONES**	**PEPTIDE-AMINE HORMONES**
Storage pools	None	Secretory vesicles
Interaction with cell membrane	Diffusion through cell membrane	Binding to receptor on cell membrane
Receptor	In cytoplasm or nucleus	On cell membrane
Action	Regulation of gene transcription (primarily)	Signal-transduction cascade(s) affect a variety of cell processes
Response time	Hours to days (primarily)	Seconds to minutes

The activated steroid receptor, binding as a dimer to SREs in the 5′ region of a gene, regulates the rate of transcription of that gene. Each response element is identifiable as a consensus sequence of nucleotides, or a region of regulatory DNA in which the nucleotide sequences are preserved through different cell types. The effect of gene regulation by activated steroid receptors binding to an SRE is dramatically illustrated by the chick ovalbumin gene. Chicks that are not exposed to estrogen have approximately four copies of the ovalbumin mRNA per cell in the oviduct. Seven days of estrogen treatment increases the number of copies of message 10,000-fold! This increase in message is due principally to an increased rate of gene transcription. However, steroid hormones can also stabilize specific mRNA molecules and increase their half-life.

The 5′ flanking region of the gene typically has one or more SREs upstream of the TATA box, a nucleotide sequence rich in adenine and thymine that is located near the starting point for transcription (p. 120). The activated steroid hormone receptors recognize these SREs from their specific consensus sequences. For example, one particular consensus sequence designates a site as a *glucocorticoid* response element if the SRE is in a cell with a glucocorticoid receptor. This same consensus sequence in a cell of the endometrium would be recognized by the activated *progesterone* receptor or, in the renal distal tubule, by the activated *mineralocorticoid* receptor. The specificity of the response thus depends on the cell's expression of particular steroid receptors, not simply the consensus sequence. For example, the renal distal tubule cell expresses relatively more mineralocorticoid receptors than it does progesterone receptors when compared with the endometrium. As a result, changes in plasma aldosterone regulate Na⁺ reabsorption in the kidney with greater sensitivity than does circulating progesterone. However, very high levels of progesterone can, like aldosterone, promote salt reabsorption.

From the foregoing it should be apparent that the specificity of response of a tissue to steroid hormones depends on the abundance of specific steroid receptors that are expressed within a cell. Because all somatic cells have the full complement of DNA with genes possessing SREs, whether a cell responds to circulating estrogen (e.g., breast), androgen (e.g., prostate), or mineralocorticoid (e.g., renal collecting duct) depends on the receptors present in the cell. This specificity raises the obvious, but as yet unanswered question of what regulates the expression of specific steroid receptors by specific tissues.

Within a given tissue a number of factors control the concentration of steroid hormone receptors. In the cytosol of all steroid-responsive tissues, steroid receptor levels usually drop dramatically immediately after exposure of the tissue to the agonist hormone. This decrease in receptor level is due to net movement of the agonist-receptor complex to the nucleus. Eventually, the cytosolic recep-

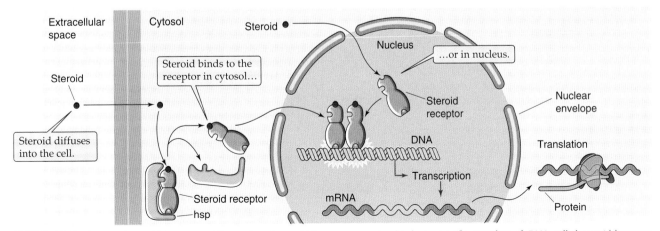

FIGURE 46–7. Action of steroid hormones. The activated steroid-hormone receptor binds to specific stretches of DNA called steroid-hormone response elements (SREs), which stimulates the transcription of appropriate genes. hsp, heat shock protein; mRNA, messenger RNA.

tors are repopulated. Depending on the tissue, this repopulation may involve new synthesis of steroid hormone receptors or simply recycling of receptors from the nucleus after dissociation of the agonist from the receptor. In addition, some steroids reduce the synthesis of their own receptor in target tissues. For example, progesterone reduces the synthesis of progesterone receptor by the uterus, thus leading to an overall net reduction or "downregulation" of progesterone receptor concentration in a target tissue. An interesting observation in this regard is that the genes for steroid receptor proteins do *not* appear to have SREs in their 5' flanking region. Thus, this regulation of receptor number probably involves *trans*-acting transcriptional factors (p. 116) other than the steroid hormones themselves.

Other factors that affect the concentration of steroid receptors in target tissues include the state of differentiation of the tissue, the presence of other hormones that affect steroid receptor synthesis, and whether the steroid hormone has previously stimulated the tissue. For example, estrogen receptor concentrations are low in an unstimulated uterus but rise dramatically in an estrogen-primed uterus (receptor upregulation). Regulation of steroid receptor number is clearly one factor that alters overall tissue sensitivity to these hormones.

Thyroid Hormones Regulate the Metabolic Rate After Binding to Intracellular Receptors, As Do Steroid Hormones

In many respects, the thyroid gland and thyroid hormone are unique among the classic endocrine axes. In Chapter 48, in which thyroid physiology is discussed in more detail, this uniqueness begins with the structure of the thyroid gland, which is composed of follicles. Each follicle is an epithelial layer of cells encircling a lake of fluid that contains a very protein-rich follicular fluid. The principal protein component of the follicular fluid is a very large protein, thyroglobulin. Neither of the two thyroid hormones—T_4 and T_3—is free in the follicular fluid. Rather, they are formed by the iodination of tyrosine residues on the thyroglobulin molecule and are thus part of the primary structure of the thyroglobulin molecule.

T_4 and T_3 remain part of the thyroglobulin molecule in the follicle lumen until thyroid secretion is stimulated. The entire thyroglobulin molecule then undergoes endocytosis by the follicular cell and is degraded within the lysosomes of these cells. Finally, the follicular cell releases the free T_4 and T_3 into the circulation. Once secreted, T_4 is tightly bound to one of several binding proteins. It is carried to its sites of action, which include nearly all the cells in the body. In the process of this transport, the liver and other tissues take up some of the T_4 and partially deiodinate it to T_3; this T_3 can then re-enter the circulation.

Both T_3 and T_4 enter target cells and bind to cytosolic and nuclear receptors. These receptors are similar to those for steroid hormones (p. 112). T_3 has higher affinity than T_4 for the thyroid hormone receptor. Even though it accounts for only approximately 5% of the circulating thy-

QUANTITATION OF STEROID RECEPTORS IN CANCER PATIENTS

The affinity of steroid molecules for their receptors can be studied in vitro in a manner analogous to that described for the radioimmunoassay of peptide hormones (Fig. 46–1). In a typical immunoassay, an antibody with high affinity for a hormone or other compound binds to a radioactively labeled hormone or other molecule. A sample containing an unknown amount of the compound to be measured is added to the antibody-labeled hormone mixture and displaces the radioisotope from the antibody in proportion to the concentration of the unknown. The amount of unknown can be quantitated by comparison to the displacing activity of known standards. For the *steroid receptors,* cell extracts containing an unknown amount of steroid receptors can be incubated with labeled steroid that binds to the receptor. Then, progressively increasing concentrations of unlabeled steroid hormone are added, and the hormone that is bound by the receptor is separated from that remaining free in the extract. The result is a saturation curve (Fig. 46–8A), provided that the tissue extract has a finite number of specific hormone receptors. This saturation curve can often be linearized by a simple arithmetic manipulation called a "Scatchard plot" (see Fig. 46–8B). This analysis allows quantitation of the affinity of the receptor for the hormone and provides an estimate of the number of receptors (actually, the *concentration* of receptors) for that particular hormone.

The technique of quantitating receptor number has found an important application in determining the number of estrogen and progesterone receptors present in breast cancer cells. The number of estrogen and progesterone receptors per milligram of breast cancer tissue (obtained by biopsy of the breast or involved lymph node) is quantitated with radiolabeled estrogen (or progesterone). For postmenopausal women with estrogen receptor–positive breast cancer (i.e., a tumor with a high level of estrogen receptors), treatment with an antiestrogen (e.g., tamoxifen) is effective therapy. For premenopausal women, an antiestrogen may be used as well, or the ovaries can be removed surgically. The woman may also be given a long-acting gonadotropin-releasing hormone (GnRH) agonist, which paradoxically blocks both luteinizing and follicle-stimulating hormone production by the anterior pituitary, thereby reducing estradiol production and accomplishing a medical oophorectomy. The continuous (as opposed to the normally pulsatile) administration of GnRH downregulates GnRH receptors in the anterior pituitary (see box on p. 1144).

These therapies are not effective in patients with cancers that do not express significant numbers of estrogen receptors. The presence of abundant estrogen and progesterone receptors in breast tumors correlates with a more favorable prognosis, possibly because of the relatively advanced state of differentiation of the tumor, as well as the tumor's responsiveness to manipulation by estrogen or progesterone therapy.

A SATURATION CURVE

B SCATCHARD PLOT

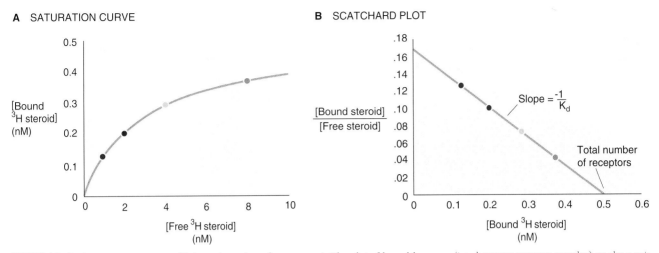

FIGURE 46–8. Quantitating receptor affinity and number of receptors. *A,* The plot of bound hormone (i.e., hormone-receptor complex) on the *y axis* versus that of free steroid concentration on the *x axis.* In this example, we have assumed that the K_d for hormone binding is 3 nM and that the maximal bound-hormone concentration is 0.5 nM. *B,* This plot is a transformation of the data in *A.* The colored points in this plot match the points of like color in *A.* Plotted on the *y axis* is the ratio of [Bound hormone]/[Free hormone]. Plotted on the *x axis* is [Bound hormone]. The slope of this relationship gives the $-1/K_d$, where K_d is the dissociation constant (3 nM). The *x-axis* intercept gives the total number of receptors (0.5 nM).

roid hormone, T_3 is probably the main effector of thyroid hormone signalling. The activated thyroid hormone receptor binds to thyroid hormone response elements in the 5′ region of responsive genes and regulates the transcription of multiple target genes.

Thyroid hormone receptors are present in many tissues, including the heart, vascular smooth muscle, skeletal muscle, liver, kidney, skin, and the CNS. A major role for thyroid hormone is overall regulation of metabolic rate. Because T_4 affects multiple tissues, individuals affected by disorders involving oversecretion or undersecretion of thyroid hormone manifest a host of varied symptoms that reflect the involvement of multiple organ systems.

REFERENCES

Books and Reviews

Berson SA, Yalow RS: Peptide hormones in plasma. Harvey Lect 62: 107–163, 1966–1967.

Farfel Z, Bourne HR, Iiri T: The expanding spectrum of G protein diseases. N Engl J Med 340:1012–1020, 1999.

Missale C, Nash SR, Robinson SW, et al: Dopamine receptors: From structure to function. Physiol Rev 78:189–225, 1998.

Scatchard G: The attraction of proteins for small molecules and ions. Ann N Y Acad Sci 51:660–672, 1949.

Sutherland EW, Robison GA: The role of cyclic-3′,5′-AMP in responses to catecholamines and other hormones. Pharmacol Rev 18:145–161, 1966.

Wilson JD, Foster DW, Kronenberg HM, Larsen PR (eds): Williams Textbook of Endocrinology, 9th ed. Philadelphia, WB Saunders, 1998.

Journal Articles

Berson SA, Yalow RS: Assay of insulin in human subjects by immunological methods. Nature 184:1948–1949, 1959.

Elgin RC, Busby WL, Clemmons DR: An insulin-like growth factor binding protein enhances the biological response to IGF-1. Proc Natl Acad Sci U S A 84:3254–3258, 1987.

Upton GV, Amatruda TT Jr: Evidence for the presence of tumor peptides with corticotropin-releasing-factor–like activity in the ectopic ACTH syndrome. N Engl J Med 285:419–424, 1971.

Yu D, Yu S, Schuster V, et al: Identification of two novel deletion mutations within the Gs alpha gene (GNAS1) in Albright hereditary osteodystrophy. J Clin Endocrinol Metab 84:3254–3259, 1999.

CHAPTER 47

The Endocrine Regulation of Growth

Eugene J. Barrett

Genes, Nutrition, and Hormones Regulate Somatic Growth

Growth from the fertilized ovum to the adult is an exceedingly complex process involving both **hyperplasia** (an increase in the number of cells) and **hypertrophy** (an increase in the size of cells) of the cellular elements of body tissues. The timing and capacity for cell division varies among tissues. In the human central nervous system (CNS), neuronal division is essentially complete by age 1, whereas bone, muscle, and fat cells continue to divide until later in childhood. Other tissues retain the capacity for hyperplasia throughout life; these include the skin, gastrointestinal epithelial cells and liver.

In humans, the genetic contribution to growth is evident from the observation that midparental height (i.e., the average of paternal and maternal height) is one of the better predictors of a child's ultimate stature. For domestic animals, breeding based on desired growth characteristics has been a mainstay of animal husbandry for millennia. The impact of environmental and nutritional factors, such as emotional or nutritional deprivation, on growth is most profound when it occurs during periods of tissue hyperplasia, most critically during the first 2 years of life.

Multiple hormones, including growth hormone (GH), insulin-like growth factors (IGF-I and -II), insulin, thyroid hormones, glucocorticoids, androgens, and estrogens contribute to the growth process in humans. Among these, GH and IGF-I have been implicated as the major determinants of growth in normal postuterine life. However, deficiencies (or excesses) of each of the other hormones can seriously affect the normal growth of the musculoskeletal system as well as the growth and maturation of other tissues.

GROWTH HORMONE

Growth Hormone, Secreted by Somatotrophs in the Anterior Pituitary, Is the Principal Endocrine Regulator of Somatic Size

Individuals with excessive GH secretion during childhood develop **gigantism**, and those with a deficiency of GH develop **pituitary dwarfism**. It is thus quite clear that GH profoundly affects somatic size. Dramatic examples of GH's somatotrophic action can be found in the descriptions of "Tom Thumb" and the "Alton giant." GH deficiency resulted in Tom

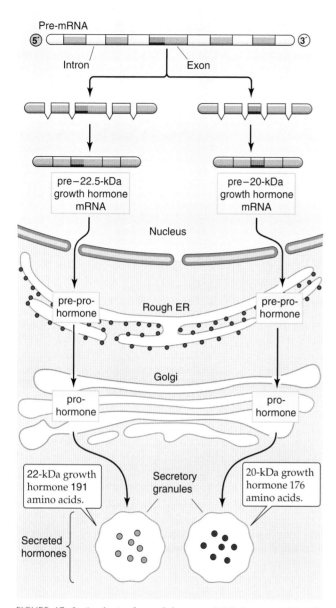

FIGURE 47–1. Synthesis of growth hormone (GH). Somatotrophic cells in the anterior pituitary are responsible for the synthesis of GH. The cell transcribes five exons to form GH messenger RNA (mRNA) for either the 22-kDa (191 amino acids) or the 20-kDa protein (176 amino acids). Alternative splicing in the third exon, which removes the RNA-encoding amino acids 32 to 46, is responsible for the two isoforms found in the pituitary. Both mRNAs have a signal sequence that causes them to be translated in the rough endoplasmic reticulum (ER) and enter the secretory pathway. Subsequent processing converts the two pre–pro-GHs first to the pro-GHs and then to the mature GHs. The cleavage of the pro-sequence and disulfide-bond formation occur during transit through the Golgi bodies. The somatotroph stores mature GH in granules until GH-releasing hormone (GHRH) stimulates the somatotroph to secrete the hormones. The 22-kDa version is the dominant form of GH.

Thumb's achieving an adult height of approximately 0.9 m. In contrast, the Alton giant had a GH-secreting pituitary tumor present from early childhood and reached an adult height of more than 2.7 m. It is important that, in both cases, the abnormality of GH secretion was present from early in life. Interestingly, children with GH defi-

ciency are of normal size at birth and only subsequently fall behind their peers in stature.

A deficiency of GH beginning in adult life does not result in any major clinical illness. However, it is now appreciated that *replacement* of GH (clinically available as a recombinant protein) in adults with **isolated GH deficiency** leads to an increased lean body mass, a decreased body fat, and perhaps an increased sense of vigor or well-being. An *excess* of GH after puberty results in the clinical syndrome of **acromegaly** (from the Greek akron = top + megas = large). This condition is characterized by the growth of bone and many other somatic tissues, including skin, muscle, heart, liver, and the gastrointestinal tract. The lengthening of long bones is not part of the syndrome because the epiphyseal growth plates close at the end of puberty. Thus, acromegaly causes a progressive thickening of bones and soft tissues of the head, hands, feet, and other parts of the body. If untreated, these somatic changes cause significant morbidity and shorten life due to joint deformity, hypertension, pulmonary insufficiency, and heart failure.

GH is made in the **somatotrophs** throughout the anterior pituitary (p. 1010). Like other peptide hormones, GH is synthesized as a larger "prehormone" (Fig. 47–1). During processing through the endoplasmic reticulum and Golgi system, several small peptides are removed. GH exists in at least three molecular forms. The predominant form is a 22-kDa polypeptide with two intramolecular sulfhydryl bonds. Alternative splicing generates a 20-kDa form of GH. Other GH forms include a 45-kDa protein, which is a dimer of the 22-kDa form, as well as larger forms that are multimers of monomeric GH. There is little information to suggest that the different principal forms of GH (i.e., the 20- and 22-kDa versions) vary in their activity, but the 20-kDa form may exert fewer of the acute metabolic actions of GH. Once synthesized, GH is stored in secretory granules in the cytosol of the somatotrophs until secreted.

Growth Hormone Is One of a Family of Homologous Hormones That Exhibit Overlap of Activity

GH appears to be a single-copy gene, but four other hormones have significant homology to GH. Most striking are three hormones made by the placenta: placental-variant GH and chorionic somatomammotropins 1 and 2 (Table 47–1). Genes for these hormones are also located in the GH gene cluster on the long arm of chromosome 17 in humans. The multiple genes in this cluster have an identical intron structure and code for proteins of similar size. There is substantial amino acid sequence homology among GH and these three other proteins. The **placental variant GH** (pvGH), like the 22-kDa GH, is a 191–amino acid peptide. It has a 93% primary sequence homology with GH, and virtually the same affinity for the hepatic GH receptor as GH. It appears able to mimic a number of the biologic actions of GH and may be an important modulator of systemic IGF-I production during pregnancy. (As we discuss later, a major action of GH is to stimulate secretion of IGF-I.) The human **chorionic so-**

TABLE 47–1

HORMONE	NUMBER OF AMINO ACIDS	HOMOLOGY (%)	CHROMOSOME
HOMOLOGY OF GROWTH HORMONE TO CHORIONIC HORMONES AND PROLACTIN			
hGH (human growth hormone)	191	100	17
pvGH (placental-variant GH)	191	93	17
hCS1 (human chorionic somatomammotropin 1)	191	84	17
hCS2 (human chorionic somatomammotropin 2)	191	84	17
hPRL (human prolactin)	199	16	6

matomammotropins (hCSs) are also called human placental lactogens (hPLs). The affinity of the two forms of hCS for the GH receptor is 100- to 1000-fold less than that of either GH or placental variant GH. As a result, they are less effective in promoting IGF-I or -II production. The somatomammotropins are primarily lactogenic, priming the breast for lactation after birth (Table 55–7).

The pituitary hormone **prolactin** (PRL; see Table 47–1) is the fourth hormone with homology to GH. It has a 16% amino acid homology with pituitary GH. PRL's principal physiological role involves promoting milk production in lactating women (p. 1187). It is made by *lactotrophs* in the anterior pituitary. Its homology to GH suggests that the two hormones, despite their divergent actions, arose from some common precursor by a gene-duplication event. The sequence homology between these proteins is underscored by the observation that GH and PRL have similar affinities for the PRL receptor. The converse is not true—that is, PRL has no significant affinity for the GH receptor and thus has no growth-promoting activity. As we discuss later, the PRL and GH receptors are coupled to an intracellular signaling system that involves stimulation of the JAK family of tyrosine kinases (p. 111) as an early postreceptor event.

Men, like women, make PRL throughout their lives. However, no physiological role for PRL in males has been defined. Interestingly, both men and women with disorders involving hypersecretion of GH or PRL can develop galactorrhea (breast milk secretion). Although GH and PRL are normally secreted by distinct cell populations in the anterior pituitary, some benign, GH-producing pituitary adenomas (i.e., tumors) secrete PRL along with GH.

Somatotrophs Secrete Growth Hormone in Pulses

It remains a paradox that whereas growth occurs slowly over months and years, the secretion of GH is highly episodic, varying on a minute-to-minute basis. Most normal children experience episodes or "bursts" of GH secretion throughout the day, most prominently within the first several hours of sleep. Underlying each peak in plasma levels of GH, illustrated for an adult in Figure 47–2, are bursts of many hundreds of pulses of GH secretion by the somatotrophs in the anterior pituitary. With the induction of slow-wave sleep, several volleys of GH pulses may occur; it is estimated that more than 70% of total daily GH secretion occurs during these periods. This pulsatile secretion underlines the prominent role of the CNS in the regulation of GH secretion and growth. The circulating GH concentrations may be up to 100-fold higher during the bursts of GH secretion (i.e., the peaks in Fig. 47–2) than during intervening periods. The pattern of bursts depends on the sleep-wake patterns, not on light-dark patterns. Exercise, stress, high-protein meals, and fasting also cause a rise in the mean GH level in humans. In circumstances in which GH secretion is stimulated—for example, fasting or a high-protein diet—the increased GH output is due to an increase in the

FIGURE 47–2. Bursts in plasma levels of growth hormone (GH), sampled in the blood plasma of a 23-year-old woman every 5 minutes over a 24-hour period. Each peak in the plasma GH concentration reflects bursts of hundreds of GH secretory pulses by the somatotrophs of the anterior pituitary. These bursts are most common during the first few hours of sleep. The integrated amount of GH secreted each day is higher during pubertal growth than in younger children or in adults. (Data from Hartman ML, Veldhuis JD, Vance ML, et al: Somatotropin pulse frequency and basal concentrations are increased in acromegaly and are reduced by successful therapy. J Clin Endocrinol Metab 70:1375, 1990.)

frequency, rather than the amplitude, of pulses of GH that the somatotrophs secrete.

Growth Hormone Secretion Is Under Hierarchical Control from Growth Hormone–Releasing Hormone and Somatostatin

The coordination of GH secretion by the somatotrophs during a secretory pulse presumably occurs in response to both positive and negative hypothalamic control signals.

GROWTH HORMONE–RELEASING HORMONE. Small-diameter neurons in the arcuate nucleus of the hypothalamus secrete **GH-releasing hormone** (GHRH), a 43–amino acid peptide that reaches the somatotrophs in the anterior pituitary via the hypophyseal portal blood (Fig. 47–3). As the name implies, this neuropeptide promotes GH secretion by the somatotrophs. GHRH is made principally in the hypothalamus, but it can also be found in neuroectodermal tissue outside the CNS; it was first isolated and purified from a pancreatic islet cell tumor of a patient with acromegaly.

SOMATOSTATIN. The hypothalamus also synthesizes **somatostatin** (SS), a 14–amino acid neuropeptide. SS is made in the periventricular region of the hypothalamus and is secreted into the hypophyseal portal blood supply. It is a potent inhibitor of GH secretion. SS is also made elsewhere in the brain and in selected tissues outside the CNS, such as the pancreatic islet δ cells (p. 1084) and D cells in the gastrointestinal tract (p. 898). Within the CNS, the 14–amino acid form of SS (SS-14) dominates. The gastrointestinal tract predominantly expresses a 28–amino acid splice variant; the N-terminal 14 amino acids of SS-28 are identical to those of SS-14.

It appears that the primary regulation of GH secretion is stimulatory, because sectioning the pituitary stalk, thereby interrupting the portal blood flow from the hypothalamus to the pituitary, leads to a decline in GH secretion. Conversely, sectioning of the stalk leads to a *rise* in PRL levels, presumably because dopamine made in the hypothalamus inhibits PRL secretion in the anterior pituitary (p. 1012). It also appears that the pulses of GH secretion are entrained by the pulsatile secretion of GHRH (as opposed to the periodic loss of SS inhibition). Such a relationship between releasing factors and pulses of pituitary hormone secretion has been directly documented in primates for the secretion of gonadotropin-releasing hormone (GnRH) and luteinizing hormone (LH), but not yet for GHRH.

GROWTH HORMONE–RELEASING HORMONE RECEPTOR. GHRH binds to a G protein–coupled receptor on the somatotrophs and activates $G_{\alpha s}$, which in turn stimulates adenylyl cyclase (p. 97). The subsequent rise in the intracellular concentration of cyclic adenosine monophosphate ($[cAMP]_i$) causes increased gene transcription and synthesis of GH. In addition, the rise in $[cAMP]_i$ opens Ca^{2+} channels in the plasma membrane, causing $[Ca^{2+}]_i$ to rise. This increase in $[Ca^{2+}]_i$ stimulates the release of preformed GH.

SOMATOSTATIN RECEPTOR. SS binds to a G protein–coupled receptor on the somatotrophs and activates $G_{\alpha i}$,

which inhibits adenylyl cyclase. As a result, $[Ca^{2+}]_i$ decreases, thereby diminishing the responsiveness of the somatotroph to GHRH. When somatotrophs are exposed to both GHRH and SS, the inhibitory action of SS prevails.

Both Growth Hormone and Insulin-Like Growth Factor I, Whose Secretion Is Stimulated by Growth Hormone, Negatively Feed Back on Growth Hormone Secretion by Somatotrophs

In addition to being controlled by GHRH and SS released from the hypothalamus, somatotroph secretion of GH is regulated by a negative feedback loop involving IGF-I. As discussed later, GH triggers the secretion of IGF-I from GH target tissues throughout the body. Indeed, IGF-I appears to mediate many of the growth-promoting actions of GH. The circulating levels of IGF-I, which produce its **endocrine** effects, largely reflect its hepatic synthesis. IGF-I synthesized in tissues such as muscle, cartilage, and bone may act more in a **paracrine** or **autocrine** fashion to promote local tissue growth. An increase in the circulating concentration of IGF-I suppresses GH secretion through both direct and indirect mechanisms (Fig. 47–4). First, circulating IGF-I exerts a *direct* action on the pituitary to suppress GH secretion by the somatotrophs, probably inhibiting GH secretion by a mechanism different from that of SS. In its peripheral target cells, IGF-I acts through a receptor tyrosine kinase (p. 110), and not by either the Ca^{2+} or cAMP messenger systems. IGF-I presumably acts by this same mechanism to inhibit GH secretion in somatotrophs.

Second, evidence also points to two *indirect* feedback pathways by which circulating IGF-I inhibits GH secretion. IGF-I appears to suppress GHRH release in the hypothalamus and to increase SS secretion. Yet another feedback system, independent of IGF-I, reduces GH secretion; GH itself appears to inhibit GH secretion in a "short-loop" feedback system.

Growth Hormone Has Acute "Anti-Insulin" Metabolic Effects As Well As Chronic Growth-Promoting Effects Mediated by Insulin-Like Growth Factor I

Once secreted, most GH circulates free in the plasma. However, a significant fraction (~40% for the 22-kDa GH) is complexed to a **GH-binding protein** formed by proteolytic cleavage of the extracellular domain of GH receptors in GH target tissues. This protein fragment binds to GH with high affinity, thereby increasing the half-life of GH and competing with GH-target tissues for GH. In the circulation, GH has a half-life of about 25 minutes.

GROWTH HORMONE RECEPTOR. GH binds to specific receptors on the surface of multiple target tissues. The monomeric GH receptor is a 620–amino acid protein with a single membrane-spanning segment. The molecular weight of the purified receptor (~130 kDa) greatly ex-

1 Neurosecretory cells in the arcuate nucleus secrete growth hormone–releasing hormone (GHRH), a 43–amino acid peptide that reaches the somatotrophs via the hypophyseal portal blood supply.

2 Cells in the periventricular region release somatostatin, a hormone that is a potent inhibitor of growth hormone (GH) secretion, into the portal blood supply.

Periventricular region

Arcuate nucleus

Hypothalamus

Released somatostatin

Released GHRH

Anterior lobe of pituitary

Somatotrophs

GHRH   GHRH receptor

Somatotroph

SS receptor

GH

(Stimulating) G-protein

AC

ATP

SS

cAMP

(Inhibitory) G-protein

Ca²⁺

Ca²⁺

PKA

3 GHRH causes somatotrophs to synthesize and release GH.

4 Somatostatin inhibits the release of GH by somatotrophs.

FIGURE 47–3. Synthesis and release of growth hormone–releasing hormone (GHRH) and somatostatin, and the control of growth hormone (GH) release. Small-bodied neurons in the arcuate nucleus of the hypothalamus secrete GHRH, a 43–amino acid peptide that reaches the somatotrophs in the anterior pituitary via the long portal veins. GHRH stimulates the somatotrophs to release GH stored in secretory granules by raising [cAMP]$_i$ and [Ca^{2+}]$_i$. Neurons in the *periventricular region* of the hypothalamus synthesize somatostatin, a 14–amino acid neuropeptide. Somatostatin, which also travels to the anterior pituitary via the long portal vessels, is a potent inhibitor of GH secretion. Somatostatin acts by inhibiting adenylyl cyclase and thus lowering [Ca^{2+}]$_i$. AC, adenylyl cyclase; ATP, adenosine triphosphate; cAMP, cyclic adenosine monophosphate; PKA, protein kinase A; SS, somatostatin.

ceeds that predicted from the amino acid composition (~70 kDa) due to extensive glycosylation. The receptor does not resemble any of the G protein–linked receptors or receptors with intrinsic tyrosine kinase activity, but is a **tyrosine kinase–*associated* receptor** that is related to several cytokine receptors (p. 111). The GH receptor forms a dimer when one GH molecule simultaneously binds to sites on two monomers and acts as a bridge. Receptor occupancy increases the activity of a tyrosine kinase (JAK 2 family) that is associated with, but is not an integral part of, the GH receptor. This tyrosine kinase

triggers a series of protein phosphorylations that modulate target cell activity.

ACUTE EFFECTS OF GROWTH HORMONE. GH has a number of acute (minutes to hours) actions on muscle, adipose tissue and liver that may not necessarily be related to the more long-term growth-promoting actions of GH. These acute metabolic effects (Table 47–2) include stimulation of lipolysis in adipose tissue, inhibition of glucose uptake by muscle, and stimulation of gluconeogenesis by hepatocytes. These actions oppose the normal effects of

4 IGF-I *indirectly* inhibits GH release by increasing secretion of somatostatin from nuclei in the periventricular region.

3 IGF-I *indirectly* inhibits GH release by suppressing GHRH release from the arcuate nucleus in the hypothalamus.

Periventricular region

Hypothalamus

Arcuate nucleus

Released somatostatin

Released GHRH

IGF-I

IGF-I

5 GH inhibits its own secretion via "short-loop" feedback on somatotrophs.

Somato-trophs

Anterior lobe of pituitary

GH

IGF-I

1 GH stimulates secretion of IGF-I from peripheral target tissue.

Target tissue

IGF-I

2 IGF-I then *directly* inhibits GH release by suppressing the somatotrophs.

FIGURE 47–4. Growth hormone (GH) and insulin-like growth factor I (IGF-I; also called somatomedin-C) negative feedback loops. Both GH and IGF-I feed back—either directly or indirectly—on the somatotrophs in the anterior pituitary to decrease GH secretion. GH itself inhibits GH secretion ("short-loop"). IGF-I, whose release is stimulated by GH, inhibits GH release by three routes, one of which is "direct" and two of which are "indirect." The direct action is for IGF-I to inhibit the somatotroph. The first indirect pathway is for IGF-I to suppress GH-releasing hormone (GHRH) release in the hypothalamus. The second is for IGF-I to increase secretion of somatostatin, which in turn inhibits the somatotroph.

TABLE 47–2

DIABETOGENIC EFFECTS OF GROWTH HORMONE	
TARGET	**EFFECT**
Muscle	↓ Glucose uptake
Fat	↑ Lipolysis
Liver	↑ Gluconeogenesis
Muscle, fat, and liver	Insulin resistance

insulin (p. 1068) on these same tissues and have been termed the "**anti-insulin**" or "**diabetogenic**" actions of GH. Chronic oversecretion of GH, such as occurs in patients with GH-producing tumors in acromegaly, is accompanied by insulin resistance and often by glucose intolerance or frank diabetes.

LONG-TERM EFFECTS OF GROWTH HORMONE VIA IGF-I. Distinct from these acute actions of GH is its action to promote tissue growth by stimulating target tissues to produce IGFs. In 1957, Salmon and Daughaday reported

FIGURE 47–5. Structure of the insulin-like growth factors (IGFs). Insulin, IGF-I, and IGF-II share three domains (A, B, and C), which share a high degree of amino acid sequence homology. The C region is cleaved from insulin (as the C peptide) during processing, but is not cleaved from either IGF-I or IGF-II. In addition, IGF-I and IGF-II also have a short D domain.

that GH itself does not have growth-promoting action on epiphyseal cartilage (the site where longitudinal bone growth occurs). In those experiments, the addition of serum from normal animals, but not from hypophysecto-mized (GH-deficient) animals, stimulated cartilage growth in vitro (assayed as incorporation of radiolabeled sulfate into cartilage). The addition of GH to GH-deficient serum did not restore the growth-promoting activity seen with normal serum. However, if the GH-deficient animals were treated in vivo with GH, then their plasma promoted cartilage growth in vitro. This led to the hypothesis that, in animals, GH provokes the secretion of another circulating factor that "mediates" the action of GH. Initially called "sulfation factor" because of how it was assayed, this intermediate was subsequently termed "**somatomedin**" because it mediates the somatic effects of GH. The responsible proteins were isolated and purified and found to be identical to two peptides with a primary structure much like that of proinsulin, and were termed insulin-like growth factors (Fig. 47–5). These peptide hormones are made in various tissues, including the liver, kidney, muscle, cartilage, and bone. They are called "insulin-like" growth factors because they exert insulin-like actions in isolated adipocytes and can produce hypoglycemia in animals and humans. The liver produces most of the IGF-I present in the circulation. IGF-I production appears to be more closely related to GH secretion than IGF-II production.

GROWTH-PROMOTING HORMONES

Insulin-Like Growth Factor I, Which Interacts with a Receptor Similar to the Insulin Receptor, Is the Principal Mediator of the Growth-Promoting Action of Growth Hormone

The synthesis of IGF-I and, to a lesser extent, IGF-II depends on circulating GH. As described earlier, the periodic nature of GH secretion results in a wide range of plasma GH concentrations. In contrast, plasma [IGF-I] does not vary by more than about 2-fold over a 24-hour period. The plasma [IGF-I] in effect "integrates" the pulsatile, highly fluctuating GH concentration. The reason for

the relatively steady plasma levels of IGF-I is that like GH—but unlike most peptide hormones—IGF-I circulates bound to several **IGF-I binding proteins**. These binding proteins are made principally in the liver, but are also manufactured by other tissues. More than 90% of IGF-I measured in the serum is bound to these proteins. At least six distinct IGF-binding proteins have been identified. In addition to providing a buffer pool in plasma of bound IGF, these proteins may also aid the transfer of IGF to the tissue receptors, thereby facilitating the action of these hormones. The local "free" fraction of IGF-I is probably the more biologically active component that binds to the receptor and stimulates tissue growth.

Like other peptide hormones, IGF-I and IGF-II are synthesized via the secretory pathway (p. 36) and are secreted into the extracellular space, where they may act locally in a paracrine fashion. In the extracellular space, the IGFs encounter binding proteins that may promote local retention of the secreted hormone by increasing the overall molecular size of the complex. This action inhibits the entry of the IGFs into the vascular system. Thus, local concentrations of the IGFs are likely to be much higher than plasma concentrations.

Whether made locally or reaching tissue through the circulation, IGF-I acts via a specific **receptor tyrosine kinase** (p. 110), a heterotetramer that is structurally related to the insulin receptor (Fig. 47–6). Like the insulin receptor (p. 1073), the IGF-I receptor has two completely extracellular α chains and two transmembrane β chains. Also like the insulin receptor, it is the β chains that have the intrinsic tyrosine kinase activity. Binding of IGF-I to its receptor enhances receptor autophosphorylation as well as phosphorylation of downstream effectors. The structural homology between the insulin and IGF-I receptors is sufficiently high that insulin can bind to the IGF-I receptor, although with an affinity that is about two orders of magnitude less than that for IGF-I. The same is true for the binding of IGF-I to insulin receptors. In fact, the homology between the insulin and IGF-I receptors is so strong that "hybrid receptors" containing one α-β chain of the insulin receptor and one α-β chain of the IGF-I receptor are present in many tissues. These hybrid receptors bind both insulin and IGF-I, but their affinity for IGF-I is greater.

Given the structural similarity between insulin and

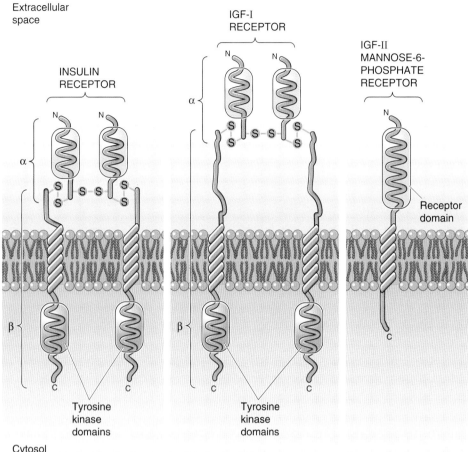

FIGURE 47–6. Comparison of insulin, insulin-like growth factor (IGF)-I, and IGF-II receptors. Both the insulin and IGF-I receptors are heterotetramers joined by disulfide bonds. For both, the cytoplasmic portion of the β subunits have tyrosine kinase domains as well as autophosphorylation sites. The IGF-II receptor (also called mannose-6-phosphate [M6P] receptor) is a single polypeptide chain with no kinase domain.

IGFs and between the insulin receptor and the IGF-I receptor, it is not surprising that IGFs can exert "insulin-like" actions in vivo. This effect has been particularly well studied for IGF-I, which, like insulin, induces hypoglycemia when injected into animals. This action is largely due to the increased uptake of glucose into muscle tissue. IGF-I is less effective in mimicking insulin's action on adipose and liver tissue; in humans, these tissues have few IGF-I receptors. In muscle, IGF-I promotes the uptake of radiolabeled amino acids and stimulates protein synthesis at concentrations that do not stimulate glucose uptake, indicating that the growth-promoting actions of IGF-I are expressed at lower circulating concentrations than those required to produce hypoglycemia.

Despite the structural similarity of their receptors, IGF-I and insulin exert different actions on tissues. IGF-I has a more marked effect on growth, and insulin has a more significant effect on glucose and lipid metabolism. However, the differences in the postreceptor signaling pathways triggered by the two hormones have not been well defined.

Insulin-Like Growth Factor II Has Actions Similar to Those of Insulin-Like Growth Factor I, but Is Less Dependent on Growth Hormone

The physiology of IGF-II differs from that of IGF-I in a number of important respects. First, as noted earlier, the

---

PLASMA INSULIN-LIKE GROWTH FACTOR I AS A MEASURE OF GROWTH HORMONE SECRETION

The plasma IGF-I concentration is a valuable measure of GH secretion. The wide swings in plasma [GH] that result from the pulsatile secretion of this hormone have confounded efforts to use GH measurements to diagnose disorders of GH deficiency or excess. However, an increased circulating concentration of IGF-I is one of the most useful clinical measures of the excess GH secretion that occurs in acromegaly (i.e., GH excess in adults) and gigantism (i.e., GH excess in children). Measurement of plasma [IGF-I] has also helped explain the genesis of a particular type of dwarfism known as "Laron dwarfism." These patients were initially identified as persons with growth failure mimicking that of typical pituitary dwarfism; however, plasma [GH] is normal or elevated, and treatment with GH is ineffective in reversing the growth failure. It was subsequently demonstrated that these individuals have mutations of their GH receptors that make the receptors nonfunctional. Thus, the mutant GH receptors cannot trigger the production of IGFs. With the availability of recombinant IGF-I, it is possible that effective treatment of these children will restore growth.

FIGURE 47–7. Serum insulin-like growth factor (IGF)-I levels and height velocity as a function of age. The *red curve* shows the mean plasma concentrations of IGF-I as a function of age in human females. The curve for males is similar, but the peak is shifted to an older age by 3 to 4 years. The *brown curve* indicates for females mean height velocity—the rate at which height increases (cm/yr). The *pubertal* peak rate of growth corresponds to the peak serum concentrations of IGF-I. (Data from Reiter EO, Rosenfeld RG: Normal and aberrant growth. In Wilson JD, Foster DW, Kronenberg HM, Larsen PR [eds]: Williams Textbook of Endocrinology, 9th ed. Philadelphia, WB Saunders, 1998, pp 1427–1507.)

synthesis of IGF-II depends less on circulating GH than that of IGF-I. In pituitary dwarfism secondary to GH deficiency, the circulating concentration of IGF-I is decreased, but that of IGF-II is not. In states of excessive GH secretion, plasma IGF-I is reliably elevated, whereas plasma IGF-II is not.

Although IGF-II also binds to the IGF-I receptor, it preferentially binds to its own so-called IGF-II receptor. This IGF-II receptor consists of a single-chain polypeptide and is structurally very distinct from the IGF-I receptor (see Fig. 47–6). The IGF-II receptor lacks a tyrosine-kinase domain and does not undergo autophosphorylation in response to the binding of either IGF-II or IGF-I. The IGF-II receptor also binds mannose-6-phosphate (M6P), but at a site different from that for IGF-II binding, and the receptor's physiological role appears to be in processing mannosylated proteins by targeting them for lysosomal degradation. Thus, the term "IGF-II receptor" is somewhat of a misnomer; the IGF-II receptor's role in the physiological action of IGF-II is not clear.

Despite these differences, IGF-II does share with IGF-I (and also with insulin) the ability to promote tissue growth and cause acute hypoglycemia. These properties appear to be due to IGF-II's structural similarity to proinsulin and its ability to bind to the IGF-I receptor.

Although Growth Rate Usually Parallels Plasma Levels of Insulin-Like Growth Factor I, the Two Diverge Both Early and Late in Life

Illustrated in Figure 47–7 is the mean concentration of total IGF-I (both free and bound) found in human serum as a function of age. Also shown is the normal rate of height increase (cm/yr). During puberty, the greatest growth rates are observed at times when plasma [IGF-I] is highest. A similar comparison can be made using GH, provided that care is taken to obtain multiple measurements at each age and thereby account for the pulsatile secretion and marked diurnal changes that occur in plasma [GH].

Whereas there is a good general concordance between growth rate and the plasma [IGF-I] during puberty, the two diverge at both younger and older ages. First, during adulthood, longitudinal growth essentially ceases, yet GH and IGF-I secretion continue to be highly regulated. As both men and women age, the circulating concentrations of both hormones decline. For a number of years, the continued secretion of these hormones in adults was considered to be largely vestigial. This belief was reinforced by the observation that cessation of GH secretion and the consequent decline of IGF-I after trauma, tumor, or surgical removal of the pituitary did not result in any clear clinical syndrome. However, with the availability of recombinant human GH, replacement of GH in GH-deficient adults has led to remarkable increases in body muscle mass, decreases in fat mass, and improved nitrogen balance (a measure of protein nutrition). These findings support the conclusion that—even after linear growth ceases after puberty—GH and IGF-I remain important regulators of body composition and appear to promote anabolic actions in muscle. Indeed, some investigators have suggested that supplementing normal adults with GH or IGF-I may reverse some of the effects of aging, including loss of muscle mass, negative nitrogen balance, and osteoporosis. Clinical studies are in progress.

A second period of life during which divergence between longitudinal growth and IGF-I occurs is very early childhood (see Fig. 47–7). This period is characterized by a very rapid growth rate, but quite low IGF-I levels. If this time frame is extended back to intrauterine life, then the discordance is even greater. Indeed, children with complete GH deficiency have very low plasma [IGF-I] levels but are of normal length and weight at birth. This observation suggests that during intrauterine life, factors other than GH and IGF-I are important regulators of growth. One of these additional factors may be insulin, as discussed later.

Another explanation for the divergence between growth rate and IGF-I levels may be IGF-II, which may be an important mediator of intrauterine growth. The plasma concentration of IGF-II is greater during fetal life than at later times, peaking just before birth. Plasma [IGF-II] plummets soon after birth, but then gradually doubles between birth and age 1 year, and remains at this level until at least age 80. Thus, IGF-II levels are at adult levels during the first several years of life, when IGF-I levels are low but growth is rapid. However, several other hormones may also contribute to somatic growth during the first several years of life.

By age 3 or 4, GH and IGF-I begin to play major roles in the regulation of growth. The concentrations of these hormones rise throughout childhood, peaking during the time of the pubertal growth spurt. The rate of long-bone growth in the pubertal growth spurt is exceeded only during intrauterine life and early childhood. The frequency of pituitary GH secretory pulses increases markedly at puberty. The factors responsible for this acceleration are not clear. However, the accompanying sexual maturation likely plays some role, as both estradiol and testosterone appear to promote GH secretion.

In addition to these humoral influences, nutritional factors also modulate both GH secretion and IGF-I production. In both children and adults, GH secretion is triggered by a high dietary protein intake. Teleologically, this is intriguing in that it might provide a linkage between the availability of amino acids to serve as substrates for body protein synthesis (growth) and the endocrine stimulus of cells to grow. This relationship is not simple, however, because the rise in GH levels in the setting of protein intake is not sufficient to fully stimulate IGF-I production. This principle is well illustrated by **fasting**, which is associated with a decline in IGF-I even with increased GH. During fasting, insulin levels are low. Increased insulin appears to be required, at least in some tissues, for GH to effectively stimulate IGF-I.

Thyroid Hormones, Steroids, and Insulin also Promote Growth

Although our discussion to this point has emphasized the action of GH and the GH-induced growth factors as modulators of somatic growth, we might regard them as necessary but not sufficient agents for normal growth. A number of other hormones, as well as a receptive growth-responsive cartilage, are required. Because growth is a difficult phenomenon to study, especially in humans (few scientists want to follow an experiment over 10 to 20 years), much of our understanding of endocrine regulation of normal growth derives from observations of abnormal growth as it occurs in clinical syndromes of endocrine excess or deficiency. Several of the more important of these endocrine influences are illustrated here. Keep in mind that the exact mechanism by which growth is regulated by these agents is not always well understood.

THYROID HORMONES. Next to GH, perhaps the most prominent among the growth-promoting hormones are the thyroid hormones thyroxine and triiodothyronine, which we discuss in Chapter 48. In many nonhuman species, thyroid hormone plays a major role in tissue growth and remodeling. For example, resorption of the tadpole tail during morphogenesis requires thyroid hormone. In humans, deficiency of thyroid hormones early

in life can cause dwarfism or cretinism (p. 1043). In children with normal thyroid function at birth, development of hypothyroidism at any time before epiphyseal fusion leads to growth retardation or arrest. Much of the loss in height that occurs can be recovered through thyroid hormone treatment, a phenomenon called "catch-up growth." However, because the diagnosis of hypothyroidism may elude detection for many months or years, delays in initiating treatment can lead to some loss of potential growth. A child's growth curve can provide a particularly sensitive early indicator of hypothyroidism.

SEX STEROIDS. As with thyroid hormones, the importance of sex steroids for growth is most readily understood by considering the effects of deficiency or excess of these hormones. Androgen or estrogen excess occurring before the pubertal growth spurt accelerates bone growth. However, the sex steroids also accelerate the rate at which the skeleton matures and thus shorten the time available for growth before epiphyseal closure occurs. Most of the time, the dominant effect of sex steroids is to narrow the growth window, thereby diminishing ultimate longitudinal bone growth. This effect is well illustrated in settings in which children are exposed to excessive sex steroid at an early age. The sex steroids can come from endogenous sources (e.g., early maturation of the hypothalamic-pituitary-gonadal axis producing a premature puberty, or tumors that secrete estrogen or androgen) or from exogenous sources (e.g., children taking sex steroids prescribed for others). Again, the growth curve is useful in that it typically shows an increase in growth rate, followed by an early leveling off of growth associated with the development of secondary sexual characteristics.

GLUCOCORTICOIDS. An *excess* of adrenal glucocorticoids inhibits growth. In children who produce too much cortisol, as a result of either adrenal or pituitary tumors (which produce adrenocorticotropic hormone [ACTH] and cause secondary increases in plasma cortisol), growth ceases. The use of synthetic glucocorticoids in treating various serious illnesses (e.g., asthma, organ transplantation, a variety of chronic autoimmune processes) also arrests growth. Restoration of normal growth does not occur until the glucocorticoid levels return toward normal. Neither GH nor IGF-I concentrations drop significantly during glucocorticoid treatment. The failure of GH administration to correct the growth retardation that occurs in glucocorticoid-treated children further confirms that GH deficiency cannot account for the growth failure associated with glucocorticoid excess. Because linear growth is related to cartilage and bone synthesis at the growth plates, glucocorticoids presumably are acting at least in part at these sites to impair growth. However, the specific biochemical locus at which glucocorticoids act remains unclear. In adults, as in children, glucocorticoid excess impairs tissue anabolism and thus may present as wasting in some tissues (e.g., bone, muscle, subcutaneous connective tissue) rather than growth failure. This tissue wasting results in some of the major clinical morbidity of glucocorticoids (i.e., osteoporosis, muscle weakness, and bruising).

In glucocorticoid *deficiency*, growth is not substantially

affected. However, other deleterious effects of cortisol deficiency (e.g., hypoglycemia; p. 1049) dominate.

INSULIN. This hormone is also an important growth factor, particularly in utero. For example, women with diabetes frequently have high blood levels of glucose during pregnancy and deliver high–birth weight babies (fetal **macrosomy**). The developing fetus, exposed to higher-than-normal glucose concentrations, secretes additional insulin. Hyperinsulinemia results in increased fetal growth. Fetal macrosomy can create significant obstetrical difficulties at the time of delivery.

Conversely, infants born with pancreatic agenesis or with one of several forms of severe insulin resistance are very small at birth. One form of this, "**leprechaunism,**" is due to a defect in the insulin receptor (see box on p. 1074). Thus it appears that insulin, acting through its own receptor, is an intrauterine growth factor.

Severe insulin deficiency produces a marked catabolic effect associated with wasting of lean body mass in both children and adults. The acute adverse effects of such deficiency (dehydration and acidosis) dominate the clinical picture. Milder degrees of insulin deficiency, seen in patients with chronically undertreated diabetes, diminishes growth in affected children. Improved diabetes management may allow restoration of normal growth rates and possibly even some transient accelerated or "catch up" growth. Thus with good care, children with diabetes can expect to achieve normal adult height.

The Musculoskeletal System Responds to Growth Stimuli of the GHRH/GH/IGF-I Axis

Longitudinal growth involves lengthening of the somatic tissues (including bone, muscle, tendons, and skin) through a combination of tissue hyperplasia and hypertrophy. Each of these tissues remodels its structure throughout life. For bone, **longitudinal growth** occurs by the hyperplasia of chondrocytes at the growth plates of the long bones, followed by endochondral ossification. The calcified cartilage is remodeled as it moves toward the metaphyses of the bone, where it is eventually replaced by true lamellar and trabecular bone (p. 1088). This process continues until epiphyseal closure occurs toward the completion of puberty.

The process of cartilage formation and longitudinal bone growth begins as the cellular elements capable of forming cartilage divide along the growth plate and then migrating toward the more mature bone. These cells synthesize the extracellular matrix of cartilage, which include type II collagen, hyaluronic acid, and mucopolysaccharides. These cells appear to respond directly to GH by proliferating and increasing production of the extracellular matrix. This response involves local generation of IGF-I within the cartilage as an early event in the growth process. As the cells more closely approach the already formed cortical and trabecular bone, ossification of the extracellular matrix begins, and eventually the cellular elements become isolated by the calcifying cartilage. However, this calcified cartilage is not structurally the same as

TABLE 47–3

OTHER GROWTH FACTORS AFFECTING GROWTH

Nerve growth factor (NGF)

Fibroblast growth factor (FGF)

Angiogenesis factor

Vascular endothelial growth factor (VEGF)

Epidermal growth factor (EGF)

Hepatocyte growth factor (HGF)

normal bone, and soon after formation it begins to be remodeled by an ingrowth of cellular elements (osteoclasts and osteoblasts) from adjacent bone. Eventually, it is replaced by normal bone, becoming part of the metaphysis of the long bone.

In most children, growth ceases within several years after completion of puberty, when the chondrocytes at the growth plates of the long bones cease dividing and calcify the previously cartilaginous surrounding matrix. After puberty, **radial growth** occurs as bones increase their *diameter* through a process of endosteal bone resorption and periosteal bone deposition. This process is not strictly compartmentalized; that is, resorption and deposition of bone occur at both the periosteal and endosteal surfaces. However, during periods of growth, the rate of periosteal deposition exceeds the rate of endosteal resorption, and the bone shafts grow in width and thickness.

As might be expected, numerous disorders disrupt the complex process of endochondral bone growth on a genetic or congenital basis (e.g., defects in collagen or mucopolysaccharide synthesis), leading to genetic forms of dwarfism. In these settings the GHRH/GH/IGF-I axis is entirely intact and appears to regulate normally. There is no apparent compensation for the short stature by increased GH secretion, suggesting that the axis is not sensitive to the growth process per se, but simply to the intermediate chemical mediator IGF-I.

GH and IGF-I clearly play important roles in mediating longitudinal bone growth and also modulate growth of other tissues. Thus, proportional growth of muscle occurs as bones elongate, and the visceral organs enlarge as the torso increases in size. The mechanisms by which GH and IGF-I coordinate this process and how other hormones or growth factors might be involved continue to be investigated. It is clear that, whereas GH and, more recently, IGF-I have been considered to be the major hormones responsible for somatic growth, other tissue growth factors play an important, albeit as-yet incompletely defined, role. Table 47–3 lists some of these growth factors. In general, the tissue growth factors have more tissue-specific actions on organogenesis and their growth-promoting activity than the IGFs, and appear to act largely in a paracrine or autocrine fashion.

REFERENCES

Books and Reviews

Argetsinger LS, Carter-Su C: Mechanism of signaling by growth hormone receptor. Physiol Rev 76:1089–1107, 1996.

Barkan AL, Jaffe CA, Padmanabhan V: In vivo investigation of hypothalamic secretory activity. Trends Endocrinol Metab 8:105–111, 1997.

Cohick WS, Clemmons DR: The insulin-like growth factors. Annu Rev Physiol 55:131–153, 1993.

Etherton TD, Bauman DE: Biology of somatotropin in growth and lactation of domestic animals. Physiol Rev 78:745–761, 1998.

Mayo KE, Godfrey PA, Suhr ST, et al: Growth hormone-releasing hormone: Synthesis and signaling. Recent Prog Horm Res 50:35–73, 1995.

Stewart CEH, Rotwein P: Growth, differentiation, and survival: Multiple physiological functions for insulin-like growth factors. Physiol Rev 76:1005–1026, 1996.

Wilson JD, Foster DW, Kronenberg HM, Larsen PR (eds): Williams Textbook of Endocrinology, 9th ed. Philadelphia, WB Saunders, 1998.

Journal Articles

Bluetpajot MT, Epelbaum J, Gourdji D, et al: Hypothalamic and hypophyseal regulation of growth hormone secretion. Cell Mol Neurobiol 18:101–123, 1998.

Daughaday WH, Trivedi B: Absence of serum growth hormone binding protein in patients with growth hormone receptor deficiency (Laron dwarfism). Proc Natl Acad Sci U S A 84:4636–4640, 1987.

Hartman ML, Clayton PE, Johnson ML, et al: A low-dose euglycemic infusion of recombinant human insulin-like growth factor I rapidly suppresses fasting-enhanced pulsatile growth hormone secretion in humans. J Clin Invest 91:2453–2462, 1993.

Thorner MO, Perryman RL, Cronin MJ, et al: Somatotroph hyperplasia: Successful treatment of acromegaly by removal of a pancreatic islet tumor secreting a growth hormone-releasing factor. Trans Assoc Am Physicians 95:177–187, 1982.

CHAPTER 48

The Thyroid Gland

Eugene J. Barrett

The thyroid gland is located in the anterior neck, lying like a small bow tie across the front of the trachea. In adults, the normal thyroid weighs approximately 20 g. It is composed of left and right lobes and a small connecting branch, or isthmus.

The thyroid gland possesses many features unique among endocrine glands, not the least of which is that it is the only endocrine gland that can be easily seen and palpated in the course of a routine clinical examination. At the biochemical level, the thyroid hormones are the only ones that require an essential trace element, iodine, for the production of active hormone. One of the rather unusual features of thyroid hormone physiology is that the hormone is stored in an extracellular site within a highly proteinaceous material called *thyroid colloid*. The major protein within this material is thyroglobulin, which contains—as part of its primary structure—the thyroid hormones thyroxine (tetraiodothyronine or T_4) and triiodothyronine (T_3). This sequestered hormone is entirely surrounded by thyroid follicular cells, which are responsible for the synthesis of thyroid hormones (Fig. 48–1).

The physiological actions of thyroid hormones also display several unique aspects. Although, like most peptide hormones, T_4 and T_3 are made as part of a larger protein, unlike peptide hormones, there are no cell-membrane receptors for these hormones. Instead, like the steroid hormones, thyroid hormones act by binding to *nuclear* receptors (p. 112) and regulate the transcription of cell proteins. The hormones secreted by the thyroid act on multiple tissues and are essential for normal development, growth, and metabolism. The thyroid makes another hormone, calcitonin, which is synthesized by the thyroid's **C cells** (parafollicular cells); these C cells are not part of the follicular unit (see Fig. 48–1). Calcitonin may play a role in Ca^{2+} and phosphate homeostasis (p. 1099). The physiology of calcitonin is discussed along with that of parathyroid hormone in Chapter 51.

SYNTHESIS OF THYROID HORMONES

Thyroid Hormones Are Made by Iodinating Tyrosine Residues on Thyroglobulin and Are Stored As Part of Thyroglobulin Molecules in Thyroid Follicles

The structures of **thyroxine** (T_4) and **triiodothyronine** (T_3), the two active thyroid hormones, are shown in Figure 48–2. T_3 is far more active than

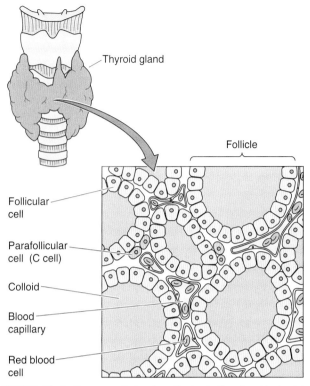

FIGURE 48–1. Structure of the thyroid gland. The thyroid gland is located anterior to the cricoid cartilage in the anterior neck. The gland comprises numerous follicles, which are filled with colloid and lined by follicular cells. These follicular cells are responsible for the trapping of iodine and the synthesis of thyroglobulin, which contains thyroid hormone as part of its primary structure. These cells also secrete thyroglobulin—the major protein of the thyroid colloid—into the lumen of the follicle. The thyroglobulin protein that is stored in the follicular lumen contains numerous iodinated tyrosines and thyronines, which are derivatives of the amino acid tyrosine. On command, the follicular cells take up the thyroglobulin and release the thyroid hormones triiodothyronine (T_3) and thyroxine, or tetraiodothyronine (T_4), into the blood.

Thyroxine (T_4) (3,5,3′,5′-tetraiodo-L-thyronine)

Triiodothyronine (T_3) (3,5,3′,-triiodo-L-thyronine)

Reverse T_3 (rT_3) (3,3′,5′ triiodothyronine)

Peptide backbone of thyroglobulin molecule

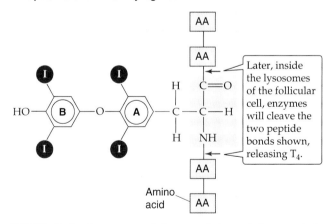

FIGURE 48–2. The structure of thyroxine (T_4), triiodothyronine (T_3), and reverse T_3 (rT_3). T_4, T_3, and rT_3 all are products of the coupling of two iodinated tyrosine derivatives. Only T_4 and T_3 are biologically active, and T_3 is far more active than T_4 because of a higher affinity for thyroid hormone receptors. Reverse T_3 forms as an iodine is removed from the inner benzyl ring (labeled "A") of T_4; rT_3 is present in approximately equal molar amounts with T_3. However, rT_3 is essentially devoid of biologic activity. As shown in the bottom panel, T_4 is part of the peptide backbone of the thyroglobulin molecule, as are T_3 and rT_3. Cleavage of the two indicated peptide bonds would release T_4.

T_4. Also shown is **reverse T_3** (rT_3), which has no known biologic activity. It has two iodines on its *outer* benzyl ring, rather than two on its *inner* ring, as is the case for T_3. All three compounds derive from the ether linkage of a tyrosine molecule to the benzyl group of a second tyrosine molecule; one or two iodine atoms are attached to each benzyl group. The *bottom panel* of Figure 48–2 shows T_4 as part of the thyroglobulin molecule.

The synthesis of thyroid hormones begins with the trapping of iodide by the thyroid gland. Iodine is essential for the formation of thyroid hormones. It exists in nature as a trace element in soil and is incorporated into many foods. The iodide anion (I^-) is rapidly absorbed by the gastrointestinal tract and is actively taken up by the thyroid gland. A specialized Na/I cotransporter is located at the basolateral membrane (i.e., facing the blood) of the thyroid **follicular cell** (Fig. 48–3). The Na/I cotransporter, termed **NIS** (for *Na Iodide Symporter*), is a 65-kDa integral membrane protein that is believed to have 12 membrane-spanning segments. NIS moves I^- into the follicular cell against the I^- electrochemical gradient, fueled by the energy of the Na^+ electrochemical gradient (p. 66). Several other anions (e.g., perchlorate, pertech-

Tyrosine

1 **Trapping:** TSH increases the activity of a Na/I cotransporter (NIS) on the basolateral membrane of the thyroid follicular cell. The result is increased iodine trapping: the ratio of follicular-cell iodine to plasma iodine (the so-called thyroid/serum or T/S ratio) increases under conditions of high TSH.

2 Iodide leaves the cell, probably via pendrin, and enters the lumen. The follicular cell also secretes thyroglobulin. Thyroid peroxidase, on the luminal surface of secretory vesicle, oxidizes I^- to I^0.

3 **Iodination:** TSH also stimulates iodination of thyroglobulin in the follicular lumen.

4 **Conjugation:** TSH stimulates the conjugation of iodinated tyrosines to form T_4 and T_3 linked to thyroglobulin.

5 **Endocytosis:** TSH stimulates the endocytosis of iodinated thyroglobulin into the follicular cells from thyroid colloid.

6 **Proteolysis:** TSH stimulates the proteolysis of the iodinated thyroglobulin, forming T_4 and T_3 in the lumen of the lysoendosome.

7 **Secretion:** TSH stimulates the secretion of T_4 and T_3 into the circulation.

Hyperplasia: Finally, TSH exerts a growth-factor effect, stimulating hyperplasia within the thyroid gland.

FIGURE 48–3. The follicular cell and its role in the synthesis of thyroxine (T_4) and triiodothyronine (T_3). The synthesis and release of T_4 and T_3 occurs in seven steps. Inside the follicular cell, a deiodinase converts some of the T_4 to T_3. Thyrotropin (or thyroid-stimulating hormone [TSH]) stimulates each of these steps except step 2. In addition, TSH exerts a growth factor or hyperplastic effect on the follicular cells. DIT, diiodotyronine; MIT, monoiodotyronine.

netate, and thiocyanate) can compete with I^- for uptake by the thyroid. Iodide leaves the follicular cell and enters the lumen of the follicle across the apical membrane, presumably via pendrin, a member of the SAT family of anion exchangers (p. 69).

In parallel with the secretion of I^- into the follicle lumen, the follicular cell secretes **thyroglobulin** into the lumen; thyroglobulin contains the tyrosyl groups to which the I^- will ultimately attach. The thyroglobulin molecule is a glycoprotein synthesized inside the follicular cell, following the secretory pathway (p. 36). Thyroglobulin is a very large protein (>600 kDa), and it accounts for approximately half of the protein content of the thyroid gland. It has relatively few tyrosyl residues (~100/mole-

cule of thyroglobulin), and only a handful of these (<20) are subject to iodination. The secretory vesicles that contain thyroglobulin also carry the enzyme **thyroid peroxidase** on their intravesicular surfaces. As the secretory vesicles fuse with the apical membrane, this enzyme faces the follicular lumen and catalyzes the oxidation of I^- to I^0. As the thyroglobulin is entering the lumen of the thyroid follicle by the process of exocytosis, its tyrosyl groups react with I^0.

One or two oxidized iodine atoms incorporate selectively into specific tyrosyl residues of thyroglobulin. Within the thyroglobulin molecule, an internal rearrangement occurs, resulting in the conjugation of two iodinated tyrosyl residues to form a single iodothyronine, as well as

IODINE DEFICIENCY

In areas where soil is relatively iodine deficient, human iodine deficiency is commonly found. Because seawater, as well as seafood, contains large amounts of iodide, iodine deficiency is more common in inland areas, particularly in locales that rely on locally grown foods. Iodine deficiency causes thyroid hormone deficiency. The pituitary responds to this deficit by increasing the synthesis of thyrotropin (thyroid-stimulating hormone; p. 1046), which in turn increases the activity of the iodine-trapping mechanism in the follicular cell in an effort to overcome the deficiency. The increased TSH also exerts a trophic effect that increases the *size* of the thyroid gland. If this trophic effect persists for sufficient time, the result is an iodine-deficient **goiter**. The term "goiter" is simply a generic term for an enlarged thyroid. If this effort at compensation is not successful (i.e., if insufficient thyroid hormone levels persist), the person develops signs and symptoms of goitrous **hypothyroidism**. When iodine deficiency occurs at critical developmental times in infancy, the effects on the CNS are particularly devastating, producing the syndrome known as **cretinism** (p. 1043). Persons so affected have a characteristic facial appearance and body habitus, and severe mental retardation. Dietary supplementation of iodine in salt and bread has all but eliminated iodine deficiency from North America. However, in many nations, and especially in mountainous and landlocked regions of developing nations, iodine deficiency remains a major cause of preventable illness.

a remnant dehydroalanine. Both remain as part of the primary structure of the iodinated thyroglobulin until it is later degraded inside the follicular cell. This coupling of two tyrosines, catalyzed by thyroid peroxidase, does not occur unless they are iodinated. Because only a minority of tyrosyl groups become iodinated, there is probably something specific about the structure of the protein near these residues that facilitates both iodination and conjugation. The thyroid hormones, although still a part of the thyroglobulin molecule, are stored as colloid in the thyroid follicle.

Follicular Cells Take Up Iodinated Thyroglobulin, Hydrolyze It, and Release T_4 and T_3 into the Blood for Binding to Thyroid-Binding Globulin and Other Proteins

While they remain attached to thyroglobulin in the thyroid follicular lumen (see Fig. 48–1), thyroid hormones remain inactive until the iodinated thyroglobulin is hydrolyzed. Before this proteolysis can begin, the follicular cells must resorb thyroglobulin from the follicular lumen by fluid-phase endocytosis (p. 42). As the endocytic vesicle containing the colloid droplet moves from the apical toward the basolateral membrane, it fuses with lysosomes, forming a lysoendosome. Inside this vesicle, lysosomal enzymes hydrolyze the thyroglobulin, forming T_4 and T_3,

as well as diiodothyronine (DIT) and monoiodothyronine (MIT). The vesicle releases both T_4 and T_3 near the basolateral membrane, and these exit the cell into the blood by an unknown mechanism. Approximately 90% of the thyroid hormone secreted by the thyroid is released as T_4, and 10% as T_3. The thyroid releases very little reverse T_3 into the blood. As is discussed in the next section, nonthyroidal tissues metabolize the T_4 released by the thyroid into T_3 and rT_3. Approximately three quarters of circulating T_3 arises from the peripheral conversion of T_4, which occurs principally in the liver and kidneys.

In the circulation, both T_4 and T_3 are highly bound to plasma proteins. **Thyroid-binding globulin** (TBG), albumin, and **transthyretin** (TTR) account for most of this binding. The affinity of these binding proteins is sufficiently high that, for T_4, over 99.98% of the hormone circulates tightly bound to protein. T_3 is bound only

FREE VERSUS BOUND THYROXINE

Most of the T_4 and T_3 in the serum is bound to proteins, the most important of which is thyroid-binding globulin (TBG). For the binding of T_4 to TBG, the reaction is

$$T_4 + TBG \overset{K}{\rightleftharpoons} T_4TBG$$

and

$$K = \frac{[T_4TBG]}{[T_4][TBG]}$$

The binding constant K is approximately 2×10^{10} M^{-1} for T_4. The comparable binding constant for T_3 is approximately 5×10^8 M^{-1}. Approximately one third of TBG's binding sites are occupied by T_4. Therefore, we have all the information we need to compute the concentration of free T_4:

$$[T_4]_{FREE} = \frac{[T_4TBG]}{K[TBG]}$$

A reasonable value for $[T_4TBG]$ would be 100 nM, and for $[TBG]$, 250 nM. Thus,

$$[T_4]_{FREE} = \frac{(100 \text{ nM})}{(2 \times 10^{10} \text{ M}^{-1}) \times (250 \text{ nM})}$$

$$= 0.20 \times 10^{-10} \text{ M}$$

$$= 20 \text{ pM}$$

Because the bound T_4 in this example is 100 nM, and the free T_4 is only 20 pM, we can conclude that only approximately 0.02% of the total T_4 in the plasma is free. Because 99.98% of the total T_4 in the plasma is bound, moderate fluctuations in the rate of T_4 release from the thyroid have only tiny effects on the level of free T_4. To simplify, we have not included the minor contribution of albumin and transthyretin in this sample calculation.

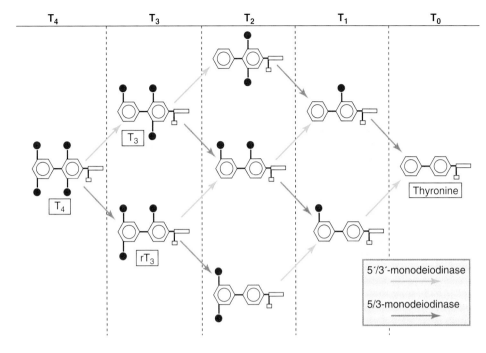

FIGURE 48–4. Peripheral metabolism of thyroxine (T_4). A 5'/3'-monodeiodinase (*green arrows*) removes I from the outer benzyl ring, whereas a 5/3-monodeiodinase (*orange arrows*) removes I from the inner benzyl ring. Thus, the action of the 5'/3'-monodeiodinase on T_4 yields triiodothyronine (T_3), whereas the action of the 5/3-monodeiodinase yields rT_3. Sequential deiodination yields T_0 (thyronine).

slightly less: About 99.5% is protein bound. Because the free or "unbound" hormone in the circulation is responsible for the actions of the thyroid hormones on their target tissues, the large amount of bound hormone has considerably confounded our ability to use simple measurements of the total amount of either T_4 or T_3 in the plasma to provide a reliable index of the adequacy of thyroid hormone secretion. For example, the amount of TBG in the serum can change substantially in different physiological states. Pregnancy, oral estrogen therapy, hepatitis, and chronic heroin abuse can all elevate the amount of TBG, and hence the *total* concentration of T_4 and T_3. Decreased levels of TBG, associated with diminished concentration of *total* T_4 and T_3, can accompany steroid usage and the nephrotic syndrome. However, despite the marked increases or decreases in the amounts of circulating TBG, the concentrations of *free* T_4 and T_3 do not change in the aforementioned examples. The box titled "Free Versus Bound Thyroxine" indicates how one can calculate levels of free T_4 or T_3, knowing the concentration of TBG and the concentration of total T_4 or total T_3.

The liver makes each of the thyroid-binding proteins. TBG is a 54-kDa glycoprotein consisting of 450 amino acids. It has the highest affinity for T_4 and T_3, and is responsible for most of the thyroid-binding capacity in the plasma. The extensive binding of thyroid hormones to plasma proteins serves several functions. It provides a large buffer pool of thyroid hormones in the circulation, so that the active concentrations of hormone in the circulation change very little on a minute-to-minute basis. The binding to plasma proteins markedly prolongs the half-lives of both T_4 and T_3. T_4 has a half-life of 8 days, and T_3, approximately 24 hours; each is longer than the half-life of the steroid or peptide hormones. Finally, because much of the T_3 in the circulation is formed by the conversion of T_4 to T_3 in extrathyroidal tissues, the presence of a large pool of T_4 in the plasma provides a reserve of prohormone available for synthesis of T_3. This reserve may be of particular importance because T_3 is responsible for most of the biologic activity of thyroid hormones.

Peripheral Tissues Deiodinate T_4 to Produce T_3

The thyroid synthesizes and stores much more T_4 than T_3, and this is reflected by the approximately 10:1 ratio of T_4/T_3 secreted by the thyroid. However, a number of tissues in the body have the capacity to selectively deiodinate T_4, producing either T_3 or rT_3. T_3 and rT_3 can each be further deiodinated to various diiodothyronines and monoiodothyronines (Fig. 48–4); both DITs and MITs are biologically inactive. Both iodine atoms on the inner ring, and at least one iodine atom on the outer ring, appear essential for biologic activity. Similarly, the loss of the amino group renders T_4 or T_3 inactive. The importance of the peripheral deiodination of T_4 to T_3 can be readily appreciated from the observation that humans whose thyroids have been removed have normal circulating concentrations of T_3 when they receive oral thyroxine (T_4) supplementation.

Inasmuch as T_3 is biologically much more active than the far more abundant T_4, the regulation of the conversion of T_4 to T_3 in peripheral tissues assumes considerable importance. Two distinct deiodinases convert T_4 to T_3 (see Fig. 48–4): The 5'/3'-deiodinase removes an I from the *outer* ring, producing T_3, whereas the 5/3-deiodinase removes an I from the *inner* ring, producing the inactive rT_3. Because the 3' and 5' positions in T_4 are equivalent stereochemically, removing either of these yields T_3. Similarly, removing the I from either the 3 or the 5 position of the inner ring of T_4 yields rT_3. Further deiodination by these two enzymes ultimately yields T_0 (i.e., thyronine).

The 5'/3'-deiodinase, which acts on the outer ring, comes in two forms. Type 1 is present in high concentra-

THE SICK EUTHYROID SYNDROME

Many hospitalized patients who are extremely ill exhibit abnormal results in thyroid function tests. However, the thyroid activity of most of these patients is actually appropriate and needs no correction. Many of these patients are in an intensive care unit (ICU) setting, and it is extremely important to distinguish true thyroid disease from this so-called *sick euthyroid syndrome*.

The sick euthyroid syndrome can take many forms, but the most common is a low or lower-than-normal total T_4 and a low T_3. In true hypothyroidism, the diminished levels of thyroid hormones decrease feedback inhibition on the pituitary gland, and lead to increased levels of thyrotropin (thyroid-stimulating hormone or TSH; p. 1046). In the sick euthyroid syndrome, the TSH level is usually normal. Although the reasons for this situation are not completely understood, at least one explanation may lie in the distinction between the type 1 deiodinase, which is found in the periphery, and the type 2 deiodinase, which is present in the pituitary. In sick euthyroid syndrome, the activity of the type 1 or peripheral 5'/3' deiodinase decreases, such that there is less conversion of peripheral T_4 to T_3, but more conversion to rT_3. As a result, peripheral T_3 levels fall. However, as was described in the main text for starvation, the type 2 deiodinase is not affected by stress nearly as much as is the type 1 deiodinase; therefore, the pituitary gland continues to sense normal levels of T_3, and it responds to what it perceives as normal levels of feedback inhibition from local T_3 on the production and release of TSH. However, other factors must also be involved, inasmuch as this mechanism does not adequately account for the decrease in total T_4.

Patients with the sick euthyroid syndrome may appear profoundly hypothyroid, exhibiting hypothermia and a sluggish sensorium, but they are not hypothyroid, and they should not receive thyroid hormone replacement. In fact, treating sick euthyroid patients with thyroid hormone yields either no improvement or a worse outcome.

tions in the liver, kidneys, and thyroid. It appears to be responsible for generating most of the T_3 that reaches the circulation. Type 2 is found predominantly in the pituitary, central nervous system (CNS), and placenta, and is involved in supplying those tissues with T_3 by local generation from plasma-derived T_4. As we show later, the type 2 enzyme in the pituitary is of particular importance because the T_3 that is generated there is responsible for the feedback inhibition of the release of thyrotropin (or thyroid-stimulating hormone, TSH).

The relative activity of the deiodinases changes in response to physiological and pathologic stimuli. Caloric restriction or severe stress inhibits the *type 1* outer ring deiodinase, thereby decreasing the conversion of T_4 to T_3—and thus decreasing the levels of T_3. On the other hand, levels of rT_3 rise by default in these situations, in part because of reduced conversion to diiodothyronines. These decreases in T_3 levels are accompanied by a decline in metabolic rate. You might think that because plasma

levels of T_3 *fall*, there would also be a compensatory *rise* in TSH, the secretion of which is inhibited by T_3. However, because *type 2* deiodinase mediates the conversion of T_4 to T_3 within the pituitary and CNS, and because caloric restriction does not affect this enzyme, local T_3 levels in the pituitary are normal. Thus, the thyrotrophs in the pituitary continue to see adequate amounts of T_3, and there is no compensatory rise in TSH. Teleologically, there is an appealing rationale to restraining calorie expenditure in settings of decreased caloric intake.

ACTION OF THYROID HORMONES

Thyroid Hormones Act via Nuclear Receptors in Target Tissues

Thyroid hormones act on many body tissues to exert both metabolic and developmental effects. Most, if not all, of the actions of thyroid hormones occur as thyroid hormones bind to and activate **nuclear receptors** (p. 112). These receptors in turn are bound to chromatin and alter the transcription of specific genes. The multitude of thyroid hormone actions are mirrored by the ubiquitous expression of thyroid hormone receptors (THRs) throughout the body's tissues. Once T_4 and T_3 leave the plasma, they enter the cell either by diffusing through the lipid of the cell membrane or by carrier-mediated transport (Fig. 48–5). Once in the cytoplasm, T_4 and T_3 bind to a number of sites in the cytosol, microsomes, and mitochondria, as well as the nucleus. This observation has prompted speculation that thyroid hormones may exert actions via mechanisms not involving transcriptional regulation. However, current evidence suggests that if these non-genomic mechanisms are operative, they are exceptions to the general schema shown in Figure 48–5, which appears to account for most of the actions of thyroid hormones.

Biologically, T_3 is much more important than T_4. This statement may be surprising inasmuch as the *total* concentration of T_4 in the circulation is 50-fold or higher than that of T_3. There are three reasons why T_3 has a greater biologic activity: First, T_4 is bound (only 0.02% is *free*) more tightly to plasma proteins than is T_3 (0.50% is *free*; i.e., a 25-fold higher ratio of free to bound). The net effect is that the amount of free T_4 in the circulation is only about twofold or more higher than the amount of free T_3. Second, because the target cell converts T_4—once it has entered the cell—to T_3, it turns out that T_4 and T_3 are present at similar concentrations in the cytoplasm of target cells. Finally, the THR in the nucleus has approximately a 10-fold greater affinity for T_3 than T_4, so that T_3 is more potent on a molar basis. As a result, T_3 is responsible for approximately 90% of the occupancy of THRs in the euthyroid state.

When T_3 or T_4 binds to the THR in the nucleus, the hormone-bound receptors either activate or repress the transcription of specific genes. As was discussed earlier (p. 131), THR preferentially binds to DNA as a heterodimer of THR and the retinoid X receptor (RXR). THR belongs to the superfamily of nuclear receptors that contains domains A through F (p. 113). Three regions are

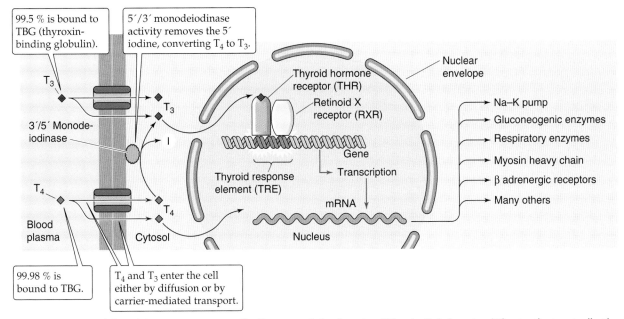

FIGURE 48-5. Action of thyroid hormones on target cells. Free extracellular thyroxine (T_4) and triiodothyronine (T_3) enter the target cell either by diffusion or by carrier-mediated transport. Once the T_4 is inside the cell, a cytoplasmic 5'/3'-monodeiodinase converts much of the T_4 to T_3, so that that cytoplasmic levels of T_4 and T_3 are about equal. Both T_4 and T_3 enter the nucleus. Thyroid hormone receptors bind to DNA at thyroid response elements in the promoter region of genes regulated by thyroid hormones. The binding of T_3 or T_4 to the receptor regulates the transcription of these genes. The receptor preferentially binds T_3. Therefore, of the total thyroid hormone bound to receptor, approximately 90% is T_3. The receptor that binds to the DNA is preferentially a heterodimer of the thyroid hormone receptor and retinoid X receptor. Thyroid hormone promotes the transcription of genes encoding a wide range of proteins. mRNA, messenger RNA.

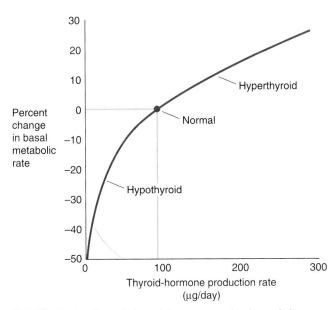

FIGURE 48-6. Effect of thyroid hormone on basal metabolic rate (BMR). This graph shows the dependence of BMR on the daily rate of thyroid hormone secretion (thyroxine [T_4] and triiodothyronine [T_3], both bound and free). We use the secretion rate because it is difficult to know whether to use free T_4 and/or free T_3. Recall that free T_4 is higher in the serum than free T_3. However, target cells convert much of the incoming T_4 to T_3. Moreover, the thyroid hormone receptor has a 10-fold–higher affinity for T_3 than for T_4. Thus, the secretion rate is a crude measure of effective thyroid hormone levels. (Data from Guyton AC, Hall JE: Textbook of Medical Physiology, 9th ed. Philadelphia, WB Saunders, 1996.)

especially important for THR: (1) The amino-terminal A/B region contains the first of two transactivation domains, which are responsible for transducing receptor binding into a conformational change in the DNA, thereby initiating transcription. (2) The middle or C region is responsible for DNA binding via two zinc fingers (p. 126), as well as dimerization between receptors. (3) The E region, toward the carboxyl terminus, is responsible for binding the ligand (T_3 or T_4), and also for dimerization.

There are actually two THR genes—α and β—that are present on chromosomes 17 and 3, respectively. The expression of these receptor genes is tissue specific and varies with time of development. The liver expresses principally the β isoform, whereas the α isoform predominates in the brain. During development, the amount of α expressed may vary 10-fold or more.

Thyroid Hormones Increase Basal Metabolic Rate by Stimulating Futile Cycles of Catabolism/Anabolism

It has long been observed that excess thyroid hormone raises the **basal metabolic rate** (BMR) as measured by either heat production (direct calorimetry) or oxygen consumption (indirect calorimetry). Conversely, thyroid hormone deficiency is accompanied by a decreased BMR. Figure 48-6 illustrates the effect of thyroid hormone levels on BMR, and Table 48-1 summarizes the effect of the thyroid hormones on several parameters. Thyroid hormones increase the BMR by stimulating both catabolic and anabolic reactions in pathways affecting fats, carbohydrates, and proteins.

TABLE 48–1

PHYSIOLOGICAL EFFECTS OF THE THYROID HORMONES (T_3 and T_4)		
PARAMETER	**LOW LEVEL OF THYROID HORMONES (HYPOTHYROID)**	**HIGH LEVEL OF THYROID HORMONES (HYPERTHYROID)**
Basal metabolic rate	↓	↑
Carbohydrate metabolism	↓ Gluconeogenesis ↓ Glycogenolysis Normal serum [glucose]	↑ Gluconeogenesis ↑ Glycogenolysis Normal serum [glucose]
Protein metabolism	↓ Synthesis ↓ Proteolysis	↑ Synthesis ↑ Proteolysis Muscle wasting
Lipid metabolism	↓ Lipogenesis ↓ Lipolysis ↑ Serum [cholesterol]	↑ Lipogenesis ↑ Lipolysis ↓ Serum [cholesterol]
Thermogenesis	↓	↑
Autonomic nervous system	Normal levels of serum catecholamines	↑ Expression of β adrenoceptors (increased sensitivity to catecholamines, which remain at normal levels)

CARBOHYDRATE METABOLISM. Thyroid hormones increase the rate of hepatic glucose production, principally by increasing hepatic gluconeogenic activity. This effect generally does not result in increases in plasma [glucose], provided the pancreas responds by increasing insulin secretion. Thyroid hormones also enhance the availability of the starting materials required for increased gluconeogenic activity (i.e., amino acids and glycerol), and specifically induces the expression of several key gluconeogenic enzymes, including phosphoenolpyruvate carboxykinase, pyruvate carboxylase, and glucose-6-phosphatase.

PROTEIN METABOLISM. The amino acids required for increased hepatic gluconeogenesis, stimulated by thyroid hormones, come from increased proteolysis, predominantly in muscle. Thyroid hormones also increase protein synthesis. Because the increases in protein degradation usually outweigh the increases in synthesis, a net loss of muscle protein occurs. The catabolic effect is exaggerated when T_3 is present in great excess, so that muscle wasting and weakness, as well as increased nitrogen loss in the urine as urea (pp. 790 and 997), can be a prominent feature of clinical thyrotoxicosis (hyperthyroidism).

LIPID METABOLISM. The glycerol required for increased hepatic gluconeogenesis, stimulated by thyroid hormones, comes from increased degradation of stored triglycerides in adipose tissue. The free fatty acids (FFAs) released along with the glycerol provide fuel for the liver to support the energy demand of gluconeogenesis. Thyroid hormones not only increase lipolysis, they also enhance lipogenesis. Indeed, modest amounts of thyroid hormones are needed for the normal synthesis of FFA by liver. Very high levels of T_3 shift the balance in favor of lipolysis, resulting in generalized fat mobilization and loss of body fat stores.

By accelerating the rates of glucose production, protein synthesis, and degradation, as well as of lipogenesis and lipolysis, the thyroid hormones stimulate energy consumption. Therefore, to the extent that thyroid hormones stimulate both synthesis and degradation, they promote **futile cycles** that contribute significantly to the increased oxygen consumption seen with thyrotoxicosis (hyperthyroidism).

How, at the molecular level, thyroid hormones affect the BMR in states of both spontaneous and experimentally induced thyroid hormone excess or deficiency has been a difficult question to answer. The changes in metabolic rate do not appear to be determined by changes in the expression of a single gene. Several specific examples of the effects of thyroid hormones on target tissues serve to illustrate their general mechanism of action.

Na-K PUMP ACTIVITY. In muscle, liver, and kidney, thyroid hormone–induced increases in oxygen consumption are paralleled by increases in the activity of the **Na-K pump** in the plasma membrane (p. 61). This increase in transport is due at least in part to an increase in the synthesis of new transporter units that are inserted into the plasma membrane. At least in some tissues, blocking the increases in Na-K pump activity with ouabain also blocks the increase in oxygen consumption. T_3 stimulates the transcription of the genes for both the α and β subunits of the Na-K pump. In addition, T_3 increases translation by stabilizing the mRNA that encodes the Na-K pump. Increases in the activity of this transporter consume additional adenosine triphosphate (ATP), and thereby consume oxygen and generate heat. Inasmuch as states of thyroid hormone excess are not accompanied by any noticeable derangement of plasma electrolyte levels, presumably the increase in Na-K pump activity is compensated in some manner by a leak of Na^+ and K^+, although such pathways have not yet been defined. Overall, the increased activity of the Na-K pump (with an accompanying cation leak) would result in a futile cycle whereby energy was consumed without useful work.

THERMOGENESIS. In rodents, thyroid hormones may affect metabolic rate and thermogenesis through another futile cycle mechanism. Brown fat in these animals expresses a mitochondrial **uncoupling protein** (UCP), or **thermogenin**, that dissociates **oxidative phosphorylation** from ATP generation. Thus, mitochondria consume O_2 and produce heat without generating ATP. Both T_3 and β-adrenergic stimulation (acting via the $β_3$ receptor) enhance respiration in brown adipose tissue by stimulating this uncoupling mechanism. We discuss thermogenin—and the vital role it plays in helping to keep newborn humans warm—on p. 1205.

Thyroid hormones also increase the BMR by increasing the thermogenic effects of other processes. An example is the effect of adrenergic stimulation on thermogenesis, discussed earlier. In humans, plasma *concentrations* of catecholamines are normal in states of both excess and deficient T_3 and T_4. However, excess thyroid hormone raises the *sensitivity* of tissues to the action of adrenergic hormones. In heart, skeletal muscle, and adipose tissue, this effect is due, at least in part, to increased expression of **β-adrenergic receptors** by these tissues. In patients who are acutely thyrotoxic, treatment with β-receptor antagonists is one of the first priorities. This treatment blunts the hypersympathetic state induced by the excess of thyroid hormones. Thyroid hormones may also exert postreceptor effects that enhance adrenergic tone. In heart, thyroid hormones also regulate the expression of specific forms of **myosin heavy chain**. Specifically, in rodents, thyroid hormone increases the expression of the myosin α chain, thereby favoring the α/α isoform of myosin heavy chain (p. 252). This isoform is associated with greater activity of both actin and Ca^{2+}-activated ATPase, more rapid fiber shortening, and greater contractility.

Thyroid Hormones Are Essential for Normal Growth and Development

In amphibians, thyroid hormone regulates the process of metamorphosis. Removing the thyroid gland from tadpoles causes development to arrest at the tadpole stage. Early administration of excess thyroid hormone can initiate premature metamorphosis. Iodothyronines are present even farther down the phylogenetic tree, at least as far as primitive chordates, although these animals lack a thyroid gland per se. However, the biologic actions of iodothyronines in many species are not known.

Thyroid hormones are essential for normal human development as well, as is starkly illustrated by the unfortunate condition of cretinism in regions of endemic iodine deficiency. **Cretinism** is characterized by profound mental retardation, short stature, delay in motor development, coarse hair, and a protuberant abdomen. Correction of iodine deficiency has essentially eliminated endemic cretinism in developed nations. Sporadic cases continue to occur, however, as a result of congenital defects in thyroid hormone synthesis. If hypothyroidism is recognized and corrected within a few days of birth, development—including mental development—can proceed almost normally. For this reason, many localities have initiated laboratory screening of newborns for hypothyroidism because

clinical recognition of the full syndrome often occurs only after the developmental abnormalities in the CNS are irreversible.

Typically overshadowed by the impaired cognitive development that occurs in cretinism is the **dwarfism** that results from the effects of thyroid hormone deficiency on human growth (Fig. 48–7). In children with normal thyroid function at birth, development of hypothyroidism at any time before the fusion of the epiphyses of the long bones leads to growth retardation or arrest. Much of the loss in height that occurs can be recovered after thyroid hormone treatment is begun, a phenomenon called "catch-up growth." If the diagnosis and treatment of hypothyroidism are delayed, loss of potential growth may occur. As is indicated in Figure 48–7, "catch-up" may not apply to mental development unless the treatment is begun very early, certainly within a few days of birth. In general, the longer the duration of congenital hypothyroidism, the more profound the mental retardation. The growth curve (i.e., a plot of the child's height and weight vs. age) can provide a particularly sensitive early indicator of hypothyroidism. An overactive thyroid is much less a

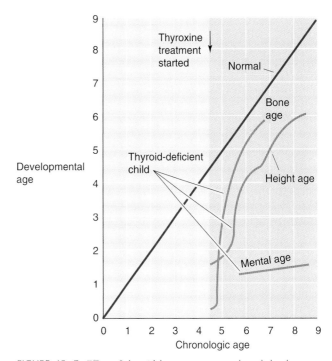

FIGURE 48–7. Effect of thyroid hormone on growth and development. This is a graph of developmental age—that is, the age that the child appears based on height, bone radiograph, and mental function—versus chronological age. For a normal child, the relationship is the straight line *(red)*, for which developmental and chronological age are identical. The three *green curves* are growth curves for a child with thyroid hormone deficiency. Notice that at age 4.5 years, before initiation of therapy, height age, bone age, and mental age are all substantially below normal. Initiating replacement therapy with thyroid hormone at age 4.5 causes a rapid increase in both height age and bone age ("catch up") but has no effect on mental age, which remains infantile. Treatment can help mental development only if the therapy is begun within a few days of birth. (Data from Wilkins L: The Diagnosis and Treatment of Endocrine Disorders of Childhood and Adolescence. Springfield, IL, Charles C Thomas, 1965.)

FIGURE 48–8. Effect of thyroid hormone on bone age. These x-rays emphasize the differences in bone development in the hand of a normal child (*A*), and a child with thyroid deficiency (*B*). Note that for the hypothyroid child, the centers of ossification in the epiphyseal regions are stippled in appearance. (From Besser GM, Thorner MO: Clinical Endocrinology. London, Mosby-Wolfe, 1994.)

problem than is an underactive thyroid with regard to its effect on growth; other signs and symptoms of an overactive thyroid predominate.

Cellular explanations of the effects of thyroid hormones on human development are incomplete. In rats, thyroid hormone induces the secretion of pituitary growth hormone (GH); thus, the growth retardation in thyroid-deficient rats might in part be due to decreased GH secretion. However, in humans, for whom there is no thyroid hormone response element in the promoter region of the GH gene, plasma [GH] is normal in hypothyroidism. Thus, the growth failure of hypothyroid human infants is not as readily explained. In humans, changes in the growth plate of the long bones are more or less characteristic of thyroid hormone deficiency (Fig. 48–8). These changes include a delay in formation of centers of ossification at the growth plate, and then the appearance of several ossification centers, which eventually merge. Radiographically, the epiphyses have a characteristic stippled appearance. Short stature in human juvenile or infantile hypothyroidism may be in part related to these abnormalities of cartilage growth and development as well as resistance to the normal action of GH to promote growth. In rodents, thyroid hormone regulates the induction of expression of several neural proteins, including myelin basic protein. How deficiencies in these proteins might result in the generalized cortical atrophy seen in infantile hypothyroidism is not clear.

THE HYPOTHALAMIC-PITUITARY-THYROID AXIS

The pituitary regulates the synthesis and secretion of thyroid hormones via the release of **thyrotropin**—also known as thyroid-stimulating hormone or TSH—from the anterior pituitary. In turn, the hypothalamus stimulates the release of TSH via **thyrotropin-releasing hor-**mone (TRH). Finally, circulating thyroid hormones exert feedback control on both TRH and TSH secretion.

Thyrotropin-Releasing Hormone from the Hypothalamus Stimulates the Thyrotrophs of the Anterior Pituitary to Secrete Thyrotropin, Which in Turn Stimulates T_4/T_3 Synthesis

THYROTROPIN-RELEASING HORMONE. TRH is a tri-peptide pyro-Glu-His-Pro containing the modified amino acid pyro-Glu. It is found in many tissues, including the cerebral cortex, multiple areas of the GI tract, and the β cells of the pancreas. However, the arcuate nucleus and the median eminence of the **hypothalamus** appear to be the major sources of the TRH that stimulates TSH synthesis and secretion (Fig. 48–9). TRH released by neurons in the hypothalamus travels to the anterior pituitary via the hypophyseal portal system (p. 1010). Hypothalamic lesions that interrupt TRH release or delivery cause a fall in basal TSH levels. Conversely, administering TRH intravenously can cause a rapid, dose-dependent release of TSH from the anterior pituitary. However, it is not clear that such bursts of TRH release and TSH secretion occur physiologically.

THYROTROPIN-RELEASING HORMONE RECEPTOR. Once it reaches the thyrotrophs in the anterior pituitary, TRH binds to the TRH receptor, a G protein–coupled receptor on the cell membranes of the thyrotrophs. TRH binding triggers the phospholipase C pathway (p. 100). The formation of diacylglycerols (DAGs) stimulates protein kinase C, leading to protein phosphorylation. The simultaneous release of inositol triphosphate (IP$_3$) triggers Ca^{2+} release from internal stores, raising [Ca^{2+}]$_i$. The result is an increase in both the synthesis and release of TSH, which is stored in secretory granules. TRH produces some of its effects by activating phospholipase A$_2$, leading to the release of arachidonic acid and the formation of a variety of

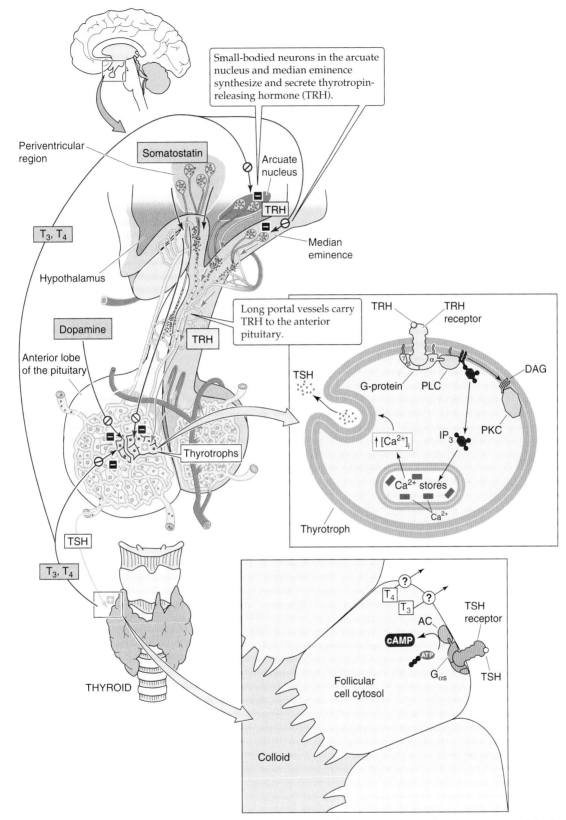

FIGURE 48–9. The hypothalamic-pituitary-thyroid axis. Small-bodied neurons in the arcuate nucleus and median eminence of the hypothalamus secrete thyrotropin-releasing hormone (TRH), a tripeptide that reaches the thyrotrophs in the anterior pituitary via the long portal veins. TRH binds to a G protein–coupled receptor on the thyrotroph membrane, triggering the DAG/IP₃ pathway, leading to protein phosphorylation and raising [Ca²⁺]ᵢ. These pathways stimulate the thyrotrophs to synthesize and release thyrotrophin (or thyroid-stimulating hormone [TSH]), which is a 28-kDa glycoprotein stored in secretory granules. The TSH binds to receptors on the basolateral membrane of thyroid follicular cells, stimulating Gαₛ, which in turn activates adenylyl cyclase and raises [cAMP]ᵢ. As outlined in Figure 48–3, TSH stimulates a number of steps in the synthesis and release of T₄ and T₃. Inside the pituitary, the type-2 form of 5′/3′-monodeiodinase converts T₄ to T₃, which negatively feeds back on the thyrotrophs as well as on the TRH-secreting neurons. Somatostatin and dopamine—released by hypothalamic neurons—inhibit TSH release and thus can influence the "set point" at which TSH is released in response to a given amount of T₃ in the pituitary. AC, adenylyl cyclase; ATP, adenosine triphosphate; cAMP, cyclic adenosine monophosphate; DAG, diacylglycerol; IP₃, inositol triphosphate; PKC, protein kinase C; PLC, phospholipase C.

GRAVES' DISEASE

Surprisingly, it is not uncommon for B lymphocytes to synthesize immune globulins that bind to and activate the TSH receptor, reproducing all the actions of TSH on the thyroid. Unfortunately, these errant lymphocytes do not regulate the production of these immunoglobulins in a manner analogous to the regulated secretion of TSH by the pituitary. As a result, iodide trapping by the thyroid increases, the synthesis and secretion of both T_3 and T_4 increase, and the thyroid grows in size, producing a goiter. Untreated, the affected individual becomes increasingly hyperthyroid. The clinical manifestations of hyperthyroidism include an increased metabolic rate with associated weight loss, sweating and heat intolerance, a rapid more forceful heartbeat, muscle weakness and wasting, tremulousness, difficulty concentrating, and changes in hair growth and skin texture. Because TSH stimulates all areas of the thyroid, the thyroid is symmetrically enlarged, and even the isthmus is frequently palpable on clinical examination.

The abnormal immunoglobulin is designated TSI for **thyroid stimulating immunoglobulin.** The constellation of symptoms noted previously, together with a symmetrically enlarged **goiter**, is called Graves' disease, after Robert Graves, who provided one of the first detailed descriptions of the disorder in the early 19th century. These antibodies are also able to stimulate connective tissue in the extraocular muscles and in the dermis of the lower extremity to synthesize mucopolysaccharides, leading to thickening of both the muscle and the dermis. Therefore, in addition to the abnormalities of thyroid growth and hyperfunction, a minority of individuals with Graves' disease develop a peculiar infiltrative abnormality in the extraocular muscles. When severe, this "infiltrative ophthalmopathy" impairs muscle function, causing diplopia (double vision) and a forward protrusion of the eyes (**exophthalmos**). Even less frequently, patients with Graves' disease develop an infiltrating dermopathy in the skin over the lower legs, called *pretibial myxedema*. This thickening of the skin occurs in localized patches and is pathologically distinct from the generalized thickening and coarsening of the skin seen in hypothyroidism (*generalized myxedema*).

biologically active eicosanoids (p. 103). In healthy humans, administering TRH also raises plasma [prolactin] by stimulating lactotrophs in the anterior pituitary (p. 1188). However, there is no evidence for a regulatory role for TRH in prolactin secretion or action.

THYROTROPIN. The thyrotrophs represent a relatively small number of cells in the **anterior pituitary**. The TSH that they release is a 28-kDa glycoprotein with α and β chains. The α chain of TSH is identical to that of the other glycoprotein hormones: the gonadotropins luteinizing hormone (LH), follicle-stimulating hormone (FSH), and human chorionic gonadotropin (hCG). The β chain is unique to TSH and confers the specificity of the hormone. Once secreted, TSH acts on the thyroid follicular cell via a specific receptor.

THYROTROPIN RECEPTOR. The TSH receptor on the thyroid follicular cells is a member of the family of G protein–coupled receptors. Like receptors for the other glycoprotein hormones (LH, FSH, and hCG), the TSH receptor activates adenylyl cyclase via $G\alpha_s$ (p. 97). This activation of the TSH receptor stimulates a diverse range of physiological processes or events, summarized in Figure 48–3:

1. Iodide uptake by the **Na/I cotransporter** (NIS) on the basolateral membrane of the thyroid follicular cell. Stimulation of this cotransporter allows for the "trapping" of dietary iodine within the thyroid gland. The ratio of follicular cell iodine to serum iodine (the so-called thyroid/serum or T/S ratio) is 30:1 in euthyroid individuals. The T/S ratio decreases under conditions of low TSH (e.g., hypophysectomy), and increases under conditions of high TSH (e.g., a TSH-secreting pituitary adenoma).
2. **Iodination** of thyroglobulin in the follicular lumen.
3. **Conjugation** of iodinated tyrosines to form T_4 and T_3 linked to thyroglobulin.
4. **Endocytosis** of iodinated thyroglobulin into the follicular cells from thyroid colloid.
5. **Proteolysis** of the iodinated thyroglobulin in the follicular cell.
6. **Secretion** of T_4 and T_3 into the circulation.
7. **Hyperplasia** of the thyroid gland because of the growth-factor effects of TSH.

T_3 Exerts Negative Feedback on Thyrotropin Secretion

Circulating *free* T_4 and T_3 inhibit both the synthesis of TRH by hypothalamic neurons, and the release of TSH by

THYROID STORM

Some patients with hyperthyroidism become extremely ill, and are said to be in *thyroid storm*. These individuals usually have a severe illness superimposed on their hyperthyroidism, and they develop high fevers, a profound tachycardia, sweating, and restlessness. Altered mental status is common. If untreated, these patients can develop severe circulatory collapse, resulting in death. Thyroid storm can be the initial presentation of hyperthyroidism or it can occur in patients already known to be hyperthyroid and treated appropriately. However, when these latter individuals experience the severe stress of a major operation, trauma, or illness, they can develop thyroid storm. This is a true emergency. Treatment consists of giving sodium iodide, which over the long term encourages thyroid hormone synthesis, but acutely blocks the release of already-synthesized thyroid hormones; a β blocker to inhibit the β adrenoceptors, whose expression is increased by the elevated levels of thyroid hormones in the blood; and a drug such as propylthiouracil (PTU), which blocks the manufacture of additional thyroid hormone by inhibiting the iodination and conjugation steps. Fluid replacement and stress doses of corticosteroids are also given to support the circulation.

HYPOTHYROIDISM

*Hypo*thyroidism is one of the most common of all endocrine illnesses—even more common than Graves' disease—affecting between 1% and 2% of all adults at some time in their lives. Women are much more commonly affected than men. Although there are several causes of hypothyroidism, the most common cause worldwide is iodine deficiency. In the United States, by far the most common cause is an autoimmune disorder called *Hashimoto's thyroiditis*. Like Graves' disease, Hashimoto's thyroiditis is caused by an abnormal immune response that includes the production of antithyroid antibodies, in this case, antibodies against the thyroid follicular cells, microsomes, and TSH receptors. Unlike the situation in Graves' disease, the antibodies in Hashimoto's thyroiditis are not stimulatory, but are part of an immune process that blocks and destroys thyroid function. The titers of these autoantibodies can reach colossal proportions.

Typically, hypothyroidism from Hashimoto's thyroiditis is an insidious, slow-developing process; indeed, many patients are diagnosed, long before striking clinical manifestations are apparent, by routine blood work revealing an elevated TSH despite normal levels of T_3 and T_4. These individuals, although not yet clinically hypothyroid, are sometimes treated with thyroid hormone replacement so that the clinical manifestations of hypothyroidism are never given a chance to develop.

In patients in whom the disease does evolve, the classical presentation consists of a painless goiter, skin changes, peripheral edema, constipation, headache, joint aches, fatigue, and, in women, anovulation. The TSH level should be checked in any female with secondary amenorrhea. In time, a subset of these patients also develop other autoimmune disorders, such as pernicious anemia, myasthenia gravis, Addison disease, diabetes mellitus, and ovarian failure.

Like patients with hyperthyroidism, who may be threatened by thyroid storm, those with hypothyroidism also have their severe, life-threatening variant, in this case called **myxedema coma**. This malady is quite rare, and occurs most commonly in elderly patients with established hypothyroidism. Patients slowly evolve hypothermia and coma, and the usual causes are failure to take prescribed thyroid hormone replacement, cold exposure, sepsis, heart failure, and alcohol abuse.

the thyrotrophs in the anterior pituitary. Plasma [TSH] is very sensitive to alteration in the levels of free T_4 and T_3; a 50% decline in free T_4 levels can cause plasma [TSH] to increase 50- to 100-fold. Conversely, as might be expected of a well-functioning feedback system, an excess of thyroid hormone leads to a decrease in plasma [TSH].

At the level of the thyrotroph, the sensor in this feedback system monitors the concentration of T_3 *inside* the thyrotroph (see Fig. 48–9). As noted earlier, either T_3 can enter directly from the blood plasma, or T_3 can form inside the thyrotroph by deiodination of T_4. The negative feedback of T_4 and T_3 on TSH release occurs at the level of the pituitary thyrotroph by both indirect and direct

mechanisms. In the **indirect feedback pathway**, intracellular T_3 decreases the number of TRH receptors on the surface of the thyrotroph. As a result, thyroid hormones *indirectly* inhibit TSH release by reducing the sensitivity of the thyrotrophs to TRH. In the **direct feedback pathway**, intracellular T_3 inhibits the synthesis of both the α and the β chains of TSH. Indeed, both the α and β TSH genes have T_3-response elements in their promoter regions. These response elements, which are *inhibitory*, differ from those found in genes that are *positively* regulated by T_3 (e.g., Na-K pump).

Free T_4 and T_3 concentrations in the plasma, which determine intracellular T_3 levels in the thyrotroph, are relatively constant over the course of 24 hours, reflecting

CLINICAL ASSESSMENT OF THYROID FUNCTION

Plasma thyrotropin levels. Direct measurements of T_4/T_3 provide a measure of *total* circulating hormone (i.e., the sum of *free* T_4 and T_3, as well as T_4 and T_3 *bound* to TBG, TTR, and albumin; p. 1038). However, these direct measurements do not allow one to distinguish between bound and free T_4/T_3. The sensitive response of TSH to changes in thyroid hormone levels provides an extremely valuable tool for assessing whether the free T_4/T_3 levels in the circulation are deficient, sufficient, or excessive. Indeed, the level of TSH reflects the amount of free, biologically active thyroid hormone in the target tissue. As a result, in recent years, measurements of plasma TSH using very sensitive immune assay methods have come to be regarded as the single best measurements of thyroid hormone status. Obviously, this approach is valid only if the thyrotrophs themselves are able to respond to T_3/T_4—that is, if there is no evidence for pituitary dysfunction.

The health of the thyrotrophs themselves can be tested by injecting a bolus of synthetic TRH and monitoring changes in plasma [TSH]. In hypothyroid patients, the subsequent rise in plasma [TSH] is more dramatic than in normal individuals. This test was of great value in confirming the diagnosis of hypothyroidism before the advent of today's sensitive assays, but it has now been largely abandoned.

Radioactive iodine uptake. Measuring the amount of a standard bolus of radioactive iodine that the thyroid can take up was also once widespread as a measure of thyroid function. A hyperactive gland would take up increased amounts of the tracer, whereas an underactive gland would take up subnormal amounts. Today, the test is mostly used for three other purposes. First, radioactive iodine uptake can show whether a solitary thyroid nodule, detected on physical examination, is "hot" (functioning) or "cold" (nonfunctioning). Cold nodules are more likely than hot ones to harbor a malignancy. Second, radioactive iodine uptake can show whether hyperthyroidism is due to thyroid inflammation (i.e., thyroiditis), in which tracer uptake is minimal, or to Graves' disease, in which tracer uptake is increased. Third, high doses of radioactive iodine are commonly used to treat patients with hyperthyroidism.

the long half-lives of both T_4 and T_3 (p. 1039). Given that the levels of T_4 and T_3 are the primary trigger in the afferent limb of the negative feedback for the hypothalamic-pituitary-thyroid axis, the feedback regulation of TSH secretion by thyroid hormones appears to be a slow process—essentially integrating thyroid hormone levels over time. Indeed, T_3 feeds back on the thyrotroph by modulating *gene transcription*, which by its very nature is a slow process.

The feedback of T_4 and T_3 on the release of TSH may also be under the control of somatostatin and dopamine, which travel from the hypothalamus to the thyrotrophs via the portal vessels (see Fig. 48–9). Somatostatin and dopamine both inhibit TSH secretion, apparently by making the thyrotroph more sensitive to inhibition by intracellular T_3—that is, shifting the set point for T_3. Thus, somatostatin and dopamine appear to counterbalance the stimulatory effect of TRH. Although these inhibitory effects are readily demonstrated with pharmacologic infusion of these agents, their physiological role in the regulation of TSH secretion appears small. In particular, with long-term administration of somatostatin or dopamine, compensatory mechanisms appear to override any inhibition.

A special example of feedback between T_3 and TSH is seen in neonates of mothers with abnormal levels of T_3. If the mother is *hyper*thyroid, both she and the fetus will have low TSH levels because T_3 crosses the placenta. After birth, the newborn rapidly metabolizes its T_3, but its TSH remains suppressed, so that the infant temporarily becomes *hypo*thyroid. Conversely, if the mother's thyroid gland has been removed and she is *hypo*thyroid because she is not receiving sufficient thyroid hormone replacement therapy, both she and the fetus will have high levels of circulating TSH. Immediately after birth, the newborn will be temporarily *hyper*thyroid.

REFERENCES

Books and Reviews

Brent GA, Moore DD, Larsen PR: Thyroid hormone regulation of gene expression. Annu Rev Physiol 53:17–35, 1991.

Cavalieri RR: Iodine metabolism and thyroid physiology: Current concepts. Thyroid 7:177–181, 1997.

Dumont JE, Lamy F, Roger P, Maenhaut C: Physiological and pathological regulation of thyroid cell proliferation and differentiation by thyrotropin and other factors. Physiol Rev 72:667–697, 1992.

Gershengorn MC, Osman R: Molecular and cellular biology of thyrotropin-releasing hormone receptors. Physiol Rev 76:175–191, 1996.

Larsen PR: Update on the human iodothyronine selenodeiodinases, the enzymes regulating the activation and inactivation of thyroid hormone. Biochem Soc Trans 25:588–592, 1997.

Orban Z, Bornstein SR, Chrousos GP: The interaction between leptin and the hypothalamic-pituitary-thyroid axis. Horm Metab Res 30:231–235, 1998.

Samuels HH, Forman BM, Horowitz ZD, Ye Z-S: Regulation of gene expression by thyroid hormone. Annu Rev Physiol 51:623–639, 1989.

Journal Articles

Arvan P, Kim PS, Kuliawat R, et al: Intracellular protein transport to the thyrocyte plasma membrane: Potential implications for thyroid physiology. Thyroid 7:89–105, 1997.

Dai G, Levy O, Carrasco N: Cloning and characterization of the thyroid iodide transporter. Nature 379:458–460, 1996.

Koenig RJ: Thyroid hormone receptor coactivators and corepressors. Thyroid 8:703–713, 1998.

CHAPTER 49

The Adrenal Gland

Eugene J. Barrett

The human adrenal glands, each weighing only about 4 g, are located above the upper pole of each kidney in the retroperitoneal space. They produce four principal hormones: cortisol, aldosterone, epinephrine (adrenaline), and norepinephrine. Each adrenal is composed of an inner medulla and an outer cortex (Fig. 49–1). Embryologically, the cortex is derived from mesoderm, whereas the medulla is derived from neural crest cells (p. 264) that migrate into the developing cortex. The cortex produces two principal steroid hormones, cortisol and aldosterone, as well as several androgenic steroids. The medulla produces epinephrine and norepinephrine.

The **adrenal cortex** can be further divided into three cellular layers: the *glomerulosa* layer near the surface, the *fasciculata* layer in the midcortex, and the *reticularis* layer near the cortical-medullary junction. **Aldosterone**, the main mineralocorticoid in humans, is made in the glomerulosa cell layer. **Cortisol**, the principal glucocorticoid, is made in the fasciculata and reticularis layers. Although both cortisol and aldosterone are made by enzymatic modification of cholesterol and are structurally quite similar, their actions on the body differ dramatically. Cortisol is considered a **glucocorticoid** because it was recognized early on to increase plasma glucose levels; deficiency of cortisol can result in hypoglycemia. Aldosterone is considered a **mineralocorticoid** because it promotes salt and water retention by the kidney. The activities of these two hormones overlap, particularly at high hormone levels, but this distinction is still very useful in identifying their most obvious functions. The adrenal cortex also synthesizes and secretes **androgenic steroids**, which to a large extent appear to be byproducts of cortisol production.

In the **adrenal medulla**, chromaffin cells produce **epinephrine** or adrenaline, a catecholamine that is synthesized from the amino acid tyrosine. Although the primary product of the medulla is epinephrine, it also produces variable amounts of the epinephrine precursor **norepinephrine**. These catecholamines are distinct from the steroid hormones both structurally and functionally.

THE ADRENAL CORTEX: CORTISOL

Cortisol Is the Primary Glucocorticoid Hormone in Humans

Steroid hormones are divided into three major classes based on their actions: glucocorticoids, mineralocorticoids, and sex steroids. **Cortisol** is

FIGURE 49–1. Anatomy of the adrenal gland. An adrenal gland sits upon each kidney. The adrenal gland is actually two glands—the cortex and the medulla. The **adrenal cortex** comprises three layers that surround the medulla. The outermost layer contains the glomerulosa cells that secrete aldosterone, and the two inner layers of cortex (fasciculata and reticularis) synthesize cortisol and sex steroids. The blood supply enters the cortex in the subcapsular region and flows through anastomotic capillary beds while coursing through both the cortex and the medulla. The **adrenal medulla** contains chromaffin cells that secrete epinephrine and a small amount of norepinephrine.

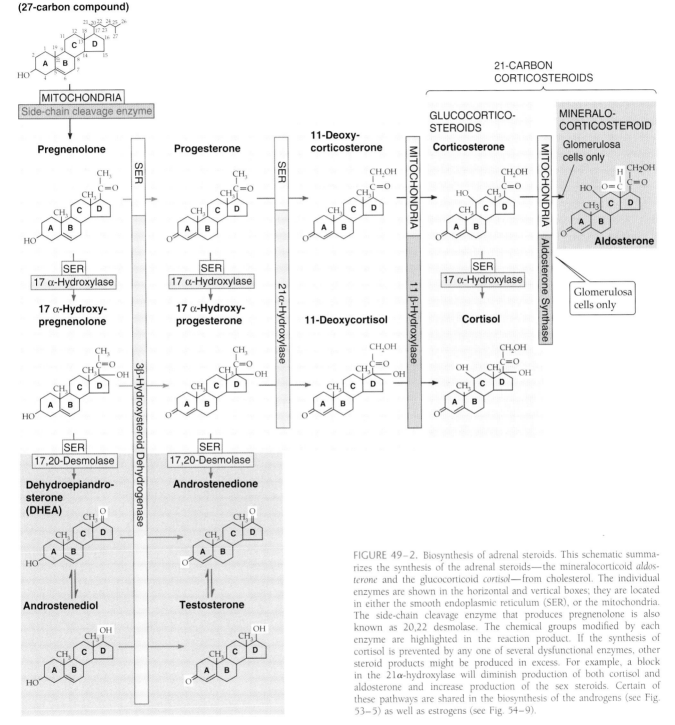

FIGURE 49–2. Biosynthesis of adrenal steroids. This schematic summarizes the synthesis of the adrenal steroids—the mineralocorticoid *aldosterone* and the glucocorticoid *cortisol*—from cholesterol. The individual enzymes are shown in the horizontal and vertical boxes; they are located in either the smooth endoplasmic reticulum (SER), or the mitochondria. The side-chain cleavage enzyme that produces pregnenolone is also known as 20,22 desmolase. The chemical groups modified by each enzyme are highlighted in the reaction product. If the synthesis of cortisol is prevented by any one of several dysfunctional enzymes, other steroid products might be produced in excess. For example, a block in the 21α-hydroxylase will diminish production of both cortisol and aldosterone and increase production of the sex steroids. Certain of these pathways are shared in the biosynthesis of the androgens (see Fig. 53–5) as well as estrogens (see Fig. 54–9).

the prototypic, naturally occurring glucocorticoid. The ability of cortisol to increase plasma [glucose] largely results from its ability to enhance mobilization of amino acids from proteins in many tissues and to enhance the ability of the liver to convert these amino acids into glucose and glycogen by activating gluconeogenesis.

Only a small difference can be seen in the structures of cortisol and aldosterone (Fig. 49–2): aldosterone lacks the -OH group at position 17 but has an aldehyde (aldo) group at position 18. Despite the seemingly minor chemical difference, aldosterone at physiologic concentrations has virtually no glucocorticoid activity.

TABLE 49–1

RELATIVE POTENCY OF GLUCOCORTICOID AND MINERALOCORTICOID ANALOGS		
COMPOUND	**GLUCO-CORTICOID EFFECT**	**MINERALO-CORTICOID EFFECT**
Cortisol	1	1
Prednisone	3–4	0.5
Methylprednisone	10	0.5
Dexamethasone	20	1
Fludrocortisone	12	125

Relative potency is determined by a combined consideration of the compound's biologic half-life and its affinity for the glucocorticoid or mineralocorticoid receptor.

TABLE 49–2

CYTOCHROME P-450 ENZYMES INVOLVED IN STEROIDOGENESIS*		
ENZYME	**SYNONYM**	**GENE**
Cholesterol side chain cleavage	$P\text{-}450_{SSC}$	*CYP11A1*
11β-Hydroxylase	$P\text{-}450_{c11}$	*CYP11B1*
17α-Hydroxylase	$P\text{-}450_{c17}$	*CYP17*
17,20-Desmolase	$P\text{-}450_{c17}$	*CYP17*
21α-Hydroxylase	$P\text{-}450_{c21}$	*CYP21A2*
Aldosterone synthase	$P\text{-}450_{aldo}$	*CYP11B2*
Aromatase	$P\text{-}450_{arom}$	*CYP19*

* $P\text{-}450_{arom}$ catalyzes a reaction essential for the production of estrogens (see Chapter 54).

TARGET TISSUES. Although classified as a "glucocorticoid," cortisol affects more than the principal glucose regulatory tissues, namely, the liver, fat, and muscle. Most body tissues, including bone, skin, other viscera, hematopoietic and lymphoid tissue, and the central nervous system (CNS), are target sites for glucocorticoid action. Although cortisol is the primary glucocorticoid in humans, in other species (e.g., the rat), corticosterone is the major glucocorticoid.

ACTIONS. Glucocorticoids have numerous actions other than their ability to raise plasma glucose levels. These actions are described later but include potent immunosuppressive and anti-inflammatory activity, effects on protein and fat metabolism, behavioral effects on the CNS, and important effects on calcium and bone metabolism. The multiple actions of glucocorticoids, in particular, their "anti-inflammatory" action on leukocytes, has led to the development of numerous synthetic analogs that are more potent, have a longer half-life, and are more selective in their specific glucocorticoid actions than are either cortisol or corticosterone. Table 49–1 lists some of these compounds and indicates their relative potency as mineralocorticoids and glucocorticoids.

The Fasciculata and Reticularis Layers of the Adrenal Cortex Synthesize Cortisol from Cholesterol

Synthesis of cortisol, as with all steroid hormones, starts with cholesterol (see Fig. 49–2). Like other cells producing steroid hormones, the adrenal gland has two sources of cholesterol (p. 1017): (1) it can import cholesterol from circulating cholesterol-containing low-density lipoprotein (LDL cholesterol) by means of LDL receptor–mediated endocytosis (p. 44), or (2) it can synthesize cholesterol de novo from acetate (see Fig. 45–16). Although both pathways provide the steroid nucleus needed for cortisol and aldosterone synthesis, circulating LDL is quantitatively more important.

In the adrenal, cholesterol is metabolized through a series of five reactions to make either cortisol or aldosterone. Except for 3β-hydroxysteroid dehydrogenase (3β-

HSD), the enzymes responsible belong to the family of cytochrome P-450 oxidases (Table 49–2) and are located within the cells in either the mitochondria or the smooth endoplasmic reticulum (SER).

1. The pathway for cortisol and aldosterone synthesis begins in the mitochondria, where the cytochrome P-450 side-chain-cleavage (SCC) enzyme (also called 20,22-desmolase or $P\text{-}450_{SSC}$) removes the long side chain (carbons 22 to 27) from the carbon at position 20 of the **cholesterol** molecule (27 carbon atoms). This enzyme, or the supply of substrate to it, appears to be the rate-limiting step for the overall process of steroid hormone synthesis.
2. The product of the SCC-catalyzed reaction is **pregnenolone** (21 carbon atoms), which exits the mitochondrion. The SER enzyme 3β-HSD (*not* a P-450 enzyme) oxidizes the hydroxyl group at position 3 of the A-ring to a ketone to form **progesterone**.
3. A P-450 enzyme in the SER, 17α-hydroxylase ($P\text{-}450_{c17}$), then adds a hydroxyl group at position 17 to form **17α-hydroxyprogesterone**. However, as shown in Figure 49–2, an alternative path to 17α-hydroxyprogesterone may be used: the 17α-hydroxylase might first add a hydroxyl group at position 17 of *pregnenolone* and form **17α-hydroxypregnenolone**, which can then be converted to 17α-hydroxyprogesterone by the aforementioned 3β-HSD.
4. In the SER, 21α-hydroxylase ($P\text{-}450_{c21}$) adds a hydroxyl at carbon 21 to produce **11-deoxycortisol**.
5. In the mitochondria, 11β-hydroxylase ($P\text{-}450_{c11}$) adds yet another hydroxyl, this time at position 11, to produce **cortisol**.

The enzymes represented by the *vertical bars* in Figure 49–2, as well as SCC, are present in all three cellular layers of the adrenal cortex. However, 17α-hydroxylase is not substantially present in the glomerulosa layer. Thus, only the fasciculata and reticularis layers can synthesize cortisol.

The cells of the fasciculata and reticularis layers of the adrenal cortex can synthesize androgens. These cells convert 17α-hydroxypregnenolone and 17α-hydroxyproges-terone into the "adrenal androgens" **dehydroepiandros-terone** and **androstenedione**. The enzyme that catalyzes this reaction is called 17,20-desmolase; however, it turns out to be the same SER enzyme as the 17α-hydroxylase that produced the 17α-hydroxypregnenolone and 17α-hydroxyprogesterone in the first place. The androgens formed by the adrenal are far less potent than either testosterone or dihydrotestosterone. However, peripheral tissue can use 17-ketosteroid reductase to convert andro-stenedione to testosterone (p. 1130). In this manner, the adrenal can contribute significant amounts of circulating androgen.

The cortisol synthesized by the adrenal cortex diffuses out of the cells and into the blood plasma. There, ap-proximately 90% of the cortisol is transported bound to **corticosteroid-binding globulin** (CBG), also known as transcortin, which is made in the liver. Transcortin is a 383–amino acid glycoprotein whose affinity for cortisol is about 30-fold higher than for aldosterone. An additional, approximately 7% of the circulating cortisol is bound to albumin. Thus, only 3% to 4% of the circulating cortisol is free.

21α-HYDROXYLASE DEFICIENCY

Mutations can affect one or more of the enzyme steps in steroid-hormone synthesis and produce unique clini-cal syndromes that are a direct result of failure to manufacture a particular hormone, accumulation of excessive amounts of precursor steroids, or both. The most common of these enzymatic disorders is 21α-hydroxylase deficiency. From Figure 49–2 we would predict that deficiency of this enzyme would lead to inadequate production of both glucocorticoid and mineralocorticoid hormones, which is indeed what oc-curs; affected infants are ill with symptoms of "salt losing" (hypotension, dehydration) and glucocorticoid deficiency (hypoglycemia). The natural reaction of the body is to attempt to overcome this deficiency by increasing the secretion of pituitary adrenocortico-tropic hormone (ACTH), which stimulates the synthesis of cortisol and aldosterone. ACTH also causes growth of the adrenal gland. However, if the mutant enzyme is totally inactive, no cortisol or aldosterone synthesis will occur. However, all other enzymes of the pathway involved in glucocorticoid and mineralocorticoid syn-thesis will be expressed in increased amounts. The re-sult is greater than normal activity of the side-chain-cleavage enzyme (SCC), 3β-hydroxysteroid dehydrogenase, 17α-hydroxylase, and 11β-hydroxy-lase, and the net effect is increased synthesis of both precursor molecules and adrenal androgens. The com-bination of inadequate production of glucocorticoids and mineralocorticoids, excessive production of andro-gens, and enhanced growth of the adrenal gland is the classic clinical syndrome of salt-losing, virilizing congenital adrenal hyperplasia. In the female, the presence of excessive adrenal androgen *in utero* results in ambiguous genitalia at birth, which should alert the pediatrician to the potential diagnosis.

Cortisol Binds to a Cytoplasmic Receptor That Translocates to the Nucleus and Modulates Transcription in Multiple Tissues

The multiple hydroxylation reactions that convert choles-terol to cortisol result in a hydrophilic compound that, unlike cholesterol, is soluble in plasma, yet lipophilic enough to cross the plasma membrane of target tissue without requiring a membrane transporter. Cortisol, like all steroid hormones, binds to intracellular receptors within target cells (p. 112). Virtually all nucleated tissues in the body contain receptors for glucocorticoids. The glucocorticoid receptor (GR) is primarily located in the cytoplasm, where in its unbound form it is complexed to a chaperone protein (i.e., the heat shock protein hsp90, among others; see Fig. 5–13A). Binding of cortisol causes the chaperone to dissociate from the GR and thus allows the cortisol-GR complex to translocate to the nucleus. There, the cortisol-receptor complex associates with **glu-cocorticoid response elements** (GREs) on the 5′ untrans-lated region of multiple genes to either enhance or dimin-ish gene expression (p. 132).

Glucocorticoid receptors are structurally similar to the receptors for mineralocorticoids, sex steroids, vitamin D, vitamin A, and thyroid hormone (p. 112). These recep-tors, either homodimers or heterodimers, belong to the superfamily of nuclear receptors that contains domains A through F (p. 113). The middle, or C, region is responsi-ble for DNA binding via two "zinc fingers" (p. 126), whereas the E region, located toward the C terminus, binds cortisol. Activity of the glucocorticoid-receptor complex requires dimerization of two identical receptor complexes (i.e., the GR functions as a *homodimer*) at the near-palindromic nucleotide site of the GRE on the chro-matin. Virtually all actions of glucocorticoids are ex-pressed via modulation of gene transcription. A possible exception to this rule is the acute feedback effect of corti-sol to block the release of preformed adrenocorticotropic hormone (ACTH) in the secretory granules of pituitary corticotrophs. This glucocorticoid effect is demonstrable within seconds to minutes and may relate to an as yet undefined effect of glucocorticoid on membrane traf-ficking.

Although glucocorticoids are named for their ability to increase hepatic glucose and glycogen synthesis, they af-fect many somatic tissues. In **liver**, cortisol induces the synthesis of enzymes that are involved in the metabolism of amino acids, thus facilitating their conversion to carbo-hydrates via gluconeogenesis. In **muscle**, cortisol stimu-lates the breakdown of muscle protein, thus providing amino acid substrate to the circulation and subsequently to the liver. Likewise, cortisol induces mobilization of fat from subcutaneous **adipose tissue**. Fatty acids supplied to the circulation afford an alternative fuel to glucose and increase the availability of glucose. Curiously, for un-known reasons, although fat is mobilized from the ex-tremities, some is also deposited centrally (see "moon facies" in the box titled Therapy with Glucocorticoids).

Cortisol has other actions that are not clearly related to its "glucocorticoid" action, including effects on the **im-mune system**, among which is an acute action to pro-mote neutrophil release from the bone marrow into the systemic circulation. In humans, cortisol also diminishes

THERAPY WITH GLUCOCORTICOIDS

The variety of glucocorticoid actions on body tissue is well illustrated by considering some of the clinically observed effects of hypercortisolism in patients receiving glucocorticoid drugs. Most strikingly, the entire body habitus changes. Body fat is centripetally distributed from the extremities to the face and trunk. This change is apparent on the trunk by an increase in supraclavicular and dorsal interscapular fat. It also causes a rounding of the face called the **"moon facies,"** which is a result of increasing subcutaneous fat in the cheeks and submandibular region. Conversely, the wasting of fat (and some supporting tissues) in the extremities produces thinning of the skin and fragility of cutaneous blood vessels. Direct effects of glucocorticoids on bone, as well as their inhibition of intestinal Ca^{2+} absorption, produce osteopenia, which can be manifested as osteoporosis, frequently with pathologic fractures. The interference with normal immune function increases both the frequency and severity of infections. Rare malignancies can develop. Wasting of muscle tissue results in a generalized weakness that is usually most prominent in the proximal muscles of the lower extremities. Finally, as would be expected from a glucocorticoid, patients are glucose intolerant. After an oral glucose challenge (p. 1070), blood glucose levels rise higher than normal because glucocorticoid antagonizes the action of insulin. Not infrequently, frank diabetes develops (see box on p. 1084). When cortisol is overproduced endogenously (from tumors producing either ACTH or cortisol), hypertension is common. The hypertension most likely results from the weak mineralocorticoid action of cortisol. Exogenous synthetic glucocorticoid therapy rarely produces hypertension because most of these drugs lack the mineralocorticoid activity of the endogenous hormone.

the circulating lymphocyte count, partly as a result of sequestration of lymphocytes in the reticuloendothelial system (spleen, thymus, and bone marrow). At high concentrations, glucocorticoids cause the lysis of lymphocytes in some species. Glucocorticoids also act on the cellular elements of trabecular bone (p. 1088) in that they decrease the ability of osteoblasts to synthesize new bone. They also interfere with absorption of Ca^{2+} from the gastrointestinal tract. In addition, glucocorticoids act on the CNS and can cause a variety of effects, including alterations in mood and cognition.

Corticotropin-Releasing Hormone from the Hypothalamus Stimulates the Corticotrophs of the Anterior Pituitary to Secrete ACTH, Which in Turn Stimulates the Adrenal Cortex to Synthesize and Secrete Cortisol

As summarized in Figure 49–3, synthesis and secretion of cortisol are stimulated by ACTH, also called corticotropin, which is released by the anterior pituitary. In turn, the release of ACTH is stimulated by corticotropin-releasing hormone (CRH), which is made in the hypothalamus.

Circulating cortisol exerts negative feedback control on the release of both ACTH and CRH.

CRH. CRH is a 41–amino-acid neuropeptide made by small-bodied neurons in the paraventricular nucleus of the **hypothalamus** (p. 1010). The structure of CRH is highly conserved among species. In humans, in addition to the hypothalamus, CRH is present in several tissues, including the pancreas and the testes, and throughout the CNS, where it serves as a neurotransmitter. The hypothalamic neurons synthesize and release CRH via the classic secretory pathway (p. 36). Neurons store CRH in secretory vesicles located in synaptic terminals in the median eminence of the hypothalamus and can release CRH acutely in the absence of new synthesis. After release into the interstitial fluid of the median eminence, CRH enters the hypophysial portal venous plexus and travels to the anterior pituitary.

CRH RECEPTOR. CRH arriving in the anterior pituitary binds to a G-protein–coupled receptor on the cell membrane of corticotroph cells. Hormone binding activates $G\alpha_s$, which in turn stimulates adenylyl cyclase and raises intracellular cyclic adenosine monophosphate levels $[cAMP]_i$ (p. 97). Subsequent stimulation of protein kinase A (PKA) activates L-type Ca^{2+} channels and thus leads to an increase in $[Ca^{2+}]_i$. This rise in $[Ca^{2+}]_i$ rapidly leads to the exocytosis of preformed ACTH. Over a much longer time frame, CRH receptor activation also leads to increased gene transcription and synthesis of the ACTH precursor (discussed later).

ARGININE VASOPRESSIN. Although CRH is the major regulator of ACTH secretion, the paraventricular nuclei also make another hormone, arginine vasopressin (AVP; see p. 1013). AVP is also a potent ACTH secretagogue. Vasopressin probably plays a physiological role in the regulation of ACTH secretion in various stress states.

ACTH. ACTH is a 39–amino-acid peptide hormone secreted by the corticotroph cells of the anterior pituitary. ACTH can also be produced by ectopic sources, particularly by small-cell carcinomas of the lung. Pituitary corti-

---

FIGURE 49–3. The hypothalamic-pituitary-adrenocortical axis. Small-bodied neurons in the paraventricular nucleus of the hypothalamus secrete corticotropin-releasing hormone (CRH), a 41–amino acid peptide that reaches the corticotrophs in the anterior pituitary via the long portal veins. CRH binds to a G protein-coupled receptor on the corticotroph membrane, triggering the adenylyl cyclase/cAMP/PKA pathway. The activation of L-type Ca^{2+} channels leads to an increase in $[Ca^{2+}]_i$ that rapidly leads to the release of preformed ACTH. CRH also increases gene transcription and synthesis of the ACTH precursor, POMC. After its release by corticotrophs, ACTH binds to **melanocortin-2 receptors** on the cell membranes in all three layers of the adrenal cortex. This receptor triggers the adenylyl cyclase/cAMP/PKA pathway, rapidly enhancing the conversion of cholesterol to pregnenolone and more slowly increasing the synthesis of several proteins that are needed for cortisol synthesis. The cerebral cortex can stimulate the hypothalamic neurons to increase their secretion of CRH. Cortisol exerts negative feedback at the level of both the pituitary and hypothalamus. In addition, ACTH produced by the corticotrophs negatively feeds back on the hypothalamic neurons in a "short loop." AC, adenylyl cyclase; ACTH, adrenocorticotropic hormone; cAMP, cyclic adenosine monophosphate; PKA, protein kinase A, POMC, pro-opiomelanocortin.

CEREBRAL CORTEX

STRESS

HYPOTHALAMUS

Diurnal rhythms

Physical

Emotional

Biochemical

Paraventricular nucleus

Small-bodied neurons in the hypothalamus synthesize and secrete corticotropin-releasing hormone (CRH).

Hypothalamus

Long portal vessels carry CRH to the anterior pituitary.

Short feedback (ACTH)

Anterior lobe of pituitary

Corticotrophs

CRH

CRH receptor

Corticotroph

ACTH

G protein

AC

ATP

cAMP

Ca²⁺

PKA

Ca²⁺

ACTH

Long feedback (cortisol)

Adrenal medulla

Adrenal cortex cell

ACTH

Melanocortin-2 receptor

G protein

AC

ATP

cAMP

PKA

↑Activity of P450$_{SCC}$

↑Synthesis of several enzymes

FIGURE 49–4. Processing of POMC. The primary gene transcript is a pre-pro-hormone called *pro-opiomelanocortin* (POMC). The processing of POMC yields a variety of peptide hormones. This processing is different in the anterior and intermediate lobes of the pituitary. In the anterior pituitary, POMC yields a long N-terminal peptide, a joining (J) peptide, ACTH, and β-LPH. In the intermediate pituitary, the same POMC yields a short N-terminal peptide, γ-MSH, J peptide, α-MSH, corticotropin-like intermediate-lobe peptide (CLIP), γ-LPH and β-END. Metabolism by the intermediate lobe is only important during fetal life and pregnancy. ACTH, adrenocorticotropic hormone; LPH, lipotropic pituitary hormone; MSH, melanocyte-stimulating hormone. (Data from Wilson JD et al: Williams Textbook of Endocrinology. Philadelphia, WB Saunders, 1998.)

cotrophs synthesize ACTH by complex post-translational processing of a large precursor protein (i.e., a preprohormone) called **pro-opiomelanocortin** (POMC). POMC is the precursor not only for ACTH but also for a variety of peptide hormones (Fig. 49–4). In the anterior pituitary, POMC yields a long N-terminal peptide, a joining (J) peptide, ACTH, and **β-lipotropin** (β-LPH). During fetal life and pregnancy, the intermediate pituitary lobe—a small wedge of tissue between the more familiar anterior and posterior lobes—processes the same POMC in a very different manner to yield a different array of peptides: a short N-terminal peptide, **γ-melanocyte–stimulating hormone** (γ-MSH), J peptide, α-MSH, corticotropin-like intermediate-lobe peptide (CLIP), γ-LPH, and β-endorphin.

α-MSH and γ-MSH act on melanocytes to increase the dispersion of pigment granules. In some patients who greatly overproduce ACTH, hyperpigmentation is a prominent clinical finding. Whether this hyperpigmentation is due to increased production of MSH, to increased production of β-LPH (which also has MSH activity), or to the melanotropic action of ACTH per se remains uncertain. β-LPH and γ-LPH mobilize lipids from adipocytes in animals, although their physiologic role in humans is unclear. **β-Endorphin** has potent opioid actions in the CNS (p. 304), but its physiologic actions (if any) in the systemic circulation are not known.

ACTH RECEPTOR. In the adrenal cortex, ACTH binds to the **melanocortin-2 receptor** on the plasma membranes of all three steroid-secreting cell types. However, because only the cells in the fasciculata and reticularis layers have the 17α-hydroxylase needed for synthesizing cortisol (see Fig. 49–2), these cells are the only ones that secrete cortisol in response to ACTH. ACTH appears to have few other actions at physiologic concentrations. The melanocortin-2 receptor is coupled to a heterotrimeric G protein and stimulates adenylyl cyclase (p. 97). The resulting increase in [cAMP]$_i$ activates PKA, which phosphorylates a

variety of proteins. A rapid effect of ACTH is to stimulate the rate-limiting step in cortisol formation, that is, the conversion of cholesterol to pregnenolone via the SCC enzyme. In addition, ACTH—over a longer time frame—increases the synthesis of several proteins needed for cortisol synthesis: (1) each of the P-450 enzymes involved in cortisol synthesis (see Fig. 49–2), (2) the LDL receptor required for the uptake of cholesterol from blood (p. 44), and (3) the 3-hydroxy-3-methylglutaryl-coenzyme A (HMG-CoA) reductase that is the rate-limiting enzyme for cholesterol synthesis by the adrenal (p. 998).

Thus, ACTH promotes the acute synthesis of cortisol—and as discussed later, aldosterone to a lesser extent—by the adrenal and increases the content of adrenal enzymes involved in steroidogenesis. In the absence of pituitary ACTH, the fasciculata and reticularis layers of the adrenal cortex atrophy. The glomerulosa layer does not atrophy under these conditions because in addition to ACTH, angiotensin II (ANG II) and high levels of K$^+$ are trophic factors that act on the glomerulosa layer. The atrophy of the fasciculata and reticularis layers occurs routinely in people treated with glucocorticoid drugs and leaves the person with an iatrogenic form of adrenal insufficiency when use of the drug is abruptly discontinued. Conversely, chronic stimulation of the adrenal by ACTH, such as can occur with pituitary tumors (Cushing disease) or with the simple physiological ACTH excess that can occur with chronic stress, can increase the weight of the adrenals several-fold.

Cortisol Exerts Negative Feedback on CRH and ACTH Secretion, Whereas Stress Acts Through Higher CNS Centers to Stimulate the Axis

Cortisol exerts negative feedback control on the very axis that stimulates its secretion (see Fig. 49–3), doing so at the level of both the anterior pituitary and hypothalamus.

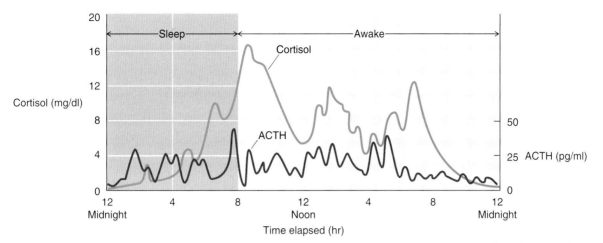

FIGURE 49–5. Rhythm of ACTH and cortisol. The corticotrophs release ACTH in a circadian rhythm, greater in the early morning hours and less late in the afternoon and early evening. Superimposed on the circadian rhythm is the effect on the corticotrophs of the pulsatile secretion of CRH by the hypothalamus. Thus, ACTH levels exhibit both circadian and pulsatile behavior. Notice that, although both ACTH and cortisol are secreted episodically, the duration of the ACTH bursts is briefer, reflecting the shorter half-life of ACTH in plasma. ACTH, adrenocorticotropic hormone; CRH, corticotropin-releasing hormone. (Data from Wilson JD et al: Williams Textbook of Endocrinology. Philadelphia, WB Saunders, 1998.)

FEEDBACK TO THE ANTERIOR PITUITARY. In the corticotrophs of the anterior pituitary, cortisol acts by binding to a cytosolic receptor, which then moves to the nucleus where it binds to GREs and modulates gene expression, thus inhibiting the synthesis of both the CRH receptor and ACTH. Even though, as seen earlier, the POMC gene yields multiple secretory products, it is *cortisol* that is the main regulator of the transcription of POMC. In addition, elevated levels of cortisol in plasma inhibit the release of presynthesized ACTH stored in vesicles.

FEEDBACK TO THE HYPOTHALAMUS. The negative feedback of cortisol on the CRH-secreting neurons of the hypothalamus is less important than that on the corticotrophs discussed earlier. Plasma cortisol decreases the mRNA and peptide levels of CRH in paraventricular hypothalamic neurons. Cortisol also inhibits the release of presynthesized CRH. Synthetic glucocorticoids have a similar action.

CONTROL BY A HIGHER CNS CENTER. CRH-secreting neurons in the hypothalamus are under higher CNS control, as illustrated by two important features of the hypothalamic-pituitary-adrenocortical axis: (1) the circadian and pulsatile nature of ACTH and cortisol secretion and (2) integration of signals from higher cortical centers that modulate the body's responses to a variety of "stressors."

The pituitary secretes ACTH with a **circadian rhythm**. The suprachiasmatic nucleus of the hypothalamus, which lies above the optic chiasm and receives input from the retina, controls the circadian rhythms of the body. Indeed, blind people loose their circadian rhythms. Input from hypothalamic nuclei to the corticotrophs—via both CRH and ADH—appears to modulate the circadian secretion of ACTH and thus the circadian secretion of cortisol as well. As is the case for other hypothalamic releasing hormones, CRH is released in pulses. As a result, superimposed on the circadian rhythm of ACTH is a **pulsatile secretion** of ACTH, as shown in Figure 49–5. The greatest ACTH secretory activity occurs in the early morning hours and diminishes late in the afternoon and early evening. The mechanism by which hypothalamic neurons generate "pulses" of secretory activity is not understood.

Other evidence of higher CNS control is the enhanced CRH secretion—and thus the enhanced ACTH secretion—that occurs in response to physical, psychological, and biochemical stress. An example of biochemical stress is hypoglycemia, which stimulates the secretion of both CRH and ACTH and thus leads to an increased release of cortisol that tends to raise blood glucose levels.

The increase in ACTH secretion that occurs nocturnally and with stress appears to be the result of an increased amplitude of the secretory CRH burst rather than an increased frequency of secretion episodes. Because the half-life of cortisol is much longer than that of ACTH, the period of the pulsatile changes in cortisol is longer and the magnitude of the excursions is damped in comparison to those of ACTH.

THE ADRENAL CORTEX: ALDOSTERONE

The mineralocorticoid **aldosterone** is the primary regulator of salt balance and extracellular volume. Aldosterone determines extracellular volume by controlling the extent to which the kidney excretes or reabsorbs the Na^+ filtered at the renal glomerulus. Sodium in the extracellular space retains water—it is the primary osmotically active particle in the extracellular space—and thus the amount of Na^+ that is present determines the volume of extracellular fluid (p. 80). The extracellular volume is itself a prime determinant of arterial blood pressure (p. 555), and therefore aldosterone plays an important role in the maintenance of blood pressure.

The effects of aldosterone on salt balance determine the extracellular volume and should not be confused with the effects of AVP (also known as antidiuretic hormone or ADH). AVP regulates the *free water* balance of the body (p. 871). Water freely passes across cell membranes and thus affects the *concentration* of Na^+ and other solutes throughout the body (p. 81). Unlike aldosterone, AVP makes only a small contribution to the maintenance of extracellular volume; instead, AVP regulates serum osmolality and hence the Na^+ concentration. Thus, to a first approximation, one can think of aldosterone as the primary regulator of extracellular volume because of its effect on renal Na^+ reabsorption, and think of AVP as the primary regulator of plasma osmolality because of its effect on free water balance.

The Glomerulosa Cells of the Adrenal Cortex Synthesize Aldosterone from Cholesterol, via Progesterone

As is the case for cortisol, the adrenal cortex synthesizes aldosterone from cholesterol by using P-450 enzymes in a series of five steps. The initial steps in the synthesis of aldosterone from cholesterol follow the same synthetic pathway that cortisol-secreting cells use to generate **progesterone** (Fig. 49–2). Because glomerulosa cells are the only ones that contain aldosterone synthase, these cells are the exclusive site of aldosterone synthesis.

1. The cytochrome P-450 **side-chain-cleavage (SCC) enzyme** (P-450$_{SSC}$) produces pregnenolone from cholesterol. This enzyme—or the supply of substrate to it—appears to be the rate-limiting step for the overall process of steroid hormone synthesis.
2. The SER enzyme 3β-HSD, which is *not* a P-450 enzyme, oxidizes pregnenolone to form **progesterone**.
3. Because *glomerulosa* cells have minimal 17α-hydroxylase (P-450$_{c17}$), they do not convert progesterone to 17α-hydroxyprogesterone. Instead, glomerulosa cells use a 21α-hydroxylase (P-450$_{c21}$) in the SER to further hydroxylate the progesterone at position 21 and produce **11-deoxycorticosterone** (DOC).
4. In the mitochondria, 11β-hydroxylase (P-450$_{c11}$) adds an -OH at position 11 to produce **corticosterone**. This pair of hydroxylations in steps 3 and 4 are catalyzed by the same two enzymes that produce cortisol from 17α-hydroxyprogesterone.
5. The glomerulosa cells—but *not* the fasciculata and reticularis cells—also have aldosterone synthase (P-450$_{aldo}$), which first adds an −OH group to the methyl at position 18 and then oxidizes this hydroxyl to an *aldehyde* group, hence the name *aldosterone*. This mitochondrial P-450 enzyme, also called 18-methyloxidase, is an isoform of the same 11β-hydroxylase (P-450$_{c11}$) that catalyzes the DOC-to-corticosterone step. In fact, aldosterone synthase can catalyze all three steps between DOC and aldosterone: 11β-hydroxylation, 18-methyl hydroxylation, and 18-methyl oxidation.

Like cortisol, no storage pool of presynthesized aldosterone is available in the glomerulosa cell for rapid secretion. Thus, secretion of aldosterone by the adrenal is limited by the rate at which the glomerulosa cells can synthesize the hormone. Although ACTH also stimulates the production of aldosterone in the glomerulosa cell, increases in extracellular [K^+] and the peptide hormone ANG II are physiologically more important secretagogues.

These secretagogues enhance secretion by increasing the activity of enzymes acting at rate-limiting steps in aldosterone synthesis. These enzymes include the SCC enzyme, which is common to all steroid-producing cells, and aldosterone synthase, which is unique to glomerulosa cells and is responsible for formation of the C-18 aldehyde.

Once secreted, about 37% of circulating aldosterone remains free in plasma. The rest weakly binds to CBG (~ 21%) and albumin (~ 42%).

Aldosterone Stimulates Na^+ Reabsorption and K^+ Excretion by the Renal Tubule

The major action of aldosterone is to stimulate the kidney to reabsorb Na^+ and water and enhance K^+ secretion. Aldosterone has similar actions on salt and water transport in the colon, salivary glands, and sweat glands. Mineralocorticoid receptors are also present in the myocardium, liver, brain, and other tissues, but the physiological role of mineralocorticoids in these latter tissues is unclear.

Aldosterone, like cortisol and all the other steroid hormones (p. 132), acts by modulating gene transcription. In the kidney, aldosterone binds to both low- and high-affinity receptors. The low-affinity receptor appears to be identical to the **glucocorticoid receptor**. The high-affinity receptor is a distinct **mineralocorticoid receptor** (MR); it has homology to the GR, particularly in the "zinc-finger" region involved in DNA binding. Surprisingly, MR in the kidney has a similar affinity for aldosterone and cortisol. Because cortisol normally circulates at much higher concentrations than does aldosterone (5 to 20 μg/dl versus 2 to 8 ng/dl), the biologic effect of aldosterone on any potential target would be expected to be greatly overshadowed by that of cortisol. (Conversely, aldosterone has essentially no significant glucocorticoid action because aldosterone binds only weakly to its low-affinity receptor—that is, the GR.)

How then do the renal tubule cells avoid sensing cortisol as a *mineralocorticoid*? The cells that are targets for aldosterone, particularly the distal convoluted tubule and the initial cortical collecting duct of the kidney, contain an enzyme, **11β-hydroxysteroid dehydrogenase**, that converts cortisol to cortisone, which has a very low affinity for the mineralocorticoid receptor (see Fig. 34–13B). As a result, locally within the target cell, the cortisol/aldosterone ratio is much smaller than the cortisol dominance seen in plasma. In other words, 11β-HSD is so effective at removing cortisol from the cytosol of aldosterone target tissues that cortisol behaves as only a weak mineralocorticoid despite the high affinity of cortisol for the so-called mineralocorticoid receptor. In this fashion the overall tissue specificity for mineralocorticoid action is conferred on aldosterone.

In the target cells of the renal tubule, aldosterone increases the activity of several key proteins involved in Na^+ transport (p. 786). It increases transcription of the Na-K pump, thus increasing distal Na^+ reabsorption. Aldosterone also increases the expression of apical Na^+ channels and an Na/K/Cl cotransporter. The net effect of these actions is to increase Na^+ reabsorption and K^+ secretion. The enhanced K^+ secretion (p. 823) appears to

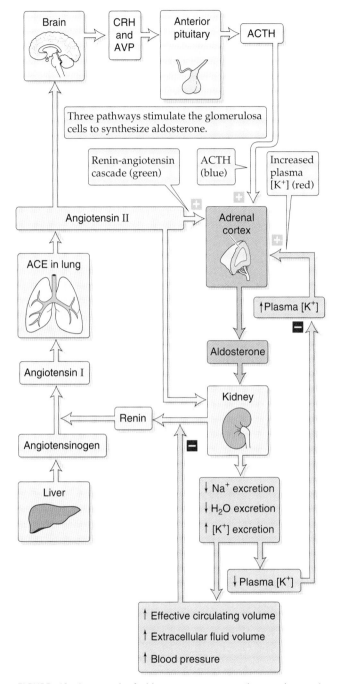

FIGURE 49-6. Control of aldosterone secretion. Three pathways (*in three different colors*) stimulate the glomerulosa cells of the adrenal cortex to secrete aldosterone. ACE, angiotensin-converting enzyme; ACTH, adrenocorticotropin hormone; AVP, arginine vasopressin; CRH, corticotropin-releasing hormone.

ing life-threatening hyperkalemia and, in the absence of other compensatory mechanisms, hypotension. Conversely, excess aldosterone secretion produces hypokalemia and hypertension.

Hyperaldosteronism is a rare cause of hypertension. Primary aldosteronism can result from either an isolated adrenal adenoma or bilateral adrenal hyperplasia; even more rarely, an adrenal carcinoma can produce excess aldosterone.

Renin-Angiotensin, Potassium, and ACTH All Stimulate Aldosterone Secretion

There are three secretagogues for the aldosterone synthesized in the glomerulosa cells of the adrenal cortex. The most important is ANG II, which is a product of the renin-angiotensin cascade. An increase in plasma [K$^+$] is also a powerful stimulus for aldosterone secretion. Third, just as ACTH promotes cortisol secretion, it also promotes the secretion of aldosterone, although this effect is weak.

RENIN-ANGIOTENSIN. We introduced the renin-angiotensin-aldosterone axis when we considered control of extracellular fluid volume on page 866. The liver synthesizes and secretes a very large protein called **angiotensinogen**, which is an α_2-globulin (Fig. 49-6). **Renin**, which is synthesized by the granular cells (or juxtaglomerular cells) of the juxtaglomerular apparatus (JGA) in the kidney (p. 743), is the enzyme that cleaves this angiotensinogen to form **angiotensin I**, a decapeptide. Finally, angiotensin-converting enzyme (ACE) cleaves the ANG I to form the octapeptide **angiotensin II**. ACE is present in both the vascular endothelium of the lung ($\sim$40%) and elsewhere ($\sim$60%). In addition to its role as a potent secretagogue for aldosterone, ANG II exerts powerful vasoconstrictor actions on vascular smooth muscle (p. 555). ANG II has a short half-life (<1 minute) because plasma aminopeptidases further cleave it to the heptapeptide ANG III.

On the plasma membrane of the glomerulosa cell, ANG II binds to the **AT$_1$ receptor** (type I ANG II receptor), which couples through the $G\alpha_q$-mediated pathway to phospholipase C (PLC). Stimulation of PLC leads to the formation of diacylglycerol (DAG) and inositol 1,4,5-triphosphate (IP$_3$; p. 100). DAG activates protein kinase C (PKC). IP$_3$ triggers the release of Ca^{2+} from intracellular stores, thus causing a rise in [Ca^{2+}]$_i$, which activates Ca^{2+}-dependent enzymes such as PKC and Ca^{2+}-calmodulin–dependent protein kinases. These changes lead to depolarization of the glomerulosa cell's plasma membrane, opening of voltage-activated Ca^{2+} channels, and a *sustained* increase in Ca^{2+} influx from the extracellular space. This rise in [Ca^{2+}]$_i$ is primarily responsible for triggering the synthesis (i.e., secretion) of aldosterone. Aldosterone secretion increases because the rise in [Ca^{2+}]$_i$ facilitates the production of pregnenolone either by directly increasing the activity of SCC or by increasing the delivery of cholesterol to the SCC enzyme in the mitochondria (see Fig. 49-2). In addition, increased [Ca^{2+}]$_i$ also stimulates aldosterone synthase and in this manner enhances the conversion of corticosterone to aldosterone.

occur as a secondary effect to the enhanced Na$^+$ reabsorption. However, the stoichiometry between Na$^+$ reabsorption and K$^+$ secretion in the distal tubule is not fixed.

Aldosterone regulates only that small fraction of renal Na$^+$ reabsorption that occurs in the distal tubule and collecting duct. Although most Na$^+$ reabsorption occurs in the proximal tubule by aldosterone-independent mechanisms, loss of aldosterone-mediated Na$^+$ reabsorption can result in significant electrolyte abnormalities, includhyperkalemia affect the cAMP pathway that is triggered by ACTH.

Aldosterone Exerts Indirect Negative Feedback on the Renin-Angiotensin Axis by Increasing Effective Circulating Volume and by Lowering Plasma [K$^+$]

The feedback regulation exerted by aldosterone is indirect and occurs through its effects of both increasing salt retention (i.e., extracellular volume) and decreasing [K$^+$]$_o$.

RENIN-ANGIOTENSIN AXIS. We have already seen in Chapter 39 that a decrease in effective circulating volume stimulates the granular cells of the JGA of the kidney to increase their synthesis and release of renin, which increases the generation of ANG II and, therefore, aldosterone (see Fig. 49–6). The **juxtaglomerular apparatus** is located at the glomerular pole of the nephron, between the afferent and efferent arterioles, where the early distal tubule comes in close proximity with its own glomerulus (Fig. 49–7). Histologically, the JGA comprises specialized epithelial cells of the distal tubule called macula-densa

---

TREATING HYPERTENSION BY ATTACKING THE RENIN-ANGIOTENSIN-ALDOSTERONE AXIS

Because the renin-angiotensin-aldosterone axis plays an important role in maintaining extracellular volume and arterial pressure, pharmacologists have sought for ways to disrupt this system to treat hypertension. Several agents acting on different parts of the axis are available. **Spironolactone** is a diuretic that directly antagonizes the effects of aldosterone on the renal tubule. It is a weak diuretic, but it is particularly useful in treating patients with ascites. For patients with hypertension or congestive heart failure, it is usually added to one of the more common thiazide diuretics (p. 779) to prevent K$^+$ wasting.

Inhibitors of angiotensin-converting enzyme (ACE) have been available for a number of years and are among the safest and best-tolerated of all antihypertensive medications. The first to be marketed in the United States was captopril, but many others, with longer half-lives that allow once-a-day dosing, are now available. These drugs also improve the quality of life and survival of patients with heart failure. More recently, drugs have been developed that specifically block the AT$_1$ receptor. These drugs offer a good alternative for those patients who cannot tolerate ACE inhibitors, usually because of a chronic cough, their most common side effect.

POTASSIUM. An increase in extracellular K$^+$ ([K$^+$]$_o$) has a more direct action on the glomerulosa cell (see Fig. 49–6). High [K$^+$]$_o$ depolarizes the plasma membrane and opens voltage-gated Ca^{2+} channels. The result is an influx of Ca^{2+} and a rise in [Ca^{2+}]$_i$ that stimulates the same two steps as ANG II—production of pregnenolone from cholesterol and conversion of corticosterone to aldosterone. Unlike the situation for ANG II, the [Ca^{2+}]$_i$ increase induced by high [K$^+$]$_o$ does not require activation of PLC or release of Ca^{2+} from the intracellular stores. Because increased [K$^+$]$_o$ and ANG II both act by raising [Ca^{2+}]$_i$, they act synergistically on the glomerulosa cell.

ACTH. ACTH has only a minor effect on aldosterone secretion by glomerulosa cells (Fig. 49–6). ACTH regulates aldosterone secretion by a pathway that is distinct from that of ANG II or high [K$^+$]$_o$. As noted earlier for the fasciculata and reticularis cells, the melanocortin-2 receptor in the glomerulosa cell is coupled via a heterotrimeric G protein to adenylyl cyclase. Increases in ACTH raise [cAMP]$_i$ and activate PKA, which phosphorylates a large number of cytosolic proteins. At some as yet undefined level, these changes stimulate Ca^{2+} influx across the plasma membrane and enhance the synthesis and secretion of aldosterone. ACTH also enhances mineralocorticoid activity by a second mechanism: stimulation of the fasciculata cells to secrete cortisol, corticosterone, and DOC, all of which have weak mineralocorticoid activity. The hypertension that is seen in individuals who oversecrete ACTH appears to be mediated by the excess synthesis of these weak mineralocorticoids. Neither ANG II nor

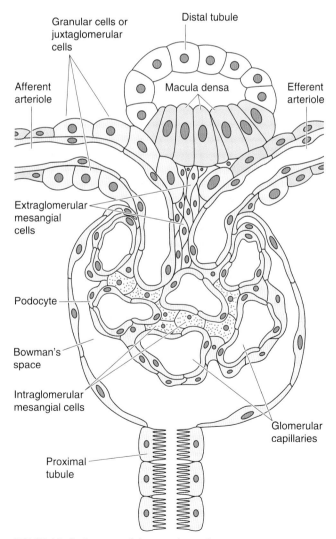

FIGURE 49–7. Structure of the juxtaglomerular apparatus.

cells, as well as specialized smooth-muscle cells of the *afferent* arteriole, which are called granular cells or juxtaglomerular cells. Macula densa cells and granular cells communicate by means of an extracellular matrix.

Decreases in effective circulating volume—or the associated decreases in systemic arterial pressure—stimulate renin release from the JGA in two ways (p. 866): first, decreased systemic arterial blood pressure stimulates the baroreceptor reflex, which triggers medullary control centers to increase sympathetic outflow to the JGA. The result of both α- and β-adrenergic stimulation is enhanced renin secretion. Second, "renal" baroreceptors in the afferent arteriole—possibly the **granular cells** themselves—respond to a fall in pressure of the afferent arteriole (i.e., decreased stretch in the arteriolar wall) by increasing the secretion of renin. Thus, both mechanisms enhance renin release and lead to increased levels of ANG II and aldosterone. ANG II negatively feeds back on renin release by directly inhibiting renin release by the kidney (short-loop feedback). ANG II also negatively feeds back on renin release by acutely increasing blood pressure (p. 555), which reduces the stimuli to the aforementioned two baroreceptor pathways. Finally, aldosterone negatively feeds back on renin release more slowly by enhancing renal Na^+ reabsorption (p. 786) and thus increasing effective circulating blood volume and blood pressure. Therefore, ANG II and aldosterone complete the regulatory feedback circuit that governs the secretion of aldosterone.

POTASSIUM. High plasma $[K^+]$ stimulates the glomerulosa cell in the adrenal cortex to synthesize and release aldosterone, which in turn stimulates the principal cells of the renal collecting duct to reabsorb more Na^+ and excrete more K^+ (see Fig. 49–6). This excretion of K^+ causes plasma $[K^+]$ to fall toward normal. As a result, stimulation of glomerulosa cells declines, aldosterone secretion falls, and the negative feedback loop is completed. This sequence of events (i.e., hyperkalemia $\rightarrow$ aldosterone secretion $\rightarrow$ K^+ excretion) probably plays a vital role in preventing wide swings in plasma $[K^+]$ in response to episodic dietary intake of large K^+ loads.

ROLE OF ALDOSTERONE IN NORMAL PHYSIOLOGY. What then is the role of aldosterone in normal physiology? Presumably, the salt- and water-retaining properties of aldosterone are of greatest value in meeting the environmental stresses that are associated with limited availability of salt, water, or both. Such conditions are not prevalent in most Western societies, but they still exist in many developing countries and were probably universal in previous periods of human evolutionary history. In healthy, normotensive humans, blockade of aldosterone generation with ACE-inhibiting drugs reduces ANG II production and markedly decreases plasma aldosterone, but causes only slight decreases in total-body Na^+ and blood pressure. Redundant mechanisms for maintaining blood pressure probably prevent a larger blood-pressure decrease. The reason for the mild effect on Na^+ balance is probably an adaptive increase in salt intake; indeed, patients with adrenal cortical insufficiency frequently crave dietary salt. In contrast to the minor effects of low aldosterone on blood pressure and *sodium* balance in normal people, the

effects of blocking aldosterone production can be catastrophic for *potassium* balance; low aldosterone can result in life-threatening hyperkalemia.

ROLE OF ALDOSTERONE IN DISEASE. Aldosterone does play important roles in several pathologic conditions. For example, in many patients with *hyper*tension, ACE inhibitors are effective in reducing blood pressure, thus implying that their renin-angiotensin-aldosterone axis was overactive. In *hypo*tension, as occurs with hemorrhage or dehydration, aldosterone secretion increases, thus increasing effective circulating volume and blood pressure.

Aldosterone secretion also increases in congestive heart failure. However, the increased salt retention in this setting is inappropriate because it results in worsening edema formation. In this case, the increase in circulating aldosterone occurs *despite* a pre-existing volume overload. The problem in congestive heart failure is that the JGA does not perceive the very real volume overload as an increase in *effective* circulating volume. Indeed, the reduced cardiac output in heart failure diminishes renal glomerular filtration, partly because of decreased arterial blood pressure and partly because of enhanced sympathetic nervous system activity, which constricts the afferent arterioles of the kidney. As a result, the kidney inappropriately assumes that the extracellular volume is decreased and stimulates the renin-angiotensin-aldosterone system.

Spontaneous increases in aldosterone synthesis can occur with tumors of the glomerulosa cell, a disorder called hyperaldosteronism or Conn syndrome. Hypertension and hypokalemia frequently develop in these patients. As would be expected from feedback regulation of the renin-angiotensin-aldosterone system, the plasma renin concentration is characteristically suppressed in this form of hypertension.

THE ADRENAL MEDULLA

The Adrenal Medulla Bridges the Endocrine and Sympathetic Nervous Systems

In Chapter 46 we described cells of the hypothalamus as "neuroendocrine" because they are part of the CNS and appear anatomically as neural tissue, yet they release peptide hormones (e.g., CRH) into the blood that act downstream on the pituitary—a classic endocrine function. The adrenal medulla is similar in many ways. The cells of the medulla, termed **chromaffin cells** because the catecholamines that they contain stain avidly with chromium, derive from neural crest cells (p. 264) and migrate into the center of the adrenal cortex, which is derived from the mesoderm. The adrenomedullary cells synthesize and secrete epinephrine and—to a lesser extent—norepinephrine; the latter is the neurotransmitter of the sympathetic division of the autonomic nervous system (p. 387). Both the norepinephrine and epinephrine made in the adrenal medulla enter the circulation and act on distal tissues just like other hormones.

Chromaffin cells are the structural and functional equivalents of the **postganglionic** neurons in the sympa-

A   CATECHOLAMINE SYNTHESIS

B   DEGRADATIVE METABOLISM OF CATECHOLAMINES

FIGURE 49–8. Synthesis and degradation of catecholamines. In A, the horizontal arrows indicate enhancement of the reaction. COMT, catecholamine-O-methyltransferase; MAO, monoamine oxidase.

thetic nervous system (p. 388). The preganglionic sympathetic fibers of the splanchnic nerves, which release acetylcholine (ACh), are the principal regulators of adrenomedullary hormone secretion.

The vascular supply to the adrenal medulla is also unusual. The medulla receives vascular input from vessels that begin in a subcapsular plexus of the adrenal cortex. The vessels then branch into a capillary network in the cortex only to merge into small venous vessels that branch into a second capillary network within the medulla. This **portal blood supply** (originating at the entrance to the adrenal) exposes the adrenal medulla to the highest concentrations of glucocorticoids and mineralocorticoids of all somatic tissues.

Chromaffin Cells of the Adrenal Medulla Are the Only Ones That Have the Enzyme for Synthesizing Epinephrine

It was first appreciated nearly a century ago that extracts of the adrenal medulla have a powerful pressor effect. Subsequent work showed that the **catecholamines**—dopa, dopamine, norepinephrine, and epinephrine—are all made in the adrenal medulla. **Norepinephrine** is found in many other somatic tissues in amounts that roughly parallel the extent of sympathetic innervation of the tissue. In other words, the norepinephrine in these other tissues is not made there but is derived from the sympathetic nerve endings in them. **Epinephrine**, the principal product of the adrenal medulla, is made *only* in the adrenal medulla.

Dopamine, norepinephrine, and epinephrine are all synthesized from the amino acid tyrosine. Figure 49–8A summarizes the reactions involved in the synthesis of epinephrine. Figure 49–9 illustrates the cellular localization of the four enzymatic reactions, as well as the three critical transport steps that shuttle the reactants and products to their proper location:

1. The activity of the first enzyme in the pathway, **tyrosine hydroxylase**, which converts tyrosine to L-dopa, is rate limiting for overall synthesis. This enzyme is located within the *cytosol* of adrenal medullary cells, as well as in sympathetic nerve terminals and in specific cells within the CNS.
2. The *cytosolic* enzyme **amino acid decarboxylase** converts L-dopa to dopamine in a number of tissues, including the adrenal medulla.
3. A catecholamine-H+ exchanger (VMAT1) moves the dopamine into membrane-enclosed dense-core vesicles called **chromaffin granules**.
4. **Dopamine β-hydroxylase** converts dopamine to norepinephrine by hydroxylating the β carbon. This β-hydroxylase is localized to the inner surface of the membrane of granules within the adrenal medulla and sympathetic nerves. In the nerve terminals of postganglionic sympathetic neurons, the synthetic pathway terminates at this step, and the granules store the norepinephrine for later secretion. However, the cells of the adrenal medulla convert the norepinephrine to epinephrine in three final steps.

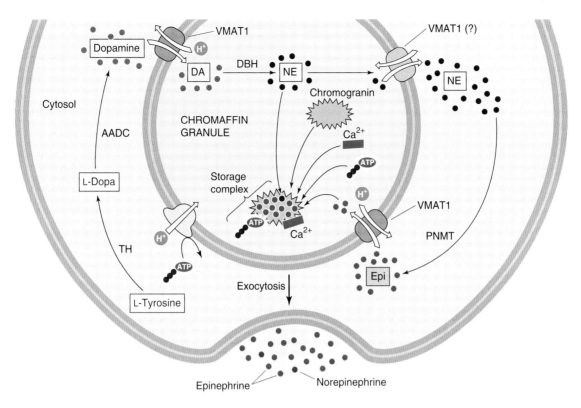

FIGURE 49–9. Cellular view of catecholamine synthesis. The chromaffin cell synthesizes and stores epinephrine in a sequence of four enzymatic and three transport steps. AADC, amino acid decarboxylase; DA, dopamine; DBH, dopamine beta-hydroxylase; Epi, epinephrine; NE, norepinephrine; PNMT, phenylethanolamine-N-methyltransferase; TH, tyrosine hydroxylase; VMAT, vesicular monoamine transporter.

5. Norepinephrine formed in the secretory granules moves out into the cytosol.

6. The cytosolic enzyme **phenylethanolamine-N-methyl-transferase** (PNMT) transfers a methyl group from S-adenosylmethionine to norepinephrine, thus creating epinephrine. This enzyme is present only in the cytosol and only in the adrenal medulla.

7. The secretory granules in the adrenal medulla take up the newly synthesized epinephrine. The same VMAT1 catecholamine-H^+ exchanger noted in step 3 appears to mediate this uptake of epinephrine. The proton gradient is maintained by an H^+ pump (i.e., a vacuolar-type H-adenosinetriphosphatase) within the secretory vesicle membrane (p. 64). Thus, in the adrenal medulla, the secretory granules store both epinephrine and norepinephrine before secretion.

Epinephrine synthesis is under control of the CRH-ACTH-cortisol axis at two levels. First, ACTH stimulates the synthesis of dopa and norepinephrine. Second, cortisol transported from the adrenal cortex by the portal circulation to the medulla upregulates PNMT in chromaffin cells. The result is synergy between the CRH-ACTH-cortisol axis and the sympathetic-epinephrine axis. Thus, the stress that is sensed and propagated by the CRH-ACTH-cortisol axis sustains the epinephrine response.

Similar to the secretory granules that are present in the postganglionic sympathetic neurons, the secretory granules of the adrenal medulla contain very high concentrations of catecholamines (up to 0.5 M). These catechol-amines—along with adenosine triphosphate (ATP) and Ca^{2+}—bind to granular proteins called **chromogranins** and thus are not osmotically active in these storage vesicles. Chromogranins are what make "dense-core vesicles" dense. In humans, the dominant chromogranin is chromogranin B. The release of catecholamines is initiated by CNS control. ACh released from preganglionic neurons in the splanchnic nerves acts on nicotinic ACh receptors to depolarize the postganglionic chromaffin cells. This depolarization triggers the opening of voltage-gated Ca^{2+} channels, which raises $[Ca^{2+}]_i$ and triggers the exocytotic release of epinephrine. The secretion of adrenal catecholamines is accompanied by the release of ATP and the granule proteins. The release of chromogranin A has been used as a marker of adrenal medullary activity. In the circulation, the catecholamines dissociate from the binding complex and are free to act on target tissues.

The early description of the "fight-or-flight" response to stress (p. 392) exemplifies the central control of adrenomedullary function. An organism faced with a severe external threat responds with centrally driven release of adrenal hormones, as well as activation of other aspects of the sympathetic division. This response includes increases in heart rate and contractility, mobilization of fuel stores from muscle and fat, piloerection, pupillary dilatation, and increased sphincter tone of the bowel and bladder. Each response is in some way adapted to successfully deal with the perceived threat. This combined neuroendocrine response is activated within seconds. The secreted catecholamines act very quickly after reaching their target tissues.

The biologic actions of catecholamines are very brief, lasting only about 10 seconds in the case of epinephrine. Circulating catecholamines are degraded first by the enzyme **catecholamine-*O*-methyltransferase** (COMT), which is present in high concentrations in endothelial cells and the heart, liver, and kidneys (see Fig. 49–8*B*). COMT converts epinephrine to metanephrine, as well as norepinephrine to normetanephrine. A second enzyme, **monoamine oxidase,** converts these metabolites to vanillylmandelic acid (VMA). The liver and also the gut then conjugate these compounds to sulfate or glucuronide (p. 987) to form derivatives that the kidney excretes in the urine. Measurement of the concentration of catecholamines, metanephrines, and VMA in the urine provides a measure of the total adrenal catecholamine production by both the adrenal medulla and the sympathetic system.

Catecholamines Bind to α and β Adrenoceptors on the Cell Surface and Act Through Heterotrimeric G Proteins

Many of the hormones that we have disccussed have a unique receptor on the cell surface (e.g., insulin, parathyroid hormone, growth hormone, thyroid-stimulating hormone) or within the cell (e.g., thyroid hormones or cortisol). Other hormones (e.g., AVP) and neurotransmitters (e.g., ACh and glutamate) may bind to more than one type of receptor, each acting via a different signal-transduction process. The situation for the catecholamines is even more complex. Epinephrine and norepinephrine can each bind to more than one type of adrenergic receptor or **adrenoceptor.** Conversely, individual adrenoceptors can generally bind both epinephrine and norepinephrine—albeit with different affinities.

About a half century ago, investigators found that epinephrine can stimulate both vasodilatory and vasoconstrictor responses in the same vascular bed, depending on the epinephrine concentration. This property, together with the observation that certain drugs could selectively block one or the other of these effects, led to the designation of "α" and "β" adrenergic receptors. This dichotomy proved to be too simple when it was observed that the actions of some drugs that have pure α or pure β activity could be blocked in some tissues but not in others; this variability in response suggested that the tissue response is determined by a *subtype* of α or β receptor.

It is now clear that there are at least three types of β and two types of α receptors (Table 49–3), as well as subtypes within these major classes. These receptors differ in primary structure and in the types of G proteins that associate with the receptor. The several β receptors are coupled to stimulatory heterotrimeric G proteins ($G\alpha_s$) that *stimulate* adenylyl cyclase and thus increase levels of cAMP (p. 97), the principal intracellular mediator of β activation. The α_2 adrenoceptors are coupled to other G proteins ($G\alpha_i$) that *inhibit* adenylyl cyclase and thus lower $[cAMP]_i$ in target tissues. The α_1 receptors are coupled to yet another heterotrimeric G protein ($G\alpha_q$) that either activates PLC or, in some cases, appears to directly alter the activity of a plasma membrane ion channel (p. 100). The net effect of α_1 stimulation is to increase the concentration of IP_3 and $[Ca^{2+}]_i$ in target tissues.

TABLE 49–3

ADRENOCEPTOR TYPES			
RECEPTOR TYPE	G PROTEIN	LINKED ENZYME	SECOND MESSENGER
α_1	$G\alpha_q$	PLC	$\uparrow$ IP_3 and Ca^{2+} DAG
α_2	$G\alpha_i$	Adenylyl cyclase	$\downarrow$ $[cAMP]_i$
β_1	$G\alpha_s$	Adenylyl cyclase	$\uparrow$ $[cAMP]_i$
β_2	$G\alpha_s$	Adenylyl cyclase	$\uparrow$ $[cAMP]_i$
β_3	$G\alpha_s$	Adenylyl cyclase	$\uparrow$ $[cAMP]_i$

cAMP, cyclic adenosine monophosphate; DAG, diacylglycerol; IP_3, inositol 1,4,5-triphosphate; PLC, phospholipase C.

The diversity of adrenoceptor subtypes has led to a panoply of pharmacologic agents that block or stimulate one or the other of these receptor subtypes. Some are nonspecific and affect several receptor subtypes; others specifically block only a single subtype. The clinical value of a particular drug depends on its spectrum of activity. Thus, for example, an agent that selectively blocks the vasoconstrictor response to norepinephrine could be a very useful antihypertensive agent, but its utility would be compromised if it also blocked the ability of bladder smooth muscle to contract.

The CNS-Epinephrine Axis Provides Integrated Control of Multiple Functions

The actions of the autonomic nervous system (see Chapter 15) in the control of blood pressure (p. 540), heart rate (p. 547), sweating (p. 1237), micturition (p. 755), and airway resistance (p. 624) are discussed in more detail in other chapters, as indicated. Here, we will mention only some of the unique actions that are attributed to adrenal catecholamine release that integrate several bodily functions as part of the stress response are mentioned. These adrenal-mediated activities do not occur in isolation but are usually accompanied by generalized noradrenergic sympathetic discharge.

In response to the stress of simple **exercise** (see Chapters 24 and 59), blood flow to muscle is increased; circulating epinephrine appears to be important in this response. Circulating epinephrine also relaxes bronchial smooth muscle to meet the demand for increased ventilation and, when combined with the increased blood flow, increases oxygen delivery to the exercising muscle. Similarly, to sustain muscular activity, particularly early in exercise, epinephrine acting via the β adrenoceptor activates the degradation of muscle glycogen to provide a ready fuel source for the contracting muscle (p. 98). Epinephrine also activates lipolysis in adipose tissue to furnish free fatty acids for more sustained muscular activity if needed. In liver, as in muscle, epinephrine activates glycogenolysis, thus maintaining the supply of glucose in the blood.

In addition to enhancing blood flow and ventilation,

PHEOCHROMOCYTOMA

The dramatic biologic effects of catecholamines are well illustrated by patients with pheochromocytoma. A **pheochromocytoma** is a relatively uncommon tumor caused by hyperplasia of either adrenal medullary tissue or extra-adrenal chromaffin tissue that failed to involute after birth. They can be benign or malignant. These tumors make catecholamines, just like the normal medulla, except in an unregulated fashion. Patients with pheochromocytomas typically have a plethora of symptoms, as might be expected from such a wide-ranging hormonal system. Paroxysmal (sudden outburst) hypertension, tachycardia, headache, episodes of sweating, anxiousness, tremor, and glucose intolerance usually dominate the clinical findings. The key to the diagnosis of this disorder is a careful history, evidence on physical examination of excessive adrenergic tone, and laboratory detection of increased amounts of urinary catecholamines and their metabolites. When chemical evaluation of the urinary metabolites confirms the presence of a pheochromocytoma, it is often possible to localize the tumor to one or the other adrenal gland and resect the tumor. Rarely, both glands will be affected and necessitate bilateral adrenalectomy. Such patients must subsequently receive glucocorticoid and mineralocorticoid replacement. Interestingly, no therapy is routinely given to replace the adrenal *medullary* function. It is not clear whether these individuals react less well to external stimuli that might trigger the fight-or-flight response.

the integrated response to exercise increases fuel availability by decreasing insulin levels. Interestingly, circulating epinephrine, acting through a β adrenoceptor, *stimulates* the secretion of insulin (p. 1071). However, during exercise, local autonomic innervation, acting by means of an α adrenoceptor of the pancreas, *inhibits* this effect so that insulin levels fall. The net effect is to promote glycogenolysis and allow muscle to increase its work while maintaining glycemia so that brain function is not impaired. The fleeing human must not only run, but know *where* to run!

Unlike other glandular tissue, no endocrine feedback loop governs the secretion of adrenal medullary hormones. Control of catecholamine secretion resides within the CNS. This principle can be illustrated by the changes in epinephrine secretion that occur with even mild **hypoglycemia**. Decreases in blood glucose below about 3.5 mM (normally, ~ 5.5 mM) are sensed by the CNS, which triggers a central sympathetic response that increases the firing of preganglionic fibers in the celiac plexus. This sympathetic outflow suppresses endogenous insulin secretion by the α-adrenergic mechanism noted earlier, thus promoting an increase in plasma [glucose]. This sympathetic outflow to the adrenal medulla also triggers a major release of epinephrine that, through β adrenoreceptors in the liver, stimulates increased hepatic glycogenolysis. This response helps restore plasma [glucose] to normal. Restoration of normoglycemia diminishes central sympathetic outflow.

REFERENCES

Books and Reviews

Autelitano DJ, Lundblad JR, Blum M, Roberts JL: Hormonal regulation of POMC gene expression. Annu Rev Physiol 51:715–726, 1989.

Burnstein KL, Cidlowski JA: Regulation of gene expression by glucocorticoids. Annu Rev Physiol 51:683–699, 1989.

Fitzsimons JT: Angiotensin, thirst, and sodium appetite. Physiol Rev 78: 583–686, 1998.

Funder JW: Glucocorticoid and mineralocorticoid receptors: Biology and clinical relevance. Annu Rev Med 48:231–240, 1997.

Young JB, Landsberg L: Catecholamines and the adrenal medulla. In Wilson JD, Foster DW, Kronenberg HM, Larsen PR (eds): Williams Textbook of Endocrinology, 9th ed. Philadelphia, WB Saunders, 1998, pp 665–728.

Journal Articles

Fevold HR: Regulation of the adrenal cortex secretory pattern by adrenocorticotropin. Science 156:1753–1755, 1967.

Gordon RD: Primary aldosteronism. J Endocrinol Invest 18:495–511, 1995.

Smith GW, Aubry JM, Dellu F, et al: Corticotropin releasing factor receptor 1–deficient mice display decreased anxiety, impaired stress response, and aberrant neuroendocrine development. Neuron 20: 1093–1102, 1998.

Turnbull AV, Rivier C: Corticotropin-releasing factor (CRF) and endocrine responses to stress: CRF receptors, binding protein, and related peptides. Proc Soc Exp Biol Med 215:1–10, 1997.

Weitzman ED, Fukushima D, Nogeire C, et al: Twenty-four hour pattern of the episodic secretion of cortisol in normal subjects. J Clin Endocrinol Metab 33:14–22, 1971.

CHAPTER 50

The Endocrine Pancreas

Eugene J. Barrett

The Islets of Langerhans Are Endocrine and Paracrine Tissues

The pancreas contains two types of glands: (1) exocrine glands, which secrete digestive enzymes and HCO_3^- into the intestinal lumen (see Chapter 42), and (2) endocrine glands, called the "islets of Langerhans."

The normal human pancreas contains between 500,000 and several million islets. Islets can be oval or spherical and measure between 50 and 300 μm in diameter. Islets contain at least four types of secretory cells—α cells, β cells, δ cells, and F cells—plus various vascular and neural elements (Fig. 50–1 and Table 50–1). **β cells** secrete insulin, proinsulin, C peptide, and a newly described protein, amylin. β cells are the most numerous type of secretory cell within the islets; they are located throughout the islet but are particularly numerous in the center. **α Cells** principally secrete glucagon, **δ cells** secrete somatostatin, and **F cells** (also called pancreatic polypeptide cells) secrete pancreatic polypeptide.

The cells within an islet receive information from the world outside the islet. These cells also can communicate with each other and influence each other's secretion. We can group these communication links into three categories:

1. **Humoral communication**. The blood supply of the islet courses outward from the center of the islet toward the periphery, carrying glucose and other secretagogues. In the rat—and less strikingly in humans—β cells are more abundant in the center of the islet, whereas α and δ cells are more abundant in the periphery. Cells within a given islet can influence the secretion of other cells as the blood supply courses outward through the islet carrying the secreted hormonal product of each cell type with it. For example, glucagon is a potent insulin secretagogue, insulin modestly inhibits glucagon release, and somatostatin potently inhibits the secretion of both insulin and glucagon (as well as the secretion of growth hormone and other nonislet hormones).
2. **Cell-cell communication**. Both gap and tight junctional structures connect islet cells with one another. Cells within an islet can communicate via gap junctions, which may be important for the regulation of both insulin and glucagon secretion.
3. **Neural communication**. Another level of regulation of islet secretion occurs via innervation from both the sympathetic and the parasympathetic divisions of the autonomic nervous system (ANS). Cholinergic

1066

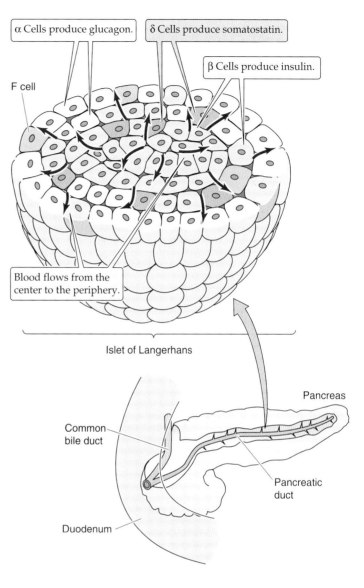

α Cells produce glucagon.

δ Cells produce somatostatin.

β Cells produce insulin.

F cell

Blood flows from the center to the periphery.

Islet of Langerhans

Pancreas

Common bile duct

Pancreatic duct

Duodenum

FIGURE 50–1. Islet of Langerhans.

stimulation augments insulin secretion. Adrenergic stimulation can have either a stimulatory or inhibitory effect, depending on whether β-adrenergic (stimulatory) or α-adrenergic (inhibitory) stimulation dominates (p. 1065).

These three communication mechanisms allow for a tight control over the synthesis and secretion of islet hormones.

INSULIN

The discovery of insulin was among the most exciting and dramatic events in the history of endocrine physiology and therapy. In the United States and Europe, insulin-dependent diabetes mellitus (IDDM), or type 1 diabetes, develops in about 1 in every 600 children in their lifetime. However, the prevalence is only about 1 in 10,000 in eastern Asia. Before 1922, all children with diabetes died within 1 or 2 years of diagnosis. It was an agonizing illness; the children lost weight despite eating well, became progressively weaker and cachectic, were

soon plagued by infections, and eventually died of overwhelming acidosis. No effective therapy was available, and few prospects were on the horizon. It was known that the blood sugar was elevated in this disease, but beyond that, there was little understanding of its pathogenesis.

In 1889, Minkowski and von Mering demonstrated that removing the pancreas from dogs caused hyperglycemia,

TABLE 50–1

PRODUCTS OF PANCREATIC ISLET CELLS

CELL TYPE	PRODUCT
α	Glucagon
β	Insulin Proinsulin C peptide Amylin
δ	Somatostatin
F	Pancreatic polypeptide

TABLE 50–2

EFFECTS OF NUTRITIONAL STATES

PARAMETER	AFTER A 24-HOUR FAST	2 HOURS AFTER A MIXED MEAL
Plasma [glucose], mg/dl	60–80	100–140
mM	3.3–4.4	5.6–7.8
Plasma [insulin], μU/ml	3–8	50–150
Plasma [glucagon], pg/ml	40–80	80–200
Liver	↑ Glycogenolysis ↑ Gluconeogenesis	↓ Glycogenolysis ↓ Gluconeogenesis ↑ Glycogen synthesis
Adipose tissue	Lipids mobilized for fuel	Lipids synthesized
Muscle	Lipids metabolized Protein degraded and amino acids exported	Glucose oxidized or stored as glycogen Protein preserved

excess urination, thirst, weight loss, and death—in short, a syndrome closely resembling type 1 diabetes. Following this lead, a group of investigators in the Department of Physiology at the University of Toronto prepared extracts of pancreas and tested the ability of these extracts to lower plasma [glucose] in pancreatectomized dogs. Despite months of failures, these investigators persisted in their belief that such extracts could be beneficial. Finally, by the winter of 1921, Banting and Best were able to demonstrate that an aqueous extract of pancreas could lower blood glucose and prolong survival in a pancreatectomized dog. Within 2 months, a more purified extract was shown to lower blood sugar in a young man with diabetes. By the end of 1923, insulin (as the islet hormone was named) was being prepared from beef and pork pancreas on an industrial scale, and patients from around the world were receiving effective treatment of their diabetes.

Since that time, the physiology of insulin synthesis, secretion, and action has been more extensively studied than that of any other hormone. Now, more than three quarters of a century later, much is known about the metabolic pathways through which insulin regulates carbohydrate, lipid, and protein metabolism in its major targets: the liver, muscle, and adipose tissue. However, the sequence of intracellular signals that triggers insulin secretion by pancreatic β cells, as well as the signal-transduction process triggered when insulin binds to a plasma membrane receptor on target tissues, and the process by which the immune system recognizes and targets β cells for destruction remain areas of intense study.

Insulin Replenishes Fuel Reserves in Muscle, Liver, and Adipose Tissue

What does insulin do? Succinctly put, insulin efficiently integrates body fuel metabolism both during periods of fasting and during feeding (Table 50–2). When an individual is *fasting*, the β cell secretes less insulin. When insulin levels decrease, lipids are mobilized from adipose tissue and amino acids are mobilized from body protein stores within muscle and other tissues. These lipids and amino acids provide fuel for oxidation and serve as precursors for hepatic ketogenesis and gluconeogenesis, respectively. With *feeding*, insulin secretion increases. Ele-

vated levels of insulin diminish the mobilization of endogenous fuel stores and stimulate carbohydrate, lipid, and amino acid uptake by specific, insulin-sensitive target tissues. In this manner, insulin directs tissues to replenish the fuel reserves that were used during periods of fasting.

As a result of its ability to carefully regulate the mobilization and storage of fuels, insulin maintains the concentration of glucose in the plasma within narrow limits. Such regulation provides the central nervous system (CNS) with a constant supply of glucose for fuel to maintain cortical function. In higher organisms, if the plasma glucose concentration declines below 2 to 3 mM (hypoglycemia) for even a brief period, confusion, seizures, and coma may result. Conversely, persistent elevations of plasma [glucose] are characteristic of the diabetic state. Severe *hyper*glycemia (plasma glucose levels above 30 to 40 mM) produces an osmotic diuresis (see box on p. 782) and can lead to severe dehydration, hypertension, and vascular collapse.

β Cells Synthesize and Secrete Insulin

THE INSULIN GENE. Insulin is made only in the β cells of the pancreatic islet. It is encoded by a single gene on

---

CLINICAL MANIFESTATIONS OF HYPOGLYCEMIA AND HYPERGLYCEMIA

Hypoglycemia: Early manifestations include palpitations, tachycardia, diaphoresis, anxiety, hyperventilation, shakiness, weakness, hunger, and nausea. For prolonged or severe hypoglycemia, manifestations include confusion, unusual behavior, hallucinations, seizures, hypothermia, focal neurologic deficits, and coma.

Hyperglycemia: Early manifestations include weakness, polyuria, polydipsia, altered vision, weight loss, and mild dehydration. For prolonged or severe hyperglycemia, manifestations include Kussmaul hyperventilation (deep, rapid breathing), stupor, coma, hypotension, and cardiac arrhythmias.

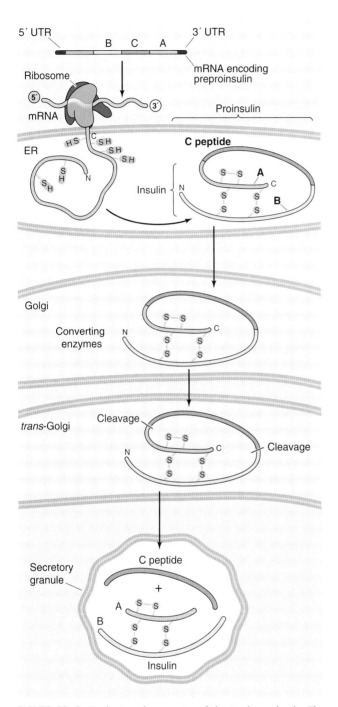

the short arm of chromosome 11. Insulin synthesis, as well as the secretion of insulin, is stimulated when islets are exposed to glucose. These effects require that glucose be metabolized. However, the molecular mechanisms by which glucose metabolites regulate insulin synthesis are not known.

INSULIN SYNTHESIS. Transcription of the insulin gene product and subsequent processing result in production of the full-length mRNA that encodes **preproinsulin**. Starting from its 5′ end, this mRNA encodes a leader sequence and then peptide domains B, C, and A. Insulin is a *secretory protein* (p. 36). As the preprohormone is synthesized, the leader sequence of approximately 24 amino acids is cleaved from the nascent peptide as it enters the rough endoplasmic reticulum. The result is **proinsulin** (Fig. 50–2), which consists of domains B, C, and A. As the *trans*-Golgi packages the proinsulin and creates secretory granules, proteases begin to slowly cleave the proinsulin molecule at two spots and thus excise the 31–amino-acid C peptide. The resulting insulin molecule has two peptide chains, designated the **A and B chains**, that are joined by two disulfide linkages. The mature insulin molecule has a total of 51 amino acids, 21 on the A chain and 30 on the B chain. In the secretory granule, the insulin associates with zinc. The secretory vesicle contains this insulin, as well as proinsulin and C peptide. All three are released into the portal blood when glucose stimulates the β cell.

SECRETION OF INSULIN, PROINSULIN, AND C PEPTIDE. C peptide has no established biologic action. However, because it is secreted in a 1:1 molar ratio with insulin, it is a useful marker for insulin secretion. Proinsulin does have modest insulin-like activities; it is approximately 1/20th as potent as insulin on a molar basis. In addition, the β cell secretes only about 5% as much proinsulin as insulin. As a result, proinsulin does not play a major role in the regulation of blood glucose.

Most of the insulin (approximately 60%) that is secreted into the portal blood is removed in a first pass through the liver. In contrast, C peptide is not extracted by the liver at all. As a result, whereas measurements of the insulin concentration in systemic blood do not quantitatively mimic the secretion of insulin, measurements of C peptide do. C peptide is eventually excreted in the urine, and measurements of the quantity of C peptide excreted in a 24-hour period therefore reflect—on a molar basis—the amount of insulin made during that time. Measurements of urinary C peptide can be used clinically to assess a person's insulin secretory capability.

FIGURE 50–2. Synthesis and processing of the insulin molecule. The mature mRNA of the insulin gene product contains a 5′ untranslated region (UTR); nucleotide sequences that encode a 24–amino acid leader sequence, as well as B, C, and A peptide domains; and a 3′ UTR. Together, the leader plus the B, C, and A domains constitute preproinsulin. During translation of the mRNA, the leader sequence is cleaved in the lumen of the rough endoplasmic reticulum. What remains is proinsulin, which consists of the B, C, and A domains. Beginning in the *trans*-Golgi, proteases cleave the proinsulin at two sites, releasing the C peptide as well as the mature insulin molecule, which consists of the B and A chains that are connected by two disulfide bonds. The secretory granule contains equimolar amounts of insulin and the C peptide, as well as a small amount of proinsulin. These components all are released into the extracellular space during secretion. ER, endoplasmic reticulum; mRNA, messenger RNA.

Glucose is the Major Regulator of Insulin Secretion

In healthy individuals, plasma [glucose] remains within a remarkably narrow range. After an overnight fast, it typically runs between 4 and 5 mM; the plasma [glucose] rises after a meal, but even with a very large meal it does not exceed 10 mM. Modest increases in plasma [glucose] provoke marked increases in insulin secretion and, thus, marked increases in the plasma [insulin] (Fig. 50–3A).

NONHUMAN AND MUTANT INSULIN

Cloning of the insulin gene has led to an important therapeutic advance, namely, the use of recombinant human insulin for the treatment of diabetes. Human insulin was the first recombinant protein available for routine clinical use. Before the availability of human insulin, either pork or beef insulin was used to treat diabetes. Pork and beef insulin differ from human insulin by one and three amino acids, respectively. The difference, although small, is sufficient to be recognized by the immune system, and antibodies to the injected insulin develop in most patients treated with beef or pork insulin; occasionally, the reaction is severe enough to cause a frank allergy to the insulin. This problem is largely avoided by using human insulin.

Sequencing of the insulin gene has not led to a major understanding of the genesis of the common forms of human diabetes. However, we have learned that rare diabetic individuals make a mutant insulin molecule. In these subjects, the abnormal insulin possesses a single amino-acid substitution in either the A or B chain. In each case that has been described, these changes lead to a less active insulin molecule (typically only about 1% as potent as insulin on a molar basis). These patients have either glucose intolerance or frank diabetes, but very high concentrations of immunoreactive insulin in their plasma. In these individuals, the immunoreactivity of insulin is not affected to the same extent as the bioactivity.

In addition to identifying these mutant types of insulin, sequencing of the insulin gene has allowed identification of a flanking polymorphic site upstream of the insulin gene that contains one of several common alleles. In some populations, one of these alleles is associated with an increased risk for the development of type 1 diabetes mellitus. The mechanism by which this increased risk is conferred is not known.

Conversely, a decline in plasma [glucose] of only 20% markedly lowers plasma [insulin]. The change in the concentration of plasma glucose that occurs in response to feeding or fasting is the main determinant of insulin secretion. In a patient with type 1 diabetes mellitus caused by destruction of pancreatic islets, an oral glucose challenge evokes either no response or a much smaller insulin response, but a much larger increment in plasma [glucose] that lasts for a much longer time (see Fig. 50–3B).

A glucose challenge given *intravenously* raises the plasma glucose concentration more rapidly than if given *orally*. Such a rapid rise in plasma glucose leads to two distinct phases of insulin secretion (see Fig. 50–3C). The acute- or first-phase insulin response lasts only 2 to 5 minutes; the duration of the second insulin response persists as long as the blood glucose level remains elevated. The insulin released during the acute-phase insulin response to intravenous glucose arises from preformed insulin that has been packaged in secretory vesicles in the cytosol of the β cell. The insulin released later comes from both preformed and newly synthesized insulin. One of the earliest detectable metabolic defects that occurs in

diabetes is loss of the first phase of insulin secretion, which can be detected experimentally by an intravenous glucose tolerance test. If a subject consumes glucose or a mixed meal, plasma [glucose] rises much more slowly—as in Figure 50–3A—because the appearance of glucose depends on intestinal absorption. Because plasma [glucose] rises so slowly, the acute-phase insulin response can no longer be distinguished from the chronic response, and only a single phase of insulin secretion is apparent.

Metabolism of Glucose by the β Cell Triggers Insulin Secretion

The pancreatic β cells take up and metabolize glucose, galactose, and mannose, and each can provoke insulin secretion by the islet. Other hexoses (for example, 3-O-methylglucose or 2-deoxyglucose) that are transported into the β cell but that cannot be metabolized do not stimulate insulin secretion. Although glucose itself is the best secretagogue, some amino acids (especially arginine and leucine) and small keto acids (α-ketoisocaproate), as well as ketohexoses (fructose), can also weakly stimulate insulin secretion. The amino acids and keto acids do not share any metabolic pathway with hexoses other than *terminal oxidation via the citric acid cycle* (p. 1220). These observations have led to the suggestion that the adenosine triphosphate (ATP) generated from the metabolism of these varied substances may be involved in insulin secretion. In the laboratory, depolarizing the islet-cell membrane by raising extracellular [K^+] provokes insulin secretion. In addition, glucagon has long been known to be a strong insulin secretagogue.

From these data has emerged a relatively unified picture of how various secretagogues trigger insulin secretion. Key to this picture is the presence in the islet of an ATP-sensitive K^+ channel and a voltage-gated Ca^{2+} channel in the plasma membrane (Fig. 50–4). Glucose triggers insulin release in a seven-step process:

1. Glucose enters the β cell via the GLUT2 glucose transporter by facilitated diffusion (p. 60). Amino acids enter via a different set of transporters.
2. In the presence of glucokinase (the rate-limiting enzyme in glycolysis), the entering glucose undergoes glycolysis and raises [ATP]$_i$ by phosphorylating adenosine diphosphate (ADP). Some amino acids also enter the citric acid cycle and produce similar changes in [ATP]$_i$ and [ADP]$_i$.
3. Either the increased [ATP]$_i$ or the increased [ATP]$_i$/[ADP]$_i$ ratio causes K_{ATP}-type K^+ channels (p. 198) to close.
4. Reducing the K^+ conductance of the cell membrane causes the β cell to depolarize (i.e., the membrane potential is less negative).
5. This depolarization activates voltage-gated Ca^{2+} channels (p. 189).
6. The increased Ca^{2+} permeability leads to increased Ca^{2+} influx and increased intracellular free Ca^{2+}. This rise in [Ca^{2+}]$_i$ additionally triggers Ca^{2+}-induced Ca^{2+} release (p. 242).
7. The increased [Ca^{2+}]$_i$, perhaps by activation of a Ca^{2+}-

A NORMAL SUBJECT RECEIVING ORAL GLUCOSE

B DIABETIC SUBJECT RECEIVING ORAL GLUCOSE

C NORMAL SUBJECT RECEIVING IV GLUCOSE

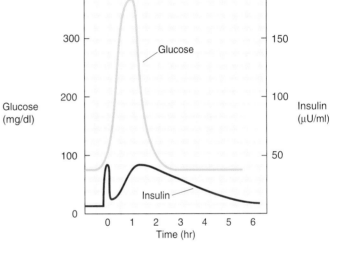

FIGURE 50–3. Glucose tolerance test. *A,* When a human consumes a load of glucose (75 g), plasma [glucose] rises slowly, reflecting the intestinal uptake of the glucose. In response, the pancreatic *β* cells secrete insulin and plasma [insulin] rises sharply. *B,* In a patient with type 1 diabetes, the same glucose load as that in *A* causes plasma [glucose] to rise to a higher level and to remain there for a longer time. The reason is that plasma [insulin] rises very little in response to the glucose challenge so that the tissues fail to dispose of the glucose load as rapidly as normal. The diagnosis of diabetes is made if the plasma glucose is above 200 mg/dl at the second hour. *C,* If the glucose challenge (0.5 g glucose/kg body weight given as a 25% glucose solution) is given intravenously, then the plasma [glucose] rises much more rapidly than it does with an oral glucose load. Sensing a rapid rise in [glucose], the *β* cells first secrete their stores of presynthesized insulin. Following this "acute-phase," the cells begin to secrete newly manufactured insulin in the "chronic phase," which lasts as long as the glucose challenge. IV, intravenous.

calmodulin phosphorylation cascade, ultimately leads to insulin release.

In addition to the pathway just outlined, other secretagogues can also modulate insulin secretion via the phospholipase C pathway (p. 100) or via the adenylyl cyclase pathway (p. 97). For example, glucagon, which stimulates insulin release, may bypass part or all of the glucose/[Ca^{2+}]$_i$ pathway by stimulating the adenylyl cyclase, raising cyclic adenosine monophosphate (cAMP) levels, and activating protein kinase A (PKA). Conversely, somatostatin, which inhibits insulin release, may act by inhibiting adenylyl cyclase.

Neural and Humoral Factors Modulate Insulin Secretion

The islet is richly innervated by both the sympathetic and the parasympathetic divisions of the ANS. Neural signals appear to play an important role in the *β*-cell response in several settings. ***β*-adrenergic** stimulation augments islet insulin secretion, whereas ***α*-adrenergic** stimulation inhib-

its it (see Fig. 50–4). Isoproterenol, a synthetic catecholamine that is a specific agonist for the *β*-adrenergic receptor, potently stimulates insulin release. In contrast, norepinephrine and synthetic *α*-adrenergic agonists suppress insulin release both basally and in response to hyperglycemia. Because the postsynaptic sympathetic neurons of the pancreas release norepinephrine, which stimulates *α* more than *β* adrenoceptors, sympathetic stimulation via the celiac nerves inhibits insulin secretion. In contrast to *α*-adrenergic stimulation, **parasympathetic** stimulation via the vagus nerve, which releases acetylcholine, causes an increase in insulin release.

EXERCISE. The effect of the sympathetic division on insulin secretion may be particularly important during exercise, when adrenergic stimulation of the islet increases. The major role for *α*-adrenergic *inhibition* of insulin secretion during exercise is to prevent hypoglycemia. Exercising muscle tissue uses glucose even when plasma [insulin] is low. If insulin levels were to rise, glucose use by the muscle would increase even further and promote hypoglycemia. Furthermore, an increase in [insulin] would

FIGURE 50–4. Mechanism of insulin secretion by the pancreatic β cell. Increased levels of extracellular glucose trigger the β cell to secrete insulin in the seven steps outlined in this figure. Metabolizable sugars (e.g., galactose and mannose) and certain amino acids (e.g., arginine and leucine) can also stimulate the fusion of vesicles that contain previously synthesized insulin. In addition to these fuel sources, certain hormones (e.g., glucagon, somatostatin, CCK) can also modulate insulin secretion. ADP, adenosine diphosphate; ATP, adenosine triphosphate; cAMP, cyclic adenosine monophosphate; CCK, cholecystokinin; DAG, diacylglycerol; ER, endoplasmic reticulum; IP₃, inositol 1,4,5-triphosphate; PIP₂, phosphatidylinositol 4,5-biphosphate; PKA, protein kinase A; PLC, phospholipase C.

SULFONYLUREAS

An entire class of drugs known as the sulfonylurea agents are used in the treatment of patients with adult-onset diabetes—also called type 2 or non–insulin-dependent diabetes mellitus (NIDDM). Patients with type 2 diabetes have two defects: (1) although their β cells are capable of making insulin, they do not respond normally to increased blood glucose levels, and (2) the target tissues are less sensitive to insulin.

The sulfonylurea agents were discovered accidentally. During the development of sulfonamide antibiotics after the Second World War, investigators noticed that the chemically related sulfonylurea agents produced hypoglycemia. These drugs turned out to have no value as antibiotics, but they did prove effective in treating the hyperglycemia of NIDDM. These drugs appeared to work in two ways: (1) the sulfonylureas enhance insulin secretion by β cells by binding to and inhibiting adenosine triphosphate–sensitive K$^+$ channels, thereby decreasing the likelihood that these channels will be open. This action enhances glucose-stimulated insulin secretion, a process in which this same channel is responsible for cell depolarization (see Figure 50–4). (2) By increasing insulin secretion and decreasing blood glucose, the sulfonylureas decrease the insulin resistance that is seen in these patients.

Unlike insulin, which must be injected, sulfonylureas can be taken orally and are therefore preferred by many patients. However, they have a therapeutic role only in type 2 diabetes (i.e., NIDDM); the β cells in patients with type 1 or juvenile-onset diabetes (i.e., insulin-dependent diabetes) are nearly all destroyed, and these patients must be treated with insulin replacement therapy.

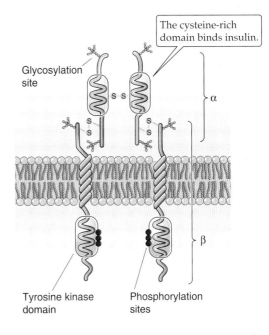

FIGURE 50–5. The insulin receptor. The insulin receptor is a heterotetramer that consists of two extracellular α chains and two membrane-spanning β chains. Insulin binding takes place on the cysteine-rich region of the α chains.

inhibit lipolysis and fatty acid release from adipocytes and thus diminish the availability of fatty acids, which the muscle can use as an alternative fuel to glucose (p. 1246). Finally, a rise in [insulin] would decrease glucose production by the liver. Suppression of insulin secretion during exercise may thus serve to prevent excessive glucose uptake by muscle, which if it were to exceed the ability of the liver to produce glucose, would lead to severe hypoglycemia, compromise the brain, and abruptly end any exercise!

FEEDING. Another important setting in which neural and humoral factors regulate insulin secretion is during feeding. Food ingestion triggers a complex series of neural, endocrine, and nutritional signals to many body tissues. The "cephalic phase" (see Chapters 41, 42, and 44) of eating, which occurs before food is ingested, results in stimulation of gastric-acid secretion and a small rise in plasma insulin. This response appears to be mediated by the vagus nerve in both cases. If no food is forthcoming, blood [glucose] declines slightly and insulin secretion is again suppressed. If food ingestion does occur, the acetylcholine released by postganglionic vagal fibers in the islet augments the insulin response of the β cell to glucose.

After a subject drinks a glucose solution, the blood glucose level rises and insulin secretion is stimulated. Moreover, the total amount of insulin secreted is greater when glucose is administered orally than when administered intravenously. This observation has led to a search for enteric factors or "incretins" that might augment the islet β-cell response to an oral glucose stimulus. Currently, two peptides, cholecystokinin and gastric inhibitory polypeptide (GIP), which are released by gut tissues in response to feeding, have been found to enhance insulin secretion. Accordingly, GIP is often called glucose-dependent insulinotropic polypeptide. Another very recently described peptide, glucagon-like peptide 1 (GLP-1), which we will discuss later, appears to play a similar role and may be the most important "incretin" yet discovered.

In the laboratory, incretins stimulate insulin secretion by isolated islets of Langerhans, and glucose increases this secretion even further. The presence of these incretins in the gut mucosa gives the islets advance notice that nutrients are being absorbed and allows them to amplify the priming of the islets that is induced by vagal stimulation.

The Insulin Receptor is a Receptor Tyrosine Kinase

Once insulin is secreted into the portal blood, it first travels to the liver, where more than half is bound and removed from the circulation. The insulin that escapes the liver is available to stimulate insulin-sensitive processes in other tissues. At each target tissue, the first action of insulin is to bind to a specific receptor tyrosine kinase (p. 110) on the plasma membrane (Fig. 50–5).

As discussed in Chapter 4, the insulin receptor—as

well as the closely related insulin-like growth factor I (IGF-I) receptor—is a heterotetramer, with two identical α chains and two identical β chains. The α and β chains are synthesized as a single polypeptide that is subsequently cleaved. The two chains are joined by disulfide linkage (reminiscent of the synthesis of the A and B chains of insulin itself) in the sequence β-α-α-β. The insulin receptor shares considerable structural similarity with the IGF-I receptor (p. 1029). The overall sequence homology is approximately 50%, and this figure rises to more than 80% in the tyrosine kinase region. This similarity is sufficient that very high concentrations of insulin can stimulate the IGF-I receptor and, conversely, high levels of IGF-I can stimulate the insulin receptor.

The insulin receptor's extracellular α chains have multiple N-glycosylation sites. The β chains have an extracellular, a membrane-spanning, and an intracellular portion. The β subunit of the receptor is glycosylated on its extracellular domains; receptor glycosylation is required for insulin binding and action. The intracellular domain of the β chain possesses tyrosine kinase activity, which increases markedly when insulin binds to sites on the α chains of the receptor. The insulin receptor can phosphorylate both itself and other intracellular substrates at tyrosine residues. This phosphorylation mechanism appears to be the major one by which insulin transmits its signal across the plasma membrane of insulin target tissues.

The insulin receptor can transmit its signals by at least three mechanisms (Fig. 50–6). First, SH2 (Src homology domain-2)-containing proteins can bind to phosphorylated tyrosine groups on the insulin receptor itself. SH2 domains on these proteins recognize specific phosphotryosine groups and activate the SH2-containing protein (p. 98). Second, the insulin receptor can tyrosine-phosphorylate—and thus activate—various cytoplasmic proteins at tyrosine residues. Third, the insulin receptor phosphorylates at tyrosine residues a family of cytosolic proteins known as **insulin-receptor substrates** (IRS-1, -2, -3 and -4), which are important links in the transduction of the insulin signal. The IGF-I receptor, which is closely related to the insulin receptor, also acts through IRS-1. The IRS proteins are *docking proteins* to which a variety of downstream effector proteins bind and thus become activated. IRS-1 has at least eight tyrosines within specific motifs that are generally recognized by SH2-containing proteins, so that a single IRS molecule simultaneously activates multiple pathways.

Figure 50–6 illustrates two major IRS-signalling pathways. The first begins with activation of phosphatidyl inositol 3-kinase (PI-3-K), which phosphorylates a membrane lipid, leading to major changes in glucose and protein metabolism. The second begins with phosphorylation of SHC (Src homology, C terminus) and activation of GRB2 (p. 134), which trigger the Ras signalling pathway, leading to increased gene expression and growth. Thus, the phosphorylation of the IRS family is only one early event in a series of parallel and diverging kinase cascades that culminates in insulin's many actions. Surprisingly, gene-deletion studies in mice show that IRS-1 deletion does not cause diabetes, but results in small mice. In contrast, IRS-2 deletion does cause diabetes, in part due to impaired insulin secretion!

THE INSULIN RECEPTOR AND RARE FORMS OF DIABETES

The ability of insulin to act on a target cell depends on three things: the number of receptors present on the target cell, the receptor's affinity for insulin, and the receptor's ability to "transduce" the insulin signal.

Several disorders have now been described in which a mutation of the insulin receptor blunts or prevents insulin's actions. One such mutation markedly affects growth *in utero,* as well as after birth. This rare disorder is called **"leprechaunism,"** and it is generally lethal within the first year of life. Other mutations of the receptor have less devastating consequences.

Some individuals make antibodies to their own insulin receptors. Insulin, produced either endogenously or administered to these individuals, does not work well because it must compete with these antibodies for sites on the receptor; as a result, the patient is hyperglycemic. Interestingly, other antibodies can be "insulin mimetic"; that is, not only to the antibodies bind to the receptor, but they also actually mimic insulin's action. This mimicry causes severe *hypo*glycemia in affected individuals.

Neither receptor mutations nor antireceptor antibodies appear to be responsible for any of the common forms of diabetes seen clinically.

High Levels of Insulin Lead to Downregulation of Insulin Receptors

The number of insulin receptors expressed on the cell surface is far greater than that needed for the maximal biologic response to insulin. In fact, in a normal individual, the glucose response to insulin is maximal when only approximately 5% of the receptors are occupied; that is, the target cells have many "spare" receptors for insulin.

The number of insulin receptors present on a target cell is determined by the balance among three factors: (1) receptor synthesis, (2) endocytosis of receptors followed by recycling of receptors back to the cell surface, and (3) endocytosis followed by degradation of receptors. Cells chronically exposed to high concentrations of insulin have fewer receptors than do those exposed to lower concentrations. This dynamic ability of cells to decrease the number of specific receptors on their surface is called "downregulation." Insulin downregulates insulin receptors by decreasing receptor synthesis and increasing degradation. Such downregulation is one mechanism by which target tissues modulate their response to hormones. Downregulation of insulin receptors results in a decrease in the sensitivity of the target tissue to insulin without diminishing insulin's maximal effect.

One example of how downregulation can affect insulin's action is shown in Figure 50–7, which illustrates the effect of increases in insulin concentration on glucose uptake in adipocytes from normal individuals or type 2 diabetics. Adipocytes from patients with type 2 diabetes (see box titled Diabetes Mellitus on p. 1084) have fewer

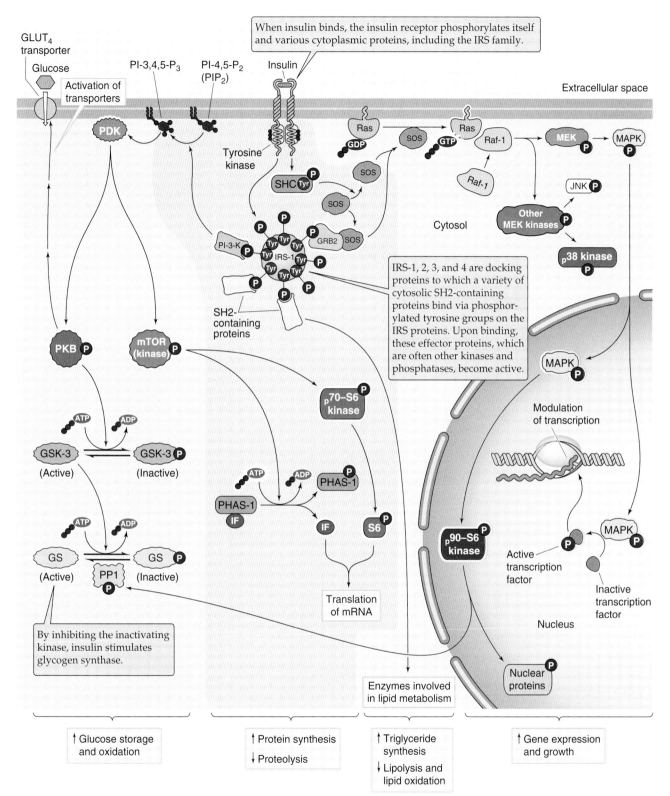

FIGURE 50–6. The insulin signal-transduction system. When insulin binds to its receptor—which is a receptor tyrosine kinase (RTK)—tyrosine kinase domains on the intracellular portion of the β chains become active. The activated receptor transduces its signals to downstream effectors by phosphorylating at tyrosine residues the receptor itself, the insulin-receptor substrate family (IRS-1, 2, 3, 4), and other cytosolic proteins (e.g., SHC). SH2-containing proteins dock onto certain phosphorylated tyrosine groups on the IRSs, and thus become activated. The figure shows two major pathways. In the first pathway, activation of phosphatidyl inositol 3-kinase (PI-3-K) phosphorylates phosphatidyl inositol-4,5-biphosphate (PIP$_2$), to form phosphatidyl inositol-3,4,5-triphosphate (PI-3,4,5-P$_3$), which in turn activates phosphatidyl inositol-dependent kinase (PDK). This Ser/Thr kinase then activates protein kinase B (PKB), which leads to the insertion of GLUT4 glucose transporters into the plasma membrane. PDK also phosphorylates and thus inactivates glycogen synthase kinase-3 (GSK-3); the net effect is reduced inactivation of glycogen synthase (GS) and enhanced glycogen synthesis. Finally PDK activates mTOR (target of rapamycin), a Ser/Thr kinase that phosphorylates the binding protein PHAS-1 and thus releases an active initiation factor (IF), promoting translation of mRNA into protein. mTOR also phosphorylates p70-S6 kinase, which phosphorylates the ribosomal S6 protein. In the second pathway, the insulin receptor phosphorylates SHC (Src homology, C terminus) at tyrosine residues, stimulating SOS. In addition, activation of GRB2 also stimulates SOS. The stimulated SOS activates the Ras pathway, as described in Fig. 5–15. The activated Raf-1, which is itself a MEK kinase, not only activates MEK, but other MEK kinases, which in turn activate JNK (a kinase) and p38 kinase. MAP kinase (MAPK) activates both a transcription factor and p90-S6 kinase. The activated p90-S6 kinase phosphorylates a variety of nuclear proteins as well as protein phosphatase 1 (PP1); the latter leads to activation of glycogen synthase.

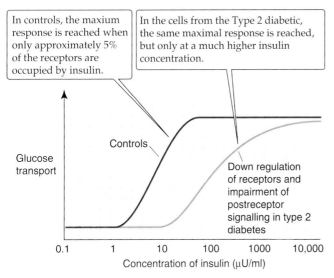

In controls, the maxium response is reached when only approximately 5% of the receptors are occupied by insulin.

In the cells from the Type 2 diabetic, the same maximal response is reached, but only at a much higher insulin concentration.

Controls

Glucose transport

Down regulation of receptors and impairment of postreceptor signalling in type 2 diabetes

0.1   1   10   100   1000   10,000
Concentration of insulin (μU/ml)

FIGURE 50–7. Response to insulin of normal and "downregulated" adipocytes.

insulin receptors per unit of surface area than do adipocytes from normal individuals. The markedly lower glucose transport across the entire physiological range of insulin concentrations in diabetic adipocytes is characteristic of "insulin resistance." In healthy controls, glucose transport is maximal when only a small fraction (~5%) of the receptors are occupied. In diabetic adipocytes, a much higher concentration of insulin is required, and a larger *fraction* of the insulin receptors is occupied. However, the major effects in type 2 diabetes are apparently not due to a decrease in receptor number, but to impairment in signalling downstream from the receptor. For example, stimulation of the GLUT4 glucose transporter requires stimulation of many steps downstream from the insulin receptor (see Fig. 50–6). It is the summation of these multiple defects, only some of which have been identified, that leads to insulin resistance.

In Liver, Insulin Promotes Storage of Glucose as Glycogen, Plus Conversion of Glucose to Triglycerides

Insulin's actions on cellular targets frequently involve a number of different enzymatic and structural processes. These effects will be illustrated as we consider—in this and the next two sections—the three principal targets for insulin action: the liver, muscle, and adipose tissue.

Because the pancreatic veins drain into the portal venous system, all hormones secreted by the pancreas must traverse the liver before entering the systemic circulation. For insulin, the liver is both a target tissue for hormone action and a major site of degradation.

The concentration of insulin in portal venous blood before extraction by the liver is three to four times greater than its concentration in the systemic circulation. The hepatocyte is therefore bathed in a relatively high concentration of insulin and is thus well positioned to respond acutely to changes in plasma [insulin].

After feeding, the plasma [insulin] rises, triggered by glucose and by neural and incretin stimulation of β cells. In liver, this insulin rise acts on four main processes

involved in fuel metabolism (Fig. 50–8). These divergent effects of insulin entail the use of multiple enzymatic control mechanisms.

GLYCOGEN SYNTHESIS AND GLYCOGENOLYSIS. Physiological increases in plasma [insulin] decrease the breakdown and utilization of glycogen and—conversely—promote the formation of glycogen from plasma glucose. Although moderately increased levels of insulin allow gluconeogenesis to persist, the hepatocytes store the newly formed glucose 6-phosphate as glycogen rather than releasing it as glucose to the bloodstream. At high concentrations, insulin can inhibit the gluconeogenic conversion of lactate/pyruvate and amino acids to glucose 6-phosphate.

Glucose enters the hepatocyte from the blood via GLUT2, which mediates the facilitated diffusion of glucose (see numbered boxes in Fig. 50–8). GLUT2 is present in abundance in the liver plasma membrane, even in the absence of insulin, and its activity is not influenced by insulin. Insulin stimulates glycogen synthesis from glucose by activating **glucokinase** (1) and **glycogen synthase** (2). The latter enzyme contains multiple serine phosphorylation sites. Insulin causes a net dephosphorylation of the protein, thus increasing the enzyme's activity. At the same time that glycogen synthase is being activated, increases in both insulin and glucose diminish **glycogen phosphorylase** activity (3). This enzyme is rate limiting for the breakdown of glycogen. The same enzyme that dephosphorylates (and thus *activates*) glycogen synthase also dephosphorylates (and thus *inhibits*) phosphorylase. Thus, insulin has opposite effects on the opposing enzymes, with the net effect that it promotes glycogen formation. Insulin also inhibits **glucose-6-phosphatase** (4), which converts glucose 6-phosphate to glucose and thus completes the conversion of glycogen to glucose. Glycogen is an important storage form of carbohydrate in both liver and muscle. The glycogen stored during the postprandial period is then available for use many hours later as a source of glucose.

GLYCOLYSIS AND GLUCONEOGENESIS. Insulin promotes the conversion of some of the glucose taken up by the liver into pyruvate and—conversely—diminishes the use of pyruvate and other three-carbon compounds for gluconeogenesis (see numbered boxes in Fig. 50–8). Insulin induces transcription of the **glucokinase** gene (1) and thus results in increased synthesis of this enzyme, which is responsible for phosphorylating glucose to glucose 6-phosphate and initiating the metabolism of glucose. In acting to promote glycolysis and diminish gluconeogenesis, insulin induces the synthesis of a glucose metabolite, fructose 2,6-bisphosphate. This compound is a potent allosteric activator of **phosphofructokinase** (5), a key regulatory enzyme in glycolysis. Insulin also stimulates **pyruvate kinase** (6), which forms pyruvate, and stimulates **pyruvate dehydrogenase** (8), which catalyzes the first step in pyruvate oxidation. Finally, insulin promotes glucose breakdown by the hexose monophosphate shunt (7).

In addition, insulin also inhibits gluconeogenesis at several steps. Insulin diminishes transcription of the **phosphoenolpyruvate carboxykinase** gene (9), thus reducing

FIGURE 50–8. Effect of insulin on hepatocytes. Insulin has four major effects on liver cells. First, insulin promotes glycogen synthesis from glucose by enhancing the transcription of **glucokinase** (*1*) and by activating **glycogen synthase** (*2*). Additionally, insulin inhibits glycogen breakdown to glucose by diminishing the activity of **glycogen phosphorylase** (*3*) and **glucose-6-phosphatase** (*4*). Glucose also inhibits the phosphorylase. Second, insulin promotes glycolysis and carbohydrate oxidation by increasing the activity of **glucokinase** (*1*), **phosphofructokinase** (*5*), and **pyruvate kinase** (*6*). Insulin also promotes glucose metabolism via the hexose monophosphate shunt (*7*). Finally, insulin promotes the oxidation of pyruvate by stimulating **pyruvate dehydrogenase** (*8*). Insulin also inhibits gluconeogenesis by inhibiting the activity of **phosphoenolpyruvate carboxykinase** (*9*), **fructose-1,6-bisphosphatase** (*10*), and **glucose-6-phosphatase** (*4*). Third, insulin promotes the synthesis and storage of fats by increasing the activity of **acetyl CoA carboxylase** (*11*) and **fatty acid synthase** (*12*) as well as the synthesis of several apoproteins packaged with VLDL. Insulin also indirectly inhibits fat oxidation because the increased levels of malonyl CoA inhibit **carnitine acyl-transferase I** (CAT I) (*13*). The inhibition of fat oxidation helps shunt free fatty acids to esterification as triglycerides and storage as VLDL or lipid droplets. Fourth, by mechanisms that are not well understood, insulin promotes protein synthesis (*14*) and inhibits protein breakdown (*15*). CoA, coenzyme A; VLDL, very low density lipoprotein.

the synthesis of a key regulatory enzyme required to form phosphoenolpyruvate from oxaloacetate early in the gluconeogenic pathway. The increased levels of fructose 2,6-bisphosphate also inhibit the activity of **fructose-1,6-bis-phosphatase** (*10*), which is likewise part of the gluconeogenic pathway.

LIPOGENESIS. Insulin promotes the storage of fats and inhibits the oxidation of free fatty acids via allosteric and covalent modification of key regulatory enzymes, as well as by transcription of new enzymes (see numbered boxes in Fig. 50–8). The pyruvate that is now available from glycolysis can be used to synthesize free fatty acids. Insulin promotes dephosphorylation of **acetyl coenzyme A (acetyl CoA) carboxylase** *(11)*, the first committed step in fatty acid synthesis in the liver. This dephosphorylation leads to increased synthesis of malonyl-CoA, which allosterically inhibits **carnitine acyltransferase** I [CAT I]. This enzyme *(13)* converts fatty acid CoA and carnitine in the intermembrane space to fatty-acid–carnitine. Thus, malonyl CoA inhibits fatty acid transport into the mitochondria, where fat oxidation occurs. At the same time, insulin stimulates **fatty acid synthase** *(12)*, which generates free fatty acids. Thus, because insulin promotes the formation of malonyl-CoA and free fatty acids but inhibits fatty acid oxidation, this hormone favors esterification of the free fatty acids with glycerol within the liver, thus forming triglycerides. The liver can either store these triglycerides in lipid droplets or export them as "very-low-density lipoprotein (VLDL) particles" (p. 998). Indeed, insulin induces the synthesis of several of the **apoproteins** that are packaged with the VLDL particle. The hepatocyte then releases these VLDLs, which leave the liver via the hepatic vein. Muscle and adipose tissue subsequently take up the lipids in these VLDL particles and either store them or oxidize them for fuel. Thus, by regulation of transcription, by allosteric activation, and by regulation of protein phosphorylation, insulin acts to promote the synthesis and storage of fat and diminish its oxidation in liver.

PROTEIN METABOLISM. Insulin stimulates the synthesis of protein and simultaneously reduces the degradation of protein within the liver (see numbered boxes in Fig. 50–8). The general mechanism by which insulin stimulates net protein synthesis *(14)* and restrains proteolysis *(15)* by the liver has not been nearly as well defined as its effects on the enzymes involved in carbohydrate and lipid metabolism. The regulatory steps in these pathways appear more complex and are less well understood.

In summary, insulin modulates the activity of multiple regulatory enzymes, which are responsible for the hepatic metabolism of carbohydrates, fat, and protein. Insulin causes the liver to take up glucose from the blood and either store the glucose as glycogen or break it down into pyruvate. The pyruvate provides the building blocks for storage of the glucose carbon atoms as fat. Insulin also diminishes the oxidation of fat, which normally supplies much of the ATP used by the liver. As a result, insulin causes the liver, as well as other body tissues, to burn carbohydrates preferentially.

In Muscle, Insulin Promotes the Uptake of Glucose and Its Storage as Glycogen

Muscle is a major insulin-sensitive tissue and the principal site of insulin-mediated glucose disposal. Insulin has four major effects on muscle. First, in muscle, unlike the liver, glucose crosses the plasma membrane principally via GLUT4, an *insulin-sensitive* glucose transporter. GLUT4, which is found virtually exclusively in striated muscle and adipose tissue, belongs to a family of proteins that mediate the facilitated diffusion of glucose (p. 60). Insulin markedly stimulates GLUT4 in both muscle and fat (see later) by a process involving "recruitment" of preformed

transporters from a membranous compartment in the cell cytosol out to the plasma membrane (Fig. 50–9). Recruitment thus places additional glucose transporters in the plasma membrane, thus increasing the V_{max} of glucose transport into muscle and increasing the flow of glucose from the interstitial fluid to the cytosol. As we saw earlier, a different glucose transporter, GLUT2, mediates glucose transport into hepatocytes (see Fig. 50–8), and insulin does *not* increase the activity of that transporter.

The second effect of insulin on muscle (see numbered boxes in Fig. 50–9) is to enhance the conversion of glucose to glycogen by activating **hexokinase** (*[1]* different from the glucokinase in liver) and **glycogen synthase** *(2)*. Third, insulin increases glucose breakdown and oxidation by increasing **phosphofructokinase** *(3)* and **pyruvate dehydrogenase** *(4)* activity. Fourth, insulin also stimulates the synthesis of protein in skeletal muscle *(5)* and slows the degradation of existing proteins *(6)*. The result is preservation of muscle protein mass, which has obvious beneficial effects in preserving strength and locomotion. The insulin-induced increase in glucose utilization permits the muscle to diminish fat utilization and allows it to store as triglycerides some of the fatty acid that it removes from the circulation. The stored triglycerides and glycogen are a major source of energy that muscle can use later when called on to exercise or generate heat.

In muscle, as in the liver, insulin directs the overall pattern of cellular fuel metabolism by acting at multiple sites. In both tissues, insulin increases the oxidation of carbohydrate, thus preserving body protein and fat stores. Carbohydrate ingested in excess of that used immediately as an oxidative fuel is either stored as glycogen in liver and muscle or converted to lipid in the liver and exported to adipose tissue and muscle.

In Adipocytes, Insulin Promotes Uptake of Glucose and Its Conversion to Triglycerides for Storage

Adipose tissue is the third major insulin-sensitive tissue involved in the regulation of body fuel. Again, insulin has several sites of action in adipocytes. All begin with the same receptor-mediated action of insulin to stimulate several cellular effector pathways. Insulin has four major actions on adipocytes: first, like muscle, adipose contains the insulin-sensitive GLUT4 glucose transporter. In insulin-stimulated cells, preformed transporters are recruited from an intracellular compartment to the cell membrane, thus markedly accelerating the entry of glucose into the cell.

Second, insulin promotes the breakdown of glucose to metabolites that will eventually be used to synthesize triglycerides (see numbered boxes in Fig. 50–10). Unlike muscle or liver, little of the glucose taken up is stored as glycogen. Instead, the adipocyte glycolytically metabolizes much of the glucose to α-glycerol phosphate, which it will use in the synthesis of triglycerides. The glucose that is not converted to α-glycerol phosphate goes on to form acetyl CoA and then malonyl-CoA and free fatty acids. Insulin enhances this flow of glucose to free fatty acids by

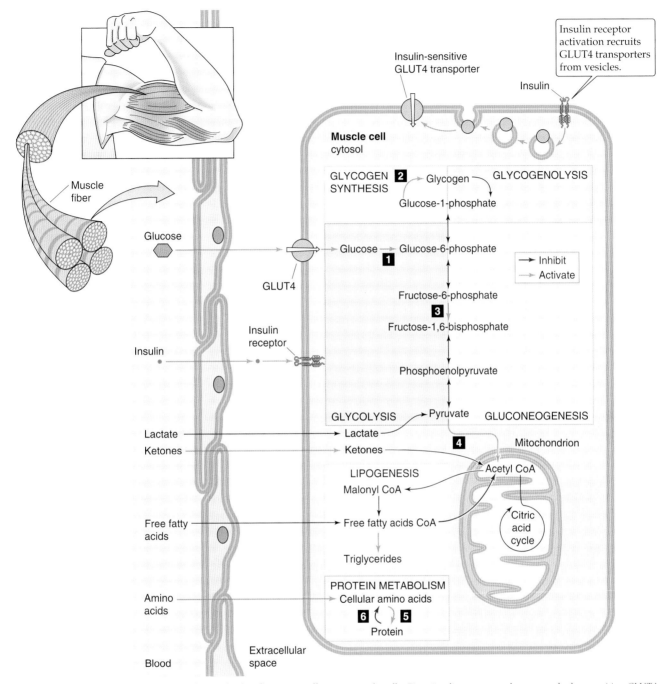

FIGURE 50–9. Effect of insulin on muscle. Insulin has four major effects on muscle cells. First, insulin promotes glucose uptake by recruiting GLUT4 transporters to the plasma membrane. Second, insulin promotes glycogen synthesis from glucose by enhancing the transcription of **hexokinase** (1) and by activating **glycogen synthase** (2). Third, insulin promotes glycolysis and carbohydrate oxidation by increasing the activity of **hexokinase** (1), **phosphofructokinase** (3), and **pyruvate dehydrogenase** (4). These actions are similar to those in liver; note that there is little or no gluconeogenesis in muscle. Fourth, insulin promotes protein synthesis (5) and inhibits protein breakdown (6).

stimulating **pyruvate dehydrogenase** (1) and **acetyl CoA carboxylase** (2).

Third, insulin promotes the formation of triglycerides by simple mass action; the increased levels of α-glycerol phosphate increase its esterification with free fatty acids (principally C-16 and C-18) to yield triglycerides. Some of the free fatty acids are a result of the glucose metabolism noted earlier. Most of the fatty acids, however, enter

the adipocyte from chylomicrons and VLDLs (see Table 45–5) in the blood (see later). The cell sequesters these triglycerides in lipid droplets, which form most of the mass of the adipose cell. Conversely, insulin restrains the activity of a **hormone-sensitive triglyceride lipase** (HSL; 3). In fat, this enzyme mediates the conversion of stored triglyceride to free fatty acids and glycerol for export to other tissues.

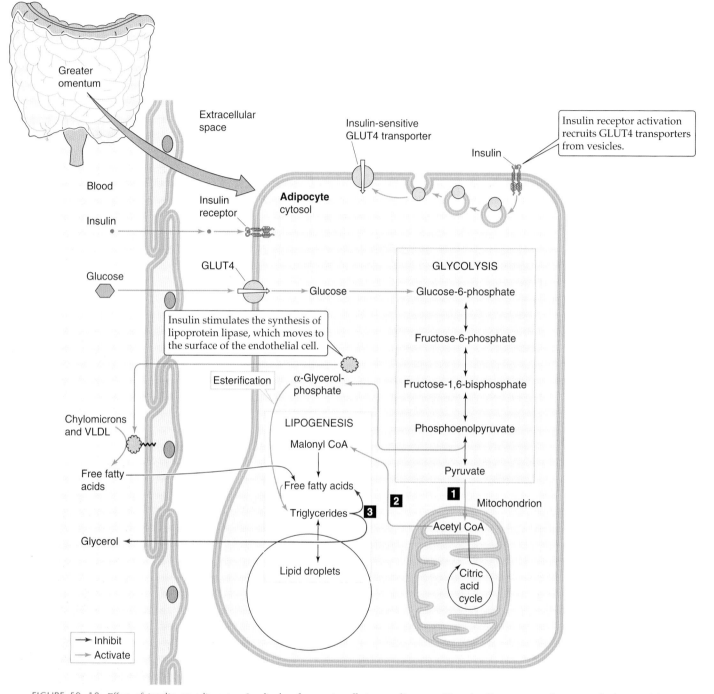

FIGURE 50–10. Effect of insulin on adipocytes. Insulin has four major effects on adipocytes. First, insulin promotes glucose uptake by recruiting GLUT4 transporters to the plasma membrane. Second, insulin promotes glycolysis, leading to the formation of α-glycerol-phosphate. Insulin also promotes the conversion of pyruvate to free fatty acids by stimulating **pyruvate dehydrogenase** (1) and **acetyl CoA carboxylase** (2). Third, insulin promotes the esterification of α-glycerol-phosphate with free fatty acids to form triglycerides, which the adipocyte stores in fat droplets. Conversely, insulin inhibits **hormone-sensitive triglyceride lipase** (3), which would otherwise break the triglycerides down into glycerol and free fatty acids. Fourth, insulin promotes the synthesis of lipoprotein lipase in the adipocyte. The adipocyte then exports this enzyme to the endothelial cell, where it breaks down the triglycerides contained in chylomicrons and VLDL, yielding free fatty acids. These free fatty acids then enter the adipocyte for esterification and storage in fat droplets as triglycerides.

Fourth, insulin induces the synthesis of a different enzyme—**lipoprotein lipase** (**LPL**). This lipase does not act on the lipid stored within the adipose cell. Rather, the adipocyte exports the LPL to the endothelial cell, where it resides on the extracellular surface of the endothelial cell, facing the blood and anchored to the plasma membrane. In this location, the LPL acts on triglycerides in chylomicrons and VLDLs and cleaves them into glycerol and free fatty acids. These free fatty acids are then available for uptake by nearby adipocytes, which esterify them with

FIGURE 50–11. The synthesis of the glucagon molecule. The proglucagon molecule includes amino acid sequences that, depending on how the peptide chain is cleaved, can yield glucagon-related polypeptide (GRPP), glucagon, IP-1, glucagon-like peptide I (GLP-1), IP-2, and GLP-2. Proteases in the pancreatic α cells cleave proglucagon at points that yield GRPP, glucagon, and a C-terminal fragment. Proteases in neuroendocrine cells in the intestine cleave proglucagon to yield glicentin, GLP-1, IP-2, and GLP-2.

glycerol phosphate to form triglycerides. This mechanism provides an efficient means by which insulin can promote the storage of lipid in adipose tissue.

GLUCAGON

Glucagon is the other major pancreatic-islet hormone that is involved in the regulation of body fuel metabolism. Ingestion of protein appears to be the major stimulus to secretion of glucagon. Glucagon's principal target tissue is the liver. Like insulin, glucagon is secreted first into the portal blood and is therefore anatomically well positioned to regulate hepatic metabolism.

Curiously, although the *amino acids* released by digestion of a protein meal appear to be the major glucagon secretagogue, glucagon's main actions on the liver appear to involve the regulation of *carbohydrate* and *lipid* metabolism. Glucagon is particularly important in stimulating glycogenolysis, gluconeogenesis, and ketogenesis. Glucagon does not act solely on the liver, but has glycogenolytic action on cardiac and skeletal muscle, has lipolytic action on adipose tissue, and promotes the breakdown of protein by several tissues. However, these latter effects appear to be more prominent when tissues are exposed to pharmacologic concentrations of glucagon. At more physiological concentration, the liver appears to be the major target tissue.

In many circumstances, the actions of glucagon antagonize those of insulin. Unlike the cellular mechanism of action of insulin, the mechanism of glucagon action is understood in considerable detail.

Pancreatic α Cells Secrete Glucagon in Response to Ingested Protein

Glucagon is a 31–amino-acid peptide (molecular weight approximately 3500) synthesized by α cells in the islets of Langerhans. In humans, the glucagon gene is located on chromosome 2. The initial gene product is the mRNA encoding preproglucagon. As is the case for insulin, a peptidase removes the signal sequence of preproglucagon during translation of the mRNA in the rough endoplasmic reticulum to yield proglucagon. Proteases in the α cells subse-

quently cleave the proglucagon (molecular weight, ~9000) into the mature glucagon molecule and several biologically active peptides (Fig. 50–11). Neuroendocrine cells (i.e., L cells) within the gut process the proglucagon differently to yield not glucagon, but GLP-1—a potent incretin—and other peptides.

PANCREATIC α CELLS. The mature glucagon molecule is the major secretory product of the α cell. Like insulin, the fully processed glucagon molecule is stored in secretory vesicles within the cell's cytosol. Although amino acids are the major secretagogues, the concentrations of amino acids required to provoke secretion of glucagon in vitro are higher than those generated in vivo. This observation suggests that other neural or humoral factors amplify the response in vivo, analogous to the effects of incretin on insulin secretion. Whereas glucose and several amino acids each stimulate insulin secretion by β cells, only amino acids stimulate glucagon secretion by α cells; glucose inhibits glucagon secretion. The signalling mechanism by which α cells recognize either amino acids or glucose is not known.

Glucagon, like the incretins, is a potent insulin secretagogue, but because most of the α cells are located downstream from the β cells (recall that the circulation of blood proceeds from the β cells and then out past the α cells), it is unlikely that glucagon exerts an important paracrine effect on insulin secretion.

INTESTINAL L CELLS. Proteases in neuroendocrine cells in the intestine process proglucagon differently than α cells do. L cells produce a peptide fragment called glicentin that contains the amino acid sequence of glucagon but does not bind to glucagon receptors. Downstream from the glucagon-coding region, the L cells generate two peptides from proglucagon called **glucagon-like peptides** 1 and 2 (GLP-1 and GLP-2). Each are "glucagon-like" in that they cross-react with some antisera directed to glucagon, but GLP-1 and GLP-2 have very weak biologic activity as glucagon analogs. However, GLP-1 is one of the most potent incretins and it stimulates insulin secretion. GLP-1 is released by the gut into the circulation in response to carbohydrate or protein ingestion. GLP-2 is not an incretin, and its biologic actions are not known.

FIGURE 50–12. Glucagon signal transduction. Glucagon generally antagonizes the effects of insulin in the liver. Glucagon binds to a $G_{\alpha s}$-coupled receptor, activating the adenylyl cyclase/cAMP/PKA cascade. Glucagon has three major effects on liver cells. First, glucagon promotes net glycogen breakdown. Glucagon inhibits glycogen synthesis by reducing the activity of **glucokinase** (1) and **glycogen synthase** (2). However, glucagon promotes glycogen breakdown by activating **glycogen phosphorylase** (3) and **glucose-6-phosphatase** (4). Second, glucagon promotes net gluconeogenesis. The hormone inhibits glycolysis and carbohydrate oxidation by reducing the activity **glucokinase** (1), **phosphofructokinase** (5), and **pyruvate kinase** (6). Glucagon also stimulates gluconeogenesis by increasing the activity of **phosphoenolpyruvate carboxykinase** (9), **fructose-1,6-bisphosphatase** (10), and **glucose-6-phosphatase** (4). Third, glucagon promotes the oxidation of fats. The hormone inhibits the activity of **acetyl-CoA carboxylase** (11). Glucagon indirectly stimulates fat oxidation because the decreased levels of malonyl CoA relieve the inhibition of malonyl CoA on **carnitine acyl-transferase** or CAT (13). The numbering scheme for these reactions is the same as that in Figure 50–8.

Glucagon, Acting Through cAMP, Promotes the Synthesis of Glucose by the Liver

Glucagon is an important regulator of hepatic glucose production and ketogenesis in the liver. As shown in Figure 50–12, glucagon binds to a receptor that activates the heterotrimeric G protein $G\alpha_s$, which stimulates membrane-bound adenylyl cyclase (p. 97). The cAMP formed by the cyclase in turn activates PKA, which phosphorylates a number of regulatory enzymes and other protein substrates, thus altering glucose and fat metabolism in the liver. Note that whereas insulin leads to the *dephosphorylation* of certain key enzymes (i.e., glycogen synthase, acetyl CoA carboxylase, phosphorylase), glucagon leads to their *phosphorylation*.

A particularly clear example of the opposing actions of

insulin and glucagon involves the activation of **glycogen-olysis**, which is discussed in Chapter 4 (see Fig 4–7). PKA phosphorylates the enzyme **phosphorylase kinase** (p. 98), thus increasing the latter's activity and allowing it to increase the phosphorylation of its substrate, **glycogen phosphorylase** *b*. The addition of a single phosphate residue to phosphorylase *b* converts it to phosphorylase *a*. Liver phosphorylase *b* has little activity in breaking the 1-4 glycosidic linkages of glycogen, but phosphorylase *a* is very active. In addition to converting phosphorylase *b* to the active phosphorylase *a* form, PKA also phosphorylates a peptide called **inhibitor I**. In its phosphorylated form, inhibitor I decreases the activity of the protein phosphatase that would normally convert phosphorylase *a* back to phosphorylase *b*. This same protein phosphatase is responsible for activating glycogen synthase. Thus, by phosphorylating inhibitor I, glucagon, acting through PKA, modulates several of the enzymes involved in hepatic glycogen metabolism to provoke *net glycogen breakdown*. As a result of similar actions on the pathways of gluconeogenesis and lipid oxidation, glucagon also stimulates these processes. Conversely, glucagon causes glycogen synthesis, glycolysis, and lipid storage to be restrained.

These actions of glucagon can be integrated with our understanding of insulin's action on the liver in a number of physiological circumstances. For example, after an overnight fast, when insulin concentrations are low, glucagon stimulates the liver to produce the glucose that is required by the brain and other tissues for their ongoing function. With ingestion of a protein meal, absorbed amino acids provoke insulin secretion, which can inhibit hepatic glucose production and promote glucose storage by liver and muscle (see earlier). If the meal lacked carbohydrate, the secreted insulin could cause hypoglycemia. However, glucagon secreted in response to a protein meal balances insulin's action on the liver and thus maintains glucose production and avoids hypoglycemia.

Glucagon Promotes the Oxidation of Fat in the Liver, Which Can Lead to the Formation of Ketone Bodies

Glucagon plays a major regulatory role in hepatic lipid metabolism. As we saw in our discussion of insulin (see Fig. 50–8), the liver can esterify free fatty acids with glycerol to form triglycerides, which it can store or export as VLDL particles. Alternatively, the liver can partially oxidize fatty acids—and form ketones—or fully oxidize them to CO_2 (p. 1220). Whereas fatty acid esterification and storage occur in the liver cytosol, oxidation and ketogenesis occur within the mitochondria.

Glucagon stimulates fat oxidation indirectly by increasing the activity of the **carnitine acyltransferase** (CAT) system, which mediates the transfer of fatty acids across the mitochondrial membrane. Glucagon produces this stimulation by inhibiting acetyl CoA carboxylase, which generates malonyl-CoA, the first committed intermediate in the synthesis of fatty acids by the liver. Malonyl-CoA is also an inhibitor of the CAT system. By inhibiting acetyl

CoA carboxylase, glucagon lowers the concentration of malonyl CoA, releases the inhibition of CAT, and allows fatty acids to be transferred into the mitochondria. These fatty acids are oxidized to furnish ATP to the liver cell. If the rate of fatty-acid transport into the mitochondria exceeds the need of the liver to phosphorylate ADP, the fatty acids will only be *partially oxidized*, and the keto acids (or "ketone bodies") **β-hydroxybutyric acid** and **acetoacetic acid** will accumulate. These keto acids can exit the mitochondria and the liver to be used by other tissues as oxidative fuel.

During fasting, the decline in insulin and the increase in glucagon promote ketogenesis; this process is of vital importance to the CNS, which can use keto acids but not free fatty acids as fuel. In the adaptation to fasting, glucagon therefore plays the important role of stimulating the conversion of fatty acids to ketones and therefore provides the brain with the fuel that is needed to allow continued function during a fast.

In addition to its effects on hepatic glucose and lipid metabolism, glucagon also has the extrahepatic actions of accelerating **lipolysis** in adipose tissue and **proteolysis** in muscle. However, these effects are generally demonstrable only with high concentrations of glucagon, and although they may be important in certain pathologic situations that are associated with greatly elevated glucagon concentrations (e.g., ketoacidosis or sepsis), they appear less important in the day-to-day actions of glucagon.

During Fasting, Falling Insulin Levels and Rising Glucagon Levels Promote the Conversion of Stored Fat to Ketone Bodies, and Promote Gluconeogenesis from Muscle Protein

Insulin and glucagon are the principal regulators of body fuel metabolism. The integrated secretion and action of insulin and glucagon are vital to fuel homeostasis. In humans, after an overnight fast, plasma [insulin] is low. The low [insulin] and the availability of glucagon result in the production of glucose by the liver from the breakdown of endogenous glycogen, as well as from the conversion of noncarbohydrate substrates into glucose (i.e., gluconeogenesis). These processes are highly regulated so that the rate at which glucose is produced by the liver matches the rate at which it is used by tissues, especially by the CNS. If the amount of glucose being provided by the liver is inadequate, plasma [glucose] will decline. The β cell, sensing this decrease, reduces the amount of insulin being secreted, whereas the α cell increases glucagon secretion. These two changes will increase glucose production by the liver and correct the plasma [glucose] toward normal. Conversely, if glucose is being overproduced and plasma [glucose] rises, insulin secretion increases and glucagon secretion is suppressed. Hepatic glucose production therefore declines and plasma [glucose] returns toward normal.

If fasting continues for several more days, insulin secretion continues to decline and glucagon secretion increases. The decline in insulin concentration allows an

DIABETES MELLITUS

Diabetes is the most common serious metabolic disease in humans. The hallmark of diabetes is an elevated blood glucose concentration, but this abnormality is just one of a number of biochemical and physiological alterations that occur. Diabetes is not one disorder, but can arise as a result of a number of defects in regulation of the synthesis, secretion, and action of insulin. The type of diabetes that most commonly affects children is called type 1 or **insulin-dependent diabetes mellitus** (IDDM). The diabetes that generally begins in adulthood and is particularly common in obese individuals is called type 2 or **non–insulin-dependent diabetes mellitus** (NIDDM).

TYPE 1 DIABETES

IDDM is caused by an immune-mediated selective destruction of the β cells of the pancreas. The other cell types present in the islet are spared. The consequence of the loss of insulin, with the preservation of glucagon, can be viewed as an accelerated form of fasting or starvation. A healthy person who is fasting for several days continues to secrete insulin at a low rate that is sufficient to balance the action of glucagon in modulating the production of glucose and ketones by the liver. However, with type 1 diabetes, insulin deficiency is severe and glucose and ketone production by the liver occur at a rate that greatly exceeds the rate at which they are being used. As a result, the concentration of these substances in blood begins to rise. Even when glucose concentrations reach levels 5 to 10 times normal, no insulin is secreted because β cells are absent. The increased glucose and ketones provide an immense solute load to the kidney that causes an osmotic diuresis. In addition, the keto acids that are produced are moderately strong organic acids (pK < 4.0), and their increased production causes a severe metabolic acidosis (p. 642). If these patients are not

treated with insulin, the acidosis and dehydration lead to death from **diabetic ketoacidosis.**

TYPE 2 DIABETES

With NIDDM, the cause of hyperglycemia is more complex. These individuals continue to make insulin. β Cells are not only present but are also frequently hyperplastic. For reasons still being defined, the β cells do not respond normally to increases in plasma glucose by increasing insulin secretion. However, altered insulin secretion is not the only problem. If we administer identical doses of insulin to the liver, muscle, and adipose tissue of a person with type 2 diabetes and a healthy control, we would find that the type 2 diabetic is resistant to the action of insulin. Thus both the metabolism of glucose in response to insulin and the secretion of insulin are abnormal in type 2 diabetics. Which problem—decreased insulin release or insulin resistance—is more important in provoking development of the diabetic state varies among individuals. Usually, these subjects make enough insulin—and it is sufficiently active—that the severe keto-acidosis described earlier for type 1 diabetic patients does not develop.

Persons with either type of diabetes appear to be at risk for chronic tissue damage from diabetes. These pathologic changes are a particular problem in the eyes, kidneys, and peripheral nerves. The problems appear to result, at least in part, from having the plasma glucose concentration elevated for a prolonged period. Recent studies have now shown that "tight" control of glucose in type 1 diabetics—use of frequent daily insulin injections or an insulin-infusion pump—can retard the development of these chronic complications, thus proving that it is the elevated glucose load itself that is probably responsible for much of the morbidity of this disease.

increased rate of proteolysis in muscle and mobilization of fatty acids from adipose tissue. The amino acids released by muscle serve as a substrate for hepatic gluconeogenesis. This response is particularly important after the first several days of fasting, when hepatic glycogen stores have been depleted and gluconeogenesis is the major pathway of hepatic glucose production. At the same time, the increased glucagon concentration stimulates ketogenesis in the liver and provides ketone bodies for the CNS. Ketones provide an alternative fuel source for the brain that allows the brain to decrease its use of glucose. Because most of the glucose comes from gluconeogenesis—and because the building blocks for gluconeogenesis come from accelerated proteolysis—the availability of ketone bodies allows the body to use the energy stored in fat and spare body protein. Because much of this body protein comes from the structural proteins in skeletal muscle and because catabolism of these proteins impairs muscle function (such as strength and mobility), it is a clear survival advantage to have the brain burn fat and not protein for fuel.

SOMATOSTATIN

Somatostatin Inhibits the Secretion of Growth Hormone, Insulin, and Other Hormones

Somatostatin is made in the δ cells of the pancreatic islets (see Fig. 50–1), as well as in the D cells of the gastrointestinal tract (p. 898), in the hypothalamus, and in a number of other sites in the CNS (p. 1026). It was first described as a hypothalamic peptide that *suppresses* the release of growth hormone—which had also been called somatotropin, thus accounting for the name "somatostatin." In both pancreatic δ cells and the hypothalamus, somatostatin exists as both 14– and 28–amino-acid peptides. In the hypothalamus, the 14–amino-acid form is predominant, whereas in the gastrointestinal tract (including the δ cells), the 28–amino-acid form predominates. The 14–amino acid form is the C-terminal portion of the 28–amino acid form. The biologic activity of somatostatin resides in these 14 amino acids.

Somatostatin inhibits the secretion of several hormones, including growth hormone, insulin, glucagon, gastrin, vasoactive intestinal peptide (VIP), and thyroid-stimulating hormone. Interestingly, the concentrations of somatostatin found in pancreatic venous drainage are sufficiently high to inhibit basal insulin secretion. Recall that blood flows from the center of each islet—which is where the bulk of the β cells are—to the periphery of the islet—which is where the δ cells tend to be located (see Fig. 50–1). This spatial arrangement minimizes the effect of somatostatin on the islet from which it is secreted. Whether somatostatin has important paracrine actions on some β cells or on α cells remains controversial.

The islet cells also make other peptides, for example, pancreatic polypeptide made in the F cells of the pancreas. Like insulin and glucagon, its secretion is altered by dietary intake of nutrients. However, whether pancreatic polypeptide has any actions in mammalian fuel metabolism is not clearly understood.

Occasionally, islet cell tumors may develop and secrete gastrin, VIP, growth hormone–releasing factor, or other hormones. Although these individual instances prove that these peptides can be made by islet tissue, they have no known normal function in the islet.

HYPOGLYCEMIA

Hypoglycemia, which can be viewed most simply as the opposite of diabetes mellitus, has many causes. Perhaps the most frequent setting is a patient with type 1 diabetes who skips a meal or fails to adjust the insulin dose when exercising. Many diabetic patients who seek to maintain tight control over their blood sugar suffer frequent hypoglycemic reactions, which they quickly learn to abort with a carbohydrate snack. Type 2 diabetic patients who take an excessive dose of sulfonylureas are subject to severe hypoglycemia, which may require continuous treatment for several days because the half-life of some of these drugs is quite long.

We saw in Chapter 49 that epinephrine—acting as a β-adrenergic agonist—is a hyperglycemic agent; that is, it promotes glycogenolysis in liver and muscle (p. 1064). Thus, β blockers can rarely cause hypoglycemia in healthy subjects, but commonly cause hypoglycemia in diabetic patients taking insulin. Another drug that can induce hypoglycemia is pentamidine, an agent used to treat *Pneumocystis carinii* pneumonia. Pentamidine is a β-cell toxin that leads to an acute, excessive release of insulin, which can be followed by hypoglycemia.

Alcoholic patients are at great risk for hypoglycemia. Ethanol suppresses gluconeogenesis, and hepatic glycogen stores may already be low because of poor nutrition. Other severe illnesses that can produce persistent hypoglycemia include liver disease, renal failure, and some large tumors that produce a hypoglycemia-inducing peptide, usually insulin-like growth factor type II. Rarely, an **insulinoma** may develop, which is an islet cell tumor (usually benign) that releases high and unregulated concentrations of insulin into the bloodstream.

Many individuals complain of postprandial hypoglycemia, frequently called "reactive hypoglycemia." Despite long years of skepticism, investigators now believe that at least some of these patients do indeed experience true symptoms of hypoglycemia within a few hours of eating. There is no absolute glucose level at which symptoms occur; many people can tolerate extremely low levels of glucose without any problems. However, a rather high *rate* of decline in the plasma glucose level after a meal may cause symptoms. One cause of postprandial hypoglycemia may be a delay in the timing of insulin release after a meal. Thus, the β cells release too much insulin too late after a meal, so the blood glucose level initially rises markedly and then rapidly falls. In some patients, this defect may herald the development of diabetes mellitus.

REFERENCES

Books and Reviews

Alberti KGMM, Zimmet P, DeFronzo RA: International Textbook of Diabetes Mellitus, 2nd ed. New York, Wiley, 1997.

Cryer PE, Polonsky KS: Glucose homeostasis and hypoglycemia. In Wilson JD, Foster DW, Kronenberg HM, Larsen PR (eds): Williams Textbook of Endocrinology, 9th ed. Philadelphia, WB Saunders, 1998, pp 939–971.

Jones PM, Persaud SJ: Protein kinases, protein phosphorylation, and the regulation of insulin secretion from pancreatic beta-cells. Endocr Rev 19:429-461, 1998.

Kimball SR, Vary TC, Jefferson LS: Regulation of protein synthesis by insulin. Annu Rev Physiol 56:321–348, 1994.

Poitout V, Robertson RP: An integrated view of beta-cell dysfunction in type-II diabetes. Annu Rev Med 47:69–83, 1996.

Journal Articles

Araki E, Lipes MA, Patti ME, et al: Alternative pathway of insulin signalling in mice with targeted disruption of the IRS-1 gene. Nature 372:186–190, 1994.

Bell GI, Pictet RL, Rutter WJ, et al: Sequence of the human insulin gene. Nature 284:26–32, 1980.

Cherrington AD: Banting Lecture 1997. Control of glucose uptake and release by the liver in vivo. Diabetes 48:1198–1214, 1999.

Gribble FM, Tucker SJ, Haug T, Ashcroft FM: MgATP activates the beta cell K_{ATP} channel by interaction with its SUR1 subunit. Proc Natl Acad Sci U S A 95:7185–7190, 1998.

Miki T, Nagashima K, Tashiro F, et al: Defective insulin secretion and enhanced insulin action in K_{ATP} channel–deficient mice. Proc Natl Acad Sci U S A 95:10402–10406, 1998.

Pilch PF, Czech MP: Hormone binding alters the conformation of the insulin receptor. Science 210:1152–1153, 1980.

CHAPTER 51

The Parathyroid Glands and Vitamin D

Eugene J. Barrett and Paula Barrett

The Gut, Kidneys, and Bone Regulate Calcium and Phosphate Balance

Calcium plays a critical role in many cellular processes, including hormone secretion, muscle contraction, nerve conduction, exocytosis, and the activation and inactivation of many enzymes. As described in Chapter 4 and elsewhere, Ca^{2+} also serves as an intracellular second messenger by carrying information from the cell membrane into the interior of the cell. It is therefore not surprising that the body very carefully regulates the plasma concentration of free ionized calcium ($[Ca^{2+}]$), the physiologically active form of the ion, and maintains plasma $[Ca^{2+}]$ within a narrow range (between 1.0 and 1.3 mM, or 4.0 and 5.2 mg/dl).

Phosphate is no less important. Because it is part of the adenosine triphosphate molecule, phosphate plays a critical role in cellular energy metabolism. It also plays crucial roles in the activation and deactivation of enzymes. However, unlike calcium, the plasma phosphate concentration is not very strictly regulated, and its levels fluctuate throughout the day, particularly after meals.

Calcium homeostasis and phosphate homeostasis are intimately tied to each other for two reasons. First, calcium and phosphate are the principal components of hydroxyapatite crystals $[Ca_{10}(PO_4)_6(OH)_2]$, which by far constitute the major portion of the mineral phase of bone. Second, they are regulated by the same hormones, primarily parathyroid hormone (PTH) and 1,25-dihydroxyvitamin D (calcitriol) and, to a lesser extent, the hormone calcitonin. These hormones act on three organ systems—the bone, the kidneys, and the gastrointestinal (GI) tract—to control the levels of these two ions in plasma. However, the actions of these hormones on calcium and phosphate are typically opposed in that a particular hormone may elevate the level of one ion while lowering that of the other.

Figure 51–1 and Figure 51–2 depict the overall daily balance of calcium and phosphate for a subject in a steady state.

CALCIUM BALANCE. Most calcium is located within bone, approximately 1 kg (see Fig. 51–1). The total amount of calcium in the extracellular pool is only a fraction of this amount, about 1 g or 1000 mg. The typical daily dietary intake of calcium is approximately 800 to 1200 mg. Dairy products are the major dietary source of calcium. Although the intestines absorb approximately one half the dietary calcium ($\sim$500 mg/day), they also secrete calcium for removal from the body ($\sim$325 mg/day), and, therefore, the *net* intestinal uptake of calcium is only approximately 175 mg/day. The

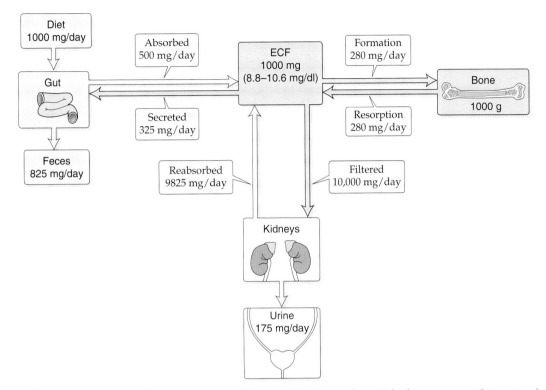

FIGURE 51–1. Calcium distribution and balance. Note that all values are for a 70-kg human, expressed in terms of elemental calcium. ECF, extracellular fluid.

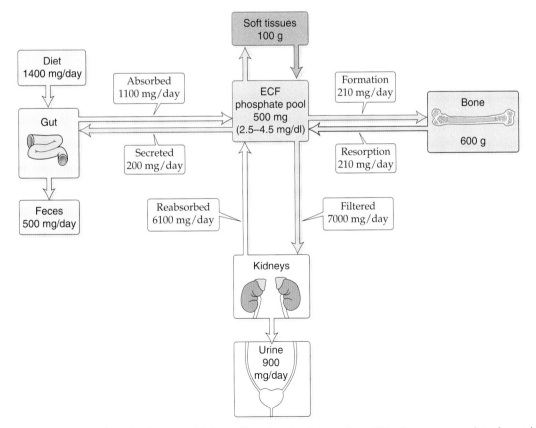

FIGURE 51–2. Phosphate distribution and balance. Note that all values are for a 70-kg human, expressed in elemental phosphorus. ECF, extracellular fluid.

second major organ governing calcium homeostasis is bone, where calcium deposition of about 280 mg/day is matched by an equal amount of calcium resorption in the steady state. The third organ system involved, the kidneys, filter about 10 times the total extracellular pool of calcium per day, about 10,000 mg/day. More than 98% of this Ca^{2+} is reabsorbed, and, therefore, the net renal excretion of Ca^{2+} is less than 2% of the filtered load (p. 807). In a person in Ca^{2+} balance, urinary excretion ($\sim$175 mg/day) is the same as net absorption by the GI tract.

In plasma, calcium exists in three physicochemical forms: (1) as a free ionized species, (2) bound to (more accurately, associated with) anionic sites on serum proteins (especially albumin), and (3) complexed with low-molecular-weight organic anions (e.g., citrate and oxalate). The **total concentration** of all three forms in the plasma is normally 2.2 to 2.7 mM (8.8 to 10.6 mg/dl). In healthy individuals, approximately 45% of calcium is free, 45% is bound to protein, and 10% is bound to small organic anions. The ionized form is the most important with regard to regulating the secretion of PTH and is involved in most of the biologic actions of calcium.

PHOSPHATE BALANCE. Most phosphate is also present in bone, approximately 0.6 kg of elemental phosphorus (see Fig. 51–2). A smaller amount of phosphorus (0.1 kg) exists in the soft tissues, mainly as organic phosphates such as phospholipids, phosphoproteins, nucleic acids, and nucleotides. An even smaller amount ($\sim$500 mg) is present in the extracellular fluid as inorganic phosphate. The daily dietary intake of phosphorus is typically 1400 mg, mostly as inorganic phosphate. Again, dairy products are the major source. The net absorption of phosphate by the intestines is approximately 900 mg/day. In the steady state, bone has relatively small phosphate turnover, about 210 mg/day. The kidneys filter approximately 14 times the total extracellular pool of phosphate per day ($\sim$7000 mg/day) and reabsorb about 6100 mg/day. Hence, the net renal excretion of phosphorus is around 900 mg/day, the same as the net absorption by the GI tract.

The concentration of total phosphate in plasma ranges from 0.8 to 1.5 mM (or 2.5 to 4.5 mg/dl of elemental phosphorus), a variation of 80%. Between 85% and 90% of the circulating phosphate is filterable by the kidneys, either ionized (50%) or complexed (40%), and only a small proportion (10% to 15%) is protein bound.

THE PHYSIOLOGY OF BONE

Dense Cortical Bone and the More Reticulated Trabecular Bone Are the Two Major Bone Types

Bone consists largely of an extracellular matrix composed of proteins and hydroxyapatite crystals, plus a small population of cells. The matrix provides strength and stability. The cellular elements continually remodel bone to accommodate growth and allow bone to reshape itself in response to varying loading stresses. Basically, bone has

three types of bone cells. **Osteoblasts** promote bone formation. **Osteoclasts** promote bone resorption and are found on the growth surfaces of bone. **Osteocytes** are found within the bony matrix and are derived from osteoblasts that have encased themselves within bone. They appear to play a role in the transfer of mineral from the interior of bone to the growth surfaces. Bone remodeling consists of a carefully coordinated interplay of osteoblastic and osteoclastic activity.

As shown in Figure 51–3, bone consists of two types of bone tissue. **Cortical** (also called "compact") bone represents about 80% of the total bone mass. Cortical bone is the outer layer (the cortex) of all bones and forms the bulk of the interior of the long bones of the body. It is a dense tissue composed mostly of bone mineral and extracellular matrix elements, interrupted only by penetrating blood vessels and a sparse population of osteocytes nested within the bone. These osteocytes are interconnected with one another and with the osteoblasts on the surface of the bone by canaliculi, through which the osteocytes extend cellular processes. These connections permit the transfer of Ca^{2+} from the interior of the bone to the surface, a process called *osteocytic osteolysis*. Dense cortical bone provides much of the strength for weight bearing by the long bones.

Trabecular (or **cancellous** or **medullary**) bone constitutes about 20% of the total bone mass. It is found in the interior of bones and is especially prominent within the vertebral bodies. It is composed of thin spicules of bone that extend from the cortex into the medullary cavity. The lacework of bone spicules is lined in many areas by osteoblasts and osteoclasts, the cells involved in bone remodeling. Trabecular bone is constantly being synthesized and resorbed by these cellular elements. Similar bone turnover occurs in cortical bone, but the fractional rate of turnover is much lower.

The Extracellular Matrix Forms the Nidus for the Nucleation of Hydroxyapatite Crystals

Collagen and the other extracellular matrix proteins that form the protein matrix of bone are called osteoid. **Osteoid** provides sites for the nucleation of hydroxyapatite crystals, the mineral component of bone. Osteoid is not a single compound, but a highly organized matrix of proteins synthesized principally by osteoblasts. Type I collagen accounts for approximately 90% of the protein mass of osteoid. It comprises a triple helix of two α1 monomers and one α2 collagen monomer. While they are still within the osteoblast, the monomers self-associate into the helical structure. After secretion from the osteoblast, the helices associate into collagen fibers; cross-linking of collagen occurs both within a fiber and between fibers. These collagen fibers are arranged in the osteoid in a highly ordered manner. The organization of collagen fibers is important for the tensile strength (i.e., the ability to resist stretch or bending) of bone. In addition to providing tensile strength, collagen also acts as a nidus for nucleation of bone mineralization. Within the collagen fibers, the crystals of hydroxyapatite are arranged with

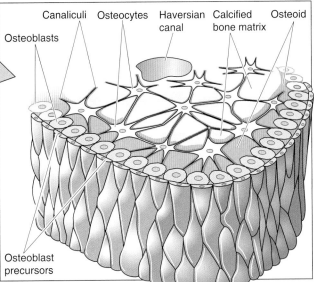

FIGURE 51–3. Cortical and trabecular bone. Under the periosteum is a layer of compact cortical bone that surrounds the more reticulated trabecular bone. The fundamental unit of cortical bone is the osteon, which is a tube-like structure that consists of a haversian canal, surrounded by ring-like lamellae. The *inset* shows a cross section through an osteon. The superficial osteogenic cells (osteoblast precursors) surround the osteoblasts, which secrete osteoid, a matrix of proteins that are the organic part of bone. Osteocytes are osteoblasts that have become surrounded by matrix. Canaliculi allow the cellular processes of osteocytes to communicate, via gap junctions, with each other and with osteoblasts on the surface. Trabecular bone has both osteoblasts and osteoclasts on its surface; this is where most bone remodeling takes place.

their long axis aligned with the long axis of the collagen fibers.

Several other osteoblast-derived proteins are important to the mineralization process, including osteocalcin and osteonectin. **Osteocalcin** is a 6-kDa protein synthesized by osteoblasts at sites of new bone formation. 1,25-Dihydroxyvitamin D induces the synthesis of osteocalcin. Osteocalcin has an unusual structure in that it possesses three γ-carboxylated glutamic acid residues. These residues are formed by posttranslation modification of glutamic acid by vitamin K–dependent enzymes. Like other proteins with γ-carboxylated glutamic acid, osteocalcin binds Ca²⁺ avidly. It binds hydroxyapatite, the crystalline mineral of bone, with even greater avidity. This observation has led to the suggestion that osteocalcin participates in the nucleation of bone mineralization at the crystal surface. **Osteonectin**, a 35-kDa protein, is another osteoblast product that binds to hydroxyapatite. It also binds to collagen fibers and facilitates the mineralization of collagen fibers in vitro. Additional proteins have been identified that appear likely to participate in the mineralization process. Some evidence indicates that the glycoproteins present extracellularly in bone may act to inhibit mineralization; removal of these glycoproteins may be necessary for bone formation to occur.

Bone Remodeling Depends on the Closely Coupled Activities of Osteoblasts and Osteoclasts

In addition to providing the proteins in osteoid, osteoblasts promote mineralization by exporting Ca^{2+} and phosphate from intracellular vesicles that have accumulated these minerals. Exocytosis of Ca^{2+} and phosphate raises the local extracellular concentration of these ions around the osteoblast to levels that are higher than in the bulk extracellular fluid, thus promoting crystal **nucleation** and growth (Fig. 51–4). Bone formation along spicules of trabecular bone appears to occur exclusively at sites of previous resorption by osteoclasts. The processes of bone resorption and synthesis are thus spatially "coupled."

Vitamin D and PTH stimulate osteoblastic cells to secrete factors—such as macrophage colony-stimulating factor (M-CSF)—that cause osteoclast precursors to proliferate (see Fig. 51–4). These precursors differentiate into mononuclear osteoclasts and then fuse to become multinucleated osteoclasts. **Osteoclasts** resorb bone in discrete areas adjacent to the "ruffled border" of the cell (Fig. 51–5). The osteoclast closely attaches to the bone matrix when integrins on its membrane attach to vitronectin in the bone matrix. The osteoclast—in reality a one-cell

FIGURE 51–4. Bone formation and resorption. Parathyroid hormone (PTH) and vitamin D stimulate osteoblastic cells to secrete factors such as M-CSF. This and other agents induce stem cells to differentiate into osteoclast precursors, mononuclear osteoclasts, and finally mature, multinucleated osteoclasts. Osteoblasts also secrete Ca^{2+} and inorganic phosphate, which nucleate on the surface of bone. PTH indirectly stimulates bone resorption by osteoclasts. Osteoclasts do not have PTH receptors. Instead, the PTH binds to receptors on osteoblasts and stimulates the release of factors, such as IL-6 and soluble RANK ligand, and the expression of membrane-bound RANK ligand. These factors promote bone resorption by osteoclasts. M-CSF, macrophage colony stimulating factor; IL, interleukin; P_i, inorganic phosphate.

epithelium—then secretes acid and proteases across its ruffled border membrane into a confined resorption space (the lacuna). The acid secretion is mediated by a V-type H^+ pump (p. 64) at the ruffled-border membrane. Abundant carbonic anhydrase provides the H^+. $Cl-HCO_3$ exchangers, located in the membrane on the opposite side of the osteoclast, remove the HCO_3^- that the carbonic anhydrase forms as a byproduct. The acidic environment beneath the osteoclast dissolves bone mineral, and acid proteases hydrolyze the matrix proteins. Having reabsorbed some of the bone in a very localized area, the osteoclast moves away from the pit or trough in the bone that it has created. Osteoblastic cells replace the osteoclast and now build new bone matrix and promote its mineralization.

A newly described protein called **osteoprotegerin ligand or RANK ligand** appears to be a major stimulator both of the differentiation of preosteoclasts to osteoclasts, and of the activity of mature osteoclasts. RANK ligand is a member of the tumor necrosis factor (TNF) cytokine family and exists both as a membrane-bound form on the surface of stromal cells and osteoblasts and as a soluble protein secreted by these same cells. RANK ligand binds to and stimulates a membrane-bound receptor of the osteoclast called **RANK** (receptor for activation of nuclear factor-κB), a member of the TNF receptor family. Osteoblastic and stromal cells also produce a soluble member of the TNF receptor family called **osteoprotegerin** (Latin for *osteo = bone + protegere = protect*). By binding

RANK ligand, osteoprotegerin protects the bone from osteoclastic activity. **Glucocorticoids** increase the production of RANK ligand by osteoblastic cells but decrease the production of osteoprotegerin. The net result is that more free RANK ligand is available to bind to RANK and thus promote bone loss. The precise role of these proteins in the development of various forms of osteoporosis and osteopetrosis is only beginning to be understood. However, the balance between the amounts of osteoprotegerin and RANK ligand produced by the osteoblast/stromal cell appears to be a very important factor.

PARATHYROID HORMONE

Plasma Ca^{2+} Regulates the Synthesis and Secretion of PTH

We have four parathyroid glands, two located on the posterior surface of the left lobe of the thyroid, and two more on the right. Combined, these four glands weigh less than 500 mg. They are composed largely of **chief cells**, which are responsible for the synthesis and secretion of PTH. These cells, like cells that secrete other peptide hormones, are highly specialized to synthesize, process, and secrete their product. The major regulator of PTH secretion is ionized plasma Ca^{2+}, although vitamin D also plays a role. Both inhibit the synthesis or release of PTH.

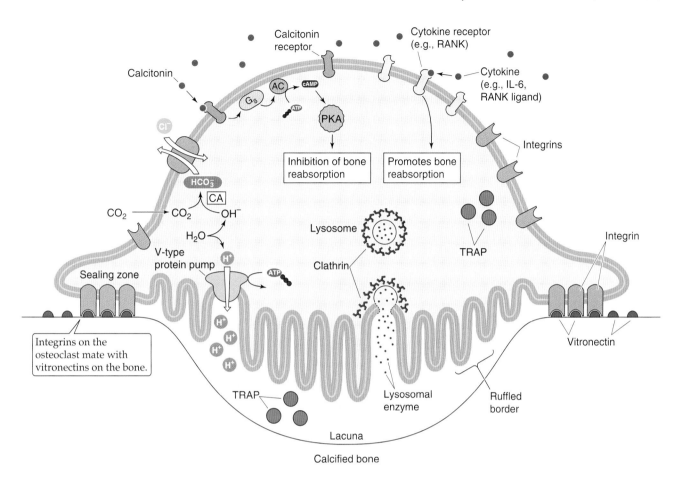

FIGURE 51–5. Bone resorption by the osteoclast. The osteoclast moves along the surface of bone and settles down sealing itself to the bone via integrins that bind to vitronectins on the bone surface. The osteoclast reabsorbs bone by secreting H^+ and acid proteases into the lacuna. Thus, the osteoclast behaves as a one-cell epithelium. The acid secretion is mediated by a V-type H^+ pump at the ruffled-border membrane facing the lacuna. Carbonic anhydrase (CA) in the cytosol supplies the H^+ to the H^+ pump and also produces HCO_3^- as a byproduct. Cl-HCO_3 exchangers—located on the membrane opposite the ruffled border—remove this HCO_3^-. AC, adenylyl cyclase; ATP, adenosine triphosphate; cAMP, cyclic adenosine monophosphate; IL, interleukin; PKA, protein kinase A; RANK, receptor for activation of NF-κB; TRAP, tartrate-resistant acid phosphatase.

PTH SYNTHESIS AND VITAMIN D. The PTH gene possesses upstream regulatory elements in the 5′ region, including both vitamin-D and vitamin-A response elements (p. 131). The vitamin-D response element binds a vitamin D receptor (VDR) when the receptor is occupied by a vitamin D metabolite, usually 1,25-dihydroxyvitamin D. The VDR is a member of the family of nuclear receptors, like the steroid hormone and thyroid hormone receptors. Like the thyroid hormone receptor, VDR forms a heterodimer with the retinoic acid X receptor (RXR) and acts as a transcription factor (see Table 5–2). The receptor has a very high affinity for the 1,25-dihydroxylated form of vitamin D ($K_d \sim 10^{-10}$ M), less affinity for the 25-hydroxy form ($K_d \sim 10^{-7}$ M), and little affinity for the parent vitamin (either D_2 or D_3, see later). Binding of the vitamin-D–VDR complex to the VDR response element *decreases* the rate of PTH transcription.

PROCESSING OF PTH. After transport of the mature PTH mRNA to the cytosol, PTH is synthesized on ribosomes of the rough endoplasmic reticulum (RER) and begins its journey through the secretory pathway (p. 36). PTH is transcribed as a pre-pro-PTH of 115 amino acids (Fig. 51–6). The 25–amino-acid "pre" fragment targets PTH for transport into the lumen of the endoplasmic reticulum. This signal sequence (p. 30) appears to be cleaved as the PTH enters the RER. During transit through the secretory pathway, the 90–amino-acid pro-PTH is further processed to the mature, active 84–amino-acid PTH. This cleavage appears quite efficient, and no pro-PTH appears in the storage granules. On the other hand, the breakdown of 1–84 or "intact" PTH into its N- and C-terminal fragments—which we discuss later—already starts in the secretory granules.

METABOLISM OF PTH. Once secreted, PTH circulates free in blood plasma and is rapidly metabolized; the half-life of 1–84 PTH is approximately 4 minutes. Beginning in the secretory granules inside the parathyroid chief cells and continuing in the circulation—predominantly in the liver—PTH is cleaved into two principal fragments, a 33– or 36–amino-acid N-terminal peptide and a larger

Pre-pro PTH
115 residues

FIGURE 51–6. Parathyroid hormone (PTH) synthesis. The synthesis of PTH begins with the production of pre-pro-PTH (115 amino acids) in the rough endoplasmic reticulum (ER). Cleavage of the signal sequence in the ER lumen yields pro-PTH (90 amino acids). During transit through the vesicular pathway, enzymes in the Golgi cleavage the "pro" sequence, yielding the mature or "intact" PTH (84 amino acids), which is stored in secretory granules. Beginning in the secretory granule, enzymes cleave PTH into two fragments. The N-terminal fragment is either 33 or 36 amino acids in length and contains all of the biologic activity.

C-terminal peptide (see Fig. 51–6). Virtually all of the known biologic activity of PTH resides in the N-terminal fragment, which is rapidly hydrolyzed, especially in the kidney. However, the half-life of the C-terminal fragment is much longer than that of either the N-terminal peptide or the intact 84–amino-acid PTH molecule. It is estimated that 70% to 80% of the PTH-derived peptide in the circulation is represented by the biologically inactive C-terminal fragment. The presence of a significant amount of antigenically recognized, but biologically inactive C-terminal fragments in the circulation has complicated the use of the usual radioimmunoassay methods for measuring PTH in both clinical and experimental settings. This problem was solved with the development of sensitive enzyme-linked immunosorbent assays that use two antibodies that react with two distinct sites on the PTH molecule. This method measures only the **intact PTH hormone** (i.e., 84 amino acids). These assays are invaluable in the diagnosis of disorders of PTH secretion, particularly when kidney function is impaired (a circumstance that further prolongs the half-life of the inactive C-terminal metabolites).

tration of ionized Ca^{2+} in the bathing medium, similar to the way that the parathyroid gland acts in vivo. Using an expression-cloning approach, investigators identified a Ca^{2+}-sensing receptor (CaSR) that resides in the plasma membrane of the parathyroid cell (Fig. 51–7A). This receptor binds Ca^{2+} in a saturable manner, with an affinity profile that is similar to the concentration dependence for PTH secretion. CaSR is a member of the G-protein–coupled receptor family (p. 92). Coupling of this Ca^{2+} receptor to $G\alpha_q$ activates phospholipase C, thus generating inositol 1,4,5-triphosphate (IP_3) and diacylglycerol (DAG) and resulting in the release of Ca^{2+} from internal stores and the activation of protein kinase C (PKC) (p. 100). Unlike most endocrine tissues, in which activation of these signalling systems promotes a secretory response, in the parathyroid, the rise in $[Ca^{2+}]_i$ and activation of PKC *inhibit* hormone secretion. (Another example is the granular cell of the juxtaglomerular apparatus, in which an increase in $[Ca^{2+}]_i$ inhibits secretion of renin; p. 867.) Thus, increasing levels of plasma $[Ca^{2+}]$ decrease PTH secretion (see Fig. 51–7B).

High Plasma [Ca²⁺] Inhibits the Synthesis and Release of Parathyroid Hormone

To a first approximation, and ignoring the contributions of vitamin D that are discussed later, regulation of PTH secretion by plasma Ca^{2+} appears to be a simple negative feedback loop. The major stimulus for PTH secretion is a *decline* in the concentration of Ca^{2+} in the blood (hypocalcemia) and extracellular fluid. Hypocalcemia also stimulates synthesis of new PTH, which is necessary because the parathyroid gland contains only enough PTH to maintain a stimulated secretory response for several hours.

The mechanism by which the parathyroid gland senses extracellular $[Ca^{2+}]$ and signals both the synthesis and secretion of PTH has only recently been clarified. Studies with cultured parathyroid chief cells have shown that these cells respond to very small decreases in the concen-

In Kidney and Bone, the Receptor Couples via G Proteins to Either Adenylyl Cyclase or Phospholipase C

The action of PTH to regulate plasma $[Ca^{2+}]$ appears to be secondary to its binding to the PTH 1R receptor. A second PTH receptor, PTH 2R, has been identified. However, its role, if any, in the regulation of plasma $[Ca^{2+}]$ is uncertain. Kidney and bone have the greatest abundance of PTH 1R receptors. Within the kidney, PTH 1R receptors are most abundant in the proximal and distal convoluted tubules. In bone, the osteoblast appears to be the important target cell. The PTH 1R receptor is a G-protein–linked receptor (p. 92). The PTH 1R receptor binds some N-terminal fragments of PTH (see Fig. 51–6), as well as the 1–84 intact PTH molecule. The PTH 1R receptor also binds parathyroid hormone–related peptide

A PARATHYROID Ca^{2+} RECEPTOR

B RESPONSE OF PARATHYROID GLAND TO CHANGES IN PLASMA [Ca^{2+}]

FIGURE 51–7. Parathyroid hormone (PTH) secretion and its dependence on ionized Ca^{2+} in the plasma. *A,* Four parathyroid glands lie on the posterior side of the thyroid. The chief cells synthesize, store, and secrete PTH. Increases in extracellular [Ca^{2+}] inhibit PTH secretion in the following manner: Ca^{2+} binds to a receptor that is coupled to a heterotrimeric G protein, Gα_q, which activates phospholipase C (PLC). This enzyme converts phosphoinositides (PIP$_2$) to inositol triphosphate (IP$_3$) and diacylglycerols (DAG). The IP$_3$ causes the release of Ca^{2+} from internal stores, whereas the DAG stimulates protein kinase C (PKC). Paradoxically, both the elevated [Ca^{2+}]$_i$ and the stimulated PKC inhibit release of granules containing PTH. Increased [Ca^{2+}]$_o$ also inhibits PTH synthesis. Thus, increased levels of plasma Ca^{2+} lower PTH release, and thus tend to lower plasma [Ca^{2+}]. *B,* Small decreases in *free* plasma [Ca^{2+}] greatly increase the rate of PTH release. About half of the total plasma Ca^{2+} is free. In patients with familial hypocalciuric hypercalcemia (FHH), the curve is shifted to the right; that is, plasma [Ca^{2+}] must rise to higher levels before inhibiting PTH secretion. As a result, the patients have normal PTH levels, but elevated plasma [Ca^{2+}]. ER, endoplasmic reticulum.

(PTHrP), which is discussed later. In contrast, the PTH 2R receptor is selectively activated by PTH.

The PTH 1R receptor appears to be coupled to two heterotrimeric G proteins and thus to two signal-transduction systems. Binding of PTH to the receptor stimulates Gα_s, which in turn activates **adenylyl cyclase** and thus releases cyclic adenosine monophosphate (cAMP) and stimulates protein kinase A (p. 97). The activated PTH receptor also stimulates Gα_q, which in turn stimulates **phospholipase C** to generate IP$_3$ and DAG (p. 100). The IP$_3$ releases Ca^{2+} from internal stores, thus increasing [Ca^{2+}]$_i$ and activating Ca^{2+}-dependent kinases. In humans, the bone PTH receptor on osteoblastic cells is identical with that present in renal cortical cells.

As discussed in the next two sections, the net effects of PTH on the kidney and bone are to increase plasma [Ca^{2+}] and lower plasma [phosphate].

In the Kidney, PTH Promotes Ca^{2+} Reabsorption, Phosphate Loss, and 1-Hydroxylation of 25-Hydroxyvitamin D

PTH exerts a spectrum of actions on target cells in the kidney (Fig. 51–8). In the renal proximal tubule, PTH receptors are located on the basolateral membrane of the polarized epithelial cell. Binding of PTH to its receptors

activates dual intracellular signalling systems and in this manner modifies several properties of the cell related to transepithelial transport.

STIMULATION OF Ca^{2+} REABSORPTION. A key action of PTH is to promote the reabsorption of Ca^{2+} in the thick ascending limb (TAL) and distal convoluted tubule of the kidney (p. 809). Most of the approximately 250 mmoles of Ca^{2+} filtered each day is reabsorbed in the proximal tubule (~65%) and TAL (~25%). The distal nephron is responsible for reabsorbing an additional 5% to 10% of the filtered load of Ca^{2+}, with about 0.5% of the filtered load left in the urine. Thus, when PTH stimulates distal Ca^{2+} reabsorption, it will greatly decrease the amount of Ca^{2+} that is excreted in the urine (usually 4 to 5 mmoles/day) and tend to raise plasma [Ca^{2+}] (see Fig. 51–8).

Greater fractional Ca^{2+} excretion occurs when either proximal or distal Ca^{2+} reabsorption is impaired, as occurs with osmotic diuresis and hypoparathyroidism, respectively. As discussed later, vitamin D has a synergistic action of promoting Ca^{2+} reabsorption in the distal convoluted tubule.

INHIBITION OF PHOSPHATE REABSORPTION. Most strikingly, PTH reduces the reabsorption of phosphate in both the proximal and distal tubule. Because most of the phosphate reabsorption occurs in the proximal tubule and

FAMILIAL HYPOCALCIURIC HYPERCALCEMIA

The Ca²⁺ receptor on the parathyroid cell is mutated in patients with the disorder **familial hypocalciuric hypercalcemia** (FHH). Serum calcium in these patients is typically elevated 10% to 30% above the normal range. These patients generally tolerate this elevated plasma [Ca²⁺] very well, and the finding of a total plasma Ca²⁺ of 3.0 to 3.3 mM (12 to 13 mg/dl)—the normal range is 2.2 to 2.7 mM (8.8 to 10.6 mg/dl)—is frequently more alarming to the physician than to the patient! Despite a plasma [Ca²⁺] that would make most people symptomatic with kidney stones, fatigue, or loss of mental concentration, these patients have remarkably few symptoms. The amount of calcium present in their urine is typically less than that seen in normal individuals (hence the designation "hypocalciuric") and much lower than that encountered in persons with hypercalcemia of other causes. Despite the high plasma [Ca²⁺], their serum parathyroid hormone (PTH) concentrations are typically normal. The normal PTH concentration suggests that regulation of PTH secretion is intact but the "set-point" at which the Ca²⁺ turns off PTH secretion is shifted toward higher plasma [Ca²⁺] (see Fig. 51–7B).

There appears to be only one allele for the Ca²⁺-sensing receptor (CaSR). FHH is an autosomal dominant disorder, and several different point mutations have been identified in different families. *Heterozygotes* express both normal and mutated Ca²⁺ receptors. Rarely, infants are born with the *homozygous* disorder (i.e., both copies of the receptor are defective). These infants have very severe hypercalcemia ([calcium], >15 mg/dl) and severe hyperparathyroidism. The condition is life threatening and characterized by markedly elevated plasma [Ca²⁺], neuronal malfunction, demineralization of bone, and calcification of soft tissues. These infants die unless the inappropriately regulated parathyroid glands are removed.

As in the case of the parathyroid gland, the distal convoluted tubule of the kidney has abundant the plasma membrane Ca²⁺ receptors. It has been suggested that serum Ca²⁺ binds to this renal Ca²⁺ receptor and inhibits Ca²⁺ reabsorption (p. 810). Thus, with a mutated receptor, renal Ca²⁺ reabsorption may not be inhibited until plasma [Ca²⁺] rises to abnormally high levels. The result would be the increased calcium reabsorption and hypocalciuria characteristic of FHH.

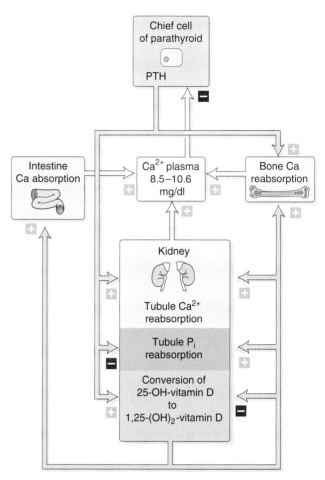

FIGURE 51–8. Feedback loops in the control of plasma Ca²⁺ levels. Parathyroid hormone (PTH) released from the parathyroid glands acts via receptors in both bone and kidney. **In kidney,** PTH has three effects. First, PTH promotes Ca²⁺ reabsorption and, thus, an increase in plasma [Ca²⁺]. Second, PTH inhibits phosphate reabsorption. Third, PTH promotes the hydroxylation of 25-hydroxy-vitamin D, creating the active metabolite 1,25-dihydroxy-vitamin D. This metabolite further promotes renal Ca²⁺ reabsorption. **In bone,** PTH promotes net bone reabsorption and, thus, an increase in plasma [Ca²⁺]. **In intestine,** the 1,25-dihydroxy-vitamin D (produced indirectly as the result of PTH) enhances Ca²⁺ absorption. Thus, net effect on bone, kidney, and gut, as far as Ca²⁺ is concerned, is to increase plasma [Ca²⁺]. The increased plasma [Ca²⁺] feeds back on the parathyroid glands, inhibiting the release of PTH.

because the effect of PTH is greatest on the proximal tubule, PTH produces a characteristic phosphaturia and tends to decrease plasma phosphate levels (see Fig. 51–8). This phosphaturia results from a PTH-induced redistribution of the Na/phosphate cotransporter (NaPi) away from the apical membrane of the renal proximal tubule and into a pool of subapical vesicles (p. 805). As discussed later, PTH stimulates bone to resorb calcium and phosphate from the hydroxyapatite crystals of bone mineral. Thus, PTH stimulates both steps in the movement of phosphate from bone to blood to urine.

Elimination of phosphate via urine plays an important

role when elevated levels of PTH liberate Ca²⁺ and phosphate from bone. At normal plasma Ca²⁺ and phosphorus concentrations, the calcium-phosphate ion product approaches the solubility product. Further PTH-induced increases in [Ca²⁺]—if accompanied by a rise in phosphate levels—could cause calcium phosphate salts to precipitate out of the soluble phase, at least partly negating the action of PTH to raise plasma [Ca²⁺]. Thus, PTH-induced phosphaturia diminishes the calcium-phosphate ion product and thus prevents precipitation when calcium mobilization is needed. It is perhaps worthwhile to recall that the body tightly regulates plasma [Ca²⁺] but allows plasma levels of phosphate to vary rather widely.

In addition to affecting phosphate reabsorption, PTH causes a decrease in proximal-tubule reabsorption of HCO₃⁻ (p. 854) and several amino acids. These actions appear to play a relatively minor role in whole-body acid-base and nitrogen metabolism, respectively.

STIMULATION OF THE LAST STEP OF SYNTHESIS OF 1,25-DIHYDROXYVITAMIN D. A third important renal action of PTH is to stimulate the 1-hydroxylation of 25-hydroxyvitamin D in the mitochondria of the proximal tubule. The resulting 1,25-dihydroxyvitamin D is the most biologically active metabolite of dietary or endogenously produced vitamin D. Its synthesis by the kidney is highly regulated, and PTH is the primary stimulus to increase 1-hydroxylation. Hypophosphatemia, either spontaneous or induced by PTH's phosphaturic action, also promotes the production of 1,25-dihydroxyvitamin D. As discussed later, the 1,25-dihydroxyvitamin D formed in the proximal tubule has three major actions: (1) enhancement of renal Ca^{2+} reabsorption, (2) enhancement of Ca^{2+} absorption by the small intestine, and (3) modulation of the movement of Ca^{2+} and phosphate in and out of bone.

In Bone, Parathyroid Hormone Promotes Net Resorption

INDIRECT STIMULATION OF OSTEOCLASTS. The second major target tissue for PTH is bone, where PTH promotes both bone resorption and bone synthesis. However, the net effect of PTH on bone is to stimulate bone *resorption*, thus increasing plasma $[Ca^{2+}]$. Osteoblasts express abundant surface receptors for PTH; osteoclasts do not. Because osteoclasts lack PTH receptors, PTH by itself cannot regulate the coupling between osteoblasts and osteoclasts. Rather, it appears that PTH acts on osteoblasts and osteoclast precursors to induce the production of several cytokines that increase both the number and the activity of bone-resorbing osteoclasts. Precisely which cytokines are involved in the physiological signalling of osteoclasts by PTH-stimulated osteoblasts in vivo is not clear. PTH causes osteoblasts to release agents such as M-CSF and stimulate the expression of RANK ligand (i.e., osteoprotegerin ligand), which promote the development of osteoclasts (see Fig. 51–4). In addition, PTH and vitamin D stimulate osteoblasts to release interleukin-6 (IL-6), which stimulates existing osteoclasts to resorb bone (see Fig. 51–5).

One of the initial clues that cytokines are important mediators of osteoclastic bone resorption came from observations on patients with multiple myeloma—a malignancy of plasma cells, which are of B lymphocyte lineage. The tumor cells produce several proteins that activate osteoclasts and enhance bone resorption. These proteins were initially called "osteoclast-activating factors." We now know that a number of lymphocyte-derived proteins strongly activate osteoclastic bone resorption; these proteins include lymphotoxin, IL-1, and TNF-α.

REDUCTION IN BONE MATRIX. PTH also changes the behavior of osteoblasts in a manner that promotes net bone resorption. For example, PTH inhibits collagen synthesis by osteoblasts and also promotes the production of proteases that digest bone matrix. Digestion of matrix is important because osteoclasts do not easily reabsorb bone mineral if the bone has an overlying layer of unmineralized osteoid.

PROMOTION OF BONE SYNTHESIS. So far, we have seen that PTH promotes bone resorption. However, PTH also promotes bone synthesis, although to a lesser extent. First, PTH promotes bone synthesis *directly* by activating Ca^{2+} channels in osteocytes, which leads to a net transfer of Ca^{2+} from bone fluid to the osteocyte. The osteocyte then transfers this Ca^{2+} via gap junctions to the osteoblasts at the bone surface. This process is called *osteocytic osteolysis*. The osteoblasts then pump this Ca^{2+} into the extracellular matrix, thus contributing to mineralization. Second, PTH stimulates bone synthesis *indirectly* in that osteoclastic bone resorption leads to the release of growth factors such as insulin-like growth factor I (IGF-I), IGF-II, and transforming growth factor β.

VITAMIN D

The Active Form of Vitamin D Is Its 1,25-Dihydroxy Metabolite

By the 1920s, it was recognized that dietary deficiency of a fat-soluble vitamin was responsible for the childhood disease **rickets**. This disorder is characterized clinically by hypocalcemia and multiple skeletal abnormalities. Dietary replacement of vitamin D corrects this disorder and has led to the practice of adding vitamin D to milk, bread, and other products. This practice has greatly reduced the prevalence of this previously common disorder.

Our understanding of how vitamin D is involved in the regulation of plasma $[Ca^{2+}]$ and skeletal physiology has been clarified only over the past two decades. Vitamin D exists in the body in two forms, vitamin D_3 and vitamin D_2 (Fig. 51–9). **Vitamin D_3** can be synthesized from the 7-dehydrocholesterol that is present in the skin, provided that sufficient ultraviolet light is absorbed. This observation explains why nutritional rickets had been a much more prevalent problem in northern countries, where clothing covers much of the skin and where individuals remain indoors much more of the year. Vitamin D_3 is also available from a number of natural sources, including cod and halibut liver, eggs, and fortified milk. **Vitamin D_2** is obtained only from the diet, largely from vegetables. Vitamins D_3 (see Fig. 51–9A) and D_2 (see Fig. 51–9B) differ only in the side chains of ring D. The side chain in vitamin D_3 (cholecalciferol) is characteristic of cholesterol, whereas that of vitamin D_2 (ergocalciferol) is characteristic of plant sterols.

Vitamin D (i.e., either D_2 or D_3) is fat soluble, but water insoluble. Its absorption from the intestine depends on its solubilization by bile salts (p. 964). In the circulation, vitamin D is found either solubilized with chylomicrons (p. 998) or associated with a plasma binding protein. Most of the body stores of vitamin D are located in body fat. The body's pools of vitamin D are large, and only 1% to 2% of the body's vitamin D is turned over each day. Therefore, several years of very low dietary intake (as well as diminished endogenous synthesis) is required before the endogenous pools are depleted and deficiency develops.

The principal active form of vitamin D is not vitamin D_2 or D_3, but rather a dihydroxylated metabolite of either.

A METABOLISM OF VITAMIN D₃

7–Dehydrocholesterol

Skin ↓ UV light

Cholecalciferol (Vitamin D₃)

Liver ↓

25–Hydroxycholecalciferol (25–OHD₃)

Kidney ↓

1,25–(OH)₂D₃

B VITAMIN D₂

Ergocalciferol (Vitamin D₂)

FIGURE 51–9. Forms of vitamin D.

Hydroxylation of vitamin D proceeds in two steps (see Fig. 51–9A). When circulating levels of 25-hydroxyvitamin D are low, adipocytes release vitamin D into the blood plasma. A cytochrome P-450 mixed-function oxidase, principally in the liver, creates the first hydroxyl group at carbon 25. The 25-hydroxylation of vitamin D does not appear to be highly regulated, but depends on the availability of vitamin D₂ or D₃. The second hydroxylation reaction occurs in the renal proximal tubule under the tight control of PTH, vitamin D itself, and phosphate. PTH stimulates this 1-hydroxylation, whereas phosphate and 1,25-dihydroxyvitamin D (the reaction product) both inhibit the process (see Fig. 51–8).

In addition to vitamins D₂ and D₃ and their respective 25-hydroxy and 1,25-dihydroxy metabolites, more than 15 other metabolites of vitamin D have been identified in plasma. However, the specific physiological function of these metabolites, if any, is unclear.

Although considered a vitamin because of its dietary requirement, vitamin D can also be considered a hormone, both because it is endogenously synthesized and because even the fraction that arises from the diet must be metabolized to a biologically active form.

Vitamin D and its metabolites, like the steroid hormones, circulate bound to a globulin binding protein, in this case a 52-kDa vitamin-D–binding protein. This binding protein appears particularly important for the carriage in the blood of vitamins D₂ and D₃, which are less soluble than their hydroxylated metabolites. Vitamin D and its metabolites arrive at target tissues and, once in the cytosol, associate with the vitamin-D receptor, a transcription factor that is in the family of nuclear receptors (p. 112). Like the thyroid hormone receptor (Table 5–2), VDR forms a heterodimer with RXR. The VDR specifically recognizes the 1,25-dihydroxyvitamin D with an affinity that is three orders of magnitude higher than that for 25-hydroxyvitamin D. However, because the circulating concentration of 25-hydroxyvitamin D is approximately 1000-fold higher than that of 1,25-dihydroxyvitamin D, both species probably contribute to the biologic actions of the hormone.

The biologic actions of 1,25-dihydroxyvitamin D appear to be expressed principally, but not exclusively via regulation of the transcription of a variety of proteins. The VDR/RXR complex associates with a regulatory site in the promoter region of the genes coding for a number of vitamin-D–regulated proteins. Thus, the occupied VDR alters the synthesis of these vitamin-D–dependent proteins. An example is PTH, which stimulates the formation of 1,25-dihydroxyvitamin D. The 5′ regulatory region of the PTH gene has a VDR consensus sequence; when occupied by the VDR complex, this element *diminishes* transcription of the PTH gene.

Vitamin D, By Acting on the Small Intestine and Kidney, Raises Plasma [Ca²⁺] and Thus Promotes Bone Mineralization

The actions of vitamin D can be grouped into two categories: actions on classic target tissues involved in regulating body mineral and skeletal homeostasis and a more general action that regulates cell growth. The actions of vita-

FIGURE 51–10. Intestinal absorption of Ca^{2+} and phosphate. *A,* The small intestine absorbs Ca^{2+} by two mechanisms. The passive, paracellular absorption of Ca^{2+} occurs throughout the small intestine. This pathway is the predominant one but is *not* under the control of vitamin D. The second mechanism—the active, transcellular absorption of Ca^{2+}—occurs only in the duodenum. Ca^{2+} enters the cell across the apical membrane via a channel. Inside the cell, the Ca^{2+} is buffered by binding proteins, such as calbindin, and is also taken up into intracellular organelles, such as the ER. The enterocyte then extrudes Ca^{2+} across the basolateral membrane via a Ca^{2+} pump and an Na-Ca exchanger. Thus, the net effect is Ca^{2+} absorption. The active form of vitamin D— 1,25-dihydroxyvitamin D—stimulates all three steps of transcellular Ca^{2+} absorption. *B,* Inorganic phosphate enters the enterocyte across the apical membrane via an Na/P_i (NaPi) cotransporter. Once inside the cell, the P_i is extruded across the basolateral membrane. Thus, the net effect is P_i absorption. ATP, adenosine triphosphate; mRNA, messenger RNA; P_i, inorganic phosphate.

min D on the small intestine, bone, and kidney serve to prevent any abnormal decline or rise in plasma $[Ca^{2+}]$.

SMALL INTESTINE. In the duodenum, 1,25-dihydroxyvitamin D increases the production of several proteins that enhance Ca^{2+} absorption. Figure 51–10*A* summarizes the intestinal absorption of Ca^{2+} (p. 971). Ca^{2+} moves from the intestinal lumen to the blood by both paracellular and transcellular routes. In the paracellular route, which occurs throughout the small intestine, Ca^{2+} moves *passively* from the lumen to the blood; 1,25-dihydroxyvitamin D does *not* regulate this pathway. The transcellular route, which occurs only in the duodenum, involves three steps. First, Ca^{2+} enters the cell across the apical membrane via Ca^{2+} channels and possibly endocytosis. Second, the en-

tering Ca^{2+} binds to several high-affinity binding proteins, particularly **calbindin**. These proteins, together with the exchangeable calcium pools in the endoplasmic reticulum and mitochondria, effectively buffer the cytosolic calcium and maintain a favorable gradient for Ca^{2+} entry across the apical membrane of the enterocyte. Thus, the intestinal cell solves the problem of absorbing relatively large amounts of Ca^{2+} while keeping its free, cytosolic $[Ca^{2+}]$ low. Third, the enterocyte extrudes Ca^{2+} across the basolateral membrane by means of both a Ca^{2+} pump and an Na-Ca exchanger.

Vitamin D promotes Ca^{2+} absorption primarily by genomic effects that involve induction of the synthesis of Ca^{2+} channels and pumps and Ca^{2+}-binding proteins, as well as other proteins (e.g., alkaline phosphatase). Although these actions probably facilitate Ca^{2+} transport by the intestine, not all steps involved in vitamin D's action to enhance transcellular Ca^{2+} transport have been well defined experimentally.

The effect of PTH to stimulate intestinal Ca^{2+} absorption is thought to be entirely indirect and mediated by increasing the renal formation of 1,25-dihydroxyvitamin D (see Fig. 51–8), which then enhances Ca^{2+} absorption.

Vitamin D also stimulates phosphate absorption by the small intestine (see Fig. 51–10*B*). The initial step is mediated by the NaPi cotransporter (p. 805) and appears to be rate limiting for transepithelial transport and subsequent delivery of phosphate to the circulation. 1,25-Dihydroxyvitamin D stimulates the synthesis of this transport protein and thus promotes phosphate entry into the mucosal cell.

KIDNEY. In the kidney, vitamin D appears to act synergistically with PTH to enhance *Ca^{2+} reabsorption* in the distal convoluted tubule (p. 810). High-affinity Ca^{2+}-binding proteins, similar to those found in the intestinal mucosa, have been specifically localized to this region of the kidney. It appears that PTH is a more potent regulator of Ca^{2+} reabsorption than vitamin D is (see Fig. 51–8). Indeed, parathyroidectomy increases the fractional excretion of Ca^{2+}, and even high doses of vitamin D cannot correct this effect. In addition, as in the intestine, vitamin D promotes *phosphate reabsorption* in the kidney. The effects of vitamin D on phosphate reabsorption, like its effects on Ca^{2+}, are less dramatic than those of PTH. Finally, 1,25-dihydroxyvitamin D directly inhibits the *1-hydroxylation* of vitamin D.

BONE. The actions of vitamin D on bone are complex and are the result of both indirect and direct actions. The overall effect of vitamin D replacement in animals with dietary-induced vitamin D deficiency is to increase the flux of Ca^{2+} into bone. However, as we will see later, these major effects of vitamin D on bone are *indirect*: vitamin D's action on both the small intestine and kidneys makes more Ca^{2+} available to mineralize previously unmineralized osteoid. The *direct* effect of vitamin D on bone is to *mobilize Ca^{2+} out of bone*. Both osteoblasts and osteoclast precursor cells have VDRs. In response to vitamin D, osteoblasts produce a number of proteins, including alkaline phosphatase, collagenase, and plasminogen activator. In addition, as noted earlier (see Fig. 51–4), vitamin D and PTH promote the development of osteoclasts from precursor cells. Thus, because vitamin D directly increases the *number* of mature osteoclasts, supplying vitamin D to bone obtained from vitamin-D–deficient animals in in vitro experiments, mobilizes Ca^{2+} from bone into the medium. Additional evidence that vitamin D directly promotes bone resorption comes from experiments on rachitic animals who are maintained on a Ca^{2+}-deficient diet. Treating these animals with vitamin D causes plasma $[Ca^{2+}]$ to rise, an indication of net bone resorption. At the same time, however, the elevated plasma $[Ca^{2+}]$ promotes the mineralization of previously unmineralized osteoid—at the expense of bone resorption from other sites.

The direct effects of vitamin D on bone, which are to mobilize Ca^{2+}, seem to be contrary to the overall effect of vitamin D on bone, which is to promote mineralization. These observations, as well as others, have led to the hypothesis, now generally accepted, that the antirachitic action of vitamin D is largely indirect. By enhancing the absorption of Ca^{2+} and phosphate from the intestine and by enhancing the reabsorption of Ca^{2+} and phosphate from the renal tubules, vitamin D raises the concentrations of both Ca^{2+} and phosphate in the blood and extracellular fluid. This increase in the calcium-phosphate ion product results in net bone mineralization. These indirect effects overshadow the direct effect of vitamin D to increase bone mobilization.

RICKETS AND OSTEOMALACIA

Deficiency of vitamin D in *children* produces the disease **rickets,** in which bone has abnormal amounts of unmineralized osteoid. Both cortical and trabecular bone are involved. The lack of mineralization diminishes bone rigidity and leads to a characteristic "bowing" of the long bones of the legs. In *adults,* vitamin D deficiency produces a disorder called **osteomalacia.** Microscopically, the bone looks very much the same in adult and childhood vitamin D deficiency. However, because the longitudinal growth of the long bones has been completed in adults, bowing of weight-bearing bones does not occur. Instead, the increased unmineralized osteoid content of bone causes a decline in bone strength. Affected individuals are more prone to the development of bone fractures. These fractures may be very small and difficult to see radiographically. As more and more of the bone surface is covered by osteoid and as recruitment of new osteoclasts is diminished, osteoclastic bone resorption is impaired and hypocalcemia develops. Hypocalcemia causes nerves to become more sensitive to depolarization. In sensory nerves, this effect leads to sensations of numbness, tingling, or burning; in motor nerves, it leads to increased spontaneous contractions, or tetany.

This same sequence of events can occur on a genetic basis when the kidney is impaired in its ability to 1-hydroxylate the 25-hydroxyvitamin D previously synthesized in the liver. An acquired version is seen in many patients with chronic renal failure, in which the activity of 1α-hydroxylase is reduced. The genetic form of the 1α-hydroxylase deficiency is a rare autosomal recessive disorder. It is called vitamin D–dependent rickets because it can be successfully treated with either 1,25-dihydroxyvitamin D or higher doses of dietary vitamin D_2 or vitamin D_3 (approximately 10- to 100-fold) than the 400 U/day used to prevent nutritional rickets.

Ca²⁺ Ingestion Lowers Levels of PTH and 1,25-Dihydroxyvitamin D, Whereas Phosphate Ingestion Raises Levels of Both PTH and 1,25-Dihydroxyvitamin D

Consider a situation in which a subject ingests a meal containing Ca^{2+}. The rise in plasma $[Ca^{2+}]$ inhibits PTH secretion. The decline in PTH causes a decrease in the resorption of Ca^{2+} and phosphorus from bone, thus limiting the postprandial increase in plasma Ca^{2+} and phosphate levels. In addition, the decrease in PTH diminishes Ca^{2+} reabsorption in the kidney and thus facilitates a calcuric response. If dietary Ca^{2+} intake remains high, the lower PTH will result in decreased 1-hydroxylation of 25-hydroxyvitamin D, which will eventually diminish the fractional absorption of Ca^{2+} from the GI tract.

If dietary Ca^{2+} intake is deficient, the body will attempt to restore Ca^{2+} toward normal by increasing plasma [PTH]. This response will help mobilize Ca^{2+} from bone, promote renal Ca^{2+} retention, and over time, increase the level of 1,25-dihydroxyvitamin D, which will enhance gut absorption of Ca^{2+}.

If one ingests phosphorus much in excess of Ca^{2+} (e.g., after drinking several colas), the rise in plasma [phosphate] will lower plasma $[Ca^{2+}]$ because the increased plasma calcium-phosphate ion product will promote the deposition of mineral in bone. The resultant decrease in plasma $[Ca^{2+}]$ will in turn increase PTH secretion. This rise in PTH will provoke a phosphaturia that will act to restore plasma [phosphate] toward normal while Ca^{2+} and phosphate are mobilized from bone by the action of PTH. Over longer time periods, the action of PTH to modulate the 1-hydroxylation of 25-hydroxyvitamin D plays an increasingly important role in defending the plasma $[Ca^{2+}]$ by increasing intestinal Ca^{2+} absorption.

CALCITONIN AND OTHER HORMONES

Calcitonin Inhibits Osteoclasts, But It Does Not Appear to be Physiologically Important in Humans

Calcitonin is a 32–amino-acid peptide hormone made by the "clear" or C cells of the thyroid gland. C cells (also called parafollicular cells) are derived from neural crest cells of the fifth branchial pouch, which in humans migrate into the evolving thyroid gland. Although it is located within the thyroid, calcitonin's major, if not sole biologic action relates to the regulation of mineral metabolism and bone turnover. The incidental nature of its relationship to the major functions of the thyroid is emphasized by the fact that in many nonhuman species, C cells are found in a body called the ultimobranchial gland and not in the thyroid at all.

Calcitonin is synthesized in the secretory pathway (p. 36) by posttranslational processing of a large procalcitonin. As illustrated in Figure 51–11, alternative splicing of the calcitonin gene product gives rise to several biologically active peptides. In the C cells, calcitonin is the only peptide made in biologically significant amounts. Within the central nervous system, calcitonin gene–related peptide (CGRP) is the principal gene product, and it appears to act as a neurotransmitter in peptidergic neurons (see Table 12–1). Calcitonin is stored in secretory vesicles within the C cells, and its release is triggered by raising the extracellular $[Ca^{2+}]$ above normal. Conversely, lowering the extracellular $[Ca^{2+}]$ diminishes calcitonin secretion. The threshold $[Ca^{2+}]$ for enhancing calcitonin secretion is in the midphysiologic range. In principle, this

secretory profile would leave calcitonin well poised to regulate body Ca^{2+} homeostasis.

The precise role for calcitonin in body Ca^{2+} homeostasis has been difficult to define. This difficulty was first apparent from the simple clinical observation that after complete thyroidectomy with removal of all calcitonin-secreting tissue, plasma $[Ca^{2+}]$ remains normal (provided that the parathyroids are not injured). Conversely, patients with a rare calcitonin-secreting tumor of the C cells frequently have plasma calcitonin concentrations that are 50 to 100 times normal, yet they maintain normal plasma levels of Ca^{2+}, vitamin D, and PTH. Nevertheless, several lines of evidence suggest that calcitonin does have biologically important actions. First, although calcitonin appears to have a minimal role in the minute-to-minute regulation of plasma $[Ca^{2+}]$ in humans, it does serve an important role in many nonmammalian species. This role is particularly clear for teleost fish. Faced with the relatively high $[Ca^{2+}]$ in sea water (and therefore in food), calcitonin, secreted in response to a rise in plasma $[Ca^{2+}]$, decreases bone resorption, thus returning the plasma $[Ca^{2+}]$ toward normal. Interestingly, salmon calcitonin, which differs from human calcitonin in 14 of its 32 amino acid residues, is roughly 10-fold more potent on a molar basis in inhibiting osteoclast function than is the human hormone.

The second line of evidence that calcitonin may have biologically important actions is the presence of calcitonin receptors. Like PTH receptors, the **calcitonin receptor** is a G-protein–coupled receptor that, depending on the target cell, may activate either adenylyl cyclase (p. 97) or phospholipase C (p. 100). Within bone, the osteoclast—which lacks PTH receptors—appears to be the principal target of calcitonin. Indeed, the presence of calcitonin receptors may be one of the most reliable methods of identifying osteoclasts. In the osteoclast, calcitonin appears to work by raising $[cAMP]_i$ and then presumably acting via one or more protein kinases. Calcitonin inhibits the resorptive activity of the osteoclast and slows the rate of bone turnover. It also appears to diminish osteocytic osteolysis, and this action—together with calcitonin's effect on the osteoclast—is responsible for the hypocalcemic effect after the acute administration of pharmacologic doses of calcitonin. The hypocalcemic action of calcitonin is particularly effective in circumstances when bone turnover is accelerated, as occurs in rapidly growing young animals and in humans with hyperparathyroidism. The antiosteoclastic activity of calcitonin is also useful in treating Paget disease (see the box titled Osteoporosis). However, within hours of exposure of osteoclasts to high concentrations of calcitonin, calcitonin's antiresorptive action begins to wane. This "escape" from the hypocalcemic effect of calcitonin has limited the use of calcitonin in the clinical treatment of hypercalcemia. The transitory nature of calcitonin's action appears to be due in part to rapid downregulation of calcitonin receptors.

In the kidney, calcitonin, like PTH, causes a mild phosphaturia by inhibiting proximal-tubule phosphate transport. Calcitonin also causes a mild natriuresis and calciuresis. These actions may contribute to the acute hypocalcemic and hypophosphatemic actions of calcitonin. However, these renal effects are of short duration

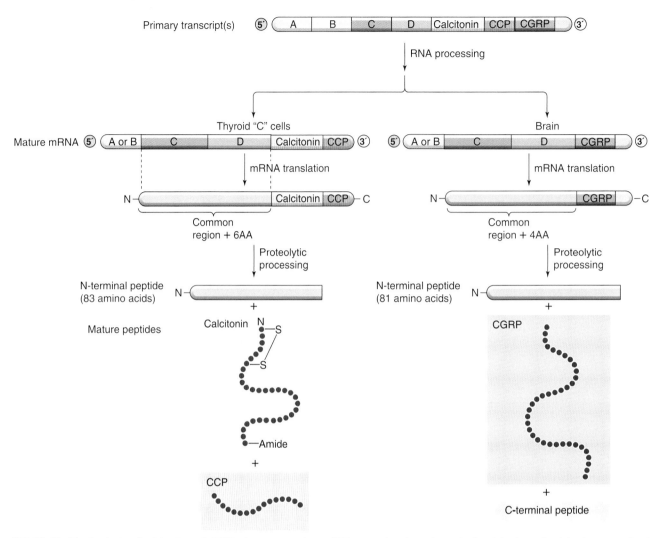

FIGURE 51–11. Synthesis of calcitonin and CGRP. A common primary RNA transcript gives rise to both calcitonin and calcitonin gene–related peptide (CGRP). In the thyroid gland, C cells produce a mature mRNA that they translate to procalcitonin. They then process this precursor to produce an N-terminal peptide, calcitonin (a 32–amino acid peptide), and CCP. In the brain, neurons produce a different mature mRNA and a different "pro" hormone. They process the peptide to produce an N-terminal peptide, CGRP and a C-terminal peptide. mRNA, messenger RNA.

and do not appear to be important in the overall renal handling of Ca^{2+}, phosphate, or Na^+.

Sex Steroid Hormones Promote Bone Deposition, Whereas Glucocorticoids Promote Resorption

Although PTH and 1,25-dihydroxyvitamin D are the principal hormones involved in modulating bone turnover, other hormones participate in this process. For example, the sex steroids **testosterone** and **estradiol** are needed for maintaining normal bone mass in males and females, respectively. The decline in estradiol that occurs postmenopausally exposes women to the risk of **osteoporosis**, that is, a decreased mass of both cortical and trabecular bone caused by a decrease in bone matrix (see the box titled Osteoporosis). Osteoporosis is less common in males because their skeletal mass tends to be greater throughout adult life and because testosterone levels in males decline slowly as they age, unlike the abrupt menopausal decline of estradiol in women.

Glucocorticoids also modulate bone mass. This action is most evident in circumstances of glucocorticoid excess, which leads to osteoporosis, as suggested by the effects of glucocorticoids on the production of osteoprotegerin and osteoprotegerin ligand (p. 1090).

The precise cellular mechanisms that mediate the action of androgens, estrogens, or glucocorticoids on bone have not been well defined. Despite the loss of bone that occurs with androgen or estrogen deficiency or glucocorticoid excess, in each case, the coupling of bone synthesis to degradation is *qualitatively* preserved. Synthesis of new bone continues to occur at sites of previous bone resorption, and no excess of unmineralized osteoid is present. Presumably, the decline in bone mass reflects a *quantitative* shift whereby the amount of new bone formed at any site is less than what was resorbed. Because this shift

OSTEOPOROSIS

Approximately 25 million Americans, mostly elderly women, are afflicted with **osteoporosis,** and between 1 and 2 million of these individuals experience a fracture related to osteoporosis every year. The cost in economic and human terms is immense. Hip fractures are responsible for much of the morbidity associated with osteoporosis, but even more concerning is the observation that as many as 20% of women with osteoporotic hip fractures will die within 1 year of their fracture.

The major risk factor for osteoporosis is the declining estrogen levels in aging women. Rarely, other endocrine disorders such as hyperthyroidism, hyperparathyroidism, and Cushing disease (hypercortisolism) are responsible. Other risk factors include inadequate dietary Ca^{2+} intake, alcoholism, cigarette smoking, and a sedentary lifestyle.

Strategies to prevent the development of osteoporosis begin in the premenopausal years. High Ca^{2+} intake and a consistent program of weight-bearing exercises are widely recommended.

A number of pharmacologic agents are now available for preventing or at least retarding the development of osteoporosis or for treating the disease once it has become established. These agents can be broadly classified into two groups: antiresorptive drugs and those that are able to stimulate bone formation.

Among the former, estrogen is by far the most widely used therapy. It is most effective when started at the onset of menopause, although it may offer benefits even in patients who are 20 or more years past

menopause. Calcitonin is generally offered to women who cannot or are unwilling to take estrogen. However, it is expensive and must be given parenterally; an intranasal spray is also available. Another class of drugs, the bisphosphonates, are becoming popular. They are powerful inhibitors of bone resorption, but some of the first agents of this class have also been found to impair mineralization. The newer bisphosphonates can be safely given in doses that decrease bone resorption without affecting mineralization.

Among the drugs that can stimulate bone formation, only vitamin D has currently won wide support. Vitamin D, often given in very high doses as 1,25-dihydroxyvitamin D (calcitriol), is often combined with Ca^{2+} therapy to increase the fractional absorption of Ca^{2+} and stimulate the activity of osteoblasts. Sodium fluoride has also begun to receive much attention. It has been shown to stimulate osteoblastic activity and thereby increase bone mass, and it appears to decrease the rate of vertebral fractures as well.

Calcitriol and the bisphosphonates have also been used successfully to treat **Paget disease,** a disorder characterized by localized regions of bone resorption and reactive sclerosis. The level of bone turnover can be extremely high. Although it remains asymptomatic in many individuals, the disease can cause pain, deformity, fractures, and vertigo and hearing loss if bony overgrowth occurs in the region of the eighth cranial nerve. The cause of Paget disease is not known.

---

occurs at multiple sites, the result is a decline in overall bone mass.

Parathyroid Hormone–Related Peptide, Which Is Encoded By a Gene That Is Entirely Distinct from That for PTH, Can Cause Hypercalcemia in Certain Malignancies

Unlike PTH, which is synthesized exclusively by the parathyroid gland, a peptide called PTHrP appears to be made in a wide variety of both normal and malignant tissues. The PTH 1R receptor in kidney and bone recognizes PTHrP with an affinity that is similar to that for intact PTH. PTHrP mimics each of the actions of PTH on kidney and bone. Thus, when present in sufficient concentrations, PTHrP causes hypercalcemia. PTHrP exists in three alternatively spliced isoforms of a single gene product. The gene encoding PTHrP is completely distinct from that for PTH. The similar actions of PTHrP and PTH arise from homology within the first 13 amino acids of PTHrP with native PTH. Only weak homology is seen between amino acids 14 and 34 (3 amino acids are identical) and essentially no homology beyond amino acid 34. This situation is an unusual example of mimicry between peptides that are structurally quite diverse.

The normal physiologic function of PTHrP is still largely undefined. Interestingly, the lactating breast secretes PTHrP, and this hormone is present in very high

concentrations in milk. PTHrP may promote the mobilization of Ca^{2+} from maternal bone during milk production. In nonlactating humans, the plasma PTHrP concentration is very low, and PTHrP does not appear to be involved in the day-to-day regulation of plasma $[Ca^{2+}]$. It appears likely that under most circumstances, PTHrP acts in a paracrine or autocrine, rather than an endocrine, regulatory fashion.

Many tumors are capable of manufacturing and secreting PTHrP, among them squamous cell tumors of the lung, head, and neck; renal and bladder carcinomas; adenocarcinomas; and lymphomas. Patients with any of these tumors are subject to severe hypercalcemia of fairly abrupt onset.

REFERENCES

Books and Reviews

Bringhurst FR, Demay MB, Kronenberg HM: Hormones and disorders of mineral metabolism. In Wilson JD, Foster DW, Kronenberg HM, Larsen PR (eds): Williams Textbook of Endocrinology, 9th ed. Philadelphia, WB Saunders, 1998, pp 1155–1209.

DeLuca HF: The transformation of a vitamin into a hormone: The vitamin D story. Harvey Lect 75:333–379, 1979–1980.

Habener JF, Rosenblatt M, Potts JT Jr: Parathyroid hormone: Biochemical aspects of biosynthesis, secretion, action, and metabolism. Physiol Rev 64:985–1053, 1984.

Jones G, Strugnell SA, DeLuca HD: Current understanding of the molecular actions of vitamin D. Physiol Rev 78:1193–1231, 1998.

Murer H, Forster I, Hilfiker H, et al: Cellular/molecular control of renal Na/Pi-cotransport. Kidney Int Suppl 65:2–10, 1998.

Stein GS, Lian JB, Stein JL, et al: Transcriptional control of osteoblast growth and differentiation. Physiol Rev 76:593–629, 1996.

Journal Articles

Broadus AE, Mangin M, Ikeda K, et al: Humoral hypercalcemia of cancer. Identification of a novel parathyroid hormone–like peptide. N Engl J Med 319:556–563, 1988.

Brown EM, Gamba G, Riccardi D, et al: Cloning and characterization of an extracellular Ca^{2+}-sensing receptor from bovine parathyroid. Nature 366:575–580, 1993.

Burgess TL, Qian Y, Kaufman S, et al: The ligand for osteoprotegerin (OPGL) directly activates mature osteoclasts. J Cell Biol 145:527–538, 1999.

IX

The
Reproductive
System

CHAPTER 52

Sexual Differentiation

Ervin E. Jones and Alan H. DeCherney

One of nature's primary goals is perpetuation of the species. All living organisms must reproduce in some manner. Nature also favors those species that are able to produce diversification among members, an attribute critical to species survival as the nature of environmental (and other) stresses changes through time. One solution to this problem is sexual differentiation, that is, the evolution of two sexually dissimilar individuals belonging to the same species, one male and one female, and each equipped with its own specific attributes necessary for its particular contribution to the process of procreation. Each sex produces its own type of sex cell (**gamete**), and the union of male and female gametes generates species-specific progeny. In addition, mechanisms, some simple, some complex, have evolved to ensure the proximity and union of the sex cells (syngamy). Thus, within each species, the relevant sexual characteristics of each partner have adapted differently to achieve the most efficient union of these progenitor cells. These differences between the sexes of one species are called **sexual dimorphism**. For example, oviparous species such as frogs release their eggs into a liquid medium only when in relative proximity to sperm. As effective as this approach is, it also typifies the wastefulness of reproduction among higher species inasmuch as most gametes go unfertilized.

Even among species that normally reproduce sexually, sexual dimorphism is not universal. For example, monoecious (i.e., hermaphroditic) species, such as cestodes and nematodes, have the capacity to produce both sperms and eggs. By definition, the ability to produce just one kind of gamete depends on sexually dimorphic differentiation.

Throughout evolution, conservation and expression of genes involved in the perpetuation of a species have clearly followed a process of "adaptation": an advantageous change in structure or function of an organ or tissue to meet the challenges of new conditions. Higher mammals normally have a single pair of **sex chromosomes** that are morphologically distinguishable from other chromosomes, the **autosomes**. Each of the sex chromosomes carries genetic information that determines the primary and secondary sexual characteristics of an individual, that is, whether the individual functions and appears as male or female. It has also become abundantly clear that genes determine gender, sexual expression, and as a result, mechanisms and patterns of reproduction.

The functional and spatial organization of all organ systems during development is genetically determined. Thus, the sex of the gonad is genetically programmed: will a female gonad (ovary) or a male gonad (testis) develop? Although germ cells of the early embryonic gonad are totipotent, these cells develop into female gametes (ova) if the gonad becomes an ovary but develop into male gametes (sperm) if the gonad becomes a testis. These two anatomically and functionally distinct gonads determine either "maleness" or "femaleness" and dictate the development of both primary and secondary sexual characteristics, as well as their function during adulthood. Endocrine and paracrine modulators that are specific for either the ovary or the testis are primarily responsible for female or male sexual differentiation and behavior and, therefore, the individual's role in procreation.

GENETIC ASPECTS OF SEXUAL DIFFERENTIATION

Meiosis, Which Occurs Only in Germ Cells, Gives Rise to Male and Female Gametes

Mitosis is the only kind of cell division that occurs in somatic cells. Mitosis results in the formation of two identical daughter cells (Fig. 52–1A), each having the same number of chromosomes (i.e., 46 in humans) and same DNA content as the original cell. Mitosis is a continuum consisting of five phases: prophase, prometaphase, metaphase, anaphase, and telophase. One reason for the genetic identity of the two daughter cells is that no exchange of genetic material occurs between homologous chromosomes, so sister chromatids (i.e., the two copies of the same DNA on a chromosome) are identical. A second reason for the genetic identity is that the sister chromatids of each chromosome split, one going to each daughter cell during anaphase of the single mitotic division.

Meiosis occurs only in germ cells. In both sexes, the production of gametes necessitates that germ cells, after having undergone several mitotic divisions, undergo two meiotic divisions (see Fig. 52–1B) to reduce the number of chromosomes from the diploid number (46) to the haploid number (23). Because of this halving of the diploid number of chromosomes, meiosis is often referred to as a "reduction division." Meiosis is a continuum composed of two phases: the homologous *chromosomes* separate during meiosis I, and the *chromatids* separate during meiosis II. As cells enter meiosis I, the chromosomes duplicate so that the cells have 23 pairs of duplicated chromosomes (i.e., each chromosome has two chromatids). During prophase of this first meiotic division, homologous pairs of chromosomes—22 pairs of autosomal chromosomes (autosomes) plus a pair of sex chromosomes—exchange genetic material. This genetic exchange is the phenomenon of "crossing over" that is responsible for the "recombination" of genetic material between maternal and paternal chromosomes. At the completion of meiosis I, the daughter cells have a haploid number (23) of duplicated, crossed-over chromosomes. During meiosis

II, no additional duplication of DNA takes place. The chromatids simply separate so that each of the daughter cells has a haploid number of unduplicated chromosomes. When two haploid gametes fuse, a mature oocyte from the mother and a mature spermatozoan from the father, a new individual is formed, a diploid zygote.

Here we will illustrate meiosis by following the production of female gametes, or ova. The analogous process of producing males gametes, or spermatozoa, is discussed on p. 1131. In the female, oocyte maturation begins in the fetal ovary. The **primordial germ cells** migrate from the hind gut to the gonadal ridge. These primordial germ cells develop into **oogonia**, or immature germ cells, which in turn proliferate in the fetal ovary by mitotic division. By 6 to 7 weeks' intrauterine life, a total of approximately 10,000 oogonia are present. This figure is the result of migration and rapid mitotic division; up until this time, no atresia occurs (p. 1157). By about 8 weeks' gestation, approximately 600,000 oogonia are present, and they may enter prophase of the first meiosis and become **primary oocytes**. From this point on, the number of germ cells is determined by three ongoing processes: mitosis, meiosis, and atresia. The number of germ cells peaks at 6 to 7 million around 20 weeks' gestation, and about 2.5 million primary oocytes are present at birth.

During prophase of the first meiosis, when the cells have a duplicated set of 23 chromosomes (22 duplicated pairs of autosomal chromosomes and one pair of duplicated X chromosomes), crossing over occurs. Meiosis is arrested in prophase I. Thus, the female germ cells are primary oocytes at birth, and they remain primary oocytes—arrested in prophase I of meiosis—until just before ovulation, many years later, when meiosis is completed and the first polar body is extruded (p. 1159). This prolonged state of meiotic arrest is known as the **dictyotene stage**.

The Genetic Sex of a Zygote Is Established at Fertilization, When an X- or Y-Bearing Sperm Fertilizes an Oocyte

The sex chromosomes that the parents contribute to the offspring determine the **genotypic sex** of that individual. The genotypic sex determines the **gonadal sex**, which in turn determines the **phenotypic sex** that becomes fully established at puberty. Thus, sex-determining mechanisms established at fertilization direct all later ontogenetic processes (processes that lead to the development of an organism) involved in male-female differentiation.

The process of fusion of a sperm and an ovum is referred to as **fertilization**, which is discussed in Chapter 55. Fusion of a sperm and egg—two haploid germ cells—results in a **zygote**, which is a diploid cell contain-

---

FIGURE 52–1. Meiosis and mitosis. *A,* In the process of mitosis, the two daughter cells are genetically identical to the mother cell. *B,* In the process of meiosis, the four daughter cells are haploid. Cell division I produces both recombination (i.e., crossing over of genetic material between homologous chromosomes) and the reduction to the haploid number of chromosomes. Cell division II separates the chromatids of each chromosome, just as in mitosis.

A MITOSIS

B MEIOSIS

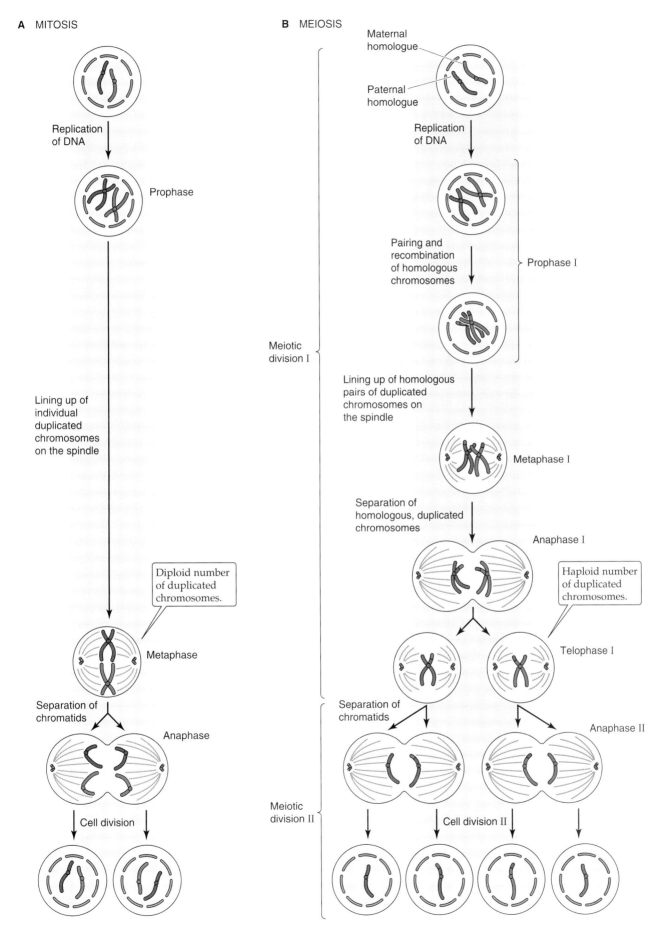

Maternal homologue

Paternal homologue

Replication of DNA

Replication of DNA

Prophase

Pairing and recombination of homologous chromosomes

Prophase I

Meiotic division I

Lining up of individual duplicated chromosomes on the spindle

Lining up of homologous pairs of duplicated chromosomes on the spindle

Metaphase I

Separation of homologous, duplicated chromosomes

Anaphase I

Diploid number of duplicated chromosomes.

Haploid number of duplicated chromosomes.

Metaphase

Telophase I

Separation of chromatids

Separation of chromatids

Anaphase

Anaphase II

Meiotic division II

Cell division

Cell division II

A   NORMAL HUMAN KARYOTYPES

FIGURE 52–2. The location of the testis-determining region of the Y chromosome and an example of translocation. *A*, The normal human has 22 pairs of autosomal chromosomes (autosomes) as well as a pair of sex chromosomes. Females have two X chromosomes, whereas males have one X and one Y chromosome. *B*, The Y chromosome is much smaller than the X chromosome. Giemsa staining of the chromosome results in alternating light and dark bands, some of which are shown here. The short or "p" arm of the Y chromosome is located above the centromere, whereas the long or "q" arm is located below. The numbers to the left of the chromosome indicate the position of bands. The testis-determining factor (TDF) is the *SRY* gene. *C*, Crossing-over events between normal X and Y chromosomes of the father can generate an X chromatid that contains a substantial portion of the TDF region and a Y chromatid that lacks its TDF. The figure shows both an equal and an unequal recombination event. If a sperm cell bearing an X chromosome with a translocated TDF fertilizes an ovum, the result is a male with a 46,XX karyotype, because one of the X chromosomes contains the TDF. Conversely, if the sperm cell carries a Y chromosome lacking its TDF, the result can be a 46,XY individual that appears to be female.

ing 46 chromosomes (Fig. 52–2A), 22 pairs of somatic chromosomes (autosomes) and a single pair of sex chromosomes. In the female, these sex chromosomes are both X chromosomes, whereas males have one X and one Y. When the karyotypes of normal females and males are compared, two differences are apparent: (1) among the 23 pairs of chromosomes in the female, 8 pairs—including the two X chromosomes—are of similar size, whereas males have only 7½ such pairs. (2) Instead of a second X chromosome, males have a Y chromosome that is small and acrocentric (i.e., the centromere is located at one end of the chromosome). This chromosome is the only such chromosome that is not present in the female.

In the offspring, 23 of the chromosomes—including 1 of the sex chromosomes—are from the mother, and 23—including the other sex chromosome—come from the father. Thus, the potential offspring has a unique complement of chromosomes differing from those of both the mother and father. The ovum provided by the mother (XX) always provides an X chromosome. Because the male is the heterogenetic (XY) sex, half the spermatozoa are X bearing whereas the other half are Y bearing. Thus, the type of sperm that fertilizes the ovum determines the sex of the zygote. X-bearing sperm produce XX zygotes that develop into females with a 46,XX karyotype,

whereas Y-bearing sperm produce XY zygotes that develop into males with a 46,XY karyotype. Thus, the genetic sex of an individual is determined at the time of fertilization. The Y chromosome appears to be the fundamental determinant of sexual development. When a Y chromosome is present, the individual develops as a male; when the Y chromosome is absent, the individual develops as a female. In embryos with abnormal sex chromosome complexes, the number of X chromosomes is apparently of little significance.

Two Intact X Chromosomes Are Required for Differentiation of the Indifferent Gonad as a Normal Ovary

The primary sex organs of an individual are the gonads. Gene complexes on sex chromosomes determine whether the indifferent gonad differentiates into a testis or an ovary. As discussed later, the Y chromosome exerts a powerful testis-determining effect on the indifferent gonad. The primary sex cords differentiate into seminiferous tubules under the influence of the Y chromosome. In the absence of a Y chromosome, the indifferent gonad develops into an ovary. The differentiated gonads in turn de-

GONADAL DYSGENESIS

The best known example of gonadal dysgenesis is a syndrome referred to as **Turner syndrome,** a disorder of the female sex characterized by short stature, primary amenorrhea, sexual infantilism, and a number of other congenital abnormalities. The cells in these individuals have a total number of 45 chromosomes and a normal karyotype, except that they lack a second sex chromosome. The karyotype is 45,XO. Examination of the gonads of individuals with Turner syndrome reveals so-called streak gonads, firm, flat, glistening streaks lying below the fallopian tubes. These glands generally do not show evidence of either germinal or secretory elements but, instead, are largely composed of connective tissue arranged in whorls suggestive of ovarian stroma. Individuals with Turner syndrome have normal female differentiation of both the internal and external genitalia, although these genitalia are usually small and immature for the patient's age.

Partial deletion of the X chromosome may also result in the full Turner phenotype, particularly if the entire short arm of the X chromosome is missing.

The so-called **ring chromosome** is an example of an abnormality of the second sex chromosome. A ring chromosome is a small round or oval chromosome that often appears as a single black dot without a central hole. It forms as a result of a deletion and subsequent joining of the two free ends of the chromosome. Formation of a ring chromosome is, in effect, a deletion of the X chromosome and produces the same characteristics as gonadal dysgenesis.

The aforementioned defects result from disordered meiosis. A central genetic lesion is an abnormality of the second sex chromosome in some or all of the cells of the person. In at least half of affected individuals, this abnormality appears to be total absence of the second X chromosome. In others, the lesion is structural, as shown by the presence of ring chromosomes that have lost some genetic material. In at least a third of cases, these lesions appear as parts of a mosaicism; that is, *some* of the germ cells carry the aberrant or absent chromosome, whereas the rest are normal.

termine the sexual differentiation of the genital ducts and external genitalia.

The indifferent gonad is composed of an outer cortex and an inner medulla. In embryos with an XX sex chromosome complement, the cortex develops into an ovary and the medulla regresses. On the other hand, in embryos with an XY chromosome complex, the medulla differentiates into a testis and the cortex regresses. Loss of a sex chromosome causes abnormal gonadal differentiation or gonadal dysgenesis. Loss of one of the X chromosomes of the XX pair results in an individual with an XO sex chromosome constitution and ovarian dysgenesis (see the box titled Gonadal Dysgenesis). Thus, two X chromosomes are necessary for normal ovarian development. In an XO individual, the gonads appear only as streaks on the pelvic sidewall in the adult. Because these streak gonads of XO individuals may contain germ cells, germ cell

migration apparently can occur during development. The absence of only some genetic material from one X chromosome in an XX individual—for example, as might occur as a result of breakage or deletion—may also cause abnormal sexual differentiation.

The Testis-Determining Gene Is Located on the Y Chromosome

It has been clearly established that a Y chromosome (see Fig. 52–2B), with rare exception (see later), is necessary for normal testicular development. Thus, it stands to reason that the gene that determines organogenesis of the testis is normally located on the Y chromosome. This so-called **testis-determining factor** (TDF) has been mapped to the short arm of the Y chromosome and, indeed, turns out to be a single gene called *SRY* (for "sex-determining region Y"). The *SRY* gene encodes a transcription factor that belongs to the high-mobility group (HMG) superfamily of transcription factors. The family to which *SRY* belongs is evolutionarily ancient. One portion of *SRY*, the 80–amino-acid HMG box, which actually binds to the DNA—is highly conserved among members of the family.

Rarely, the TDF may also be found translocated on other chromosomes. One example is an XX male (see Fig. 52–2C), an individual whose sex chromosome complement is XX but whose phenotype is male. During normal male meiosis, human X and Y chromosomes pair and recombine at the distal end of their short arms. It appears that most XX males arise as a result of an aberrant exchange of genetic material between X and Y chromosomes in the father; in such cases, the TDF is transferred from a Y chromatid to an X chromatid. If the sperm cell that fertilizes the ovum contains such an X chromosome with a TDF, the resultant individual will be an XX male.

Phenotypic Differentiation Is Modulated by Endocrine and Paracrine Messengers

Just as an individual's genes determine whether the indifferent gonad develops into an ovary or a testis, so does the sex of the gonad dictate the gonad's endocrine and paracrine functions. Normally, chemical messengers—both endocrine and paracrine—produced by the gonad determine the primary and secondary sexual phenotypes of the individual. However, if the gonads fail to produce the proper messengers, if other organs (e.g., the adrenal glands) produce abnormal levels of sex steroids, or if the mother is exposed to chemical agents (e.g., synthetic progestins, testosterone) during pregnancy, sexual development of the fetus may deviate from that programmed by the genotype. Therefore, genetic determination of sexual differentiation is not irrevocable; numerous internal and external influences during development may modify or completely reverse the phenotype of the individual, whatever the genotypic sex.

An abnormal chemical environment can affect sexual differentiation at the level of either the genital ducts or the development of secondary sex characteristics. Higher vertebrates, including humans, have evolved highly elaborate systems of glands and ducts for transporting gametes.

DISCORDANCE BETWEEN GENOTYPE AND GONADAL PHENOTYPE

A group of patients have been reported who have no recognizable Y chromosome but do have testes. Some of these individuals are 46,XX and are **true hermaphrodites;** that is, they possess both male and female sex organs. Other patients have **mixed gonadal dysgenesis**—a testis plus a streak ovary—and a 45,XO karyotype. Some are **pseudohermaphrodites;** that is, affected individuals have only one type of gonadal tissue, but morphologic characteristics of both sexes. All these patterns can result from mosaicisms (e.g., 46,XY/46,XX) or from translocation of the SRY gene (Fig. 52–2C)—which normally resides on the Y chromosome—to either an X chromosome or an autosome. A "normal" testis in the absence of a Y chromosome has never been reported.

Another group of individuals with a sex chromosome complex of 46,XY have **pure gonadal dysgenesis**—streak gonads, but no somatic features of XO. In the past it has been assumed that these individuals possess an abnormal Y chromosome. Perhaps the SRY gene is absent or its expression is somehow blocked.

This system of glands and conduits collectively comprises the **accessory sex organs**. Together with the gonads, these accessory sex organs constitute the primary sex characteristics. The gonads produce and secrete hormones that condition and develop these accessory sex organs and, to a large extent, influence phenotypic sexual differentiation; that is, they induce either "maleness" or "femaleness" and influence the psychobiologic phenomena involved in sex behavior.

Secondary sex characteristics are external specializations that are not essential for the production and movement of gametes; instead, they are primarily concerned with sex behavior and with the birth and nutrition of offspring. Examples include the development of pubic hair and breasts. Not only do the sex steroids produced by the gonads affect the accessory sex organs, they also modulate the physiologic state of the secondary sex characteristics toward "maleness" in the case of the testes and "femaleness" in the case of the ovaries.

DIFFERENTIATION OF THE GONADS

After the Migration of Germ Cells from the Yolk Sac, the Undifferentiated Primordial Gonad Develops into Either a Testis or an Ovary

The **primordial germ cells** do not originate in the gonad; instead, they migrate to the gonad from the yolk sac along the mesentery of the hindgut at about the fifth week of embryo development (Fig. 52–3A, B). The primordial germ cells of humans are first found in the endodermal epithelium of the yolk sac in the vicinity of the allantoic stalk, and from there the germ cells migrate into the adjoining mesenchyme. They eventually take up their position embedded in the gonadal ridges. Gonadal development fails to progress normally in the absence of germ cells. Thus, any event that interferes with germ cell migration may cause abnormal gonadal differentiation.

The gonad forms from a portion of the coelomic epithelium, the underlying mesenchyme, and the primordial germ cells that migrate from the yolk sac. At 5 weeks' development, a thickened area of coelomic epithelium develops on the medial aspect of the urogenital ridge as a result of proliferation of both the coelomic epithelium and cells of the underlying mesenchyme. This prominence, which forms on the medial aspect of the mesonephros, is known as the **gonadal ridge** (see Fig. 52–3B, C).

Migration of the primordial germ cells to the gonadal ridge establishes the "anlagen" for the primordial gonad. The primordial gonad at this early stage of development consists of both a peripheral cortex and a central medulla (see Fig. 52–3C) and has the capacity to develop into either an ovary or a testis. As discussed later, the cortex and medulla have different fates in the male and female. The germ cells themselves seem to direct the sexual development of the gonad. An embryo with an XY chromosome complement undergoes development of the medullary portion of the gonad to become a testis and the cortex regresses. On the other hand, XX germ cells appear to stimulate development of the cortex of the early gonad to become an ovary and the medulla regresses.

DEVELOPMENT OF THE PRIMITIVE TESTIS. In male embryos, primordial germ cells migrate from the cortex of the gonad, in which they were originally embedded, into the primitive sex cords of the medulla (see Fig. 52–3D). The primitive sex cords become hollowed out and develop into the **seminiferous tubules**. The primordial germ cells give rise to spermatogonia, the first cells in the pathway to mature sperm (p. 1131). The sex cords give rise to Sertoli cells. The **rete testis** is a system of thin, interconnected tubules that develop in the dorsal part of the gonad; they drain the seminiferous tubules. The contents of the rete testes flow into the **efferent ductules**, which—as we will see later—develop from the adjoining tubules of the mesonephros. These tubular structures establish a pathway from the male gonad to the mesonephric duct, which—as we will also see later—evolves into the outlet for sperm. The cortex of the primordial gonad is a thin epithelial layer covering the coelomic surface of the testis.

DEVELOPMENT OF THE PRIMITIVE OVARY. In female embryos, the medulla of the gonad regresses, the primary sex cords are resorbed, and the interior of the gonad is filled with a loose mesenchyme that is highly permeated by blood vessels. However, the cortex greatly increases in thickness, with the primordial germ cells remaining embedded within (see Fig. 52–3E). Masses of cortical cells are split up on the inner surface of the cortex into groups and strands of cells, or secondary sex cords, surrounding one or several primordial germ cells, or oogonia, during

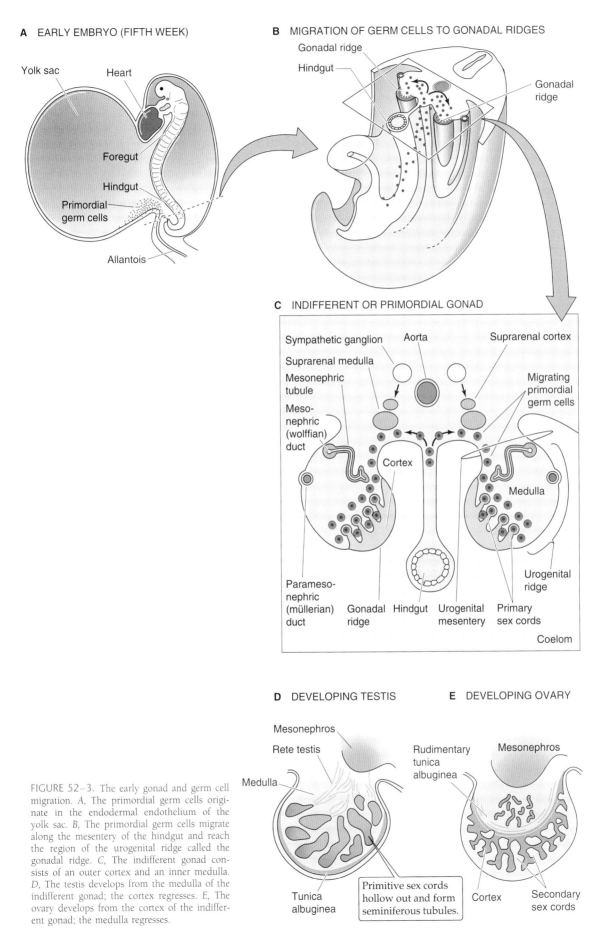

A EARLY EMBRYO (FIFTH WEEK)

Yolk sac

Heart

Foregut

Hindgut

Primordial germ cells

Allantois

B MIGRATION OF GERM CELLS TO GONADAL RIDGES

Gonadal ridge

Hindgut

Gonadal ridge

C INDIFFERENT OR PRIMORDIAL GONAD

Sympathetic ganglion

Suprarenal medulla

Mesonephric tubule

Meso-nephric (wolffian) duct

Aorta

Suprarenal cortex

Migrating primordial germ cells

Cortex

Medulla

Urogenital ridge

Parameso-nephric (müllerian) duct

Gonadal ridge

Hindgut

Urogenital mesentery

Primary sex cords

Coelom

D DEVELOPING TESTIS

Mesonephros

Rete testis

Medulla

Tunica albuginea

Primitive sex cords hollow out and form seminiferous tubules.

E DEVELOPING OVARY

Rudimentary tunica albuginea

Mesonephros

Cortex

Secondary sex cords

FIGURE 52–3. The early gonad and germ cell migration. *A*, The primordial germ cells originate in the endodermal endothelium of the yolk sac. *B*, The primordial germ cells migrate along the mesentery of the hindgut and reach the region of the urogenital ridge called the gonadal ridge. *C*, The indifferent gonad consists of an outer cortex and an inner medulla. *D*, The testis develops from the medulla of the indifferent gonad; the cortex regresses. *E*, The ovary develops from the cortex of the indifferent gonad; the medulla regresses.

growth of the gonad. These germ cells become primary oocytes that enter the initial stages of oogenesis.

The Embryonic Gonad Has Local Effects on Development of the Internal Genitalia and Also Determines the External Sexual Phenotype

As discussed in the following subchapter, several products of the developing male or female gonad have profound effects on differentiation of the internal sex ducts, as well as on development of the external genitalia. Thus, just as genetic sex determines the gonadal phenotype, products of the gonad primarily determine the sexual phenotype. Androgens produced by the developing testis cause development of the mesonephric or **wolffian ducts**. The paramesonephric or müllerian ducts degenerate in the male under the influence of antimüllerian hormone (AMH). In the female embryo, the **müllerian ducts** develop whereas the wolffian ducts degenerate. In the absence of a functioning testis, the left and right müllerian ducts develop

according to the female phenotype, that is, as the fallopian tubes (oviducts), the uterus, and the upper third of the vagina (see the next section).

Just as the absence of male hormones or androgens causes the *internal* genital ducts to follow a female pattern of differentiation, the absence of androgens causes the *external* genital development to be female. Conversely, testosterone and dihydrotestosterone (DHT) cause masculinization of the external genitalia (see the subchapter titled Differentiation of the External Genitalia).

DIFFERENTIATION OF THE INTERNAL GENITAL DUCTS

The genital ducts are an essential part of the genital organs and are the means by which the sex cells—ova and spermatozoa—are transported to a location where fertilization occurs. As discussed in the previous section, embryos of both sexes have a double set of genital ducts (Fig. 52–4A): the mesonephric or **wolffian ducts**, which

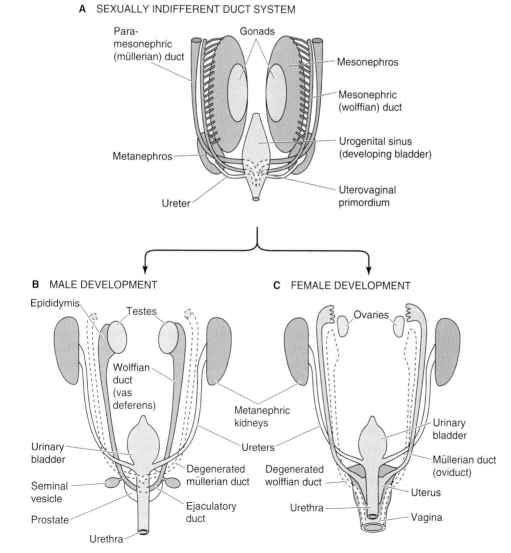

FIGURE 52–4. Transformation of the genital ducts. *A,* At the time that the gonad is still indifferent, it is closly associated with the mesonephros as well as the excretory duct (mesonephric or wolffian duct) that leads from the mesonephros to the urogenital sinus. Parallel to the wolffian ducts are the paramesonephric or müllerian ducts, which merge caudally to form the uterovaginal primordium. *B,* In males, the mesonephros develops into the epididymis. The wolffian duct develops into the vas deferens, seminal vesicles, and ejaculatory duct. The müllerian ducts degenerate. *C,* In females, the mesonephros as well as the wolffian (mesonephric) ducts degenerate. The paramesonephric or müllerian ducts develop into the fallopian tubes, the uterus, the cervix, and the upper one third of the vagina.

in males develop into the vas deferens and other structures, and the paramesonephric or **müllerian ducts**, which in females become the oviducts, uterus, and upper third of the vagina.

It is perhaps worth recalling that during mammalian development, three sets of kidneys develop, two of which are transient. The **pronephric kidney**, which develops first, is so rudimentary that it never functions. However, the duct that connects the pronephric kidney to the urogenital sinus—the pronephric duct—eventually serves the same purpose for the second kidney, the **mesonephric kidney** or mesonephros, as it develops embryologically. Unlike the pronephric kidney, the mesonephros functions transiently as a kidney. It has glomeruli and renal tubules; these tubules empty into the mesonephric duct (see Fig. 52–4A), which in turn carries fluid to the urogenital sinus. As discussed later, the mesonephros and its mesonephric duct will—depending on the sex of the developing embryo—either degenerate or develop into other reproductive structures. In addition to the mesonephric ducts, a second pair of genital ducts, the paramesonephric or müllerian ducts, develop as invaginations of the coelomic epithelium on the lateral aspects of the mesonephros. These paramesonephric ducts run caudally and parallel to the mesonephric ducts. In the caudal region, they cross ventral to the mesonephric ducts and fuse to form a cylindrical structure, the uterovaginal canal. The third or **metanephric kidney** becomes the permanent mammalian kidney. Its excretory duct is the ureter.

In the Male, the Mesonephros Gives Rise to the Epididymis, and the Mesonephric (Wolffian) Ducts Give Rise to the Vas Deferens, Seminal Vesicles, and Ejaculatory Duct

During development, the **mesonephros** ceases to be an excretory organ in both sexes. The only part that remains functional is the portion—in males—that develops into the most proximal end of the epididymis, the **efferent ductules**. As the mesonephros degenerates, persisting mesonephric tubules develop into many parallel efferent ductules that connect the upstream rete testes to the head of the epididymis, which serves as a reservoir for sperm.

The **mesonephric ducts** develop into the channels through which the spermatozoa exit the testes (see Fig. 52–4B). The most proximal portion of the mesonephric duct becomes the head, the body, and the tail of the epididymis. The tail of the epididymis connects to the **vas deferens**, which also arises from the wolffian duct. A lateral outgrowth from the distal end of the mesonephric duct forms the **seminal vesicle**. The portion of the mesonephric duct between the seminal vesicle and the point where the mesonephric duct joins the urethra becomes the **ejaculatory duct**. At about the level where the ejaculatory duct joins with the urethra, multiple outgrowths of the urethra grow into the underlying mesenchyme and form the **prostate gland**. The mesenchyme of the prostate gives rise to the stroma of the prostate, whereas the prostatic glands develop from endodermal cells of the prostatic urethra.

In the Female, the Paramesonephric (Müllerian) Ducts Give Rise to the Fallopian Tubes, the Uterus, and the Upper Third of the Vagina

In female embryos, both the mesonephros and the wolffian (mesonephric) ducts degenerate. The müllerian ducts establish three functional regions (see Fig. 52–4C). The cranial portions of the müllerian ducts remain separate and give rise to the fallopian tubes. The upper end of the duct gains a fringe, which will become the fimbria, by adding a series of minor pits or müllerian tunnels. The midportions of the left and right müllerian ducts fuse and give rise to the fundus and corpus of the uterus. The most distal portions of the bilateral müllerian ducts had previously fused as the **uterovaginal primordium**. The cranial portion of this common tube gives rise to the cervix and remains the longest portion of the uterus until puberty. The caudal portion of this common tube becomes the upper third of the vagina.

In Males, Development of the Wolffian Ducts Requires Testosterone, Whereas Regression of the Müllerian Ducts Requires Some Other Testicular Product

As we have already noted, the developing embryo has two precursor duct systems (Fig. 52–5A). In a normal male (see Fig. 52–5B), the wolffian ducts develop whereas the müllerian ducts regress. In a normal female (see Fig. 52–5C), the müllerian ducts develop whereas the wolffian ducts regress. It appears that maturation of one of these systems and degeneration of the other depend on local factors produced by the developing gonad.

A classic series of experiments performed by Alfred Jost in 1953 revealed that masculine genital development requires factors produced by fetal testicular tissue. The experimental approach was to castrate rabbit fetuses at various stages of development and allow the pregnancies to continue. Castrating a male fetus before maturation of the wolffian ducts caused the müllerian ducts to persist (i.e., fail to regress) and induced the development of female internal and external genitalia (see Fig. 52–5D). However, castrating female fetuses at a comparable stage in development had no appreciable effect, with müllerian development continuing along normal female lines (see Fig. 52–5E). Thus, although normal male development requires the testes, development of the fallopian tubes and uterus does *not* require the ovaries.

Unilateral removal of the testis resulted in female duct development on the same (ipsilateral) side as the castration, but virilization of the external genitalia proceeded normally (see Fig. 52–5F). Removing *both* testes—and administering testosterone—resulted in essentially normal development of the wolffian ducts, but no müllerian regression was seen (see Fig. 52–5G). Thus, although testosterone can support wolffian development, it is unable

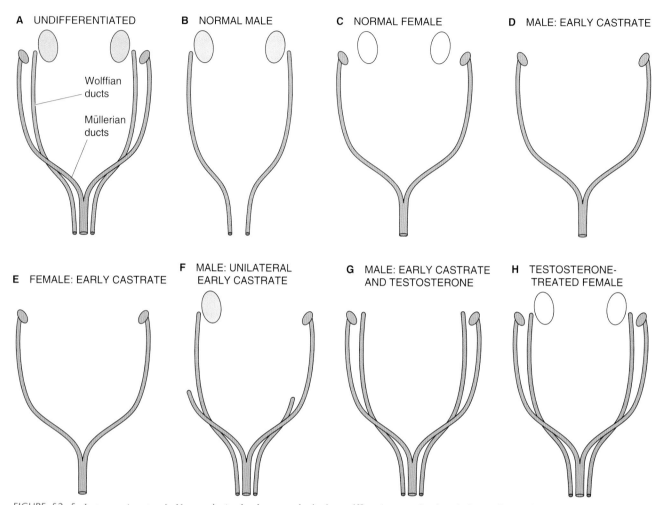

A UNDIFFERENTIATED

Wolffian ducts

Müllerian ducts

B NORMAL MALE

C NORMAL FEMALE

D MALE: EARLY CASTRATE

E FEMALE: EARLY CASTRATE

F MALE: UNILATERAL EARLY CASTRATE

G MALE: EARLY CASTRATE AND TESTOSTERONE

H TESTOSTERONE-TREATED FEMALE

FIGURE 52–5. Jost experiments. *A,* Very early in development, both the wolffian (mesonephric) and the müllerian (paramesonephric) ducts are present in parallel. *B,* The wolffian duct develops into the vas deferens, the seminal vesicles, and the ejaculatory duct. The müllerian ducts degenerate. *C,* The paramesonephric or müllerian ducts develop into the fallopian tubes, the uterus, the cervix and the upper one third of the vagina. The wolffian (mesonephric) ducts degenerate. *D,* Bilateral removal of the testes deprives the embryo of both anti-müllerian hormone ([AMH] also known as müllerian-inhibiting substance [MIS]) and testosterone, which are both testicular products. As a result of the absence of AMH, the müllerian ducts follow the female pattern of development. In the absence of testosterone, the wolffian ducts degenerate. Thus, the genetically male fetus develops female internal and external genitalia. *E,* After bilateral removal of the ovaries, müllerian development continues along normal female lines. Thus, the ovary is not required for female duct development. *F,* Unilateral removal of the testis results in female duct development on the same (ipsilateral) side as the castration. Duct development follows the male pattern on the side with the remaining testis. Virilization of the external genitalia proceeds normally. *G,* In the absence of both testes, administering testosterone preserves development of the wolffian ducts. However, because of the absence of AMH—which is a product of the testis—there is no müllerian regression. *H,* In the presence of both ovaries, the testosterone promotes development of the wolffian ducts. Because there are no testes—and therefore no AMH—the müllerian ducts develop normally.

to cause müllerian regression. It became clear that a testicular product other than testosterone is necessary for regression of the müllerian ducts. Following this reasoning, one would predict that treating a normal female with testosterone would lead to preservation of the wolffian ducts, as well as the müllerian ducts. This pattern of dual ducts is indeed observed (see Fig. 52–5*H*).

Antimüllerian Hormone (Müllerian-Inhibiting Substance) Causes Regression of the Müllerian Ducts

After Jost, other investigators performed experiments indicating that the Sertoli cells of the testis produce a non-

steroid macromolecule—**antimüllerian hormone (AMH)** or **müllerian-inhibiting substance** (MIS)—that causes müllerian degeneration in the male fetus. AMH, a growth-inhibitory glycoprotein, is a member of the transforming growth factor β (TGF-β) superfamily of glycoproteins involved in the regulation of growth and differentiation (p. 110). Besides TGF-β, this gene superfamily includes the inhibins and activins (p. 1151). The proteins produced via this gene family are all synthesized as dimeric precursors and undergo post-translational processing for activation. AMH is glycosylated and secreted as a 140-kDa dimer consisting of two identical disulfide-linked subunits. The antimitogenic activity and müllerian duct bioactivity of AMH reside primarily in its C-terminal domain.

The human AMH gene is located on chromosome 19, and AMH is one of the earliest sexually dimorphic genes expressed during development. The transcription factor SRY, which represents the TDF, may be involved in initiating the transcription of AMH. The sequential timing of SRY and AMH expression is consistent with activation of AMH by SRY, a series of events that may control sexual dimorphism.

Although the exact mechanism of AMH action has not been completely clarified, it is thought to involve receptor-mediated *de*phosphorylation. AMH appears to act directly on mesenchymal cells of the müllerian duct and, indirectly through the mesenchyme, on müllerian duct epithelial cells. AMH binding has been localized to the mesenchymal cells surrounding the müllerian duct and to the developing oocytes in preantral follicles.

During embryogenesis in males, AMH—which is secreted by the Sertoli cells in the testis—causes involution of the müllerian ducts, whereas testosterone—which is secreted by the Leydig cells of the testis—stimulates differentiation of the wolffian ducts. In females, the müllerian ducts differentiate spontaneously in the absence of AMH, and the wolffian ducts involute spontaneously in the absence of testosterone.

DIFFERENTIATION OF THE EXTERNAL GENITALIA

The Urogenital Sinus Develops into the Urinary Bladder, the Urethra, and, in the Female, the Vestibule of the Vagina

Early in embryologic development, a tubular structure called the cloaca is the common termination of the urogenital and gastrointestinal systems (Fig. 52–6A). The cloacal membrane separates the cloaca from the amniotic fluid. Eventually, a wedge of mesenchymal tissue separates the cloaca into a dorsal and a ventral cavity (see Fig. 52–6B). The dorsal cavity is the rectum. The ventral compartment is the **urogenital sinus**. You will recall that both the wolffian and the müllerian ducts empty into this urogenital sinus (see Fig. 52–4A).

The urogenital sinus can be divided into three regions: the vesicle part, the pelvic part, and the phallic part. In the male (see Fig. 52–6C), the vesicle part becomes the urinary bladder, the pelvic part becomes the prostatic part of the urethra, and the phallic part becomes the initial portion of the penile urethra.

In the female (see Fig. 52–6D), the vesicle part of the urogenital sinus also develops into the urinary bladder. The pelvic part becomes the entire female urethra. The phallic portion of the urogenital sinus develops into the vestibule of the vagina; into this vestibule empty the urethra, the vagina, and the ducts of the greater vestibular glands of Bartholin.

As we noted earlier, fusion of the caudal portion of the müllerian ducts produces the uterovaginal primordium. As this primordium contacts the dorsal wall of the urogenital sinus, it induces the development of paired sino-vaginal bulbs, which grow into the urogenital sinus and then fuse to form a solid core of tissue called the **vaginal plate**. This plate grows caudally to the phallic portion of the urogenital sinus. Resorption of the center of the vaginal plate creates the vaginal lumen. The remaining cells of the vaginal plate appear to form the vaginal epithelium. During early fetal development, a thin membrane, the **hymen**, separates the lumen of the vagina from the cavity of the urogenital sinus. Usually, the hymen partially opens during the prenatal period. Occasionally, the hymenal membrane persists completely, does not allow escape of the menstrual effluvium at menarche, and gives rise to a condition known clinically as hematocolpos.

In the male, the vagina disappears when the müllerian ducts are resorbed. However, remnants of the vagina sometimes persist as a prostatic utricle.

The External Genitalia of Both Sexes Develop from Common Anlagen

Although anatomically separate precursors give rise to the internal genitalia, a common anlagen gives rise to the external genitalia of the two sexes (Fig. 52–7A). Knowledge of the common origins of the external genitalia during normal development facilitates understanding of the ambiguities of abnormal sexual development.

The **genital tubercle** (see Fig. 52–7B) develops during the fourth week on the ventral side of the cloacal membrane. As a result of elongation of the genital tubercle, a phallus develops in both sexes. The genital tubercle of the primitive embryo develops into the **glans penis** in the male (see Fig. 52–7C) and the **clitoris** in the female (see Fig. 52–7D). Until about the end of the first trimester of pregnancy, the external genitalia of males and females are anatomically difficult to distinguish. The phallus undergoes rapid growth in the female initially, but its growth slows, and in the absence of androgens, the phallus becomes the relatively small clitoris in the female.

The paired **urogenital folds** give rise to the ventral aspect of the penis in the male (see Fig. 52–7C) and the labia minora in the female (see Fig. 52–7D). After formation of the urogenital opening, a groove—the urethral groove—forms on the ventral side of the phallus; this groove is continuous with the urogenital opening. The bilateral urogenital folds fuse over the urethral groove to form an enclosed spongy urethra; the line of fusion is the penile raphe. As the urogenital folds fuse to form the ventral covering of the penis, they do so in a posterior-to-anterior direction, thus displacing the urethral orifice to the tip of the penis. Elongation of the genital tubercle and fusion of the genital folds occur at the 12th to the 14th week of gestation. However, in the female, the urogenital folds normally remain separate as the labia minora.

In the male, **the genital or labioscrotal swellings** fuse to give rise to the scrotum. In females, however, the labioscrotal swellings fuse anteriorly to give rise to the mons pubis and posteriorly to form the posterior labial commissure. The unfused labioscrotal swellings give rise to the labia majora.

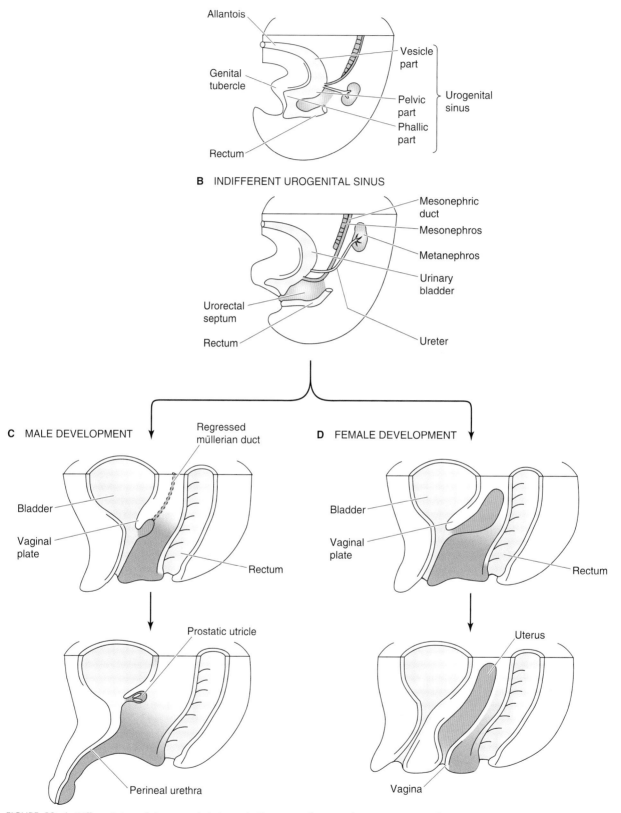

A PARTITIONING OF CLOACA

Allantois

Genital tubercle

Vesicle part

Pelvic part

Phallic part

Urogenital sinus

Rectum

B INDIFFERENT UROGENITAL SINUS

Mesonephric duct

Mesonephros

Metanephros

Urinary bladder

Urorectal septum

Rectum

Ureter

C MALE DEVELOPMENT

Regressed müllerian duct

Bladder

Vaginal plate

Rectum

Prostatic utricle

Perineal urethra

D FEMALE DEVELOPMENT

Bladder

Vaginal plate

Rectum

Uterus

Vagina

FIGURE 52–6. Differentiation of the urogenital sinus. *A,* The urorectal septum begins to separate the rectum (dorsal) from the urogenital sinus (ventral). The urogenital sinus is divided into a vesicle (i.e., urinary bladder) part, a pelvic part, and a phallic part. The common space into which the rectum and urogenital sinus empty, the cloaca, is closed by the cloacal membrane. *B,* At this stage, the rectum and the urogenital sinus are fully separated. The urogenital membrane separates the urogenital sinus from the outside of the embryo. *C,* The male has a common opening for the reproductive and urinary tracts. The prostatic utricle, which is the male homologue of the vagina, empties into the prostatic urethra. *D,* A solid core of tissue called the *vaginal plate* grows caudally from the posterior wall of the urogenital sinus. The lumen of the vagina forms as the center of this plate resorbs. Thus, the female has separate openings for the urinary and reproductive systems.

A   EARLY INDIFFERENT STAGE

Genital fold

Genital swelling

B   LATE INDIFFERENT STAGE

Genital tubercle

Cloacal membrane

C   MALE DEVELOPMENT

D   FEMALE DEVELOPMENT

Glans

Fused urogenital folds

Urethral groove

Fused labioscrotal swellings

Perineum

Anus

Glans penis

Glans clitoridis

Urethral groove

Labium minus

Scrotum

Labium majus

Posterior labial commissure

Anus

Prepuce

Mons pubis

Urethral orifice

Clitoris

Body of penis

Scrotum

Urethral orifice

Vestibule of the vagina

Hymen

Posterior labial commissure

Scrotal raphe (line of fusion of labioscrotal swellings)

ENDOCRINE AND PARACRINE CONTROL MECHANISMS IN SEXUAL DIFFERENTIATION

The *SRY* Gene Triggers Development of the Testis, Which Then Makes Androgens and Antimüllerian Hormone Necessary for the Male Pattern of Sexual Differentiation

We have already noted that the female pattern of sexual differentiation occurs in the absence of testes. In fact, the embryo follows the female pattern even in the absence of all gonadal tissue. It thus appears that it is the male pattern of sexual differentiation that is directed by endocrine and paracrine control mechanisms. Therefore, we will successively examine the control of testicular development, the development of the male internal system of genital ducts, and the development of the male urogenital sinus and external genitalia.

Testicular development proceeds in the presence of TDF—the gene product of the *SRY* gene—before 9 weeks of gestation. If TDF is not present or if TDF is present only after the critical window of 9 weeks has passed, an ovary will develop instead of a testis. Further male-pattern sexual differentiation depends on the presence of three hormones, testosterone, DHT, and AMH. The testis directly produces both testosterone and AMH. Peripheral tissues convert testosterone to DHT.

TESTOSTERONE PRODUCTION. The primary sex steroid produced by both the fetal and the postnatal testis is testosterone. The testes also produce DHT and estradiol, although in lesser amounts. **Leydig cells** are the source of sex-steroid production in the testes. The Leydig cells differentiate from mesenchymal tissue that surround the testicular cords. This tissue makes up greater than half the testicular volume by 60 days of gestation. The early increase in the number of Leydig cells and secretion of testosterone in humans could depend on either maternal chorionic gonadotropin (hCG) or fetal luteinizing hormone (LH). The human testis has its greatest abundance of side-chain-cleavage enzyme—which catalyzes the first committed step in steroid synthesis (see Fig. 49–2)—at 14 to 15 weeks of gestation and low values by 26 weeks of gestation. Because hCG follows a similar temporal pattern, it may be hCG that supports *early* testosterone production. Late regulation of testosterone production by fetal LH is supported by the finding that the testes of anencephalic fetuses (see box on p. 266) at term have few Leydig cells.

FIGURE 52–7. Development of the external genitalia. *A,* Genital folds and genital swellings surround the cloacal membrane. *B,* Early in the fourth week of development—in both sexes—the genital tubercle begins to enlarge to form the phallus. *C,* In males, the genital tubercle becomes the glans penis. The urogenital folds fuse to form the shaft of the penis. The labioscrotal swellings become the scrotum. *D,* In females, the genital tubercle becomes the clitoris. The urogenital folds remain separate as the labia minora. The labioscrotal swellings become the labia majora where they remain unfused. Ventrally, the labioscrotal swellings fuse to form the mons pubis. Dorsally they fuse to form the posterior labial commissure.

CONGENITAL ADRENAL HYPERPLASIA

Ambiguous genitalia in genotypic females may be due to disorders of adrenal function. Several forms of **congenital adrenal hyperplasia** have been described, including the deficiency of several enzymes involved in steroid synthesis (see Fig. 49–2): the side-chain-cleavage enzyme, 17α-hydroxylase, 21α-hydroxylase, 11β-hydroxylase, and 3β-hydroxysteroid dehydrogenase. Deficiencies in 21α-hydroxylase, 11β-hydroxylase, and 3β-hydroxysteroid dehydrogenase all lead to virilization in females—and thus ambiguous genitalia—as a result of the hypersecretion of adrenal androgens. **21α-Hydroxylase deficiency,** by far the most common, accounts for approximately 95% of cases. We discuss some of the consequences of this deficiency in the box on 21α-hydroxylase deficiency on p. 1053.

As summarized in Figure 49–2, 21α-hydroxylase deficiency reduces the conversion of progesterone to 11-deoxycorticosterone—which goes on to form aldosterone—and also reduces the conversion of 17α-hydroxyprogesterone to 11-deoxycortisol—which is the precursor of cortisol. As a result, adrenal steroid precursors are shunted into androgen pathways. In female infants, the result is sometimes called the adrenogenital syndrome. The external genitalia are difficult to distinguish from male genitalia on visual inspection. The clitoris is enlarged and resembles a penis, and the labioscrotal folds are enlarged and fused and resemble a scrotum. The genitalia thus have a male phenotype in an otherwise normal female infant.

THE ANDROGEN RECEPTOR. Androgens diffuse into target cells and act by binding to androgen receptors, which are present in genital tissues. In the absence of adequate androgen production or functioning androgen receptors, sexual ambiguity occurs. The androgen receptor functions as a homodimer (AR/AR) and is a member of the family of nuclear receptors (p. 112). The AR/AR receptor complex is a transcription factor that binds to hormone-response elements on DNA located 5′ from the genes that the androgens control (see Table 5–2). Interaction between the receptor-steroid complex and nuclear chromatin causes increased transcription of structural genes, the appearance of mRNA, and subsequent translation and production of new proteins. Congenital absence of the androgen receptor, or the production of abnormal androgen receptor, leads to a syndrome known as testicular feminization (see the box titled Impaired Androgen Action in Target Tissues).

DIHYDROTESTOSTERONE FORMATION. In certain target tissues, cytoplasmic 5α-reductase converts testosterone to DHT (see Fig. 53–5), which binds to the same androgen receptor as testosterone does. However, DHT binds to the androgen receptor with an affinity that is about 100-fold greater than the binding of testosterone to the androgen receptor. Moreover, the DHT-receptor complex binds to chromatin more tightly than does the testosterone-receptor complex.

ANTIMÜLLERIAN HORMONE. As noted earlier, the Sertoli cells of the testis produce AMH, also known as MIS. AMH is a homodimer of two monomeric glycoprotein subunits that are linked by disulfide bonds.

Androgens Direct the Male Pattern of Sexual Differentiation of the Internal Ducts, the Urogenital Sinus, and the External Genitalia

Androgens play two major roles in male phenotypic differentiation: (1) they trigger conversion of the wolffian ducts to the male ejaculatory system and (2) they direct the differentiation of the urogenital sinus and external genitalia. The wolffian phase of male sexual differentiation is regulated by testosterone itself and does not require conversion of testosterone to DHT. In contrast, virilization

ANDROGEN DEPENDENCE OF TESTICULAR DESCENT

In preparation for descent, the testes enlarge. In addition, the mesonephric kidneys and wolffian (mesonephric) ducts atrophy, which frees the testes for their future move down the posterior abdominal wall and across the abdomen to the deep inguinal rings. Testicular descent occurs in three phases during the last two thirds of gestation. During the first stage of testicular descent, rapid growth of the abdominopelvic region causes a *relative* movement of the testes down to the inguinal region (Fig. 52–8A). The role of the gubernaculum—the ligament attaching the inferior part of the testes to the lower segment of the labioscrotal fold—is uncertain. However, the gubernaculum shortens and appears to guide the testis to its place of ultimate functional residence in the scrotum. The second stage of testicular descent is herniation of the abdominal wall adjacent to the gubernaculum (Fig. 52–8B). This herniation, which occurs as a result of increasing abdominal pressure, forms the processus vaginalis; the processus vaginalis then folds around the gubernaculum and creates the inguinal canal. In the third stage, the gubernaculum increases to the approximate diameter of the testis. As its proximal portion degenerates, the gubernaculum draws the testis into the scrotum through the processus vaginalis (Fig. 52–8C).

The testes usually complete their descent by the seventh month of gestation; approximately 97.5% of full-term infants and 79% of premature infants have fully descended testes at birth. At 9 months of age, only 0.8% of male infants have undescended testes. The incidence of undescended testes in young adult males is 0.2%.

Testicular descent is an androgen-dependent process, and development of the structures involved in testicular descent is dependent on testosterone. Thus, in testosterone-deficient states caused by inadequate secretion or disordered androgen action, the testes of genetic males often fail to descend. This abnormality can be seen in individuals with both 5α-reductase deficiency and complete androgen resistance (i.e., testicular feminization syndrome).

IMPAIRED ANDROGEN ACTION IN TARGET TISSUES

We have seen that in the absence of androgens, male embryos follow a typically female pattern of sexual development. However, such a female developmental pattern can occur even if testosterone levels are normal or elevated. Any defect in the mechanisms by which androgens *act* on target tissues—in genotypic males—may lead to a syndrome of **male pseudohermaphroditism.** Affected individuals have a normal male karyotype (46,XY) and unambiguous male gonads but ambiguous external genitalia or may phenotypically appear as females. In principle, impaired androgen action could result from a deficiency of the enzyme that converts testosterone to dihydrotestosterone (DHT) in target tissues, absent androgen receptors, qualitatively abnormal receptors, a quantitative deficiency in receptor levels, or postreceptor defects. The two major forms that have been identified clinically are defects in the conversion of testosterone to DHT (5α-reductase deficiency) and androgen receptor defects.

5α-REDUCTASE DEFICIENCY

The activity of 5α-reductase, which is necessary for the conversion of testosterone to DHT, is either low or absent in fibroblasts taken from the genital region and other tissues of these individuals. The testosterone concentration is either normal or increased. On the other hand, the concentration of DHT is low, which explains why testosterone-dependent development occurs (e.g., differentiation of the wolffian duct) whereas DHT-dependent development does not (e.g., male-pattern development of the urogenital sinus and external genitalia). This disorder is transmitted as an autosomal recessive gene that is phenotypically manifested only in genetic males. At birth, these children have ambiguous genitalia, with a blind vaginal pouch and a small phallus that is bound ventrally and covered by a hood; they also have hypospadias (i.e., the urethral orifice is located too low on the undersurface of the penis). Wolffian duct development (which depends on testosterone) occurs, and müllerian regression (which depends on antimüllerian hormone [AMH]) is normal. These individuals may be raised as females.

At the time of puberty, marked, though selective, virilization occurs. The testes descend from their intra-abdominal position. These individuals also undergo other signs of masculinization, including deepening of the voice, muscular development, and phallic enlargement.

The cause for virilization at puberty in these individuals is unknown. However, it may be that the large quantities of testosterone produced at puberty are able to sufficiently stimulate androgen receptors in DHT-dependent tissues or that even relatively low levels of 5α-reductase activity are able to generate sufficient DHT in the presence of high levels of substrate (i.e., testosterone). However, masculine features that depend on DHT—such as beard growth, acne, and temporal balding—fail to occur.

COMPLETE ANDROGEN RESISTANCE OR ANDROGEN INSENSITIVITY SYNDROME OR TESTICULAR FEMINIZATION

Individuals with this disorder have normal levels of testosterone and DHT. Moreover, the pathways of testosterone metabolism and half-life are normal. However, androgen receptors are defective or absent. As a result, either androgens do not bind to receptors at high levels, or the androgen-receptor complex does not bind properly to DNA. Because target cells behave as though androgens were not present at all, androgen-dependent sexual development does not occur. As a result, the wolffian ducts degenerate, and the urogenital sinus and external genitalia all develop according to the female pattern. However, the normal levels of AMH suppress müllerian development. Although a rudimentary uterus and fallopian tubes are sometimes found, their growth and development have obviously been inhibited.

The term **testicular feminization,** which is no longer used, was introduced by J.M. Morris in 1953 to describe a group of patients with a distinctive form of male pseudohermaphroditism. This X-linked disorder has a prevalence of 1 in 20,000 live male births. These individuals are genetic males—their sex chromosome complex is XY—but phenotypic females. They appear normal at birth with the exception of the presence of an inguinal hernia. The testis is either intra-abdominal, located in an inguinal hernia, or in the labia majora. They have unambiguous female external genitalia. However, the labia majora are underdeveloped, the vagina is shallow and ends blindly, and the uterus is at most rudimentary. The clitoris is normal or small. Development and growth of individuals with complete androgen resistance usually follow the normal female pattern. At puberty, breast development occurs at the expected time. However, these individuals have a significant deficiency or total lack of pubic and axillary hair and failure to menstruate.

of the urogenital sinus, the prostate, the penile urethra, and the external genitalia during embryogenesis requires DHT, as does sexual maturation at puberty.

DIFFERENTIATION OF THE DUCT SYSTEM. After formation of the testicular cords, the Sertoli cells produce AMH, which causes the müllerian ducts to regress. The cranial end of the müllerian duct becomes the vestigial appendix testis at the superior pole of the testis. Shortly after the initiation of AMH production, the fetal Leydig cells begin producing testosterone. The embryonic mesenchyme contains androgen receptors and is the first site of androgen action during formation of the male urogenital tract. The

Sertoli cells also produce a substance referred to as **androgen-binding protein** (ABP). It is possible that ABP binds and maintains a high concentration of testosterone locally. These high local levels of testosterone stimulate growth and differentiation of the medulla of the gonad into the rete testes, as well as differentiation of the wolffian ducts into the epididymis, the vas deferens, the seminal vesicles, and the ejaculatory duct. Testosterone also promotes development of the prostate from a series of endodermal buds located at the proximal aspect of the urethra. Cells of the wolffian ducts lack 5α-reductase and therefore cannot convert testosterone to DHT. Thus, the internal male ducts respond to testosterone per se and do not require the conversion of testosterone to DHT. In the absence of testosterone, the wolffian system remains rudimentary, and normal male internal ductal development does not occur.

DIFFERENTIATION OF THE UROGENITAL SINUS AND EXTERNAL GENITALIA. The cells of the urogenital sinus and external genitalia, unlike those of the wolffian duct, contain 5α-reductase and are thus capable of converting testosterone to DHT. Indeed, conversion of testosterone to DHT is required for normal male development of the external genitalia. Congenital absence of 5α-reductase (see the box titled Impaired Androgen Action in Target Tissues) is associated with normal development of the wolffian duct system but impaired virilization of the external genitalia.

At about 9 weeks' gestation, soon after virilization of the internal genital ducts of the male, development of the external genitalia commences. It is completed by 13 weeks of gestation. In the presence of high intracellular concentrations of DHT, the genital tubercle, the bipotential predecessor to either a clitoris or a penis, elongates to become the glans penis, the corpus spongiosum, and the two corpora cavernosa. Formation of the penis and scrotum is complete by approximately 13 weeks, and even extremely high concentrations of testosterone after this time fail to cause midline fusion of the urethral groove or scrotum, although the clitoris will enlarge. The urogenital sinus gives rise to the prostrate and the bulbourethral glands, also under the influence of DHT.

In the absence of androgen secretion by the fetal testis—or abnormal extragonadal sources—the indifferent external genitalia remain unfused and follow the female pattern of differentiation.

Androgens and Estrogens Influence Sexual Differentiation of the Brain

Anatomically sexually dimorphic nuclei have been identified in the diencephalons of rodents and lower primates. Gonadal steroids influence the development of these sexually dimorphic nuclei. Androgens do not act directly on the hypothalamus and other areas of the brain having to do with sex behavior and control of gonadotropin secretion. Rather, aromatase—which catalyzes the formation of estrone and estradiol (see Fig. 54–9)—converts androgens to estrogens in the brain. Thus, androgens in the brain serve as prohormones for estrogens. Therefore, it is estrogens that are derived from androgens that appear to directly masculinize sexually dimorphic nuclei in the brain. It is not clear why, in females, estrogens do not *masculinize* the brain.

Gonadal steroids affect sex behavior in both males and females. In rodents, lordosis behavior in females plus mounting behavior in males is one example of sex behavior. An example of functional sexual dimorphism in the human brain is the manner in which gonadotropin is released. Gonadotropin release has been described as "cyclic" in the female and "tonic" in the male inasmuch as females have midcycle cyclic release of gonadotropin before ovulation whereas males seem to have a continuous tonic pattern of gonadotropin release.

Although controversy continues over the role of prenatal virilization in the determination of sexual dimorphism, sex steroids clearly have an impact on sexual behavior and sexual reference in humans.

The Secondary Sex Characteristics that Appear at Puberty Represent the Completion of Sexual Differentiation and Development

Although at birth humans have the primary and secondary sex organs necessary for procreation, final sexual maturity occurs only at puberty. Profound alterations in hormone secretion during the peripubertal period cause changes in the primary and secondary sex organs. The events occurring in puberty are discussed in more detail for both the male (see Chapter 53) and the female (see Chapter 54).

In the female, the vagina reflects the effects of estrogens on the vaginal mucosa. The uterus and cervix enlarge, and their secretory functions increase under the influence of estrogen. The uterine glands increase in number and length, and the endometrium and stroma proliferate in

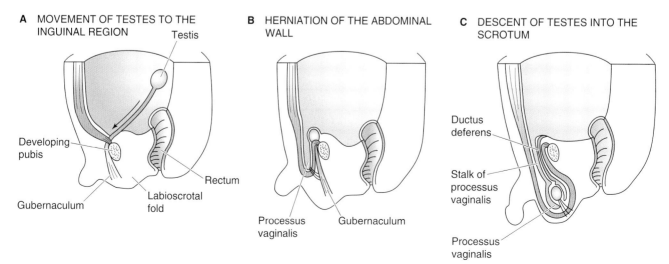

A MOVEMENT OF TESTES TO THE INGUINAL REGION

Testis

Developing pubis

Gubernaculum

Labioscrotal fold

Rectum

B HERNIATION OF THE ABDOMINAL WALL

Processus vaginalis

Gubernaculum

C DESCENT OF TESTES INTO THE SCROTUM

Ductus deferens

Stalk of processus vaginalis

Processus vaginalis

FIGURE 52–8. Testicular descent.

response to estrogen secretion. The cervical glands produce increasing quantities of cervical mucus, which serves to lubricate the vaginal vault. The mucous membranes of the female urogenital tract are made of stratified squamous epithelium; these membranes respond to hormones, particularly estrogens. Estrogen levels increase and cause increased epithelial proliferation with the formation of successive intermediate and superficial layers. The cells of the vaginal mucosa are transformed into superficial cells, and the thickness of the vaginal mucosa increases. Development of the breasts occurs under the influence of a complex of hormones. Progesterone is primarily responsible for development of the alveoli, which are analogous to the acini of other exocrine glands. Estrogen is the primary stimulus for development of the duct system that connects the alveoli to the exterior. Insulin, growth hormone, glucocorticoids, and thyroxin contribute to breast development, but they are incapable of causing breast growth by themselves. Lactation is discussed on p. 1185.

In the male, the penis undergoes rapid growth under the influence of testosterone secreted by the testes. The testes also increase dramatically in size in response to increasing androgen secretion at puberty.

REFERENCES

Books and Reviews

Donahoe PK, Budzik GP, Trelstad R, et al: Mullerian-inhibiting substance. An update. Recent Prog Horm Res 38:279, 1982.

Grumbach MM, Conte FA: Disorders of sex differentiation. In Wilson JD, Foster DW, Kronenberg HM, Larsen PR (eds): Williams Textbook of Endocrinology, 9th ed. Philadelphia, WB Saunders, 1998, pp 1303–1425.

Haqq CM, Donahoe PK: Regulation of sexual dimorphism in mammals. Physiol Rev 78:1–33, 1998.

Jost A, Vigier B, Prepin J, Perchellet JP: Studies on sex differentiation in mammals. Recent Prog Horm Res 29:1–41, 1973.

Lee MM, Donahoe PK: Müllerian inhibiting substance: A gonadal hormone with multiple functions. Endocr Rev 14:152–164, 1993.

Naftolin F, Ryan KJ, Davie KJ, et al: The formation of estrogens by central neuroendocrine tissues. Recent Prog Horm Res 31:295–319, 1975.

Rebar RW: Normal and abnormal sexual differentiation and pubertal development. In Moore TR, Reiter RC, Rebar RW, Baker VV (eds): Gynecology & Obstetrics. A Longitudinal Approach. New York, Churchill Livingstone, 1993, pp 97–146.

Journal Articles

Griffin JE, Wilson JD: The syndromes of androgen resistance. N Engl J Med 302:198–209, 1980.

Judd HL, Hamilton CR, Barlow JJ, et al: Androgen and gonadotropin dynamics in testicular feminization syndrome. J Clin Endocrinol Metab 34:229–234, 1972.

New MI, Dupont B, Pang S, et al: An update of congenital adrenal hyperplasia. Recent Prog Horm Res 37:105–181, 1981.

Sinclair AH, Berta P, Palmer MS, et al: A gene from the human sex-determining region encodes a protein with homology to a conserved DNA-binding motif. Nature 346:240–244, 1990.

Turner HH: A syndrome of infantilism, congenital webbed neck, and cubitus valgus. Endocrinology 23:566–574, 1938.

Wilkins L: Masculinization of the female fetus due to the use of orally given progestins. JAMA 172:1028–1032, 1960.

CHAPTER 53

The Male Reproductive System

Ervin E. Jones and Alan H. DeCherney

The male reproductive system (Fig. 53–1A) consists of two essential elements: the *gonads* and the complex array of glands and conduits that constitute the **sex accessories**.

The **gonads** in males are the testes, and they are responsible for the production of gametes, the haploid cells (spermatozoa) necessary for sexual reproduction. The gonads also synthesize and secrete the hormones that are necessary for functional conditioning of the sex organs, control of gonadotropin secretion, and modulation of sexual behavior.

The testis (Fig. 53–1B, C) is largely composed of seminiferous tubules and the interstitial cells of Leydig, located in the spaces between the tubules. The seminiferous tubules are lined by seminiferous epithelium, which rests on the inner surface of a basement membrane (Fig. 53–1D). The basement membrane is supported by a thin lamina propria externa.

The **sex accessories** in the male include the paired epididymides, the vas deferens, the seminal vesicles, and the ejaculatory ducts. Also included among the sex accessories are the prostate, the bulbourethral (Cowper's) glands, the urethra, and the penis. The primary role of the male sex accessory glands and ducts is to store and transport spermatozoa to the exterior at the proper time, thus enabling them to come in contact with and fertilize female gametes.

PUBERTAL DEVELOPMENT AND MALE SECONDARY SEXUAL CHARACTERISTICS

Puberty Occurs in Five Defined Stages

During the final month of fetal life, the testes descend (see the box titled Androgen Dependence of Testicular Descent on p. 1118) into an integumentary pouch called the scrotum. The inguinal canals through which the testes descend are sealed off shortly after birth. Because the internal temperature of the testicle must be closely regulated for optimum function, localization of the testes within the scrotum appears to be a necessary adaptation for testicular function. Aberrant retention of the testes in the abdominal cavity (cryptorchidism) causes marked damage to the seminiferous tubules and diminished testicular function.

The range of onset of normal male puberty extends from 9 to 14 years. Boys complete pubertal development within 2 to 4½ years. In a normal male, the first sign of puberty (stage 2) is enlargement of the testes to greater than 2.5 cm. Testicular enlargement is mainly a result of growth of

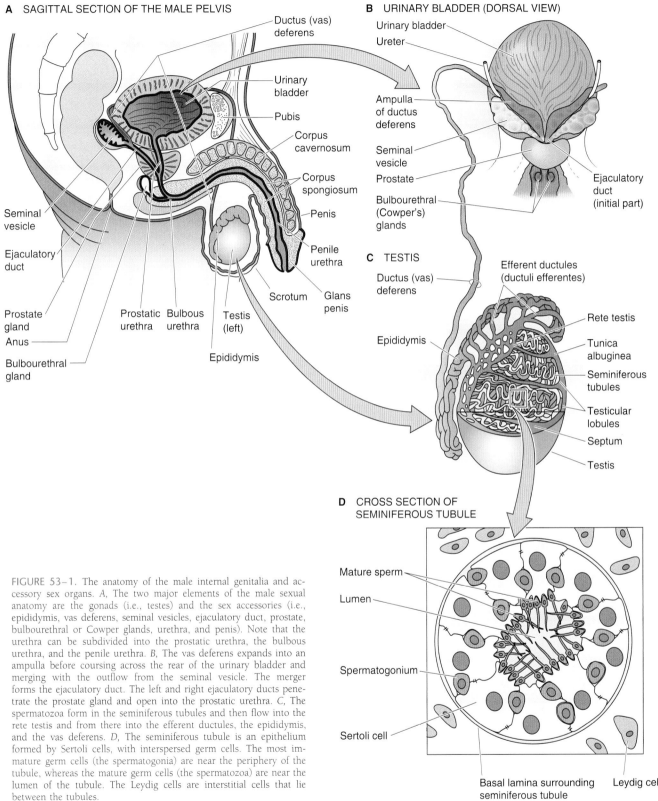

A   SAGITTAL SECTION OF THE MALE PELVIS

Ductus (vas) deferens

Urinary bladder

Pubis

Corpus cavernosum

Corpus spongiosum

Penis

Penile urethra

Glans penis

Scrotum

Testis (left)

Epididymis

Seminal vesicle

Ejaculatory duct

Prostate gland

Anus

Bulbourethral gland

Prostatic urethra

Bulbous urethra

B   URINARY BLADDER (DORSAL VIEW)

Urinary bladder

Ureter

Ampulla of ductus deferens

Seminal vesicle

Prostate

Bulbourethral (Cowper's) glands

Ejaculatory duct (initial part)

C   TESTIS

Ductus (vas) deferens

Epididymis

Efferent ductules (ductuli efferentes)

Rete testis

Tunica albuginea

Seminiferous tubules

Testicular lobules

Septum

Testis

D   CROSS SECTION OF SEMINIFEROUS TUBULE

Mature sperm

Lumen

Spermatogonium

Sertoli cell

Basal lamina surrounding seminiferous tubule

Leydig cell

FIGURE 53–1. The anatomy of the male internal genitalia and accessory sex organs. *A*, The two major elements of the male sexual anatomy are the gonads (i.e., testes) and the sex accessories (i.e., epididymis, vas deferens, seminal vesicles, ejaculatory duct, prostate, bulbourethral or Cowper glands, urethra, and penis). Note that the urethra can be subdivided into the prostatic urethra, the bulbous urethra, and the penile urethra. *B*, The vas deferens expands into an ampulla before coursing across the rear of the urinary bladder and merging with the outflow from the seminal vesicle. The merger forms the ejaculatory duct. The left and right ejaculatory ducts penetrate the prostate gland and open into the prostatic urethra. *C*, The spermatozoa form in the seminiferous tubules and then flow into the rete testis and from there into the efferent ductules, the epididymis, and the vas deferens. *D*, The seminiferous tubule is an epithelium formed by Sertoli cells, with interspersed germ cells. The most immature germ cells (the spermatogonia) are near the periphery of the tubule, whereas the mature germ cells (the spermatozoa) are near the lumen of the tubule. The Leydig cells are interstitial cells that lie between the tubules.

the seminiferous tubules, but Leydig cell enlargement contributes as well. Androgens from the testes are the driving force behind secondary sexual development, although adrenal androgens play a role in normal puberty. The Tanner method of describing the stages of pubertal development is widely accepted. Genital development and growth of pubic hair are best described separately, as indicated by the two columns in Table 53–1. Thus, it is possible for an adolescent boy to be at genital stage 3, pubic hair stage 2.

Testicular size is generally determined by using a ruler or calipers. It is expected that a length greater than 2.5 cm is compatible with the onset of normal pubertal development. The **testicular volume index** is defined as the sum of the length × width product for the left and right testes. An orchidometer allows direct comparison of the patient's testes with an oval of measured volume. A popular method uses the Prader orchidometer, a set of solid or hollow ovals encompassing the range from infancy to adulthood (1 to 25 ml). The volumes of the testes are then recorded; a volume of 3 ml closely correlates with the onset of pubertal development.

Spermarchy, or the first appearance of spermatozoa in early morning urine, occurs at a mean age of about 13.4 years and corresponds to genital stages 3 to 4 and pubic hair stages 2 to 4. The **pubertal spurt**, a marked increase in growth rate (total body size), occurs late in puberty in boys, at genital stages 3 to 4. The acceleration of growth appears to be partly a result of increased secretion of growth hormone at puberty and partially a result of testosterone production. Boys experience, on average, 28 cm of growth during the pubertal spurt. The 10-cm mean difference in adult stature between men and women is due to a greater pubertal growth spurt in boys and to greater height at the onset of peak height velocity in boys versus girls. Before puberty, boys and girls have the same mean body mass, skeletal mass, and body fat. However, men have 150% of the average woman's lean and skeletal body mass, and women have 200% of the body fat of men. Men have twice the number of muscle cells that women have and 1.5 times the muscle mass.

Androgens Determine Male Secondary Sexual Characteristics

The male sex steroids, which are known as androgens, affect nearly every tissue in the body, including the brain. The development of both the external and the internal genitalia depends on male sex hormones (p. 1118). Androgens stimulate adult maturation of the external genitalia and accessory sexual organs, including the penis, the scrotum, the prostate, and the seminal vesicles. Androgens also determine the male secondary sexual characteristics, which include deepening of the voice, as well as evolving male patterns of hair growth. The effects on the voice are a result of androgen-dependent effects on the size of the larynx, as well as the length and thickness of the vocal cords. In boys, the length of the vocal cords increases by about 50% during puberty, whereas girls have little increase in vocal cord length. The surfaces of the human body that bear secondary sexual hair include the face (particularly the upper lip, chin, and the sideburn areas), the axilla, and the pubic region. Temporal hair recession and male-pattern balding are also androgen-dependent phenomena.

Muscle Development and Growth Are Androgen-Dependent Processes

Androgens have anabolic effects, including stimulation of linear body growth, nitrogen retention, and muscular development in the adolescent and mature male. The biologic effects of testosterone and its metabolites have been classified according to their tissue sites of action. Effects that relate to growth of the male reproductive tract or development of secondary sexual characteristics are referred to as **androgenic**, whereas the growth-promoting effects on somatic tissue are called **anabolic**. These androgenic and anabolic effects are two independent biologic actions of the same class of steroids. Experimental evidence, however, indicates that these responses are organ specific and that the molecular mechanisms that initiate

TABLE 53–1

STAGES IN MALE PUBERTY

STAGE	GENITAL DEVELOPMENT	PUBIC HAIR
1	Preadolescent. The penis, scrotum, and testes are the same size—relative to body size—as in a young child	Preadolescent. No pubic hair is present, only vellus hair, as on the abdomen
2	Scrotum and testes are enlarged	Pubic hair is sparse, mainly at the base of the penis
3	Penis is enlarged, predominantly in length. Scrotum and testes are further enlarged	Pubic hair is darker, coarser, and curlier and spreads above the pubis
4	Penis is further enlarged in length and also in diameter. Scrotum and testes are further enlarged	Pubic hair is of the adult type, but covers an area smaller than in most adults
5	Adult pattern	Adult pattern

androgenic responses are the same as those that stimulate anabolic activity.

HYPOTHALAMIC-PITUITARY-GONADAL AXIS AND CONTROL OF MALE SEXUAL FUNCTIONS

The male hypothalamic-pituitary-gonadal axis (Fig. 53–2) controls two primary functions: (1) production of male gametes (spermatogenesis) in the seminiferous tubules and (2) androgen biosynthesis in the Leydig cells in the testes. The hypothalamus produces gonadotropin-releasing hormone (GnRH), which stimulates the gonadotrophs in the anterior pituitary to secrete the two gonadotropins, luteinizing hormone (LH) and follicle stimulating hormone (FSH). As discussed in Chapter 54, the names of these hormones reflect their function in the female reproductive system. LH and FSH control, respectively, the Leydig and Sertoli cells of the testes.

The Hypothalamus Secretes GnRH, Which Acts on Gonadotrophs in the Anterior Pituitary

GnRH, which is synthesized by small-bodied peptidergic neurons in the hypothalamus, stimulates the synthesis, storage, and secretion of gonadotropins by gonadotroph cells in the anterior pituitary. The hypothalamic-pituitary-portal system (p. 1010) describes the route by which GnRH and other releasing hormones emanating from the hypothalamus reach the anterior pituitary gland. The neurons that synthesize, store, and release GnRH are dispersed throughout the hypothalamus but are principally located in the arcuate nucleus and preoptic area. Studies involving both rats and primates have shown that extrahypothalamic sites (e.g., the limbic system) of GnRH production can also participate in the control of sex behavior. Neuronal systems originating from other areas of the brain impinge on the hypothalamic GnRH-releasing neurons and thus form a functional neuronal network.

GnRH is a decapeptide hormone that the aforementioned hypothalamic neurons synthesize in the secretory pathway (p. 36). Like many other peptide hormones, GnRH is synthesized as a prohormone—69 amino acids long in this case—from which the mature GnRH is generated by enzymatic cleavage. The synthesis of GnRH is discussed in more detail on p. 1146. The neurons release GnRH into the extracellular space, to be carried to the anterior pituitary via the long portal vessels.

GnRH stimulates the release of both FSH and LH from the gonadotroph cells of the anterior pituitary. FSH and LH are the primary gonadotropins; in males, they stimulate testicular function. The cell surface of the pituitary gonadotrophs is the site of high-affinity membrane receptors for GnRH. These receptors are coupled to the G protein $G\alpha_q$, which activates phospholipase C (PLC; p. 100). PLC acts on membrane phosphoinositides to liberate inositol 1,4,5-triphosphate (IP_3), which triggers Ca^{2+} release from internal stores, and diacylglycerol (DAG), which stimulates protein kinase C. The result is the syn-

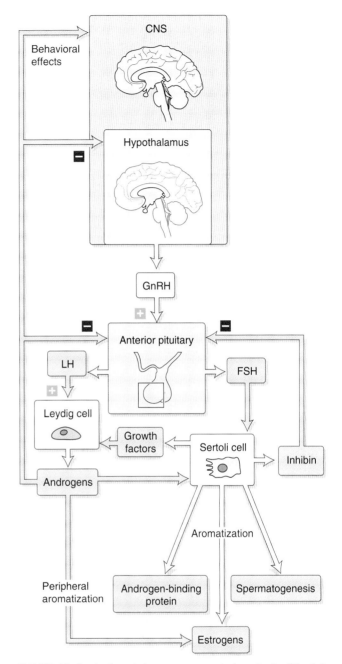

FIGURE 53–2. The hypothalamic-pituitary-testicular axis. Small-bodied neurons in the arcuate nucleus and preoptic area of the hypothalamus secrete gonadotropin-releasing hormone (GnRH), a decapeptide that reaches the gonadotrophs in the anterior pituitary via the long portal veins. Stimulation by GnRH causes the gonadotrophs to synthesize and release follicle stimulating hormone (FSH) and luteinizing hormone (LH). The LH binds to receptors on Leydig cells, stimulating the transcription of several proteins that are involved in the biosynthesis of testosterone. FSH binds to receptors on the basolateral membrane of Sertoli cells, stimulating gene transcription and protein synthesis. These proteins include androgen-binding protein, aromatase, growth factors, and inhibin. Negative feedback on the hypothalamic-pituitary-testicular axis occurs by two routes. First, testosterone inhibits the pulsatile release of GnRH by the hypothalamic neurons and the release of LH by the gonadotrophs in the anterior pituitary. Second, inhibin inhibits the release of FSH by the gonadotrophs in the anterior pituitary. CNS, central nervous system.

thesis and release of both LH and FSH from the gonado-trophs. Because secretion of GnRH into the portal system is pulsatile, secretion of both LH and FSH by the gonado-trophs is also episodic. The frequency of pulsatile LH discharge in men is approximately 8 to 14 pulses over a 24-hour period. FSH pulses are not as prominent as LH pulses, both because of their lower amplitude and because of the longer half-life of FSH in the circulation.

Although pulsatile GnRH discharge elicits a corresponding pulsatile release of LH and FSH, *continuous* administration of GnRH—or intermittent administration of high doses of GnRH analogues—suppresses the release of gonadotropins. As described in the box titled Therapeutic Uses of GnRH on p. 1149, the mechanism is inhibition of the replenishment of GnRH receptors so that insufficient receptors are available for GnRH function. A clinical application of this principle is in prostatic cancer, where the administration of GnRH analogues lowers LH and FSH levels, thus lowering testosterone production (i.e., chemical castration).

Products of the testes, particularly sex steroids and inhibin (see later), exert negative feedback control on hypothalamic and anterior-pituitary function. Neural elements in the arcuate nucleus respond to sex steroids. Sex steroids alter the frequency and amplitude of the LH secretory pulses in both men and women. Androgens also exert powerful influences on higher brain function, as evidenced by alterations in sex behavior.

Under the Control of GnRH, Gonadotrophs in the Anterior Pituitary Secrete LH and FSH

LH and FSH, which are secreted by the gonadotrophs of the anterior pituitary, are the primary regulators of testicular function. LH and FSH are members of the same family of hormones as human chorionic gonadotropin (hCG; p. 1172) and thyroid-stimulating hormone (TSH; p. 1046). All these glycoprotein hormones are composed of two polypeptide chains designated α and β. Both subunits, α and β, are required for full biologic activity. The α subunits of LH and FSH, as well as the α subunits of hCG and TSH, are identical. In humans, the common α subunit has 92 amino acids and a molecular weight of approximately 20 kDa. It is the β subunits that differ among these four hormones and thus confer specific functional and immunologic characteristics to the intact molecules.

The unique β subunits of FSH and LH are each 115 amino acids in length. The β subunits of LH and hCG are identical, except that the β subunit of hCG has an additional 24 amino acids and additional glycosylation sites at the C terminus. hCG is secreted by the placenta, and some reports have described small amounts of this substance being made in the testes, pituitary gland, and other nonplacental tissue. The biologic activities of LH and hCG are very similar. Indeed, in most clinical uses (e.g., in an attempt to initiate spermatogenesis in oligo-spermic males), hCG is substituted for LH because hCG is much more readily available.

The specific gonadotropin and the relative proportions of each gonadotropin released from the anterior pituitary

depend on the developmental age, as well as the existing hormonal milieu. The pituitary gland of the male fetus contains functional gonadotrophs by the end of the first trimester of gestation. Thereafter, gonadotropin secretion rises rapidly and then plateaus. Gonadotropin secretion begins to decline in utero during late fetal life and increases again during the early postnatal period.

Male primates release LH in response to GnRH administration at 1 to 3 months of age, indicative of functional competence of the anterior pituitary gland. Also during this time, a short-lived postnatal surge of LH and testosterone secretion occurs in males. Although the etiology of this short-lived surge of gonadotropins remains to be understood, it is clearly independent of sex steroids. The sensitivity of the gonadotrophs to stimulation subsequently diminishes, and the system remains quiescent until just before puberty.

Release of FSH is greater than that of LH during the prepubertal period, a pattern that is reversed after puberty. GnRH preferentially triggers LH release in an adult human male. This preferential release of LH may reflect maturation of the testes, which secrete inhibin, a specific inhibitor of FSH secretion at the level of the anterior pituitary gland. Increased sensitivity of the pituitary to increasing gonadal steroid production may also be responsible for the diminished secretion of FSH.

Luteinizing Hormone Stimulates the Leydig (Interstitial) Cells of the Testis to Produce Testosterone

LH derives its name from effects observed in the female, that is, from the ability to stimulate luteal function. The comparable substance in the male was originally referred to as interstitial cell–stimulating hormone (ICSH). Subsequently, it was realized that LH and ICSH are the same, and the common name became LH.

Testosterone production decreases in males after hypophysectomy. This observation led to our current understanding that LH secreted by the anterior pituitary gland is essential for testosterone production by the testis. The interstitial cells of the testis, the **Leydig cells**, are the primary source of testosterone production in the male. Leydig cells synthesize androgens from cholesterol by using a series of enzymes that are part of the steroid biosynthetic pathways (see later).

LH binds to specific high-affinity cell-surface receptors on the plasma membrane of Leydig cells (Fig. 53–3). Binding of LH to this G-protein–coupled receptor on the Leydig cell stimulates membrane-bound adenylyl cyclase (p. 97), which catalyzes the formation of cyclic adenosine monophosphate (cAMP) and thus activates protein kinase A (PKA). Activated PKA modulates gene transcription (p. 133) and increases the synthesis of enzymes and other proteins necessary for the biosynthesis of testosterone. Indeed, the action of LH on steroidogenesis in Leydig cells requires the synthesis of new protein. New mRNA is necessary for the synthesis of these proteins inasmuch as their synthesis is inhibited by the transcription inhibitor actinomycin D. The net effect of LH on Leydig cells is to stimulate the synthesis of testosterone.

FIGURE 53–3. Leydig- and Sertoli-cell physiology. The Leydig cell (*left*) has receptors for LH. The binding of LH increases testosterone synthesis. The Sertoli cell (*right*) has receptors for FSH. (Useful mnemonics: "L" for LH and Leydig, "S" for FSH and Sertoli.) FSH promotes the synthesis of androgen-binding protein (ABP), aromatase, growth factors, and inhibin. There is crosstalk between Leydig cells and Sertoli cells. The Leydig cells make testosterone, which acts on Sertoli cells. Conversely, the Sertoli cells convert some of this testosterone to estradiol (because of the presence of aromatase), which can act on the Leydig cells. Sertoli cells also generate growth factors that act on the Leydig cells. ATP, adenosine triphosphate; cAMP, cyclic adenosine monophosphate; FSH, follicle stimulating hormone; PKA, protein kinase A.

In addition to the enzymes specifically involved in steroidogenesis, LH stimulates the synthesis of other proteins, including sterol-carrier protein (SCP) and sterol-activating protein (SAP). **Sterol-carrier protein** (SCP-2), a 13.5-kDa protein, appears to contribute to the transport of cholesterol from the outer mitochondrial membrane to the inner mitochondrial membrane, where the side-chain-cleavage enzyme is located. This process is thus necessary for the first step of steroidogenesis, the synthesis of pregnenolone. A 3.2-kDa protein referred to as **sterol-activating protein** also activates steroidogenesis. SAP was originally isolated from adrenal cells and has been found in the Leydig cell as well.

Follicle-Stimulating Hormone Stimulates Sertoli Cells to Synthesize a Number of Products Needed by Both Leydig Cells and Developing Spermatogonia

The Sertoli cells seem to be the primary testicular site of FSH action (Fig. 53–3), as has become clear from experiments involving suppression of LH secretion. FSH also regulates Leydig-cell physiology via effects on Sertoli cells. The early biochemical events after FSH binding are similar to those described for LH on the Leydig cell. Thus, binding of FSH to a G-protein–coupled receptor initiates a series of reactions involving stimulation of adenylyl cyclase, increase in [cAMP]ᵢ, stimulation of PKA, transcription of specific genes, and increased protein synthesis. Several proteins are synthesized in response to FSH. Some are important for steroid action:

First, FSH leads to the synthesis of **androgen-binding protein** (ABP), which is secreted into the luminal space of the seminiferous tubule, near the developing sperm cells. ABP helps keep local testosterone levels high (p. 1119).

Second, FSH causes the synthesis of a **P-450 aromatase** (P-450$_{arom}$, p. 1153). Inside the Sertoli cells, this enzyme converts testosterone, which diffuses from the Leydig cells to the Sertoli cells, into estradiol.

Third, FSH leads to the production of a number of **growth factors** and other products by Sertoli cells that support sperm cells and spermatogenesis. These substances significantly increase the number of spermatogonia, spermatocytes, and spermatids in the testis. Therefore, it appears that the stimulatory effect of FSH on spermatogenesis is not a direct action of FSH on the spermatogonia; instead, stimulation of spermatogenesis occurs via the action of FSH on Sertoli cells. FSH may also increase the fertility potential of sperm; it appears that this effect of FSH is due to stimulation of motility rather than an increase in the absolute number of sperm.

Fourth, FSH causes Sertoli cells to synthesize **inhibins**. The inhibins are members of the so-called transforming growth factor β (TGF-β) gene family, which also includes the activins and antimüllerian hormone (p. 1114). Inhibins are glycoprotein heterodimers consisting of one α and one β subunit that are covalently linked. The granulosa cells in the ovary and the Sertoli cells in the testis are the primary sources of inhibin in humans, other primates, and the lower vertebrates. We discuss the biology of inhibins and activins in more detail on p. 1151. Inhibins are secreted into the seminiferous tubule fluid and into the interstitial fluid of the testicle. Inhibins have both paracrine and endocrine actions. Locally, the inhibins are

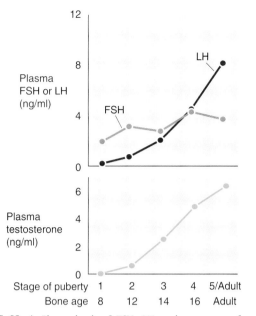

FIGURE 53–4. Plasma levels of FSH, LH, and testosterone from puberty to adulthood. Plasma levels of biologically active LH and FSH and of testosterone increase during puberty, expressed in terms of both the stages of puberty (see Table 53–1) and bone age. FSH, follicle stimulating hormone; LH, luteinizing hormone. (*Upper panel* data from Reiter EO, Beitins IZ, Ostrea TR, et al: Bioassayable luteinizing hormone during childhood and adolescence and in patients with delayed pubertal development. J Clin Endocrinol Metab 54:155–161, 1982 and Beitins IZ, Padmanabhan V, Kasa-Vubu J, et al: Serum bioactive follicle-stimulating hormone concentrations from prepuberty to adulthood: A cross-sectional study. J Clin Endocrinol Metab 71:1022–1027, 1990. *Lower panel* data from Grumbach MM, Styne DM: Puberty: ontogeny, neuroendocrinology, physiology, and disorders. In Wilson JD, Foster, DW, Kronenberg HM, Larsen PR: Williams Textbook of Endocrinology, 9th ed. Philadelphia, WB Saunders, 1998; pp. 1509–1625.)

some of the growth factors secreted by Sertoli cells that are thought to act on Leydig cells. More importantly, inhibins in the male play an important feedback role in the hypothalamic-pituitary-testicular axis (see later).

Interestingly, Leydig cells and Sertoli cells engage in **crosstalk**. For example, Leydig cells make testosterone that acts on Sertoli cells. In the rat, β-endorphin produced by fetal Leydig cells binds to opiate receptors in Sertoli cells and inhibits their multiplication. Synthesis of β-endorphins could represent a local feedback mechanism by which Leydig cells modulate Sertoli cell numbers. Conversely, Sertoli cells also have an effect on Leydig cells. For example, Sertoli cells convert testosterone—manufactured by Leydig cells—to estradiol, which then acts on the Leydig cells. In addition, FSH acting on Sertoli cells produces growth factors that may increase the number of LH receptors on Leydig cells during development and thus result in an increase in steroidogenesis (i.e., an increase in testosterone production).

What then is required for optimal spermatogenesis to occur? It appears that two testicular cell types (Leydig cells and Sertoli cells) are required, as well as two gonadotropins (LH and FSH) and one androgen (testosterone). First, LH and Leydig cells are required to produce testosterone. Thus, LH, or rather its substitute hCG, is used therapeutically to initiate spermatogenesis in azoospermic or oligospermic men. Second, FSH and Sertoli cells are important for the nursing of developing sperm cells and

for the production of inhibin and growth factors, which affect the Leydig cells. Thus, FSH plays a primary role in regulating development of the appropriate number of Leydig cells such that adequate testosterone levels are available for spermatogenesis.

During early puberty in boys, both FSH and LH levels increase while, simultaneously, the Leydig cells proliferate and plasma levels of testosterone increase (Fig. 53–4).

The Hypothalamic-Pituitary-Testicular Axis Is Under Reciprocal Inhibition by Testicular Hormones and Inhibin

The hypothalamic-pituitary axis not only generates testosterone and inhibin but also receives negative feedback from these substances (see Fig. 53–2). Normal circulating levels of both testosterone and estradiol exert inhibitory effects on LH secretion in males. Testosterone inhibits the pulsatile release of LH, presumably by inhibiting the pulsatile release of GnRH by the hypothalamus. Testosterone also appears to have negative feedback action on LH secretion at the level of the pituitary gonadotrophs.

A testicular hormone also feeds back on FSH secretion. Evidence for negative feedback by a testicular substance on FSH secretion is that plasma FSH concentrations increase in proportion to the loss of germinal elements in the testis. The FSH-inhibiting substance—inhibin—is a nonsteroid present in both the testis and cultures of Sertoli cells. Thus, FSH specifically stimulates Sertoli cells to produce inhibin, and inhibin "inhibits" FSH secretion. The preponderance of evidence indicates that inhibin diminishes FSH secretion by acting at the level of the anterior pituitary gland (not at the level of the hypothalamus).

THE PRODUCTION, METABOLISM, AND ACTION OF TESTOSTERONE

The Leydig Cells of the Testis Synthesize and Secrete Testosterone

Cholesterol is the obligate precursor for androgens, as well as other steroids produced by the testis. The Leydig cell can synthesize cholesterol de novo from acetyl coenzyme A or take it up as low-density lipoproteins from the extracellular fluid by receptor-mediated endocytosis (p. 44). The two sources appear to be equally important in humans.

The **Leydig cell** uses a series of five enzymes to convert cholesterol to testosterone. Three of these enzymes are P-450 enzymes (see Table 49–2). As summarized in Figure 53–5, because 3β-hydroxysteroid dehydrogenase (3β-HSD) can oxidize the A ring of four intermediates, testosterone synthesis from cholesterol can take four pathways; we follow the "preferred" pathway:

1. The pathway for testosterone synthesis begins in the mitochondria, where the cytochrome P-450 side-chain-cleavage (SCC) enzyme (also called 20,22-desmolase or P-450$_{SCC}$) removes the long side chain (carbons 22 to

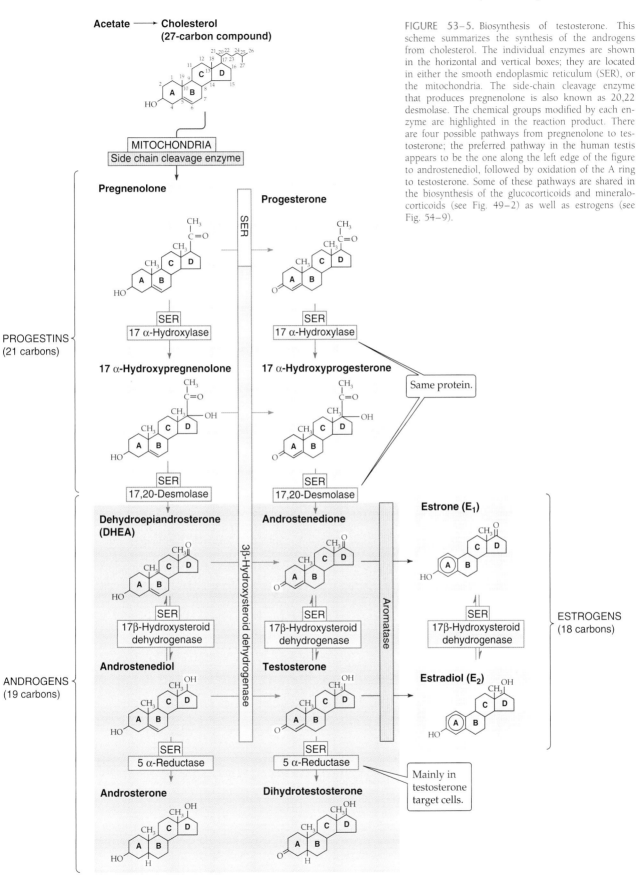

FIGURE 53–5. Biosynthesis of testosterone. This scheme summarizes the synthesis of the androgens from cholesterol. The individual enzymes are shown in the horizontal and vertical boxes; they are located in either the smooth endoplasmic reticulum (SER), or the mitochondria. The side-chain cleavage enzyme that produces pregnenolone is also known as 20,22 desmolase. The chemical groups modified by each enzyme are highlighted in the reaction product. There are four possible pathways from pregnenolone to testosterone; the preferred pathway in the human testis appears to be the one along the left edge of the figure to androstenediol, followed by oxidation of the A ring to testosterone. Some of these pathways are shared in the biosynthesis of the glucocorticoids and mineralocorticoids (see Fig. 49–2) as well as estrogens (see Fig. 54–9).

27) from the carbon at position 20 of the **cholesterol** molecule (27 carbon atoms). The rate-limiting step in the biosynthesis of testosterone, as for other steroid hormones, is the conversion of cholesterol to pregnenolone. LH stimulates this reaction and is the primary regulator of the overall rate of testosterone synthesis by the Leydig cell. LH appears to promote pregnenolone synthesis in two ways. First, it increases the affinity of the enzyme for cholesterol. Second, LH has long-term action in which it increases steroidogenesis in the testis by stimulating synthesis of the SCC enzyme.

2. The product of the SCC-catalyzed reaction is **pregnenolone** (21 carbon atoms). In the smooth endoplasmic reticulum (SER), 17α-hydroxylase (P-450$_{c17}$) then adds a hydroxyl group at position 17 to form **17α-hydroxypregnenolone**.

3. In the SER, the 17,20-desmolase (a different activity of the *same* P-450$_{c17}$ whose 17α-hydroxylase activity catalyzes the previous step) removes the side chain from carbon 17 of 17α-hydroxypregnenolone. That side chain begins with carbon 20. The result is a 19-carbon steroid called **dehydroepiandrosterone** (DHEA).

4. In the SER of the Leydig cell, a 17β-hydroxysteroid dehydrogenase (17β-HSD, which is *not* a P-450 enzyme) converts the ketone at position 17 to a hydroxyl group to form **androstenediol**.

5. Finally, 3β-HSD (*not* a P-450 enzyme) oxidizes the hydroxyl group at position 3 of the A ring to a ketone to form **testosterone**.

In addition, the testis can also use 5α-reductase, which is located in the SER, to convert testosterone to dihydrotestosterone (DHT). However, it is extratesticular tissue that is responsible for most of the production of DHT. The conversion of testosterone to DHT is especially important in certain testosterone target cells (p. 1118).

The Leydig cells of the testes make about 95% of the circulating testosterone. Although testosterone is the major secretory product, the testis also secretes pregnenolone, progesterone, 17-hydroxyprogesterone, androstenedione, androsterone, and DHT. Androstenedione is of major importance because it serves as a precursor for extraglandular estrogen formation.

Other Organs—Such as Adipose Tissue, Skin, and the Adrenal Cortex—also Produce Testosterone and Other Androgens

In men who are between the ages of 25 and 70 years, the rate of testosterone production remains relatively constant (Table 53–2). Figure 53–6 summarizes the changes in plasma testosterone levels as a function of age in human males.

Several tissues besides the testes—including adipose tissue, brain, muscle, skin, and adrenal cortex—produce testosterone and several other androgens. These substances may be synthesized de novo or produced by peripheral conversion of precursors. Moreover, the peripheral organs and tissues may convert sex steroids to less active forms (see Fig. 53–5). Notable sites of extragona-

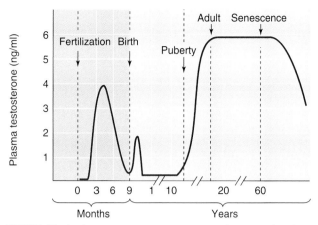

FIGURE 53–6. Plasma testosterone versus age in human males. (Data from Griffin JE, et al: The testis. In Bondy PK, Rosenberg LE: Metabolic Control and Disease. Philadelphia, WB Saunders, 1980; and Winter JS, Hughes IA, Reyes FI, Faiman C: Pituitary-gonadal relations in infancy: 2. Patterns of serum gonadal steroid concentrations in man from birth to two years of age. J Clin Endocrinol Metab 42:679–686, 1976.)

dal conversion include the skin and adipose tissue. Androstenedione is converted to testosterone in peripheral tissues. In this case, **androstenedione** is the precursor for the hormone testosterone. Testosterone can be converted to estradiol or DHT or go "backward" by reversible interconversion to androstenedione. Thus, a potent hormone such as testosterone may also serve as a precursor for a weaker hormone (androstenedione), a hormone with different activities (estradiol), or a more potent hormone having similar activities (DHT). This last example may be illustrated by the effects of DHT on hair follicles, sebaceous glands, and the sex accessories.

The adrenal gland (p. 1053) is another source of androgen production in both males and females. Normal human adrenal glands synthesize and secrete the androgens DHEA, conjugated DHEA sulfate, and androstenedione. Essentially, all the DHEA in male plasma is of adrenal origin. However, less than 1% of the total testosterone in plasma is derived from DHEA. As summarized in Table 53–2, the plasma concentration of androstenedione in males is only about 25% that of testosterone. About 20% of androstenedione is generated by peripheral metabolism of other steroids. Although the adrenal gland contributes significantly to the total androgen milieu in males, it does not appear to have significant effects on stimulation and growth of the male accessory organs.

Testosterone Acts on Target Organs by Binding to a Nuclear Receptor

Most testosterone in the circulation is bound to specific binding proteins. About 45% of plasma testosterone is bound to **sex hormone–binding globulin** (SHBG)—also called testosterone-binding globulin (TeBG), whereas about 55% is bound to serum albumin and corticosteroid-binding globulin (CBG) (p. 1053). A small fraction (~2%) of the total circulating testosterone circulates free, or unbound, in plasma. It is the free form of testosterone that enters the cell by passive diffusion and subsequently

TABLE 53-2

ANDROGEN PRODUCTION AND TURNOVER		
STEROID	**BLOOD PRODUCTION RATE—HORMONE DELIVERED TO THE BLOOD (μg/day)**	**PLASMA CONCENTRATION (μg/liter)**
Testosterone	6500	6.5
Androstenedione	2000–6000	1.5
Dihydrotestosterone	300	0.5

exerts biologic actions or undergoes metabolism by other organs such as the prostrate, liver, and intestines (see the next section). The quantity of testosterone entering a cell is determined by the plasma concentration and by the intracellular milieu of enzymes and binding proteins.

Once it diffuses into the cell, testosterone either binds to a high affinity-androgen receptor in the nucleus or is converted to DHT, which also binds to the androgen receptor. The androgen receptor functions as a homodimer (AR/AR) and is a member of the family of nuclear receptors (see Table 5–2) that includes receptors for glucocorticoids, mineralocorticoids, progestins, estrogens, vitamin D, thyroid hormone, and retinoic acid. The gene coding for the androgen receptor is located on the X chromosome. The androgen receptor is a protein with a molecular weight of approximately 110 kDa. The androgen-AR complex is a transcription factor that binds to hormone response elements on DNA located 5′ from the genes that the androgens control. Interaction between the androgen-AR complex and nuclear chromatin causes marked increases in transcription, ultimately leading to the synthesis of specific proteins. As a result of these synthetic processes, specific cell functions ensue, including growth and development. The presence of the androgen receptor in a cell or tissue determines whether that tissue can respond to androgens.

Whether the active compound in any tissue is DHT or testosterone depends on the presence or absence in that tissue of the microsomal enzyme **5α-reductase**, which converts testosterone to DHT. The biologic activity of DHT is 30 to 50 times higher than that of testosterone.

Non-genomic effects of androgens have also been described. For example, androgens may stimulate hepatic microsomal protein synthesis by a mechanism independent of binding to the androgen receptor. In other tissues, including the brain, testosterone is aromatized to estradiol, and thus the action of this metabolite occurs via the estrogen receptor. Other evidence indicates that the action of androgens on the prostate gland may occur via the adenylyl cyclase/PKA system (p. 97) and could result in gene activation under some circumstances.

Metabolism of Testosterone Occurs Primarily in the Liver and Prostate

Only small amounts of testosterone enter the urine without metabolism; this urinary testosterone represents less than 2% of the daily testosterone production. The large remaining balance of testosterone and other androgens is converted in the liver to 17-ketosteroids, and in the prostate to DHT. The degradation products of testosterone are primarily excreted in the urine as water-soluble conjugates of either sulfuric acid or glucuronic acid. These conjugated testosterone metabolites are also excreted in the feces.

TESTOSTERONE AND THE AGING MALE

For a long time, the abrupt hormonal alterations that signal the dramatic changes of female menopause were believed to have no correlate in males. We now know that men do experience a gradual decline in their serum testosterone levels (see Fig. 53–6) and that this decline is closely correlated with many of the changes that accompany aging: decreased bone formation, muscle mass, growth of facial hair, appetite, and libido. The blood hematocrit also decreases. Testosterone replacement can reverse many of these changes by restoring muscle and bone mass and correcting the anemia.

Although the levels of both total and free testosterone decline with age, levels of luteinizing hormone are frequently not elevated. This finding is believed to indicate that some degree of hypothalamic-pituitary dysfunction accompanies aging.

BIOLOGY OF SPERMATOGENESIS AND SEMEN

Spermatogenesis Includes the Mitotic Divisions of Spermatogonia, the Meiotic Divisions of Spermatocytes to Haploid Spermatids, and Maturation to Spermatozoa

Mature spermatozoa are derived from germ cells through a series of complex transformations. When seminiferous tubules are viewed in cross section (see Fig. 53–1D), the least mature cells are located adjacent to the basement membrane, whereas the most differentiated germ cells are located nearest the lumen.

As discussed in Chapter 52, the primordial germ cells migrate into the gonad during embryogenesis; these cells become immature germ cells, or **spermatogonia** (Fig. 53–7). Beginning at puberty and continuing thereafter throughout life, these spermatogonia, which lie next to the basement membrane of the stratified epithelium lining the seminiferous tubules, divide mitotically (Fig. 53–8).

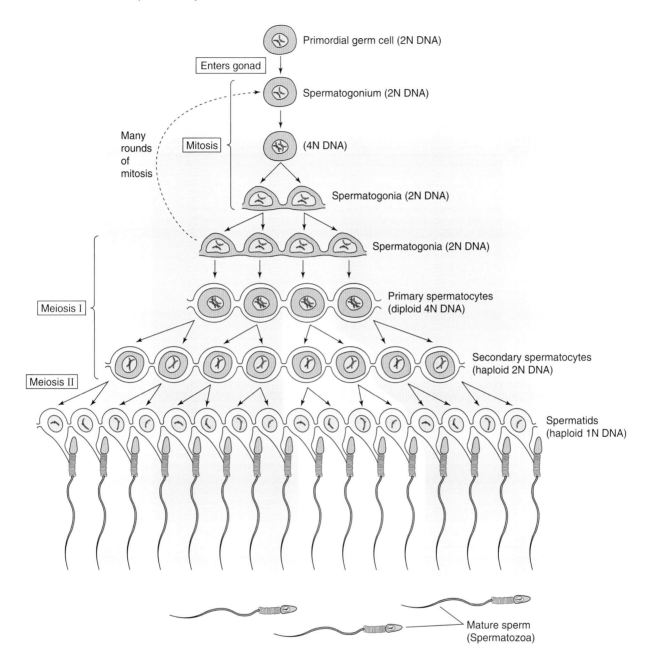

FIGURE 53–7. Schematic of spermatogenesis. Early during embryogenesis, the primordial germ cells migrate to the gonad, where they become spermatogonia. Beginning at puberty, the spermatogonia undergo many rounds of mitotic division. Some of these spermatogonia (2N DNA) enter the first meiotic division, at which time they are referred to as *primary spermatocytes*. During prophase, each primary spermatocyte has a full complement of duplicated chromosomes (4N DNA). Each primary spermatocyte divides into two secondary spermatocytes, each with a haploid number of duplicated chromosomes (2N DNA). The secondary spermatocyte enters the second meiotic division, producing two spermatids, each of which has a haploid number of unduplicated chromosomes (1N DNA). Further maturation of the spermatids yields the spermatozoa (mature sperm). Note that one primary spermatocyte yields four spermatozoa.

The spermatogonia have the normal diploid complement of 46 chromosomes (2N): 22 pairs of autosomal chromosomes plus one X and one Y chromosome.

Some of the spermatogonia enter into their first meiotic division and become **primary spermatocytes**. At the prophase of this first meiotic division, the chromosomes undergo crossing over (see Fig. 52–1). At this stage, each cell has a duplicated set of 46 chromosomes (4N): 22 pairs of duplicated autosomal chromosomes, a duplicated

X chromosome, and a duplicated Y chromosome. After completing this first meiotic division, the daughter cells become **secondary spermatocytes**, which have a haploid number of duplicated chromosomes (2N): 22 duplicated autosomal chromosomes and either a duplicated X or a duplicated Y chromosome. These secondary spermatocytes enter their second meiotic division almost immediately. This division results in smaller cells called spermatids, which have a *haploid* number of *unduplicated* chromo-

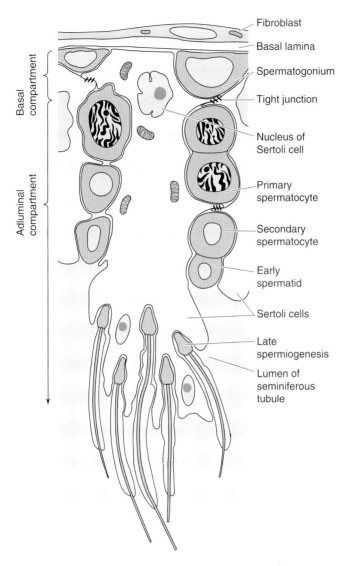

Fibroblast

Basal lamina

Spermatogonium

Tight junction

Nucleus of
Sertoli cell

Primary
spermatocyte

Secondary
spermatocyte

Early
spermatid

Sertoli cells

Late
spermiogenesis

Lumen of
seminiferous
tubule

Basal
compartment

Adluminal
compartment

FIGURE 53-8. Interaction of Sertoli cells and sperm. This figure is an idealized high-magnification view of a portion of the wall of a seminiferous tubule (see Fig. 53-1C). A single Sertoli cell spans from the basal lamina to the lumen of the seminiferous tubule. Adjacent Sertoli cells are connected by tight junctions and surround developing germ cells. From the basal lamina to the lumen of the tubule, there is a gradual maturation of the germ cells.

development undergo mitosis simultaneously. Transformation of spermatogonia into functional spermatozoa requires approximately 74 days. Each stage of spermatogenesis has a specific duration. In humans, the life span of the germ cells is 16 to 18 days for spermatogonia, 23 days for primary spermatocytes, 1 day for secondary spermatocytes, and approximately 23 days for spermatids. The rate of spermatogenesis is constant and cannot be accelerated by hormones such as gonadotropins or androgens. Germ cells must move forward in their differentiation; if the environment is unfavorable and makes it impossible for them to pursue their differentiation at the normal rate, they degenerate and are eliminated.

The most reliable expression of the sperm-production rate is the daily number of sperm cells produced per gram of testicular parenchyma. In 20-year-old men, the production rate is approximately 6.5 million sperm per gram per day. The rate falls progressively with age and averages around 3.8 million sperm per gram per day in men 50 to 90 years old. This decrease is probably related to the high rate of degeneration of germ cells during meiotic prophase. Among fertile men, those aged 51 to 90 years exhibit a significant decrease in the percentage of morphologically normal and motile spermatozoa.

In summary, three processes occur concurrently in the seminiferous epithelium: (1) an increase in the number of cells by mitosis, (2) a reduction in the number of chromosomes by meiosis, and (3) the production of mature sperm from spermatids by spermiogenesis. Thus, spermatogenesis is a regular, ordered, sequential process resulting in the production of mature male gametes.

It is instructive to consider how spermatogenesis in the male differs from oogenesis in the female. In fact, the two processes differ in each of the three steps just noted: (1) in the female, the *mitotic* proliferation of germ cells takes place entirely before birth. In the male, spermatogonia proliferate only after puberty and then throughout life. (2) The *meiotic* divisions of a primary oocyte in the female produce only one mature ovum. In the male, the meiotic divisions of a primary spermatocyte produce four mature spermatozoa. (3) In the female, the second meiotic division is completed only upon fertilization (p. 1169). Thus, no further development of the cell takes place after the completion of meiosis. In the male, the products of meiosis (the spermatids) undergo substantial further differentiation to produce mature spermatozoa.

The Sertoli Cells Support Spermatogenesis

The Sertoli cells are generally regarded as support or "nurse" cells for the spermatids (see Fig. 53-8). **Sertoli cells** are large polyhedral cells extending from the basement membrane toward the lumen of the seminiferous tubule. Spermatids are located adjacent to the lumen of the seminiferous tubules during the early stages of spermiogenesis and are surrounded by processes of Sertoli-cell cytoplasm. Tight junctions connect adjacent Sertoli cells. In addition, gap junctions between the Sertoli cells and developing spermatozoa may represent a mechanism for transferring material between these two types of cells. Release of the spermatozoa from the Sertoli cell has been

somes (1N). **Spermatids** form the inner layer of the epithelium and are found in rather discrete aggregates inasmuch as the cells derived from a single spermatogonium tend to remain together and differentiate synchronously. Spermatids transform into **spermatozoa** in a process called **spermiogenesis**, which involves cytoplasmic reduction and differentiation of the tail pieces. Thus, as maturation progresses, developing male gametes decrease in volume. Conversely, maturation leads to an increase in cell number, with each primary spermatocyte producing four spermatozoa, two with an X chromosome and two with a Y.

As additional generations of spermatogonia mature, the advanced cells are displaced toward the lumen of the tubule. Groups of spermatogonia at comparable stages of called **spermiation**. Spermatids progressively move toward the lumen of the tubule and eventually lose all contact with the Sertoli cell after spermiation.

Sperm Maturation Occurs in the Epididymis

The seminiferous tubules open into a network of tubules, the **rete testes**, which serves as a reservoir for sperm. The rete testes are connected to the epididymis via the **efferent ductules** (p. 1113), which are located near the superior pole of the testicle. The epididymis is a highly convoluted single long duct, 4 to 5 m in total length, on the posterior aspect of the testis. The epididymis can be divided anatomically into three regions: the head (the segment closest to the testis), the body, and the tail.

Spermatozoa are essentially immotile on completion of spermiogenesis. Thus, transfer of spermatozoa from the seminiferous tubule to the rete testes is passive. Secretions flow from the testes through the epididymis, with assistance by ciliary action of the luminal epithelium and contractility of the smooth-muscle elements of the efferent duct wall. Thus, sperm transport through this ductal system is also primarily passive. As noted earlier, about 74 days is required to produce spermatozoa, about 50 days of which is spent in the seminiferous tubule. After leaving the testes, sperm take 12 to 26 days to travel through the epididymis and appear in the ejaculate. The epididymal transit time for men between the ages of 20 and 80 years does not differ significantly.

Sperm are stored in the epididymis, where they undergo a process of maturation before they are capable of progressive motility and fertilization (Table 53–3). Spermatozoa released at ejaculation are fully motile and capa-

TABLE 53–3

SPERM MATURATION IN THE EPIDIDYMIS
Progressive increase in forward motility
Increased ability to fertilize
Maturation of acrosome
Molecular reorganization of the plasma membrane:
Lipids (stabilization of plasma membrane)
Proteins (shedding as well as acquisition of new proteins)
Ability to bind to zona pellucida
Acquisition of receptors for proteins of the zona pellucida
Increased disulfide bonds between cysteine residues in sperm nucleoproteins
Topographic regionalization of glycosidic residues
Accumulation of mannosylated residues on the periacrosomal plasma membrane
Decreased cytoplasm and cell volume

ble of fertilization, whereas spermatozoa obtained directly from the testis are functionally immature insofar as they cannot penetrate an ovum. However, these immature spermatozoa can fertilize if injected into an ovum. During maturation in the epididymis, spermatozoa undergo changes in motility, metabolism, and morphology. Spermatozoa derived from the head (caput) of the epididymis are often unable to fertilize ova, whereas a larger proportion of spermatozoa captured from the body (corpus) are fertile. Spermatozoa obtained from the tail (cauda) of the epididymis, or from the vas deferens, are almost always capable of fertilization.

The epididymis empties into the **vas deferens**, which is responsible for the movement of sperm along the tract. The vas deferens contains well-developed muscle layers that facilitate sperm movement. The vas deferens passes through the inguinal canal, traverses over the ureter, and continues medially to the posterior and inferior aspect of the urinary bladder, where it is joined by the duct arising from the **seminal vesicle**; together, they form the ejaculatory duct. The **ejaculatory duct** enters the prostatic portion of the urethra after passing through the prostate. Sperm are stored in the epididymis as well as in the proximal end of the vas deferens. All these accessory structures depend on androgens secreted by the testis for full functional development.

The Accessory Male Sex Glands—the Seminal Vesicles, Prostate, and Bulbourethral Glands—Produce the Seminal Plasma

Only 10% of the volume of **semen** (i.e., seminal fluid) is sperm cells. The normal concentration of sperm cells is greater than 20 million/ml, and the typical ejaculate vol-

---

SERTOLI CELL–ONLY SYNDROME

A group of normally virilized males have been described whose testes are small bilaterally and whose ejaculates contain no sperm cells (azoospermia). The seminiferous tubules of these men are lined by Sertoli cells, but they show a complete absence of germ cells. Sertoli cell–only syndrome (or germinal cell aplasia) accounts for 10% to 30% of male infertility secondary to azoospermia and can either be caused by a single-gene defect or be acquired (e.g., as a result of orchitis, alcoholism, toxic agents). Leydig cell function is usually preserved. Plasma testosterone and luteinizing hormone levels are usually normal, whereas follicle stimulating hormone (FSH) levels are often, but not always, elevated. It is not entirely clear why FSH levels are elevated in these men. It may be due to the absence of germ cells or to suboptimal secretion of inhibin by the Sertoli cells, inasmuch as inhibin is a powerful inhibitor of FSH secretion at the level of the anterior pituitary gland. Segments of Sertoli cell–only tubules may be observed in conditions such as orchitis or exposure to other agents that are toxic to the gonads. However, these individuals generally have functional spermatogenesis in the other seminiferous tubules.

ume is greater than 2 ml. The typical ejaculate content varies between 150 and 600 million spermatozoa.

Aside from the sperm cells, the remainder of the semen (i.e., 90%) is **seminal plasma**, the extracellular fluid of semen (Table 53–4). Very little seminal plasma accompanies the spermatozoa as they move through the testes and epididymis. The seminal plasma is derived primarily from the accessory glands (the seminal vesicles, prostate gland, and the bulbourethral glands). The seminal vesicles contribute approximately 70% of the volume of semen. Aside from the sperm, the remaining approximately 20% represents epididymal fluids, as well as secretions of the prostate gland and bulbourethral glands. However, the composition of the fluid exiting the urethral meatus during ejaculation is not uniform. The first fluid to exit is a mixture of prostatic secretions and spermatozoa with epididymal fluid. Subsequent emissions are composed of

TABLE 53–4

NORMAL VALUES FOR SEMEN

PARAMETER	VALUE
Volume	2–6 ml
Viscosity	Liquefaction in 1 hr
pH	7–8
Count	$\geq$20 million/ml
Motility	$\geq$50%
Morphology	60% normal

CONGENITAL AND ACQUIRED DUCTAL OBSTRUCTION

Genital duct obstruction may be congenital and result from ductal absence or structural abnormality, or it may be acquired as a result of stricture, infection, or vasectomy. Genital duct obstruction is found in approximately 7% of infertile men. An uncommon cause of male infertility is congenital **absence of the vas deferens,** which accounts for as many as 50% of cases of congenital ductal obstruction. These patients generally have azoospermic ejaculates with low volume. Congenital absence of the vas deferens is common in males with cystic fibrosis (CF) and is sometimes the only manifestation of CF.

Epididymal abnormalities range from the presence of an incomplete epididymis to the presence of only small portions of the epididymis; in addition, the seminal vesicles are often absent. Spermatogenesis is thought to be normal inasmuch as testicular biopsy specimens demonstrate germ cells in several stages of development. Obstruction of the epididymis may also occur as a result of gonococcal or tuberculous epididymitis. Smallpox and filariasis are common causes of ductal obstruction in areas where these diseases are endemic. Inspissated secretions may occlude the epididymis in men with Young syndrome or cystic fibrosis.

Elective vasectomy, a simple surgical procedure in which a small segment of the vas deferens is removed to ensure male infertility, is currently the leading cause of ductal obstruction.

Azoospermia in men with normal testes is the hallmark of genital duct obstruction. However, when specimens of testicles from men who have had vasectomies are examined microscopically, interstitial fibrosis has been found in as many as 20% of cases. It is this group that exhibits low fertility after elective reversal of their vasectomies. When the seminiferous tubules are examined, increased thickness of the tubule wall, an increase in cross-sectional tubular area, and decreased numbers of Sertoli cells are usually noted. Testosterone and gonadotropin levels are normal in most patients with ductal obstruction.

mainly secretions derived from the seminal vesicle. The first portion of the ejaculate contains the highest density of sperm; it also usually contains a higher percentage of motile sperm cells.

The seminal plasma is isotonic. The pH in the lumen of the epididymis is approximately 7.0. Addition of the relatively alkaline secretions of the seminal vesicles raises the final pH of seminal plasma to between 7.3 and 7.7. The quiescence of epididymal sperm is not well correlated with pH. Spermatozoa generally tolerate alkalinity better than acidity. A pH near neutrality or slightly higher is optimal for the motility and survival of sperm cells in humans and in other species as well.

Seminal plasma contains a plethora of sugars and ions. Fructose and citric acid are contributed to the seminal plasma by the accessory glands, and their concentrations vary with the volume of semen ejaculated. The **fructose** is produced in the seminal vesicles. In a man with oligospermia (i.e., a low daily sperm output) and a low ejaculate volume (recall that more than half of the ejaculate comes from the seminal vesicles), the absence of fructose suggests obstruction or atresia of the seminal vesicles. Ascorbic acid and traces of B vitamins are also found in human seminal plasma. The prostate gland releases a factor—which contains sugars, sulfate, and a vitamin E derivative—that acts to prevent the clumping of sperm heads. In addition, human semen also contains high concentrations of choline and spermine, although their roles remain to be clarified.

Seminal plasma is also rich in Ca^{2+}, Na^+, Mg^{2+}, K^+, Cl^-, and phosphate. Concentrations of Zn^{2+} and Ca^{2+} are higher in semen than in any other fluid and most other tissues. Calcium ions stimulate the motility of immature epididymal spermatozoa, but inhibit the motility of spermatozoa in ejaculates obtained from humans. It appears that the diminished response of sperm to Ca^{2+} and the acquisition of progressive motility are functions of epididymal maturation.

Semen also contains low-molecular-weight polypeptides and proteins. The free amino acids probably arise from the breakdown of protein after the semen is ejaculated. The amino acids may protect spermatozoa by binding heavy metals, which may be toxic, or by preventing the agglutination of proteins.

Human semen coagulates immediately after ejaculation. Coagulation is followed by liquefaction, which is apparently caused by proteolytic enzymes, which are contained in prostatic secretions. Prostatic secretion is rich in acid phosphatase. The natural substrate for acid phosphatase is phosphorylcholine, which is contributed by the seminal vesicles. Hyaluronidase is also present in human semen, although its functional role remains to be clarified. Hyaluronidase is not a product of the accessory glands; rather, it is contained within the sperm cell cytoplasm and is rapidly released into the seminal plasma. Hyaluronidase might perform a role in facilitating penetration of the oocyte by the sperm cell because of the ability of hyaluronidase to depolymerize hyaluronic acid.

MALE SEX ACT

Sex steroids influence the central nervous system, even in utero, and play important roles in determining and regulating complex patterns of sexual behavior. However, reproductive behavior is extraordinarily complex and influenced by numerous factors other than sex steroids, such as one's genetic constitution, social contacts, and the age at which hormones exert their effects. In this subchapter we describe the neurophysiology of the male sex act.

The Sympathetic and Parasympathetic Divisions of the Autonomic Nervous System Control the Male Genital System

The testes, epididymis, male accessory glands, and erectile tissue of the penis receive dual innervation from the sympathetic and parasympathetic branches of the autonomic nervous system (ANS). The penis also receives both somatic efferent (i.e., motor) and afferent (i.e., sensory) innervation via the pudendal nerve (S2 through S4).

SYMPATHETIC DIVISION OF THE ANS. As described in Chapter 15, the preganglionic **sympathetic neurons** originate in the thoracolumbar segments of the spinal cord (T1 through T12, L1 through L3; see Fig. 15–4). For the lower portion of the sympathetic chain (T5 and below), the preganglionic fibers may pass through the paravertebral sympathetic trunk and then pass via splanchnic nerves to a series of prevertebral plexuses and ganglia (see later). Once within one of these plexuses or ganglia, the preganglionic fiber may either (1) synapse with the postganglionic fiber or (2) pass on to a more caudal plexus or ganglion without synapsing.

The sympathetic efferent (motor) nerve fibers that are supplied to the male sex organs emanate from five primary prevertebral nerve plexuses (Fig. 53–9): the celiac, superior mesenteric, inferior mesenteric, superior hypogastric, and inferior hypogastric or pelvic plexuses. The **celiac plexus** is of interest in a discussion of male sex organs only because preganglionic sympathetic fibers pass through this plexus on their way to more caudal plexuses. The **superior mesenteric** plexus lies on the ventral aspect of the aorta. Preganglionic fibers from the celiac plexus pass through the superior mesenteric plexus on their way to more caudal plexuses.

Most of the preganglionic sympathetic fibers pass from the superior mesenteric plexus to the **inferior mesenteric** plexus, although some of the nerves pass directly to the hypogastric plexus. The **superior hypogastric plexus** is a network of nerves located distal to the bifurcation of the aorta. The **inferior hypogastric** or **pelvic plexus** receives sympathetic supply from the hypogastric nerve.

In addition to these five plexuses, two other small ganglia are of interest. The **spermatic ganglion** is located near the origin of the testicular artery from the aorta. The spermatic ganglion receives fibers directly from the lumbar sympathetic nerves and from branches of several other ganglia. The **hypogastric** (or pelvic) **ganglion** is located at the junction of the hypogastric and pelvic nerve trunks.

PARASYMPATHETIC DIVISION OF THE ANS. The preganglionic **parasympathetic neurons** relating to the male reproductive system originate in the sacral segments of the spinal cord (S2 through S4; see Fig. 15–4). These fibers pass via the pelvic nerve to the pelvic plexus, where they synapse with the postganglionic parasympathetic neurons.

VISCERAL AFFERENTS. Sensory fibers are present in all the nerve tracts described (see Fig. 15–2). These fibers either travel (1) with the pelvic nerves to the dorsal root of the spinal cord, (2) with the sacral nerves to the sympathetic trunk and then rising in the sympathetic trunk to the spinal cord, or (3) with the hypogastric nerve and ascending to more rostral prevertebral plexuses and then to the spinal cord.

The principal functions of motor innervation to the male accessory glands include control of smooth-muscle contraction, vascular tone, and epithelial secretory activity.

Erection Is Primarily Under Parasympathetic Control

The two corpora cavernosa and the corpus spongiosum are usually coordinated in their erection (i.e., tumescence) and detumescence. However, they may act independently inasmuch as their vascular and neuroeffector systems are relatively independent. During erection, relaxation of the smooth muscles of the corpora allows increased inflow of blood to fill the corporal interstices and results in an increase in volume and rigidity. Vascular actions of the smooth muscles of the corpora and the perineal striated muscles are coordinated. For example, contraction of the striated muscles overlying the vascular reservoirs of the penile bulb increases the pressure of the blood in the corpora and promotes increased rigidity. The three major efferent (i.e., motor) pathways for the regulation of penile erection are parasympathetic (pelvic nerve), sympathetic (hypogastric nerve), and somatic (pudendal nerve).

PARASYMPATHETIC INNERVATION. The first and most important pathway for erection is the parasympathetic division of the ANS. These fibers derive from the lumbar and sacral portions of the spinal cord and travel via the *pelvic nerve*, the *pelvic plexus*, and the *cavernous nerve* to the penile corpora and vasculature (see Fig. 53–9). This pathway is almost entirely parasympathetic, but apparently also carries some sympathetic fibers (see later). The

A SYMPATHETIC INNERVATION

B SAGITTAL SECTION SHOWING INNERVATION OF MALE GENITAL SYSTEM

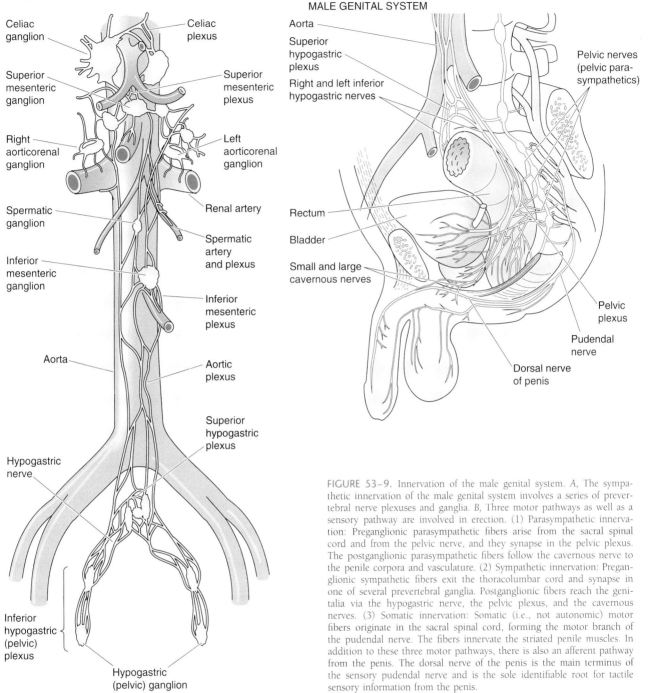

FIGURE 53–9. Innervation of the male genital system. *A,* The sympathetic innervation of the male genital system involves a series of prevertebral nerve plexuses and ganglia. *B,* Three motor pathways as well as a sensory pathway are involved in erection. (1) Parasympathetic innervation: Preganglionic parasympathetic fibers arise from the sacral spinal cord and from the pelvic nerve, and they synapse in the pelvic plexus. The postganglionic parasympathetic fibers follow the cavernous nerve to the penile corpora and vasculature. (2) Sympathetic innervation: Preganglionic sympathetic fibers exit the thoracolumbar cord and synapse in one of several prevertebral ganglia. Postganglionic fibers reach the genitalia via the hypogastric nerve, the pelvic plexus, and the cavernous nerves. (3) Somatic innervation: Somatic (i.e., not autonomic) motor fibers originate in the sacral spinal cord, forming the motor branch of the pudendal nerve. The fibers innervate the striated penile muscles. In addition to these three motor pathways, there is also an afferent pathway from the penis. The dorsal nerve of the penis is the main terminus of the sensory pudendal nerve and is the sole identifiable root for tactile sensory information from the penis.

parasympathetic activity results in vasodilatation of the penile blood vessels, thus increasing blood flow to the cavernous tissue and engorging the organ with blood. In erectile tissue, parasympathetic postganglionic terminals release acetylcholine (ACh) and nitric oxide (NO), similar to the system we discussed in Chapter 15 (see Fig. 15–11). First, ACh may bind to M_3 muscarinic receptors on endothelial cells. Via $G\alpha_q$, these receptors would then lead to stimulation of PLC, increased $[Ca^{2+}]_i$, activation of NO synthase, and local release of NO (p. 110). Second, the nerve terminals may also directly release NO. Regardless of the source of NO, this gas diffuses to the vascular smooth-muscle cell, where it stimulates guanylyl cyclase to generate cyclic guanosine monophosphate, which in turn causes vasodilation (p. 545). See the box titled Erectile Dysfunction.

SYMPATHETIC INNERVATION. The second pathway, which is thought to be entirely **sympathetic**, exits the thoracolumbar cord. The preganglionic fibers then course via the least splanchnic nerve, the sympathetic chain, and the inferior mesenteric ganglion. The postganglionic fibers reach the genitalia via the *hypogastric nerve,* the *pelvic plexus,* and the *cavernous nerves* (see earlier). Tonic sympathetic activity contributes to penile *flaccidity.* During erection, a decrease in this sympathetic tone allows relaxation of the corpora and thus contributes to tumescence.

SOMATIC INNERVATION. The third pathway is the motor branch of the pudendal nerve. It has primarily **somatic** (i.e., not autonomic) fibers, originates in the sacral cord, and innervates the striated penile muscles. Contraction of the striated ischiocavernosus muscle during the final phase of erection increases pressure inside the corpora cavernosa to values that are even higher than systemic arterial pressure. Contraction of the striated bulbospongiosus muscle increases engorgement of the corpus spongiosum, and thus the glans penis, by pumping blood up from the penile bulb underlying this muscle. Humans are apparently less dependent on their striated penile muscle for achieving and maintaining erection. However, these muscles are active during ejaculation and contribute to the force of seminal expulsion.

Postganglionic neurons release other so-called nonadrenergic, noncholinergic neurotransmitters (p. 545)—including NO—that also contribute to the erectile process.

AFFERENT INNERVATION. The penis also has an afferent pathway. The dorsal nerve of the penis is the main terminus of the sensory pudendal nerve and is the sole identifiable root for tactile sensory information from the penis.

Emission Is Primarily Under Sympathetic Control

The term seminal **emission** refers to movement of the ejaculate into the prostatic or proximal part of the urethra. Under some conditions, seminal fluid escapes episodically or continuously from the penile urethra; this action is also referred to as emission. Emission is the result of peristaltic contractions of the ampullary portion of the vas deferens, the seminal vesicles, and the prostatic smooth muscles. These actions are accompanied by constriction of the internal sphincter of the bladder, which is under sympathetic control (p. 754), thus preventing retrograde ejaculation of sperm into the urinary bladder (see the box titled Ejaculatory Dysfunction—Retrograde Ejaculation).

The rhythmic contractions that are involved in emission are due to contraction of smooth muscle. In contrast to other visceral organ systems, the smooth-muscle cells of the male ducts and accessory glands fail to establish close contact with one another and show limited electrotonic coupling. In the male accessory glands, individual smooth-muscle cells are directly innervated and have only limited spontaneous activity (i.e., "multiunit smooth muscle"; p. 231). This combination allows a fast, powerful, and coordinated response to neural stimulation.

ERECTILE DYSFUNCTION

Sildenafil (**Viagra**®) is a reasonably well tolerated oral treatment for erectile dysfunction. Men with erectile dysfunction experience significant improvement in rigidity and duration of erections when treated with oral sildenafil.

As indicated in the text, the smooth-muscle tone of the human corpus cavernosum is regulated by the synthesis and release of nitric oxide, which raises the intracellular concentration of cyclic guanosine monophosphate ($[cGMP]_i$) in vascular smooth-muscle cells and thereby leads to vasodilatation and erection. Breakdown of cGMP by cGMP-specific phosphodiesterase type 5 limits the degree of vasodilation and, in the case of the penis, limits erection. Sildenafil is a highly selective, high-affinity inhibitor of cGMP-specific phosphodiesterase type 5 and thereby raises $[cGMP]_i$. Orally administered sildenafil thus increases $[cGMP]_i$ in smooth muscle and in this manner improves erection in men with erectile dysfunction.

This new therapy is attractive because sildenafil is the first pill (for oral use) with established efficacy that benefits most men with insufficient erection. This medication stimulates erection only during sexual arousal and thus has a rather natural effect. Sildenafil does not need to be taken daily, but it may be taken when needed, 1 hour before planned sexual activity.

Interestingly, one of the side effects of sildenafil is "blue vision," a consequence of the effect of inhibiting cGMP-specific phosphodiesterase in the retina. In individuals taking other vasodilators, sildenafil can lead to sudden death. In women, sildenafil may improve sexual function by increasing blood flow to the accessory secretory glands (p. 1143 and p. 1162).

MOTOR ACTIVITY OF THE DUCT SYSTEM. A gradation between two forms of smooth-muscle activity occurs along the male duct system. The efferent ducts and proximal regions of the epididymis are sparsely innervated, but display spontaneous contractions that can be increased via adrenergic agents acting on α-adrenergic receptors. In contrast, the distal end of the epididymis and the vas deferens are normally quiescent until neural stimulation is received during the ejaculatory process. Contraction of the smooth muscle of the distal epididymis, vas deferens, and accessory sex glands occurs in response to stimulation of the *sympathetic* fibers in the hypogastric nerve and release of norepinephrine. Indeed, an intravenous injection of epinephrine or norepinephrine can induce seminal emission, whereas selective chemical sympathectomy or an adrenergic antagonist can inhibit seminal emission. The role of *parasympathetic* innervation to the musculature of these ducts and accessory glands in the male is not entirely clear. Parasympathetic fibers may be preferentially involved in basal muscular activity during erection (i.e., before ejaculation) and during urination.

SECRETORY ACTIVITY OF THE ACCESSORY GLANDS. The effect of autonomic innervation on the secretory activity of the epithelia of the male accessory glands has been studied extensively. Electrical stimulation of the pelvic nerves (parasympathetic) induces copious secretions. The secretory rate depends on the frequency of stimulation and can be blocked with atropine, a competitive inhibitor of muscarinic ACh receptors. Cholinergic drugs induce the formation of copious amounts of secretions when administered systemically. Secretions from the bulbourethral glands also contribute to the ejaculate. The bulbourethral glands do not store secretions but produce them during coitus. The secretory activity of the bulbourethral glands also appears to be under cholinergic control inasmuch as administration of atropine causes marked inhibition of secretion from these glands.

Control of the motor activity of the ducts and the secretory activity of the accessory glands is complex and involves both the sympathetic and the parasympathetic divisions of the ANS. The central nervous system initiates and coordinates all these activities.

Ejaculation Is Under Control of a Spinal Reflex

As discussed, seminal emission transports semen to the proximal (posterior) part of the urethra. **Ejaculation** is the forceful expulsion of this semen from the urethra. Ejaculation is normally a reflex reaction triggered by the

---

EJACULATORY DYSFUNCTION— RETROGRADE EJACULATION

As noted in the text, emission is normally accompanied by constriction of the internal urethral sphincter. Retrograde ejaculation occurs when this sphincter fails to constrict. As a result, the semen enters the urinary bladder rather than passing down the urethra. Retrograde ejaculation should be suspected in patients who report absent or small-volume ejaculation after orgasm. The presence of greater than 15 sperm per high-power field in urine specimens obtained after ejaculation confirms the presence of retrograde ejaculation.

Lack of emission or retrograde ejaculation may result from any process that interferes with innervation of the vas deferens and bladder neck. Several medical illnesses, such as diabetes mellitus (which can cause peripheral neuropathy) and multiple sclerosis, or the use of pharmaceutical agents that interfere with sympathetic tone can lead to retrograde ejaculation. Retrograde ejaculation may also occur as a result of nerve damage associated with certain surgical procedures, including bladder neck surgery, transurethral resection of the prostate, colorectal surgery, and retroperitoneal lymph node dissection. Retrograde ejaculation from causes other than surgery involving the bladder neck may be treated with pharmacologic therapy. Sympathomimetic drugs such as phentolamine (an α-adrenergic agonist), ephedrine (which enhances norepinephrine release), and imipramine (which inhibits norepinephrine re-uptake by presynaptic terminals) may promote normal (i.e., anterograde) ejaculation by increasing the tone of the vas deferens (propelling the seminal fluid) and the internal sphincter (preventing retrograde movement).

NEURONAL LESIONS AFFECTING ERECTION AND EJACULATION

Erectile dysfunction is often associated with disorders of the central and peripheral nervous systems. Spinal cord disease and peripheral neuropathies are of particular interest, and spinal-cord injuries have been studied in some detail. Erectile capacity is usually preserved in men with lesions of the premotor neurons (neurons that project from the brain to the spinal cord; see Table 53–5). In these men, reflexogenic erections occur in 90% to 100% of cases, whereas psychogenic erections do not occur because the pathways from the brain are blocked. Ejaculation is more significantly impaired in upper than in lower motor neuron lesions, presumably because of loss of the psychogenic component.

A clinically important feature of the spinal segmentation of nerve roots for generating erection (i.e., thoracolumbar and lumbosacral) is that spinal or peripheral nerve damage may affect only one of the effector systems. Because the lumbosacral system also carries most of the penile afferents, erection in response to penile stimulation (reflexogenic) will be most affected by damage to the lower spinal cord or the nerves that project there. Evidence from men with spinal injuries in the T10 through T12 region has implicated the sympathetic thoracolumbar pathway in mediating erections resulting from sexual stimuli received via the cranial nerves or generated within the brain as memories, fantasies, or dreams. In men with lower–motor-neuron lesions, reflexogenic erections are absent. However, psychogenic erections still occur in most men with incomplete lesions and in about one quarter of men with complete lesions. It remains uncertain whether this sympathetic pathway is normally the principal route for psychogenic erections or whether it just assumes the role when lumbosacral parasympathetic pathways are damaged.

---

entry of semen from the prostatic urethra into the bulbous urethra. Thus, emission sets the stage for ejaculation. The ejaculatory process is a spinal-cord reflex, although it is also under considerable cerebral control. The afferent (i.e., sensory) impulses reach the sacral spinal cord (S2 through S4) and trigger efferent activity in the somatic motor neurons that travel via the pudendal nerve. The resulting rhythmic contractions of the striated muscles of the perineal area—including the muscles of the pelvic floor, as well as the ischiocavernosus and bulbospongiosus muscles—forcefully propel the semen via the urethra through the external meatus. In addition, spasmodic contractions of the muscles of the hips and the anal sphincter generally accompany ejaculation.

Orgasm is a term best restricted to the culmination of sexual excitation, as generally applied to both men and women. Orgasm is the cognitive correlation of ejaculation in the human male. Although orgasm, the pleasurable sensation that accompanies ejaculation, is not well understood, clearly, it is as much a central phenomenon as it is a peripheral one.

TABLE 53–5

EFFECTS OF NEURAL LESIONS ON ERECTION AND EJACULATION

LESION	REFLEXOGENIC ERECTION	PSYCHOGENIC ERECTION	EFFECT ON EJACULATION
Upper motor neuron	Present	Absent	Significantly impaired
Lower motor neuron	Absent	Present	Less impaired

REFERENCES

Books and Reviews

Ackland JF, Schwartz NB, Mayo KE, Dodson RE: Nonsteroidal signals originating in the gonads. Physiol Rev 72:731–787, 1992.

Andersson K-E, Wagner G: Physiology of penile erection. Physiol Rev 75:191–236, 1995.

Hecht NB: Molecular mechanisms of male germ cell differentiation. Bioessays 20:555–561, 1998.

Mather JP, Moore A, Li RH: Activins, inhibins, and follistatins: Further thoughts on a growing family of regulators. Proc Soc Exp Biol Med 215:209–222, 1997.

Skinner MK: Cell-cell interaction in the testis. Endocr Rev 12:45–77, 1991.

Wilson JD, Foster DW, Kronenberg HM, Larsen PR (eds): Williams Textbook of Endocrinology, 9th ed. Philadelphia, WB Saunders, 1998.

Journal Articles

Beitins IZ, Padmanabhan V, Kasa-Vubu J, et al: Serum bioactive follicle-stimulating hormone concentrations from prepuberty to adulthood: A cross-sectional study. J Clin Endocrinol Metab 71:1022–1027, 1990.

Carter AJ, Ballard SA, Naylor AM: Effect of the selective phosphodiesterase type 5 inhibitor sildenafil on erectile dysfunction in the anesthetized dog. J Urol 160:242–246, 1998.

Koraitim M, Schafer W, Melchior H, Lutzeyer W: Dynamic activity of bladder neck and external sphincter in ejaculation. Urology 10:130–132, 1977.

Ludwig DG: The effect of androgen on spermatogenesis. Endocrinology 46:453–481, 1950.

Reiter EO, Beitins IZ, Ostrea TR, Gutai JP: Bioassayable luteinizing hormone during childhood and adolescence and in patients with delayed pubertal development. J Clin Endocrinol Metab 54:155–161, 1982.

CHAPTER 54

The Female Reproductive System

Ervin E. Jones and Alan H. DeCherney

Reproductive Function in the Human Female Is Inherently Cyclic

Reproductive function in human females is controlled by hormones that emanate from the hypothalamic-pituitary-gonadal axis (p. 1010). The release of a mature ovum from an ovary, known as **ovulation**, is the dominant event of the **menstrual cycle**. Whereas ovulation in some mammals is triggered by mating, ovulation in the human female is spontaneous and regulated by *cyclic functional interactions* among signals coming from the hypothalamus, the anterior pituitary, and the ovaries. Although many aspects of female reproduction are cyclic, maturation and atresia of the functional units of the ovaries—the ovarian follicles—are continuous processes that occur throughout reproductive life.

The ovaries are not the only female organs that undergo rhythmic changes. Alterations in cervical and uterine function are controlled by changes in the circulating concentrations of ovarian hormones, that is, the estrogens and progestins. For example, the uterine endometrium thickens under the influence of ovarian hormones and deteriorates and sloughs at the end of the cycle when ovarian estrogen and progestin secretion diminishes. Menstruation reflects this periodic shedding of the endometrium. Menstrual cycles are generally repetitive unless they are interrupted by pregnancy or terminated by menopause. All the cyclic physiological changes prepare the female reproductive tract for sperm and ovum transport, fertilization, implantation, and pregnancy.

Female Reproductive Organs Include the Ovaries and Accessory Sex Organs

The ovaries lie on the sides of the pelvic cavity (Fig. 54–1A). A layer of mesothelial cells covers the surface of the ovary. The ovary itself consists of an inner medulla and an outer zone, or cortex, that surrounds the medulla except at the hilar area. The **cortex** of the ovary in a mature female contains developing follicles and corpora lutea in various stages of development (see Fig. 54–1B). These elements are interspersed throughout the stroma, which includes connective tissue, interstitial cells, and blood vessels. The **medulla** comprises large blood vessels and other stromal elements.

The female **accessory sex organs** include the fallopian tubes, the uterus,

A OBLIQUE VIEW OF THE INTERNAL FEMALE SEX ORGANS

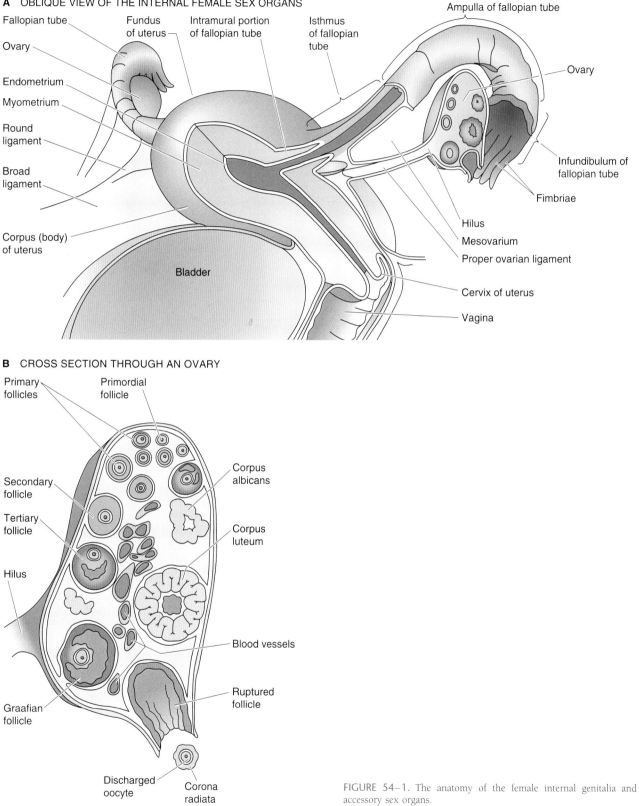

B CROSS SECTION THROUGH AN OVARY

FIGURE 54–1. The anatomy of the female internal genitalia and accessory sex organs.

the vagina, and the external genitalia. The **fallopian tube** provides a pathway for the transport of ova from the ovary to the uterus. The distal end of the fallopian tube expands as the infundibulum, which ends in multiple fimbriae. The infundibulum is lined with epithelial cells that have cilia that beat toward the uterus. The activity of these cilia and the contractions of the wall of the fallopian tube, particularly around the time of ovulation, facilitate transport of the ovum.

The **uterus** is a complex, pear-shaped, muscular organ that is suspended by a series of supporting ligaments. It is composed of a fundus, a corpus, and a narrow caudal portion that is called the **cervix**. The external surface of the uterus is covered by serosa, whereas the interior, or endometrium, of the uterus consists of complex glandular tissue and stroma. The uterus is continuous with the vagina via the cervical canal. The cervix is composed of dense fibrous connective tissue and muscle cells. The cervical glands lining the cervical canal produce a sugar-rich secretion, the viscosity of which is conditioned by estrogen and progesterone.

The human **vagina** is about 10 cm in length and is a single, expandable tube. The vagina is lined by stratified epithelium and is surrounded by a thin muscular layer. During development, the lower end of the vagina is covered by the membranous hymen, which is partially perforated during fetal life. In some instances, the hymen remains continuous. The **external genitalia** include the clitoris, the labia majora, and the labia minora, as well as the accessory secretory glands (including the glands of Bartholin), which open into the vestibule. The **clitoris** is an erectile organ, which is homologous to the penis (p. 1120) and mirrors the cavernous ends of the glans penis.

TABLE 54–1

STAGES IN FEMALE PUBERTY

STAGE	BREAST DEVELOPMENT	PUBIC HAIR
1	Preadolescent. Only papillae are elevated	Preadolescent. No pubic hair is present, only vellus hair, as on the abdomen
2	Breasts and papillae are both elevated, and the diameter of the areolae increases	Pubic hair is sparse, mainly along the labia majora
3	The breasts and areolae further enlarge	Pubic hair is darker, coarser, and curlier and spreads over the pubis
4	The areolae and papillae project out beyond the level of the expanding breast tissue	The pubic hair is of adult type, but covers an area smaller than in most adults
5	With further enlargement of the breast, the areolae are now on the same level as the rest of the breast. Only the papillae project. Adult pattern	Adult pattern

PUBERTY

Puberty Marks the Transition to Cyclic, Adult Reproductive Function

Puberty is the transition from a noncyclic, relatively quiescent reproductive endocrine system to a state of cyclic reproductive function that allows procreation. Puberty involves the beginning of menstrual cycles (**menarche**), breast development (**thelarche**), and an increase in adrenal androgen secretion (**adrenarche**). Table 54–1 summarizes the stages of puberty in the female.

The precise cause of the onset of puberty is not completely understood, although multiple intrinsic and extrinsic factors play a role. Genetic factors are major determinants of pubertal onset. Other factors, such as nutrition, geographic location, and exposure to light, also play a role. Over the last century, the age of girls at menarche in the United States and Europe has gradually decreased. Although the reason that menarche now occurs at a younger age remains incompletely understood, it is probably because of improved nutritional status. However, better nutritional status alone cannot completely explain the decreased age of pubertal onset. Distance from the equator and lower altitudes are associated with early onset of puberty. A loose correlation is also seen between the onset of menarche in the mother and the onset of

menarche in the daughter. The onset of puberty is also related to body composition and to fat deposition. Severe obesity and heavy exercise delay puberty.

Gonadotropin Levels Are Low During Childhood

As shown in Figure 54–2A, a surge in the levels of the pituitary gonadotropins, luteinizing hormone (LH) and follicle-stimulating hormone (FSH), occurs during intra-uterine life. A second peak takes place in the immediate postnatal period. However, gonadotropin levels tend to decrease at approximately 4 months of age; thereafter, they decline and remain low until just before puberty. Gonadotropin levels are lowest between 6 and 8 years of age. Although the reason for low gonadotropin secretion by the pituitary in childhood remains unknown, it was once thought to be due to feedback inhibition by *high levels* of gonadal steroids. However, an experiment of nature has revealed that such is not the case. Indeed, girls with gonadal dysgenesis, like normal girls, have low levels of LH and FSH, even though their ovaries produce *low levels* of steroids. Thus, it is likely that the low levels of gonadotropins in the prepubertal period do not reflect high levels of steroids, but rather a *high sensitivity* to feedback inhibition of the hypothalamic-pituitary system by these steroids. We discuss this feedback mechanism in the next section.

A   PATTERNS OF GONADOTROPIN LEVELS THROUGHOUT THE LIFE OF A FEMALE

B   NEGATIVE FEEDBACK OF ESTROGENS
ON GONADOTROPIN RELEASE

C   AGE DEPENDENCE OF FEEDBACK SENSITIVITY

FIGURE 54–2. Gonadotropin function during life. *A*, The levels of both luteinizing hormone (LH) and follicle stimulating hormone (FSH) peak during fetal life and again during early infancy, before falling to low levels throughout the rest of childhood. At the onset of puberty, LH and FSH levels slowly rise and then begin to oscillate at regular monthly intervals. At menopause, gonadotropin levels rise to very high levels. The four *insets* show daily changes in gonadotropin levels. *B*, This is a highly schematic plot of how estrogen levels negatively feed back on gonadotropin secretion by the gonadotroph cells of the anterior pituitary. In childhood, even very low estrogen levels are sufficient to fully suppress gonadotropin output. In adolescence, higher levels of estrogens are required. In the adult woman, estrogens must be at very high levels to suppress gonadotropin release. *C*, This is a plot—versus age—of the midpoints of curves such as those in *B*.

During Puberty, GnRH Secretion Becomes Pulsatile, and the Sensitivity of the Gonadotrophs to Feedback Inhibition by Estrogens Decreases

As shown by the *insets* to Figure 54–2*A*, one of the earliest events of puberty is the onset of pulsatile gonadotropin secretion from the pituitary during rapid eye movement (REM) sleep; this pulsatile gonadotropin secretion reflects the pulsatile release of gonadotropin-releasing hormone (GnRH) from the hypothalamus. The development of secondary sexual characteristics follows the onset of sleep-associated pulsatility. With maturation, these

pulses occur throughout the day. It is not understood why pulsatile behavior should occur initially only during REM sleep. The precipitating event that is responsible for initiating pulsatile GnRH release is also unknown, although it may reflect the maturation of hypothalamic neurons. Once a pulsatile pattern of gonadotropin secretion is established, it continues throughout reproductive life into menopause.

The increased pulsatility of GnRH release eventually leads to a marked increase in plasma LH levels—the **LH surge** that marks the initiation of the first menstrual cycle. During early pubescence, the LH surges do not occur in a regular pattern, so menstrual cycles are generally irregular. As the reproductive system matures, the LH surges gradually come at regular intervals, and cyclic reproductive function becomes firmly established.

The appearance of GnRH pulsatility early in puberty is associated with decreased sensitivity of the hypothalamic-pituitary system to circulating sex steroids. In young girls, even low levels of sex steroids are sufficient to feed back on the hypothalamic-pituitary system and block the release of gonadotropins (see Fig. 54–2B). As a girl goes through puberty, the levels of steroids required to block gonadotropin release progressively become higher and higher. At about the same time, the levels of sex steroids also rise. Eventually, a situation is reached in which the monthly oscillations in sex-steroid levels produce the full range of feedback inhibition of gonadotropin release. Thus, during maturation, the sensitivity of the hypothalamic-pituitary system to inhibition by sex steroids falls to reach the low level that is characteristic of the adult (see Fig. 54–2C). As discussed later, in addition to the negative feedback of sex steroids on gonadotropin release, *positive* feedback also occurs near the midpoint of the menstrual cycle.

During puberty, basal levels of LH and FSH increase (see Fig. 54–2A). Concentrations of androgens and estrogens also increase manyfold as a result of gonadal stimulation by FSH and LH. The LH surge that occurs at midcycle is thus superimposed on an already high basal level of circulating LH.

HYPOTHALAMIC-PITUITARY-GONADAL AXIS AND CONTROL OF THE FEMALE MENSTRUAL RHYTHM

The menstrual cycle reflects a complex interplay between the brain, the pituitary gland, and the ovary. Although menstrual cycles are generally regular during the reproductive years, the length of the menstrual cycle may be highly variable because of disturbances in neuroendocrine function. The mean menstrual cycle is 28 days long, but considerable variation occurs during both the early reproductive years and the premenopausal period. Irregular menses during adolescence and the premenopausal period occur primarily because of the increased frequency of anovulatory cycles.

The hypothalamic-pituitary-ovarian axis drives the menstrual cycle. The hypothalamus exerts the highest level of control. As discussed later, neurons in the hypothalamus synthesize, store, and release **gonadotropin-releasing hormone**. Long portal vessels carry the GnRH to the anterior pituitary, where the hormone binds to receptors on the surface of gonadotrophs. The result is the synthesis and release of both **follicle-stimulating hormone** and **luteinizing hormone** from the gonadotrophs.

These trophic hormones, LH and FSH, stimulate the ovary to synthesize and secrete the sex steroids **estrogens** and **progestins**. The ovaries also produce peptides called **inhibins** and **activins**. Together, these ovarian steroids and peptides exert both negative and positive feedback on both the hypothalamus and the anterior pituitary. This complex interaction is unique among the endocrine systems of the body inasmuch as it generates a monthly pattern of hormone fluctuations. Because the cyclic secretion of estrogens and progestins primarily controls endometrial maturation, menstruation reflects these cyclic changes in hormone secretion.

Cyclic Changes in Ovarian Steroid Secretion Produce Changes in the Endometrium That Are Responsible for the Menstrual Rhythm

The "menstrual cycle" actually involves cyclic changes in two organs: the ovary and the uterus (Fig. 54–3). The **ovarian cycle** includes the follicular phase and the luteal phase, separated by ovulation. The **endometrial cycle** includes the menstrual, the proliferative, and the secretory phases.

The first phase of the *ovarian cycle* is the **follicular phase**, which begins with the initiation of menstruation and averages about 14 days in length. The duration of the follicular phase is the most variable of the cycle. FSH levels start to rise in the late luteal phase of the preceding cycle. Shortly thereafter, early in the follicular phase, LH levels rise as well. Increased FSH secretion is important for recruitment of a cohort of ovarian follicles. After the initiation of follicle development (i.e., folliculogenesis), the granulosa cells of the follicles increase production of the estrogen **estradiol**. Under the influence of the rise in estradiol secretion by the ovary, the endometrium of the uterus undergoes rapid and continuous growth and maturation. This period is the **proliferative phase** of the *endometrial cycle*. As estrogen secretion rises during the midfollicular phase, FSH secretion slowly decreases as a result of a *negative* feedback effect that is discussed later. Just before ovulation, the rise in estradiol secretion becomes more rapid and, by a *positive* feedback effect on the anterior pituitary, triggers a surge in LH, which causes **ovulation**. Also occurring just before ovulation is a smaller FSH surge that is triggered by a rise in progesterone as well as activin.

After ovulation, the follicle, having released its ovum, transforms into a corpus luteum. The second half of the *ovarian cycle* is called the **luteal phase**. The follicle's remaining granulosa and theca cells are anatomically and physiologically transformed into luteal cells, and they begin to produce a progestin called **progesterone**. The corpus luteum also produces significant quantities of estrogen and **inhibin**. Estrogens and progestins, acting in concert, stimulate further endometrial growth and development. This period is the **secretory phase** of the *endometrial cycle*. The high levels of progesterone, estrogens, and inhibins maximally suppress the hypothalamic-pituitary system. The result is that FSH and LH levels fall. As LH levels fall, the target of LH, the corpus luteum, rapidly diminishes its production of estrogen and progestins. This withdrawal of estrogen and progestins, just before menses, has two effects. First, it induces a catastrophic degeneration of the endometrium that leads to menstrual bleeding. This period is the **menstrual phase** of the *endometrial cycle*. Second, the fall in estrogen and progestin levels diminishes the feedback inhibition on the hypotha-

FIGURE 54-3. Hormonal changes during the menstrual cycle. The menstrual cycle is a cycle of the hypothalamic-pituitary-ovarian axis, as well as a cycle of the targets of the ovarian hormones: the endometrium of the uterus. Therefore, the menstrual cycle includes both an ovarian cycle—which includes the follicular phase, ovulation, and the luteal phase—and the endometrial cycle—which includes the menstrual, the proliferative, and the secretory phases. FSH, follicle stimulating hormone; LH, luteinizing hormone.

lamic-pituitary system, and gonadotropin secretion rises once again, thus beginning the next menstrual cycle.

Neurons in the Hypothalamus Release GnRH in a Pulsatile Fashion

The highest level of control in the hypothalamic-pituitary-ovarian axis (Fig. 54–4) is at the hypothalamus. Neurons in the arcuate nucleus and the preoptic area of the hypothalamus synthesize GnRH and transport it to their nerve terminals for storage and subsequent release. As we shall see later, each of the aforementioned two groups of neurons is responsible for a very different kind of rhythm of GnRH secretion. Axons of the GnRH neurons project directly to the median eminence, the extreme basal portion of the hypothalamus, and terminate near portal vessels. These vessels carry GnRH to the gonadotrophs in the anterior pituitary.

The gene encoding GnRH is located on chromosome 9 (Fig. 54–5). The mature mRNA for GnRH encodes a preprohormone that is composed of 92 amino acids. After removing the 23–amino-acid signal sequence (residues −23 to −1), the neuron produces a prohormone (residues 1 to 69). Cleavage of this prohormone yields the decapeptide GnRH (residues 1 to 10), a 56–amino-acid peptide (residues 14 to 69) referred to as GnRH-associ-

TABLE 54-2

BENEFITS AND RISKS OF ORAL CONTRACEPTIVES

Oral Contraceptives Decrease the Risk of

Ovarian cancer

Endometrial cancer

Ovarian retention cysts

Ectopic pregnancy

Pelvic inflammatory disease

Benign breast disease

Oral Contraceptives Increase the Risk of

Benign liver tumors

Cholelithiasis (gallstones)

Hypertension

Heart attack

Stroke

Deep vein thrombosis

Pulmonary embolus

THE BIRTH CONTROL PILL

Hormonal contraception is the most commonly used method of contraception in the United States, with about 30% of sexually active women taking the oral contraceptive pill (OCP). A number of combination (i.e., estrogen and progestin) oral contraceptives and progestin-only pills are available. The estrogens and progestins used in oral contraceptives have varying potencies. In the United States, two estrogen compounds are approved for oral contraceptive use: ethinyl estradiol and mestranol. The progestins used in oral contraceptive pills are modified steroids in which the methyl at position 19 (Fig. 54–9) is removed; these progestins include norethindrone, norgestrel, norethynodrel, norethindrone acetate, and ethnodiol diacetate. A new generation of progestins—including gestodene and norgestimate—have reduced androgenic effects.

The woman takes the oral contraceptive daily for 21 days out of the 28-day cycle; she takes no pill, a placebo, or an iron pill during days 22 to 28. No medication is usually given during this fourth week to allow withdrawal bleeding to occur. Three regimens of contraceptive steroid administration are used:

1. **Monophasic or fixed-combination oral contraceptives.** The pills taken for the first 21 days of the cycle are identical.
2. **Multiphasic or varying-dose pills.** The pills contain two or three different amounts of the same estrogen and progestin, the dosages of which vary at specific intervals during the 21-day medication period. Multiphasic oral contraceptives generally maintain a low dose of estrogen throughout the cycle, combined with varying amounts of progestin. The rationale for this type of formulation is that the woman takes a lower total dose of steroid but is not at increased risk of breakthrough endometrial bleeding.
3. **Progestin-only oral contraceptive pills** ("mini-pill"). The woman takes these estrogen-free pills daily for 3 weeks of a 4-week cycle. This regimen may be associated with irregular, low-grade, breakthrough endometrial bleeding. The progestin-only pill is a good option for nursing mothers, as well as women for whom estrogens are contraindicated (e.g., those with thromboembolic disease, cerebral vascular incidents, and hypertension).

BIOLOGIC ACTION OF ORAL CONTRACEPTIVES
The contraceptive effectiveness of OCPs accrues from several actions. Like natural ovarian steroids, contraceptive steroids feed back both directly at the level of the hypothalamus (decreasing secretion of gonadotropin releasing hormone) and at the level of the gonadotrophs in the anterior pituitary (Fig. 54–4). The net effect is suppressed secretion of the gonadotropins, follicle-stimulating hormone (FSH), and luteinizing hormone (LH). The low FSH levels are insufficient to stimulate normal folliculogenesis; the low LH levels obviate the LH surge and therefore inhibit ovulation. However, in the commonly used doses, contraceptive steroids do not completely abolish either gonadotropin secretion or ovarian function.

The progestin effect of the OCP causes the cervical mucus to thicken and become viscid and scanty. These actions inhibit sperm penetration into the uterus. The progestins also impair the motility of the uterus and oviducts and therefore decrease transport of both ova and sperm to the normal site of fertilization in the distal fallopian tube (p. 1167). Progestins also produce changes in the endometrium that are not conducive for implantation of the embryo. These changes include decreased glandular production of glycogen and thus diminished energy for the blastocyst to survive in the uterus.

Progestin-only pills do not effectively inhibit ovulation, as do the combination pills. However, they do produce the other actions: mucus thickening, reduced motility, and impaired implantation. Because they are inconsistent inhibitors of ovulation, the progestin-only pills have a substantially higher failure rate than the combined type of pill does.

Side effects from the compounds in oral contraceptives are those associated with estrogens and progestins and include nausea, edema, headaches, and weight gain. Side effects from progestins include depression, mastodynia, acne, and hirsutism. Many of the side effects associated with the progestin component of the pill are due to the androgenic actions of the progestins used, particularly the acne and hirsutism. The potential benefits of the newer progestins include decreased androgenic effects, such as increased sex hormone–binding globulin, improved glucose tolerance (p. 1070), and increased high- and decreased low-density lipoprotein cholesterol (p. 1000). The clinical impact of these changes remains to be determined. Table 54–2 lists the major benefits and risks of OCPs.

---

ated peptide (**GAP**), and three amino acids that link the two. The neuron transports both GnRH and GAP down the axon for secretion into the portal circulation. The importance of GAP is unknown, but it may inhibit prolactin secretion.

GnRH is present in the hypothalamus at 14 to 16 weeks' gestation, and its target, the gonadotropin-containing cells (gonadotrophs), are present in the anterior pituitary gland as early as 10 weeks' gestation. The hypothalamic-pituitary system is functionally competent by approximately 23 weeks' gestation, at which time fetal tissues release GnRH.

The GnRH neurons do not release GnRH continuously, but in rhythmic pulses (Fig. 54–6). GnRH is released in bursts into the portal vessels about once per hour, intermittently stimulating the gonadotrophs in the anterior pituitary. Because the half-life of GnRH in blood is only 2 to 4 minutes, these hourly bursts of GnRH cause clearly discernible oscillations in portal-plasma GnRH levels that result in hourly surges in release of the gonadotropins LH

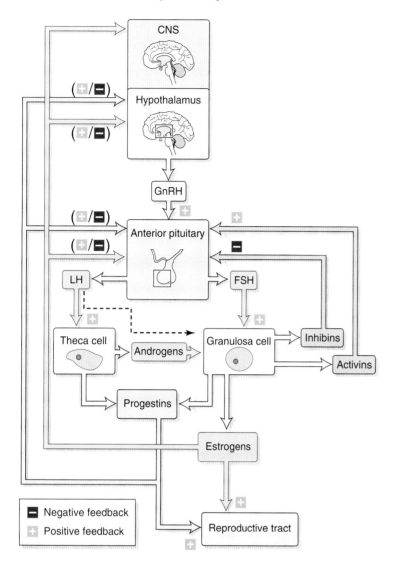

FIGURE 54–4. Hypothalamic-pituitary-ovarian axis. Small-bodied neurons in the arcuate nucleus and the preoptic area of the hypothalamus secrete gonadotropin-releasing hormone (GnRH), a decapeptide that reaches the gonadotrophs in the anterior pituitary via the long portal veins. GnRH binds to a G-protein–coupled receptor on the gonadotroph membrane, triggering the IP$_3$/DAG pathway, raising [Ca^{2+}]$_i$ and phosphorylation. Stimulation causes the gonadotrophs to synthesize and release two gonadotropins—follicle stimulating hormone (FSH) and luteinizing hormone (LH)—that are stored in secretory granules. Both FSH and LH are glycoprotein heterodimers comprising common α-subunits and unique β subunits. The LH binds to receptors on theca cells, stimulating Gα_s, which in turn activates adenylyl cyclase. The resultant rise in [cAMP]$_i$ stimulates protein kinase A (PKA), which increases the transcription of several proteins that are involved in the biosynthesis of progestins and androgens. The androgens enter granulosa cells, which convert the androgens to estrogens. The *dashed arrow* indicates that the granulosa cells also have LH receptors. FSH binds to receptors on the basolateral membrane of granulosa cells, also activating PKA, stimulating gene transcription and synthesis of the relevant enzymes (e.g., aromatase), activins, and inhibins. Negative feedback on the hypothalamic-pituitary-ovarian axis occurs by several routes. The activins and inhibins act only on the anterior pituitary. The estrogens and progestins act on both the anterior pituitary and on the hypothalamic neurons, exerting both positive and negative feedback controls. cAMP, cyclic adenosine monophosphate; CNS, central nervous system; DAG, diacylglycerol; FSH, follicle stimulating hormone; LH, luteinizing hormone.

and FSH. Early in the follicular phase of the cycle, when the gonadotrophs are not very GnRH sensitive, each burst of GnRH elicits only a small rise in LH (see Fig. 54–6A). Later in the follicular phase, when the gonadotrophs in the anterior pituitary become much more sensitive to the GnRH in the portal blood, each burst of GnRH triggers a much larger release of LH (see Fig. 54–6B).

Although the mechanisms controlling the hourly pulses

FIGURE 54–5. Map of the gonadotropin-releasing–hormone gene. The mature mRNA encodes a preprohormone with 92 amino acids. Removal of the 23–amino-acid signal sequence yields the 69–amino-acid prohormone. Cleavage of this prohormone yields GnRH, gonadotropin-releasing hormone.

of GnRH remain unclear, the pulse generator for GnRH is thought to be located in the **arcuate nucleus** of the medial basal hypothalamus, where one group of GnRH neurons resides. In rodents, bursts of nerve impulses from neurons in these nuclei correspond in time with the pulsatile release of GnRH from the hypothalamus and with the episodic release of LH from the anterior pituitary. These data suggest that a built-in system within the hypothalamus controls the pulsatile discharge of GnRH from nerve terminals. The pulse-generating mechanism is key to control of cyclic reproductive function and to regulation of the menstrual cycle. The *frequency* of GnRH release determines the specific response of the gonad. Pulses spaced 60 to 90 minutes apart upregulate the gonadotrophs' GnRH receptors and thus stimulate the release of gonadotropins. However, continuous administration of GnRH (or an analogue) causes downregulation of the gonadotrophs' GnRH receptors, thus suppressing gonadotropin release and gonadal function (see the box titled Therapeutic Uses of GnRH).

In addition to the hourly rhythm of GnRH secretion, orchestrated by the arcuate nucleus, a monthly rhythm of

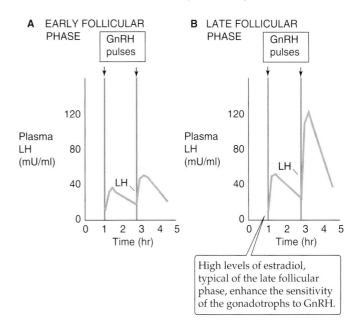

FIGURE 54-6. Pulsatile release of GnRH and pulsatile secretion of LH. (Data from Wang CF, Lasley BL, Lein A, Yen SS: The functional changes of the pituitary gonadotrophs during the menstrual cycle. J Clin Endocrinol Metab 42:718–728, 1976.)

GnRH secretion also occurs—in rhesus monkeys. A massive increase in GnRH secretion at midcycle is, in part, responsible for the LH surge, which in turn leads to ovulation. Which neurons produce the massive surge in GnRH that leads to the LH surge? These are not the GnRH neurons in the arcuate nucleus but, rather, those in the preoptic area. The preoptic GnRH neurons have inhibitory γ-aminobutyric acid (GABA) receptors, whereas the arcuate GnRH neurons have inhibitory opioid receptors. Later in this chapter, we discuss how these two sets of GnRH neurons may underlie the negative and positive feedback produced by estrogens.

THERAPEUTIC USES OF GnRH

Continuous administration of gonadotropin-releasing hormone (GnRH) leads to downregulation (suppression) of gonadotropin secretion, whereas pulsatile release of GnRH causes upregulation (stimulation) of follicle-stimulating hormone and luteinizing hormone secretion. Clinical problems requiring upregulation of gonadotropin secretion, which leads to stimulation of the gonads, are therefore best treated by a *pulsatile* mode of GnRH administration. On the other hand, when the patient requires gonadal inhibition, a *continuous* mode of administration is necessary.

An example of a disease requiring *pulsatile* GnRH administration is **Kallmann syndrome.** Disordered migration of GnRH cells during embryologic development causes Kallmann syndrome, which in adults results in **hypogonadotropic hypogonadism** and **anosmia** (loss of sense of smell). Normally, primordial GnRH cells originate in the nasal placode during embryologic development. These primitive cells then migrate through the forebrain to the diencephalon, where they become specific neuronal groups within the medial-basal hypothalamus and preoptic area. In certain individuals, both male and female, proper migration of GnRH cells fails to occur. The etiology of Kallmann syndrome was confirmed in humans when researchers studied a 19-week-gestation fetus that had complete deletion of the X-linked Kallmann locus. The GnRH cells were found along their known migration route, but not in the brain. Females with Kallmann syndrome generally have amenorrhea (no men-

strual cycles). However, the pituitary and gonads of these individuals can function properly when appropriately stimulated. Thus, females treated with exogenous gonadotropins or GnRH analogues—*pulsatile administration* with a programmed infusion pump—can have normal folliculogenesis, ovulation, and pregnancy.

An example of a disease requiring *continuous* GnRH administration to downregulate gonadal function is endometriosis. **Endometriosis** is a common condition caused by the aberrant presence of endometrial tissue outside the uterine cavity. This tissue responds to estrogens during the menstrual cycle and is a source of pain and other problems, including infertility. In patients with endometriosis, *continuous administration* of GnRH analogue inhibits replenishment of the receptor for GnRH in the gonadotrophs in the anterior pituitary. As a result, insufficient numbers of GnRH receptors are available for optimum GnRH action, thereby diminishing gonadotropin secretion and producing relative hypoestrogenism. Because estrogen stimulates the endometrium, continuous administration of GnRH or GnRH analogues causes involution and diminution of endometriotic tissue.

Leiomyomas (a smooth-muscle tumor) of the uterus (also called a uterine "fibroid") are also estrogen dependent. When estrogen levels are decreased, the proliferation of these lesions is decreased. Therefore, leiomyomas of the uterus can also be effectively treated by *continuous* administration of GnRH analogues.

GnRH Stimulates Gonadotrophs in the Anterior Pituitary to Secrete FSH and LH, Which Stimulate Ovarian Cells to Secrete Estrogens and Progestins

GnRH enters the anterior pituitary via the portal system and binds to GnRH receptors on the surface of the gonadotroph, thus initiating a series of cellular events that result in the synthesis and secretion of gonadotropins (Fig. 54–7). GnRH binds to a G-protein–linked receptor coupled to $G\alpha_q$. The result is activation of phospholipase C (PLC), which in turn hydrolyzes phosphatidylinositol 4,5-biphosphonate (PIP$_2$) to inositol 1,4,5-triphosphate (IP$_3$), and diacylglycerol (DAG) (p. 100). Both IP$_3$ and DAG are second messengers. Release of Ca^{2+} from the endoplasmic reticulum by IP$_3$ causes an increase in $[Ca^{2+}]_i$. This Ca^{2+} induces the Ca^{2+} channels at the cell membrane to open and allow an influx of extracellular Ca^{2+} that sustains the elevated $[Ca^{2+}]_i$. The rise in $[Ca^{2+}]_i$ triggers exocytosis and gonadotropin release.

In addition to the IP$_3$ pathway, GnRH also acts through the DAG pathway. The DAG formed by PLC stimulates protein kinase C, which indirectly leads to increases in gene transcription. The net effect is an increase in synthe-sis of the gonadotropins FSH and LH. In addition, GnRH increases mRNA levels for a number of immediate early response genes (e.g., *c-Fos*, *c-Jun*, and *JunB*).

The GnRH receptor is internalized and partially degraded in the lysosomes. However, a portion of the GnRH receptor is shuttled back to the cell surface. Return of the GnRH receptor to the cell membrane is referred to as **receptor replenishment** and is related to the upregulation of receptor activity discussed earlier. The mechanism through which GnRH receptor replenishment occurs remains unclear.

FSH and LH are in the same family as thyroid-stimulating hormone (TSH; p. 1046) and human chorionic gonadotropin (hCG; p. 1172). All four are glycoprotein hormones with α and β chains. The α chains of all four of these hormones are identical; in humans, they have 92 amino acids and a molecular weight of approximately 20 kDa. The β chains of FSH and LH are unique and confer the specificity of the hormones. The rhythm of GnRH secretion influences the relative rates of expression for genes encoding the synthesis of the α, β_{FSH}, and β_{LH} subunits of FSH and LH. GnRH pulsatility also determines the dimerization of the α and β_{FSH} subunits, or α and β_{LH}, as well as their glycosylation.

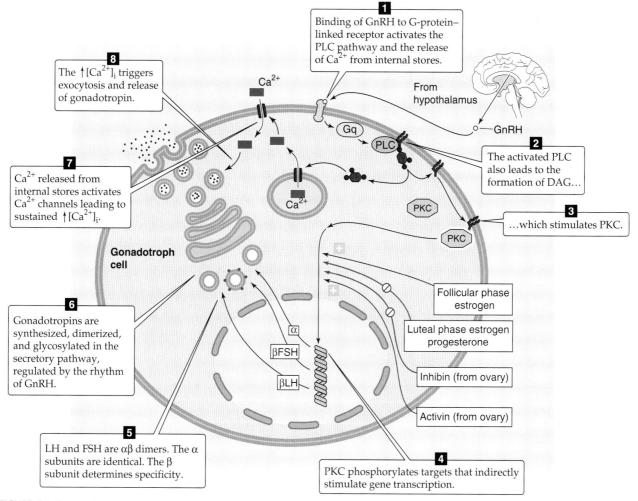

FIGURE 54–7. Gonadotropin secretion. FSH, follicle stimulating hormone; GnRH, gonadotropin-releasing hormone; LH, luteinizing hormone; PKC, protein kinase C; PLC, phospholipase C.

Differential secretion of FSH and LH is also affected by several other hormonal mediators, including ovarian steroids, inhibins, and activins. We discuss the role of these agents in the section on feedback control of the hypothalamic-pituitary-ovarian axis. Thus, depending on the specific hormonal milieu produced by different physiologic circumstances, the gonadotroph produces and secretes the α and β subunits of FSH and LH at different rates. The secretion of LH and FSH is further modulated by neuropeptides, amino acids such as aspartate, neuropeptide Y, corticotropin-releasing hormone (CRH), and endogenous opioids.

Before ovulation, the LH and FSH secreted by the gonadotrophs act on cells of the developing follicle. The **theca cells** of the follicle have LH receptors, whereas the **granulosa cells** have both LH and FSH receptors. Both LH and FSH are required for estrogen production because neither the theca cell nor the granulosa cell can carry out all the required steps. After ovulation, LH acts on the cells of the corpus luteum; recall that after ovulation, the cells of the follicle give rise to the corpus luteum.

LH and FSH bind to specific receptors on the surface of their target cells. Both the LH and the FSH receptors are coupled via $G\alpha_s$ to adenylyl cyclase (p. 97), which catalyzes the conversion of adenosine triphosphate (ATP) to cyclic adenosine monophosphate (cAMP). cAMP stimulates protein kinase A, which not only stimulates the enzymes involved in steroid biosynthesis but also induces the synthesis of certain proteins and increases cell division. Among the proteins whose synthesis is promoted by gonadotropins is the low-density lipoprotein (LDL) receptor required for cholesterol uptake and the aromatase required for estrogen synthesis.

Ovaries Also Produce Peptide Hormones: Inhibins, Which Inhibit FSH Secretion, and Activins, Which Activate It

The inhibins and the activins are peptides that modulate FSH secretion by the gonadotrophs. The transforming growth factor β (TGF-β) supergene family is a group of molecules that are structurally related and include TGF-β, antimüllerian hormone (AMH; p. 1114), the activins, the inhibins, and other glycoproteins. These growth factors modulate growth and differentiation during development. The inhibins and activins are dimers that are constructed from a related set of building blocks: a glycosylated 20-kDa α subunit and two nonglycosylated 12-kDa β subunits, one called β_A and the other called β_B (Fig. 54–8). The *inhibins* are always composed of one α subunit and either a β_A or a β_B subunit; the α and β subunits are linked by disulfide bridges. The α-β_A dimer is called inhibin A, whereas the α-β_B dimer is called inhibin B. The *activins*, however, are composed of two β-type subunits. Thus, there are three kinds of activins: β_A-β_A, β_B-β_B, and the heterodimer β_A-β_B.

The **inhibins** are produced by the granulosa cells of the follicle, as well as other tissues, including the pituitary, the brain, the adrenal gland, the kidney, the bone marrow, the corpus luteum, and the placenta. It is specifically FSH that stimulates the granulosa cells to produce

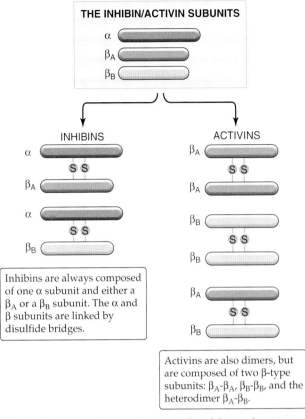

THE INHIBIN/ACTIVIN SUBUNITS

Inhibins are always composed of one α subunit and either a β_A or a β_B subunit. The α and β subunits are linked by disulfide bridges.

Activins are also dimers, but are composed of two β-type subunits: β_A-β_A, β_B-β_B, and the heterodimer β_A-β_B.

FIGURE 54–8. The inhibins and activins. The inhibins and activins are peptide hormones that are made up of a common set of building blocks. For both the inhibins and the activins, disulfide bonds link the two subunits.

inhibins. Also involved in the regulation of inhibin production are a number of other factors, including hormones and growth-stimulating factors. Estradiol may stimulate inhibin production via an intraovarian mechanism. Just before ovulation, after the granulosa cells acquire LH receptors, LH also stimulates the production of inhibin by granulosa cells. The biologic action of the inhibins is primarily confined to the reproductive system. As discussed later, the inhibins inhibit FSH production by gonadotrophs.

The **activins** are produced in the same tissues as the inhibins, but they *stimulate*—rather than inhibit—FSH release from pituitary cells.

Both the Ovarian Steroids (Estrogens and Progestins) and Peptides (Inhibins and Activins) Feed Back on the Hypothalamic-Pituitary Axis

As summarized in Figure 54–4, the ovarian steroids—the estrogens and progestins—exert both negative and positive feedback on the hypothalamic-pituitary axis. Whether the feedback is negative or positive depends on both the concentration of the gonadal steroids and the duration of the exposure to these steroids (i.e., the time in the menstrual cycle). In addition, the ovarian peptides—the inhibins and activins—also feed back on the anterior pituitary.

NEGATIVE FEEDBACK BY OVARIAN STEROIDS. Throughout most of the menstrual cycle, the estrogens and progestins that are produced by the ovary feed back negatively on both the hypothalamus and the gonadotrophs of the anterior pituitary. The net effect is to reduce the release of both LH and FSH. The estrogens exert negative feedback at both low and high concentrations, whereas the progestins are effective only at high concentrations.

Although estrogens inhibit the GnRH neurons in the arcuate nucleus and preoptic area of the hypothalamus, this inhibition is not direct. Rather, the estrogens stimulate interneurons that inhibit the GnRH neurons. In the arcuate nucleus, these inhibitory neurons exert their inhibition via opiates. However, in the preoptic area, the inhibitory neurons exert their inhibitory effect via GABA, a classic inhibitory neurotransmitter (p. 308).

POSITIVE FEEDBACK BY OVARIAN STEROIDS. Although ovarian steroids feed back negatively on the hypothalamic-pituitary axis during most of the menstrual cycle, they have the opposite effect at the end of the follicular phase. **Estrogen** levels gradually rise during the follicular phase of the ovarian cycle (see Fig. 54–3). After the estradiol levels reach a certain threshold for a minimum of 2 days, the hypothalamic-pituitary axis reverses its sensitivity to estrogens. That is, estrogens feed back *positively* on the axis. One manifestation of this positive feedback is that estrogens now *increase* the sensitivity of the gonadotrophs in the anterior pituitary gland to GnRH. As discussed in the next section, this switch to positive feedback promotes the LH surge. Indeed, pituitary cells that are cultured in the absence of estrogen have suboptimal responses to GnRH. Once high levels of estrogens have properly conditioned the gonadotrophs, rising levels of **progesterone** during the late follicular phase also produce a positive feedback response and thus facilitate the LH surge.

NEGATIVE FEEDBACK BY THE INHIBINS. The inhibins inhibit FSH secretion by the gonadotrophs of the anterior pituitary (hence the name "inhibin") in a classic negative feedback arrangement. The initial action of inhibin appears to be beyond the Ca^{2+}-mobilization step in FSH secretion. In cultured pituitary cells, even very small amounts of inhibin markedly reduce mRNA levels for both the $\alpha_{LH/FSH}$ and the β_{FSH} subunits. As a result, inhibins suppress FSH secretion. In contrast, inhibins have no effect on the mRNA levels of β_{LH}. In addition to their actions on the anterior pituitary, the inhibins also have the intraovarian effect of decreasing androgen production, which can have secondary effects on intrafollicular estrogen production.

POSITIVE FEEDBACK BY THE ACTIVINS. Activins promote marked increases in β_{FSH} mRNA and FSH release, with no change in β_{LH} formation. The stimulatory effect of activins on FSH release is independent of GnRH action. Like the inhibins, the activins also have the intraovarian action of stimulating the synthesis of estrogens. Thus, by their actions on both the gonadotrophs and the ovaries, the activins and inhibins regulate the activity of the follicular cells during the menstrual cycle.

Modulation of Gonadotropin Secretion by Positive and Negative Ovarian Feedback Produces the Normal Menstrual Rhythm

We have seen that the pulsatile release of GnRH from the hypothalamus, generally occurring every 60 to 90 minutes, triggers a corresponding pulsatile release of LH and FSH from the gonadotrophs of the anterior pituitary. Because the gonadotropins elicit the release of ovarian steroids, and these steroids modulate the hypothalamic-pituitary axis, the interaction between the ovarian steroids and gonadotropin release is an example of feedback. This feedback is especially interesting because it is bidirectional in that it elicits *negative* feedback throughout most of the menstrual cycle but *positive* feedback immediately before ovulation.

When compared with the luteal phase, as discussed later, the **follicular phase** is characterized by a relatively high frequency of GnRH—and thus LH—pulses. Early in the follicular phase, when levels of estradiol are low but rising, the frequency of LH pulses remains unchanged, but their amplitude gradually *increases* with time. We see this increase in amplitude in Figure 54–6, in which the "early" and the "late" follicular phases are compared. Later in the follicular phase of the menstrual cycle, the higher estrogen levels cause both the frequency and the amplitude of the LH pulses to increase gradually. During this time of high estradiol levels, the ovarian steroids are beginning to feed back positively on the hypothalamic-pituitary axis. Late in the follicular phase, the net effect of this increased frequency and amplitude of LH and FSH pulses is an increase in the time-averaged level of circulating LH, as seen in Figure 54–3.

The **LH surge** is an abrupt and dramatic rise in the LH level that occurs around the 13th to 14th day of the follicular phase in the average woman. The LH surge peaks approximately 12 hours after its initiation and lasts for approximately 48 hours. The peak concentration of LH during the surge is about three-fold greater than the presurge concentration. The LH surge is superimposed on the smaller FSH surge. Positive feedback of estrogens, progestins, and activins on the hypothalamic-pituitary axis is involved in the induction of this LH surge. The primary trigger of the gonadotropin surge is a rise in **estradiol** to very high "threshold" levels just before the LH surge. The rise in estrogen levels has two effects. First, the accelerated rate of increase in estradiol levels in the preovulatory phase sensitizes the gonadotrophs in the anterior pituitary to GnRH pulses (see Fig. 54–6). Second, the increasing estrogen levels also modulate hypothalamic neuronal activity and induce a GnRH surge, presumably via GnRH neurons in the preoptic area of the hypothalamus. Thus, the powerful *positive* feedback action of estradiol induces the midcycle surge of LH and, to a lesser extent, FSH. Gradually rising levels of the activins—secreted by granulosa cells—also act in a positive feedback manner to contribute to the FSH surge. In addition, gradually increasing levels of LH trigger the preovulatory follicle to increase its secretion of progesterone. These increasing—but still "low"—levels of **progesterone** also have a positive feedback effect on the hypothalamic-pituitary axis that is synergistic with the positive feedback effect of the estrogens. Thus, although progesterone is not the primary trigger for the LH surge, it augments the effects of estradiol.

The gonadotropin surge causes ovulation and luteinization. The ovarian follicle ruptures, probably because of weakening of the follicular wall, and expels the oocyte and with it the surrounding cumulus and corona cells. This process is known as **ovulation**, and it is discussed in more detail in Chapter 55. As discussed later, a physiological change—**luteinization**—in the granulosa cells of the follicle causes them to secrete progesterone rather than estradiol. The granulosa and theca cells undergo structural changes that transform them into luteal cells, a process known as luteinization. The pulsatile rhythm of GnRH release and gonadotropin secretion is maintained throughout the gonadotropin surge.

As the **luteal phase** of the menstrual cycle begins, circulating levels of LH and FSH rapidly decrease (see Fig. 54–3). This fall-off in gonadotropin levels reflects *negative* feedback by three ovarian hormones—estradiol, progesterone, and inhibin. Moreover, as gonadotropin levels fall, the levels of ovarian steroids also fall. Thus, immediately after ovulation we see more or less concurrent decreases in the levels of both gonadotropins and ovarian hormones.

Later, during the luteal phase, the luteal cells of the corpus luteum gradually increase their synthesis of estradiol, progesterone, and inhibin (see Fig. 54–3). The rise in concentration of these hormones causes—in typical negative feedback fashion—the continued decrease of gonadotropin levels midway through the luteal phase. One of the mechanisms of this negative feedback is the effect of progesterone on the hypothalamic-pituitary axis. Recall that at the peak of the LH surge, both the frequency and the amplitude of LH pulses are high. Progesterone levels rise, and high levels stimulate inhibitory opioidergic interneurons in the hypothalamus, thus inhibiting the GnRH neurons. This inhibition decreases the frequency of LH pulses, although the amplitude remains rather high.

By approximately 48 hours before onset of the menses, the pulsatile rhythm of LH secretion has decreased to one pulse every 3 to 4 hours. As a result, circulating levels of LH slowly fall during the luteal phase. During the late luteal phase, the gradual demise of the corpus luteum leads to decreases in the levels of progesterone, estradiol, and inhibin (see Fig. 54–3). After the onset of menstruation, the hypothalamic-pituitary axis returns to a follicular-phase pattern of LH secretion (i.e., a gradual increase in the frequency of GnRH pulses).

THE OVARIAN STEROIDS

Starting From Cholesterol, the Ovary Synthesizes Estradiol, the Major Estrogen, and Progesterone, the Major Progestin

Estrogens in the female are derived from the ovary and the adrenal gland and from peripheral conversion in adipose tissue. In a *nonpregnant* female, estradiol, the primary circulating estrogen, is secreted principally by the ovary. The precursor for the biosynthesis of the ovarian

steroids, as it is for all other steroid hormones produced elsewhere in the body, is cholesterol. Cholesterol is a 27-carbon sterol that is both ingested in the diet and synthesized in the liver from acetate (p. 998). Ovarian cells can synthesize their own cholesterol de novo. Alternatively, cholesterol can enter cells in the form of LDL cholesterol and bind to LDL receptors.

As shown in Figure 54–9, a P-450 enzyme (Table 49–2) known as the "side-chain-cleavage" enzyme (or 20,22-desmolase) catalyzes the conversion of cholesterol to **pregnenolone**. This reaction is the rate-limiting step in estrogen production. Ovarian cells then convert pregnenolone to progestins and estrogens. The initial steps of estrogen biosynthesis from pregnenolone follow the same steps as synthesis of the two so-called adrenal androgens **dehydroepiandrosterone** (DHEA) and **androstenedione**, both of which have 19 carbon atoms. We discussed these steps in connection with both Figure 49–2 and Figure 53–5. The Leydig cells in the testis can use either of two pathways to convert these weak androgens to **testosterone**. Cells in the ovaries are different because as shown in Figure 54–9, they have an aromatase that can convert androstenedione to estrone and testosterone to estradiol. This aromatization also results in loss of the 19-methyl group (thus, the estrogens have only 18 carbons), as well as conversion of the ketone at position 3 to a hydroxyl in the A ring of the androgen precursor. Once formed, **estrone** can be converted into the more powerful estrogen **estradiol**, and vice versa, by 17β-hydroxysteroid dehydrogenase (17β-HSD). Finally, the liver can convert both estradiol and estrone into the weak estrogen **estriol**.

The two major **progestins**, **progesterone** and **17α-hydroxyprogesterone**, are formed even earlier in the biosynthetic pathway than the "adrenal androgens." Functionally, progesterone is the more important progestin, and it has higher circulating levels.

Estrogen Biosynthesis Requires Two Ovarian Cells and Two Gonadotropins, Whereas Progestin Synthesis Requires Only a Single Cell

In the follicular phase of the menstrual cycle, the follicle synthesizes estrogens, whereas in the luteal phase, the corpus luteum does the synthesis. A unique aspect of estradiol synthesis is that it requires the contribution of two distinct cell types: the theca and granulosa cells within the follicle and the theca-lutein and granulosa-lutein cells within the corpus luteum (Fig. 54–10). We discuss these cells—as well as development of the follicle and corpus luteum—in the next subchapter.

The superficial **theca cells** and theca-lutein cells can take up cholesterol and produce the "adrenal androgens," but they do not have the aromatase necessary for estrogen production. However, the deeper **granulosa cells** and granulosa-lutein cells have the aromatase, but they lack the 17α-hydroxylase and 17,20-desmolase (which are the same protein) necessary for making the "adrenal androgens." Another difference between the two cell types is that—in the follicle—the superficial theca cell is near blood vessels and is hence a source of LDL cholesterol.

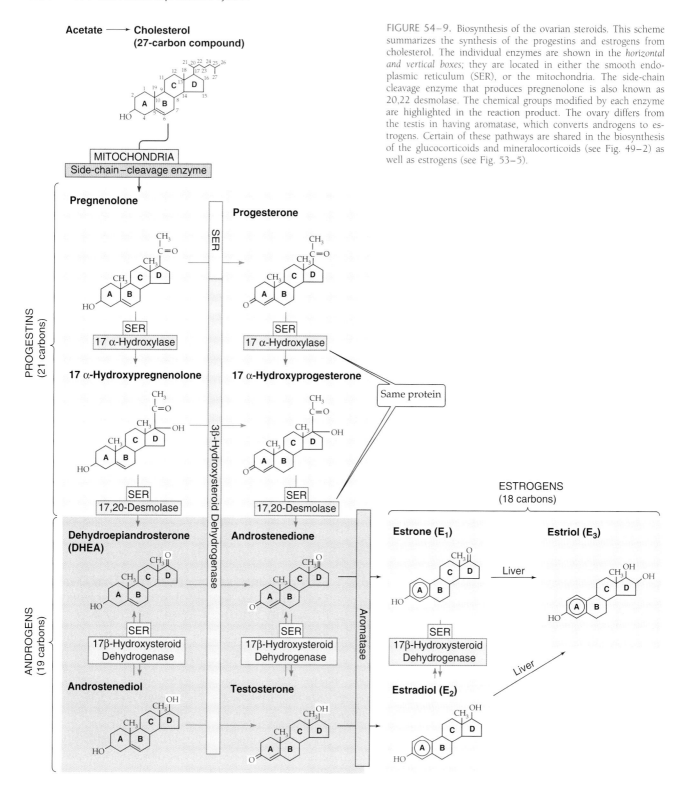

FIGURE 54–9. Biosynthesis of the ovarian steroids. This scheme summarizes the synthesis of the progestins and estrogens from cholesterol. The individual enzymes are shown in the *horizontal and vertical boxes;* they are located in either the smooth endoplasmic reticulum (SER), or the mitochondria. The side-chain cleavage enzyme that produces pregnenolone is also known as 20,22 desmolase. The chemical groups modified by each enzyme are highlighted in the reaction product. The ovary differs from the testis in having aromatase, which converts androgens to estrogens. Certain of these pathways are shared in the biosynthesis of the glucocorticoids and mineralocorticoids (see Fig. 49–2) as well as estrogens (see Fig. 53–5).

The granulosa cell, on the other hand, is far from blood vessels and, instead, is surrounded by LDL-poor follicular fluid. Thus, in the follicular stage, the granulosa cells obtain most of their cholesterol by de novo synthesis. However, after formation of the corpus luteum, the accompanying vascularization makes it possible for the granulosa-lutein cell to take up LDL cholesterol from the blood and to thus synthesize large amounts of progesterone. A final difference between the two cell types is that theca cells have LH receptors and granulosa cells have both LH and FSH receptors.

Because of their unique physiological properties, neither the theca/theca-lutein cells nor the granulosa/granulosa-lutein cells can make estrogens by themselves. Ac-

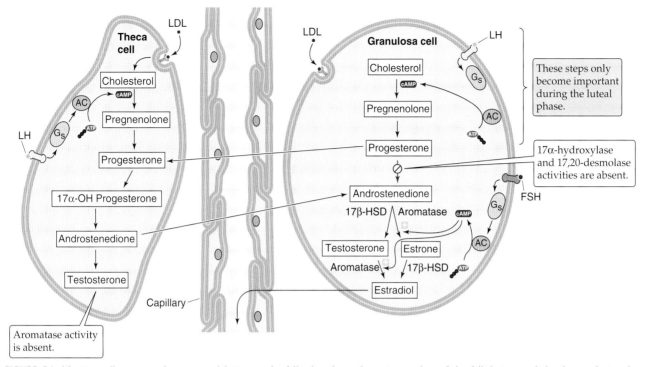

FIGURE 54–10. Two-cell, two-gonadotropin model. During the follicular phase, the major product of the follicle is estradiol, whereas during the luteal phase, the major products of the corpus luteum are the progestins, although estradiol synthesis is still substantial. In the follicular phase, LH primes the theca cell to convert cholesterol to androstenedione. Because the theca cell lacks aromatase, it cannot generate estradiol from this androstenedione. Instead, the androstenedione diffuses to the granulosa cell, whose aromatase activity has been stimulated by FSH. The aromatase converts the androstenedione to estradiol. In the luteal phase, the vascularization of the corpus luteum makes LDL available to the granulosa-lutein cells. Thus, both the theca-lutein and the granulosa-lutein cells can produce progesterone, the major product of the corpus luteum. For production of 17α-hydroxyprogesterone (17α-OH progesterone), some of the progesterone diffuses into the theca-lutein cell, which has the 17α-hydroxylase activity needed for converting the progesterone to 17α-hydroxyprogesterone. The theca-lutein cell can also generate the androstenedione, which diffuses into the granulosa-lutein cell for estradiol synthesis. AC, adenylyl cyclase; ATP, adenosine triphosphate; cAMP, cyclic adenosine monophosphate; FSH, follicle stimulating hormone; HSD, hydroxysteroid dehydrogenase; LDL, low density lipoprotein; LH, luteinizing hormone.

cording to the **two-cell, two-gonadotropin hypothesis**, estrogen synthesis occurs in the following steps:

Step 1: LH stimulates the theca cell, via the adenylyl cyclase pathway, to increase its synthesis of LDL receptors and the side-chain-cleavage enzyme.

Step 2: Thus stimulated, the theca cell increases its synthesis of androstenedione.

Step 3: The androstenedione synthesized in the theca cells freely diffuses to the granulosa cells.

Step 4: FSH, also acting via the adenylyl cyclase pathway, stimulates the granulosa cell to produce aromatase.

Step 5: The aromatase converts androstenedione to estrone (see Fig. 54–9). 17β-HSD then converts the estrone to estradiol. Alternatively, 17β-HSD can first convert the same androstenedione to testosterone, and then the aromatase can convert this product to estradiol. By these pathways, theca-derived androgens are converted to estrogens in the granulosa cell.

Step 6: The estradiol diffuses into the blood vessels.

At low concentrations, the weak androgens produced by the theca cells are substrates for estrogen synthesis by the granulosa cells, in addition to enhancing the aromatase activity of granulosa cells. However, at high concentrations, conversion of androgens to estrogens is diminished. Instead, the weak androgens are preferentially converted by 5α-reductase (see Fig. 53–5) to more potent androgens, such as **dihydrotestosterone**, a substance that cannot be converted to estrogen. Furthermore, these 5α-reduced androgens inhibit aromatase activity. Thus, the net effect of a high-androgen environment in the follicle is to decrease estrogen production. These androgens also inhibit LH receptor formation on follicular cells.

In the luteal phase of the cycle, luteinization of the follicle substantially changes the biochemistry of the theca and granulosa cells. As part of the formation of the corpus luteum, blood vessels invade deep toward the granulosa-lutein cells. Recall that in the follicle, the granulosa cells had been surrounded by follicular fluid, which is poor in LDL cholesterol. The increased vascularity facilitates the delivery of LDL cholesterol to the granulosa-lutein cells. In addition, LH stimulates the granulosa-lutein cell to take up and process cholesterol—as it does in theca cells. The net effect is the increased progesterone biosynthesis that is characteristic of the midluteal phase. Indeed, the major products of the corpus luteum are **progesterone** and 17α-hydroxyprogesterone, although the corpus luteum also produces estradiol. As indicated in Figure 54–10, the granulosa-lutein cell cannot make either 17α-hydroxyprogesterone or estradiol directly because these cells lack the protein that has dual activity for 17α-hydroxylase and 17,20-desmolase (see Fig. 54–9). Thus, 17α-hydroxyprogesterone synthesis necessitates that progesterone first moves to the theca-lutein cell (see Fig. 54–10), which can convert progesterone to **17α-hydroxy-progesterone**, as well as androstenedione. Furthermore, estradiol synthesis necessitates that androstenedione from the theca-lutein cell moves to the granulosa-lutein cell for aromatization and formation of **estradiol**.

The Principal Function of Estrogens Is Stimulation of Cellular Proliferation and Growth of Sex Organs and Other Tissues Related to Reproduction

Most estrogens in blood plasma are bound to carrier proteins, as are testosterone and other steroid hormones. In the case of estradiol, 60% is bound to **albumin** and 38% to **sex-hormone binding globulin** (SHBG)—also known as testosterone-binding globulin (TeBG; p. 1130). The latter name is doubly a misnomer; not only does "TeBG" bind estradiol, but "TeBG" levels are twice as high in women as they are in men. At least one reason for the higher levels in women is that estrogens (including birth control pills) stimulate the synthesis of SHBG. Only 2% of total plasma estradiol circulates as the free hormone. Because of their lipid solubility, estrogens readily cross cell membranes. Although it was once believed that estrogens bind to cytoplasmic receptors, it has recently become clear that the receptor for estradiol resides in the cell nucleus (p. 113). The estrogen receptor functions as a homodimer (Table 5–2). The estrogen–estrogen receptor complex interacts with steroid-response elements on chromatin and rapidly induces the transcription of specific genes to produce mRNA. The RNA enters the cytoplasm and increases protein synthesis, which modulates numerous cellular functions. Over the next several hours, DNA synthesis increases, and the mitogenic action of estrogens becomes apparent. Estrogens almost exclusively affect particular target sex organs that have the estrogen receptor. These organs include the uterus and the breasts.

The **progestins**, particularly progesterone, stimulate glandular secretion in reproductive tissue and promote the maturation of certain estrogen-stimulated tissue. One of the most prominent actions of progesterone is the induction of secretory changes in the endometrium. The endometrium must be conditioned by estrogen for progesterone to act effectively. During the latter half of the menstrual cycle, progesterone induces final maturation of the uterine endometrium for reception and implantation of the fertilized ovum.

THE OVARIAN CYCLE: FOLLICULOGENESIS, OVULATION, AND FORMATION OF THE CORPUS LUTEUM

Follicles Mature in Stages from Primordial to Graafian (or Preovulatory) Follicles

Oogonia undergo many rounds of *mitotic* division in early fetal life (p. 1106). By middle fetal life, all the mitotic divisions of the female germ cells have been completed and oogonia enter their first *meiotic* division. These cells—now called **primary oocytes**—arrest in the prophase of their first meiotic division, where crossing over occurs (see Fig. 52–1B). Primary oocytes have a diploid number (i.e., 46) of duplicated chromosomes. During the remainder of fetal life and childhood, the number of primary oocytes gradually declines to about 2 to 2.5 million at birth and to about 400,000 just before puberty. The minority of primary oocytes that have survived are those that are surrounded by flat, spindle-shaped follicular or **pregranulosa cells** (Fig. 54–11). This oocyte–pregranulosa cell complex is enclosed by a basement lamina. At this stage of development, the primary oocyte with its surrounding single layer of pregranulosa cells is called a **primordial follicle**. Primordial follicles are 30 to 60 μm in diameter. The first primordial follicle usually appears about 16 weeks into intrauterine life, and the generation of primordial follicles is complete by about 6 months after birth.

The ovarian follicle is the primary functional unit of the ovary. Throughout reproductive life, some 90% to 95% of all follicles are primordial (i.e., "nongrowing") follicles. The growing follicles that are recruited from this pool of primordial follicles undergo a striking series of changes in size, morphology, and physiology. The first step in follicular growth is that a primordial follicle becomes a primary follicle, followed by the transition to a secondary and a tertiary follicle and finally a preovulatory or graafian follicle (see Fig. 54–11). This follicular development, as well as the subsequent ovulation, is central to control of the menstrual cycle. The primordial, primary, and secondary follicles are solid masses of cells that lack an "antrum"; they are therefore referred to as *preantral* follicles. The tertiary and graafian follicles have a fluid-filled "antrum."

The **primary follicle** forms as the spindle cells of the primordial follicle become cuboidal cells. In addition, the oocyte enlarges. Thus, the primary follicle contains a larger primary oocyte that is surrounded by a single layer of cuboidal granulosa cells.

The **secondary follicle** contains a primary oocyte surrounded by *several* layers of cuboidal granulosa cells. The granulosa cells of a primary follicle proliferate and give rise to several layers of cells. In addition, stromal cells differentiate, surround the follicle, and become the theca cells. These theca cells are on the outside of the follicle's basement membrane. The oocyte increases in size to a diameter of approximately 120 μm. As the developing follicle increases in size, the number of granulosa cells increases to about 600 and the theca cells show increasing differentiation. The progression to secondary follicles also entails the formation of capillaries and an increase in the vascular supply to developing follicular units.

As the increasingly abundant granulosa cells secrete fluid into the center of the follicle, they create a fluid-filled space called the **antrum**. At this stage, the follicle is now a **tertiary follicle**, the first of the two antral stages. Gap junctions are located among both theca cells and granulosa cells. In addition, tight junctions and desmosomes exist between adjacent cells. Gap junctions may also exist between the oocyte and the granulosa cells closest to the oocyte and may function as thoroughfares to transport nutrients and information from the granulosa

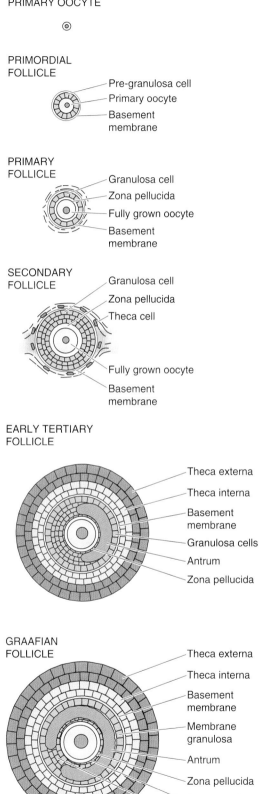

PRIMARY OOCYTE

PRIMORDIAL
FOLLICLE

- Pre-granulosa cell
- Primary oocyte
- Basement
  membrane

PRIMARY
FOLLICLE

- Granulosa cell
- Zona pellucida
- Fully grown oocyte
- Basement
  membrane

SECONDARY
FOLLICLE

- Granulosa cell
- Zona pellucida
- Theca cell
- Fully grown oocyte
- Basement
  membrane

EARLY TERTIARY
FOLLICLE

- Theca externa
- Theca interna
- Basement
  membrane
- Granulosa cells
- Antrum
- Zona pellucida

GRAAFIAN
FOLLICLE

- Theca externa
- Theca interna
- Basement
  membrane
- Membrane
  granulosa
- Antrum
- Zona pellucida
- Corona radiata
- Cumulus oophorus

FIGURE 54–11. The maturation of the ovarian follicle.

cells to the oocyte and vice versa. The granulosa cells closest to the oocyte also secrete the mucopolysaccharides that form the **zona pellucida** immediately surrounding the oocyte.

As the antrum enlarges, it eventually encircles the preovulatory or **graafian follicle**, except for a small "mound" or cumulus that attaches the oocyte to the rest of the follicle. At the same time, the follicle's diameter increases to 20 to 33 mm. The granulosa cells of the tertiary and graafian follicles are of three types: mural granulosa cells, antral granulosa cells, and cumulus cells. **Mural granulosa cells**, which are the farthest from the center of the follicle, are the most metabolically active and contain large quantities of LH receptors and enzymes that are necessary for the synthesis of steroids. **Cumulus granulosa cells** are shed with the oocyte at the time of ovulation. **Antral granulosa cells**, which face the antrum, are left behind within the follicle to become the large luteal cells of the corpus luteum. The capacity of the three types of granulosa cells to generate steroids differs. Cumulus cells contain neither the side-chain-cleavage enzyme (P-450_{scc}) nor aromatase (P-450_{arom}) and therefore cannot generate estrogens. Moreover, cumulus cells respond less to LH and have a low overall LH receptor content. The exact role of the cumulus layer has not been definitively established, although it has been postulated that the cumulus layer may function as a feeder layer and provide stem cells that differentiate into other follicular cell types.

Both FSH and LH Stimulate Follicular Growth

Even in fetal life and childhood, some primordial follicles can develop all the way to the antral stage. However, these follicles all undergo atresia (death of the ovum, followed by collapse of the follicle and scarring) at some stage in their development. At the time of puberty, the increase in levels of gonadotropins and ovarian steroids produces a marked increase in the rate of follicular development. During the luteal phase of each cycle, a cohort of primordial follicles is recruited for further development into graafian follicles, which occurs during the follicular phase of the next cycle. Thus, primordial follicles may remain in a nongrowing state for 50 years before developing into primary follicles. All along the course of this development, follicular units undergo atresia until only one dominant graafian follicle remains at the time of ovulation. There is some controversy about how long this developmental process takes. Some believe that the entire developmental process takes three to four monthly cycles. However, the predominant view is that a cohort of primary follicles is recruited during the end of one cycle and that from among these follicles, one develops into the dominant graafian follicle.

PRIMARY FOLLICLES. Appropriate structural and functional development of the follicle necessitates that the follicle is exposed to the appropriate sequence of three hormones: FSH, estradiol, and LH. FSH secretion occurs during early fetal life, and FSH can be detected as early as 5 months into gestation (see Fig. 54–2). Three pieces of evidence suggest that gonadotropins and estrogens are essential for early follicular growth, that is, for the progression from *primordial* to *primary follicles*. First, hypophysectomy (i.e., removal of the pituitary) causes depletion of *primordial* follicular units in primates. Thus, with the absence of gonadotropins—as well as other pituitary hormones—and a reduction in estrogens, no follicular development takes place in females. Second, patients with "resistant ovary syndrome" have a normal complement of *primordial* follicles, but the follicles do not develop beyond the primordial stage. Although these patients have high circulating levels of FSH, they have no receptors for FSH and LH in their ovaries. Thus, FSH or LH must be able to act on the ovary for follicular development to occur. Third, in individuals with 17α-hydroxylase deficiency—and thus low estrogen levels—follicular development does not progress beyond the *primordial* stage. Circulating levels of LH in these individuals are normal or high. These three lines of evidence suggest that removing either the gonadotropins, the gonadotropin receptors, or the estrogens halts early follicular growth.

SECONDARY FOLLICLES. As primary follicles form secondary follicles, the theca cells proliferate and acquire LH receptors, as well as the ability to synthesize steroids. Moreover, the granulosa cells acquire receptors for FSH, androgens, and estrogens. When the granulosa cells acquire FSH receptors, the follicular unit becomes a functional steroid-producing entity.

TERTIARY FOLLICLES. Formation of the antrum, which leads to the development of a tertiary follicle, also requires gonadotropins. FSH, acting in concert with estrogens, causes the proliferation of granulosa cells after development of the antrum, and as a result, the total number of receptors for FSH is increased. FSH, along with estradiol, also induces the proliferation of LH receptors in granulosa cells.

GRAAFIAN FOLLICLES. When human granulosa cells from graafian follicles are studied in vitro, the mitotic and steroid-synthesizing characteristics of these cells reflect the hormonal condition of the follicle from which they came. Both FSH and estradiol are needed for mitosis to occur in granulosa cells. FSH, LH, and estradiol are necessary for maximum progesterone production by granulosa cells. Premature exposure of developing follicles to LH *inhibits* mitosis, as well as steroidogenesis. Therefore, the follicle must be exposed to the appropriate sequence of hormones (e.g., FSH, followed by estradiol and then LH) for appropriate maturational and functional development.

Each Month, A Cohort of Follicles Is Recruited, One of Which Achieves Dominance

The consensus is that the monthly cycle of folliculogenesis actually begins from the primary-follicle stage 2 to 3 days before onset of the menses of the previous cycle. At this time, FSH levels begin to increase (see Fig. 54–3) because of decreasing inhibin concentrations, thus inducing folliculogenesis, which is completed in the next cycle.

Although we do not understand why some primordial follicles—and not others—join a developing cohort of follicles, FSH is thought to be at least partly responsible for continued development of a cohort of follicles each cycle. The number of follicles in a cohort depends on the residual pool of remaining follicles in the ovary. As the cycle continues, only a portion of the cohort of follicles continues to develop in response to gonadotropin secretion. The other members of the cohort of follicles undergo atresia.

The one follicle destined to ovulate is recruited during the early days of the current menstrual cycle and eventually achieves dominance. Although the mechanism of selection of the dominant follicle is not completely understood, it is thought to be caused by estrogen-induced events within the follicles. As estrogen levels rise during the follicular phase of the cycle, the pituitary gradually lowers its secretion of FSH (see Fig. 54–3). Rising inhibin levels also feed back on the anterior pituitary to decrease FSH secretion. Peak inhibin levels correlate with the number of follicles present and rise in parallel with circulating estradiol levels.

Decreased levels of FSH cause a decline in FSH-dependent aromatase activity in granulosa cells. As a result, estrogen production decreases in the less mature follicles. On the other hand, estrogen *increases* the effectiveness of FSH in the more mature follicles by increasing the number of FSH receptors. Although the dominant follicle continues to be dependent on FSH, it has more FSH receptors, a greater rate of granulosa cell proliferation, more FSH-dependent aromatase activity, and more estrogen production than the less dominant follicles. Because the less dominant follicles have less aromatase activity, the androstenedione in the theca cells cannot be converted so readily to estrogens in the granulosa cell. Instead, the androstenedione either builds up or is converted to other androgens. As a result, the less dominant follicles undergo atresia under the influence of androgens in their local environment. In contrast, the production of estrogens and inhibins allows the dominant follicle to become prominent and gain an even greater edge over its competitors. The vascular supply to the thecal layer of the dominant follicle increases rapidly so that during the late follicular phase, the vasculature of the dominant follicle is severalfold greater than that of other follicles in the cohort. Increased vascularity may allow greater FSH delivery to the dominant follicle, thus helping maintain dominance of the follicle selected for ovulation.

Estradiol Secretion by the Dominant Follicle Triggers the LH Surge, Which in Turn Signals Ovulation

Ovulation occurs at the midpoint of every normal menstrual cycle and is triggered by the LH surge, which in turn is stimulated by rapidly rising levels of estradiol. Estradiol secretion by the dominant follicle increases rapidly near the end of the late follicular phase (see Fig. 54–3). This dramatic rise in circulating estradiol exerts positive feedback on the anterior pituitary and sensitizes it to GnRH. The net effect of a rising estradiol level is induction of the LH surge. The LH surge is generally initiated 24 to 36 hours after peak estradiol secretion is achieved, and ovulation usually occurs approximately 36 hours after onset of the LH surge and about 12 hours after its peak. Thus, it appears that the developing follicle, via its increased estradiol secretion, signals the hypothalamic-pituitary system that follicular maturation is complete and that the hypothalamic-pituitary axis can now release a bolus of gonadotropin to induce ovulation. The LH surge appears to terminate in part as a result of rising levels of progesterone, via negative feedback, and in part as a result of loss of the positive feedback that is derived from estradiol. Depletion of gonadotropin stores in the anterior pituitary gland may also contribute to termination of the LH surge.

At the time of the LH surge, the oocyte, which had been arrested in the prophase of its first meiotic division since fetal life (p. 1106), now resumes meiosis and completes its first meiotic division several hours before ovulation. The result of this first meiotic division is a small **first polar body**, which degenerates or divides to form nonfunctional cells, and a much larger **secondary oocyte**. Both the first polar body and the secondary oocyte, like secondary spermatocytes (p. 1132), have a haploid number of duplicated chromosomes: 22 duplicated somatic chromosomes and one duplicated X chromosome. This secondary oocyte begins its second meiotic division, but becomes arrested in metaphase until the time of fertilization (p. 1169). The secondary oocyte is surrounded by the zona pellucida and one or more layers of follicular cells, the **corona radiata**. Before ovulation, the **cumulus oophorus** expands under the influence of LH, and eventually a complex consisting of the cumulus, the oocyte, and its surrounding cells breaks free with its "stalk" and floats inside the antrum, surrounded by follicular fluid. Breaking away of the oocyte-cumulus complex is probably facilitated by increased hyaluronidase synthesis that is stimulated by FSH.

Release of the oocyte from the follicle—**ovulation**—follows thinning and weakening of the follicular wall, probably under the influence of both LH and progesterone. Both LH and progesterone enhance the activity of proteolytic enzymes (e.g., collagenase) within the follicle and thus lead to the digestion of connective tissue in the follicular wall. Just before ovulation, FSH and, to a lesser extent, LH stimulate the release of **plasminogen activator** from granulosa cells; plasminogen activator promotes the conversion of plasminogen in the follicular fluid to plasmin, which is a protease that dissolves blood clots. Prostaglandins, particularly those in the E and F series, are also believed to be involved in ovulation. Although the mechanisms by which prostaglandins induce ovulation remain unclear, it is believed that prostaglandins cause the release of lysosomal enzymes that digest the follicular wall. Ultimately, a **stigma**—or spot—forms on the surface of the dominant follicle (see Fig. 54–11). As this stigma balloons out and forms a vesicle, it ruptures and the oocyte is expelled. Ovulation is apparently facilitated by increased intrafollicular pressure and contraction of smooth muscle in the theca as a result of prostaglandin stimulation.

The expelled oocyte, with its investment of follicular cells, is picked up by the fimbriae of the fallopian tube (see Fig. 54–1) as they move over the surface of the ovary. The oocyte is then transported through the infundibulum into the ampulla by means of ciliary movement of the tubal epithelium, as well as by muscular contrac-tions of the tube. Fertilization, if it occurs, takes place in the ampullary portion of the fallopian tube. The resulting zygote subsequently resides there for approximately 72 hours, followed by rapid transport through the isthmus to the uterine cavity, where it floats free for an additional 2 to 3 days before attaching to the endometrium.

After Ovulation, the Theca and Granulosa Cells of the Follicle Differentiate into the Theca-Lutein and Granulosa-Lutein Cells of the Highly Vascularized Corpus Luteum

After expulsion of the oocyte, the granulosa and theca cells are thrown up into folds that occupy the follicular cavity and form the **corpus luteum**, a temporary endocrine organ whose major product is progesterone. The corpus luteum is highly vascularized, and surrounding blood vessels penetrate the theca and granulosa layers. Blood accumulates in the resealed antral cavity of the corpus luteum soon after ovulation. Formation of the corpus luteum occurs as a result of transformation of the granulosa and theca cells under the influence of LH (see Fig. 54–11). The theca cells at the periphery of the follicle differentiate into stroma and give rise to **theca-lutein cells**—also known as small luteal cells. The granulosa cells, on the other hand, enlarge and give rise to **granulosa-lutein cells**—also known as large luteal cells. Therefore, the mature corpus luteum is composed of two cell types, theca-lutein and granulosa-lutein cells.

During the luteal phase of the menstrual cycle, estrogens and progestins inhibit folliculogenesis. Luteal function begins to decrease approximately 11 days after ovulation. The mechanisms responsible for luteal regression—or **luteolysis**—remain open to speculation. One school of thought postulates that withdrawal of trophic support results in demise of the corpus luteum, whereas the second school maintains that local factors induce luteal regression. For example, prostaglandin $F_{2\alpha}$ inhibits luteal function and terminates the life of the corpus luteum.

Growth and Involution of the Corpus Luteum Produce the Rise and Fall in Progestins and Estrogens During the Luteal Phase of the Menstrual Cycle

Although the corpus luteum produces both estrogen and progesterone, the luteal phase is primarily dominated by progesterone secretion. Estrogen production by the corpus luteum is largely a function of the theca-lutein or the small cells, which also produce androgens. Progestin production in the corpus luteum is primarily a function of the granulosa-lutein or large cells (see Fig. 54–10), which also produce estrogens.

As shown earlier in Figure 54–3, **progesterone** production rises before follicular rupture. After ovulation, progesterone levels rise sharply and peak in about 7 days. Progesterone acts locally to inhibit follicular growth during the luteal phase. In addition, progesterone may act centrally by inhibiting gonadotropin secretion. Progestins are also antiestrogens. As a result, progestins acting locally may downregulate estrogen receptors and reduce the effectiveness of estradiol. Therefore, increasing progesterone production may have adverse effects on folliculogenesis.

Estradiol levels also rise during the luteal phase (see Fig. 54–3) and reflect production by the corpus luteum. The estradiol produced during the luteal phase is necessary for the occurrence of progesterone-induced changes in the endometrium.

Unless rescued by hCG, luteal production of progesterone ceases toward the end of the menstrual cycle. Chorionic gonadotropin produced by the developing conceptus maintains steroidogenic function of the corpus luteum until approximately the 9th week of gestation, at which time placental function is well established. If not rescued by pregnancy, the hormone-producing cells of the corpus luteum degenerate and leave behind a fibrotic **corpus albicans**.

THE ENDOMETRIAL CYCLE

In the human female fetus, the uterine mucosa is capable of responding to steroid hormones by 20 weeks' gestation. Indeed, some of the uterine glands begin secreting material by the 22nd week of gestation. Endometrial development in utero apparently occurs in response to estrogens derived from the maternal placenta. At approximately 32 weeks' gestation, glycogen deposition and stromal edema are present in the endometrium. As estro-

genic stimulation is withdrawn after delivery, the endometrium regresses, and at about 4 weeks after birth, the glands are atrophic and lack vascularization. The endometrium remains in this state until puberty.

The Ovarian Hormones Drive the Morphologic and Functional Changes of the Endometrium During the Monthly Cycle

The ovarian steroids—estrogens and progestins—control the cyclic monthly growth and breakdown of the endometrium. The three major phases in the endometrial cycle are the menstrual, proliferative, and secretory phases.

THE MENSTRUAL PHASE. If the oocyte was not fertilized and pregnancy did not occur in the previous cycle, a sudden diminution in estrogen and progesterone secretion signals the demise of the corpus luteum. As hormonal support of the endometrium is withdrawn, the vascular and glandular integrity of the endometrium degenerates, the tissue breaks down, and menstrual bleeding ensues, which is defined as day 1 of the menstrual cycle (Fig. 54–12). After menstruation, all that remains on the inner surface of most of the uterus is a thin layer of *nonepithelial* stromal cells and some remnant glands. However, epithelial cells remain in the lower uterine segments, as well as regions close to the fallopian tubes.

THE PROLIFERATIVE PHASE. After menstruation, the endometrium is restored by about the fifth day of the cycle

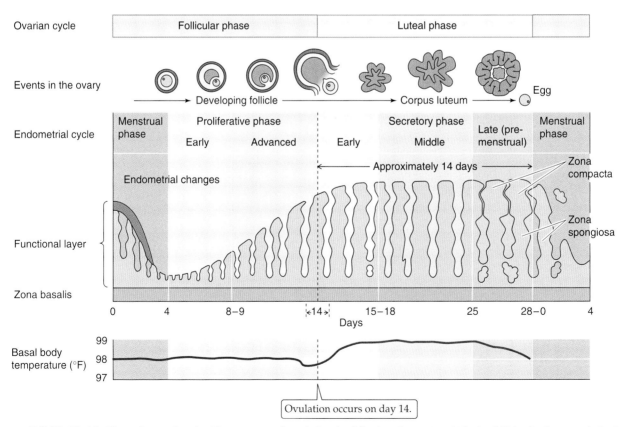

FIGURE 54–12. The endometrial cycle. The ovarian cycle includes the follicular phase—in which the follicle develops—and the luteal phase—in which the remaining follicular cells develop into the corpus luteum. The endometrial cycle has three parts: the menstrual, the proliferative, and the secretory phases.

(see Fig. 54–12) as a result of proliferation of the basal stromal cells on the denuded surface of the uterus (the *zona basalis*), as well as the proliferation of epithelial cells from other parts of the uterus. The stroma gives rise to the connective tissue components of the endometrium. Increased mitotic activity of the stromal and glandular epithelium continues throughout the follicular phase of the cycle and beyond, until approximately 3 days after ovulation. Cellular hyperplasia and increased extracellular matrix result in thickening of the endometrium during the late proliferative phase. The thickness of the endometrium increases from about 0.5 to as much as 5 mm during the proliferative phase.

Proliferation and differentiation of the endometrium are stimulated by estrogen that is secreted by the developing follicles. Levels of estrogen rise early in the follicular phase and peak just before ovulation (see Fig. 54–3). Estrogen *receptor* levels in the endometrium also increase during the follicular phase of the menstrual cycle. Levels of endometrial estrogen receptor are highest during the proliferative phase and decline after ovulation in response to changing levels of progesterone. As we have already seen, estradiol binds to a nuclear receptor on the endometrial cell, and the activated receptor interacts with the hormone-response elements of specific genes and modulates their transcription rates.

It is believed that estrogen acts on the endometrium in part via its effect on the expression of proto-oncogenes (p. 111) that are involved in the expression of certain genes. Part of the effect of estrogens is to induce the synthesis of growth factors such as the insulin-like growth factors (IGFs, also called somatomedins; p. 1029), TGFs, and epidermal growth factor (EGF). These autocrine and paracrine mediators are necessary for maturation and growth of the endometrium. Estrogen causes the stromal components of the endometrium to become highly developed. Estrogen also induces the synthesis of progestin receptors in endometrial tissue. Levels of progestin receptors peak at ovulation, when estrogen levels are highest, to prepare the cells for the high progestin levels of the luteal phase of the cycle.

Progesterone, on the other hand, opposes the action of estrogen on the epithelial cells of the endometrium and functions as an antiestrogen. Although progesterone inhibits *epithelial* cell proliferation, it promotes proliferation of the endometrial *stroma*. Progesterone exerts its primary antiestrogen effects by stimulating 17β-HSD and sulfotransferase, enzymes that convert estradiol to weaker compounds. Thus, 17β-HSD may convert the estradiol captured from the extracellular environment to estrone (see Fig. 54–9), and sulfotransferase may conjugate estrogens to sulfate and produce derivatives such as estradiol 3-sulfate. Estrone is far less active than estradiol, and sulfated estrogens are by themselves biologically inactive.

THE SECRETORY PHASE. During the early luteal phase of the ovarian cycle, progesterone further stimulates the 17β-HSD and sulfation reactions. These antiestrogenic effects halt the proliferative phase of the endometrial cycle. Progesterone also stimulates the glandular components of the endometrium and thus induces secretory changes in the endometrium. The epithelial cells exhibit a marked increase in secretory activity, as indicated by increased amounts of endoplasmic reticulum and mitochondria. These increases in synthetic activity occur in anticipation of the arrival and implantation of the blastocyst. The **early secretory phase** of the menstrual cycle (see Fig. 54–12) is characterized by the development of a network of interdigitating tubes within the nucleolus of the endometrial epithelial cells. These tubes are referred to as the **nucleolar channel system**, and progesterone apparently stimulates their development. The cytoplasm invaginates near the nucleolar channel system, although it remains unclear whether actual connections exist between the channel system and the cytoplasm. The nucleolar channel system may provide a route of transport for mRNA to the cytoplasm.

During the **middle to late secretory phase**, evidence of increased secretory capacity of the endometrial glands becomes more apparent. Vascularization of the endometrium increases, the glycogen content increases, and the thickness of the endometrium increases to 5 to 6 mm. The endometrial glands become engorged with secretions. They are no longer straight; instead, they become tortuous and achieve maximal secretory activity at approximately day 20 or 21 of the menstrual cycle.

The changes in the endometrium are not limited to the glands; they also occur in the stromal cells between the glands. Beginning 9 to 10 days after ovulation, stromal cells that surround the spiral arteries of the uterus enlarge and develop eosinophilic cytoplasm, with a prominent Golgi and endoplasmic reticulum. This process is referred to as **predecidualization**. The rounded **decidual cells** differentiate from spindle-shaped fibroblast-like stromal cells under the influence of progesterone. As the stromal cells differentiate into decidual cells, their biochemical activity changes and they form secretory products typical of decidual cells. Laminin, fibronectin, heparin sulfate, and type IV collagen surround matrices of decidualizing cells. Multiple foci of these decidual cells spread throughout the upper layer of the endometrium and form a dense layer called the **zona compacta** (see Fig. 54–12). This spreading is so extensive that the glandular structures of the zona compacta become inconspicuous. Inflammatory cells accumulate around glands and blood vessels. Edema of the midzone of the endometrium distinguishes the compact area from the underlying **zona spongiosa**, where the endometrial glands become more prominent.

Together, the superficial *zona compacta* and the mid-level *zona spongiosa* make up the so-called **functional layer** of the endometrium. This functional layer is the region that proliferates early in the monthly endometrial cycle, that later interacts with the embryo during pregnancy, that is shed after pregnancy, and that is also shed each month during menstruation. The deepest layer of the endometrium—the **zona basalis**—is the layer left behind after parturition or menstruation. It is the cells of the zona basalis that give rise to the proliferation at the beginning of the next endometrial cycle.

During the late luteal phase of the menstrual cycle, just before the next menstruation, levels of both estrogens and progestins diminish, and these decreased ovarian steroid levels lead to eventual demise of the upper two thirds of the endometrium. During this period, the spiral arteries rhythmically go into spasm and then relax. This period of the cycle is sometimes referred to as the **ischemic phase**. As cells begin to die, hydrolases are released from lysosomes and cause further breakdown of the endometrium. Prostaglandin production increases as a result of the action of phospholipases liberated from lysosomes. Necrosis of vascular cells leads to microhemorrhage. The average loss of blood, tissues, and serous fluid amounts to approximately 30 ml. Menstrual blood does not clot because of the presence of fibrolysins released from necrotic endometrial tissue.

The Effective Implantation Window is 3 to 4 Days

From studies of embryo transfer to recipient mothers in oocyte donation programs (see box on p. 1170), when both the age of the donated embryo and the time of the endometrial cycle of the recipient are known, it is estimated that the period of endometrial receptivity for implantation of the embryo extends from as early as day 16 to as late as day 19 of the menstrual cycle. Of course, because implantation must normally follow the ovulation that occurs on day 14 and because fertilization normally occurs within 1 day of ovulation, the effective window is less than 4 days, from day 16 to day 19. In contrast, when embryos are transferred on cycle days 20 through 24, no pregnancies are achieved.

Although the mechanisms underlying endometrial receptivity remain unclear, several changes in the endometrium are believed to be associated with increased receptivity of the endometrium for the embryo. The formation of microvilli and pinopods (i.e., protrusions of endometrial cells near gland openings) during the midluteal phase and the secretion of extracellular matrix composed of such materials as glycoproteins, laminin, and fibronectin may provide a surface that facilitates attachment of the embryo (p. 1173).

THE FEMALE SEX ACT

Female sexual desire—**libido**—is a complex phenomenon that consists of physical and psychological effects, all modulated by circulating sex steroids. Libido varies during the ovarian cycle, with the frequency of female sexual activity increasing around the time of ovulation. There may also be an increase in the rate of initiation of sexual activity by the female around the time of ovulation. These changes may in part reflect the increased secretion of androgenic steroids that occurs just before and during ovulation secondary to the LH surge.

The Female Sex Response, Which Is Elicited by Physical, Psychic, and Hormonal Stimuli, Occurs in Four Distinct Phases

Although sexual function has a strong physiological basis, it is not possible to separate sexual response from the other emotional and contributing factors that are involved in sexual relationships. Masters and Johnson published, in their now classic work *Human Sexual Response*, a discussion of data obtained on the sexual cycles of 700 subjects. Our current understanding of the female sexual response is based on their findings. Masters and Johnson described four stages of the sex response in females: the excitement or seduction phase, plateau, orgasm, and resolution. Following is a brief description of each phase.

EXCITEMENT. The excitement or arousal phase of the female sex response may be initiated by a multitude of internal or external stimuli, including psychological factors, such as thoughts and emotions, and physical factors, such as sight and tactile stimuli. Table 54–3 summarizes the responses of the excitement phase, many of which reflect activity of the parasympathetic division of the autonomic nervous system (ANS). Sexual intensity rises in crescendo fashion.

PLATEAU. The plateau stage is the culmination of the excitement phase as it reaches its peak. It is associated with a marked degree of vasocongestion throughout the body.

ORGASM. During orgasm, the sexual tension that has built up in the entire body is released. The climax, or orgasm, is intense and includes a myotonic response throughout the body. Muscle contractions start 2 to 4 seconds after the woman begins to experience orgasm, and they repeat at 0.8-second intervals. The actual number of contractions, as well as their intensity, varies from woman to woman. Some women observed to have orgasmic contractions are not aware that they are having an orgasm. Masters and Johnson suggested that prolonged stimulation during the excitement phase leads to more pronounced orgasmic activity. Whereas the excitement phase is under the influence of the parasympathetic division of the ANS, as is the erection phase in the male, orgasm seems to be related to the sympathetic division, as is the emission phase in the male (p. 1138).

RESOLUTION. The last phase of the female sex response is a return of the woman's physiological state to the preexcitement level. During the resolution phase, the woman generally experiences a feeling of personal satisfaction, well-being, and relaxation of sexual desire. A new sexual excitement cycle may be initiated at any time after orgasm without the refractory phase that occurs in the male.

Both the Sympathetic and the Parasympathetic Divisions Control the Female Sex Response

Much of the response in the excitement phase is due to stimulation of the **parasympathetic fibers** of the ANS. In some cases, anticholinergic drugs may interfere with a full response in this stage. Dilatation of blood vessels in the erectile tissues causes engorgement with blood and erection of the clitoris, as well as distention of the periintroital tissues and subsequent narrowing of the lower third of the vagina. Parasympathetic fibers emanating from the sacral plexus (p. 381) innervate these erectile tissues, just as in the male (p. 1136). In addition, the parasympathetic system innervates the Bartholin's glands,

TABLE 54–3

FEMALE SEXUAL RESPONSE CYCLE

Excitement

Warmth and erotic feelings

Increased sexual tension

Deep breathing

Increased heart rate

Increased blood pressure

Generalized vasocongestion

Skin flush

Breast engorgement

Nipple erection (myotonic effect)

Engorgement of labia and clitoris

Vaginal "sweating" (transudative lubrication)

Secretions from Bartholin glands

Uterine tenting into pelvis

Plateau

Marked vasocongestion

"Sex flush" (maculopapular rash on breasts, chest, and epigastrium)

Nipple erection

Engorgement of the labia

Engorgement of lower third of the vagina, with narrowing of diameter

Dilation of upper two thirds of vagina

Clitoral swelling and erection

Vaginal "sweating"

Uterine tenting

Orgasm

Release of tension

Generalized, rhythmic myotonic contractions

Contractions of perivaginal muscles and anal sphincter

Uterine contractions

Resolution

Return to pre-excitement state

Personal satisfaction and well-being

New excitement cycles may be initiated

which empty into the introitus, as well as the vaginal glands. Adequate lubrication is necessary to minimize the friction of intercourse and thus maximize the stimulation to achieve orgasm.

Both physical stimulation and psychic stimuli are important for female orgasm. Psychic stimuli are coordinated via the cerebrum, which causes the generalized tension throughout the body, as discussed earlier, and also modulates the autonomic response. The female orgasm is also coordinated via a spinal cord reflex that results in rhythmic contractions of the perineal muscles. The afferent pathways for this spinal cord reflex follow the pudendal nerves, which emanate via sacral segments 2 to 4 and are the primary innervation to the perineum and the external genitalia of the female. This spinal-cord reflex is similar to that observed in the male.

The Female Sex Response Facilitates Sperm Transport Through the Female Reproductive Tract

The spinal reflexes previously discussed may also increase uterine and cervical activity and thus promote transport of gametes. The cervix dilates during orgasm, thus facilitating sperm transport into the upper part of the reproductive tract. The release of oxytocin at the time of orgasm stimulates uterine contractility, which also facilitates gamete transport. Although 150 to 600 million sperm cells (p. 1135) are normally deposited in the vagina during sexual intercourse, about 100,000 reach the cavity of the uterus and only 50 to 100 viable sperm reach the distal fallopian tube where fertilization occurs. Aside from the one or more sperm that fertilize the ovum (or ova), most sperm degenerate, to be disposed of by the female genital tract. Sperm transport is accomplished by swimming movements of the sperm tail through the mucus of the cervical canal. The sperm reach the ampulla of the fallopian tubes within 5 minutes of ejaculation. Clearly, this rapid rate of transport could not be achieved by the swimming activity of the sperm alone. Therefore, uterine or tubal activity must serve a major role in sperm transport.

MENOPAUSE

Menopause, or the climacteric, signals the termination of reproductive function in the female. Cyclic reproductive function ceases, menstruation comes to an end, and childbearing is generally no longer possible. Also occurring are significant physiological changes (Table 54–4) that have a major impact on health.

Only a Few Functioning Follicles Remain in the Ovaries of a Menopausal Woman

Progressive loss of ovarian follicular units occurs throughout life. About 6 to 7 million germ cells are present in the two ovaries of the developing female fetus at 20 weeks' gestation. At birth, only about 1 to 2 million follicular units remain in the ovaries. At puberty about 400,000 remain, again reflecting the continued process of atresia during the prepubertal years. Puberty generally occurs in American girls at about 12.5 years of age. The average age of menopause in American women is 51.5 years. Thus, it is estimated that more than 400 oocytes are ovulated during the reproductive life of a woman. At

TABLE 54–4

THE MENOPAUSAL SYNDROME AND PHYSICAL CHANGES IN MENOPAUSE

MENOPAUSAL SYNDROME	PHYSICAL CHANGES IN MENOPAUSE
Vasomotor instability	Atrophy of the vaginal epithelium
Hot flashes	Changes in vaginal pH
Night sweats	Decrease in vaginal secretions
Mood changes	Decrease in circulation to vagina and uterus
Short-term memory loss	Pelvic relaxation
Sleep disturbances	Loss of vaginal tone
Headaches	
Loss of libido	Cardiovascular disease
	Osteoporosis
	Alzheimer's disease

menopause and during the ensuing 5 years, the ovary contains only an occasional secondary follicle and a few primary follicles in a prominent stroma. The massive loss of oocytes over the reproductive life of a woman—from 400,000 at puberty to virtually none at menopause—is due to the rapid, continuous process of atresia during reproductive life. During each cycle, a large cohort (about 10 to 30) of follicles are recruited, but only one reaches dominance and ovulates. The others become atretic. However, even if we multiply the number of follicles in a cohort by the total number of menstrual cycles, we cannot account for all 400,000 of the prepubertal units. Thus, most of the primordial and primary ovarian follicles are lost as a result of atresia during the reproductive life of the individual.

During Menopause, Levels of the Ovarian Steroids Fall, Whereas Gonadotropin Levels Rise

The loss of functional ovarian follicles is primarily responsible for menopause in primates. Even before the onset of menopause, significant hormonal changes occur very early during reproductive life. Because of a gradual decline in the number of follicles, the decreased ovarian production of estrogen reduces the negative feedback to the anterior pituitary and leads to increased levels of FSH. Increased levels of FSH are seen as early as 35 years of age, even though cyclic reproductive function continues. When compared with younger women, older—but premenopausal—women have diminished estradiol production and decreased luteal function during natural cycles. Diminished inhibin production by the aging ovary may also contribute to the sharp rise in FSH levels that occurs in the perimenopausal period of life.

During menopause, estradiol levels are generally less than 30 pg/ml, and progesterone levels are often less than 1 ng/ml of plasma. Both these values are somewhat less

HORMONE REPLACEMENT THERAPY DURING MENOPAUSE

Although the mean age at menopause is approximately 51.5 years, changes in hormone secretion patterns are seen much earlier. Increases in levels of follicle stimulating hormone occur as early as age 35. The mechanisms responsible for this change remain to be elucidated. However, it is clear that ovarian function begins to diminish far in advance of a woman's last menstrual period. The increase in gonadotropin secretion is probably a result of decreased folliculogenesis leading to decreased secretion of sex steroids and inhibin and thus lowered negative feedback on the gonadotrophs during the perimenopausal period.

The characteristic changes associated with menopause are due primarily to low circulating estrogen levels. Estrogen is a very important regulatory hormone in females. In addition to the role of estrogen in reproductive processes, it has profound effects on several other physiological systems (Table 54–4).

Hormone replacement therapy is indicated during menopause to alleviate the menopausal syndrome and to prevent or diminish the physical changes that occur as a result of estrogen deficiency. Menopausal hormone replacement therapy consists of estrogen and progestin administration. The reason for administering progestins is that the endometrium is at significant risk of neoplasia from the unopposed actions of estrogens. Thus, progestins are not generally administered to women who have had hysterectomies. Estrogen replacement is very effective against the menopausal syndrome, as well as osteoporosis and cardiovascular disease. However, because of side effects (e.g., menstruation) and concern about endometrial and breast cancer, compliance with hormone replacement therapy is often compromised.

The selective estrogen receptor modulators (**SERMS**) are a group of structurally dissimilar compounds that interact with estrogen receptors. However, they act as either estrogen agonists or estrogen antagonists depending on the target tissue and hormonal status of the individual. The exact mechanisms through which SERMS elicit their effects in specific tissues remain unclear and constitute an area of active research. The estrogen antagonist effects of SERMS may be mediated by classic competition for the estrogen receptor. SERMS such as tamoxifen and raloxifene have beneficial effects, similar to those of estrogens, on bone and the cardiovacular system, whereas they antagonize estrogen in reproductive tissue. Clearly, the ideal SERM would have all the beneficial effects of estrogen without the negative and potentially dangerous side effects. For example, the perfect SERM would alleviate the menopausal syndrome, protect against cardiovascular and Alzheimer disease, and act as estrogen agonists in certain reproductive tissues and as antagonists in others.

than the lowest levels seen during the menstrual cycle of a younger woman (see Fig. 54–3). Ovarian production of androstenedione is minimal during menopause, although androstenedione production by the adrenal cortex remains normal.

Because the output of estrogens, progestins, and inhibins from the ovaries falls to very low levels during menopause, negative feedback on the hypothalamic-pituitary-ovarian axis (see Fig. 54–4) becomes minimal. As a result, levels of FSH and LH may be higher than those seen during the midcycle surge in premenopausal women—the futile attempt of the axis to stimulate follicular development and production of the female sex steroids. During menopause, the anterior pituitary still secretes FSH and LH in pulses, presumably after cyclic release of GnRH from the hypothalamus (see Fig. 54–2*A*). Although gonadotropins cannot generally stimulate the postmenopausal ovary, it appears that the gonadotrophs in the anterior pituitary can respond to exogenous GnRH.

REFERENCES

Books and Reviews

Adashi EY, Rock JA, Rosenwaks Z (eds): Reproductive Endocrinology, Surgery and Technology. Philadelphia, Lippincott-Raven, 1996.

de Kretser DM, Robertson DM, Risbridger GP: Recent advances in the physiology of human inhibin. J Endocrinol Invest 13:611–624, 1990.
Dufau ML: The luteinizing hormone receptor. Annu Rev Physiol 60: 461–496, 1998.
Marshall WA, Tanner JM: Puberty. In Falkner F, Tanner JM (eds): Human Growth, Vol 2. New York, Plenum, 1986, pp 171–209.
Masters WH, Johnson VE: Human Sexual Response. Boston, Little, Brown, 1966.
Wilson JD, Foster DW, Kronenberg HM, Larsen PR (eds): Williams Textbook of Endocrinology, 9th ed. Philadelphia, WB Saunders, 1998.
Woodruff TK, Mather JP: Inhibin, activin and the female reproductive axis. Annu Rev Physiol 57:214–244, 1995.

Journal Articles

Erickson GF, Wang C, Hsueh AJW: FSH induction of functional LH receptors in granulosa cells cultured in a chemically defined medium. Nature 279:336–338, 1979.
Fiddes JC, Goodman HM: The gene encoding the common alpha subunit of the four human glycoprotein hormones. J Mol Appl Genet 1: 3–18, 1981.
Ryan KJ: Granulosa-thecal cell interaction in ovarian steroidogenesis. J Steroid Biochem 11:799–800, 1979.
Schwanzel-Fukuda M, Pfaff DW: Origin of luteinizing hormone–releasing hormone neurons. Nature 338:161–164, 1989.
Veldhuis JD, Dufau ML: Estradiol modulates the pulsatile secretion of bioactive luteinizing hormone in vivo. J Clin Invest 80:631–638, 1987.

CHAPTER 55

Fertilization, Pregnancy, and Lactation

Ervin E. Jones and Alan H. DeCherney

TRANSPORT OF GAMETES AND FERTILIZATION

The Action of Cilia and Smooth Muscle Controls the Transport of Gametes and Conceptus within the Female Genital Tract

The human male deposits 150 to 600 million sperm into the vagina of the female at the time of ejaculation. Only 50 to 100 actually reach the ampullary portion of the fallopian tube, where fertilization normally occurs. However, the sperm get there very quickly, within approximately 5 minutes of ejaculation. The swimming motion of the sperm alone cannot account for such rapid transport. Forceful contractions of the uterus, cervix, and fallopian tubes propel the sperm into the upper reproductive tract during female orgasm. Prostaglandins in the seminal plasma may induce further contractile activity.

As the fimbria of the fallopian tube sweep over the ovarian surface, they pick up the oocyte, surrounded by its complement of granulosa cells, the cumulus oophorus, and corona radiata (p. 1159). Shortly after ovulation, movements of the cilia and the fallopian tube propel the oocyte-cumulus complex toward the uterus. The egg normally comes into contact with the sperm in the ampullary portion of the tube, where fertilization usually occurs several hours after ovulation. The fertilized ovum then resides in the fallopian tube for approximately 3 days, during which time it develops to the **morula** stage (i.e., a mulberry-shaped solid mass of 12 or more cells), receiving nourishment from fallopian-tube secretions. During these three days, smooth-muscle contractions of the isthmus prevent advancement of the conceptus into the uterus while the endometrium is preparing for implantation. The mechanisms by which the ovum is later propelled through the isthmus of the fallopian tube to the uterus probably include beating of the cilia of the tubal epithelium and contraction of the fallopian tube.

After the morula rapidly moves through the isthmus to the uterine cavity, it floats freely in the lumen of the uterus, and transforms into a blastocyst. A **blastocyst** is a ball-like structure with a fluid-filled inner cavity. Surrounding this cavity is a thin layer of **trophoectoderm** cells that forms the trophoblast, which develops into a variety of supporting structures, including the amnion, the yolk sac, and the fetal portion of the placenta. On one side of the cavity, attached to the trophoblast, is an **inner cell mass**, which develops into the embryo proper. The conceptus floats freely in the uterine cavity for approximately 72 hours before it attaches to the endometrium. Thus, implantation of the human blastocyst normally occurs 6 to 7 days following ovulation. Numerous maturational events occur in the conceptus as it travels to the uterus. The embryo must be prepared to draw nutrients from the endometrium on arrival in the uterine cavity, and the endometrium must be prepared to sustain the implantation of the blastocyst.

The "Capacitation" of the Spermatozoa that Occurs in the Female Genital Tract Enhances the Ability of the Sperm Cell to Fertilize the Ovum

As discussed earlier, sperm begin to mature while they are stored in the epididymis (p. 1134). In most species, neither freshly ejaculated sperm cells nor sperm cells that are removed from the epididymis are capable of fertilizing the egg until they have undergone further maturation ("capacitation") in the female reproductive tract. **Capacitation** is a poorly understood physiologic process by which spermatozoa acquire the ability to penetrate the zona pellucida of the ovum. The removal or modification of a protective protein coat from the sperm cell membrane appears to be an important molecular event in the capacitation.

In the human female, sperm do not need to pass through the cervix and uterus to achieve capacitation. Successful pregnancy can occur with gamete intrafallopian transfer (GIFT), in which spermatozoa and oocytes are placed directly into the ampulla of the fallopian tube, and also with direct ultrasound-guided intraperitoneal insemination, in which the sperm are deposited in the peritoneum, near the fimbria. Thus, capacitation of sperm in the reproductive tract is not strictly organ specific. As evidenced by the success of in vitro fertilization (see the box on In Vitro Fertilization and Embryo Transfer), capacitation is feasible even if the sperm does not make contact with the female reproductive tract.

Fertilization Begins as the Sperm Cell Attaches to the Zona Pellucida and Undergoes the Acrosomal Reaction, and it Ends with the Fusion of the Male and Female Pronuclei

After ovulation, the egg is in a semidormant state. If it remains unfertilized, the ripe egg remains quiescent for some time and eventually degenerates. However, if it is fertilized by a sperm cell, the egg awakens ("**activation**") to initiate a series of morphologic and biochemical events that lead to cell division and differentiation. **Fertilization** occurs in eight steps:

Step 1: The sperm head weaves its way past the follicular cells and attaches to the *zona pellucida* that surrounds the oocyte (Fig. 55–1). The zona pellucida is composed of three glycoproteins; ZP1 crosslinks the filamentous ZP2 and ZP3 into a latticework. Receptors on the plasma membrane of the sperm cell bind to **ZP3**, initiating a signal-transduction cascade.

Step 2: As a result of the sperm-ZP3 interaction, the sperm cell undergoes the **acrosomal reaction**, a prelude to the migration of the sperm cell through the mucus-like zona pellucida. The acrosome is a unique sperm organelle, essentially a large secretory vesicle, that originates from the Golgi complex in the spermatid (p. 1133). The acrosome contains hydrolyzing enzymes that are necessary for the sperm to penetrate the zona pellucida. The acrosome lies in front of and around the anterior two thirds of the sperm nucleus, much like a motorcycle helmet fits over one's head. During the acrosomal reaction, an increase in $[Ca^{2+}]_i$ triggers fusion of the *outer* acrosomal membrane with the sperm cell's plasma membrane, resulting in the exocytosis of most of the acrosomal contents.

Step 3: The spermatozoon penetrates through the zona pellucida. One mechanism of this penetration is the action of the acrosomal enzymes. Protease inhibitors can block the penetration of spermatozoa through the zona pellucida. The sperm cell also penetrates the zona pellucida by mechanical action. The sperm head rapidly oscillates about a fulcrum that is situated in the neck region. This rapid, vigorous, rocking action occurs with a frequency of approximately 6 to 8 oscillations/s. The sperm penetrates the zona pellucida at an angle, creating a tangential cleavage slit and leaving the sperm head lying sideways against the oocyte membrane.

Step 4: The cell membranes of the sperm and the oocyte fuse. Microvilli on the oocyte surface envelop the sperm cell, which probably binds to the oocyte membrane via specific proteins on the surfaces of the two cells. The posterior membrane of the acrosome—which remains part of the sperm cell after the acrosomal reaction—is the first portion of the sperm to fuse with the plasma membrane of the egg. The sperm cell per se does not enter the oocyte. Rather, the cytoplasmic portions of the head and tail enter the oocyte, leaving the sperm-cell plasma membrane behind, similar to a snake crawling out of its skin.

Step 5: The oocyte undergoes the cortical reaction. As the spermatozoon penetrates the oocyte's plasma membrane, it initiates formation of IP_3, causing Ca^{2+} release from internal stores (p. 100), an increase in $[Ca^{2+}]_i$ and $[Ca^{2+}]_i$ waves. This rise in $[Ca^{2+}]_i$ in turn triggers the oocyte's second meiotic division—discussed later—and the cortical reaction. In the **cortical reaction**, small electron-dense granules that lie just beneath the plasma membrane fuse with the oocyte's plasma membrane. Exocytosis of these granules releases enzymes that act on glycoproteins in the zona pellucida, causing them to harden. In the process, polysaccharides are liberated from these glycoproteins. From a teleologic perspective, the cortical granule reaction prevents **polyspermy**. Polyspermic embryos are abnormal because they are polyploid. They do not develop beyond the early cleavage stages.

Step 6: The oocyte completes its second meiotic division. The oocyte, which had been arrested in the prophase of its first meiotic division since fetal life (p. 1106), completed its first meiotic division at the time of the surge of luteinizing hormone (LH), which occurred several hours before ovulation (p. 1159). The result was the first polar body and a secondary oocyte with a

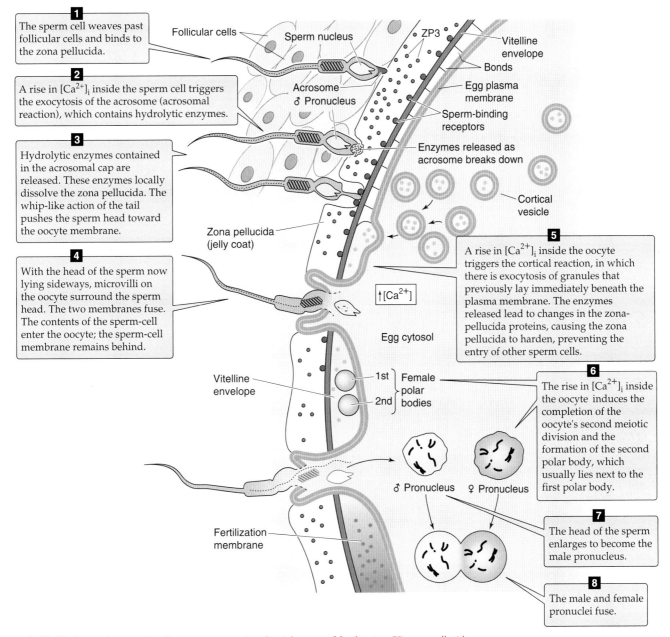

1 The sperm cell weaves past follicular cells and binds to the zona pellucida.

2 A rise in $[Ca^{2+}]_i$ inside the sperm cell triggers the exocytosis of the acrosome (acrosomal reaction), which contains hydrolytic enzymes.

3 Hydrolytic enzymes contained in the acrosomal cap are released. These enzymes locally dissolve the zona pellucida. The whip-like action of the tail pushes the sperm head toward the oocyte membrane.

4 With the head of the sperm now lying sideways, microvilli on the oocyte surround the sperm head. The two membranes fuse. The contents of the sperm-cell enter the oocyte; the sperm-cell membrane remains behind.

5 A rise in $[Ca^{2+}]_i$ inside the oocyte triggers the cortical reaction, in which there is exocytosis of granules that previously lay immediately beneath the plasma membrane. The enzymes released lead to changes in the zona-pellucida proteins, causing the zona pellucida to harden, preventing the entry of other sperm cells.

6 The rise in $[Ca^{2+}]_i$ inside the oocyte induces the completion of the oocyte's second meiotic division and the formation of the second polar body, which usually lies next to the first polar body.

7 The head of the sperm enlarges to become the male pronucleus.

8 The male and female pronuclei fuse.

Follicular cells — Sperm nucleus — ZP3 — Vitelline envelope — Bonds — Egg plasma membrane — Sperm-binding receptors — Enzymes released as acrosome breaks down — Cortical vesicle — Acrosome — ♂ Pronucleus — Zona pellucida (jelly coat) — $\uparrow[Ca^{2+}]$ — Egg cytosol — Vitelline envelope — 1st / 2nd Female polar bodies — ♂ Pronucleus — ♀ Pronucleus — Fertilization membrane

FIGURE 55–1. Fertilization. The illustration summarizes the eight steps of fertilization. ZP, zona pellucida.

haploid number of duplicated chromosomes (see Fig. 52–1). Before fertilization, this secondary oocyte had begun a second meiotic division, which was arrested in metaphase. The rise in $[Ca^{2+}]_i$ inside the oocyte—which the sperm cell triggers, as noted earlier—not only causes the cortical reaction, but also the completion of the oocyte's second meiotic division. One result is the formation of the **second polar body**, which contains a haploid number of unduplicated maternal chromosomes. The oocyte extrudes the chromosomes of the second polar body, together with a small amount of ooplasm, into a space that is immediately below the zona pellucida; the second polar body usually lies close to the first polar body. The nucleus of the oocyte also contains a haploid number of unduplicated chromo-

somes. As its chromosomes decondense, the nucleus of this mature ovum becomes the **female pronucleus**.

Step 7: The sperm nucleus decondenses and transforms into the **male pronucleus**, which, like the female pronucleus, contains a haploid number of unduplicated chromosomes (see Fig. 53–7). The cytoplasmic portion of the sperm's tail degenerates.

Step 8: The male and female pronuclei fuse, forming a new cell, the **zygote**. The mingling of chromosomes (syngamy) can be considered as the end of fertilization and the beginning of embryonic development. Thus, fertilization results in a conceptus that bears 46 chromosomes, 23 from the maternal gamete and 23 from the paternal gamete. As noted in Chapter 52, fertilization of the ovum by a sperm bearing an X chromo-

IN VITRO FERTILIZATION AND EMBRYO TRANSFER (IVF-ET)

In vitro fertilization is a procedure in which an oocyte or oocytes are removed from a woman and then fertilized with sperm under laboratory conditions. Early development of the embryo also proceeds under laboratory conditions. Finally, the physician transfers one or more embryos to the uterine cavity, where the embryo will hopefully implant and develop.

Indications for IVF-ET. Indications for IVF-ET include disorders that impair the normal meeting of the sperm and the egg in the distal portion of the fallopian tube. These disorders include ovulatory dysfunction, uterine or tubal factors (including adhesions or endometriosis), or other disease processes of the female peritoneal cavity. In addition, IVF-ET is indicated in some cases of male-factor infertility (abnormalities in male reproductive function) or unexplained infertility.

Ovarian stimulation. Because the success rates are less than 100% for each of the stages of IVF-ET, the physician needs several oocytes, all obtained in a single ovarian cycle. However, the human female normally develops a single dominant follicle each cycle (p. 1159). Thus, to obtain the *multiple* oocytes for IVF-ET, the physician must stimulate the development of multiple follicles in the woman by controlled ovarian hyperstimulation. Although this procedure qualitatively mimics the hormonal control of the normal cycle, the high dose of gonadotropins triggers the development of *many* follicles. The physician administers some combination of follicle-stimulating hormone (FSH) and luteinizing hormone (LH) or pure FSH preparations, either intramuscularly or subcutaneously. Because exogenous gonadotropins stimulate the ovaries directly, GnRH analogues (see box on p. 1149) are often used to downregulate the hypothalamic-pituitary axis during controlled ovarian stimulation. One usually administers these GnRH analogues prior to initiating gonadotropin therapy, primarily to prevent a premature LH surge and ovulation.

Cycle monitoring. After administering the gonadotropins, the physician monitors the simulated follicular growth in the ovaries, using sonographic imaging. Size, number, and serial growth of ovarian follicles may be assessed daily or at other appropriate intervals. Serum estradiol levels provide an additional measure of follicular growth and function. When estradiol levels and follicular growth indicate—by established criteria—appropriate folliculogenesis, the physician simulates a natural LH surge by injecting human chorionic gonadotropin (hCG), which is a close relative of LH (p. 1150). However, in this case, the simulated LH surge completes the final maturation of *multiple* follicles and oocytes. As we already know (p. 1158), ovulation usually occurs 36 to 39 hours following the beginning of the LH surge. Thus, the physician plans oocyte retrieval in such a way to allow maximal follicular maturation, but still to harvest the oocytes *prior* to ovulation. Thus, retrievals are scheduled for 34 to 36 hours following the administration of hCG.

Oocyte retrieval. The physician retrieves oocytes by aspirating them from individual follicles, under sonographic guidance. With the patient under conscious sedation, and after applying a local anesthetic to the posterior vaginal wall, the physician inserts a probe, equipped with a needle guide, into the vagina. After inserting a 16 to 18 gauge needle though the vaginal wall, the specialist aspirates the follicular fluid from each mature follicle and collects it in a test tube containing a small amount of culture medium. The eggs are identified in the follicular fluid, separated from the fluid and other follicular cells, and then washed and prepared for insemination. This procedure normally yields 8 to 15 oocytes.

Insemination. The sperm sample is subjected to a number of washes, followed by column chromatography to separate the sperm cells from the other cells and debris found in the ejaculate. Each egg is inseminated with 50,000 to 300,000 motile sperm in a drop of culture medium, and incubated overnight. Fertilization can usually be detected by the presence of two pronuclei in the egg cytoplasm after 16 to 20 hours. Fertilization rates generally range from 60% to 85%. Embryo development is allowed to continue in vitro for another 48 to 120 hours until embryos are transferred to the uterus.

Among couples in which the male partner has very low numbers of motile sperm, high fertilization rates can be achieved using **intracytoplasmic sperm injection** (ICSI). Micromanipulation techniques are used to inject a sperm cell into the cytoplasm of each egg in vitro. Fertilization rates after ICSI are generally 60% to 70%, or approximately equivalent to conventional insemination in vitro.

Embryo transfer. After culturing the cells for 48 to 120 hours, the physician transfers three to four embryos to the uterus at the 4- to 8-cell stage (after 2 days) or fewer embryos at the blastocyst stage (after 5 days). Embryos are selected and loaded into a thin flexible catheter, which is inserted into the uterine cavity to the desired depth under ultrasonic guidance. The woman usually receives supplemental progesterone to support implantation and pregnancy. In certain cases, the embryos are transferred to the fallopian tube during laparoscopy. This procedure is referred to as **tubal embryo transfer** (TET). The rationale for this procedure is that the fallopian tube contributes to the early development of the embryo as it travels down the tube to the uterus.

Success rates. Implantation rates usually range from 8% to 15% per embryo transferred. In the United States, the mean live birth rate per embryo-transfer procedure is approximately 33%.

GIFT. In certain cases of infertility, the physician collects the oocytes and sperm cells in much the same way as described earlier for IVF-ET, but directly transfers the gametes to the fallopian tube, where fertilization occurs. The gamete intrafallopian transfer (GIFT) is accomplished using laparoscopic techniques.

some produces a zygote with XX sex chromosomes; this develops into a female. Fertilization with a Y-bearing sperm produces an XY zygote, which develops into a male. Therefore, chromosomal sex is established at fertilization.

IMPLANTATION OF THE DEVELOPING EMBRYO

As discussed, the ovum is fertilized in the ampullary portion of the fallopian tube several hours after ovulation, and the conceptus remains in the fallopian tube for approximately 72 hours. The embryo spends an additional approximately 72 hours in the uterus before actual implantation. Because there is a specific window in time during which implantation can occur, temporal relationships between embryonic and endometrial maturation assume extreme importance.

The Presence of an Embryo Leads to Decidualization, a Completion of the Predecidualization of the Endometrium that Was Initiated During the Late Secretory Phase of the Endometrial Cycle

During the middle to late secretory phase of the normal endometrial cycle, the endometrium becomes more vascularized, increases in thickness, and the endometrial glands become tortuous and engorged with secretions (p. 1161). These changes, driven by progesterone from the corpus luteum, peak at approximately 7 days after ovulation. Additionally, beginning 9 to 10 days after ovulation, a process known as **predecidualization** (p. 1161) begins near the spiral arteries. During predecidualization, stromal cells transform into rounded decidual cells, and these spread across the superficial layer of the endometrium making it more compact (zona compacta) and separating it from the deeper, more spongy layer (zona spongiosa; see Fig. 54–12). If conception fails to occur, the secretory activity of the endometrial glands decreases, followed by regression of the glands 8 to 9 days after ovulation, which is ultimately followed by menstruation.

When pregnancy occurs, the predecidual changes in the endometrium are sustained and extended, completing the process of **decidualization**. The **decidua** is the specialized endometrium of pregnancy. Its original name was "membrana decidua," referring to the "membranes" of the endometrium that are shed following pregnancy, like the leaves of a "deciduous" tree. Because the degree of decidualization is considerably greater in conception cycles than in nonconception cycles, it is likely that the blastocyst itself promotes decidualization. Indeed, either the presence of the embryo or a traumatic stimulus that mimics the embryo's invasion of the endometrium induces changes in the endometrium.

The area underneath the implanting embryo becomes the **decidua basalis** (Fig. 55–2). Other portions of the decidua that become prominent later in pregnancy are the **decidua capsularis**, which overlies the embryo,

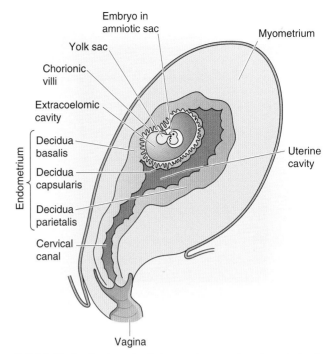

FIGURE 55–2. The three decidual zones during early embryonic development. The figure shows a sagittal section through a pregnant uterus, with the anterior side to the right.

and the **decidua parietalis**, which covers the remainder of the uterine surface. The upper zona compacta layer and the middle zona spongiosa layer of the nonpregnant endometrium are still recognizable in the decidualized endometrium of pregnancy. The glandular epithelium within the zona spongiosa continues its secretory activity during the first trimester. Some of the glands take on a hypersecretory appearance in what has been referred to as the *Arias-Stella* phenomenon of early pregnancy—named after the pathologist Javier Arias-Stella. Although the decidualized endometrium is most prominent during the first trimester, prior to the establishment of the definitive placenta, elements of decidualization persist throughout gestation.

Uterine Secretions Nourish the Pre-Implantation Embryo, Promote Growth, and Prepare It for Implantation

Before the embryo implants in the endometrium and establishes an indirect lifeline between the mother's blood and its own, it must receive its nourishment from uterine secretions. Following conception, the endometrium is primarily controlled by progesterone, which initially comes from the corpus luteum (p. 1153). The uterine glandular epithelium synthesizes and secretes several steroid-dependent proteins (Table 55–1) that are thought to be important for the nourishment, growth, and implantation of the embryo. The endometrium secretes cholesterol, steroids, and various nutrients, including iron and fat-soluble vitamins. It also synthesizes matrix substances, adhesion molecules, and surface receptors for matrix proteins, all of which may be important for implantation.

Pinopodes appear as small, finger-like protrusions on endometrial cells between day 19 (about the time the embryo would arrive in the uterus) and day 21 (about the time of implantation) of the menstrual cycle; they persist for only 2 to 3 days. Pinopode formation appears to be progesterone dependent, and it is inhibited by estrogens. Pinopodes endocytose macromolecules and uterine fluid and absorb most of the fluid in the lumen of the uterus during the early stages of embryo implantation. By removing uterine luminal fluid, the pinopodes may allow the embryo and the uterine epithelium to approximate one another more closely. Because apposition and adhesion of the embryo to the uterus are the first events of implantation, the presence and action of pinopodes may determine the extent of the implantation window.

The Blastocyst Secretes Substances that Facilitate Implantation

If the blastocyst is to survive, it must avoid rejection by the maternal cellular immune system. It does so by releasing immunosuppressive agents (Table 55–2). The embryo also synthesizes and secretes macromolecules that promote implantation, the development of the placenta, and the maintenance of pregnancy.

Both short-range and long-range embryonic signals may be necessary for implantation, although the nature of some of these signals remains enigmatic. One short-range signal from the blastocyst may stimulate local changes in the endometrium at the time of its apposition to the endometrium. A long-range signal that is secreted by the early blastocyst is **human chorionic gonadotropin** (hCG), which is closely related to LH (p. 1150) and sustains the corpus luteum in the face of rapidly falling levels of maternal LH.

hCG is one of the most important of the factors secreted by the trophoblast of the blastocyst, both pre-implantation and postimplantation. Besides rescuing the corpus luteum, hCG acts as an immunosuppressive agent, has growth-promoting activity, and acts as an autocrine growth factor that promotes trophoblast growth and placental development. Thus, hCG may have a role in the adhesion of the trophoblast to the epithelia of the endometrium. hCG has protease activity, and hCG levels are high in the area where the trophoblast faces the endometrium.

TABLE 55–1

ENDOMETRIAL PROTEINS, GLYCOPROTEINS, AND PEPTIDES SECRETED BY THE ENDOMETRIAL GLANDS DURING PREGNANCY

Mucins

Prolactin

Insulin-like growth factor binding protein-1 (IGFBP-1)

Placental protein 14 (PP14) or glycodelin

Pregnancy-associated endometrial α_2-globulin (α_2-PEG)

Endometrial protein 15

Fibronectin

Laminin

Entactin

Collagen IV

Heparin sulfate

Proteoglycan

Integrins

Albumin

β-Lipoprotein

Relaxin

Acidic fibroblast growth factor

Basic fibroblast growth factor

Pregnancy-associated plasma protein A (PAPP-A)

Stress response protein 27 (SRP-27)

CA-125

β-Endorphin

Leu-enkephalin

Diamine oxidase

Plasminogen activator (PA)

Plasminogen activator inhibitor

Renin

Progesterone-dependent carbonic anhydrase

Lactoferrin

During Implantation, the Blastocyst Apposes Itself to the Endometrium, Adheres to Epithelial Cells, and then Finally Breaks Through the Basement Membrane and Invades the Stroma

As noted earlier, the conceptus lies unattached in the uterine cavity for approximately 72 hours. About halfway through this period (i.e., 5–6 days after ovulation), the morula transforms into the blastocyst (Fig. 55–3A). Prior to the initiation of implantation, the zona pellucida that surrounds the blastocyst degenerates. This process, known as "**hatching**" of the embryo, occurs 6 to 7 days after ovulation. Lytic factor(s) in the endometrial cavity appear to be essential for the dissolution of the zona pellucida. The blastocyst probably also participates in the process of zona lysis and hatching; when an *unfertilized*

TABLE 55–2

SUBSTANCES SECRETED BY THE BLASTOCYST

Immunosuppressive agents
Platelet-activating factor (PAF)

Human chorionic gonadotropin (hCG)

Early pregnancy factor

Immunosuppressive factor

Prostaglandin E_2

Interleukins 1α and 6

Interferon-α

Leukemia inhibitory factor

Colony-stimulating factor

Metalloproteases (facilitate invasion of trophoblast into the endometrium)
Collagenases: digest collagen types I, II, III, VII, and X

Gelatinases: 2 forms, digest collagen type IV and gelatin

Stromelysins: digest fibronectin, laminin, and collagens IV, V, and VII

Serine proteases (facilitate invasion of trophoblast into the endometrium)

Other factors or actions
Ovum factor

Early pregnancy factor

Embryo-derived histamine-releasing factor

hCG: autocrine growth factor

Plasminogen activator and its inhibitors

Insulin-like growth factor type II (IGF-II): promotes trophoblast invasiveness

Estradiol

β_1 Integrin

Fibroblast growth factor (FGF)

Transforming growth factor-α (TGF-α)

Inhibins

egg is placed in the uterus under the same conditions, its zona remains intact. A factor produced by the blastocyst may activate a lytic factor that is derived from a uterine precursor. Plasmin, produced from plasminogen, is a plausible candidate for this uterine factor, because plasmin exhibits a lytic effect on the zona pellucida in vitro, and inhibitors of plasmin block in vitro hatching of rat blastocysts.

Implantation occurs in three stages: (1) apposition, (2) adhesion, and (3) invasion.

APPOSITION. The earliest contact between the blastocyst wall, the trophoectoderm, and the endometrial epithelium is a loose connection called *apposition* (see Fig. 55–3B).

Apposition usually occurs in a crypt in the endometrium. From the standpoint of the blastocyst, it appears that apposition occurs at a site where the zona pellucida is ruptured or lysed and where it is possible for the cell membranes of the trophoblast to make direct contact with the cell membranes of the endometrium. Although the pre-implantation blastocyst is asymmetric, it seems that the entire trophoectoderm has the potential to interact with the endometrium, and that the final correct orientation—with the inner cell mass pointing toward the endometrium—occurs by free rotation of the inner cell mass within the sphere of overlying trophoectoderm cells.

ADHESION. The trophoblast appears to attach to the uterine epithelium via the microvilli of the trophoblast; ligand-receptor interactions are probably involved in adhesion (see Fig. 55–3C). The receptors for these ligand-receptor interactions are often members of the **integrin family** (p. 19) and can be either on the blastocyst or on the endometrium. Integrins are bifunctional integral membrane proteins; on their intracellular side, they interact with the cytoskeleton, whereas on their extracellular side, they have receptors for **matrix proteins** such as collagen, laminin, fibronectin, and vitronectin. There are, therefore, two possible orientations for ligand-receptor interactions. For the first, the extracellular surface of the *trophoblast* has integrins for binding fibronectins, laminin, and collagen IV. Thus, during implantation, the trophoblast binds to the laminin that is distributed around the stromal ("decidual") cells of the endometrium. Fibronectin, a component of the basement membrane, probably guides the implanting embryo (see later) and is subsequently broken down by the trophoblast.

For the second orientation of matrix-integrin interactions, the extracellular surface of the *glandular epithelium* also expresses integrins on days 20 to 24 of the menstrual cycle, the implantation window (p. 1162). The expression of receptors for fibronectin and vitronectin (i.e., integrins) may serve as markers of the endometrial capacity for implantation. Small peptides containing sequences that are homologous to specific sequences of fibronectin block blastocyst attachment and outgrowth on fibronectin.

In addition to the integrin-matrix interactions, another important class of ligand-receptor interactions appears to be between heparin or heparan sulfate proteoglycans (p. 40), which are attached to the surface of the blastocyst and surface receptors on the uterine epithelial cell. These endometrial proteoglycan receptors increase as the time of implantation approaches.

Any of the above ligand-receptor interactions can lead to cytoskeletal changes. Thus, adhesion of the trophoblast via ligand-receptor interactions may dislodge the uterine epithelial cells from their basal lamina, facilitating access of the trophoblast to the basal lamina for penetration.

INVASION. As the blastocyst attaches to the endometrial epithelium, the trophoblastic cells rapidly proliferate, and the trophoblast differentiates into two layers: an inner **cytotrophoblast** and an outer syncytiotrophoblast (see

A HATCHING

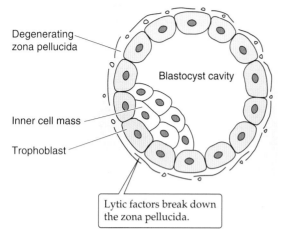

Degenerating zona pellucida

Blastocyst cavity

Inner cell mass

Trophoblast

Lytic factors break down the zona pellucida.

B APPOSITION

Endometrial capillary

Endometrial gland

Endometrial epithelium

Inner cell mass

Embryonic pole

Trophoblast

Blastocyst cavity

C ADHESION

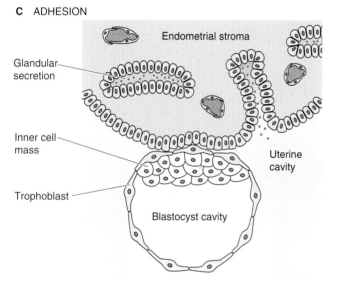

Endometrial stroma

Glandular secretion

Inner cell mass

Uterine cavity

Trophoblast

Blastocyst cavity

D INVASION

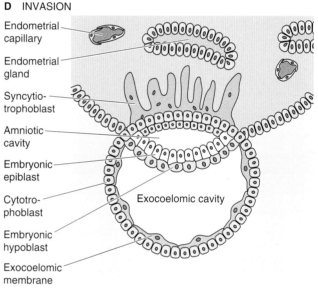

Endometrial capillary

Endometrial gland

Syncytio-trophoblast

Amniotic cavity

Embryonic epiblast

Cytotro-phoblast

Embryonic hypoblast

Exocoelomic membrane

Exocoelomic cavity

FIGURE 55–3. Embryo hatching, apposition, adhesion, and invasion.

Fig. 55–3D). The **syncytiotrophoblast** is a multinucleated mass without cellular boundaries. During implantation, long protrusions from the syncytiotrophoblast extend between the uterine epithelial cells. The protrusions dissociate these endometrial cells by secreting tumor necrosis factor-α (TNF-α), which interferes with the expression of cadherins (cell-adhesion molecules; p. 19) and β-catenin (an intracellular protein that helps anchor cadherins to the cytoskeleton). The syncytiotrophoblast protrusions then penetrate the basement membrane of the uterine epithelial cells and ultimately reach the uterine stroma.

The trophoblast secretes several autocrine factors, which appear to stimulate invasion of the endometrial epithelium, as well as proteases (Table 55–2). By degrading the extracellular matrix, metalloproteases and serine proteases may control both the proliferation and the invasion of the trophoblast into the endometrium.

Around the site of penetration of the syncytiotrophoblast, uterine stromal cells take on a polyhedral shape and become laden with lipids and glycogen. These are the **decidual cells** discussed earlier. The decidual cells degenerate in the region of the invading syncytiotrophoblast, providing nutrients to the developing embryo. The blastocyst superficially implants in the zona compacta of the endometrium, and eventually becomes completely embedded in the decidua. As the finger-like projections of the syncytiotrophoblast invade the endometrium, they reach the maternal blood supply and represent a primordial form of the chorionic villus of the mature placenta, which we discuss in the next subchapter.

PHYSIOLOGY OF THE PLACENTA

Eventually, almost all the materials that are necessary for fetal growth and development move from the maternal circulation to the fetal circulation across the placenta,

FIGURE 55-4. Development of the placenta. *A,* Shortly after the blastocyst has implanted (6 to 7 days after fertilization), the syncytiotrophoblast invades the stroma of the uterus (i.e., the decidua). Within the syncytiotrophoblast are lacunae. *B,* The invading syncytiotrophoblast breaks through into endometrial veins first, and then later into the arteries, creating direct communication between lacunae and maternal vessels. In addition, the proliferation of cytotrophoblasts creates small mounds known as *primary chorionic villi. C,* The primary chorionic villus continues to grow with the proliferation of cytotrophoblastic cells. In addition, mesenchyme from the extraembryonic coelom invades the villus, forming the secondary chorionic villus. Eventually, these mesenchymal cells form fetal capillaries; at this time, the villus is known as a tertiary chorionic villus. The lacunae also enlarge by merging with one another. *D,* With further development, the outer surface of the mature chorionic villus is covered with a thin layer of syncytiotrophoblast. Under this are cytotrophoblasts, mesenchyme, and fetal blood vessels. The lacunae into which the villi project gradually merge into one massive intervillous space. Maternal blood is trapped in this intervillous space, between the endometrium on the maternal side and the villi on the fetal side. In the mature placenta (*shown here*), "spiral" arteries from the mother empty directly into the intervillous space, which is drained by maternal veins. The villi look like a thick forest of trees arising from the "chorionic plate," which is the analog of the soil from which the trees sprout.

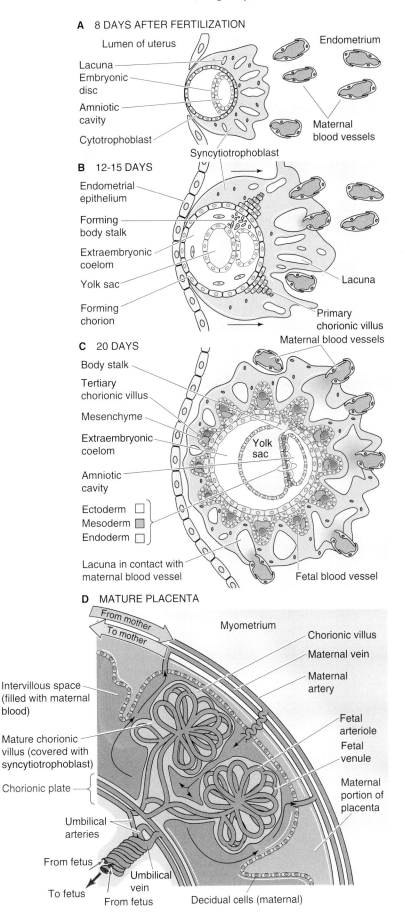

either by passive diffusion or by active transport. Except for CO_2, waste products are largely excreted via the amniotic fluid.

At the Placenta, the Space Between the Fetus's Chorionic Villi and the Mother's Endometrial Wall Contains a Continuously Renewed Pool of Extravasated Maternal Blood

Within the syncytium of the invading syncytiotrophoblast, fluid-filled holes called **lacunae** develop 8 to 9 days after fertilization (Fig. 55–4A). Twelve to fifteen days after fertilization, the finger-like projections of the syncytiotrophoblast finally penetrate the endothelial layer of small veins of the endometrium. Later, these projections also penetrate the small spiral arteries. The result is a free communication between the lacunae of the syncytiotrophoblast and the lumens of maternal blood vessels (see Fig. 55–4B). Within 12 to 15 days after fertilization, some cytotrophoblasts proliferate and invade the syncytiotrophoblast, forming finger-like projections that are the **primary chorionic villi**.

With further development, mesenchymal cells from the extraembryonic mesoderm invade the primary chorionic villi, which now are known as **secondary chorionic villi**. Eventually, these mesenchymal cells form fetal blood vessels de novo, at which point the villi are known as **tertiary chorionic villi** (see Fig. 55–4C). Continued differentiation and amplification of the surface area of the fetal tissue that is protruding into the maternal blood creates mature chorionic villi. The outer surface of each villus is lined with a very thin layer of syncytiotrophoblast, which has prominent microvilli ("brush border") that face the maternal blood. Underneath the syncytiotrophoblast lie sparse cytotrophoblasts, mesenchyme, and fetal blood vessels. The lacunae, filled with maternal blood, eventually merge with one another, creating one massive, intercommunicating **intervillous space** (see Fig. 55–4D). The fetal villi protruding into this space resemble a thick forest of trees arising from the "chorionic plate," which is the analog of the soil from which the trees sprout. Thus, in the mature placenta, fetal blood is separated from maternal blood only by the fetal capillary endothelium, some mesenchyme and cytotrophoblasts, and a thin layer of syncytiotrophoblast.

MATERNAL BLOOD FLOW. The maternal arterial blood is discharged from approximately 120 spiral arteries; these arteries may have multiple openings, not all of which need be open at the same time. Blood enters in pulsatile spurts through the wall of the uterus and moves in discrete streams into the intervillous space toward the chorionic plate (see Fig. 55–4D). Small lakes of blood near the chorionic plate dissipate the force of the arterial spurts and reduce blood velocity. The maternal blood spreads laterally and then reverses direction and cascades over the closely packed villi. Blood flow slows even more, allowing adequate time for exchange. After bathing the chorionic villi, the maternal blood drains through venous orifices in the basal plate, enters the larger maternal pla-

cental veins, and ultimately flows into the uterine and other pelvic veins. Note that there are no capillaries between the maternal arterioles and venules; the intervillous space is the functional capillary. Because the intervillous spaces are very narrow, and the arterial and venous orifices are randomly scattered over the entire base of the placenta, the maternal blood moves efficiently among the chorionic villi and avoids arteriovenous shunts.

The spiral arteries are generally perpendicular, and the veins are generally parallel to the uterine wall. Thus, because of both the geometry of the maternal blood vessels and the difference between maternal arterial and venous pressure, the uterine contractions that occur periodically during pregnancy, as well as during delivery, attenuate arterial inflow and completely interrupt venous drainage. Thus, the volume of blood in the intervillous space actually increases, providing continual, albeit reduced, exchange. The principal factors that regulate the flow of maternal blood in the intervillous space are maternal arterial blood pressure, intra-uterine pressure, and the pattern of uterine contraction.

FETAL BLOOD FLOW. The fetal blood originates from two **umbilical arteries**. Unlike *systemic* arteries after birth, umbilical arteries carry *deoxygenated* blood. As these umbilical arteries approach the placenta, they branch repeatedly beneath the amnion, penetrate the chorionic plate, and then branch again within the chorionic villi, forming a capillary network. Blood that has obtained a significantly higher O_2 and nutrient content returns to the fetus from the placenta through the single **umbilical vein**.

The **amniotic fluid** that fills the amniotic cavity serves two important functions. First, it serves as a mechanical buffer, and thus protects the fetus from external, physical insults. Second, it serves as a mechanism by which the fetus excretes many waste products. The water in the amniotic fluid turns over at least once a day. After the fetal kidneys mature (10–12 weeks), the fetus's renal excretions are the major source of amniotic-fluid production (~75%), with pulmonary secretions accounting for the rest. Fluid removal occurs through the actions of the fetal gastrointestinal tract (~55%), amnion (~30%), and lungs (~15%).

Gases and Other Solutes Move Across the Placenta Via Simple Diffusion, Facilitated Diffusion, Secondary Active Transport, and Endocytosis

The placenta is the major lifeline between the mother and the fetus. It provides nutrients and O_2 to the fetus, and it removes CO_2 and certain wastes from the fetus.

O_2 AND CO_2 TRANSPORT. The maternal blood coming into the intervillous space has a gas composition that is similar to that of systemic arterial blood: a partial pressure of oxygen (P_{O_2}) of approximately 100 mm Hg (Table 55–3), a P_{CO_2} of approximately 40 mm Hg, and a pH of 7.40. However, the diffusion of O_2 from the maternal blood into the chorionic villi of the fetus causes the P_{O_2}

TABLE 55–3

MATERNAL AND FETAL OXYGEN LEVELS

SITE	Po$_2$ (mm Hg)	HEMOGLOBIN SATURATION (%)
Maternal values Uterine artery	100	97.5
Intervillous space	30–35	57–67
Uterine vein	30	57
Fetal values Umbilical arteries	23	60
Umbilical vein	30	85

of blood in the intervillous space to fall, so that the average Po$_2$ is 30 to 35 mm Hg. Given the O$_2$ dissociation curve of maternal (i.e., adult) hemoglobin (Hb), this Po$_2$ translates to an O$_2$ saturation of approximately 65% (p. 656). The Po$_2$ of blood in the umbilical vein is even less. Despite the relatively low Po$_2$ of the maternal blood in the intervillous space, the fetus does not suffer from a lack of O$_2$. Because fetal Hb has a much higher affinity for O$_2$ than does maternal Hb (p. 663), the fetal Hb can extract O$_2$ from the maternal Hb. Thus, a Po$_2$ of 30 to 35 mm Hg, which yields an Hb saturation of approximately 65% in the intervillous space in the mother's blood, produces an Hb saturation of approximately 85% in the umbilical vein of the fetus (see Table 55–3), assuming that the O$_2$ fully equilibrates between intervillous and fetal blood. Other mechanisms of ensuring adequate fetal oxygenation include: (1) the relatively high cardiac output per unit body weight of the fetus, and (2) the O$_2$-carrying capacity of fetal blood late in pregnancy increases as the Hb concentration rises to a level that is 50% higher than that of the adult.

The transfer of CO$_2$ from the fetus to the mother is driven by a concentration gradient between the blood in the umbilical arteries and that in the intervillous space. Near the end of pregnancy, the Pco$_2$ in the umbilical arteries is approximately 48 mm Hg, and the Pco$_2$ in the intervillous space is approximately 43 mm Hg, a gradient of approximately 5 mm Hg. The fetal blood also has a somewhat lower affinity for CO$_2$ than does maternal blood, thus favoring the transfer of CO$_2$ from the fetus to mother.

OTHER SOLUTES. A variety of other solutes besides O$_2$ and CO$_2$ move across the placenta between the mother and the fetus, availing themselves of a variety of transport mechanisms. Some of these solutes, such as the waste products urea and creatinine, probably move passively from fetus to mother. The lipid-soluble steroid hormones shuttle among the mother, the placenta, and the fetus by simple diffusion. Glucose moves from the mother to the fetus by facilitated diffusion (p. 60), and amino acids, by

secondary active transport (p. 61). The placenta also transports several other essential substances, such as vitamins and minerals, that are needed for fetal growth and development. Many substances are present in the fetal circulation at concentrations higher than in the maternal blood, and must be actively transported against concentration or electrochemical gradients. The necessary energy (i.e., adenosine triphosphate [ATP]) is derived from glycolysis and the citric acid cycle, for which the enzymes are present in the human placenta at term. Also present are the enzymes for the pentose phosphate pathway, an alternative pathway for the oxidation of glucose, which provides the nicotinamide adenine dinucleotide phosphate [NADPH] that is necessary for several synthetic pathways that need reducing equivalents in the human placenta at term.

The placenta takes up large molecules from the mother through receptor-mediated endocytosis (p. 42). The uptake of substances such as low-density lipoproteins (LDL), transferrin, hormones (e.g., insulin), and antibodies (e.g., immunoglobulin G) increases throughout gestation until just before birth.

TABLE 55–4

HORMONES MADE BY THE PLACENTA

Peptide Hormones and Neuropeptides
  Human chorionic gonadotropin (hCG)

  Thyrotropin (thyroid-stimulating hormone [TSH])

  Placental-variant growth hormone

  Human chorionic somatomammotropins 1 and 2 (hCS1 and hCS2), also known as human placental lactogen (hPL: hPL1 and hPL2)

  Placental proteins PP12 and PP14

  Thyrotropin-releasing hormone (TRH)

  Corticotropin-releasing hormone (CRH)

  Growth hormone–releasing hormone (GHRH)

  Gonadotropin-releasing hormone (GnRH)

  Substance P

  Neurotensin

  Somatostatin

  Neuropeptide Y

  Adrenocorticotropic hormone (ACTH)-related peptide

  The inhibins

Steroid Hormones
  Progesterone

  Estrone

  Estradiol

  Estriol

The Placenta Makes a Variety of Peptide Hormones, Including Human Chorionic Gonadotropin and Human Chorionic Somatomammotropin

The placenta plays a key role in steroid synthesis, which is discussed in the next subchapter. In addition, the placenta manufactures a number of amines, polypeptides (including peptide hormones and neuropeptides), proteins, glycoproteins, and steroids (Table 55–4). Among these peptides are the placental variants of all known releasing hormones, which are produced by the hypothalamus (p. 1010). These placental releasing hormones may act in a paracrine fashion, controlling the release of local placental hormones, or they may enter the maternal or fetal circulations. In addition, several proteases are also present in the placenta. Although the placenta synthesizes a wide variety of substances, the significance of many of these is not clear.

The most important of the placental peptide hormones is **hCG**. In the developing blastocyst, and later in the mature placenta, it is the syncytiotrophoblast cells that synthesize hCG, perhaps under the direction of progesterone and estrogens. The placenta also produces two **human chorionic somatomammotropins**, hCS 1 and hCS 2, also called *human placental lactogen* (hPL). hCS 1 and 2 are polypeptide hormones that are structurally related to growth hormone and placental-variant growth hormone, as well as to prolactin (see Table 47–1). They play a role in the conversion of glucose to fatty acids and ketones, thus coordinating the fuel economy of the fetoplacental unit. The fetus and placenta use fatty acids and ketones as energy sources and store them as fuels in preparation for the early neonatal period, when a considerable reservoir of energy is necessary for the transition from intrauterine life to life outside the uterus. hCS 1 and 2 also promote development of maternal mammary glands during pregnancy.

In addition to its secretory functions, the placenta also stores vast amounts of proteins, polypeptides, glycogen, and iron. Many of these stored substances can be used at times of poor maternal nutrition and also at the transition from intra- to extra-uterine life.

THE MATERNAL-PLACENTAL-FETAL UNIT

During Pregnancy, Progesterone and Estrogens Rise to Levels that Are Substantially Higher than their Peaks in a Normal Cycle

Following ovulation during a "normal" or nonconception cycle, the cells of the ovarian follicle functionally transform into luteal cells, which mainly produce progesterone, but also produce estrogens (p. 1145). However, the corpus luteum has a finite life span, which lasts only about 12 days before it begins its demise in the face of declining LH levels. As a consequence of luteal demise, levels of both progesterone and estrogens decline.

In contrast, during pregnancy, maternal levels of pro-

gesterone and estrogens (estradiol, estrone, estriol) all increase, reaching levels that are substantially higher than those achieved during a normal menstrual cycle (Fig. 55–5). These elevated levels are necessary for maintaining the pregnancy. For example, progesterone reduces uterine motility and inhibits propagation of contractions. How are these elevated levels of female steroids achieved? Early in the first trimester, hCG that is manufactured by the syncytiotrophoblast rescues the corpus luteum, which is the major source of progesterone and estrogens. This function of the corpus luteum in the ovary continues well into early pregnancy. However, by itself, the corpus luteum is not adequate to generate the very high steroid levels that are characteristic of late pregnancy. The developing placenta itself augments its production of progesterone and estrogens so that by 8 weeks of gestation the placenta has become the major source of these steroids. The placenta continues to produce large quantities of estrogens, progestins, and other hormones throughout gestation. **Estriol,** which is not important in nonpregnant women, is a major estrogen during pregnancy (see Fig. 55–5).

After Eight Weeks of Gestation, the Coordinated Biosynthetic Activity of the Maternal-Placental-Fetal Unit Maintains High Levels of Progesterone and Estrogens

Although it emerges as the major source of progesterone and estrogens (Table 55–5A), the placenta cannot synthe-

FIGURE 55–5. Maternal levels of progesterone and the estrogens just before and during pregnancy. The y-axis scale is logarithmic. The zero point on the x axis is the time of fertilization. The progesterone spikes near −8 and −4 weeks refer to the two menstrual cycles before the one that resulted in the pregnancy. (Data from Wilson JD, et al: Williams Textbook of Endocrinology. Philadelphia: WB Saunders, 1998.)

TABLE 55–5

ROLES OF THE MOTHER, PLACENTA, AND FETUS IN STEROID BIOSYNTHESIS

	NEEDS	CONTRIBUTES	LACKS
Mother	Progesterone Estrone Estradiol Estriol	LDL cholesterol	Adequate synthetic capacity for progesterone and estrogens
Placenta		3β-Hydroxysteroid dehydrogenase Aromatase (P-450$_{arom}$)	Adequate cholesterol-synthesizing capacity 17α-Hydroxylase (P-450$_{c17}$; needed to synthesize estrone and estradiol) 17,20-Desmolase (P-450$_{c17}$; needed to synthesize estrone and estradiol) 16α-Hydroxylase (needed to synthesize estriol)
Fetus		17α-Hydroxylase (P-450$_{c17}$; needed to synthesize estrone and estradiol) 17,20-Desmolase (P-450$_{c17}$; needed to synthesize estrone and estradiol) 16α-Hydroxylase (needed to synthesize estriol)	3β-Hydroxysteroid dehydrogenase Aromatase (P-450$_{arom}$)

LDL, low-density lipoprotein.

size these hormones by itself; it requires the assistance of both mother and fetus. This joint effort in steroid biosynthesis has led to the concept of the **maternal-placental-fetal unit**. Figure 55–6—which is similar to the road maps describing the synthesis of glucocorticoids, mineralocorticoids (see Fig. 49–2), male steroids (see Fig. 53–5), and female steroids (see Fig. 54–9)—illustrates the pathways that the maternal-placental-fetal unit uses to synthesize progesterone and the estrogens. Figure 55–7 summarizes the exchange of synthetic intermediates among the three members of the maternal-placental-fetal unit.

Unlike the corpus luteum, which manufactures progesterone, estrone, and estradiol early in pregnancy (p. 1153), the placenta is an imperfect endocrine organ. First, the placenta cannot manufacture adequate cholesterol, the precursor for steroid synthesis. Second, the placenta lacks two crucial enzymes that are needed for synthesizing estrone and estradiol. Third, the placenta lacks a third enzyme that is needed to synthesize estriol. The enzymes "missing" from the placenta are listed in Table 55–5, and also are indicated with a *brown background* in Figure 55–6 and Figure 55–7.

The maternal-placental-fetal unit overcomes these placental shortcomings in two ways. First, the mother supplies most of the cholesterol as LDL particles (p. 1000). With this supply of maternal cholesterol, the placenta can generate large amounts of progesterone and export it to the mother, thus solving the problem of maintaining maternal progesterone levels after the corpus luteum becomes inadequate. Second, the fetal adrenal gland and liver supply the three enzymes that the placenta lacks. The fetal adrenal glands are up to this metabolic task; at term, the fetal adrenals are as large as those of an adult.

The fetus does not synthesize estrogens without assistance for two reasons. First, it *cannot*, because the fetus lacks the enzymes that catalyze the last two steps in the production of estrone, the precursor of estradiol. These two enzymes are also necessary to synthesize estriol. The enzymes that are missing from the fetus are listed in Table 55–5, and they also are indicated with a *blue background* in Figure 55–6 and Figure 55–7. Second, the fetus *should not* synthesize estrogens without assistance. If the fetus were to carry out the complete, classic biosynthesis of progesterone and the estrogens, it would expose itself to dangerously high levels of hormones that are needed not by the fetus, but by the mother.

The fetus and its placenta use three strategies to extricate themselves from this conundrum. First, because the fetus lacks the two enzymes noted above, it never makes anything beyond dehydroepiandrosterone (DHEA) and 16α-hydroxy-DHEA (see Fig. 55–6). In particular, the fetus cannot make progesterone or any of the three key estrogens. Second, the placenta is a massive sink for the weak androgens that the fetus does synthesize, thus preventing the masculinization of female fetuses. Third, the fetus conjugates the necessary steroid intermediates to sulfate, which greatly reduces their biological activity (see Fig. 55–7). Thus, as pregnenolone moves from the placenta to the fetus, it is sulfated. The products of fetal pregnenolone metabolism are also sulfated (DHEA-S and 16α-hydroxy-DHEA-S) as long as they reside inside the fetus. It is only when DHEA-S and 16α-hydroxy-DHEA-S finally move to the placenta that a sulfatase removes the sulfate groups, and thus the placenta can complete the process of steroidogenesis and export the hormones to the mother.

FIGURE 55–6. Synthesis of progesterone and the estrogens by the maternal-placental-fetal unit. Individual enzymes are shown in horizontal and vertical boxes. See Figures 49–2, 53–5, and 54–9 for cellular localizations of enzymes. Chemical groups modified by each enzyme are highlighted in reaction product. The fetus lacks 3β-hydroxysteroid dehydrogenase and aromatase (P450$_{arom}$), shown on blue background. Placenta lacks 17α-hydroxylase and 17,20-desmolase activity (contributed by the same protein, P450$_{c17}$) and 16α-hydroxylase; shown on brown background. Blue/brown color coding of enzymes distinguishes fetus from placenta, whereas color coding in previous steroidogenesis figures indicated subcellular localization.

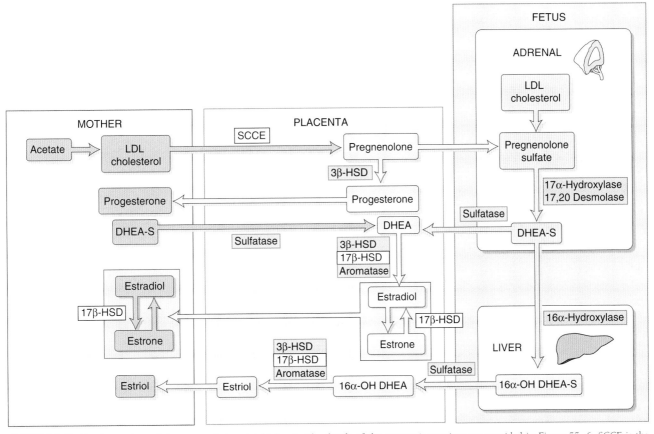

FIGURE 55–7. The interactions of the maternal-placental-fetal unit. The details of the enzymatic reactions are provided in Figure 55–6. SCCE is the side-chain-cleavage enzyme; the S in DHEA-S and 16α-OH DHEA-S represents sulfate. 17β-HSD is 17β-hydroxysteroid dehydrogenase, and 3β-HSD is 3β-hydroxysteroid dehydrogenase. LDL, low-density lipoprotein.

RESPONSE OF THE MOTHER TO PREGNANCY

The mean duration of pregnancy is approximately 266 days (38 weeks) from the time of ovulation or 280 days (40 weeks) from the first day of the last menstrual period. During this time, the mother experiences numerous and profound adaptive changes in her cardiovascular system, fluid volume, respiration, fuel metabolism, and nutrition. These orderly changes reflect the effects of various hormones, as well as the increase in the size of the pregnant uterus.

Both Maternal Cardiac Output and Blood Volume Increase During Pregnancy

The maternal **blood volume** starts to increase during the first trimester, expands rapidly during the second trimester, and rises at a much lower rate during the third trimester, and finally achieves a plateau during the last several weeks of pregnancy. Maternal blood volume may have increased by as much as 45% near term in singleton pregnancies and up to 75% to 100% in twin/triplet pregnancies. The ultimate increase in blood volume results from an increase in the volume of both the plasma and erythrocytes. However, the rise in plasma volume begins earlier and is ultimately greater (~50%) than the rise in total erythrocyte volume (~33%). A proposed mechanism for the increase in plasma volume is that elevated progesterone and estrogens cause a vasodilation that decreases peripheral vascular resistance and thus renal perfusion. One mechanism of this effect is refractoriness to the pressor effects of angiotensin II. The renin-angiotensin-aldosterone axis responds by increasing aldosterone (p. 866), which augments renal reabsorption of salt and water. In addition, pregnancy causes a leftward shift of the relationship between arginine vasopressin (AVP) release and plasma osmolality (p. 873). Immediately after the delivery of the placenta, with the attendant decreases in progesterone and estrogen levels, the mother commences a vigorous diuresis.

The increase in blood volume is needed to meet the demands of the enlarged pregnant uterus with its greatly hypertrophied vascular system. It also protects mother and fetus against the deleterious effects of impaired venous return in the supine and erect positions, and it safeguards the mother against the adverse effects of the blood loss that is associated with parturition.

Cardiac output increases appreciably during the first trimester of pregnancy (by 35%–40%), but increases only slightly during the second and third trimesters (~45% at term). The increase in cardiac output, which reflects mainly an increase in stroke volume but also heart rate, is highly targeted. Renal blood flow increases 40%. Uterine blood flow rises from just 1% to 15% of cardiac output. The blood flow to the heart (to support increased cardiac output), skin (to increase heat radiation), and breasts (to support mammary development) also increase. However, there is no change in blood flow to the brain, gut, or skeleton. The increase in cardiac output with physical activity is greater in pregnant women (for most of the pregnancy) than it is in nonpregnant women.

Despite the large increase in plasma volume, **mean arterial pressure** (MAP) usually decreases during mid-pregnancy and then rises during the third trimester, although it normally remains at or below normal. The reason for this initial fall in MAP is a decrease in peripheral vascular resistance, possibly reflecting—in part—the vasodilating effects of progesterone and estradiol.

Posture has a major effect on cardiac output (p. 577). In late pregnancy, cardiac output is typically higher when the mother is in the lateral recumbent position than when she is in the supine position. In the supine position, the fundus of the enlarged uterus rests on the inferior vena cava near L5, impeding venous return to the heart. The posture of the pregnant woman also affects arterial blood pressure. Typically, blood pressure in the brachial artery is highest when sitting, lowest in the lateral recumbent position, and intermediate when the mother is supine.

Increased Levels of Progesterone During Pregnancy Increase Alveolar Ventilation

During pregnancy, hormonal and mechanical factors lead to several anatomic changes that have the net effect of increasing alveolar ventilation. The level of the diaphragm rises approximately 4 cm, probably reflecting the relaxing effects of progesterone on the diaphragm muscle and fascia. At the same time, the costovertebral angle widens appreciably as the transverse diameter of the thoracic cage increases about 2 cm. Although these two changes have opposite effects on the residual volume (RV) of air in the lungs (p. 607), the elevation of the diaphragm dominates, causing a net decrease in RV and functional residual capacity (FRC). Vital capacity (VC), maximal pulmonary ventilation, and pulmonary compliance do not change appreciably. Total pulmonary resistance falls, facilitating airflow. Because of the increased size of the abdominal contents during pregnancy, the abdominal muscles are less effective in aiding forced expirations.

Although pregnancy has little effect on respiratory rate, it increases tidal volume (V_T) markedly—by approximately 40%—and thereby increases **alveolar ventilation** ($\dot{V}_A$; p. 687). These increases in V_T and $\dot{V}_A$ are some of the earliest physiologic changes during pregnancy, beginning 6 weeks after fertilization. They may reflect, at least in part, a direct stimulatory effect of progesterone and, to a lesser extent, estrogen on the medullary respiratory centers. The physiological effect of the increased $\dot{V}_A$ during pregnancy is a fall in maternal arterial P_{CO_2}, which typically decreases from a pre-pregnancy value of approxi-

mately 40 mm Hg to approximately 32 mm Hg, despite the net increase in CO_2 production that reflects fetal metabolism. A side effect is a mild respiratory alkalosis for which the kidneys compensate by lowering plasma $[HCO_3^-]$ modestly (p. 648).

Pregnancy Increases the Demand for Dietary Protein, Iron, and Folic Acid

During pregnancy, an additional 30 grams of protein are needed each day to meet the demand of the growing fetus, placenta, uterus, and breasts, as well as the increased maternal blood volume. Most protein should come from animal sources, such as meat, milk, eggs, cheese, poultry, and fish, because these foods furnish amino acids in optimal combinations.

Almost any diet that includes iodized salt and adequate caloric intake to support the pregnancy also contains enough minerals, except for **iron** (see Table 57–5). Pregnancy necessitates a net gain of approximately 800 mg of circulating iron to support the expanding maternal hemoglobin mass, the placenta, and the fetus. Most of this iron is utilized during the latter half of pregnancy. A *non-pregnant* woman of reproductive age needs to *absorb* approximately 1.5 mg/day of iron in a diet that contains 15 to 20 mg/day (p. 973). In contrast, during pregnancy, the average required iron uptake rises to approximately 7 mg/day. Very few women have adequate iron stores to supply this amount of iron, and a typical diet seldom contains sufficient iron. Thus, the recommended supplementation of elemental iron is 60 mg/day, taken in the form of a simple ferrous iron salt.

Maternal **folate** requirements increase significantly during pregnancy, in part reflecting an increased demand for producing blood cells. This increased demand can lead to lowered plasma folate levels or, in extreme cases, to maternal megaloblastic anemia (p. 967). Folate deficiency may cause neural-tube defects in the developing fetus. Because oral supplementation of 400 to 800 μg/day of folic acid produces a vigorous hematologic response in pregnant women with severe megaloblastic anemia, this dose would almost certainly provide very effective prophylaxis.

Less than One Third of the Total Maternal Weight Gain During Pregnancy Represents the Fetus

The recommended weight gain during a singleton pregnancy for a woman with a normal weight/height ratio (i.e., "body mass index") is 11.5 to 16 kg. This figure is greater for women with a low body mass index. A weight gain of 14 kg would include 5 kg for intrauterine contents—the fetus (3.3 kg), placenta/membranes (0.7 kg), and amniotic fluid (1 kg). The maternal contribution of 9 kg would include increases in the weight of the uterus (0.7 kg), the blood (1.3 kg), and the breasts (2.0 kg), as well as adipose tissue and interstitial fluid (5.0 kg). The interstitial-fluid expansion may be in part due to increased venous pressure that is created by the large pregnant uterus.

For a woman whose weight is normal before pregnancy, a weight gain in the recommended range correlates well with a favorable outcome of the pregnancy. Most pregnant women can achieve an adequate weight gain by eating—according to appetite—a diet that is adequate in calories, protein, minerals, and vitamins. Seldom, if ever, should maternal weight gain be deliberately restricted below this level. Failure to gain weight is an ominous sign; birth weight parallels maternal weight, and neonatal mortality rises with low birth weight, particularly for babies who weigh fewer than 2500 grams.

PARTURITION

Throughout most of pregnancy, the uterus is quiescent. Both progesterone and relaxin may promote this inactivity. Weak and irregular uterine contractions occur throughout the last month of pregnancy. Eventually, a series of regular, rhythmic, and forceful contractions—"labor"—develop (Table 55–6). These may last for several hours, a day, or even longer and eventually result in the expulsion of the fetus, placenta, and membranes. Although not all of the factors leading to the initiation of labor are known, endocrine, paracrine, and mechanical stretching of the uterus all play a role. Once labor is initiated, it is sustained by a series of positive-feedback mechanisms.

Signals from the Placenta or Fetus May Initiate Labor

In rabbits, withdrawal of progesterone, made primarily in the *placenta*, results in prompt evacuation of the uterus; administration of progesterone delays the onset of labor. However, most human studies have failed to provide evidence that progesterone levels fall *before* the onset of labor. Nonetheless, it appears that progesterone plays an important role in maintaining the length of gestation in primates.

Other studies point to the importance of the *fetal* hypothalamic-pituitary-adrenal axis in the preparation for, or initiation of, parturition. In the fetal lamb, transection of the hypothalamic portal vessels prolongs gestation. In the human, an equivalent disruption of the fetal hypothalamic-pituitary-adrenal axis occurs in anencephalic fetuses, in which the cerebral hemispheres are absent and the rest of the brain is severely malformed. Indeed, gestation is prolonged in human pregnancies with anencephalic fetuses.

Infusing adrenocorticotropic hormone (ACTH) into fetal lambs with intact adrenal glands, or directly infusing cortisol, causes premature parturition. Although the theory that cortisol plays a role in initiating parturition remains attractive, several naturally occurring instances of failure of cortisol production in the human fetus do not prolong gestation. As discussed in the next section, prostaglandins appear to play a crucial role in the initiation of labor.

Prostaglandins Initiate Uterine Contractions, and Both Prostaglandins and Oxytocin Sustain Labor

Whereas hormones (particularly oxytocin) and paracrine factors (particularly prostaglandins) play an important role in stimulating the uterine contractions that sustain labor, only the prostaglandins are believed to have a key role in the initiation of labor.

PROSTAGLANDINS. The uterus, as well as the placenta and fetal membranes, synthesize and release prostaglandins (p. 104). Prostaglandins from the uterine decidual cells, particularly $PGF_{2\alpha}$ and PGE_2, act by a paracrine mechanism on uterine smooth-muscle cells. Oxytocin (see later) stimulates uterine decidual cells to increase their $PGF_{2\alpha}$ synthesis. Arachidonic acid, the precursor of prostaglandins, is present in very high concentrations in the fetal membranes near term.

Prostaglandins have three major effects. First, prostaglandins strongly stimulate the contraction of uterine smooth-muscle cells. Second, $PGF_{2\alpha}$ potentiates the contractions induced by oxytocin by promoting formation of **gap junctions** between uterine smooth-muscle cells; es-

TABLE 55–6

STAGES OF LABOR		
STAGE	**CHARACTERISTICS**	**PHYSIOLOGICAL CHANGES**
0	"Uterine tranquility and refractoriness to contraction"	
1	"Uterine awakening," initiation of parturition, extending to complete cervical dilatation	Increase in the number of gap junctions between myometrial cells. Increase in the number of OT receptors
2	"Active labor," from complete cervical dilatation to delivery of the newborn	
3	From delivery of the fetus to expulsion of the placenta and "final uterine contraction"	

OT, oxytocin.
Adapted from Casey ML, MacDonald PC: Endocrine changes of pregnancy. In Wilson JD, Foster DW, Kronenberg HM, Larsen PR (eds): Williams Textbook of Endocrinology. Philadelphia, WB Saunders, 1998.

tradiol also increases the number of gap junctions (p. 254). These gap junctions permit a synchronous contraction of the uterine smooth-muscle cells, reminiscent of the contraction of the ventricles of the heart. Third, prostaglandins also cause softening, dilatation, and thinning out ("effacement") of the cervix, which occurs early during labor. This softening is akin to an inflammatory reaction in that it is associated with an invasion by polymorphonuclear leukocytes (e.g., neutrophils). Because of these effects, prostaglandins are used to induce labor and delivery in a number of clinical settings.

Prostaglandins may physiologically initiate labor. Both $PGF_{2\alpha}$ and PGE_2 evoke myometrial contractions at *any* stage of gestation, regardless of the route of administration. The levels of prostaglandins or their metabolic products naturally increase in the blood and amniotic fluid just before and during labor. Arachidonic acid instilled into the amniotic cavity causes the uterus to contract and expel its contents. Aspirin, which inhibits the enzyme COX (p. 104), reduces the formation of $PGF_{2\alpha}$ and PGE_2, thus inhibiting labor and prolonging gestation.

OXYTOCIN. The nonapeptide oxytocin (OT) is closely related to vasopressin (Fig. 55–8). The two hormones apparently evolved from vasotocin, the single neurohypophyseal hormone in nonmammalian vertebrates. OT and AVP, which both differ from vasotocin by a single amino acid, are synthesized in the cell bodies of the neurons in the supraoptic and paraventricular nuclei of the hypothalamus. Both OT and AVP then move by fast axonal transport to the posterior pituitary gland, where they are stored in the nerve terminals until released in response to the appropriate stimuli. Both OT and AVP are closely associated with—and released with—peptides known as neurophysins.

Circulating oxytocin binds to $G\alpha_q$-coupled **oxytocin receptors** on the plasma membrane of uterine smooth-muscle cells, triggering the phospholipase C cascade (p. 100). Presumably, formation of IP_3 leads to Ca^{2+} release from internal stores and to an increase in $[Ca^{2+}]_i$. The rise in $[Ca^{2+}]_i$ activates calmodulin, which stimulates myosin light-chain kinase to phosphorylate the regulatory light chain, causing contraction of uterine smooth-muscle cell (p. 238) and increased intrauterine pressure. Oxytocin also binds to a receptor on decidual cells, stimulating $PGF_{2\alpha}$ production, as discussed earlier.

Estrogen increases the *number* of oxytocin receptors in the myometrial and decidual tissue of pregnant women. The uterus actually remains *in*sensitive to oxytocin until approximately 20 weeks gestation, at which time the number of oxytocin receptors increases progressively to 80-fold above baseline values by approximately 36 weeks, plateaus just before labor, then rises again to 200-fold during early labor. The time course of the expression of oxytocin receptors may account for the increase in spontaneous myometrial contractions even in the absence of increased plasma oxytocin levels. Note that, whereas the uterus is sensitive to oxytocin only at the end of pregnancy, it is susceptible to prostaglandins throughout pregnancy.

Although the prevailing view is that oxytocin of *maternal* origin is not involved in initiating labor in humans, maternal oxytocin may help maintain labor. Oxytocin of *fetal* origin, which moves to the maternal circulation, could be involved in the onset of labor, because fetal plasma oxytocin levels rise during the first stage of labor (Table 55–6). However, infusing oxytocin into the circulation of the fetal lamb only stimulates uterine contractions at pharmacologic doses. Therefore, normal levels of fetal oxytocin probably have little influence on labor.

Once labor is initiated (stage 1), **maternal oxytocin** is released in bursts, and the frequency of these bursts increases as labor progresses. The primary stimulus for the release of maternal oxytocin appears to be distention of the cervix; this effect is known as the **Ferguson reflex**. Oxytocin is an important stimulator of myometrial contraction late in labor. During the second stage of labor, oxytocin release may play a synergistic role in the expulsion of the fetus by virtue of its ability to stimulate prostaglandin release.

During the third stage of labor, uterine contractions induced by oxytocin are also important for constricting uterine blood vessels at the site where the placenta used to be, thus promoting hemostasis (i.e., blood coagulation). Basal maternal plasma oxytocin levels are unchanged after delivery. Fetal plasma oxytocin levels are higher after vaginal delivery than after delivery by cesarean section, presumably because the maternal oxytocin triggered by the Ferguson reflex crosses the placenta into the fetus.

RELAXIN. This 48-amino-acid polypeptide hormone, structurally related to insulin, is produced by the corpus luteum, the placenta, and the decidua. Relaxin may play a role in keeping the uterus in a quiet state during pregnancy. Production and release of relaxin increases during labor, when it may soften and thus help dilate the cervix.

MECHANICAL FACTORS. Mechanical stretch placed on the uterine muscle may lead to the rhythmic contractions of labor. Thus, the increase in the size of the uterine

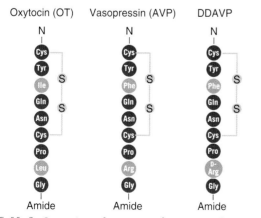

FIGURE 55–8. Comparison of structures of oxytocin and vasopressin. DDAVP is a synthetic AVP in which an L-Arg is replaced with a D-Arg (see upper box on page 843).

contents to a critical level may stimulate uterine contractions, leading to initiation of labor.

POSITIVE FEEDBACK. Once labor is initiated, several positive-feedback loops involving prostaglandins and oxytocin help sustain it. First, uterine contractions stimulate prostaglandin release, which itself increases the intensity of uterine contractions. Second, uterine activity stretches the cervix, stimulating oxytocin release via the Ferguson reflex. Because oxytocin stimulates further uterine contractions, they become self-perpetuating.

Involution of the Uterus Is Due Primarily to a Changing Endocrine Milieu

Almost immediately following delivery of the newborn, marked changes occur in the endocrine status of the mother. During pregnancy, many hormones are secreted in massive quantities. Estrogens are mitogenic, causing considerable hypertrophy of the uterine muscle cells during gestation. As the levels of these hormones fall abruptly, stimulation ceases, and uterine smooth-muscle cells decrease in size. The vasculature of the uterus regresses and blood flow to the uterus is significantly curtailed, leading to further involution of this organ.

LACTATION

The fundamental secretory unit of the breast (Fig. 55–9A) is the alveolus (see Fig. 55–9B,C), which is surrounded by contractile myoepithelial cells and adipose cells. These alveoli are organized into lobules, each of which drains into a ductule. A group of 15 to 20 ductules drain into a duct, which widens at the ampulla—a small reservoir. The lactiferous duct carries the secretions to the outside.

Breast development at puberty depends on several hormones, but primarily on the estrogens and progesterone. During pregnancy, gradual increases in levels of prolactin (PRL) and human chorionic somatomammotropin, as well as very high levels of estrogens and progesterone, lead to full development of the breasts.

As summarized in Table 55–7, hormones affecting the breast are **mammogenic** (promoting the proliferation of alveolar and duct cells), **lactogenic** (promoting initiation of milk production by alveolar cells), **galactokinetic** (promoting contraction of myoepithelial cells, and thus milk ejection) or **galactopoietic** (maintaining milk production after it has been established).

The Epithelial Alveolar Cells of the Mammary Gland Secrete the Complex Mixture of Sugars, Proteins, Lipids, and Other Substances that Constitute Milk

Milk is an emulsion of fats in an aqueous solution containing sugar (lactose), proteins (lactalbumin and casein), and several cations (K^+, Ca^{2+}, and Na^+) and anions (Cl^- and phosphate). The composition of human milk differs

TABLE 55–7

HORMONES AFFECTING THE MAMMARY GLAND DURING PREGNANCY AND BREAST-FEEDING

Mammogenic hormones (promote cell proliferation)
  Lobuloalveolar growth
    Estrogen
    Growth hormone (IGF-I)
    Cortisol
    Prolactin
    Relaxin?
  Ductal growth
    Estrogen
    Growth hormone
    Cortisol
    Relaxin

Lactogenic hormones (promote initiation of milk production by alveolar cells)
  Prolactin
  hCS (or hPL)
  Cortisol
  Insulin (IGF-I)
  Thyroid hormones
  Growth hormone?
  Withdrawal of estrogens and progesterone

Galactokinetic hormones (promote contraction of myoepithelial cells, and thus milk ejection)
  Oxytocin
  Vasopressin (1%–20% as powerful as OT)

Galactopoietic hormones (maintain milk production after it has been established)
  Prolactin (primary)
  Cortisol and other metabolic hormones (permissive)

hCS, human chorionic somatomammotropin; hPL, human placental lactogen; IGF-I, insulin-like growth factor type I; OT, oxytocin.

from that of human **colostrum** (the thin, yellowish, milk-like substance secreted during the first several days after parturition) and cow's milk (Table 55–8). Cow's milk has nearly three times more protein than human milk, almost exclusively a result of its much higher casein concentration. It also has a higher electrolyte content. The difference in composition between human and cow's milk is important because a newborn, with its delicate gastrointestinal tract, may not tolerate the more concentrated cow's milk.

The epithelial cells in the alveoli of the mammary gland secrete the complex mixture of constituents that make up milk by five major routes (see Fig. 55–9D).

1. **Secretory pathway.** The milk proteins **lactalbumin** and **casein** are synthesized in the endoplasmic reticulum and sorted to the Golgi apparatus (p. 36). Here alveolar cells add Ca^{2+} and **phosphate** to the lumen. Lactose synthetase in the lumen of the Golgi catalyzes synthesis of **lactose**, the major carbohydrate. Lactose synthetase has two components, a galactosyl transferase and lactalbumin, both made in the endoplasmic reticulum. Water enters the secretory vesicle by osmo-

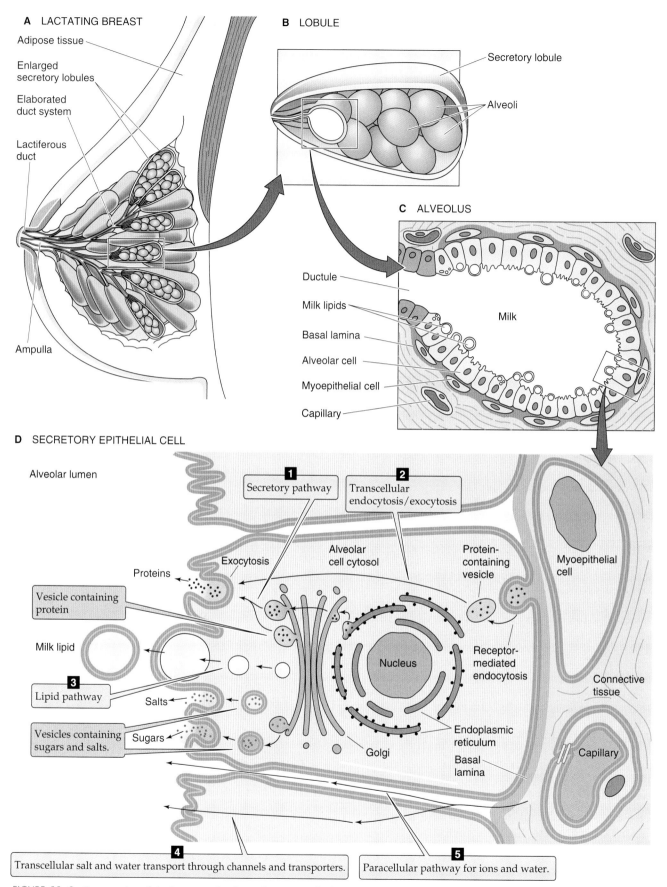

A LACTATING BREAST

Adipose tissue

Enlarged secretory lobules

Elaborated duct system

Lactiferous duct

Ampulla

B LOBULE

Secretory lobule

Alveoli

C ALVEOLUS

Ductule

Milk lipids

Basal lamina

Alveolar cell

Myoepithelial cell

Capillary

Milk

D SECRETORY EPITHELIAL CELL

Alveolar lumen

1 Secretory pathway

2 Transcellular endocytosis/exocytosis

Exocytosis

Proteins

Vesicle containing protein

Milk lipid

3 Lipid pathway

Salts

Vesicles containing sugars and salts.

Sugars

Alveolar cell cytosol

Protein-containing vesicle

Myoepithelial cell

Receptor-mediated endocytosis

Nucleus

Endoplasmic reticulum

Golgi

Basal lamina

Connective tissue

Capillary

4 Transcellular salt and water transport through channels and transporters.

5 Paracellular pathway for ions and water.

FIGURE 55–9. Cross section of the breasts and milk production. *A,* The breast consists of a series of secretory lobules, which empty into ductules. The ductules from 15 to 20 lobules combine into a duct, which widens at the ampulla—a small reservoir. The lactiferous duct carries the secretions to the outside. *B,* The lobule is made up of many alveoli, the fundamental secretory units. *C,* Each alveolus consists of secretory epithelial cells (alveolar cells) that actually secrete the milk, as well as contractile myoepithelial cells, which are in turn surrounded by adipose cells. *D,* The alveolar cell secretes the components of milk via five pathways.

1186

TABLE 55–8

COMPOSITION OF HUMAN COLOSTRUM, HUMAN MILK, AND COW'S MILK (PER DECILITER OF FLUID)

COMPONENT	HUMAN COLOSTRUM	HUMAN MILK	COW'S MILK
Total protein (g)	2.7	0.9	3.3
Casein (% of total protein)	44	44	82
Total fat (g)	2.9	4.5	3.7
Lactose (g)	5.7	7.1	4.8
Caloric content (kcal)	54	70	69
Calcium (mg)	31	33	125
Iron (μg)	10	50	50
Phosphorus (mg)	14	15	96
Cells (macrophages, neutrophils and lymphocytes)	$7–8 \times 10^6$	$1–2 \times 10^6$	—

sis. Finally, exocytosis discharges the contents of the vesicle into the lumen of the alveolus.

2. **Transcellular endocytosis/exocytosis.** The basolateral membrane takes up maternal immunoglobulins by receptor-mediated endocytosis (p. 42). Following transcellular transport of these vesicles to the apical membrane, the cell secretes these immunoglobulins (primarily IgA) by exocytosis. The GI tract of the infant takes up these immunoglobulins (p. 956), which are important for conferring immunity before the infant's own immune system matures.

3. **Lipid pathway.** Epithelial cells synthesize short-chain fatty acids. However, the longer chain fatty acids (>16 carbons) that predominate in milk originate primarily from the diet or from fat stores. The fatty acids form into lipid droplets and move to the apical membrane. As the apical membrane surrounds the droplets and pinches off, it secretes the **milk lipids** into the lumen in a membrane-bound sac.

4. **Transcellular salt and water transport.** A variety of transport processes at the apical and basolateral membranes move small electrolytes from the interstitial fluid into the lumen of the alveolus. Water follows an osmotic gradient generated primarily by lactose (present at a final concentration of ~200 mM) and, to a lesser extent, by the electrolytes.

5. **Paracellular pathway.** Salt and water can also move into the lumen of the alveolus via the tight junctions (p. 82). In addition, cells, primarily leukocytes, also squeeze between cells and enter the milk.

Prolactin Is Essential for Milk Production, and Suckling Is a Powerful Stimulus for Prolactin Secretion

Prolactin is a polypeptide hormone that is structurally related to growth hormone (GH), placental-variant growth hormone, and hCS 1 and hCS 2 (see Table 47–1). Like GH, PRL is made and released in the anterior pituitary; however, lactotrophs rather than somatotrophs are responsible for PRL synthesis. Another difference is that, whereas growth hormone–releasing hormone *stimulates* somatotrophs to release GH, dopamine (DA) *inhibits* the release of PRL from lactotrophs. Thus, it is the removal of inhibition that promotes PRL release.

The actions of prolactin on the mammary glands (see Table 55–7) include the promotion of mammary growth (mammogenic effect), initiation of milk secretion (lactogenic effect), and maintenance of milk production once it has been established (galactopoietic effect). Although the initiation of lactation requires the coordinated action of several hormones, prolactin is the classic lactogenic hormone. Initiating milk production also necessitates the abrupt fall in estrogens and progesterone that accompanies parturition. Prolactin is also the primary hormone responsible for maintaining milk production once it has been initiated.

PRL binds to a tyrosine-kinase-associated receptor (p. 111) in the same family of receptors as the GH receptor. PRL receptors, which have equal affinities for GH, are present in tissues such as breast, ovary, and liver. Presumably via pathways initiated by protein phosphorylation at tyrosine residues, PRL stimulates transcription of the genes that encode several milk proteins, including lactalbumin and casein.

Suckling is the most powerful physiologic stimulus for prolactin release. Nipple stimulation triggers prolactin secretion via an afferent neural pathway through the spinal cord, inhibiting dopaminergic neurons in the median eminence of the hypothalamus (Fig. 55–10). Because **dopamine** normally inhibits PRL release from the lactotrophs, it is called a **prolactin inhibitory factor** (PIF). Thus, because suckling decreases dopamine delivery via the portal vessels, it relieves the inhibition on the lactotrophs in the anterior pituitary and stimulates bursts of PRL release. Treating women with dopamine-receptor agonists rapidly inhibits prolactin secretion and milk production.

Several factors act as **prolactin releasing factors** (PRFs): thyrotropin-releasing hormone (TRH), angiotensin

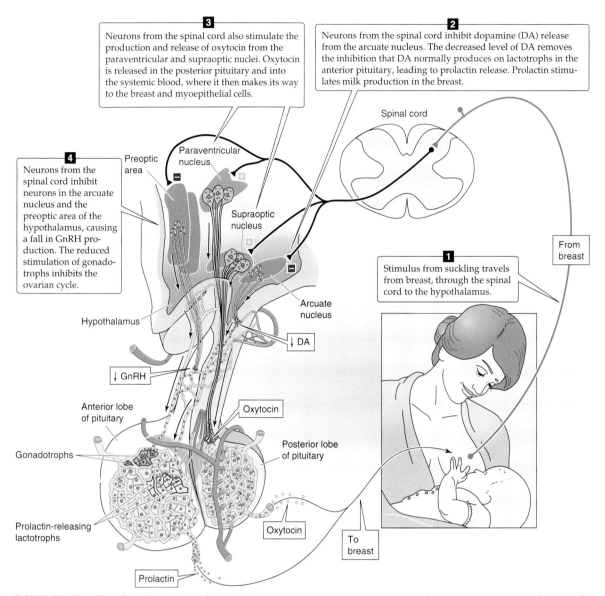

3 Neurons from the spinal cord also stimulate the production and release of oxytocin from the paraventricular and supraoptic nuclei. Oxytocin is released in the posterior pituitary and into the systemic blood, where it then makes its way to the breast and myoepithelial cells.

2 Neurons from the spinal cord inhibit dopamine (DA) release from the arcuate nucleus. The decreased level of DA removes the inhibition that DA normally produces on lactotrophs in the anterior pituitary, leading to prolactin release. Prolactin stimulates milk production in the breast.

4 Neurons from the spinal cord inhibit neurons in the arcuate nucleus and the preoptic area of the hypothalamus, causing a fall in GnRH production. The reduced stimulation of gonadotrophs inhibits the ovarian cycle.

1 Stimulus from suckling travels from breast, through the spinal cord to the hypothalamus.

Spinal cord

From breast

Preoptic area

Paraventricular nucleus

Supraoptic nucleus

Arcuate nucleus

Hypothalamus

↓ DA

↓ GnRH

Anterior lobe of pituitary

Oxytocin

Posterior lobe of pituitary

Gonadotrophs

Prolactin-releasing lactotrophs

Oxytocin

To breast

Prolactin

FIGURE 55–10. Effect of suckling on the release of prolactin, oxytocin, and gonadotropin-releasing hormone (GnRH). Suckling has four effects. First, it stimulates sensory nerves, which carry the signal from the breast to the spinal cord where they synapse with neurons that carry the signal to the brain. Second, in the arcuate nucleus of the hypothalamus, the afferent input from the nipple inhibits neurons that release dopamine (DA). DA normally travels via the hypothalamic-portal system to the anterior pituitary where it inhibits prolactin (PRL) release by lactotrophs. Thus, inhibition of DA release leads to an increase in PRL release. Third, in the supraoptic and paraventricular nuclei of the hypothalamus, the afferent input from the nipple triggers the production and release of oxytocin in the posterior pituitary. Fourth, in the preoptic area and arcuate nucleus, the afferent input from the nipple inhibits GnRH release. GnRH normally travels via the hypothalamic-portal system to the anterior pituitary, where it stimulates the synthesis and release of follicle-stimulating hormone (FSH) and luteinizing hormone (LH). Thus, inhibiting GnRH release inhibits FSH and LH release, and thereby inhibits the ovarian cycle.

II, substance P, β-endorphin, and vasopressin. In the rat, suckling stimulates the release of **TRH** from the hypothalamus. In lactating women, TRH leads to increased milk production. **Estradiol** modulates prolactin release in two ways. First, estradiol increases the sensitivity of the lactotroph to stimulation by TRH. Second, estradiol decreases the sensitivity of the lactotroph to inhibition by dopamine.

During the first 3 weeks of the neonatal period, maternal prolactin levels remain tonically elevated. Thereafter, prolactin levels decrease to a constant baseline level that is higher than that observed in women who are not pregnant. If the mother does *not* nurse her young, prolactin levels generally fall to nonpregnant levels after 1 to 2 weeks. If the mother *does* breast feed, increased prolactin secretion is maintained for as long as suckling continues. Suckling causes episodic increases in prolactin secretion with each feeding, thus producing peaks in prolactin levels that are superimposed on the elevated baseline prolactin levels. After the infant completes a session of nursing, prolactin levels return to their elevated baseline and remain there until the infant nurses again.

Oxytocin and Psychic Stimuli Initiate Milk Ejection ("Let-down")

Oxytocin, which can promote uterine contraction, also promotes milk ejection by stimulating the contraction of the network of myoepithelial cells surrounding the alveoli and ducts of the breast (galactokinetic effect). Nursing can sometimes cause uterine cramps. During nursing, suckling stimulates nerve endings in the nipple and triggers rapid bursts of oxytocin release (see Fig. 55–10). This neurogenic reflex is transmitted thorough the spinal cord, the midbrain, and the hypothalamus, where it stimulates neurons in the paraventricular and supraoptic nuclei that release oxytocin from their nerve endings in the *posterior pituitary*. From the posterior pituitary, oxytocin enters the systemic circulation, eventually reaching the myoepithelial cells that are arranged longitudinally on the lactiferous ducts and around the alveoli in the breast (see Fig. 55–9C,D). Because these cells have oxytocin receptors, oxytocin causes them to contract by mechanisms that are similar to those for the contraction of uterine smooth muscle, described earlier. The result is to promote the release of pre-existing milk, known as the **"let-down" reflex**.

In addition to the suckling stimulus, a vast array of psychic stimuli emanating from the infant, as well as neuroendocrine factors, also promote oxytocin release. The site or sound of an infant may trigger milk "let-down," a phenomenon that is observed in many mammals. Thus, the posterior pituitary releases oxytocin episodically even in anticipation of suckling. This psychogenic reflex is suppressed when fear, anger, or other stresses are encountered, thus inhibiting oxytocin release and suppressing milk outflow.

Suckling Inhibits the Ovarian Cycle

Lactation generally inhibits cyclic ovulatory function. Suckling likely reduces the release of gonadotropin-releasing hormone (GnRH) by neurons in the arcuate nucleus and the preoptic area of the hypothalamus (see Fig. 55–10). Normally, GnRH travels via the portal vessels to the gonadotrophs in the anterior pituitary. Thus, decreased GnRH release that is induced by suckling reduces the secretion of follicle-stimulating hormone (FSH) and LH and has a negative effect on ovarian function. As a result, breast-feeding delays ovulation and normal menstrual cy-

cles. However, if the mother continues to nurse her infant for a prolonged period, ovulatory cycles eventually resume. Suckling intensity and frequency, which decrease with the introduction of supplementary foods to the infant, determine the duration of anovulation and amenorrhea in well-nourished women. In breast-feeding Bangladesh women, the period of anovulation averages 18 to 24 months. If the mother does *not* nurse her young after delivery, ovulatory cycles resume, on average, 8 to 10 weeks after delivery, with a range of up to 18 weeks.

REFERENCES

Books and Reviews

Fuchs A-R: Physiology and endocrinology of lactation. In Gabbe SG, Niebyl JR, Simpson JL (eds): Obstetrics: Normal and Problem Pregnancies, 3rd ed. New York, Churchill Livingstone, 1996, pp. 137–157.

Lamberts SWJ, Macleod RM: Regulation of prolactin secretion at the level of the lactotroph. Physiol Rev 70:279–318, 1990.

Moore TR, Reiter RC, Rebar RW, Baker VV (eds): Gynecology and Obstetrics: A Longitudinal Approach. New York, Churchill Livingstone, 1993.

Ramsey EM, Eonner MW: Placental vasculature and circulation. Philadelphia, WB Saunders, 1980.

Stulc J: Placental transfer of inorganic ions and water. Physiol Rev 77: 805–836, 1997.

Vonderhaar BK, Ziska SE: Hormonal regulation of milk protein gene expression. Annu Rev Physiol 51:641–652, 1989.

Wilson JD, Foster DW, Kronenberg HM, Larsen PR (eds): Williams Textbook of Endocrinology, 9th ed. Philadelphia, WB Saunders, 1998.

Yen SSC, Jaffe RB (eds): Reproductive Endocrinology. Philadelphia, WB Saunders, 1986.

Journal Articles

Fuch AR, Fuchs F, Husslein P, et al: Oxytocin receptors and human parturition: A dual role for oxytocin in the initiation of labor. Science 215:1396–1398, 1982.

Goebelsmann U, Jaffe RB: Oestriol metabolism in pregnant women. Acta Endocrinol 66:679–693, 1971.

Liggins GC: Initiation of parturition. Br Med Bull 35:145–150, 1979.

Perez A, Vela P, Masnick GS, Potter RG: First ovulation after childbirth: The effect of breast feeding. Am J Obstet Gynecol 114:1041–1047, 1972.

Tabibzadeh S, Babaknia A: The signals and molecular pathways involved in implantation, a symbiotic interaction between blastocyst and endometrium involving adhesion and tissue invasion. Hum Reprod 10: 1579–1602, 1995.

Wigglesworth JS: Vascular organization of the human placenta. Nature 216:1120–1121, 1967.

Wilkening RB, Meschia G: Fetal oxygen uptake, oxygenation, and acid-base balance as a function of uterine blood flow. Am J Physiol 244: H749–H755, 1983.

Fetal and Neonatal Physiology

Ervin E. Jones and Alan H. DeCherney

Growth of the fetus begins soon after fertilization, when the first cell division occurs. Cell division, hypertrophy, and differentiation are highly coordinated events that result in the growth and development of specialized organ systems. The fetus, fetal membranes, and placenta develop and function as a unit throughout pregnancy, and their development is interdependent. The growth trajectory of fetal mass is relatively flat during the first trimester, increases linearly at the beginning of the second trimester, and rises rapidly during the third trimester.

BIOLOGY OF FETAL GROWTH

Growth Occurs by Hyperplasia and Hypertrophy

The growth of an organ occurs as a result of an increase in cell number (**hyperplasia**), an increase in cell size (**hypertrophy**), or both. We can define three sequential phases of growth: (1) pure hyperplasia, (2) hyperplasia and concomitant hypertrophy, and (3) hypertrophy alone. The time courses of the three phases of growth are organ specific. For example, the **placenta** goes through all three phases of growth, but these phases are compressed because placental life span is relatively short. Moreover, simple hypertrophy is the primary form of placental growth. Thus, the weight, RNA content and protein content of human placenta increase linearly until term, but cell number does not increase during the third trimester.

In contrast to placental growth and development, growth of the **fetus** occurs almost entirely by hyperplasia. Thus, DNA content increases linearly in all fetal organs beginning early in the second trimester. Stimuli that either increase or decrease cell number, cell size, or both may accelerate or retard the growth of the whole fetus or of individual organs. The phase of growth during which the stimulus acts determines the response of the organ. For example, malnutrition occurring during the period of *hyperplasia* retards cell division, causing a deficiency in cell number. Therefore, adequacy of nutrition early in life may determine the number of cells in any organ. This effect on cell number may be irreversible, even if normal nutrition is restored later. Conversely, malnutrition occurring during the period of *hypertrophy* causes a reduction in cell size. However, this effect can be reversed, and normal cell size can be achieved if adequate nutrition is restored. Thus, reversibility depends on the timing of the stimulus.

Genetic Factors Primarily Determine Growth During the First Half of Gestation and Epigenetic Factors, During the Second Half

The fertilized egg contains the genetic material that directs cell multiplication and differentiation and guides development of the human phenotype. For specific developmental events to occur at precise times (Table 56–1), a programmed sequence of gene activation and suppression is necessary. Ignoring apoptosis, the fertilized egg must undergo an average of approximately 42 divisions to reach newborn size. A fertilized ovum, weighing less than 1 ng, gives rise to a newborn weighing slightly more than 3 kg (an increase of more than 10^{12} fold)! Not only must the total cell number in a term fetus lie within relatively narrow limits, but also the developmental program must trigger cell differentiation after a specified number of cell divisions. After birth, only about five additional divisions are necessary for the net increase in mass that is necessary to achieve adult size. Obviously, many tissues (e.g., gastrointestinal tract, skin, blood cells) must continually undergo cell division to replenish cells lost by apoptosis.

TABLE 56–1

CHRONOLOGIC DEVELOPMENT OF ORGANS, SYSTEMS, AND BODY FORM

ORGAN	CHRONOLOGY OF DEVELOPMENT
Bronchial apparatus and pharyngeal pouches	4th week, ridges and grooves appear over the future neck region
Thyroid gland	4th week, endoderm appears over the floor of the pharynx
Tongue	4th week, primordia appear in the floor of the pharynx
Face	End of 4th week, primordia appear
Palate	Begins in the 5th week
Upper respiratory system	4th week, laryngotracheal groove appears
Digestive system	4th week, primitive gut forms

Foregut derivatives
    Pharynx and its derivatives
    Lower respiratory tract
    Esophagus, stomach, proximal duodenum (from stomach to entry of the common bile duct)
    Liver, biliary tract, gallbladder, pancreas
	4th week, formation of midgut derivatives begins

Midgut derivatives
    Small intestine, except proximal duodenum
    Cecum, appendix
    Ascending colon and proximal half of transverse colon
	6th week, primordia appear, midgut elongates

Hindgut derivatives
    Distal half of transverse colon
    Descending and sigmoid colon
    Rectum and upper portion of anal canal
    Part of the urogenital system
	End of 7th week, anal canal has formed

Kidneys, urinary bladder, urethra	5th week, permanent adult kidney begins to develop
Adrenal glands	5th week, primordia of adrenal glands develop
Gonads, genital ducts, external genitalia	5th week, gonadal ridges form
Heart	3rd week, development of the heart begins
Atria	5th week, the atria are formed
Ventricles	5th week, the ventricles form
Fetal circulation	3rd week, embryonic blood vessels develop
Brain and spinal cord	End of 4th week, primary vesicles form and walls of the neural tube thicken to form the spinal cord
Pituitary	6th week, connection of Rathke's with oral cavity disappears
Limbs	End of 4th week, limb buds appear
Skull	7th week, paired cartilages begin to fuse to form the cranium

TABLE 56–2

DETERMINANTS OF BIRTH WEIGHT

FACTOR	CONTRIBUTION TO FINAL BIRTH WEIGHT (%)
Maternal environment	30
Maternal genotype	20
Paternal genotype	20
Fetal genotype (excluding gender)	15
Fetal gender	2
Multifactorial (gestational age at delivery, multiple gestation, etc.)	13

Although the genetic makeup of the fetus principally determines its growth and development, other influences—both stimulatory and inhibitory—are superimposed on the genetic program. During the first half of pregnancy, the fetus's own genetic program is the primary determinant of growth, constraining patterns of growth. During the second half, the patterns of growth and development are more variable. The four primary epigenetic factors at work during the second half of pregnancy are placental, hormonal, environmental (e.g., maternal nutrition, disease, drugs, altitude) and metabolic (e.g., diabetes). We discuss the first two (placental and hormonal) in the next two sections.

Studies of birth weights in families reveal that both parental and fetal genotypes affect birth weight (Table 56–2). The mother contributes to birth weight both through her influence on the environment that she provides for the fetus (~30%), as well as through the genes that she passes on to the fetus (~20%). The mother's contribution to the fetal environment includes maternal health and nutritional status, environment, life style, age (e.g., adolescents and older women have infants with lower birth weight), parity, pre-pregnancy weight and prenatal weight gain, early fat deposition, height, chronic diseases, infection, and stress. The father contributes to birth weight only through the genes that he passes on to his offspring (~20%). The unique fetal genotype—the interaction of the alleles provided by the parents (e.g., dominant vs. recessive genes) considered apart from the individual contributions of the two parents—contributes approximately 15%. The gender of the fetus contributes approximately 2%. The remaining approximately 13% of the contribution to birth weight is multifactorial and may include variations in such factors as gestational age at delivery and multiple gestation (e.g., twinning).

Increases in Placental Mass Parallel Periods of Rapid Fetal Growth

The placenta plays several important roles in fetal growth and development. In addition to its transport and storage functions, the placenta is involved in a variety of biosynthetic activities. These include the synthesis of steroids, such as estrogen and progesterone, and protein hormones, such as human chorionic gonadotropin (hCG) and the human chorionic somatomammotropins (hCS) (p. 1178).

Fetal growth closely correlates with placental weight. During periods of rapid fetal growth, placental weight increases. As the placental mass increases, the total surface area of the placental villi (p. 1176) increases to sustain gas transport and fetal nutrition. Moreover, maternal blood flow to the uterus and fetal blood flow to the placenta also increase in parallel with the increase in placental mass. Placental growth increases linearly until approximately 4 weeks before birth. **Intrauterine growth retardation** (see the box on p. 1193) may occur as a result of decreased "placental reserve" caused by any insult. Adequate placental reserve is particularly important during the third trimester, when fetal growth is very rapid. For example, mothers who smoke during pregnancy tend to have small placentas and are at high risk of delivering a low birth weight baby.

Insulin, the IGFs, and Thyroxin Stimulate Fetal Growth

In Chapter 47 we discuss several hormones—including glucocorticoids, insulin, growth hormone, the insulin-like growth factors, and thyroid hormones—that are important for achieving final adult mass.

GLUCOCORTICOIDS AND INSULIN. As its major energy source, the growing fetus uses glucose, which moves across the placenta by facilitated diffusion. Unlike the adult, which uses sophisticated hormonal systems to control blood-glucose levels (p. 1068), the fetus is passive: the exchange of glucose across the placenta controls fetal blood-glucose levels. The fetus normally has little need for gluconeogenesis, and the levels of gluconeogenic enzymes in the fetal liver are low. **Glucocorticoids** in the fetus promote the storage of glucose as glycogen in the fetal liver, a process that increases greatly during the final month of gestation in preparation for the increased glycolytic activity required during and immediately after delivery. Near term, when fetal glucose metabolism becomes sensitive to **insulin,** this hormone contributes to the storage of glucose as glycogen, as well as to the uptake and utilization of amino acids, and lipogenesis (see Chapter 50). Transient increases in maternal blood-glucose levels after meals are closely mirrored by increases in fetal blood-glucose levels. This transient fetal hyperglycemia leads to increased fetal production of insulin. Note that maternal insulin cannot cross the placenta.

In a mother with poorly controlled diabetes (see the box on Diabetes on p. 1084), sustained maternal hyperglycemia leads to sustained fetal hyperglycemia, and therefore fetal hyperinsulinemia. The resulting high levels of fetal insulin, which is a growth factor (p. 1033), cause an increased size of fetal organs (organomegaly) and increased fetal body mass (macrosomia). During the last half of the third trimester, fetal weight in poorly controlled diabetic pregnancies generally exceeds that in normal pregnancies. In some cases, large fetal size leads to problems at delivery. Indeed the frequency of cesarean

GROWTH RETARDATION

Intrauterine growth retardation (IUGR) is an abnormality of fetal growth and development that affects 3% to 7% of all pregnancies. IUGR has been variously defined as a birth weight below the 3rd, 5th, or 10th percentile for gestational age, or a birth weight that is more than two standard deviations below the mean for gestational age.

The growth-retarded fetus is at substantial risk of morbidity and mortality. The risks include birth asphyxia, neonatal hypoglycemia, hypocalcemia, meconium aspiration, persistent fetal circulation, pulmonary hemorrhage, thrombocytopenia, polycythemia, delayed neurologic development, and hypothermia. Ultrasound methods offer objective, reliable means for identifying retarded intrauterine fetal growth. Intrauterine measurements of biparietal diameter (distance between the two parietal eminences of the head) and abdominal circumference predict IUGR in as many as 90% of the cases.

The three recognized categories of IUGR are related to the time of onset of the pathologic process.

Type I or **symmetric IUGR** refers to the infant with decreased growth potential. Type I IUGR accounts for 20% to 30% of growth retarded fetuses. The entire fetus is small for gestational age. Length, weight, and abdominal and head circumferences are all below the 10th percentile for gestational age. Type I IUGR results from growth inhibition during early stages of fetal development (4–20 weeks gestation), which is referred to as the *hyperplastic stage* of fetal development. Thus, the pathologic result is fewer cells in the fetus. Causes include intrauterine infections (e.g., rubella, cytomegalovirus), chromosomal disorders, congenital malformations, maternal drug ingestion, and smoking. Of fetuses with a severe, early onset of growth retardation, approximately 25% have aneuploidy (i.e., abnormal number of chromosomes). Uniformly (or "symmetrically") diminished growth of these fetuses may result from inhibition of mitosis during early development.

Type II or **asymmetric IUGR** refers to the infant with restricted growth, most frequently due to utero-placental insufficiency, and accounts for 70% to 80% of growth-retarded fetuses. This type of growth retardation results from an insult that occurs later in gestation than those in type I IUGR, usually after 28 weeks' gestation. Here, late in the second trimester, hypertrophy dominates. There is rapid increase in cell size and increases in the formation of fat, muscle, bone, and other tissues. Fetuses with type II IUGR have a normal total number of cells, but these cells are smaller than normal. The distinguishing feature of the fetus with asymmetric IUGR is that the fetus has a normal length and head circumference (brain-sparing effect), but abdominal growth slows during the late 2nd and early 3rd trimester. Redistribution of fetal cardiac output occurs, with increased flow to the brain, heart, and adrenals and decreased glycogen storage and liver mass. This form of IUGR is most often associated with maternal disease such as kidney disease, chronic hypertension, diabetes mellitus, and others.

Intermediate intrauterine growth retardation is a combination of types I and II IUGR and accounts for 5% to 10% of all growth-retarded fetuses. It probably occurs during the middle phase of fetal growth (20–28 weeks), between the hyperplastic and hypertrophic phases. During this middle period, mitotic rate decreases and overall cell size increases progressively. Chronic hypertension, lupus nephritis, or other maternal vascular diseases that are severe and begin early in the second trimester may result in an intermediate IUGR, with symmetric growth and no significant brain-sparing effect.

---

section is much higher in deliveries of fetuses born to diabetic mothers.

INSULIN-LIKE GROWTH FACTORS. Postnatally, **growth hormone** acts by binding to growth hormone (GH) receptors, primarily in the liver, and triggering the production of the "somatomedin" or insulin-like growth factor I (IGF-I). IGF-II is not so much under the control of GH. The IGF-I receptor is similar, but not identical, to the insulin receptor and can bind both IGF-I and IGF-II, as well as insulin (p. 1029). In the fetus, both IGF-I and IGF-II, which are mitogenic peptides, are extremely important for growth. IGF-I and IGF-II are present in the fetal circulation from the end of the first trimester, and increase thereafter in both mother and fetus. Birth weight correlates positively with IGF levels. However, both relative levels of the IGFs and control of the IGFs are very different in the fetal stage than they are postnatally. First, fetal IGF-II levels are much higher than IGF-I levels; IGF-I/IGF-II levels become adult-like soon after birth. Second, in the fetus, IGF-I as well as IGF-II levels correlate poorly with GH levels. Indeed, it appears that GH may have only a minimal effect on fetal growth. For example, anencephalic fetuses (see box on p. 266), which have low GH levels, generally grow normally. Moreover, unlike the adult liver, the fetal liver has relatively few GH receptors.

EPIDERMAL GROWTH FACTOR. The fetus has abundant epidermal growth factor (EGF) receptors (p. 110), and EGF is well known for its mitogenic properties, especially with regard to development of ectodermal and mesodermal structures. However, the fetus has no detectable mRNA encoding EGF. Thus, transforming growth factor α (TGFα), another potent mitogen, which binds to EGF receptors on target cells, may act as a ligand for the EGF receptor.

THYROID HORMONES. The thyroid hormones are obligatory for normal growth and development (p. 1043). Before the second trimester, most of the T_4 in the fetus is maternal. Fetal production of thyrotropin (TSH) and the thyroid hormone T_4 begin to increase in the second trimester, concurrent with development of the hypothalamic-pituitary portal system. Hypothyroidism has adverse effects on fetal growth, generally reflected as a reduction in the size of organs such as the heart, kidney, liver, muscle and spleen.

PEPTIDE HORMONES. Peptide hormones secreted by the placenta (see Table 55–4) can act via endocrine, paracrine, and autocrine mechanisms to stimulate growth and differentiation in several organ systems.

Many Fetal Tissues Produce Red Blood Cells Early in Gestation

Early during gestation, production of red blood cells (erythropoiesis) occurs in many tissues not normally thought of as erythropoietic in the adult. Erythropoiesis begins during the third week of fetal development in the yolk sac and placenta. At about the fourth week of gestation, the endothelium of blood vessels as well as the mesenchyme also begin to contribute to the erythrocyte pool, shortly followed by the liver. The bone marrow, spleen, and other lymphoid tissues begin to produce red blood cells only near the end of the first trimester. All of these organ systems except bone marrow gradually lose their ability to manufacture blood cells, and by the third trimester, the marrow becomes the dominant source of blood cells.

The erythrocytes formed early in gestation are nucleated, but as fetal development progresses, more and more of the circulatory erythrocytes are non-nucleated. The blood volume in the common circulation of the fetoplacental unit increases as the fetus grows. The fraction of total erythrocytes that are "reticulocytes" (immature, non-nucleated erythrocytes with residual polyribosomes) is high in the young fetus, but decreases to only approximately 5% at term. In the adult, the reticulocyte count is normally less than 1%. The life span of fetal erythrocytes depends on the age of the fetus; in a term fetus, it is approximately 80 days, or two thirds that in an adult. The life span of erythrocytes of less mature fetuses is much shorter.

The hemoglobin (Hb) content of the fetal blood rises to approximately 15 g/dl by midgestation, equivalent to the level in normal adult males. The Hb concentration of fetal blood at term is higher than the Hb concentration of maternal blood, which may be only approximately 12 g/dl. Embryonic Hb with different combinations of α-type and β-type chains (see Table 28–1) are present very early in gestation. A genetic program of development governs the eventual transition to HbF, which predominates at birth (see Fig. 5–5). HbA and a small amount of HbA$_2$ gradually replace HbF during the first 12 months of life, culminating in the adult pattern of Hb expression (see Table 28–2).

The Fetal Gastrointestinal and Urinary Systems Excrete Products into the Amniotic Fluid by Midpregnancy

The fetus imbibes considerable quantities of amniotic fluid by 20 weeks' gestation. However, it is not until the final 12 weeks that fetal gastrointestinal function is similar to that of the normal infant at term. The fetal gastrointestinal tract continuously excretes small amounts of meconium into the amniotic fluid. **Meconium** consists of excretory products from the gastrointestinal mucosa and glands, along with unabsorbed residua from the imbibed amniotic fluid.

By the beginning of the second trimester, the fetus also

begins to urinate. Fetal urine constitutes approximately 75% of the amniotic-fluid production (p. 1176). The fetal renal system does not acquire the capacity to regulate fluid, electrolyte, and acid-base balance until the beginning of the third trimester. Full development of the renal system does not occur until several months following delivery.

A Surge in Protein Synthesis, with an Increase in Muscle Mass, Is a Major Factor in the Rapid Fetal Weight Gain During the Third Trimester

Fetal tissues constantly synthesize and break down proteins. Protein synthesis predominates throughout gestation, especially during the third trimester, when fetal protein synthesis—primarily in muscle and liver—increases three- to four-fold. The number of ribosomes per cell increases throughout gestation and early postnatal life. The efficiency of ribosomes at translating mRNA may also improve during gestation. Substrate availability (i.e., amino acids) and modulation of the synthetic apparatus by endocrine and other factors play important roles in regulating protein synthesis during gestation.

The formation of each peptide bond requires four molecules of adenosine triphosphate (ATP), so that the energy cost of protein synthesis is 0.86 kcal/g. Protein synthesis comprises 15% to 20% of fetal metabolic expenditure in the third trimester. At equivalent phases of development, fetuses across several species invest similar fractions of total energy in protein synthesis. Because glucose is the major metabolic fuel, a shortfall of oxidized metabolic substrates (e.g., glucose and lactate) has a direct negative impact on protein synthesis.

Increases in skeletal-muscle mass account for 25% to 50% of fetal weight gain during the second half of gestation, when the number of muscle cells increases eight-fold and cell volume increases approximately 2.6-fold. Although skeletal-muscle fibers are not differentiated in the first half of gestation, distinct type I and type II muscle fibers (p. 251) appear in equal amounts between 20 and 26 weeks of gestation.

Fetal Lipid Stores Increase Rapidly During the Third Trimester

Fetal fat stores account for only 1% of fetal body weight during the first trimester. By the third trimester, as much as 15% of fetal body weight is fat. At birth, humans have more fat than other warm-blooded animals (e.g., the newborn cat has 2%; the guinea pig, 9.5%; the rat, 11%), with the exception of hibernating mammals and migratory birds.

About half the increase in body fat reflects increased lipid transport across the placenta, and the other half reflects increased fatty acid synthesis in the fetal liver. Blood levels of fetal lipids (i.e., triglycerides, fatty acids, and ketone bodies) remain low prior to 32 weeks' gestation. In the last 2 months, the fetus increases its lipid storage as triglycerides in white and brown adipose tissue as well as in liver. During this period, both subcutaneous fat (i.e., white fat) and deep fat (i.e., white and brown) increase exponentially. The stored fat ensures adequate fuel stores for postnatal survival, and also provides thermal insulation to the newborn. In addition, brown fat is important for thermogenesis in the postnatal period.

Several factors are responsible for increased lipid stores in the near-term fetus. Increases in fetal albumin facilitate fatty-acid transfer across the placenta. Insulin acts on fetal hepatocytes to stimulate lipogenesis. Insulin also promotes the availability of substrates, including glucose and lactate, which in turn increase the synthesis of fat (p. 1078).

DEVELOPMENT AND MATURATION OF THE CARDIOPULMONARY SYSTEM

Fetal Lung Development Involves Repetitive Branching of Both the Bronchial Tree and the Pulmonary Arterial Tree

The fetal lung begins as an outpouching of the foregut at approximately 24 days' gestation. Several days later, this lung bud branches into two tubular structures, the precursors of the main bronchi. At 4 to 6 weeks gestation, the bronchial tree begins to branch repetitively. The further maturation of the lungs occurs in four overlapping phases: (1) pseudoglandular period, (2) canalicular period, (3) terminal-sac period, and (4) alveolar period.

During the **pseudoglandular period** (5–17 weeks), the lung "airways" resemble branching exocrine glands.

The **canalicular period** is characterized by canalization of the airways (16–25 weeks) and is complete when approximately 17 generations of airways have formed, including the respiratory bronchioles. Each respiratory bronchiole gives rise to as many as six alveolar ducts, which give rise to the primitive alveoli during the second trimester. The branching of the pulmonary *arterial* tree parallels, both temporally and spatially, the branching of the *bronchial* tree. However, at approximately 24 weeks' gestation, considerable interstitial tissue separates the capillaries from the respiratory epithelium. Thus, if the fetus were born at this stage of its development, the premature infant would have a very low diffusing capacity (p. 670) owing to the great distance between the edge of the alveolar lumen and the edge of the capillary lumen.

During the **terminal-sac period** (24 weeks to birth), the respiratory epithelium thins out greatly, and the capillaries push into the alveolar sacs. The potential for gas exchange improves after approximately 24 weeks' gestation, when capillaries proliferate and come into closer proximity to the thin type I alveolar pneumocytes (p. 603). During this period, surfactant synthesis and storage begins (although not extensively) in the differentiated type II cells.

In the **alveolar period** of lung development (late fetal life to 8 years of age), final alveolar growth occurs. Alveolar-like structures are present at approximately 32 weeks' gestation, and at 34 to 36 weeks' gestation, 10% to 15% of the adult number of alveoli are present. Alveolar number continues to increase until as late as eight years of age.

An Increase in Cortisol, in Conjunction with other Hormones, Triggers Production of Surfactant by Type II Alveolar Pneumocytes in the Third Trimester

Hormones play a major role in controlling fetal lung growth and development in preparation for *ex utero* function. A key target is surfactant (p. 618), which increases lung compliance. A number of hormones stimulate surfactant biosynthesis, including glucocorticoids, thyroid hormone, thyrotropin-releasing hormone, and prolactin, as well as growth factors such as EGF. Glucocorticoids in particular play an essential role in stimulating fetal lung maturation by increasing the number of both type II alveolar pneumocytes and lamellar bodies (p. 619) within these cells. Glucocorticoid receptors are probably present in lung tissue at mid-term. Fetal cortisol levels rise steadily during the third trimester and surge just before birth. Two thirds of this cortisol is of fetal origin; the rest crosses the placenta from the mother.

The predominant phospholipid in surfactant is **dipalmitoylphosphatidylcholine** (DPPC). Glycogen serves as a primary energy and carbon source for the fatty acids involved in phospholipid synthesis (Fig. 56–1). The free fatty acids used in the synthesis of surfactant enter the type II cells directly from the bloodstream. The condensation of diacylglycerol with cytosine diphosphate choline ultimately leads to the production of DPPC. At approximately 32 weeks' gestation, increases in cortisol and the other hormones mentioned previously stimulate several regulatory enzymes, including **fatty acid synthase** and **phosphocholine transferase**. Thus, the net effect is a vastly increased production of pulmonary surfactant late in gestation. Coincident with increased surfactant synthesis is a large increase in lung distensibility and stability on inflation.

Fetal Respiratory Movements Begin Near the End of the First Trimester but Wane Just Before Birth

Fetal breathing movements have been confirmed in humans by both Doppler ultrasound and tocodynamometer (an external device that records uterine movements), commencing near the end of the first trimester. It appears that hypoxia and tactile stimulation of the fetus promote these breathing movements, which occupy less than half of any 24-hour period. Near term, breathing movements are regular, similar to those found after birth. However, just prior to labor, fetal breathing decreases.

The fetal lung undergoes many changes in preparation for birth. *In utero*, the alveoli and airways of the fetal lung are filled with a volume of fluid approximating the functional residual capacity (p. 608) of the neonatal lung. The onset of labor is accompanied by increases in catecholamines and arginine vasopressin, which decrease fluid production by the fetal lung and initiate its active reabsorption. The pulmonary circulation absorbs the majority of the fluid, and the pulmonary lymphatics absorb some as well. A small portion of the lung fluid is forced out of the trachea as the fetus passes thorough the birth canal.

FIGURE 56–1. Synthesis of DPPC. Before birth, cortisol upregulates several enzymes that are important for the synthesis of surfactant, including fatty-acid synthase and phosphocholine transferase. ADP, adenosine diphosphate; ATP, adenosine triphosphate; CoA, coenzyme A; CMP, cytidine monophosphate.

FETAL ASPHYXIA

Any insult that interferes with the ability of the placenta to exchange O_2 and CO_2 between the maternal and fetal circulations may lead to "fetal asphyxia." Common causes include **maternal hypotension**, **abruptio placentae** (i.e., "breaking away" of a portion of the placenta from the uterine wall), and a **prolapsed umbilical cord** (i.e., the umbilical cord "falls" into the birth canal "in front of" the head or other part of the fetus). The result is low fetal P_{O_2}, high P_{CO_2}, and acidosis. These effects can decrease myocardial function, lowering cardiac output and further compromising O_2 delivery to the tissues, creating a vicious cycle.

In the brain, asphyxia produces substantial alterations in cerebral intracellular metabolism. As the brain is forced to shift from aerobic to anaerobic metabolism, high-energy phosphate compounds (e.g., ATP) decrease in concentration and their breakdown products (e.g., ADP and inorganic phosphate) increase. Lactic acid accumulates. Changes in P_{O_2}, P_{CO_2}, pH, and metabolism can profoundly affect neurotransmitter release and re-uptake, and thus concentrations of various ions in neurons, glia, and the brain extracellular fluid (p. 408). Asphyxia also may lead to accumulation of prostaglandins and leukotrienes, vasoactive compounds that can dilate microvessels in critical areas of the brain, permitting the generation of free radicals that in turn lead to cell damage.

Fetuses experiencing chronic O_2 deficiency in utero are at increased risk of delayed breathing immediately after birth, in part because their energy reserves are already low, so that fetal hypoxia can lead to neonatal hypoxia. The metabolic derangements of asphyxia remain evident for as long as 24 hours after birth.

The Fetal Circulation Has Four Unique Shunts: The Placenta, the Ductus Venosus, the Foramen Ovale, and the Ductus Arteriosus

The circulatory system differentiates from the mesoderm of the embryo. The fetal heart begins to beat in the fourth week of gestation. The major difference between the circulatory system of the fetus and that of the adult is the presence of the placenta. The placenta performs for the fetus functions that—at least in part—are performed by four organ systems in extrauterine life: (1) the lungs (gas exchange); (2) gastrointestinal tract (nutrition); (3) liver (nutrition, waste removal); and (4) kidneys (fluid/electrolyte balance, waste removal). Thus, the fetal heart pumps large quantities of blood through the placenta and smaller amounts of blood through the other four organ systems. The key principle governing the unique pattern of blood flow in the fetus is the presence of four **shunts**, that is, pathways that allow blood to bypass the future postnatal route.

We illustrate these shunts in Figure 56–2. Because, to a large extent, the right and left hearts of the fetus pump in *parallel* rather than in *series*, and because their inputs and outputs mix, we define the **combined cardiac output** (CCO) as the sum of the outputs of the right and left ventricles. Figure 56–2A shows the fraction of the CCO that flows through the fetal circulatory system at important checkpoints. Figure 56–2B shows values for P_{O_2} and the percent saturation of fetal hemoglobin at these same checkpoints. The numerical values in Figure 56–2 are reasonable values for a healthy fetus.

PLACENTA. The first of these shunts is the placenta itself. Of the combined cardiac output late in gestation, approximately 69% reaches the thoracic aorta (Fig. 56–2A). Half of the CCO enters the placenta as deoxygenated blood through the *paired* umbilical arteries, which arise from the two common iliac arteries. This massive blood flow to the placenta not only shunts blood away from the lower trunk, but also lowers effective blood flow to all abdominal viscera, including the kidneys. The umbilical arteries branch repeatedly under the amnion, ultimately forming dense capillary networks within the terminal villi (p. 1176). The *single* umbilical vein returns oxygenated blood (which has a P_{O_2} of 30–35 mm Hg) back to the fetus from the placenta. This blood enters the ductus venosus, which then merges with the inferior vena cava.

DUCTUS VENOSUS. This second shunt bypasses the liver, which is largely nonfunctional. The ductus venosus allows blood from the umbilical vein, approximately 50% of CCO, to enter the inferior vena cava directly, without ever entering the liver. In addition, some blood from the portal circulation may enter the ductus venosus. Blood from the ductus venosus then combines with blood from the inferior vena cava, approximately 19% of CCO, which drains the lower body and liver. Thus, approximately 69% of the CCO ($P_{O_2} \cong 27$ mm Hg) enters the right atrium.

FORAMEN OVALE. The third major shunt is blood entering the right atrium and then crossing the foramen ovale to enter the *left* atrium. The foramen ovale is an oval hole in the septum dividing the atria, located in the posterior aspect of the right atrium. Of the 69% of the CCO that enters the right atrium via the inferior vena cava, approximately 27% shunts through the foramen ovale directly into the left atrium. This movement represents a **right-to-left shunt**. Therefore, the left side of the heart receives relatively well oxygenated blood ($P_{O_2} \cong 27$ mm Hg) from the inferior vena cava. In addition, the left atrium receives 7% of the CCO as poorly oxygenated blood ($P_{O_2} \cong 20$ mm Hg) from the nonfunctional lungs. Thus, the left ventricle pumps a total of 27% + 7% = 34% of the CCO ($P_{O_2} \cong 25$ mm Hg). Because this blood enters the aorta upstream from the ductus arteriosus, it primarily flows to the head and forelimbs.

Returning now to the *right* atrium, 69% − 27% = 42% of the CCO entering the right atrium from the inferior vena cava does not shunt through the foramen ovale. This relatively well-oxygenated blood ($P_{O_2} \cong 27$ mm Hg) joins the relatively poorly oxygenated 21% of the CCO ($P_{O_2} \cong 17$ mm Hg) that enters the right atrium from the superior vena cava and another 3% from the coronary vessels. Because of the valve-like nature of the septum surrounding the foramen ovale, none of the incoming

**A   BLOOD FLOW EXPRESSED AS PERCENT
OF COMBINED CARDIAC OUTPUT**

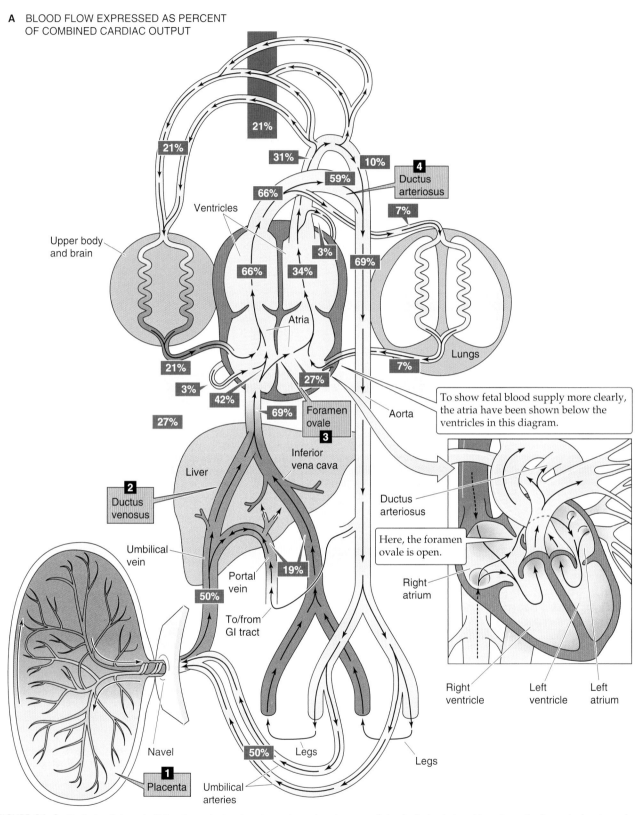

21%

21%

31%

10%

59%

4 Ductus
arteriosus

66%

7%

Ventricles

Upper body
and brain

66%   34%

3%

69%

Lungs

Atria

7%

21%

27%

3%

Aorta

42%

To show fetal blood supply more clearly,
the atria have been shown below the
ventricles in this diagram.

69%

Foramen
ovale

27%

3

Inferior
vena cava

Liver

Ductus
arteriosus

2

Ductus
venosus

Here, the foramen
ovale is open.

Umbilical
vein

Right
atrium

Portal
vein

19%

50%

To/from
GI tract

Right
ventricle

Left
ventricle

Left
atrium

Navel

50%   Legs

Legs

1

Placenta

Umbilical
arteries

FIGURE 56–2. Fetal circulation. *A,* This schematic drawing shows the major elements of the fetal circulation. Note that—in the *main drawing*—the heart is upside-down, for the sake of presenting the blood flow as simply as possible. The heart is right-side-up in the *inset.* Because the inputs and outputs of the right and left hearts mix, we define the combined cardiac output as the sum of the outputs of the right and left ventricles. The percent of the combined cardiac output that passes various checkpoints is represented as a number in a black box. Note that combined cardiac outputs of the right ventricle (66%) and the left ventricle (34%) add up to 100%. The fetal circulation has four major shunts: the placenta, the ductus venosus, the foramen ovale, and the ductus arteriosus.

B   OXYGEN SATURATION / P$_{O_2}$

FIGURE 56–2. *Continued. B,* The schematic drawing is the same as in *A,* except that—at each checkpoint—we show the O$_2$ saturation of fetal hemoglobin against a *black background,* and the P$_{O_2}$ (in mm Hg) against a *white background.* The relationship between the O$_2$-saturation and P$_{O_2}$ figures is based on the O$_2$-saturation curve for fetal hemoglobin (similar to the curve labeled "Hb + CO$_2$" in Fig. 28–7).

blood from the superior vena cava or coronary vessels shunts through the foramen ovale. Rather, it goes through the tricuspid valve to the right ventricle. Thus, the right ventricle receives 42% + 21% + 3% = 66% of the CCO (P_{O_2} = 18 to 22 mm Hg). Note that the P_{O_2} in the fetal right ventricle is somewhat lower than that in the left ventricle. The blood from the right ventricle then enters the trunk of the pulmonary artery.

DUCTUS ARTERIOSUS. The fourth major shunt, also a right-to-left shunt, directs blood from the pulmonary artery to the aorta via the **ductus arteriosus**. The ductus arteriosus contains substantial smooth muscle in its vessel wall. The patency of this vessel is due to *active relaxation* of this smooth muscle, mediated by prostaglandins, particularly PGE_2. Fetal PGE_2 levels are as much as five-fold higher than adult levels are. Administering prostaglandin inhibitors to an experimental fetal animal causes the ductus arteriosus to vasoconstrict.

Although 66% of the CCO enters the pulmonary artery, only 7% of the CCO perfuses the unventilated fetal lungs, reflecting the high resistance of the pulmonary vasculature in the fetus. This high resistance is the result of hypoxic vasoconstriction and acidosis (p. 699), the collapsed state of the airways, and perhaps leukotrienes (particularly LTD_4). The rest of the blood entering the pulmonary artery, 66% − 7% = 59% of the CCO ($P_{O_2} \cong 22$ mm Hg), enters the descending aorta via the ductus arteriosus and mixes with the blood from the aortic arch, 10% of CCO, that did not perfuse the head and upper body ($P_{O_2} \cong 25$ mm Hg). Thus, the descending aorta receives 59% + 10% = 69% of the CCO ($P_{O_2} \cong 23$ mm Hg). The placenta receives blood with a P_{O_2} of 23 mm Hg, and returns blood to the fetus with a P_{O_2} of 30 to 35 mm Hg.

CARDIOPULMONARY ADJUSTMENTS AT BIRTH

As the newborn exits the birth canal, it takes its first breath, which not only expands the lungs, but also triggers a series of changes in the circulatory system. At the same time, the newborn loses its nutritional connection to the mother and apprehends a cold new world. Three major changes in metabolism accompany birth: *hypoxia*, *hypoglycemia*, and *hypothermia*. We discuss the adaptations of the respiratory and cardiovascular systems in this subchapter, and adjustments of other organ systems in the next.

Loss of the Placental Circulation Requires the Newborn to Breathe on its Own

Although separation of the placenta does not occur until several minutes after birth, vasoconstriction in the umbilical *arteries* terminates the ability of the placenta to deliver oxygenated blood to the newborn immediately upon birth. Thus, even though the newborn may remain attached to its placenta during the first few moments of life, it is essential that the baby begins to breathe immediately. Umbilical vasoconstriction has two origins. First, stretching the umbilical arteries during delivery stimulates

them to constrict. Second, the sudden rise in the systemic arterial P_{O_2} in the newborn also stimulates and maintains vasoconstriction in the umbilical arteries. Birth may also be associated with an "autotransfusion" as blood in the placental circulation preferentially moves into the body of the emerging baby. Because the umbilical *veins* do not constrict, as do the umbilical arteries, blood flows from placenta to newborn if the newborn is below the level of the placenta, and if the umbilical cord is not clamped. This autotransfusion may constitute 75 to 100 ml, which is a substantial fraction of the newborn's total blood volume of approximately 300 ml.

At birth, the newborn must transform its circulatory system from one that supports gas exchange in the placenta to one that supports O_2 and CO_2 exchange in the lungs. In addition, other circulatory adjustments must occur as the gastrointestinal tract, liver, and kidneys assume their normal roles. As the lungs become functional at birth, the pulmonary and systemic circulations shift from interconnected and *parallel* systems to separate entities that function in *series*.

Mild Hypoxia and Hypercapnia, as well as Tactile Stimuli and Cold Skin, Trigger the First Breath

The first breath is the defining event for the newborn. Not only does it inflate the lungs, but also—as discussed later—it triggers circulatory changes that convert the fetal pattern of blood flow to the adult pattern. The functional capabilities of the lungs depend on their surface area available for gas exchange, the ability of surfactant to maximize lung compliance, neural mechanisms that control breathing and the aforementioned circulatory changes.

The first breath is normally also the most difficult inspiration of a lifetime. A considerable negative pressure within the intrapleural space is necessary to overcome the effects of surface tension (p. 616). The infant's first inspiratory effort requires a transpulmonary pressure (P_{TP})—the pressure difference between the intrapleural space and alveolar air spaces (p. 614)—of 60 cm H_2O to increase the lung volume by approximately 40 ml. In contrast, a typical adult only needs to change P_{TP} by approximately 2.5 cm H_2O during a typical tidal volume of 500 ml (p. 615). The newborn's first ventilatory effort creates an air-water interface for the first time, opening the alveoli. Breathing becomes far easier once the alveoli are open and the type-II alveolar pneumocytes deliver surfactant to the air-water interface. Thus, the second inspiration might require a P_{TP} of only 40 cm H_2O. The newborn may not achieve the adult level of relative lung compliance until one hour after birth. Very immature neonates, who lack adequate surfactant (box on Respiratory Distress Syndrome), may have difficulty expanding the lungs.

The rapid onset of breathing immediately after delivery appears to be induced by a temporary state of **hypoxia** and **hypercapnia**. In most normal deliveries, these changes in P_{O_2} and P_{CO_2} result from the partial occlusion of the umbilical cord. Tactile stimulation and decreased skin temperature also promote the onset of breathing. When newborns do not begin to breathe immediately,

RESPIRATORY DISTRESS SYNDROME

Respiratory distress syndrome (RDS) affects 10% to 15% of infants born prematurely. In very immature infants, delivered at fewer than 30 weeks of gestation, cyanosis, tachypnea, nasal flaring, intercostal and sub-costal retractions, the use of accessory musculature, and grunting may be immediately apparent in the delivery room. In more mature preterm infants, these symptoms may evolve over several hours. A chest radiograph reveals atelectasis with air bronchograms (i.e., air-filled bronchi standing out against the white background of collapsed lung tissue). Infants with severe RDS may develop edema and respiratory failure that requires mechanical ventilation. Uncomplicated cases usually resolve spontaneously. Because RDS occurs in premature infants, the course is often confounded by coexistence of a patent ductus arteriosus. This combination of problems raises the risk for short- and long-term complications, such as alveolar rupture with pneumothorax and pulmonary interstitial emphysema, necrotizing enterocolitis, intraventricular hemorrhage, and chronic lung disease.

RDS is caused by a deficiency of pulmonary surfactant. Although prematurity is by far the single most important risk factor for developing RDS, others include male sex, cesarean section, perinatal asphyxia, second twin pregnancy, and maternal diabetes. Surfactant insufficiency can result from abnormalities of surfactant synthesis, secretion, or reutilization. Decreased lung compliance and atelectasis result from both structural immaturity and surfactant deficiency, promoting airway collapse. The resulting right-to-left shunting of blood past poorly ventilated alveoli results in hypoxemia, which—at the level of the alveoli—causes capillary damage and leakage of plasma proteins into the alveolar space. These proteins may inactivate surfactant, thus exacerbating the underlying condition.

The discovery that a deficiency of surfactant is the underlying problem in infants with RDS led investigators to look for ways of assessing fetal lung maturity and adequacy of surfactant production before delivery, so that elective induction and cesarean section could be timed successfully in infants who need to be delivered prematurely. Clinical tests for assessing lung maturity exploit the knowledge that the major surfactant lipids are phosphatidyl cholines (i.e., "lecithins"), and that phosphatidyl glycerol (PG) is also over-represented (p. 618). A lecithin/sphingomyelin (L/S) ratio that is greater than 2.0 in the amniotic fluid is consistent with mature lungs, as is a positive PG assay. An analysis of amniotic fluid to assess surfactant is now routine in all cases of elective delivery of a preterm infant. For fetuses predicted to have immature lung function, mothers receive glucocorticoids, which accelerate lung maturation and surfactant production. In the newborn who develops signs of RDS soon after birth, surfactant is instilled into the trachea, markedly reducing the course and morbidity of the respiratory insufficiency.

hypercapnia and hypoxia increase and provide further simulation for the infant to breathe.

The peripheral and central chemoreceptors (p. 723) are responsible for sensing the blood-gas parameters (i.e., low P_{O_2}, high P_{CO_2}, and low pH) characteristic of the asphyxia that accompanies birth. In addition, increased sympathetic tone may stimulate breathing at the time of birth by constricting vessels to the peripheral chemoreceptors (p. 723), thereby lowering the local P_{O_2} in the microenvironment of the glomus cells (p. 725), and mimicking an even more severe hypoxia. Finally, independent of the initial stimuli that trigger breathing, other CNS mechanisms may help to sustain breathing in the newborn.

The neonate's ability to control its blood-gas parameters depends on the sensitivity of the lung's mechanical (i.e., stretch) reflexes, sensitivity of the central and peripheral chemoreceptors, gestational and postnatal age, the ability of the respiratory muscles to resist fatigue, and effects of the sleep state.

Newborns tend to have respiratory variability from breath to breath, including periods of apnea. This variability is greater during active sleep than during quiet sleep. In addition, the fraction of time spent in apnea is greater in the preterm than in the term infant. During sleep, the breathing pattern in preterm infants may change from "periodic" (i.e., periods of breathing interspersed with apnea) to "regular." Having the infant breathe air with a low level of CO_2 (recall that inspired air normally contains negligible CO_2) can mimic this switch from a periodic to a regular pattern, indicating that chemoreceptor responses in the newborn play a major role in controlling ventilation.

At Birth, Removal of the Placental Circulation Increases Systemic Vascular Resistance, Whereas Pulmonary Expansion Decreases Pulmonary Vascular Resistance

As we noted earlier, the fetal circulation has four unique shunts absent in the adult: the placental circulation, ductus venosus, foramen ovale and ductus arteriosus. At or around birth, these shunts disappear. In addition, the pulmonary circulation, which received only approximately 7% of the combined cardiac output in the fetus, now accepts the entire cardiac output. In this and the next three sections, we discuss the closure of each of these four shunts.

CLOSURE OF PLACENTAL CIRCULATION. In the fetus, the placental circulation receives approximately 50% of the CCO (see Fig. 56–2A). Thus, the placental circulation represents a major parallel path in the systemic circulation, accounting for the low vascular resistance of the fetal systemic circulation. As the placental circulation disappears at birth, the total peripheral resistance doubles. Because blood flow through the descending aorta is essentially unchanged, aortic pressure must increase, causing upstream pressure in the left ventricle to increase as well.

OPENING OF PULMONARY CIRCULATION. As noted earlier, during fetal life, pulmonary vascular resistance is high as the result of hypoxic vasoconstriction, acidosis, the collapsed state of the airways, and perhaps agents such as LTD_4 (p. 1200). As a result, only approximately 7% of the CCO of the term fetus flows through the lungs, a figure corresponding to approximately 11% of its right ventricular output. At birth, expansion of the lungs by itself markedly decreases pulmonary vascular resistance, perhaps by triggering the release of prostaglandin I_2 (PGI_2 or prostacyclin). In addition, the increase in PO_2 and pH that occurs with breathing leads to pulmonary vasodilation. Together, these changes reduce pulmonary vascular resistance more than five-fold (Fig. 56–3). Because the blood flow through the pulmonary vasculature increases by a slightly smaller factor, pressure in the pulmonary artery decreases. As a result, upstream pressure in the right ventricle also falls.

Closure of the Ductus Venosus within the First Three Hours of Life Forces Portal Blood to Perfuse the Liver

During fetal life, a large fraction of the blood in the portal vein bypasses the liver by entering the ductus venosus and merging with blood from the umbilical vein (see Fig. 56–2A). Although blood flow through the umbilical vein ceases soon after birth, the majority of the portal blood continues to flow through the ductus venosus. Thus, immediately after birth, portal flow through the liver remains low. Within approximately 3 hours after birth, however, constriction of the vascular smooth muscle within the ductus venosus completely occludes this shunt pathway. As a result, pressure in the portal vein increases markedly, diverting blood into the liver. The mechanisms underlying the contraction of the muscular walls of the ductus venosus remain unknown.

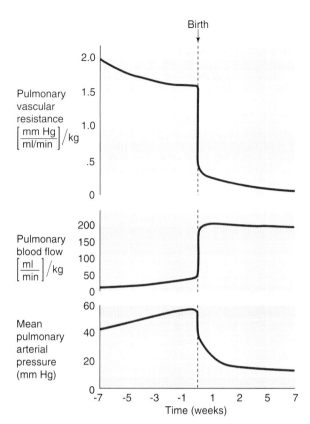

FIGURE 56–3. Effect of birth on pulmonary vascular resistance, blood flow, and mean arterial pressure. In the fetus, pulmonary vascular resistance is high, pulmonary blood flow is low, and mean pulmonary arterial pressure is high. At birth, each of these three situations rapidly reverses. The primary event is the fall in resistance, which occurs because: (1) the pulmonary blood vessels are no longer being crushed; (2) breathing causes an increased PO_2, which in turn causes vasodilation; and (3) local prostaglandins cause vasodilation. The reason that pressure falls after birth is that the fall in pulmonary vascular resistance is greater than the rise in blood flow. (Data from Rudolf AM: Congenital Diseases of the Heart: Clinical-Physiological Considerations. Armonk NY, Futura, 2001.)

At Birth, Left Atrial Pressure Begins to Exceed Right Atrial Pressure, Causing the Foramen Ovale to Close

In the fetus, blood from the inferior vena cava moves preferentially from the right atrium across the **foramen ovale** into the left atrium (see Fig. 56–2A). After entering the left ventricle, this well-oxygenated blood moves into the ascending aorta and primarily perfuses the head, neck and coronary arteries. At birth, the decrease in the pulmonary vascular resistance increases blood flow through the lungs, increasing venous return to the left atrium, elevating **left-atrial pressure**. At the same time, the venous return to the right atrium falls from 69% + 21% + 3% = 93% of the combined cardiac output of *both* ventricles in the fetus to 100% of the cardiac output of a *single* ventricle at birth. Thus, **right-atrial pressure** falls. The net effect is a reversal of the pressure gradient across the atrial septum, pushing the foramen ovale's "valve"—situated on the "left" side of the septum—against the opening of the foramen ovale (Fig. 56–4A). Closing this valve usually prevents what would otherwise be movement of blood from the left to the right atrium of the

newborn. The left side of the heart now receives blood only from the lungs.

Gradually a *permanent seal* forms between the valve and the wall of the septum, a process that can take as little as a few months or as long as a few years. In some newborns, the valve does not completely seal to the septum, leaving a remnant potential pathway between the two atria. However, the 15% to 20% of adults with this condition do not have left-to-right shunting, because the foramen ovale's valve is effective even if not completely sealed. However, if right atrial pressure should increase above left atrial pressure for some pathological reason (e.g., pulmonary hypertension), then a right-to-left shunt between the atria would occur.

Closure of the Ductus Arteriosus Completes the Separation Between Pulmonary and Systemic Circulations

During fetal life, blood flows from the pulmonary artery, through the ductus arteriosus, and into the aorta (see Fig. 56–2A). Prostaglandins maintain the patency of the duc-

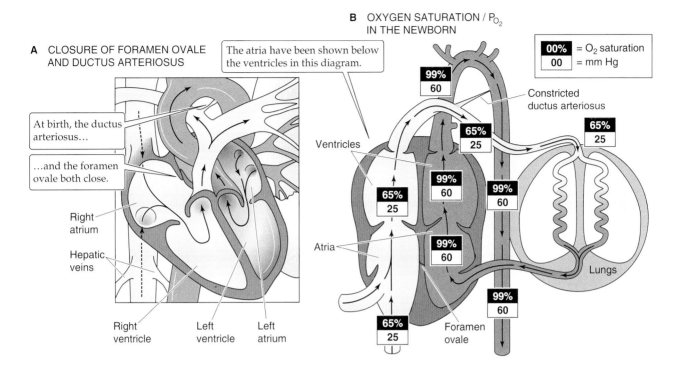

B OXYGEN SATURATION / P$_{O_2}$ IN THE NEWBORN

A CLOSURE OF FORAMEN OVALE AND DUCTUS ARTERIOSUS

The atria have been shown below the ventricles in this diagram.

At birth, the ductus arteriosus...

...and the foramen ovale both close.

Right atrium

Hepatic veins

Right ventricle   Left ventricle   Left atrium

Constricted ductus arteriosus

Ventricles

Atria

Foramen ovale

Lungs

00% = O$_2$ saturation
00 = mm Hg

FIGURE 56–4. Changes in the circulation at and around birth. *A,* The closure of these two shunts establish separate right and left circulatory systems. As the pressure in the left atrium rises above the pressure in the right atrium—due to the large decrease in pulmonary vascular resistance—the flap of the foramen ovale pushes against the septum, preventing blood flow from the left to the right atrium. Eventually this flap seals shut. As aortic pressure exceeds the pressure of the pulmonary artery, blood flow through the ductus arteriosus reverses. Well-oxygenated aortic blood now flows through the ductus arteriosus. This high P$_{O_2}$ causes vasoconstriction, which functionally closes the ductus arteriosus within a few hours. Falling prostaglandin levels also contribute to the rapid closure. Eventually, the lumen of the ductus becomes anatomically obliterated. *B,* The elimination of the fetal shunts and the oxygenation of blood in the lungs lead to major increases in the O$_2$ saturation and P$_{O_2}$ in the circulation.

tus arteriosus during fetal life. Immediately after birth, the ductus arteriosus remains open. However, it now conducts blood in the direction *opposite* from that of the fetus: from the aorta to the pulmonary artery. This reversal of blood flow is the result of the increased systemic resistance (which elevates aortic pressure) and decreased pulmonary vascular resistance (which lowers pulmonary-arterial pressure).

Obviously, the open ductus arteriosus during the first few hours of postnatal life constitutes an undesirable left-to-right shunt. Fortunately, within a few hours after birth, the ductus arteriosus closes *functionally* because its muscular wall constricts (see Fig. 56–4A). Usually all blood flow through the ductus arteriosus ceases within 1 week after birth. Within a month or so, the lumen becomes obliterated *anatomically* because of thrombosis (i.e., blood clot within the lumen), proliferation of the vessel's intimal layer, and growth of fibrous tissue. Occasionally, the ductus arteriosus fails to close. The incidence of patent ductus arteriosus is one in several thousand.

The relatively rapid *functional* closure of the ductus arteriosus is primarily the result of the increased P$_{O_2}$ of the blood perfusing this vessel immediately after birth. As the P$_{O_2}$ of blood flowing through the ductus arteriosus rises from 18 to 22 torr *in utero* to approximately 60 torr a few hours after birth, the smooth muscle in the wall of the ductus arteriosus contracts. In newborns who are hy-

poxemic, the low P$_{O_2}$ has three effects: (1) pulmonary vascular resistance and pressure remain high; (2) the ductus arteriosus remains patent; and (3) the patent ductus arteriosus maintains a right-to-left shunt. In these infants, the administration of 100% O$_2$ closes the ductus arteriosus. If these infants are allowed to breathe room air again too quickly, the ductus arteriosus reopens.

Other factors, in addition to a high P$_{O_2}$, contribute to the rapid functional closure of the ductus arteriosus. Shortly after birth, circulating levels of *prostaglandins* fall quickly, relieving the ductus arteriosus of their vasodilating influence. Pre-term infants tend to maintain high circulating prostaglandin levels, which may account for their tendency to maintain a patent ductus arteriosus. Treating such infants with indomethacin (a nonsteroidal anti-inflammatory drug that inhibits COX, reducing prostaglandin synthesis) (see box on p. 106) induces closure of the ductus arteriosus, even at a low P$_{O_2}$. Norepinephrine, acetylcholine, and bradykinin also produce constrictor responses.

The closure of the ductus arteriosus completes the separation of the right and left circulations initiated with closure of the foramen ovale. Whereas the ventricles functioned in *parallel* in the fetus, now they function in *series* in the neonate. As a result, the O$_2$ saturation of the newborn's hemoglobin is similar to the adult's (see Fig. 56–4B). However, because the O$_2$ saturation curve of *fetal* hemoglobin is relatively left shifted (p. 663), the newborn achieves these O_2 saturations at lower P_{O_2} values. In the neonate, the sum of the ventricular outputs of the two ventricles (i.e., twice the "cardiac output") is larger than the CCO in the fetus, a result primarily of a marked rise in the output of the left ventricle, which doubles its stroke volume. Compared with the adult, the newborn has a markedly lower systemic vascular resistance, and thus can achieve a relatively high blood flow with a relatively low perfusion pressure.

NEONATAL PHYSIOLOGY

In humans, the neonatal period is defined as the first 4 weeks of life. The newborn's ability to survive during this period depends on the adequate development and maturation of various fetal organ systems, as well as on adaptations of these organ systems to extra-uterine life. As the newborn loses its nutritional link with the placenta, it must now rely on its own gastrointestinal tract. Moreover, other functions normally carried out by the placenta are now entrusted to the liver and kidneys. Finally, upon exiting its uterine "incubator," the newborn must stabilize its body temperature.

Breast Milk from a Mother with a Balanced Diet Satisfies all of the Infant's Nutritional Requirements During the First Several Months of Life

Provided the mother's diet is adequate during pregnancy, the newborn is in complete nutritional balance at birth. The newborn's natural nutrition for the first few days of life is **colostrum** (a milk-like substance secreted by the mammary glands) and, thereafter, **breast milk** (see Table 55–8 for compositions), both of which the newborn's gastrointestinal tract is prepared to digest. If the infant is breastfed, and if the mother's nutritional status is good, colostrum and breast milk meet all of the newborn's nutritional needs. Moreover, colostrum and breast milk make important contributions to the newborn's immune status. Both contain high concentrations of immunoglobulin A (or "secretory") antibodies directed against bacteria and viruses, and also contain macrophages. Breast milk contains factors that promote the growth of lactobacilli, which colonize the colon and may protect the infant from some virulent strains of *Escherichia coli*. Barring complications or contraindications, pediatricians recommend that mothers breast feed their infants for several months to a year.

If the mother's dietary intake of iron was adequate during pregnancy, the infant's hepatic stores of **iron** are adequate for hematopoiesis for 6 to 9 months following delivery. Administering medicinal iron or providing iron-fortified milk can prevent iron-deficiency anemia.

The **calcium** in breast milk can meet the infant's needs for the rapid calcification of bones and teeth. However, fluoride for minimizing tooth decay must be provided as a supplement. Although the supply of calcium per se is unlikely to be a problem, **vitamin D** is necessary for the proper absorption of calcium by the intestines (p. 1097). Vitamin D supplementation may be necessary if the newborn or the mother is not exposed to sufficient sunlight to generate vitamin D in the skin (p. 1095). Supplementation may also be required in formula-fed infants and in infants born prematurely. **Rickets** (see box on p. 1098) can develop rapidly in a vitamin-D–deficient infant.

Vitamin C (ascorbic acid) is necessary for the synthesis of hydroxyproline in collagen and chondroitin sulfate (see Table 57–6) in cartilage, bone, and other connective tissues. The neonate is normally born with sufficient stores of vitamin C and receives adequate amounts of this vitamin in breast milk. If the breast milk or formula is vitamin C deficient, the infant may develop **scurvy**, which can be prevented with vitamin C supplements for the mother or infant.

The Neonate Mobilizes Glucose and Fatty Acids Soon After Delivery

CARBOHYDRATE METABOLISM. Elimination of the placental circulation at birth means that the newborn now has to forage for its own food. However, the newborn may not start suckling for approximately 6 hours. During late fetal life, glucocorticoids promote rapid accumulation of glycogen through their action on glycogen synthase. In its first few hours, the neonate uses glycogenolysis to mobilize its hepatic glycogen stores, releasing glucose into the bloodstream. The two enzymes needed for breaking down hepatic glycogen, phosphorylase, and glucose-6-phosphatase (p. 1218) are present in the fetus but do not become active until soon after birth.

The newborn depletes its hepatic glycogen stores in the first 12 hours of life. Stores of glycogen in cardiac muscle are 10 times those in the adult, and those in the skeletal muscle are three to five times those in the adult, but the fetus mainly uses the glycogen stored in these tissues to provide glucose for local use. The net effect is that during the first day of life, blood glucose levels may decline to 40 to 50 mg/dl, though they soon rise to near adult values once nutrition becomes adequate.

Infants born of **diabetic mothers** run a very high risk of having a pathologic hypoglycemia (i.e., <35 mg/dl). The high maternal blood-glucose levels translate to high fetal blood-glucose levels, causing hyperplasia of β cells in the fetal pancreatic islets and hyperinsulinism in the fetus. Insulin levels remain high after birth, producing extreme symptomatic hypoglycemia. Blood-glucose levels tend to reach their low point within a few hours after birth and begin to recover spontaneously within 6 hours.

Even in the normal newborn, low levels of blood glucose in the immediate postnatal period lead to a decrease in blood levels of **insulin** (p. 1069) and a reciprocal increase of **glucagon** (p. 1081). This hormonal milieu promotes the net release of glucose by the liver. In the liver, glucagon acts through cyclic adenosine monophosphate (cAMP) to stimulate glycogenolysis, inhibit glycogen synthesis, stimulate gluconeogenesis, and initiate synthesis of some gluconeogenic enzymes. All of these actions promote formation of glucose for release into the bloodstream (see Fig. 50–12). In contrast to the adult, in whom phosphorylation is the main mechanism for regulating the enzymes involved in glycogen metabolism, in the fetus, the relative *concentration* of the enzymes may be more important.

Epinephrine also promotes glucose mobilization (see Chapter 4) in the immediate postnatal period, using the same cAMP pathway as glucagon. Hypoxia, hypoglycemia, and hypothermia all stimulate the release of epinephrine from the adrenal medulla.

FAT METABOLISM. During the final 2 months of gestation, the fetus stores approximately 500 g of fat (i.e., approximately 15% of body weight), an important source of energy for the neonate. Decreased blood glucose just after birth raises levels of glucagon and epinephrine, which stimulate hormone-sensitive lipase in adipose tissue via cAMP (p. 1218). This lipase breaks down triglycerides into glycerol and free fatty acids (FFAs), which enter the bloodstream. The liver can take up glycerol and ultimately synthesize glucose (i.e., gluconeogenesis). The liver can also take up FFAs and generate ketone bodies, which are important as the newborn deals with glycogen depletion.

Because of its High Rates of Fluid Turnover and Acid Production, the Neonate Is at Special Risk to Develop Fluid and Acid-Base Imbalances

The newborn normally loses 6% to 10% of its body weight during the first week of life, reflecting a decrease in both interstitial and intravascular volume. After about a week, the rate of fluid intake begins to exceed that rate of loss, and term infants return close to birth weight by 1½ weeks.

The newborn's total body water is approximately 75% of body weight compared with 60% for men and 50% for women (see Table 3–1). Once the newborn is in a steady state, daily turnover of body water is 100 to 120 ml/kg, which is 3- to 4-fold higher than in adults. Thus, even small changes in the balance between fluid intake and loss can lead to rapid and profound disturbances in body-fluid compartments. The sick newborn can have a very difficult time maintaining fluid status, and requires very careful management.

The immaturity of the neonate's **kidneys** further complicates matters. For example, glomerular filtration rate (GFR; see Chapter 34) is extremely low at birth and increases rapidly during the first 2 weeks of life. However, even when normalized for body weight, GFR does not reach adult levels until about 1 year of age. Moreover, the concentrating ability of the newborn kidney (i.e., a maximal urine osmolality of $\sim$450 mOsm) is substantially less than that of an adult ($\sim$1200 mOsm).

The neonate's **metabolic rate**—expressed per kilogram of body weight—is much higher than that of the adult. Immediately after birth, the neonate's daily metabolic rate is approximately 55 kcal/kg and rises to approximately 100 kcal/kg after about a week. These figures compare with approximately 30 kcal/kg for the resting metabolic rate in a healthy young adult. Because of its relatively high metabolic rate, the neonate's cardiac output and ventilation are also correspondingly higher than those of the adult. Metabolism generates fixed acids (p. 845), and the newborn's relative acid load is also greater. The immature state of neonatal kidneys with respect to acid excretion puts the neonate at risk for developing metabolic acidosis (p. 642).

Although the Newborn Is Prone to Hypothermia, Nonshivering Thermogenesis in Brown Fat Helps Keep the Neonate Warm

The body loses heat to its environment by radiation, conduction, convection, and evaporation (p. 1234). Their relative importance depends on the circumstances. For instance, at birth the infant moves from a warm and liquid environment to cool and dry surroundings. Hence, evaporation is the main source of heat loss immediately after delivery. However, even after the newborn's skin is dry, the infant is at risk for losing body heat by each of the previously discussed mechanisms. The major reasons are the newborn's: (1) large skin surface area relative to its small body mass (i.e., large surface-to-volume ratio); (2) limited ability to generate heat through muscle contraction (e.g., shivering thermogenesis); (3) poor thermal insulation from the environment by adipose tissue; and (4) inability to adjust his or her own protection (e.g., put on warmer clothes) from the thermal stress of the environment or to modify that environment (e.g., turn up the thermostat). Premature and growth-retarded infants are at an even higher risk for heat loss and hypothermia.

Fortunately, the newborn has one important asset for fighting hypothermia: **nonshivering thermogenesis**, a process that occurs primarily in liver, brain, and brown fat (Fig. 56–5). Cold stress triggers an increase in the levels of epinephrine and thyroid-stimulating hormone (TSH). **TSH** stimulates the release of the thyroid hormones, predominantly T_4 (p. 1038). Working in parallel, **epinephrine** activates, particularly in brown fat, the 5′/3′-monodeiodinase responsible for the peripheral conversion of circulating T_4 to the far more active T_3. T_3 acts locally in brown fat to uncouple mitochondrial oxidation from phosphorylation and thereby increase heat production.

Brown fat differs from white fat in having a high density of mitochondria; the cytochromes in these mitochondria give the brown-fat cells their brown color. Newborns have particularly high levels of brown fat in the neck and midline of the upper back. In brown fat, the locally generated T_3 upregulates a protein called uncoupling protein (UCP) or **thermogenin**. This protein is an H^+ channel located in the inner mitochondrial membrane. Normally, intracellular purine nucleotides (e.g., ATP, guanosine diphosphate [GDP]) inhibit thermogenin. However, epinephrine, acting through a cAMP pathway, activates the lipase that liberates free fatty acids from triglycerides. These FFAs relieve the inhibition of the H^+ channel and increase its conduction of protons. The result

is that the protons generated by electron transport enter the mitochondrion through thermogenin that dissipates the H⁺ gradient needed by the H⁺-translocating ATP synthase (p. 64). Thus, the mitochondria in brown fat can produce heat without producing useful energy in the form of ATP. The oxidation of fatty acids in brown fat generates approximately 27 kcal/kg of body weight each day, contributing a large fraction of the neonate's high metabolic rate.

Humoral and Cellular Immune Responses Begin at Early Stages of Development in the Fetus

Maternal **antibodies** play a key role in protecting the infant from infection both *in utero* and during the first several months after birth.

FETUS. The placenta actively transports the small IgG immunoglobulins from mother to fetus, so that fetal IgG levels are even higher than those in the mother. These maternal IgG antibodies ward off infection by viruses and some bacteria. However, maternal IgA (which is primarily present in secretions), IgE, and IgM antibodies generally do not cross the placenta in appreciable amounts, and the baby is generally born with very low levels of these other immunoglobulins.

The fetus begins to develop its own immune capabilities at very early stages of development. However, because the fetus is isolated from antigens, the fetal immune system normally does not make large amounts of antibodies. Nevertheless, the fetus can respond to intra-uterine infections by generating IgM antibodies. In addition, the fetus also begins to produce other proteins that help protect against bacterial and viral infections. Among these are (1) the components of the **complement** pathway; (2) **lysozyme**, an enzyme found in secretions such as tears and mucus, which digests the cell walls of bacteria and fungi; and (3) **γ-interferon**, which is produced by T lymphocytes and which activates B lymphocytes, macrophages, and endothelial cells.

NEONATE. In addition to its high prenatal levels of maternal IgG, the newborn receives copious amounts of secretory IgA antibodies in colostrum and breast milk. However, the blood levels of *maternal* IgG antibodies progressively fall, and IgG levels in the infant's blood reach a nadir at about 3 months of age. After that time, the infant's own production of IgG antibodies causes total IgG levels to gradually increase. However, even at 1 year of age, IgG levels—as well as the levels of IgA, IgM, and IgE—are still only half of the adult level.

Antibodies obtained *in utero* from the mother protect against most childhood diseases, including **diphtheria**, **measles**, and **polio**. The persistence of antibodies—at levels high enough for protection—vary considerably from one disease to another. For example, maternal measles antibodies are so persistent that vaccinations against measles often fail if attempted before 15 months of age. On the other hand, maternal antibodies against **whooping cough** (pertussis) are generally inadequate to protect the infant beyond 1 to 2 months. The infant normally receives its first DTP immunization (diphtheria, tetanus, and pertussis), as well as the first polio immunization, at 2 months of age.

The Premature Newborn has Especially Immature Organ Systems and Homeostatic Control Mechanisms, Exacerbating Postnatal Risks

According to the World Health Organization, a **premature infant** is defined as one born fewer than 37 weeks after its mother's last menstrual period, compared with the normal 40 weeks (p. 1181). For the premature infant whose birth weight is *appropriate for its gestational age*, the only problem is that the uterus was unable to retain the fetus for the appropriate term for any of a variety of reasons (e.g., premature rupture of the membranes, incompetent cervix). **Intra-uterine growth retardation** (IUGR; see box on p. 1193) describes a newborn that not only has a low birth weight, but is also *small for its gestational age*. Virtually all of the challenges to the health of the neonate are made more severe in prematurity or IUGR, conditions that are therefore associated with reduced chances of survival. These problems generally reflect either immaturity of certain organ systems (e.g., lungs, intestines, liver, kidneys) or immaturity of the homeostatic mechanisms (e.g., thermoregulation).

REFERENCES

Books and Reviews

Ballard PL: Hormonal regulation of pulmonary surfactant. Endocrine Rev 10:165–181, 1989.

Benirschke K: Normal embryologic development. In Moore TR, Reiter RC, Rebar RW, Baker VV (eds): Gynecology and Obstetrics: A Longitudinal Approach. New York, Churchill Livingstone, 1993, pp. 37–53.

Furon J-C, Skoll A: Fetal cardiovascular physiology and response to stress conditions. In Reece A, Hobbins J (eds): Medicine of the fetus and mother. Philadelphia, WB Saunders, 1998, pp. 115–130.

Strang LB: Fetal lung liquid: Secretion and reabsorption. Physiol Rev 71: 991–1016, 1991.

Warshaw JB: Fatty acid metabolism during development. Semin Perinatol 3:131–139, 1979.

Journal Articles

Avery ME, Mead J: Surface properties in relation to atelectasis and hyaline membrane disease. Am J Dis Child 97:517, 1959.

FIGURE 56–5. Nonshivering thermogenesis in brown fat. AC, adenylyl cyclase; ADP, adenosine diphosphate; ATP, adenosine triphosphate; cAMP, cyclic adenosine monophosphate; GTP, guanosine triphosphate; P$_i$, inorganic phosphate; RXR, retinoid X receptor; THR, thyroid hormone receptor; TRE, thyroid response element.

Gluck K, Kulovich M: Lecithin/sphingomyelin ratios in amniotic fluid in normal and abnormal pregnancy. Am J Obstet Gynecol 115–539, 1973.

Goldenberg RL, Cutter GR, Hoffman HJ, et al: Intrauterine growth retardation: Standards for diagnosis. Am J Obstet Gynecol 161:271–277, 1989.

Gross I: Regulation of fetal lung maturation. Am J Physiol 259:L337–L344, 1990.

Kari MA, Hallman M, Eronen M, et al: Prenatal dexamethasone treatment in conjunction with human surfactant therapy, a randomized placebo-controlled multicenter study. Pediatrics 94:730–736, 1994.

Wilkening RB, Meschia G: Fetal oxygen uptake, oxygenation, and acid-base balance as a function of uterine blood flow. Am J Physiol 244:H749–H755, 1983.

X

The Physiology of Everyday Life

CHAPTER 57

Metabolism and Nutrition

Ethan Nadel

The body's metabolism encompasses all of the chemical processes involved in energy production, energy release, and growth. These processes can be **anabolic** (formation of substances) or **catabolic** (breakdown). Ultimately, all energy contained in ingested nutrients manifests itself as either heat, work done on the environment, or growth. A healthy young man requires approximately 30 kcal per kg body weight to sustain resting metabolism for one day. Thus, a 70-kg man requires 2100 kcal/day, which is known as the **resting metabolic rate** (RMR). The amount of calories increases with increased activity, illness, or other stress. The **basal metabolic rate** (BMR) is a clinical definition for metabolism that is measured under standardized conditions in which the subject: (1) has had a full night of restful sleep, (2) has been fasting for 12 hours, (3) is in a neutral thermal environment (p. 1234), (4) has been resting physically for 1 hour, and (5) is free of psychic and physical stimuli. The BMR (*units:* kcal per hour and per square meter of body surface area) in adults is approximately 5% higher for males than for females and falls with age. The BMR is less than the RMR.

The body's nutritional status influences the effectiveness of metabolic processes. Numerous vitamins, minerals, and other cofactors, along with water, contribute to the environment for cellular metabolism to function effectively and efficiently.

ENERGY BALANCE

Energy Input to the Body is the Sum of Energy Output and Storage

The **first law of thermodynamics** states that energy can neither be created nor destroyed; in a closed system, total energy is constant. This concept is illustrated in Figure 57–1. Humans acquire almost all their energy from ingested food, store it in different forms, and expend it in different ways. In the steady state, energy uptake must equal energy output.

The gastrointestinal (GI) tract breaks down ingested carbohydrates, fats, and proteins into smaller components and then absorbs them into the bloodstream for transport to sites of metabolism. For example, the GI tract reduces ingested carbohydrates to simple sugars (e.g., glucose), which are then transported to muscle cells and either oxidized to release energy or converted to glycogen for storage. Oxidation of fuels not only generates free energy but also waste products and heat (thermal energy).

FIGURE 57–1. Energy balance.

The body's energy *inputs* must balance the sum of its energy *outputs* and the energy *stored*. When the body takes in more energy than it expends, the person is in **positive energy balance** and will gain weight. Healthy children are in positive energy balance during growth periods. Conversely, when energy intake is less than expenditure, this **negative energy balance** leads to weight loss. A person in negative energy balance preferentially uses stored fat as fuel.

A person can gain or lose weight by manipulating energy intake or output. An optimal strategy to encourage weight loss involves both increasing energy output as well as reducing energy intake. In most people, a substantial decrease in energy intake alone leads to inadequate nutrient intake, which can compromise bodily function.

Because of the Inefficiency of Chemical Reactions, the Body's Total Free Energy Falls

The **second law of thermodynamics** states that chemical transformations always result in a loss of free energy. The total internal energy (E) of the human body is the sum of the disposable or "good" energy (i.e., the **Gibbs free energy, G**) plus the unavailable or "wasted" energy (i.e., the product of absolute temperature, *T*, and entropy, *S*):

$$E = G + T \cdot S$$
Equation 57–1

Imagine that you eat some glucose, which increases

your total internal energy by a small amount (ΔE). Some of this energy will be stored as glycogen (ΔG), and some will waste as heat ($T \cdot \Delta S$). According to Equation 1, as long as the temperature is constant, the change in total internal energy will have two components:

Equation 57–2
$$\Delta E \quad = \quad \Delta G \quad + \quad T \cdot \Delta S$$

| Energy of ingested glucose | Energy stored as glycogen | Energy wasted as heat |

Thus, some of the increased total energy (ΔE) will be stored as glycogen (ΔG). However, because of the inefficiencies of the chemical reactions that convert glucose to glycogen, some of the ΔE is wasted as heat ($T \cdot \Delta S$). Another way of stating the second law is that $T \cdot \Delta S$ can never be zero or negative, and chemical reactions can never be 100% efficient.

If we add *no energy* to the body (i.e., ΔE is zero), the body's total free energy must decline (i.e., ΔG is negative). This decline in G matches precisely the rise in $T \cdot S$, reflecting inefficiencies inherent in chemical transformations. Consider, for example, what would happen if you took 1 mole of glucose (180 g), put it into a bomb calorimeter with O_2, and completely burned the glucose to CO_2 and H_2O. This combustion would yield 686 kcal in the form of heat but conserve no usable energy. Now consider what happens if your body burns this same 1 mole of glucose. In contrast to the bomb calorimeter, your mitochondria not only oxidize glucose to CO_2 and H_2O but also conserve part of the free energy in the form of adenosine triphosphate (ATP). Each of the many chemical-conversion steps from glucose to CO_2 and H_2O makes available a small amount of the total energy contained in glucose. Converting 1 mole of adenosine diphosphate (ADP) and inorganic phosphate (P_i) to 1 mole of ATP under the conditions prevailing in a cell consumes approximately 11.5 kcal/mole. Therefore, if a particular step in glucose oxidation releases *at least* 11.5 kcal/mole, it can be coupled to ATP synthesis. The conversion of the lower-energy ADP to the higher-energy ATP traps energy in the system, conserving it for later use. The cellular oxidation of 1 mole of glucose conserves approximately 400 kcal of the potential 686 kcal/mole; the remaining 286 kcal/mole are liberated as heat. Because the body cannot reconvert this heat to energy, the body's total free energy falls.

Free Energy, Conserved as High-Energy Bonds in ATP, is Released in a Controlled Manner to Provide the Energy for Cellular Functions

ATP consists of a nitrogenous ring (adenine), a five-carbon sugar (ribose), and three phosphate groups (Fig. 57–2). The last two phosphates are connected to the rest of the molecule by high-energy bonds. The same is true for a related nucleotide, guanosine triphosphate (GTP). If we compare the free energies of phosphate bonds of various molecules, we see that the "high-energy" phosphate bonds of ATP lie toward the middle of the free-energy scale. Thus, in the presence of P_i, ADP can accept energy from compounds that are higher on the free-energy scale (e.g., phosphocreatine), whereas ATP can release energy in the formation of compounds that are lower on the free-energy scale (e.g., glucose-6-phosphate [G6P]). Thus, ATP can *store* energy derived from energy-releasing reactions and *release* energy needed to drive other chemical reactions.

Examples of the chemical reactions fueled by converting ATP to ADP and P_i include the formation of peptide bonds in protein synthesis, bridge formation between actin and myosin during muscle contraction, and pumping Ca^{2+} against its concentration gradient during muscle re-

laxation. Although the conversion of ATP to ADP and P_i is often referred to as a "hydrolysis reaction," because the traditional representation is ATP + H_2O → ADP + P_i + H^+, the reaction actually occurs in two steps. The first typically involves transfer of a part of the phosphate group to an intermediate molecule, thus increasing the intermediate's free-energy content. The second step involves displacing the phosphate moiety, releasing P_i and energy. In contrast, true hydrolysis reactions merely release heat, which cannot be trapped to drive chemical processes.

ENERGY STORAGE (ANABOLISM)

The Body Can Store Nearly All of the Energy Contained in Foodstuffs as Glycogen or Triglycerides

Because energy acquisition by the body is intermittent, whereas energy expenditure is continuous, the body needs to store and then parcel out energy. Ingested foodstuffs contain carbohydrates, lipids, proteins, and small quantities of minerals and vitamins. The GI tract digests (hydrolyzes) these substances and absorbs the products. In this section, we examine how the body handles and stores these assimilated foodstuffs.

Carbohydrates have the chemical makeup $(CH_2O)_n$. Dietary carbohydrates include the *monomers* glucose, fructose, and galactose; *dimers* such as sucrose and lactose; complex but *digestible polymers* such as starches; and *indigestible polymers* such as cellulose. The GI tract breaks down the digestible carbohydrates and then absorbs the products as monomers (see Fig. 44–3). After reaching the portal blood, these carbohydrates are stored in the liver and skeletal muscle. In either case, the predominant storage form is glycogen, a complex polymer of glucose.

The synthesis of glycogen from glucose starts with the transport of glucose across the plasma membrane of either a hepatocyte or muscle cell. This uptake is promoted after a meal by the elevation of blood glucose and the subsequent increase in insulin concentration. Insulin potentiates glucose transport in muscle by binding to the insulin receptor on the cell surface, which causes translocation of the GLUT4 glucose transporter (p. 1078) from cytoplasmic vesicles to the cell's surface. Once glu-

FIGURE 57–2. Hydrolysis of ATP to ADP, inorganic phosphate, and H^+. ADP, adenosine diphosphate; ATP, adenosine triphosphate.

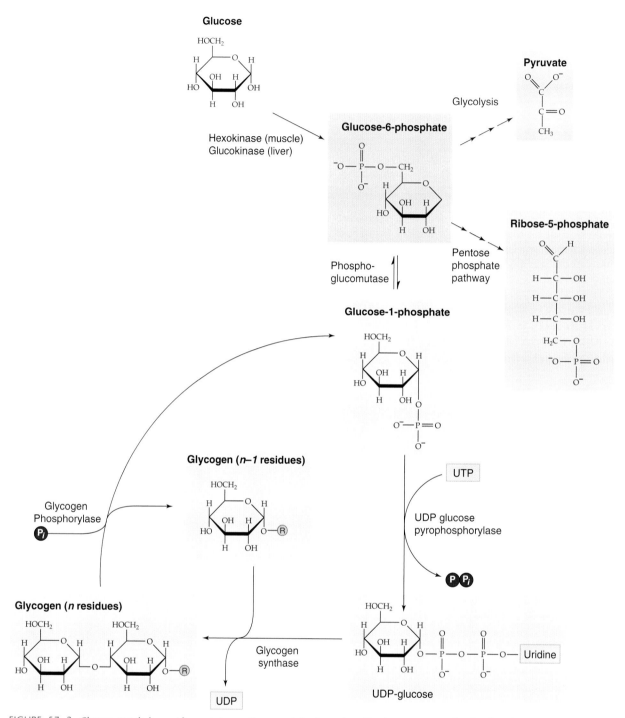

FIGURE 57–3. Glucose metabolism. After entering a liver or skeletal-muscle cell, glucose is immediately phosphorylated to glucose-6-phosphate, which can have three fates: glycolysis, breakdown via the pentose phosphate shunt, and glycogen synthesis. ATP, adenosine triphosphate; NADPH, nicotinamide adenine dinucleotide phosphate; UDP, uridine diphosphate; UTP, uridine triphosphate.

cose moves across the plasma membrane through the GLUT4 transporter, it is phosphorylated to G6P in the cytosol. If the metabolic demand is low, G6P is converted to glycogen by action of the enzyme glycogen synthase (Fig. 57–3). We discussed the hormonal control of glycogen metabolism in Chapter 50 (see Figs. 50–8 and 50–9).

Glycogen is made up of glucose molecules linked together by α-1,4 linkages in the straight portions of the polymer, and by α-1,6 linkages at the frequent branch points. Thus, glycogen resembles the starch amylopectin (see Fig. 44–3), except that glycogen is more highly branched. The molecular weight of glycogen typically averages more than 5000 kDa, thus providing a handy storage depot for low molecular-weight compounds (monosaccharides) without affecting the osmotic pressure of the intracellular space. Glycogen is found in "granules," which also contain the enzymes needed for glycogen synthesis and degradation.

Lipids are dietary substances that are soluble in organic solvents but not in water. The GI tract breaks down ingested triglycerides into free fatty acids and 2-monoglycerides (or glycerol). **Fatty acids** are composed of long carbon chains (14–24) with a carboxyl terminus, and have the general form CH_3-$(CH_2)_n$-COOH. The fatty acid chains can be either *saturated* with hydrogen atoms or *unsaturated* (i.e., double bonds may connect one or more pairs of carbon atoms). A 2-monoglyceride is a glycerol molecule esterified to a fatty acid in its 2 position. The enterocyte takes up fatty acids and 2-monoglycerides across its apical membrane (p. 966) and re-esterifies these building blocks to reconstruct triglycerides ("**monoglyceride pathway**") (Fig. 57–4A). Alternatively, the enterocyte can esterify free fatty acids to glycerol-3-phosphate, a byproduct of glucose metabolism, thus generating phosphatidic acid and, subsequently, either triglycerides ("**phosphatidic acid pathway**") or phospholipids. The enterocyte packages triglycerides, cholesterol, phospholipid, and apolipoprotein into extremely large aggregates called **chylomicrons**, which enter the lymph and ultimately the blood (p. 966).

After a meal, chylomicrons find their way to the endothelial surface of capillaries of adipose tissue, skeletal muscle, and heart (see Fig. 57–4B). There, they encounter **lipoprotein lipase** (LPL; p. 998), which hydrolyzes triglycerides in the chylomicrons to fatty acids and glycerol, leaving behind "remnant" chylomicrons.

The **fatty acids** enter adipocytes, muscle, and also hepatocytes. Adipocytes and muscle esterify the fatty acids to glycerol-3-phosphate to form monoglycerides, diglycerides, and **triglycerides**. Lipids are stored primarily as triglycerides in adipose tissue and skeletal muscle but also in all cell membranes as **phospholipids**. Hepatocytes either β oxidize the fatty acids (p. 1220), which does not contribute to energy storage, or convert them to triglycerides for storage. The **glycerol** released by the action of lipoprotein lipase (LPL) enters the hepatocytes, which convert glycerol to glucose by gluconeogenesis or break glycerol down to pyruvate by glycolysis.

The final products of LPL hydrolysis are triglyceride-depleted chylomicrons, shrunk to form **remnant chylomicrons**. Hepatocytes take up these remnant chylomicrons via receptor-mediated endocytosis. The hepatocytes then hydrolyze the dietary fats in these remnant chylomicrons and use them as fuel or convert them to very-low-density lipoproteins (VLDLs) for carriage in the blood to extrahepatic tissues.

LPL on the surface of endothelial cells is distinct from the hormone-sensitive lipase (HSL) that is *inside* the adipocyte (p. 1218). We discuss this intracellular lipase later in connection with the breakdown of triglycerides stored in adipocytes. Insulin enhances LPL synthesis (see Fig. 50–10) and thus ensures the manufacture of fatty acids and glycerol for energy storage. However, as discussed later, insulin inhibits the hormone-sensitive lipase that would otherwise break down the stored triglycerides.

Proteins are linear polymers of L-amino acids (Fig. 57–5), which have the general molecular structure ^+H_3N-HC(R)-COO$^-$. Different functional "R" groups distinguish the 20 amino acids incorporated into nascent proteins during messenger RNA (mRNA) translation. In addition, four other amino acids are present in mature proteins: γ-carboxyglutamic acid, hydroxylysine, 4-hydroxyproline, and 3-hydroxyproline. However, these amino acids result from post-translational modification of amino acids that are already in the polypeptide chain. In α-amino acids, the amino group (-NH_3^+), the carboxyl group (-COO$^-$), and R are all attached to the central or α carbon atom. In proteins, the amino acids are linked together by peptide bonds that are formed between the α amino group of one amino acid and the α carboxyl group of another. Nine of the amino acids are termed **essential amino acids** because they cannot be synthesized at rates sufficient to sustain growth and maintenance of function, and thus must be obtained in the diet (Table 57–1).

Proteins are stored in all tissues and can be structural or functional. Structural proteins make up skin, collagen, ligaments, and tendons. Functional proteins include enzymes that catalyze reactions, muscle filaments such as myosin and actin, and various hormones. There is a constant breakdown of proteins to amino acids, and vice versa, allowing the cells to change their make-up of proteins as the demands change.

Interconversions among dietary foodstuffs enable an excess intake of carbohydrate, for example, to be stored in the form of triglycerides in adipose tissue (lipogenesis). Excess intake of amino acids can be converted to either triglycerides or to glucose (gluconeogenesis) and then to glycogen for storage. In contrast, excess lipid intake is stored in adipose tissue in the form of triglycerides because humans cannot convert fatty acids to either glycogen or protein.

The Available Energy Stored in Fat Greatly Exceeds that Stored in Carbohydrates and Proteins

Energy-storage does not come for free, although it is relatively inexpensive from a total-energy standpoint. The process of digesting a mixed meal in the GI tract elevates whole-body metabolic rate by 20% to 25% above the

TABLE 57–1

ESSENTIAL AND NONESSENTIAL α-AMINO ACIDS	
ESSENTIAL	**NONESSENTIAL**
Histidine	Alanine
Isoleucine	Arginine
Leucine	Asparagine
Lysine	Aspartate
Methionine	Cysteine
Phenylalanine	Glutamate
Threonine	Glutamine
Tryptophan	Glycine
Valine	Proline
	Serine
	Tyrosine

A INTESTINAL ABSORPTION AND RE-ESTERIFICATION OF TRIGLYCERIDES

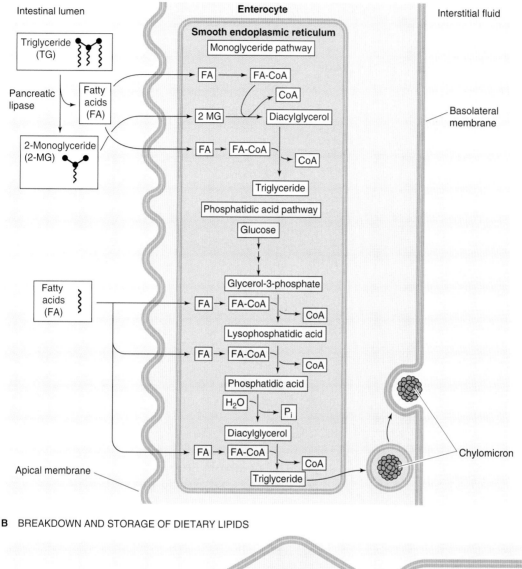

B BREAKDOWN AND STORAGE OF DIETARY LIPIDS

FIGURE 57–4. Digestion, absorption, and storage of triglycerides. In *A*), Pancreatic lipase breaks down triglycerides (TGs) into fatty acids (FA) and 2-monoglycerides (2-MG) in the lumen of the small intestine. These products enter the enterocyte, which uses either the monoglyceride or the phosphatidic-acid pathway to re-esterify them. The resulting triglycerides are packaged into chylomicrons, which enter the lymph and, ultimately, the blood. In *B*), Lipoprotein lipase (LPL) in capillaries hydrolyzes TGs in chylomicrons to FA and glycerol. Adipocytes re-esterify the FAs to TGs for storage in fat droplets. Hepatocytes take up remnant chylomicrons by receptor-mediated endocytosis, glycerol, and some FA.

BMR for approximately 90 minutes following a meal. In addition to this cost of digestion and absorption, the energy cost of *storing* dietary carbohydrate as glycogen or dietary lipid as triglyceride is 3% to 7% of the energy taken in. The cost of storing amino acids as protein is nearly 25% of the energy taken in. Moreover, storage after *interconversions* among dietary categories is particularly expensive. The cost of storing dietary carbohydrate as triglyceride, or of storing amino acids as glycogen, is nearly 25% of the intake energy.

Lipids are the most concentrated depot of energy storage because they represent, on average, 9.4 kcal/g, and because they are in an anhydrous state. Thus, fat has evolved to be the storage depot of choice. Most of the body's fat depots exist in the subcutaneous adipose tissue layers, although fat also exists to a small extent in muscle and in visceral (deeper) depots in obese and older people. A typical 70-kg human with 20% fat (14 kg) thus carries 131,600 kcal of energy stored in adipose tissue. Assuming an RMR of 2100 kcal/day and 100% efficiency of converting the fat to energy, mobilization and subsequent oxidation of this entire depot could theoretically sustain the body's entire resting metabolic requirement for nearly 63 days.

Carbohydrates contain only 4.1 kcal/g or less than half the energy of lipids per unit mass. The liver normally contains 75 to 100 g of glycogen but can store up to 120 grams (8% of its weight) as glycogen. Skeletal muscle normally contains 300 to 400 g, but can store up to 600 g of glycogen (3% of its weight). A typical 70-kg human has up to approximately 700 g of glycogen (~1% of body weight). Thus, the total energy stored in the body in the form of glycogen can be as great as 3000 kcal, which is still only a tiny fraction of that stored in the form of lipid, enough to supply resting metabolism for less than a day and a half, assuming 100% efficiency. Nonetheless, carbohydrate stores are essential because certain tissues, particularly the brain, rely heavily on carbohydrates for their fuel.

Proteins contain 4.3 kcal/g, about the same as carbohydrates. A typical 70-kg human with 14% protein (9.8 kg)—only about half of which can be mobilized as a fuel source—can thus store approximately 20,000 kcal in the form of available protein. Generally, proteins are far more important as structural or functional components than as energy stores. Thus, it is not surprising that protein catabolism makes only a small contribution—much less than 5%—to resting energy requirements. On the other hand, during starvation, when carbohydrate reserves are exhausted, protein catabolism can contribute as much as

15% of the energy necessary to sustain the resting metabolic requirements.

Nitrogen balance, an indication of the *change* in whole-body protein stores, is estimated from dietary protein intake and urinary nitrogen (i.e., urea) excretion. Children eating a balanced diet are in positive nitrogen balance because they store amino acids as protein in the process of growth. Patients who have suffered burns or trauma are usually in negative nitrogen balance, indicating the loss of lean body mass.

ENERGY LIBERATION (CATABOLISM)

When energy use exceeds the energy available from the diet, the body draws on its stored energy to meet its requirements. A shortfall of energy intake compared with output occurs either when energy intake is too low (e.g., starvation) or when energy liberation is elevated (e.g., hyperthyroidism; see box on p. 1046) or during sustained physical activity (e.g., running a marathon). In reality, the body constantly cycles energy between storage and mobilization, with the balance favoring one or the other, depending on the instantaneous energy requirement. The general principle in energy catabolism is that the body first breaks down a complex storage polymer (e.g., glycogen or triglycerides) to simpler compounds (e.g., glucose, fatty acids plus glycerol) that cells can then burn.

The First Step in Energy Catabolism is to Break Down Glycogen or Triglycerides to Simpler Compounds

SKELETAL MUSCLE. Skeletal muscle liberates stored **carbohydrate** by converting glycogen to glucose-1-phosphate (**glycogenolysis**), a reaction catalyzed by glycogen phosphorylase (see Fig. 57–6A). **Epinephrine** triggers glycogenolysis by binding to a β-adrenergic receptor, promoting the formation of cyclic adenosine monophosphate (cAMP; p. 97). The cAMP activates protein kinase A (PKA), which in turn phosphorylates phosphorylase kinase (PK; see p. 98). The now active form of PK then converts the inactive glycogen phosphorylase b (GPb) to the active **glycogen phosphorylase a** (GPa). In skeletal muscle, a second way of activating GPb is for it to bind AMP allosterically; $[AMP]_i$ increases during muscle activity owing to increased turnover of ATP. Conversely, ATP competes with AMP for this nucleotide-binding site, and thus inhibits GPb. Yet a third way of activating GPb is for

FIGURE 57–5. Structure of proteins. The chemistry of R determines the identity of the amino acid.

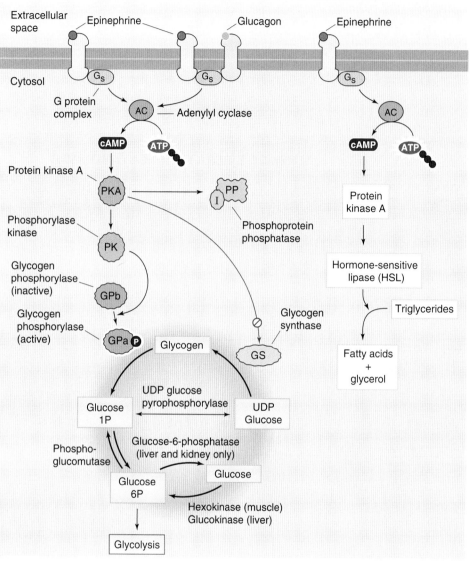

FIGURE 57–6. Mobilization of energy stores. In *A*, epinephrine activates glycogen phosphorylase, which breaks down glycogen in muscle. Because glucose-6-phosphatase is absent from muscle, the end product is glucose-6-phosphate, which cannot leave the cell and thus must be consumed locally. In *B*, glucagon triggers glycogen breakdown, yielding glucose-6-phosphate in hepatocytes. Because they have glucose-6-phosphatase, hepatocytes can generate glucose and export it to the blood. In *C*, epinephrine activates hormone-sensitive lipase, which hydrolyzes triglycerides to glycerol and fatty acids, which leave the adipocytes and enter the blood. ATP, adenosine triphosphate; cAMP, cyclic adenosine monophosphate; GS, glycogen synthase; UDP, uridine diphosphate.

Ca^{2+} to activate PK allosterically. Thus, during intense activity of skeletal muscle, the accompanying increase in $[Ca^{2+}]_i$ directly promotes muscle glycogenolysis. Skeletal muscle converts the G1P generated from glycogen breakdown to G6P, which in turn enters the glycolytic pathway within the muscle cell.

LIVER. As is the case in muscle, hepatocytes make stored **carbohydrate** available by using glycogen phosphorylase to convert glycogen to G1P. The mechanism for determining the ratio of GPa to GPb is the same as in muscle, except that in the liver it is **glucagon** (and to a lesser extent, epinephrine) that triggers the increase in $[cAMP]_i$ (see Fig. 57–6*B*). In the presence of glucagon, the liver converts glycogen to G1P and this, as in muscle, to G6P (p. 1082). However, unlike muscle, liver contains the enzyme G6Pase, which cleaves the phosphate from G6P, yielding glucose, which is free to enter the bloodstream. Thus, whereas glycogenolysis in skeletal muscle

serves to meet *local* energy demands by releasing G6P, glycogenolysis in the liver serves to meet whole-body energy demands by releasing glucose to the *blood*. After an overnight fast, glycogenolysis accounts for about half of hepatic glucose release. The remainder of hepatic glucose release reflects gluconeogenesis (i.e., de novo generation of glucose), starting primarily from certain amino acids, but also lactate, glycerol, and pyruvate.

ADIPOCYTES. Adipocytes release stored **lipids** by using hormone-sensitive lipase (HSL) to hydrolyze triglycerides to free fatty acids (FFAs) and glycerol. Nearly all (95%) of the available energy of triacylglycerols resides in the FFA moieties. Two hormones can stimulate lipolysis: **epinephrine**, which the adrenal medulla secretes under conditions of low blood glucose, and also growth hormone (p. 1027). As in skeletal muscle and hepatocytes, epinephrine acts through cAMP (see Fig. 57–6*C*). The result is activation of HSL, which hydrolyzes the ester linkages of triac-

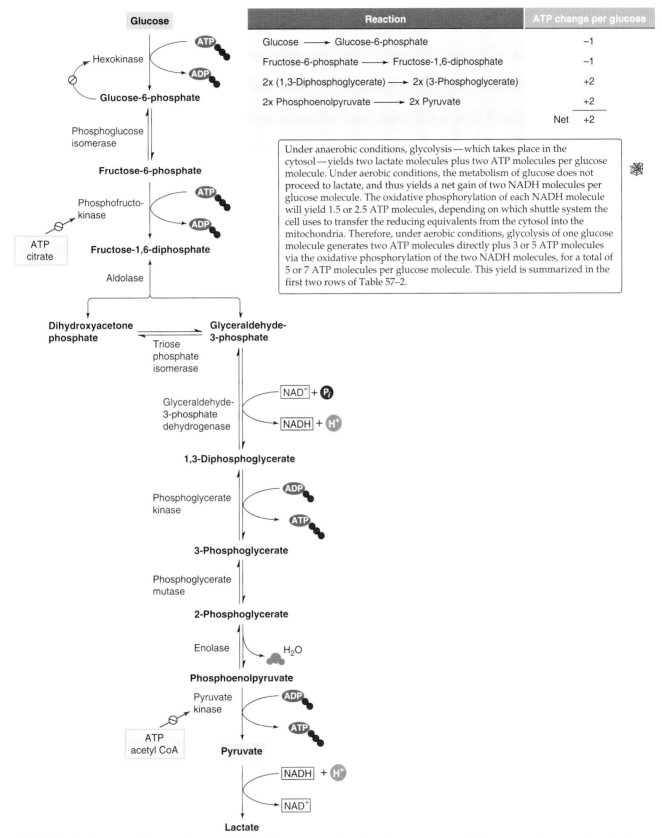

Reaction	ATP change per glucose
Glucose $\longrightarrow$ Glucose-6-phosphate	−1
Fructose-6-phosphate $\longrightarrow$ Fructose-1,6-diphosphate	−1
2x (1,3-Diphosphoglycerate) $\longrightarrow$ 2x (3-Phosphoglycerate)	+2
2x Phosphoenolpyruvate $\longrightarrow$ 2x Pyruvate	+2
Net	+2

Under anaerobic conditions, glycolysis—which takes place in the cytosol—yields two lactate molecules plus two ATP molecules per glucose molecule. Under aerobic conditions, the metabolism of glucose does not proceed to lactate, and thus yields a net gain of two NADH molecules per glucose molecule. The oxidative phosphorylation of each NADH molecule will yield 1.5 or 2.5 ATP molecules, depending on which shuttle system the cell uses to transfer the reducing equivalents from the cytosol into the mitochondria. Therefore, under aerobic conditions, glycolysis of one glucose molecule generates two ATP molecules directly plus 3 or 5 ATP molecules via the oxidative phosphorylation of the two NADH molecules, for a total of 5 or 7 ATP molecules per glucose molecule. This yield is summarized in the first two rows of Table 57–2.

FIGURE 57–7. Glycolysis. ADP, adenosine diphosphate; ATP, adenosine triphosphate; CoA, coenzyme A; NAD, nicotinamide adenine dinucleotide.

ylglycerol molecules, releasing FFAs, which diffuse out of the adipocytes into the bloodstream. There, the poorly soluble FFAs bind to circulating **albumin**, which releases them at the sites of energy demand.

The Second Step in Carbohydrate Catabolism Is Glycolysis

The degradation of glucose to pyruvate by the process known as glycolysis (Fig. 57–7) generates energy even in the absence of O_2 (**anaerobic catabolism**). This process yields 47 kcal of free energy per mole of glucose. Of this energy, the cell can trap enough to yield directly 2 ATP molecules. Under *aerobic* conditions, the mitochondria can generate an additional 3 to 5 ATP molecules per glucose from two reduced nicotinamide adenine dinucleotide (NADH) molecules. Cells that contain few mitochondria (e.g., fast-twitch muscle fibers; p. 251) or no mitochondria (i.e., erythrocytes) rely exclusively on anaerobic glycolysis for energy. In mixed skeletal muscle (p. 252), glycolysis can support the high energy demand of rhythmic contractions for only a few minutes at most, because glycolysis is quite inefficient compared with the aerobic regeneration of ATP.

In 1861, Pasteur recognized that glycolysis by yeast occurs faster in anaerobic conditions than in aerobic conditions. This **Pasteur effect** reflects the cell's attempt to maintain a constant $[ATP]_i$ by controlling the rate at which glycolysis breaks down glucose to generate ATP. The key is the **allosteric regulation** of enzymes that catalyze the three reactions in the glycolytic pathway that are essentially irreversible: hexokinase, phosphofructokinase, and pyruvate kinase (Fig. 57–7). In each case, either the direct reaction product (i.e., G6P in the case of hexokinase) or downstream metabolic products (e.g. ATP in the case of the other two) inhibit the enzyme. If glycolysis should temporarily outstrip the cell's need for ATP, the buildup of products slows down glycolysis. The basis of the Pasteur effect thus becomes more clear: introducing O_2 activates the citric acid cycle, which, as we shall see, raises $[ATP]_i$, inhibiting phosphofructokinase and pyruvate kinase, and slowing glycolysis.

Under anaerobic conditions, cells may convert pyruvate to lactate, accompanied by the accumulation of H^+ (**lactic acidosis**). The decreased muscle-cell pH impedes force generation by inhibiting both certain enzymes that regulate cross-bridge turnover and certain key glycolytic enzymes that are needed for ATP synthesis. Thus, sustained skeletal-muscle activity must depend on the aerobic metabolism of pyruvate.

The Second Step in Triglyceride Catabolism is the β Oxidation of Fatty Acids

β oxidation is a multi-step process that removes a two-carbon fragment from the end of an acyl coenzyme A (**acyl CoA**; i.e., the fatty-acid chain coupled to CoA), releasing the fragment as an acetyl CoA (Fig. 57–8, lower right). The process also releases one $FADH_2$, one NADH, and the remainder of the acyl chain (beginning with the original "β" carbon), which serves as the starting

point for the next cycle. β oxidation continues until it consumes the entire fatty acid chain. For a fatty-acid chain containing n carbons, the number of cycles is $([n/2]-1)$. The final cycle generates two acetyl CoA molecules. Unlike the breakdown of glucose, which can yield ATP even in the absence of O_2 (via glycolysis), the catabolism of free fatty acids yields energy only in the presence of O_2.

The Final Common Pathway in the Complete Oxidation of Carbohydrates, Triglycerides, and Proteins Is the Citric Acid Cycle and Oxidative Phosphorylation

Under aerobic conditions, cells containing mitochondria typically convert most of the pyruvate they generate from carbohydrate metabolism to acetyl CoA, rather than lactate. Pyruvate—a three-carbon piece of glucose's carbon skeleton—moves from the cytoplasm into the mitochondrial matrix (Fig. 57–9). There, pyruvate is oxidatively decarboxylated to **acetyl CoA**, releasing CO_2 as well as an NADH. Acetyl CoA also forms in the mitochondria as the end product of the β oxidation of fatty acids, as well as amino-acid breakdown. The metabolism of the acetate moiety of acetyl CoA, as well as the oxidation of NADH and $FADH_2$, is the final common pathway of **aerobic catabolism**, releasing CO_2, H_2O, ATP, and heat.

CITRIC ACID CYCLE. Acetyl CoA—representing a two-carbon fragment of glucose, a fatty acid, or an amino acid—enters the citric-acid-cycle phase of catabolism, also called "internal respiration" (p. 594) or "oxidative decarboxylation" because the two-carbon fragment ends up as two CO_2 molecules (Fig. 57–9). The citric acid cycle conserves the liberated energy as GTP and the reduced electron carriers NADH and $FADH_2$.

Cells tightly control the citric acid cycle by three *mechanisms* that limit substrate flux through the citric acid cycle: substrate availability, product accumulation, and feedback inhibition of key enzymes. Cells regulate the citric acid cycle at four *sites*. The two entry-point enzymes, pyruvate dehydrogenase and citrate synthase, are the most important. **Pyruvate dehydrogenase** is inhibited allosterically by two of its immediate products (NADH and acetyl CoA) and one downstream product (ATP). The second primary site of regulation in the citric acid cycle is **citrate synthase**, which is under feedback inhibition of a downstream product (ATP). The citrate produced in this reaction feeds back negatively on phosphofructokinase, as discussed earlier, effectively coupling glycolysis and oxidative metabolism (see Fig. 57–7). Two other enzymes, isocitrate dehydrogenase and α-ketoglutarate dehydrogenase, may also be rate limiting for the citric acid cycle under the right conditions.

Oxidative phosphorylation is the process by which mitochondria retrieve energy from $FADH_2$ and NADH. These reduced nucleotides are products of glycolysis (see Fig. 57–7), β oxidation (see Fig. 57–8) conversion of pyruvate to acetyl CoA (see Fig. 57–9), and the citric acid cycle. Oxidative phosphorylation involves the transfer of electrons along a chain of molecules, ultimately trapping the releasing energy in the formation of 1.5 ATP

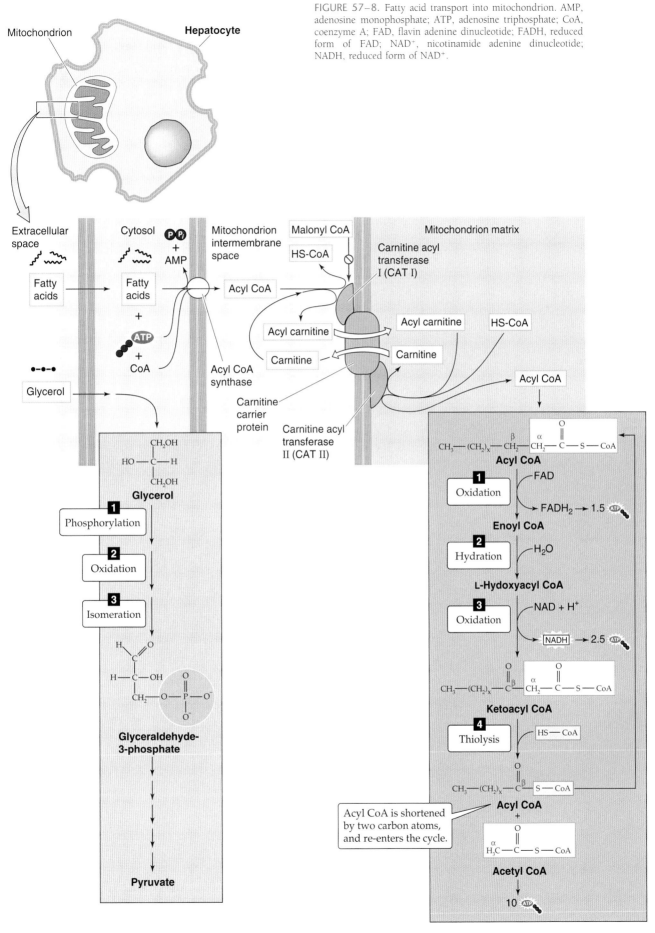

FIGURE 57–8. Fatty acid transport into mitochondrion. AMP, adenosine monophosphate; ATP, adenosine triphosphate; CoA, coenzyme A; FAD, flavin adenine dinucleotide; FADH, reduced form of FAD; NAD⁺, nicotinamide adenine dinucleotide; NADH, reduced form of NAD⁺.

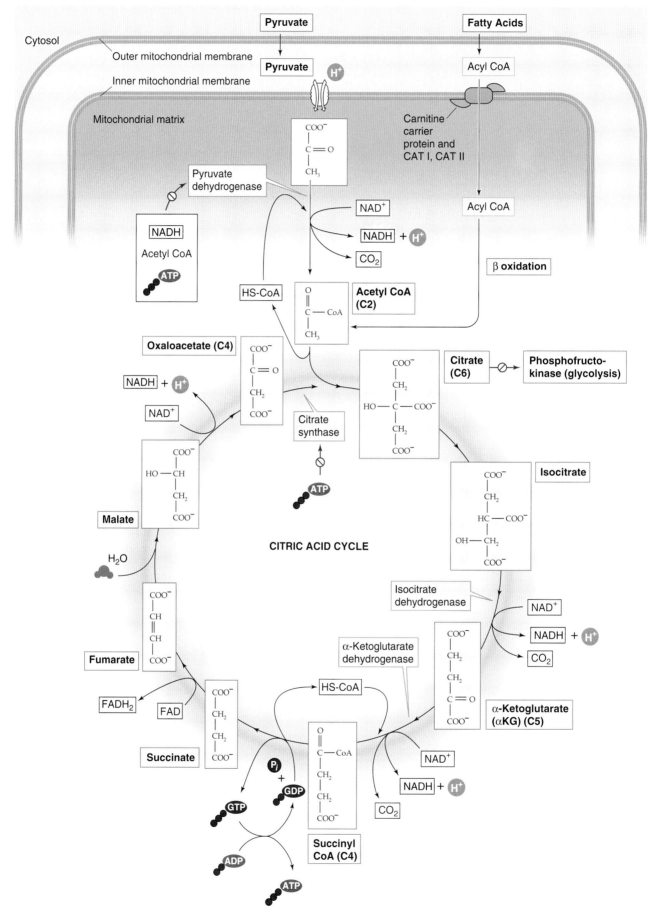

FIGURE 57–9. Citric acid cycle. ADP, adenosine diphosphate; ATP, adenosine triphosphate; CoA, coenzyme A; FAD, flavin adenine dinucleotide; FADH₂, reduced form of FAD; GDP, guanosine diphosphate; GTP, guanosine triphosphate; NAD⁺, nicotinamide adenine dinucleotide, NADH, reduced form of NAD⁺.

TABLE 57–2

GENERATION OF ATP FROM THE COMPLETE OXIDATION OF GLUCOSE*

Glycolysis $\xrightarrow{\text{direct}}$	2 ATP
Glycolysis → 2 × 1 NADH $\xrightarrow{\text{Ox. Phos.}}$	3 or 5 ATP
2 × (Pyruvate → acetyl-CoA) → 2 NADH $\xrightarrow{\text{Ox. Phos.}}$	5 ATP
Citric acid cycle → 2 × 1 GTP $\xrightarrow{\text{direct}}$	2 ATP
Citric acid cycle → 2 × 3 = 6 NADH $\xrightarrow{\text{Ox. Phos.}}$	15 ATP
Citric acid cycle → 2 × 1 = 2 FADH$_2$ $\xrightarrow{\text{Ox. Phos.}}$	3 ATP
Total:	30 or 32 ATP per glucose

*The calculation in this table assumes that the oxidative phosphorylation of each NADH molecule produced in the cytosol (row 2) will yield 1.5 or 2.5 ATP molecules, depending on which shuttle system that the cell uses to transfer the reducing equivalents from the cytosol into the mitochondria. The calculation also assumes that the oxidative phosphorylation of each NADH produced in the mitochondria (rows 3 and 5) yields 2.5 ATPs, and the oxidative phosphorylation of each FADH$_2$ produced in the mitochondria (row 6) yields 1.5 ATPs.

ATP, adenosine triphosphate; FADH$_2$, reduced flavin adenine dinucleotide; GTP, guanosine triphosphate; NADH, reduced nicotinamide adenine dinucleotide; ox. phos., oxidative phosphorylation.

molecules per FADH$_2$ and 2.5 ATP molecules per NADH (see Fig. 3–9).

Oxidizing Different Fuels Yields Similar Amounts of Energy Per Unit O$_2$ Consumed

The complete oxidation of different energy sources (i.e., carbohydrate, lipid, protein) in a bomb calorimeter may yield different amounts of energy. The source with the greatest energy density (kcal/g) is saturated fatty acid chains, which have a high density of the carbon and hydrogen oxidized to CO$_2$ and H$_2$O. Accordingly, the complete combustion of 1 g of an energy-rich fuel (i.e.,

lipid) requires more O$_2$. However, the energy yield per O$_2$ is similar among fuels, because about the same amount of O$_2$ is needed to oxidize each carbon and hydrogen. The energy yield per unit of O$_2$ is only slightly greater for carbohydrate (5.0 kcal/liter of O$_2$) than lipid (4.7 kcal/liter O$_2$). Carbohydrate, with its greater energy yield per O$_2$, is the body's preferred fuel for combustion during maximal exercise when O$_2$ availability is limiting. However, fat is the preferred fuel during prolonged activity, when O$_2$ is available and fuel sources are abundant.

Cells are not interested in how much *total* energy is in a molecule but how much *free* energy they can trap as ATP. In the case of glucose catabolism, complete oxidation of 1 molecule of glucose to CO$_2$ and H$_2$O via oxidative metabolism traps 30 or 32 molecules of ATP (Table 57–2). The efficiency of *aerobic* catabolism is far greater than that of *anaerobic* catabolism (a net of 30 or 32 vs. only 2 molecules of ATP per molecule of glucose), conserving approximately 60% of the potential energy of glucose for later use.

In the case of fatty-acid metabolism (see Fig. 57–8), each cycle of β oxidation yields a total of 14 ATP molecules (Table 57–3). The total number of ATP molecules generated from a fatty acid depends on the number of carbon atoms in the fatty-acid chain. For example, palmitic acid, a 16-carbon fatty acid, needs seven β oxidation cycles to form eight acetyl CoA molecules. The seven cycles generate 7 × 14 = 98 ATPs. The left-over acetyl CoA represents an additional 10, for a total of 108 ATPs. Because the initial activation of the palmitate to palmitoyl CoA involves converting an ATP to AMP plus pyrophosphate—and regenerating ATP from AMP requires forming two high-energy phosphate bonds—the net ATP production is 108 − 2 = 106 ATPs per palmitate oxidized.

Table 57–4 provides the energy equivalents of the primary fuel sources as well as the **respiratory quotient** (RQ), or ratio of moles of CO$_2$ produced per mole of O$_2$ consumed at the tissue level, for each. The RQ is merely the consequence of the density of oxygen atoms in the fuel source. For example, with carbohydrates, the cell needs to supply only enough external O$_2$ to oxidize the carbon atoms to CO$_2$. The H$_2$O is already built in to the carbohydrate molecule, which has an H-to-O ratio of 2 to 1.

TABLE 57–3

GENERATION OF ATP IN ONE CYCLE OF β OXIDATION OF A FATTY ACID*

(Acyl CoA → Enoyl CoA) → 1 FADH$_2$ $\xrightarrow{\text{Ox. Phos.}}$	1.5 ATP
(L-Hydroxyacyl CoA → Ketoacyl CoA) → 1 NADH $\xrightarrow{\text{Ox. Phos.}}$	2.5 ATP
1 Acetyl CoA → Citric acid cycle $\xrightarrow{\text{direct}}$ 1 GTP →	1 ATP
Citric acid cycle → 3 NADH $\xrightarrow{\text{Ox. Phos.}}$	7.5 ATP
Citric acid cycle → 1 FADH$_2$ $\xrightarrow{\text{Ox. Phos.}}$	1.5 ATP
Total:	14 ATP per cycle

*The above calculation assumes that oxidative phosphorylation generates 2.5 ATP/NADH, and 1.5 ATP/FADH$_2$.

TABLE 57–4

ENERGY EQUIVALENTS OF THE MAJOR FOODSTUFFS		
	ENERGY YIELD (kcal/g)	**RESPIRATORY QUOTIENT**
Carbohydrate	4.1	1.00
Protein	4.3	0.80–0.85
Lipid	9.4	0.70

Carbohydrate Oxidation

Equation 57–3

$C_6H_{12}O_6$ + 6 O_2 + 30 or 32 ADP + 30 or 32 P_i ⟶
Glucose

6 CO_2 + 6 H_2O + 30 or 32 ATP + heat
$RQ = 6\ CO_2/6\ O_2 = 1.00$

However, because lipids contain so many fewer oxygen atoms, more external O_2 is needed to oxidize both carbon and hydrogen atoms:

Lipid oxidation:

Equation 57–4

$C_{15}H_{31}COOH$ + 23 O_2 + 106 ADP + 106 P_i ⟶
Palmitic acid

16 CO_2 + 16 H_2O + 106 ATP + heat
$RQ = 16\ CO_2/23\ O_2 = 0.70$

The RQ for protein oxidation is 0.80–0.85.

Protein oxidation constitutes a very minor fraction of the total fuel oxidation in any tissue. Certain tissues (e.g., brain) use carbohydrate nearly exclusively and have an RQ of 1.0. Most tissues oxidize both carbohydrate and fat, and the RQ reflects this mixture. The whole-body RQ is approximately 0.8 for people eating a typical Western diet; individuals with less lipid intake have a higher RQ (i.e., approaching the value of 1 for carbohydrates).

NUTRITIONAL REQUIREMENTS

There Is No Absolute Daily Requirement for Carbohydrate or Fat Intake

Nutritionists recommend that the daily intake of carbohydrate versus fat should not differ with age, gender, or activity level. Of the total caloric intake in a Western diet, 55% to 60% is typically carbohydrate, 25% to 30% is fat, and the remaining 10% to 15% is protein.

The requirements for **total** caloric intake vary among individuals and depend on a number of factors, including a person's ability to use and store energy (efficiency) and the daily activity level. Differences in the efficiency of energy use among individuals are due in part to variations in muscle mass but also to genetic factors. Because adipose tissue has a low metabolic rate, people with a

large fat mass require less caloric intake per kg of body weight. Stated differently, the requirement for energy intake is greater per kg of *lean* body mass than per kg of *total* body mass (which includes fat). Thus, men generally require a greater daily caloric intake per kg of body weight than do women, who have relatively less muscle and more fat.

Activity level is the primary factor determining the daily energy requirement, assuming a stable body weight. For example, in a steady state, athletes must consume more than nonathletes not only because of a higher muscle-fat ratio but also because of a higher energy expenditure. Manual labor necessitates a greater energy intake than does sedentary activity, again to maintain energy balance and body weight. Excess intake over output causes weight gain over time. Using the conversion of 9.4 kcal/g, one kg of fat stores 9400 kcal, sufficient energy to carry the BMR for 4 days.

Eating a low-carbohydrate diet (e.g., the Atkins diet) leads to an accelerated breakdown of tissue protein, and thus to the wasting of muscle and other vital tissues, as well as the breakdown of fat. The breakdown of both protein and fat leads to an accumulation of ketone bodies in the blood (from the conversion of amino acids and fatty acids to acetyl CoA).

In addition to serving as a source of energy, fatty acids are also important for membrane structure (p. 10), as well as signal transduction by pathways such as those involving diacylglycerols (p. 100) and arachidonic acid (p. 103). In mammalian cells, fatty acid synthase produces two major fatty acids: palmitic and oleic acids. Palmitic acid, which has 16 carbons and is fully saturated, is referred to as 16:0. Oleic acid has 18 carbons and a single *cis* double bond between carbons 9 and 10. This unsaturated fatty acid is referred to as 18:1 *cis*-Δ^9. Because mammals cannot insert double bonds beyond carbon 9, they need two fatty acids in the diet: linoleate (18:2 *cis*-Δ^9 Δ^{12}) and linolenate (18:3 *cis*-Δ^9 Δ^{12} Δ^{15}). These **essential fatty acids** serve as precursors for other unsaturated fatty acids, including arachidonic acid, which is a precursor to prostaglandins, leukotrienes, and thromboxanes.

The current recommendations favoring low-fat intake are based on the view that a high fat intake is associated with chronic diseases such as atherosclerosis and non–insulin-dependent diabetes (see box on p. 1073). However, fats have a positive side. In addition to the roles we have discussed in this chapter, fats enhance satiety and aid in the absorption of certain vitamins (p. 960). Finally, the so-called ω-3 polyunsaturated fatty acids—in which the first double bond is three carbons from the terminal methyl group (or "ω carbon")—appear to protect against cardiovascular disease and some forms of cancer.

The Daily Protein Requirement for Adult Humans Is Typically 0.8 g/kg Body Weight, but Is Higher in Pregnant Women, Postsurgical Patients, and Athletes

The diet must contain the nine essential amino acids (see Table 57–1) because the body cannot synthesize them (see Chapter 45). Eleven other amino acids are necessary for protein synthesis, but the body can synthesize their carbon skeletons from intermediates of carbohydrate metabolism. **Vegetarian diets** can meet the protein needs of the body, provided the protein contains adequate amounts of essential amino acids. Food protein is "scored" based on its content of essential amino acids, compared with that of a reference protein, usually egg protein, which is given a score of 100. For example, a food containing protein with a score of 40 for threonine, 80 for phenylalanine, and 100 for lysine—all three of which are essential amino acids—receives a protein score of 40 because, relative to the standard, threonine is present in the lowest amount.

Protein intake is most important to meet the needs for tissue maintenance and repair, for muscle and neural function, and to maintain host defense mechanisms. The daily requirement for protein intake depends on one's nutritional status. The average human needs approximately 0.6 g of protein per kg of body weight per day to maintain nitrogen balance. The recommended dietary allowance (RDA) of protein is approximately 0.8 g/kg of body weight for adults, approximately 1 g/kg for adolescents, and approximately 2 g/kg in the first 6 months of life. Pregnant and lactating women require extra protein intake to ensure adequate fetal development and milk production. Athletes require more than 1 g/kg to maintain a greater lean body mass and to fuel a highly active metabolism. Well-balanced but larger meals usually provide adequate protein for those with a greater need. Burn victims, patients recovering from surgery, and patients with disorders of protein absorption all require increased daily protein intake.

The distribution of amino acids required for protein accretion by growing infants and children is different than that for tissue maintenance. Moreover, the requirements change throughout development. The child uses 25% of amino-acid intake for protein accretion at 6 months of age but only 10% by 18 months of age. Over 40% of a child's protein intake must consist of essential amino acids versus only 20% for an adult.

Proteins play a key role in host defenses. For example, proteins provide the structural backbone for skin and mucus. Protein synthesis is essential for phagocytes and lymphocytes that are responsible for antibody and cell-mediated immunity. The skin, lungs, and intestinal tract are the main structural defenses against invading organisms. In both the lungs and the GI tract, mucus (containing glycoproteins) coats the surface of these passageways and aids in defending against disease by catching most foreign particles. Protein-depleted individuals, regardless of age, have impaired immune competence. Protein depletion limits the availability of amino acids for synthesis of the cellular proteins of the immune system, including glutathione, mucus glycoproteins, and metallothreonine. The acute-phase response to invading organisms is suboptimal in a protein-deficient state.

The impaired immune competence of AIDS patients is a function of poor nutrition in addition to the effects of the virus itself. During infection, the body mobilizes amino acids to synthesize proteins for defense against invading organisms. Thus, improving protein and energy intake may be beneficial for some AIDS patients.

Aside from being the backbone of proteins, amino acids play a variety of physiologic roles. For example, arginine is a precursor to **nitric oxide** (p. 110). Glutamate is a major **excitatory neurotransmitter** in the brain (p. 307), whereas glycine is a major **inhibitory neurotransmitter** (p. 308). Glutamine is a major source of NH_3 **production** in the kidney (p. 854) and also regulates **protein turnover** in muscle. The decrease in muscle glutamine concentration that occurs during trauma and infection is associated with a general decline of muscle function. Research on anorectic patients shows that the most important factor affecting muscle function is insufficient nutrient intake. Increasing total nutrient intake in these subjects by total parenteral nutrition increases muscle function before having a measurable effect on muscle mass.

TABLE 57–5

ESSENTIAL MINERALS

MINERAL	ROLE	RDA
Ca	Bone (p. 1086), intracellular signaling (p. 102)	800–1200 mg
Cr	Possibly a cofactor in metabolism of carbohydrates, protein, lipids	50–200 μg
Cu	Enzyme cofactor (e.g., superoxide dismutase)	1.5–3 mg
Fe	Hemoglobin and cytochromes (p. 655 and 986)	Male: 10 mg Female (child bearing age): 15 mg
I	Thyroid hormones (p. 1035)	150 μg
Mg	Complexes with ATP (p. 972)	Male: ~350 mg Female: ~280 mg
Mn	Antioxidant	2–5 mg
Mo	Cofactor in carbon, nitrogen, and sulfur metabolism	75–250 μg
P	Bone (p. 1088)	800–1000 mg
Se	Antioxidant	Male: 70 μg Female: 55 μg
Zn	Antioxidant Enzyme cofactor (p. 126 & box on p. 637)	Male: 15 mg Female: 12 mg

RDA, recommended dietary allowance.

Minerals and Vitamins Are Not Energy Sources, but Are Necessary for Certain Enzymatic Reactions, for Protein Complexes, or as Precursors for Biomolecules

Vitamins and minerals do not provide energy but are essential for such functions as metabolism, immune competence, muscle-force production, and blood clotting.

MINERALS. Table 57–5 lists the essential minerals. The current recommendations for daily mineral intake are based on a mix of "balance studies" and usual dietary intakes in the United States. The recommendation for copper, for example, is based on balance studies, whereas

those for manganese, chromium, and molybdenum are based on dietary intakes.

Assigning daily mineral intakes is problematic because some methods of determining mineral status do not always expose functional deficiencies. For example, a frank deficiency in calcium intake leads to bone loss even though blood calcium levels remain normal. Iron deficiency is difficult to detect because no clinical signs appear until iron stores are depleted. It is difficult to base recommendations simply on absorption because, for some minerals, absorption varies with intake. For example, copper deficiency or toxicity is unlikely in humans because absorption is *inversely* related to intake. Furthermore, in-

TABLE 57–6

VITAMINS			
MINERAL	**ROLE**	**RDA**	**DEFICIENCY**
A	Retinal pigment	Male: 1000 μg Female: 800 μg	Follicular hyperkeratosis, night blindness
B$_1$ (thiamine)	Coenzyme in decarboxylation of pyruvate and α-keto acids	Male: 1.5 mg Female: 1.1 mg	Beriberi
B$_2$ (riboflavin)	Coenzymes FAD and FMN, H carriers in mitochondria	Male: 1.7 mg Female: 1.3 mg	Hyperemia of nasopharyngeal mucosa, normocytic anemia
B$_3$ niacin (nicotinic acid)	Coenzymes NAD and NADP, H carriers in mitochondria	Male: 19 mg Female: 15 mg	Pellagra
B$_6$ (pyridoxine)	Coenzyme in transmination for synthesis of amino acids	Male: 2 mg Female: 1.6 mg	Stomatitis, glossitis, normocytic anemia
B$_{12}$ (cobalamin)	Coenzyme in reduction of ribonucleotides to deoxyribonucleotides. Promotes formation of erythrocytes, myelin (p. 970)	2 μg	Pernicious anemia (a megaloblastic anemia)
C (ascorbic acid)	Coenzyme in formation of hydroxyproline used in collagen	60 mg	Scurvy
D (1,25-cholecalciferol)	Ca^{2+} absorption (p. 1096)	5–10 μg	Rickets
E (α-tocopherol)	Antioxidant: thought to prevent oxidation of unsaturated fatty acids	Male: 10 mg Female: 8 mg	Peripheral neuropathy
K (K$_1$ = phylloquinone, K$_2$ = various menaquinones)	Clotting: necessary for synthesis by liver of prothrombin and factors VII, IX and X	Male: 70–80 μg Female: 60–65 μg	Hemorrhagic disease
Folate	Backbone used to synthesize purines and thymine (p. 967)	Male: 200 μg Female: 180 μg Pregnancy: 400 μg	Megaloblastic anemia
Biotin	Coenzyme in carboxylation reactions	30–100 μg*	Neurologic changes
Pantothenic acid	Coenzyme A (CoA). Necessary for carbohydrate and fat metabolism involving acetyl-CoA; amino acid synthesis	4–7 mg*	Abdominal pain, vomiting, neurologic signs

*Safe and allowable range.

FAD, flavin adenine dinucleotide; FMN, flavin mononucleotide; NAD, nicotinamide adenine dinucleotide; RDA, recommended dietary allowance.

teractions among minerals must be taken into account when establishing recommendations.

The goal is to base recommendations on scientific evidence. Radioisotopes can be used to monitor storage, absorption, and excretion. Another approach is to establish the physiologic role of the mineral and then determine the mineral intake required for maintaining that physiologic role. However, because of redundancy in function, it is often difficult to assess which mineral is deficient when function is compromised. For example, both iron and copper are involved in energy metabolism at the level of the electron transport chain. The blood clotting cascade involves calcium, copper, and vitamin K. Zinc, selenium, and manganese all have antioxidant activities.

VITAMINS. Even though vitamins are not energy sources themselves, they play an integral role as cofactors in many metabolic processes. Some vitamins are involved in group-transfer reactions, such as decarboxylations and carboxylations in fatty-acid and glucose metabolism, and transaminations in amino-acid metabolism. Vitamins act as oxidizing and reducing agents in the generation of ATP, as well as antioxidants to quench free radicals produced as a byproduct of oxidation.

Of the 13 identified vitamins, RDAs have been established for 11 (Table 57–6). Safe and allowable ranges are estimated for the remaining two—biotin and pantothenic acid. Recommendations differ widely among countries. Lower recommendations are generally based on scientific evidence. For each vitamin, a person's nutritional *status* falls into one of five categories: deficient, marginal, satisfactory, excessive, and toxic. Although "marginal" and "excessive" are not usually associated with overt clinical signs, people whose vitamin status falls into one of these categories are at increased risk for various diseases.

In the past, recommendations for the intake of vitamins and minerals was based largely on levels necessary to promote normal growth and development. However, the role of vitamins and minerals in optimizing body function and promoting longevity is becoming an area of intense interest both to researchers and to the general public. Older people generally have a less vigorous immune response than do young people, in large part because of deficiencies in iron, zinc, and vitamin C. Correcting these improves immune competence significantly. In addition, older people with poor dietary habits may have inadequate intake of calcium, vitamin D, and other nutrients involved in bone deposition and strength (see Chapter 51), putting them at greater risk for hip fracture.

Mineral deficiencies usually do not occur without extreme abnormalities in diet, and even then, a mineral deficiency may not impair function (see Table 57–5). However, deficiencies of almost every vitamin can cause functional impairment (see Table 57–6).

Excessive Intake of Vitamins and Minerals Has Mixed Effects on Bodily Function

A current controversy surrounds the use of so-called "mega-doses" of certain vitamins and minerals. Such excessive intake has mixed effects. Slight excesses of vita-

mins A and E, zinc, and selenium are associated with an enhanced immune response, especially for burn, trauma, and sepsis patients. In these conditions, "excess" intake may not be an excess at all but rather the intake that meets the greater need. Increased intake of fruits and vegetables—which contain a variety of vitamins as well as "fiber"—clearly decreases the risk of various cancers. However, efforts to link these effects specifically to dietary carotenoid levels have failed to show a correlation; indeed, the excessive intake of β-carotene supplements may even increase the risk of some cancers. Antioxidants (e.g., β-carotene, vitamins C and E) quench peroxyl radicals, suppress tumor growth, and decrease atherosclerotic lesions in rabbits. Enhanced vitamin E intake lowers the risk for coronary heart disease, by nearly one half.

The excessive intake of certain minerals and vitamins may compromise the immune response. Excess vitamin E intake in infants may increase the risk of infection, possibly by quenching superoxide radicals that are important for killing bacteria. Excess lipids can impair the immune response, too. A high intake of saturated and polyunsaturated fatty acids leads to decreases in cell-mediated immunity. Excessive calcium intake interferes with the ability to use iron, zinc, and magnesium, while high dietary copper affects zinc absorption and excretion.

Because the kidneys readily excrete water-soluble vitamins in the urine, toxicity from excessive intake is not common. Because fat-soluble vitamins are not easily excreted in the urine, it is easier to develop toxicity for these vitamins. In particular, polar-bear liver, a component of the Inuit diet, contains extraordinarily high levels of vitamin A (35,000 IU/g vs. the RDA of 5000 IU), which can lead to acute hypervitaminosis A and death.

REGULATION OF FOOD INTAKE

It is the balance between food intake and energy expenditure that determines overall body weight. Food intake is primarily under the control of the hypothalamus, although higher CNS centers and other areas also play roles. Hypothalamic centers respond to two major kinds of afferent input: short-term factors that reflect daily meal activity and long-term factors that reflect whole-body energy stores.

Hypothalamic Centers Control the Sensations of Satiety and Hunger

Classic studies—in which investigators made lesions in, or electrically stimulated, specific brain regions—identified two areas in the hypothalamus that are important for controlling eating. The "**satiety center**" is located in the ventromedial nucleus (VMN; see Fig. 46–3). Electrical stimulation of the satiety center elicits sensations of satiety, even when an animal is in the presence of food. Conversely, a lesion of the satiety center causes continuous food intake (*hyperphagia*) even in the absence of

TABLE 57–7

HYPOTHALAMIC FACTORS THAT CONTROL APPETITE	
ANOREXIGENIC (INHIBIT FEEDING)	**OREXIGENIC (STIMULATE FEEDING)**
Corticotropin-releasing hormone (CRH)	Neuropeptide Y (NPY)
Glucagon-like peptide I (GLP-I)	Norepinephrine (NE)
α-Melanocyte-stimulating hormone (α-MSH)	Gamma-aminobutyric acid (GABA)
Cocaine- and amphetamine-regulated transcript (CART)	Galanin (GAL)
	Ghrelin
	Endogenous opioid peptides (EOP)
	Orexin-A, -B

Modified from Kalra SP, Dube MG, Pu S, et al: Interacting appetite-regulating pathways in the hypothalamic regulation of body weight. *Endocr Rev* 20:68–100, 1999.

need. The **hunger** (or feeding) **center** is located in the lateral hypothalamic area (LHA) (see Fig. 46–3). Electrical stimulation of the LHA elicits a voracious appetite, even after the animal has ingested adequate amounts of food. A lesion of the hunger center causes a complete and lasting cessation of food intake (*aphagia*).

A vast array of neurotransmitters within the hypothalamus appear to modulate food intake. These neurotransmitters fall into two major groups (Table 57–7). Injecting orexigenic (Greek *orexis*, "appetite") substances stimulates feeding, whereas injecting anorexigenic substances into the brain inhibits feeding. Investigators have identified areas within the hypothalamus that synthesize these neurotransmitters or store them in relatively high concentrations. Other studies have identified and localized receptors for these neurotransmitters. However, these molecular-localization studies have not yet led to a wiring diagram for the hypothalamic neurons that regulate appetite. In general, orexigenic factors are associated with the LHA (hunger center), whereas anorexigenic factors are associated with the VMN (satiety center).

Among the **orexigenic factors** (Fig. 57–10), neuropeptide Y (NPY) appears to play a central role. NPY-containing neurons in the arcuate nucleus project to the paraventricular nucleus, which makes corticotropin-releasing hormone (CRH). Exciting new orexigenic factors are the peptides orexin A and orexin B, which are present in neurons in the LHA. The orexin receptor is G-protein linked and signals the cell by opening Ca^{2+} channels and raising $[Ca^{2+}]_i$. Consistent with their roles as orexigenic factors, both NPY and prepro-orexin mRNA levels increase with fasting. Among the **anorexigenic factors**, one of the most important seems to be CRH (p. 1054), which is made in the paraventricular nucleus of the hypothalamus. A recent addition to the list of anorexigenic factors is a peptide called "cocaine- and amphetamine-regulated

transcript" (CART). Food deprivation decreases mRNA levels of CART in the arcuate nucleus.

Short-Term Factors That Regulate Feeding Include Plasma "Nutrient" Levels and Gastrointestinal Hormones Such as Cholecystokinin

Investigators have proposed various theories to explain the *short-term* regulation of food intake, including models focusing on the regulation of levels of blood glucose (glucostatic), amino acids (aminostatic), or lipid (lipostatic). For example, hypoglycemia produces hunger and also increases the firing rate of glucose-sensitive neurons in the hunger center, but decreases the firing rate of glucose-sensitive neurons in the satiety center. Hypoglycemia also activates orexin-containing neurons in the LHA.

Feedback from the GI tract also controls the short-term desire for food (Fig. 57–10). GI distention triggers vagal afferents that suppress the hunger center. Peripherally administering any of several "GI peptides" normally released in response to a meal—gastrin-releasing peptide (GRP), glucagon, somatostatin, and cholecystokinin (CCK)—reduces meal size. The most important is CCK, which is more effective when injected directly into the peritoneal cavity; this effect requires an intact vagus nerve. Therefore, CCK may act by stimulating vagal afferents, which then transmit the signal to the hypothalamus. Additionally, an oropharyngeal reflex responds to chewing and swallowing; it may meter food intake, inhibiting further eating after a threshold.

A Long-Term Factor That Suppresses Appetite Is Leptin, a Protein Secreted by Adipocytes That Binds to Hypothalamic Receptors

In addition to the short-term regulatory pathways, the body has long-term mechanisms for controlling hunger. One such long-term regulator is leptin, the plasma levels of which seem to reflect whole-body fat stores. Research on a strain of obese mice led to the discovery of the mutant *ob* gene that accounts for their obesity. The normal gene encodes a 167–amino-acid polypeptide hormone called **leptin** (Greek *leptos*, "thin"), which adipocytes produce. Mice that are homozygous (*ob/ob*) for a missense leptin mutation are severely obese, hyperphagic, and hypoactive. Administering leptin to ob/ob mice reverses the symptoms. Because leptin is particularly effective when injected directly into the brain, leptin secreted into the blood by adipocytes may feed back on the brain to produce satiety (see Fig. 57–10). In the brain, leptin binds to tyrosine-kinase–associated receptors (p. 111) and inhibits expression of NPY (orexigenic), but stimulates expression of CART (anorexigenic). Mice that are homozygous for a mutation that deletes a portion of the leptin *receptor* also become obese and are resistant to treatment with exogenous leptin.

Plasma leptin levels reflect total-body fat *stores* (i.e., a long-term signal). Over a wide range of body-fat mass, more fat is associated with higher plasma leptin levels. In

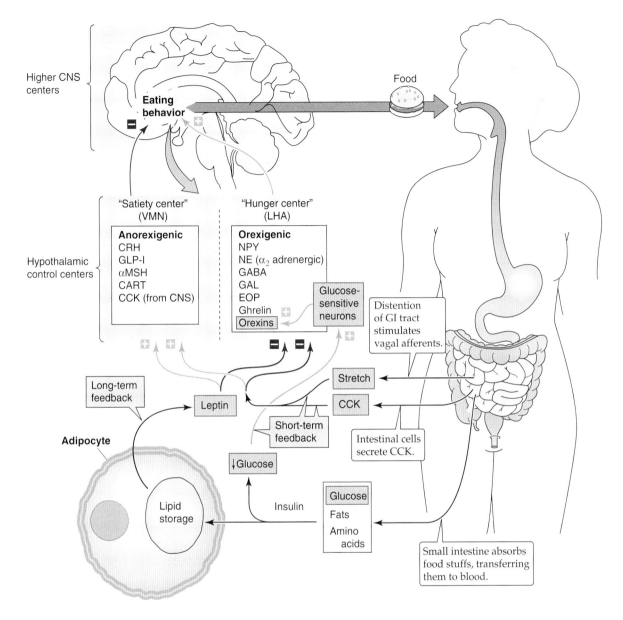

FIGURE 57–10. Control of appetite. Table 57–7 defines the abbreviations of the anorexigenic and orexigenic factors.

addition, leptin levels reflect the *fed/fasting state* (i.e., short-term signal). Thus, even in obese animals, which have high baseline leptin levels, fasting decreases plasma leptin levels.

Obesity Reflects a Chronic Excess of Energy Intake Over Expenditure

The regulation of food intake does not work effectively in everyone. **Obesity** is a condition in which energy intake exceeds energy output over time, and body fat becomes greater than 30% of ideal body weight. The development of obesity requires months and years to occur because the storage of one kg of fat represents an excess energy intake (over output) of 9,400 kcal. Because the average caloric

expenditure of a sedentary person is approximately 2100 kcal/day, a sedentary person ingesting an excess of 1000 kcal/day (i.e., a diet of 3100 kcal/day) would require 9 to 10 days to store 1 kg of fat.

Fat stores are not limited in the same manner as carbohydrate and protein stores. Adipocytes can increase in number (hyperplasia) or in size (hypertrophy) during the evolution of obesity. **Hyperplastic obesity** usually develops during the first few years of life and is maintained thereafter. The rate of formation of new adipocytes is greatest during these first years of life, and the absolute number of adipocytes becomes fixed during this period. Individuals who became obese in early childhood may not respond well to weight reduction regimes as adults, because the number of fat cells contributes in some way to the hypothalamic feedback control of fat storage. **Hypertrophic obesity**, in contrast, first occurs in adulthood and is most often associated with diabetes and other age-related metabolic alterations. Adult-onset obesity may be caused by a reduction in the hormone-sensitive lipase in adipose tissue, making it more difficult to mobilize the fat deposited there. Hormone-sensitive lipase activity depends on physical activity as well as factors associated with aging, so adult-onset obesity can be reversed by caloric restriction and increased activity.

In contrast to the *ob* mice, most obese humans produce large quantities of leptin but are insensitive to its effects. Thus, obese people may have defective leptin receptors, reduced numbers of leptin receptors, defective post-receptor signal transduction, or another factor that overrides the leptin satiety signal.

Obesity is probably a multifactorial condition, involving both genetic and environmental factors. For example, a significant proportion of obese patients scores high on tests for measuring mental depression. In addition, obese patients consistently underestimate the number of calories they consume each day. Because obesity is a major risk factor for major chronic diseases (e.g., cardiovascular disease, adult-onset diabetes, cancer), investigators have invested much effort searching for ways to minimize fat storage, especially in older people who are at greater risk.

Starvation Depletes Body Carbohydrate Stores Immediately, Fat Stores Thereafter, and Protein Stores Last

The average 70-kg adult uses approximately 2100 kcal/day to support resting metabolic needs. During starvation, all of this energy must come from body stores. The total energy stored as glycogen in liver and skeletal muscle is at most approximately 3000 kcal. The body uses this glycogen preferentially during starvation, depleting it within 1.5 days. The average 70-kg adult also has fat stores of approximately 131,000 kcal. Mobilization and subsequent oxidation of this entire fat depot could theoretically sustain the body's resting metabolic requirement for approximately 2 months. In addition, the body can mobilize about half of its protein store, representing another approximately 20,000 kcal, sufficient for an additional 10 days. In reality, people seldom survive for 2 months without nutrition (even assuming unlimited water availability), because vitamin deficiencies and their associated effects begin to appear after a week or two and compromise body function.

During starvation, fat becomes the fuel of choice once carbohydrate stores are expended. Fatty-acid oxidation continues at a constant rate throughout starvation. Ketone bodies form as a byproduct of fatty-acid oxidation during starvation and in diabetes mellitus (when lack of insulin

inhibits glucose utilization; see the box on diabetes mellitus on p. 1084). The liver releases the major keto-acids (acetoacetic and β-hydroxybutyric acid) into the circulation, thus lowering blood pH and creating a condition known as **ketoacidosis**. Acetone, another ketone produced by the liver, is eliminated in the expired air, accompanied by the fruity smell characteristic of ketosis. Ketone bodies can cross the blood-brain barrier and serve as the primary fuel for the CNS when glycogen stores are depleted and the only means for generating glucose is by transamination of amino acids (gluconeogenesis) in the liver.

Protein oxidation is rapid during the initial stage of starvation due to its use as a precursor for glucose in transamination reactions in the liver. Once easily mobilized protein has been consumed, the rate of gluconeogenesis falls markedly, and the body's protein stores are relatively conserved during starvation. Finally, during the latter stage of starvation, when the body has used most of its fat stores, protein becomes the only source of energy left, forcing the body to draw on these stores as a last gasp for survival.

REFERENCES

Books and Reviews

Auwerx J, Staels B: Leptin. Lancet. 351:737–742, 1998.

Hillgartner FB, Salati LM, AG Goodridge: Physiological and molecular mechanisms involved in nutritional regulation of fatty acid synthesis. Physiol Rev 75:47–76, 1995.

Jequier E, Tappy J: Regulation of body weight in humans. Physiol Rev 79:451–480, 1999.

Kalra SP, Dube MG, Pu S, et al: Interacting appetite-regulating pathways in the hypothalamic regulation of body weight. Endocrine Rev 20:68–100, 1999.

Koretsky AP: Insights into cellular energy metabolism from transgenic mice. Physiol Rev 75:667–688, 1995.

Shulman GI, Landau BR: Pathways of glycogen repletion. Physiol Rev 72:1019–1035, 1992.

Wilson JD, DW Foster, HM Kronenberg, Larsen PR (eds): Williams Textbook of Endocrinology, 9th ed. Philadelphia, WB Saunders, 1998.

Journal Articles

Kristensen P, Judge ME, Thim L, et al: Hypothalamic CART is a new anorectic peptide regulated by leptin. Nature 393:72–76, 1998.

Moriguchi T, Sakurai T, Nambu T, et al: Neurons containing orexin in the lateral hypothalamic area of the adult rat brain are activated by insulin-induced acute hypoglycemia. Neurosci Lett 264:101–104, 1999.

Pelleymounter MA, Cullen MJ, Baker MB, et al: Effects of the obese gene product on body weight regulation in *ob/ob* mice. Science 269:540–543, 1995.

Sakurai T, Amemiya A, Ishii M, et al: Orexins and orexin receptors: A family of hypothalamic neuropeptides and G protein-coupled receptors that regulate feeding behavior Cell. 92:573–585, 1998.

van den Pol AN, Gao XB, Obrietan K, et al: Presynaptic and postsynaptic actions and modulation of neuroendocrine neurons by a new hypothalamic peptide, hypocretin/orexin. J Neurosci 18:7962–7971, 1998.

CHAPTER 58

Regulation of Body Temperature

Ethan Nadel

HEAT AND TEMPERATURE: THE ADVANTAGES OF HOMEOTHERMY

Homeothermy Enables an Organism to Maintain Its Activity Over a Wide Range of Environmental Temperatures

The ability to regulate internal body temperature has provided higher organisms independence from the environment. Because the rates of most physical and chemical reactions depend on temperature, most physiological functions are sensitive to temperature changes. Thus, the activity levels of **poikilotherms** (species that do not regulate internal body temperature) by and large depend on environmental temperature, whereas those of **homeotherms** (species that do regulate internal body temperature) are relatively stable over a broad range of ambient conditions. A lizard, for example, is capable of relatively less movement away from its lair on a cold, overcast day than on a hot, sunny day, whereas a prairie dog may be equally mobile on either day. An arctic fox acclimatizes to the extreme cold of winter by growing a thick, insulating coat that enables it to resist body cooling and minimize the necessity to increase metabolic heat generation, which requires increased food intake.

The thermoregulatory mechanism of homeotherms creates an internal environment in which reaction rates are relatively high and optimal. At the same time, an effective thermoregulatory system avoids the pathologic consequences of wide deviations in body temperature (Table 58–1). The thermoregulatory system incorporates both anticipatory controls and negative-feedback controls. The components of this system are: (1) thermal sensors, (2) afferent pathways, (3) an integration system in the central nervous system (CNS), (4) efferent pathways, and (5) target organs that control heat generation and transfer, such as skeletal muscle (e.g., shivering to generate heat), circulation to the skin (to dissipate heat), and the sweat glands (to dissipate heat).

The focus of this chapter is temperature regulation in homeotherms. We examine the physical aspects of heat transfer both within the body and between body and environment, as well as the physiological mechanisms that are involved in altering the rates of transfer. Lastly, we look at the consequences of extreme challenges to the thermoregulatory mechanism, such as hypothermia and dehydration.

TABLE 58–1

CONSEQUENCES OF DEVIATIONS IN BODY TEMPERATURE	
TEMPERATURE (°C)	**CONSEQUENCE**
40–44	**Heat stroke, brain lesions**
38–40	**Fever or exercise**
36–38	**Normal range**
34–36	**Mild hypothermia**
30–34	**Impairment of temperature regulation**
27–29	**Cardiac fibrillation**

Body Core Temperature Depends on Time of Day, Physical Activity, Time in the Menstrual Cycle, and Age

Temperature scales are relative scales of heat content. The centigrade scale is divided into equal increments, referenced to the freezing (0°C) and boiling (100°C) points of water. The "normal" body temperature of an adult human is approximately 37°C (i.e., 98.6°F) but may be as low as 36°C or as high as 37.5°C in active, healthy people. "Body temperature" usually refers to the temperature of the body *core*, measured under the tongue (sublingually), in the ear canal, or in the rectum. For clinical purposes, the most reliable (although the least practical) among these three is the last, because it is least influenced by air temperature. Measurement devices range from traditional mercury-in-glass thermometers to electronic, digital read-out thermistors. Nearly all such instruments are accurate to 0.1°C.

Body core temperature depends on the time of day, the stage of the menstrual cycle in women, the level of the person's activity, and the individual's age.

All homeotherms maintain a circadian (24-h cycle) body-temperature rhythm, with variations of approximately 1°C. In humans, body temperature is usually lowest between 3:00 to 6:00 a.m., and peaks at 3:00 to 6:00 p.m. This circadian rhythmicity is inherent in the autonomic nervous system, independent of the sleep-wakefulness cycle, but entrained by light-dark cues to a 24-h cycle.

In many women, body temperature increases approximately 0.5°C during the post-ovulatory phase of the menstrual cycle (p. 1159). An abrupt increase in body temperature of 0.3°C to 0.5°C accompanies ovulation and may be useful as a fertility guide.

Physical activity generates excess heat as a byproduct of elevated metabolic rate. A portion of this excess heat remains in the body, causing core temperature to rise and triggering appropriate heat-loss responses. Core temperature remains elevated during activity and for an extended period during recovery.

Infants and older people are less able to maintain a "normal" body temperature than are the rest of the population, particularly in the face of an external challenge. Newborns do not readily shiver or sweat and thus are more like poikilotherms than like homeotherms. These properties, along with a high surface-to-mass ratio, render infants more susceptible to fluctuations in core temperature when exposed to a hot or cold environment. Older people are also subject to greater fluctuations in core temperature. Aging is associated with a progressive deficit in the ability to sense heat and cold, and also reduced ability to generate heat (reduced metabolic rate and metabolic potential due to lower muscle mass) and to dissipate heat (reduced cardiovascular reserve and sweat-gland atrophy from disuse).

The Body's Rate of Heat Production Can Vary From Approximately 80 kcal/h at Rest to 600 kcal/h During Jogging

The body's rate of heat production is closely linked to the rate of metabolism; minor variations occur depending on the mixture of fuels (foods) being oxidized. Because of their inherent inefficiency, metabolic transformations generate heat (p. 1212). Ultimately, all of the energy contained in fuels appears as either heat, mass storage/growth, or physical work done on the environment.

The body's metabolic rate, and thus its rate of heat production, is not constant. The **resting metabolic rate** (RMR; see p. 1211) is the rate necessary to maintain the functions of resting cells; these functions include active transport as well as cardiac and respiratory-muscle activity. Voluntary or involuntary (e.g., shivering) muscular activity adds to the overall metabolic heat production. Even digesting a meal increases the metabolic rate (p. 1215). An increase in tissue temperature itself raises the metabolic rate, according to the van't Hoff relation (i.e., a 10°C increase in tissue temperature more than doubles the metabolic rate). Furthermore, certain hormones, notably thyroxine and epinephrine, increase the cellular metabolic rate. Because the body's heat-production rate is variable, the rate of heat loss must match it if the body temperature is to remain constant.

Under sedentary (i.e., RMR) conditions, when the body's energy requirements are low, the rate of heat production is approximately 80 kcal/h (~90 watts) in an adult of average size. During physical exercise, the rate of energy production—and hence, heat generation—increases in proportion to the intensity of exercise. An average adult can comfortably sustain an energy-production rate of 400 to 600 kcal/h for extended periods (e.g., a fast walk or a modest jog). Nearly all of this increased heat generation occurs in active skeletal muscle, although a portion arises from increased cardiac and respiratory-muscle activity. A thermal load of this magnitude would raise core temperature by 1.0°C every 8 to 10 minutes if the extra heat could not escape the body. Physical activity would be limited to 25 to 30 minutes, at which time the effects of excessive hyperthermia (>40°C) would begin to impair body function. This impairment, of course, does not occur, primarily because of the efficiency of the thermoregulatory system. Within a relatively short period, the body increases its rate of heat dissipation to match heat production. Thereafter, the body maintains a new, elevated steady temperature until exercise ceases.

MODES OF HEAT TRANSFER

Heat Generated by Metabolism Moves from Heat Sources to the "Body Core" by Convection

In simplest analysis, the rate of heat transfer from any tissue to the blood depends on (1) the rate of tissue energy production, (2) temperature of the tissue, (3) temperature of the incoming blood, and (4) blood flow through the tissue.

Inactive skeletal muscle, for example, has a low blood flow and a correspondingly low rate of metabolism. The rate of O_2 consumption ($\dot{V}o_2$)—a measure of metabolic rate—averages 1.5 to 2.0 ml of O_2 consumed per minute for each kg muscle tissue. Because the temperature of resting muscle (33°C–35°C) is lower than that of the body core (i.e., 37°C), heat flows from arterial blood to inactive skeletal muscle. A similar analysis shows that heat moves from a highly active tissue such as the liver (~38°C) to the blood, which distributes the heat to the other tissues of the body core.

The body's greatest *potential* heat source is skeletal muscle, which has a relatively large mass and can increase its rate of heat production more than 100-fold. Because skeletal muscle has such potential, it is useful for modeling heat transfer and changes in tissue temperature (Fig. 58–1). The **energy balance equation** for skeletal muscle is:

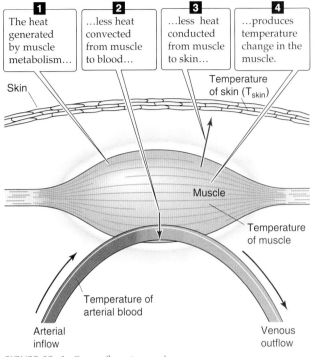

FIGURE 58–1. Energy flows in muscle.

Equation 58–1

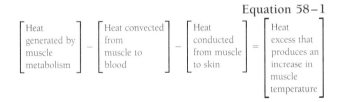

The three terms on the left describe all the heat that the muscle gains or loses. If they add up to a positive number, muscle temperature increases. In the steady state, these three terms add up to zero, and muscle temperature is stable.

During the onset of exercise, the heat produced by metabolism increases rapidly. If the three terms on the left side of the equation sum to a very positive number (implying a large energy excess), muscle temperature rises rapidly. However, the dramatic increase in the rate of warming is relatively short-lived because of two factors: (1) The increase in muscle temperature reverses the temperature gradient between muscle and the blood perfusing it, so that heat now flows from muscle to blood. (2) Muscle vascular resistance decreases and cardiac output increases rapidly (p. 583), so that blood flow through the muscle increases proportionally with the intensity of exercise. These adjustments are relatively complete within a few minutes. Increases of up to 30-fold in blood flow account for a proportional increase in heat transfer from active muscle to blood.

As exercise continues, muscle temperature increases to a new steady-state level, causing more heat transfer from muscle to blood. The result is an increase in core temperature as warm venous blood leaving the muscles enters the body core.

Heat Moves from the Body Core to the Skin, Primarily by Convection

Now that the blood has carried the excess heat away from active tissue, such as muscle, to the body core, we need to ask how the body prevents the core from overheating. The answer is that the core transfers this heat to a heat sink. The organ serving as the body's greatest potential heat sink is the relatively cool skin, which is the largest organ in the body. Only a minor amount of the body's generated heat flows *directly* from the body core to the skin by **conduction** across the body tissues. Most of the generated body heat flows to the skin by **convection** in the blood, and blood flow to the skin can increase markedly. Afterward, nearly all of the heat transferred to the skin must flow to the environment, facilitated by the skin's large surface area.

The transfer of heat from core to skin occurs by two routes:

Equation 58–2

FIGURE 58–2. Model of energy transfer from the body to environment.

tract. The evaporative rate is primarily a function of the rate of pulmonary ventilation (p. 686), which in turn increases linearly with the metabolic rate over a wide range of exercise intensities.

Heat Moves from the Skin to the Environment by Radiation, Conduction, Convection, and Evaporation

Figure 58–2 summarizes heat transfer from the body core to the skin, and between skin to environment. Heat transfer from skin to environment can occur by radiation, conduction, convection, and evaporation.

RADIATION. Heat transfer by radiation occurs between the skin and solid bodies in the environment. The infrared portion of the electromagnetic energy spectrum carries this energy, which is why infrared cameras can detect warm bodies at night. The body gains or loses heat by radiation at a rate that is proportional to the temperature difference between the skin and the radiating body:

Equation 58–3

Rate of radiative heat loss	*Radiative* heat-transfer coefficient	Mean skin temp	Radiant temp of another object	Body surface area available for *radiative* heat exchange
R	=	$H_{radiative}$	$\overbrace{(\overline{T}_{skin} - T_{radiant})}$	$A_{radiative}$
$\dfrac{kcal}{h}$		$\dfrac{kcal}{m^2 h\,°C}$	(°C)	(m^2)

Note that R is positive when the body loses heat and negative when it gains heat.

Radiative heat fluxes to and from the body are often subtle, particularly when the $T_{radiant}$ differs from the ambient environmental temperature ($T_{ambient}$). Indoors, $T_{radiant}$ is the same as $T_{ambient}$ because surrounding objects thermally equilibrate with one another. Outdoors, radiating bodies may be at widely different temperatures. The **radiant heat load** from the sun to the body on a summer day in the desert may exceed the RMR by a considerable amount. The radiant heat load from a fire or a radiant lamp can provide substantial warming of bodies in the radiant field. Conversely, on a winter evening, the **radiant heat loss** from the body to a cloudless, dark sky—which has a low radiant temperature—may exceed RMR. Thus, one may feel a sudden chill when walking past an uncurtained window. This chill is caused by the sudden fall in skin temperature owing to radiant heat loss. Radiation of heat from the body accounts for approximately 60% of heat lost when the body is at rest in a neutral thermal indoor environment. A **neutral thermal environment** is a set of conditions (air temperature, air flow and humidity, and temperatures of surrounding radiating surfaces) in which the temperature of the naked body does not change when the subject is "at rest" (i.e., RMR) and not shivering.

CONDUCTION. Heat transfer by conduction occurs when the body touches a solid material of different temperature. For example, lying on the hot sand will cause one to gain heat by conduction. Conversely, placing an ice pack on a

Both the conduction and convection terms in the previous equation are proportional to the temperature gradient from core to skin ($T_{core} - \overline{T}_{skin}$), where $\overline{T}_{skin}$ is the average temperature of at least four skin sites. The "proportionality constant" for passive conduction across the subcutaneous fat (the body's insulation) is relatively fixed. However, the proportionality constant for convection by blood is a rather variable term, reflecting the variable blood flow to the skin. The ability to alter skin blood flow, under physiological control, is therefore the primary determinant of heat flow from core to skin. The capacity to *limit* blood flow to the skin is an essential defense against body cooling (hypothermia). Just as importantly, the capacity to *elevate* skin blood flow is an essential defense against hyperthermia. On very hot days when skin temperature may be very high and close to body core temperature, even a high skin blood flow may not be adequate to transfer sufficient heat to allow body core temperature to stabilize.

Although most of the heat leaving the core is transferred to the skin, some is also transferred from the body core by the evaporation of water from the respiratory sore muscle causes heat loss by conduction. However, under most circumstances (i.e., when one is fully clothed), heat gain/loss by conduction is minimal.

CONVECTION. Heat transfer by convection occurs when a fluid such as air or water carries the heat between the body and the environment. The convective heat loss is proportional to the difference between skin and ambient temperature:

Equation 58–4

Rate of convective heat loss	*Convective* heat-transfer coefficient	Mean skin temp	Ambient temp	Body surface area available for *convective* heat exchange
C	=	$h_{convective}$	$\underbrace{(\bar{T}_{skin} - T_{ambient})}_{(°C)}$	$A_{convective}$
$\dfrac{kcal}{h}$		$\dfrac{kcal}{m^2 h °C}$		(m^2)

Note that C is positive when the body loses heat, and negative when it gains heat.

Whereas the radiative heat transfer coefficient ($h_{radiative}$) is constant, the convective coefficient ($h_{convective}$) is variable and can increase up to five-fold when air velocity is high. Thus, even when ($\bar{T}_{skin} - T_{ambient}$) is fixed, convective heat loss increases markedly as wind speed increases (i.e., "wind chill" factor). In the absence of air movement, the air immediately overlying the skin warms as heat leaves the skin, thus reducing the effective temperature gradient that drives heat loss. With air movement, cooler "ambient" air constantly replaces the warmer air overlying the skin, which increases the effective temperature gradient.

EVAPORATION. Humans can dissipate nearly all of the heat produced during exercise by evaporating sweat from the skin surface. The evaporative rate is independent of the temperature gradient between skin and environment. Instead, it is proportional to the water vapor–pressure gradient between skin and environment:

Equation 58–5

Rate of evaporative heat loss	*Evaporative* heat-transfer coefficient	H_2O vapor pressure of skin	H_2O vapor pressure of environment	Body surface area available for *radioactive* heat exchange
E	=	$h_{evaporative}$	$\underbrace{(P_{skin} - P_{ambient})}_{(mm\ Hg)}$	$A_{evaporative}$
$\dfrac{kcal}{h}$		$\dfrac{kcal}{m^2 h\ mm\ Hg}$		(m^2)

Note that E is positive when the body loses heat by evaporation and negative when it gains heat by condensation.

The evaporation of 1 g of water removes approximately 0.6 kcal from the body. Because the body's sweat glands can deliver up to 30 g of fluid per minute (approaching 2 liters/h) to the skin surface, evaporation can remove 0.6 × 30 or 18 kcal/min. Thus, nearly all of the heat produced during heavy exercise could theoretically be removed by evaporation under ideal conditions (i.e., when ambient humidity is sufficiently low to allow efficient evaporation). As with convection, air movement increases

the effective vapor-pressure gradient between skin and the overlying air.

The efficiency of heat transfer from the skin to the environment depends on both physiological and environmental factors. If ambient humidity is high, the water vapor–pressure gradient between skin and air will be low, slowing evaporation and increasing the body's tendency to accumulate excess heat produced during exercise. This phenomenon underlies the temperature-humidity index ("heat index"). Conversely, if ambient humidity is low, as in the desert, net heat loss from the body by evaporation occurs readily, even when ambient temperature exceeds skin temperature and the body gains heat by radiation and convection.

When the body is immersed in water, nearly all heat exchange occurs by convection, as essentially no exchanges can occur by radiation or evaporation. Because of the high conductivity and thermal capacity of water, the heat-transfer coefficient is approximately 100 times greater than that of air. Thus, rates of heat exchange underwater are much greater than they are in air. It is not surprising that nearly all the deaths in the *Titanic* shipwreck disaster were due to hypothermia rather than drowning.

With a knowledge of the transfer coefficients, and the gradients of temperature and water vapor–pressure between the skin and environment, it becomes possible to predict the body heat flux and thus the change in core temperature. For the athlete, all of these factors are important because dissipating the thermal load is essential for prolonging exercise. The clinician must understand these principles to treat thermally related illnesses. For example, excessive heat exposure can lead to **heat exhaustion**, in which core temperature rises to as high as 39°C because the body cannot dissipate the heat load. The mechanisms are dehydration (which reduces sweating) and hypovolemia (which reduces blood flow from muscle to core to skin). Heat exhaustion is the most common temperature-related abnormality in athletes. In more severe cases, excessive heat can lead to **heat stroke**, in which core temperature rises to 41°C or more, due to impaired thermoregulatory mechanisms.

When Heat Loss from the Body Balances Heat Production, Core Temperature Is Constant

Unless metabolically generated heat moves from the tissues to the core to the skin to the environment, core temperature will increase. Just as we wrote an energy balance equation for skeletal muscle (see Equation 58–1), we can write a comparable equation for the whole body:

Equation 58–6

Heat generated by *metabolism*		Radiative heat loss		Convective heat loss		Evaporative heat loss		Rate of heat storage
M	−	R	−	C	−	E	=	S

(kcal/h) for all terms

When the rate of metabolic heat production equals the rate of heat loss (i.e., three "negative" terms in Equation 58–6), the rate of heat storage is nil and core temperature is constant. Of course, core temperature rises when the rate of heat storage is positive, as is the case with exercise, prolonged immersion in warm water, and excessive heat exposure:

$$\underbrace{\frac{\Delta \overline{T}_{body}}{\Delta t}}_{\substack{\text{Rate of} \\ \text{temperature} \\ \text{increase}}} = \frac{\text{Rate of heat storage}}{\underbrace{0.83}_{\substack{\text{Specific} \\ \text{heat of} \\ \text{body} \\ \text{tissues}}} \cdot \underbrace{BW}_{\substack{\text{Body} \\ \text{weight}}}}$$

Equation 58–7

$$\frac{°C}{h} = \frac{\text{kcal/h}}{\text{kcal/(kg °C)} \times \text{kg}}$$

🕸 $\overline{T}_{body}$ is the mean body temperature.

Clothing Insulates the Body from the Environment and Limits Heat Transfer from the Body to the Environment

Placing one or more layers of clothing between the skin and the environment insulates the body and retards heat transfer between core and environment. In the presence of clothing, heat transfer from a warmer body to a cooler environment occurs by the same means as without clothing (i.e., radiation, conduction, convection, and evaporation), but from the clothing surface rather than the skin surface. The insulating effect of clothing is described by the **clo unit**. By definition, one clo is the insulation necessary to maintain a resting person at a thermal steady state in comfort at 21°C with minimal air movement. Obviously, clo units increase with greater skin coverage or thicker clothing.

ACTIVE REGULATION OF HEAT TRANSFER

The body regulates its temperature by a feedback system that includes temperature sensors, afferent nerve fibers that carry sensory information to the brain, a hypothalamic control center, efferent nerve fibers that are principally part of the autonomic nervous system, and thermal effectors that either control heat transfer between the body and environment or regulate the body's rate of heat production.

Thermal Sensors Over the Skin Surface and in the Preoptic Anterior Hypothalamus Respond to Changes in Local Temperature

The body has specialized sensors that provide the CNS with information about the body's thermal condition. The thermosensitive elements are free nerve endings that are distributed over the entire skin surface; they are also in

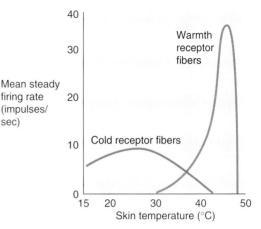

FIGURE 58–3. Response of warmth and cold receptors to temperature change.

high concentration in the preoptic anterior hypothalamus (see Fig. 46–3).

SKIN THERMORECEPTORS. The skin has anatomically distinct warmth and cold receptors (p. 355). Increasing local temperature, up to 44–46°C, causes **warmth receptors** to increase their steady firing rate (Fig. 58–3). **Cold receptors** characteristically increase their steady firing rate as local temperature decreases from approximately 40°C to 24–28°C. In either case, a sustained temperature change (see Fig. 13–25) may cause a stable change in the sensor's firing rate (i.e., *tonic* or static response), or a temporary change (i.e., *phasic* or dynamic response).

Skin thermoreceptors provide the hypothalamic thermoregulatory center with information about *ambient temperature*, and thus serve as an early-warning system in conditions of rapidly changing ambient temperature. Information from skin thermoreceptors also travels via thalamic pathways to the cerebral cortex, providing the basis for conscious perception of the thermal environment and estimation of thermal comfort.

HYPOTHALAMIC THERMORECEPTORS. In the hypothalamus (p. 393), approximately 10% of hypothalamic neurons show a positive temperature coefficient when local temperature is cycled over a range of 2°C to 4°C about the mean. Hypothalamic thermoreceptors are especially important during exercise, which is one of the few conditions in which the body's heat production and dissipation rates can differ dramatically, leading to rapid changes in core temperature. Hypothalamic warmth receptors greatly outnumber cold receptors.

The Hypothalamic Center Integrates Thermal Information and Directs Changes in Efferent Activity to Modify Heat Transfer Rates

Cooling or warming of the skin alters both the tonic and the phasic components of cold- or warmth-receptor activity. The neural activity of these skin thermoreceptors travels via the spinal cord to the hypothalamus, which integrates thermal information from other parts of the body, including the hypothalamus, compares the prevailing thermal status with an idealized set of thermal conditions, and directs efferent commands to alter the rate of heat generation and modify heat transfer rates within and from the body.

The skin receptors provide information about environmental temperature, which affects the body's heat-loss rate and could ultimately cause core temperature to change if the body did not initiate the appropriate thermoregulatory responses to skin cooling or warming. Thus, reflex responses to changes in the average skin temperature may be thought of as **anticipatory**. These anticipatory reflexes are essential elements for an effective thermoregulatory system, because the body's thermal inertia is too great to rely on central receptors alone. Conversely, thermoregulatory responses to changes in core (i.e., hypothalamic) temperature, such as those that occur during exercise, are **negative feedback** in nature, inasmuch as they modify heat transfer rates that restore the core temperature to its regulated level. These negative feedback reflexes are also essential because they minimize changes in core temperature and consequent changes in metabolic activity.

Figure 58–4 is a conceptual model that describes the role of core and skin temperature receptors in modulating thermoregulatory output from the hypothalamic control center. This model includes both anticipatory and negative-feedback elements, as well as effector organs that together act to regulate core temperature about a constant level. The hypothalamic integration center interprets increases in the firing rate of either skin or hypothalamic *cold receptors* as an error signal, and therefore an offset from the idealized or **set-point temperature** that would lead to body cooling if no compensatory alterations in heat flux occurred. Conversely, the hypothalamic integration center interprets increases in the firing rate of either skin or hypothalamic *warmth receptors* as an error signal that would otherwise lead to body heating. The so-called set-point temperature has no neuroanatomical basis but reflects the integrated response of the multiple components of the regulatory system.

The Thermal Effectors Include the Cutaneous Circulation, the Sweat Glands, and the Skeletal Muscles That Are Responsible for Shivering

Adjusting the smooth-muscle tone of cutaneous arterioles controls **blood flow**, and therefore heat flow, from the core to the skin surface, the primary site of heat dissipation to the environment. Over most of the skin, the autonomic nervous system controls cutaneous blood flow (p. 572). Active vasodilation can increase cutaneous blood flow up to 10-fold above the resting level. Cutaneous vasoconstriction, mediated by sympathetic nerves, can elicit a relatively minor reduction in cutaneous blood flow, to half the resting rate.

With a moderate heat load, the autonomic response primarily increases the heat transfer rate from core to skin by increasing cutaneous blood flow. However, if the heat load is sufficiently great, the autonomic nervous system also activates the **eccrine sweat glands**, which secrete sweat onto the skin surface, thus elevating the partial pressure of water vapor there and promoting increased evaporation. The innervation of the secretory segment of the sweat gland is sympathetic, but it is unusual in that acetylcholine is the neurotransmitter (p. 388).

If a cold stress is sufficiently great, the physiologic response includes increasing heat production by involuntary rhythmic contractions of skeletal muscle. This **shivering** can double the metabolic rate for extended periods (hours) before fatigue occurs; for brief intervals, shivering can triple or quadruple the metabolic rate. Nonshivering thermogenesis in newborn infants and hibernating animals can also produce substantial amounts of heat, primarily in brown-fat cells (p. 1205).

Over the years, many investigators have examined the control of skin blood flow, sweating, and shivering. Their work has led to models of how the CNS controller evaluates thermal information and directs efferent activity. Experiments in which investigators heated or cooled the preoptic anterior hypothalamus led to the conclusion that functional hypothalamic thermosensitivity is about nine times greater than functional average cutaneous thermosensitivity. That is, a one-degree change in core temperature produces a nine-fold greater thermoeffector response than does a one-degree change in mean skin temperature. Furthermore, skin thermosensitivity is approximately three times greater on the face than on the extremities.

The model in Figure 58–4, which combines the lumped thermoeffector responses of skin blood flow, sweating, and shivering, is known as the **proportional-control** model:

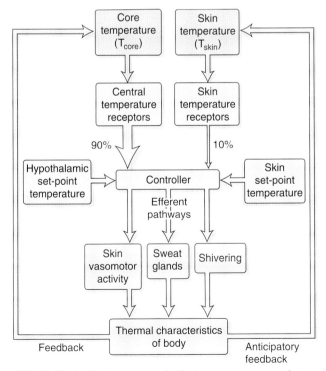

FIGURE 58–4. Model of negative feedback in temperature regulation.

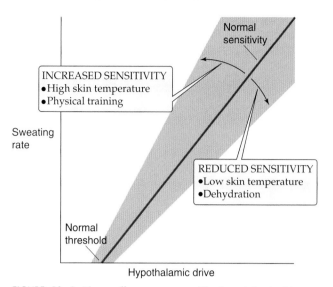

FIGURE 58–5. Thermoeffector responses. The hypothalamic drive on the x-axis is the output of the "controller" in Fig. 58–4.

Equation 58–8
$$\text{Thermoeffector Response} = 0.9\ \alpha\ (T_{core} - 37.0\ ^\circ C) + 0.1\ \alpha\ (\overline{T}_{skin} - 34.0\ ^\circ C)$$

The proportional-control model is an oversimplification. As shown in Figure 58–5, *skin* temperature and other factors can modulate the effector response (i.e., sweating rate) to changes in core temperature (i.e., hypothalamic drive). Under normal conditions, the response increases linearly with an increase in hypothalamic drive. Increasing mean skin temperature has two effects: (1) shifting the threshold downward, and (2) increasing the sensitivity (i.e., slope) of the response. Training produces similar effects in an athlete—increasing heat loss for a given hypothalamic drive. On the other hand, lowering mean skin temperature shifts the threshold upward and decreases the sensitivity (i.e., slope). Dehydration, which limits the ability to sweat, has similar effects.

HYPERTHERMIA, HYPOTHERMIA, AND FEVER

Exercise Increases Temperature, Which Stimulates Sweating and Gradually Brings Heat Dissipation Into Balance With Heat Production—But at the Cost of a Persisting Hyperthermia of Exercise

At the onset of muscular exercise, the rate of heat production increases in proportion to the exercise intensity and exceeds the current rate of heat dissipation, causing heat storage and a rise in core temperature (Fig. 58–6). Hypothalamic thermoreceptors sense this increase in core temperature. The hypothalamic integrator compares this

temperature signal with a reference signal, detects an error between the two, and directs neural output that activates heat dissipation (see Fig. 58–4). As a result, skin blood flow and sweating increase as core temperature rises, promoting an increase in the rate of heat transfer from core to environment and slowing the rate of temperature rise. At some point, the rising rate of heat dissipation equals the rate of heat production and the rate of heat storage falls to zero. However, the now-elevated steady-state core temperature persists.

The steady-state core temperature during exercise is not "regulated" at the elevated level; rather, the hyperthermia of exercise is the consequence of the initial imbalance between rate of heat production and dissipation. This imbalance is unavoidable because temperature must increase to provide the error signal that culminates in increased heat dissipation and because the response is not instantaneous. In Figure 58–6, metabolic heat production rises rapidly to its maximal level. However, evaporative heat loss increases only after a delay and then rises slowly to its maximal level. Physical training (see Fig. 58–5) reduces the hyperthermia of exercise by reducing the threshold for sweating (so that sweating will begin earlier) and increasing sweating sensitivity (so that a given hypothalamic drive produces more sweating), thus providing a greater margin of safety between operating and limiting temperatures for exercise. To the extent that training enhances sweat-gland function (evaporative heat loss), one reduces reliance on cutaneous circulation (convective heat loss), thus preserving blood flow for perfusion of muscle.

FIGURE 58–6. Whole-body heat balance during exercise.

The relative dehydration caused by continuous water losses during prolonged exercise elevates the temperature threshold for sweating and reduces the sensitivity (see Fig. 58–5). The result is a higher core temperature during exercise.

Progressive Hyperthermia and Hypothermia Occur When the Heat-Transfer Potential of the Environment Overwhelms the Body's Regulatory Capacity

Although the body's temperature-regulating machinery is impressive, its capabilities are not limitless. Any factor that causes sufficiently large shifts—either positive or negative—in the rate of heat storage (Equation 58–6) could result in progressive hyper- or hypothermia (Equation 58–7). Because humans must operate within a fairly narrow core-temperature range, such temperature changes could become life-threatening.

The most common environmental condition that results in excessive **hyperthermia** is prolonged exposure to heat and high ambient humidity, particularly when accompanied by physical activity (i.e., elevated heat-production rate). The ability to dissipate heat by *radiation* falls as the radiant temperature of nearby objects increases (Equation 58–3), and the ability to dissipate heat by *convection* falls as ambient temperature increases (Equation 58–4). When ambient temperature reaches the mid-30s (°C), evaporation becomes the only effective avenue for heat dissipation. However, high ambient humidity reduces the skin-to-environment gradient for water vapor pressure, reducing *evaporation* (Equation 58–5). The combined reduction of heat loss by these three pathways can markedly increase the rate of heat storage (Equation 58–6), causing progressive hyperthermia.

It is uncommon for radiative or convective heat gain to cause hyperthermia under conditions of low ambient humidity, because the body has a high capacity for dissipating the absorbed heat by evaporation. Radiative heat gain can be excessively high during full exposure to the desert sun or during exposure to heat sources such as large furnaces. The most obvious protections against radiative hyperthermia are avoiding radiant sources (e.g., sitting in the shade) or covering the skin with loose clothing. The latter screens the radiation while allowing air movement underneath the clothing and maintaining evaporative and convective losses.

The most common environmental condition causing excessive **hypothermia** is prolonged immersion in cold water. Water has a specific heat per unit volume that is approximately 4000 times that of air and a thermal conductivity that is approximately 25 times that of air. Both contribute to a convective heat-transfer coefficient ($h_{convective}$ in Equation 58–4) that is approximately 100-fold greater in water than it is in air. The $h_{convective}$ is approximately 200 kcal/($m^2h°C$) at rest in still water but approximately 500 kcal/($m^2h°C$) while swimming. The body's physiological defenses against hypothermia include peripheral vasoconstriction (increasing insulation) and shivering (increasing heat production), but even these will

not prevent hypothermia during prolonged exposure because of water's high thermal conductivity. A thick layer of insulating fat retards heat loss to the water and postpones or even prevents hypothermia during prolonged exposures. Endurance swimmers use this knowledge to protect themselves, as they apply a thick layer of grease to the skin surface prior to an event. Herman Melville noted this principle nearly 150 years ago, when he referred to the low thermal conductivity of fat:

> *For the whale is indeed wrapt up in his blubber as in a real blanket. . . . It is by reason of this cozy blanketing that the whale is enabled to keep himself comfortable in all seas. . . . this great monster, to whom corporeal warmth is as indispensable as it is to man. . . .*
>
> — *Moby Dick*

Like blubber, clothing adds insulation between skin and environment, thus reducing heat loss during exposure to the cold. The more skin one covers, the more one reduces the surface area for direct heat loss from skin to environment by convection and radiation. Adding *layers* of clothing increases the resistance of heat flow by trapping air, which is an excellent insulator. During heat exposure, the major avenue for heat loss is evaporation of sweat. Because evaporation also depends on the surface area available, the amount of clothing should be minimized. Wetting the clothing increases the rate of heat loss from the skin because water is a better conductor than air is. Water also can evaporate from the clothing surface, removing heat from the outer layers and increasing the temperature gradient (and rate of heat loss) from skin to clothing.

HEAT STROKE

As body core temperature rises, excessive cutaneous vasodilation can lead to a fall in arterial pressure (p. 579) and, therefore, to a decrease in brain perfusion. As core temperature approaches 41°C, confusion and, ultimately, loss of consciousness occur. Excessive hyperthermia (> 41°C) leads to the clinical condition known as **heat stroke**. High temperature can cause fibrinolysis and consumption of clotting factors and thus disseminated intravascular coagulation (DIC), which results in uncontrolled vascular thrombosis and hemorrhage. Heat-induced damage to the cell membranes of skeletal and myocardial muscle leads to rhabdomyolysis (in which disrupted muscle cells release their intracellular contents, including myoglobin, into the circulation) and myocardial necrosis. Cell damage may also cause acute hepatic insufficiency and pancreatitis. Renal function, already compromised by low renal blood flow, may be further disrupted by the high plasma levels of myoglobin. Ultimately, the central nervous system is affected by the combination of high brain temperature, DIC, and metabolic disturbances.

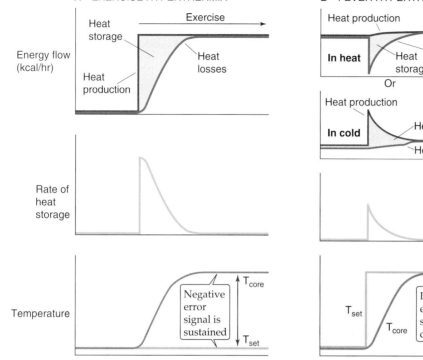

FIGURE 58–7. Exercise hyperthermia versus fever. *A,* The *top panel* shows how, during exercise, heat production temporarily exceeds heat loss, resulting in net heat storage. The *middle panel* shows that the rate of heat storage is highest initially and falls to zero in the new steady state. Finally, the *bottom panel* shows that as body core temperature rises away from the set point, the error signal gradually increases. In the new steady state, the error signal is maximal and sustained. *B,* The *top pair of panels* show how, during fever, net heat storage can occur because of either reduced heat loss or increased heat production. The *third panel* shows that, as in exercise, the rate of heat storage is highest initially. The *bottom panel* shows that as body-core temperature rises, it approaches the new elevated set point. Thus, the error signal is initially maximal and gradually decreases to zero in the new steady state.

Fever Differs From Other Types of Hyperthermia in that it Represents an Increase in the Set Point for Temperature Regulation

Fever is a *regulated* elevation of core temperature due to effects associated with infection or disease. Fever is caused by the action of circulating cytokines called **pyrogens**, which are low-molecular-weight polypeptides produced by cells of the immune system. As for the hyperthermia of exercise, fever begins when heat production temporarily exceeds heat dissipation. However, fever differs from other hyperthermias in that the hypothalamus actively regulates core temperature to an elevated set point.

Figure 58–7 illustrates the basic differences between the events leading to exercise hyperthermia and those leading to a fever. During the genesis of exercise hyperthermia (see Fig. 58–7A), the rate of heat production increases above the rate of heat dissipation for a period, causing net heat storage. Moreover, the temperature set point (T_{set}) is unchanged, and thus the error signal gradually increases to a new, sustained level. During the genesis of a fever (see Fig. 58–7B), T_{set} suddenly increases to a value that is above the normal temperature, so that the integrator "sees" the normal temperature as being below the new T_{set}. The fever is an appropriate response to this condition and develops as the heat-loss rate from the body falls or the heat-production rate rises until such time as core temperature increases to the new "regulated" level. Thus, the error signal is initially large but becomes smaller as the fever develops. In the new steady state, core temperature remains elevated until the signals responsible for the fever (i.e., pyrogens) subside and T_{set} returns to normal.

The subjective assessments of thermal comfort support this description. During exercise, one perceives the rise in core temperature as body heating and may choose to remove clothing to cool the body. During the onset of a fever, however, the individual feels cold and may choose to put on additional clothing and warm the body. If fever strikes when the patient is in a warm environment in which the cutaneous vessels are dilated (see Fig. 58–7B, *top panel*), the response to the T_{set} increase is to vasoconstrict, which decreases heat loss. On the other hand, if the patient is in a cold environment in which the cutaneous vessels are already constricted (see Fig. 58-7B, *second panel*), the response is to shiver.

Figure 58–8 summarizes the responses to fever-producing stimuli. Macrophages and, to a lesser extent, lymphocytes release cytokines into the circulation in response to a variety of infectious and inflammatory stimuli. Cytokines, the messenger molecules of the immune system, are a diverse group of proteins that are involved in numerous tasks in the host-defense response. The first is the *immune response* to foreign substances including stimulation of T-lymphocyte proliferation, natural killer cells, and antibody production. The second is the *acute-phase response* to foreign substances, a diffuse collection of nonspecific host reactions to infection or trauma. Finally, cytokines may act as endogenous pyrogens (Table 58–2). However, no one cytokine, administered experimentally, can fully mimic the temperature increase that occurs during fever. Fever production may occur through a cascade that is initiated when interleukin (IL-1β), for example, interacts with the endothelial cells in a leaky portion of the blood-brain barrier (p. 409) located in the capillary bed of the *organum vasculosum laminae terminalis* (OVLT). The OVLT is highly vascular tissue that lies in the wall of the third ventricle (above the optic chiasm) in the brain.

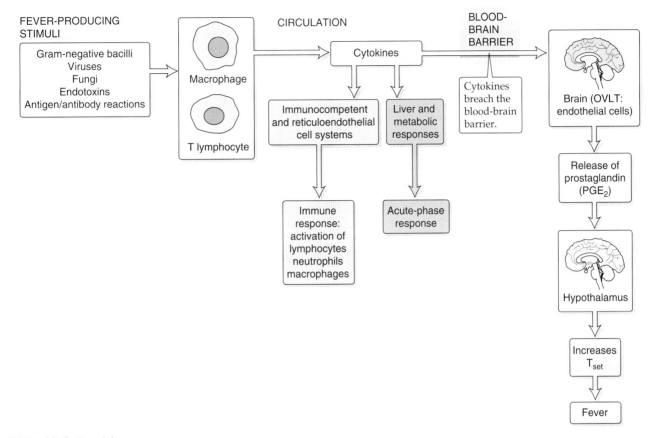

FIGURE 58–8. Host-defense response.

TABLE 58–2

ENDOGENOUS PYROGENS

PYROGEN	SYMBOL
Interleukin-1α	IL-1α
Interleukin-1β	IL-1β
Interleukin-6	IL-6
Interleukin-8	IL-8
Tumor necrosis factor α	TNF-α
Tumor necrosis factor β	TNF-β
Macrophage inflammatory protein 1α	MIP-1α
Macrophage inflammatory protein 1β	MIP-1β
Interferon-α	INF-α
Interferon-β	INF-β
Interferon-γ	INF-γ

IL-1β triggers endothelial cells within the OVLT to release prostaglandin E$_2$ (p. 104), which then diffuses into the adjacent hypothalamus and—in a manner not yet understood—elevates T$_{set}$ and initiates the febrile response.

The value of fever in fighting infection is still debated. A popular hypothesis is that the elevated temperature enhances the host's response to infection. This view is supported by the in vitro observation that the rate of T-lymphocyte proliferation in response to interleukins is many-fold higher at 39°C than it is at 37°C.

REFERENCES

Blatteis CM, Sehic E: Fever: How may circulating pyrogens signal the brain? News Physiol Sci 12:1–9, 1997.

Block BA: Thermogenesis in muscle. Annu Rev Physiol 56:535–577, 1994.

Horowitz M. Do cellular heat acclimation responses modulate central thermoregulatory activity? News Physiol Sci 13:218–225, 1998.

Lee-Chiong TL, Stitt JT Jr: Disorders of temperature regulation: Comprehensive Therapy 21:697–704, 1995.

Simon HB: Current concepts: Hyperthermia. N Engl J Med 329:483–487, 1993.

CHAPTER 59

Exercise Physiology and Sports Science

Ethan Nadel

Physical exercise is the most extreme stress that the body encounters during everyday life. During an acute bout of exercise, the body must make rapid and integrated cellular and organ-system adjustments to meet the body's metabolic, thermal, and fluid demands. Also important are the slower *adaptations* to physical training, which occur over weeks and months of repeated bouts of physical activity.

Exercise physiology is the study of the physical and chemical events that provide for the conversion of chemical energy to mechanical work. Both the contraction and the relaxation processes in skeletal muscle require energy (see Chapter 9). Because the free energy supply in skeletal muscle is extremely small, and because the demands of contracting skeletal muscles are large relative to their resting demands, sustained activity requires an integrated cellular and organ-system response that increases the rates of fuel and O_2 delivery to the muscles. The study of exercise physiology uncovers the control processes that are responsible for making energy available to skeletal muscles during acute exercise and for slower adaptations during training.

MUSCLE WORK AND FATIGUE

Total muscle tension (or force) is the sum of both passive and active tensions (Fig. 9–12C,D). Stretching inactive muscle tissue increases *passive* tension monotonically, in the same way that stretching a rubber band increases its tension. However, as a skeletal muscle is stretched, the *active* tension reaches a maximum at a point where the thick and thin filaments optimally overlap. Interestingly, maximally developed **stress** (force per unit cross-sectional area) is a constant for all mammalian muscles, despite wide variations in size, activities of energy-releasing enzymes, and intrinsic speed of shortening among different muscles.

An **isometric** contraction is a static contraction in which the muscle does not shorten (p. 245). An **isotonic** contraction is one in which the force of contraction remains constant throughout the shortening. Isotonic contractions can be concentric or eccentric. A **concentric** contraction of skeletal muscle occurs when shortening a muscle (e.g., quadriceps femoris) while exerting a **force** (e.g., walking *up* stairs). An **eccentric** contraction occurs when lengthening a muscle (e.g., quadriceps femoris) while resisting an external load (e.g., walking *down* stairs). The **series elastic component** of skeletal muscle, which allows the muscle to stretch by 2% to 3% of its resting length on application of a load, gives the muscle spring-like characteristics that are rigid enough to transform shortening into external power production and yet flexible enough to withstand sudden changes in length without breaking.

The movement of limbs, which requires energy release in skeletal muscle, can impart mechanical **work**, which is the product of force and the distance over which the force is applied (*units:* newton × meter = joule). **Power** is work per unit time (*units:* joule/s = watt). During activity that involves *concentric* muscle contractions, work is imparted to the environment, whereas during activity involving *eccentric* muscle contractions, the environment works on the muscle. Because of inherent inefficiencies in both biochemical reactions (p. 1212) and biomechanical transfers, cells can convert only approximately 24% of stored chemical energy to mechanical work during concentric contractions; the remainder appears as heat. At any given power output, eccentric muscle contraction requires much less energy release than do concentric contractions, which require much more cross-bridge cycling.

Fast-Twitch (Type II) Muscle Fibers Shorten More Rapidly Than Do Slow-Twitch (Type I) Fibers

During concentric muscle contractions, the velocity of shortening declines rapidly with an increasing load or force (Fig. 59–1). Stated another way, muscles shorten more slowly against a heavy load than against a light load. In the extreme case in which the velocity of shortening is zero (i.e., isometric contraction), the muscle produces maximal force. Unlike the velocity of shortening, power reaches a maximum with intermediate load. In a mixed (slow and fast twitch fibers) muscle, maximal power production occurs when velocity is about half maximal.

We discussed differences between slow- and fast-twitch muscle fibers on p. 251. Slow-twitch (oxidative or **type I**) muscle fibers have lower velocities of shortening than do fast-twitch (glycolytic or **type II**) muscle fibers at a given normalized load. The maximum velocity of shortening in

these different fibers depends on myosin-adenosine triphosphatase activity (see Table 9–1), which determines the maximal rate of unloaded cross-bridge cycling.

During the Contraction of a Mixed Muscle, the First Motor Units Recruited Are Small and Have Slow-Twitch Fibers

A **motor unit** consists of a single motor nerve and all of the muscle fibers it innervates (p. 249). The motor unit is the functional unit of muscle contraction because all fibers in a unit contract simultaneously when the motor neuron fires. In general, small, precision-control muscles have relatively few muscle fibers per motor unit, whereas large muscles that are involved in posture or locomotion may have as many as several hundred. Muscle fibers belonging to a single motor unit are all of the same type and may interdigitate with those from other motor units.

The body can increase the intensity of whole-muscle contraction by increasing the frequency of firing or by increasing the number of motor units that fire simultaneously (p. 249). The interdigitation noted above, together with the recruitment of motor units, permits a graded response that is evenly distributed through the cross section of the muscle. A relatively low excitatory input to the motor-neuron pool will depolarize neurons with smaller cell bodies first. These small-sized, relatively excitable motor neurons have relatively low axon diameters and, because of their cable properties, relatively low conduction velocities. They also innervate relatively small motor units that consist of slow-twitch (type I) fibers. Thus, during muscle activation, the brain first recruits smaller motor units, which generate less force. As excitatory input increases, larger motor units are recruited and force generation increases accordingly. Because the larger motor units contain fast-twitch (type II) muscle fibers, and because the effective load on each fiber is less when more muscle fibers participate in contraction against a given load, recruitment of more units increases the velocity of muscle contraction. This pattern of force generation, in which smaller motor units are recruited first, is known as the **size principle**.

The size principle explains two observations. First, the force of a voluntary contraction increases smoothly as one makes more effort. Second, one can sustain moderate tensions (dominated by slow-twitch fibers) for extended periods, but one can sustain maximal tensions (dominated by fast-twitch fibers) for only a brief period. The latter are limited by the rapid fuel depletion of the glycogen-dependent fast-twitch muscle fibers.

Fatigue Is the Inability to Maintain Muscle Force Generation

Fatigue is defined as the inability to maintain a particular force or power output. Central fatigue is a failure at any link in the chain of command for muscular activity that originates in the brain and traverses the spinal cord before involving the muscle. Other potential causes of fatigue include impaired neuromuscular transmission at the

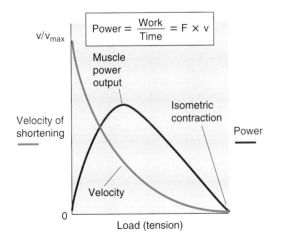

FIGURE 59–1. Load-velocity and power relationships for skeletal muscle.

motor end plate, impaired action potential generation in the muscle cell, abnormal electrolyte distribution, impaired excitation-contraction coupling, or inability to generate energy at a rate that is sufficient to meet the energy requirement due to the reduced availability of O_2 or fuel.

As we see in the next two sections, the fatigue that develops from a maximum voluntary contraction, such as lifting a heavy weight, is very different from that which develops during repeated moderate contractions, such as running at a comfortable pace.

High-Frequency Fatigue Occurs During Maximal Contraction, Which Recruits All Fibers in the Muscle Group—Including Fast-Twitch Fibers

To develop *maximal* contraction of a skeletal muscle group, the excitatory input must be sufficiently high to recruit the entire motor-neuron pool (p. 250), and thus all of the fibers in the muscle, and to excite them at a sufficiently high frequency. In fast-twitch or type II (glycolytic) fibers, fatigue sets in rapidly, on the order of tens of seconds or minutes (Fig. 59–2, *blue curve*). This fatigue probably reflects the inability of the type II fibers to maintain tension owing to several factors, including the rapid decline in glycogen and a decrease in local pH. Also contributing may be an associated impairment in the conduction of action potentials along the muscle fiber as a result of accumulation of extracellular K^+ in the transverse tubular system. High-frequency fatigue is of relatively short duration; the fiber can develop a maximal contraction within moments after terminating the previous one.

Training does not markedly increase resistance to high-frequency fatigue. Activities such as weightlifting promote increased strength and thus an ability to generate a greater force but do not enhance resistance to high-frequency fatigue. Maximal muscle glycogen storage increases after repeated bouts of anaerobic training, but this adaptation has little effect on maximal effort.

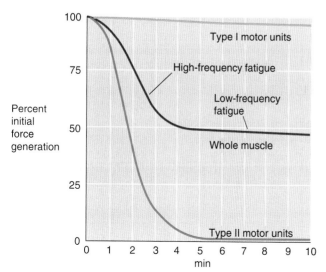

FIGURE 59–2. Fatigue of skeletal muscle.

Low-Frequency Fatigue Occurs During Repeated Moderate Muscle Contractions, Which Recruit Primarily Slow-Twitch Fibers

Exercise involving repeated *moderate* contractions, in which muscle shortening results primarily from activating slow-twitch or type I (oxidative) fibers, requires a motor-neuron discharge frequency much lower than that needed for maximal contraction. In such conditions, fatigue develops more slowly—on the order of tens of minutes or even hours (see Fig. 59–2, *orange curve*). Low-frequency fatigue is probably due to impaired excitation-contraction coupling (p. 241). The impairment itself may reflect a critical depletion of the intracellular Ca^{2+}, which plays an essential role in contraction. This pattern of fatigue is probably attributable to the distinctive mechanics of force generation during prolonged exercise. As low-frequency fatigue develops in type I fibers, the brain increasingly recruits type II fibers. Once maximal recruitment occurs, power output begins to decline because no additional recruitment is possible to compensate for the decline in the activity of type I fibers.

The functional adaptations that increase resistance to low-frequency fatigue promote increased endurance and thus a greater ability to maintain a given submaximal power output.

In a whole muscle, which contains both type I and type II motor units, fatigue occurs in two phases (see Fig. 59–2, *red curve*). The high-frequency fatigue of type II fibers causes a rapid decrease in force production, whereas low-frequency fatigue of type I fibers causes a much slower decrease.

CONVERSION OF CHEMICAL ENERGY TO MECHANICAL WORK

During the Contraction and Relaxation of Skeletal Muscle, Energy Conversion Can Exceed 100 Times the Basal Rate

Resting skeletal muscle has a low resting metabolic rate ($\dot{V}_{O_2}$) relative to most other tissues, 1.5 to 2 ml O_2/(min · kg). During physical activity, when the skeletal muscle metabolic rate can exceed 150 ml O_2/(min · kg), a ready supply of energy is necessary to support both the contraction and the relaxation processes. This energy is released within the muscle cell by breakdown of adenosine triphosphate (ATP) and by regeneration of ATP from the high-energy phosphocreatine (PCr). Because skeletal muscle stores these high-energy compounds in quantities that are capable of supporting rhythmic contractions for no more than a few seconds, the cells must regenerate ATP from other sources. As discussed later, the *anaerobic* regeneration of ATP, while rapid, is inefficient and self-limiting. Under *aerobic* conditions, skeletal muscle can sustain physical activity at light levels only by the high rate of ATP regeneration that is made possible by the oxidation of glucose (Table 57–2), free fatty acids (Table 57–3), and ketone bodies (Fig. 59–3). The high rate of ATP regeneration that is necessary to sustain light muscular activity occurs in the mitochondria of type I (slow-

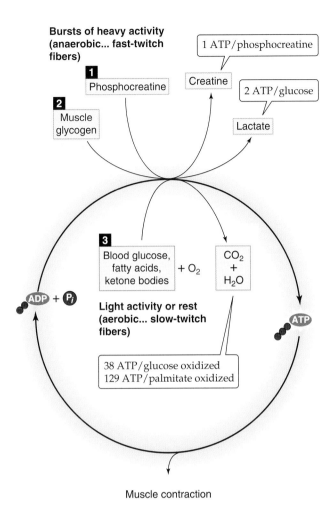

Bursts of heavy activity (anaerobic... fast-twitch fibers)

1 ATP/phosphocreatine

1 Phosphocreatine → Creatine

2 Muscle glycogen

2 ATP/glucose

Lactate

3 Blood glucose, fatty acids, ketone bodies + O_2 → CO_2 + H_2O

Light activity or rest (aerobic... slow-twitch fibers)

38 ATP/glucose oxidized
129 ATP/palmitate oxidized

ADP + P_i → ATP

Muscle contraction

FIGURE 59–3. Energy conversion in skeletal muscle. During light activity, slow-twitch (oxidative) fibers burn fatty acids, ketone bodies, and blood glucose. This oxidation generates large amounts of ATP. During bursts of heavy activity, the fibers—including the fast-twitch (glycolytic) fibers—consume phosphocreatine and glycogen anaerobically, generating far less ATP. ADP, adenosine diphosphate; ATP, adenosine triphosphate; P_i, inorganic phosphate.

twitch) fibers as a consequence of the complete oxidation of carbohydrates and fats. The catabolism of protein also can generate ATP, but this means of energy production is relatively minor during physical activity. The integrated physiological response to activity involves the delivery of sufficient O_2 and fuel to ensure that adenosine diphosphate (ADP) is re-energized into ATP at a rate that is equivalent to that at which ATP is hydrolyzed. Indeed, muscle precisely regulates the ATP/ADP ratio even when ATP turnover rate increases more than three orders of magnitude.

When Oxygen Is Not Available, Glycolysis and Phosphocreatine Are Limited Sources of ATP

If O_2 availability to active muscle is inadequate for any reason—such as occurs at the very onset of exercise, during increasingly heavy exercise, or in a hypoxic environment—muscle can regenerate ATP anaerobically either from phosphocreatine or from glycolysis (see Fig. 59–3).

PHOSPHOCREATINE. Muscle can regenerate ATP by the creatine phosphokinase reaction, which transfers the high-energy phosphate from PCr to ATP:

Equation 59–1

$$PCr + ADP \longrightarrow ATP + Cr$$

This reaction protects us against entering into muscle rigor by maintaining $[ATP]_i$ at the expense of PCr.

GLYCOLYSIS. Both type I and II muscle fibers can regenerate ATP to some extent by glycolysis, which can convert glucose to pyruvate (p. 1220). In the absence of O_2, the cell converts pyruvate to lactate:

Equation 59–2

$$\overbrace{C_6H_{12}O_6}^{Glucose} + 2\ ADP + P_i \longrightarrow 2\ ATP + 2\ \underbrace{C_3H_5O_3^-}_{Lactate} + 2\ H^+ + heat$$

However, glycolysis by itself can support rhythmic contractions for only a brief period at best. Glycolysis is inefficient compared with the aerobic regeneration of ATP, and it is accompanied by the accumulation of lactic acid and thus a decrease of intracellular pH (pH_i). This lactic acidosis (p. 1220) impedes force generation. After exhaustive exercise, muscle pH_i may be as low as 6.4—an extreme drop from the normal value of 7.1. Thus, low pH_i may be the common regulator for the maximal rates at which the muscle can hydrolyze ATP. This speculation is consistent with the observation that even at the peak of exhaustion, the ATP content in muscles is only reduced by approximately 25%. Thus, the byproducts of anaerobic metabolism appear to be directly responsible for the progressive impairment of the contractile process and are therefore the likely specific components of fatigue. Muscular activity cannot continue beyond a certain accumulation of these products.

The progressive slowing of the contractile process with an increasing accumulation of glycolytic byproducts serves as a built-in protective device that prevents the muscle from depleting its ATP supply and, as a consequence, entering into rigor (p. 238).

When Oxygen Is Available, The Regeneration of ATP Initially Comes from Oxidation of Local Glycogen

Although the body can store only a small amount of O_2, most humans carry sufficient fuel to supply a long-distance run of more than 1600 km. Most of this stored energy is in the form of triglycerides, located in adipocytes. The average 70-kg person carries approximately 130,000 kcal of potential energy in adipose tissue (p. 1217) and an additional approximately 8000 kcal of potential energy as intramuscular lipid stores. These intramuscular stores of fatty acids may be as important as the supply from adipose tissue in providing for the total fatty-acid oxidation during prolonged muscular exertion. In spite of the relatively large energy stores in triglycerides, the ability to oxidize fatty acids during exercise is restricted to approximately 70% of the muscle's maximal fuel-oxidation rate, owing to limitations in the transport rate from blood into the mitochondrial matrix and the contribution of glycogen to aerobic energy production (see p. 1247).

The other primary store of energy is glycogen. Muscle can contain 300 to 400 g of glycogen, which represents 1200 to 1600 kcal of potential energy. Liver normally contains 75 to 100 g of glycogen, which represents 300 to 400 kcal. Although the body has an abundant supply of stored fuel (i.e., lipids and glycogen), this supply is of little use for muscular contraction until it is made available to the muscle cells.

At the onset of exercise under aerobic conditions, the immediate fuel sources are ATP and phosphocreatine, which are stored in the muscle cells themselves, followed almost instantaneously by the glycogen that is stored in the muscle (see the previous section). Studies involving rhythmic forearm exercise, in which the entire arterial and venous circulations serving the forearm muscle can be isolated and sampled, reveal that the muscle respiratory quotient (ratio of CO_2 produced to O_2 consumed, p. 1223) during the first minutes is close to 1.0, which is characteristic of glucose oxidation. (Fatty-acid oxidation would have yielded a respiratory quotient of 0.7.) Muscle also releases lactic acid during this initial period as glycogenolysis rapidly liberates glucose, and glycolysis forms pyruvate faster than the muscle can oxidize it. After the initial minutes, the muscle takes up glucose from the blood, and the release of lactic acid diminishes (assuming a moderate intensity of exercise that is supported aerobically).

During exercise at relatively high intensities (>65% of maximal aerobic power), fatigue develops on the order of tens of minutes and is due to the inability of the O_2-delivery systems to meet the O_2 requirement of muscle. During exercise at relatively low intensities, which well-trained athletes can maintain for hours, the onset of low-frequency fatigue is largely attributable to the development of a critically low fuel availability to the active muscles. Although this explanation seems incongruous in light of the potential energy stored throughout the body, the combined delivery rates of blood-borne fatty acid and glucose and intramuscular fatty acid are inadequate to accommodate the energy requirement during prolonged exercise when stores of muscle glycogen become relatively depleted.

In the Steady State, Active Muscle Relies Heavily on Glucose Arriving from the Liver and from the Fatty Acids That Arrive from Adipose Tissue

During the initial transition of moderate to heavy exercise, muscle glycogen is the primary fuel for the contracting muscle. As summarized in Figure 59–4, elevated levels of epinephrine, acting through cyclic adenosine monophosphate (cAMP), promote the breakdown of muscle glycogen but inhibit glycogen synthesis in skeletal muscle (see Fig. 4–7). However, as the duration of exercise increases, a larger portion of the carbohydrate that is oxidized comes via the blood from the liver, which generates glucose by glycogenolysis and gluconeogenesis. During the

steady state of exercise, the oxidation of glucose, both from muscle glycogen and blood-borne glucose, accounts for 40% to 50% of the energy release in active skeletal muscle, with fatty acid oxidation accounting for the remainder.

GLUCOSE. As presented earlier in Equation 57–3, the overall reaction describing glucose oxidation is:

Equation 59–3

Glucose

$$\overbrace{C_6H_{12}O_6} + 6\ O_2 + 38\ ADP + 38\ P_i \longrightarrow$$
$$6\ CO_2 + 6\ H_2O + 38\ ATP + heat$$
$$RQ = 6\ CO_2/6\ O_2 = 1.00$$

During exercise of up to 1 hour, increased glucose release from the liver balances the glucose uptake from the blood by active muscle, thus stabilizing the blood glucose concentration. In situations when O_2 is limited in muscle, the muscle cells capture energy from carbohydrates as they break glycogen and glucose down to lactate (see Fig. 59–4). The lactate then enters the blood and travels to the liver, where hepatocytes use energy to convert the lactate to glucose (i.e., gluconeogenesis). The first step in gluconeogenesis, the oxidation of the entering lactate to pyruvate, is favored by the low $NADH/NAD^+$ ratio in hepatocytes. This hepatic glucose can then enter the blood and reach the muscle, completing the so-called **Cori cycle**, in which the *liver* converts the metabolic end product of anaerobic *muscle* metabolism (i.e., lactate) to a fuel that muscle can use anaerobically (i.e., glucose).

Increased hepatic glucose production is primarily the consequence of increased glycogenolysis. However, gluconeogenesis also plays a role and becomes increasingly important as exercise is prolonged beyond an hour. Enhanced hepatic glucose output during exercise probably reflects decreased blood levels of **insulin** and increased levels of **glucagon** (in particular) and **epinephrine** (see Fig. 50–12). Glucagon and epinephrine bind to receptors on the hepatocyte plasma membrane (see Fig. 59–4), raise $[cAMP]_i$, and ultimately stimulate glycogenolysis and inhibit glycogen synthase. In addition, the arrival of lactate and alanine from contracting muscle also enhances hepatic gluconeogenesis by "mass action."

FATTY ACIDS. Free fatty acids provide important fuel during prolonged exercise, accounting for up to 60% of the oxidized fuel supply of the muscle. As presented earlier in Equation 57–4, the overall reaction describing the oxidation of fatty acids (using palmitic acid as an example) is:

Equation 59–4

Palmitic acid

$$\overbrace{C_{15}H_{31}COOH} + 23\ O_2 + 129\ ADP + 129\ P_i \longrightarrow$$
$$16\ CO_2 + 16\ H_2O + 129\ ATP + heat$$
$$RQ = 16\ CO_2/23\ O_2 = 0.70$$

Early during exercise, increased blood levels of epinephrine, acting through cAMP, stimulate hormone-sensitive lipase in adipocytes (see Figure 59–4). This enzyme

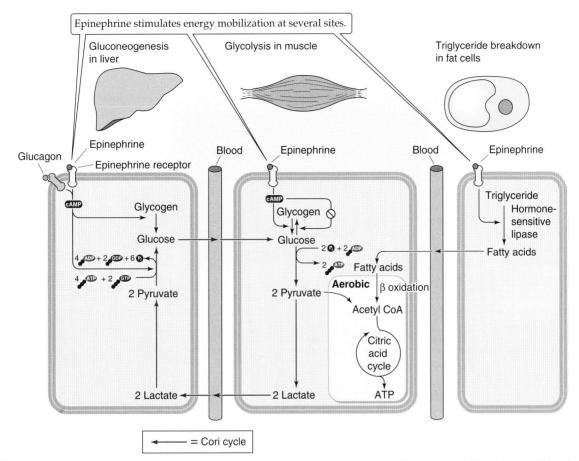

FIGURE 59–4. Steady-state energy supply to muscle from energy stores in muscle, liver, and adipose tissue. ADP, adenosine diphosphate; ATP, adenosine triphosphate; cAMP, cyclic adenosine monophosphate; GDP, guanosine diphosphate; GTP, guanosine triphosphate; P_i, inorganic phosphate.

converts triglycerides to free fatty acids (p. 1218), which enter the blood and bind to albumin for delivery to exercising muscle. During prolonged exercise, elevated growth hormone in the blood plays an increasing role in the mobilization of free fatty acids (p. 1027). The greater the levels of fatty acids in arterial blood, the greater their uptake and oxidation by exercising muscle, independent of any hormonal influence. Consequently, at a given metabolic demand, increased availability of fatty acids translates to lower rates of glucose oxidation and muscle glycogenolysis.

Fatigue During Prolonged Exercise Reflects Decreased Muscle Glycogen Levels

During prolonged exercise of moderate intensity in which O_2 transport is well maintained, the eventual decrease in muscle-fuel availability will decrease power output (e.g., running speed decreases), contributing to the development of fatigue. Long-distance runners describe this phenomenon as "hitting the wall." Exercise performance depends on the absolute amount of glycogen stored in the large leg muscles before exercise, which is measured by muscle biopsy or magnetic resonance spectroscopy. Running pace deteriorates in a long-distance race when glycogen concentration in the quadriceps muscle drops below 3 g/kg wet muscle weight.

The precise reason for this type of fatigue is not clear,

although some have speculated that the type II muscle fibers can no longer be recruited when local supplies become exhausted, and thus, power output declines. Assuming an average glycogen concentration in rested muscle to be 18 g/kg wet muscle weight, and assuming an average glycogenolysis rate during a distance race to be 0.5 g/(kg wet muscle weight · km), muscle glycogen will fall to 3 g/kg wet muscle weight—and thus the typical runner will "hit the wall"—at 30 km. To resist the fatigue associated with muscle glycogen depletion, the runner must either begin the event with an elevated level of muscle glycogen or race more slowly. Because glycogen storage is primarily a function of diet, a carbohydrate-rich diet will increase resting muscle glycogen concentration and postpone the onset of fatigue. Adaptations to aerobic exercise spare muscle glycogen by shifting the mix of fuels being oxidized toward free fatty acids.

FACTORS LIMITING MAXIMAL O_2 UPTAKE

The O_2 required for oxidative metabolism by exercising muscle travels from the atmosphere to the muscle mitochondria in three discrete steps:

1. The **uptake** of O_2 by the lungs depends on pulmonary ventilation.

2. The **delivery** of O_2 to muscle depends on blood flow and O_2 content.
3. The **extraction** of O_2 from blood by muscle depends on O_2 delivery and the Po_2 gradient between blood and mitochondria.

Maximal O_2 Uptake Can Be More Than 20 Times Resting O_2 Uptake

Although the body can easily match O_2 delivery to muscle demand at moderate exercise intensities, as exercise intensity progressively increases, the body eventually reaches a point at which the capacity of the O_2-transport systems can no longer keep pace with demand. At rest, the O_2 uptake by the lungs ($\dot{V}o_2$) is approximately 250 ml/min for a 70-kg person (p. 655), which amounts to a $\dot{V}o_2$ of approximately 3.6 ml O_2/(min · kg body weight). Maximal oxygen uptake by the lungs ($\dot{V}o_{2max}$) is an objective index of the functional capacity of the body's ability to generate power. In people who have a deficiency in any part of the O_2-transport system (e.g., chronic obstructive pulmonary disease or advanced heart disease), $\dot{V}o_{2max}$ can be as low as 10 to 20 ml O_2/(min · kg body weight). The range for mildly active middle-aged adults is 30 to 40 ml O_2/(min · kg body weight); for people in this category, a 3-month program of physical conditioning can increase $\dot{V}o_{2max}$ by 20%. In elite endurance athletes, $\dot{V}o_{2max}$ may be as high as 80 to 90 ml O_2/(min · kg body weight), a 20-fold elevation above the resting $\dot{V}o_2$. Hemorrhage or high-altitude decreases $\dot{V}o_{2max}$, whereas a blood transfusion or training increases it.

The typical method for determining $\dot{V}o_{2max}$ is an incremental exercise test on a stationary cycle ergometer or treadmill. Such tests assess training status, predict performance in athletes, and provide an index of functional impairment in patients. During the test, the technician monitors the Po_2 and Pco_2 of the subject's expired air, as well as total ventilation. The criteria for achieving $\dot{V}o_{2max}$ include: (1) an inability to continue pace at the prescribed power requirement; (2) a leveling off of $\dot{V}o_2$ with increasing power requirement; and (3) a "respiratory exchange ratio" ($\dot{V}co_2/\dot{V}o_2$) that is greater than 1.15. This $\dot{V}co_2/\dot{V}o_2$ is a transient/non–steady-state occurrence (i.e., not a real respiratory quotient) (p. 1223) and indicates that a significant hyperventilation, triggered by low blood pH (p. 723), is reducing the body's CO_2 stores.

Figure 59–5 shows the results of $\dot{V}o_{2max}$ tests on two athletes with nearly identical $\dot{V}o_{2max}$ values. Each data point is the average $\dot{V}o_2$ during the steady state at a given power output, and the slopes of the blue and red lines represent **mechanical efficiency**. Thus, Athlete 1 was considerably more efficient than Athlete 2 (27% versus 20%) in generating mechanical power from stored energy. In other words, despite the similar maximal capacities of their O_2 transport systems, Athlete 1 has a greater maximal power output than does Athlete 2. Mechanical efficiency ranges rather widely among skilled athletes (18% to 34%), implying that $\dot{V}o_{2max}$ is not a unique predictor of performance. The major reason for the large range in efficiency among individuals may be genetically determined differences in the metabolic machinery associated

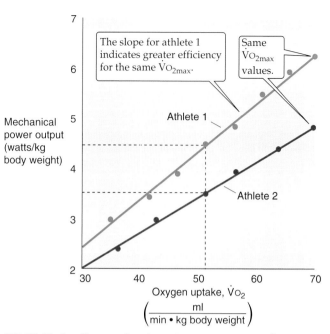

FIGURE 59–5. Efficiency of mechanical power output. At a $\dot{V}o_2$ of 50 ml/min/kg body weight, the more efficient athlete generates 4.5 watts/kg body weight, whereas the less efficient athlete produces only 3.6 watts/kg body weight. (Data from Nadel, E.R. Physiological adaptations to aerobic training. Am. Scientist 73:334–343, 1985.)

with the distribution of muscle-fiber types. Indeed, the velocity of muscle shortening, and therefore the economy of muscle-tension development, depends on myosin ATPase (see Table 9–1). Other differences in efficiency may reflect subtle actions of antagonist and postural muscles or subtle differences in aerobic enzyme kinetics, induced over years of training. Thus, in assessing athletic potential, it is essential to measure both $\dot{V}o_{2max}$ and efficiency (i.e., maximal mechanical power output).

O_2 Usage by Muscle Depends on Muscle Blood Flow and O_2 Extraction

The body's store of O_2 is approximately only one liter (mainly in the form of O_2 bound to hemoglobin), a volume that can support moderate exercise for 30 seconds at best, heavy exercise for not more than 15 seconds, and maximal exercise for less than 5 seconds. If activity is to persist, the body must transport O_2 from the ambient air to the muscle mitochondria at a rate that is equivalent to the O_2 utilization by the muscle. This increased O_2 transport is accomplished by increasing alveolar ventilation to maintain alveolar Po_2 levels that are sufficient to saturate arterial blood fully (p. 692) and by increasing cardiac output to ensure a sufficiently high flow of oxygenated blood to the muscles (p. 466). The integrated organ-system response to the new, elevated metabolic load involves the close coupling of the pulmonary and the cardiovascular O_2-delivery systems to the O_2-acceptor mechanisms in the muscle; the response includes sophisticated reflexes to ensure matching of the two processes.

The convective O_2-delivery rate is the product of cardiac output (i.e., heart rate · stroke volume) and arterial O_2 content:

Equation 59–5

Arterial O_2 delivery rate to whole body		Heart rate	Cardiac stroke volume	Arterial O_2 content
$\dot{Q}a_{O_2}$	=	HR	· SV	· Ca_{O_2}
$\dfrac{ml\ O_2}{min}$		$\dfrac{beats}{min}$	$\dfrac{ml\ blood}{beat}$	$\dfrac{ml\ O_2}{ml\ blood}$

The rate of O_2 uptake by skeletal muscle ($\dot{Q}o_2$) depends on both the O_2 delivery to skeletal muscle and the **extraction** of oxygen by the muscle. According to the Fick equation (p. 442), $\dot{Q}o_2$ is the product of blood flow to muscle (F) and the arteriovenous difference for O_2

Equation 59–6

Rate of O_2 uptake by skeletal muscle		Blood flow to skeletal muscle	A-V difference of O_2 content
$\dot{Q}a_{O_2}$	=	F	· $(Ca_{O_2} - Cv_{O_2})$
$\dfrac{ml\ O_2}{min}$		$\dfrac{ml\ blood}{min}$	$\dfrac{ml\ O_2}{ml\ blood}$

The $\dot{Q}o_2$, established by the rate of cross-bridge cycling and thus ATP turnover in muscle, requires an adequate and appropriate rate of O_2 delivery to the active muscle. Exercise triggers a complicated series of changes in the cardiovascular system that has the net effect of increasing F (p. 582). Increased O_2 extraction from the blood by active skeletal muscle occurs at the onset of exercise, owing to the low intracellular Po_2 in exercising muscle, which increases the gradient for O_2 diffusion from blood to mitochondria.

At the onset of exercise, $[Ca_{O_2}]$ actually increases somewhat (e.g., from 19 to 20 ml O_2/ml blood) secondary to the increase in alveolar ventilation—an anticipatory response called "striking"—triggered by the central nervous system (p. 395). Also as a consequence of the anticipatory hyperventilation, Pco_2 actually falls with the onset of exercise. Possible mechanisms of this ventilatory increase include a response to: mechanoreceptors in joints and muscles; descending cortical input; or resetting of peripheral chemoreceptors by a reduction in their blood supply (p. 725). The increase in ventilation in anticipation of future needs is enhanced in well-trained athletes.

The Cardiovascular System Is the Limiting Step for Maximal O_2 Utilization

For years, exercise and sports scientists have debated over the factors that limit $\dot{V}o_{2max}$ and thus contribute to performance limitations. As noted earlier, the transport of O_2 from atmosphere to muscle mitochondria occurs in three steps: uptake, delivery, and extraction. A limitation in any step could be rate limiting for maximal O_2 utilization by muscle.

LIMITED O_2 UPTAKE BY LUNGS. One view is that the lungs limit $\dot{V}o_{2max}$. An inability of alveolar O_2 diffusion to saturate arterial blood fully occurs (p. 682) in a subset of elite athletes (also in race horses). Thus, a decrease in Ca_{O_2} occurs at maximal effort on an incremental test. The inability to saturate arterial blood in athletes could be the consequence of a ventilation-perfusion mismatch at very high cardiac outputs (see Chapter 30).

LIMITED O_2 DELIVERY BY CARDIOVASCULAR SYSTEM. According to the prevalent view, a limitation in O_2 transport by the cardiovascular system determines $\dot{V}o_{2max}$. That is, according to the **convective flow model**, maximal cardiac output, and hence O_2 delivery, is the limiting step. Support for this view comes from the observation that training can considerably augment maximal cardiac output and muscle blood flow (see the following section). Moreover, $\dot{V}o_{2max}$ largely increases in parallel with such augmentations (Fig. 59–6).

LIMITED O_2 EXTRACTION BY MUSCLE. A third point of view is that, with increasing demand, muscle's extraction of O_2 from blood becomes inadequate despite adequate O_2 delivery. According to this **diffusive flow model**, a major limitation in O_2 transport is the kinetics of O_2 diffusion from hemoglobin in the red cell to the muscle mitochondrial matrix. Anything that lowers either the muscle diffusing capacity for O_2 or the Po_2 gradient between hemoglobin and mitochondria reduces $\dot{V}o_{2max}$.

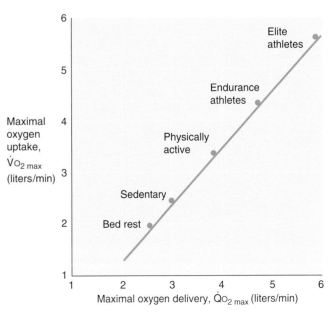

FIGURE 59–6. Dependence of maximal oxygen utilization on oxygen delivery. The *graph* illustrates the relationship between maximal O_2 delivery to the peripheral tissues ($\dot{Q}_{O_{2max}}$) and maximal O_2 uptake by lungs ($\dot{V}_{O_{2max}}$) for five individuals with different life styles. Training increases both O_2 delivery and O_2 uptake. (Data from B. Saltin and S. Strange. Maximal oxygen uptake: old and new arguments for a cardiovascular limitation. Med. Sci. Sports Ex. 24:30–37, 1992.)

INTERACTION BETWEEN EXERCISE AND CONTROL OF EFFECTIVE CIRCULATING VOLUME AND TEMPERATURE

During Exercise, Maintaining an Adequate Effective Circulating Volume Can Take Precedence Over Maintaining Cutaneous Blood Flow for Temperature Regulation

When we exercise in the heat, our circulatory systems must simultaneously support a large blood flow to both the skin (p. 1236) and contracting muscles, thus taxing the cardiac output and effective circulating volume. During exercise, the ability to maintain both arterial blood pressure and body core temperature within acceptable physiological limits depends on maintaining an adequate effective circulating volume (p. 864). Effective circulating volume depends on total blood volume, which in turn depends on extracellular fluid volume, and overall vasomotor (primarily venomotor) tone, which is important for distributing blood between central and peripheral pools.

Effective circulating volume tends to fall during prolonged exercise, especially exercise in the heat, for three reasons (Fig. 59–7). First, exercise causes a **shift in plasma water** from the intravascular to the interstitial space. This transcapillary movement of fluid during exercise reflects primarily an increased capillary hydrostatic pressure (p. 471). In addition, an increased osmolality within muscle cells removes water from the extracellular space. When exercise intensity exceeds 40% of $\dot{V}_{O_{2max}}$, this loss of plasma water is proportional to the exercise intensity. In extreme conditions, this loss of plasma water can amount to more than 500 ml of plasma water or about one sixth of the total plasma volume.

The second reason that effective circulating volume falls during exercise is loss of total-body water by **evaporation of perspiration**. To the extent that this perspiration is "free water" (p. 79), it is ultimately derived from all body fluid compartments, including the blood. It is not unusual for an individual to lose up to 2 liters/hour of perspiration in a hot environment (p. 1235). This water loss provides an evaporative rate in excess of 1000 kcal/h, but costs the body an important fraction of its total water if exercise is prolonged. A loss of body water in excess of 3% of body weight is associated with early signs of heat-related illness, including lightheadedness and disorientation, and constitutes **clinical dehydration**.

The third factor that acts to reduce effective circulating

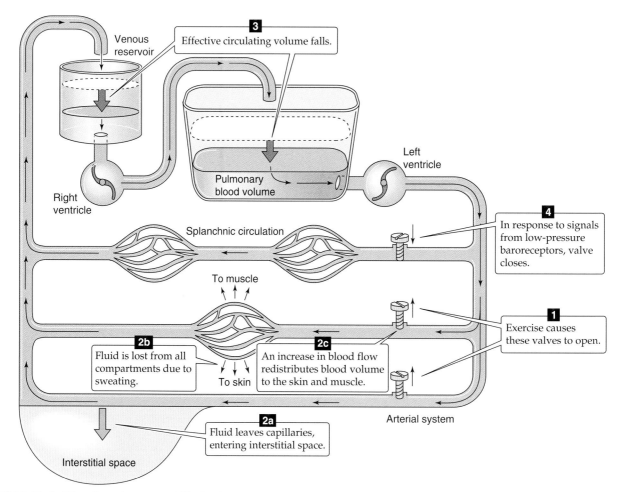

FIGURE 59–7. Effect of exercise on central blood volume.

blood volume during exercise is **redistribution of blood volume** to the skin because of the increase in cutaneous blood flow in response to body heating. Venous volume *in the skin* increases as a result of the increased pressure in the compliant vessels as blood flow to the skin rises. No compensatory venoconstriction occurs in the skin because of the overriding action of the temperature-control system.

In response to this decrease in effective circulating volume that occurs during exercise, the cardiopulmonary, low-pressure baroreceptors (p. 548) initiate compensatory responses to increase total vascular resistance (see Fig. 59–7). This resistance increase is accomplished by:

1. Increasing the splanchnic vascular resistance.
2. Offsetting some of the vasodilatory drive to the skin initiated by the temperature-control system.
3. Offsetting some of the vasodilatory drive to the active skeletal muscles (in extreme conditions).

Although limiting peripheral blood flow has the benefit of helping maintain arterial blood pressure and effective circulating volume, it carries two liabilities. First, it reduces convective heat transfer from core to skin because of the reduced skin blood flow, contributing to excessive heat storage. Second, the limitation of blood flow to active muscle may compromise O_2 delivery.

In conditions of low thermal and metabolic demand, no serious conflict arises among the systems that regulate effective circulating volume, arterial blood pressure, and body temperature. The cutaneous circulation is capable of handling the heat transfer requirements of the temperature regulatory mechanism without impairing muscle blood flow or cardiac filling pressure. However, in conditions of heavier thermal and metabolic demand, signals related to the decreased effective circulating volume may compromise temperature regulation and muscle blood flow, as noted in the previous paragraph.

A Dilute (Hypotonic) Perspiration Preserves Extracellular NaCl, and, Therefore, Blood Volume

The rate of perspiration increases with body core temperature (see Fig. 58–5), which in turn increases during exercise (p. 1238) and exposure to heat. The rate of water loss from the skin can exceed 30 ml/min under extreme conditions. The rate of water loss from the pulmonary system can add an additional 2 ml/min during heavy exercise. Thus, assuming that water comprises 60% of the body mass, a 70-kg adult could lose almost 2 liters or 5% of water content each hour. The water lost from the body comes from all body-fluid compartments, including the blood compartment.

Perspiration is hypotonic with respect to blood plasma. The concentration of the different electrolytes in perspiration varies widely (1) among individuals, (2) at different rates of perspiration, and (3) according to the individual's level of heat acclimatization and physical fitness. The concentrations of Na^+ and Cl^-, the major ions in perspiration, average 40 to 60 mM and 30 to 45 mM, respectively, which are approximately one third of their concentrations in plasma. The $[K^+]$ of perspiration is 5 to 10 mM, somewhat higher than its plasma concentration. The difference between the volume of the hypotonic perspiration and the volume of isotonic plasma that would contain the same electrolytes as the perspiration is called the **free water loss**.

Because of the hypotonicity of perspiration, the body loses relatively more water than salt during conditions of body heating, causing the extracellular fluid to become both reduced in volume and relatively hypertonic. Following the increase in extracellular-fluid osmolality, water moves out of the cells down an osmotic gradient, resulting in a decrease in intracellular fluid volume and an increase in intracellular osmolality (p. 76). This water movement helps maintain the extracellular fluid volume.

It is not surprising that among the benefits of physical training and heat acclimatization is the development of a more dilute perspiration, which conserves NaCl during dehydration. In turn, the NaCl content of the extracellular fluids is a major determinant of plasma volume (p. 80). If perspiration were isotonic with plasma, perspiring would deplete extracellular fluid volume, leaving behind an isotonic extracellular fluid. In such a case, just as in hemorrhage, plasma osmolality would not transiently increase and no water would move from the intracellular to the extracellular compartment. Thus, the result of perspiring a large volume of *isotonic* fluid would be a decrease in extracellular fluid and plasma volume, and ultimately hypovolemic shock.

Ingesting Salt with Water Is the Best Way to Recover Total-Body Water Following Dehydration from Heat Exposure or Exercise

Restoring body-fluid volume following dehydration is often delayed in humans despite the consumption of fluids. The reason for this delay is that dehydrated humans drink free water, which reduces the osmolality of the extracellular fluid and reduces the osmotic drive for drinking (p. 871). This consumed free water distributes into—and dilutes—the cells as well as the extracellular space. In addition, the reduced plasma osmolality leads to decreased secretion of arginine vasopressin (i.e., antidiuretic hormone), increasing free-water excretion by the kidney (p. 840).

A more effective means of restoring body fluid volume is to ingest NaCl with water. When Na^+ is taken with water, as when certain commercially available "exercise drinks" are consumed, plasma $[Na^+]$ remains elevated throughout a greater duration of the rehydration period and is significantly higher than when water alone is ingested. In such conditions, the salt-dependent thirst drive is maintained and the stimulation of urine production is delayed, leading to a more complete restoration of body water content. A better recovery of body fluid status provides a better ability to regulate body temperature, particularly in conditions of thermal stress.

AEROBIC TRAINING

Training Increases the Resistance to Fatigue

Aerobic conditioning increases the resistance to fatigue at all exercise intensities. As already noted, training increases $\dot{V}o_{2max}$ (p. 1248) as well as the body's ability to eliminate excess heat that is produced during exercise (see Fig. 58–5).

The increased $\dot{V}o_{2max}$ that occurs with training has obvious practical benefits. As the requirement for energy release in active muscle approaches $\dot{V}o_{2max}$, anaerobic processes become increasingly important in maintaining ATP production. Increasing one's $\dot{V}o_{2max}$ allows a given rate of ATP production to occur relatively more aerobically, all other factors being equal. When $\dot{V}o_2$ is less than 50% of the maximum, essentially all of the net energy release in active muscle is aerobic. In this condition, the O_2 transport via the pulmonary and circulatory systems matches the O_2 demand in the muscle, avoiding disturbances in acid-base balance.

When O_2 uptake exceeds 60% of $\dot{V}o_{2\,max}$, muscle anaerobiosis increases roughly in proportion to the increase in relative power output. In addition, the muscle produces *excess lactic acid* and protons, and these byproducts diffuse into the bloodstream. The body partially compensates for the resulting decrease in blood pH by hyperventilation (p. 723). Increasing the $\dot{V}o_{2\,max}$ thus raises the threshold of exercise intensity at which lactic acid appears, suggesting that physical training alters both the O_2-transport and O_2-acceptance systems.

Aerobic Training Increases Maximal O_2 Delivery By Increasing Plasma Volume, Thereby Increasing Maximal Cardiac Output

Maximal O_2 uptake could increase as the result of either optimizing O_2 delivery to active muscle or optimizing O_2 extraction by active muscle, as demonstrated in the following modification of Equation 59–6:

Equation 59–7

Maximal rate of O_2 uptake	Optimized heart rate	Optimized stroke volume	Maximal A-V difference of O_2 content

$$\dot{Q}a_{O_2} = \underbrace{HR_{opt} \cdot SV_{opt}}_{\substack{\text{Maximal} \\ \text{cardiac output}}} \cdot (Ca_{O_2} - Cv_{O_2})_{max}$$

In fact, aerobic training improves both O_2 delivery and extraction; the problem for physiologists has been to determine to what extent each system contributes to the whole-body response. For example, an increase in the circulatory system's capacity to deliver O_2 could reflect an increase in either the maximal arterial O_2 content or the maximal cardiac output, or both.

MAXIMIZING ARTERIAL O$_2$ CONTENT. Several factors could theoretically contribute to maximizing Ca_{O_2}:

1. Increasing the maximal alveolar ventilation enhances the driving force for O_2 uptake by the lungs (see Fig. 30–4).
2. Increasing the capacity for gases to diffuse across the alveolar-capillary barrier in the lungs could enhance O_2 uptake at very high cardiac output, particularly at high altitude (see Fig. 26–8).
3. Improving the matching of pulmonary ventilation to perfusion increases arterial Po_2 and increases the saturation of hemoglobin (p. 705).
4. Increasing the concentration of hemoglobin enables a given volume of arterial blood to carry a greater amount of O_2 (p. 656).

In nearly all conditions of exercise, the pulmonary system maintains alveolar Po_2 at levels that are sufficiently high to ensure nearly complete (i.e., $\sim 97\%$) O_2 saturation of hemoglobin, even at maximal power output. Thus, it is unlikely that an increase in the maximal alveolar ventilation or pulmonary diffusing capacity could explain the large increase in $\dot{V}o_{2\,max}$ that occurs with training.

Ca_{O_2} would be increased by elevating the blood's hemoglobin concentration. However, there is no evidence that physical training induces such an increase. To the contrary, [hemoglobin] tends to be slightly lower in endurance athletes, a phenomenon called "sports anemia," which reflects an expansion of the plasma compartment (see later). Whereas increasing [hemoglobin] provides a greater O_2-carrying capacity in blood, the maximal O_2 transport does not necessarily increase accordingly because blood viscosity, and therefore total vascular resistance, would also increase. The heart would be required to develop a higher arterial pressure to generate an equivalent cardiac output. The resultant increased cardiac work would thus be counterproductive to the overall adaptive response.

MAXIMIZING CARDIAC OUTPUT. Factors that contribute to increasing maximal cardiac output include optimizing the increases in heart rate and cardiac stroke volume so that their product (i.e., cardiac output) is maximal (see Equation 59–7).

Figure 59–8 illustrates how conditioning affects cardiac output and the arteriovenous difference for O_2 content. Compared with a control situation (*blue curves*), prolonged bed rest (*red curves*) has little effect on maximal heart rate, diminishes maximal stroke volume, and greatly reduces maximal cardiac output. However, training (*green curves*) increases maximal stroke volume, slightly decreases maximal heart rate, but greatly increases maximal cardiac output. Neither training nor bed rest has a substantial effect on $(Ca_{O_2} - Cv_{O_2})_{max}$ (i.e., maximal O_2 extraction).

Because training produces no dramatic increase in either maximal heart rate or maximal O_2 extraction, nearly all of the increase in $\dot{V}o_{2\,max}$ that occurs with training must be due to an increase in maximal cardiac output, the product of optimal heart rate and optimal stroke vol-

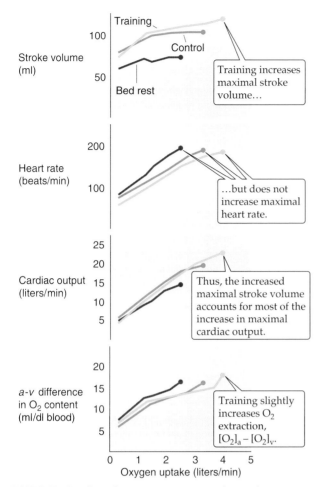

FIGURE 59–8. Effect of training on various cardiovascular parameters. The four *graphs* show changes in four cardiovascular parameters at different levels of O_2 uptake (i.e., different intensities of exercise). The four *blue curves* represent mean values for five untrained subjects. The *purple curves* summarize similar data for the same five subjects after 20 days of bed rest. The *green curves* summarize data after 50 days of physical training. (Data from Saltin B, Blomqvist G, Mitchell JH, et al: Response to submaximal and maximal exercise after bed rest and training. Circulation 38(Suppl. 7):1968.)

*Labels within figure:*

Stroke volume (ml) — Training; Control; Bed rest; "Training increases maximal stroke volume…"

Heart rate (beats/min) — "…but does not increase maximal heart rate."

Cardiac output (liters/min) — "Thus, the increased maximal stroke volume accounts for most of the increase in maximal cardiac output."

a-v difference in O_2 content (ml/dl blood) — "Training slightly increases O_2 extraction, $[O_2]_a - [O_2]_v$."

Oxygen uptake (liters/min)

ume in Equation 59–7. The athlete achieves this increased cardiac output by increasing **maximal cardiac stroke volume**. Maximal cardiac output can increase by approximately 40% during physical conditioning that also increases maximal aerobic power by 50%. The difference between 40% and 50% is accounted for by an increased extraction, $(Ca_{O_2} - Cv_{O_2})_{max}$. The latter is the consequence of capillary proliferation and of elevating key oxidative enzymes in the mitochondria of type I muscle fibers, creating a greater O_2 sink under maximal conditions (see the next section).

Maximal cardiac stroke volume increases during aerobic training because expansion of the plasma compartment increases the heart's preload (p. 528). An increase in preload increases ventricular filling and proportionally increases stroke volume (Starling's law of the heart), elevating maximal cardiac output accordingly. An additional benefit is that a trained athlete achieves a given cardiac output at a lower cardiac frequency, both at rest and

during moderate exercise. Because it is more efficient to increase stroke volume than heart rate, increasing stroke volume reduces the myocardial metabolic load for any particular level of activity.

The expansion of plasma volume probably reflects an increase in albumin content (1 g albumin is dissolved in 18 g of plasma H_2O). This increase appears to be due both to translocation (by an unknown mechanism) from the interstitial compartment and to increased synthesis by the liver. The result is increased colloid osmotic pressure in the capillaries, promoting a shift of fluid from the interstitium to the blood. Although the total volume of red blood cells increases with aerobic training, the plasma-volume expansion is greater than the red-cell expansion, thus reducing the hemoglobin concentration; hence, the **sports anemia**.

The increased blood volume has another beneficial effect: it enhances the ability to maintain a high skin blood flow in potentially compromising conditions (e.g., heavy exercise in the heat), thus providing a greater heat transport from core to skin and thus a relatively lower storage of heat (p. 1233).

Training Enhances Diffusion of O_2 into Muscle

Whereas an increase in maximal cardiac output accounts for most of the increased delivery of O_2 to muscle with training, a lesser fraction reflects increased O_2 extraction from blood. Fick's law describes the diffusion of O_2 between the alveolar air and pulmonary capillary blood (see Equation 29–7). A similar relationship, shown in Equation 58–8, describes the diffusion of O_2 from the systemic capillary blood to the mitochondria.

The factors that contribute to D_{O_2} are analogous to those that affect the diffusing capacity in the lung. Trained muscle can accommodate a greater maximal blood flow (and therefore an increased blood volume) because of the growth of new capillaries. Indeed, well-conditioned people have a 60% greater number of capillaries for a given cross-sectional area of muscle fiber than sedentary people do. This increased capillary density increases D_{O_2}, thus providing a greater surface area for diffusion. Increased capillary density also reduces the diffusion distance for O_2 between the capillary and muscle fibers (see Fig. 19–4).

Another consequence of increased capillary density (and perhaps increased capillary length as well) is that at a given blood flow the mean transit time of blood in muscle increases. Because the blood lingers for a longer time in the muscle capillaries, O_2 extraction increases. However, training also increases maximal skeletal-muscle blood flow, reflecting an increase in maximal cardiac output and the greater number of parallel vessels in muscle. The increase in blood flow through active skeletal muscle minimizes the decay in capillary P_{O_2} that tends to occur along the vessel as the result of increased D_{O_2} and capillary density. This preservation of capillary P_{O_2} maintains the blood-to-mitochondrion P_{O_2} gradient, enhancing O_2 diffusion.

Equation 59–8

Rate of O_2 uptake by skeletal muscle	O_2 diffusion capacity for skeletal muscle	P_{O_2} in blood of muscle capillary	P_{O_2} in muscle mitochondria
$\dot{Q}O_2$	$= D_{O_2}$	$(P_{O_2\ cap}$	$- P_{O_2\ mito})$
ml O_2/(min · kg)	ml O_2/(min · kg · mm Hg)		(mm Hg)

Aerobic Training Also Increases the Expression of Key Mitochondrial Enzymes

Another factor that accounts for the increased uptake of O_2 by muscle in trained people is elevated oxidative enzyme activity in the muscle mitochondria (Fig. 59–9). Levels of mRNA increase for specific enzymes, implying increased transcription owing to signals associated with the exercise stimulus (e.g., elevated hormones, altered plasma osmolality). Prolonged aerobic conditioning increases levels of succinic dehydrogenase, NADH dehydrogenase, and cytochrome oxidase.

Increased oxidative enzyme activity increases the muscle Po_2 sink (i.e., decreases $Po_{2\ mito}$ as illustrated in Equation 59–8), enhancing O_2 diffusion from capillary to mitochondrion. This increased diffusion is also the reason why $(Ca_{O_2} - Cv_{O_2})_{max}$ in Equation 59–7 remained approximately constant with training, even though blood flow increased markedly. If O_2 diffusion had *not* increased, $[O_2]_V$ would have risen, and $(Ca_{O_2} - Cv_{O_2})_{max}$ would have *decreased*.

Trained athletes mobilize free fatty acids more rapidly during exercise. Increasing mitochondrial oxidative enzyme activity provides an increased ability to oxidize these free fatty acids during a demand for fuel delivery.

This change is accompanied by an adaptive *decrease* in the activity of glycolytic rate-limiting enzymes. These adaptations conserve muscle glycogen and thus delay glycogen depletion during a given demand for fuel.

Aerobically trained people have a decreased tissue sensitivity to insulin during exercise, in contrast to the increase that occurs during exercise in the general (untrained) population. A decreased insulin sensitivity slows glucose transport into muscle, increasing the reliance on the oxidation of free fatty acids, and further sparing muscle glycogen.

REFERENCES

Books and Reviews

Booth FW, Thomason DB: Molecular and cellular adaptation of muscle in response to exercise: Perspectives of various models. Physiol Rev 71:541–585, 1991.

Fitts RH: Cellular mechanisms of muscle fatigue. Physiol Rev 74:49–94, 1994.

Jones JH, Lindstedt SL: Limits to maximal performance. Annu Rev Physiol 55:547–569, 1993.

Lehmann MJ, Lormes W, Opitz-Gress A, et al: Training and overtraining: An overview and experimental results in endurance sports. J Sports Med Phys Fitness 37:7–17, 1997.

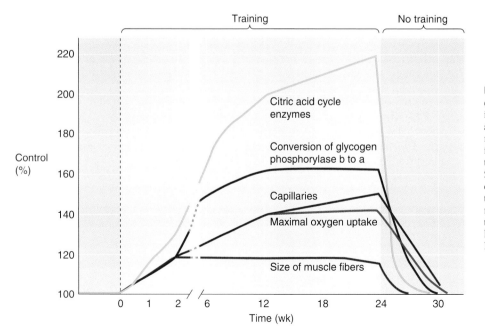

FIGURE 59–9. Enzyme adaptation during training. Training causes a slow increase in the level of several enzymes, as well as in the number of capillaries, maximal O_2 uptake, and size of muscle fibers. These changes reverse rapidly on the cessation of training. (Data from Saltin B, Henriksson J, Nygaard E, Andersen P: Fiber types and metabolic potentials of skeletal muscles in sedentary man and endurance runners. The Marathon: Physiological, Medical, Epidemiological, and Psychological Studies. Ann NY Acad Sci 301:3–29, 1977.)

Nadel ER: Physiological adaptations to aerobic training. Am Scientist 73: 334–343, 1985.

Saltin B, Strange S: Maximal oxygen uptake: Old and new arguments for a cardiovascular limitation. Med Sci Sports Ex 24:30–37, 1992.

Wagner PD: Determinants of maximal oxygen transport and utilization. Annu Rev Physiol 58:21–50, 1996.

Journal Articles

Gollnick PD, Armstrong RB, Saubert CW IV, et al: Enzyme activity and fiber composition in skeletal muscle of untrained and trained men. J Appl Physiol 33:312–319, 1972.

Nadel ER, Bussolari SR: The Daedalus Project: Physiological problems and solutions. Am Scientist 76:351–360, 1988.

Saltin B, Blomqvist G, Mitchell JH, et al: Response to submaximal and maximal exercise after bed rest and training. Circulation 38(Suppl 7): 1–78, 1968.

CHAPTER 60

Environmental Physiology
Diving, Altitude, and Space

Ethan Nadel

The earth and its atmosphere provide environments that are compatible with an extraordinary number of diverse life forms, each adapted to its particular ecologic niche. However, not all of the earth's surface is equally friendly for *human* survival, let alone comfort and function. Mountain climbers and deep-sea divers know the profound effects of **barometric pressure** on human physiology, and astronauts quickly learn how the physically equivalent forces of **gravity** and **acceleration** affect the body. Humans can adapt to changes in barometric pressure and gravity up to a point, but survival under extreme conditions requires special equipment; otherwise, our physiological limitations would restrict our occupancy of this planet to its lowland surfaces.

The Ideal Gas Law Describes How Increases in Barometric Pressure or Decreases in Absolute Temperature Decrease Gas Volume

In the mid-17th century, Robert Boyle demonstrated that the relation between the pressure (*P*) and volume (*V*) of a *real* gas at a fixed temperature is essentially hyperbolic. **Boyle's law** states that *P* and *V* for an *ideal* gas vary inversely:

Equation 60–1

$$PV = \textit{Constant \#1}$$

At the molecular level, the pressure exerted by a fixed number of gas molecules—the total force of gas per unit surface area of the container—reflects the number of collisions molecules make with the walls of the container. If we reduce the container's volume by half, the number of collisions doubles for each square centimeter of the container's walls and, therefore, pressure doubles.

A century after Boyle's work, Jacques Charles found that the volume of a gas varies linearly with absolute temperature (*T*, in °K) if pressure is constant:

Equation 60–2

$$V = (\textit{Constant \#2}) \cdot T$$
$$or$$
$$V/T = \textit{Constant \#2}$$

At the molecular level, **Charles' law** states that increasing the temperature increases the velocity of gas molecules, forcing the perfectly compliant container to increase in size.

Combining these two laws yields the so-called **Boyle-Charles law**:

Equation 60–3

$$PV/T = Constant \ \#3$$

For an ideal gas, "Constant #3" is nothing more than $n \cdot R$, where n is the number of moles and R is the universal gas constant. Incorporating n and R into Equation 60–3 yields the **ideal gas law**:

Equation 60–4

$$PV = nRT$$

If we compare the relationship among pressure, volume, and temperature for a fixed number of moles of the gas under two conditions, we see that

Equation 60–5

$$\frac{P_1 \cdot V_1}{T_1} = \frac{P_2 \cdot V_2}{T_2}$$

With this simple equation, one better appreciates what happens when barometric pressure increases during diving or decreases during ascent to high altitude.

The barometric pressure (P_B) is the sum of the **partial pressures** of the individual gases in the air mixture (**Dalton's law**) (see box on p. 597). Thus, in the case of ordinary *dry* air (see Table 25–1), most of the sea-level P_B of 760 mm Hg is due to N_2 (~593 mm Hg) and O_2 (~159 mm Hg), with smaller contributions from trace gases such as argon (~7 mm Hg) and CO_2 (~0.2 mm Hg). Thus, as P_B increases during diving beneath the water, or as P_B decreases during ascent to high altitude, the partial pressure of each constituent gas will change in proportion to the change in P_B. This relationship is important for O_2 delivery to tissues, because a key variable that determines the O_2 saturation of hemoglobin (Hb) is P_{O_2} in the inspired air (p. 692).

The conducting airways humidify inspired air so that it becomes fully saturated with H_2O vapor at body temperature (see box on p. 595). The H_2O vapor then occupies part of the space in the lungs. At a body temperature of 37°C, P_{H_2O} is 47 mm Hg. If P_B is 760 mm Hg, only $760 - 47 = 713$ mm Hg is available for the sum of P_{O_2}, P_{N_2}, and P_{CO_2}. Because H_2O readily evaporates from (or condenses into) liquid water, its partial pressure does not change with changes in P_B.

DIVING PHYSIOLOGY

For Every 10 Meters of Depth of Immersion, Barometric Pressure Increases by One Atmosphere, Thereby Compressing Gases in the Lungs

The average P_B at sea level is 760 mm Hg. In other words, if you stand at sea level, the column of air extending from your feet upward for several tens of kilometers through the atmosphere exerts a pressure of "1 atmosphere (atm)." It is only when diving under the water surface that humans experience a significant *increase* in

P_B. A column of fresh water 10.3 m high exerts a pressure of 760 mm Hg, the average P_B at sea level; the same is true for a column of water extending from the surface of a lake to a depth of 10.3 m. For seawater, which has a density approximately 2.5% greater than that of fresh water, the column must be only 10 m to exert 1 atm of pressure. P_B increases linearly with the height (weight) of the column of water (Fig. 60–1A). Ten meters below the surface of the sea, P_B is 2 atm, 1 atm for the atmospheric pressure and 1 atm for the column of water. As the depth increases to 20 m and then to 30 m, P_B increases to 3 atm, then 4 atm, and so on.

The body's fluid and solid components are relatively resistant to compression by increased external water pressure. However, external pressure compresses the body's air compartments to an extent that is determined by the compliance of the particular compartment. According to Boyle's law (Equation 60–1), P and V vary inversely with each other. Thus, if the chest wall were perfectly compliant, a breath-holding dive to 10 m below the surface would double the pressure and compress the air held in the lungs to half its original volume.

The human record for a breath-hold dive is an amazing 70 m below the surface, and animals dive to far greater depths. Whales, for example, can extend a breath-hold dive for up to 2 hours, descending to depths as great as 900 m (91 atm) without suffering any ill effects.

As P_B increases with depth, so will the partial pressures of each constituent gas, such as O_2 and N_2. Increasing alveolar P_{O_2} increases the volume of the O_2 that is physically dissolved in blood. Similarly, the increased alveolar P_{N_2} forces larger amounts of even poorly soluble N_2 from alveoli into blood. As discussed later, increasing inspired P_{O_2} and P_{N_2} for an extended period is potentially harmful.

The increase in P_B will also increase alveolar P_{CO_2}. Descending far enough to double the P_B will increase alveolar P_{CO_2} to 80 mm Hg, which is substantially above the P_{CO_2} of mixed-venous blood at sea level (46 mm Hg), causing CO_2 to enter the blood and increase arterial P_{CO_2}. In addition, metabolically generated CO_2 accumulates in the blood during a breath-holding dive, eventually raising mixed-venous P_{CO_2} above alveolar P_{CO_2}. The increase in arterial P_{CO_2} can reduce the duration of the dive by stimulating the chemoreceptors (p. 723) and increasing the drive to ventilate. During the ascent phase of the dive, alveolar P_{CO_2} falls below the P_{CO_2} of mixed-venous blood, favoring CO_2 exit from the blood.

Diving also compresses the air that is held in air spaces other than the airways (e.g., the gastrointestinal tract). In relatively stiff cavities, or in cavities that cannot equilibrate readily with external pressure, increases of external pressure can distort the cavity wall, resulting in pain or damage. For example, if the eustachian tube is blocked, the middle-ear pressure cannot equilibrate with external pressure, and the tympanic membrane can rupture.

Divers Breathe Compressed Air to Keep Their Lungs Fully Expanded

Early techniques enabled divers to remain beneath the water surface for periods greater than that permitted by a single breath-hold. One of the earliest such devices was a

A PRESSURES AT INCREASING DEPTH

Breathing a mixture of O_2 and helium to "saturation" at this depth requires nearly 4 days for decompression.

Human record for breath-hold dive.

Breathing air for 2–4 h ("saturation") at this depth requires 40 h for decompression.

B DIVING BELL

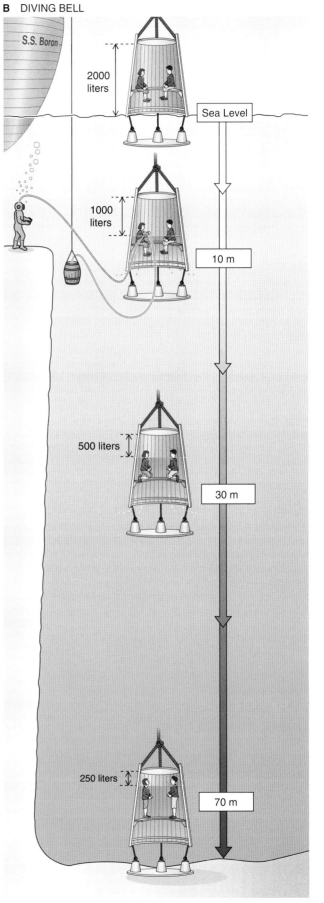

S.S. Boron

2000 liters

Sea Level

1000 liters

10 m

500 liters

30 m

250 liters

70 m

FIGURE 60–1. Effects of descending to increased depth. *A*, The pressure at the surface of the ocean is 1 atm and increases by 1 atm for each 10 m of immersion in sea water. In fresh water, which has a lower density, the pressure is 1 atm for each 10.3 m. *B*, In 1690, Halley, the astronomer who gave his name to the comet, designed and built a wooden diving bell with an open bottom. Because the bell was at a relatively shallow depth, the water level only rose partly into the bell. In Halley's system, the air was replenished from a barrel. This design was in use for a century, until a practical pump was available for pumping air directly from the surface. The *lower part* of the figure illustrates what would have happened if Halley's bell had been lowered to much larger depths. The greater the depth, the greater the water pressure. Because the air pressure inside the bell must be the same as the water pressure, the air volume progressively decreases at greater depths, and the water level rises inside the bell.

diving bell that surrounded the diver on all sides except the bottom. Such a bell was reportedly used by Alexander the Great in 330 BC and then improved by Sir Edmund Halley in 1690 (see Fig. 60–1B). By the early 19th century, pumping compressed air from above the water surface through a hose to the space underneath the bell kept water out of the bell. In all of these cases, the diver breathed air at the same pressure as the surrounding water. Although the pressures both surrounding the diver's chest and inside the airways were far higher than at sea level, the pressure *gradient* across the chest wall was normal. Thus, the lungs were normally expanded.

The conditions are essentially the same in a modern-day **caisson**, a massive, hollow, pressurized structure that functions like a large diving bell. Once again, the pressure inside the caisson (3–4 atm) has to be high enough to prevent water at the bottom of the caisson from entering. Several workers ("sand-hogs") at the bottom of the caisson might excavate material from the bottom of a river for constructing tunnels or foundations of bridges. Eventually, individual divers wore diving suits with spherical helmets over their heads (Fig. 60–2A). Of course, the air inside these helmets needed to be pressurized to match exactly the pressure of the water in which they were diving.

In 1943, Jacques Cousteau perfected the "self-contained underwater breathing apparatus," or **SCUBA**, that replaced cumbersome gear and increased the mobility and convenience of an underwater dive (see Fig. 60–2B). The SCUBA system consists of five major elements:

1. A tank of gas compressed to a pressure that exceeds the highest pressures that the diver would encounter during the dive.

2. A reducing valve that delivers gas from the tanks to the diver's hose at a pressure of 6 to 7 atm.

3. A "demand" breathing valve for inspiration, triggered to open by the slight decrease in pressure caused by the diver's inspiration. This valve delivers the air mixture to the diver at the ambient pressure.

4. An exhaust valve that allows expired air to be released at a pressure that is slightly higher than ambient.

5. A face mask or mouthpiece with a gas-delivery system that has a small ventilatory dead space (p. 687).

These techniques permit deep dives for extended periods of time. However, for reasons that will become apparent, use of any of these techniques while breathing *room air* carries certain hazards, including nitrogen narcosis, oxygen toxicity, and problems with decompression. Advances in understanding the physiology of gases at high pressures has led to approaches and equipment that allow for safe, prolonged exposures at depth.

Increasing Alveolar P_{N_2} Can Cause Narcosis

Descending beneath the water causes the inspired P_{N_2}—nearly 600 mm Hg at sea level (see Table 25–1)—to increase as P_B increases. Thus, according to Henry's law (box on p. 597), the increased P_{N_2} will cause more N_2 to dissolve in the body's tissues. Because of its high lipid solubility, N_2 dissolves readily in adipocytes and in membrane lipids. A high P_{N_2} reduces the ion conductance of membranes, and therefore neuronal excitability, by mechanisms that are similar to those contributing to the narcotizing effect of gas anesthetics. Diving to increased depths (e.g., 4–5 atm) while breathing compressed air causes **nitrogen narcosis**. Mild nitrogen narcosis resembles alco-

A DIVING HELMET

Air from surface

Air hose

Diving helmet

B SCUBA SYSTEM

Hose

Reducing valve

Air cylinder

Demand and exhaust valve

FIGURE 60–2. Devices for breathing under water. *A*, Compressed air, pumped from the surface to the diver, keeps the pressure inside the helmet slightly higher than that of the surrounding water. *B*, SCUBA is an acronym for "self-contained underwater breathing apparatus."

hol intoxication (e.g., loss of psychosocial inhibitions). According to "Martini's law," each 15 m of depth has the effects of drinking an additional martini! Progressive narcosis occurs with increasing depth or time of the dive and is accompanied by lethargy and drowsiness, rapid onset of fatigue, and, eventually, a loss of consciousness. Because it develops insidiously, nitrogen narcosis poses a real threat to divers who are not aware of the risks. The consequences under the water can prove fatal.

Increasing Alveolar P_{O_2} Can Lead to Oxygen Toxicity

At sea level, dry inspired air has a P_{O_2} of 159 mm Hg. However, the *alveolar* P_{O_2} of a healthy person at sea-level air is approximately 101 mm Hg, reduced from 159 mm Hg by humidification in the airways and removal of O_2 by alveolar gas exchange (p. 693). Arterial P_{O_2} at sea level is very close to alveolar P_{O_2} (i.e., ~10 mm Hg) and nearly saturates Hb, yielding an arterial O_2 content of approximately 20 ml/dl blood (Fig. 60–3, *red curve*). As P_B —and therefore arterial P_{O_2}—increases at greater depths, the O_2 bound to Hb increases very little, whereas the O_2 that is physically dissolved in the water of blood increases linearly (*black line*). Thus, the increment of total O_2 content at depth reflects dissolved O_2 (*blue curve*).

During a breath-holding dive to 5 atm, or in a hyperbaric chamber pressurized to 5 atm, arterial P_{O_2} increases to approximately 700 mm Hg, slightly higher than breathing 100% O_2 at sea level. Exposure to such a high P_{O_2} has no ill effects up to several hours. However, prolonged exposure damages the airway epithelium and smooth muscle, causing bronchiolar and alveolar membrane inflammation and, ultimately, pulmonary edema, atelectasis, fibrin formation, and lung consolidation. These effects are the result of inactivating several structural repair enzymes and oxidizing certain cellular constituents.

A prolonged, elevated P_{O_2} also has detrimental effects on nonpulmonary tissues, including the central nervous system (CNS). Exposure to an ambient P_{O_2} of approximately 1500 mm Hg (e.g., breathing room air at ~10 atm) for as little as 30 to 45 minutes can cause seizures and coma (see Fig. 60–3). Preliminary symptoms of **oxygen toxicity** include muscle twitching, nausea, disorientation, and irritability. The toxic effects of O_2 occur because oxygen free radicals (e.g., superoxide and peroxide free radicals) oxidize the polyunsaturated fatty acid component of cell membranes as well as the enzymes that are involved in energy metabolism. At the more modest P_{O_2} levels that normally prevail at sea level, scavenger enzymes (e.g., superoxide dismutase, peroxidase, and catalase) eliminate the relatively few radicals formed.

In Long-Term Deep Dives, Replacing N_2 in the Inspired Air with Helium Avoids Nitrogen Narcosis, and Lowering the Fractional O_2 in the Inspired Air Avoids Oxygen Toxicity

Several occupations require people to spend extended periods at a P_B greater than that at sea level.

FIGURE 60–3. O_2 content of blood at high pressures. The *red curve* is the same hemoglobin-O_2 dissociation curve as that in Figure 28–3, except that the range is extended to very high values of P_{O_2}.

DEEP MINING. In deep mining, workers descend down a shaft to depths as great as 2.4 km below the surface. Just as P_B falls with ascent to a high altitude, it rises with descent to a great depth in a mine, doubling approximately every 5.5 km of depth. Nevertheless, 2.4 km below the earth's surface, P_B is only approximately 1.4 atm, presenting little problem to the miner. The greatest health hazards for the deep miner are from exposure to high temperature (ambient temperature increases by 1°C every ~300 m), from humidity (miners use a fine water spray to minimize dust), and from inspiring particulates.

CAISSON WORK. Caisson workers rarely experience more than 3 or 4 atm, and only for relatively brief periods. Because nitrogen narcosis begins to appear only at approximately 5 atm of room air after more than an hour, and because oxygen toxicity only begins to appear at approximately 10 atm of room air after more than 30 min, caisson workers can avoid the adverse effects of increased P_B while they are *in* the caisson. However, caisson workers may have major difficulties caused by decompression when *exiting* the caisson.

DEEP DIVING WORK. Divers may spend hours, days, or even weeks at depths between 60 m and 300 m below the water surface. They wear diving suits when working and live in compression chambers when at "leisure." Deep divers who spend days or weeks at high P_B must breathe special gas mixtures to avoid nitrogen narcosis and oxygen toxicity.

During an extended dive (one exceeding several hours), the body's tissues gradually equilibrate with the high-pressure gases that one has been breathing. After such a **saturation**, the diver must rise to the surface slowly (no faster than ~3 m/h) to allow enough time for the circulatory system to carry the dissolved N_2 to the alveoli. At sea level, the human body normally contains approximately 1 liter of dissolved N_2, equally distributed between the body's water and fat compartments. As P_{N_2} rises, the N_2 equilibrates only slowly with the body's lipid stores because adipose tissue is relatively underperfused. Although a deep dive of several minutes does not provide sufficient time to equilibrate the fat with N_2, one of several hours' duration does. At equilibrium, the volume of N_2 dissolved in the tissues is proportional to alveolar P_{N_2}. Thus, if the body normally dissolves 1 liter of N_2 at a P_B of 1 atm, it will ultimately dissolve 10 liters of N_2 at a P_B of 10 atm. These same principles apply to O_2, although the degree to which O_2 dissolves in various tissues, and the speed at which equilibration takes place, is different.

The adverse effects of N_2 and O_2 depend on the amount of gas that is dissolved in tissues. The amount, in turn, increases with the dive's depth (i.e., partial pressure of the gas) and duration (i.e., how close the gas is to achieving equilibrium with various tissues). Thus, the length of time that a diver can spend safely under water is inversely proportional to the depth of the dive.

To prevent **N_2 narcosis** in saturation-diving conditions, divers must partly or completely replace N_2 with another inert gas. Helium is the replacement gas of choice for four reasons: First, helium has only a fraction of the narcotizing effect of nitrogen. Second, helium dissolves in the tissues to a lesser extent than N_2. Third, helium has a lower density than N_2 does, which lowers effective airway resistance. However, the low density of helium facilitates convective "air" cooling around the body, increasing heat

loss. Thus, ambient temperature must be higher in a high-helium compression chamber. Fourth, during the decompression phase of a dive, helium diffuses out of the tissues more rapidly than does N_2, thereby reducing most of the problems associated with decompression.

To prevent **O_2 toxicity** in saturation-diving conditions, divers must reduce the $F_{I_{O_2}}$ (i.e., fraction of inspired air that is O_2) in the compressed-gas mixture. Thus, at a P_B of 10 atm, a mixture of 2% O_2 in helium will provide the same inspired P_{O_2} as room air does at sea level (i.e., ~20% O_2 at a P_B of 1 atm).

Following an Extended Dive, a Diver Must Decompress Slowly to Avoid the "Chokes" or the "Bends"

Although we have focused on problems divers face *while* at great depths, serious difficulties also arise if a diver returns to the surface too quickly *after* a deep dive. Too rapid an ascent causes the N_2 in the tissues—previously dissolved under high pressure—to leave solution and form bubbles as the P_B falls. This process is identical to the formation of gas bubbles when one opens a bottle of a carbonated beverage that had been capped under high pressure. During decompression, if the ascent occurs too rapidly, bubble formation will occur in any tissue in which N_2 has previously dissolved. Bubble formation can lead to **decompression sickness**, which has three major components. First, a bubble can form an embolus in the blood, which can carry it along until it becomes wedged and obstructs a vessel. Gas emboli in small blood vessels can cause tissue ischemia in the peripheral or pulmonary circulation (the "**chokes**"). Second, bubble formation in the myelin sheath of axons can compromise nerve conduction. Symptoms may range from dizziness to paralysis. Third, and most commonly, bubbles may form in muscles and joints, causing an intense pain called the "**bends**." The victim usually feels the pain most severely in the limbs and abdomen. Fourth, if air is trapped behind an

FIGURE 60–4. The need for decompression as a function of depth and duration of dive. If the dive is sufficiently brief or sufficiently shallow, no decompression is required *(teal area)*. For deeper depths or longer durations, a decompression protocol is required *(salmon area)*. (Data from Duffner GJ: Medical problems in involved in underwater compression and decompression. Ciba Clin Symp 10:99–117, 1958.)

Depth of submersion (m)

No decompression required

Decompression required

Duration of submersion (h)

obstructed bronchus, as it expands it can tear the lung tissue, enter an artery, and lodge in the brain. The results can be catastrophic unless the victim receives immediate recompression treatment.

Imagine that a diver has breathed compressed air at 4 atm for 2 hours, long enough to achieve equilibration with the tissues. Because the tissues normally dissolve 1 liter of N_2 at 1 atm, they will dissolve 4 liters of N_2 at 4 atm. As the diver now ascends to *sea level*, the "excess" N_2 moves from the tissues to lungs. However, because N_2 exits from water much faster than it does from fat, the total elimination of N_2 has two components: some compartments empty quickly (e.g., blood) and some empty slowly (e.g., joints, fat, eyeballs).

Figure 60–4 shows how long a diver can spend at various depths—breathing room air—without having to undergo a decompression protocol during the ascent. For example, a dive to 8 m can last indefinitely without any ill effects during the ascent. A dive of 25 min will not provide sufficient time to saturate the tissues unless the dive exceeds 40 m. However, a longer dive at 40 m will require a decompression program. For instance, a 20-min dive to a depth of 90 m requires nearly 3 hours of decompression time. Thus, the rate at which a diver should ascend to avoid decompression sickness depends on both the depth and the duration of the dive. Divers use detailed tables to plan their rate of ascent from a deep dive.

The best treatment for decompression sickness is to *recompress* the diver in a hyperbaric chamber. Recompression places the gases back under high pressure, forcing them to re-dissolve in the tissues, which instantly relieves symptoms. Once the diver is placed under high pressure, decompression can be carried out at a deliberate and supervised pace.

HIGH-ALTITUDE PHYSIOLOGY

The Barometric Pressure and, Therefore, the Ambient P_{O_2} at the Peak of Mount Everest Are Each About One Third of Their Respective Values at Sea Level

Unlike a column of water, which is relatively noncompressible and has a uniform density, the column of air in the atmosphere does not have the same density at all altitudes. The density of air decreases exponentially ascending from sea level. Half of the mass of the earth's atmosphere is contained in the lowest 5500 m. The next quarter is contained in the next 5500 m (i.e., 5500 m–11,000 m of altitude). In other words, at higher and higher altitudes, the number of gas molecules pressing down on a mountain climber also falls exponentially, with P_B falling by half for each approximately 5500 m of ascent (Fig. 60–5).

The peak of Mount Everest is the highest point of land on the earth's surface, measuring 8848 m above sea level. P_B at the peak is approximately 255 mm Hg, about one third that at sea level, and the ambient P_{O_2} is only approximately 53 mm Hg. For a climber at the peak of Everest, the P_{O_2} of the *humidified* inspired air entering the alveoli is even lower, because of the effects of water vapor ($P_{H_2O} = 47$ mm Hg at 37°C), so that the inspired $P_{O_2} = 21\% \times (255 - 47) = 44$ mm Hg, compared with 149 mm Hg at sea level (see Table 25–1). Hypoxia is thus a major problem at the summit of Mount Everest.

At an altitude of 5500 m—which also happens to be the altitude of the first "base camp" used in the ascent of Mount Everest—the ambient P_{O_2} is half the value at sea level, or approximately 80 mm Hg. At this altitude, arte-

FIGURE 60–5. Dependence of barometric pressure (P_B) on altitude.

rial O_2 delivery (arterial-blood O_2 content × cardiac output) can still meet O_2 demands in most healthy, active persons, even during mild physical activity. However, the body's compensatory responses to reduced ambient PO_2 at high altitude are different in different people. Thus, exposure to an altitude of 5500 m is problematic for a significant portion of the population.

Up to an Altitude of Approximately 3100 M, Arterial O_2 Content Falls More Slowly Than Does P_B Because of the Shape of the Hemoglobin-O_2 Dissociation Curve

Although P_B and ambient PO_2 decrease by the same fraction with increasing altitude, the O_2 saturation of hemoglobin in arterial blood decreases relatively little at altitudes up to approximately 3100 m. The reason is that at this altitude, arterial PO_2 is 60 to 70 mm Hg, which corresponds to the relatively flat portion of the O_2-Hb dissociation curve (see Fig. 28–3), where almost all of the O_2 in blood is bound to Hb. Decreasing arterial PO_2 has relatively little effect on arterial O_2 *content* until arterial PO_2 falls below this "flat" portion. Thus, the characteristics of Hb protect the arterial O_2 content, despite modest reductions of PO_2.

Although the amount of O_2 in the blood leaving the lung is important, even more important is the amount of O_2 that the systemic tissues take up. This uptake is the product of cardiac output and the arteriovenous (a−v) difference in O_2 content (p. 658). At sea level, arterial PO_2 is approximately 100 mm Hg, corresponding to an Hb saturation of approximately 97.5%, whereas the mixed-venous PO_2 is approximately 40 mm Hg, corresponding to an Hb saturation of approximately 75%. The difference between the arterial and the venous O_2 contents is approximately 22.5% of hemoglobin's maximal carrying capacity for O_2. However, at an altitude of 3100 m, arterial PO_2 is only approximately 60 mm Hg, which may correspond to an Hb saturation of only 88%. This reduction in blood O_2 content is called **hypoxemia**. Assuming everything else remains the same (e.g., O_2 utilization by the tissues, hematocrit, 2,3-DPG levels, pH, cardiac output), then the mixed arteriovenous (a−v) difference in Hb saturation must still be 22.5%. Thus, the mixed-venous blood at 3100 m must have an Hb saturation of 88% − 22.5% = 65.5%, which corresponds to a PO_2 of approximately 33 mm Hg. As a result, the a−v difference of O_2 *partial pressure* is much larger at sea level (100 − 40 = 60 mm Hg) than at 3100 m (60 − 33 = 27 mm Hg), even though the a−v difference in O_2 *content* is the same. The reason for the discrepancy is that the O_2-Hb dissociation curve is steeper in the region covered by the PO_2 values at high altitude.

At very high altitudes, still another factor comes into play. The uptake of O_2 by pulmonary-capillary blood slows at high altitudes, reflecting the smaller O_2 gradient from alveolus to blood (see Figure 29–8D). As a result, at sufficiently high altitudes, particularly during exercise, O_2 may no longer reach diffusion equilibrium between alveolar air and pulmonary-capillary blood by the time the blood reaches the end of the capillary. Thus, at in-

creasing altitude, not only does alveolar PO_2—and thus the maximal attainable arterial PO_2—fall in a predictable way, but the actual arterial PO_2 may fall to even a greater extent because of a failure of pulmonary capillary blood to equilibrate with alveolar air.

During the First Few Days, Compensatory Adjustments to Hypoxemia Include Tachycardia and Hyperventilation

A reduction in arterial PO_2 stimulates the peripheral chemoreceptors (p. 723), causing an immediate increase in ventilation. Increased ventilation has two effects. First, it brings alveolar PO_2 (and thus arterial PO_2) closer to the ambient PO_2. Second, hyperventilation blows off CO_2, producing a respiratory alkalosis (p. 692) that inhibits the peripheral but especially the central chemoreceptors (p. 726), decreasing ventilatory drive. Thus, total ventilation during an acute exposure to 4500 m is only about twice that at sea level, whereas the hypoxia by itself would have produced a much larger stimulation. Accompanying the increased ventilatory drive during acute altitude exposure is an increase in heart rate, probably owing to the increased sympathetic drive that accompanies acute hypoxemia (p. 546). The resultant increase in cardiac output enhances O_2 delivery.

During the next few days to weeks at an elevation of 4500 m, **acclimatization** causes ventilation to increase progressively by about the same amount as the acute response. As a result, PO_2 continues to improve and PCO_2 falls. There appear to be two mechanisms for this slower phase of increased ventilation. First, the pH of the cerebrospinal fluid (CSF) decreases, counteracting the respiratory alkalosis induced by the increase in ventilation and thus offsetting the inhibition of central chemoreceptors. However, the time course of the pH increase in CSF does not correlate tightly with the time course of the increase in ventilation. The pH at the actual site of the central chemoreceptors may fall with the appropriate time course. However, long-term hypoxia appears to increase the sensitivity of the peripheral chemoreceptors to hypoxia, and this effect may better account for acclimatization.

In the second mechanism for acclimatization, the kidneys respond over a period of several days to the respiratory alkalosis by decreasing their rate of acid secretion (p. 856) so that blood pH decreases toward normal (i.e., metabolic compensation for respiratory alkalosis). Another result of this compensation is spillage of HCO_3^- into the urine, which produces an osmotic diuresis and an alkaline urine. The consequence of reducing both CSF and plasma pH is to remove part of the inhibition caused by alkaline pH, allowing hypoxia to drive ventilation to higher values.

An extreme case of adaptation to high altitude occurs in people climbing very high mountains. In 1981, a team of physiologists ascended to the peak of Mount Everest while making various physiological measurements. Climbers at the summit obtained alveolar gas samples, trapping exhaled air in a specially designed, evacuated metal container. The alveolar PCO_2 at the summit was a minuscule

7 to 8 mm Hg, or approximately one fifth the value of 40 mm Hg at sea level. Thus, assuming a normal rate of CO_2 production, the climber's alveolar ventilation must have been fivefold higher than normal (p. 691). Because the work of heavy breathing and increased cardiac output at the summit (driven by hypoxia) would increase CO_2 production substantially, the increase in alveolar ventilation must have been substantially greater than fivefold.

The alveolar PO_2 at the peak of Mount Everest was approximately 28 mm Hg, which is marginally adequate to provide a sufficient O_2 content in the arterial blood to sustain the "resting" metabolic requirement at the summit. However, the term "resting" is somewhat of a misnomer, because the work of breathing and the cardiac output are markedly elevated.

Long-Term Adaptations to Altitude Include Increases in Hematocrit, Pulmonary Diffusing Capacity, Capillarity, and Oxidative Enzymes

Although the increases in ventilation and cardiac output help to maintain O_2 delivery during acute hypoxia, they are costly from an energy standpoint and cannot be sustained for extended periods. During prolonged residence at a high altitude, the reduced arterial PO_2 triggers profound adaptations. These changes enhance O_2 delivery to tissues at a cost that is lower than that exacted by the short-term compensatory strategies. Many of these adaptations are mediated by an increase **in hypoxia-inducible factor 1** (HIF-1), which is a transcription factor that activates genes involved in erythropoiesis, angiogenesis, and other processes.

HEMATOCRIT. Red-blood cell mass slowly increases with prolonged hypoxemia. The hemoglobin concentration of blood increases from a sea-level value of 14 to 15 g/dl to more than 18 g/dl, and hematocrit increases from 40% to 45% to more than 55%. Normally, the body regulates red-blood cell mass within fairly tight limits. However, renal hypoxia, and also norepinephrine, stimulate production and release of **erythropoietin** (EPO) from fibroblast-like cells in the kidney (see box on p. 664). EPO is a growth factor that stimulates the production of proerythroblasts in the bone marrow and also promotes accelerated development of red cells from their progenitor cells.

PULMONARY DIFFUSING CAPACITY. Acclimatization to high altitude also causes a two- to threefold increase in pulmonary diffusing capacity (p. 670). Much of this increase appears to be due to an increase in the blood volume of pulmonary capillaries (p. 674) and to the associated increase in capillary surface area available for diffusion. This surface area expands even further because hypoxia stimulates an increase in the depth of inspiration. Finally, right-ventricular hypertrophy increases pulmonary arterial pressure, increasing the perfusion to the upper, well-ventilated regions of the lungs (p. 693).

CAPILLARY DENSITY. Hypoxia causes a dramatic increase in tissue vascularity. Tissue **angiogenesis** (p. 481) occurs within days of exposure to hypoxia, triggered by

growth factors that hypoxic tissues release. Among these angiogenic factors are vascular endothelial growth factor (VEGF), fibroblast growth factor (FGF), and angiogenin.

OXIDATIVE ENZYMES. Hypoxia promotes expression of oxidative enzymes in the mitochondria, thereby enhancing the tissues' ability to extract O_2 from the blood (p. 1254). Thus, acclimatization to high altitude not only increases O_2 delivery to the periphery, but also increases O_2 uptake by the tissues.

Ascent to Altitude Leads to Fatigue, Nausea, and Decreased Cognition in Most People and to Acute or Chronic Mountain Sickness in Susceptible Individuals

The first documented evidence of the ill effects of high altitude was in 35 BC, when Chinese travelers called the Himalayas the "Headache Mountains." Recreational mountain climbing first became popular in the mid-19th century, and with modern rapid transportation, many people can now travel rapidly to mountain resorts. In fact, it is possible to ascend passively from sea level to high altitude in a matter of minutes to hours (e.g., in a balloon). A rapid ascent may precipitate a constellation of relatively *mild symptoms*: drowsiness, fatigue, headache, nausea, and a gradual decline in cognition. These uncomfortable effects of acute hypoxia are progressive with increasing altitude. They occur in some people at altitudes as low as 2100 m and occur in most people at altitudes that are above 3500 m. Initially, these symptoms reflect an inadequate compensatory response to hypoxemia (i.e., vasodilation), resulting in reduced O_2 delivery to the brain. In the longer term, symptoms may stem from mild *cerebral edema*, which probably results from dilation of the cerebral arterioles, leading to increased capillary filtration pressure and enhanced transudation (p. 469).

Some people who ascend rapidly to altitudes as seemingly moderate as 3000 m to 3500 m develop **acute mountain sickness (AMS)**. The symptoms—which include headache, fatigue, dizziness, dyspnea, sleep disturbance, peripheral edema, nausea, and vomiting—usually develop within the first day and last for 3 to 5 days. The primary problem in AMS is hypoxia, and the symptoms probably have two causes. The first is thought to be a progressive, more severe case of *cerebral edema*. The second cause for the symptoms is *pulmonary edema*, which occurs as hypoxia leads to hypoxic pulmonary vasoconstriction (p. 699), which in turn increases total pulmonary vascular resistance, pulmonary-capillary pressure, and transudation. Certain people have an exaggerated pulmonary-vascular response to hypoxia, and they are especially susceptible to AMS. Cerebral or pulmonary edema can be fatal if the exposure to hypoxia is not rapidly reversed, first by providing supplemental O_2 to breathe, then by removing the individual from the high altitude.

Although being physically fit provides some protection against AMS, the most important factor is an undefined constitutional difference. Those least likely to develop symptoms ventilate more in response to the hypoxia and, therefore, tend to have a higher P_{O_2} and a lower P_{CO_2}. The higher P_{O_2} and lower P_{CO_2} lead to less cerebral vasodilation, and the higher P_{O_2} minimizes pulmonary vasoconstriction.

Chronic mountain sickness occurs after prolonged residence at high altitude. The etiology of this disorder is an overproduction of red blood cells—an exaggerated response to hypoxia. In such conditions, the hematocrit can exceed 60% (i.e., polycythemia), thereby dramatically increasing blood viscosity and vascular resistance, and increasing the risk of intravascular thrombosis. The combination of pulmonary hypoxic vasoconstriction and increased blood viscosity is especially onerous for the right side of the heart, which experiences a greatly increased load. These conditions eventually lead to *congestive heart failure* of the right ventricle.

FLIGHT AND SPACE PHYSIOLOGY

Acceleration in One Direction Shifts the Blood Volume in the Opposite Direction

Newton's **first law of motion** establishes the concept of *inertia*: an object at rest remains at rest, and a body in motion remains in motion—at the same velocity—unless acted upon by an external force.

The **second law of motion** deals with changes in *momentum*, which is the product of mass and velocity. Because velocity has both magnitude and direction, so does momentum. When an external force (which also has magnitude and direction) acts on a body, the change in the body's momentum is in the direction of the force. Furthermore, momentum changes at a rate that is proportional to the magnitude of the force. Thus, the change in the momentum (i.e., velocity) of a spacecraft depends on the magnitude, direction, and duration of the force (i.e., thrust) exerted by the engine.

The **third law of motion** establishes that applying an external force generates an equivalent, but opposing, inertial force ("for every action, there is an equal and opposite reaction").

To accelerate a rocket from rest, we must apply enough force to overcome its inertial force (i.e., its weight, the product of its mass, and the acceleration due to gravity) as well as the frictional forces of the environment. This requirement is merely a restatement of the *second law* of motion. With the rocket accelerating vertically, astronauts inside experience an inertial "G force," as required by the *third law*, pressing them into their seats in the direction opposite to the rocket's acceleration. This G force is a dimensionless number that describes the magnitude of the acceleration force (a) experienced by an astronaut, relative to the force the astronaut experiences due to the earth's gravity at sea level (g_0):

Equation 60–6

$$G = \frac{a}{g_0}$$

Before liftoff, an astronaut experiences only the force of gravity, $+1G$. As a rocket blasts off from earth, the astronaut experiences higher G forces. In early rockets, astro-

FIGURE 60–6. G forces during ascent into space on the space shuttle. Before liftoff, astronauts experience $+1G$, the acceleration that is due to earth's gravity. After liftoff, the solid rockets burn for about 2 minutes, during which time the G force ramps up to slightly more than $+3G$. After the solid-rocket burn, the G force falls back to $+1G$. Thereafter, the main engine gradually builds up the G force to about $+4G$ before engine cut-off. These G-force data were generated in a human centrifuge to simulate the profile of a shuttle launch. (Data from Buckey JC, Goble RL, Blomqvist CG: A new device for continuous ambulatory central venous pressure measurement. Medical Instrumentation 87:238–243, 1987.)

nauts sometimes experienced G forces as high as $+10G$, although maximal G forces in the modern Space Shuttle are only about $+4G$ (Fig. 60–6). Similarly, pilots of high-performance aircraft experience *positive* G forces as they pull out of a dive, and we all experience *negative* G forces when an aircraft hits turbulence and suddenly loses altitude, lifting us out of our seats. Although G forces can frequently have potentially large effects on aircraft pilots, they affect astronauts only during the liftoff and re-entry phases of spaceflight. To ensure that acceleration effects have a minimal influence on body function, astronauts sit with their backs perpendicular to the direction of the accelerating force, so that the G force acts across the chest from front to back.

G forces propel the body's tissues in the direction opposite the direction of acceleration, compressing soft tissues against underlying structural elements (e.g., bone) or pulling these tissues away from overlying structural elements. In addition, G forces tend to shift the blood volume away from the direction of acceleration, adding to the other component forces that determine blood pressure (p. 426).

In high-performance aircraft, the rapid motions associated with changes in flight direction or altitude produce G forces that can be considerable for several minutes, exceeding 8 Gs. Even in relatively primitive aircraft, aerobatic maneuvers can shift blood volume away from the head, resulting in transient reductions in cerebral blood flow and O_2 delivery. If these reductions are sufficiently large, they can result in a loss of consciousness. The early warnings of such an event are narrowing of the visual field (i.e., loss of peripheral vision) and loss of color perception as the retina is deprived of O_2, a phenomenon called **gray-out**. The term **blackout** describes a total loss of consciousness that occurs during acceleration that lasts for tens of seconds or minutes. Pilots experiencing gray-out or blackout are at extreme risk. As early as World War II, fighter pilots used G-suits that provided counterpressure to the lower extremities when making repeated tight maneuvers during dogfights. The counterpressure opposed the pooling of blood in the extremities and maintained sufficient cardiac filling, cardiac output, and blood flow to the brain, thereby eliminating the tendency toward gray-out.

"Weightlessness" Causes a Cephalad Shift of the Blood Volume

An astronaut in an orbiting spacecraft experiences "weightlessness," a state of near-zero G force, also called a **microgravity** environment. Although an astronaut at an altitude of 200 km still experiences approximately 94% of the force of the earth's gravity at sea level (i.e., the astronaut truly has weight), the centrifugal force of the spacecraft's orbital trajectory balances the earth's gravitational force, and the astronaut experiences no net acceleration forces and, thus, has the sensation of weightlessness. This weightlessness, however, differs from the true near-zero-gravity environment in "outer space."

Because we are adapted to life at +1G, arteriolar tone in the lower extremities prevents pooling of blood in the capacitance vessels (p. 578), ensuring adequate venous return to the right heart. The acute effects of microgravity on the circulatory system are exactly what you would expect for a system designed to oppose the effect of gravity in a standing person: blood volume redistributes toward the head. This cephalad shift of blood volume—away from the capacitance vessels of the legs—expands the central blood *volume*, increasing the cardiac preload and increasing the filtration of plasma water into the interstitium of the facial region. The resulting edema explains the dramatically bloated facial appearance of astronauts in microgravity within 24 hours of the launch. From this discussion, you might think that the central venous *pressure* (CVP) is higher in space. However, such an increase in CVP has been difficult to confirm.

In laboratory studies involving prolonged head-down tilt (i.e., a model intended to simulate microgravity exposure), the cephalad shift of blood volume produces the expected increase in CVP and rapid reflex responses to the apparent volume overload. First, the increased stretch on the right atrium causes release of **atrial natriuretic peptide** (ANP) (p. 555). Second, stimulation of the low-pressure baroreceptors inhibits secretion of **arginine vasopressin** or antidiuretic hormone from the posterior pituitary (p. 549). These two events increase excretion of salt and water by the kidneys (p. 864), tending to correct the perceived volume overload and explaining the tendency for astronauts to remain relatively underhydrated during space flight.

In orbiting spacecraft, the cephalad shift of blood volume, even without an increase in CVP, causes a small increase in cerebral arterial pressure and thus in blood flow to the brain. Such regional alterations in blood volume and flow do not substantially impact *total* peripheral resistance in space. Thus, mean arterial pressure and cardiac output are not significantly different from their values on the earth's surface.

Space Flight Leads to Motion Sickness as Well as to Decreases in Muscle and Bone Mass

Despite training (e.g., in three-dimensional motion simulators), more than half of all astronauts experience motion sickness during the initial days of microgravity. **Motion sickness** (i.e., nausea and vomiting) results from conflicting sensory input to the brain regarding the position of the body. In space flight, motion sickness is the consequence of altered inertial stimulation of the vestibular system in the absence of normal gravitational forces. Nearly all cases of motion sickness resolve within the first 96 hours of microgravity exposure as the vestibular system or the CNS accommodates to the novel input.

The increased cerebral blood flow and blood volume in microgravity, accompanied by increased capillary filtration of fluid from the intravascular space, contribute to the increased incidence of headache, nausea, and motion sickness, at least during the transition period to microgravity. These symptoms reduce performance. Astronauts attempt to minimize these effects by restricting water intake prior to launch.

Numerous other changes occur during prolonged residence in microgravity, many of which are related to the markedly diminished aerobic power output in space, where the force of gravity does not oppose muscle contraction. The major physiological alterations include reductions in body-water content, plasma and red cell volume, total-body nitrogen stores, muscle mass, and total-body calcium and phosphate (associated with a loss in bone mass). The bone loss appears to be continuous with time in a weightless environment, whereas the other changes occur only during the first weeks in space. The reductions in plasma and red-cell volumes result in a marked decrease in *maximum* cardiac output (p. 1252), a determinant of maximal aerobic power. The reduction of muscle mass decreases the maximal force developed by muscle. The reduction in bone mass likewise decreases bone strength. Although these changes are appropriate adaptations to a microgravity environment, in which there is little inherent value to great strength and high aerobic capacity, they are decidedly disadvantageous on return to the earth's surface.

Exercise Partially Overcomes the "Deconditioning" of Muscles During Spaceflight

The intermittent loading of muscles, bone, and the cardiovascular system prevents—to some extent—the "deconditioning" effects of spaceflight on muscle mass and performance. Astronauts have used bungee (i.e., elastic) cords and ergometric (i.e., "work-measuring") stationary bicycles to provide a resistance against which to exert force. The most effective exercise regime appears to be walking on a motor-driven treadmill with the lower body encased in a **negative-pressure chamber**. Reducing the chamber pressure to 100 mm Hg below ambient pressure creates transmural pressure differences—across the blood vessels in the feet—that are similar to those that exist when standing upright on the earth's surface. However, this arrangement greatly exaggerates transmural pressure differences near the waist. For this reason, these astronauts also wear positive-pressure pants that compress the tissues by 70 mm Hg at the level of the waist and—decrementally—by 0 mm Hg at the feet. The net effect of the negative-pressure chamber and the graded positive-pressure pants is to create a physiological toe-to-waist gradient of transmural pressures across the blood vessels of the lower body. The aerobic activity, the impact of the feet on the treadmill, and the generation of physiological transmural pressure gradients appear to be sufficient to simulate exercise at +1G. This regimen can reduce or even eliminate the deconditioning effects of space flight.

The Return to Earth Requires Special Measures to Ensure Maintenance of Arterial Blood Pressure

The problems associated with "re-entry" reflect a return to full gravity on earth's surface. The most dramatic effects are due to reduced blood volume and decreased tone of the leg vessels. Both factors contribute to reductions in cardiac preload, orthostatic tolerance, and exercise capacity. It has been common practice to shield astronauts from public view immediately after return to the earth's surface, until they have regained a good orthostatic response.

In recent years, astronauts have employed various strategies just prior to re-entry to counter the adaptations to microgravity. The countermeasure to orthostatic intolerance is restoration of blood volume prior to re-entry. One means of attenuating the reduction of blood volume in space flight is an exercise program. Even a brief period (e.g., 30 min) of intense exercise expands plasma albumin content (p. 1253), increasing plasma oncotic pressure and plasma volume by 10% within 24 hours. The problems with exercise programs are difficulties in logistics and the astronauts' lack of motivation. A second means of minimizing the reduced blood volume is increasing salt and fluid intake. However, this has proven difficult to implement because of the consequent increase in urine flow. Currently, astronauts are educated about the effects of prolonged space flight and then maintained under continuous scrutiny after re-entry until they have regained a normal orthostatic response. This usually occurs within hours, and certainly within one day, of re-entry.

REFERENCES

Books and Reviews

Bunn HF, Poyton RO: Oxygen sensing and molecular adaptation to hypoxia. Physiol Rev 76:839–885, 1996.
Crystal RG, West JB: The Lung. New York, Raven, 1991.
Duffner GJ: Medical problems involved in underwater compression and decompression. Ciba Clin Symp 10:99–117, 1958.
Krakauer J: Into thin air. New York, Anchor Books-Doubleday, 1997.
Monge C: Chronic mountain sickness. Physiol Rev 23:166–184, 1943.
West JB: Man in space. News in Physiol Sci 1:189–192, 1986.

Journal Articles

Cain SM, Dunn JE II: Low doses of acetazolamide to aid the accommodation of men to altitude. J Appl Physiol 21:1195–1200, 1966.
Schoene RB, Lahiri S, Hackett PH, et al: Relationship of hypoxic ventilatory response to exercise performance on Mount Everest. J Appl Physiol 56:1478–1483, 1984.
West JB: Human physiology at extreme altitudes on Mount Everest. Science 223:784–788, 1984.

Index

Note: Page numbers followed by f indicate figures; those followed by t indicate tables; and those followed by b indicate boxed material.